Body Mass Index

BMI	Normal						Overweight					Obese										Extreme Obesity														
	19	20	21	22	23	24	25	26	27	28	29	30	31	32	33	34	35	36	37	38	39	40	41	42	43	44	45	46	47	48	49	50	51	52	53	54
Height (inches)	Body Weight (pounds)																																			
58	91	96	100	105	110	115	119	124	129	134	138	143	148	153	158	162	167	172	177	181	186	191	196	201	205	210	215	220	224	229	234	239	244	248	253	258
59	94	99	104	109	114	119	124	128	133	138	143	148	153	158	163	168	173	178	183	188	193	198	203	208	212	217	222	227	232	237	242	247	252	257	262	267
60	97	102	107	112	118	123	128	133	138	143	148	153	158	163	168	174	179	184	189	194	199	204	209	215	220	225	230	235	240	245	250	255	261	266	271	276
61	100	106	111	116	122	127	132	137	143	148	153	158	164	169	174	180	185	190	195	201	206	211	217	222	227	232	238	243	248	254	259	264	269	275	280	285
62	104	109	115	120	126	131	136	142	147	153	158	164	169	175	180	186	191	196	202	207	213	218	224	229	235	240	246	251	256	262	267	273	278	284	289	295
63	107	113	118	124	130	135	141	146	152	158	163	169	175	180	186	191	197	203	208	214	220	225	231	237	242	248	254	259	265	270	276	282	287	293	299	304
64	110	116	122	128	134	140	145	151	157	163	169	174	180	186	192	197	204	209	215	221	227	232	238	244	250	256	262	267	273	279	285	291	296	302	308	314
65	114	120	126	132	138	144	150	156	162	168	174	180	186	192	198	204	210	216	222	228	234	240	246	252	258	264	270	276	282	288	294	300	306	312	318	324
66	118	124	130	136	142	148	155	161	167	173	179	186	192	198	204	210	216	223	229	235	241	247	253	260	266	272	278	284	291	297	303	309	315	322	328	334
67	121	127	134	140	146	153	159	166	172	178	185	191	198	204	211	217	223	230	236	242	249	255	261	268	274	280	287	293	299	306	312	319	325	331	338	344
68	125	131	138	144	151	158	164	171	177	184	190	197	203	210	216	223	230	236	243	249	256	262	269	276	282	289	295	302	308	315	322	328	335	341	348	354
69	128	135	142	149	155	162	169	176	182	189	196	203	209	216	223	230	236	243	250	257	263	270	277	284	291	297	304	311	318	324	331	338	345	351	358	365
70	132	139	146	153	160	167	174	181	188	195	202	209	216	222	229	236	243	250	257	264	271	278	285	292	299	306	313	320	327	334	341	348	355	362	369	376
71	136	143	150	157	165	172	179	186	193	200	208	215	222	229	236	243	250	257	265	272	279	286	293	301	308	315	322	329	338	343	351	358	365	372	379	386
72	140	147	154	162	169	177	184	191	199	206	213	221	228	235	242	250	258	265	272	279	287	294	302	309	316	324	331	338	346	353	361	368	375	383	390	397
73	144	151	159	166	174	182	189	197	204	212	219	227	235	242	250	257	265	272	280	288	295	302	310	318	325	333	340	348	355	363	371	378	386	393	401	408
74	148	155	163	171	179	186	194	202	210	218	225	233	241	249	256	264	272	280	287	295	303	311	319	326	334	342	350	358	365	373	381	389	396	404	412	420
75	152	160	168	176	184	192	200	208	216	224	232	240	248	256	264	272	279	287	295	303	311	319	327	335	343	351	359	367	375	383	391	399	407	415	423	431
76	156	164	172	180	189	197	205	213	221	230	238	246	254	263	271	279	287	295	304	312	320	328	336	344	353	361	369	377	385	394	402	410	418	426	435	443

Source: Adapted from National Heart, Lung, and Blood Institute: Clinical Guidelines on the Identification, Evaluation, and Treatment of Overweight and Obesity in Adults: the Evidence Report.
See http://www.nhlbi.nih.gov/guidelines/obesity/bmi_tbl.pdf

CONN'S CURRENT THERAPY 2024

CONN'S CURRENT THERAPY 2024

RICK D. KELLERMAN, MD
Professor and Chair
Department of Family and Community Medicine
University of Kansas School of Medicine–Wichita
Wichita, Kansas

DAVID P. RAKEL, MD
Esther Millard Endowed Professor and Chair
Department of Family Medicine and Community Health
University of Wisconsin School of Medicine and Public Health
Madison, Wisconsin

JOEL J. HEIDELBAUGH, MD
Professor
Departments of Family Medicine and Urology
University of Michigan Medical School
Ann Arbor, Michigan

ERNESTINE M. LEE, MD, MPH
Associate Professor
Department of Community and Family Medicine
Geisel School of Medicine
Dartmouth College
Hanover, New Hampshire

ELSEVIER

Elsevier
1600 John F. Kennedy Blvd.
Ste 1800
Philadelphia, PA 19103-2899

CONN'S CURRENT THERAPY 2024   ISBN-13: 978-0-443-12151-7

Notice

ISBN-13: 978-0-443-12151-7

Senior Content Strategist: Charlotta Kryhl
Content Development Manager: Meghan Andress
Content Development Specialist: Kevin Travers
Publishing Services Manager: Catherine Albright Jackson
Senior Project Manager: Doug Turner
Designer: Renee Duenow

Printed in Canada

Last digit is the print number: 9   8   7   6   5   4   3   2   1

Contributors

Mustafa Abdul-Hussein, MD, MSCR
Physician, Gastroenterology and Hepatology, St. Anthony Hospital, Oklahoma City, Oklahoma
Gastroesophageal Reflux Disease (GERD)

Sunil Abhyankar, MD
Professor, Internal Medicine, University of Kansas Medical Center, Kansas City, Kansas
Stem Cell Therapy

Rodney D. Adam, MD
Professor, Pathology and Medicine, Aga Khan University, Nairobi, Kenya
Giardiasis

T.M. Ayodele Adesanya, MD, PhD
Instructor, Family and Community Medicine, The Ohio State University College of Medicine, Columbus, Ohio
Premature Beats

Nelson Iván Agudelo Higuita, MD
Associate Professor, Internal Medicine, University of Oklahoma Health Sciences Center, Oklahoma City, Oklahoma
Plague

Mehwish Ahmed, MD
Fellow, Gastroenterology and Hepatology, University of Michigan Medical School, Ann Arbor, Michigan
Inflammatory Bowel Disease: Crohn Disease and Ulcerative Colitis

Lee Akst, MD
Director, Laryngology, Johns Hopkins Medical Institutes, Baltimore, Maryland
Hoarseness and Laryngitis

Ethan Alexander, MD
Assistant Professor, Endocrinology, Diabetes, Metabolism, Clinical Pharmacology, University of Kansas Medical Center, Kansas City, Kansas
Diabetes Mellitus in Adults

Patrick L. Allen, MD
Clinical Assistant Professor, Family and Community Medicine, University of Kansas School of Medicine–Wichita, Wichita, Kansas
Brucellosis

Kelley P. Anderson, MD
Clinical Adjunct Professor of Medicine, Researcher Emeritus, Marshfield Clinic Research Institute, University of Wisconsin School of Medicine and Public Health, Marshfield, Wisconsin
Heart Block

Paul Andre, MD
Assistant Professor, Internal Medicine, University of New Mexico School of Medicine, Albuquerque, New Mexico
Tachycardias

Gregory Anstead, MD, PhD
Staff Physician, Medicine, Audie L. Murphy Memorial Veterans Affairs Hospital; Professor, Medicine, University of Texas Health, San Antonio, Texas
Coccidioidomycosis

Ann M. Aring, MD
Clinical Assistant Professor, Family Medicine, The Ohio State University College of Medicine; Associate Program Director, Family Medicine Residency, Riverside Methodist Hospital, Columbus, Ohio
Drug Hypersensitivity Reactions; Rhinosinusitis

Cheryl A. Armstrong, MD
Professor, Dermatology, University of Colorado School of Medicine, Aurora, Colorado; Dermatology Division Chief, Medicine, Denver Health Medical Center, Denver, Colorado
Viral Diseases of the Skin

Arash Arshi, MD
Interventional Cardiologist, Cardiology, OhioHealth, Columbus, Ohio
Valvular Heart Disease

Cecilio R. Azar, MD
Gastroenterologist and Hepatologist, Clinical Associate, Gastroenterology, American University Beruit, Medical Center, Beirut, Lebanon
Bleeding Esophageal Varices

Amir Azarbal, MD
Interventional Cardiologist, Monongahela Valley Hospital, Monroeville, Pennsylvania
Pericarditis

Jihoon Baang, MD
Assistant Professor of Clinical Medicine, Internal Medicine, University of Michigan Medical School, Ann Arbor, Michigan
Toxoplasmosis; Histoplasmosis

Zachary Baeseman, MD, MPH
Associate Chief Medical Officer, Leadership Development and Clinical Transformation, ThedaCare Physicians, ThedaCare, Neenah, Wisconsin; Adjunct Professor, Family Medicine, Medical College of Wisconsin, Milwaukee, Wisconsin
Vaginal Bleeding in Pregnancy

Justin Bailey, MD
Associate Professor, Family Medicine, University of Washington School of Medicine; Director, Procedures Institute, Family Medicine Residency of Idaho, Boise, Idaho
Gaseousness, Indigestion, Nausea, and Vomiting; Palpitations

Mandeep Bajaj, MD
Professor, Medicine, Baylor College of Medicine, Houston, Texas
Hyperlipidemia

Juliana Bakk, MD
Fellow, Maternal Fetal Medicine, The University of Kansas Medical Center, Kansas City, Kansas
Hypertensive Disorders in Pregnancy

Dana M. Bakula, PhD
Assistant Professor, Pediatrics, Children's Mercy Kansas City; Assistant Professor, Pediatrics, University of Missouri-Kansas City School of Medicine, Kansas City, Missouri
Infant and Children Feeding Problems

Federico Balagué, MD
Physician, Rheumatology, HFR Fribourg-Hôpital Cantonal, Fribourg, Switzerland
Spine Pain

Bradley E. Barth, MD
Professor, Emergency Medicine, University of Kansas Medical Center, Kansas City, Missouri
Burns

Gina M. Basello, DO
Vice Chair and Residency Program Director, Family Medicine, Jamaica Hospital Medical Center, Jamaica, New York; Assistant Clinical Professor, Family and Social Medicine, Albert Einstein College of Medicine, Bronx, New York
Fever

Renee Bassaly, DO
Associate Professor, Female Pelvic Medicine and Reconstructive Surgery, University of South Florida College of Medicine, Tampa, Florida
Urinary Incontinence

Adel Bassily-Marcus, MD
Associate Professor, Surgery, Mount Sinai Medical Center, New York, New York
Targeted Temperature Management (Therapeutic Hypothermia)

Julie M. Baughn, MD
Consultant, Sleep Medicine, Mayo Clinic, Rochester, Minnesota
Pediatric Sleep Disorders

Aleksandr Belakovskiy, MD
Assistant Professor, Family Medicine, University of Michigan Medical School, Ann Arbor, Michigan
Erectile Dysfunction

Ronen M. Ben-Ami, MD
Head, Infectious Diseases Department, Tel Aviv Sourasky Medical Center, Tel Aviv, Israel
Cat Scratch Disease

David I. Bernstein, MD
Professor-Affiliate, Division of Immunology, Allergy, and Rheumatology, University of Cincinnati College of Medicine, Cincinnati, Ohio
Hypersensitivity Pneumonitis

Jonathan A. Bernstein, MD
Professor, Internal Medicine, University of Cincinnati College of Medicine, Cincinnati, Ohio
Anaphylaxis

Caroline Beyer
Physician, Los Angeles LGBT Center, Los Angeles, California
Palpitations

Mitchell Birt, MD
Faculty Professor, Orthopedic Surgery, University of Kansas School of Medicine-Kansas City; Faculty Professor, Orthopedic Surgery, Kansas City VA, Kansas City, Missouri
Osteomyelitis

Yooni Blair, MD
Assistant Professor, Urology, University of Michigan Medical School, Ann Arbor, Michigan
Trauma to the Genitourinary Tract

Natalie Blonien, PT, DPT
Faculty Associate, University of Wisconsin School of Medicine and Public Health, Madison, Wisconsin
Rehabilitation of the Stroke Patient

Diana Bolotin, MD, PhD
Associate Professor, Dermatology, University of Chicago Pritzker School of Medicine, Chicago, Illinois
Nonmelanoma Cancer of the Skin

Rachel A. Bonnema, MD, MS
Associate Professor, Internal Medicine, UT Southwestern Medical Center, Dallas, Texas
Contraception

David Borenstein, MD
Clinical Professor of Medicine, Rheumatology, The George Washington University Medical Center, Potomac, Maryland; Partner, Arthritis and Rheumatism Associates, Washington, District of Columbia
Spine Pain

Nicole Boschuetz, MD
Assistant Clinical Professor, Gastroenterology and Hepatology, University of Wisconsin Hospital and Clinics, Madison, Wisconsin
Nonalcoholic Fatty Liver Disease (NAFLD)

Christopher Bossart, MD
Assistant Professor, Emergency Medicine, University of New Mexico School of Medicine, Albuquerque, New Mexico
Osteoarthritis

Deidra Bowman, MD
Fellow, Infectious Diseases, University of Oklahoma Health Sciences Center, Oklahoma City, Oklahoma
Plague

Dee Ann Bragg, MD
Clinical Assistant Professor, Family and Community Medicine, University of Kansas School of Medicine–Wichita Residency Program at Via Christi Hospitals, Wichita, Kansas
Rubella and Congenital Rubella

Scott Bragg, PharmD
Associate Professor, Clinical Pharmacy and Outcomes Science, Family Medicine, Medical University of South Carolina, Charleston, South Carolina
Osteoporosis

Sylvia L. Brice, MD
Clinical Professor, Dermatology, University of Colorado School of Medicine, Aurora, Colorado
Viral Diseases of the Skin

Allyson M. Briggs, MD
Clinical Instructor, Emergency Medicine, University of Kansas Medical Center, Kansas City, Kansas
Burns

John Brill, MD, MPH
Vice President, Population Health, Advocate Aurora Health, Milwaukee, Wisconsin
Gonorrhea

Rachel Brown, MBBS
Professor and Chair, Psychiatry and Behavioral Sciences, University of Kansas School of Medicine–Wichita, Wichita, Kansas
Autism

Peter F. Buckley, MD
Dean, School of Medicine, Virginia Commonwealth University School of Medicine, Richmond, Virginia
Schizophrenia

Sarah Burns, DO, MS
Associate Professor, Hospital Medicine–Internal Medicine, University of New Mexico School of Medicine, Albuquerque, New Mexico
Acute Kidney Injury

Kenneth Byrd, DO
Assistant Professor, Internal Medicine–Hematologic Malignancies and Cellular Therapeutics, University of Kansas Medical Center, Kansas City, Kansas
Disseminated Intravascular Coagulation

Diego Cadavid, MD
Chief Medical Officer, Clinical Development, Verge Genomics, South San Francisco, California; Affiliate Instructor, Neurology, UMass Chan Medical School, Worcester, Massachusetts
Relapsing Fever

Thomas Caraccio, PharmD
Clinical Pharmacist/Toxicologist, Pharmacy Department, NYU Winthrop Hospital, Mineola/New York, New York
Medical Toxicology

Peter Carek, MD, MS
Professor and Chair, Family Medicine, Prisma Health, Greenville, South Carolina
Osteoporosis

Andres F. Carrion, MD
Associate Professor, Digestive Health and Liver Diseases, University of Miami Miller School of Medicine, Miami, Florida
Cirrhosis

Carlos Anthony Casillas, MD, MPH
Hospital Medicine Fellow, Hospital Medicine, Cincinnati Children's Hospital Medical Center, Cincinnati, Ohio
Viral Meningitis

Amanda S. Cass, PharmD
Clinical Pharmacist Specialist, Thoracic Oncology, Pharmaceutical Services, Vanderbilt University Medical Center, Nashville, Tennessee
Lung Cancer

Anthony P. Catinella, MD, MPH
Department Chair, Family Medicine, Texas Tech University Health Sciences Center El Paso, El Paso, Texas
Pulmonary Hypertension

William E. Cayley Jr., MD, MDiv
Clinical Professor, Family Medicine and Community Health, University of Wisconsin School of Medicine and Public Health, Eau Claire, Wisconsin, Family Physician, Prevea Family Medicine Residency Program–Augusta, Augusta, Wisconsin
Chest Pain

Kristine L. Cece, MD, PhD
Assistant Professor, Family Medicine, Michigan Medicine, Ann Arbor, Michigan
Hiccups

Sonia Cerquozzi, MD
Clinical Assistant Professor, Internal Medicine, Hematology, University of Calgary Cumming School of Medicine, Calgary, Alberta, Canada
Polycythemia Vera

Alvaro Cervera, MD, PhD
Consultant Neurologist, Neurology, Royal Darwin Hospital, Darwin, Northern Territory, Australia
Ischemic Cerebrovascular Disease

Filomena Cetani, MD, PhD
Physician, Endocrinology, University Hospital of Pisa, Pisa, Italy
Hyperparathyroidism and Hypoparathyroidism

Rachel Chamberlain, MD
Associate Program Director, Sports Medicine Fellowship; Assistant Professor, Family and Community Medicine, University of New Mexico School of Medicine, Albuquerque, New Mexico
Osteoarthritis

Lawrence Chan, MD
Distinguished Emeritus Professor, Medicine, Molecular & Cellular Biology, Biochemistry & Molecular Biology, Molecular & Human Genetics, Baylor College of Medicine, Houston, Texas
Hyperaldosteronism; Hyperlipidemia; Hyperprolactinemia

Miriam Chan, PharmD
Program Director of Quality and Safety, Medical Education, OhioHealth; Adjunct Assistant Professor, Family Medicine, The Ohio State University College of Medicine, Columbus, Ohio; Clinical Assistant Professor, Pharmacology, Ohio University, Athens, Ohio
Drug Hypersensitivity Reactions; Popular Herbs and Nutritional Supplements

Divya Chandramohan, MD
Fellow, Infectious Diseases, UT Health-San Antonio, San Antonio, Texas
Coccidioidomycosis

Zenas Chang, MD
Assistant Professor, Clinical Obstetrics and Gynecology, Gynecologic Oncology, Indiana University School of Medicine, Indianapolis, Indiana
Ovarian Cancer

Jimmy Chen, MD
Assistant Professor, Pediatrics, University of Florida College of Medicine-Jacksonville, Jacksonville, Florida
Parenteral Fluid Therapy for Infants and Children

Lin Yee Chen, MBBS, MS
Professor, Medicine/Cardiology, University of Minnesota Medical School, Minneapolis, Minnesota
Atrial Fibrillation

Shingo Chihara, MD
Physician, Infectious Disease, Virginia Mason Medical Center, Seattle, Washington
Anthrax

Meera Chitlur, MD
Professor, Pediatric Hematology/Oncology, Central Michigan University/Children's Hospital of Michigan; Barnhart-Lusher Hemostasis Research Endowed Chair, Pediatrics, Wayne State University School of Medicine, Detroit, Michigan
Hemophilia and Related Conditions

Saima Chohan, MD
Clinical Assistant Professor, Rheumatology, University of Arizona College of Medicine, Phoenix, Arizona
Gout and Hyperuricemia

Jacob Christensen, DO
Physician, Primary Care Sports Medicine, University of Idaho, Moscow, Idaho
Osteoarthritis

Kuang-Yuh Chyu, MD, PhD
Associate Director, Coronary Intensive Care Unit, Cardiology, Cedars-Sinai Medical Center; Health Science Clinical Professor, Medicine, David Geffen School of Medicine at UCLA, Los Angeles, California
Acute Myocardial Infarction

Joaquin E. Cigarroa, MD
Division Head of Cardiology, Professor, Medicine, Knight Cardiovascular Institute, Oregon Health and Sciences University, Portland, Oregon
Congenital Heart Disease

Paul Cleland, MD
Clinical Assistant Professor, Family and Community Medicine, University of Kansas School of Medicine–Wichita, Wichita, Kansas
Heat Illness

Matthew K. Cline, MD
Affiliate Professor, Family Medicine, Medical University of South Carolina, Charleston, South Carolina
Antepartum Care

Laura C. Coates, MBChB, PhD
Senior Clinical Research Fellow, Orthopaedics, Rheumatology, and Musculoskeletal Sciences, University of Oxford, Oxford, United Kingdom
Psoriatic Arthritis

August Colenbrander, MD
Affiliate Senior Scientist, RERC, Smith-Kettlewell Eye Research Institute, San Francisco, California
Vision Rehabilitation

Christine Conageski, MD
Associate Professor, Obstetrics and Gynecology, University of Colorado School of Medicine, Aurora, Colorado
Vulvar Neoplasia

John M. Conly, MD
Medical Officer, Infection Prevention and Control, Foothills Medical Center; Professor, Medicine; Medical Director, Ward of the 21st Century, Cummings School of Medicine; Co-Director, Snyder Institute for Chronic Diseases, University of Calgary, Calgary, Alberta, Canada
Methicillin-Resistant Staphylococcus aureus

Ashley Cooper, MD
Associate Professor, Pediatrics, Children's Mercy Kansas City/University of Missouri, Kansas City, Missouri
Juvenile Idiopathic Arthritis

Stacy Cooper, MD
Assistant Professor, Oncology, Johns Hopkins University School of Medicine, Baltimore, Maryland
Acute Leukemia in Children

Allison Cormier, MD
Assistant Professor, Infectious Disease, Tulane University School of Medicine, New Orleans, Louisiana
Human Immunodeficiency Virus: Treatment and Prevention

Burke A. Cunha, MD
Physician, Infectious Disease, NYU Winthrop Hospital, Mineola, New York
Babesiosis; Viral and Mycoplasmal Pneumonias

Cheston B. Cunha, MD
Medical Director, Antimicrobial Stewardship, Infectious Disease, Warren Alpert Medical School of Brown University, Providence, Rhode Island
Babesiosis; Viral and Mycoplasmal Pneumonias

Thomas Curran, MD, MPH
Assistant Professor, Surgery, Medical University of South Carolina, Charleston, South Carolina
Tumors of the Colon and Rectum

Amy Curry, MD
Clinical Associate Professor, Family and Community Medicine, University of Kansas School of Medicine–Wichita, Wichita, Kansas
Pelvic Inflammatory Disease

Cori L. Daines, MD
Professor and Division Chief, Pediatric Pulmonary and Sleep Medicine, Pediatrics, University of Arizona College of Medicine, Tucson, Arizona
Cystic Fibrosis

Beth Damitz, MD
Professor, Family and Community Medicine; Associate Program Director, All Saints Family Medicine Residency Program, Medical College of Wisconsin, Milwaukee, Wisconsin
Immunization Practices

Nandini Datta, PhD
Clinical Instructor, Child and Adolescent Psychiatry, Stanford University School of Medicine, Stanford, California
Eating Disorders

Natalie C. Dattilo, PhD
Director of Psychology, Psychiatry, Brigham and Women's Hospital, Boston, Massachusetts
Generalized Anxiety Disorder; Posttraumatic Stress Disorder

Raul Davaro, MD
Associate Professor, Clinical Medicine, University of Massachusetts Medical School, Worcester, Massachusetts
Smallpox; Whooping Cough (Pertussis)

Kevin A. David, MD
Physician, Blood Disorders, Rutgers Cancer Institute of New Jersey, Rutgers University, New Brunswick, New Jersey
Non-Hodgkin Lymphoma

Joshua Davis, MD
Assistant Medical Director, Emergency Medicine, Vituity; Clinical Instructor, Medicine, University of Kansas School of Medicine–Wichita, Wichita, Kansas
Acute Diarrhea

Alexei O. DeCastro, MD
Associate Professor, Family Medicine, Medical University of South Carolina, Charleston, South Carolina
Osteoporosis

Katharine C. DeGeorge, MD, MS
Associate Professor, Family Medicine, University of Virginia School of Medicine, Charlottesville, Virginia
Bacterial Pneumonia; Asthma in Children

Thomas G. DeLoughery, MD
Professor, Hematology, Oregon Health & Science University, Portland, Oregon
Hemolytic Anemias

Atul A. Deodhar, MD
Professor of Medicine, Arthritis, and Rheumatic Diseases, Oregon Health & Science University, Portland, Oregon
Axial Spondyloarthritis

Urmi Desai, MD, MS
Assistant Professor, Medicine, Center for Family and Community Medicine; Director, Foundations of Clinical Medicine Clerkships, Columbia University Irving Medical Center, New York, New York
Vulvovaginitis

Clio Dessinioti, MD, PhD
Dermatologist, A. Sygros Hospital, Athens, Greece
Parasitic Diseases of the Skin

Mahua Dey, MD
Director of Surgical Neuro-oncology, Neurosurgery, University of Wisconsin School of Medicine and Public Health, Madison, Wisconsin
Central Nervous System Neoplasms

Michael P. Diamond, MD
Senior Vice President for Research, Obstetrics/Gynecology, Augusta University Medical College of Georgia, Augusta, Georgia
Infertility

Christopher Dion, DO
Medical Toxicology Fellow, Medical Toxicology, Banner–University Medical Center Phoenix, Phoenix, Arizona
Venomous Snakebite

Thomas E. Dobbs, MD, MPH
Dean, School of Population Health, University of Mississippi Medical Center; Physician, Communicable Diseases, Mississippi State Department of Health, Jackson, Mississippi
COVID-19

Margaret Dobson, MD
Assistant Professor, Family Medicine, University of Michigan Medical School, Ann Arbor, Michigan
Pruritus

Colleen A. Donahue, MD
Assistant Professor, Department of Surgery, Medical University of South Carolina, Charleston, South Carolina
Tumors of the Colon and Rectum

Geoffrey A. Donnan, MD
Professor of Neurology, Director, The Florey Institute of Neuroscience and Mental Health, The University of Melbourne, Melbourne, Australia
Ischemic Cerebrovascular Disease

John N. Dorsch, MD
Professor Emeritus, Department of Family and Community Medicine, University of Kansas School of Medicine–Wichita, Wichita, Kansas
Red Eye

Michael Dougan, MD, PhD
Assistant Professor, Medicine/Gastroenterology, Massachusetts General Hospital, Boston, Massachusetts
Monoclonal Antibodies; Fungal Infections of the Skin

Chad Douglas, MD, PharmD
Assistant Professor, Family and Preventive Medicine, University of Oklahoma Health Sciences Center, Oklahoma City, Oklahoma
Erythema Multiforme

Dar Dowlatshahi, MD, PhD
Professor, Medicine, University of Ottawa Faculty of Medicine, Ottawa, Ontario, Canada
Intracerebral Hemorrhage

Shannon Dowler, MD
Adjunct Associate Professor, Family Medicine, University of North Carolina School of Medicine Asheville, Asheville, North Carolina
Non-Gonococcal Urethritis

Douglas A. Drevets, MD
Regents' Professor, Chief, Infectious Diseases, Medicine, University of Oklahoma Health Sciences Center, Oklahoma City, Oklahoma
Plague

Samuel Dudley, MD, PhD
Professor, Medicine, University of Minnesota Medical School, Minneapolis, Minnesota
Atrial Fibrillation

Peter R. Duggan, MD
Clinical Associate Professor, Medicine, University of Calgary Cumming School of Medicine, Calgary, Alberta, Canada
Polycythemia Vera

Kim Eagle, MD
Albion Walter Hewlett Professor of Internal Medicine, Cardiovascular Medicine, University of Michigan Medical School, Ann Arbor, Michigan
Angina Pectoris

Leigh M. Eck, MD
Professor, Medicine, University of Kansas Medical Center, Kansas City, Kansas
Thyroiditis

Sarah Edwards, DO
Pediatric Gastroenterologist, Pediatrics, Children's Mercy Kansas City, University of Missouri-Kansas City School of Medicine, Kansas City, Missouri
Infant and Children Feeding Problems

Wissam I. El Atrouni, MD, MSc
Associate Professor, Internal Medicine, University of Kansas School of Medicine, Kansas City, Kansas
Osteomyelitis

Dirk M. Elston, MD
Professor and Chair, Department of Dermatology, Medical University of South Carolina, Charleston, South Carolina
Diseases of the Hair

John M. Embil, MD
Professor, Medicine, University of Manitoba College of Medicine, Winnipeg, Manitoba, Canada
Blastomycosis

Scott K. Epstein, MD
Professor, Medicine, Tufts University School of Medicine, Boston, Massachusetts
Acute Respiratory Failure

Susan Evans, MD
Assistant Professor, Family Medicine, University of Nebraska Medical Center, Omaha, Nebraska
Iron Deficiency Anemia

Andrew M. Evens, DO, MBA, MSc
Professor, Medicine; Chief, Division of Hematology/Oncology, Rutgers Cancer Institute of New Jersey, Rutgers University, New Brunswick, New Jersey
Non-Hodgkin Lymphoma

Mark Fairweather, MD, PhD
Associate Surgeon, Brigham and Women's Hospital; Assistant Professor, Surgery, Harvard Medical School, Boston, Massachusetts
Tumors of the Stomach

Marni J. Falk, MD
Executive Director, Mitochondrial Medicine Frontier Program, Division of Human Genetics, Department of Pediatrics, The Children's Hospital of Philadelphia; Associate Professor, Pediatrics, University of Pennsylvania Perelman School of Medicine, Philadelphia, Pennsylvania
Mitochondrial Disease

Anna Faris, MD
Resident Physician, Urology, University of Michigan Medical School, Ann Arbor, Michigan
Trauma to the Genitourinary Tract

Francis A. Farraye, MD, MS
Director, Inflammatory Bowel Disease Center, Mayo Clinic, Jacksonville, Florida
Inflammatory Bowel Disease: Crohn Disease and Ulcerative Colitis

Anthony J. Faugno III, MD
Assistant Professor, Pulmonary, Critical Care, and Sleep, Tufts Medical Center, Boston. Massachusetts
Acute Respiratory Failure

Hilary Faust, MD
Assistant Professor, Medicine, University of Wisconsin School of Medicine and Public Health, Madison, Wisconsin
Sepsis

Kinder Fayssoux, MD
Faculty, Center for Family Medicine, Eisenhower Medical Associates, La Quinta, California
Bacterial Infections of the Urinary Tract in Women

Ian D. Ferguson, MD
Associate Professor, Pediatrics, Yale School of Medicine, New Haven, Connecticut
Post-COVID-19 Multisystem Inflammatory Syndrome in Children

Terry D. Fife, MD
Director, Otoneurology & Balance Disorders, Neurology, Barrow Neurological Institute; Professor
Neurology, University of Arizona College of Medicine, Phoenix, Arizona
Ménière's Disease

David J. Finley, MD
Chief, Thoracic Surgery, Dartmouth-Hitchcock Medical Center, Lebanon, New Hampshire; Associate Professor, Surgery, Geisel School of Medicine at Dartmouth, Hanover, New Hampshire
Pleural Effusion and Empyema

Jonathon Firnhaber, MD, MAEd, MBA
Residency Program Director, Family Medicine, East Carolina University Brody School of Medicine, Greenville, North Carolina
Diseases of the Nail

Lynn Fisher, MD
Assistant Professor, Family and Community Medicine, University of Kansas School of Medicine–Wichita, Wichita, Kansas
Red Eye

William E. Fisher, MD
Professor, Surgery, Baylor College of Medicine, Houston, Texas
Acute and Chronic Pancreatitis

Maria Fleseriu, MD
Professor, Medicine and Neurological Surgery, Oregon Health & Science University, Director, Pituitary Center, Portland, Oregon
Adrenocortical Insufficiency; Hypopituitarism

Donald C. Fletcher, MD
Adjunct Associate Professor, Ophthalmology, University of Kansas School of Medicine, Kansas City Kansas; Medical Director, Low Vision Rehabilitation, Envision, Wichita, Kansas; Senior Scientist, Smith-Kettlewell Eye Research Institute, Medical Director, Frank Stein and Paul S May Center for Low Vision Rehabilitation, Ophthalmology, California Pacific Medical Center, San Francisco, California
Vision Rehabilitation

Jeffrey Michael Foster, DO
Clinical Assistant Professor, Anesthesiology, University of Missouri at Kansas City; Anesthesiology and Interventional Pain Medicine, Saint Luke's Hospital of Kansas City, Kansas City, Missouri
Fibromyalgia

Jennifer Frank, MD
Family Physician, Family Medicine, Advocate Aurora, Oshkosh, Wisconsin
Syphilis

Ellen W. Freeman, PhD
Research Professor, Obstetrics/Gynecology and Psychiatry (retired), University of Pennsylvania Perelman School of Medicine, Philadelphia, Pennsylvania
Premenstrual Syndrome

David A. Frenz, MD
Adjunct Clinical Assistant Professor, Family Medicine and Community Health, University of Minnesota Medical School, Minneapolis, Minnesota
Alcohol Use Disorder

Ruchi Gaba, MD
Associate Professor, Endocrinology, Diabetes and Metabolism, Baylor College of Medicine, Houston, Texas
Hyperaldosteronism

Melissa Gaines, MD
Physician, Cox Senior Health, Cox Health; Volunteer Faculty, University of Missouri School of Medicine Springfield Campus, Springfield, Missouri
Constipation

Mark E. Garcia, MD
Assistant Professor, Internal Medicine, Cardiology, University of New Mexico Health Sciences Center, University of New Mexico, Albuquerque, New Mexico
Congestive Heart Failure

Virgilio V. George, MD
Director, Division of Colorectal Surgery, Medical University of South Carolina, Charleston, South Carolina
Tumors of the Colon and Rectum

Marc G. Ghany, MD, MHSc
Senior Investigator, Liver Diseases Branch, National Institute of Diabetes and Digestive and Kidney Diseases, National Institutes of Health, Bethesda, Maryland
Hepatitis A, B, D, and E

Muhammad Ahmad Ghazi, MD
Consulting Associate, Family and Community Medicine, Duke University School of Medicine, Raleigh, North Carolina
Pruritus Ani and Vulvae

Geoffrey T. Gibney, MD
Co-Leader Melanoma Program, Lombardi Comprehensive Cancer Center, Medstar Georgetown University Hospital, Washington, District of Columbia
Melanoma

Donald L. Gilbert, MD
Professor, Pediatrics, Cincinnati Children's Hospital Medical Center, Cincinnati, Ohio
Gilles de la Tourette Syndrome

Karissa Gilchrist, MD
Assistant Professor, Family and Community Medicine, University of Kansas School of Medicine–Wichita, Wichita, Kansas
Bacterial Diseases of the Skin

Erin A. Gillaspie, MD, MPH
Assistant Professor, Thoracic Surgery; Head of Thoracic Surgery Robotics, Vanderbilt University Medical Center, Nashville, Tennessee
Lung Cancer

Tarvinder Gilotra, MD
Consultant Physician, Infectious Disease, Catholic Health, Buffalo, New York
Intestinal Parasites

Mark T. Gladwin, MD
Jack D. Myers Professor and Chair, Medicine, University of Pittsburgh School of Medicine, Pittsburgh, Pennsylvania
Sickle Cell Disease

Stephen J. Gluckman, MD
Professor, Medicine, University of Pennsylvania Perelman School of Medicine; Clinical Director, Penn Global Medicine; Medical Director, Travel Medicine Clinic, Philadelphia, Pennsylvania
Myalgic Encephalomyelitis/Chronic Fatigue Syndrome

Andrew W. Goddard, MD
Professor, Psychiatry, University of California San Francisco Fresno, Fresno, California
Generalized Anxiety Disorder

Kyle Goerl, MD
Associate Professor, Family Medicine, University of Colorado School of Medicine, Aurora Colorado; Team Physician, CU Athletics, Boulder, Colorado
Bursitis and Tendinopathy

Mark S. Gold, MD
Professor, Psychiatry, Washington University, St. Louis, Missouri
Drug Use Disorders

Amy Goldstein, MD
Associate Professor, Pediatrics, University of Pennsylvania Perelman School of Medicine; Clinical Director, Mitochondrial Medicine Frontier Program, Division of Human Genetics, Department of Pediatrics, Children's Hospital of Philadelphia, Philadelphia, Pennsylvania
Mitochondrial Disease

Gregory Goodwin, MD
Assistant Professor, Pediatrics, Harvard Medical School; Senior Associate Physician in Pediatrics, Boston Childrens Hospital, Boston, Massachusetts
Diabetes Mellitus in Children

Daniel Gorelik, MD
Resident Physician, Otolaryngology-Head and Neck Surgery, Houston Methodist Hospital, Houston, Texas
Rhinitis; Obstructive Sleep Apnea

Aidar R. Gosmanov, MD, PhD, DMSc
Section Chief, Endocrinology, Stratton VAMC; Professor, Endocrinology, Albany Medical College, Albany, New York
Diabetic Ketoacidosis

Luigi Gradoni, PhD
Former Research Director, Vector-Borne Diseases, Istituto Superiore di Sanità, Rome, Italy
Leishmaniasis

Timothy P. Graham, MD, MHPE
Chief Medical Officer, Administration, Mount Carmel St. Ann's, Westerville, Ohio
Hypertension

Jane M. Grant-Kels, MD
Professor and Founding Chair Emeritus, Vice Chair, Founding Director, Cutaneous Oncology Center and Melanoma Program, Dermatology, University of Connecticut Health Center, Farmington, Connecticut; Adjunct Professor, Dermatology, University of Florida College of Medicine, Gainesville, Florida
Nevi

Kristine Grdinovac, MD
Assistant Professor, Endocrinology, Metabolism, and Genetics, Director, Cray Diabetes Self-Management Center, University of Kansas Medical Center, Kansas City, Kansas
Diabetes Mellitus in Adults

Leslie A. Greenberg, MD
Family Physician; Associate Professor, Family and Community Medicine, University of Nevada Reno School of Medicine, Reno, Nevada
Chronic Diarrhea; Keloids

William M. Greene, MD
Associate Professor, Psychiatry, University of Florida College of Medicine, Gainesville, Florida
Drug Use Disorders

Joseph Greensher, MD
Professor, Pediatrics, Renaissance School of Medicine at Stony Brook University, Stony Brook, New York; Medical Director and Associate Chair, Department of Pediatrics, Long Island Regional Poison and Drug Information Center, Winthrop-University Hospital, Mineola, New York
Medical Toxicology

David S. Gregory, MD
Professor, Family and Community Medicine, Virginia Tech Carilion School of Medicine, Roanoke, Virginia
Resuscitation of the Newborn

Justin Greiwe, MD
Partner, Bernstein Allergy Group, Inc.; Clinical Assistant Professor, Immunology, Allergy, and Rheumatology, University of Cincinnati College of Medicine, Cincinnati, Ohio
Anaphylaxis

Melissa Hague, MD
Clinical Associate Professor, Obstetrics and Gynecology, University of Kansas School of Medicine–Wichita, Wichita, Kansas
Female Sexual Dysfunction

Rebat M. Halder, MD
Professor Emeritus and Chairman Emeritus, Dermatology, Howard University College of Medicine, Washington, District of Columbia
Pigmentary Disorders

Alan M. Hall, MD
Associate Professor, Internal Medicine and Pediatrics, University of Kentucky College of Medicine, Lexington, Kentucky
Parenteral Fluid Therapy for Infants and Children

Kari R. Harris, MD
Associate Professor, Pediatrics, University of Kansas School of Medicine–Wichita, Wichita, Kansas
Adolescent Health

Taylor B. Harrison, MD
Associate Professor, Neurology, Emory University School of Medicine, Atlanta, Georgia
Myasthenia Gravis

Adam L. Hartman, MD
Program Director, Division of Clinical Research, National Institute of Neurological Disorders and Stroke/National Institutes of Health, Rockville, Maryland
Epilepsy in Infants and Children

Erin Hayes, MD
Associate Clinical Professor, Child and Adolescent Psychiatry, Medical University of South Carolina, Charleston, South Carolina
Attention-Deficit/Hyperactivity Disorder

James W. Haynes, MD
Interim Dean, University of Tennessee College of Medicine Chattanooga, Chair of the Department of Family Medicine, Chattanooga, Tennessee
Uterine Leiomyoma

Joel J. Heidelbaugh, MD
Clinical Professor, Family Medicine, University of Michigan Medical School, Ann Arbor, Michigan
Erectile Dysfunction

Molly A. Hinshaw, MD
Associate Professor and Chief of Dermatopathology, University of Wisconsin School of Medicine and Public Health, Madison, Wisconsin
Connective Tissue Disorders; Cutaneous Vasculitis

Brandon Hockenberry, MD
Renown Health, Reno, Nevada
Sports-Related Head Injuries

Raymond J. Hohl, MD, PhD
Director, Penn State Cancer Institute; Professor, Medicine and Pharmacology, Milton S. Hershey Medical Center, University Professorship in Medicine, Penn State University, Hershey, Pennsylvania
Thalassemia

Therese Holguin, MD
Assistant Professor, Dermatology, University of New Mexico School of Medicine, Albuquerque, New Mexico
Fungal Infections of the Skin

Sarah A. Holstein, MD, PhD
Professor, Internal Medicine, University of Nebraska Medical Center, Omaha, Nebraska
Thalassemia

Michael Holyoak, DO
Physician, Idaho Endocrinology, Meridian, Idaho
Thyroid Cancer

Gretchen Homan, MD
Associate Professor, Pediatrics, The University of Kansas School of Medicine–Wichita, Wichita, Kansas
Pediatric Failure to Thrive

Kevin Hommema, BSME
Principal Research Scientist, Battelle, Columbus, Ohio
Biologic Agents Reference Chart; Toxic Chemical Agents Reference Chart

Laurie A.M. Hommema, MD
Associate Program Director, Family Medicine Residency, Riverside Methodist Hospital; Medical Director, Provider and Associate Well-Being, Quality and Patient Safety, OhioHealth, Columbus, Ohio
Biologic Agents Reference Chart; Toxic Chemical Agents Reference Chart

Ahmad Reza Hossani-Madani, MD, MD
Dermatologist, Kaiser Permanente, Upper Marlboro, Maryland
Pigmentary Disorders

Steven A. House, MD, HMDC
Professor, Family and Geriatric Medicine, University of Louisville/Glasgow Family Medicine Residency Program, Glasgow, Kentucky
Pain; Palliative and End-of-Life Care

Sarah Houssayni, MD
Pediatrics, Ascension Via Christi Clinic Family Medicine, Wichita, Kansas
Encopresis

Bethany Howlett, MD, MHS
Assistant Professor, Family Medicine and Community Health, University of Wisconsin School of Medicine and Public Health, Madison, Wisconsin
High-Altitude Illness

William J. Hueston, MD
Adjunct Professor, Family and Community Medicine, Medical College of Wisconsin, Waukesha, Wisconsin
Hyperthyroidism; Hypothyroidism

Richard Huettemann, MD
Chairman, Department of Pediatrics, Children's Medical Group Providence Hospital, Mobile, Alabama
Tumors of the Colon and Rectum

Alison N. Huffstetler, MD
Medical Director, Health Services Research, Robert Graham Center; Assistant Professor, Family Medicine, Georgetown University School of Medicine, Washington, District of Columbia; Assistant Professor, Family Medicine and Population Health, Virginia Commonwealth University School of Medicine, Richmond, Virginia
Bacterial Pneumonia

Anthony Hunter, MD
Assistant Professor, Hematology and Medical Oncology, Winship Cancer Institute of Emory University, Atlanta, Georgia
Acute Leukemia in Adults

Jacqueline Huynh, MD
Associate Program Director, Family and Community Medicine, Dignity Health East Valley Family Medicine Residency Program, Gilbert, Arizona
Chronic Diarrhea

Oyetokunbo Ibidapo-Obe, MD
Assistant Professor, Director Women's Health, Family Medicine, University of Texas Medical Board at Galveston, Galveston, Texas
Infective Endocarditis

Alice M. Ing, MD
Assistant Professor, Psychiatry, Yale School of Medicine, New Haven, Connecticut
Depressive, Bipolar, and Related Mood Disorders

Gretchen Irwin, MD, MBA
Associate Professor, Family and Community Medicine; Associate Dean of Graduate Medical Education, University of Kansas School of Medicine–Wichita, Wichita, Kansas
Otitis Media

Daniel Isaac, DO
Assistant Professor, Medicine, Michigan State University College of Human Medicine, East Lansing, Michigan
Chronic Leukemias

Alan C. Jackson, MD
Neurologist, Medicine, Thompson General Hospital, Thompson, Manitoba, Canada; Neurologist, Medicine, Lake of the Woods District Hospital, Kenora, Ontario, Canada
Rabies

Caitlin Jackson-Tarlton, MD
Assistant Professor, Medicine, Dalhousie University Faculty of Medicine; Neurologist, Medicine, Nova Scotia Health; Assistant Director, Multiple Sclerosis Clinic, NS Health, Halifax, Nova Scotia, Canada
Multiple Sclerosis

Kurt M. Jacobson, MD
Associate Professor, Cardiovascular Medicine, University of Wisconsin School of Medicine and Public Health, Madison, Wisconsin
Mitral Valve Prolapse

Jose A. Jaller, MD
Dermatology, Albert Einstein College of Medicine, Bronx, New York
Venous Ulcers

W. Ennis James, MD
Associate Professor, Pulmonary and Critical Care Medicine, Medical University of South Carolina, Charleston, South Carolina
Sarcoidosis

Lauren Jeang, MD
Assistant Professor, Ophthalmology, University of Florida College of Medicine, Gainesville, Florida
Dry Eye Syndrome

Abhishek Jha, MBBS
Visiting Postdoctoral Fellow, Medical Neuroendocrinology, Eunice Kennedy Shriver National Institute of Child Health and Human Development, National Institutes of Health, Bethesda, Maryland
Pheochromocytoma

Xiaoming Jia, MD
Instructor, Medicine, Baylor College of Medicine, Houston, Texas
Hyperlipidemia

Lisa M. Johnson, MD
Associate Professor, Family Medicine; Assistant Dean, Office of Diversity, Equity, and Inclusion, University of Cincinnati College of Medicine, Cincinnati, Ohio
Acne Vulgaris; Rosacea

Joshua S. Jolissaint, MD
General Surgeon, Brigham and Women's Hospital, Harvard Medical School, Boston, Massachusetts
Pancreatic Cancer; Atelectasis

Tamilarasu Kadhiravan, MD
Professor, Medicine, Jawaharlal Institute of Postgraduate Medical Education and Research, Puducherry, India
Typhoid Fever

Farah Kaiksow, MD, MPP
Assistant Professor, Medicine, University of Wisconsin School of Medicine and Public Health, Madison, Wisconsin
Chronic Obstructive Pulmonary Disease

Rachna Kalia, MD
Clinical Assistant Professor, Psychiatry and Behavioral Sciences, University of Kansas School of Medicine–Wichita, Wichita, Kansas
Obsessive-Compulsive Disorder

Sagar Kamprath, MD
Associate Professor, Family Medicine, The University of Texas Medical Branch at Galveston, Galveston, Texas
Post-Acute COVID Syndrome

Jessica Rachel Kanter, MD
Resident, Obstetrics and Gynecology, Augusta University Medical College of Georgia, Augusta, Georgia
Infertility

Dilip R. Karnad, MD
Consultant in Critical Care, Jupiter Hospital, Thane, Maharashtra, India
Tetanus

Rudruidee Karnchanasorn, MD
Associate Professor, Internal Medicine, The University of Kansas Medical Center, Kansas City, Kansas
Thyroid Cancer

Andreas Katsambas, MD, PhD
Professor, Dermatology-Venereology, University of Athens; Professor, Dermatology, Hygeia Hospital, Athens, Greece
Parasitic Diseases of the Skin

Ben Z. Katz, MD
Professor, Pediatrics, Northwestern University Feinberg School of Medicine; Attending Physician, Division of Infectious Diseases, Ann & Robert H. Lurie Children's Hospital of Chicago, Chicago, Illinois
Infectious Mononucleosis

Rebecca Katzman, MD
Clinical Assistant Professor, Family Medicine, University of Washington School of Medicine, Seattle, Washington
Palpitations

Andrew M. Kaunitz, MD
Professor and Associate Chairman, Obstetrics and Gynecology, University of Florida College of Medicine-Jacksonville, Jacksonville, Florida
Menopause

Rick Kellerman, MD
Professor and Chair, Department of Family and Community Medicine, University of Kansas School of Medicine–Wichita, Wichita, Kansas
Chikungunya; Mpox; Zika Virus Disease

Scott Kellermann, MD, MPH
Adjunct Professor, Public Health and Tropical Medicine, Tulane University School of Medicine, New Orleans, Louisiana; Clinical Professor, Clinical Sciences, California Northstate College of Medicine, Elk Grove, California; Adjunct Professor, Clinical Sciences, University of San Francisco School of Medicine, San Francisco, California
Chikungunya; Mpox; Zika Virus Disease

Christina M. Kelly, MD
Assistant Professor, Family Medicine, Uniformed Services University of the Health Sciences, Bethesda, Maryland
Ectopic Pregnancy

Sheevaun Khaki, MD
Associate Professor, Pediatrics, Oregon Health and Science University, Portland, Oregon
Infant Hyperbilirubinemia

Arthur Y. Kim, MD
Associate Professor, Medicine, Harvard Medical School, Boston, Massachusetts
Hepatitis C

Haejin Kim, MD
Senior Staff Allergist, Allergy and Clinical Immunology, Henry Ford Health System; Clinical Assistant Professor, Wayne State University School of Medicine, Detroit, Michigan
Hypersensitivity Pneumonitis

Jami A. Kinnucan, MD
Senior Associate Consultant; Chair, GI Clinical Practice, Gastroenterology & Hepatology, Mayo Clinic, Jacksonville, Florida
Inflammatory Bowel Disease: Crohn Disease and Ulcerative Colitis

Robert S. Kirsner, MD, PhD
Chair and Harvey Blank Professor, Dr. Phillip Frost Department of Dermatology and Cutaneous Surgery, University of Miami Miller School of Medicine, Miami, Florida
Venous Ulcers

Sonam R. Kiwalkar, MBBS
Assistant Professor, Rheumatology, Washington State University; Associate Program Director, Legacy Salmon Creek; Rheumatologist, The Vancouver Clinic, Vancouver, Washington
Axial Spondyloarthritis

Janice Knoefel, MD, MPH
Professor, Neurology and Internal Medicine (Geriatrics), University of New Mexico School of Medicine, Albuquerque, New Mexico
Alzheimer's Disease

Amanda Kolb, MD
Family Medicine, University of Vermont Larner College of Medicine, Burlington, Vermont
Asthma in Children

Bhanu Prakash Kolla, MD
Center for Sleep Medicine, Mayo Clinic, Rochester, Minnesota
Sleep Disorders

Frederick Korley, MD
Robert E. Meyerhoff Assistant Professor of Emergency Medicine, The Johns Hopkins University School of Medicine; Staff, Johns Hopkins Medicine, Baltimore, Maryland
Disturbances Due to Cold

Mark Kraemer, MD
Resident, Neurosurgery, University of Wisconsin Hospitals and Clinics, Madison, Wisconsin
Central Nervous System Neoplasms

Megan Krause, MD
Assistant Professor, Allergy, Clinical Immunology, and Rheumatology, University of Kansas School of Medicine, Kansas City, Kansas
Rheumatoid Arthritis

Eric H. Kraut, MD
Professor, Internal Medicine, The Ohio State University College of Medicine, Columbus, Ohio
Platelet-Mediated Bleeding Disorders

Lakshmanan Krishnamurti, MD
Chief of Pediatric Hematology, Oncology, and Bone Marrow Transplant, Yale School of Medicine, New Haven, Connecticut
Sickle Cell Disease

Kumar Krishnan, MD
Assistant Professor, Internal Medicine, Harvard Medical School, Boston, Massachusetts
Dysphagia and Esophageal Obstruction

Zachary Kuhlmann, DO
Program Director, Clinical Professor, Obstetrics and Gynecology, University of Kansas School of Medicine–Wichita, Wichita, Kansas
Endometriosis

Roshni Kulkarni, MD
Professor and Director Emerita, MSU Center for Bleeding and Clotting Disorders, Pediatrics and Human Development, Michigan State University College of Human Medicine, East Lansing, Michigan
Hemophilia and Related Conditions

Seema Kumar, MD
Professor, Pediatric and Adolescent Medicine, Mayo Clinic, Rochester, Minnesota
Obesity in Children

Mary R. Kwaan, MD, MPH
Health Sciences Clinical Professor, Surgery, David Geffen School of Medicine at UCLA, Los Angeles, California
Hemorrhoids, Anal Fissure, and Anorectal Abscess and Fistula

Robert A. Kyle, MD
Hematology, Mayo Clinic, Rochester, Minnesota
Multiple Myeloma

Matthew Lambert, MD
Clinical Instructor, Infectious Disease, University of Wisconsin School of Medicine and Public Health, Madison, Wisconsin
Travel Medicine

Lucius Marion Lampton, MD
Clinical Associate Professor, Family and Community Medicine, Tulane University School of Medicine, New Orleans, Louisiana; Clinical Professor, Family Medicine, William Carey University, Hattiesburg, Mississippi
COVID-19; Yellow Fever

Richard A. Lange, MD, MBA
President, Department of Medicine; Dean, Paul L. Foster School of Medicine, Texas Tech University Health Sciences Center El Paso, El Paso, Texas
Congenital Heart Disease

Fabienne Langlois, MD
Assistant Professor, Medicine, Endocrinology, Centre Hospitalier Universitaire de Sherbrooke, Sherbrooke, Quebec, Canada
Adrenocortical Insufficiency; Hypopituitarism

Christine L. Lau, MD
George Minor Professor of Surgery, University of Virginia Health System, Charlottesville, Virginia
Atelectasis

Susan Lawrence-Hylland, MD
Clinical Assistant Professor, Rheumatology, University of Wisconsin Hospital and Clinics, Madison, Wisconsin
Connective Tissue Disorders; Cutaneous Vasculitis

Jake Lazaroff, MD
Micrographic Surgery and Dermatologic Oncology Fellow, MD Anderson Cancer Center, Houston, Texas
Nonmelanoma Cancer of the Skin

Lydia U. Lee, MD
Clinical Lecturer, Family Medicine, University of Michigan Medical School, Ann Arbor, Michigan
Postpartum Depression

Jerrold B. Leikin, MD
Consultant, Illinois Health and Hospital Association, Illinois Poison Center, Chicago, Illinois; Professor, Medicine, Rosalind Franklin University/Chicago Medical School, North Chicago, Illinois
Disturbances Due to Cold

Scott Leikin, DO
Assistant Professor, Anesthesia and Critical Care Medicine, Baylor College of Medicine, Houston, Texas
Targeted Temperature Management (Therapeutic Hypothermia); Disturbances Due to Cold

Alexander K.C. Leung, MBBS
Clinical Professor, Pediatrics, University of Calgary Cumming School of Medicine; Pediatric Consultant; Pediatrics, Alberta Children's Hospital, Calgary, Alberta, Canada
Nocturnal Enuresis

Grace Levy-Clarke, MD
Associate Professor, Ophthalmology, West Virginia University School of Medicine, Morgantown, West Virginia
Uveitis

Martin M. LeWinter, MD
Professor, Medicine and Molecular Physiology & Biophysics, University of Vermont Larner College of Medicine; Attending Cardiologist, University of Vermont Medical Center, Burlington, Vermont
Pericarditis

Ming Li, MD, PhD
Staff Physician, Medicine, Phoenix VA Medical Center; Clinical Assistant Professor, Medicine, University of Arizona College of Medicine, Phoenix, Arizona
Hyperlipidemia; Hyperprolactinemia

Tyler Liebenstein, PharmD
Clinical Pharmacist, Pharmacy, William S. Middleton Memorial Veterans Hospital, Madison, Wisconsin
Human Immunodeficiency Virus: Treatment and Prevention

Albert P. Lin, MD
Assistant Professor, Ophthalmology, Baylor College of Medicine, Staff Physician, Eye Care Line, Michael E. DeBakey Veterans Affairs Medical Center, Houston, Texas
Glaucoma

Jeffrey A. Linder, MD, MPH
Professor and Chief, General Internal Medicine, Northwestern University Feinberg School of Medicine, Chicago, Illinois
Influenza

James Lock, MD, PhD
Professor, Psychiatry, Stanford University School of Medicine, Stanford, California
Eating Disorders

M. Chantel Long, MD
Clinical Assistant Professor, Family and Community Medicine, University of Kansas School of Medicine–Wichita; Staff Physician, Concierge Primary Care Clinic, Ascension Via Christi, Wichita, Kansas
Condylomata Acuminata; Warts (Verrucae)

Colleen Loo-Gross, MD, MPH
Assistant Professor, Family and Community Medicine, University of Kansas School of Medicine–Wichita, Wichita, Kansas
Amenorrhea

Julia R. Lubsen, MD
Assistant Professor, Family Medicine and Community Health, University of Wisconsin School of Medicine and Public Health, Madison, Wisconsin
Pyelonephritis

Ronda Lun, MD
Resident Physician, Neurology, The Ottawa Hospital, Ottawa, Ontario, Canada
Intracerebral Hemorrhage

David (Sasha) Mahvi, MD
Surgical Resident, Brigham and Women's Hospital, Boston, Massachusetts
Tumors of the Stomach

RosaMarie Maiorella, MD
Assistant Professor, Pediatrics, University of Cincinnati College of Medicine, Cincinnati, Ohio
Viral Meningitis

Jonathan Maldonado, MD
Clinical Instructor, Urology, Kansas University Medical Center, Kansas City, Missouri
Hematuria

Uma Malhotra, MD
Clinical Professor, Infectious Diseases, University of Washington School of Medicine, Seattle, Washington
Ebola Virus Disease

Emily Manlove, MD
Adjunct Clinical Assistant Professor, Family Medicine, Indiana University, Bloomington, Indiana
Cough

JoAnn E. Manson, MD, DrPH
Chief, Division of Preventive Medicine Brigham and Women's Hospital; Professor of Medicine and the Michael and Lee Bell Professor of Women's Health, Harvard Medical School, Boston, Massachusetts
Menopause

Meghna P. Mansukhani, MD
Professor, Center for Sleep Medicine, Mayo Clinic, Rochester, Minnesota
Sleep Disorders

Claudio Marcocci, MD
Professor, Endocrinology, Clinical and Experimental Medicine, University of Pisa, Pisa, Italy
Hyperparathyroidism and Hypoparathyroidism

Curtis E. Margo, MD, MPH
Clinical Professor, Pathology & Cell Biology and Ophthalmology, University of South Florida Morsani College of Medicine, Tampa, Florida
Uveitis

Jason E. Marker, MD, MPA
Associate Director, Memorial Family Medicine Residency, Memorial Hospital, South Bend, Indiana
Neurofibromatosis (Type 1)

Paul Martin, MD
Chief, Gastroenterology/Hepatology, University of Miami Miller School of Medicine, Miami, Florida
Cirrhosis

Samuel Mathis, MD
Assistant Professor, Family Medicine, University of Texas Medical Branch at Galveston, Galveston, Texas
Infective Endocarditis

Mark A. Matza, MD, MBA
Physician, Rheumatology, Massachusetts General Hospital, Boston, Massachusetts
Polymyalgia Rheumatica and Giant Cell Arteritis

Pinckney J. Maxwell IV, MD
Associate Professor, Colon and Rectal Surgery, Medical University of South Carolina, Charleston, South Carolina
Tumors of the Colon and Rectum

Danica May, MD
Assistant Professor, Urologic Oncology and Urology, University of Kansas Medical Center, Kansas City, Kansas
Malignant Tumors of the Urogenital Tract

Marshall Mazepa, MD
Assistant Professor, Hematology, Oncology, and Transplantation, University of Minnesota Medical School, Minneapolis, Minnesota
Porphyrias

Molly McClain, MD, MPH
Assistant Professor; Program Director, Family and Community Medicine, University of New Mexico School of Medicine, Albuquerque, New Mexico
Gender Affirming Care

Christopher McGrew, MD
Professor, Family and Community Medicine, Orthopedics and Rehabilitation, Sports Medicine, University of New Mexico Health Sciences Center, Albuquerque, New Mexico
Sports-Related Head Injuries

Christopher C. McGuigan, MBChB, MPH
Honorary Senior Lecturer, Public Health Medicine, University of Aberdeen, Aberdeen, Scotland, United Kingdom
Psittacosis

†Michael McGuigan, MD
Medical Toxicology

Meetal Mehta, MD
Nutrition Support Service Attending, Surgery; Obesity Medicine Physician, Endocrinology, Diabetes, and Hypertension, Brigham and Women's Hospital, Boston, Massachusetts
Parenteral Nutrition in Adults

Mick S. Meiselman, MD
Director, Advanced Therapeutic Endoscopy, Gastroenterology; Director, Advanced Therapeutic Endoscopy, Dignity Health Central Coast, San Luis Obispo, California
Calculous Biliary Disease

Moises Mercado, MD
Director, Endocrine Research Unit, Hospital de Especialidades, Centro Medico Nacional S.XXI, IOMSS; Professor, Medicine, Faculty of Medicine, Universidad Nacional Autónoma de Mexico, Mexico City, Mexico
Acromegaly

Steven L. Meyers, MD
Vice Chair, Quality and Informatics, Neurology, NorthShore University Health System, Evanston, Illinois
Acute Facial Paralysis

William Michael, MD
Assistant Professor, Family Medicine and Community Health, University of Wisconsin School of Medicine and Public Health, Madison, Wisconsin
Peripheral Artery Disease

Brian J. Miller, MD, PhD, MPH
Professor, Psychiatry and Health Behavior, Augusta University Medical College of Georgia, Augusta, Georgia
Schizophrenia

Timothy M. Millington, MD
Assistant Professor, Surgery, Dartmouth-Hitchcock Medical Center, Lebanon, New Hampshire
Pleural Effusion and Empyema

Moben Mirza, MD
Professor, Urology, University of Kansas Medical Center, Kansas City, Kansas
Hematuria; Malignant Tumors of the Urogenital Tract

Kriti Mishra, MD
Resident Physician, Dermatology, University of New Mexico School of Medicine, Albuquerque, New Mexico
Fungal Infections of the Skin

Howard C. Mofenson, MD
Professor of Pharmacology and Toxicology, New York College of Osteopathic Medicine, Old Westbury, New York; Professor of Pediatrics and Emergency Medicine, Renaissance School of Medicine at Stony Brook University, Stony Brook, New York
Medical Toxicology

Kris M. Mogensen, MS
Team Leader Dietitian Specialist, Nutrition, Brigham and Women's Hospital, Boston, Massachusetts
Parenteral Nutrition in Adults

Michael L. Moritz, MD
Professor, Pediatrics, UPMC Children's Hospital of Pittsburgh, Pittsburgh, Pennsylvania
Parenteral Fluid Therapy for Infants and Children

Rami Mortada, MD
Physician, Endocrine Center of Kansas, Wichita, Kansas
Diabetes Insipidus

Parisa Mortaji, MD
Instructor, Medicine, University of Colorado School of Medicine, Aurora, Colorado
Tuberculosis and Other Mycobacterial Diseases

Heather E. Moss, MD, PhD
Assistant Professor, Ophthalmology & Neurology and Neurological Sciences, Stanford University School of Medicine, Stanford, California
Optic Neuritis

Salama Mostafa, MBBCH
Fellow, Pediatric Endocrinology, Mayo Clinic, Rochester, Minnesota
Obesity in Children

Judd W. Moul, MD
James H. Semans, MD Professor of Surgery, Urologic Surgery, Duke University School of Medicine, Durham, North Carolina
Benign Prostatic Hyperplasia

Martha Muller, MD
Professor, Pediatrics, University of New Mexico School of Medicine, Albuquerque, New Mexico
Bacterial Meningitis

Natalia Murinova, MD
Clinical Professor; Director Headache Clinic, Neurology, University of Washington School of Medicine, Seattle, Washington
Migraine

Michael Murphy, MD
Dermatopathologist, Dermatology, UConn Health, Farmington, Connecticut
Nevi

Arjun Muthusubramanian, MD, MPH
Attending Physician, Landmark Health, Optum, Richmond, Virginia
Bacterial Pneumonia

Alykhan S. Nagji, MD
Assistant Professor, Thoracic Surgery, University of Kansas Medical Center, Kansas City, Kansas
Atelectasis

Brian James Nagle, MD, MPH
Assistant Professor, Neurology, University of Wisconsin School of Medicine and Public Health, Madison, Wisconsin
Parkinson Disease

Laura Naranjo, MD
Senior Medical Affairs Manager, Vaccines CARICAM, GlaxoSmithKline Panamá, Inestigador Nacional 1 SNI-Senacyt, Panamá, Panama
Malaria

Rabab Nasim, MD
Pulmonary and Critical Care Medicine, University of Wisconsin School of Medicine and Public Health, Madison, Wisconsin
Sepsis

Matthew Nazari, MD
Clinical Researcher, Eunice Kennedy Shriver National Institute of Child Health and Human Development, National Institutes of Health, Bethesda, Maryland
Pheochromocytoma

Moniba Nazeef, MD
Assistant Professor, Hematology and Oncology, University of Wisconsin School of Medicine and Public Health, Madison, Wisconsin
Venous Thromboembolism

Viswanathan K. Neelakantan, MD
Senior Professor of Medicine, Consultant in Tropical Medicine, Faculty of Medicine, Sri Manakula Vinayagar Medical College Hospital, Pondicherry, India
Foodborne Illnesses

Donald A. Neff, MD
Assistant Professor, Urology, University of Kansas School of Medicine, Kansas City, Kansas
Urinary Tract Infections in the Male

Tara J. Neil, MD
Clinical Associate Professor, Family and Community Medicine, University of Kansas School of Medicine–Wichita, Wichita, Kansas
Postpartum Care

William G. Nelson, MD, PhD
Professor and Director, Sidney Kimmel Comprehensive Cancer Center, Johns Hopkins University School of Medicine, Baltimore, Maryland
Prostate Cancer

David G. Neschis, MD
Clinical Associate Professor, Surgery, The Maryland Vascular Center, University of Maryland Baltimore Washington Medical Center, Glen Burnie, Maryland
Aortic Disease: Aneurysm and Dissection

Theresa Nester, MD
Professor, Laboratory Medicine and Pathology, University of Washington Medical Center, Medical Director of Integrated Transfusion Services, Bloodworks Northwest, Seattle, Washington
Blood Component Therapy and Transfusion Reactions

Tam T. Nguyen, MD
Clinician and Instructor, Family Medicine, Washington Township Medical Group, Fremont, California
Papulosquamous Eruptions

Andrea L. Nicol, MD, MSc
Associate Professor, Anesthesiology, University of Kansas School of Medicine, Kansas City, Kansas
Fibromyalgia

Lucybeth Nieves-Arriba, MD
Assistant Professor, Gynecology Oncology, Zimmer Cancer Center, Wilmington, North Carolina
Cancer of the Uterine Cervix

Crystal M. North, MD, MPH
Physician, Pulmonary and Critical Care Medicine, Massachusetts General Hospital; Instructor, Medicine, Harvard Medical School, Boston, Massachusetts
Monoclonal Antibodies

Andrei Novac, MD, DFAPA
Clinical Professor, Psychiatry, Director, Traumatic Stress Program, Department of Psychiatry, University of California, Irvine, School of Medicine, Irvine, California
Depressive, Bipolar, and Related Mood Disorders

Enrico M. Novelli, MD
Associate Professor, Medicine, University of Pittsburgh School of Medicine, Pittsburgh, Pennsylvania
Sickle Cell Disease

Lauren Nye, MD
Associate Professor, Medical Oncology, University of Kansas School of Medicine, Kansas City, Kansas
Benign Breast Disease; Breast Cancer

Andrea T. Obi, MD
Assistant Professor, Surgery, University of Michigan Medical School, Ann Arbor, Michigan
Venous Thrombosis

Jeffrey P. Okeson, DMD
Professor and Dean, Oral Health Science, University of Kentucky, Lexington, Kentucky
Temporomandibular Disorders

Carlos R. Oliveira, MD, PhD
Assistant Professor, Pediatrics, Yale School of Medicine; Assistant Professor, Biostatistics, Yale School of Public Health, New Haven, Connecticut
Lyme Disease and Post-Treatment Lyme Disease Syndrome

Peck Y. Ong, MD
Associate Professor, Pediatrics, USC/Children's Hospital Los Angeles, Los Angeles, California
Atopic Dermatitis

Daniel S. Oram, MD
Adjunct Assistant Professor, Family Medicine, University of Michigan Medical School, Ann Arbor, Michigan
Postpartum Depression

David D. Ortiz, MD
Director, Medical Residency Programs, National Health Institute, Asunción, Paraguay
Leg Edema and Venous Stasis

Sabah Osmani, BA
Resident, Dermatology, University of North Carolina School of Medicine, Chapel Hill, North Carolina
Fungal Infections of the Skin

Bulent Ozgonenel, MD
Associate Professor, Pediatric Hematology Oncology, Children's Hospital of Michigan, Detroit, Michigan
Hemophilia and Related Conditions

Karel Pacak, MD, PhD, DSc
Chief, Section on Medical Neuroendocrinology, Eunice Kennedy Shriver National Institute of Child Health and Human Development, National Institutes of Health, Bethesda, Maryland
Pheochromocytoma

Jose A. Padin-Rosado, MD
Associate Professor, Neurology; Medical Director, Neurodiagnostic Laboratory, University of New Mexico School of Medicine, Albuquerque, New Mexico
Seizures and Epilepsy in Adolescents and Adults

Tanyatuth Padungkiatsagul, MD
Associate Professor, Ophthalmology, Faculty of Medicine Ramathibodi Hospital, Mahidol University, Bangkok, Thailand
Optic Neuritis

Contributors

Heather L. Paladine, MD, MEd
Assistant Professor, Medicine, Columbia University Medical Center, Center for Family and Community Medicine, Columbia College of Physicians and Surgeons, New York, New York
Vulvovaginitis

John E. Pandolfino, MD
Hans Popper Professor of Medicine, Northwestern University Feinberg School of Medicine, Chicago, Illinois
Dysphagia and Esophageal Obstruction

Marc Parrish, DO
Associate Professor, Obstetrics and Gynecology; Division Director, Maternal-Fetal Medicine; Fellowship Director, Maternal-Fetal Medicine, The University of Kansas Medical Center, Kansas City, Kansas
Hypertensive Disorders in Pregnancy

Deval Patel, MD
Pediatric Hospitalist, Hospital Pediatrics, Nemours Children's Specialty Care; Associate Program Director, Department of Pediatrics, University of Florida College of Medicine-Jacksonville, Jacksonville, Florida
Parenteral Fluid Therapy for Infants and Children

Hirenkumar Patel, MD
Assistant Professor, Pediatric Neonatology, Virginia Tech Carilion School of Medicine; Assistant Medical Director, Pediatric Neonatology, Pediatrix Medical Group, Roanoke, Virginia
Resuscitation of the Newborn

Simon Patton, MD
Physician, Female Pelvic Medicine and Reconstructive Surgery, Ascension Via Christi, Wichita, Kansas
Urinary Incontinence

Gerson O. Penna, PhD
Medical and Senior Researcher of the Tropical Medicine Centre, University of Brazil, Brasilia, Brazil
Leprosy

Maria Lucia Penna, MD, PhD
Professor, Epidemiology and Biostatistics, Universidade Federal Fluminense, Niteroi, Rio de Janeiro, Brazil
Leprosy

Allen Perkins, MD, MPH
Professor and Chair, Family Medicine, University of South Alabama College of Medicine, Mobile, Alabama
Marine Poisonings, Envenomations, and Trauma

Vesna M. Petronic-Rosic, MD, MSc, MBA
Physician, Dermatology, Cook County Health, Chicago, Illinois
Melanoma

Hanna Phan, PharmD
Clinical Associate Professor, Clinical Pharmacy, University of Michigan; Clinical Pharmacist Specialist, Pediatric Pulmonary; Pharmacy Innovations and Partnerships, C.S. Mott Children's, Michigan Medicine; Faculty Affiliate, Susan B. Meister Child Health Evaluation and Research Center, University of Michigan, Ann Arbor, Michigan
Cystic Fibrosis

Hiep Phan, MD
Internal Medicine, University of Wisconsin Health, Madison, Wisconsin
Nonalcoholic Fatty Liver Disease (NAFLD)

Mark Pietroni, MD, MBA
Medical Director, Medical Directorate, Gloucestershire Hospitals NHS FT, Gloucester, United Kingdom
Cholera

Gregory A. Plotnikoff, MD, MTS
Medical Director, Internal Medicine and Pediatrics, Minnesota Personalized Medicine, Minneapolis, Minnesota
Genomic Testing

Susan M. Pollart, MD, MS
Ruth E. Murdaugh Professor, Family Medicine; Senior Associate Dean for Faculty Affairs and Faculty Development, Office of the Dean, University of Virginia School of Medicine, Charlottesville, Virginia
Asthma in Children

Jennifer K. Poon, MD
Professor, Pediatrics, Augusta University Medical College of Georgia, Augusta, Georgia
Attention-Deficit/Hyperactivity Disorder

Andrew S.T. Porter, DO
Director of Sports Medicine Fellowship; Clinical Associate Professor, Family and Community Medicine; University of Kansas School of Medicine–Wichita, Wichita, Kansas
Common Sports Injuries

Charles Powell, MD
Associate Professor, Urology, Indiana University School of Medicine, Indianapolis, Indiana
Prostatitis

Margaret Pusateri, MD
Sports Medicine, Emergency Medicine, Pittsburgh, Pennsylvania
Sports-Related Head Injuries

James M. Quinn, MD
Associate Program Director, Allergy/Immunology, San Antonio Uniformed Service Health Education Consortium, San Antonio, Texas; Professor, Medicine, Uniformed Services University of the Health Sciences, Bethesda, Maryland
Allergic Reactions to Insect Stings

Peter S. Rahko, MD
Professor, Medicine, University of Wisconsin School of Medicine and Public Health; Director, Adult Echocardiography Laboratory, University of Wisconsin Hospital, Madison, Wisconsin
Mitral Valve Prolapse

S. Vincent Rajkumar, MD
Edward W. and Betty Knight Scripps Professor of Medicine, Hematology, Mayo Clinic, Rochester, Minnesota
Multiple Myeloma

Anand Rajpara, MD
Associate Professor and Founding Chair, Department of Dermatology, University Health/University of Missouri School of Medicine, Kansas City, Missouri
Autoimmune Bullous Diseases; Pyoderma Gangrenosum

Kalyanakrishnan Ramakrishnan, MD
Professor, Family and Preventive Medicine, University of Oklahoma Health Sciences Center, Oklahoma City, Oklahoma
Necrotizing Skin and Soft-Tissue Infections

Jatin Rana, MD
Assistant Professor, Hematology/Oncology, Michigan State University College of Human Medicine, East Lansing, Michigan
Chronic Leukemias

Matthew A. Rank, MD
Professor, Allergy, Asthma, and Clinical Immunology, Mayo Clinic, Scottsdale, Arizona
Asthma in Adolescents and Adults

Didier Raoult, MD, PhD
Unite de Recherche Sur les Maladies Infectieuses Tropicales, Aix-Marseille Universite, Marseille, France
Q Fever

Alwyn Rapose, MD
Consultant, Infectious Diseases, Reliant Medical Group; Assistant Professor, Medicine, UMass Chan Medical School, Worcester, Massachusetts
Toxic Shock Syndrome

Rachel E. Rau, MD
Associate Professor, Pediatrics, Baylor College of Medicine, Houston, Texas
Acute Leukemia in Children

Anita Devi K. Ravindran, MD
Physician, Microbiology, Manipal University College Melaka, Melaka Tengah, Malaysia
Foodborne Illnesses

Jared Regehr, MD
Assistant Professor, Family and Community Medicine, University of Kansas School of Medicine–Wichita, Wichita, Kansas
Fatigue

Ian R. Reid, MBChB, MD
Distinguished Professor, Medicine, University of Auckland Faculty of Medical and Health Sciences, Auckland, New Zealand
Paget's Disease of Bone

Elissa Rennert-May, MD, MSc
Infectious Diseases Physician, Medicine, University of Calgary Cumming School of Medicine, Calgary, Canada
Methicillin-Resistant Staphylococcus aureus

Karl Rew, MD
Associate Professor, Family Medicine and Urology, University of Michigan Medical School, Ann Arbor, Michigan
Erectile Dysfunction

Amanda Rhyne, MD
Clinical Assistant Professor, Family and Community Medicine, University of Kansas School of Medicine–Wichita, Salina, Kansas
Serum Sickness

Martha Riese, MD
Clinical Assistant Professor, Family and Community Medicine, University of Kansas School of Medicine–Wichita, Salina, Kansas
Varicella (Chickenpox)

David C. Robbins, MD, MPH
Professor, Medicine; Director, University of Kansas Diabetes Institute; Bud and Sally Cray Professor of Diabetes, University of Kansas School of Medicine, Kansas City, Kansas
Diabetes Mellitus in Adults

Sophie Robert, PharmD
Clinical Pharmacy Specialist, Psychiatry; Affiliate Faculty, Psychiatry & Behavioral Sciences, Medical University of South Carolina, Charleston, South Carolina
Attention-Deficit/Hyperactivity Disorder

Amy Robertson, PharmD
Assistant Professor, Pharmacy Practice, University of Arkansas–Northwest Campus; Clinical Pharmacist, Family Medicine, UAMS Health Family Medical Center Fayetteville, Fayetteville, Arkansas
Serum Sickness

Malcolm K. Robinson, MD
Assistant Professor, Surgery, Harvard Medical School; Attending Physician, Metabolic Support Service, Brigham and Women's Hospital, Boston, Massachusetts
Parenteral Nutrition in Adults

William P. Roche, MD
Neuromuscular Division, Emory University, Atlanta, Georgia
Myasthenia Gravis

Tessa E. Rohrberg, MD
Assistant Professor, Family and Community Medicine, University of Kansas School of Medicine–Wichita, Wichita, Kansas
Delirium

Candice E. Rose, MD, MS
Assistant Professor, Internal Medicine, The University of Kansas Health System, Kansas City, Kansas
Diabetes Mellitus in Adults

Peter G. Rose, MD
Staff Physician, Gynecological Oncology, The Cleveland Clinic, Cleveland, Ohio
Cancer of the Uterine Cervix

Stephen Ross, MD
Professor and Vice Chair, Neurology, Penn State University, Hershey, Pennsylvania
Nonmigraine Headache

Alan R. Roth, DO
Chairman, Family Medicine and Ambulatory Care, Jamaica Hospital Medical Center, Jamaica, New York; Assistant Professor, Family and Social Medicine, Albert Einstein College of Medicine, Bronx, New York; Professor, Family Medicine, NYIT College of Osteopathic Medicine, Old Westbury, New York; Chief, Integrative Pain and Palliative Care, Medisys Health Network, Jamaica, New York
Fever

Anne-Michelle Ruha, MD
Chair, Medical Toxicology, Banner–University Medical Center Phoenix; Professor, Internal Medicine and Emergency Medicine, University of Arizona College of Medicine, Phoenix, Arizona
Spider Bites and Scorpion Stings; Venomous Snakebite

Kristen Rundell, MS, MD
Professor and Chair, Department of Family and Community Medicine, University of Arizona College of Medicine, Tucson, Arizona
Drug Hypersensitivity Reactions, Mumps

Adnan Said, MD, MS
Professor, Medicine, Gastroenterology and Hepatology, University of Wisconsin School of Medicine and Public Health, Madison, Wisconsin
Nonalcoholic Fatty Liver Disease (NAFLD)

Tomoko Sairenji, MD, MS
Associate Professor, Family Medicine, University of Washington School of Medicine, Seattle, Washington
Acute Bronchitis and Other Viral Respiratory Infections

Susan L. Samson, MD, PhD
Chair, Medicine/Endocrinology, Mayo Clinic, Jacksonville, Florida
Hyponatremia

Carlos E. Sanchez, MD
Faculty, Interventional Cardiology and Advanced Structural Heart Disease, Internal Medicine, Riverside Methodist Hospital, Columbus, Ohio
Valvular Heart Disease

Sandeep Sangodkar, DO
Cardiologist, Cardiology Specialists Medical Group; Assistant Clinical Professor, Internal Medicine/Cardiology, University of California, Riverside, School of Medicine, Riverside, California; Clinical Assistant Professor, Internal Medicine/Cardiology, Western University, Pomona, California
Hypertrophic Cardiomyopathy

Arelis Santana, MD, MPH
Assistant Professor, Infectious Diseases, University of New Mexico School of Medicine, Albuquerque, New Mexico
Salmonellosis

Ravi Sarode, MD
Director, Division of Transfusion and Hemostasis, Pathology, UT Southwestern Medical Center, Dallas, Texas
Thrombotic Thrombocytopenic Purpura

Michael Schatz, MD, MS
Staff Physician, Allergy, Kaiser Permanente; Clinical Professor, Medicine, University of California San Diego School of Medicine, San Diego, California
Asthma in Adolescents and Adults

Alex Schevchuck, MD, MS
Associate Professor, Internal Medicine/Cardiology, University of New Mexico School of Medicine, Albuquerque, New Mexico
Congestive Heart Failure; Tachycardias

Lawrence R. Schiller, MD
Chair, Institutional Review Boards, Baylor Scott & White Research Institute, Baylor University Medical Center, Clinical Professor, Medical Education, Texas A&M School of Medicine, Dallas Campus, Dallas, Texas
Malabsorption

Kristin Schmid Biggerstaff, MD
Associate Professor, Ophthalmology, Baylor College of Medicine; Glaucoma Staff, Eye Care Line, Michael E. DeBakey Veterans Affairs Medical Center, Houston, Texas
Glaucoma

Darren Schmidt, MD
Assistant Professor, Medicine; Clinical Nephrologist, University of New Mexico Health Sciences Center, Albuquerque, New Mexico
Chronic Kidney Disease

Sarina Schrager, MD, MS
Professor, Family Medicine, University of Wisconsin School of Medicine and Public Health, Madison, Wisconsin
Abnormal Uterine Bleeding

Dan Schuller, MD
Professor, Medicine, Texas Tech University Health Science Center; Chair, Department of Medicine-Transmoutain, Texas Tech University Health Sciences Center. El Paso, Texas
Lung Abscess; Pulmonary Hypertension

Teresa Sciortino, MD
Fellow Physician, Endocrinology, Diabetes and Clinical Pharmacology, University of Kansas Medical Center, Kansas City, Kansas
Thyroid Cancer

Justin Seashore, MD
Physician, Pulmonary and Critical Care, Kaiser Permanente, Vacaville, California
Post-Acute COVID Syndrome

Wafik G. Sedhom, MD
Hematology/Oncology, McGaw Medical Center of Northwestern University, Chicago, Illinois
Myelodysplastic Syndromes

†Steven Seifert, MD
Professor, Emergency Medicine, University of New Mexico School of Medicine; Medical Director, New Mexico Poison and Drug Information Center, University of New Mexico Health Sciences Center, Albuquerque, New Mexico
Venomous Snakebite

Jeffery D. Semel, MD
Physician, Infectious Diseases, Medicine, NorthShore University Healthsystem, Evanston, Illinois; Associate Professor of Clinical Medicine, University of Chicago Pritzker School of Medicine, Chicago, Illinois
Clostridioides difficile Colitis

Saeed Kamran Shaffi, MD, MS
Associate Professor, Internal Medicine/Nephrology, University of New Mexico School of Medicine, Albuquerque, New Mexico
Primary Glomerular Disease

Beejal Shah, MD
Endocrinologist, Bay Pines VA, Bay Pines, Florida
Hyponatremia

Meera Shah, MBChB, MRCP (Edin)
Consultant, Endocrinology, Diabetes, and Nutrition, Mayo Clinic, Rochester, Minnesota
Obesity in Adults

Prediman K. Shah, MD
Professor, Medicine, University of California Los Angeles Cedars-Sinai Medical Center; Shapell and Webb Chair in Clinical Cardiology, Director of Oppenheimer Atherosclerosis Research Center and Atherosclerosis Prevention and Treatment Center, Smidt Heart Institute, Cedars-Sinai Medical Center, Los Angeles, California
Acute Myocardial Infarction

Shenil Shah, MD
Cardiology Fellow, Cardiovascular Medicine, University of Wisconsin Hospitals and Clinics, Madison, Wisconsin
Mitral Valve Prolapse

Jamile M. Shammo, MD
Professor, Medicine, Hematology Oncology, and Stem Cell Transplant, Rush University Medical Center, Chicago, Illinois
Myelodysplastic Syndromes

Kathleen Mary Shannon, MD
Professor and Chair, Department of Neurology, University of Wisconsin School of Medicine and Public Health, Madison, Wisconsin
Parkinson Disease

---

†Deceased.

Eugene D. Shapiro, MD
Professor, Pediatrics, Epidemiology of Microbial Diseases, and Investigative Medicine, Yale School of Medicine, New Haven, Connecticut
Lyme Disease and Post-Treatment Lyme Disease Syndrome

Ala I. Sharara, MD
Professor, Internal Medicine, American University of Beirut Medical Center, Beirut, Lebanon
Bleeding Esophageal Varices

Sonal Sharma, MD
Pediatric Neurologist, Mitochondrial Medicine Frontier Program, Children's Hospital of Philadelphia, Philadelphia, Pennsylvania
Mitochondrial Disease

John P. Sheehan, MD
Professor, Medicine/Hematology-Oncology, University of Wisconsin School of Medicine and Public Health; Medical Director, UW Health Comprehensive Bleeding Disorders Program, University of Wisconsin Hospital and Clinics; Medical Director, UWHC Special Coagulation Laboratory, UW Health, Madison, Wisconsin
Venous Thromboembolism

Kamille Sherman, MD
Assistant Professor, Family and Community Medicine, University of North Dakota School of Medicine and Health Sciences, Grand Forks, North Dakota
Sunburn

Laura Elyse Shevy, MD
Associate Professor, Infectious Diseases, University of New Mexico Health Sciences Center, Albuquerque, New Mexico
Tuberculosis and Other Mycobacterial Diseases

Sable Shew, MD
Physician, Urology, University of Kansas School of Medicine, Kansas City, Kansas
Urethral Stricture Disease

Victor S. Sierpina, MD
Professor, Family and Integrative Medicine, University of Texas Medical Branch at Galveston, Galveston, Texas
Post-Acute COVID Syndrome

Karlynn Sievers, MD
Associate Program Director, Family Medicine, St. Mary's Family Medicine Residency, Grand Junction, Colorado
Trigeminal Neuralgia

Hugh Silk, MD, MPH
Professor, Family Medicine and Community Health, UMass Chan Medical School, Worcester, Massachusetts
Trigeminal Neuralgia; Diseases of the Mouth

Lisa Simon, MD, DMD
Fellow, Oral Health Policy and Epidemiology, Harvard Medical School, Boston, Massachusetts
Diseases of the Mouth

Aaron D. Sinclair, MD
Associate Professor, Family and Community Medicine, University of Kansas School of Medicine–Wichita, Wichita, Kansas
Diverticula of the Alimentary Tract

Dawd S. Siraj, MD, MPH, TM
Professor, Infectious Diseases, University of Wisconsin School of Medicine and Public Health, Madison, Wisconsin
Travel Medicine

Jeannina Smith, MD
Associate Professor, Medicine, University of Wisconsin School of Medicine and Public Health, Madison, Wisconsin
Sepsis

Zachary L. Smith, DO
Assistant Professor, Gastroenterology and Liver Disease, Case Western Reserve University, Cleveland, Ohio
Calculous Biliary Disease

Rupal Soder, PhD
Project Director, Midwest Stem Cell Therapy Center, University of Kansas Medical Center, Kansas City, Kansas
Stem Cell Therapy

John Sojka, MD
Director of Orthopaedic Trauma, Orthopaedic Surgery, University of Kansas Health System, Lake Quivira, Kansas
Osteomyelitis

William J. Somers, MD
Physician, Urology, Columbus VA Ambulatory Care Center, Columbus, Ohio
Nephrolithiasis

Mihae Song, MD
Assistant Professor, Gynecologic Oncology, City of Hope, Duarte, California
Ovarian Cancer

Nestor Sosa, MD, MS
Infectious Diseases Division Chief, Internal Medicine, University of New Mexico School of Medicine, Albuquerque, New Mexico
Malaria

Timothy Sowder, MD
Assistant Professor, Pain Medicine, University of Kansas Health System, Kansas City, Kansas
Fibromyalgia

Linda Speer, MD
Professor and Chair, Family Medicine, University of Toledo College of Medicine and Life Sciences, Toledo, Ohio
Dysmenorrhea

Erik Kent St. Louis, MD
Professor, Neurology and Medicine, Mayo Clinic, Rochester, Minnesota
Sleep Disorders

Todd Stephens, MD, DTM&H
Clinical Associate Professor, Family and Community Medicine, University of Kansas School of Medicine–Wichita, Wichita, Kansas
Genital Ulcer Disease: Chancroid, Granuloma Inguinale, and Lymphogranuloma

Melissa Stiles, MD
Professor, Family Medicine, University of Wisconsin School of Medicine and Public Health, Madison, Wisconsin
Pyelonephritis

Constantine Stratakis, MD, PhD
Scientific Director, Eunice Kennedy Shriver National Institute of Child Health and Human Development,, National Institutes of Health, Bethesda, Maryland
Cushing's Syndrome

Daniel Stulberg, MD
Professor and Chair, Family and Community Medicine, Western Michigan University Homer Stryker M.D. School of Medicine, Kalamazoo, Michigan; Emeritus Professor, Family and Community Medicine, University of New Mexico School of Medicine, Albuquerque, New Mexico
Premalignant Skin Lesions

Jose D. Suarez, MD
Tropical Medicine Advisor, Pediatric Infectious Disease, Clinical Research Unit; Instituto Conmemorativo Gorgas, Panamá, Panama, Investigator SNI, Secretaría Nacional de Ciencia, Tecnología e Innovación, Panamá, Panama
Malaria

Masayoshi Takashima, MD
Chairman, Otolaryngology–Head and Neck Surgery, Houston Methodist Hospital, Houston, Texas
Rhinitis; Obstructive Sleep Apnea

Varun Takyar, MD
Staff Gastroenterologist/Hepatologist, Sutter Health East Bay Medical Foundation, Berkeley, California
Hepatitis A, B, D, and E

Carolina Talhari, MD, PhD
Adjunct Professor, Dermatology, State University of Amazonas; Dermatologist, Alfredo da Matta Foundation, Manaus, Brazil
Leprosy

Jie Tang, MD
Associate Professor, Kidney Diseases and Hypertension, Warren Alpert Medical School of Brown University, Providence, Rhode Island
Hypokalemia and Hyperkalemia

Emma Taylor-Salmon, MD
Clinical Fellow, Pediatrics, Yale School of Medicine, New Haven, Connecticut
Lyme Disease and Post-Treatment Lyme Disease Syndrome

Kimberly Templeton, MD
Professor, Orthopaedic Surgery, University of Kansas Medical Center, Kansas City, Kansas
Osteomyelitis

Joyce M.C. Teng, MD, PhD
Professor, Dermatology and Pediatrics, Stanford University School of Medicine, Stanford, California
Urticaria and Angioedema

Jill Thein-Nissenbaum, PT, DSc
Professor, Sports Medicine Physical Therapy, Staff Physical Therapist, University of Wisconsin Athletics, University of Wisconsin, Madison, Wisconsin
High-Altitude Illness

Daniel R. Tilden, MD, MPH
Assistant Professor, Endocrinology, Diabetes, and Clinical Genetics, University of Kansas Medical Center, Kansas City, Kansas
Diabetes Mellitus in Adults

William Tillett, MBChB, PhD
Rheumatologist, Royal National Hospital for Rheumatic Diseases; Senior Lecturer, Pharmacy and Pharmacology, University of Bath, Bath, United Kingdom
Psoriatic Arthritis

Kenneth Tobin, DO
Clinical Assistant Professor, Cardiovascular Disease, University of Michigan Medical School, Ann Arbor, Michigan
Angina Pectoris

Theodore T. Tsaltas, MD
Assistant Professor, Obstetrics and Gynecology, University of Tennessee College of Medicine–Chattanooga, Chattanooga, Tennessee
Uterine Leiomyoma

Katherine Turner, MD
Clinical Assistant Professor, Family Medicine, University of Michigan Medical School, Ann Arbor, Michigan
Pruritis

Sebastian H. Unizony, MD
Assistant, Medicine, Massachusetts General Hospital; Instructor, Rheumatology, Allergy, and Immunology, Massachusetts General Hospital, Harvard Medical School, Boston, Massachusetts
Polymyalgia Rheumatica and Giant Cell Arteritis

Mark Unruh, MD
Chair, Department of Internal Medicine, University of New Mexico School of Medicine, Albuquerque, New Mexico
Chronic Kidney Disease

Locke Uppendahl, MD
Clinical Instructor, Gynecologic Oncologist, Obstetrics and Gynecology, University of Kansas School of Medicine–Wichita, Wichita, Kansas
Cancer of the Endometrium

Colin Vale, MD
Assistant Professor, Hematology and Medical Oncology, Emory University School of Medicine, Atlanta, Georgia
Acute Leukemia in Adults

Anusha Vallurupalli, MBBS
Assistant Professor, Medicine, Oregon Health Science University, Portland, Oregon
Hodgkin Lymphoma; Pernicious Anemia/Megaloblastic Anemia

George Van Buren II, MD
Associate Professor, Surgery, Baylor College of Medicine, Houston, Texas
Acute and Chronic Pancreatitis

†Daniel J. Van Durme, MD, MPH
Senior Associate Dean for Clinical and Community Affairs, Family Medicine and Rural Health, Florida State University College of Medicine, Tallahassee, Florida
Acne Vulgaris; Rosacea

Kristi VanDerKolk, MD
Family Medicine Residency Program Director, Department of Family and Community Medicine, Western Michigan University Homer Stryker M.D. School of Medicine, Kalamazoo, Michigan
Premalignant Skin Lesions

Elena V. Varlamov, MD
Assistant Professor, Medicine and Neurological Surgery, Oregon Health and Science University, Portland, Oregon
Adrenocortical Insufficiency; Hypopituitarism

---

†Deceased.

Megan Veglia, MD
Fellow, Pulmonary and Critical Care, Medical University of South Carolina, Charleston, South Carolina

Christopher Vélez, MD
Assistant in Medicine, Massachusetts General Hospital, Boston, Massachusetts
Dysphagia and Esophageal Obstruction

Gregory Vercellotti, MD
Professor, Medicine, University of Minnesota Medical School, Minneapolis, Minnesota
Porphyrias

Kyle Vincent, MD
Clinical Associate Professor, Surgery, University of Kansas School of Medicine–Wichita, Wichita, Kansas
Gastritis and Peptic Ulcer Disease

Donald C. Vinh, MD
Director, Center of Excellence for Genetic Research in Infection and Immunity, McGill University Health Center; Associate Professor, Clinician-Scientist, Medical Microbiology, McGill University Health Center, Montreal, Quebec, Canada
Blastomycosis

Jatin M. Vyas, MD, PhD
Associate Professor, Medicine, Massachusetts General Hospital; Associate Professor, Medicine, Harvard Medical School, Boston, Massachusetts
Rat-Bite Fever

Tamara Wagner, MD
Associate Professor, Pediatrics, Oregon & Health Science University, Portland, Oregon
Bronchiolitis

Thomas W. Wakefield, MD
Professor, Vascular Surgery, University of Michigan Medical School, Ann Arbor, Michigan
Venous Thrombosis

Arnold Wald, MD
Professor, Gastroenterology and Hepatology, University of Wisconsin School of Medicine and Public Health, Madison, Wisconsin
Irritable Bowel Syndrome

Ellen R. Wald, MD
Professor, Pediatrics, University of Wisconsin School of Medicine and Public Health; Physician; Infectious Diseases/Pediatrics, American Family Children's Hospital, Madison, Wisconsin
Urinary Tract Infections in Infants and Children

Sargun Walia, MD
Nonmigraine Headache

Robin A. Walker, MD
Clinical Assistant Professor, Family and Community Medicine, University of Kansas School of Medicine–Wichita, Wichita, Kansas
Epididymitis and Orchitis

Ernest Wang, MD
Clinical Professor, Emergency Medicine; Assistant Dean for Medical Education, Office of Academic Affairs, NorthShore University HealthSystem, Evanston, Illinois
Disturbances Due to Cold

Jennifer Wang, DO
Physician, Institute for Critical Care Medicine, Surgery, Mount Sinai Hospital, New York, New York
Targeted Temperature Management (Therapeutic Hypothermia)

Koji Watanabe, MD, PhD
Staff Doctor, AIDS Clinical Center, National Center for Global Health and Medicine, Tokyo, Japan
Amebiasis

Alexis Waters, PA
Physician Assistant, Hospital Medicine, UW Health, Madison, Wisconsin
Chronic Obstructive Pulmonary Disease

Ruth Weber, MD, MSEd
Clinical Associate Professor, Family and Community Medicine, Medical University of South Carolina, Charleston, South Carolina
Pharyngitis

Cheryl Wehler, MD
Assistant Professor, Psychiatry and Behavioral Sciences, University of Kansas School of Medicine–Wichita, Wichita, Kansas
Panic Disorder

Alice C. Wei, MD, MSc
Associate Attending Surgeon, Memorial Sloan Kettering Cancer Center; Associate Professor, Surgery; Weill Medical College of Cornell University, New York, New York
Pancreatic Cancer

Jane A. Weida, MD
Professor, Department Chair, Director of Clinical Affairs, Family, Internal, and Rural Medicine, University of Alabama, Tuscaloosa, Alabama
Measles (Rubeola)

David N. Weissman, MD
Director, Respiratory Health Division, National Institute for Occupational Safety and Health, Morgantown, West Virginia
Pneumoconiosis: Asbestosis and Silicosis

Robert C. Welliver Sr., MD
Professor, Pediatrics; Senior Scientist, Heartland Vaccines LLC, Stillwater, Oklahoma; Emeritus Professor, Pediatric Infectious Diseases, SUNY at Buffalo and Children's Hospital, Buffalo, New York
Viral Respiratory Infections

Rebecca M. Wester, MD
Adjunctive Associate Professor, Family Medicine-Geriatrics, University of Nebraska Medical Center, Omaha, Nebraska
Pressure Injury

Randell Wexler, MD, MPH
Professor and Clinical Vice Chair, Family Medicine, The Ohio State University College of Medicine, Columbus, Ohio
Premature Beats

Katarzyna Wilamowska, MD, PhD
Research Volunteer, Center for Memory and Aging, University of New Mexico School of Medicine, Albuquerque, New Mexico
Alzheimer's Disease

Kimberly Williams, MD
Clinical Assistant Professor, Family and Community Medicine, University of Kansas School of Medicine–Wichita, Salina, Kansas
Otitis Externa

Tracy L. Williams, MD
Associate Professor, Family and Community Medicine, University of Kansas School of Medicine–Wichita, Wichita, Kansas
Chlamydia Trachomatis

Boris Winterhoff, MD
Associate Professor, Gynecologic Oncology, University of Minnesota Medical School, Minneapolis, Minnesota
Cancer of the Endometrium

Jennifer Wipperman, MD, MPH
Associate Professor, Family and Community Medicine, University of Kansas School of Medicine–Wichita, Wichita, Kansas
Dizziness and Vertigo

Mark Wirtz, MD
Assistant Professor, Family Medicine and Community Health, University of Wisconsin School of Medicine and Public Health, Madison, Wisconsin
Pyelonephritis

Robert Wittler, MD
Professor, Pediatrics, University of Kansas School of Medicine–Wichita, Wichita, Kansas
Tickborne Rickettsial Diseases (Rocky Mountain Spotted Fever and Other Spotted Fever Group Rickettsioses, Ehrlichioses, and Anaplasmosis)

Gary S. Wood, MD
Professor Emeritus and Founding Chair, Dermatology, University of Wisconsin School of Medicine and Public Health; Physician, Medicine (Dermatology), Middleton VA Medical Center, Madison, Wisconsin
Cutaneous T-Cell Lymphomas, Including Mycosis Fungoides and Sézary Syndrome

Scott Worswick, MD
Associate Professor, Dermatology, USC Keck School of Medicine, Los Angeles, California
Stevens-Johnson Syndrome and Toxic Epidermal Necrolysis

Dominic J. Wu, MD
Autoimmune Bullous Diseases; Pyoderma Gangrenosum

Steve W. Wu, MD
Associate Professor, Neurology, Cincinnati Children's Hospital Medical Center, Cincinnati, Ohio
Gilles de la Tourette Syndrome

Hadley Wyre, MD
Associate Professor, Urology, University of Kansas School of Medicine, Kansas City, Kansas
Urethral Stricture Disease

Cathy Xie, DO
Post-Acute COVID Syndrome

Marita Yaghi, MD
Research Fellow, Dermatology, University of Miami Miller School of Medicine, Miami, Florida
Venous Ulcers

Steven J. Yakubov, MD
Director, Advanced Structural Heart Disease, Cardiology, Riverside Methodist Hospital, Columbus, Ohio
Valvular Heart Disease

Yul W. Yang, MD, PhD
Consultant, Dermatology, Mayo Clinic, Scottsdale, Arizona
Contact Dermatitis

Kenneth S. Yew, MD, MPH
Faculty, Gundersen Medical Foundation Family Medicine Residency Program, Gundersen Medical Center, La Crosse, Wisconsin
Tinnitus

James A. Yiannias, MD
Associate Professor, Dermatology, Mayo Clinic, Scottsdale, Arizona
Contact Dermatitis

Natawadee Young, MD
Affiliate Professor, Clinical Director, Family Medicine, AnMed Health Family Medicine Residency Program, Anderson, South Carolina
Antepartum Care

Alonso G. Zea Vera, MD
Neurologist, Children's National Hospital, Washington, District of Columbia
Gilles de la Tourette Syndrome

Shiwei Zhou, MD
Clinical Assistant Professor, Internal Medicine, University of Michigan Medical School, Ann Arbor, Michigan
Legionellosis (Legionnaire's Disease and Pontiac Fever)

Heinz Zoller, MD
Professor, Hepatology, Head, Christian Doppler Laboratory on Iron and Phosphate Biology, Medical University of Innsbruck, Innsbruck, Austria
Hemochromatosis

Preface

The anonymous quote, "Ask yourself if what you are doing today is getting you closer to where you want to be tomorrow," has a multitude of meanings and interpretations. In the realm of clinical medical practice, this quote drives us to ponder what we know, what we think we know, what we need to know, and how to advance our fund of knowledge in a rapidly changing field. Most practicing clinicians will admit that they likely know enough to survive tomorrow but fear that the rapid evolution of medical practice that looms after that may be overwhelming and insurmountable.

So ask yourself now, how do you stay current in medicine? What resources do you use? How many journals a week do you read? The editorial team at *Conn's Current Therapy* respects the challenges of managing vast amounts of new information while maintaining the core knowledge germane to our practices. Our perennial mission is to provide an easy-to-use and knowledge-forward reference to guide clinicians, even as the incidence of chronic diseases is climbing and life expectancy for men and women in the United States has declined for the fifth consecutive year after a catastrophic and massive modern day pandemic.

Our authors have the formidable task of ensuring that they deliver cogent synopses across each organ system, incorporating new references and key points that affirm and potentially change primary care practice. We are indebted to our returning authors who continue to provide updated chapters and to our new authors who lend their expertise and energy to developing new content. They all work diligently to revise, update, and create efficient chapters filled with information that is ready to use.

We, the editors of *Conn's Current Therapy 2024*, the 76th edition of this publication, have many people to thank for contributing to and ensuring the success and impactful magnitude of this annual publication. We would like to first thank our faithful readers for their continued interest in this book, as well as our many new readers, as it is *you* who drive us to raise the standard of excellence in providing a meaningful and educational guide for your clinical practices. We collectively dedicate this volume to our readers who against fatigue, burnout, various adversities, and information overload have always risen to the challenge and opportunity to provide outstanding healthcare to patients in need. We sincerely hope that this textbook provides a foundation for you to achieve success in the arena of optimal healthcare delivery.

In no particular order, we must acknowledge the phenomenal contributions of several people. This book does not move forward, develop, or get processed and published on time without the tireless and meticulous efforts of our Senior Content Development

Manager Katie DeFrancesco and our Content Development Specialist Kevin Travers. They do the "heavy lifting" and are actively involved in the onerous task of time management—which means keeping the editors on pace—to deliver a textbook comprising more than 335 chapters, 1500 pages, and 500 authors during an annual 8-month publication cycle window. We are honored to consider them as true partners in this project; we greatly value their organizational skills and appreciate their dedication to this textbook.

The real "behind the scenes" people whom we should never take for granted are the medical copyeditors who perfect the final product by ensuring accuracy and consistency in spelling, phrasing, grammar, and punctuation of the English language in this text. It is these individuals who allow for *Conn's Current Therapy* to maintain its cohesive style in readability and diction.

We greatly acknowledge Miriam Chan, PharmD, as a co-author and an authority who reviews every drug referenced in this textbook for FDA approval status and accurate dosing guidelines. This is a vast undertaking that requires substantial time and energy, as well as great attention to detail given the ever-changing and evolving field of pharmacology.

Charlotta "Lotta" Kryhl, our Senior Content Specialist, is truly the one who "steers the ship" and keeps the editorial team honest in our mission. She is a wealth of knowledge regarding the opportunities and challenges within the publication industry and provides us with guidance on how to plan for this publication year over year. She remains a champion of our passion to bring this updated textbook to you on an annual basis. Simply stated, without Lotta, we have no *Conn's Current Therapy*.

Doug Turner is our Senior Project Manager who oversees the final stages of production, including preparation for hard copy and electronic publication. Renee Duenow, our Senior Book Designer, creates the attractiveness and marketability of the layout, including the front and back cover design; we're *loving* the purple cover this year!

We are indebted to those above and to many others who contributed to this massive undertaking. Mostly, we are indebted to our readers and welcome feedback on how *Conn's Current Therapy* can continue to evolve in the coming years to meet your needs as busy clinicians.

Rick D. Kellerman, MD
David P. Rakel, MD
Joel J. Heidelbaugh, MD
Ernestine M. Lee, MD, MPH

Contents

SECTION 4
Digestive System

SECTION 5
Endocrine and Metabolic Disorders

Contents

SECTION 6
Hematology

SECTION 7
Head and Neck

SECTION 8
Infectious Diseases

Contents

†Deceased.

SECTION 18
Pregnancy and Antepartum Care

SECTION 19
Children's Health

Contents

† Deceased.

***Conn's Current Therapy 2024* uses a standardized system of footnotes:**

1. Not FDA approved for this indication.
2. Not available in the United States.
3. Exceeds dosage recommended by the manufacturer.
4. Not yet approved for use in the United States.
5. Investigational drug in the United States.
6. May be compounded by pharmacists.
7. Available as dietary supplement.
8. Orphan drug in the United States.
9. Available as homeopathic remedy.
10. Available in the United States from the Centers for Disease Control and Prevention.

Contents

xxxvii

1 Symptomatic Care Pending Diagnosis

CHEST PAIN

Method of
William E. Cayley Jr., MD, MDiv

CURRENT DIAGNOSIS

- Initial evaluation of chest pain should include evaluation of clinical stability, a concise history and physical examination, and a chest x-ray and electrocardiogram (ECG) unless the cause is clearly not life-threatening.
- Chest pain described as exertional, radiating to one or both arms, similar to or worse than prior cardiac chest pain, or associated with nausea, vomiting, or diaphoresis indicates high risk for acute coronary syndrome. ECG identifies ST-elevation myocardial infarction (STEMI); cardiac biomarkers are essential for further evaluation of suspected chest pain in the absence of STEMI.
- The Wells, Geneva, and Pisa clinical prediction rules and the pulmonary embolism rule-out criteria can help stratify a patient's risk of pulmonary embolism.
- Aortic dissection is an uncommon cause of chest pain, but patients with abrupt or instantaneous chest pain that is ripping, tearing, or stabbing should be evaluated for dissection with chest x-ray, computed tomography (CT), or magnetic resonance imaging.
- Chest pain associated with dyspnea or painful inspiration and tachycardia or friction rub on auscultation may indicate pericarditis or myocarditis.
- Esophageal rupture may be suspected in patients with pain, dyspnea, and shock after a forceful emesis, and prompt imaging with CT or esophagography is essential.
- Patients who have suspected tension pneumothorax and who are clinically stable should have a chest x-ray for confirmation before needle decompression is attempted.

CURRENT THERAPY

- Patients with ST-elevation myocardial infarction (STEMI) require urgent reperfusion, and those with unstable angina or non–NSTEMI require admission for further monitoring and evaluation.
- Most patients with pulmonary embolism require admission for monitoring and anticoagulation, although outpatient treatment may be possible for low-risk patients after initial evaluation and anticoagulation.
- Prompt surgical consultation is required for patients with confirmed or suspected aortic dissection or esophageal rupture.
- Clinically unstable patients with suspected tension pneumothorax need immediate needle decompression.

Epidemiology

Chest pain is the chief complaint in 1% to 2% of all outpatient primary care visits. More than 50% of emergency department (ED) visits for chest pain are for serious cardiovascular conditions such as acute coronary syndrome (ACS) or pulmonary embolism (PE), but these account for less than 15% of outpatient primary care encounters for chest pain, and up to 15% of chest pain episodes never reach a definitive diagnosis. Other potentially life-threatening etiologies for chest pain include PE, dissecting aortic aneurysm, esophageal rupture, and tension pneumothorax. In outpatient primary care, the most common causes of chest pain are musculoskeletal, gastrointestinal, angina caused by stable coronary artery disease (CAD), anxiety or other psychiatric conditions, and pulmonary disease.

Initial Assessment

In the initial evaluation of chest pain, it is important to obtain a clear history of the onset and evolution of the pain, especially details such as location, quality, duration, and aggravating or alleviating factors. Initial physical examination should include vital signs, assessment of the patient's overall general condition, and examination of the heart and lungs. If there are any clinical signs of instability (altered mental status, hypotension, marked dyspnea, or other signs of shock), initial stabilization and diagnosis must be addressed simultaneously, consistent with current guidelines for emergency cardiovascular care. Unless the history and physical examination suggest an obviously nonthreatening cause of chest discomfort, most adults with chest pain should at least have basic diagnostic testing with an electrocardiogram (ECG) and a chest x-ray. Several clinical prediction rules are available to help confirm or exclude some common causes of chest pain (Box 1).

Diagnosis and Treatment

Acute Coronary Syndrome

ACS includes acute myocardial infarction (MI) (ST-segment elevation and depression, and Q wave and non–Q wave) and unstable angina. Findings on the history and physical examination that increase the likelihood of ACS include radiation of pain to the right arm or shoulder, to both arms or shoulders, or to the left arm; pain associated with exertion, diaphoresis, nausea, or vomiting; pain described as pressure or as "worse than previous angina or similar to a previous MI"; or the presence of hypotension or an S3 on cardiac auscultation. Elements of the history and examination that decrease the likelihood of ACS are pleuritic, positional, or sharp chest pain; pain in an inframammary location; pain not associated with exertion; pain lasting just seconds or lasting more than 24 hours; or chest pain reproducible with palpation. A low-risk score on the Marburg Heart Score (MHS) or the INTERCHEST Clinical Prediction Rule can help exclude CAD in primary care patients with chest pain, and use of the MHS when evaluating primary care patients with chest pain has been shown to improve clinical diagnostic accuracy (Table 1). Recent studies have demonstrated that the presence or absence of typical cardiac risk factors (e.g., gender, diabetes, hypertension, smoking, high cholesterol, family history) have little diagnostic

BOX 1 · Clinical Prediction Rules for Evaluating Patients With Chest Pain

Acute Coronary Syndrome
- Diagnosing cardiac ischemia with exercise treadmill testing: Duke Treadmill score: https://www.mdcalc.com/duke-treadmill-score
- Assessing the risk of a major cardiac event in the next 6 weeks: HEART score: https://www.mdcalc.com/heart-score-major-cardiac-events
- Assessing the risk of ACS in someone with chest pain: Marburg Heart Score: https://www.mdcalc.com/marburg-heart-score-mhs
- Assessing the risk of ACS in someone with chest pain: INTERCHEST Clinical Prediction Rule: https://www.mdcalc.com/interchest-clinical-prediction-rule-chest-pain-primary-care
- Assessing long-term risk in those with ACS: GRACE ACS risk calculator: http://www.outcomes-umassmed.org/grace/
- Estimating mortality for patients with unstable angina and NSTEMI: TIMI Risk Score: https://timi.org/calculators/timi-risk-score-calculator-for-ua-nstemi/

Pulmonary Embolism
- Geneva score for predicting risk of PE: https://www.mdcalc.com/geneva-score-revised-pulmonary-embolism
- Pisa clinical model for predicting the probability of PE: https://ebmcalc.com/PulmonaryEmbRiskPisaCXR.htm
- Wells scoring system for risk of PE: https://www.mdcalc.com/wells-criteria-pulmonary-embolism
- Pulmonary embolism rule-out criteria: https://www.mdcalc.com/perc-rule-pulmonary-embolism

Thoracic Aortic Dissection
- Aortic dissection detection risk score: https://www.mdcalc.com/aortic-dissection-detection-risk-score-add-rs

Pneumonia
- Diehr diagnostic rule for pneumonia in adults with acute cough: http://www.soapnote.org/infectious/diehr-rule/

ACS, Acute coronary syndrome; *GRACE,* Global Registry of Acute Coronary Events; *NSTMI,* non–ST elevation myocardial infarction; *PE,* pulmonary embolism; *TIMI,* Thrombolysis in Myocardial Infarction Study Group.

TABLE 1 · Marburg Heart Score*

FINDING	POINTS
Women >64 years, men >54 years	1
Known CAD, cerebrovascular disease, or peripheral vascular disease	1
Pain worse with exercise	1
Pain not reproducible with palpation	1
Patient assumes pain is cardiac	1

*Approximately 23% of patients with an MHS score of ≥3 will have CAD. Approximately 97% of patients with an MHS score of ≤2 will not have CAD.
CAD, Coronary artery disease.
Modified from Haasenritter J, Bösner S, Vaucher P, et al. Ruling out coronary heart disease in primary care: External validation of a clinical prediction rule. *Br J Gen Pract.* 2021;62(599):e415-e421.

value for determining the likelihood of ACS in patients older than 40 years, and the absence of risk factors should not preclude further cardiac evaluation in patients with concerning symptoms.

An ECG should be obtained promptly for any patient with suspected ACS. ST-segment elevation in two or more contiguous leads or a presumed new left bundle branch block is diagnostic of ST-elevation myocardial infarction (STEMI) and requires urgent revascularization with thrombolysis or angioplasty at an appropriate facility. Ischemic ST-segment depression of more than 0.5 mm in leads V2 to V3 or more than 1 mm in all other leads, dynamic T-wave inversion with chest discomfort, or transient ST-segment elevation of 0.5 mm or more is classified as unstable angina or non–ST-elevation myocardial infarction (NSTEMI). However, none of these findings is sensitive enough that its absence can exclude MI, and patients whose chest pain is not low risk still require further assessment for ACS.

In patients with high-risk chest pain but without STEMI, elevated cardiac troponin (cTn) I or T levels distinguish NSTEMI from unstable angina. High-sensitivity cardiac troponin assays (hs-cTn I or hs-cTn T) have higher sensitivity and better negative predictive values than standard troponin measurements. Initial management of NSTEMI includes hospital admission for antiplatelet, antithrombin, and antianginal therapy. Patients with unstable angina should also be hospitalized for observation, and those with either NSTEMI or unstable angina require risk stratification using the Thrombolysis in Myocardial Infarction Study Group (TIMI) or Global Registry of Acute Coronary Events (GRACE) risk scores (see Box 1).

Patients with chest pain suspicious for CAD but no definite initial diagnosis of STEMI or NSTEMI on initial presentation are often admitted to the hospital for overnight observation and serial cardiac biomarker measurements to "rule out MI." However, numerous clinical decision pathways have been developed integrating history, ECG findings, and cardiac biomarkers to determine who is at sufficiently low risk of major adverse cardiac events (MACE) to allow discharge for close follow-up. hs-cTn assays may be used to guide disposition of chest pain with repeat sampling at 1, 2, or 3 hours from ED arrival using the pattern of rise or fall (i.e., delta) and the repeat value itself, based on assay-specific diagnostic thresholds; however, when using conventional cTn assays, the sampling time frame is extended to 3 to 6 hours from ED arrival. Recent evidence suggests that the HEART score may outperform TIMI and GRACE in determining which patients are at low risk (see Box 1). The combination of a low-risk HEART score (0–3) plus a single normal troponin value may predict sufficiently low risk of ACS to allow discharge from the ED with short-term outpatient follow-up, and a recent retrospective observational study of 1989 patients seen in emergency rooms for chest pain found that those with intermediate-risk HEART scores (4–6) may be at sufficiently low risk of MACE to allow discharge if clinical follow-up can be arranged within 1 week.

Patients at low risk for ACS or MI can usually defer further testing unless there are other risk factors in their family or past medical history markedly increasing the likelihood of CAD. Current recommendations are that all other patients with chest pain suggestive of CAD should have further noninvasive testing within 7 days. However, a retrospective analysis of 7988 ED patients with chest pain who were discharged to complete diagnostic testing found no difference in MACE between those who had testing within 3 days and those who had testing between 4 and 30 days from discharge.

Patients who can exercise and have no left bundle branch block, preexcitation, or significant resting ST-segment depression on an ECG can be evaluated with an exercise stress ECG, and the Duke Treadmill Score (DTS) can then be used to further quantify cardiac risk (see Box 1). The ability to attain a low-risk DTS (≥5) and the ability to achieve 10 metabolic equivalents of exercise are both associated with very low rates of cardiovascular death or nonfatal MI. Patients with baseline ECG abnormalities should have perfusion imaging performed along with a stress ECG, and those who cannot exercise may be evaluated with a pharmacologic stress or vasodilator test (e.g., dobutamine [Dobutrex][1] or

---

[1] Not FDA approved for this indication.

TABLE 2 Simplified Wells Scoring System for Pulmonary Embolism

CLINICAL FINDING	SCORE
Symptoms of DVT	3.0
No alternative diagnosis more likely than PE	3.0
Heart rate > 100 beats/min	1.5
Immobilization >3 days or surgery in past 4 weeks	1.5
Previous objectively diagnosed DVT or PE	1.5
Hemoptysis	1.0
Malignancy	1.0
Probability of PE: <2 points = low, 2–6 points = moderate, >6 points = high	

DVT, Deep vein thrombosis; *PE*, pulmonary embolism.
Modified from Miniati M, Bottai M, Monti S. Comparison of 3 clinical models for predicting the probability of pulmonary embolism. *Medicine (Baltimore)*. 2005;84(2):107-114; Torbicki A, Perrier A, Konstantinides S, et al. Guidelines on the diagnosis and management of acute pulmonary embolism: the Task Force for the Diagnosis and Management of Acute Pulmonary Embolism of the European Society of Cardiology (ESC). *Eur Heart J*. 2008;29(18):2276-2315.

TABLE 3 Pulmonary Embolism Rule-Out Criteria

Criteria (Excludes PE if all criteria are met and pretest probability is estimated at <15%)
Age < 50 years
Heart rate < 100 beats/min
Pulse oximetry on room air > 95%
No unilateral leg swelling
No hemoptysis
No surgery or trauma in the last 4 weeks
No prior DVT or PE
No hormone use

DVT, Deep vein thrombosis; *PE*, pulmonary embolism.
Modified from Kline JA, Mitchell AM, Kabrhel C, et al. Clinical criteria to prevent unnecessary diagnostic testing in emergency department patients with suspected pulmonary embolism. *J Thromb Haemost*. 2004;2(8):1247-1255.

adenosine [Adenocard]). Patients at high risk for CAD or those with NSTEMI should generally proceed directly to angiography, which enables definitive assessment of the coronary artery anatomy.

Pulmonary Embolism

There are no individual symptoms or physical examination findings that reliably diagnose or exclude PE, but four clinical prediction rules have all been validated for use in determining the likelihood of PE and therefore whether further testing is needed (see Box 1). The Pisa rule may be the most accurate, but it is also the most mathematically complicated and depends on clinical, ECG, and x-ray findings. The Geneva rule requires blood gas and chest x-ray findings. The Wells rule (Table 2) is based on the simplest combination of history and examination findings, and a comparison between the Wells and Geneva rules found that the Wells rule has a lower failure rate. With the Wells and Geneva prediction rules, the likelihood of PE is approximately 10% in the low-probability category, 30% in the moderate-probability category, and 65% in the high-probability category. If a patient is clinically suspected to be at low risk for PE (<15% pretest probability) and meets all of the pulmonary embolism rule-out criteria (Table 3), the risk of PE is less than 2%, and no further testing is needed.

Routine tests done for patients with chest pain are not particularly helpful in diagnosing or excluding PE. The chest x-ray may be abnormal, but findings that typically occur with PE (atelectasis, effusion, or elevation of a hemidiaphragm) are nonspecific. ECG signs of right ventricular strain (S wave in lead I, Q wave, and inverted T wave in lead III) may be helpful if present, but their absence does not exclude PE. Hypoxia may be present, but up to 20% of patients with PE have a normal alveolar-arterial oxygen gradient.

Additional tests recommended for evaluating patients with suspected PE include D-dimer testing, compression ultrasonography, and pulmonary imaging with ventilation-perfusion (VQ) scintigraphy or computed tomography (CT) angiography. Although CT may be more sensitive than VQ scanning, CT is also associated with higher radiation doses; for younger patients with suspected PE and a normal chest x-ray, VQ scanning may be preferable to limit overall radiation exposure. The use of adjusted D-dimer levels based on age or clinical setting has been studied, but none of these approaches have been standardized. Patients with suspected high-risk PE (i.e., those with shock or hypotension) should have immediate imaging and treatment for PE if the imaging is positive, although an echocardiographic finding of right ventricular overload may be used to justify treatment for PE in the unstable patient with high clinical suspicion for PE when imaging is not available. Patients who have suspected PE and are not at high risk (i.e., no shock or hypotension) and have a high clinical probability (based on Wells, Geneva, or Pisa scoring) should also proceed directly to imaging, with appropriate treatment if the scan is positive. Patients with a low clinical probability of PE (based on one of the validated clinical prediction rules) do not need further D-dimer testing or imaging. Patients with intermediate clinical probability should initially have D-dimer testing; further testing or treatment for PE is unnecessary if the D-dimer is negative, and imaging should be performed if the D-dimer is positive.

Anticoagulation, with thrombolysis in high-risk patients, is the foundation of treatment for PE. Patients with shock or hypotension are at high risk and require hemodynamic and respiratory support, thrombolysis, or embolectomy, followed by appropriate attention to anticoagulation. Normotensive patients with echocardiographic evidence of right ventricular dysfunction or serologic evidence of myocardial injury (elevated cTn I or T) have intermediate risk and should be admitted for anticoagulation. Normotensive patients who have normal results on echocardiography and testing for myocardial injury are at low risk and often may be discharged early for management at home after initiation of anticoagulation. Anticoagulation for PE should be started at the time of diagnosis. Apixaban (Eliquis) or rivaroxaban (Xarelto) may be used without prior oral anticoagulation; alternatively, unfractionated heparin, low-molecular-weight heparin, or fondaparinux (Arixtra) may be started and continued for 5 to 10 days with simultaneous initiation of dabigatran (Pradaxa), edoxaban (Savaysa or Lixiana), or warfarin (Coumadin) titrated to maintain an international normalized ratio between 2.0 and 3.0.

Thoracic Aortic Dissection

Thoracic aortic dissection is a much less common cause of chest pain; prevalence estimates are 2.0 to 3.5 cases per 100,000 person-years. Up to 40% of patients die immediately, and 5% to 20% die during or shortly after surgery. Risk factors for acute thoracic aortic dissection include hypertension, presence of a pheochromocytoma, cocaine use, weightlifting, trauma or a rapid deceleration event, coarctation of the aorta, and certain genetic abnormalities. Pain caused by acute aortic dissection is perceived as abrupt and severe in 84% to 90% of cases, and more than 50% of patients describe the pain as sharp or stabbing. No physical findings are sensitive or specific for detecting aortic dissection because approximately equal percentages of patients are hypertensive or normotensive or have hypotension or shock. The most common physical findings (a murmur of aortic insufficiency or a pulse deficit) occur in less than one-half of patients.

In any patient with severe chest pain that is abrupt or instantaneous in onset or has a ripping, tearing, or stabbing quality, acute thoracic aortic dissection should be suspected. Physical examination should assess for a pulse deficit, a systolic pressure differential between limbs of greater than 20 mm Hg, a focal neurologic deficit, or a new aortic regurgitation murmur. It is also important to ask about a family history of connective tissue disease (including Marfan syndrome), about any family or personal history of aortic dissection or thoracic aneurysm, and about any known aortic valve disease or recent aortic interventions. D-dimer testing has been proposed as a way to screen for aortic dissection, but it is more important to obtain prompt imaging and surgical intervention for those in whom dissection is confirmed. A low-risk aortic dissection detection risk score (see Box 1) can help exclude the diagnosis of aortic dissection, whereas patients with a high-risk score require further evaluation.

An ECG should be obtained in all patients with suspected aortic dissection to exclude STEMI (which can manifest with similar symptoms). In all low- and intermediate-risk patients, a prompt chest x-ray can help by either confirming an alternative diagnosis or confirming the presence of thoracic aortic disease. High-risk patients should have prompt imaging with CT or MRI, and those who are in shock or clinically unstable may be evaluated by bedside transesophageal echocardiography. If thoracic aortic dissection is confirmed on imaging, urgent surgical consultation is required. Medical therapy should be started with intravenous β-blockers. Patients with dissection of the ascending aorta require urgent surgery, whereas those with descending thoracic aortic dissection may be managed medically unless hypotension or other complications develop.

Pericarditis and Myocarditis

Acute pericarditis is an inflammatory syndrome of the pericardium (with or without effusion), and myocarditis is an inflammation of the myocardium; some patients may have an inflammatory myopericarditis. Viral infections are the most common identified cause of pericarditis (although most cases are idiopathic). Myocarditis may also be caused by a viral infection (including COVID-19) or secondary to systemic disease (e.g., rheumatoid arthritis or sarcoidosis) or toxin exposure (e.g., alcohol). Pericarditis or myocarditis should be suspected in patients with acute substernal chest pain that is associated with dyspnea or painful inspiration and tachycardia or friction rub on auscultation; myocarditis should also be suspected in any patient with heart failure and no clear underlying cause. Diagnostic testing should include ECG, cTn, and echocardiography. Supportive care and electrocardiographic monitoring are important for any patient with hemodynamic compromise. Pericarditis is typically treated with nonsteroidal antiinflammatory drugs (NSAIDs) plus colchicine,[1] whereas treatment of myocarditis generally involves addressing treatment of any identified causes.

Esophageal Rupture

Esophageal rupture, or Boerhaave syndrome, has a high mortality rate. Esophageal rupture is rare; the most common cause is endoscopically induced injury, but it can happen in other settings as well. Common misdiagnoses include perforated ulcer, MI, PE, dissecting aneurysm, and pancreatitis. The "classic" presentation has been described as pain, dyspnea, and shock associated with forceful emesis, but the history and physical examination are commonly nonspecific. Up to 45% of patients with Boerhaave syndrome have no history of vomiting, and esophageal perforation can develop with any cause of sudden increased intraesophageal pressure, including childbirth, seizure, prolonged coughing or laughing, or extreme exertion. Diagnosis most commonly is made by contrast esophagography or CT of the chest.

Patients whose rupture is diagnosed less than 48 hours after symptom onset are typically treated surgically (especially if sepsis is present) or endoscopically; however, nonoperative management may be considered in patients with evidence of a contained leak within the cervical esophagus or mediastinum. Those who present more than 48 hours after symptom onset may be considered for conservative treatment with hyperalimentation, antibiotics, and nasogastric suction.

Tension Pneumothorax

Tension pneumothorax is relatively rare among patients presenting with chest pain, but it is potentially life-threatening if not treated properly. Common symptoms and physical findings include chest pain, respiratory distress, decreased ipsilateral air entry, and tachycardia; hypoxia, tracheal deviation, and hypotension are less common.

Emergency needle decompression is usually recommended if tension pneumothorax is suspected, but this is ineffective in some cases and is associated with risks to the patient of pain, bleeding, infection, and cardiac tamponade. However, waiting for radiographic confirmation of the diagnosis is associated with up to a fourfold increase in mortality because of delay in decompression of the pneumothorax, and prompt needle decompression is associated with a 9% absolute risk reduction of mortality at 24 hours in trauma patients with tension pneumothorax. Patients most likely to benefit from an immediate attempt at needle decompression are those with an oxygen saturation below 92% while on oxygen, a decreased level of consciousness while on oxygen, a systolic blood pressure less than 90 mm Hg, or a respiratory rate less than 10 breaths/min. Patients without signs of instability may be better managed by waiting for chest imaging to confirm or exclude the presence of a pneumothorax. Although plain chest x-rays have typically been used for diagnosing a pneumothorax, pleural ultrasonography may have higher sensitivity. A metaanalysis of eight trials with 1342 patients found that for spontaneous pneumothorax there may be no difference in clinical success rates between conservative and interventional treatment.

Other Causes of Chest Pain

A patient with chest pain and cough, fever, egophony, or dullness to percussion might have pneumonia, but none of these individual findings is specific enough to confirm the diagnosis. However, adults with an acute respiratory infection who have normal vital signs and a normal pulmonary examination are very unlikely to have community-acquired pneumonia. A large study in 1984 developed a decision rule (Table 4) using seven clinical findings to predict the likelihood of pneumonia. There is ongoing debate over the reliability of pneumonia diagnosis based solely on history and physical examination; chest x-ray is usually considered the reference standard. However, a 2013 Cochrane review found two trials suggesting that routine chest radiography does not affect the clinical outcomes in adults and children whose presentations are suggestive of a lower respiratory tract infection. Thus at least for clinically stable outpatients, treatment for pneumonia based on appropriate clinical findings alone may be reasonable.

Heart failure alone is an uncommon cause of chest pain, but it may accompany ACS or cardiac valve disease. A displaced apical impulse and a prior history of CAD support this diagnosis, and because virtually all patients with heart failure have exertional dyspnea, its absence is very helpful in excluding this diagnosis. An abnormal ECG and cardiomegaly on chest x-ray can increase the likelihood of heart failure among patients with chest pain, and B-natriuretic peptide (BNP) or N-terminal pro-B-type natriuretic peptide (NT-proBNP) are now commonly used for detecting heart failure in patients presenting with acute dyspnea. Point-of-care ultrasonography may have high sensitivity and specificity for diagnosing acute cardiogenic pulmonary edema.

---

[1]Not FDA approved for this indication.

TABLE 4	Signs and Symptoms

FINDING	POINTS
Rhinorrhea	−2
Sore throat	−1
Night sweats	1
Myalgia	1
Sputum all day	1
Respiratory rate > 25 breaths/min	2
Temperature > 100°F	2

Interpretation

SCORE	PROBABILITY OF PNEUMONIA
−3	5
−1	12
0	21
1	30
3	37

Modified from Cayley WE Jr. Diagnosing the cause of chest pain. *Am Fam Physician* 2005;72:2012-2021.

Panic and anxiety are a common cause of chest pain in those at low risk for heart disease. There is good evidence that psychological interventions such as cognitive behavioral therapy and breathing exercises can improve chest pain symptoms for patients with nonspecific chest pain who do not have CAD. However, even in patients with possible panic disorder, further cardiac testing should be done if there are significant cardiac risk factors.

Gastrointestinal disease can cause chest pain, but the history and physical examination are relatively inaccurate for diagnosing or excluding serious gastrointestinal pathology. However, if life-threatening cardiovascular or pulmonary causes of chest pain have been excluded, it is appropriate to try a short course of a high-dose proton pump inhibitor (omeprazole [Prilosec] 40 mg daily, lansoprazole [Prevacid] 30 mg daily, or esomeprazole [Nexium] 40 mg daily) to evaluate for undiagnosed gastroesophageal reflux disease (GERD) as the cause of chest pain (even for patients without typical GERD symptoms).

Chest wall pain can usually be diagnosed by history and examination if other etiologies have been excluded, and such pain is more likely if the patient's pain is reproducible by palpation. Measurement of the sedimentation rate is not generally helpful in making the diagnosis, although in unusual situations radiography may be helpful. Typical management options include heat, NSAIDs, topical lidocaine, physical therapy, or acupuncture.

References

Bhatt DL, Lopes RD, Harrington RA: Diagnosis and treatment of acute coronary syndromes: a review, *JAMA* 327(7):662–675, 2022.

Basso C: Myocarditis, *N Engl J Med* 387(16):1488–1500, 2022, https://doi.org/10.1056/NEJMra2114478. PMID: 36260793. https://www.nejm.org/doi/full/10.1056/NEJMra2114478.

Cao AM, Choy JP, Mohanakrishnan LN, et al: Chest radiographs for acute lower respiratory tract infections, *Cochrane Database Syst Rev* 12:CD009119, 2013.

Cayley WE Jr: Diagnosing the cause of chest pain, *Am Fam Physician* 72:2012–2021, 2005.

Chiabrando JG, et al: Management of acute and recurrent pericarditis: JACC state-of-the-art review, *J Am Coll Cardiol* 75(1):76–92, 2020, https://doi.org/10.1016/j.jacc.2019.11.021PMID: 31918837.

DeVivo A, Sheng AY, Koyfman A, Long B: High risk and low prevalence diseases: esophageal perforation, *Am J Emerg Med* 53:29–36, 2022, https://doi.org/10.1016/j.ajem.2021.12.017. Epub 2021 Dec 18. PMID: 34971919. https://pubmed.ncbi.nlm.nih.gov/34971919/.

Eriksson D, Khoshnood A, Larsson D, et al: Diagnostic accuracy of history and physical examination for predicting major adverse cardiac events within 30 days in patients with acute chest pain, *J Emerg Med* 58(1): 1–10, 2020. https://doi.org/10.1016/j.jemermed.2019.09.044.

Harskamp RE, Laeven SC, Himmelreich JC, et al: Chest pain in general practice: a systematic review of prediction rules, *BMJ Open* 9(2):e027081, 2019.

Hendriksen JM, Geersing GJ, Lucassen WA, et al: Diagnostic prediction models for suspected pulmonary embolism: systematic review and independent external validation in primary care, *BMJ* 8(351):h4438, 2015.

Hiratzka LF, Bakris GL, Beckman JA, et al: 2010 ACCF/AHA/AATS/ACR/ASA/SCA/SCAI/SIR/STS/SVM guidelines for the diagnosis and management of patients with thoracic aortic disease: a report of the American College of Cardiology foundation/American Heart Association Task Force on Practice Guidelines, *Circulation* 121:e266–e369, 2010. *Erratum in Circulation* 122(4):e410, 2010.

Katz PO, Dunbar KB, Schnoll-Sussman FH, Greer KB, Yadlapati R, Spechler SJ: ACG clinical guideline for the diagnosis and management of gastroesophageal reflux disease, *Am J Gastroenterol* 117(1):27–56, 2022, https://doi.org/10.14309/ajg.0000000000001538. PMID: 34807007; PMCID: PMC8754510. https://pubmed.ncbi.nlm.nih.gov/34807007/.

Kisely SR, Campbell LA, Yelland MJ, Paydar A: Psychological interventions for symptomatic management of non-specific chest pain in patients with normal coronary anatomy, *Cochrane Database Syst Rev* 6:CD004101, 2015.

Lam Y, Hwang DS, Mounsey A: Tips and tools to help refine your approach to chest pain, *J Fam Pract* 70(9):420–430, 2021, https://doi.org/10.12788/jfp.0301. PMID: 34818149.

Leigh-Smith S, Harris T: Tension pneumothorax–time for a re-think? *Emerg Med J* 22(8–16), 2005.

Liu WL, Lv K, Deng HS, Hong QC: Comparison of efficiency and safety of conservative versus interventional management for primary spontaneous pneumothorax: a meta-analysis, *Am J Emerg Med* 45:352–357, 2021, https://doi.org/10.1016/j.ajem.2020.08.092. Epub 2020 Sep 6. PMID: 33046307. https://pubmed.ncbi.nlm.nih.gov/33046307/.

McConaghy JR, Sharma M, Patel H: Acute chest pain in adults: outpatient evaluation, *Am Fam Physician* 102(12):721–727, 2020.

Mott T, Jones G, Roman K: Costochondritis: rapid evidence review, *Am Fam Physician* 104(1):73–78, 2021. PMID: 34264599.

Moustapha A, Mah AC, Roberts L, et al: Can ED chest pain patients with intermediate HEART scores be managed as outpatients?, *CJEM* 24(7):770–779, 2022, https://doi.org/10.1007/s43678-022-00355-4. Epub 2022 Sep 21. PMID: 36129627. https://pubmed.ncbi.nlm.nih.gov/36129627/.

Nienaber CA, Clough RE: Management of acute aortic dissection, *Lancet* 385(9970):800–811, 2015.

Gulati M, et al: 2021 AHA/ACC/ASE/CHEST/SAEM/SCCT/SCMR guideline for the evaluation and diagnosis of chest pain: a report of the American College of Cardiology/American Heart Association Joint Committee on Clinical Practice Guidelines, *Circulation* 144(22):e368–e454, 2021, https://doi.org/10.1161/CIR.0000000000001029. Epub 2021 Oct 28. Erratum in: *Circulation*. 144(22):e455, 2021. PMID: 34709879.

Raja AS, Greenberg JO, Qaseem A, et al: Clinical Guidelines Committee of the American College of Physicians. Evaluation of patients with suspected acute pulmonary embolism: best practice advice from the clinical guidelines committee of the American College of Physicians, *Ann Intern Med* 163(9):701–711, 2015.

Reinhardt SW, Lin CJ, Novak E, Brown DL: Noninvasive cardiac testing vs clinical evaluation alone in acute chest pain: a secondary analysis of the ROMICAT-II randomized clinical trial, *JAMA Intern Med* 178(2):212–219, 2018.

Swap CJ, Nagurney JT: Value and limitations of chest pain history in the evaluation of patients with suspected acute coronary syndromes, *J Am Med Assoc* 294:2623–2629, 2005.

Wassie M, Lee MS, Sun BC, et al: Single vs serial measurements of cardiac troponin level in the evaluation of patients in the emergency department with suspected acute myocardial infarction, *JAMA Netw Open* 4(2):e2037930, 2021, https://doi.org/10.1001/jamanetworkopen.2020.37930. PMID: 33620444; PMCID: PMC7903256. https://pubmed.ncbi.nlm.nih.gov/33620444/.

Wong BC: Is proton pump inhibitor testing an effective approach to diagnose gastroesophageal reflux disease in patients with noncardiac chest pain?: a meta-analysis, *Arch Intern Med* 165(11):1222–1228, 2005.

CONSTIPATION

Method of
Melissa Gaines, MD

CURRENT DIAGNOSIS

- Although constipation is a benign process, it is important to recognize signs of a serious condition.
- Classification of normal transit constipation, slow transit constipation, or pelvic floor dysfunction guides therapy.
- Clinical testing has low benefit, but colonoscopy or imaging can assess organic causes.

CURRENT THERAPY

- Initial therapy includes soluble dietary fiber to improve symptoms in chronic constipation.
- Osmotic laxatives are preferred while using stimulant laxatives as rescue agents.
- Surgery is reserved for pelvic floor dysfunction after optimal therapies have failed.

Epidemiology

Constipation is common, with a prevalence of 1.9% to 27.2%, but the description of symptoms is variable. A thorough history and focused physical examination aids diagnosis. Treatment is directed toward relief of symptoms, alleviation of precipitating factors, and prevention of recurrence. Although constipation is a benign process, it is important to recognize concerning signs for a more serious medical condition such as malignancy.

Risk Factors

Vulnerable populations include female, elderly, neurodegenerative disease, low-fiber diet, painful rectal disorders, hypothyroidism, and diabetes mellitus.

Pathophysiology

With aging, there is decreased rectal compliance, diminished rectal sensation, and decreased resting anal pressures, while colonic transit time is preserved. Normal transit constipation is a component of irritable bowel syndrome with normal transit time and stool frequency. Slow transit constipation is a condition with colonic dysmotility resulting from altered enteric nervous system. Defecatory disorders include structural disturbances of the pelvic floor. Pelvic floor dysfunction is the paradoxical contraction of the external anal sphincter and puborectalis muscles during defecation. Secondary causes of constipation are listed in Table 1.

Prevention

Provide an environment of privacy and comfort to allow for natural defecation. Prescribe an adequate fluid and fiber intake with specific amounts that vary depending on the patient's condition. Encourage physical activity, with a low to moderate level of exercise depending on the patient's functional status. Develop a routine for defecation with a prompt response to a call to defecate urgently. Recurrent fecal impaction can be prevented with polyethylene glycol (PEG, MiraLAX).

Clinical Manifestations

Patients will complain using qualitative terms of hard stools, a feeling of incomplete voiding, straining, prolonged time for laxation, the need for additional maneuvers, abdominal bloating, and abdominal pain (Table 2). A change in bowel habit differentiates the current complaint from a serious medical condition. Red flags include acute onset, weight loss, abdominal pain or cramping, rectal bleeding, nausea or vomiting, rectal pain, fever, or a change in stool caliber. Infants with abdominal distension and failure to pass meconium within 24 hours indicate Hirschsprung disease. Patients should be asked if they have had loose stools or bowel incontinence to assess for fecal impaction. A medication review is required (see Table 1). Classification of patients with normal transit constipation, slow transit constipation, or pelvic floor dysfunction/defecatory disorders guides therapy.

Diagnosis

Diagnostic criteria have been established because the symptoms can vary (see Table 2). Conduct a physical examination that includes an assessment of vital signs, weight, volume status, auscultation of bowel sounds, abdominal percussion for tympani, and abdominal palpation for tenderness or mass. A rectal examination can detect resting rectal tone, fecal impaction, anorectal disorders, or rectal mass. Defecatory disorders show an increased resistance to the insertion of the examiner's finger with an impaired relaxation of the sphincter complex and reduced perineal descent during a Valsalva maneuver. Conduct laboratory testing on electrolytes, hemoglobin, thyroid-stimulating hormone, and fecal occult after initial measures fail. Red flag symptoms require imaging with computed tomography (CT) of the abdomen and pelvis or an endoscopy to diagnose malignancy or fecal impaction. Anorectal testing with manometry and a rectal balloon expulsion test is appropriate for pelvic floor dysfunction or defecatory disorders. Hirschsprung disease is diagnosed with barium enema, rectal manometry, or a rectal suction biopsy. Colonic transit rates with radiopaque markers (Sitz) on serial abdominal radiographs over 4 to 7 days diagnose slow transit constipation disorders.

Treatment

Nonpharmacologic therapies have limited benefit. Unless there are signs of dehydration, increasing fluid intake is not indicated. Moderate-intensity exercise improves symptoms of irritable bowel syndrome. Probiotics are not beneficial.

There is moderate evidence for pharmacologic agents (Table 3). Normal transit constipation responds to soluble dietary fiber supplements (e.g., psyllium [Metamucil]); however, these should not be used in the case of slow transit constipation or drug-induced constipation. Osmotic agents with PEG (MiraLAX) or lactulose (Chronulac) can be dose increased for soft stools. Stimulant laxatives are used as rescue therapy if patients do not have a bowel movement for 2 days.

TABLE 1	Causes of Constipation
Dietary	Low-fiber diet, dementia, depression, anorexia, dehydration
Metabolic	Diabetes mellitus, hypercalcemia, hypokalemia, hypothyroidism, systemic sclerosis
Neurologic	Parkinson disease, spinal cord disorder, multiple sclerosis, cerebrovascular disease (stroke)
Iatrogenic	Antacids, iron, anticholinergics, antidepressants, antipsychotics, opiates, antiepileptics
Painful anorectal condition	Anal fissure, hemorrhoids, abscess, fistula, pelvic floor dysfunction, malignancy

TABLE 2	Rome III Criteria

More than two present:
1. Straining in more than 25% of defecations
2. Hard or lumpy stool in more than 25% of defecations
3. Sensation of incomplete evacuation
4. Sensation of anorectal blockage
5. Manual maneuvers
6. Fewer than three defecations per week

Loose stools are rare without laxative use

Insufficient criteria for irritable bowel syndrome

Symptoms for 3 months with onset 6 months before diagnosis

New classes of drugs to manage constipation include intestinal secretagogues, serotonin 5-HT$_4$ receptor antagonists, and opiate antagonists. Lubiprostone (Amitiza) requires a negative pregnancy test with contraception. Linaclotide (Linzess) is a 14–amino acid peptide similar to heat-stable enterotoxins that cause diarrhea. Lubiprostone and linaclotide are US Food and Drug Administration (FDA)-approved for chronic idiopathic constipation (CIC) and irritable bowel syndrome with constipation (IBS-C). Lubiprostone is also indicated for treatment of opioid-induced constipation (OIC). Plecanatide (Trulance) is an approved drug for treatment of CIC and IBS-C in adults. It is a guanylate cyclase-C agonist that increases fluid secretion into the upper intestine. Methylnaltrexone (Relistor) and naloxegol (Movantik) are opiate receptor antagonists that can cause laxation in patients on chronic opiate therapy with number needed to treat (NNT) of 5.

Pelvic floor dysfunction or defecatory disorders respond to biofeedback therapy by using manometry and visual or auditory feedback. Patients practice expelling a balloon and improve pelvic floor muscle coordination with Kegel exercises. Surgical intervention with subtotal colectomy with ileorectal anastomosis is indicated for slow transit constipation or defecatory disorders after failure of optimal medical management.

Complications

Fecal impaction is a complication and a large bowel obstruction with colonic perforation has high mortality. Pediatric and geriatric patients are most susceptible with signs and symptoms of fecal incontinence, abdominal pain, abdominal distention, anorexia, weight loss, and delirium. Treatments for adults include a large-volume tap-water enema (500 to 1000 mL), local anesthetics administered topically with abdominal massage, a colonoscopy, or surgery. The prevention of recurrence requires maintenance bowel regimen with osmotic agents such as PEG (MiraLAX).

TABLE 3 Drug Dosing and Adverse Effects

CLASS	DRUG NAME (BRAND)	ADULT DOSING	MECHANISM OF ACTION	TIME TO ONSET (H)	ADVERSE EFFECT
Fiber	Bran Psyllium (Metamucil) Methylcellulose (Citrucel) Calcium polycarbophil (FiberCon)	1 cup/day 1 tsp 1 tbsp or 1 tab twice daily 2–4 tabs/day	Increase water content and bulk of stool decreasing transit time	Unknown	Bloating excessive gas
Hyperosmolar agent	Sorbitol 70% Lactulose (Chronulac)	15–30 mL twice daily	Disaccharide metabolized by colonic bacteria into acetic acid and short-chain fatty acids	24–48	Sweet tasting, transient abdominal cramps, flatulence
Hyperosmolar agent	PEG-ES (GoLytely,[1] CoLyte[1]) PEG (MiraLAX)	8–32 oz daily 17 g (1 tbsp) qd	Osmotic effect increasing intraluminal fluids	0.5–1	Incontinence
Guanylate cyclase-C agonist	Plecanatide (Trulance) Linaclotide (Linzess)	CIC and IBS-C: 3 mg once daily CIC: 72–145 mcg once daily IBS-C: 290 mcg once daily	Osmotic effect increasing intraluminal fluids, increase transit time	Cannot be calculated	Diarrhea Abdominal pain, diarrhea
Chloride channel activator	Lubiprostone (Amitiza)	CIC and OIC: 24 mcg twice daily IBS-C in women ≥18 y: 8 mcg twice daily	Increase intestinal fluid secretion and improve fecal transit	Unknown	Headache, nausea, diarrhea
Stimulant	Glycerin suppository Bisacodyl (Dulcolax) Senna (Senokot, Perdiem) Senna/docusate (Peri-Colace)	1 daily 10 mg suppository or 5–10 mg PO 3 times a week 2–4 tabs twice daily	Local rectal stimulation, secretory and prokinetic effect	8–12	Degeneration of Meissner and Auerbach plexus
Enemas	Mineral oil retention enema Tap water enema Sodium phosphate enema (Fleet)	199–250 mL daily PR 500–1000 mL PR 1 unit PR	Evacuation induced by distended colon and mechanical lavage	6–8 for a mineral oil enema 5–15 min for all other enemas	Mechanical trauma, incontinence, rectal damage
Opioid antagonist	Methylnaltrexone (Relistor)	8–12 mg 1 dose SC every other day as needed for OIC with advanced illness. 450 mg PO once daily or 12 mg SC once daily for OIC with chronic noncancer pain.	Opioid mu receptor antagonist in gut decreasing transit time	4	Diarrhea, intestinal perforation
Opioid antagonist	Naloxegol (Movantik)	12.5–25 mg PO daily	Same as Relistor	6–36	Abdominal pain, opioid withdrawal reported

[1]Not US Food and Drug Administration (FDA) approved for this indication.
CIC, Chronic idiopathic constipation; *IBS-C,* irritable bowel syndrome with constipation; *OIC,* opioid-induced constipation; *PEG-ES,* polyethylene glycol and electrolyte solution; *PO,* by mouth; *PR,* per rectum; *SC,* subcutaneously.

References

Arshad A, Powell C: Easily missed? Hirschsprung's disease, *Br Med J* 345:e5521, 2012.

Barish DF, Crozier RA, Griffin PH: Long-term treatment with plecanatide was safe and tolerable in patients with irritable bowel syndrome with constipation, *Curr Med Res Opin* 1–5, 2018.

Bharucha AE, Pemberton JH, Locke GR: American Gastroenterological Association technical review on constipation, *Gastroenterology* 144:218–238, 2013.

Gallagher PF, O'Mahony D, Quigley EM: Management of chronic constipation in the elderly, *Drugs Aging* 25:807–821, 2008.

Gastroenterology: Rome criteria. Available at http://www.romecriteria.org/.

Higgins PD, Johanson JF: Epidemiology of constipation in North America: a systematic review, *Am J Gastroenterol* 99:750–759, 2004.

Larkin PJ, Sykes NP, Centeno C, et al: The management of constipation in palliative care: Clinical practice recommendations, *Palliat Med* 22:796–807, 2008.

McCallum IJ, Ong S, Mercer-Jones M: Chronic constipation in adults, *Br Med J* 338:b831, 2009.

Nee J, et al: Efficacy of treatments for opioid-induced constipation: a systemic review and meta-analysis, *Clin Gastroenterol Hepatol*, 2018 Jan 25.

Schoenfeld P, et al: Low-Dose linaclotide (72ug) for chronic idiopathic constipation: A 12-week, randomized, double-blind, placebo-controlled trial, *Am J Gastroenterol*, 2018, 113-105–114. https://doi.org/10.1038/ajg.2017.230.

Thomas J, Karver S, Cooney GA, et al: Methylnaltrexone for opioid-induced constipation in advanced illness, *N Engl J Med* 358:2332–2343, 2008.

Wald A: Management and prevention of fecal impaction, *Curr Gastroenterol Rep* 10:299–501, 2008.

Wald A: Constipation: Advances in diagnosis and treatment, *JAMA* 315(2):185–191, 2016 Jan 12.

COUGH

Method of
Emily Manlove, MD

CURRENT DIAGNOSIS

- Acute cough
  - Noninfectious
    - Chronic obstructive pulmonary disease exacerbation
    - Asthma exacerbation
    - Congestive heart failure exacerbation
    - Pulmonary embolism
  - Infectious
    - Viral rhinosinusitis (the common cold)
    - Acute bacterial sinusitis
    - Acute bronchitis (chest cold)
    - Pneumonia
    - COVID-19 pertussis (whooping cough)
    - Bronchiolitis (infants)
- Chronic cough
  - First, evaluate/rule out
    - Tobacco smoking and risk for lung cancer
    - Angiotensin-converting enzyme (ACE) inhibitor–associated cough
  - Next, evaluate for the three most common etiologies
    - Chronic upper airway cough syndrome
    - Cough variant asthma/nonasthmatic eosinophilic bronchitis
    - Gastroesophageal reflux disease
  - Last, consider other causes and more advanced testing (bronchoscopy, high-resolution computed tomography [CT], referral), and consider earlier if history, physical examination, or chest x-ray suggests an alternative diagnosis
    - Oral pharyngeal dysphagia
    - Lung tumors
    - Interstitial pulmonary diseases
    - Bronchiectasis
    - Occupational and environmental exposures
    - Sarcoidosis
    - Tuberculosis
    - Somatic cough syndrome
    - Tic cough

CURRENT THERAPY

- Acute cough caused by viral rhinosinusitis
  - Dextromethorphan (Delsym) 30 mg PO every 6 to 8 hours × 1 week
  - Diphenhydramine (Benadryl) 25 mg PO every 4 hours × 1 week
  - Nasal saline irrigation twice daily × 1 week
- Acute or subacute cough caused by *Bordetella pertussis*
  - Azithromycin (Z-Pak)[1] 500 mg PO on day 1 followed by 250 mg PO daily on days 2 to 5
- Treatment of unexplained chronic cough
  - Multimodality speech pathology therapy
  - Gabapentin (Neurontin) 300 mg PO daily, can be titrated up to a maximum daily dose of 1800 mg a day in two divided doses (off-label use)

[1]Not FDA approved for this indication.

Acute Cough

Acute cough is a cough that lasts fewer than 3 weeks. It is a common presenting complaint in the primary care physician's office and also in the emergency department. The key goal is to differentiate between patients whose cough has a benign cause and those who may be at risk for more serious illness. Infectious causes of cough are most common, but noninfectious causes should also be considered. Exacerbations of preexisting pulmonary conditions such as asthma and chronic obstructive pulmonary disease (COPD) can be associated with cough, therefore a thorough medical history should be obtained. Cough can also be associated with decompensated heart failure; in fact, cough is present in 70% of congestive heart failure (CHF) exacerbations. Also, 30% to 40% of patients with acute pulmonary embolism (PE) have a new cough at presentation of symptoms, and the classic signs and symptoms of chest pain, dyspnea, and hypoxia may not always accompany the cough.

Upper respiratory tract infections are a common cause of benign acute cough. Viral rhinosinusitis (the common cold) is probably the most common cause of acute cough. The lung examination is normal. If fever is present, it is low grade and is only present on the first or second day of illness. Most symptoms begin to resolve by 7 to 10 days, but cigarette smokers may be ill for twice as long. Symptomatic treatment is the mainstay of therapy. Antihistamine-decongestant-analgesics can provide some symptomatic benefit but may also cause side effects. Second-generation antihistamines are not effective in the treatment of cough associated with viral rhinosinusitis; it is likely that first-generation antihistamines are effective because of their anticholinergic properties. Other treatments that may be helpful include nasal saline irrigation, nasal glucocorticoids, and nasal decongestants. It is necessary to distinguish viral rhinosinusitis from acute bacterial rhinosinusitis, which may also be associated with cough. Less than 2% of all rhinosinusitis has a bacterial cause. Acute bacterial rhinosinusitis should not be diagnosed in the first week of symptoms unless the patient displays severe symptoms such as high fever. Sinus imaging studies are unlikely to be helpful, as both viral and bacterial sinusitis will have radiologic evidence of inflammation.

It is also necessary to distinguish acute cough caused by an upper respiratory tract infection from that caused by a lower respiratory tract infection. Furthermore, it is necessary to distinguish between acute bronchitis, which almost always has a viral cause, versus pneumonia, which may be bacterial. Both illnesses often have a presenting symptom of cough, which may be productive. If there is any derangement in vital signs or evidence of pulmonary consolidation on the lung examination, a chest x-ray should be performed. Infectious Diseases Society of America (IDSA) guidelines require the presence of consolidation on chest x-ray to diagnose pneumonia. Influenza and COVID-19 should also be considered for patients who have fever and cough. An elevated procalcitonin level may help guide the physician in his or her decision to prescribe antibiotics. Inhaled beta agonists should not be routinely used to alleviate cough in acute viral bronchitis, but they may be helpful to alleviate wheezing and are more likely to benefit patients with airflow obstruction at baseline.

In pediatric patients, bronchiolitis should be considered as a cause of cough and fever. It is the most common cause of hospitalization in those younger than 1 year of age. Laboratory testing (including viral swabs), radiographic imaging, and treatment with beta agonists, epinephrine, or glucocorticoids do not change the course of illness. Exclusive breastfeeding for the first 6 months of infancy can decrease the morbidity of respiratory infections. *Bordetella pertussis* can cause severe illness with cough and apnea in infants. Adults have subtle symptoms and lack the classic "whooping cough" and posttussive emesis seen in children. The physician should have suspicion for pertussis in adult patients who have a cough lasting longer than 2 weeks and paroxysms of coughing; the cough can last up to 2 months. The diagnosis can be confirmed with polymerase chain reaction (PCR). Antibiotics do not alter the course of illness but reduce the spread of infection; azithromycin (Zithromax)[1] should be given for 3 to 5 days. Pregnant women should be vaccinated with each pregnancy, and other adults should replace 1 dose of Td at the earliest convenience.

Chronic Cough

A chronic cough is a cough lasting more than 8 weeks. Patients may have a presenting symptom of a cough that has been present for more than 3 weeks but fewer than 8 weeks; this is considered a subacute cough. In this case, the physician should illicit a history of respiratory infection; the patient is likely suffering from a postinfectious cough, which is related to inflammation of the airway epithelium, mucus hypersecretion, and/or increased cough reflex sensitivity. Inhaled corticosteroids may provide some benefit. If there is no history of recent infection, then the cough should be managed as a chronic cough. Chest x-ray can be considered during this time frame, but if no red flags are present (fever, unintended weight loss, night sweats, dysphagia, odynophagia, hemoptysis), the physician and patient together can decide to wait on radiography.

Chronic cough must be approached in a systematic manner, which is more likely to identify the causative agent of the cough and provide alleviation of symptoms. All of the common causes of chronic cough (see later) must be considered as the associated symptoms and the patient's description of the cough do not alter the diagnostic algorithm. It is important to confirm compliance throughout the treatment course and identify barriers to compliance with the patient. Failure to respond to empiric treatment does not necessarily rule out a diagnosis as the patient may have two diagnoses. Therefore it is prudent to continue any partially effective treatment for chronic cough.

First, it must be determined if the patient smokes. If so, the differential diagnosis is altered. The physician must determine if the smoke is a simple smoker's cough, chronic bronchitis, or possibly lung cancer; cough is the most common presenting symptom of lung cancer. Smokers are less likely to seek help for a cough and may not see a physician until a more serious problem has advanced. It is possible for a cough to worsen initially after smoking cessation, but a cough persisting more than 1 month after cessation should be investigated. Any change in a smoker's cough, a new cough, and cough with hemoptysis should be investigated. Physicians should consider low-dose CT scanning as screening for lung cancer in qualifying smokers. The second factor to rule out in all chronic cough cases is cough induced by an angiotensin-converting enzyme (ACE) inhibitor. All patients with chronic cough should stop taking an ACE inhibitor. The medication is more likely to cause a cough if it was started in the prior year, and the cough should resolve within 1 month after cessation of the ACE inhibitor. The next step to determining the cause of a chronic cough is to rule out the three most common causes of cough (see next). Last, all patients with a cough lasting more than 8 weeks should be evaluated with chest radiography to identify any obvious causative factors.

Upper Airway Cough Syndrome

Upper airway cough syndrome (UACS), previously called *postnasal drip syndrome,* is likely caused by activation of cough receptors in the hypopharynx or larynx and increased sensitivity of these receptors. It is likely the most common cause of chronic cough. UACS is almost always associated with rhinosinusitis, which can be caused by a number of factors (allergic rhinitis, postinfectious rhinitis, perennial nonallergic rhinitis, rhinitis resulting from chemical irritants, rhinitis medicamentosa, pregnancy-associated rhinitis, bacterial sinusitis, allergic fungal sinusitis). The patient may complain of frequently needing to clear the throat or a sensation of "dripping" in the back of the throat; however, absence of these symptoms does not rule out UACS, nor does a history of wheezing. The physical examination may reveal mucus in the posterior oropharynx and cobblestoning of the mucosa. If the cause of rhinitis is obvious, it should be specifically treated. Otherwise, a trial of a first-generation antihistamine should be started; improvement should be seen in 2 weeks. If the side effects of this therapy are intolerable, a nasal antihistamine, nasal anticholinergic, or nasal corticosteroid can be used. If the diagnosis of UACS is highly suspected but the patient does not respond to empiric therapy, sinus CT imaging may be necessary to guide diagnosis and treatment.

Cough Variant Asthma and Nonasthmatic Eosinophilic Bronchitis

Cough-variant asthma and nonasthmatic eosinophilic bronchitis (NAEB) both primarily present with a cough, and the patient may have few other symptoms. Patients with cough-variant asthma will have abnormal spirometry, whereas those with NAEB will not. When spirometry is performed, bronchoprovocation testing with methacholine should be performed as it increases the negative predicative value of the test. If spirometry is negative, the sputum should be evaluated for eosinophils, which are present in both diseases. Both diseases are treated as asthma; an inhaled corticosteroid should be started and long-acting beta agonists and leukotriene receptor antagonists can be considered as adjunctive therapy. A positive response should be expected within 2 weeks.

Gastroesophageal Reflux Disease

Gastroesophageal reflux disease (GERD) is common, but not all patients with GERD have an associated cough; therefore, the presence of GERD does not ensure that it is the source of the patient's cough. However, patients whose cough is clearly not caused by UACS, cough-variant asthma, or NAEB are very likely to have a GERD-induced cough. Cough can be caused by acidic and nonacidic reflux, so a proton pump inhibitor (PPI) may not always be beneficial. A pH probe can be performed in cases when it is unclear whether reflux is occurring. All patients should utilize lifestyle changes to attenuate reflux, such as smoking cessation, avoidance of alcohol and acidic foods, weight loss, and treatment of sleep apnea. It may take 3 to 6 months of treatment to see improvement in cough. If the patient does not improve and GERD is highly suspected, referral to a surgeon may be necessary for fundoplication.

Other Causes of Chronic Cough

In patients who still suffer from chronic cough and the above causes have been ruled out, further investigation should be sought. Referral to a pulmonologist may be necessary in addition to high-resolution CT scanning and bronchoscopy. Causative factors may include oral pharyngeal dysphagia, lung tumors, interstitial pulmonary diseases, bronchiectasis, occupational and environmental exposures, sarcoidosis, and tuberculosis. Somatic cough syndrome (previously referred to as *psychogenic cough*) and tic cough

---

[1] Not FDA approved for this indication.

(previously referred to as *habit cough*) may be considered in some patients. Treatment options include speech language pathology intervention, empiric gabapentin, and/or referral to a cough clinic.

References

Chung KF, Pavord ID: Prevalence, pathogenesis, and causes of chronic cough, *Lancet* 371(9621):1364–1374, 2008.

Côté A, Russell RJ, Boulet LP, et al: Managing chronic cough due to asthma and NAEB in adults and adolescents: CHEST guideline and expert panel report, *Chest* 158(1):68–96, 2020.

De Sutter AI, Eriksson L, van Driel ML: Oral antihistamine–decongestant–analgesic combinations for the common cold, *Cochrane Database Syst Rev* 1(1):CD004976, 2022.

Gibson P, Wang G, McGarvey L, et al: Treatment of unexplained chronic cough: CHEST guideline and expert panel report, *Chest* 149(1):27–44, 2016.

Irwin RS, French CL, Chang AB, et al: Classification of cough as a symptom in adults and management algorithms: CHEST guideline and expert panel report, *Chest* 153(1):196–209, 2018.

Michaudet C, Malaty JJ: Chronic cough: evaluation and management, *Am Fam Physician* 96(9):575–580, 2017.

Ralston SL, Lieberthal AS, Meissner HC, et al.: Clinical practice guideline: the diagnosis, management, and prevention of bronchiolitis, *Pediatrics* 134(5):e1474–1502, 2014.

DIZZINESS AND VERTIGO

Method of
Jennifer Wipperman, MD, MPH

CURRENT DIAGNOSIS

- Benign paroxysmal positional vertigo
  - Repeated, brief episodes lasting less than 1 minute
  - Triggered by changes in head position
  - Positive Dix-Hallpike or Supine Roll Test
- Vestibular neuritis
  - Single, severe, constant episode lasting days
  - Subacute onset
  - Positive head impulse test
  - Nystagmus is unidirectional and horizontal
- Vestibular migraine
  - Recurrent episodes lasting hours to days
  - Includes features of migraine headache
  - Responds to traditional migraine treatment
- Ménière's disease
  - Recurrent episodes of vertigo lasting hours
  - May have hearing loss, tinnitus, or ear fullness
- Red flags for stroke include:
  - Sudden onset
  - Risk factors for stroke
  - Bidirectional or purely vertical nystagmus
  - Abnormal HINTS exam
  - Focal neurologic signs
  - Inability to walk

CURRENT THERAPY

- Benign paroxysmal positional vertigo
  - The canalith repositioning procedure (Epley maneuver) is the most effective treatment.
  - Avoid vestibular suppressant medications
  - Observation with close follow-up is optional if a patient will not tolerate the canalith repositioning procedure and if symptoms are mild
- Vestibular neuritis
  - Brief symptomatic care with benzodiazepines, antiemetics, and antihistamines
  - Early vestibular rehabilitation speeds recovery.
  - Use of corticosteroids is controversial.

The "dizzy" patient is often a frustrating phenomenon in clinical medicine. However, after a careful history and physical examination, most patients can be diagnosed and serious causes excluded. Peripheral causes of vertigo are usually benign and include vestibular neuritis and benign paroxysmal positional vertigo (BPPV). Life-threatening central causes include stroke, demyelinating disease, and an intracranial mass. The first step in evaluating vertigo is differentiating among the four types of dizziness: near syncope or light-headedness, disequilibrium, psychogenic dizziness, and true vertigo. True vertigo is a false sense of motion, and patients often report that "the room is spinning." This chapter will focus on the two most common causes of episodic vertigo: BPPV and vestibular neuritis.

Epidemiology

Vertigo is a common office complaint. Every year, millions of Americans are evaluated for dizziness in ambulatory care settings, and approximately 50% of these cases are vertigo. BPPV and vestibular neuritis are two of the most common causes of vertigo seen in the office setting.

Risk Factors

BPPV is seven times more likely in individuals over age 60, and it is also more common in women. A history of prior head trauma and other vestibular disorders increases risk of BPPV. There are no identified risk factors for vestibular neuritis.

Pathophysiology

BPPV is thought to occur when calcium carbonate debris (otoconia) are dislodged and float freely in the semicircular canals of the inner ear. The posterior canal is most often involved. During head movement, loose otoconia move in the canal and cause a continued sense of motion for a few seconds until they settle. The pathophysiology of vestibular neuritis is uncertain. Limited evidence supports a viral infection, which causes inflammation of the eighth cranial nerve. When hearing loss accompanies vertigo, the condition is called *acute labrynthitis*.

Clinical Manifestations

The history and physical examination are fundamental in the evaluation of vertigo. Key questions include the frequency and duration of attacks, triggers such as positional or pressure changes, prior head trauma, associated neurologic symptoms, hearing loss, and headache. A personal history of diabetes, hypertension, and hyperlipidemia are risk factors for stroke. BPPV, stroke, and migraine can have a familial preponderance. Many medications, including anticonvulsants and antihypertensives, cause dizziness.

BPPV causes brief, recurrent episodes that last less than 1 minute and are brought on by changes in head movement or position. Nausea and vomiting may be associated. Vestibular neuritis usually has a subacute onset over several hours, peaks in intensity for 1 to 2 days, and then gradually subsides over the next few weeks. Symptoms of vertigo are constant, and nausea and vomiting can be severe during the first few days. Patients with vestibular neuritis may have difficulty standing and veer toward the affected side. Although changes in position worsen the vertigo in vestibular neuritis, vertigo is always present at baseline. In BPPV, patients have no vertigo between attacks.

General physical examination should include a thorough cardiovascular, ear, nose, throat, and neurologic examination. The neurologic examination can differentiate between benign (peripheral) and life-threatening (central) causes based on the ability to walk, type of nystagmus, results of the head impulse test, and presence of associated neurologic signs (Table 1).

Patients with vestibular neuritis may have difficulty walking, but the inability to walk is a red flag for a central lesion. Nystagmus is unidirectional (always beats in the same direction) and horizontal in vestibular neuritis, and is suppressed by visual fixation. Having a patient focus on an object in the room will stop the nystagmus, which reappears if a blank sheet of paper is placed a few inches in front of the patient's face. Nystagmus in central causes is not suppressed by visual fixation and may be direction-changing (nystagmus beats to

	PERIPHERAL CAUSES		
	BPPV	**VESTIBULAR NEURITIS**	**CENTRAL CAUSES**
History	Brief, recurrent attacks of vertigo lasting less than 1 minute Triggered by positional changes No vertigo between attacks	Subacute onset Constant and severe vertigo lasting days Nausea and vomiting may be severe	Sudden onset Risk factors for stroke May have severe headache
Nystagmus	Up-beating and torsional	Horizontal and unidirectional	Bidirectional Pure vertical Pure torsional
Gait	Unaffected between episodes	May veer towards affected side	Unable to walk
Specialized physical examination tests	Positive Dix-Hallpike or Positive supine roll test	Positive head impulse test Visual fixation stops nystagmus	HINTS exam abnormal Visual fixation does not stop nystagmus
Additional neurologic signs	Rare	Rare	Common (e.g., dysarthria, aphasia, incoordination, weakness, or numbness)

TABLE 1 Differentiating Peripheral and Central Causes of Vertigo

Abbreviation: BPPV = benign paroxysmal positional vertigo.

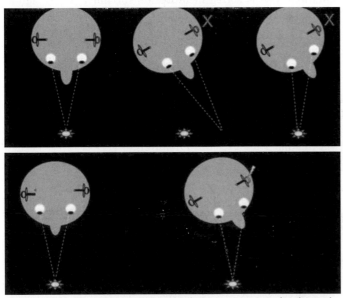

Figure 1 Head impulse test. Top panel shows a positive head impulse test. The examiner moves the patient's head quickly 10 degrees to the side, in this case to the patient's left. A catch-up saccade is observed when the patient looks away and then refixes on the visual target, indicating a peripheral lesion on the left. Lower figure shows a normal head impulse test. The patient maintains visual fixation during head movement. Adapted from Seemungal BM, Bronstein AM. A practical approach to acute vertigo. *Pract Neurol* 2008; 8:211–21.

Figure 2 Treatment maneuver for posterior canal benign paroxysmal positional vertigo affecting the right ear. To treat the left ear, the procedure is reversed. The drawing of the labyrinth in the center shows the position of the particle as it moves around the posterior semicircular canal (PSC) and into the utricle (UT). The patient is seated upright, with head facing the examiner, who is standing on the right. A, The patient is rapidly moved to head-hanging right position (Dix-Hallpike test). This position is maintained until the nystagmus ceases. B, The examiner moves to the head of the table, repositioning hands as shown. C, The head is rotated quickly to the left with right ear upward. This position is maintained for 30 seconds. D, The patient rolls onto the left side while the examiner rapidly rotates the head leftward until the nose is directed toward the floor. This position is then held for 30 seconds. E, The patient is rapidly lifted into the sitting position, now facing left. The entire sequence should be repeated until no nystagmus can be elicited. After the maneuver, the patient is instructed to avoid head-hanging positions to prevent the particles from reentering the posterior canal. Reprinted with permission from Rakel RE. *Conn's Current Therapy 1995.* Philadelphia, WB Saunders, 1995, p 839.

the right when the patient looks right, and beats to the left when the patient looks left) or purely vertical. The head impulse test (Figure 1) is positive in peripheral causes like vestibular neuritis. The examiner holds the patient's head while the patient fixes her eyes on the examiner's nose, and then the examiner quickly moves the patient's head 10 degrees to the right and left. If a saccade (the eyes look away and then re-fixate on the examiner's nose) is found, this indicates a peripheral lesion on the side that the head is turned toward. Central lesions will not cause saccades, and the head impulse test will be negative. HINTS (Head Impulse test, Nystagmus, Test of Skew), which combines three physical examination findings, has been found to have a 97% sensitivity and 99% specificity for a central cause of vertigo in the acute setting and to be more accurate than MRI in the initial 24 hours after symptom onset. If one or more of the tests indicate a central cause, (e.g., a negative head impulse test, direction-changing horizontal nystagmus, or vertical eye misalignment grossly

observed or detected on cover-uncover test), then the HINTS test is considered positive for a central cause and imaging should be obtained. A negative HINTS exam is an excellent rule-out test for stroke, with a negative likelihood ratio of 0.02.

The Dix-Hallpike maneuver is diagnostic of posterior canal BPPV (Figure 2). The patient should be warned that nausea and vomiting may occur. After the patient is placed in the head-hanging position, there is a 5- to 20-second latency period before the nystagmus and symptoms appear. Both the nystagmus and vertigo will increase in severity and then resolve within 60 seconds. The nystagmus observed is up-beating and torsional. If nystagmus is constant for as long as the head is in the hanging position, the patient should be evaluated for a central cause. The maneuver should be repeated with the head held to the opposite side. The side that elicits the symptoms and nystagmus diagnoses BPPV in the ipsilateral ear. If both sides elicit symptoms, the patient may have bilateral BPPV. If the test is negative and BPPV is strongly suspected, the patient should lie supine and the examiner can turn the head to each side (supine roll test; Figure 3). This maneuver will cause vertigo and nystagmus in patients with horizontal canal BPPV.

Diagnosis

BPPV and vestibular neuritis are diagnosed clinically. Further diagnostic testing is indicated if the diagnosis is uncertain or a central cause is suspected. Audiometry may be abnormal in Ménière's disease. MRI is the best imaging test for central lesions because it includes the posterior fossa and is most sensitive for stroke. Vestibular function testing is useful if the diagnosis is unclear or in cases of refractory vertigo. Vestibular function testing evaluates the ocular and vestibular response to position changes and caloric stimulation. Video-oculographic recordings of nystagmus can magnify the eye and allow for repeated viewings for further study. Some patients with BPPV may have additional vestibular disorders causing vertigo that vestibular function testing can elucidate.

Differential Diagnosis

Ménière's disease is suspected in patients with the triad of tinnitus, fluctuating hearing loss, and vertigo. Episodes usually last hours, are disabling, and are recurrent over years, over time leading to permanent dysfunction. Migrainous vertigo features episodes lasting hours to days in patients with other migraine symptoms such as headache, photophobia, phonophobia, or aura. Central lesions such as stroke or intracranial mass are most concerning. Red flags for stroke include sudden onset, risk factors for stroke, associated neurologic signs, inability

to walk, abnormal HINTS exam, severe associated headache, and characteristic nystagmus. Posttraumatic vertigo may occur in patients after head trauma who present with vertigo, tinnitus, and headache. A perilymphatic fistula is rare, but may be suspected in a patient with episodic vertigo after head trauma, heavy lifting, or barotrauma. Pressure changes with sneezing or coughing trigger vertigo attacks. Postural hypotension should be ruled out in all patients. An acoustic neuroma presents with slowly progressive, unilateral sensorineural hearing loss and tinnitus. Many patients may have an unsteady gait, but true vertigo is rare.

Treatment

Posterior canal BPPV is best treated with the *canalith repositioning procedure (CRP)*, such as the Epley maneuver (Figure 2). Studies have shown the procedure is safe and effective with an odds ratio of 4.2 (95% CI. 2.3-11.4) for symptom resolution. Patients should be warned that nausea or vomiting may occur during the procedure, and may be pretreated with an antiemetic medication. The procedure can be repeated immediately if unsuccessful, and the majority of patients will respond after three attempts. Posttreatment activity restrictions are unnecessary. Horizontal canal BPPV can be treated with the barbeque roll maneuver (Figure 4). Vestibular rehabilitation (VR) is a treatment option for BPPV but is significantly less effective than the canalith repositioning procedure. VR is helpful in patients with chronic, nonspecific dizziness after successful treatment with CRP and for improving gait stability in those with increased fall risk, such as the elderly. Observation is an option if symptoms are mild and if a patient will not tolerate the canalith repositioning procedure. However, time to resolution with observation is 1–3 months, and recurrence rates are higher compared to treatment with CRP. Vestibular-suppressant medications such as antihistamines and benzodiazepines are discouraged because they increase fall risk and treatment with CRP is effective. Surgery is rarely needed for BPPV, but may be helpful in refractory cases.

Vestibular neuritis is primarily treated with rest, vestibular suppressant medications, and vestibular rehabilitation. Patients may

Figure 3 Supine roll test. Patient begins lying supine facing upward. The patient's head is rotated to one side laterally 90 degrees and the examiner observes for nystagmus and vertigo. Once symptoms resolve, the patient's head is rotated back to midline. Next, the patient's head is rotated 90 degrees laterally to the opposite side and the examiner observes for nystagmus and vertigo. The side with the worst symptoms indicates the involved ear. (From Kerber KA, et al: Benign paroxysmal positional vertigo in the acute care setting. NCL, Elsevier, 2015.)

Figure 4 Barbecue roll (Lempert maneuver). Patient begins lying supine facing upward (A). Head is rotated laterally 90 degrees toward the affected ear (B). Next, the head is rotated another 90 degrees laterally back to midline (B). Next, the head is rotated laterally 90 degrees toward the opposite side (C). Next, the head is rotated laterally 90 degrees in the same direction (D). Finally, with the patient's head in the same position, the patient is brought into a seated position (E). Each position is held 30 to 60 seconds, long enough for symptoms to occur and then resolve. Once resolved, the patient is moved into the next position. (From Moseley L, Cueco RT: Essential guide to the cervical spine - Volume 2: Clinical Syndromes and Manipulative Treatment. Elsevier, 2016.)

initially be hospitalized if symptoms, such as nausea and vomiting, are severe or if stroke is suspected. Treatment with antihistamines (dimenhydrinate [Dramamine][1] 50 mg every 6 hours), antiemetics (promethazine [Phenergan][1] 25 mg every 6 hours), or benzodiazepines (lorazepam [Ativan][1] 1 to 2 mg every 4 hours) may be used to treat severe symptoms. However, these should not be continued for more than 2 to 3 days because they inhibit central compensation. In vestibular neuritis, patients' vertigo improves not due to return of vestibular nerve function, but due to central compensation for the peripheral deficit. Using vestibular suppressants blocks central compensation and lengthens the course of the disease. The use of corticosteroids is controversial due to the lack of high quality evidence to support symptomatic improvement. Finally, antiviral medications have not been proven effective for vestibular neuritis.

---

[1]Not FDA approved for this indication.

For patients with vestibular neuritis, vestibular rehabilitation should be started as soon as symptoms improve and a patient can tolerate the exercises. Exercises include balance and gait training as well as coordination of head and eye movements. Vestibular rehabilitation hastens recovery and improves balance, gait, and vision by increasing central compensation for vestibular dysfunction. Exercises may be home-based for compliant patients with mild symptoms, whereas formal referral may be more beneficial for patients with severe symptoms, or for the elderly.

Monitoring

Patients diagnosed with BPPV should be reassessed in 1 month regardless of treatment. Failure to improve warrants further evaluation for other etiologies, including central causes. Similarly, patients with vestibular neuritis should slowly improve over several weeks, and failure to do so suggests alternative diagnoses.

Complications

Patients with BPPV are at increased risk for falls. Thirty percent of elderly patients with BPPV have multiple falls in a year. Thus patients should be assessed for fall risk, functional mobility, and balance. Home safety evaluation and home supervision should be considered. BPPV often recurs, with an estimated rate of 15% per year. Counseling patients about recurrence can lead to earlier recognition, earlier treatment, and avoidance of falls. Patients with vestibular neuritis are at increased risk for BPPV and Ménière's disease. Vestibular neuritis rarely recurs.

References

Baloh RW: Vestibular neuritis, *N Engl J Med* 348:1027–1032, 2003.
Bhattacharyya N, Gubbels SP, Schwartz SR, et al: Clinical practice guideline: benign paroxysmal positional vertigo (update), *Otolaryngol Head Neck Surg* 156(Supp 3):S1–S47, 2017.
Chan Y: Differential diagnosis of dizziness, *Otolaryngol Head Neck Surg* 17:200–203, 2009.
Epley JM: The canalith repositioning procedure: for treatment of benign paroxysmal positional vertigo, *Otolaryngol Head Neck Surg* 107:399–404, 1992.
Fishman JM, Burgess C, Waddell A: Corticosteroids for the treatment of idiopathic acute vestibular dysfunction (vestibular neuritis), *Cochran Database Syst Rev* 5, CD008607, 2011. Review.
Hilton MP, Pinder DK: The Epley (canalith repositioning) manoeuvre for benign paroxysmal positional vertigo, *Cochrane Database Syst Rev* 12, CD003162, 2014.
Kerber KA: Vertigo and dizziness in the emergency department, *Emerg Med Clin North Am* 27:39–50, 2009.
McDonnell MN, Hillier SL: Vestibular rehabilitation for unilateral peripheral vestibular dysfunction, *Cochrane Database Syst Rev* 1, CD005397, 2015.
Newman-Toker DE, Kerber KA, Hsieh YH, et al: HINTS outperforms ABCD2 to screen for stroke in acute continuous vertigo and dizziness, *Acad Emerg Med* 20(10):986–996, 2013.
Seemungal BM, Bronstein AM: A practical approach to acute vertigo, *Pract Neurol* 8:211–221, 2008.

FATIGUE

Method of
Jared Regehr, MD

CURRENT DIAGNOSIS

- It is important to evaluate for potential causes of fatigue with a thorough history and physical exam. Basic lab work is also important to evaluate for organic etiologies of fatigue.
- Most cases of fatigue do not have an identifiable underlying etiology.
- A broad differential is important as clinicians evaluate patients with fatigue.

CURRENT THERAPY

- Identifying the underlying cause of fatigue is the most important step in treatment, and any discovered cause should be treated promptly.
- Good sleep hygiene, physical activity, regularly scheduled follow-up visits, and cognitive behavioral therapy have all been shown to improve symptoms of fatigue.
- Short naps are proven performance enhancers.

Epidemiology

Fatigue is a common concern for patients and is the primary complaint for 5% to 10% of patient encounters in the primary care setting. Certain risk factors predispose patients to fatigue. Female sex (1.5 times more likely to report fatigue than males), increased age, and coexisting depression are all associated with higher rates of fatigue. While fatigue can be a normal physiologic response to prolonged activity or stressors, pathologic fatigue has a significant negative impact on patients each year. Individuals with fatigue report decreased quality of life, along with social and emotional dysfunction. Furthermore, it is estimated that fatigue costs US employers $126 billion each year due to decreased production and lost work days.

Prevention

Prevention of fatigue is very similar to the treatment of fatigue. Good sleep hygiene, regular physical exercise, and stress reduction all help with preventing fatigue. Additionally, regularly scheduled follow-up for health maintenance examinations with primary care physicians helps patients avoid comorbidities that may exacerbate fatigue.

Clinical Manifestations

Patients with fatigue often present with lack of energy, delayed recovery after activity, poor muscle endurance, mental exhaustion, and nonrestorative sleep. There is a wide spectrum of severity of disease from a general nuisance to debilitating symptoms.

Diagnosis

Fatigue can be classified based on duration: recent (<1 month), prolonged (1–6 months), and chronic (>6 months). Notably, these timeframes are arbitrary based on the continuous nature of fatigue. For most clinicians, having a broad differential is more helpful in identifying a cause than categorizing fatigue based on time. Even so, identifying the underlying etiology of fatigue can be a challenging and frustrating diagnosis for primary care physicians to make because of vague symptoms and the overlap with comorbidities. A thorough history and physical examination along with appropriate laboratory tests can aid in the diagnosis. There is much debate about the extent of initial laboratory workup, but a reasonable approach includes a complete blood count, basic metabolic panel, hepatic function testing, erythrocyte sedimentation rate, thyroid-stimulating hormone, ferritin, pregnancy test in women of childbearing age, and screening for HIV and hepatitis C in at-risk populations. These tests are useful to help identify "can't miss" diagnoses, but results of laboratory studies only affect management in about 5% of cases. Therefore the importance of a thorough history and physical examination is paramount. It is essential to remember that the information collected from the patient does not need to be limited to the time spent together in the office; a symptom diary with close follow-up can be an extremely beneficial tool as the physician–patient dyad works to find a cause.

TABLE 1	Common Causes of Fatigue: DEAD TIRED
D	Depression
E	Endocrine
A	Anemia, apnea
D	Diabetes
T	Thyroid, tumors
I	Infection, insomnia
R	Rheumatologic
E	Endocarditis/cardiovascular
D	Drugs

The causes of fatigue are extensive and oftentimes coexisting. The most common causes are encompassed in the mnemonic DEAD TIRED (Table 1). Most of these categories have multiple subcategories. As with all chief complaints, it is imperative to allow patients the opportunity to lead the physician to the diagnosis by letting them speak without interruption. Depression is a common cause of fatigue. Medically unexplained symptoms of fatigue are associated with depressive disorders in 50% to 75% of patients, and patients are nearly 11 times more likely to have a lifetime diagnosis of depression than nonfatigued individuals. Importantly, fatigue may be the first presenting symptom for patients who do not yet meet the *Diagnostic and Statistical Manual of Mental Disorders* (DSM) criteria for depression, so close monitoring for other depressive symptoms is vital for prompt recognition and treatment. In most of these cases, there are often other lifestyle factors that contribute to patients' feelings of fatigue. It is important to ask about sleep hygiene, physical exercise, and home/social stressors, as suboptimal functioning in these areas can exacerbate symptoms of fatigue.

Other common secondary causes of fatigue include anemia, endocrine abnormalities, sleep apnea, and medication use. If anemia is noted on initial laboratory evaluation, further workup is usually patient-specific. Markers such as mean corpuscular volume (MCV), ferritin, iron profile, B12, folate, lactate dehydrogenase, and haptoglobin can help guide decision making as clinicians consider causes of anemia. Gastrointestinal bleeding secondary to ulcers, colon cancer, inflammatory bowel disease, or diverticulosis are critical to rule out. Lack of sufficient dietary vitamin intake may be a simple reason for anemia. Endocrine abnormalities that can lead to fatigue include thyroid dysfunction, diabetes mellitus, and adrenal insufficiency. If patients describe persistent daytime sleepiness, evaluation for obstructive sleep apnea is useful, especially in the setting of risk factors (obesity, snoring, hypertension). Additionally, medication usage can cause fatigue. An in-depth review of the legion of medications that can cause fatigue is beyond the scope of this article, but prescription, over-the-counter, and illicit drugs should be considered in the evaluation of fatigue.

Infection is a cause of fatigue, and the most frequent infectious etiology associated with fatigue is of viral origin. Any one of several viruses can cause fatigue, including hepatitis A, B, and C; Epstein-Barr virus; human immunodeficiency virus; and as of recently, COVID-19. Certainly not every patient presenting with fatigue necessitates laboratory evaluation for each of these causes, but if the history or examination suggests an infectious cause, further workup is prudent. Even after recovery from COVID-19, 72.8% of patients report persistent fatigue, by far the most common long-term symptom

reported by survivors of COVID-19. This is an important consideration even months after patients have otherwise recovered from the disease. Postinfluenza asthenia refers to the prolonged fatigue some patients experience after a bout of influenza.

Finally, rheumatologic, cardiovascular, and neoplastic causes should be considered when appropriate in the evaluation of fatigue. Although there are innumerable reports of fatigue in patients with rheumatologic, cardiovascular, oncologic, and hematologic disorders, isolated fatigue as the presenting complaint is not well documented in current medical literature. Additionally, multiple neurologic and autoimmune disorders can have associated fatigue. If the rest of the history and examination warrants further workup for these causes, then evaluation should be pursued. However, an extensive workup based on an isolated complaint of fatigue is not likely to yield beneficial results.

Therapy

Treatment for fatigue should be directed at managing the underlying cause of fatigue when an etiology can be identified based on the history, physical, and laboratory evaluation. However, when no organic cause is identified, there are still ways to help patients get relief. Importantly, ordering more tests is not one of them. In a systemic review of patients with fatigue in which there was a low level of clinical concern for serious illness, the degree of patient reassurance was not increased with additional laboratory testing. Instead, the clinician should start with having an honest conversation with the patient regarding ways to move forward. It is imperative to acknowledge the patient's symptoms and the negative effects on the patient's life, discuss consistent follow-up, and discuss assessment of any new symptoms that may develop. Additionally, there is evidence that sleep hygiene, physical activity, and cognitive behavioral therapy may be helpful in these settings of nondiagnostic fatigue. Short naps have also proven to be helpful and may be a possible solution for some patients.

Monitoring

Monitoring patients with persistent fatigue in the primary care setting can be accomplished by administering a Fatigue Severity Scale (FSS). This method assesses the impact of fatigue on patients' daily lives with a nine-item survey that incorporates a Likert-type rating scale. The FSS has been validated in multiple studies as a reliable tool to assess fatigue. Although there is no generally agreed upon timing for frequency of monitoring, it is reasonable to start with monthly assessments and utilize shared decision making with each patient to individualize a management plan.

References

Corfield E, Martin N, Nyholt D: Co-occurrence and symptomatology of fatigue and depression, *Compr Psychiatry* 71:1–10, 2016.

Finsterer J, Zarrouk-Mahjoub S: Fatigue in health and diseased individuals, *Am J Hosp Palliat Med* 31(5):562–575, 2014.

Friedberg F, Napoli A, Coronel J, et al: Chronic fatigue self-management in primary care: a randomized trial, *Psychosom Med* 75(7):650–657, 2013.

Kamal M, Abo Omirah M, Hussein A, Saeed H: Assessment and characterisation of post–COVID-19 manifestations, *Int J Clin Pract*, 2020. Available at: https://doi-org.proxy.kumc.edu/10.1111/ijcp.13746. Accessed December 31, 2020.

Morelli V: Toward a comprehensive differential diagnosis and clinical approach to fatigue in the elderly, *Clin Geriatr Med* 27(4):687–692, 2011.

O'Connor K, Wright J: Fatigue, *Med Clin North Am* 98(3):597–608, 2014.

Rosenthal T, Majeroni B, Pretorius R, Malik K. Fatigue: an overview. *Am Fam Physician*. 15;78(10):1173–1179

Valko P, Bassetti C, Bloch K, Held U, Baumann C: Validation of the fatigue severity scale in a swiss cohort, *Sleep* 31(11):1601–1607, 2008.

Zhang XY, Huang HJ, Zhuang DL, et al: Biological, clinical and epidemiological features of COVID-19, SARS and MERS and AutoDock simulation of ACE2, *Infect Dis Poverty* 9, 2020. Available at: https://doi.org/10.1186/s40249-020-00691-6. Accessed December 31, 2020.

FEVER

Method of
Alan R. Roth, DO; and Gina M. Basello, DO

CURRENT DIAGNOSIS

- Numerous endogenous and exogenous factors play a role in determining body temperature. Current standards define *fever* as an oral temperature of ≥100.4°F (≥38°C).
- Though temperature varies with measurement technique, in clinical practice, most recommendations refer to oral, rectal, and axillary temperature measurements, with rectal temperature being the standard of care in infants and young children.
- Tympanic thermometers should not be used in young children.
- Fever is not an illness. It is the body's physiologic response to a disease process and has beneficial effects in fighting infection.
- All neonates with a fever should be admitted to the hospital for a sepsis evaluation. For infants between 1 and 3 months of age, evidence-based guidelines, along with clinical evaluation, determine the diagnostic and therapeutic approach.
- For well-appearing term infants 29 to 60 days of age with fever ≥38.0°C and no evident infection source, diagnostic testing should include urinalysis, blood cultures, and inflammatory markers (e.g., procalcitonin and absolute neutrophil count [ANC]).
- With widespread immunization use, the incidence of bacteremia and bacterial meningitis in young infants has significantly decreased, and UTI is now the most prevalent bacterial infection, with the most common etiologic pathogen being *E. coli* for both.
- The possibility of infection with the SARS-CoV-2 virus must be considered in all patients presenting with fever and tested for appropriately. Global health considerations may necessitate additional testing in returning travelers (e.g., monkeypox, polio).
- Urine leukocyte esterase has emerged as a highly accurate diagnostic test for UTI in febrile infants with greater than 95% sensitivity.
- FUO requires a systematic, thoughtful, and thorough evaluation based on the age of the patient and the existing clinical evidence, with repeated clinical assessments being essential.
- Hyperthermia is an unregulated, significant elevation of core body temperature above the normal diurnal range due to failure of thermoregulation from a hypothalamic insult, not a pyogenic source, and is considered a medical emergency. It is not synonymous with fever and often requires immediate intervention to avoid deleterious central nervous system (CNS) effects.

CURRENT THERAPY

- Treating a fever significantly increases the patient's level of comfort, activity, and oral feeding and fluid intake, in addition to decreasing the body temperature.
- Multiple randomized, controlled trials reveal that treating fever does not shorten or prolong the overall duration of illness or reduce the occurrence of febrile seizures.
- Many clinical recommendations state that a temperature less than 102.2°F (39°C) in healthy children does not require treatment. Antipyretics are known to provide comfort to children and their caregivers.
- Antipyretic treatment for children includes acetaminophen (Tylenol) 10 to 15 mg/kg every 4 to 6 hours or ibuprofen (Advil, Motrin) 10 mg/kg every 6 hours.
- Ibuprofen and acetaminophen have both been shown to reduce fever effectively and safely. Combination therapy has been shown in some studies to have an added benefit in both reduction of temperature and comfort without an increase in side effects, though caution should be taken to avoid dosing errors.
- Antipyretic therapy for adults and adolescents includes acetaminophen 650 to 1000 mg orally (PO) every 6 hours to a maximum of 3 g per day, ibuprofen 200 to 400 mg PO every 6 hours, or aspirin (ASA) 325 to 650 mg every 6 hours as needed (PRN) for fever.
- ASA should not be used in children due to the risk of Reye's syndrome.
- Sponge bathing should be done with tepid water and no alcohol. Recommendation: sponge bathing and other home remedies should not be used as sole treatment.

Fever is one of the most common clinical presentations encountered by primary care physicians and the most common complaint of acute visits for children in the ambulatory or emergency department setting. Fever is a symptom and one of the most reliable signs of illness rather than a disease process itself. Most causes of fever are secondary to acute viral illnesses such as upper respiratory infections (URIs), which account for 50 million visits to primary care providers annually. Less commonly, bacterial infections may cause pharyngitis, otitis, sinusitis, pneumonia, and urinary tract infections (UTIs). A cost-effective, evidence-based approach using clinical protocols, guidelines, and consensus recommendations to the diagnosis and management of febrile illness, including the appropriate use of antibiotic therapy, is the cornerstone of quality medical care for this presentation. Fever produces significant anxiety for patients, parents, and health care providers, which can lead to overtreatment. Typically, fever is transient and only requires treatment to provide patient comfort.

Definitions

The definition of fever is dependent on numerous endogenous and exogenous factors that play a role in determining body temperature, including age, time of day, site, and measuring device, as well as operator variables. Fever is an elevation of body temperature due to the adjustment of the hypothalamic-pituitary set point. This usually occurs in response to a pathologic stimulus. Fever is a beneficial physiologic mechanism that helps to promote an augmented immunologic response.

Despite individual variability, core body temperature is maintained at about 98.6°F (37°C). Diurnal variation results in lower body temperatures in the early morning and a temperature higher in the late afternoon or early evening, which is consistent with what is encountered in clinical practice.

In adults, a morning oral temperature of 98.9°F (37.2°C) or higher, or an evening temperature of 99.9°F (37.7°C) or higher defines a fever. Rectal temperatures are generally considered to be 0.7°F (0.4°C) higher than oral readings.

In infants and young children, rectal temperatures are still considered the standard of care and a rectal temperature greater than 100.4°F (38°C) is considered a fever.

Axillary temperatures of greater than 98.6°F (37°C) are regarded as a fever, though this measurement site is generally considered less accurate. An accurate measurement of body temperature is dependent on site, measuring device, and the clinical skills of the operator. Site selection should be determined by the age of the patient.

Young infants and older adults often have a diminished febrile response due to physiologic factors, thereby warranting the use of other clinical factors to guide diagnosis.

Recent technologic advances, including electronic devices, tympanic membrane scanning, and temporal artery scanning, have replaced the older mercury-in-glass thermometers. These devices offer faster results and minimal inconvenience to the patient and are becoming increasingly reliable. Chemical content or liquid crystal thermometers applied to the skin are neither accurate nor cost-effective.

Hyperthermia is an uncontrolled elevation of core body temperature that exceeds the body's ability to lose heat. In hyperthermia, the setting of the hypothalamic thermoregulatory center is unchanged, in contrast to fever. Hyperthermia requires urgent medical intervention because it could be rapidly fatal and does not respond to antipyretics. Common etiologies include heat stroke, neuromalignant syndrome, serotonin syndrome, malignant hyperthermia, endocrinopathy, and CNS damage.

Classic *fever of unknown origin* (FUO) is defined as a disorder with temperatures ≥100.9 °F (38.3 °C) that have persisted for at least 3 weeks, with no definitive cause elucidated after initial comprehensive inpatient or outpatient workup. The etiologies of FUO generally fall into four diagnostic categories: infectious, autoimmune or inflammatory, neoplastic, and miscellaneous.

Pathophysiology

Fever occurs as part of an inflammatory response to an inciting stimulus. The response includes the production of various cytokines that ultimately increase the production of prostaglandin E_2 (PGE_2), which resets the hypothalamic thermoregulatory set point at a higher level. Important pyogenic cytokines include interleukin-1 (IL-1), interleukin-6 (IL-6), tumor necrosis factor α (TNF-α), interferon-β (IFN-β), and interferon-γ (IFN-γ).

Risks and Benefits of Fever

Fever is known to enhance the immunologic response while suppressing the growth and replication of bacterial and viral infections. Though often uncomfortable for patients, caregivers, and health care providers, evidence supports the notion that fever is beneficial and ultimately protects against the development of asthma and other allergic disorders. In most instances, fever is not harmful. It does increase cardiac demand and metabolic needs, resulting in the common associated signs and symptoms of tachycardia, tachypnea, shivering, malaise, and diaphoresis.

The use of antipyretic agents has not been shown to either prolong or shorten the duration of illness. Febrile seizures cause significant anxiety for parents. They occur most commonly in children between the ages of 6 months and 6 years. Most febrile seizures are uncomplicated and have not been shown to be associated with significant bacteremia or to lead to the development of seizure disorder in older children. Antipyretic agents have not been shown to decrease the incidence of febrile seizures.

Diagnostic Evaluation of Fever

In most cases, the etiology of a febrile illness is a self-limiting viral infection. From 5% to 10% of fevers may be associated with a more serious bacterial infection such as pneumonia, UTI, bacteremia, meningitis, or bone and joint infections. At times, these conditions may be challenging to distinguish, and a thoughtful, systematic, evidence-based approach to the diagnostic evaluation will be most cost-effective while avoiding the inappropriate use of antibiotics.

Although the most common clinical presentation of COVID is fever with respiratory symptoms, a significant proportion of patients will present with fever alone or atypically. Considering this, COVID testing is indicated for all patients presenting with fever.

All infants less than 28 days old with a fever should be admitted to the hospital for a full sepsis workup and empiric intravenous antibiotic therapy.

Young infants, 1 to 3 months of age, with a febrile illness can be especially challenging. Numerous studies addressing this challenging population have led to the development of multiple guidelines and clinical protocols that utilize risk stratification criteria. The use of these age-specific stratification criteria, along with clinical treatment guidelines, helps guide the clinician in the evaluation of febrile illness. Clinical judgment remains the cornerstone of good clinical care.

With the widespread use of *Haemophilus influenzae* type B (Hib) and pneumococcal vaccinations, the incidence of bacteremic illness has decreased significantly. UTI has emerged as the most prevalent bacterial infection. The increased use of rapid viral testing in the office and emergency department settings may alleviate the need for more invasive testing and antibiotic use because the risk of concurrent bacterial infection has been reported to be negligible.

In this age group, an initial workup that reveals a white blood cell (WBC) count of less than 5000 or greater than 15,000 indicates an increased likelihood of a significant bacterial illness (SBI). Blood cultures, urinalysis, urine culture, and cerebrospinal fluid (CSF) evaluation should then be obtained and accompanied by intravenous antibiotic therapy. When considering the use of inflammatory markers diagnostically, procalcitonin has emerged as the most accurate inflammatory marker, followed by (in descending order) C-reactive protein, absolute neutrophil count, and white blood cell count. Incorporating urine concentration when interpreting urine analyses can help in the differentiation of infants at higher risk of UTI.

Children age 3 to 36 months, who appear well and do not have any underlying medical history, require only a comprehensive clinical evaluation and do not warrant antibiotic therapy or diagnostic testing in most instances. Septic or ill-appearing children need a more aggressive evaluation, including complete blood count (CBC), inflammatory markers, urinalysis, urine culture, blood cultures, and a chest x-ray. High-risk children in this age group require empiric antibiotic therapy, and clinical judgment should guide the decision to hospitalize.

Classic FUO is defined as a disorder with temperatures greater than 100.9 °F (38.3 °C) that has persisted for at least 3 weeks with no clear etiology determined after 3 days of hospital evaluation or three outpatient visits. Common etiologic categories include infectious, neoplastic, inflammatory, and miscellaneous causes, of which drug fever has been shown to be the most prevalent.

The initial approach includes a thorough history, physical examination, and appropriate laboratory testing. The initial choice of imaging should be guided by clinical findings and most commonly includes a chest x-ray and a CAT scan of the abdomen and pelvis. If the etiology remains elusive, positron emission tomography (PET) scanning or invasive diagnostic testing should then be considered.

Differential Diagnosis

Hyperthermia is an unregulated, significant elevation of core body temperature above the normal diurnal range due to failure of thermoregulation from a hypothalamic insult, not a pyogenic source, and is considered a medical emergency. It is not synonymous with fever and often requires immediate intervention to avoid deleterious CNS effects. Since the hypothalamic set point remains unchanged, antipyretics are ineffective in hyperthermia. The most common etiology is the inability to regulate or dissipate excess body heat. Hyperthermia is a medical emergency that requires immediate treatment to prevent excessive morbidity and mortality.

Treatment

Though controversy exists regarding the necessity of lowering fever, antipyretics have been shown to effectively and safely reduce temperature and improve symptoms with minimal side effects. Acetaminophen (Tylenol) is available in many formulations. Dosing should be based on body weight and not age of the patient. The dose is 10 to 15 mg/kg every 4 to 6 hours, not to exceed 3 g daily or 2 g in patients with renal or hepatic impairment. Ibuprofen (Advil, Motrin) is a nonsteroidal antiinflammatory drug (NSAID) that has both antiinflammatory and antipyretic effects. Dosing is 10 mg/kg every 6 to 8 hours in children and 200 to 400 mg every 6 hours in adolescents and adults. Ibuprofen is also available in multiple formulations, including a newer intravenous preparation (ibuprofen [Caldolor]) that may be beneficial in oral-intolerant hospitalized patients. Some studies suggest that ibuprofen may be a more effective antipyretic agent than acetaminophen.

In adults, aspirin (ASA) remains a therapeutic alternative for lowering fever at a dose of 325 to 650 mg every 4 to 6 hours. It should not be used in children with a febrile illness due to the risk of Reye's syndrome.

A combination of acetaminophen and ibuprofen in alternating doses has been shown in some studies to have an added benefit in both reduction of temperature and comfort without an increase in side effects, though caution should be taken to avoid dosing errors.

Nonpharmacologic therapies such as sponge bathing with tepid water and other environmental measures to control temperature, including adjusting room temperatures and sipping cool fluids to avoid dehydration, are used commonly and do provide symptom relief and comfort. These measures should never be used as the sole therapy for fever reduction.

References

Cunha BA: Fever of unknown origin: focused diagnostic approach based on clinical clues from the history, physical examination, and laboratory tests, *Infect Dis Clin North Am* 21:1137–1187, 2007.

Dorney K, Bachur RG: Febrile infant update, *Curr Opin Pediatr* 29:280–285, 2017.

Herzog L, Phillips S: Addressing concerns about fever, *Clin Pediatr* 50:383–390, 2011.

Huppler AR, Eickhoff JC, Wald ER: Performance of low-risk criteria in the evaluation of young infants with fever: review of the literature, *Pediatrics* 125:228, 2010.

Jhavier R, Byington C, Klein J, Shapiro E: Management of the non-toxic appearing acutely febrile child: a 21st century approach, *J Pediatr* 159:181–185, 2011.

Makoni M, Mukundan D: Fever, *Curr Opin Pediatr* 22:100–106, 2010.

Pantell RH, Roberts KB, Adams WG, et.al.: Clinical practice guideline: evaluation and management of well-appearing febrile infants 8 to 60 days old. *Pediatrics* 148(2):e2021052228, 2021.

Pantell RH, Roberts KB, Greenhow TL, Pantell MS: Advances in the diagnosis and management of febrile infants: challenging tradition, *Adv Pediatr* 65(1):173–208, 2018.

Roth AR, Basello GM: Fever. In Paulman PM, Harrison JD, Paulman MD, et al, *Signs and Symptoms in Family Medicine*, Philadelphia, 2012, Mosby, pp 317–326.

Roth AR, Basello GM: Approach to the adult patient with fever of unknown origin, *Am Fam Physician* 68:2223–2228, 2003.

Struyf T, Deeks, Dinnes J, et al; Cochrane COVID-19 Diagnostic Test Accuracy Group: Signs and symptoms to determine if a patient presenting in primary care or hospital outpatient settings has COVID-19. *Cochrane Database of Systematic Reviews* 2021, Issue 2. Art. No.: CD013665.

Sullivan J, Farrar HC: Clinical report: fever and antipyretic use in children, *Pediatrics* 127:580–587, 2011.

Van den Bruel A, Thompson MJ, Haj-Hassan, et al: Diagnostic value of laboratory tests in identifying serious infections in febrile children; systematic review, *BMJ* 342:382, 2011.

GASEOUSNESS, INDIGESTION, NAUSEA, AND VOMITING

Method of
Justin Bailey, MD

Nausea is a vague, subjective feeling that vomiting (forceful expulsion of gastric contents) is imminent. Dyspepsia (based on Rome III criteria) can include postprandial fullness, early satiety, epigastric pain, burning, and reflux (return of gastric content to the lower esophagus or mouth, accompanied by a sour taste or "heartburn" sensation). Gaseousness can present with a variety of complaints, including belching, bloating, abdominal pain, or flatulence.

Epidemiology

Nausea and vomiting (ICD-10 Code R11.2) is one of the top reasons patients see a primary care provider. Infectious diseases causing nausea and vomiting, gastroenteritis, diarrhea, and dehydration are leading causes of death in developing countries, and of sick days and reduction of employee productivity in the United States. Nausea and vomiting postoperatively and during cancer chemotherapy add significant costs, pain, and discomfort to hospital and ambulatory treatment. Dyspepsia occurs in an estimated 25% of the US population every year, many of whom do not seek care. Gaseousness is ubiquitous in the population and is troubling to a small portion.

Risk Factors

Previous gastrointestinal (GI) surgery, certain medications, chemotherapeutic regimens, substance abuse, pregnancy, infectious diseases, medical conditions, and central nervous system disorders increase the risk for nausea and vomiting symptoms. Dyspepsia risk is increased significantly with ingestion of nonsteroidal antiinflammatory drugs (NSAIDs), tobacco use, *Helicobacter pylori* infection, obesity, anxiety, somatization, neuroticism, depression, and unemployment. Increased upper GI gaseousness can be seen with air swallowing from gum chewing and eating quickly, as well as consumption of foods that relax the lower esophageal sphincter (e.g., chocolate, fats, mints). Ingestion of lactose, fructose, sorbitol, undigested starches (e.g., bran), and carbonated beverages can all increase the risk of bloating and flatulence.

Pathophysiology

The pathophysiologic regulation of nausea and vomiting is complex and incompletely understood. Multiple neurotransmitters are involved, including acetylcholine, dopamine, histamine, and serotonin. The therapeutic action of antiemetics is often based on blocking the action of these neurotransmitters. Neurologic regulation of nausea and vomiting involves the chemoreceptor triggers in the fourth ventricle, the nucleus tractus solitarius in the medulla, motor nuclei that control the vomiting reflex, and vagal afferent nerves from the GI tract. The sympathetic and parasympathetic nervous systems are involved in conjunction with the smooth muscle cells and the enteric brain within the wall of the stomach and intestine.

The pathophysiology of dyspepsia is unclear but probably has multiple causes. Delayed gastric motility can occur in up to 30% of patients with dyspepsia. In addition, decreased gastric compliance, alteration in gut microbiome, duodenal inflammation, and psychosocial dysfunction can also be associated with dyspeptic patients.

Sensations of lower tract gaseousness result from one of three different mechanisms: excess gas production, abnormal intestinal transit, and increased visceral sensitivity. Gas production caused by carbohydrate maldigestion, (e.g., lactose intolerance, poorly absorbed starches) results in bloating and a sensation of fullness. High-fiber diets, celiac disease, and small intestine bacterial overgrowth can increase gas production. Dysmotility associated with diabetes mellitus, scleroderma, amyloidosis, and endocrine disease may result in gastroparesis and chronic intestinal pseudo-obstruction. In addition, previous Nissen fundoplication, fat intolerance, and various familial conditions may cause dysmotility. Increased visceral sensitivity is thought to be a main cause of pain and fullness in patients with functional bowel disorders such as irritable bowel syndrome (IBS) and functional dyspepsia.

Prevention

Once the diagnosis has been established, appropriate treatment of the underlying cause of the symptoms can be instituted. When the cause of nausea and vomiting is related to medication, the dose can be adjusted or the medication changed as appropriate.

Upper GI bloating and fullness is almost exclusively caused by excess air swallow and can be improved with altering behaviors such as gulping food and gum chewing. Lower GI symptoms can be prevented by avoiding problem foods such as milk products in patients with lactose intolerance.

Clinical Manifestations

Nausea and vomiting are extremely common and are associated with many conditions. Associated symptoms are helpful in sorting out causes. Many common historical associations are listed in Table 1.

The diagnosis of dyspepsia is based mainly on clinical symptoms. The Rome III criteria are listed in the opening paragraph. Alarm symptoms that should raise suspicions for gastric cancer include unintended weight loss, persistent vomiting, progressive dysphasia, odynophagia, unexplained anemia, iron deficiency, hematemesis, palpable abdominal mass, lymphadenopathy, family history of gastric cancer, previous gastric surgery, or jaundice.

Gaseousness usually presents with abdominal fullness and bloating. Pain associated with the fullness is often relieved with eructation or flatulence (see Table 1).

Diagnosis

The first step in the assessment of patients with abdominal complaints is complete history of the duration of symptoms, the frequency of episodes, work environment, recent travel, household member illness, association of symptoms with certain foods or beverages (i.e., pain relief or worsening with food), and determination of the success or failure of what the patient has tried to alleviate the symptoms, all of which may offer diagnostic clues. Focused inquiries into surgeries, sexual activity, and other elements of a review of symptoms may be helpful. A complete review of medication usage, with particular attention to GI-irritating medications such as NSAIDs and over-the-counter medications, illicit drugs, and herbal products is important. Physical examination and diagnostic work-up can help isolate the cause (Table 2).

In patients with acute (<24 hours) nausea and vomiting, a laboratory work-up is often unnecessary. Patients with the most commonly identified acute causes, such as acute gastroenteritis, vestibular neuritis, chemotherapy, medication, and alcohol ingestion, and those who are postoperative, can be started on symptomatic therapy. For persistent symptoms of nausea and vomiting, laboratory work-up is guided by the history and physical examination and can include a complete blood count and differential, serum chemistries, renal function, liver function tests, serum protein and albumin, thyroid-stimulating hormone, amylase or lipase, drug screen, and a pregnancy test in women of childbearing age. Imaging should not be routine but should be directed by the history and physical findings as well as pertinent laboratory results. Useful studies may include acute abdominal series (chest x-ray, flat

TABLE 1	Key Symptoms and Differential Vomiting, Dyspepsia, and Bloating
SYMPTOMS	**DIFFERENTIAL**
Abdominal Pain ± N/V • RUQ • Epigastric • RLQ • LLQ • Pelvic	Organic etiologies • Cholelithiasis, cholecystitis • Dyspepsia, pancreatitis, GERD, gastritis, MI • Appendicitis • Diverticulitis • PID, ovarian torsion, ectopic pregnancy
Abdominal pain + distention + N/V	Bowel obstruction
Abdominal distention associated with foods (lactose, wheat-based products, bran, legumes)	Lactose intolerance Celiac disease Carbohydrate malabsorption, Oligosaccharide fermentation (legumes)
Vomiting several hours after eating + succussion splash + N/V	Gastric obstruction Gastroparesis
Heartburn ± N/V	GERD, dyspepsia
Early morning + N/V	Pregnancy
Feculent vomiting + N/V	Intestinal obstruction Gastrocolic fistula
Vertigo + nystagmus + N/V	Vestibular neuritis
Dental erosions, parotid gland enlargement, lanugo-like hair, callus on dorsal surface of hands	Bulimia
Positional N/V	Neurogenic
N/V relieved with hot shower or bath	Cannabis hyperemesis

GERD, Gastroesophageal reflux disease; LLQ, left lower quadrant; MI, myocardial infarction; N/V, nausea and vomiting; PID, pelvic inflammatory disease; RLQ, right lower quadrant; RUQ, right upper quadrant.

TABLE 2	Physical Examination: Nausea, Vomiting, Dyspepsia, and Gaseousness
FINDINGS	**POSSIBLE ETIOLOGY**
Fever	Infectious
Tachycardia, hypotension	Dehydration, volume depletion, sepsis (infectious), ectopic pregnancy, myocardial infarction, aortic aneurysm
Exophthalmos	Hyperthyroid
Papilledema	Increased intracranial pressure (tumors, subdural hemorrhage)
Bulging tympanic membrane	Otitis media, effusion
Thyromegaly	Hypothyroid
Lymphadenopathy	Infection, malignancy
Dry mucous membranes	Dehydration, volume depletion
Dental erosions	Bulimia
Abdominal distention	Obstruction, ileus, gastroparesis, irritable bowel, hepatic/splenic flexure syndrome, postoperative gas-bloat syndrome
Absent bowel sounds	Ileus, perforation
Sense of abdominal distention without bloating	Irritable bowel syndrome
Abdominal bloating	Irritable bowel syndrome, obstruction
RUQ abdominal pain/guarding	Cholecystitis, cholelithiasis
RLQ/LLQ abdominal pain/guarding	Appendicitis (RLQ), ovarian torsion, diverticulitis, ectopic pregnancy
Cervical motion tenderness	Pelvic inflammatory disease, endometriosis
Bladder tenderness	Urinary tract infection
Testicular pain	Torsion, epididymitis
Abnormal rectal examination	Fecal impaction, prostatitis, appendicitis, ovarian tumor, ectopic pregnancy, endometriosis
Delayed cap refill, poor skin turgor	Dehydration
Jaundice	Gallbladder disease, biliary obstruction

LLQ, Left lower quadrant; RLQ, right lower quadrant; RUQ, right upper quadrant.

and upright views of the abdomen), abdominal computed tomography (CT), and abdominal ultrasound.

Similarly, in patients with dyspetic symptoms, laboratory tests should be obtained based on the history and physical examination. Many therapies, such as discontinuing offending medications (e.g., NSAIDs) or acid suppression in patients without alarm symptoms, may be started without a laboratory work-up. Blood count chemistries and *H. pylori* testing can be considered if warranted. Alarm symptoms may warrant further imaging or direct visualization with esophagogastroduodenoscopy (EGD).

In gaseousness and bloating, the most sensitive work-up is the history and physical examination. Further work-up should be directed by initial findings. Patients with alarm symptoms such as weight loss, diarrhea, abdominal pain, distention, and anorexia may benefit from a malabsorption work-up including lactose tolerance test, stool fat, ova and parasites, stool culture, *Clostridium difficile*, acute abdominal series, or EGD. A hydrogen breath test may be beneficial in selected patients to assess the relationship between specific foods and symptoms. Other blood work, tests, and imaging, such as CT, magnetic resonance imaging (MRI), and EGD are guided by availability of testing and the history, examination, and laboratory findings.

Differential Diagnosis

Tables 3, 4, and 5 summarize the wide differential diagnoses of nausea and vomiting, dyspepsia, and gaseousness.

Treatment

Antiemetics, hydration, and dietary changes are the first line treatments for acute episodes of nausea and vomiting. Controlling the symptoms is often all that is necessary in acute, self-limited bouts of nausea and vomiting symptoms. If patients are dehydrated, oral rehydration can be accomplished by encouraging the patient to take small amounts (6 ounces or less) of cool water or electrolyte solutions on a frequent basis. If patients are unable to accomplish this, parenteral rehydration and antiemetics may be warranted.

Table 6 lists the common antiemetics agent, indications, dosages, side effects, and relative cost of medications.

Location of the cause with directed treatment is most effective for gaseousness. If no cause is found, it can be difficult to treat. Avoiding foods that are contributory, such as those containing lactose, fructose, sorbitol, high fiber, and starches, may be all that is necessary. Symptoms associated with increased sensitivity to normal levels of gas (i.e., IBS) can be difficult to treat. Therapeutic relationships, education, and dietary modification are the mainstays of IBS treatment. For moderate to severe symptoms, short-term treatment with antispasmodics, tricyclic antidepressants, and antidiarrheal agents may have some benefit. Medical treatments for bloating are listed in Table 7.

For most patients with dyspepsia, information can be powerful. Validation of symptoms and working toward a goal of management rather than cure are therapeutic. In patients with dyspepsia in which a concern for *H. pylori* exists, a test-and-treatment strategy can be effective. In other patients, proton pump inhibitors, H-2 receptor antagonists, prokinetic agents, and peppermint oil are all effective short-term therapies.

Monitoring

For patients who have complications related to nausea and vomiting, monitoring serum electrolytes, renal function, nutritional status, and other parameters may be necessary until hydration improves, electrolytes are replaced, and laboratory results and clinical status return to normal.

Further testing is needed in patients with dyspepsia and alarm symptoms; however, in patients without alarm symptoms, no further testing is needed.

Complications

The complications of prolonged nausea and vomiting are dehydration, electrolyte disturbances (e.g., hypokalemia, hypophosphatemia,

TABLE 3	Differential Diagnosis for Nausea and Vomiting
Central Nervous System	**Psychiatric**
Multiple sclerosis, tumor, intracranial bleeding, infarction, abscess, meningitis, trauma, labyrinthitis, Ménière disease, vestibular neuritis, motion sickness	Anorexia, anxiety, bulimia, depression
Migraine headaches, seizure disorders	**Medication Related** Acetaminophen (Tylenol) Acyclovir (Zovirax) Alcohol abuse
Gastrointestinal Disorders	Antibiotics: azithromycin (Zithromax), sulfasalazine (Azulfidine), erythromycin, metronidazole (Flagyl), sulfonamides (e.g., sulfamethoxazole-trimethoprim [Bactrim]), tetracycline
Appendicitis, gastric bypass, gastroparesis, hepatobiliary disease, cholecystitis, hepatitis, neoplasia	
Ileus	Antidepressants: Selective serotonin reuptake inhibitors (SSRIs)
Crohn disease, ulcerative colitis	
Irritable bowel syndrome	Antihypertensives: β-blockers (atenolol [Tenormin], metoprolol [Lopressor]), calcium channel blockers, diuretics (hydrochlorothiazide)
Ischemia: mesenteric, small bowel	
Obstruction: scarring/adhesions from previous surgeries, small bowel obstruction, esophageal spasm	Cannabis Chemotherapeutic agents: cisplatinum (Cisplatin [Platinol]), cyclophosphamide (Cytoxan), nitrogen mustard (Mustargen), dacarbazine (DTIC-Dome), methotrexate (Trexall), vinblastine (Velban)
Pancreatitis	
Peptic ulcer disease: esophagitis, gastritis, gastroesophageal reflux	
Peritonitis	Diabetes treatment: metformin (Glucophage), sulfonylureas
Endocrine	Digoxin (Lanoxin)
Addison disease, diabetes (ketoacidosis, gastroparesis), hyperthyroidism, hypothyroidism, hyperparathyroidism, hypoparathyroidism, porphyria	Ergotamines: dihydroergotamine (Migranal), methysergide (Sansert)[2]
	Ferrous gluconate, ferrous sulfate
Genitourinary	Gout treatment: allopurinol (Zyloprim)
Nephritis, nephrolithiasis, torsion (ovary, testicle), uremia, kidney stone	Hormones: estrogen, progesterone, and oral and injected contraceptives
Infectious Etiologies	Levodopa (L-dopa), carbidopa (Lodosyn)
Bacterial: Campylobacter, Salmonella, Shigella, Enterogenic Escherichia coli	Nicotine (patch, gum, smokeless tobacco, cigarette/pipe/cigar)
Viral: rotavirus, influenza	Nonsteroidal antiinflammatory: aspirin, ibuprofen (Motrin), naproxen (Naprosyn)
Otitis media: bacterial or viral	
Sexually transmitted infection: cervicitis, epididymitis, pelvic inflammatory disease, prostatitis, urethritis; multiple organisms including gonorrhea and chlamydia	Opioids: codeine, heroin, hydrocodone, oxycodone, morphine, buprenorphine/naloxone (Suboxone)
Urinary tract infection: lower (cystitis) or upper (pyelonephritis)	Prednisone Seizure medications: phenobarbital, phenytoin (Dilantin)
Pregnancy	
Morning sickness, hyperemesis gravidarum, intrauterine and ectopic pregnancies	Theophylline (Uniphyl)

[2]Not available in the United States.

and hypomagnesemia), depletion of vitamins and trace elements, metabolic alkalosis, and malnutrition. Usually these can be corrected with oral or intravenous hydration, correction of electrolyte deficiencies, and treatment of the underlying cause. In patients whose nausea and vomiting are accompanied by gastroenteritis, symptoms and clinical status may not return to baseline unless all electrolytes such as potassium, magnesium, phosphorus, and trace elements such as zinc are replaced.

Dyspeptic patients without alarm symptoms rarely have complications. In patients with chronic bloating, complications are uncommon.

TABLE 4 Differential Diagnosis of Dyspepsia

Gastrointestinal Disorders	Medications
Functional or nonulcer (most common)	NSAIDs
Peptic ulcer disease	Antibiotics (macrolides and metronidazole)
Gastroesophageal reflux	Corticosteroids
Gastritis	Digoxin
Pancreatitis	Narcotics
Gastroparesis	Theophylline
Gastric cancer	**Respiratory**
Intestinal ischemia	Pneumonia
Esophageal rupture	**Cardiac**
Malabsorption	Myocardial ischemia or pericarditis
Lactase deficiency	**Musculoskeletal**
Celiac	Abdominal hernia
Infectious	**Psychiatric**
Parasite infection	Physical sexual abuse
Helicobacter pylori	
Pregnancy	

NSAIDs, Nonsteroidal antiinflammatory drugs.

TABLE 5 Differential Diagnosis of Bloating and Gaseousness

Upper Gastrointestinal	Gas-Producing Foods
Air swallowing	Beans, peas, lentils, broccoli, Brussels sprouts, cauliflower, cabbage, parsnips, leeks, onions, beer, coffee, pork
Small Bowel	
Pneumatosis cystoides intestinalis	**Infectious**
Carbohydrate Malabsorption	Parasites
Lactase deficiency	*Helicobacter pylori*
Legumes (indigestible oligosaccharides)	Bacterial overgrowth
Fructose malabsorption	**Malabsorption**
Undigested starch (bran)	Celiac
Irritable Bowel Syndrome	Crohn disease

TABLE 6 Medications for Nausea and Vomiting

DRUG	USE	SIDE EFFECTS	DOSAGE
Anticholinergics Act as antimuscarinic agents		Sedation, dry mouth, dizziness, hallucinations, confusion, exacerbate narrow angle glaucoma, blurred vision.	
Scopalamine	Nausea associated with motion sickness		1–1.5 mg patch TD q3d
Antihistamines		Sedation, dry mouth, confusion, urinary retention, blurred vision	
Diphenhydramine (Benadryl)	Nausea associated with motion sickness		50 mg PO q6h or 10–50 mg IV or IM
Doxylamine (Unisom)[1]	Nausea associated with pregnancy		5–10 mg PO qd
Hydroxyzine (Vistaril)[1]	Nausea associated with motion sickness		25–100 mg q6h
Meclizine (Antivert)	Nausea associated with motion sickness		25–50 mg q6h
Promethazine (Phenergan)	Nausea associated with motion sickness		12.5–25 mg (PO, IM, IV, PR) q4–6h
Benzamides: Prokinetic agents; work on peripheral and central dopamine, weak hydroxytryptamine type 3 (5-HT$_3$)		Sedation, hypotension, extrapyramidal effects, diarrhea, neuroleptic syndrome, supraventricular tachycardia, CNS depression	
Metoclopramide (Reglan)	Second line therapy for chemotherapy-induced nausea		10 mg (PO, IM, IV) q6h
Trimethobenzamide (Tigan)[1]	Chemotherapy-induced nausea		300 mg PO q6h
Butyrophenones: Dopamine antagonists		Sedation, hypotension, extrapyramidal effects, tachycardia, dizziness, QT prolongation and torsades de pointes, neuroleptic malignant syndrome	
Droperidol (Inapsine)	Postoperative nausea/vomiting		0.625–1.25 mg (IM, IV) q4h
Haloperidol (Haldol)[1]			0.5–5 mg (PO, IM, IV) q8h
Phenothiazines: Dopamine antagonists		Sedation, hypotension, extrapyramidal effects, neuroleptic malignant syndrome, cholestatic jaundice	
Chlorpromazine (Thorazine)	Generalized nausea		10–25 mg (PO, IM, PR) q6h
Prochlorperazine (Compazine)	Generalized nausea		10 mg (PO, IM, IV) q6h; 25 mg q12h PR

TABLE 6	Medications for Nausea and Vomiting—cont'd		
DRUG	**USE**	**SIDE EFFECTS**	**DOSAGE**
5-HT3: Serotonin Antagonists		Fever, constipation, diarrhea, dizziness, sedation, nervousness, altered liver function tests, headache, fatigue	
Dolasetron (Anzemet)	Chemotherapy-induced nausea		100 mg (PO, IV) q24h
Granisetron (Kytril)	Chemotherapy-induced nausea		2 mg (PO, IV) q24h
Ondansetron (Zofran)	Chemotherapy-induced nausea		4–8 mg (PO, IV) q8–12h
Palonosetron (Aloxi)	Prevention of chemotherapy-induced nausea		0.5 mg PO or 0.25 mg IV ×1
Neurokinin Receptor Antagonists		Headache, site reaction	
Aprepitant capsule (Emend)	Prevention of postoperative nausea and vomiting (POV)		40 mg PO × 1 prior to anesthesia
Fosaprepitant (Emend IV)	Prevention of chemotherapy-induced nausea		115 mg IV × 1, 125 mg PO ×1[3]
Steroids		GI upset, anxiety, euphoria, flushing, insomnia	
Dexamethasone (Decadron)[1]	Prophylaxis of chemotherapy-related nausea and vomiting		4 mg–10 mg (PO, IM, IV) q6–12h
Methylprednisolone (Medrol)[1]			40–100 mg (PO, IM, IV) q24h
Cannabinoids		Vertigo, xerostomia, hypotension, dysphoria	
Dronabinol (Marinol)	Chronic or chemotherapy-induced nausea and vomiting		5 mg/m^2 PO q2-4h; 4–6 doses per day
Miscellaneous			
Erythromycin[1]	Nausea associated with gastroparesis		250 mg PO q8h × 5–7 d
Ginger[7]	Nausea associated with pregnancy		250 mg PO q6h or 1 g qd
Pyridoxine (vitamin B6)[1]	Nausea associated with pregnancy (traditionally combined with doxylamine)		10 mg q6h
Aromatherapy-Isopropyl Alcohol[1]	Nausea	None	Swab held under nose and inhaled.

CNS, central nervous system; IM, intramuscular; IV, intravenous; PO, by mouth; PR, per rectum
[1]Not US Food and Drug Administration (FDA) approved for this indication.
[3]Exceeds dosage recommended by the manufacturer.
[7]Available as dietary supplement.

TABLE 7	Medications for Treatment of Gaseousness and Bloating	
MEDICATION	**INDICATION**	**DOSE**
Rifaximin (Xifaxan)[1]	Bloating (flatulence) from suspected bacterial overgrowth	200 mg PO tid × 7 days
Probiotics (multi-component)[7]	Bloating (flatulence)	Varies by preparation
Alpha-galactosidase (Bean-o)	Bloating associated with gas-producing foods	300–1200 mg with meals high in fermentable carbs
Simethicone	Bloating (flatulence) (indicated but not found to be effective)	80–120 mg qid prn
Bismuth subsalicylate	Odor from flatus	525 mg PO qid prn
Odor-neutralizing devices (briefs, pillows)	Odor from flatus	prn

[1]Not US Food and Drug Administration (FDA) approved for this indication.
[7]Available as dietary supplement

References

Abraczinskas D: Intestinal gas and bloating. Available http://www.uptodate.com, December 2018. [Accessed 3 February 2020].

ACOG Practice Bulletin No: 189: American College of Obstetrics and Gynecology: nausea and vomiting in pregnancy, *Obstet Gynecol* 131:e15–e30, 2018.

Bailey J: Effective management of flatulence, *Am Fam Phys* 79:1098–1100, 2009.

Flake ZA, Linn B, Hornecker J: Practical selection of antiemetics in an ambulatory care setting, *Am Fam Phys* 91(15):293–296, 2015 Mar 1.

Kraft R: Nausea and vomiting. In Bope ET, Rakel RE, Kellerman R, editors: *Conn's Current Therapy 2010*, Philadelphia, 2010, Saunders, pp 5–9.

Lacy B, Parkman H, Camilleri M: Chronic Nausea and Vomiting, Evaluation and Treatment, *Am J Gastroenterology* 113:647–659, 2018.

Longstreth GF: Functional dyspepsia in adults. Available at http://www.uptodate.com, December 2019. [Accessed 3 February 2020].

Longstreth GF: Approach to the patient with dyspepsia. Available at http://www.uptodate.com, December, 2019. [Accessed 3 February 2020].

Owings S: Gaseousness and dyspepsia. In Bope ET, Rakel RE, Kellerman R, editors: *Conn's Current Therapy 2010*, Philadelphia, 2010, Saunders, pp 9–11.

Talley NJ, Vakil NB, Moayyedi P: 2005 American Gastroenterological Association technical review on the evaluation of dyspepsia, *Gastroenterology* 125:1756–1780, 2005.

HEMATURIA

Method of
Jonathan Maldonado, MD; and Moben Mirza, MD

CURRENT DIAGNOSIS

- Hematuria is defined as the presence of red blood cells in the urine.
- Hematuria can be gross (readily visible) or microscopic (detected by dipstick or microscopy).
- In the adult population, any unexplained hematuria should be presumed to be of malignant origin until proven otherwise.
- Urologic evaluation of the upper and lower urinary tract is compulsory for patients with gross hematuria.
- Patients with asymptomatic microscopic hematuria (≥3 RBC/HPF) should have a careful history and physical examination performed to rule out benign causes of hematuria as well as to assess overall risk of urologic malignancy.
- Following patient risk stratification, further diagnostic evaluation with repeat urinalysis, cystoscopy, and upper tract imaging (renal ultrasound or multiphasic computed tomography) may be indicated.
- Concurrent nephrologic evaluation should occur in select cases.

Epidemiology

Hematuria is a common clinical finding in adults. The prevalence of hematuria ranges from 2.4% to 31.1%. Prevalence varies based on age, gender, frequency of testing, threshold used to define hematuria, and study group characteristics. Transient microscopic hematuria may occur in up to 40% of patients; however, persistent microscopic hematuria in greater than three evaluated urine samples is limited to 2% of the population. A wide range of causes can result in hematuria. Transient hematuria may be caused by vigorous exercise, sexual intercourse, mild trauma, menstrual contamination, and instrumentation. Patients with underlying urinary tract disease can have transient or persistent hematuria. The presence of gross hematuria carries a higher likelihood of significant pathology compared with microscopic hematuria. For example, approximately 5% of patients with microscopic hematuria in contrast to 40% of patients with gross hematuria are found to have urologic malignancy on evaluation. The most common cause of gross hematuria in adults older than age 50 is bladder cancer.

Risk Factors

Given the wide range of etiologies for hematuria, the risk factors are dependent on the etiology itself. The most concerning etiology of hematuria is urothelial malignancy. Smoking is the best-established and the most significant risk factor for the development of urothelial malignancies of the kidney, ureter, and bladder.

Pathophysiology

The presence of blood in the urine can be separated into glomerular and nonglomerular origin. Normal urine contains less than three red blood cells per high-power field. The kidney does not excrete red blood cells under physiologic conditions. Therefore, the presence of blood in the urine is due to pathology at the glomerulus (glomerular hematuria), allowing excretion of red blood cells into the urine or pathology in the urinary tract distal to the glomerulus (nonglomerular hematuria), which results in blood mixing into the already excreted urine. Nonglomerular hematuria can be further divided into medical and surgical disorders. Except for renal tumors, nonglomerular hematuria of medical/renal origin is due to tubulointerstitial, renovascular, or systemic disorders. Surgical nonglomerular hematuria or essential hematuria includes urologic tumors, stones, and urinary tract infections.

The urine dipstick, commonly used for the detection of blood in the urine, is dependent on the peroxidase-like activity of hemoglobin, which catalyzes the reaction and causes oxidation of the chromogen indicator. False positives can occur in states of hemoglobinuria and myoglobinuria, and microscopic examination of the urine for red blood cells can distinguish hematuria. Glomerular hematuria is suggested when dysmorphic erythrocytes, red blood cell casts, and proteinuria are present. Nonglomerular hematuria can be distinguished from glomerular hematuria in the presence of circular erythrocytes and the absence of erythrocyte casts. In the surgical and medical subcategories of nonglomerular hematuria, surgical hematuria is suggested by the absence of significant proteinuria.

Anticoagulation at normal therapeutic levels does not predispose patients to hematuria. Therefore patients who have hematuria while receiving either anticoagulation or antiplatelet therapy should undergo evaluation similarly to patients who are not receiving these therapies. In fact, supratherapeutic anticoagulation may serve to unmask underlying pathology.

Prevention

As previously mentioned, hematuria can be caused by a spectrum of causes. Prevention can be achieved by the avoidance of what results in the pathologic state. For example, smoking is a modifiable risk factor in urothelial malignancy. Patients who have never smoked are at low risk for bladder cancer. Smoking cessation can also reduce the risk of developing bladder cancer. Liberal fluid intake and balanced sodium and protein intake can help prevent urolithiasis. Urinary tract infections can also be prevented by good voiding habits, facilitation of complete bladder emptying, and use of vaginal estrogen cream[1] in postmenopausal women.

Clinical Manifestations

The presentation of hematuria is often dependent on the cause. Certain characteristics of the presentation can help in the investigation. Is the hematuria gross or microscopic? Is the hematuria associated with pain? Are there any irritative voiding symptoms? Is there a presence of blood clots? Is it related to exercise? Is there any family history? Is there a presence of rash, arthritis, hemoptysis, upper respiratory infection, or skin infection? Is there a history of radiation, diabetes, or analgesic abuse? Is there a history of smoking or occupational exposures? Table 1 highlights findings in etiologies of hematuria. Patients with bladder cancer generally present with gross painless hematuria.

Diagnosis

The diagnosis and evaluation of hematuria starts with a careful history, physical examination, and microscopic urinalysis. The cause in an adult patient is urologic malignancy until proven otherwise.

---

[1] Not FDA approved for this indication

TABLE 1	Differential Diagnosis and Findings in Etiologies of Hematuria	
DIAGNOSIS	**FINDINGS**	**OTHER**
Glomerular		
Familial hematuria	Abnormal urinalysis	Family history
Systemic lupus erythematous	Elevated C3, C4, ANA	Rash, arthritis
Goodpasture syndrome	Microcytic anemia	Hemoptysis, bleeding tendency
Poststreptococcal glomerulonephritis	Elevated ASO titer, C3	Recent upper respiratory infection, rash
IgA nephropathy	Normal ASO and C3, renal biopsy positive for IgA, IgG	Related to exercise
Nonglomerular Medical		
Exercise-induced hematuria	Abnormal urine analysis	After strenuous exercise
Papillary necrosis	Gross hematuria, absence of urolithiasis on CT	Flank pain, African American, analgesic abuse, diabetes
Medullary sponge kidney, polycystic kidney disease	Abnormal CT	Family history of renal cystic disease
Renovascular disease	Renal artery embolus, vein thrombus, AV fistula	Atrial fibrillation, dehydration, bruit
Nonglomerular Surgical		
Urinary tract infection	Urine dip with LCE, Nit. positive urine culture, elevated WBC	Dysuria, fever
Urolithiasis (renal, ureteral, or bladder stone)	Demonstrated on imaging such as CT, ultrasound, KUB	Flank pain, pelvic pain, vomiting, infection, renal obstruction
Urologic tumor (kidney, ureter, bladder, urethra)	Demonstrated on CT, cystoscopy, ureteropyeloscopy	Constitutional, irritative symptoms, pain if obstructed, blood clots
Enlarged prostate or benign prostatic hyperplasia	Enlarged prostate on examination or cystoscopy	Irritative and obstructive voiding symptoms
Radiation cystitis	Generally gross hematuria, friable tissue on cystoscopy	Irritative voiding symptoms, history of pelvic radiation
Urothelial strictures (ureter or urethra)	Demonstrated on ureteroscopy, pyelography, cystoscopy, or urethrography	Flank pain, renal insufficiency, bladder outlet obstruction

ANA, Antinuclear antibodies; *ASO,* antistreptolysin O; *AV,* atrioventricular; *CT,* computed tomography; *Ig,* immunoglobulin; *KUB kidney, ureter, bladder radiograph, LCE leukocyte esterase, WBC,* white blood cell.

Some important questions are outlined in the section, Clinical Manifestations. The physical exam should first focus on blood pressure and a cardiovascular examination. An abdominal examination should evaluate for the presence of a palpable mass or costovertebral angle tenderness, followed by a complete genitourinary examination including a prostate examination in males and a vaginal examination in the females. The assessment should help rule out causes such as infection, menstruation, vigorous exercise, medical renal disease, viral illness, trauma, or recent urologic procedures.

A urine specimen should be collected as a midstream sample, and patients should be instructed to discard the initial 10 mL. The sample should be collected in a sterile cup after gently cleaning the urethral meatus with a sterilization towelette. Uncircumcised men should retract the foreskin before collection. Female patients should be asked to spread the labia adequately to allow cleansing of the urethral meatus and avoid introital contamination.

The following patients may require catheterization for collection: menstruating women, obese patients, patient with a nonintact urinary tract, patients who do intermittent catheterization, or have an indwelling urinary catheter (Foley or suprapubic tube). Additionally, a urine sample with excessive squamous cells is a sign of contamination, and catheterization may be required for an adequate specimen. A urine dipstick can be performed in the office setting, but all samples should be sent for microscopic analysis. As mentioned previously, attention should be paid to dysmorphic erythrocytes, red blood cell casts, and the presence of protein. A urine culture should be performed based on the clinical presentation and findings of urinalysis. Urine cytology should not be used in the initial evaluation of microscopic hematuria but may have clinical utility in evaluating patients with irritative voiding symptoms or persistent microhematuria after a comprehensive urologic evaluation. The laboratory workup should include an evaluation of the serum creatinine. Additional helpful tests are serum electrolytes and a complete blood count.

Patients with a urinary tract infection should be treated appropriately and should have a urinalysis repeated in 2 to 6 weeks after treatment. Patients with an identified etiology such as urolithiasis should have a reevaluation of urine after the stone has been passed or treated.

A urologic evaluation of the upper and lower urinary tract is compulsory for patients with gross hematuria. Given the high prevalence of asymptomatic microscopic hematuria (≥ 3 RBC/HPF) and lower rate of malignancy in this population, risk stratification should be performed to guide diagnostic evaluation and limit the potential for patient harm. This microhematuria risk stratification has been found to be clinically meaningful and helps differentiate the need for more aggressive diagnostic work-ups based on the likelihoods of bladder cancer within each risk group. Patients should be categorized as low, intermediate, or high risk

TABLE 2	Microhematuria Risk Stratification		
LOW RISK (ALL OF THE FOLLOWING):	**INTERMEDIATE RISK (ANY OF THE FOLLOWING):**	**HIGH RISK (ANY OF THE FOLLOWING):**
Women age <50 y ears	Women age 50–59 years	Women and men age _60 years
Men ag e <40 years	Men age 40–59 years	>30 pack-years
Never smoker or <10 pack-years	10–30 pack-years	>25 RBC/HPF on one UA
3–10 RBC/HPF on one UA	11–25 RBC/HPF on one UA	History of gross hematuria
No prior episodes of microscopic hematuria	Previously low risk, no prior evaluation, and 3–25 RBC/HPF on repeat UA	Previously low risk, no prior evaluation, and >25 RBC/HPF on repeat UA
No additional risk factors for urothelial cancer*	Any additional risk factors for urothelial cancer*	

*Irritative voiding symptoms, history of cyclophosphamide or ifosamide chemotherapy, family history of urothelial carcinoma or Lynch syndrome, occupational exposures to benzene chemicals or aromatic amines, history of chronic indwelling foreign object in urinary tract
UA, Urinalysis.
Adapted from Barocas D, Boorjian S, Alvarez R, et al: Microhematuria: AUA/SUFU guideline, J Urol 204:778–786, 2020.

based on factors in Table 2. Low-risk patients should undergo cystoscopy and renal ultrasound or repeat urinalysis within 6 months to assess for persistence of the microscopic hematuria. An abnormal repeat urinalysis should prompt reclassification as intermediate or high risk and full evaluation should be performed. Cystoscopy and renal ultrasound (intermediate risk) or multiphasic computed tomography (high risk) are indicated for the evaluation of these risk groups. While contrasted computed tomography is preferred for evaluation of the upper tracts, a contraindication may exist for some patients due to allergy or renal insufficiency. In this scenario, a urologist can determine whether magnetic resonance imaging or retrograde pyelography is appropriate.

Differential Diagnosis

The differential diagnosis of hematuria includes glomerular diseases, nonglomerular medical diseases, and nonglomerular surgical diseases. Table 1 shows a differential diagnosis for hematuria.

Hematuria is considered to be from a malignant source until proven otherwise.

Therapy, Monitoring, and Complications

Therapy, monitoring, and complications for hematuria are dependent on the etiology. It is important that hematuria not be ignored even when treated empirically. For example, it is important to recheck a urinalysis after a course of antibiotics for a presumed urinary tract infection. Often, the transient nature of hematuria misleads clinicians into thinking that an intervention or observation without the appropriate workup is adequate. Unfortunately, this can result in significant morbidity from the progression of disease, especially in the case of urothelial malignancies.

References

Barocas D, Boorjian S, Alvarez R, et al: Microhematuria: AUA/SUFU Guideline, J Urol 204:778–786, 2020.
Davis R, Jones SJ, Barocas D, et al: Diagnosis, evaluation and follow-up of asymptomatic microscopic hematuria (AMH) in adults. AUA guideline, J Urol 188(Suppl 6):2473, 2012.
Gerber GS, Brendler CB: Evaluation of the urologic patient: History, physical, and urinalysis. In Wein Campbell-Walsh Urology, ed 10, Philadelphia, 2011, Saunders, pp 73–98.
Khadra MH, Pickard RS, Charlton M, et al: A prospective analysis of 1,930 patients with hematuria to evaluate current diagnostic practice, J Urol 163:524, 2000.
Masahito J: Evaluation and management of hematuria, Prim Care 37:461, 2010.
Sudakoff GS, Dunn DP, Guralnick ML, et al: Multidetector computerized tomography urography as the primary imaging modality for detecting urinary tract neoplasms in patients with asymptomatic hematuria, J Urol 179:862, 2008.
Woldu SL, Ng CK, Loo RK, et al: Evaluation of the new American Urological Association guidelines risk classification for hematuria, J Urol 205(5):1387–1393, 2021.

HICCUPS

Kristine L. Cece, MD, PhD

CURRENT DIAGNOSIS

- Hiccups result from involuntary contractions of the diaphragm and intercostal muscles, forcing rapid inspiration that is interrupted by the closure of the glottis. This pathway is mediated by a poorly understood reflex arc, with central processing taking place in the midbrain (medulla).
- Hiccups lasting longer than 48 hours are considered to be persistent, and those lasting longer than 1 month are labeled as intractable.
- Hiccups are a symptom of another underlying diagnosis; a thorough history, physical examination, basic laboratory workup, and chest x-ray are indicated in most patients with intractable hiccups. Advanced imaging and diagnostic procedures are warranted on a case-by-case basis depending on the suspected etiology.

CURRENT THERAPY

- Nonpharmacologic treatment including oropharyngeal stimulation (intranasal vinegar, ingestion of ice water, use of smelling salts), vagal maneuvers, and self-induced hypercapnia via paper bag breathing may be useful for treatment of transient hiccups.
- Hiccups are commonly seen in patients with gastroesophageal reflux disease, and therefore a trial of omeprazole (Prilosec)[1] is reasonable first-line therapy.
- Although few high-quality studies have examined use of these medications, the available data support use of baclofen (Lioresal),[1] gabapentin (Neurontin),[1] and metoclopramide (Reglan)[1] for treatment of hiccups.
- The side effect profile must be considered when choosing a pharmacologic intervention for hiccups.
- In cases that are refractory to medications, patients may benefit from physical interventions such as phrenic nerve blockade or acupuncture.

[1]Not FDA approved for this indication.

Pathophysiology

Hiccups (Lat. *singultus*) are a common occurrence that result from involuntary and repetitive contractions of the inspiratory musculature including the diaphragm and intercostal muscles. Rapid inspiration of air is then interrupted by closure of the glottis, generating the characteristic "hic" sound for which this disorder is named. The pathophysiology behind these involuntary contractions is poorly understood but is generally thought to be related to stimulation of a reflex arc that includes peripheral pathways and central midbrain modulation. The afferent component of the reflex arc includes phrenic, vagus, and sympathetic nerves that transmit somatic and visceral sensory information to the midbrain (medulla). Multiple neurotransmitters play a role regulating rhythmic breathing in the midbrain, including dopamine, glutamate, glycine, gamma-aminobutyric acid (GABA), and serotonin. The efferent component of the reflex arc includes motor nerves that communicate via the phrenic nerve to the diaphragm and intercostals. Stimulation of this pathway can occur via many mechanisms including but not limited to neoplastic processes, vascular disease, gastroesophageal reflux disease (GERD), medications, procedural instrumentation, and infection. Hiccups are not thought to serve a physiologic purpose.

Prevention

There are currently no reliable preventative measures for hiccups.

Clinical Manifestations

Virtually all people will experience hiccups during their lifetime. For many, this is a brief and self-limited nuisance. For others, hiccups can be long-lasting and lead to serious morbidity, including insomnia, exhaustion, malnutrition, dehydration, and wound dehiscence. Hiccups can occur 4 to 60 times per minute. Transient hiccups tend to last minutes to hours and are often triggered by eating quickly or in excess, spicy foods, carbonated drinks, or ingesting hot or cold food or beverages. Hiccups lasting longer than 48 hours are considered to be persistent, whereas those lasting more than 1 month are labeled intractable.

Hiccups are observed in utero, most frequently in the third trimester, and are thought to be a mechanism of training the inspiratory muscles for respiration after birth. Intractable hiccups occur more commonly in men (91%) than women, and the incidence increases with age (most often in those over age 50). Hiccups are also frequently experienced by patients with gastrointestinal and central nervous system disorders, including 10% of patients with GERD and 20% of patients with Parkinson disease.

Diagnosis

Hiccups are a symptom of another underlying diagnosis that can be organic, psychogenic, or idiopathic. Persistent and intractable hiccups warrant further workup to identify their etiology, though there is no strong consensus on what that workup entails. A basic evaluation should include a thorough history, physical examination, and laboratory/diagnostic studies.

History

When taking the patient's history, it is important to identify any triggers or comorbid disease processes such as gastrointestinal or neurologic disorders. Understanding frequency, duration, and palliative treatments or maneuvers can also be helpful. Additionally, a thorough medication review is essential, as many common medications have been associated with persistent or intractable hiccups, including aripiprazole (Abilify), antibiotics including azithromycin (Zithromax) and sulfonamides, donepezil (Aricept), benzodiazepines including chlordiazepoxide (Librium) and diazepam (Valium), steroids, barbiturates, opioids, methyldopa, L-dopa, dopamine, and cisplatin. Alcohol has also been identified as a hiccup inducer. In cases in which a medication is the cause of hiccups, symptoms typically resolve once the offending agent is stopped.

Physical Examination

A head-to-toe physical examination looking for signs of neoplasm or infection is warranted. A thorough neurologic exam to rule out stroke or temporal arteritis, a cardiovascular exam to evaluate for pericardial friction rub, and an abdominal exam to identify epigastric tenderness are also helpful. Additionally, foreign body irritation of the tympanic membrane can induce hiccups, so a head, eyes, ears, nose, and throat exam should be performed.

Laboratory/Diagnostic Workup

Basic laboratory studies should include a metabolic panel to look for electrolyte imbalances and uremia, a complete blood cell count to look for infection, an electrocardiogram, and a chest x-ray. Advanced imaging and endoscopy may also be warranted on a case-by-case basis.

Treatment

Nonpharmacologic Interventions

Physical maneuvers are considered first-line for treatment of transient hiccups and can be effective at shortening acute attacks. These maneuvers include nasopharyngeal stimulation by intranasal application of vinegar, use of smelling salts, or ingestion of ice water. Vagal stimulation can also help resolve symptoms, including application of a cold compress to the face, carotid massage, Valsalva, and induced fright or vomiting. Finally, respiratory maneuvers including breath holding, paper bag rebreathing (inducing hypercapnia), and continuous positive airway pressure can be used as well, though clinical trial data on all of these approaches are lacking. None of these maneuvers is thought to be helpful for treatment of persistent or intractable hiccups.

Pharmacologic Interventions

The approach to pharmacologic management of persistent or intractable hiccups should first consider treatment of all identified reversible causes. If no etiology is identified after the history, physical exam, and diagnostic testing discussed above, it is reasonable to start with empiric treatment for GERD given the prevalence of the disease (an estimated 20% of adults in Western culture) and association with hiccups as a prominent symptom. A trial of a proton pump inhibitor such as omeprazole[1] (Prilosec, 20–40 mg once or twice daily) should be initiated for a minimum of 7 days. If no response, other pharmacologic treatments can be considered.

Although data are limited and large-scale studies have not been conducted, pharmacologic therapies shown to be most efficacious in treating intractable hiccups act on dopamine and GABA-ergic receptors. There are two medications that are supported by data from randomized controlled trials: baclofen (Lioresal)[1] and metoclopramide (Reglan).[1] Baclofen, a GABA$_B$ agonist, administered at a dosage of 10 mg three times daily for 5 days, was shown to be effective in treating persistent hiccups in stroke patients compared with placebo. Although this study reported no adverse side effects to baclofen use, this medication is known to cause muscle

---

[1]Not FDA approved for this indication.

weakness, confusion, and sedation in some patients, and particular care must be taken in patients with renal impairment to avoid accumulation and toxicity. Metoclopramide, a dopamine receptor antagonist and serotonin agonist, was also shown in a small randomized controlled trial to improve hiccup symptoms at a dose of 10 mg every 8 hours for 15 days. Although no adverse effects were observed in this study, one must weigh the known risks of tardive dyskinesia associated with metoclopramide use, which renders this medication more of a second-line therapy.

Several case series have reported use of gabapentin (Neurontin)[1] alone or in conjunction with other medications such as omeprazole as an effective treatment for hiccups, particularly in cases where a central etiology is suspected. These studies looked at doses ranging from 300 to 600 mg three times daily, and durations of therapy from 1 day to indefinite. The side effect profile is generally acceptable, with sedation, dizziness, and vision changes most commonly reported. Other antiepileptics are sometimes used to treat hiccups as well, though evidence to support their use is lacking and they are associated with weight gain, mood, and neurologic disturbance. These include carbamazepine[1] (Tegretol, 100–300 mg three times daily), phenytoin[1] (Dilantin, 100 mg three times daily), and valproic acid[1] (Depakote, 20 mg/kg/day).

Antipsychotic medications have historically been widely used for treatment of hiccups since the 1950s, though have fallen out of favor in more recent years due to their modest benefit and unfavorable side effect profile. Interestingly, chlorpromazine (Thorazine, 10–50 mg three times daily) is the only medication that has been FDA approved for treatment of hiccups. Haloperidol[1] (Haldol, 1–4 mg every 24 hours) is another common antipsychotic that is reached for in cases of intractable hiccups. Both medications act as dopamine receptor antagonists in the brain and should be used with extreme caution due to the risk of sedation, hypotension, dystonia, and tardive dyskinesia.

The use of benzodiazepines is generally not recommended for treatment of intractable hiccups, and, in fact, this class of medications can actually trigger episodes of hiccups when given at low doses. One exception is the use of midazolam (Versed)[1] in patients with terminal illness. Several case reports describe the use of midazolam (10–60 mg every 24 hours subcutaneously) at the end of life to effectively suppress the hiccup reflex.

Limited data from a small case series support the use of nifedipine (Adalat)[1] at doses of 20 to 60 mg/day, which partially or totally resolved intractable hiccups in five of seven patients studied. There was a noted high recurrence rate after stopping the medication. Known side effects of nifedipine use include hypotension and reflex tachycardia.

Amitriptyline (Elavil),[1] which is a tricyclic antidepressant, has been shown to be effective in a small number of patients at doses of 25 to 100 mg nightly. Although amitriptyline is known to increase the neurotransmitters serotonin and norepinephrine in the neuronal synapses, its mechanism of action in reducing hiccup symptomatology is not well understood, though may relate to its sodium channel–blocking properties.

Other medications that have been suggested as potential therapeutic agents for hiccups despite a lack of consistent data supporting their efficacy include lidocaine (Xylocaine),[1] methylphenidate (Ritalin),[1] and ondansetron (Zofran).[1] Interestingly, ondansetron has been noted to worsen hiccups in some cases.

Physical Interventions

Case reports of ultrasound-guided phrenic nerve blockade of the efferent limb of the reflex arc have shown some promise in the treatment of persistent hiccups in cases that were refractory to pharmacologic therapy. In a case where phrenic nerve blockade was unsuccessful, afferent vagal blockade was shown to have some efficacy in alleviating symptoms. Ultrasound-guided ablation of the phrenic nerve can also be effective; however, this runs the risk of respiratory complications.

A common home remedy for hiccups is paper bag rebreathing, which induces hypercapnia. One study reported that use of an airtight plastic bag was more efficacious because CO_2 levels need to increase substantially for suppression of the hiccup reflex arc.

Other physical maneuvers are patient specific; for example, in hiccups that are thought to be due to abdominal distension, placement of a nasogastric tube for decompression may help alleviate symptoms. In patients who are ventilated, inducing a mechanical Valsalva maneuver by increasing positive end-expiratory pressure may be helpful.

Finally, acupuncture may be helpful as an adjunct to medical therapy in patients suffering from intractable hiccups, though, again, data from randomized controlled trials are lacking.

Monitoring

No ongoing monitoring for recurrence of hiccups is necessary as patients will undoubtedly be aware of a return of symptoms. Posttreatment monitoring after pharmacologic therapy should primarily focus on adverse reactions to the medications discussed above. In cases in which phrenic or vagus nerve block or phrenic nerve destruction have been performed, the patient should be monitored for respiratory compromise.

Complications

Complications of untreated intractable hiccups include malnutrition, weight loss, sleep deprivation, wound dehiscence, and depression.

---

[1]Not FDA approved for this indication.

References

Brañuelas Quiroga J, Urbano García J, Bolaños Guedes J: Hiccups: a common problem with some unusual causes and cures, *Br J Gen Pract* 66(652):584–586, 2016.

Chang FY, Lu CL: Hiccup: mystery, nature and treatment, *J Neurogastroenterol Motil* 18(2):123–130, 2012.

Jeon YS, Kearney AM, Baker PG: Management of hiccups in palliative care patients, *BMJ Support Palliat Care* 8(1):1–6, 2018.

Nausheen F, Mohsin H, Lakhan SE: Neurotransmitters in hiccups, *Springerplus* 5(1):1357, 2016.

Obuchi T, Shimamura S, Miyahara N, et al: CO_2 retention: the key to stopping hiccups, *Clin Respir J* 12(8):2340–2345, 2018.

Polito NB, Fellows SE: Pharmacologic interventions for intractable and persistent hiccups: a systematic review, *J Emerg Med* 53(4):540–549, 2017.

Steger M, Schneemann M, Fox M: Systematic review: the pathogenesis and pharmacological treatment of hiccups, *Aliment Pharmacol Ther* 42(9):1037–1050, 2015.

---

[1]Not FDA approved for this indication.

HOARSENESS AND LARYNGITIS

Method of
Lee Akst, MD

CURRENT DIAGNOSIS

- The general term to describe vocal difficulty is dysphonia. Hoarseness is a specific term for rough voice quality, which is one type of dysphonia. Laryngitis signifies laryngeal inflammation, which is one possible cause of dysphonia.
- An accurate history and physical examination guide the diagnosis of voice complaints. Although many portions of the examination for dysphonia can be done in a general setting, videostroboscopy is often necessary for diagnosis and may be available only in specialized laryngology offices.
- The most common cause of acute hoarseness is viral laryngitis. Symptoms are self-limited and usually resolve within 2 weeks.
- Dysphonia persisting for longer than 2 weeks suggests the possibility of another diagnosis, such as vocal cord paralysis, neoplasm, phonotraumatic lesion, or chronic laryngitis.
- Indications for referral of a patient with voice complaints to an otolaryngologist include dysphonia that persists for longer than 2 weeks, that is of acute onset during voicing, or that is accompanied by other symptoms such as otalgia, dysphagia, or difficulty breathing.

CURRENT THERAPY

- Appropriate treatment of voice complaints depends on accurate diagnosis.
- Supportive therapy is all that is necessary for most cases of acute laryngitis associated with viral upper respiratory tract infections.
- Laryngopharyngeal reflux is a common cause of chronic laryngitis, and appropriate therapy often requires twice-daily administration of proton pump inhibitors for at least 2 months.
- Microlaryngeal phonosurgery may be indicated for some patients with benign phonotraumatic lesions.
- Vocal cord medialization can rehabilitate the voice in a patient with unilateral vocal cord paralysis.
- Many patients with dysphonia benefit from voice therapy, alone or in combination with other treatment strategies.

Voice is an essential component of communication. Vocal difficulty is very distressing to patients and can have a negative impact on physical, social, and emotional qualities of life. To understand the pathophysiology, evaluation, and treatment of voice complaints, it is important to understand the anatomy and physiology of normal voice production. Looking first at how good voice quality is achieved makes it readily apparent how alterations in vocal fold vibration, symmetry, or closure can lead to various vocal difficulties.

To aid discussion of voice complaints, clarification of terminology is necessary. Although "hoarseness" is a term that most patients use to describe any type of voice complaint and "laryngitis" is the presumptive explanation that many patients provide for their symptoms, each of these terms has a more precise meaning. Dysphonia is the general term for vocal difficulty. Hoarseness implies a rough or raspy change in voice quality and is one type of dysphonia. Other categories include limited vocal projection, strained vocal effort, and change in pitch—each of which may

occur with or without vocal roughness. The term "laryngitis" specifically describes inflammation of the larynx. This inflammation may be acute or chronic, and again it describes some but certainly not all cases of dysphonia. This distinction will be made clear as the evaluation and management of dysphonia are described.

Normal Laryngeal Function

The larynx plays a central role in voice production by serving as a vibrating instrument that turns airflow from the lungs into sound. The sound is shaped into intelligible speech through the resonating and articulating functions of the pharynx and oral cavity. The ability of the larynx to create vibration and serve as a sound source is a function of its complex, layered microanatomy. The deeper layers of the vocal fold include the thyroarytenoid muscle and the vocal ligament, which position the more superficial layers of the superficial lamina propria and epithelium during phonation. Compared with the fibrous nature of the vocal ligament, the superficial lamina propria is a loose gelatinous layer whose pliability allows for voice production.

During inspiration (Figure 1A), the vocal folds are abducted so that air can move past the larynx without resistance. During phonation (Figure 1B), the vocal folds are held in an adducted position while the lungs drive air toward the larynx. Air pressure builds in the subglottis, beneath the vocal folds, until it overcomes the forces of vocal fold closure, pushes past the vocal folds, and generates negative pressure in its wake as it moves past the larynx. A combination of the vocal folds' intrinsic viscoelasticity and the negative pressure created through Bernoulli's effect draws the vocal fold edges back together, allowing subglottic pressure to rebuild and the cycle to repeat. Repeated cycles of opening and closing at the level of the vocal fold edges generate a so-called mucosal wave, which travels from the inferior edge of each vocal fold up across the medial and superior edges (Figure 1C). These waves may repeat hundreds of times each second, depending on pitch. This cycled opening and closing of the vocal folds during phonation imparts pressure waves to the air column that moves the vocal folds, generating sound. The ability of vocal folds to vibrate easily and symmetrically in this very rapid fashion allows for clear, smooth voicing.

Evaluation of Dysphonia

Central to the evaluation of dysphonia is the understanding that any disruption of vocal fold closure, symmetry, or vibration impairs the ability of the vocal folds to generate a clear sound source. Most voice complaints arise from anatomic or functional limitations in glottal closure or mucosal wave formation, although other parts of the respiratory tree are also responsible for components of the voice. General points concerning evaluation of dysphonia are discussed in this section, with specific causes discussed afterward.

History

A careful history can provide many clues that point toward the proper diagnosis in patients with dysphonia. Although many patients offer the complaint of "hoarseness" as a general term, a careful historian distinguishes between complaints related to voice quality, vocal projection, vocal effort or strain, vocal fatigue, and so on. Two questions that can help a patient organize his or her own thoughts related to poor voice are "What abnormal things does your voice do now that it did not do before?" and "What normal things did your voice do before that it no longer can do?" The acuteness of onset, duration, severity, and progression of any complaint should be determined.

The history should also determine what other factors or events might have caused or exacerbated the dysphonia. Recent sources of laryngeal inflammation might include intubation, excessive voice use, or upper respiratory tract infection. Baseline conditions that foster chronic laryngeal inflammation include environmental allergies, rhinitis, and laryngopharyngeal reflux. Laryngopharyngeal reflux can exist in the absence of heartburn, with reflux-associated inflammation of the larynx and pharynx providing symptoms of globus pharyngeus, throat clearing, nonproductive cough, effortful swallowing, and even mild dysphagia in association with dysphonia.

Figure 1 A, Normal vocal folds in abducted position for inspiration. B, Normal vocal folds in adducted position for phonation. C, Displacement of the vocal fold medial edges creates mucosal wave propagation during phonation and produces voice.

Concerning the possibility of laryngeal malignancy, any patient with dysphonia should be asked about smoking and alcohol use, because these are risk factors for squamous cell carcinoma. Another important question in distinguishing inflammatory dysphonia from a mass lesion of the vocal fold concerns whether there are any periods of normal voice or the dysphonia is constant—inflammation may wax and wane, but dysphonia associated with mass lesions is usually progressive and unremitting. Finally, the history should elicit other possible head and neck complaints, including dyspnea, stridor, dysphagia, odynophagia, otalgia, sore throat, and pain with speaking (odynophonia). If hoarseness is associated with some of these symptoms for longer than 2 weeks, the suspicion of malignancy is increased.

Physical Examination

The physical examination for patients with dysphonia includes a complete head and neck evaluation with focus on the larynx and laryngeal function. Although much of the head and neck examination can be performed in a general setting, some portions of the laryngeal examination require specialized equipment found only in some otolaryngology offices that specialize in voice care. Routine head and neck evaluation should include systematic examination of the ears, nose, oral cavity, oropharynx, and neck.

Complaint of otalgia in the setting of an unremarkable ear examination suggests a possibility of referred pain from a lesion of the larynx or pharynx, and is concerning for possible malignancy. Edematous and erythematous nasal mucosa suggests rhinitis, with the possibility of postnasal drip contributing to laryngeal inflammation. Tremor of the tongue or palate might suggest neurologic disorder, whereas pharyngeal erythema and exudate suggest possible acute infection. Pachydermia (cobblestoning) of the posterior pharyngeal wall suggests the possibility of laryngopharyngeal reflux. Tenderness with manipulation of the hyoid bone suggests tension of the strap muscles and correlates closely with complaint of odynophonia and the possibility of muscle tension dysphonia. A neck mass might represent either metastatic lymphadenopathy from a laryngeal malignancy or a primary lesion which itself compresses the recurrent laryngeal nerve and causes paralytic dysphonia. Surgical scarring along the neck suggests the possibility that prior thyroid surgery, carotid endarterectomy, or anterior approach to the cervical spine might have led to vocal fold paralysis.

Laryngeal Examination

Beyond a general examination of the head and neck, there should be directed evaluation of the larynx and laryngeal function. The examiner should listen to the voice carefully, because vocal characteristics such as roughness, breathiness, strain, vocal breaks, and diplophonia (pitch instability, with two different pitches present simultaneously) can help guide the differential diagnosis of dysphonia. Visual examination of the larynx has many forms, ranging from mirror examination to flexible fiberoptic laryngoscopy to videostrobolaryngoscopy.

Mirror examination offers an adequate view of the vocal folds in many patients but may be limited by patient tolerance,

physician inexperience, and the inherently limited ability of this technique to brightly illuminate the larynx or record the examination for later review. Flexible laryngoscopy is routinely available in almost all otolaryngology offices, is well tolerated by patients, and offers good views of the larynx that can be recorded with appropriate equipment. Mirror examination and flexible laryngoscopy are limited to observation of vocal fold motion and anatomy but cannot observe laryngeal function because they do not visualize vibration of the vocal folds. To examine vocal fold vibration, videostroboscopy uses a strobe light to create the impression of slow-motion analysis of mucosal waves. Stroboscopy is typically available only in selected otolaryngology practices in which laryngologists specialize in the treatment of voice disorders.

Other Testing

Videostroboscopic evaluation, combined with a thorough history and routine physical examination, can establish the diagnosis for almost all patients with voice complaints, but further testing is sometimes indicated. For instance, electromyography is used by some laryngologists for further evaluation of vocal fold paralysis or paresis. More commonly, radiographic studies are used for further evaluation of some voice complaints. Computed tomography (CT) scans are ordered most often in the evaluation of suspected laryngeal neoplasms and for patients with vocal fold paralysis.

In the case of neoplasm, CT scanning is useful to assess the extent of the primary lesion and to evaluate possible metastatic cervical lymphadenopathy. In patients with laryngeal malignancy, chest radiography is also important to assess for pulmonary metastases. For patients with vocal fold paralysis who do not have a clear history of surgical injury of the recurrent laryngeal nerve, a CT scan from skull base to thoracic inlet identifies possible lesions along the course of the recurrent laryngeal nerve. Central problems are less likely, but if they are suspected as a cause of vocal fold paralysis, then magnetic resonance imaging of the brain may be indicated as well.

Types of Dysphonia

Although not comprehensive, the conditions discussed here account for the vast majority of voice complaints. Some patients with voice complaints have more than one condition, and not every patient will fit neatly into a single category. Nevertheless, understanding how each of these conditions creates dysphonia, and knowing which particular history and physical examination findings might be associated with each cause, can help a physician to appropriately diagnose and manage voice complaints.

Acute Laryngitis

Acute laryngitis is the most common cause of hoarseness and dysphonia. It is most often viral in nature, and onset of laryngeal symptoms may be associated with other symptoms of upper respiratory tract infection, including fever, myalgia, sore throat, and rhinorrhea. Viral inflammation of the vocal folds leads to diminished and more effortful vocal fold vibration, yielding a voice characterized by increased effort and a harsh, strained quality with decreased projection. Characteristic findings on laryngoscopy include vocal fold edema and erythema with decreased amplitude of the mucosal wave. Treatment of acute viral laryngitis is supportive, with counseling for hydration, humidification, and mucolytics. Symptoms generally are self-limited and resolve within 2 weeks. During this time, patients should be instructed to use the voice in a comfortable fashion, rather than straining or pushing to get loudness, because pushing behaviors may lead to the development of persistent muscle tension dysphonia.

Bacterial or fungal infections also cause acute laryngitis in rare cases. With appropriate physical findings and in the right clinical setting, antibiotic or antifungal therapy may be used to treat these conditions. Amoxicillin-clavulanate (Augmentin) is often the antibiotic of choice, and fluconazole (Diflucan) is a commonly used antifungal agent.

Chronic Laryngitis

Chronic laryngitis is the nonspecific condition of prolonged laryngeal inflammation; the term itself does not indicate an etiology for the inflammation. Among the many possible sources for this inflammation are mechanical irritation from traumatic coughing or prolonged speaking, chemical irritation from environmental irritants (e.g., smoking, inhaled medications), and irritation from postnasal drip or laryngopharyngeal reflux. More than one cause may exist simultaneously. Issues related to cigarette use, excessive voice use, medication effect, and rhinitis can be identified with careful history taking. Laryngopharyngeal reflux is a very common source of chronic laryngitis. It may manifest with several nonspecific symptoms, such as throat irritation, globus pharyngeus, frequent throat clearing, and nonproductive cough, with or without accompanying heartburn. Because vocal fold inflammation increases with continued mechanical trauma, the hoarseness of chronic laryngitis typically gets worse with prolonged voice use and improves with voice rest. Examination findings in chronic laryngitis include generalized laryngeal edema and erythema, and careful inspection may also reveal interarytenoid hyperplasia, subglottic edema, laryngeal ventricular obliteration, and an increase in thick glottic secretions.

Treatment of chronic laryngitis is tailored to the cause of the inflammation. Vocal hygiene with moderate voice use and instructions to reduce throat clearing and coughing may diminish mechanical irritation, and smoking cessation is recommended to any smoker with laryngeal complaints. Several studies have suggested that an appropriate trial of proton pump inhibitors for treatment of laryngopharyngeal reflux includes twice-daily therapy for at least 2 months, in contrast to the once-daily dosing often used for typical heartburn complaints. Lifestyle counseling to limit consumption of caffeine, carbonation, alcohol, and acidic foods can improve reflux, and attention to hydration and humidification decreases the viscosity of glottic secretions. For patients who are troubled by vocal difficulties associated with chronic laryngitis, referral to a speech–language pathologist for voice therapy can improve compliance with suggested lifestyle changes and help foster vocal improvement.

Vocal Fold Paralysis

The dysphonia in cases of vocal fold paralysis usually relates to poor vocal fold closure (Figure 2). The result is a breathy voice with limited projection and increased vocal effort. The farther from midline the immobile vocal fold, the more air leaks through the incompetent glottal valve without being turned into sound. Patients whose immobile vocal fold sits in a lateral position may have severely weak and breathy voices, whereas patients whose immobile vocal fold sits near midline may have a perceptually near-normal conversational voice and complain only of mild increase in effort, vocal fatigue, or problems with loud projection. Because of their glottal insufficiency, patients may complain of "running out of air" with prolonged speech. Impaired glottal closure may also decrease airway protection during swallowing, so patients with vocal fold paralysis need to be questioned about aspiration as well. Whereas rehabilitation of poor voice may be elective, patients with increased aspiration risk need prompt therapy.

Figure 2 Vocal fold paralysis prevents the right vocal fold from closing to midline and creates dysphonia.

Evaluation of vocal fold paralysis includes identification of the cause of paralysis. Surgical injury to the recurrent laryngeal nerve accounts for almost half of all cases of unilateral vocal fold paralysis, and cervical or thoracic neoplasm and idiopathic paralysis account for most of the remaining cases. In a patient without a clear surgical history explaining the paralysis, CT scanning from skull base to mediastinum can identify any possible lesions along the course of the recurrent laryngeal nerve. In those patients whose histories suggest other possible causes (e.g., central neurologic injury, Lyme disease), further investigations, such as magnetic resonance imaging of the brain or blood work may be indicated as well. Some physicians perform laryngeal electromyography to help with the prognosis of paralysis or to differentiate neurologic injury from cricoarytenoid joint fixation; however, this study is neither standardized nor routine in many practices. Although flexible laryngoscopy alone may be satisfactory to document vocal fold immobility, stroboscopy can be added to investigate the impact of glottal insufficiency on vocal cord vibration and possible vocal fold flutter.

Treatment of vocal fold paralysis might include any combination of voice therapy, injection laryngoplasty, transcervical medialization laryngoplasty, and laryngeal reinnervation. Depending on the cause of the paralysis, some patients experience gradual recovery with synkinetic reinnervation or recovery of purposeful vocal fold motion over a period of several months. Based on the degree of voice and swallowing handicap, treatment of patients with vocal fold paralysis may be optional rather than necessary. Voice therapy can help teach patients to produce a stronger voice despite the paralysis, but by itself will not help a paralyzed vocal cord to recover motion. Various medialization techniques have been developed to help reposition an immobile vocal fold in the midline, where the contralateral mobile vocal fold can provide for complete glottal closure and lead to improved voice and swallowing. Injection medialization can be performed in the office or in the operating room, with temporary or permanent materials; if recovery of vocal fold motion is thought possible, then temporary injection is preferred. Transcervical medialization is a permanent but reversible surgical technique performed by otolaryngologists that repositions an immobile vocal fold in the midline. Laryngeal reinnervation offers the possibility of midline positioning of the immobile vocal fold with restored tone and bulk of the vocal fold musculature; however, because results may not mature for several months, this technique is less commonly performed than either injection or transcervical medialization.

Phonotraumatic Lesions: Nodules, Polyps, and Cysts

During vibration, vocal folds are subject to the shearing stresses of vibration. Although vocal fold structure is designed to accommodate these stresses in most circumstances, patients with vocal abuse or excessive voice use are at risk for development of lesions as the result of cumulative phonotrauma. Depending on the location and nature of these lesions, they are categorized as nodules, polyps, or cysts.

Figure 3 A large right hemorrhagic polyp, which can impair vocal fold vibration.

Figure 4 Symmetrical polypoid degeneration of the bilateral vocal folds, characteristic of Reinke's edema.

Vocal fold nodules are areas of fibrovascular scarring that are located just beneath the epithelium, at the level of the basement membrane and superficial lamina propria. They are typically bilateral and symmetrical, sitting at the junction of the anterior one third and the posterior two thirds of each vocal fold. Polyps are typically unilateral lesions that may be edematous or fibrous in nature and may contain hemorrhage (Figure 3). They usually are exophytic and extend outward from the vocal fold epithelium, although the fibrous base of a polyp may extend into the superficial lamina propria of a vocal fold. In contrast to an epithelial-based lesion such as a polyp, a vocal fold cyst is a subepithelial encapsulated lesion that sits entirely within the vocal fold; its size may exert a mass effect that deforms the medial edge of the involved vocal fold. These cysts are occasionally noted as congenital lesions in children, but in adults they are more often caused by traumatic occlusion of the ducts of the seromucinous glands within the larynx.

Nodules, polyps, and cysts cause dysphonia by disturbing vocal fold vibration, leading to rough voice quality. These lesions get larger as traumatic voice use accumulates, and vocal roughness usually becomes more severe and more constant as the lesions progress. Because vibration is more easily disturbed at high pitch, performers with these lesions may notice that high pitch is affected first. Effort of phonation often increases, but projection remains intact. Lesions large enough to limit vocal fold closure may also cause a slightly breathy voice quality. Because patients with excessive voice use are at risk for these lesions, a history of social and occupational voice demands is valuable in cases of suspected phonotrauma.

Treatment for these lesions always begins with voice therapy designed to modify the patient's voice use so as to diminish trauma. Voice therapy may be all that is necessary to allow resolution of some early traumatic changes, particularly in the case of edematous nodules. If dysphonia persists despite voice therapy and other conservative measures, surgery may be considered. Surgery with the goal of voice preservation and restoration (phonosurgery) is typically performed by otolaryngologists who specialize in the care of persons with vocal difficulties. The goal of phonosurgery for these lesions is to remove the lesion that impairs vibration while preserving as much of the remaining, pliable superficial lamina propria as possible, so that vocal fold vibration can be restored.

Reinke's Edema
Reinke's edema, also known as polypoid corditis, is a benign swelling of the vocal folds that is most commonly seen in patients with a long-term smoking history. The edema, a reaction to long-term irritation, accumulates within the superficial lamina propria. The edema is most often bilateral and occurs diffusely along the entire length of the vocal fold, rather than being limited to a more discrete area, as is seen with phonotraumatic polyps (Figure 4). As vocal fold mass increases with disease progression, the pitch

of the voice decreases, and this is the change in voice most associated with Reinke's edema. A classic presentation of this condition is a female in her fifth or sixth decade of life who provides a long history of smoking and progressive deepening of her voice. In rare circumstances, the vocal folds gradually accumulate enough edema to compromise the airway, so breathing complaints should be evaluated as well.

Because a significant smoking history is also a risk factor for vocal fold leukoplakia and malignancy, good visualization of the vocal folds is necessary to evaluate for other lesions in these patients. If benign edema of the vocal folds is truly the only lesion noted, management depends on the degree to which voice quality is disturbing to the patient or the degree to which the airway is narrowed. Smoking cessation can lead to stabilization of pitch at its current level, and phonosurgery to remove excess vocal fold mass can help lead to normalization of pitch and improve the airway. Phonosurgery may be performed with cold instruments or with the pulsed photoangiolytic lasers, an emerging therapy; in either case, there is a risk of creating a vocal fold scar that might limit vocal fold vibration even as vocal fold contours are improved.

Recurrent Respiratory Papillomatosis
Recurrent respiratory papillomatosis (Figure 5) is a benign laryngeal neoplasm that is caused by the human papilloma virus. It is the most common source of hoarseness in children, although adults also may be affected. As the lesions grow on the laryngeal epithelium, they create hoarseness and sometimes effortful voice by disrupting vocal fold vibration, particularly if the lesions are located along the medial edge of either vocal fold. Large and bulky lesions may lead to airway compromise, and advanced disease may spread throughout the mucosa of the upper aerodigestive tract rather than being limited to the larynx. Although accurate diagnosis depends on histopathologic analysis, a diagnosis of benign papilloma can be suspected from the characteristic appearance of the vascular fronds, which can be seen under magnified visualization in the office or in the operating room.

Treatment of recurrent respiratory papillomatosis is surgery, which is performed with a carbon dioxide laser, microdebrider, cold instruments, or the emerging technology of pulsed potassium titanyl phosphate (KTP) laser. As its name implies, the condition is recurrent: Even though surgery may reduce or remove the papilloma temporarily, the tissue continues to harbor the papilloma virus, and the disease usually grows back. Because repeated surgeries are expected, the goal of any single procedure is to remove as much disease as possible while limiting surgical scarring of the vocal folds. Scarring created as a result of surgery is cumulative, and over time patients develop persistent dysphonia caused as much by repeated surgeries as by recurrence of the disease. An ability to treat epithelial lesions while limiting scarring at the level of the superficial lamina propria is one main advantage of pulsed laser photoangiolysis; that these pulsed laser procedures can be

- Reassure, work to manage anxiety.
- Behavioral approaches: relaxation, distraction, hypnosis.
- Limit the number of people in the room.
- Open window.
- Eliminate environmental irritants.
- Keep line of sight clear to outside.
- Reduce room temperature, but avoid chilling the patient.
- Introduce humidity.
- Reposition, elevate the head of the bed, keep patient turned.
- Educate and support the family.

is preferred in the elderly because it does not cross the blood-brain barrier. For nonpharmacologic interventions, see Box 1.

Nausea/Vomiting

The treatment of nausea and vomiting depends on the underlying cause. For chemotherapy-related nausea/vomiting, the 5HT3 receptor antagonists are far more effective than other classes of antiemetics. The 5HT3 class includes ondansetron (Zofran), granisetron (Sancuso, Sustol), dolasetron (Anzemet), and palonosetron (Aloxi). In addition, there is a combination of netupitant/palonosetron (Akynzeo), which combines a 5HT3 antagonist for acute-phase nausea/vomiting and a substance P/neurokinin-1 receptor antagonist (NK1RA) for the delayed phase, and it should be given with dexamethasone (Decadron)[1]. Its only indication is for prophylaxis of chemotherapy-related nausea/vomiting, especially with highly emetogenic chemotherapy. The combination demonstrated superiority over palonosetron alone. Rolapitant (Varubi), another NK1RA, has a longer half-life than netupitant, with fewer drug interactions. Aprepitant (Emend) is an NK1RA with fosaprepitant (Emend injection) as its IV alternative. Olanzapine (Zyprexa)[1] was more effective than aprepitant and noninferior to fosaprepitant in the setting of highly emetogenic chemotherapy, whereas it is far more cost-effective than either NK1RA and serves as a better acute antiemetic than metoclopramide (Reglan). Prochlorperazine (Compazine) was found to be superior to promethazine (Phenergan) for uncomplicated nausea/vomiting (Table 2).

Constipation

Constipation is quite common in palliative care, and it is easier to prevent than to treat. It is one of the primary side effects of opioids that does not attenuate with time. For routine constipation, almost any laxative will do. Polyethylene glycol 3350 (MiraLax, GlycoLax) daily with as-needed sennosides (Senokot) or bisacodyl (Dulcolax) is one example of a simple regimen. If the patient is taking medications that have constipation as a side effect, such as anticholinergic medications or calcium channel blockers, they should be discontinued if possible. Opioid-induced constipation is due to the interaction of opioids with the mu receptors in the gut, thus leading to poor motility. It can be prevented for the most part if a stimulant laxative is initiated simultaneously with the opioid. Senna is safe for long-term use, but bisacodyl can damage the myenteric plexus over time. The chloride-channel activator lubiprostone (Amitiza) and the guanylate cyclase activator linaclotide (Linzess)[1] increase intestinal fluid secretion and motility, and the peripheral mu antagonists methylnaltrexone (Relistor), naldemidine (Symproic), and naloxegol (Movantik) are indicated for use by the FDA to treat refractory opioid-induced constipation. Alvimopan (Entereg)[1] is another peripheral mu antagonist, but its primary indication is for ileus, especially postoperatively. Fiber and bulking agents should be avoided because they can worsen the problem (Table 3).

Anxiety

There are numerous reasons for patients receiving palliative care to be anxious, whether undergoing painful/unpleasant but curative interventions, suffering uncontrolled pain or dyspnea, or progressing toward hospice. Fear and uncertainty about the future are common causes, and they can be related to physical, psychological, social, spiritual, or practical (finances, managing home responsibilities) issues. Excessive alcohol or caffeine use can exacerbate anxiety, which may present with agitation, insomnia, restlessness, sweating, tachycardia, hyperventilation, panic disorder, worry, tension, and/or psychosomatic symptoms. For patients with expectation of cure or longer survival, SSRI or serotonin and norepinephrine reuptake inhibitor (SNRI) antidepressants can be beneficial. Venlafaxine (Effexor ER) has the shortest half-life, and steady state can be reached in 4 to 7 days. Benzodiazepines are helpful for shorter life expectancy, or they can be used until the antidepressants take effect. Diazepam (Valium) has a long duration of action due to numerous active metabolites, but it is slower in onset, as is clonazepam (Klonopin)[1]. Alprazolam (Xanax) has very rapid onset but short duration of action. Lorazepam (Ativan) strikes a happy medium between speed of onset and duration of action. Counseling and cognitive behavioral therapy are effective, especially in combination with medications.

Delirium

Delirium is a waxing/waning state of confusion that can be characterized by anxiety, disorientation, cognitive dysfunction, and hallucinations. There is also a catatonic variety of delirium. This condition can be caused by many things, but a short list would include constipation/impaction, hypoxemia, infection, electrolyte abnormalities, medications (including benzodiazepines and opioids), and pain. If a cause is identified and corrected but the patient is still symptomatic, haloperidol (Haldol)[1], chlorpromazine (Thorazine)[1], or olanzapine (Zyprexa)[1] can be helpful; however, haloperidol is by far the cheapest alternative and a good place to start. It can be given intravenously or orally, or it can be given subcutaneously (off-label).

Hiccups

Hiccups (singultus) is a common nuisance that can become quite distressing, especially if persistent (>48 hours) or intractable (>1 month). For patients with pain in the chest or abdominal regions, hiccups can make pain difficult to control in addition to being a bothersome symptom that can significantly decrease quality of life. Chlorpromazine, at 25 to 50 mg PO up to four times per day prn, is the only FDA-approved medication for hiccups, but haloperidol[1] is a viable and much cheaper alternative, as is metoclopramide (Reglan)[1]. Gabapentin (Neurontin)[1] and phenytoin (Dilantin)[1] have been used with some success, notably in cases with a central nervous system etiology. Many other medications, including baclofen (Lioresal)[1], have been tried without much success (i.e., some improvement in symptoms but did not eliminate the hiccups). Nonpharmacologic methods (e.g., breath holding, hyperventilation, gargling) are worth trying, but evidence is lacking for any particular intervention.

Monitoring

Patients should be reevaluated routinely for the adequacy of pain and symptom control, as well as for their ability to cope with the underlying disease, symptom burden, and functional decline. The family needs to be assessed for additional stressors and coping mechanisms, as the family's adjustment, or lack thereof, can be detrimental to the patient's condition. If opioids or benzodiazepines are being used, the supply needs to be monitored for any signs of aberrant use by the patient and/or the family and visitors. In addition, patients can be monitored for excessive sedation or respiratory depression, especially when using methadone with or without a benzodiazepine. The FDA has issued a warning regarding coadministration of benzodiazepines or gabapentinoids with opioids as

---

[1] Not FDA approved for this indication

[1] Not FDA approved for this indication

TABLE 2 — Antiemetics

Antipsychotics/Dopamine Antagonists

Chlorpromazine (Thorazine) 10–25 mg PO q4h prn. Can use 25–50 mg IM q3h prn, but change to PO as soon as possible. Also available as 25 mg or 100 mg (can be halved) suppositories that can be given every 6 hours as needed.
Haloperidol (Haldol) 0.5–5 mg PO/IV bid–tid prn (off-label for nausea/vomiting); maximum 100 mg/d, but use lowest effective dose. Good choice when also managing delirium.
Metoclopramide (Reglan) 5–10 mg PO/IV q6h prn (contraindicated in bowel obstructions)
Olanzapine (Zyprexa) 5–10 mg PO daily–bid prn (off-label for nausea/vomiting)
Prochlorperazine (Compazine) 5–10 mg PO/IM/IV q6h prn; maximum 10 mg/dose, 40 mg/d. Suppository, 25 mg PR q12h prn

Antihistamines

Hydroxyzine (Atarax, Vistaril) 25–100 mg PO q6h prn or IM q4h prn
Meclizine (Antivert, Bonine) 25–100 mg/d PO divided bid–tid prn (off-label)
Promethazine (Phenergan) 12.5–25 mg PO/PR/IM/IV q4h prn. Use with caution IV: can cause necrosis and gangrene.

Antiserotonin (5HT3 Antagonists)

Granisetron (Granisol, Sancuso [transdermal], Sustol [sustained release SC injection]) 2 mg PO ×1 or 1 mg PO q12h ×2 doses given within an hour before chemotherapy. If IV, 10 mcg/kg IV ×1 within 30 min before chemotherapy. Transdermal, apply 1 patch (3.1 mg/24 h) ×1 24 h before chemotherapy and leave on for up to 7 days. If SC, 10 mg SC q 7 days (give with dexamethasone [Decadron][1]).
Ondansetron (Zuplenz, Zofran, Zofran ODT) 8 mg PO q8h for nausea/vomiting; 24 mg PO ×1 30 min before highly emetogenic chemotherapy.
Palonosetron (Aloxi) 0.25 mg IV ×1 or 0.5 mg PO[2] ×1 30 min before chemotherapy.

Antineurokinin (NK1 RA)

Aprepitant (Emend), fosaprepitant (Emend injection) 125 mg PO ×1 day 1 of chemotherapy, then 80 mg PO daily ×2 days. Or 150 mg IV ×1 30 min before chemotherapy.
Netupitant/palonosetron (Akynzeo), fosnetupitant/palonosetron (Akynzeo IV) 300/0.5 mg, 1 capsule 1 h before highly emetogenic chemotherapy or 235 mg/0.25 mg IV x 1 dose, 30 min before chemotherapy (use w/corticosteroid).
Rolapitant (Varubi) 180 mg PO ×1, 1–2 h before chemotherapy.
All NK1RAs should be given with an HT3RA and dexamethasone[1] before highly emetogenic chemotherapy.

Cannabinoid Receptor Agonists

Dronabinol (Marinol, Syndros) 2.5–10 mg PO bid prn. Syndros is available as a 5 mg/mL solution.
Dronabinol is indicated for chemotherapy-related nausea/vomiting refractory to other drugs and AIDS-associated anorexia and weight loss. Significant psychiatric adverse events are possible.

Unknown Mechanism

Trimethobenzamide (Tigan) 300 mg PO or 200 mg IM q6h prn

[1]Not FDA approved for this indication.
[2]Not available in the United States.
bid, Two times per day; *IM*, intramuscular; *IV*, intravenous; *q4h*, every four hours; *q6h*, every 6 hours; *q8h*, every 8 hours; *qAC*, before meals; *qd*, daily; *qHS*, at bedtime; *po*, by mouth; *pr*, per rectum; *prn*, as needed; *SC*, subcutaneous; *tid*, three times per day.

TABLE 3 — Laxatives

Osmotic

Lactulose (Kristalose) 10 g per 15 mL; 15–30 mL daily or BID, maximum 60 mL/day (40 g/day)
Magnesium citrate (1.745 g/30 mL) 195–300 mL/d PO daily or divided bid; maximum: 300 mL/d
Magnesium hydroxide (milk of magnesia), 400 mg/5 mL; 30–60 mL (2400–4800 mg) PO daily PRN. Maximum 60 mL/day, can be divided 2–4 doses per day.
Polyethylene glycol 3350 (MiraLax), 17 g in 8 oz. liquid PO daily

Stimulant

Bisacodyl (Dulcolax) 5 mg tabs 1–3 PO daily prn or 10 mg suppository PR daily prn
Sennosides (Senna) 8.6 mg tabs; 2–4 tabs PO bid; maximum: 4 tabs PO bid

Secretory

Linaclotide (Linzess)[1] 145 mcg PO daily. Stimulates cGMP production to increase intestinal fluid secretion and motility.
Lubiprostone (Amitiza) 24 mcg PO bid. Activates chloride channel to increase intestinal fluid secretion and motility.
Plecanatide (Trulance)[1] 3 mg PO daily. Stimulates cGMP production to increase intestinal fluid secretion and motility.

Peripheral Mu-Receptor Antagonists

Methylnaltrexone (Relistor) 8–12 mg SC qod prn (or 0.15 mg/kg SC qod prn). Maximum: 1 dose/24 h
Naldemedine (Symproic) 0.2 mg PO daily
Naloxegol (Movantik) 25 mg PO daily

[1]Not US Food and Drug Administration approved for this indication.
bid, Two times per day; *IM*, intramuscular; *IV*, intravenous; *q4h*, every four hours; *q6h*, every 6 hours; *q8h*, every 8 hours; *qAC*, before meals; *qd*, daily; *qHS*, at bedtime; *po*, by mouth; *pr*, per rectum; *prn*, as needed; *SC*, subcutaneous; *tid*, three times per day.

systemic etiology because the itch-scratch cycle can damage skin and/or nerves. Acute pruritis may have a readily identifiable cause, whereas chronic pruritis can be more difficult to diagnose and manage. Initial investigations for pruritis of unknown etiology should include comprehensive metabolic panel, complete blood count (CBC) with platelets, and thyroid-stimulating hormone. Abnormalities in hemoglobin, renal function, hepatic function, or thyroid function can help suggest the etiology.

Prevention

The standard approach to preventing pruritis is to avoid dryness of the skin. Specific preventive measures should be directed at the underlying cause.

Therapy

Treatment of pruritis depends on the underlying etiology if known. For general management, and for unknown etiology, avoid development of dry skin by using a minimal amount of hypoallergenic soap, showering in warm (not hot) water, limiting the time immersed in water or in the shower, frequent application of a neutral hydrating emollient, and limiting hot or spicy foods. Table 1 summarizes conditions, clinical clues, diagnostic measures, and management by the grouping classification mentioned above.

Topical Therapies
Corticosteroids

Topical corticosteroids aid in improvement of pruritis by decreasing the localized inflammation at the area of application. They do not have inherent antipruritic properties. Strength of corticosteroids should be targeted to the primary etiology of pruritis. Topical corticosteroids are most beneficial for pruritis due to group 1 conditions. Overuse of topical steroids can lead to skin atrophy, hypopigmentation, and rebound symptoms.

Capsaicin

Topical capsaicin[1] provides antipruritic treatment by antagonizing histamine receptors at peripheral nerves. It is most beneficial for neuropathic pruritis. It often requires multiple applications per day at higher doses for efficacy. This, as well as local skin irritation, often limits use. It should be avoided in actively inflamed skin because of the irritation it can cause.

Coolants

Topical coolants such as methanol and camphor activate afferent cooling nerves and thus provide antipruritic effects. They can be particularly beneficial for neuropathic itch and can help with infectious pruritis. They can cause skin irritation.

Doxepin

Doxepin 5% (Prudoxin, Zonalon) cream provides pruritis relief as an antihistamine. Its benefit has been demonstrated clinically for atopic dermatitis. In the elderly, it can cause drowsiness with widespread application of more than 10% of body surface area.

Calcineurin Inhibitors

The topical calcineurin inhibitor tacrolimus (Protopic) can improve pruritis by decreasing local inflammation. The efficacy of calcineurin inhibitors has been documented for dermatologic conditions such as some eczema, psoriasis, and seborrheic dermatitis. The most common side effect is a burning sensation, which can improve with continued use.

Anesthetics

Topical anesthetics, including lidocaine, prilocaine, and pramoxine, are useful for uremic and neuropathic itch. Pramoxine is more effective if stored in a cool area. Anesthetics work by

---

[1] Not FDA approved for this indication.

TABLE 1   Causes of Pruritis

GROUP 1: PRURITIS OF PRIMARY INFLAMED, DISEASED SKIN			
CONDITION	**CLINICAL CLUES**	**DIAGNOSTIC MEASURES**	**MANAGEMENT**
Inflammatory: dry skin, atopic dermatitis, contact dermatitis, psoriasis, lichen planus, drug reactions	Physical exam consistent with disease, exposures to common contact allergens (cosmetics, plants, fragrances, jewelry), medication use	Auspitz sign (scraping reveals punctate bleeding, points to psoriasis or AK), punch biopsy	Antihistamines, topical corticosteroids, topical doxepin (Prudoxin, Zonalon), topical calcineurin inhibitors, oral corticosteroids, immunosuppressants. Referral to dermatology often appropriate if not responsive to initial measures
Infections: scabies, mosquito bite, parasites, viral or bacterial infection, fungal infections	Exposure suggested in history suggests exposure, appearance of lesion	Can perform scraping with microscopy or send sample to pathology for evaluation	Antiinfective agents directed at infectious etiology. Symptomatic pruritis treated with antihistamines, coolants, topical corticosteroids
Autoimmune: bullous dermatoses, dermatomyositis	Cutaneous findings consistent with diagnosis; muscle weakness, pain; known or suspected malignancy	Punch biopsy	Topical corticosteroids, topical calcineurin inhibitors, immunosuppressants, dermatology referral for consideration of immune modulator
Dermatoses of pregnancy: polymorphic eruption of pregnancy, pemphigoid gestationis, pustular psoriasis of pregnancy, atopic eruption of pregnancy	Pregnant patients with cutaneous findings consistent with diagnosis	Often not necessary for diagnosis, may consider punch biopsy if diagnosis is uncertain	Topical corticosteroids. Pustular psoriasis of pregnancy associated with adverse pregnancy outcomes, requiring oral corticosteroids or immunosuppressants, dermatology referral (if uncertain diagnosis), and maternal-fetal medicine referral (for associated monitoring)

TABLE 1 Causes of Pruritis—cont'd

GROUP 2: PRURITIS OF PRIMARY NONINFLAMED, NONDISEASED SKIN

CONDITION	CLINICAL CLUES	DIAGNOSTIC STUDY	MANAGEMENT
Endocrine and metabolic diseases: chronic renal failure, chronic liver disease, hyperthyroidism, malabsorption, perimenopausal pruritis	Systemic symptoms: confusion, jaundice, palpitations, hot flashes, menstrual changes	CMP (uremia, transaminitis, hypoalbuminemia, electrolyte disturbances), TSH	Topical anesthetics, anticonvulsants, SSRIs
Hematologic diseases: polycythemia, Hodgkin and non-Hodgkin lymphoma, iron deficiency, lymphoproliferative diseases	Unintentional weight loss, thrombosis, dyspnea, chronic cough, sleep apnea, smoking	CBC with differential	Anticonvulsants, antidepressants
Infectious diseases: HIV, parasites, helminths	Systemic symptoms: nausea, diarrhea, unintentional weight loss, cough, fevers History: travel, exposure, multiple sex partners, IV drug use	CBC (lymphopenia, eosinophilia), CMP (transaminitis, hypoalbuminemia)	Topical corticosteroids, coolants, antihistamines
Neoplasms: cervix, colon, prostate, carcinoid syndrome	Unintentional weight loss; abnormal uterine bleeding; melena or hematochezia, constipation or diarrhea, urinary hesitancy; flushing, palpitations	Routine screening up to date with additional testing based on history Pap smear/HPV testing; colonoscopy; PSA; urinary 5-hydroxyindoleacetic acid	Treat underlying cancer; for pruritic symptoms: capsaicin, topical anesthetics, SSRIs, mirtazapine (Remeron), anticonvulsants
Pregnancy: pruritis of pregnancy, ICP	Xeroderma; pruritis, particularly of palms and soles, without cutaneous findings	Bile acids, CMP	Ursodeoxycholic acid (ursodiol) for ICP; cholestyramine (Questran), if refractory ICP is associated with adverse fetal outcomes, so referral to maternal-fetal medicine may be appropriate
Drug-induced pruritis: opioids, ACE inhibitors, amiodarone, hydrochlorothiazide, estrogens, simvastatin, allopurinol, trimethoprim-sulfamethoxazole, calcium-channel blockers, heparin	Exposure to offending medication	Often not necessary for diagnosis	Switch offending agent

GROUP 3: PRURITIS WITH CHRONIC SECONDARY SCRATCH LESIONS

CONDITION	CLINICAL CLUES	DIAGNOSTIC STUDY	MANAGEMENT
Neurogenic origin: multiple sclerosis, postherpetic neuralgia, cerebral infarcts, spinal infarcts, vulvodynia, neuropathy	Neurologic deficits; prior dermatologic infection; vulvar pain, dyspareunia	Often not necessary for diagnosis	Topical anesthetics, capsaicin, coolants, anticonvulsants, antidepressants
Somatoform pruritis: psychogenic itch, obsessive-compulsive disorder	Psychiatric history, hallucinations	Often not necessary for diagnosis	Behavioral therapy, anticonvulsants, antidepressants

ACE, Angiotensin-converting enzyme; *AK,* actinic keratosis; *CBC,* complete blood cell count; *CMP,* comprehensive metabolic panel; *HPV,* human papilloma virus; *ICP,* intrahepatic cholestasis of pregnancy; *IV,* intravenous; *PSA,* prostate-specific antigen; *SSRIs,* selective serotonin reuptake inhibitors; *TSH,* thyroid-stimulating hormone.

antagonizing sodium channels in the nerves. Vectors for administration include creams, patches, and lotions.

Systemic Therapies
Antihistamines
Both first- and second-generation antihistamines can provide pruritis relief by blocking histamine receptors. They are also most effective in acute itch with urticaria because that etiology is primarily mediated by histamine. First-generation antihistamines are more effective than second generation for chronic itch because their sedating effects can help alter neurotransmission in the somatosensory cortex. Long-term use of antihistamines can increase dementia risk. Their use should be limited in the elderly due to their anticholinergic properties.

Immunosuppressants
A variety of immunosuppressive agents (methotrexate, mycophenolate [CellCept],[1] azathioprine [Imuran],[1] cyclosporine [Neoral], prednisone) have demonstrated efficacy in the treatment of primary dermatologic conditions such as atopic dermatitis, psoriasis, dermatomyositis, lupus, and scleroderma. Choice of agent should be directed at the underlying cause. Their use is limited in patients with pruritis of unknown origin but could be beneficial for those with greater than 4% eosinophils on CBC differential. Medications can cause gastrointestinal side effects, myelosuppression,

---

[1] Not FDA approved for this indication.

hepatotoxicity, and stomatitis and can increase risks for infections. Patients with acute infections should not take immunosuppressants. Use of medications is limited in patients with underlying hepatic dysfunction, hypersensitivity, immunodeficiency, or underlying blood dyscrasias. Patients whose condition would benefit from the use of immunosuppressants should be referred to a dermatologist.

Anticonvulsants

The gamma-aminobutyric acid inhibitors gabapentin (Neurontin)[1] and pregabalin (Lyrica)[1] improve pruritis by decreasing the pruritis sensation at the dorsal root ganglia and spinal cord. Their sedating side effects often limit use. There have been some documented benefits in treatment of pruritis of unknown origin, neuropathic pruritis, paraneoplastic pruritis, and uremic pruritis. Use with caution in the elderly because of sedating properties and ataxia.

Antidepressants

The tricyclic antidepressants amitriptyline[1] and doxepin[1] are beneficial for neuropathic or psychogenic pruritis. They have antihistamine properties, which help treat pruritis. However, their anticholinergic side effects limit use, particularly in the elderly. Several selective serotonin reuptake inhibitors such as fluoxetine (Prozac),[1] fluvoxamine,[1] paroxetine (Paxil),[1] and sertraline (Zoloft)[1] also may help with psychogenic, paraneoplastic, or cholestatic pruritis. Serotonin acts as a neurotransmitter in the skin to trigger the sensation of pruritis. Mirtazapine (Remeron)[1] may also help with pruritis from malignancy or nocturnal pruritis.

Monitoring

Assess response to therapy and consider further treatment options or diagnostic workup.

Complications

Severe itching can result in disruption of the skin integrity and can lead to complex, chronic itching–related skin conditions including prurigo nodularis or extensive excoriations at risk for infection and cellulitis. Chronic itching can be emotionally debilitating, affecting quality of life similar to chronic pain.

---

[1]Not FDA approved for this indication.

References

Abu Hassan F, Hafiz S, Dweik A, Alhussain E, Walker J: Decompensated heart failure presenting as severe pruritis, *Am J Med Sci*, 2023.

Cho J, Chiou D, Patil P, Hyder S: Pruritis & dysphagia: gastrointestinal manifestations of lichen planus, *Am Coll Gastroenterol*, 2020.

Grabnar M, Tiwari M, Vallabh J: Brachioradial pruritis due to cervical spine pathology, *JMIR Dermatology* 5(3):e39863, 2022.

Huang AH, Kaffenberger BH, Reich A, Szepietowski JC, Ständer S, Kwatra SG: Pruritus associated with commonly prescribed medications in a tertiary care center, *Medicines (Basel)* 6(3):84, 2019.

Kini SP, DeLong LK, Veledar E, McKenzie-Brown AM, Schaufele M, Chen SC: The impact of pruritus on quality of life: the skin equivalent of pain, *Arch Dermatol* 147(10):1153–1156, 2011.

Sutaria N, Adawi W, Goldberg R, et al: Itch: pathogenesis and treatment, *J Am Acad Dermatol* 86:17–34, 2022.

Yosipovitch G, Bernhard J: Chronic pruritis, *N Engl J Med* 368:1625–1634, 2013.

Voicu C, Tebeica T, Zanardelli M, et al: Lichen simplex chronicus as an essential part of the dermatologic masquerade, *Open Access Maced J Med Sci* 5(4):556–557, 2017. https://www.itchforum.net/general-info/itch/.

◼ RHINITIS

Method of
Masayoshi Takashima, MD; and Daniel Gorelik, MD

Introduction

Rhinitis is defined as inflammation of the nasal mucous membranes. Despite the definition of rhinitis, there are both inflammatory and noninflammatory forms of rhinitis. Rhinitis presents as one or more of the symptoms of nasal congestion, sneezing, itching, rhinorrhea, and/or postnasal drainage. It can be divided into allergic rhinitis (AR) and nonallergic rhinitis (NAR). Often patients will have a mixed rhinitis, which has components of both allergic and nonallergic disease. AR is nasal inflammation that is mediated by immunoglobulin (Ig)E to environmental allergens. NAR is defined by non–IgE-mediated perennial symptoms. NAR shares symptoms with AR but is only distinguishable by negative allergy tests. NAR includes a broad group of diseases including vasomotor rhinitis, gustatory rhinitis, NAR with eosinophilia syndrome (NARES), occupational rhinitis, hormonal rhinitis, drug-induced rhinitis, atrophic rhinitis, and infectious rhinitis.

Most research still classifies AR according to its seasonality or its perennial nature. Seasonal AR is commonly caused by pollen allergens; perennial AR is mainly caused by dust mites and animal dander. AR can be further classified as mild or moderate/severe. Mild rhinitis is rhinitis that does not impair work, school, daily functioning, or sleep. Moderate to severe rhinitis interferes with activities of daily living, quality of life, and/or sleep. Episodic AR occurs with sporadic inhalant aeroallergen exposure not typically encountered by the patient's usual indoor and outdoor environments. Both AR and NAR can also be classified based on symptom frequency, intermittent (<4 days/week or <4 consecutive weeks/year) versus persistent (>4 days/week and >4 consecutive weeks/year).

Local allergic rhinitis (LAR) is a newly defined entity found in nonatopic patients. LAR is characterized by local inflammatory reactions including local eosinophils and localized IgE in response to aeroallergens. LAR does not show significant skin-prick testing reactions, and patients have negative systemic IgE reactions to aeroallergens.

Rhinitis may be viewed by some as a trivial disease, but it places a significant financial burden on society. The estimated direct and indirect costs to society of rhinitis were around $11.58 billion in 2002. There is a significant loss of work and school days and decreased productivity and school performance. It is estimated at least 20% to 33% decrease in productivity when patients with AR have an exacerbation of their symptoms. Patients also report significant decreased quality of life related to their rhinitis symptoms including disturbed sleep, daytime somnolence, fatigue, irritability, depression, impairment of physical and social functioning, impairment of attention and memory, and learning deficits. Appropriate recognition, diagnosis, and treatment can help alleviate these economic and societal costs.

Epidemiology/Risk Factors

The National Health and Nutrition Survey (NHANES II and III) suggests that the overall prevalence of IgE sensitivity might be increasing. Of the patients evaluated for rhinitis in the United States, 43% (58 million people) have allergic disease, 23% (19 million people) have nonallergic disease, and 34% (26 million people) have mixed rhinitis. It is estimated the prevalence of physician-diagnosed AR is up to 20% of the population and 17% to 52% for NAR. Seventy percent of allergic patients develop the disease in childhood (20 years and younger) as opposed to NAR patients, 70% of whom develop disease in adulthood. Approximately two-thirds of NAR patients have vasomotor rhinitis, and one-third have NARES. NAR has a female predominance.

Pathophysiology

Allergic

Allergic rhinitis is the result of an IgE-mediated, type I hypersensitivity allergic reaction in response to an inhaled allergen. Allergens are proteins derived from airborne particulate matter, including dust mite feces, pollens, animal dander, and cockroach particles. Antigen presenting cells (APCs) engulf allergens, break them down, and then present these peptides to T cells (THO). These cells differentiate into the TH2 subtype and generate cytokines that regulate B lymphocytes and sequester inflammatory cells (including eosinophils). B lymphocytes produce IgE, which attach to mast cells and basophils and render them sensitized. When mast cells and basophils are exposed to the specific allergen, they degranulate and release a host of inflammatory mediators including histamine and prostaglandin. Histamine stimulates histamine type I (H1) receptors on nerve endings that cause pruritus, sneezing, and increased secretions, which constitute the early phase response of AR (minutes to 1 hour).

Eosinophils produce interleukin (IL)-5, which acts to promote activation and survival of other eosinophils. Eosinophils also produce toxic products, which damages the mucosal cells and causes nasal congestion. This damage occurs several hours after allergen exposure and constitutes the late phase.

Nonallergic Rhinitis

The nasal mucosa has two major functions: One is trapping inhaled particles through mucus production and the second is humidifying inhaled air through a complex vascular system. The mucus glands and the vascular system are regulated by the parasympathetic and the adrenergic nervous systems. Sensory nerves are stimulated by irritants in the nose through the use of a sensory receptor called a nociceptor. The nociceptive signal generates a neural reflex in the central nervous system (CNS) controlling sympathetic and parasympathetic tone in the nasal mucosa. Parasympathetic stimulation results in mucus production. Sympathetic stimulation causes vasoconstriction, which empties venous cavities. Lack of sympathetic tone causes venous engorgement and nasal congestion.

Symptomatic NAR is an exaggeration of a normal defensive mechanism. Inflammation in the nose causes an upregulation of this neural activity, resulting in the exaggerated response (also known as neural hyperresponsiveness). Hyperresponsive parasympathetic efferent nerves trigger glandular activation in the nasal mucosa, leading to vasodilation and mucus production. Excessive mucus production anteriorly causes rhinorrhea and posteriorly causes postnasal drip. This hyperresponsiveness can be due to structural or functional components of the nasal mucosa altered through genetic or pathologic factors. NAR is often associated with hyperreactivity of the nasal mucosa but the exact mechanisms is often different based on the specific type of NAR. Broadly speaking, NAR is defined as rhinitis independent of an IgE-mediated mechanism.

Infectious Rhinitis

Most infectious causes of rhinitis occur as a viral upper respiratory infection. Viruses may account for more than 95% of acute rhinitis infections, but it can be difficult to distinguish viral from bacterial infections. Viral rhinitis infections often cause nasal mucosal edema, impairment of the ciliary movement, and often obstruction of the sinonasal cavities. Duration of symptoms greater than 7 to 10 days is used clinically to distinguish viral from bacterial rhinitis/rhinosinusitis.

Clinical History

The best diagnostic tool in the evaluation of rhinitis is the clinical history. Information regarding previous evaluation and treatment should be elicited. A positive family history of rhinitis points toward allergic disease. The history of symptoms should include questions regarding congestion; sneezing; rhinorrhea; sore throat; dry throat; cough; itchy, red, or tearing eyes; voice changes; sinus symptoms of drainage; pressure or pain; snoring; ear pain or loss of hearing; and smelling difficulty.

When gathering the details of each symptom, evaluate the onset (such as those in childhood), frequency (episodic vs. persistent), pattern (seasonality), characteristics of secretions, triggers, severity (to include quality of life evaluation), and associated geographic location or environment (home vs. work). Once a trigger is identified, history needs to be gathered even further to evaluate the possibility of modifying the exposure.

Physical Examination

As with any disease process, the physical examination provides clues into the diagnosis (Table 1). Although the physical examination in rhinitis patients should focus on the nasal mucosa, other body areas should be examined to rule out other processes. For example, the tympanic membranes should be examined for mobility, retraction, erythema, and Eustachian tube dysfunction.

TABLE 1	Clinical Manifestations of Rhinitis
TYPE OF RHINITIS	**CLINICAL FINDINGS**
Allergic rhinitis	• Symptoms of palatal itching, nasal itching, ocular symptoms, or sneezing • Allergic shiners, allergic salute, bluish boggy turbinates, mucosal stranding
Vasomotor rhinitis	• Predominantly intermittent nasal obstruction and rhinorrhea • Symptoms triggered by temperature, exercise, and environmental stimuli (odors, smoke, and dust).
NARES	• More intense symptoms, paroxysms of flares including sneezing, watery rhinorrhea, nasal itching, congestion, and hyposmia • Eosinophils on a nasal smear, but lack other allergic evidence by skin-prick testing
Gustatory rhinitis	• Nasal congestion and rhinorrhea associated with ingestion of foods and, sometimes, alcoholic beverages
Atrophic rhinitis	• Nasal crusting, dryness, and fetor due to glandular cell atrophy • Patients may have abnormally wide nasal cavities with associated squamous metaplasia
Occupational rhinitis	• Symptoms of nasal congestion and rhinorrhea triggered by an occupational exposure • Symptoms improve when away from occupation • Common substances leading to symptoms include irritating chemicals, grain dust, ozone, laboratory animal antigens, and wood
Hormonal rhinitis	• Symptoms of nasal congestion and rhinorrhea associated with pregnancy and/or menstrual cycle • Resolves 2 weeks postdelivery
Drug-induced rhinitis	• Symptoms of rhinorrhea and congestion caused by certain medications including ACE inhibitors, phosphodiesterase-5 selective inhibitors, alpha-receptor antagonists, and phentolamine
Rhinitis Medicamentosa	• Symptoms of severe rebound nasal congestion caused by prolonged and repetitive use of topical nasal decongestants
Infectious rhinitis	• Symptoms of acute-onset nasal congestion and rhinorrhea most often caused by virus. Bacterial overgrowth from virus-induced inflammation can lead to bacterial rhinosinusitis

ACE, Angiotensin-converting enzyme; *NARES,* nonallergic rhinitis with eosinophilia syndrome.

Examination of the eyes in AR might show conjunctival edema, erythema, and/or cobblestoning with excessive lacrimation. Patients with AR may also have darkening of the skin of the lower eyelids, which is also called "allergic shiners."

A nasal examination is essential for the diagnosis of rhinitis. Otolaryngologists will often use nasal endoscopy to evaluate the sinonasal cavity, but it is not necessary to diagnose different forms of rhinitis. Allergic and nonallergic nasal mucosa often will have a similar appearance with boggy, enlarged, and erythematous inferior turbinates. Bluish turbinates with allergic stranding are more common in AR. Evidence of excessive watery-clear mucus and postnasal drainage are also common findings to rhinitis. Other examination findings, which can occur in conjunction with rhinitis, are nasal polyps, sinusitis, septal deviation, septal perforation, and crusting. Looking for elongated facies, mouth breathing, and a high arch in the palate may provide a clue to the severity of the nasal obstruction in children. The tonsils and adenoids should be examined for enlargement. Posterior nasal drainage and cobblestoning in the oropharynx are common findings in rhinitis patients.

The skin examination provides useful information in the patient with AR. Atopic dermatitis or urticaria may be findings associated with allergic disease. The skin should be evaluated for dermatographism because these patients will not be able to be evaluated for allergic disease using skin-prick testing.

Diagnosis

The diagnosis of AR, NAR, and infectious rhinitis is based largely on history and physical examination. Other diagnostic testing can be performed to aid in providing a more definitive diagnosis or to rule out other causes.

AR is confirmed by IgE reactivity to environmental allergen sensitivity through skin-prick testing. When skin-prick testing is difficult to interpret or if it is not feasible, serum–allergen-specific IgE testing can be used. Nasal smears looking for eosinophils are not recommended for routine use in the diagnosis of AR. Other testing available for evaluation of rhinitis includes nasal endoscopy and radiologic imaging. Nasal endoscopy is reserved for those with atypical symptoms or an inadequate response to treatment. Radiologic imaging, such as computed tomography (CT) and magnetic resonance imaging (MRI), is used to evaluate anatomic structure and for evidence of concomitant rhinosinusitis but it is not recommended for the diagnosis of AR. If a provider suspects a cerebrospinal fluid (CSF) leak, the rhinorrhea can be evaluated for beta transferrin protein, which is present only in CSF.

Differential Diagnosis

The differential for chronic rhinitis symptoms includes AR, NAR and the many subtypes described earlier, and mixed rhinitis. Many different pathologic conditions can present similarly to rhinitis including chronic sinusitis with and without nasal polyps; ciliary dyskinesia syndrome; anatomic abnormalities such as deviated septum or septal perforation; sinonasal tumors; nasal turbinate hypertrophy; cerebrospinal fluid rhinorrhea; pharyngonasal reflux; systemic disorders such as vasculitis, sarcoidosis, and autoimmune disorders; aspirin intolerance, and other medication side effects.

Treatment
Overall

Current guidelines in treatment of rhinitis do not take cost into consideration. However, the individual treatment goals should be based on factors such as age, route of administration preference (i.e., nasal vs. oral), severity, seasonality, side effects, cost, benefit to comorbid conditions, and onset of action. For example, onset of action is an important consideration for an individual who has more episodic symptoms. Also, individual patients respond differently to treatment regimens within a given group.

Avoidance

Due to the lack of high-quality evidence, implementation of avoidance measures is largely based on panel recommendations. In addition, the ubiquitous nature of allergens may limit the effectiveness of the avoidance measures. For dust mites, encasing pillows and bedding in dust mite–resistant materials may be beneficial. Pollen is seasonal and can be minimized by keeping the windows closed, using air conditioning, and limiting outdoor exposure. Using particulate filters in the home can also assist in reducing overall allergen load of pollens and dust. Avoiding basements and lowering household humidity may reduce the amount of mold exposure patients receive. Pet avoidance can only be reached by ridding the house of the pet altogether. Other, less effective measures include limiting exposure of the pet to the house and/or bedroom.

Oral Medications
Oral Antihistamine

Oral antihistamines block H1 receptors, thereby reducing nasal and palatal itching, rhinorrhea, sneezing, conjunctivitis, and urticaria. They are recommended in the treatment of AR. However, nasal congestion is not treated well with oral antihistamines. First-generation oral antihistamines are poorly selective for H1 receptors. The sedative effects of these antihistamines result from crossing the blood–brain barrier; they have been linked to industrial accidents and contribute to loss of function at work and school. Given there is no evidence of increased efficacy over second-generation antihistamines, it is not recommended to use these medications. Second-generation H1 antagonists (e.g., cetirizine [Zyrtec, generic], levocetirizine [Xyzal, generic], fexofenadine [Allegra, generic], loratadine [Claritin, generic], desloratadine [Clarinex, generic]) have excellent evidence for therapeutic efficacy and are considered first line in the treatment of AR. They particularly help the systemic symptoms associated with AR. These medications may have some role in the treatment of NAR because of their anticholinergic properties, but consideration must be given to these systemic properties, including dry mucous membranes, blurry vision, constipation, tachycardia, and urinary retention. A combination of intranasal corticosteroid treatment with oral antihistamines may be effective for sneezing and rhinorrhea in NARES.

Leukotriene Receptor Antagonists

Currently leukotriene receptor antagonists (LTRAs) are not recommended as first-line treatment for AR and are only recommended if other first-line treatments have failed. These medications were originally found to have benefits in the treatment of asthma and thus are prescribed for concomitant asthma and AR. Montelukast (Singulair, generic) is the only US Food and Drug Administration (FDA) approved form of LTRA that is clinically efficacious in perennial and seasonal AR and asthma. Montelukast is approved for children 6 months and older and has a pregnancy category B rating. However, because of the potential rare neuropsychiatric side effects including sleep disturbances, depression, anxiety, aggression, psychotic reactions, and suicidal behavior this class of medications are used as second line. Currently LTRAs have no role in the treatment of NAR.

Oral Decongestants

Oral decongestants such as pseudoephedrine reduce nasal congestion and can temporarily relieve symptoms. They can cause significant side effects including insomnia, anorexia, irritability, palpitations, and elevation in blood pressure. They are not routinely used for the treatment for AR and NAR but can help temporarily alleviate symptoms of nasal congestion in severe disease in conjunction with oral antihistamines.

Systemic Corticosteroids

Systemic corticosteroids are only recommended for the treatment of severe or intractable AR. A short 5-to 7-day course is recommended in severe cases to help decrease inflammation to allow better penetration via intranasal therapy and improve symptoms. A prolonged course greater than 3 weeks can lead to serious side effects including adrenal suppression. They have no role in the treatment of NAR.

Intranasal Medications

Intranasal Corticosteroid. Intranasal corticosteroids (INCs) are first-line treatment for moderate to severe AR and most NAR conditions. They penetrate the nasal mucosa with the result of decreased neutrophil chemotaxis, decreased eosinophil chemotaxis, reduced mast cell mediator release, and reduced basophil mediator release. Fluticasone (Flonase, generic) and beclomethasone (Beconase AQ) are the only two topical INCs approved by the FDA for NAR. In general, this class of medications are well tolerated with minimal systemic side effects.

INC side effects include irritation, bleeding, and perforation of the nasal septum; rarely, local candidiasis is seen with INC use. No single INC preparation is more efficacious than, or has any relevant difference from, any other. INC has negligible hypothalamic-pituitary-adrenal axis suppression, and systemic burden is clinically insignificant.

Intranasal Antihistamine. Azelastine (Astepro, generic) and olapatadine (Patanase, generic) are nasal sprays approved by the FDA for AR and NAR. Azelastine, considered a first-line treatment for AR, is available in 0.1% and 0.15% formulations and is thought to improve symptoms because of its antiinflammatory properties. This medication has been shown to diminish eosinophil activation and adhesion molecule expression and suppresses generation of inflammatory cytokines. Azelastine may also reduce neurogenic excitation from olfactory stimuli. These medications have a faster onset of action than INCs and are as effective in the treatment of nasal symptoms. They are more effective and have a faster onset of action than oral antihistamines for the treatment of nasal symptoms associated with AR. Intranasal antihistamine (INA) does not produce a significant amount of sedation, but side effects include headache, epistaxis, bitter taste, and nasal irritation.

Combination Intranasal Antihistamine and Intranasal Corticosteroids. The combined use of INCs and intranasal topical antihistamines is considered to be an effective treatment for both AR and NAR. It is more effective than either medication alone. The combination of the two medications can be given separately or through a combined spray with azelastine (137 mcg) and fluticasone propionate (50 mcg) called Dymista. It is currently recommended to use combination INAs and INCs for moderate to severe AR or NAR[1] that is resistant to monotherapy. The combination therapy is more effective in relieving total nasal symptom score including nasal congestion and obstruction than either drug alone.

Intranasal Anticholinergic. Ipratropium bromide (Atrovent) is the only FDA approved intranasal anticholinergic that inhibits parasympathetic function in the nasal mucosa. The parasympathetic blockade reduces the output of secretions from seromucous glands in the nose. It is mainly used in the treatment of anterior watery rhinorrhea but has a very limited role in reducing postnasal drip, nasal congestion, or sneezing. This medication is especially helpful in gustatory rhinitis and vasomotor rhinitis where there is a specific trigger for the onset of rhinorrhea. Patients can take this medication prophylactically prior to exposure of the known trigger or irritant to help control symptoms.

Nasal Cromolyn. Cromolyn (NasalCrom, generic) is a mast cell stabilizer and inhibits the release of mast cell mediators that promote IgE-mediated AR. It should be given prophylactically prior to allergen exposure in order to reduce symptoms of AR from episodic allergen exposure. It has a favorable safety profile and is considered if first-line treatments are not effective. Cromolyn has very limited usefulness for NAR conditions.

Nasal Saline. Using nasal saline to irrigate the nasal cavities helps remove mucus, enhance ciliary movement, remove allergic and irritant particles, and moisturize the dry nasal passages. There are multiple delivery methods including nose spray, bottle, pump, irrigation, or nebulizer. However, the delivery method, volume, and isotonic or hypertonic use has not been established for the treatment of AR. There is evidence that saline irrigation for AR may reduce patient-reported disease severity compared with no saline irrigation at 3 months of treatment.

Topical Decongestants. Topical decongestants reduce congestion but have no effect on itching, sneezing, or rhinorrhea. Oxymetazoline (Afrin, generic), a common topical decongestant, causes nasal vasoconstriction and can be used as a rescue medication for severe nasal congestion symptoms. There is risk for rebound congestion with prolonged use greater than 2 to 3 days and is not routinely recommended for the treatment of AR and NAR.

Surgery and Procedures for Allergic and Nonallergic Rhinitis
The role of surgery in the treatment and management of both AR and NAR is to improve symptoms that occur as a result of the disease processes rather than treat the underlying disease. Patients with symptoms of nasal obstruction and congestion will get improvement with septoplasty (if deviated and causing obstruction) and turbinate reduction. There are multiple methods to reduce the inferior turbinate, which include minimally invasive radiofrequency ablations to partial resection of the turbinate. Recently there is evidence that reduction of enlarged nasal septal swell body and nasal vestibular swell bodies can improve symptoms of nasal congestion.

Traditionally, patients with vasomotor rhinitis can also be treated with endoscopic Vidian or posterior nasal neurectomy, which improves rhinorrhea and nasal obstruction in 90% of patients. There are risks involved in this surgery including dry eye and cheek and palate numbness, which usually resolve within 6 months of the procedure. This surgery has fallen out of favor to newer in-office techniques including cryoablation and radiofrequency ablation of the posterior nasal nerve (Clarifix and Rhinaer). These procedures can be done under local anesthesia and have shown to significantly improve total nasal symptom score including nasal congestion and rhinorrhea. They are FDA approved for the treatment of chronic rhinitis and vasomotor rhinitis. There is a growing body of evidence that in-office posterior nasal nerve ablation is effective for the treatment of allergic rhinitis. It is important to consider nasal anatomy, given the differences in efficacy due to anatomic variations in nasal structures and the extensive branching of the posterior nasal nerves.

Anti-IgE Therapy
Omalizumab (Xolair) is a monoclonal antibody available for the treatment of poorly controlled asthma, but it might have a role in the treatment of AR.[1] Omalizumab binds to IgE, hindering its relationship with inflammatory cells. Omalizumab only binds to circulating IgE and not bound IgE. Due to its high cost, reports of anaphylaxis, and its injectable-only formulation, omalizumab has a limited role in AR treatment.

Immunotherapy
Allergen extract immunotherapy has been used in the treatment of respiratory allergic disease since 1911, and its efficacy has been documented since the 1970s. The amount of allergen in each immunotherapy dose is slowly increased with each dose until a maintenance phase is reached. Immunotherapy is an effective treatment for AR and is the only treatment proven to alter the course of allergic disease. Debate exists regarding which form of immunotherapy is superior (subcutaneous vs. sublingual). Contraindications to immunotherapy include beta blocker use, due to complications in treating anaphylaxis, and uncontrolled underlying diseases, such as uncontrolled asthma.

Subcutaneous immunotherapy uses the injectable form of allergen extract. Adequate treatment usually consists of a 3- to 5-year course of immunotherapy. Subcutaneous immunotherapy is indicated in those patients for whom medications and avoidance measures are inadequate, as well as those with only a few relevant allergens. The inherent risk of subcutaneous immunotherapy is systemic anaphylaxis; therefore it is dosed in the physician's office. The rate of local reactions in subcutaneous immunotherapy is 0.6% to 58% and systemic reactions is 0.06% to 0.9%. Subcutaneous immunotherapy is covered by most insurance plans.

Studies for local-route immunotherapy (noninjected), many of which were carried out in Europe, have only been undertaken in adults. Local routes of immunotherapy include sublingual, local nasal, oral, and bronchial.

Sublingual immunotherapy was approved by the FDA in April 2014. The risk profile is low and therefore can be dosed at home. The rate of local reactions with sublingual immunotherapy is 0.2% to 97% and systemic reactions is 0.056%. Multiple large meta-analyses have found noninferiority when comparing sublingual to subcutaneous immunotherapy. Some medical allergy providers use subcutaneous extracts (aqueous) as sublingual therapy, but this is an off-label use.

---

[1]Not FDA approved for this indication.

[1]Not FDA approved for this indication.

Alternative Treatments

Acupuncture. Acupuncture aims to address AR symptoms, including nasal congestion, and is widely offered as a complementary therapy to pharmacotherapy. This is considered a safe therapy with minimal adverse reactions, although multiple sessions are required for effect. Electroacupuncture involves directing small electrical pulses through needles and can interfere with implantable devices, so this needs to be considered. The mechanism of action for acupuncture remains poorly understood despite its widespread use, but it may have a role in modulating IgE and IL-10 levels. Several systematic reviews have reported equivocal data as to the true effect of acupuncture, but given its low-risk profile, it is supported as an adjunct option to existing therapies.

Monitoring

The provider should consider stepping down treatment when the patient's symptoms have been controlled. The Total Nasal Symptom Score (TNSS) is a subjective assessment of the patient's specific symptoms, including rhinorrhea, nasal congestion, sneezing, and pruritus, and can be used to assess effectiveness of medications. The Rhinoconjunctivitis Quality of Life Questionnaire can also be used. Consideration for referral to an allergist might be extended to patients who have had a prolonged course, secondary infections, polyps, or other comorbid conditions including chronic sinusitis and asthma, or if immunotherapy is a consideration.

References

Brinkhaus B, Witt CM, Jena S, Liecker B, Wegscheider K, Willich SN. Acupuncture in patients with allergic rhinitis: a pragmatic randomized trial. *Ann Allergy Asthma Immunol.* 101(5):535-543, 2008.

Brozek J, Bousquet J, Baena-Cagnani C, et al: Allergic rhinitis and its impact on asthma (ARIA) guidelines: 2010 revision, *J Allergy Clin Immunol* 126:466–476, 2010.

Chaaban M, Corey J: Pharmacotherapy of rhinitis and rhinosinusitis, *Facial Plast Surg Clin North Am* 20:61–71, 2012.

Cox L, Compalati E, Canonica W: Will sublingual immunotherapy become an approved treatment method in the United States? *Curr Allergy Asthma Rep* 11:4–6, 2011.

Davies C, Gorelik D, Lane AP, Takashima M, Ahmed OG. Is posterior nasal nerve ablation effective in treating symptoms of allergic rhinitis?. *Laryngoscope.* 132(12):2295-2298, 2022.

Dykewicz M: Management of rhinitis: guidelines, evidence basis, and systematic clinical approach for what we do, *Immunol Allergy Clin North Am* 31:619–634, 2011.

Dykewicz MS, Wallace DV, Amrol DJ, et al: Rhinitis 2020: a practice parameter update, *J Allergy Clin Immunol* 146(4):721–767, 2020, https://doi.org/10.1016/j.jaci.2020.07.007. Epub 2020 Jul 22. Review.

Fan T, Chandna M, Gorelik D, et al. Correlation between middle turbinate insertion in relation to sphenopalatine foramen and failure rates of cryotherapy and radiofrequency treatment for chronic rhinitis. *Int Forum Allergy Rhinol.* 13(1):88-91, 2023.

Greiner A, Meltzer E: Overview of the treatment of allergic rhinitis and nonallergic rhinopathy, *Proc Am Thorac Soc* 8:121–131, 2011.

Hellings PW, Klimek L, Cingi C, et al: Non-allergic rhinitis: position paper of the European Academy of Allergy and Clinical Immunology, 72:1657–1665, 2017.

Meltzer EO, LaForce C, Ratner P, et al: MP29-02 (a novel intranasal formulation of azelastine hydrochloride and fluticasone propionate) in the treatment of seasonal allergic rhinitis: a randomized, double-blind, placebo-controlled trial of efficacy and safety, 33:324–332, 2012.

Rondon C, Campo P, Galindo L, et al: Prevalence and clinic relevance of local allergic rhinitis, *Allergy* 67:1282–1288, 2012, https://doi.org/10.1111/all.12002.

Seidman MD, Schwartz SR, Bonner JR, et al: Clinical practice guideline: allergic rhinitis, *Otolaryngol Head Neck Surg* 152(1 Suppl):S1–S43, 2015.

Sertel S, Bergmann Z, Ratzlaff K, Baumann I, Greten HJ, Plinkert PK. Acupuncture for nasal congestion: a prospective, randomized, double-blind, placebo-controlled clinical pilot study. *Am J Rhinol Allergy.* 23(6):e23-e28, 2009.

Settipane R, Charnock D: Epidemiology of rhinitis: allergic and nonallergic, *Clin Allergy Immunol* 19:23–34, 2007.

Sin B, Togias A: Pathophysiology of allergic and nonallergic rhinitis, *Proc Am Thorac Soc* 8:106–114, 2011.

van Cauwenberge P, Bachert C, Passalacqua G, et al: Consensus statement on the treatment of allergic rhinitis. European Academy of Allergology and Clinical Immunology, *Allergy* 55:116–134, 2000.

Wallace D, Dykewicz M: The diagnosis and management of rhinitis: an updated practice parameter, *J Allergy Clin Immunol* 122:S1–S84, 2008. Young-Yuen.

Wise SK, Damask C, Roland LT, et al. International consensus statement on allergy and rhinology: allergic rhinitis - 2023 [published online ahead of print, 2023 Mar 6]. *Int Forum Allergy Rhinol.* 2023.

Wu A: Immunotherapy: vaccines for allergic disease, *J Thorac Dis* 4:198–202, 2012.

Yan CH, Hwang PH: Surgical management of nonallergic rhinitis, *Otolaryngol Clin North Am* 51(5):945–955, 2018.

SPINE PAIN

Method of
David Borenstein, MD; and Federico Balagué, MD

CURRENT DIAGNOSIS

- Most spine pain is mechanical in origin in 95% or more of patients.
- Symptoms of mechanical acute spine pain resolve in most patients in 1 to 8 weeks.
- Most patients with spine pain do not require laboratory tests or radiographs to achieve resolution of their symptom of spine pain.

CURRENT THERAPY

- Localized neck or low back pain
  - Encouragement to remain active out of bed
  - Patient education about the natural history to improvement
  - Reassurance about the incidence of resolution
  - Effective oral drug therapy: nonsteroidal antiinflammatory drugs (NSAIDs), analgesics, muscle relaxants
  - Physical therapy with exercise program
- Radicular pain
  - Encouragement to remain active out of bed
  - Patient education about the potential for improvement
  - Efficacy of oral drug therapy: NSAIDs, analgesics, muscle relaxants, corticosteroids, antiseizure medication, epidural corticosteroid injections
  - Physical therapy: Mackenzie exercises for disk herniation (https://sportsrehab.ucsf.edu/sites/sportsrehab.ucsf.edu/files/Mckenzie%20Back%20Protocol.pdf)
- Surgical decompression for cauda equina, progressive motor weakness, or intractable pain

Spine pain is a common symptom that is diagnosed and treated by a wide variety of healthcare professionals. The interest in this medical problem is not limited to its incidence as a patient problem but also stems from the likelihood of spine pain being experienced by the treating physician as well. The good news about spine pain is that the vast majority of patients (about 90%) improve over 2 months with minimal intervention, but relapses are frequent. The bad news is that the smaller number of patients who develop chronic spine pain use more than the majority of health resources expended on this expensive medical problem. The goal of therapy is to relieve spine pain while it is acute so that chronic pain does not develop.

The axial skeleton may be divided into cervical, thoracic, lumbar, sacral, and coccygeal locations. The lumbar and cervical areas are the most mobile and at greatest risk for damage. These two areas will be the primary subjects of this article.

Epidemiology

Spine pain is the most common musculoskeletal complaint worldwide and produces direct and indirect costs of hundreds of billions of dollars each year in the United States. More than 80% of the world's population at some time during their lives will have an episode of low back pain. An estimated 20% of the US population has back pain every year. Neck pain occurs at a variable rate ranging from 0.055/1000 person-years (disk herniation with radiculopathy) to 213/1000 person-years (self-reported neck pain). Thoracic spine pain is relatively rare compared with the incidence of pain in the other two locations in the axial skeleton.

Persons of all ages develop spine pain. Younger people are at risk for developmental problems (idiopathic scoliosis, spondylolysis, spondylolisthesis), and older patients develop disorders associated with degeneration of spinal structures (osteoarthritis, spinal stenosis).

Risk Factors

Psychosocial factors are stronger predictors of incident low back pain than mechanical factors in adolescent populations. In adults, psychosocial difficulties are risk factors for chronicity more strongly related to outcome than any clinical or mechanical variables. Previous episodes of spine pain are strong predictors of future ones.

Studies of cohorts of twins have shown that nonspecific low back pain is more than 60% genetically determined, and work and leisure-time physical activities play a minor role. Other environmental factors, such as smoking and obesity, have not been shown to be a predictor of the development of spine pain on a consistent basis.

Pathophysiology

Most of the structures of the axial skeleton receive sensory input. The presence of anatomic alterations in these structures is not sufficient to predict the presence of pain. In general, spine pain is referred to as nonspecific because no definite pain generator can be identified. The nociceptive inputs generated by musculoskeletal structures are referred to as *somatic pain*.

In the first few decades of life, muscular sprains and strains of the paraspinous muscles in the lumbar and cervical regions are the most likely source of spinal pain. These muscular injuries occur when lifting in a position that places stress on paraspinous structures. Often the spine is in an awkward position and is mechanically disadvantaged. The subsequent muscle injury results in reflexive muscular contraction that can recruit muscles in the same myotome. Tonic contraction approximates the damaged components of the muscle but results in relative anoxia that causes the production of anaerobic metabolites that stimulate nociceptors. The number of recruited muscles may be extensive, manifested by severe spinal stiffness and limitation of motion. Most of these soft-tissue injuries to the muscle heal spontaneously without any long-term structural alterations.

Simultaneously, as people age, intervertebral disks become flatter as the nucleus pulposus loses its absorbency and the annulus fibrosus fissures and degenerates. The process results in the loss of disk integrity. Degeneration of normal biomechanical and biochemical disk properties results. Biomechanical insufficiency inevitably results in a transfer of stresses posterior to the facet joints and ligaments that are ill suited to assume compressive, tensile, and shear loads. Osteophytes form in response to these abnormal pressures, compromising the space for the neural elements. Disk degeneration itself might not be a painful process until alterations in facet joint alignment result in the onset of articular pain.

Spondylolysis is a developmental abnormality associated with a stress fracture in the growth plate of the pars interarticularis. This abnormality may be discovered as a radiographic abnormality in an asymptomatic patient. An increased risk of low back pain occurs with spondylolisthesis, the abnormality associated with instability of spinal elements in the setting of spondylolysis.

Pain generation in the axial skeleton may be somatic or neuropathic in origin. The joints, ligaments, muscles, fascia, blood vessels, and disks can be the source of localized somatic spine pain. Somatic pain, when it does radiate, tends to be less focused in distribution and exacerbated by specific positions of the spine.

Neuropathic or radicular pain is the sensation generated by damage of neural elements. Intervertebral disk herniation with compression of spinal nerve roots causes neural inflammation resulting in neuropathic and radicular pain. Radicular pain follows the path of the corresponding spinal nerve root. In addition to pain, sensory deficits and muscle weakness can occur, depending on the intensity of the nerve compression. In the setting of chronic low back pain, the role of the central nervous system in mediating persistent symptoms has been highlighted increasingly in the medical literature.

Prevention

Since the turn of the century, epidemiologic studies in adolescents have reported nonspecific spine pain at an incidence similar to that in adult populations. This finding suggests that primary prevention must be given at a very early age to have any chance of efficacy.

Among papers reporting on primary prevention, only exercise has shown effectiveness, with effect sizes ranging from 0.39 to 0.69. Other techniques, such as stress management, shoe inserts, back supports, education, and reduced lifting, were found ineffective. Some evidence in favor of occupational interventions (exercise with or without educational component) has been recently reported.

Clinical Manifestations

The most common symptoms of spinal disorders are regional pain and decreased range of motion associated in a minority of patients with radiating pain. For the majority of patients, pain has mechanical characteristics: Its intensity increases with physical activity, movements, or some postures and decreases with rest. However, it has been demonstrated that nocturnal pain is not uncommon in the absence of serious, specific spinal disorders. The precise topography of pain is often difficult for the patient to describe, and its interpretation is difficult owing to the overlap of the cutaneous projections between adjacent spinal levels and the similarities between dermatomes, myotomes, and sclerotomes.

Diagnosis

The diagnosis of spine pain is based upon the patient's history and physical examination. The history and physical examination should include a description of the pain that is as detailed as possible (e.g., past episodes, precise location, beginning of symptoms, factors increasing or decreasing pain intensity, radiating pain, neurologic symptoms, systemic symptoms), patient's medical history (e.g., past spinal surgery, neoplasia, corticosteroid treatments), and a limited physical examination focused on the posture of the spine, range of motion, muscle contraction, pain on palpation or percussion, and a brief neurologic examination.

Besides the high rate of false-positive results and financial costs, imaging studies have a negative effect on a patient's quality of life. Therefore unless there is a clear-cut surgical indication or a suspicion of an underlying life-threatening disorder, no imaging studies should be ordered on the first encounter for a patient with acute nonspecific low back or neck pain. Similarly, laboratory testing is not required unless a patient presents with clinical symptoms that suggest a systemic illness (e.g., fever, weight loss).

Differential Diagnosis

A number of guidelines are available in the literature to help a clinician in the diagnosis and treatment of patients with spine pain. The purpose of these approaches is to differentiate the vast majority of patients with mechanical disorders who will improve with noninvasive therapy without the need for radiographic or laboratory investigation from the small minority with a specific cause of spinal pain.

Traditionally, red flags have been used to identify patients with a systemic disorder causing spine pain. The red flags have included questions regarding prior history of cancer, weight loss, prolonged morning stiffness, bladder dysfunction, and bowel dysfunction. The presence of these findings suggests a diagnosis of malignancy, infection, spondyloarthropathy, or cauda equina syndrome, respectively. A study has reported

TABLE 1	Mechanical Low Back Pain					
FEATURE	**MUSCLE STRAIN**	**HERNIATED NUCLE-US PULPOSUS**	**OSTEOARTHRITIS**	**SPINAL STENO-SIS**	**SPONDYLOLISTHESIS**	**SCOLIOSIS**
Age (year)	20–40	30–50	> 50	> 60	20	30
Pain Pattern						
Location	Back (unilateral)	Back/leg (unilateral)	Back (unilateral)	Leg (bilateral)	Back	Back
Onset	Acute	Acute (previous episodes)	Insidious	Insidious	Insidious	Insidious
Standing	↑	↓	↑	↑	↑	↑
Sitting	↓	↑	↓	↓	↓	↓
Bending	↑	↑	↓	↓	↑	↑
Straight leg	–	+	–	+ (stress)	–	–
Plain radiograph*	–	–	+	+	+	+

↑, Increased; ↓, decreased; +, present; –, absent.
*Possibility of seeing the abnormality, not a recommendation to get radiographs.
Reprinted with permission from Mechanical low back pain. In Borenstein DG, Wiesel SW, Boden SD (eds): Low back and neck pain, 3rd ed., Philadelphia, Saunders, 2004.

TABLE 2	Mechanical Neck Pain				
FEATURE	**NECK STRAIN**	**HERNIATED NUCLEUS PULPOSUS**	**OSTEOARTHRITIS**	**MYELOPATHY**	**WHIPLASH**
Age (year)	20–40	30–50	> 50	> 60	30–40
Pain Pattern					
Location	Neck	Neck/arm	Neck	Arm/leg	Neck
Onset	Acute	Acute	Insidious	Insidious	Acute
Flexion	+	+	–	–	+
Extension	–	+/–	+	+	+
Plain radiograph*	–	–	+	+	–

+, Present; –, absent.
*Possibility of seeing the abnormality, not a recommendation to get radiographs.
Reprinted with permission from Mechanical neck pain. In Borenstein DG, Wiesel SW, Boden SD (eds): Low back and neck pain, 3rd ed., Philadelphia, Saunders, 2004.

that red-flag disorders occur so infrequently and have so many false-positive findings as not to be helpful in the primary care setting at the initial visit. The one exception was spine pain associated with osteoporotic vertebral compression fractures.

Despite the findings of this one report, clinicians need to be mindful of patients who would be harmed to a significant degree by delayed therapy. The disorders that require expeditious evaluation and treatment are intraabdominal vascular disorders with tearing pain and hemodynamic instability (expanding aortic aneurysm); cauda equina syndrome with bilateral sciatica; saddle anesthesia; bladder or bowel incontinence (lumbar space-occupying compressive lesions); and cervical myelopathy with balance difficulties, autonomic dysfunction, and hyperreflexia with spasticity and Babinski's sign (cervical space-occupying compressive lesions). These disorders require expeditious vessel repair or decompression surgery.

The differential diagnosis of mechanical low back pain (Table 1) and mechanical neck pain (Table 2) includes disorders ranging from muscle strain and herniated disk to scoliosis and whiplash injuries. The age of patients, pain pattern with exacerbating and mitigating factors, tension signs, and findings of plain radiographs can help differentiate among these common causes of spine pain.

Nonspecific is a term used commonly to describe the pain associated with mechanical disorders. On occasion, physicians have confused the use of "nonspecific" as meaning an absence of pathology

causing pain associated with mechanical disorders. The "nonspecific" designation refers to the inability to identify the specific pain-generating anatomic structure, not the absence of somatic pain.

Therapy

Many mechanical disorders of the spine are self-limited in duration, with a vast majority of patients improving gradually over time (Box 1). This progression to "natural healing" makes placebo look efficacious in many clinical trials investigating therapies for spine pain. This situation results in evidence-based reviews of spine pain therapies revealing very few categories that have a clinically significant impact on improvement. Nonetheless, physicians need to make therapeutic choices for their patients despite this relative paucity of evidence. Therapy for spine pain includes controlled physical activity, nonsteroidal antiinflammatory drugs (NSAIDs), skeletal muscle relaxants, local and epidural corticosteroid injections, and long-term pain therapy. Surgical intervention is reserved for patients who have surgically correctable abnormalities and who have cauda equina syndrome, increasing motor weakness, spasticity, or intractable pain.

The treatment of an individual patient has to be tailored based on the patient's expectations and preferences. Goals of the treatment should be clearly defined, and the patient should be informed about the expected benefits and side effects of the treatment at the first encounter. A short trial limited to a few days may be a good start.

Self-management with education of the patient about maintaining physical activities as tolerated has been encouraged for neck and low back pain. Information on nonpharmacologic pain-management strategies and daily life activities may be provided by healthcare providers, but patients adhere more to the former than to the latter.

Exercises are slightly effective for pain and function in patients with chronic low back pain. No specific form of exercise is clearly better than others. Simply walking has shown an efficacy similar to exercising.

The use of manipulative physical techniques in the care of patients with spine pain remains controversial. The absence of clear-cut distinctions between manipulative techniques with or without thrust adds to the confusion when one analyzes the efficacy of manual therapy treatments. Overall there is some clinical trial evidence in favor of spinal manipulation for acute low back pain.

NSAIDs have short-term efficacy for both acute and chronic low back pain; however, the effect sizes are not very large. The efficacy of these drugs for patients with radicular pain has not been evaluated well enough to make general recommendations. No single class of NSAIDs has superiority to another. Cyclooxygenase 2 (COX-2) inhibitors have a better gastrointestinal (GI) safety profile but no greater efficacy. A patient's response cannot be predicted, and a trial-and-error approach is often necessary.

Opiates have not demonstrated any favorable influence in the outcome of low back pain patients. Side effects are quite common and the risk of addiction is real. When these kinds of drugs are effective, the improvement is more important in pain intensity than in terms of function. Muscle relaxants do have some efficacy

for acute and chronic low back pain, but the effect size is limited. Long-term use of muscle relaxants can effect cognitive function due to their strong anticholinergic effects.

Antidepressants are not generally prescribed owing to an inconsistent improvement of patients. For patients with chronic low back pain and depression, an optimized antidepressant treatment shows a better effect on depression than on pain and functional capacity. Duloxetine (Cymbalta), a serotonin and norepinephrine reuptake inhibitor, is approved by the US Food and Drug Administration for the indication of chronic low back pain.

Evidence is lacking to support the prescription of systemic corticosteroids. However, corticosteroids have the advantage of not being toxic to the kidneys. Oral corticosteroids may be considered in patients with radicular pain from a herniated disk or spinal stenosis where epidural injections are relatively contraindicated (chronic warfarin therapy).

Some patients will have persistent neuropathic pain despite surgical decompression or as a result of postsurgical fibrosis. Opioid therapy is ineffective in many patients with chronic neuropathic pain. Antiseizure medicines, such as gabapentin (Neurontin)[1] and pregabalin (Lyrica), have efficacy in peripheral neuropathic pain. These same medicines are prescribed in patients with chronic neuropathic radicular pain with the hope that the mechanisms that work with peripheral neuropathy will also work for spine pain patients. Although the evidence of benefit for nonperipheral neuropathy pain has been limited. Other medicines including antidepressants (duloxetine [Cymbalta],[1] tricyclic antidepressants) have been tried when other drugs have been ineffective.

Epidural, selective nerve root, or facet joint injections have not shown adequate efficacy to be recommended on a regular basis. However, a limited number (two or three) of spinal injections may be attempted for patients with radicular pain who do not improve with oral medication.

Spinal surgery is indicated for disk herniation with radicular compromise, cervical or lumbar spinal stenosis with myelopathy or neurogenic claudication, and unstable spondylolisthesis. Controversy remains, however, concerning the relative benefit of surgical versus medical therapy for radiculopathy. Diskectomy significantly shortens (by about 8 weeks) the acute phase of pain associated with radiculopathy. However, studies with longer follow-up periods have never shown a clear difference between conservative and surgical therapies. Some studies have shown that intensive, multidisciplinary, conservative programs can be compared with surgical fusion procedures for patients with spinal instability.

For the most chronically disabled spine pain patients only, intensive multidisciplinary programs including, among others, physical reconditioning and cognitive-behavioral methods, have shown effectiveness.

Monitoring

From the standpoint of monitoring the efficacy of the treatment, five main dimensions have been recommended to evaluate the outcome of patients with spine pain. The intensity of pain is relevant but so is the perceived functional capacity, generic health status, work disability, and satisfaction with treatment. Many tools are available for the evaluation of each specific dimension. The clinician who decides to start using any specific tool needs to know, among other information, the minimal clinically meaningful changes for each tool, because differences that may be statistically significant when comparing two groups of patients may be irrelevant at the individual patient level. For example, in terms of intensity of pain, the threshold usually accepted is 3.5 to 4.7 and 2.5 to 4.5 out of 10 for patients with acute and chronic pain, respectively.

Precisely evaluating several domains with specific tools is rather time consuming. However, for busy clinicians, there are

---

[1]Not FDA approved for this indication.

brief instruments (core set of measures) with roughly seven or eight questions that include all the previously mentioned dimensions and that have been properly validated. One example is the Core Outcome Measure Index (COMI).

Complications

The clinician should inform the patient about the possible side effects of therapies as they are initiated. At subsequent visits, specific questions regarding the potential side effects are asked. For example, the presence of hypertension, peripheral edema, and hepatic and renal dysfunction need to be evaluated in patients who are taking chronic NSAID therapy.

In addition, a majority of NSAIDs have potential GI toxicity including mild mucosal irritation, ulcers, and perforations. Hematologic and neurologic toxicity are quite variable depending on the prescribed drug. Cardiovascular toxicity may clearly be an issue, particularly for long-term treatments. The benefit of persistent use of NSAIDs for patients with chronic spine pain needs to be weighed against the increased risk of toxicities.

Besides the risks of addiction or death, the use of opiates induces constipation and urinary retention that may be a serious problem for some patients. These drugs can also produce drowsiness, headache, nausea, or vomiting.

Antidepressants also produce drowsiness and anticholinergic symptoms during the first couple of weeks of use. These drugs have specific side effects including tachycardia, weight gain, or sexual problems.

References

Balague F, Mannion AF, Pellise F, Cedraschi C: Seminar on nonspecific low back pain, *Lancet* 379(9814):482–491, 2012.
Borenstein D: Mechanical low back pain—a rheumatologist's view, *Nat Rev Rheumatol* 9:643–653, 2013.
Borenstein D, Balague F: Low back pain in adolescent and geriatric populations, *Rheum Dis Clin N Am* 47:149–163, 2021.
Briggs AM, Smith AJ, Straker LM, Bragge P: Thoracic spine pain in the general population: prevalence, incidence and associated factors in children, adolescents and adults. a systematic review, *BMC Musculoskelet Disord* 10:77, 2009.
Bulloch L, Thompson K, Spector L: Cauda equina syndrome, *Orthop Clin N Am* 53:247–254, 2022.
Chou R, Baisden J, Carragee EJ, et al: Surgery for low back pain: a review of the evidence for an American Pain Society Clinical Practice Guideline, *Spine* 34(10):1094–1109, 2009.
Chou R, Deyo R, Firedly J, et al: Systematoic pharmacologic therapies for low back pain: a systematic review for an American College of Physicians Clinical Practice Guideline, *Ann Intern Med* 166:480–492, 2017.
Cohen SP: Epidemiology, diagnosis and treatment of neck pain, *Mayo Clin Proc* 90:284–299, 2015.
Coombs DM, Machado GC, Richards B, et al: Clinical course of patients with low back pain following an emergency department presentation: a systematic review, *Emerg Med J* 2020. https://doi.org/10.1136/emermed-2019-20929.
Deyo RA, Mirza SK: Herniated lumbar intervertebral disk, *N Engl J Med* 374:1763–1772, 2016.
Deyo RA, Von Korff M, Duhrkoop D: Opioids for low back pain, *BMJ* 350:g6380, 2015. https://doi.org/10.1136/bmj.g6380.
Enomoto H, Fujikoshi S, Funa J, et al: Assessment of direct analgesic effect of duloxetine for chronic low back pain: post hoc path analysis of double-blind, placebo-controlled studies, *J Pain Res* 10:1357–1368, 2017.
Fritz JM, Lane E, McFadden M, et al: Physical therapy referral from primary care for acute back pain with sciatica: a randomized controlled trial, *Ann Intern Med* 174:8–17, 2021.
Hooten WM, Cohen SP: Evaluation and treatment of low back pain: a clnically focused review for primary care specialists, *Mayo Clin Proc* 90:1699–1718, 2015.
Karran EL, McAuley JH, Traeger AC, et al: Can screening instruments accurately determine poor outcome risk in adults with recent onset low back pain? A systematic review and meta-analysis, *BMC Med* 15(1):13, 2017. Erratum reported in BMC Med. 2017 Feb 17;15(1):44.
Katz JN, Zimmerman BS, Mass H, Makhni MC: Diagnosis and management of lumbar spinal stenosis: a review, *JAMA* 327:1688–1699, 2022.
Maher C, Underwood M, Buchbinder R: Non-specific low back pain, *Lancet* 389(10070):736–747, 2017.
Qaseem A, Wilt TJ, McLean RM, et al: Noninvasive treatments for acute, subacute, and chronic low back pain: a clinical practice guideline from the American College of Physicians, *Ann Intern Med* 166:514–530, 2017.
Rubinstein SM, de Zoete A, van Middelkoop M, et al: Benefits and harms of spinal manipulative therapy for the treatment of chronic low back pain: systematic review and meta-analysis of randomised controlled trials, *BMJ* 364:l689, 2019. https://doi.org/10.1136/bmjl689.
Sowah D, Boyko R, Antle D, et al: Occupational interventions for the prevention of back pain: overview of systematic reviews, *J Safety Res* 66:39–59, 2018.
Steffens D, Maher CG, Pereira, et al: Prevention of low back pain: a systematic review and meta-analysis, *JAMA Intern Med* 176:199–2087, 2016.
Theodore N: Degenerative cervical spondylosis, *N Engl J Med* 383:159–168, 2020.
Tsiang JT, Kinzy TG, Thompson N, et al: Sensitivity and specificity of patient-entered red flags for lower back pain, *Spine J* 19(2):293–300, 2019.
Vanti C, Andreatta S, Borghi S, et al: The effectiveness of walking versus exercise on pain and function in chronic low back pain: a systematic review and meta-analysis of randomized trials, *Disabil Rehabil* 41(6):622–632, 2019.
William J, Roehmer C, Mansy L, Kennedy DJ: Epidural steroid injections, *Phys Med Rehabil Clin N Am* 33:215-231, 2022.

TINNITUS

Method of
Kenneth S. Yew, MD, MPH

CURRENT DIAGNOSIS

- Tinnitus is most commonly associated with hearing loss or exposure to loud noise.
- In addition to history and examination, most patients will benefit from an audiogram.
- Unilateral or pulsatile tinnitus, focal neurologic or otologic findings, and tinnitus with vertigo warrant imaging and further evaluation.
- Patients should be evaluated for distress from tinnitus, insomnia, depression, and anxiety.

CURRENT THERAPY

- Although no cure exists for tinnitus, education and support at initial diagnosis will help alleviate fears, dispel misconceptions, and guide expectations of treatment.
- Hearing amplification for patients with significant hearing loss can frequently resolve tinnitus.
- Cognitive behavioral therapy—either online or in person—can relieve distress in patients with chronic tinnitus.
- Tinnitus distress should be monitored, and comorbid insomnia, depression, and anxiety should be treated.

Definition and Epidemiology

Tinnitus is defined as a perceived sound without an external cause. It can be classified in several ways. By a traditional method of classification, the most common type of tinnitus is subjective, defined as tinnitus without a corresponding sound on auscultation. Objective tinnitus, on the other hand, can be heard by the examiner and the patient. The 2014 American Academy of Otolaryngology–Head and Neck Surgery Foundation (AAO-HNSF) tinnitus guideline classifies tinnitus as primary or idiopathic if, after investigation, no cause other than the presence of sensorineural hearing loss (SNHL) can be determined and secondary if it is "associated with a specific underlying cause (other than SNHL) or an identifiable organic condition." Both the traditional and AAO-HNSF classifications see tinnitus from the perspective of the examiner or investigator. Another common classification is dual, based on whether the patient has nonpulsatile or pulsatile tinnitus. Tinnitus that can be modulated by movement of the head, neck, jaw, or a limb is considered to have a somatosensory component, which is detectable in up to 83% of patients with tinnitus.

Prevalence of "any tinnitus" in adults is 14.4% (95% confidence interval [CI], 12.6%–16.5%). The estimate for children and adolescents (≤17 years) is similar at 13.6% (95% CI, 8.5%–21.0%) but more uncertain because of variability in how studies asked children about their symptoms. Prevalence increases from

9.7% in young adulthood (18–44 years) to 13.7% in middle age (45–64 years) and to 23.6% in older age (≥65 years). Prevalence of severe tinnitus is similar in adults and children at 2.3% and 2.7%, respectively, but increased with age to 6.9% in people 65 and older. In the largest review to date, tinnitus prevalence did not vary by sex. Limited adult data suggest a 9.8% prevalence of chronic tinnitus and an annual tinnitus incidence of 1%. Pulsatile tinnitus represents less than 10% of all presentations.

Risk Factors and Etiologies

The most common causes of subjective tinnitus are SNHL and occupational noise exposure. Other etiologies of subjective tinnitus include the following:

- Otologic—Conductive hearing loss, cholesteatoma, Meniere disease, vestibular schwannoma (VS), otitis media, traumatic cerumen removal
- Somatic—Temporomandibular joint (TMJ) dysfunction
- Ototoxic drugs—Antiinflammatory agents (aspirin, nonsteroidals), antimalarials (quinine, chloroquine), antimicrobials (aminoglycosides, macrolides, tetracyclines, other), antineoplastic agents, loop diuretics, local anesthetics, and other
- Genetic—Moderate genetic component noted in chronic tinnitus
- Infectious
- Metabolic/cardiovascular—Association with hyperlipidemia, hypertension, diabetes mellitus, or obesity not shown by the best current epidemiologic data
- Neurologic—Multiple sclerosis, vestibular migraine, tension headache, type I Chiari malformation, spontaneous intracranial hypotension, and brainstem stroke
- Psychiatric—Stress: association between chronic tinnitus and depression found by most studies; greater likelihood of depression and/or anxiety associated with more severe tinnitus; neither depression nor anxiety demonstrated to cause tinnitus. (Data partially adapted from Yew, 2014.)

The most common causes of pulsatile tinnitus include idiopathic, neoplasms, arterial, venous, and middle ear pathology. Specific causes include the following:

- Neoplasm—Paraganglioma, VS, meningioma, dermoid tumor
- Arterial—Dural arteriovenous fistula, arteriovenous malformation, tortuosity or aneurysm, atherosclerotic plaque, congenital abnormality, fibromuscular dysplasia
- Venous—Idiopathic intracranial hypertension, sigmoid sinus dehiscence or diverticulum, jugular or sigmoid sinus venous thrombosis, venous hum
- Otologic—Superior canal dehiscence, patulous eustachian tube, otosclerosis
- Myoclonus—Stapedius, tensor tympani or palatal muscles
- Hyperdynamic states or increased bone vascularity—pregnancy, anemia, thyrotoxicosis, Paget disease, bone-invading tumors or hemangiomas
- Somatosensory

Pathophysiology

Tinnitus is thought to arise from an intricate interaction between peripheral and central mechanisms. Although the inciting event for tinnitus may be hearing loss or cochlear damage, the actual generation and maintenance of tinnitus occurs centrally, involving both auditory and nonauditory pathways. Decreased input from the peripheral auditory system alters the excitatory/inhibitory balance within the central auditory processing system. This, in turn, may cause signal hyperactivity and increased synchrony between neural centers as the brain tries to maintain its pre–hearing loss state, a process called "homeostatic plasticity." These processes may account for a phenomenon called *central gain,* in which the central auditory system becomes hypersensitive. Human and animal studies suggest a role for the brain's emotional/cognitive areas—including the temporal, parietal, sensorimotor, and limbic cortices—in the pathogenesis of tinnitus. Limbic nonauditory and auditory pathway interactions have been found in tinnitus patients using multiple functional imaging modalities, but not all investigators have confirmed differences between patients with and without tinnitus. Frontostriatal circuits

appear to be critical in the development and maintenance of both tinnitus and chronic pain, consistent with the view that tinnitus, phantom limb pain, and central pain sensitization may share common pathways. The perception of tinnitus also seems to reside in somatic memory. The medial geniculate body in the thalamus is posited as the site of connection between sound perception, the auditory cortex, and the limbic system. A number of theoretical models of tinnitus psychopathology exist, but as yet none have been found to account for all findings in patients with tinnitus.

Prevention

Hearing conservation and careful use of ototoxic drugs should help prevent tinnitus. As industrial hearing conservation programs are well established, leisure time noise exposure is now estimated to be associated with more hearing loss than occupational exposure. The use of hearing protection while firing weapons and using power tools should be encouraged. Personal listening devices (PLDs) represent the greatest current risk to hearing. A recent systematic review of studies examining short- and long-term hearing effects in PLD users found evidence of significantly poorer hearing thresholds in long-term PLD users compared with nonusers. Keeping volume settings to no more than 60% or 70% of maximum should comply with current World Health Organization guidelines to limit leisure noise to less than 70 dB for continuous exposure and less than 85 dB for up to 2 hours/day, respectively.

Clinical Manifestations

Patients report an abrupt or insidious onset of a sound in one or both ears that is continuous or intermittent. The sound may be a ringing, buzzing, roaring, or clicking; it may be high or low pitched. The tinnitus may have a pulsatile quality. Its severity and persistence may vary from transient and mild to chronic and severe. If sought carefully, the pitch or loudness of the tinnitus may be modulated by moving the head, neck, or jaw. Other otologic symptoms include preexisting hearing loss, hearing loss or ear fullness during tinnitus, vertigo, noise annoyance, or ear pain. How bothersome tinnitus is to patients varies by its severity and the presence of coexisting depression or anxiety symptoms.

Diagnosis

The evaluation of patients presenting with tinnitus in a primary care setting includes a thorough history and focused examination. Most patients need an audiogram, and some will require imaging or standardized tinnitus impact investigations.

History

- Description—Onset, pitch, quality, unilateral/bilateral, loudness, continuous/intermittent, pulsatile/nonpulsatile
- Associated symptoms—Hearing loss, vertigo, otalgia, ear fullness, hyperacusis, headache, neck or TMJ pain, visual disturbance, gait problem, weakness, or paresthesia
- Provocative/palliative factors—Stress; change in tinnitus with head, neck, or jaw movement
- Past history—Prior tinnitus; hearing loss; occupational/leisure noise exposure; recent head, neck, or ear injury; bruxism; current or recent medications; or medical history
- Family history—Chronic tinnitus, Meniere disease, or otosclerosis
- Impact—Degree of tinnitus distress, insomnia, or lifestyle interference

Examination

- General—Blood pressure, body mass index
- Head—Masticatory muscle or TMJ tenderness; tinnitus changed by head, face, or jaw movement or contraction
- Eye—Nystagmus if vertigo history and papilledema if headache history
- Ear—Cerumen impaction, otorrhea, cholesteatoma, retrotympanic mass (refer for microscopic otologic exam before imaging if retrotympanic mass suspected)

- Neck—Neck mass, tenderness
- Neurologic—Cranial nerves; neurologic exam if neurologic symptoms, headache, vertigo, or pulsatile tinnitus
- Psychologic—Screen for depression and anxiety if mood symptoms or bothersome tinnitus
- For pulsatile tinnitus
  - Palpate pulse—Ask patient to tap out the tinnitus frequency
  - Pulse asynchronous—Consider patulous eustachian tube or myoclonic etiologies
  - Pulse synchronous—Ausculate for bruits over mastoid, preauricular area, temple, orbits, carotids, and for cardiac murmurs

Although SNHL is the most common etiology for tinnitus, it is important to evaluate for other etiologies during the initial evaluation. Brief, intermittent, nonpulsatile tinnitus without associated headache, neurologic symptoms, hearing loss, or vertigo may be observed without further evaluation. Patients with recent onset of nonbothersome pulsatile tinnitus without history of hypertension, obesity, new vision changes, ipsilateral subjective or objective hearing loss, and normal otoscopic findings may be considered for a month or two of observation. If symptoms persist or worsen, pursue imaging and/or specialty referral. Recent loud noise exposure or use of an ototoxic medication can inform the diagnosis and guide both therapy and prognosis. Headache should prompt a careful search for findings suggestive of vestibular migraine, idiopathic intracranial hypertension, or spontaneous intracranial hypotension. Unilateral tinnitus with vertiginous symptoms with or without hearing loss suggests vestibular migraine, Meniere disease, or VS. An abrupt onset is more often seen in somatosensory tinnitus, migraine, Meniere disease, and brainstem stroke or transient ischemic attack.

Tinnitus with a somatosensory component is suggested if the patient is able to change the tinnitus by movement or muscle contraction, especially if there is a history of coincident onset of musculoskeletal pain and tinnitus, bruxism, or TMJ pain.

An audiogram should be obtained for patients with unilateral or pulsatile tinnitus, suspicion of hearing loss, or tinnitus lasting over 6 months. It is an option for patients with tinnitus of less than 6 months. A criterion for asymmetric hearing loss to optimize sensitivity for VS is an average 10 dB difference over the frequencies 1 to 8 kHz.

No reviewed guideline recommends laboratory testing to evaluate patients with tinnitus. Laboratory investigation in patients presenting with tinnitus can be guided by clinical suspicion and existing preventive services screening guidelines.

Table 1 lists imaging options for patients with tinnitus. Specialty consultation is helpful to evaluate the myriad causes of pulsatile tinnitus. Magnetic resonance imaging may be uncomfortable for patients with tinnitus with noise sensitivity. In such cases, contrast-enhanced computed tomography is an alternative.

Patients should be asked how bothered they are by their tinnitus. If bothersome tinnitus is endorsed, then it is helpful to learn how the tinnitus is interfering with the patient's sleep, work, concentration, mood, and quality of life. This understanding will guide subsequent education, support, evaluation, and therapy. Validated questionnaires to assess tinnitus impact and monitor therapeutic response include the Tinnitus Handicap Inventory (THI), screening THI, and Tinnitus Functional Index (TFI). The National Institute for Health and Care Excellence tinnitus guideline highlights the TFI as it assesses global tinnitus impact, hearing acuity, sleep, anxiety, and depression. The TFI is available at https://apps.ohsu.edu/research/tech-portal/technology/view/1004796.

Differential Diagnosis

Brief spontaneous tinnitus, also called "transient ear noise," is a benign, fleeting, high-pitched, unilateral sound of unknown cause sometimes accompanied by a sensation of hearing loss. The tonal quality of tinnitus must be distinguished from the voices or music heard in an auditory or musical hallucination. Musical hallucinations can be experienced by people with SNHL or more rarely as a manifestation of epilepsy.

Treatment

Goals for treating patients with tinnitus are to help them understand that tinnitus is common, normally benign, and can improve over time; if it is chronic, therapies exist to help such patients live well with it. Table 2 lists evidence-based tinnitus therapies. Observation with support and education after negative diagnostic workup can be sufficient if tinnitus is not bothersome. In a recent observational study of patients with intrusive tinnitus, the provision of a standardized bundle of tinnitus information to all patients was associated with a nearly a fourfold drop in patients who requested further formal treatment for their tinnitus. Patient interview studies document that tinnitus support and education is beneficial at every stage of care. However, as many as 82.6% of patients with tinnitus surveyed worldwide felt that their tinnitus was managed "not very effectively" or "not at all." As there is still no cure for tinnitus, part of this dissatisfaction may stem from their expectations of therapy. When U.S. audiologists and their patients were asked about treatment goals, audiologists endorsed reduced tinnitus awareness, stress, and anxiety, whereas

TABLE 1	Imaging for Patients With Tinnitus	
PRESENTATION OF TINNITUS	**IMAGING CHOICE**	**COMMENT**
Uncomplicated, bilateral, and nonpulsatile	None	Hearing loss symmetric if present. No other indications for imaging, such as stroke/TIA symptoms, acute vestibular syndrome, focal neurologic exam, or retrotympanic mass.
Bilateral and nonpulsatile with asymmetric hearing loss by audiogram or unilateral and nonpulsatile	MRI of head and IAC	VS risk ~2% if asymmetric hearing loss by audiogram.
Pulsatile	MRI with contrast/MRA of head or CT of head/IAC without contrast and CTA	If negative and there is concern for dAVF, consider 4D-CTA if available or DSA. Add MRV if concern for venous etiologies or IIH. MRI more sensitive for neoplasms.
Pulsatile with suspicion of retrotympanic mass by microscopic examination or temporal bone disease	CTA of head and IAC with temporal bone reconstruction	

CT, Computed tomography; *4D-CTA*, dynamic computed tomographic angiography; *dAVF*, dural arteriovenous fistula; *DSA*, digital subtraction angiography; *IAC*, internal auditory canal; *IIH*, idiopathic intracranial hypertension; *MRA*, magnetic resonance angiography; *MRI*, magnetic resonance imaging; *MRV*, magnetic resonance venography; *TIA*, transient ischemic attack; *VS*, vestibular schwannoma.

TABLE 2	Treatment for Patients With Chronic Tinnitus
TREATMENT	**COMMENT**
Support and education—Teaching at time of evaluation provided in addition to printed or online materials	Help patients understand what tinnitus is and that it is typically benign. Explain that tinnitus is a result of, not a cause for, hearing loss. Reassure that it may persist but can improve over time. Discuss the potential for medications to cause or worsen tinnitus. Discuss prevention of tinnitus. Discuss no cures at present but management helpful to relieve distress. Review beneficial treatments and treatments unlikely to benefit.
Amplification	Offer amplification if hearing loss is affecting communication and consider for hearing loss without communication difficulties. Do not offer without documented hearing loss.
Sound therapy—via an in-ear or wearable device, environmental sound, smartphone, etc.	Option to offer, but limited current evidence of efficacy.
Medications	Avoid medications. Currently there is no evidence for efficacy of any medication to improve tinnitus. Medication may help with insomnia, depression, or anxiety, if present.
Psychological therapies	CBT is the most effective therapy for reducing tinnitus distress and severity. The NICE guideline suggests a stepped approach beginning with online CBT, then group therapy, then individual CBT.
Combination therapies—Tinnitus retraining therapy with amplification, with or without sound therapy	Current evidence does not support additional efficacy of this widely practiced approach beyond usual care.
Neuromodulation—rTMS, tDCS, tVNS, acoustic neuromodulation therapy, and others	Neuromodulation is experimental. There is insufficient evidence of efficacy from small, short-term studies.
Other therapies—Acupuncture, herbal, vitamins, minerals, and other dietary supplements	Other therapies are ineffective or inconclusive.
Treatments for somatosensory tinnitus	There is some evidence for oromyofascial therapy, dental occlusal splints, physical therapy, and relaxation training.

AAO-HNSF, American Academy of Otolaryngology–Head and Neck Surgery Foundation; *CBT,* cognitive behavioral therapy; *NICE,* National Institute for Health and Care Excellence; *rTMS,* repetitive transcranial magnetic stimulation; *tDCS,* transcranial direct current stimulation, *tVNS,* transcutaneous vagal nerve stimulation.
Data from NICE, AAO-HNSF, and European tinnitus guidelines.

their patients wanted reduced tinnitus loudness or its elimination. Accurate, supportive education about tinnitus and its treatment is essential to help patients develop informed expectations. Table 3 lists selected patient education resources for tinnitus.

Aside from hearing amplification and cognitive behavior therapy (CBT), no other therapy has proven effectiveness for tinnitus. Sound therapy to help distract from or mask tinnitus may be helpful for individual patients, but evidence of its overall efficacy is limited. Tinnitus retraining therapy (TRT) classically combines sound-enrichment therapy and directive counseling. It can be combined with amplification. Although its individual components may be beneficial, combined TRT has not proven superior in reducing tinnitus distress compared with usual care. Many medications and mineral and herbal supplements have been studied for the treatment of tinnitus, but none have proven beneficial. Available studies of acupuncture for tinnitus treatment are limited by methodologic flaws, precluding its recommendation as an effective tinnitus therapy. A variety of neuromodulation techniques to treat tinnitus have been studied; however, the studies have been small and relatively brief, with heterogeneous results. Patients with a somatosensory component to their tinnitus may experience relief from physical or dental splint therapies.

CBT targets thoughts and emotions to affect behavior. Drawing attention to inaccurate thoughts and thought patterns aided by a skilled therapist can help patients develop a more beneficial response to their tinnitus. Other cognitive-based approaches that have been studied for tinnitus include mindfulness-based CBT and acceptance and commitment therapy (ACT). All of these therapies have been shown to decrease the severity and distress of tinnitus but have not improved quality of life or mitigated tinnitus annoyance or loudness,

depression, anxiety, or sleep. The exceptions are ACT, which decreases tinnitus-associated depression, and cognitive behavioral therapy for insomnia, which improved insomnia related to tinnitus in one trial. Limited access to CBT therapists is an issue for many patients. Online CBT and ACT effectively reduces tinnitus severity and distress, although in-person therapy tends to have a larger effect.

Monitoring
Response to therapy can be assessed by clinical impression or a validated instrument like the TFI. As tinnitus can be associated with depression, use of a depression screening instrument such as the PHQ-9 and inquiring about suicidal ideation is recommended, especially for patients with at least moderately distressing tinnitus. If distress from tinnitus is not improving or worsens, review the completeness of the workup and discuss with the patient a referral for CBT or tinnitus specialty evaluation. Fortunately, although the severity of tinnitus may fluctuate, over time it tends not to worsen and may improve.

Complications
Carefully monitoring the level of a patient's distress from tinnitus, diagnosing treatable etiologies, and recognizing and treating comorbid conditions such as depression, insomnia, and anxiety will help avoid most complications. Care to ensure follow-up and consultation for patients presenting with pulsatile tinnitus is important, as up to one-third of them can have an underlying neoplasm or vascular etiology with potential for complications including vision loss, stroke, or hemorrhage. It is unknown if tinnitus is a risk factor for future dementia in a person with SNHL or if screening for dementia in this setting will improve outcome.

TABLE 3	Education Resources for Patients
SPONSORING ORGANIZATION	**INTERNET ADDRESS**
American Tinnitus Association—podcasts, tinnitus education and support	https://www.ata.org Tinnitus Patient Navigator: https://www.ata.org/managing-your-tinnitus/tinnitus-patient-navigator
Tinnitus UK (formerly BTA)—a wealth of information and support for people with tinnitus	https://www.tinnitus.org.uk
"Take on Tinnitus"—free, self-paced, brief modules from Tinnitus UK designed to help patients get information "quickly and easily"	https://www.takeontinnitus.co.uk
Tinnitus information from the Hearing Health Foundation	https://hearinghealthfoundation.org/what-is-tinnitus
How to Manage Your Tinnitus: A Step-by-Step Workbook, 3rd ed—Handbook produced by the U.S. Veterans Administration incorporating sound therapy and cognitive behavioral therapy	https://www.ncrar.research.va.gov/Documents/HowToManageYourTinnitus-abbrev-web.pdf
Hyperacusis Network—Extensive support and education about hyperacusis and tinnitus	http://www.hyperacusis.net

BTA, British Tinnitus Association.

References

Biswas R, Genitsaridi E, Trpchevska N, et al: Low evidence for tinnitus risk factors: a systematic review and meta-analysis, *J Assoc Res Otolaryngol* 24(1):81–94, 2023. Available at https://link.springer.com/content/pdf/10.1007/s10162-022-00874-y.pdf.

Cima RFF, Mazurek B, Haider H, et al: A multidisciplinary European guideline for tinnitus: diagnostics, assessment, and treatment, *HNO* 67(Suppl 1):10–42, 2019.

Haider HF, Bojic T, Ribeiro SF, et al: Pathophysiology of subjective tinnitus: triggers and maintenance, *Front Neurosci* 12:866, 2018. Available at https://www.ncbi.nlm.nih.gov/pmc/articles/PMC6277522/pdf/fnins-12-00866.pdf.

Hassaan A, Trinidade A: The tinnitus patient information pack: usefulness in intrusive tinnitus, *Int J Health Care Qual Assur* 32(2):360–365, 2019.

Jarach CM, Lugo A, Scala M, et al: Global prevalence and incidence of tinnitus: a systematic review and meta-analysis, *JAMA Neurol* 79(9):888–900, 2022. Available at https://jamanetwork.com/journals/jamaneurology/articlepdf/2795168/jamaneurology_jarach_2022_oi_220043_1667512347.25045.pdf.

Lynch P, Mitton T, Killeen DE, et al: Diagnosing pulsatile tinnitus: a review of 251 patients, *Otol Neurotol* 43(1):128–136, 2022.

Marks E, Hallsworth C, Vogt F, et al: Cognitive behavioural therapy for insomnia (CBTi) as a treatment for tinnitus-related insomnia: a randomised controlled trial, *Cogn Behav Ther* 52(2):91–109, 2023. Available at https://www.tandfonline.com/doi/epdf/10.1080/16506073.2022.2084155?needAccess=true&role=button.

McFerran DJ, Stockdale D, Holme R, et al: Why is there no cure for tinnitus?, *Front Neurosci* 13:802, 2019. Available at https://www.ncbi.nlm.nih.gov/pmc/articles/PMC6691100/pdf/fnins-13-00802.pdf.

Scherer RW, Formby C, Group TRTTR: Effect of tinnitus retraining therapy vs standard of care on tinnitus-related quality of life: a randomized clinical trial, *JAMA Otolaryngol Head Neck Surg* 145(7):597–608, 2019.

Tinnitus: assessment and management (NG155): *National Institute for Health and Care Excellence.* Available at https://www.nice.org.uk/guidance/ng155, 2020. [Accessed 4/1/20].

Trevis KJ, McLachlan NM, Wilson SJ: A systematic review and meta-analysis of psychological functioning in chronic tinnitus, *Clin Psychol Rev* 60:62–86, 2018.

Tunkel DE, Bauer CA, Sun GH, et al: Clinical practice guideline: tinnitus, *Otolaryngol Head Neck Surg* 151(2 Suppl):S1–S40, 2014.

Yew KS: Diagnostic approach to patients with tinnitus, *Am Fam Physician* 89(2):106–113, 2014.

You S, Kong TH, Han W: The effects of short-term and long-term hearing changes on music exposure: a systematic review and meta-analysis, *Int J Environ Res Public Health* 17(6):2091, 2020. Available at: https://www.mdpi.com/1660-4601/17/6/2091/htm.

Allergy

ALLERGIC REACTIONS TO INSECT STINGS

Method of
James M. Quinn, MD

CURRENT DIAGNOSIS

Classify reaction based upon clinical manifestations
- Local reactions
  - Uncomplicated "usual" local reaction—mild redness, pain, and swelling limited to area of sting
  - Large local reaction—redness, pain, and swelling extending beyond area of sting
- Systemic reactions
  - Cutaneous only—flushing, urticaria, angioedema (excluding tongue, throat, larynx)
  - Anaphylaxis (cutaneous symptoms and/or respiratory symptoms, gastrointestinal symptoms, cardiovascular symptoms, uterine cramping, etc.)

CURRENT THERAPY

- Local reactions
  - Uncomplicated local reaction
    - H1 antihistamines, analgesics, cold compress
    - Discuss avoidance measures
  - Large local reaction
    - H1 antihistamines, analgesics, cold compress, avoidance measures
    - Discuss avoidance measures
    - Further evaluation, testing, epinephrine autoinjectors optional
- Systemic reactions
  - Cutaneous only
    - Based upon clinical situation and prior history
    - H1 antihistamines, epinephrine in some circumstances
    - Discuss avoidance measures
    - Further evaluation, testing, epinephrine autoinjectors optional
  - Anaphylaxis
    - Epinephrine intramuscularly
    - Consider adjunctive therapy—antihistamines, bronchodilators, intravenous fluids, vasopressors, oxygen, other supportive measures.
    - Provide epinephrine autoinjectors
    - Discuss avoidance measures
    - Consider further evaluation, testing, consideration of immunotherapy

Pathophysiology

The pathophysiology of insect sting reactions varies based upon the classification. Uncomplicated local reactions are due to direct toxic effects of the venoms. Venom components include enzymes, vasoactive amines, peptides, and other contents that directly lead to local cell death, tissue destruction, vasodilatation, altered hemostasis, and inflammation.

Fire ant stings initially follow the pattern of the uncomplicated local reactions described. Fire ant venom is unique in containing highly basic pH piperidine alkaloids. Piperidine alkaloids lead to local tissue necrosis and a pathognomonic sterile pseudopustule at the center of an otherwise uncomplicated local reaction.

Large local reactions result from an immunologic response rather than simply direct toxic effects. The reaction is a broader and more sustained immunologic late-phase response to specific antigens in the venom. It is often (up to 80% of cases) associated with and possibly mediated by venom-specific immunoglobulin E (IgE).

Systemic reactions are characterized by signs and symptoms occurring distantly from the sting site. Onset is generally rapid and can include cutaneous, respiratory, cardiovascular, gastrointestinal, and/or other symptoms. Systemic reactions are the result of mast cell degranulation from venom specific-IgE binding. Mast cells release a wide array of vasoactive amines, prostaglandins, leukotrienes, platelet activating factor, and other cytokines. These lead to vasodilatation, capillary leak, edema, bronchospasm, etc.

There are clinical situations when patients should be suspected of having an underlying mast cell disorder as a pathophysiologic contributor. These include very severe anaphylaxis, hypotension, severe anaphylaxis without cutaneous symptoms, and patients without detectable IgE.

Prevention

Prevention focuses on avoidance of stings. General strategies that may be effective include using professional exterminators for known nests with periodic reinspections; wearing fully closed-toe shoes or sandals outdoors (include socks for fire ant prevention); use of caution when or avoidance of eating or drinking outdoors, especially drinking from closed or opaque containers or straws; vigilance in wooded areas, around flowering plants, and garbage; and wearing shoes, socks, long pants, long sleeves, and hats when gardening or performing other "at-risk" outdoor activity. If the history of the sting or diagnostic testing identifies the suspected insect, teach patients about the habits and nesting of the specific insect.

Stinging insects are the Hymenoptera order and include the Apidae (bee) family of honeybees and bumblebees; the Vespidae (wasp) family of hornets, yellow jackets, and paper wasps; and the Formicidae (ant) family of the imported fire ant. Honeybees and bumblebees are generally not aggressive. They feed on nectar from flowering plants and will sting only in self-defense such as stepping barefoot on a bee in a field or with an accidental close encounter. Bees will also sting after a direct threat to their nests. Bees nests can be found in commercial hives, tree hollows, old logs, or, less commonly, in the walls of buildings. Africanized honeybees, found primarily in the southern third of the United States, differ only in that they are far more aggressive in defense of their hives. Massive and persistent retaliation can result simply from the vibration of lawn equipment several yards from their hive. The stingers of bees are barbed and often result in retention of the stinger and venom sac at the sting site. A retained stinger can occur, although less commonly, with wasps.

Yellow jackets are scavengers, seeking food wherever available—at picnics, around garbage containers, in soda cans, etc. They are highly aggressive and may sting even if unprovoked. Their nests are found underground, in rotted wood, or in wall spaces. In many areas of the country, yellow jackets are the most common cause of stings.

Hornets and paper wasps generally are not aggressive and do not sting unless defending their nests. Paper wasp nests are classically thin, paper-like honeycomb structures found under the eaves of homes, windowsills, and railings. Hornet nests are typically grayish paper mâché structures hanging from tree limbs. There are several species of hornets and wasps that have black and yellow coloring that can make them difficult to distinguish from yellow jackets and bees, making simple visual identification unreliable.

Imported fire ants are extremely aggressive, especially in defense of their nest. Fire ants are endemic to the southern United States. Fire ant nests are built underground and generally capped by a mound of overlying loose soil. Individual ants can sting multiple times and the disturbed mound easily spills out hundreds to thousands of workers prepared to sting in defense of the nest.

Clinical Manifestations

Classification of insect sting reactions based upon the clinical manifestations is important to the diagnostic and therapeutic approach. Most insect sting reactions can be classified as local or systemic. Local reactions are further subdivided as uncomplicated local reactions or as large local reactions. Systemic reactions can be further subdivided as cutaneous only or as anaphylaxis.

Uncomplicated local reactions are the expected usual reaction and are characterized by mild redness, pain, itching, and swelling limited to the area of sting generally not larger than 5 to 10 cm. These local reactions begin immediately after the sting and generally resolve over several hours but may linger up to 48 hours. Uncommonly, the pain, burning, or itch of an isolated fire ant sting goes unnoticed, but the sterile pseudopustule appears within 24 hours of the sting.

Large local reactions occur in approximately 5% to 15% of insect stings. These reactions are generally defined as larger than 10 cm or a patient's palm and can progress, involving an entire limb. Large local reactions generally begin within 6 to 12 hours, peak within 24 to 48 hours, and resolve within 3 to 10 days. Large local reactions commonly recur with repeat stings.

Systemic reactions occur in approximately 1% to 7% of stings. Systemic cutaneous-only reactions are limited to flushing, urticaria, and angioedema (excluding the airway—tongue, throat, larynx). Most systemic reactions in children are cutaneous only, whereas most systemic reactions in adults are anaphylactic.

Systemic anaphylaxis occurs in 1% to 3% of stings. Anaphylaxis is defined as the acute onset (minutes to several hours) of symptoms after a sting and include two or more of the following organ systems: cutaneous (pruritus, flushing, urticaria, angioedema), respiratory (shortness of breath, chest tightness, cough, stridor, wheezing), cardiovascular (light headedness, syncope, tachycardia, hypotension), or gastrointestinal (abdominal pain, nausea, vomiting, diarrhea). In addition, anaphylaxis can be defined as the acute onset of hypotension after exposure to a known allergen for the patient.

Toxic reactions can occur due to large numbers of stings (>20 to 50 flying Hymenoptera stings in an adult). Toxic signs and symptoms are often delayed and can include myalgia, fevers/chills, headache, rhabdomyolysis, renal failure, hemolysis, diffuse intravascular coagulation, acute respiratory distress syndrome, and death. The lethal dose for a 60-kg adult has been estimated at more than 1100 honeybee stings.

There are also unusual and rare reactions of unknown pathophysiology that include glomerulonephritis, Guillain-Barré syndrome, seizures, and serum sickness.

Diagnosis

Categorizing the type of reaction is essential for risk assessment, diagnostic evaluation, and treatment planning. History of the event, signs and symptoms, and response to therapy are important and will allow the reaction to be accurately categorized as uncomplicated local, large local, systemic cutaneous-only, or systemic anaphylaxis.

Patients experiencing uncomplicated local reactions are not at increased risk of anaphylaxis and do not require additional diagnostic evaluation.

Patients experiencing large local reactions generally do not require additional diagnostic evaluation because they have a small relative risk of future anaphylaxis. Despite the common occurrence of venom specific IgE, only 4% to 10% of patients with a history of large local reactions go on to develop a systemic reaction, and only less than 5% go on to develop anaphylaxis after repeat stings.

Patients with systemic cutaneous-only reactions generally do not require additional diagnostic evaluation because they also have a small relative risk of future anaphylaxis. Only 10% to 15% of children with systemic cutaneous-only reactions have recurrent cutaneous-only reactions and less than 3% go on to have anaphylaxis. For adults with cutaneous-only reactions, there is a less than 3% to 5% risk of progression to anaphylaxis after resting.

There may be special situations when patients with large local or systemic cutaneous-only reactions are at increased risk and would benefit from referral to consider additional diagnostic testing, epinephrine autoinjectors, and possible immunotherapy. Special situations include frequent stings, high-risk medical conditions, at-risk medications (β-blockers, angiotensin-converting enzyme [ACE] inhibitors), impaired quality of life, and/or imported fire ant stings. Data regarding future risk of repeat fire ant stings are not robust, and multiple sting attack rates are high. In these patients, the decision regarding evaluation and therapy is based on a risk-benefit discussion with the patient.

Patients with systemic anaphylaxis after stings should undergo referral for further diagnostic testing. Patients with systemic reactions to stings have a 25% to 75% chance of another systemic reaction with the highest rates of recurrence seen with more severe reactions. Systemic anaphylaxis to insect stings can be fatal. Insect stings account for up to 20% of all fatalities due to anaphylaxis and estimates are that 40 (and likely more) patients die annually from insect sting anaphylaxis in the United States.

Additional diagnostic testing may commonly include prick and intradermal skin testing, serologic assessment of specific IgE, and serum tryptase.

Therapy and Monitoring

Uncomplicated local reaction should be cleaned, and any retained stinger carefully removed. Symptomatic therapy with antihistamines, analgesics, and cold compresses can be administered. Patients should also be given advice regarding avoidance measures to prevent future stings. In the case of fire ant stings, the pseudopustule is sterile and bacteriostatic; it should not be unroofed or opened.

Large local reactions should be approached similarly to uncomplicated local reactions with symptomatic therapy. For patients with frequent painful and/or debilitating large local reactions, the unstudied method of a short burst of oral corticosteroids for 3 to 7 days is sometimes used. Efficacy with immunotherapy for large local reactions has been demonstrated in early trials, but further study is needed. Unneeded antibiotic therapy for cellulitis should be avoided. Cellulitis is unlikely at 24 to 48 hours when patients commonly present. Later presentations of large local reactions can make distinguishing cellulitis more difficult. However, after 48 hours, many large, local reactions are plateauing or improving while infection would be expected to worsen. In addition, presence of fever would suggest infection.

Systemic cutaneous-only reactions (flushing, urticaria, angioedema not involving the airway) may require a more nuanced approach. Because of the low risk of developing additional symptoms, patients with a history of prior cutaneous-only reactions can be appropriately treated with antihistamines and close observation if they present again with cutaneous-only reactions. On the other hand, patients with a history of anaphylaxis who may initially present with cutaneous-only symptoms should immediately be treated with injectable epinephrine because of the significant risk that additional symptoms will develop.

Those patients with large local reactions or systemic cutaneous-only reactions and in whom special situations exist may be given epinephrine autoinjectors, recommended to wear medical identification information, and referred to an allergist/immunologist for consideration of further evaluation.

Systemic anaphylaxis to insect stings should be treated acutely in the same way as anaphylaxis from any cause. The drug of choice, epinephrine 1 mg/mL (1:1000), should be injected intramuscularly preferentially in the lateral thigh with 0.3 to 0.5 mg in adults and 0.01 mg/kg up to 0.3 mg in children without delay. Transport to a fully capable emergency medical facility should be undertaken as soon as practicable. As available, adjunctive therapies with antihistamines, bronchodilators, intravenous fluids, vasopressors, oxygen, and other supportive measures can be considered after the administration of epinephrine based on the clinical scenario. These adjunctive therapies should not be used as a substitute for possible repeat doses of epinephrine if additional epinephrine is available and indicated. Epinephrine administration should not be delayed because delayed use of epinephrine has been associated with fatal reactions in humans. In addition, animal models demonstrate that advanced anaphylaxis can become refractory to epinephrine. Patients with a rapid and complete response to initial therapy should generally be observed for 3 to 6 hours. Prolonged observation or admission should be considered for patients with severe, prolonged, or refractory symptoms.

After acute treatment but before discharge, patients should be given an epinephrine autoinjector (Auvi-Q, EpiPen) and instructed in the proper technique for use. Patients should be instructed in basic avoidance strategies to prevent future stings and offered medical identification information. Patients should understand the significant risk of recurrence and the need to follow up for additional testing and consideration for immunotherapy. If additional evaluation identifies specific IgE to the stinging insect, immunotherapy can be offered. Immunotherapy to stinging insects is quite effective in reducing the risk of a systemic reaction while on immunotherapy and provides longer lasting risk reduction for many years after completing 3 to 5 years of immunotherapy.

References

Freeman TM: Hypersensitivity to hymenoptera stings, *N Engl J Med* 351:1978–1984, 2004.

Golden DBK: Large local reactions to insect stings, *J Allergy Clin Immunol* 3:331–334, 2015.

Golden DBK, Demain J, Freeman TM, et al: Stinging insect hypersensitivity: a practice parameter update 2016, *Ann Allergy Asthma Immunol* 118:28–54, 2017.

Jacobson RS: Entomological aspects of insect sting allergy. In Freeman TM, Tracy JM, editors: *Stinging Insect Allergy*, Switzerland, 2017, Springer, pp 17–42.

Rueff F, Przybilla M, Bilo MB, et al: Predictors of severe systemic anaphylactic reactions in patients with hymenoptera venom allergy: importance of baseline serum tryptase, *J Allergy Clin Immunol* 124:1047–1054, 2009.

Sampson HA, Munoz-Furlong A, Campbell RL, et al: Second symposium on the definition and management of anaphylaxis: summary report, *J Allergy Clin Immunol* 117:391–397, 2006.

Tracy JM, Demain JG, Quinn JM, et al: The natural history of the exposure to the imported fire ant (solenopsis invicta), *J Allergy Clin Immunol* 95:824–828, 1995.

ANAPHYLAXIS

Method of
Justin Greiwe, MD; and Jonathan A. Bernstein, MD

CURRENT DIAGNOSIS

- There is no universal agreement on the definition of anaphylaxis or the criteria for diagnosis.
- A comprehensive clinical history of the events surrounding the reaction provides the most valuable data along with a detailed review of current medications, recently ingested foods and/or drugs, insect stings, and physical activities before or after the event.
- While anaphylaxis remains primarily a clinical diagnosis, measurement of selected biomarkers (most commonly serum tryptase) has been used in research and clinical settings to assist in confirming this reaction.
- Cutaneous or serum-specific immunologic testing should only be performed to confirm or exclude a suspected agent under the supervision of an allergy specialist trained to interpret the meaning of the test results. Random testing to a large panel of foods or other allergens without a specific history has low diagnostic utility.

CURRENT THERAPY

- Prompt administration of intramuscular epinephrine is the gold-standard first-line medication for the treatment of anaphylaxis. Delay in treatment with epinephrine has been associated with increased morbidity and mortality.
- Patients with severe reactions can have massive fluid shifts that can occur rapidly due to increased vascular permeability which require aggressive fluid resuscitation.
- Additional treatments are considered supportive and include the addition of H1 and H2 antihistamines for itching, urticaria, and gastrointestinal complaints; albuterol for bronchospasm; oxygen; and placing the patient in the Trendelenburg position.
- Corticosteroids are not useful for the acute treatment of anaphylaxis since these medications take 4 to 6 hours to reach maximum effectiveness and there is a lack compelling evidence that corticosteroids reduce anaphylaxis severity or prevent biphasic reactions.

Introduction

Anaphylaxis is an acute, potentially life-threatening multisystem reaction caused by the sudden systemic release of preformed mediators from mast cells and basophils which include histamine, tryptase, chymase, heparin, histamine-releasing factor, and platelet-activating factor (PAF). Cellular activation also stimulates the production of lipid-derived newly formed mediators, such as prostaglandins and cysteinyl leukotrienes. These reactions are frequently, but not always, mediated by an immunologic mechanism involving two or more organs and/or are associated with hypotension or upper respiratory compromise. Other clinical manifestations include flushing, pruritus, urticaria, angioedema, shortness of breath, wheezing, nausea, vomiting, and diarrhea. Risk of death is mainly from cardiovascular collapse or asphyxiation caused by laryngeal edema. Drugs (nonsteroidal antiinflammatory drugs [NSAIDs]/antibiotics), foods, and Hymenoptera venom stings are the most common triggers; however any agent capable of inciting a sudden, systemic degranulation of mast cells can lead to anaphylaxis.

Various organizations have attempted to clarify the definition of anaphylaxis but with no consensus agreement. Experts from the

TABLE 1	Comorbidities and Risk Factors for the Development of Anaphylaxis

Age: infants are at risk because manifestations might not be detected; teenagers are at risk because of "risky behavior"; elderly are at risk because of medical comorbidities and increased use of medications such as β-blockers leading to more severe cardiovascular symptoms at presentation

Gender: anaphylaxis is more common overall in females

Drugs: medications may impact severity of symptoms and response to treatment (see Table 2)

Comorbid Conditions: asthma, other respiratory diseases (e.g., chronic obstructive pulmonary disease, interstitial lung disease), cardiovascular disease, mast cell disorder (e.g., systemic mastocytosis)

Route of Administration: oral antigens are less likely to trigger anaphylaxis than parenteral antigens

Geography: prescription rates for self-injectable epinephrine devices are greater in northern than in southern states; living in a rural environment may affect incidence

Atopy: risk factor for anaphylactic and anaphylactoid reactions in general

Exposure History: the longer the interval since previous antigen exposure, the less likely a reaction will occur; previous anaphylactic reaction

Other Factors: active infections (e.g., upper respiratory tract infection, fever), physical exertion, premenstrual status, delayed administration of epinephrine, substance abuse (impairs judgement and can diminish recognition of symptoms), mental illness not well controlled

TABLE 2	Concurrent Medications That May Impact Severity of Symptoms and Response to Treatment

Possibly put patient at risk for more serious, treatment resistant anaphylaxis*

- β-adrenergic blockers
- α-adrenergic blockers
- Angiotensin-converting enzyme (ACE) inhibitors
- Angiotensin II receptor blockers
- Some tricyclic antidepressants (e.g., amitriptyline)
- Monoamine oxidase inhibitors

Potentially affect recognition of anaphylaxis

- Sedatives, hypnotics, antidepressants, ethanol, recreational drugs

Exacerbate anaphylaxis symptoms by causing nonimmunologic mast cell activation

- Ethanol, opiates, nonsteroidal anti-inflammatory drugs

Evidence of impact for most of these medications are still controversial/debatable, and expert opinion continues to shift with regard to the safety of these medications in anaphylaxis, especially with regard to concurrent use during aeroallergen and venom immunotherapy. A recent systematic review and meta-analysis of studies that assess the influence of β-blockers and ACE inhibitors on anaphylaxis suggest that the quality of evidence showing that the use of these medications increases the severity of anaphylaxis is low owing to differences in the control of confounders arising from the concomitant presence of cardiovascular diseases

National Institute of Allergy and Infectious Disease (NIAID) and Food Allergy and Anaphylaxis Network (FAAN) met in 2005 and published diagnostic criteria for anaphylaxis. Controversy arose shortly thereafter with the World Allergy Organization (WAO) claiming that the published definition of anaphylaxis might exclude patients with clinical manifestations expressed by a single system only. Subsequent criteria published by Sampson et al. attempted to address this concern by adding single system caveats. Regardless of the continuing debate, the NIAID/FAAN criteria has been validated in real-world emergency room settings, establishing an accurate diagnosis of anaphylaxis with a sensitivity of 95% and a specificity of 71%.

Epidemiology

The prevalence of anaphylaxis in industrialized countries is estimated to range between 1.6% to 5.1%; however, rates seem to be increasing. In one study the majority (80.2%) of anaphylaxis cases were triggered by food, principally peanut and tree nut, indicating that increased rates of anaphylaxis might coincide with increasing rates of food allergy worldwide. Given increased prevalence rates, accurate recognition and management of anaphylactic episodes is of the utmost importance as a delay in treatment can lead to increased morbidity and mortality. In this regard, several consensus guidelines, including the American, European, and WAO guidelines, have been published to simplify this task.

Risk Factors

Anaphylactic reactions are becoming increasingly more common with an estimated 1500 fatalities/year caused by anaphylaxis in the United States. Comorbidities and concurrent medications may impact the severity of symptoms and response to treatment in patients experiencing anaphylaxis. Risk factors for the development of anaphylaxis and medications that may impact severity of symptoms and response to treatment are reviewed in Tables 1 and 2. Risk factors for fatal reactions include adolescence, a history of a previous anaphylactic reaction, allergy to peanut or tree nuts, history of asthma, absence of cutaneous symptoms, and delayed administration of epinephrine.

While rare and typically limited to hempseed ingestion, anaphylaxis to cannabis or marijuana has been increasingly reported as these products gain more traction in the medical community and through legalization. Multiple cannabis allergens have been sequenced, four of which are accepted by the WHO/IUIS Allergen Nomenclature Subcommittee (Can s 2, Can s 3, Can s 4, Can s 5). Allergic sensitization can result from inhaling, smoking, touching, and eating cannabis, with increased risk for those who work in the industrial manufacture of these products. Hempseed exposures can be inadvertent as it can be found hidden in foods and drinks, and there have been reports of cross-reactivity between marijuana and certain foods including cherry, tangerine, peach, tomato, and hazelnut. However, the importance and relevance of these allergens have not been well established.

Pathophysiology

Most anaphylactic reactions are mediated by immunoglobulin E (IgE); however, not all episodes can be attributed to this mechanism. The WAO uses the term "immunologic anaphylaxis" to describe IgE-mediated, IgG-mediated, and immune complex/complement-mediated reactions. "Nonimmunologic anaphylaxis" (previously referred to as anaphylactoid reactions) is caused by agents or events that induce sudden degranulation of mast cells or basophils without the involvement of immunoglobulins like IgE.

Prevention

Avoidance of the confirmed trigger is the best way to prevent recurrence of anaphylaxis. For foods, this means educating patients about reading food labels, informing family and friends about these reactions, and being vigilant about avoiding the food(s) when eating in public establishments. Other triggers are more difficult to avoid such as venomous stinging insects or not possible in the case of idiopathic anaphylaxis (IA). In rare instances, an infection may require treatment with an antibiotic known to cause anaphylaxis in a patient. If there are no equally efficacious alternatives (i.e., penicillin for syphilis), an allergist/immunologist may perform skin testing to penicillin major and if available, minor determinants to confirm the allergy, and if positive, perform penicillin desensitization. This procedure involves relatively rapid administration of increasing amounts of the antibiotic under carefully controlled conditions by trained personnel with emergency therapy readily available until the target dose is reached. Thus desensitization results in tolerance which allows the allergic patient to take the medication without a reaction.

Immunologic changes associated with immunotherapy are complicated, but the goal is to induce immune tolerance. The mechanism for inducing tolerance for different antigens is still poorly elucidated but is believed to occur by increasing regulatory T cells resulting in increased production of inhibitory cytokines like interleukin (IL)-10, transforming growth factor β (TGF-β), or both. IL-10 and TGF-β encourage the shift of antibody production from IgE toward the noninflammatory isotypes IgG4 and IgA, respectively. IL-10 is also involved in the reduction of proinflammatory cytokine release from mast cells, eosinophils, and T cells, as well as elicitation of tolerance in T cells by means of selective inhibition of the CD28 costimulatory pathway which effectively reduces lymphoproliferative responses to allergens. There also seems to be a shift in the immune response from a Th2 to a Th1 cytokine profile later in the immunotherapy course possibly mediated by the increased production of IL-12.

Long-term preventive measures include venom immunotherapy for Hymenoptera stinging insects (honey bee, wasp, yellow jacket, yellow hornet, white faced hornet) and food immunotherapy (oral, sublingual) for IgE-mediated food allergies. It is essential to recognize and manage poorly controlled comorbid conditions such as asthma and other respiratory diseases, cardiovascular disease, mastocytosis, and mast cell activation syndrome that may increase the risk for anaphylaxis. Administration of certain medications such as β-blockers and possibly angiotensin-converting enzyme (ACE) inhibitors (see Table 2) are associated with a greater risk for severe anaphylaxis by interfering with the therapeutic response to epinephrine and should be avoided if possible. This is especially true for the administration of therapeutics that place the patient at increased risk for anaphylaxis such as allergen immunotherapy (i.e., subcutaneous, sublingual, and venom immunotherapy).

Clinical Manifestations

Anaphylaxis is an acute multiorgan system reaction that generally begins within seconds to minutes but can be delayed occurring anywhere from 1 to 24 hours later after exposure to a trigger. The most common organ system involved is the skin or mucous membranes with >90% of patients presenting with some combination of pruritus, urticaria, and/or angioedema and erythema. Anaphylaxis, by nature, is unpredictable and heterogeneous in its presentation so it may be mild and resolve spontaneously or it may be severe and progress to significant respiratory or cardiovascular compromise. To help classify the severity of anaphylactic reactions, the WAO developed a universal 5-stage grading system. It was intended to more accurately assess when epinephrine should be administered during subcutaneous immunotherapy (SCIT), but has since been used to better classify all forms of systemic reactions. Each grade is based on the organ system involved defined as cutaneous, conjunctival, upper respiratory, lower respiratory, gastrointestinal, cardiovascular, or other, and the severity is based on clinical judgement (Table 3).

Anaphylaxis can present as a uniphasic response, biphasic response, or as being refractory to treatment, all of which need to be considered and recognized by the clinician evaluating these patients. Biphasic anaphylaxis is defined as a potentially life-threatening recurrence of symptoms after the resolution of the initial immediate anaphylactic episode without re-exposure to the causative agent. The delayed portion of the biphasic reaction typically occurs within 12 hours but has been reported to occur up to 72 hours after resolution of initial symptoms. Biphasic reactions have been reported to develop in up to 21% of anaphylactic episodes (all ages) and in up to 15% of children. Biphasic reactions seem to be associated with the severity of the initial anaphylactic episode. Rarely, the onset of anaphylaxis will be delayed beginning hours rather than minutes after exposure to the causative agent. This is especially true for red meat allergy, also called mammalian meat allergy or α-gal allergy. This condition is characterized by development of an IgE antibody directed against a mammalian oligosaccharide epitope, galactose-α-1,3-galactose ("α-gal") after a lone star tick bite which contains the α-gal protein. Patients typically do not develop symptoms until several hours (4 to 6 hours or even longer) after eating red meat.

TABLE 3 World Allergy Organization Subcutaneous Immunotherapy Systemic Reaction Grading System

Grade 1:
Symptom(s)/sign(s) of 1 organ system present
Cutaneous: generalized pruritus, urticaria, flushing, or sensation of heat or warmth
or
Angioedema (not laryngeal, tongue or uvular)
or
Upper respiratory: rhinitis (e.g., sneezing, rhinorrhea, nasal pruritus, and/or nasal congestion)
or
Throat-clearing (itchy throat)
or
Cough perceived to originate in the upper airway, not the lung, larynx, or trachea
or
Conjunctival: erythema, pruritus, or tearing
Other: nausea, metallic taste, or headache

Grade 2:
Symptom(s)/sign(s) of more than 1 organ system present
or
Lower respiratory: asthma: cough, wheezing, shortness of breath (e.g., less than 40% PEF or FEV1 drop, responding to an inhaled bronchodilator)
or
Gastrointestinal: abdominal cramps, vomiting, or diarrhea
or
Other: uterine cramps

Grade 3:
Lower respiratory: asthma (e.g., 40% PEF or FEV1 drop NOT responding to an inhaled bronchodilator)
or
Upper respiratory: laryngeal, uvula, or tongue edema with or without stridor

Grade 4:
Lower or upper respiratory: respiratory failure with or loss of consciousness
or
Cardiovascular: hypotension with or without loss of consciousness

Grade 5: Death

FEV1, forced expiratory volume in one second; *PEF*, peak expiratory flow.

Diagnosis

There is no universal agreement on the definition of anaphylaxis or the criteria for diagnosis. Table 4 summarizes the NIAID/FAAN criteria established in 2005 which continues to be generally accepted today.

While anaphylaxis remains primarily a clinical diagnosis, measurement of selected biomarkers has been used in research and clinical settings to assist in confirming this reaction. Plasma histamine, platelet activating factor, and serum tryptase can be obtained in certain situations; however, there are specific collection timeframes that need to be strictly adhered to for the result to be valid. Serum tryptase is the most commonly used biomarker to distinguish anaphylaxis from other conditions with a similar presentation (i.e., carcinoid syndrome, vasovagal reactions, seizures). Acute elevation of serum tryptase secondary to mast cell degranulation can occur through an IgE-mediated mechanism (i.e., venom and drug allergy) or direct degranulation of mast cells through a non-IgE mediated mechanism (i.e., NSAIDs or opiates). Tryptase can rise in serum or plasma as early as 15 minutes after clinical onset of anaphylaxis and should be collected between 30 minutes and 2 hours after symptom-onset if possible. Samples collected before or after this window are less accurate due to diminished sensitivity. Previous studies have questioned the sensitivity of serum tryptase in food-induced reactions; however a recent prospective study suggests that serum tryptase is a valuable tool in food allergic reactions as well

TABLE 4	Diagnostic Criteria for Anaphylaxis

Anaphylaxis is highly likely when any 1 of the following 3 criteria is met:

1. Sudden onset of symptoms (minutes to several hours) with involvement of skin and/or mucosa (e.g., generalized hives, itching or flushing, swollen lips/tongue/uvula), AND at least one of the following:
   • Respiratory symptoms or signs (e.g., shortness of breath, wheezing, cough, hypoxemia)
   • Hypotension or other symptoms of target-organ dysfunction (e.g., collapse, incontinence)

2. Sudden onset of 2 or more of the following after exposure to a likely allergen or other trigger for that patient (minutes to several hours):
   • Skin or mucosal membrane symptoms
   • Respiratory symptoms
   • Hypotension or other symptoms of target-organ dysfunction
   • Gastrointestinal symptoms such as abdominal pain or vomiting

3. Hypotension occurring acutely (minutes to several hours) after exposure to a known or established allergen for that patient. Hypotension is defined as the following:
   • Adults: Systolic blood pressure < 90 mm Hg, or a decrease > 30% from patient's baseline
   • Infants and children: Low systolic blood pressure (age-specific) or a decrease > 30% in systolic pressure

Modified from Weller KN, Hsieh FH: Anaphylaxis: highlights from the practice parameter update, *Cleve Clin J Med* 89(2):106–111, 2022.

and correlates with symptom severity. There is still debate on how serum tryptase can be used effectively in diagnosing anaphylaxis or mast cell activation with different studies quoting different cutoff values. Data on cutoffs specifically for food allergy are even harder to come by (Table 5).

According to this study comparing peak tryptase reaction levels at 2 hours with baseline is essential in correct interpretation, and a rise in tryptase of 30% above baseline is associated with a food allergic reaction. It is important to note that a normal serum tryptase level does not exclude anaphylaxis as the diagnosis.

A comprehensive clinical history of the events surrounding the reaction provides the most valuable data along with a detailed review of current medications, recently ingested foods and/or drugs, insect stings, and physical activities before or after the event. This approach oftentimes uncovers the appropriate trigger; however, in many cases no clear trigger can be identified. More accurate diagnostic testing can be utilized in some cases when the patient or clinician suspects a specific antigen as the triggering agent. Cutaneous or serum specific immunologic testing should only be performed to confirm or exclude a suspected agent under the supervision of an allergy specialist trained to interpret the meaning of the test results. Random testing to a large panel of foods or other allergens (i.e., venoms) without a specific history has a low diagnostic utility and can result in more questions rather than answers given the high rate of false positive reactions reported, especially for foods. If diagnostic skin testing is performed, it should be delayed for at least 3 to 4 weeks after the event to obtain an accurate test result in order to allow for recovery of skin mast cells. In certain cases there may be no validated cutaneous or in vitro test to detect the potential for an IgE-mediated reaction. In these circumstances, a graded challenge or provocation test can safely be carried out under the supervision of an experienced allergist in a setting that is fully equipped to respond to any potential medical emergency including anaphylaxis. Unlike desensitization, graded challenges do not work by modifying the allergic response to the agent. Therefore patients who tolerate a graded challenge is an indication that they are not allergic to the specific agent administered.

Differential Diagnosis

Anaphylaxis can sometimes be difficult to recognize because it can mimic other conditions and is variable in its presentation. Common conditions that mimic anaphylaxis are included in Table 6. It is beyond the scope of this review to discuss in detail clonal and nonclonal mast cell disorders, but these conditions should be considered in a patient presenting with anaphylaxis, especially in the context of a stinging insect venom allergic reaction.

Therapy (or Treatment)

Prompt administration of intramuscular epinephrine is the gold-standard first-line medication for the treatment of anaphylaxis. Delay in treatment with epinephrine has been associated with increased morbidity and mortality. Epinephrine autoinjectors (EAI [Auvi-Q (kaléo, Richmond, VA), EpiPen Jr, EpiPen (Mylan Inc, Canonsberg, PA)]) are commercially available in three different concentrations in the United States: 0.1 mg (7.5 to 14 kg body weight), 0.15 mg (15 to 30 kg), and 0.3 mg (>30 kg). Epinephrine can be administered intramuscularly (preferred) or subcutaneously every 5 to 15 minutes but can be given more frequently if deemed appropriate. The recommended adult dose of 1:1000 (1 mg/mL) epinephrine is 0.2 to 0.5 mg (mL), whereas the pediatric dose is 0.01 mg/kg (0.01 mL/kg/dose of 1 mg/mL solution), with a maximum dose of 0.3 mg. If not administered through an autoinjector, the epinephrine dose should be drawn up using a 1 mL syringe and injected intramuscularly into the mid-outer thigh. A higher dose (e.g., 0.5 mL) within the recommended dose range should be considered in patients with severe anaphylaxis.

Patients with severe reactions can have massive fluid shifts that can occur rapidly due to increased vascular permeability which require aggressive fluid resuscitation. Additional treatments are considered supportive and include the addition of H1 and H2 antihistamines for itching, urticaria, and gastrointestinal complaints; albuterol for bronchospasm; oxygen; and placing the patient in the Trendelenburg position. Corticosteroids are not useful for the acute treatment of anaphylaxis since these medications take 4 to 6 hours to reach maximum effectiveness. Despite this, corticosteroids are often used in the emergency treatment of anaphylaxis under the assumption that these medications may be beneficial in preventing biphasic reactions. A comprehensive literature review of 31 studies recently reported that biphasic reactions were more likely to occur in moderate to severe anaphylaxis or when anaphylaxis was not treated with timely epinephrine. Due to the potential adverse effects of corticosteroids and lack of compelling evidence demonstrating an effective role in reducing anaphylaxis severity or preventing biphasic anaphylaxis, the authors do not advocate their routine use for treatment of anaphylaxis. The appropriate observation period after an anaphylactic event often depends on the severity and duration of the initial reaction as well as the patient's response to treatment, previous reaction history, associated comorbidities, and access to medical care. Patients with moderate to severe anaphylaxis should be observed for a minimum of 4 to 8 hours; however, milder presentations can be observed for a shorter time period. All patients with a history of anaphylaxis should be given a prescription for an EAI along with instructions for self-administration and an allergy action plan specific to their trigger.

Monitoring

The main tenants of anaphylaxis management and prevention are simple in theory but difficult in practice. Complete avoidance of the triggering agent provides protection from future episodes however, accidental exposures can occur, especially for food induced anaphylaxis. Other conditions like IA occur randomly with no known triggers making avoidance impossible. While episodes of IA tend to decline in frequency over time, patients experiencing more frequent attacks often benefit from daily prophylactic treatment with H1 and/or H2 antihistamines, leukotriene receptor antagonist (LTRA), and oral prednisone as needed. In refractory cases omalizumab (Xolair)[1] has been shown to be effective as well.

---

[1] Not FDA approved for this indication.

TABLE 5	Proposed Optimal Cutoffs for Tryptase Elevations Signifying Mast Cell Activation or Anaphylaxis	
AUTHOR	**CRITERIA FOR TRYPTASE INCREASE**	**CRITERIA IDENTIFY**
Phadia AB, 2008	Values above 11.4 ng/mL (upper 95th percentile)	Raised tryptase
Valent et al., 2012	20% plus 2 ng/mL over baseline level	Mast cell activation
Enrique et al., 1999	Levels >8.23 ng/mL	Anaphylaxis
Brown et al., 2009	Increase of 2 µg/L	Anaphylaxis
Egner et al, 2016	Threshold increment of 20%	Mast cell mediator release
Wongkaewpothong et al., 2014	Delta tryptase 0.8 µg/L	Anaphylaxis

TABLE 6	Differential Diagnosis of Anaphylaxis
SYSTEM	**DIFFERENTIAL DIAGNOSIS**
Cutaneous	acute generalized urticaria, acute angioedema, ACE inhibitor angioedema, hereditary/acquired angioedema, carcinoid syndrome, postmenopause, Red man syndrome
Cardiac	vasovagal syncope, myocardial infarction, arrhythmia, shock
Respiratory	asthma or COPD exacerbation, vocal cord dysfunction syndrome, laryngospasm, pulmonary embolism, inhaled foreign body (infants/toddlers)
Psychological	panic attacks or acute anxiety, Munchausen syndrome
Other	mastocytosis and mast cell activation syndrome, pheochromocytoma, capillary leak syndrome, scombroid fish ingestion, hypoadrenergic or hyperadrenergic paroxysmal orthostatic tachycardia (POTS), hereditary alpha tryptasemia

ACE, Angiotensin-converting enzyme; *COPD,* chronic obstructive pulmonary disorder.

Carrying an EAI at all times provides patients with quick access to life-saving treatment; however, adherence has historically been poor. The predicament of poor adherence to medical treatment is a well-recognized problem; however in anaphylaxis the consequences of nonadherence can be fatal. One study from 2008 demonstrated that 48% of children prescribed an EAI did not have the device available at school, and of those with the medication on site, 78% of the autoinjectors were kept in the nurse's office or by another administrator not in close proximity to the child. Real-world data from a 2018 survey also demonstrated a poor level of adherence in patients and caregivers to anaphylaxis treatment guidelines which recommend carrying more than one EAI at all times. Most (82%) did not carry two EAIs at all times, mainly due to keeping one EAI in another location; 84% respondents said they kept at least one EAI at home; however, few patients and caregivers kept more than one. More than half of the respondents (64%) said they received counseling with an emphasis on always having one EAI and keeping another in a different location, but only 27% reported counseling that emphasized always having two EAIs available. It is important to recognize that a second epinephrine dose may be required in 16% to 36% of patients; therefore a more concerted effort should be made by physicians to properly educate patients and caregivers on the importance of following standard treatment guidelines. According to a 2018 study, only 26% of milk-allergic children in the U.S. had a current EAI prescription, the lowest reported rate among the top nine food allergies.

While poor patient adherence deserves some of the blame, evidence suggests that prescribers are equally responsible for this omission. Among 208 patients identified with anaphylaxis, 64.4% were seen in the emergency department and discharged home, but only 36.6% were prescribed an EAI, and only 31.3% were referred to an allergy specialist for further evaluation. Another retrospective cross-sectional descriptive study of patients 21 years old or younger who received care for anaphylaxis reported that EAIs were prescribed to only 63%, and referral to an allergist was recommended to only 33%. Both of these studies suggest that emergency department physicians may be missing an important opportunity to empower patients with the ability to self-administer treatment for a recurrent episode and to prevent future anaphylactic reactions by not referring patients for specialized follow-up care. Finally, a comprehensive analysis of 10,184 anaphylaxis incidents using the European anaphylaxis register revealed that in the early 2000s 27.1% of patients with anaphylaxis treated by a health professional received epinephrine while only 14.7% of lay or self-treated cases were treated with an EAI. Progress was tracked over the next decade and epinephrine administration from a health professional almost doubled to 30.6% in 2015–2017 but no significant change was found in the lay emergency respondents group.

Failing to follow published guidelines for the treatment of anaphylaxis is another barrier to timely and appropriate treatment. Oftentimes antihistamines are used as first-line agents in the treatment of an anaphylactic reaction and is the most common reason providers report for not using epinephrine, leaving patients at increased risk for life-threatening sequelae. It should be reiterated that antihistamines have no effect on arresting true anaphylactic reactions and should only be used for symptomatic relief of associated pruritus and urticaria.

Reasons for patients and caregivers not to carry or use their EAIs or to delay administration are multifaceted and complex. Teenagers and young adults are at highest risk of fatal anaphylaxis-related reactions due to delayed epinephrine injection. Cost can be a difficult barrier for patients to overcome either related to having no insurance, high insurance co-pays, and/or deductibles. The cost of the best-known autoinjector, EpiPen, made headline news in recent years when pricing rose to more than $600/2-pak by 2016. Bad press followed by public outcry led the manufacturer to produce a generic version for half the cost. Potential barriers for not carrying an EAI are summarized in Table 7.

Since many patients who have been prescribed an EAI do not routinely carry one, and emergency rooms fail to prescribe them, it is essential that life-saving EAIs be readily available in community spaces and public venues. To improve access to life-saving treatment, there is an increasing effort to distribute nonspecific EAIs to public locations including schools, parks, pools, airports, public venues, and shopping malls. In 2013, President Obama signed the "School Access to Emergency Epinephrine Act," which encouraged, but did not require, all states to adopt stock epinephrine regulations for schools. Several drug companies like Mylan Specialty (EpiPen-4Schools) and Kaléo ("Q Your School") are providing free stock EAIs for schools to help improve access to epinephrine in the event a person experiences anaphylaxis in an academic setting. According to a recent EpiPen4Schools survey sponsored by Mylan Specialty, in each academic year, one in every six U.S. schools will have a student or staff member experience anaphylaxis. About 1140 episodes of anaphylaxis occurred across 6574 U.S. schools with most (89.5%) incidents involving students. More reactions were seen in high school students, who tend to be at higher risk, and food was the trigger for a majority (60%) of the reactions. Other triggers include

| TABLE 7 | Reasons for Patients and Caregivers Not to Carry or Use Their Epinephrine Autoinjectors or to Delay Administration |

- Never prescribed
- Cost
- Inconvenience
- Lack of perception of need of the medication
  - many do not use device for years so may not think it is essential or forget how to use it properly
- Poor knowledge of appropriate use
- Lack of familiarity with different brands of autoinjectors
- Mistakenly believe EAI might be available for emergency use in many public spaces
- History of mild allergic reaction
  - might think they are not at risk for a potentially fatal reaction
- Emotional/behavioral
  - embarrassment, feeling different
- Having been OK after a past reaction without treatment
- Wait for antihistamine to work
- Rely on other medications
- Don't want to go to the emergency department
- Needle phobia

EAI, Epinephrine autoinjectors.

environmental, medication, and insect stings or bites; however, 22% of severe reactions were from unknown triggers. EAIs (both stock and personal) were used to treat 77% of anaphylactic events reported. Overall this survey revealed that not only are anaphylactic events a relatively common occurrence in schools, but also that the risk extends beyond those with diagnosed allergies. A quarter of the individuals who experienced anaphylaxis in a school setting had no known allergies. The previously stated data tend to further support the need for stock EAIs in schools, and training for staff on when and how to use them.

With increased availability of epinephrine in public settings there needs to be a focus on increased educational initiatives for the people administering life-saving treatment. Just having epinephrine available does not improve outcomes during an anaphylactic event. Healthcare professionals, first responders, and the general public need to be able to recognize classic anaphylactic symptoms and know how to properly initiate treatment. Unfortunately, when these groups are surveyed, anaphylaxis is still underrecognized and undertreated (Table 8).

Recent anaphylaxis guidelines published in the 2020 Practice Parameter Update answered five PICO questions using GRADE methodology. The first question addressed the risk of developing a biphasic reaction related to anaphylaxis and what is an appropriate observation time in the ED to monitor for a biphasic reaction. The recommendation was to take the severity of the initial anaphylaxis reaction and/or the use of one or more doses of epinephrine into account in determining the risk for a biphasic reaction and to have an extended observation period in patients considered high risk for a biphasic reaction. The second question addressed the treatment of an anaphylaxis reaction with antihistamines and glucocorticoids to prevent a biphasic reaction and recommended against this approach as epinephrine is considered more effective in this regard. The third and fourth questions asked whether patients with a history of chemotherapeutic or radiocontrast reactions should be treated with antihistamines and glucocorticoids to prevent subsequent reactions. With respect to chemotherapeutic agents this treatment was recommended; however, for radiocontrast reactions it was not, as evidence suggests using a low or iso-osmolar agent is sufficient for preventing a subsequent reaction. Finally the fifth question asked whether pretreatment with antihistamines and glucocorticoids should be used for patients undergoing rush allergen immunotherapy and the recommendation was in favor of this approach. It is important to emphasize that all of these recommendations were conditional, and the rating of evidence was very low, emphasizing the need for well designed studies to investigate best practices for the management of anaphylaxis.

| TABLE 8 | Are Healthcare Professionals and First Responders Able to Appropriately Recognize and Treat Anaphylaxis? |

SURVEY	RESULTS
1114 pediatric emergency medicine physicians	• 93.5% correctly identified epinephrine as the treatment of choice for anaphylaxis • 66.9% used the intramuscular (IM) route of administration • 37.4% admitted affected patients for observation • Many discharge patients home after an abbreviated period
468 pediatricians (41%) responded to the survey	• 70% agreed that the clinical scenario was consistent with anaphylaxis • 72% chose to administer epinephrine • 56% of respondents agreed with both the diagnosis of anaphylaxis and treating with epinephrine • 70% did not recognize that a 30-min observation period after anaphylaxis was too short
7822 physicians, allied health, medical students, and other health professionals	• 80% of responders correctly identified the case of anaphylaxis with prominent skin and respiratory symptoms • 55% correctly recognized the case without skin symptoms as anaphylaxis • 23% of responders correctly selected risk factors for anaphylaxis

3537 paramedics	• 98.9% correctly recognized a case of classic anaphylaxis
	• 2.9% correctly identified the atypical presentation
	• 46.2% identified epinephrine as the initial drug of choice
	• 38.9% chose the IM route of administration
	  • 60.5% identified the deltoid as the preferred location
	  • 11.6% correctly identified the thigh
	• ~98% were confident they could recognize and manage anaphylaxis
	  • 39.5% carry EAIs on response vehicles
	• 95.4% were confident they could use an EAI
	  • 36.2% stated that there were contraindications to epinephrine administration in anaphylactic shock

EAI, Epinephrine autoinjectors.

In general, good clinical practice requires consideration of risk versus benefit of treatment and should take into account patient preference when appropriate.

Management of Complications

In general, anaphylactic reactions resolve without any major complications. Even though the prevalence rates of anaphylaxis seem to be increasing, fatal outcomes are rare, making up less than 1% of total mortality risk. In older patients, cardiovascular complications like atrial fibrillation and myocardial infarction can arise during anaphylaxis, but these events are also infrequent.

COVID-19 Vaccines and Anaphylaxis

Since the onset of the pandemic caused by severe acute respiratory syndrome coronavirus 2 (SARS-CoV-2), three vaccines have been utilized in the United States to help curb the spread of this extremely infectious virus. The Pfizer-BioNTech and Moderna COVID-19 vaccines are messenger RNA vaccines, also called mRNA vaccines, and the Johnson & Johnson/Janssen COVID-19 vaccine is a viral vector vaccine. As with all vaccines, there is a low but recognizable risk of anaphylaxis. Given the circumstances with which these vaccinations were released, the safety and efficacy of these novel products have been under intense scrutiny since their implementation and have been monitored closely by the national Vaccine Adverse Event Reporting System (VAERS). Soon after vaccination programs were started, cases of anaphylaxis following administration of the Moderna and Pfizer-BioNTech vaccines began to be reported. Early accounts in the United States, gathered through January 18, 2021, demonstrated low risks of anaphylaxis for both vaccines: 4.7 cases/million for the Pfizer-BioNTech vaccine and 2.5 cases/million for the Moderna vaccine. Continued safety monitoring of all three COVID-19 vaccines has confirmed that anaphylaxis following vaccination is a rare event, with a recent study ranking COVID-19 vaccines fifth in reported anaphylaxis rates (10.67 cases/106 doses) behind rabies, tick-borne encephalitis, measles-mumps-rubella-varicella, and human papillomavirus vaccines (70.77, 20, 19.8, and 13.65 cases per 106 vaccine doses, respectively). The CDC's current estimate for anaphylaxis rate in the United States is approximately 5 people/million vaccinated. Although rates of anaphylaxis to COVID-19 vaccines are low, locations administering these vaccines are required to adhere to CDC guidelines, including screening recipients for contraindications and precautions, having necessary supplies and staff members available to manage anaphylaxis, implementing recommended postvaccination observation periods, and immediately treating suspected anaphylaxis with intramuscular epinephrine injection.

Conclusion

Anaphylaxis is a common medical condition affecting both adult and pediatric populations and its incidence and prevalence continue to increase. Prompt recognition and treatment with epinephrine administered in a timely manner remains the mainstay of treatment for anaphylaxis. Preventive measures including patient education, immunotherapy when appropriate, antigen avoidance, and optimal management of comorbid conditions is important in preventing recurrences. There is a concerning lack of knowledge and preparedness for management of anaphylaxis at all care levels that needs to be better addressed.

Readings

Brown SGA, Blackman KE, Heddle RJ: Can serum mast cell tryptase help diagnose anaphylaxis? *Emerg Med Australas* 16:120–124, 2004.

Campbell RL, Kelso JM: Anaphylaxis: Acute diagnosis. Walls RM, ed. UpToDate. Waltham, MA: UpToDate Inc. http://www.uptodate.com (Accessed on December 04, 2018.)

CDC COVID-19 Response Team; Food and Drug Administration: Allergic reactions including anaphylaxis after receipt of the first dose of Moderna COVID-19 vaccine—United States, December 21, 2020-January 10, 2021, *MMWR Morb Mortal Wkly Rep* 70(4):125–129, 2021.

Centers for Disease Control and Prevention: Interim clinical considerations for use of COVID-19 vaccines currently authorized in the United States. Updated March 5, 2021. Accessed March 8, 2021. https://www.cdc.gov/vaccines/covid-19/info-by-product/clinical-considerations.html#:~:text=CDC%20considers%20a%20history%20of,of%20the%20COVID%2D19%20vaccine.

Centers for Disease Control and Prevention: Checklist of best practices for vaccination clinics held at satellite, temporary, or off-site locations. Updated August 18, 2020. https://www.cdc.gov/flu/business/hosting-vaccination-clinic.htm. Accessed 8 March 2021.

Commins SP, Jerath MR, Cox K, et al: Delayed anaphylaxis to alpha-gal, an oligosaccharide in mammalian meat, *Allergol Int* 65:16, 2016.

Dua S, Dowey J, Foley L: Diagnostic value of tryptase in food allergic reactions: a prospective study of 160 adult peanut challenges, *J Allergy Clin Immunol Pract* 6(5):1692–1698, 2018 Sep - Oct.

Egner W, Sargur R, Shrimpton A, et al: 17-year experience in perioperative anaphylaxis 1998-2015: harmonizing optimal detection of mast cell mediator release, *Clin Exp Allergy* 46:1465–1473, 2016.

Enrique E, García-Ortega P, Sotorra O, Gaig P, Richart C: Usefulness of UniCAP-Tryptase fluoroimmunoassay in the diagnosis of anaphylaxis, *Allergy* 54:602–606, 1999.

Grabenhenrich LB, Dölle S, Rueff F, et al: Epinephrine in severe allergic reactions: the European anaphylaxis register, *J Allergy Clin Immunol Pract* 6(6):1898–1906, 2018 Nov - Dec.

Greenhawt M, Abrams EM, Shaker M, et al: The risk of allergic reaction to SARS-CoV-2 vaccines and recommended evaluation and management: a systematic review, meta-analysis, GRADE assessment, and international consensus approach, *J Allergy Clin Immunol Pract* 10(9):3546–3567, 2021.

Grossman SL, Baumann BM, Garcia Peña BM, et al: Anaphylaxis knowledge and practice preferences of pediatric emergency medicine physicians: a national survey, *J Pediatr* 163(3):841–846, 2013.

Jackson B, Cleto E, Jeimy S: An emerging allergen: cannabis sativa allergy in a climate of recent legalization, *Allergy Asthma Clin Immunol* 16:53, 2020.

Jacobsen RC, Toy S, Bonham AJ, et al: Anaphylaxis knowledge among paramedics: results of a national survey, *Prehosp Emerg Care* 16(4):527–534, 2012.

Krugman SD, Chiaramonte DR, Matsui EC: Diagnosis and management of food-induced anaphylaxis: a national survey of pediatricians, *Pediatrics* 118(3):e554–e560, 2006.

Lee S, Bellolio MF, Hess EP, et al: Time of onset and predictors of biphasic anaphylactic reactions: a systematic review and meta-analysis, *J Allergy Clin Immunol Pract* 3:408, 2015.

Lieberman P, Nicklas RA, Randolph C, et al: Anaphylaxis--a practice parameter update 2015, *Ann Allergy Asthma Immunol* 115:341, 2015.

Maltezou HC, Anastassopoulou C, Hatziantoniou S, et al: Anaphylaxis rates associated with COVID-19 vaccines are comparable to those of other vaccines, *Vaccine* 40(2):183–186, 2022.Phadia AB: *ImmunoCAP Tryptase. Directions for Use*, Uppsala, Sweden: Phadia AB; 2008.

Shaker MS, Wallace DV, Golden DB, et al: Anaphylaxis - a 2020 Practice Parameter Update, Systematic Review and GRADE Analysis, *J Allergy Clin Immunol* 145(4):1082–1123, 2020.

Shimabukuro TT, Cole M, Su JR: Reports of anaphylaxis after receipt of mRNA COVID-19 vaccines in the US—December 14, 2020-January 18, 2021, *JAMA*. Published online February 12, 2021.

Shimabukuro T, Nair N: Allergic reactions including anaphylaxis after receipt of the first dose of Pfizer-BioNTech COVID-19 vaccine, *JAMA*. Published online January 21, 2021.

Simons FE, Frew AJ, Ansotegui IJ, et al: Risk assessment in anaphylaxis: current and future approaches, *J Allergy Clin Immunol* 120(suppl 1):S2–S24, 2007.

Skypala IJ, Jeimy S, Brucker H, et al: Cannabis-related allergies: an international overview and consensus recommendations, *Allergy* 77(7):2038–2052, 2022.

Tejedor-Alonso MA, Farias-Aquino E, Pérez-Fernández E, et al: Relationship between anaphylaxis and use of beta-blockers and angiotensin-converting enzyme inhibitors: a systematic review and meta-analysis of observational studies, *J Allergy Clin Immunol Pract* 7(3):879–897, 2019 Mar.

Turner PJ, Jerschow E, Umasunthar T: Fatal anaphylaxis: mortality rate and risk factors, *J Allergy Clin Immunol Pract* 5(5):1169–1178, 2017.

Valent P, Akin C, Arock M, et al: Definitions, criteria and global classification of mast cell disorders with special reference to mast cell activation syndromes: a consensus proposal, *Int Arch Allergy Immunol* 157:215–225, 2012.

Wang J, Young MC, Nowak-Węgrzyn A: International survey of knowledge of food-induced anaphylaxis, *Pediatr Allergy Immunol* 25(7):644–650, 2014.

DRUG HYPERSENSITIVITY REACTIONS

Method of
Miriam Chan, PharmD; Ann M. Aring, MD; and Kristen Rundell, MS, MD

CURRENT DIAGNOSIS

- Detailed history should include past medical history; current diagnosis; previous and current medication use, including over-the-counter drugs and herbals as well as other nonprescribed medications; duration of the medication use; any similar reactions in the past.
- Physical examination should include vitals, temperature, and skin examination for rash.
- Laboratory testing should be conducted based on symptoms that may include complete blood count (CBC) with differential, eosinophils, sedimentation rate, liver enzymes, international normalized ratio (INR), C-reactive protein (CRP), and diagnostic skin biopsy or testing.

CURRENT THERAPY

- For life-threatening anaphylaxis reaction, start basic life support using pneumonic ACB (airway, compression, breathing) and give epinephrine immediately.
- Discontinue the offending drug if medically possible. Try drug substitution if warranted.
- An alternative option is to reduce the dose or frequency of the drug.
- Start symptomatic treatment based on the type of reaction and the offending medication.
- Some reactions may respond to treatment with antihistamines, H_2 blockers, or steroids.

TABLE 1 Classification of Drug Hypersensitivity Reactions

TYPE	MECHANISM	CLINICAL FEATURES	TIMING OF REACTIONS	EXAMPLES
Type 1 (IgE mediated)	Drug-IgE complex binds to mast cells	Urticaria, angioedema, bronchospasm, pruritus, GI symptoms, anaphylaxis	Immediate (minutes to hours after drug exposure, depending on the route of administration)	β-lactam antibiotic
Type II (cytotoxic)	Specific IgG or IgM antibodies directed at drug-hapten–coated cells	Hemolytic anemia, neutropenia, thrombocytopenia	Variable	Penicillin (hemolytic anemia), heparin (thrombocytopenia)
Type III (immune complex)	Antigen-antibody complexes	Serum sickness, vasculitis, drug fever	1–3 weeks after drug exposure	Penicillin (serum sickness), sulfonamides (vasculitis), azathioprine (drug fever)
Type IV (delayed, cell mediated)	Activation and expansion of drug-specific T cell	Prominent skin findings: Contact dermatitis, morbilliform eruptions	2–7 days after exposure	Topical antihistamine, penicillin, sulfonamides

Epidemiology

Drug hypersensitivity reactions are one of the many different types of adverse drug reactions (ADRs). ADRs are common, yet the more severe reactions have been estimated to cause 3% to 6% of hospital admissions. More than 100,000 deaths annually are caused by serious ADRs, making these reactions one of the leading causes of death in the United States. Early detection of all ADRs can potentially improve patient outcomes and lower health care costs.

Classifications

An ADR is a broad term that refers to any predictable or unpredictable reaction to a medication. A predictable (type A) reaction is dose dependent and is related to the known pharmacologic properties of the drug. Predictable reactions account for about 80% of all ADRs. An example of a type A reaction is gastritis that results from taking nonsteroidal antiinflammatory drugs (NSAIDs). The remaining 20% of ADRs are caused by unpredictable (type B) reactions. Type B reactions occur in susceptible individuals. These are hypersensitivity reactions that are different from the pharmacologic actions of the drug; they are results of interactions between the drug and the individual human immune system. Type B reactions can be further divided into drug intolerance, drug idiosyncrasy, drug allergy (immunologically medicated), and pseudoallergic reactions (anaphylactoid reactions). This chapter will focus on these type B drug hypersensitivity reactions.

Pathophysiology

Several mechanisms may play a role in the underlying etiology of immunologic drug reactions. The Gell and Coombs classification system was the original system to describe four predominant immune mechanisms. These four reaction types are listed as type I reactions (IgE medicated), type II reactions (cytotoxic), type III reactions (immune complex), and type IV reactions (delayed, cell mediated). Table 1 provides a detailed description of this classification. Type I and IV reactions are more common than type II and III reactions. Most drugs cause one type of reaction, whereas certain drugs, such as penicillin, can induce all four types of reactions.

The Gell and Coombs classification has recently been revised to reflect the functional heterogeneity of T cells. Under the new system, type IV reactions are further subclassified into four categories: IVa (macrophage activation), IVb (eosinophils), IVc (CD4+ or CD8+ T cells), and IVd (neutrophils). Nevertheless, many common hypersensitivity reactions cannot be classified in this system because of the lack of knowledge of their immune mechanism or a mixed mechanism.

A new concept of drug interaction with immune receptors has recently been developed by Pichler and colleagues. It is called the *p-i concept* (pharmacologic interaction with immune receptors). In this concept, a drug binds noncovalently to a T-cell receptor and stimulates an immune response, which can cause inflammatory reactions of different types. The stimulation of the T cell is enhanced by the additional interaction with the major histocompatibility complex molecule. This is direct stimulation of memory and effector T cells, and no sensitization is required. The skin has a high concentration of effector memory T cells, which can be rapidly stimulated by antigen penetration. The skin also possesses a dense network of dendritic cells that act as antigen-presenting cells and increase hypersensitivity reactions. As a result, clinical symptoms by p-i drugs may appear more rapidly. Some severe reactions—such as Stevens-Johnson syndrome (SJS), toxic epidermal necrolysis (TEN), the drug rash with eosinophilia and systemic symptoms (DRESS) syndrome, or hypersensitivity syndrome—are believed to be p-i related. Examples are abacavir (Ziagen) hypersensitivity syndrome and SJS/TEN from carbamazepine (Tegretol).

Risk Factors for Hypersensitivity Drug Reactions

The chemical structure and molecular weight of the drug may help predict the type of hypersensitivity reaction. Larger drugs with greater structural complexity are more likely to be immunogenic. However, drugs with small molecular weight (< 1000 Da) can elicit hypersensitivity reactions by coupling with carrier proteins to form hapten-carrier complexes. Other drug-related factors include the dose, route of administration, duration of treatment, repetitive exposure to the drug, and concurrent illness. Topical and intravenous drug administrations are more likely to cause hypersensitivity reactions than are oral medications.

Patient risk factors include age, female gender, HIV infection or immunocompromised, atopy, specific genetic polymorphisms, previous drug hypersensitivity reactions, and inherent predisposition to react to multiple unrelated drugs.

Clinical Manifestations

Drug hypersensitivity reactions can manifest in a great variety of clinical symptoms and diseases. While some reactions are mild and often unnoticed, others, such as anaphylaxis, can be severe and even fatal. Dermatologic symptoms are the most common physical manifestation of allergic drug reactions. Drug hypersensitivity reactions can also affect various internal organs, causing diseases such as hepatitis, nephritis, and pneumonitis. The noncutaneous physical findings are generally nonspecific and may not be helpful and even delay the diagnosis and management decisions.

Dermatologic Symptoms

The most common allergic drug reactions affect the skin and can cause a variety of different exanthems. The most common skin reaction is the classic "drug rash," which is a morbilliform eruption originating on the trunk. Other dermatologic symptoms include urticaria, angioedema, acne, bullous eruptions, fixed drug eruptions, erythema multiforme, lupus erythematosus, photosensitivity, psoriasis, purpura, vasculitis, and pruritus. The most severe forms of cutaneous drug reactions are Stevens-Johnson syndrome (SJS), toxic epidermal necrolysis (TEN), and drug rash with eosinophilia and systemic symptoms (DRESS) syndrome.

Stevens-Johnson Syndrome

SJS is a systemic disorder that has cutaneous manifestations. SJS was previously thought to be synonymous with erythema multiforme major. There are now criteria that separate the two disorders. In contrast to erythema multiforme, the target lesions associated with SJS have only two rings. The inner ring may have urticaria, pustules, or necrotic lesions surrounded by macular erythema. It is a T-cell–mediated toxic reaction to the basement membrane of the epidermal cells. There is massive and widespread apoptosis, for which there are several associated cytokines. The recent theories suggest that there are two pathways, one that consists of granule-medicated exocytosis (perforin and granzyme B), and one that consists of Fas-Fas ligand interaction associated apoptosis for the keratinocytes. More recent data suggest that granulysin, which is a cationic cytolytic protein released by T lymphocytes, may play a role as well.

Interestingly, HLA genotype may predispose patients to SJS or TEN. Those patients with the HLA-B1502 found among the Han Chinese population may be associated with increased risk for developing SJS/TEN and use of carbamazepine.

SJS and TEN are on the same continuum. The definition of epidermal detachment and desquamation of epidermal cells is less than 10% of the body surface area for SJS and more than 30% for TEN. There is an overlapping diagnosis of SJS/TEN for the 10% to 30% category. To help differentiate from other ADRs, there is often a prodromal period in which a patient may have a cough and a fever. The lesions may occur up to 4 weeks after exposure to the drug. In addition, the lesions may be limited to the trunk; however, they more commonly involve the palmar surface of the hands and the dorsum of the feet, as well as the mucous membranes.

The most common drug classes associated with SJS and TENs are sulfonamides, cephalosporins, imidazole agents, and oxicam derivatives. Drugs such as carbamazepine, phenytoin (Dilantin), valproic acid (Depakote), lamotrigine (Lamictal), allopurinol (Zyloprim), nevirapine (Viramune), peramivir (Rapivab), and quinolones have been reported to cause SJS/TEN. In a retrospective chart review of 64 patients who had a diagnosis of SJS/TEN, Miliszewski et al. identified allopurinol as the single most common offending agent (20% of cases). According to the US Food and Drug Administration (FDA) Safety Alerts in 2013, acetaminophen has been associated with SJS, TEN, and acute generalized exanthematous pustulosis (AGEP). The evidence supporting causality primarily comes from a small number of cases reported in the medical literature.

The treatment is immediate cessation of the culprit drug and symptomatic treatment. Glucocorticoids are controversial and depend on the course and extent of the disease.

Toxic Epidermal Necrolysis

As previously stated, TEN is the cell-mediated disorder that involves more than 30% of the body surface. This is the more-severe form of the ADR: the mortality rates may be as high as 50%, mostly from sepsis. Patients are usually admitted to the burn unit for electrolyte and infection management. Glucocorticoids are contraindicated. There have been mixed results using IV immunoglobulin (IVIG)[1] in these patients. The IVIG is believed to inhibit the Fas-Fas ligand, which is the underlying mechanism for the basement membrane separation.

Drug Rash with Eosinophilia and Systemic Symptoms

DRESS syndrome or drug-induced hypersensitivity syndrome (DIHS) is a rare, life-threatening drug-induced reaction with a mortality rate of 10%. Therefore it is important to recognize the signs and symptoms early to initiate treatment. Most patients will have fever, lymphadenopathy (75%), eosinophilia, and an erythematous morbilliform rash on the face and body in addition to liver and multiorgan damage. The symptoms can occur 2 to 6

weeks after the drug administration. There are many drugs that can cause DRESS syndrome such as allopurinol, sulfonamides, and psychotropic medications. Based on literature review, DRESS syndrome is increasingly being recognized by psychiatrists. Carbamazepine is the most frequently reported etiology; however, DRESS syndrome is also seen with lamotrigine, phenytoin, valproate, and phenobarbital. The treatment is drug withdrawal, systemic corticosteroids, topical treatment for lesions, and supportive care, often in the ICU or burn unit.

Acute Generalized Exanthematous Pustulosis

Acute generalized exanthematous pustulosis (AGEP) is a rare ADR that presents as a fever and small nonfollicular pustules on a widespread erythematous background. AGEP may closely mimic pustular psoriasis clinically. The presence of acanthuses and papillomatosis and a personal or family history of psoriasis favor a diagnosis of pustular psoriasis. Exposure to medication, especially antibiotics with a short latency from the initiation of the drug, favors AGEP. The eruption usually occurs within 24 hours of the initiation of the drug, and healing occurs quickly after the discontinuation of the drug. Lesions heal within 2 weeks of discontinuation without scarring. The exact mechanism of drug-specific T lymphocytes is unknown, yet IL-3 and IL-8 may be the trigger for neutrophil-activating cytokines in the skin.

Acute Interstitial Nephritis

Acute interstitial nephritis (AIN) is an important cause of acute kidney injury (AKI). More than two thirds of AIN cases are caused by drug hypersensitivity reactions. Drugs most commonly associated with AIN include antibiotics (particularly β-lactam, fluoroquinolones, and rifampicin), NSAIDs, proton pump inhibitors, phenytoin, allopurinol, and 5-aminosalicylates.

The clinical presentation of drug-induced AIN is highly variable and depends on the class of drug involved. Patients with AIN may be asymptomatic with elevation in creatinine or blood urea nitrogen or abnormal urinary sediment. When present, symptoms are nonspecific. The "classic" triad of fever, rash, and eosinophilia is present in less than 5% to 10% of patients. Each individual component of the triad also occurs at various rates.

A diagnosis of AIN should be considered in any patients with unexplained AKI, clinical manifestations of a hypersensitivity reaction, and a history of exposure to any drug associated with AIN. A definitive diagnosis of AIN is established by kidney biopsy. AIN is characterized by interstitial inflammation, tubulitis, edema, and, in some cases, eventual interstitial fibrosis. The precise disease mechanism is unclear, but the presence of T lymphocytes in the inflammatory infiltrate suggests a type IV hypersensitivity response.

Early recognition is crucial as patients can ultimately develop chronic kidney disease. The mainstay of therapy is timely discontinuation of the causative agent. If AIN persists, corticosteroids may be used to improve kidney function. However, available data on corticosteroids are inconclusive, and randomized controlled trials are needed to confirm the benefits of corticosteroids in the treatment of AIN.

Evaluation

Because the history is essential for determining whether a patient is experiencing a drug hypersensitivity reaction, it is important to review all medications and the timeline of exposure. This includes any over-the-counter medications, herbal supplements, or occasional-use medications. Occasional-use medications may include NSAIDs, acetaminophen, cold medications, and so forth. It is important to establish a temporal relationship to the onset of the medication and the initiation of the symptoms. Oftentimes, the medication may have been discontinued before the appearance of the first symptom, so a review of medications from several weeks before the symptoms is also important. In addition, because the host immune response plays a role in some of the IgE-mediated reactions, it is important to review any immunocompromising chronic or acute illnesses or states that the patient may have or is currently experiencing. This includes HIV, chronic obstructive

---

[1]Not FDA approved for this indication.

pulmonary disease (COPD), asthma, chemotherapy, and pregnancy. For some ADRs, HLA type may be important. A patient's known genetic predisposition needs to be taken into account as well. A thorough history will also need to include any organ system or symptom that may be related to the suspected ADR.

A physical examination should augment and help to establish the working diagnosis of the type of ADR and the potentially offending drug. This should include vital signs of temperature, respiratory, and hydration status. The skin examination is important, as are appropriate evaluation and documentation of the type of lesion or lesions present. An examination of the oral mucosa and the conjunctiva of the eye should be done. Any lymphadenopathy, petechiae, or pallor should be noted.

Laboratory testing may be obtained to confirm or rule out a diagnosis. This may include a chest x-ray, CBC with differential, possible skin biopsy, liver function testing, creatinine, and electrolyte testing. A sedimentation rate and CRP testing may also be useful. Although additional autoimmune or antibody testing may be done, caution is suggested. There may not be a high yield on these tests, and they can be quite costly for patients.

Management
Anaphylaxis
Anaphylaxis can be a fatal drug hypersensitivity reaction because of its rapid onset. It is often underrecognized and undertreated because it can mimic other conditions and is variable in its presentation. However, respiratory compromise and cardiovascular collapse are of greatest concern, because they are the most common causes of death. Urticaria and angioedema are the most common manifestations but may be delayed or absent. The more quickly anaphylaxis occurs after exposure to the offending agent, the more likely the reaction is to be severe and potentially life threatening.

Most anaphylaxis episodes are IgE-mediated reactions resulting in a sudden mast cell and basophil degranulation. This sudden release of mediators affects the cutaneous, pulmonary, cardiac, GI, vascular, and neurologic systems. Medications are a common trigger of anaphylaxis in adults. Most cases of IgE-mediated drug anaphylaxis in the United States are due to penicillins and cephalosporins. Antibiotics are also the most common cause of perioperative anaphylaxis because skin eruptions may be missed in patients who are draped during surgery. Some anaphylaxis reactions involve other immunologic mechanisms. Administration of blood products (e.g., IVIG, animal antiserum) can cause an anaphylactoid reaction due, at least in part, to complement activation. Activation of the complement cascade can cause mast cell/basophil degranulation. Anaphylaxis episodes can also occur independently of any immunologic mechanism. Certain drugs, such as opioids, dextrans, and protamine, can cause a direct release of histamine and other mediators from mast cells and basophils. Finally, there are acute systemic reactions without any obvious triggers or mechanisms (idiopathic anaphylaxis).

Anaphylaxis is a clinical diagnosis with a short window of treatment time available. Therefore laboratory testing is limited and may not be of much value. Initially, the patient will describe flushing, pruritus, and a sense of impending doom. Some patients will have dyspnea, dizziness, syncope, or GI symptoms of diarrhea and abdominal cramping. Most patients will have cutaneous symptoms of flushing, urticaria, or angioedema. Some patients will progress to respiratory or cardiovascular complications.

The goal of therapy should be early recognition and treatment with epinephrine to prevent a progression to life-threatening respiratory or cardiovascular failure. The immediate intervention should include stopping the offending drug if possible, epinephrine injection, basic life support, high-flow oxygen, cardiac monitoring, and IV access. Epinephrine is the drug of choice for anaphylaxis. The therapeutic actions of epinephrine include α-1-adrenergic vasoconstrictor effects (decreases mucosal edema, thereby relieving upper airway obstruction, and increases blood pressure to prevent shock), β-1 adrenergic effects (increases rate and force of cardiac contractions), and β-2 effects (increases bronchodilation and decreases release of mediators of inflammation from mast cells/basophils).

Delayed epinephrine administration has been associated with fatalities. Intramuscular epinephrine in the thigh results in high-plasma concentrations and is preferred in the setting of anaphylaxis. The recommended dose of epinephrine is 0.3 mg (1 mg/mL) IM every 5 minutes. Typically, only one or two additional doses are needed. Patients in shock should receive epinephrine by slow IV infusion at 2 to 10 mcg/min with the rate titrated according to response and the presence of continuous hemodynamic monitoring. Patients taking beta-blockers may be resistant to treatment with epinephrine. In this case, glucagon[1] 1 to 5 mg IV over 5 minutes should be administered because its cardiac effects are not mediated through beta-receptors.

Adjunctive therapies for the treatment of anaphylaxis include antihistamines and corticosteroids. Consider an inhaled beta-agonist if wheezing. Diphenhydramine (Benadryl), an H_1 antihistamine, may be given intravenously at the dose of 25 to 50 mg. If an H_2 blocker is considered, give ranitidine (Zantac)[1] 50 mg/20 mL as an IV infusion over 5 minutes. Use of both diphenhydramine and ranitidine is superior to diphenhydramine alone. Corticosteroids are used to prevent a potential late-phase reaction that may occur in up to 23% of adults with anaphylaxis. There is no proven best dose or route of steroid therapy. The most common dosage is prednisone 20 to 60 mg daily for 3 to 5 days.

Angioedema
Angioedema is characterized by a deep dermal, subcutaneous, mucosal swelling. Many patients present with both urticaria and angioedema. Angioedema can progress rapidly from a mild swelling of the oral mucosal to a life-threatening laryngeal edema. With this rapid sequence of events, the most important part of treatment is obtaining and maintaining a patent airway. Epinephrine 0.3 mg IM every 10 minutes should be administered to patients who present with anaphylaxis, respiratory distress, or severe laryngeal edema. Once the airway is patent, the patient should be treated with H_1 antihistamines, H_2 blockers, and steroids. The milder cases may be treated similarly to other allergic reactions. H_1 antihistamines such as diphenhydramine and hydroxyzine (Atarax) are effective in relieving pruritus but can cause significant sedation. Therefore second-generation H_1 antihistamines[1] (loratadine [Claritin], cetirizine [Zyrtec], desloratadine [Clarinex], fexofenadine [Allegra]) are often chosen for outpatient therapy. Doxepin (Sinequan),[1] a tricyclic antidepressant with potent H_1 and H_2 blocker activities, can be used as an alternative to H_1 antihistamines. However, it should not be used as first-line treatment for acute urticaria and angioedema because of its significant side effects of severe sedation, dry mouth, and weight gain. Corticosteroids are used in patients who are not responsive to antihistamines. For most patients, a short course of oral prednisone is adequate.

In drug-induced angioedema, the offending drug should be stopped and avoided. Further trial of the medication is not recommended, because the patient will respond more quickly and with more severe symptoms on reintroduction. The patient should be counseled, and epinephrine 0.3 mg in an auto-injectable device (EpiPen, Auvi-Q, Adrenaclick) may be prescribed in case of recurrence in the future.

Specific Drugs
Almost all drugs can cause a drug hypersensitivity reaction. However, certain drugs are more frequently associated with specific types of reactions. Some of the more commonly used drugs are discussed here in more detail.

Antibiotics
Penicillin
Penicillin allergy is the most well-known drug allergy and also the most costly ADR. Although most drugs usually have type I and type IV reactions, penicillin may cause all four types of allergic drug reactions. The rate of penicillin-induced anaphylaxis after intravenous administration is approximately 1 to 2 per 10,000 treated patients.

---

[1] Not FDA approved for this indication.

Only about 10% of patients who report a penicillin drug allergy actually have a true immunologic response. IgE antibodies in patients with documented IgE-mediated acute penicillin reaction decline with time, resulting in 80% patients tolerating penicillin after 10 years. Patients with a penicillin allergy label are more likely to be treated with broad-spectrum or second-line antibiotics. Inappropriate use of antibiotics is linked to increased antibiotic resistance and adverse health outcomes. There is an increasing focus on penicillin allergy delabeling as an integral part of antimicrobial stewardship. Algorithms are available to clarify a patient's allergy status and expedite the evaluation for true penicillin allergy. Trubiano et al. recently developed a clinical decision tool, PEN-FAST, to aid risk stratification of patients with penicillin allergy and facilitate appropriate delabeling and prescribing strategies.

Penicillin skin testing is the best method for diagnosing an IgE-mediated penicillin allergy. A commercially available product, PRE-PEN, contains benzylpenicilloyl polylysine (PPL), which is a major antigenic determinant of penicillin. Minor determinants are metabolic derivatives of penicillin that may also produce an immune response. The current recommendations for penicillin skin testing are to administer both the major determinant (PPL) and the minor determinants (penicillin G). These two tests identify approximately 90% to 97% of the currently allergic patients. Patients with a history of penicillin allergy but negative skin test should be given an oral 250-mg amoxicillin challenge and observed for 1 hour following the skin test. If the skin test and oral challenge are both negative, the risk for Ig-E-mediated anaphylaxis is almost zero.

In general, patients who report symptoms consistent with an immediate or type I reaction or are skin-test positive to penicillin should not receive penicillin. Desensitization should be considered if penicillin is the treatment of choice for an infection and no acceptable nonpenicillin alternatives are available. Patients should be desensitized in a hospital setting. Desensitization involves administering incremental doses of oral penicillin every 15 minutes for a total of 4 to 12 hours, after which time the first dose of penicillin is given. For intravenous desensitization, three drug concentrations of penicillin are infused in 12 steps. Penicillin desensitization protocols are available in the review article by Castells et al. Desensitization is temporary and only lasts for two dosing intervals of the drug before the desensitization needs to be repeated.

Penicillin and Cephalosporin Cross-Reactivity

The rate of cross-reactivity between penicillin and cephalosporins has been historically cited to be as high as 10%. Recent data suggest that the rate may be much lower. The degree of cross-reactivity is highest between penicillins and first-generation cephalosporins, which have identical R-group side chains. In this case amoxicillin would be cross-reactive with cefadroxil (Duricef) and cefprozil (Cefzil), whereas ampicillin would be with cefaclor and cephalexin. Because of the differences in the chemical structures, second- and third-generation cephalosporins (cefdinir [Omnicef], cefuroxime [Ceftin], cefpodoxime [Vantin], and ceftriaxone [Rocephin]) are unlikely to be associated with cross-reactivity with penicillin. According to the latest guidelines for acute otitis media from the American Academy of Pediatrics and American Academy of Family Physicians, alternative initial antibiotics in patients with penicillin allergy include cefdinir, cefuroxime, cefpodoxime, or ceftriaxone.

Patients with penicillin allergy who have a negative skin-test result to penicillin (major and minor determinants) may safely receive cephalosporins. Cephalosporin treatment of patients with penicillin allergy who did not have a severe or recent penicillin reaction history shows a reaction rate of 0.1%. Use cephalosporin with caution in patients who report an immediate or accelerated penicillin allergy or those with a positive skin test to penicillin.

Sulfonamides (Sulfa Drugs)

Beside penicillins, sulfonamide antibiotics are the second most common cause of drug-induced allergic reactions. They commonly cause a delayed maculopapular/morbilliform eruption. Acute urticarial reactions (IgE mediated) to sulfamethoxazole

(SMX) or trimethoprim (TMP) are relatively infrequent; the incidence of skin rash resulting from SMX-TMP (Bactrim) in healthy subjects is estimated to be 3%. Sulfonamides are also the most common cause of SJS and TEN.

Patients with HIV have the greatest risk of sulfonamide-induced allergic reactions. The typical reaction to SMX-TMP in patients with HIV is a generalized maculopapular eruption that occurs during the second week of treatment and is usually accompanied by pruritus and fever. Because SMX-TMP is the drug of choice for a number of HIV-associated infections such as *Pneumocystis carinii* pneumonia and spontaneous bacterial peritonitis, several methods of desensitization have been devised to administer SMX-TMP to patients with HIV with a history of allergic reaction to the drug.

There are three classes of sulfonamides based on chemical structure: sulfonylarylamines (including sulfa antibiotics), nonsulfonylarylamines, and sulfonamide-moiety-containing drugs. A sulfonylarylamine has a sulfonamide moiety directly attached to a benzene ring with an amine ($-NH_2$) moiety at the N4 position. A nonsulfonylarylamine also has a sulfonamide moiety attached to a benzene ring, but it does not have an amine group at the N4 position. A sulfonamide-moiety–containing drug has a sulfonamide group that is not connected to a benzene ring. Table 2 presents a list of sulfonamide-containing drugs based on their chemical structure.

The N4 amine is critical for the development of delayed reactions to sulfa antibiotics. Given the important chemical differences between drugs containing sulfa antibiotics and sulfa in nonantibiotics, the risk of cross-reactivity is extremely unlikely. A retrospective cohort study by Strom and colleagues showed that approximately 90% of patients with sulfa antibiotic allergy did not have a reaction to a sulfonamide nonantibiotic. Patients with allergic reactions to sulfa antibiotics are also more likely to

TABLE 2	Classification of Sulfonamides Based on Chemical Structure
Drug	

Sulfonylarylamines

Antibiotics:	*Antiinflammatory:*
Sulfadiazine	Sulfasalazine (Azulfidine)
Sulfamethoxazole	Protease Inhibitors:
Sulfisoxazole	Darunavir (Prezista)
Sulfapyridine	Fosamprenavir (Lexiva)

Nonsulfonylarylamines

Carbonic Anhydrase Inhibitors:	*Sulfonylureas:*
Acetazolamide (Diamox)	Chlorpropamide
Brinzolamide (Azopt)	Glimepiride (Amaryl)
Dorzolamide (Trusopt)	Glipizide (Glucotrol)
Methazolamide (Neptazane)	Glyburide (Diabeta)
Cyclooxygenase 2 (COX-2) Inhibitors:	Tolbutamide
Celecoxib (Celebrex)	Tolazamide (Tolinase)
Loop Diuretics:	Other Agents:
Bumetanide (Bumex)	Mafenide (Sulfamylon)
Furosemide (Lasix)	Probenecid
Torsemide (Demadex)	Tamsulosin (Flomax)
Thiazides Diuretics:	Tipranavir (Aptivus)
Chlorothiazide (Diuril)	
Chlorthalidone	
Hydrochlorothiazide	
Indapamide (Lozol)	
Metolazone (Zaroxolyn)	

Sulfonamide-Moiety-Containing Drugs

5-HT Agonists:	*Other Agents:*
Naratriptan (Amerge)	Ibutilide (Corvert)
Sumatriptan (Imitrex)	Simeprevir (Olysio)
	Sotalol (Betapace)
	Topiramate (Topamax)
	Zonisamide (Zonegran)

experience allergic reactions to the other types of sulfonamides, but this is not because of cross-sensitivity. There is no reliable skin test to rule out or confirm sulfa allergy. Some experts recommend avoiding all classes of sulfonamides in patients with serious reactions such as SJS, TEN, or anaphylaxis to any one sulfonamide.

Most diuretics are sulfonamide derivatives. The only diuretics that are not in this group are the potassium-sparing diuretics (triamterene [Dyrenium], spironolactone [Aldactone], amiloride [Midamor]) and ethacrynic acid (Edecrin). Dapsone is a sulfone that is chemically unrelated to sulfonamides. *It should also be noted that sulfates, sulfur, and sulfites are chemically unrelated to sulfonamides and do not cross-react.*

Angiotensin-Converting Enzyme Inhibitors

Angiotensin-converting enzyme inhibitors (ACEIs) have two major adverse effects: cough and angioedema. The cough is typically dry and nonproductive. The incidence of ACEI-induced cough has been reported to be 5% to 35%. Cough occurs more commonly in women, African-Americans, and Asians. The onset of cough ranges from within hours of the first dose to months after the initiation of therapy. The diagnosis is confirmed by the resolution of cough, usually within 1 to 4 weeks after discontinuation of the ACEI; however, the cough can linger for up to 3 months. The cause for ACEI-induced cough is unclear but might be related to bradykinin, substance P, or another mechanism. Angiotensin II receptor blockers (ARBs) are not associated with an increased incidence of cough and can be used as an alternative to ACEIs. Because the cough may persist for several months after stopping the ACEI, starting the ARB is not a contraindication at this time, yet the cough may persist through the initiation of the new drug.

The incidence of angioedema with ACEIs is approximately 0.1% to 0.7%. With the widespread use of ACEIs, angioedema has become a growing problem. ACEI-induced angioedema is more common in patients who are over age 65, black, or female. Angioedema frequently involves swelling of the face or upper airway and can be life threatening or fatal. It can occur within days, months, or even years after the start of treatment. However, nearly 60% of cases occur within the first week of therapy. ACEIs cause angioedema by direct interference with the degradation of bradykinin, thereby increasing bradykinin levels and leading to increased vascular permeability, inflammation, and activation of nociceptors. Bradykinin is also a prominent mediator in hereditary angioedema. Therefore ACEIs are contraindicated in patients with hereditary angioedema.

ARBs directly inhibit the angiotensin receptor and do not interfere with bradykinin degradation. Theoretically, they can be relatively safe alternatives for patients with a previous history of ACEI-associated angioedema. However, some reports of ARB-induced angioedema have recently been published. The mechanism of how ARBs cause angioedema is unclear. A meta-analysis suggests that for patients who developed angioedema when taking an ACEI, the risk of persistent angioedema when subsequently switched to an ARB is less than 10%. Therefore ARBs may be an alternative only for patients with a high therapeutic need for angiotensin inhibition. ARB treatment should be started with observation. Patients should be educated on the signs of angioedema and provided with proper emergency instructions on how to proceed if angioedema should occur.

The direct renin inhibitor aliskiren (Tekturna) does not alter local or circulating bradykinin and is believed to be an alternative in patients with ACEI- and ARB-related angioedema. However, cases of angioedema have been reported with aliskiren. As with ARBs, renin inhibitors should be used with caution in patients who previously experienced angioedema to ACEIs.

Aspirin and NSAIDs

Aspirin (ASA) and NSAIDs can cause several types of hypersensitivity reactions. The four most-common types of reactions are based on the drug pathways. Aspirin-exacerbated respiratory disease (AERD) is a serious reaction induced by ASA and NSAIDs in patients with asthma and chronic rhinosinusitis. AERD does not fit precisely into a specific type of ADR and is often referred to as a type of pseudoallergic reaction. AERD affects up to 20% of adults with asthma. It is more common in women. The usual age of onset is around 30 years. The pathophysiology of AERD is related to aberrant arachidonic acid metabolism. Patients with AERD also have increased respiratory tract expression of cysteinyl leukotriene 1 receptor and heightened responsiveness to inhaled leukotriene E_4. Administration of aspirin or an NSAID to these patients leads to inhibition of cyclooxygenase 1 (COX-1), resulting in a decrease in prostaglandin E_2 levels. Prostaglandin E_2 normally inhibits 5-lipooxygenase. As a result of decreased prostaglandin E_2 levels, arachidonic acid is preferentially metabolized in the 5-lipooxygenase pathway, leading to increased production of cysteinyl leukotrienes.

Patients with AERD typically have both rhinoconjunctivitis and bronchospasm within minutes of ingestion of a dose of ASA or NSAID. The bronchospasm can be severe and result in respiratory failure, which may require intubation and mechanical ventilation. Management of patients with AERD involves treatment of the patient's asthma and chronic rhinosinusitis and avoidance of aspirin and NSAIDs. Desensitization is available in cases when the patient has a specific therapeutic need for regular ASA or NSAID therapy. Selective COX-2 inhibitors very rarely cause reactions in patients with AERD and can be taken safely.

The second type of ASA and NSAID hypersensitivity reaction is an exacerbation of urticaria or angioedema in patients with chronic idiopathic urticaria. Approximately 20% to 40% of patients with chronic urticaria may have this drug-induced reaction. The mechanism of this reaction is related to COX-1 inhibition. The exacerbating effects are usually dose dependent. All drugs that inhibit COX-1 cross-react to cause this reaction. Selective COX-2 inhibitors are generally considered safe to take in patients with chronic idiopathic urticaria.

The third type of hypersensitivity reaction is an anaphylactic or immediate urticarial reaction or angioedema appearing soon after the intake of a specific NSAID. Other NSAIDs from other groups or even an NSAID from the same group with a slightly different chemical structure is tolerated by the patient. An IgE-mediated mechanism is implicated only in some instances. The diagnosis is made mainly by exclusion. Further research is needed in this topic.

The fourth type of hypersensitivity reaction is urticaria or angioedema caused by ASA or any NSAID that inhibits COX-1 in patients without chronic urticaria. These reactions may be either drug specific or cross-reactive to other NSAIDs. Rarely, patients may have combined respiratory and cutaneous reactions that cannot be classified into one of the four reaction types described.

Corticosteroids

Corticosteroids are the most frequently used drugs for the treatment of allergic conditions, yet they can also induce hypersensitivity reactions. Most hypersensitivity reactions to steroids can be classified into type I (immediate, IgE-mediated) and type IV (delayed, cell-mediated) mechanisms. Type I reactions are characterized by the presence of urticaria and anaphylaxis. Type IV reactions can be presented as maculopapular exanthema and delayed urticaria.

Allergic contact dermatitis (type IV reaction) caused by topical administration of steroids is the most common type of allergic reaction induced by this class of drugs, occurring at the rate of 3% to 6%. Usually this is seen as a failure to improve or a worsening of an existing dermatitis that is being treated with topical steroid. Keep in mind that the reaction can also be due to other constituents of the creams, such as neomycin or cetostearyl alcohol. The diagnosis can be done using patch testing, which detects more than 90% of allergic patients. The topical steroids most frequently involved are nonfluorinated, such as hydrocortisone and budesonide.

Inhaled and intranasal steroids can induce both local and systemic reactions. Local reactions include contact dermatitis, pruritus, nasal congestion, erythema, and dry cough and are quite often irritant in nature. Systemic reactions include eczematous lesions, particularly on the face, exanthema, and urticaria. The most frequently involved steroid is budesonide. The actual mechanism of this reaction is not clear, but it may be a T-cell–mediated reaction.

Hypersensitivity reactions to systemically administered steroids seldom occur. Most of the data come from case reports. Both immediate and delayed reactions have been described, ranging from urticaria to sudden cardiovascular collapse and death. Most immediate reactions are caused by intravenous methylprednisolone and hydrocortisone. In a few cases, the reactions can be induced by salts, such as succinate, or rarely by certain diluents such as carboxymethylcellulose or metabisulfite. Non-immediate reactions are mainly mild, such as delayed urticaria or maculopapular exanthema. The drug involved most often is betamethasone.

Cross-reactivity between steroids is difficult to assess. Based on corticosteroid patch test results and their chemical structure, Coopman and colleagues divided the steroids into four groups: A (hydrocortisone type), B (triamcinolone acetonide type), C (betamethasone type), and D (hydrocortisone-17-butyrate type). Group D can be subdivided into D1 and D2 depending on the presence or absence of a C16 methyl substitution and/or halogenations on the C9 of the B ring. Table 3 provides the listing of the four groups. High cross-reactivity exists between corticosteroids in each group, as well as between group D2 and groups A and B, with group D1 exhibiting quite low cross-reactivity with the other groups.

Local Anesthetics

The most common immunologic reaction to local anesthetic is allergic contact dermatitis (type IV). IgE-mediated reactions (type I) to local anesthetics are very rare. Most adverse reactions are due to nonallergic factors such as vasovagal response, anxiety, dysrhythmias, and toxic reactions resulting from inadvertent IV epinephrine effects.

Any patient who presents with a history of an allergic reaction to local anesthetics should be carefully evaluated. Skin testing and graded challenge can be performed in patients who present with a history suggestive of a possible IgE-mediated allergic reaction to these drugs. A local anesthetic that does not contain epinephrine or other additives, such as parabens or sulfites, is preferred in this situation.

It is necessary to identify the type of local anesthetics to be used. Local anesthetics are classified as esters or amides based on their chemical structure. Drugs in the esters group include benzocaine (Americaine, Dermoplast, Lanacane, Hurricaine), chloroprocaine, cocaine, procaine (Novocaine), proparacaine (Alcaine, Opthaine), and tetracaine (Tetcaine). Most allergic reactions reported in the literature have been caused by agents in the esters group, which are derivatives of para-aminobenzoic acid (PABA), a known allergen. Cross-reactivity occurs among members of the ester group, but the esters do not cross-react with the amides. Agents in the amides group include bupivacaine (Marcaine), lidocaine, mepivacaine (Polocaine), prilocaine (Citanest), and ropivacaine (Naropin). Amide local anesthetics generally do not cross-react with other amides or with the esters.

Radiocontrast Media

There are two types of radiocontrast media (RCM): ionic high osmolality and nonionic low osmolality. Both of these agents contain iodine. The nonionic RCMs are much more widely used today than the ionic agents.

Allergic reactions to RCM are common and can range from mild to life threatening. Anaphylactoid reactions and severe life-threatening reactions occur in 1% to 3% and 0.22% of patients who receive ionic RCM, respectively. Less than 0.5% and 0.04% of patients who receive nonionic agents have anaphylactoid reactions and severe reactions, respectively. The fatality rate is approximately 1 to 2 per 100,000 procedures, and it is similar for both ionic and nonionic agents. RCM reactions are typically not mediated by IgE antibodies. RCM acts directly on mast cells and basophils, resulting in the release of histamine and other systemic mediators, which cause the anaphylactoid reactions. Patients at greater risk for more serious anaphylactoid reactions include females; those with asthma, heart disease, and a history of previous anaphylactoid reaction to RCM; and those taking beta-blockers. People who have seafood allergy are not at increased risk for reactions to RCM compared with the general population. The pathogenesis of anaphylactoid reactions is also not related to iodine.

Management of patients with previous RCM reactions include the use of a nonionic, low-osmolarity agent and a pretreatment regimen. One common regimen consists of prednisone (50 mg PO at 13, 7, and 1 hour before the procedure), diphenhydramine (50 mg at 1 hour before the procedure), and a histamine H_2-receptor antagonist (1 hour before the procedure). This will significantly reduce the risk for anaphylactoid reaction with reexposure to RCM.

Delayed reactions to RCM occur 1 hour to 1 week after RCM administration. Approximately 2% of patients have delayed reactions to RCM. These reactions are generally mild, self-limited cutaneous eruptions. The mechanism is usually T-cell mediated. Rarely, more serious and life-threatening delayed reactions such as SJS, TEN, and DRESS syndrome have been reported.

Chlorhexidine

Chlorhexidine gluconate is an antiseptic agent. It is commonly available in OTC products as a skin and wound disinfectant (e.g., Betasept, Hibiclens). Hypersensitivity reactions to chlorhexidine include contact dermatitis, pruritus, urticaria, dyspnea, and anaphylaxis. Prescription chlorhexidine gluconate mouthwashes and

GROUP	TYPE	DRUGS
A	Hydrocortisone	Hydrocortisone (acetate, succinate, phosphate) Methylprednisolone (acetate, succinate, phosphate) Prednisolone, prednisolone acetate Tixocortol pivalate*
B	Triamcinolone acetonide	Amcinonide (Cyclocort) Budesonide (Pulmicort, Rhinocort, Entocort) Desonide (Desonate, DesOwen) Flunisolide Fluocinolone acetonide (Synalar) Fluocinolone Halcinonide (Halog) Triamcinolone Triamcinolone acetonide (Kenalog)
C	Betamethasone	Betamethasone (Celestone) Desoxymethasone Dexamethasone Paramethasone* Fluocortolone*
D1	Hydrocortisone-17-butyrate	Beclomethasone dipropionate (QVAR) Betamethasone valerate Betamethasone dipropionate Clobethasone 17-butyrate* Clobetasol 17-propyonate (Clobex)
D2	Hydrocortisone-17-butyrate	Fluticasone (Flonase) Mometasone Prednicarbate (Dermatop) Hydrocortisone 17-butyrate (Locoid) Hydrocortisone 17-propionate* Methylprednisolone aceponate*

TABLE 3 Coopman Classification of Cross-Reactivity in Corticosteroids

*Not available in the United States.
From Torres and Canto (2010).

oral chips used for gum disease contain a warning about the rare but serious allergic reactions in their labels. According to a recent FDA Drug Safety Communication, the number of reports of serious allergic reactions to chlorhexidine-containing products has increased over the last several years. As a result, an anaphylaxis warning is now added to the OTC product labels under Drug Facts.

Several case reports have suggested that some patients with prior exposure to chlorhexidine and patients with chlorhexidine-induced contact dermatitis may be susceptible to anaphylaxis caused by chlorhexidine sensitization. Since chlorhexidine is the standard skin disinfectant used before surgery or invasive procedures, the exposure to the agent becomes more widespread. Even though severe anaphylaxis to chlorhexidine has been estimated to be rare, the actual rate may be higher than reported. Such reports remind clinicians to be vigilant about chlorhexidine as a hidden allergen, especially in surgical patients.

Herbal Supplements

There is a perception that herbal supplements are "natural" and therefore safe. In fact, severe allergic reactions including asthma and anaphylaxis have been well documented in patients using bee pollen products and echinacea. Echinacea is an herb belonging to a group of flowering plants known as Asteraceae. Asteraceae-derived pollens are an important cause of hay fever and asthma. Asteraceae may cause contact allergic dermatitis. Cross-reactivity exists between members of the Asteraceae family, such as ragweed, dandelion, daisy, chamomile, echinacea, feverfew, and milk thistle.

A lack of quality control has been a major concern in the herbal supplement industry. Chinese herbal products may be adulterated with synthetic medications not listed on the label. Contaminated supplements may be a potential risk for systemic contact dermatitis in nickel- and mercury-allergic patients. Because of the widespread use of herbal supplements and the underreporting of adverse events to herbs, all patients should be questioned about the use of herbal supplements when being evaluated for hypersensitivity reactions.

Conclusion

Drug hypersensitivity reactions are common; fortunately, severe and often fatal reactions are not. It is important for the clinician to have a working knowledge of common drug-induced hypersensitive reactions as well as the ability to identify and document common dermatologic findings. With that background knowledge, a thorough history and physical examination should enable the clinician to diagnose the majority of these types of reactions. A timely and appropriate management plan can then be implemented. As always, it is important to educate patients regarding their drug hypersensitivity history and the potential for future reactions.

References

American Academy of Pediatrics: Clinical practice guideline: The diagnosis and management of acute otitis media, *Pediatrics* 131:e964–e969, 2013.
Bommersbach TJ, Lapid MI, Leung JG, et al: Management of psychotropic drug-induced DRESS syndrome: A systematic review, *Mayo Clin Proc* 91(6):787–801, 2016.
Castells M, Khan DA, Phillips EJ: Penicillin allergy, *N Engl J Med* 381:2338–2351, 2019.
CDC: Sexually transmitted disease treatment guidelines 2021, *MMWR* 70(4):1–192, 2021.
Fernando SL: Acute generalized exanthematous pustulosis, *Australas J Dermatol* 53:87–92, 2012.
Harr T, French L: Toxic epidermal necrolysis and Stevens-Johnson syndrome, *Orphanet J Rare Dis* 5:39, 2010. Available at http://www.ojrd.com/content/5/1/39.
Haymore BR, Yoon J, Mikita CP, et al: Risk of angioedema with angiotensin receptor blockers in patients with prior angioedema associated with angiotensin-converting enzyme inhibitors: A meta-analysis, *Ann Allergy Asthma Immunol* 101:495–499, 2008.
Husain Z, Reddy BY, Schwartz RA: DRESS syndrome, part I. Clinical perspectives, *J Am Acad Dermatol* 68:693.e1–693.e14, 2013.
Inomata N: Recent advances in drug-induced angioedema, *Allergol Int* 61:545–557, 2012.
Joint Task Force on Practice Parameters, AAAAI, ACAAI: Drug allergy: An updated practice parameter, *Ann Allergy Asthma Immunol* 105:259–273, 2010.
Khan DA, Solensky R: Drug allergy, *J Allergy Clin Immunol* 125:S126–S137, 2010.
Lieberman P, Nicklas RA, Opperheimer J, et al: The diagnosis and management of anaphylaxis practice parameter: 2010 update, *J Allergy Clin Immunol* 126:477–480, 2010.
Miliszewski MA, Kirchhof MG, Sikora S, et al: Stevens-Johnson syndrome and toxic epidermal necrolysis: An analysis of triggers and implications for improving prevention, *Am J Med* 129(11):1221–1225, 2016.
Moka E, Argyra E, Siafaka I, Vadalouca A: Chlorhexidine: Hypersensitivity and anaphylactic reactions in the perioperative setting, *J Anaesthesiol Clin Pharmacol* 31(2):145–148, 2015.
Murata J, Abe R: Soluble Fas ligand: Is it a critical mediator of toxic epidermal necrolysis and Stevens-Johnson syndrome? *J Invest Dermatol* 127:744–745, 2007.
Perazella MA, Markowitz GS: Drug-induced acute interstitial nephritis, *Nat Rev Nephrol* 6(8):461–470, 2010.
Philips JF, Yates AB, Deshazo RD: Approach to patients with suspected hypersensitivity to local anesthetics, *Am J Med Sci* 334:190–196, 2007.
Pichler WJ: Consequences of drug binding to immune receptors: Immune stimulation following pharmacological interaction with immune receptors (T-cell receptor for antigen or human leukocyte antigen) with altered peptide-human leukocyte antigen or peptide, *Dermatol Sin* 31:181–190, 2013.
Ponka D: Approach to managing patients with sulfa allergy. Use of antibiotic and nonantibiotic sulfonamides, *Can Fam Physician* 52:1434–1438, 2006.
Sharma P, Nagarajan V: Can an ARB be given to patients who have had angioedema on an ACE inhibitor? *Cleve Clin J Med* 80:755–757, 2013.
Shenoy ES, Macy E, Rowe T, Blumenthal KG: Evaluation and management of penicillin allergy: a review. *JAMA* 321:188–99, 2019.
Torres MJ, Canto G: Hypersensitivity reactions to corticosteroids, *Curr Opin Allergy Clin Immunol* 10:273–279, 2010.
Trubiano JA, Vogrin S, Chua KY, et al: Development and validation of a penicillin allergy clinical decision rule, *JAMA Intern Med* 180(5):745–752, 2020.

SERUM SICKNESS

Method of
Amy Robertson, PharmD; and Amanda Rhyne, MD

CURRENT DIAGNOSIS

- Identified by: fever, rash, joint pain (in combination or isolated)
- 7–14 days after exposure to offending agent
- Most frequently in the adult female population
- There are no disease defining labs, although complement tests may be elevated

CURRENT THERAPY

- Identify and discontinue offending agent
- Symptomatic relief with analgesics and antihistamines, as needed
- Those with severe disease may be treated with oral or intravenous corticosteroids for 10–14 days
- If symptoms reappear after discontinuation of corticosteroid, reinitiate with a slow taper

Pathophysiology

Serum sickness is classified as a type III delayed immune-complex–mediated hypersensitivity reaction. It was first noted by Von Pirquet in the early 1900s after administration of equine antisera. The mechanism consists of exposure to an antigen (often a large protein) that leads to formation of an antigen-antibody complex. The immune complex load becomes too high to be appropriately excreted from the body, causing deposition in joints, tissues, and vascular endothelium. It also leads to activation of the complement pathway, which prompts mast cell and basophil degranulation with vasoactive amine release. The deposition of immune complexes and release of inflammatory mediators (histamine, serotonin) leads to the common symptoms of urticarial rash, joint pain, and fever.

Serum sickness–like reaction is not as well defined as true serum sickness. It is postulated that a non-protein drug binds to a serum protein to make a complete antigen. The newly formed antigen goes on to become an antigen-antibody complex. These complexes mimic the inflammatory cascade and symptomatic response of a true serum sickness reaction.

Epidemiology

Serum sickness is most common in the adult female population. A systematic review involving 33 cases of rituximab (Rituxan)-induced serum sickness (RISS) showed 76.7% female predominance with a mean age of 39.1 years. The majority of cases occurred in patients with an autoimmune condition, specifically immune thrombocytopenic purpura and Sjogren. Due to a lack of clear diagnostic tools and varying symptoms that can closely mimic a flare of an underlying rheumatologic illness, these reactions are often poorly documented or not identified. A study of Australian snake antivenom showed that the incidence of serum sickness was 29% (N = 32/109). Further research will need to be done to determine current incidence with the increasing treatment of rheumatologic disorders with immunologic medications.

Risk Factors

Risk factors for serum sickness include parenteral and cutaneous administration of chemicals, especially those with large molecular weights (e.g., proteins, serum). Heterologous (animal-derived) proteins, in particular, are associated with a high risk for a delayed immune response. Historically, equine-derived antisera and antitoxins were common causes and now includes murine and chimeric monoclonal antibodies such as rituximab (Rituxan) and infliximab (Remicade). Fewer adverse events have been reported with adalimumab (Humira), a humanized monoclonal antibody. Additional risk factors include administration of large doses, repeated dosing, and longer administration times. Patients with autoimmune disorders, circulating histamine-releasing factors, and atopy are also at an increased risk.

Serum sickness–like reactions are associated with a wider variety of molecules, including non-protein medications (e.g., antibiotics), vaccines, allergy extracts, hormones, and enzymes. See Table 1 for a list of agents commonly associated with serum sickness and serum sickness–like reactions.

Clinical Manifestations

Common manifestations of serum sickness include fever, pruritic rash (not involving mucosal membranes), and arthralgia of the metacarpophalangeal joints, knees, wrists, ankles, and shoulders. The timing of these symptoms occurs 7 to 14 days after exposure to the offending agent and can happen more promptly if there has been previous exposure. Urticaria has been reported as the most prominent symptom, present in 90% of cases. In a study of 33 cases of RISS: 78.8% presented with fever, 72.7% with arthralgia, and 69.7% with rash. The triad of fever, rash, and arthralgia were present in 48.5% of the cases. There are many less prominent manifestations of serum sickness, including headache, gastrointestinal (GI) bloating, cramps, diarrhea, and nephropathy.

Diagnosis

Recommended workup includes complete blood count (CBC), erythrocyte sedimentation rate (ESR), C-reactive protein (CRP), urinalysis (UA), and comprehensive metabolic panel (CMP). Although lab work can help to differentiate from other causes, diagnosis is made clinically. Attempts have been made to link serum sickness to elevated levels of rheumatoid factor, complement, and antibody levels without success.

Differential Diagnosis

The differential diagnoses for serum sickness include: serum sickness–like reaction, other hypersensitivity reactions, viral illness, rheumatologic disease, tick-borne disease, reactive arthritis, Stevens-Johnson syndrome, rheumatic fever, and lupus.

TABLE 1	Medications Associated With Serum Sickness and Serum Sickness–Like Reactions

Serum Sickness

Heterologous (animal-derived) proteins:
- Antivenom for snake bites: Crotalidae polyvalent immune fab, North and South American snake antivenom (CroFab)
- Chimeric (murine/human) monoclonal antibodies: rituximab (Rituxan), infliximab (Remicade)
- Equine serum heptavalent botulism antitoxin
- Equine-derived antivenom for spider bites
- Equine-derived diphtheria antitoxin
- Murine monoclonal antibodies
- Polyclonal antibodies: equine or rabbit anti-thymocyte globulin (Atgam, Thymoglobulin)

Homologous (human-derived) proteins:
- Anti-D (Rho[D]) immune globulin (RhoGAM)
- Humanized monoclonal antibodies: adalimumab (Humira), omalizumab (Xolair), natalizumab (Tysabri), alemtuzumab (Lemtrada)
- Intravenous immune globulin (Carimune NF, Gamunex-C)

Serum Sickness–like Reactions
- Allopurinol (Zyloprim)
- Antimicrobials
  - Cephalosporins (especially cefaclor [Ceclor])
  - Ciprofloxacin (Cipro)
  - Griseofulvin (Gris-PEG)
  - Isoniazid (Nydrazid, INH)
  - Minocycline (Minocin)
  - Penicillins (Pen-Vee K)
  - Streptomycin (Agri-mycin-17, Agrept)
  - Sulfonamides
- Barbiturates
- Bupropion (Wellbutrin)
- Captopril (Capoten)
- Hydantoins
- Hydralazine (Apresoline)
- Iodides
- Methyldopa (Aldomet)
- Phenytoin (Dilantin)
- Procainamide (Pronestyl, Procan-SR, Procanbid)
- Quinidine (Cardioquine)
- Thiouracils (e.g., methimazole [Tapazole])

Treatment

Treatment of serum sickness and serum sickness–like reactions are similar. Discontinuation and avoidance of the offending agent is recommended and usually leads to spontaneous resolution within several weeks. Due to the self-limiting nature and generally mild presentation, treatment is symptom driven. Low-grade fever and/or arthralgias can be treated with analgesics (e.g., acetaminophen [Tylenol]) or nonsteroidal anti-inflammatory drugs. Antihistamines and corticosteroids are commonly used, but there are limited data to support their efficacy. Antihistamines may be used to treat urticarial symptoms. Those with more severe disease (e.g., temperature >38.5°C, severe arthralgias, extensive rashes) can be treated with a short course of corticosteroids (e.g., prednisone [Deltasone] 40 to 60 mg by mouth daily). Generally oral corticosteroids are sufficient, but intravenous agents may be appropriate for some patients (e.g., methylprednisolone [Solu-Medrol] 1 to 2 mg/kg in one or two divided doses intravenously). A systematic review revealed intravenous methylprednisolone (Solu-Medrol) as the most common treatment of RISS. Other treatment options identified were intravenous betamethasone (Celestone Soluspan), intravenous hydrocortisone (Solu-Cortef), oral prednisone (Deltasone), and oral prednisolone (Millipred). This study demonstrated a mean treatment duration of 9 days with complete resolution of symptoms in all cases. Some studies recommend tapering corticosteroids over 2 weeks to avoid rebound symptoms. There are currently no evidence-based guidelines available to guide dosing or duration of therapy.

Plasmapheresis or plasma exchange is another treatment option used to eliminate immune complexes. One study reports the use of plasmapheresis in five patients post–renal transplant who experienced anti-thymocyte globulin-induced serum sickness with no improvement after administration of oral prednisone (Deltasone) 1 mg/kg/d or intravenous prednisolone (Millipred) 2 mg/kg/d. This treatment method is generally reserved for refractory cases that do not respond to corticosteroid therapy due to limited evidence of its safety and efficacy.

References

de Silva HA, Ryan NM, de Silva HJ: Adverse reactions to snake antivenom, and their prevention and treatment, *Br J Clin Pharmacol* 81(3):446–452, 2015.

Erffmeyer JE: Serum sickness, *Ann Allergy* 56:105–109, 1986.

Karmacharya P, Poudel DR, Pathak R, et al: Rituximab-induced serum sickness: a systematic review, *Semin Arthritis Rheum* 45:334–340, 2015.

Lawley TJ, Bielory L, Gascon P, et al: A prospective clinical and immunologic analysis of patients with serum sickness, *N Engl J Med* 311:1407–1413, 1984.

Lin RY: Serum sickness syndrome, *Am Fam Physician* 33(1):157–162, 1986.

Lundquist AL, Chari RS, Wood JH, et al: Serum sickness following rabbit antithymocyte-globulin induction in a liver transplant recipient: case report and literature review, *Liver Transpl* 13:647–650, 2007.

Naguwa SM, Nelson BL: Human serum sickness, *Clin Rev Allergy* 3:117–126, 1985.

Ryan NM, Kearney RT, Brown S, et al: Incidence of serum sickness after the administration of Australian snake antivenom (ASP-22), *Clin Toxicol* 54(1):27–33, 2016.

Solensky R, Khan DA, et al: Drug allergy: an updated practice parameter, *Ann Allergy Clin Immunol* 105:259–273, 2010.

Tatum AJ, Ditto AM, Patterson R: Severe serum sickness-like reaction to oral penicillin drugs: three case reports, *Ann Allergy Asthma Immunol* 86:330–334, 2011.

Tanriover B, Chuang P, Fishbach B, et al: Polyclonal antibody-induced serum sickness in renal transplant recipients: treatment with therapeutic plasma exchange, *Transplantation* 80:279–281, 2005.

3 Cardiovascular System

ACUTE MYOCARDIAL INFARCTION

Method of
Kuang-Yuh Chyu, MD, PhD; and Prediman K. Shah, MD

CURRENT DIAGNOSIS

- Patients are encouraged to seek medical evaluation as soon as possible when chest pain or angina-equivalent symptoms occur.
- Early presentation leads to early recognition, diagnosis, and treatment of acute myocardial infarction.
- The diagnosis of acute myocardial infarction relies on detailed history, electrocardiogram (ECG) changes consistent with myocardial ischemia, and elevation of serum biomarkers.
- Although echocardiogram is not essential to diagnose acute myocardial infarction, it is useful in diagnosing mechanical complications or other complications, such as left ventricular (LV) dysfunction with congestive heart failure, from acute myocardial infarction and guiding management.

CURRENT THERAPY

- Timely reperfusion of occluded coronary artery is essential in managing ST-elevation myocardial infarction (STEMI).
- Early reperfusion therapy (percutaneous coronary intervention [PCI] or coronary artery bypass grafting [CABG]) in patients with non-ST-elevation myocardial infarction (NSTEMI) with high-risk features such as congestive heart failure or with dynamic ECG changes such as ST-segment depression, arrhythmia, and refractory angina is beneficial.
- Medical therapy and lifestyle modification strategies are important to reduce long-term atherosclerotic cardiovascular events.

Coronary heart disease results from atherosclerotic coronary artery disease (CAD), and its acute manifestation is acute coronary syndrome (ACS). Based on the presenting symptoms, characteristic ECG changes, and cardiac biomarkers (e.g., high-sensitivity troponin), ACS can be further subdivided into unstable angina, non-ST-elevation myocardial infarction (NSTEMI), or ST-elevation myocardial infarction (STEMI). Most patients with ACS have similar underlying pathophysiology: atherosclerotic plaque formation leading to narrowing of coronary arteries with plaque rupture or erosion and superimposed thrombus formation resulting in an acute presentation. A small portion of ACS cases can be owing to conditions such as coronary artery spasm, spontaneous coronary artery dissection, coronary embolization, or cocaine use. Stress-induced acute cardiomyopathy, without angiographic signs of severely occlusive disease, can closely simulate atherothrombotic STEMI.

Although the three ACS entities share similar pathophysiology, their presentations vary widely. The initial recognition, diagnostic testing, and management strategies for these entities are similar and applicable to all patients with ACS. Diagnostically, patients with STEMI, as a whole, reflect a more homogeneous group of patients compared with patients with unstable angina or NSTEMI, and patients with STEMI carry the highest risk regarding acute morbidity and mortality. The major difference in managing these three groups of patients lies in the decision for and timing of acute reperfusion of occluded coronary arteries.

In the past 3 decades, there has been a steady decline in the incidence of STEMI and significant improvement in the outcomes of patients with STEMI with the introduction of early coronary reperfusion strategies. Improved adjunctive pharmacologic therapies, adoption of guideline-directed treatments such as lipid lowering, strict control of hypertension and diabetes mellitus, and cigarette smoking cessation are risk factors that are effective to modify. Currently, the in-hospital mortality of STEMI has reached as low as 7%.

Diagnosis

Electrocardiogram

ECG is the most important diagnostic test to detect STEMI because clinical features, physical examination, and CAD risk factor profile only have modest sensitivity and specificity in diagnosing STEMI. In the absence of LV hypertrophy or left bundle branch block (LBBB), current guidelines define ST elevation as new ST elevation at the J point in at least 2 contiguous leads of 2 mm (0.2 mV) in men or 1.5 mm (0.15 mV) in women in leads V2–V3 and/or of 1 mm (0.1 mV) in other contiguous chest leads or the limb leads. Other ECG abnormalities, such as paced rhythm, drug or electrolyte (hyperkalemia) effects, or Brugada syndrome, also reduce the sensitivity and specificity of STEMI ECG interpretation.

Some patients present with ECG changes, although not with typical ST elevation, indicating equivalent clinical risk to STEMI, and should be treated as having a true STEMI. These STEMI-equivalent ECG patterns include (1) isolated ST depression in two or more precordial leads (V1 to V4), indicating true posterior wall STEMI; (2) ST depression in multiple leads with ST elevation in aVR, indicating left main or triple-vessel CAD; (3) Wellens sign with symmetric deep T-wave inversions in anterior precordial leads V2 and V3; (4) LBBB or paced ventricular beats meeting Sgarbossa, modified Sgarbossa, or Barcelona criteria; and (5) de Winter sign showing ST depression and peaked T waves in the precordial leads. Occasionally, patients with left circumflex artery occlusion can present with a normal or near-normal ECG.

Serum Biomarkers

Serum biomarkers of myocardial necrosis, such as cardiac-specific high-sensitivity troponin T and I levels, are complementary to diagnosing STEMI. In clinical practice, STEMI is often diagnosed with ECG alone before the laboratory result of biomarkers is available. The troponin level typically rises 4 to 6 hours after the onset of symptoms and peaks within 12 to 24 hours if reperfusion therapy succeeds in reperfusing the occluded coronary artery and patients present early in the course of STEMI; its level tends to peak after 24 hours if reperfusion therapy fails or in patients who receive no reperfusion therapy. After STEMI, successfully reperfused or not, the troponin level remains elevated for 7 to 10 days.

For patients suspected of having recurrent ACS within a week after the index STEMI, given that the troponin level remains elevated, creatine kinase (CK) and the MB isoform of CK (CK-MB) levels can be used as biomarkers to establish additional myocardial necrosis from a recurrent event because CK and CK-MB levels usually return to normal 48 to 72 hours after the initial index event. For patients with symptoms of ACS but without ST elevation on ECG, normal levels of serial high-sensitivity troponin using the 0/3-hour algorithm has a negative predictive value of approximately 99% to exclude ACS. Shorter 0/1-hour or 0/2-hour algorithms have also been validated and included in the 2020 ESC NSTEMI guideline.

Imaging

STEMI is commonly accompanied with wall motion abnormalities on echocardiogram, but echocardiogram is not essential to diagnose STEMI. Echocardiogram is extremely useful in managing patients with STEMI, especially when they present with acute complications from STEMI such as acute congestive heart failure, acute mitral regurgitation, free wall or ventricular septal rupture, pericardial effusion, cardiogenic shock, or LV thrombus.

Management of STEMI

The principal concept of managing STEMI is "time is muscle"; hence, it is important for patients to recognize symptoms for early presentation and for the medical community to administer suitable reperfusion therapy in a timely manner.

Prehospital Phase

Current guidelines recommend that patients with STEMI receive reperfusion therapy as soon as possible but within 12 hours of symptom onset to achieve optimal myocardial salvage to reduce mortality and morbidity. In daily clinical practice, a substantial number of patients still present late and miss the golden window of reperfusion. Common reasons for late presentation include (1) patients' lack of knowledge to recognize symptoms, (2) patients' reluctance to seek medical care, (3) patients' lack of access to medical care, and (4) atypical symptoms that lead patients or medical care providers to consider noncardiac problems.

Patients with suspicious myocardial ischemic symptoms are encouraged to call emergency medical services (EMS) immediately for help, leading to the following benefits: (1) patients can receive early treatment, (2) patients can receive immediate resuscitation should STEMI complications such as cardiac arrest occur en route to the hospital, and (3) an early prehospital ECG and communication with a hospital capable of PCI by EMS significantly reduce reperfusion time and improve outcomes. A recent Lifeline STEMI Accelerator Study reported that only 55% of patients with STEMI were transported via EMS. Improving this requires public education to enhance recognition of symptoms, implementation of an efficient EMS system, and infrastructures with standardized treatment algorithms for STEMI.

Initial management by EMS or outpatient clinic usually includes pain relief by morphine and administration of nitroglycerin,[1] oxygen, and nonenteric-coated aspirin (162 to 325 mg) unless contraindicated. The role of routine oxygen supplementation to patients with STEMI studied in a randomized clinical trial (Air Versus Oxygen in Myocardial Infarction trial) suggested that supplemental oxygen therapy (8 L/min via face mask) in patients with STEMI without hypoxia (oxygen saturation >94%) may increase early myocardial injury and is associated with larger myocardial infarction size at 6 months.

Once STEMI is identified by a prehospital ECG performed by EMS, an assessment of candidacy for and availability of reperfusion therapy is an important next step of management to ensure

[1] Not FDA approved for this indication.

immediate reperfusion and administration of its adjunctive therapy to maintain culprit coronary artery patency, limit infarct size and adverse LV remodeling, and improve outcome. To achieve the best outcome from reperfusion therapy, patients with STEMI should receive suitable reperfusion therapy within 12 hours of symptom onset—the earlier the better. Current reperfusion therapy options for STEMI include primary percutaneous coronary intervention (PPCI) or fibrinolysis. PPCI is the treatment of choice for STEMI because it confers a beneficial reduction in mortality and recurrent ischemia compared with fibrinolysis. Hence, current guidelines recommend EMS to transport patients to a PCI-capable hospital and PPCI as the preferred method of reperfusion therapy with a system goal of less than 90 minutes from first medical contact (FMC) to device time. Such timely reperfusion is even more important for patients with STEMI with cardiogenic shock, but without out-of-hospital cardiac arrest, because every 10-minute treatment delay between 60 to 180 minutes from the first medical contact leads to 3.3 additional deaths per 100 PCI-treated patients (FITT-STEMI trial).

Not every hospital is capable of performing PCI. If a patient is sent to or arrives at a non-PCI-capable hospital, guidelines recommend transferring that patient to a PCI-capable hospital for PPCI with a system goal of less than 120 minutes from FMC to device time. If there is an anticipated delay of FMC to device time of 120 minutes or more, a fibrinolytic agent can be given within 30 minutes of hospital arrival if the patient has no contraindications for fibrinolysis (Box 1). Prehospital fibrinolysis, administered by EMS with physician supervision, has been shown to be feasible

| BOX 1 | Contraindications and Cautions for Fibrinolytic Therapy in STEMI* |

Absolute Contraindications
- Any prior ICH
- Known structural cerebral vascular lesion (e.g., arteriovenous malformation)
- Known malignant intracranial neoplasm (primary or metastatic)
- Ischemic stroke within 3 months; selected patients with acute ischemic stroke presented within 4.5 hours can receive thrombolytic therapy
- Suspected aortic dissection
- Active bleeding or bleeding diathesis (excluding menses)
- Significant closed-head or facial trauma within 3 months
- Intracranial or intraspinal surgery within 2 months
- Severe uncontrolled hypertension (unresponsive to emergency therapy)
- For streptokinase, prior treatment within the previous 6 months

Relative Contraindications
- History of chronic, severe, poorly controlled hypertension
- Significant hypertension on presentation (SBP >180 mm Hg or DBP >110 mm Hg)
- History of prior ischemic stroke >3 months
- Dementia
- Known intracranial pathology not covered in absolute contraindications
- Traumatic or prolonged CPR (>10 min)
- Major surgery (<3 weeks)
- Recent (within 2–4 weeks) internal bleeding
- Noncompressible vascular punctures
- Pregnancy
- Active peptic ulcer
- Oral anticoagulant therapy

*Viewed as advisory for clinical decision making and may not be all-inclusive or definitive.
CPR, Cardiopulmonary resuscitation; *DBP,* diastolic blood pressure; *ICH,* intracranial hemorrhage; *SBP,* systolic blood pressure; *STEMI,* ST-elevation myocardial infarction.

and safe, with a shortened reperfusion time and reduced mortality. Such a strategy, however, is not used in the United States.

In real-world clinical practice, sometimes it is not possible to achieve strict time goals because of uncertainty of the initial diagnosis, necessity to treat concomitant comorbidities or complications, patient preference or consent issues, and local factors delaying transport. Therefore emphasis should be on delivering reperfusion therapy to eligible patients as rapidly as possible.

In-Hospital Reperfusion Strategy
Primary Percutaneous Coronary Intervention
PPCI performed in a high-volume hospital by experienced operators achieves a higher patency rate of infarct-related artery (IRA) and lower rate of recurrent ischemia, reinfarction, hemorrhagic stroke, and death compared with fibrinolysis. In particular, PPCI has the greatest benefit in high-risk patients such as those with cardiogenic shock. Hence, PPCI, with the system goal of 90 to 120 minutes, is the preferred method of reperfusion whenever possible.

The reperfusion technique used in PPCI has evolved greatly in the past few decades, from balloon angioplasty, bare-metal stent (BMS), and drug-eluting stent (DES) to bioresorbable vascular scaffolds (BVSs). Compared with balloon angioplasty, BMS used in PPCI confers reduced risk for subsequent target vessel revascularization but does not reduce the mortality rate. Compared with BMS, DES used in PPCI decreases the restenosis rate and need for reintervention without reduction in reinfarction and death. BVS is a new stent technology with a hope of better restoration of vasomotion, less lumen loss, and reduction of target lesion revascularization in the stented vessels compared with metallic DES. However, polymer-based ABSORB BVS failed to demonstrate such benefits; instead, it caused a concerning hazard of device thrombosis. A newer generation of metallic BVS (Magmaris, Biotronik) also increased late lumen loss and target lesion revascularization in patients with STEMI compared with a sirolimus-eluting stent in a recently published MAGSTEMI trial.

Fibrinolysis
The currently available intravenous fibrinolytic agents are tenecteplase (TNKase), reteplase (Retavase), and alteplase (Activase) (Table 1). A fibrinolytic agent should be administered to eligible patients without contraindication within 30 minutes of arrival at the emergency department. It is important to evaluate the risk–benefit ratio for each individual patient before administering fibrinolytic therapy because it carries a small but fatal risk of hemorrhage stroke (about 1%). The ideal patient to receive a fibrinolytic agent would be one with symptom onset within 1 to 2 hours, low bleeding risk, and age younger than 65 years.

Although fibrinolysis achieves a reasonable patency rate of IRA (see Table 1), a substantial portion of patients fail to achieve successful reperfusion as defined by the following clinical criteria: (1) resolution of chest pain, (2) reduction of >50% of the initial ST-segment elevation pattern on follow-up ECG 60 to 90 minutes after initiation of fibrinolysis, and (3) occurrence of reperfusion arrhythmia (accelerated idioventricular rhythm). If fibrinolysis does not achieve resolution of ST elevation by at least 50% in the worst lead at 60 to 90 minutes, rescue PCI (transfer to PCI-capable hospital if necessary) should be strongly considered.

Percutaneous Intervention After Fibrinolysis
Approximately 40% of patients with STEMI who receive fibrinolysis fail to achieve successful reperfusion and require emergent rescue PCI. Other indications for rescue PCI include severe heart failure, cardiogenic shock, persistent chest pain, or electrical instability. Hence, these patients should be transferred to a PCI-capable hospital immediately if fibrinolysis has been administered in a non-PCI capable hospital.

Otherwise, stable patients after successful fibrinolysis can undergo coronary angiography with an intent to revascularize as soon as logistically feasible, ideally between 3 and 24 hours after fibrinolysis (so-called pharmaco-invasive strategy). In patients older than 75 years, if a pharmaco-invasive strategy is chosen as the reperfusion strategy, a fibrinolytic agent at half dose (such as the half dose of tenecteplase used in the STREAM trial) should be used to reduce bleeding risks because patients will receive concomitant antiplatelets and anticoagulants for PCI. The EARLY-MYO trial confirmed that the efficacy of a pharmaco-invasive strategy using half-dose alteplase followed by PCI within 3 to 24 hours was noninferior to primary PCI in 30-day rates of total death, reinfarction, heart failure, or major bleeding but had a higher rate of minor bleeding. Very early PCI after successful fibrinolysis (<2 to 3 hours) is not recommended.

Facilitated Percutaneous Intervention
This strategy refers to a full or partial dose of fibrinolysis plus a glycoprotein IIb/IIIa antagonist or antithrombotic followed by immediate PCI if there is no evidence of reperfusion failure. Current guidelines do not recommend this strategy owing to potential harms, such as an increase in ischemic events, bleeding, and mortality.

Patients With STEMI and Multivessel Coronary Artery Disease
About 40% to 65% of patients with STEMI undergoing PPCI for culprit IRA have multivessel CAD. Significant multivessel CAD, if left unrevascularized, is associated with a worse clinical prognosis. For patients with STEMI with multivessel CAD and cardiogenic shock, conventional paradigm deemed it reasonable to perform multivessel PPCI (or emergency CABG in selected patients) to achieve as complete a revascularization as possible.

TABLE 1	Comparison of Fibrinolytic Agents		
	ALTEPLASE (t-PA) (ACTIVASE)	RETEPLASE (r-PA) (RETAVASE)	Tenecteplase (TNK-tPA) (TNKase)
Dose	Up to 100 mg in 90 min (weight based)	10 U + 10 U IV boluses given 30 min apart	30–50 mg based on weight as a single bolus
Bolus administration	No	Yes	Yes
Antigenic	No	No	No
Allergic reaction	No	No	No
Fibrin specificity	++	++	++++
90-min TIMI 2 or 3 patency rate (%)	73–84	84	85
TIMI 3 flow (%)	54	60	63

IV, Intravenous; *TIMI*, thrombolysis in myocardial infarction.
Modified from 2013 ACCF/AHA STEMI guideline.

However, the CULPRIT-SHOCK trial showed that initial revascularization of the culprit vessel only by PCI in patients with acute myocardial infarction (MI) and multivessel CAD with cardiogenic shock resulted in a lower 30-day risk of death or renal replacement therapy compared with a strategy of immediate multivessel PCI.

For stable patients, randomized clinical trials have demonstrated the feasibility of performing multivessel PPCI in acute settings. This approach has the following advantages: complete revascularization leading to improved LV function and prognosis, decreased vascular complications from repeated procedures, and reduced length of stay and medical costs. However, the procedure will be longer, with higher radiation exposure; larger contrast load, leading to higher risk for contrast nephropathy; risk of compromising viable myocardium supplied by the nonculprit coronary artery owing to procedure complications; and unnecessary stenting to the nonculprit artery without objective evidence of ischemia.

Many guidelines published by the professional cardiology societies in North America and Europe support multivessel PCI, either at the time of PCI to the STEMI culprit vessel or as a staged procedure in selected hemodynamically stable patients. A recent COMPLETE trial further confirmed the efficacy of reducing new myocardial infarction or ischemia-driven revascularization in the complete revascularization group than in the culprit lesion PCI group but without mortality benefit. Interventional cardiologists should integrate clinical data, characteristics of lesions and procedures, clinical risks, and complications from procedures to determine the best timing and strategy to achieve the optimal benefit.

Patients With STEMI Older Than 75 Years

Patients older than 75 years are usually underrepresented in STEMI clinical trials; however, revascularization with PCI still confers beneficial clinical outcomes compared with no revascularization despite age, frailty, and comorbidities. Hence, PCI as a revascularization strategy for STEMI in the elderly is encouraged whenever patients' conditions allow. In the United States, the utilization of PCI for patients with STEMI older than 70 years has increased from 11% in 1998 to 35.7% in 2013 based on data from the National Inpatient Sample Database. When taking care of this group of patients, cardiologists need to pay particular attention to minimize bleeding complication by using radial access, monitoring patients' nonverbal responses because many patients have difficulty communicating with caregivers effectively, and identifying and treating comorbid conditions early given that many elderly patients lack functional reserves in many organ systems and are prone to adverse effects of drug interactions.

Patients With STEMI Who Present Later Than 12 Hours After Symptom Onset

Irrespective of time of presentation, patients with STEMI who present with hemodynamic or electrical instability should undergo coronary angiography with an intent to revascularize the jeopardized myocardium as soon as possible.

Patients with STEMI who present between 12 hours and 2 days after symptom onset without unstable symptoms or signs are no longer eligible for fibrinolysis but are still eligible for PPCI to salvage myocardium, which confers the benefit of reduced infarct size compared with conventional therapy guided by a pre-discharge symptom-limited exercise test or with unplanned PCI guided by clinical instability, as demonstrated in the Beyond 12 Hours Reperfusion Alternative Evaluation trial. For patients with STEMI who present more than 48 hours after symptom onset without clinical instability, a strategy of symptom-limited stress test first or coronary angiography first to delineate high-risk features of coronary anatomy is reasonable with an intent to revascularize high-risk coronary anatomy. If patients are clinically stable without high-risk coronary anatomy noted by angiography and present between 3 and 28 days after symptom onset, PCI to open the occluded IRA does not confer clinical benefits in

reducing mortality, congestive heart failure, or nonfatal myocardial infarction compared with medical therapy, as demonstrated in the Occluded Artery Trial.

Figure 1 summarizes current pathways of managing patients with STEMI based on their time of presentation, their clinical status, and the availability of reperfusion therapy.

Adjunct Therapy
Antiplatelet Therapy
Aspirin
Unless contraindicated, 162 to 325 mg of aspirin should be administered as a loading dose immediately followed by at least 81 to 325 mg daily in all patients with STEMI, with 81 mg being the preferred maintenance dose. Patients with a history of aspirin allergy can be given clopidogrel (Plavix) instead.

P2Y$_{12}$ Receptor Inhibitors
Clopidogrel is a second-generation thienopyridine and irreversibly blocks the platelet P2Y$_{12}$ receptor to inhibit platelet activation and aggregation. Current guidelines support the use of clopidogrel during fibrinolysis or PPCI. For patients undergoing fibrinolytic therapy, a loading dose of 300 mg followed by a maintenance dose of 75 mg daily has been recommended for patients younger than 75 years. For patients older than 75 years, only the maintenance dose of 75 mg should be given. Prasugrel (Effient) and ticagrelor (Brilinta) have not been studied and hence are not recommended in the setting of fibrinolysis as reperfusion therapy. For patients undergoing PPCI, depending on whether they are receiving a fibrinolytic agent and the timing of subsequent PCI, a different dosing regimen of clopidogrel may be recommended (Figure 2).

Prasugrel is a third-generation thienopyridine P2Y$_{12}$ receptor inhibitor. It is metabolized to its active form more quickly than clopidogrel and hence confers a more potent effect. In a subset of patients with STEMI in the TRITON-TIMI 38 trial, prasugrel was more efficacious in preventing composite endpoints of cardiovascular (CV) death, myocardial infarction, and stroke compared with clopidogrel, but it had a higher major bleeding rate. Prasugrel is also contraindicated in patients older than 75 years, with body weight less than 60 kg, or with prior history of stroke or transient ischemic attack.

Ticagrelor is a direct reversible P2Y$_{12}$ receptor inhibitor with a more potent, faster-acting property compared with clopidogrel or prasugrel. In the pivotal Platelet Inhibition and Patient Outcomes trial, ticagrelor lowered composite CV death, myocardial infarction, and stroke compared with clopidogrel but with an increase in non-procedure-related bleeding.

Biotransformation of clopidogrel into active metabolites requires CYP2C19, whereas prasugrel mainly relies on CYP3A4, CYP2B6, and, to a lesser extent, CYP2C19 to form active metabolites. Ticagrelor is an active P2Y$_{12}$ inhibitor, and its metabolite via CYP3A4 carries equal antiplatelet potency. About 30% of the U.S. population carries one or two CYP2C19 loss-of-function alleles, rendering them less responsive to the antiplatelet effect of clopidogrel. Hence, genotyping CYP2C19 polymorphism could potentially affect the selection of P2Y$_{12}$ receptor inhibitor. In STEMI populations, a recent study demonstrated that a genotype-guided strategy—that is, patients without loss of function of CYP2C19 were treated with clopidogrel, whereas patients with loss of function received ticagrelor or prasugrel—was not inferior to a standard treatment with ticagrelor or prasugrel in the control group with respect to thrombotic events at 12 months. It was associated with lower risk of bleeding.

Clopidogrel, prasugrel, and ticagrelor require several hours to achieve maximal platelet inhibition. Additionally, in the setting of STEMI, the bioavailability of these oral agents may be hampered by clinical factors such as nausea, vomiting, and cardiogenic shock, leading to poor gastrointestinal absorption and leaving patients not adequately protected by platelet inhibition during

Figure 1 Pathways of managing ST-elevation myocardial infarction *(STEMI)*. *FMC*, First medical contact; *LHC*, left heart catheterization; *PCI*, percutaneous intervention; *PPCI*, primary percutaneous coronary intervention.

*Congestive heart failure, cardiogenic shock, presence of mechanical complications, ventricular arrhythmia, ongoing symptoms suggesting myocardial ischemia.

immediate PPCI. Cangrelor (Kengreal) is a fast-acting, reversible adenosine diphosphate receptor inhibitor that is administered intravenously to achieve $P2Y_{12}$ inhibition within 2 minutes. Its plasma half-life is 3 to 6 minutes, and platelet function returns to normal within 60 minutes after discontinuation of infusion. The U.S. Food and Drug Administration (FDA) has approved cangrelor to be used as an adjunct therapy during PCI to reduce repeat coronary revascularization and stent thrombosis in patients who have not been pretreated with an oral $P2Y_{12}$ inhibitor and are not receiving a glycoprotein IIb/IIIa receptor antagonist. How to transition from cangrelor to an oral $P2Y_{12}$ inhibitor after PCI depends on which oral $P2Y_{12}$ inhibitor a patient is being transitioned to. Based on the CHAMPION PHOENIX trial, to transition to clopidogrel, 600 mg clopidogrel loading is necessary immediately after discontinuation of cangrelor infusion. Based on pharmacodynamic data, prasugrel 60 mg should be administered immediately after stopping cangrelor infusion, whereas ticagrelor 180 mg can be given anytime during cangrelor infusion or immediately after infusion ends.

Use and duration of antiplatelet therapy

Current guidelines recommend giving aspirin and one of the potent $P2Y_{12}$ inhibitors (ticagrelor or prasugrel) prior to primary PCI for patients with STEMI. When potent $P2Y_{12}$ inhibitors are not available or contraindicated, clopidogrel can be given instead. For patients with NSTEMI in whom coronary artery anatomy is not known and an early invasive management is planned, routine administration of $P2Y_{12}$ inhibitors is not recommended. This recommendation is based on the aggregated results from several clinical trials and registries, including ACCOAST, ISAR-REACT 5, DUBIUS, ARIAM-Andalucia registry, and SCAAR. Once coronary anatomy is defined and PCI is deemed necessary, a $P2Y_{12}$ inhibitor can be administered. This approach has the benefit of

reducing unnecessary bleeding risk in patients whose NSTEMI diagnosis is disproved by coronary angiogram, reducing the wait time for patients with suitable coronary anatomy for bypass surgery.

Current American and European guidelines recommend 12 months of dual antiplatelet therapy (DAPT) in patients with ACS (STEMI or NSTEMI) after stent implantation. If bleeding risk is high (such as with PRECISE DAPT >25), duration of DAPT can be shortened to 6 months, followed by discontinuation of the $P2Y_{12}$ inhibitor (American guideline) or aspirin (European guideline). Shorter duration of DAPT (3 months), followed by aspirin, may be considered in patients with high bleeding risk (European guideline). Continuation of DAPT beyond 12 months is reasonable in patients who tolerate DAPT, do not have bleeding complications, and are not at high bleeding risk (prior bleeding on DAPT, coagulopathy, or oral anticoagulant use).

The use and duration of DAPT becomes more complicated in patients taking oral anticoagulation therapy for a variety of reasons. Guidelines and consensus documents from North America recommend the default approach of administering triple therapy (DAPT + anticoagulation) during PCI procedure and in hospital for up to 1 week followed by clopidogrel and oral anticoagulant for 12 months. If patients are at high risk for an ischemic event, the default approach is modified to use triple therapy for 1 month and discontinue acetylsalicylic acid (ASA; aspirin) afterward. If patients have high bleeding risk, the default approach is modified to use triple therapy for up to 1 week, followed by oral anticoagulant and clopidogrel, with discontinuation of clopidogrel after 6 months. A non-vitamin K oral anticoagulant is preferred to a vitamin K antagonist as an oral anticoagulant unless the clinical condition prohibits the use of non-vitamin K oral anticoagulants. Oral anticoagulant alone can be used after 12 months of treatment with an additional single antiplatelet

Figure 2 Oral regimen of different P2Y$_{12}$ receptor inhibitors based on reperfusion strategies. *PCI*, Percutaneous intervention. Modified from 2013 ACCF/AHA STEMI guideline.

agent based on individual clinical circumstance. Other strategies, including use of a radial artery approach as vascular access, use of proton pump inhibitors, avoidance of glycoprotein (GP) IIb/IIIa inhibitors unless for periprocedural complications, and avoidance of nonsteroidal antiinflammatory drugs, should also be used.

Glycoprotein IIb/IIIa Receptor Antagonists

Glycoprotein IIb/IIIa receptor antagonists include abciximab (ReoPro, a chimeric monoclonal antibody), eptifibatide (Integrilin, a synthetic peptidic inhibitor), and tirofiban (Aggrastat, a nonpeptidic inhibitor). The benefit of intravenous GP IIb/IIIa receptor antagonists in patients with STEMI was largely established before the era of oral DAPT. With current use of DAPT, contemporary trials fail to show benefit with upstream administration of GP IIb/IIIa receptor antagonists before PPCI with either unfractionated heparin (UFH)[1] or bivalirudin (Angiomax). Current U.S. and European guidelines recommend using GP IIb/IIIa receptor antagonists for bailout situations after a large thrombus burden, no reflow or slow flow, or inadequate P2Y$_{12}$ receptor antagonist loading during PCI.

Anticoagulants

UFH,[1] low-molecular-weight heparin with enoxaparin (Lovenox) as a prototype, fondaparinux (Arixtra),[1] and bivalirudin (Angiomax) are widely used in reperfusion therapy to limit thrombus propagation, reduce reocclusion and reinfarction, and improve vessel patency unless contraindicated. The choice of individual agent and its dose and duration of use depend on the choice of

reperfusion therapy, concomitant use of other antiplatelet agents, and renal function (Table 2).

Given that PPCI is the preferred method of reperfusion and occurs early after presentation, and given physicians' familiarity with UFH, intravenous UFH is the preferred anticoagulant agent for PPCI. In patients with high bleeding risk, bivalirudin with DAPT is a reasonable alternative to UFH (whether the patient was pretreated with UFH) when avoidance of GP IIb/IIIa receptor antagonists is desired during PPCI.

For patients with STEMI who receive fibrinolysis as initial reperfusion therapy, UFH, enoxaparin, and fondaparinux[1] all receive a class I recommendation based on American College of Cardiology/American Heart Association (ACC/AHA) guidelines. UFH is preferred since a pharmaco-invasive strategy is common

or for patients who may need rescue PCI. Bivalirudin may be used after fibrinolysis in patients who develop heparin-induced thrombocytopenia and require continued anticoagulation.

Guideline-Directed Medical Therapy

Beta Blockers

Beta blocker therapy decreases myocardial oxygen demand and improves myocardial remodeling with the benefits of reducing angina, infarct size, and mortality. Current guidelines recommend initiating oral beta blockers in the first 24 hours in patients with STEMI who are without contraindications such as congestive heart failure; evidence of a low output state, or increased risk for cardiogenic shock, heart block, or reactive airway disease. If not given in the first 24 hours owing to contraindications, physicians need to reevaluate patients to determine their subsequent

---

[1] Not FDA approved for this indication.

[1] Not FDA approved for this indication.

	REPERFUSION THERAPY	
	FIBRINOLYSIS	**PRIMARY PCI**
Unfractionated heparin	• IV bolus of 60 U/kg (maximum 4000 U) followed by an infusion of 12 U/kg/h (maximum 1000 U) initially, adjusted to maintain aPTT at 1.5–2.0 times control (approximately 50–70 s) for 48 h or until revascularization	• With GPI planned, 50–70 U/kg IV bolus, to achieve ACT 200–250 s • Without GPI planned, 70–100 U/kg IV bolus to achieve ACT 250–300 s with HemoTec or 300–350 s with Hemochron
Low-molecular-weight heparin (enoxaparin [Lovenox])	• If age <75 years: 30-mg IV bolus, followed in 15 min by 1 mg/kg subcutaneously every 12 h (maximum 100 mg for the first 2 doses) • If age ≥75 years: no bolus, 0.75 mg/kg subcutaneously every 12 h (maximum 75 mg for the first 2 doses) • Regardless of age, if CrCl <30 mL/min: 1 mg/kg subcutaneously every 24 h • Duration: For the index hospitalization, up to 8 days or until revascularization	No information
Bivalirudin (Angiomax)	No information	• With or without prior heparin: 0.75 mg/kg bolus, 1.75 mg/kg/h infusion to the end of PCI. Additional bolus of 0.3 mg/kg if needed • Reduce infusion to 1 mg/kg/h if estimated CrCl <30 mL/min • Prefer over heparin and GPI in high-risk cases of bleeding
Fondaparinux (Arixtra)	• Initial dose 2.5 mg IV, then 2.5 mg subcutaneously daily starting the following day, for the index hospitalization up to 8 days or until revascularization • Contraindicated if CrCl <30 mL/min	Not recommended as sole anticoagulant

ACT, Activated clotting time; *aPTT,* activated partial thromboplastin time; *CrCl,* creatinine clearance; *GPI,* glycoprotein IIb/IIIa inhibitors; *IV,* intravenous; *PCI,* percutaneous intervention; *STEMI,* ST-elevation myocardial infarction.
Modified from 2013 ACCF/AHA STEMI guideline.

eligibility. Oral beta blockers should be continued for 3 years after MI, as recommended by the ACC/AHA secondary prevention guideline, and longer if there are other indications (such as systolic LV dysfunction). Commonly used beta blocker regimens are (1) metoprolol tartrate (Lopressor) 25 to 50 mg every 6 to 12 hours orally, transitioned over the next 2 to 3 days to twice-daily dosing of metoprolol tartrate or to daily metoprolol succinate (Toprol XL) and then titrated to a daily dose of 200 mg as tolerated and (2) carvedilol (Coreg)[1] 6.25 mg twice daily, titrated to 25 mg twice daily as tolerated.

Current guidelines recommend intravenous beta blockers only for patients with refractory hypertension or ongoing ischemia without contraindications. Several small randomized clinical trials have suggested that early use of intravenous metoprolol tartrate in selected patients with STEMI with Killip class I to II and no atrioventricular (AV) block before PPCI may reduce infarct size with a higher LV ejection fraction (LVEF) or reduce the incidence of malignant arrhythmia in the acute phase without an excess of adverse events.

Angiotensin-Converting Enzyme Inhibitors or Angiotensin II Receptor Blockers

Angiotensin-converting enzyme inhibitors (ACEIs) and angiotensin II receptor blockers (ARBs) reduce afterload and decrease myocardial remodeling. Either ACEIs or ARBs should be started within 24 hours if there are no contraindications such as worsening renal function, advanced kidney disease, bilateral renal artery stenosis, hyperkalemia, or hypotension. These agents have the largest benefit in patients with anterior STEMI, congestive heart failure, or LVEF less than 40%. ACEIs may be given routinely to all patients without contraindication, whereas ARBs are an alternative for patients intolerant to ACEIs. There is no additional benefit, only more harm, if ACEIs and ARBs are given concomitantly.

Commonly used ACEI regimens are (1) captopril 6.25 to 12.5 mg three times per day to start, titrated to 25 to 50 mg three times per day as tolerated; (2) lisinopril (Prinivil) 2.5 to 5 mg/day to start, titrated to 10 mg/day or higher as tolerated; (3) ramipril (Altace) 2.5 mg twice daily to start, titrated to 5 mg twice daily as tolerated; and (4) trandolapril (Mavik) test dose 0.5 mg, titrated up to 4 mg daily as tolerated. A commonly used ARB regimen is valsartan (Diovan) 20 mg twice daily to start, titrated to 160 mg twice daily as tolerated.

Angiotensin Receptor-Neprilysin Inhibitors

Valsartan/sacubitril (Entresto) has been shown to confer mortality and heart failure admission benefit in symptomatic heart failure patients with EF less than 40% compared with enalapril in the PARADIGM-HF trial. However, its use in patients with acute MI with pulmonary congestion and EF <40% did not confer similar benefit compared with ramipril in a 2021 PARADISE-MI trial.

3-Hydroxy-3-Methylglutaryl Coenzyme A Reductase Inhibitors (Statins)

Treatment with statins after ACS lowers the risk of CV mortality, recurrent MI, stroke, and the need for coronary revascularization. All patients with ACS should have a nonfasting lipid panel obtained as early as possible, with lipoprotein(a) level to be included if not known previously for overall risk assessment and high-intensity statins to be initiated as early as possible to improve compliance. Although current guidelines do not endorse a specific low-density lipoprotein cholesterol (LDL-C) level as a treatment goal, it is recommended to reduce LDL-C level at least 50% from baseline, with a goal of LDL-C less than 55 mg/dL.

A commonly used high-intensity statin regimen is atorvastatin (Lipitor) 40 to 80 mg or rosuvastatin (Crestor) 20 to 40 mg daily as tolerated. Statins need to be used cautiously with drugs metabolized via CYP3A4 and fibrates, with frequent monitoring for myopathy and hepatic toxicity. Statin use needs to be combined with diet and therapeutic lifestyle therapies. In patients who cannot achieve LDL-C level <70 mg/dL on adequate statin treatment, addition of a PCSK9 antibody, such as alirocumab (Praluent) or evolocumab (Repatha), can further reduce the LDL-C level and risk of recurrent cardiovascular events. This stepwise approach is now being questioned because observational data indicated that there are few dose adjustment or lipid-lowering agents prescribed, leading to the LDL-C goal not being met in a majority of patients. A recent European consensus statement advocated dual lipid-lowering agents (high-intensity statin + ezetimibe [Zetia][1]) to be initiated as early as possible, even before coronary angiography. For patients with additional CAD high-risk features, such as multivessel CAD, polyvascular disease, familial hypercholesterolemia, premature CAD, or recurrent events, PCSK9 inhibitors can be added in the acute phase of ACS.

Aldosterone Antagonists

Eplerenone (Inspra) improves myocardial remodeling and may reduce all-cause and CV mortality and rehospitalization. The 2013 ACC/AHA STEMI guideline recommends starting this medication 3 to 14 days after STEMI in eligible patients (creatinine ≤2.5 mg/dL in men and ≤2.0 mg/dL in women, potassium ≤5.0 mEq/L) with heart failure and LVEF less than 35% to 40% and who are already on adequate doses of beta blockers and ACEIs or ARBs. However, earlier administration (<7 days) is preferable to achieve mortality and rehospitalization benefits, as suggested by a post hoc analysis of the Eplerenone Post-Acute Myocardial Infarction Heart Failure Efficacy and Survival Study trial.

Implantable Cardioverter-Defibrillator

Patients who develop ventricular tachycardia (VT) or fibrillation more than 48 hours after STEMI have the highest risk of sudden cardiac death (SCD) and hence are eligible for an implantable cardioverter-defibrillator as a secondary prevention measure for SCD. For primary prevention, multiple trials have established the efficacy of prevention of SCD by implantable cardioverter-defibrillator implantation in patients with LVEF less than 35% and New York Heart Association class II or III symptoms (or LVEF <30% with New York Heart Association class I symptoms) despite optimal medical therapy 40 days after index STEMI and expectation of at least 1-year survival.

Other Medical Therapy

Morphine

Morphine is a time-honored medication used to reduce pain and anxiety, especially in patients with pulmonary edema during acute presentation of STEMI. However, analysis of results from several clinical trials and a large meta-analysis involving more than 69,000 patients with ACS suggested that a morphine/P2Y$_{12}$ inhibitor interaction exists, which could lead to adverse clinical consequences. Several pharmacokinetic studies in healthy volunteers have shown that intravenous morphine administration can reduce the level of active metabolites of clopidogrel and delay the maximal inhibition of platelet aggregation. A similar effect of morphine on ticagrelor was also reported. Given the current trend of using oral P2Y$_{12}$ receptor inhibitors before PPCI for STEMI, careful selection of patients and judicious administration of morphine with P2Y$_{12}$ receptor inhibitors deserves careful consideration.

Nitrate

Nitroglycerin reduces LV preload, increases coronary blood flow, and relieves chest pain symptoms. However, it plays no role in decreasing myocardial injury from coronary artery occlusion in STEMI. Its use in STEMI is mostly for congestive heart failure, hypertension, or rare cases of coronary spasm. It is contraindicated in patients with hypotension (systolic blood pressure [SBP]

<90 mm Hg or SBP >30 mm Hg below baseline), right ventricular infarction from right coronary artery occlusion, or use of phosphodiesterase-5 inhibitors within 24 to 48 hours.

Complications of STEMI

Cardiogenic Shock

Cardiogenic shock is defined as an SBP less than 90 mm Hg for longer than 1 hour that is (1) not responsive to fluid administration alone, (2) secondary to cardiac dysfunction, or (3) associated with signs of hypoperfusion or cardiac index less than 2.2 L/min per m^2 and pulmonary capillary wedge pressure greater than 18 mm Hg. It occurs in fewer than 10% of patients with STEMI (2.4% in the 1986 GISSI-1 trial; 6.5% in the German ALKK-PCI registry as reported in 2013).

Almost 75% to 80% of cases of cardiogenic shock are owing to severe LV systolic dysfunction; right ventricular infarction, mechanical complications from ventricular septal rupture, acute mitral regurgitation, and free wall rupture leading to tamponade account for the rest. Other uncommon causes of shock from noncardiac etiology after STEMI are bleeding, systemic inflammatory response syndrome, infection, bowel ischemia, or iatrogenic reasons (such as due to medication).

Cardiogenic shock due to mechanical complications after STEMI occurs in a bimodal fashion, with most cases occurring within 24 hours. Risk factors for mechanical complication include female sex, older age, and late or no reperfusion in the infarcted territory. An early echocardiogram is extremely helpful to delineate the etiology of cardiogenic shock to guide subsequent definitive treatment. Cardiogenic shock carries a high in-hospital mortality, approaching 50%, and is higher in patients older than 75 years. These high-mortality patients require immediate stabilization to prevent end-stage organ damage followed by emergency coronary angiography and revascularization (Box 2).

Electrical Complications

Ventricular Arrhythmia

Lethal ventricular arrhythmia (VT, or ventricular fibrillation [VF]) is the most common cause of out-of-hospital cardiac arrest in STEMI. For hospitalized patients, VT/VF occurs in fewer than 10% of cases in the era of reperfusion therapy, and most cases occur within 48 hours of presentation. VT/VF is often associated with congestive heart failure, cardiogenic shock, or failed reperfusion of an occluded coronary artery. Hence, correction of electrolyte and acid-base disturbance, adequate reperfusion to reduce myocardial ischemia, and treatment of heart failure or shock are important preventive measures. Early administration of beta blockers within 24 hours to patients without contraindications reduces the incidence of VF. If VT/VF occurs, treatment includes immediate defibrillation or cardioversion and an antiarrhythmic agent such as amiodarone (Cordarone). Isolated premature ventricular contractions, nonsustained VT without hemodynamic instability, and accelerated idioventricular rhythm do not generally require specific treatment.

Supraventricular Arrhythmia

Common supraventricular arrhythmias after STEMI include atrial fibrillation, atrial flutter, and sinus tachycardia. They are usually the consequence of or are triggered by congestive heart failure, atrial infarction, pericarditis, hypoxia, or other underlying systemic problems (such as chronic obstructive pulmonary disease, bleeding, anemia, or infection). Treatment is directed to the underlying causes. For atrial fibrillation/flutter, physicians should pay special attention to anticoagulation use given the frequent concomitant use of DAPT and antithrombotics and the rate versus rhythm control strategy.

Bradycardia and Heart Block

Sinus bradycardia may occur after inferior STEMI. Because it is generally mediated through increased vagal tone, close monitoring usually suffices. High-grade AV block (second or third degree) can occur after inferior or anterior STEMI, with a worse

---

[1]Not FDA approved for this indication.

BOX 2 — Management Measures for Cardiogenic Shock

Immediate Stabilization of Patients to Prevent End-Stage Organ Damage

Maintain adequate mean arterial blood pressure with norepinephrine (Levophed), dopamine, or dobutamine with intraarterial pressure monitoring; norepinephrine preferred over dopamine for less arrhythmogenic effect

Hemodynamic monitoring with Swan-Ganz catheter to guide inotrope or fluid management

Selective use of mechanical circulatory support* if patient cannot be stabilized by previous measures

Early echocardiography to define etiology of cardiogenic shock

Early mechanical ventilation

Management of hemodynamically significant arrhythmia

Fibrinolysis in STEMI if delay to PCI >2 h

Early Coronary Angiography and Revascularization

Early transfer to regional tertiary care hospital for revascularization

Prophylactic IABP placement before transfer

PCI often the treatment of choice

CABG (with correction of mechanical complications if present) in cardiogenic shock if feasible

---

CABG, Coronary artery bypass grafting; *IABP,* intraaortic balloon pump; *PCI,* percutaneous intervention; *STEMI,* ST-elevation myocardial infarction.

*IABP is more readily available; limited experience with other LV assist devices such as Impella and TandemHeart device.

---

prognosis after anterior STEMI owing to a greater degree of myocardial injury. High-grade AV block after inferior STEMI usually is transient and with a narrow complex escape rhythm, which subsides within 2 weeks. Occasionally, temporary pacemaker placement may be necessary if bradycardia causes hemodynamic instability. High-grade AV block from anterior STEMI usually requires placement of a prophylactic temporary pacing system because it is commonly associated with hemodynamic instability.

References

Bainey KR, Armstrong PW: Transatlantic comparison of ST-segment elevation myocardial infarction guidelines: Insights from the United States and Europe, *J Am Coll Cardiol* 67(2):216–219, 2016.

Bates ER, Tamis-Holland JE, Bittl JA: PCI strategies in patients with ST-segment elevation myocardial infarction and multivessel coronary artery disease, *J Am Coll Cardiol* 68(10):1066–1081, 2016.

Cannon CP, de Lemos JA, Rosenson RS, et al: Use of lipid-lowering therapies over 2 years in GOULD, a registry of patients with atherosclerotic cardiovascular disease in the US, *JAMA Cardiol* 16;6(9):1–9, 2021.

Capodanno D, Huber K, Mehran R, et al: Management of antithrombotic therapy in atrial fibrillation patients undergoing PCI: JACC state-of-the-art review, *J Am Coll Cardiol* 74(1):83–99, 2019.

Capodanno D, Angiolillo DJ: Timing, selection, modulation, and duration of P2Y12 inhibitors for patients with acute coronary syndromes undergoing PCI, *JACC Cardiovasc Interv* 6(1):1–18, 2023.

Cassese S, Byrne RA, Ndrepepa G: Everolimus-eluting bioresorbable vascular scaffolds versus everolimus-eluting metallic stents: a meta-analysis of randomized controlled trials, *Lancet* 387(1018):537–544, 2016.

Chandrasekhar J, Mehran R: The ideal anticoagulation strategy in ST-elevation myocardial infarction, *Prog Cardiovasc Dis* 58:247–259, 2015.

Claassens DMF, Vos GJA, Bergmeijer TO: A genotype-guided strategy for oral P2Y12 inhibitors in primary PCI, *N Engl J Med* 381(17):1621–1631, 2019.

Collet JP, Thiele H, Barbato E, et al: 2020 ESC Guidelines for the management of acute coronary syndromes in patients presenting without persistent ST-segment elevation: the Task Force for the management of acute coronary syndromes in patients presenting without persistent ST-segment elevation of the European Society of Cardiology, *Eur Heart J* 42(14):1289–1367, 2021.

Damluji AA, Forman DE, van Diepen S: Older adults in the cardiac intensive care unit: factoring geriatric syndromes in the management, prognosis, and process of care. A scientific statement from the American Heart Association, *Circulation* 141:e6–e32, 2020.

Di Pasquale G, Filippini E, Pavesi PC: Complete versus culprit-only revascularization in ST-elevation myocardial infarction and multivessel disease, *Intern Emerg Med* 11(4):499–506, 2016.

Duarte GS, Nunes-Ferreira A, Rodrigues FB: Morphine in acute coronary syndrome: systematic review and meta-analysis, *BMJ Open* 9:e025232, 2019.

Elbadawi A, Elgendy IY, Ha LD: National trends and outcomes of percutaneous coronary intervention in patients > 70 years of age with acute coronary syndrome (from the National Inpatient Sample Database), *Am J Cardiol* 123(1):25–32, 2019.

Ellis SG, Kereiakes DJ, Metzger DC: Everolimus-eluting bioresorbable scaffolds for coronary artery disease, *N Eng J Med* 373(20):1905–1915, 2015.

Frampton F, Devries JT, Welch TD: Modern management of ST-segment elevation myocardial infarction, *Curr Probl Cardiol* 45(3):100393, 2020.

Guedeney P, Collet JP: Diagnosis and management of acute coronary syndrome: what is new and why? Insight from the 2020 European society of cardiology guidelines, *J Clin Med* 9(11):3474, 2020.

Halvorsen S, Jortveit J, Hasvold P, et al: Initiation of and long-term adherence to secondary preventive drugs after acute myocardial infarction, *BMC Cardiovasc Disord* 16:115, 2016.

Hochman JS, Lamas GA, Buller CE: Coronary intervention for persistent occlusion after myocardial infarction, *N Engl J Med* 355:2395–2407, 2006.

Ibanez B, Macaya C, SÆnchez-Brunete V: Effect of early metoprolol on infarct size in ST-segment-elevation myocardial infarction patients undergoing primary percutaneous coronary intervention: the Effect of Metoprolol in Cardioprotection during an Acute Myocardial Infarction (METOCARD-CNIC) trial, *Circulation* 128(14):1495–1503, 2013.

Kragholm K, Lu D, Chiswell K: Improvement in care and outcomes for emergency medical service-transported patients with ST-elevation myocardial infarction (STEMI) with and without prehospital cardiac arrest: a mission:lifeline STEMI accelerator study, *J Am Heart Assoc* 6:e005717, 2017.

Krychtiuk KA, Ahrens I, Drexel H, et al: Acute LDL-C reduction post ACS: strike early and strike strong: from evidence to clinical practice. A clinical consensus statement of the association for acute CardioVascular care (ACVC), in collaboration with the European association of preventive cardiology (EAPC) and the European society of cardiology working group on cardiovascular pharmacotherapy, *Eur Heart J Acute Cardiovasc Care* 11(12):939–949, 2022. 27.

Kubica J, Kubica A, Jilma B: Impact of morphine on antiplatelet effects of oral P2Y12 receptor inhibitors, *Int J Cardiol* 215:201–208, 2016.

Mehta SR, Wood DA, Storey RF: Complete revascularization with multivessel PCI for myocardial infarction, *N Engl J Med* 381(15):1411–1421, 2019.

Pfeffer MA, Claggett B, Lewis EF, et al: Angiotensin receptor-neprilysin inhibition in acute myocardial infarction, *N Engl J Med* 385(20):1845–1855, 2021.

Pu J, Ding S, Ge H: Efficacy and safety of a pharmaco-invasive strategy with half-dose alteplase versus primary angioplasty in ST-segment-elevation myocardial infarction: EARLY-MYO trial (early routine catheterization after alteplase fibrinolysis versus primary PCI in acute ST-segment-elevation myocardial infarction), *Circulation* 136:1462–1473, 2017.

Qamar A, Bhatt DL: Current status of data on cangrelor, *Pharmacol Ther* 159:102–109, 2016.

Roolvink V, IbÆæez B, Ottervanger JP: Early intravenous beta-blockers in patients with ST-segment elevation myocardial infarction before primary percutaneous coronary intervention, *J Am Coll Cardiol* 67(23):2705–2715, 2016.

Sabate M, Alfonso F, Cequier A: Magnesium-based resorbable scaffold versus permanent metallic sirolimus-eluting stent in patients with ST segment elevation myocardial infarction: the MAGSTEMI randomized clinical trial, *Circulation* 140(23):1904–1916, 2019.

Scholz KH, Maier SKG, Maier LS, et al: Impact of treatment delay on mortality in ST-segment elevation myocardial infarction (STEMI) patients presenting with and without haemodynamic instability: results from the German prospective, multicentre FITT-STEMI trial, *Eur Heart J* 39(13):1065–1074, 2018.

Schomig A, Mehilli J, Antoniucci D: Mechanical reperfusion in patients with acute myocardial infarction presenting more than 12 hours from symptom onset: a randomized controlled trial, *JAMA* 293(23):2865–2872, 2005.

Schwartz GG, Steg PG, Szarek M, et al: Alirocuman and cardiovascular outcomes after acute coronary syndrome, *N Engl J Med* 379(22):2097–2107, 2018.

Serruys PW, Chevalier B, Sotomi Y: Comparison of an everolimus-eluting bioresorbable scaffold with an everolimus- eluting metallic stent for the treatment of coronary artery stenosis (ABSORB II): a 3 year, randomised, controlled, single- blind, multicentre clinical trial, *Lancet* 388(10059):2479–2491, 2016.

Shah RU, Henry TD, Rutten-Ramos S: Increasing percutaneous coronary interventions for ST-segment elevation myocardial infarction in the United States: progress and opportunity, *JACC Cardiovasc Interv* 8:139–146, 2015.

Thiele H, Akin I, Sandri M: PCI strategies in patients with acute myocardial infarction and cardiogenic shock, *N Engl J Med* 377(25):2419–2432, 2017.

Yerasi C, Case BC, Forrestal BJ, et al: Optimizing monotherapy selection, aspirin versus P2Y12 inhibitors, following percutaneous coronary intervention, *Am J Cardiol* 135:154–165, 2020.

ANGINA PECTORIS

Method of
Kenneth Tobin, DO; and Kim Eagle, MD

CURRENT DIAGNOSIS

- The clinical diagnosis of angina depends largely on the accurate assessment of a patient's risk factor profile for coronary artery disease and the typicality of the symptom complex.
- The most common symptom of angina pectoris is left-sided chest pain or pressure, with or without associated radiation of pain or pressure to the jaw or left arm, occurring with exertion and relieved with rest or sublingual nitroglycerin.
- Women may present with atypical symptoms such as sharp, nonexertional chest pain, generalized fatigue, shortness of breath, or right-sided chest pain.
- Basic screening tests (e.g., 12-lead electrocardiogram, laboratory data, chest radiograph) are normal in most cases.
- For an initial diagnosis, appropriate noninvasive testing or coronary angiography, or both, is important to define the amount of ischemic myocardium and an overall treatment plan.
- Even when invasive procedures are clinically indicated, aggressive medical therapy with high-dose statins, attainment of appropriate blood pressure levels, smoking cessation, and use of antiplatelet therapy is of paramount importance.
- Patients who have clinical evidence of unstable angina and laboratory evidence of myocardial ischemia most often benefit from early invasive treatment strategies.

CURRENT THERAPY

Stable Angina Pectoris
- Treatment includes β-blockers, nitrates, and calcium channel blockers for symptom control.
- Consider the addition of ranolazine (Ranexa) if symptoms are not adequately controlled.

Aggressive Cholesterol Treatment Based on the American College of Cardiology (ACC)-American Hearth Association (AHA) Blood Cholesterol Guidelines
- Blood pressure management
- Antiplatelet therapy
- Lifestyle modifications:
  - Smoking cessation
  - Exercise prescription
  - Mediterranean, plant-based diet
  - Depression assessment

Unstable Angina
- With positive biomarkers for myocardial ischemia, consider coronary angiography.
- With negative biomarkers for myocardial ischemia, consider noninvasive assessment once symptoms are controlled.
- With a substantial ischemic burden identified, consider coronary angiography.
- With no or minimal ischemia identified, consider increasing medical therapy.
- With persistent symptoms, consider other treatment modalities.

Angina pectoris is defined as cardiac-induced pain that is a direct result of a mismatch between myocardial oxygen supply and demand. The initial presentation of ischemic heart disease is chronic stable angina in approximately 50% of patients; it is estimated that 16.5 million Americans are being diagnosed with this condition. Ischemic heart disease is the leading cause of death in the United States.

Stable angina refers to predictable chest discomfort during various levels of exertional activity that is predictably resolved with rest or administration of sublingual nitroglycerin (Nitrostat). Unstable angina is an acute ischemic event; this diagnosis includes patients with new-onset cardiac chest pain, angina at rest, postmyocardial infarction angina, or an accelerating pattern of previously stable angina. The terms unstable angina and non–Q wave myocardial infarction are often used interchangeably and should be further defined on the basis of myocardial necrosis as measured by serum biomarkers.

The clinical sensation of angina pectoris is caused by stimulation of chemosensitive and mechanosensitive receptors of unmyelinated nerve cells found within cardiac muscle fibers and around the coronary vessels. This stimulation cascade is thought to occur when lactate, serotonin, bradykinin, histamine, reactive oxygen species, and adenosine are released into the coronary circulation during periods of lactic acidosis. Nerve stimulation via the sympathetic ganglia occurs most commonly between the seventh cervical and fourth thoracic portions of the spinal cord. This explains from an anatomic standpoint why the most commonly recognized pain patterns for angina pectoris involve discomfort in the chest, neck, jaw, and left arm.

The most common cause of angina pectoris is coronary atherosclerosis. As plaque is initially deposited within a coronary vessel, there may be no significant internal luminal compromise during the early positive remodeling phase. However, at the point at which this compensatory mechanism fails, internal luminal compromise ensues. As long as the coronary artery segment distal to the stenosis retains the ability to vasodilate in response to increasing blood flow demands, coronary homeostasis is maintained. Once the critical threshold is passed, the blood supply cannot accommodate this demand, and angina may occur. The four major factors that determine myocardial oxygen demand are heart rate, systolic blood pressure, myocardial wall tension, and myocardial contractility.

Clinical Features

For patients with documented coronary artery disease (CAD) who have predictable episodes of classic symptoms, the diagnosis of angina pectoris is straightforward. Most patients are aware of the levels of exertion that typically induce angina symptoms. Most describe a pain or heaviness across their middle chest that may or may not radiate to the jaw or left arm. Some patients deny chest pain symptoms altogether and instead complain of exertional dyspnea or diaphoresis. Environmental situations such as cold exposure, emotional stress, or heavy meals can induce angina. The Canadian Cardiovascular Society and the New York Heart Association classification systems are used to define angina severity. Both systems use a I through IV scale, with mild angina (class I) referring to episodes that occur with extreme exertion and severe angina (class IV) to episodes that occur with minimal or no exertion. These classification systems are useful for risk stratification and for assessing medical therapy efficacy.

There are clear gender differences in the clinical presentations of angina. Pleuritic, musculoskeletal-type pain, nonexertional pain, and nocturnal pains have been reported as anginal equivalents in women. Fatigue is one of the most common presenting symptoms for CAD in women. The key to the diagnosis in men and women lies in a thorough history, which should always include the quality, location, provoking activities, and duration of pain and factors that relieve the pain. Based on a detailed clinical history, the many diagnoses that can masquerade as angina may be eliminated (Table 1).

Diagnostic Testing

A baseline electrocardiogram (ECG) is often one of the initial tests obtained in a patient with the complaint of chest pain. A normal tracing does not exclude the diagnosis of ischemic heart

TABLE 1	Differential Diagnosis of Chest Pain
Cardiac ischemia	
Angina	
Myocardial infarction	
Vasospastic angina	
Pericarditis	
Aortic dissection (new-onset chest pain and new aortic insufficiency noted on auscultation is an aortic dissection until proven otherwise)	
Pulmonary embolism	
Esophageal spasm	
Gastroesophageal reflux disease	
Musculoskeletal pain	
Biliary colic	
Acute pneumonia	

disease. More than 50% of patients with diagnosed angina have a normal ECG at rest. The baseline ECG may, however, show evidence of pathologic Q waves or left ventricular hypertrophy, either of which increases the statistical probability of significant CAD. Baseline laboratory data should include a fasting lipid panel to help define the patient's risk factor profile.

Stress testing is an appropriate screening tool for the initial diagnosis of CAD, risk stratification after acute ischemic syndrome, and assessment of treatment efficacy. Whenever feasible, it is more advantageous to obtain an exercise stress test rather than a pharmacologically based study. The additional prognostic data obtained through exercise include blood pressure response, heart rate response, heart rate recovery, metabolic equivalent level attained, and ECG assessment of the ST segment. There are several validated exercise protocols that provide additional risk stratification measures to the test results.

The predictive value of exercise treadmill stress testing ranges from 40% for single-vessel disease to 90% for three-vessel disease. A baseline left bundle branch block, paced rhythm, poorly controlled atrial arrhythmia, or left ventricular hypertrophy with secondary ischemic changes often renders the test inconclusive when assessing for ischemic changes. However, if stress testing is being performed for attainment of hemodynamic responses and achievable metabolic equivalent levels, these baseline ECG abnormalities may be overlooked.

Stress test accuracy is markedly improved by the addition of an imaging modality such as echocardiography or nuclear perfusion scanning. The sensitivity and specificity of stress echocardiography and stress nuclear imaging are 85% to 90%. Stress echocardiography is believed to be more specific, and stress nuclear imaging is thought to be more sensitive. A stress echocardiogram also allows assessment of left ventricular systolic function and valvular function and prediction of right ventricular pressure. In deciding on which stress test to perform, one should rely on the expertise of the testing facility and the individual patient's circumstance.

Risk Factor Management
Hypertension
Hypertension is a commonly occurring, well-established, major cardiovascular risk factor. Initial treatment of hypertension in patients with ischemic heart disease should always include lifestyle management. Appropriate weight loss with a goal of achieving a body mass index <25 kg/m^2 can improve hypertension control. A reduction in dietary salt intake can also have positive effects on a patient's blood pressure. Following a heart healthy diet and increased physical activity with a structured exercise program are also very important.

Discord has resulted from the publication of several recent hypertension guidelines by various medical societies, as well as the 2014 Evidence-Based Guideline for the Management of High Blood Pressure in Adults Report from the Panel Members Appointed to the Eighth Joint National Committee. It has been shown that cardiovascular risk progressively increases at blood pressures greater than 115/75 mm Hg. A meta-analysis of 61 prospective observational trials of hypertension involving 1 million adults with no known vascular disease at baseline revealed several interesting findings. Patient outcomes were related per decade of age to the usual blood pressure at the start of that decade. For example, from ages 40 to 69 years, for each increase in 20 mm Hg systolic blood pressure, a twofold increase in cardiovascular death rate occurred. These findings were much more pronounced in patients who were between 80 and 89 years old than in the youngest cohort, 40 to 49 years old. Although the relative risk was much higher in the younger group, the absolute risk was greatest among the octogenarians. These increased cardiovascular risks were not confined to subjects with blood pressures greater than 140/90 mm Hg; rather, there was a threshold of risk shown all the way down to 115/75 mm Hg. Even small reductions in blood pressure can have a significant positive impact on cardiovascular disease. Blood pressure reductions of 4 mm Hg systolic and 3 mm Hg diastolic were shown to reduce cardiovascular events by 15% in a cohort of 20,888 patients.

The Heart Outcomes Prevention Evaluation study asked the question whether all patients with atherosclerosis, regardless of blood pressure, should be treated with an angiotensin-converting enzyme inhibitor. Although many subsequent editorials implied that all patients with CAD could benefit from this therapy, a closer look at the data suggests a different interpretation. The mean blood pressure was 139/79 mm Hg, suggesting that a significant portion of the 9297 participants had a baseline blood pressure higher than this value. Compared with placebo, the treatment group had a 22% reduction in the primary outcome composite of myocardial infarction, stroke, or cardiovascular death. A small substudy using 24-hour ambulatory blood pressure monitoring showed blood pressure differences of 11 mm Hg systolic and 4 mm Hg diastolic in the treatment group compared with the placebo group, which may explain the cardiovascular event reductions reported.

The Systolic Blood Pressure Intervention Trial (SPRINT) studied cardiovascular outcomes in patients with increased cardiovascular risk (excluding diabetes) and randomized the more than 9000 participants to either intensive blood pressure control of <120 mm Hg or a standard blood pressure goal of <140 mm Hg. The trial was halted early because of the significant benefits seen in the intensive blood pressure arm. The intensive group had a 25% relative risk reduction for the primary composite endpoint compared to the standard care group. The blood pressure goal for treatment of hypertension in patients at high cardiovascular risk should be <130/80 mm Hg. High cardiovascular risk is defined as a history of clinical cardiovascular (CV) disease (established coronary artery disease, heart failure, or stroke), or an estimated 10-year atherosclerosis CV disease of ≥10%. (One must be careful with aggressive diastolic blood pressure management, as some studies have shown a J-shaped curve relationship between diastolic blood pressures and coronary events.)

Hyperlipidemia
Dyslipidemia is an important risk factor for atherosclerotic cardiovascular disease, and the lowering of low density lipoprotein (LDL)-cholesterol has been shown to correlate with reductions in cardiovascular disease event rates. Previously published cholesterol treatment guidelines recommended achieving less than 70 mg/dL LDL-cholesterol levels in CAD patients. The current guidelines published by the ACC-AHA depart from these specific values, and instead recommend using high-intensity 3-hydroxy-3-methylglutaryl coenzyme reductase inhibitors (statins) to reduce the LDL-cholesterol levels by more than 50%. These agents have been shown to be well tolerated and have positive nonlipid pleiotropic effects, as well as the ability to dramatically lower LDL levels.

Observational evidence suggests that regardless of how cholesterol is lowered, a reduction in atherosclerotic cardiovascular disease will result. However, to achieve meaningful reductions in cardiovascular mortality, the recommended choice for lowering LDL-cholesterol levels among the currently available pharmacology are the statins. These agents have been studied exclusively using fixed-dose combinations and not dose-titrated to achieve various LDL-C levels; therefore currently available data do not support specific LDL target goals.

The Cholesterol Treatment Trialists' meta-analysis, including 90,056 subjects from 14 trials, showed a 12% reduction in all-cause mortality per 38.6 mg/dL (1 mmol/L) reduction in LDL-cholesterol, with a 19% reduction in coronary mortality, a 24% reduction in need for revascularization, a 17% reduction in stroke incidence, and a 21% reduction in any major vascular event during a mean follow-up period of 5 years. These benefits were observed in different age groups, across genders, at different baseline cholesterol levels, and equally among those with and without prior CAD and cardiovascular risk factors.

The Heart Protection Study showed that in patients with established CAD, other atherosclerotic vascular disease, or diabetes, statin therapy reduced cardiovascular events regardless of the baseline LDL-cholesterol level. The trial, which enrolled 20,536 patients aged 40 to 80 years, showed a 24% reduction in major cardiovascular events, a 25% reduction in stroke, and a 13% reduction in overall mortality with statin therapy.

Patients with a recent acute ischemic syndrome were enrolled in the Pravastatin or Atorvastatin Evaluation and Infection Therapy trial, known as Thrombolysis in Myocardial Infarction 22, which compared 80 mg atorvastatin (Lipitor) with 40 mg of pravastatin (Pravachol). The atorvastatin group achieved a median LDL level of 62 mg/dL, compared with 96 mg/dL in the pravastatin group. The relative risk reduction for this reduced LDL level was 16%. A substudy looking at the LDL-cholesterol levels achieved with atorvastatin showed that those subjects achieving a level of 40 to 60 mg/dL had a 22% reduction in events, compared with those achieving a level of 80 to 100 mg/dL. Therefore, it appears that high-dose statin therapy and aggressive LDL-lowering in this patient population lead to reduced cardiovascular events.

The Treating to New Targets trial was the first to compare a more intensely treated group with a less intensely treated group using the same agent. The design of this 10,000-patient study eliminated concerns that outcome differences were induced by dissimilar statin preparations. The mean LDL level achieved was 101 mg/dL with 10 mg atorvastatin, and 77 mg/dL with the 80 mg dose. This LDL reduction was associated with a relative risk reduction of 27% for the primary endpoint of the first major cardiovascular event.

There is an increased risk of myopathy and rhabdomyolysis in patients taking 80 mg simvastatin (Zocor), according to the Study of the Effectiveness of Additional Reductions in Cholesterol and Homocysteine (SEARCH). The US Food and Drug Administration (FDA) has subsequently restricted high-dose simvastatin to patients who have been on this dose for longer than 12 months without evidence of myopathy, and the agency has recommended that new patients should not be started on this particular dose.

To effectively achieve a greater than 50% LDL-cholesterol reduction in CAD patients utilizing currently available pharmacologic agents, the most recent treatment guidelines suggest either atorvastatin 40 to 80 mg or rosuvastatin (Crestor) 20 to 40 mg. In other patient populations that require moderate-intensity statin therapy, there are several statin choices. Because there is no currently available evidence to suggest that nonstatin lipid-altering agents effectively reduce cardiovascular mortality, these medications should not be routinely prescribed.

It is apparent from both primary and secondary prevention lipid trials that achieving lower LDL levels reduces cardiovascular event rates. Because there is no high-quality clinical evidence to support achieving specific LDL levels in patients with diagnosed CAD, high-dose statin therapy should be the mainstay of pharmacologically based therapy, if tolerated.

Although statins are the standard pharmacologic approach for primary and secondary prevention of atherosclerotic cardiovascular disease, as many as 20% of patients may be intolerant. The numbers may be even higher if medication adherence is included. For secondary prevention in patients whose cholesterol levels are not adequately achieved on a statin or other cholesterol-lowering medication, a proprotein convertase subtilisin kexin type 9 (PCSK9) inhibitor is an FDA-approved option. PCSK9 inhibitors can also be considered for those with familial hypercholesterolemia and can be prescribed with or without a statin. The FOURIER Cardiovascular Outcomes trial studied more than 27,000 patients with stable atherosclerotic cardiovascular disease and showed that evolocumab (Repatha) reduced the primary endpoint of atherosclerotic events by 15%, without significant safety differences between treatment groups. Subgroup analyses suggested that greater benefits were seen in patients with longer exposure to evolocumab, recent acute coronary syndrome, multiple myocardial infarctions, multivessel coronary artery disease, peripheral arterial disease, as well as the subgroup who achieved very low low-density lipoprotein-cholesterol levels of below 0.3 mmol/L (10 mg/dL).

Omega-3 Fatty Acids

Omega-3 polyunsaturated fatty acids (PUFAs) are a well known part of a heart healthy diet, and are also an effective treatment for patients with elevated triglyceride levels. The Reduce-it trial studied a prescription strength omega-3 PUFA in well-controlled statin-treated patients with elevated triglycerides and either documented coronary artery disease, diabetes mellitus, or other cardiovascular risk factors. Seventy percent of the 8179 patients enrolled had a previous diagnosis of ischemic heart disease.

Patients were randomly assigned to receive 2 g of icosapent ethyl twice daily or placebo. The primary end point included cardiovascular death, nonfatal myocardial infarction, nonfatal stroke, coronary revascularization, or unstable angina. Patients treated with icosapent ethyl had a 25% risk reduction in cardiovascular events, and a 20% reduction in death due to cardiovascular causes.

This preparation of omega PUFA, icosapent ethyl (Vascepa), is pure eicosapentaenoic acid (EPA) which differs from agents used in other similar trials that contain both EPA and docosahexaenoic acid (DHA). This may explain the strongly positive outcomes that have not been shown in other similar trials.

Metabolic Syndrome

The combined presence of insulin resistance, hypertension, dyslipidemia, and abdominal obesity define metabolic syndrome. There is debate about whether this is a true syndrome or simply a clustering of cardiovascular risk factors in a particular individual. The key concept is that the concomitant presence of these particular cardiovascular risk factors markedly increases a patient's chances of developing diabetes mellitus and coronary atherosclerosis. The approach to treatment for this syndrome is no different from that for the individual components. Recognition of the components is key to the treatment of this disorder.

Smoking

Cigarette smoking is probably the most important of the identified modifiable cardiovascular risk factors. The incidence of CAD is two to four times higher in smokers than in nonsmokers. The pathophysiologic process that leads to atherosclerosis from smoking stems from induced platelet dysfunction, endothelial dysfunction, smooth muscle cell proliferation, and attenuated high-density lipoprotein cholesterol levels. Smoking cessation must be sought for every CAD patient.

Diet

Lifestyle changes for patients with CAD must incorporate healthy eating habits. The Mediterranean diet has been shown to positively affect cardiovascular disease, and conversely, a diet high in saturated fats has been shown to negatively influence multiple cardiac risk factors. Patients should be encouraged to incorporate high proportions of fruits and vegetables into their diet, along with olive oil and regular servings of fish coupled with a reduced amount of red meats and excess sugar.

Other Lifestyle Changes

Exercise should be encouraged in patients with stable angina, once all appropriate invasive and noninvasive tests have been completed and a stable medical regimen has been established.

Increasing a patient's aerobic capacity can lower the body's oxygen requirement for a given workload, which can lead to increased exercise tolerance and reduced anginal symptoms. Aerobic exercise can improve endothelial function and positively affect baroreflex sensitivity and heart rate variability in patients with CAD.

Endorphins released during exercise are thought to be mood enhancers, as well as effective muscle relaxants. Exercise itself improves sleep patterns. Cortisol levels are reduced with regular exercise, which may attenuate the body's sensation of stress and anxiety. For these reasons, appropriate exercise programs for patients with stable angina have far-reaching positive benefits. Exercise guidelines for CAD patients have been published and should be reviewed before patients begin aggressive secondary prevention efforts.

Major depression affects approximately 25% of people recovering from a myocardial infarction, and another 40% suffer from mild depression. In any given year, one of every three long-term acute ischemic syndrome survivors will develop depression. The Heart and Soul Study examined 1017 patients with stable CAD over a period of 4.8 years. Patients identified with depression were twice as likely to experience recurrent cardiovascular events. Physical inactivity was associated with a 44% greater rate of cardiovascular events. Patients with symptoms of depression were less likely to follow dietary, exercise, and medication recommendations.

Approach to Treatment

Medical Therapy

Medications used to treat angina pectoris and typical dosages are listed in Table 2.

Nitrates

Nitrates provide an exogenous source of nitric oxide, which serves to relax smooth muscle and inhibit platelet aggregation. Nitrates exert their antianginal effect by reducing myocardial oxygen demand through coronary and systemic vasodilation. Nitrates are strong venodilators, and in higher doses they can also induce arterial dilation. Reducing the preload through venodilation reduces myocardial oxygen demand. Coronary artery dilatation of stenotic vessels and intracoronary collaterals directly increases myocardial oxygen delivery. Through these mechanisms, nitrates have been shown to prevent recurrent episodes of angina and to increase exercise tolerance.

There are several nitrate preparations; they differ mainly in route of administration, onset of action, and effective half-life. Nitrate tolerance can occur with long-term use of any nitrate preparation and can be avoided by providing a 10- to 12-hour nitrate-free interval. Nitrates should be used with caution in patients with a diagnosis of hypertrophic obstructive cardiomyopathy.

β-Blockers

β-Blockers competitively inhibit catecholamines from binding to β-receptors. Over time, β-blocker therapy leads to an increase in β-receptor density. Because of receptor upregulation, acute β-blocker withdrawal may lead to a transient supersensitivity to catecholamines and subsequent angina or even myocardial infarction. There are three classes of β-receptors. Some β-blockers are receptor specific, and some exert an effect over all three receptors. However, at higher doses, even β-selective agents have cross-reactivity for all β-receptors. β-Blockers reduce myocardial oxygen demand through a negative inotropic effect, a chronotropic effect, and a reduction in left ventricular wall stress.

TABLE 2	Medications Used for the Treatment of Angina Pectoris
NAME	**DOSAGE**
β-Blockers	
Atenolol (Tenormin)	25–200 mg PO qd
Metoprolol tartrate (Lopressor)	25–200 mg bid
Metoprolol succinate (Toprol XL)	25–200 mg qd
Carvedilol (Coreg)[1]	6.25–25 mg PO bid
Carvedilol phosphate (Coreg CR)[1]	20–80 mg PO qd
Propranolol (Inderal)	80–320 mg/d, divided bid or tid
Propranolol (Inderal LA)	80–160 mg PO qd
Labetalol (Trandate, Normodyne)[1]	200–800 mg bid
Nitrates	
Isosorbide dinitrate (Isordil)	10–40 mg PO bid or tid
Isosorbide mononitrate (Imdur)	30–240 mg PO qd
Nitroglycerin (Nitrostat)	0.4 mg SL q5min
Nitroglycerin transdermal (Nitro-Dur)	0.2–0.8 mg/h 12–14 h patch
Calcium Channel Blockers	
Dihydropyridines	
Amlodipine (Norvasc)	2.5–10 mg PO qd
Felodipine (Plendil)[1]	2.5–10 mg PO qd
Nifedipine (Procardia XL)	30–90 mg PO qd
Nondihydropyridines	
Verapamil (Calan)	80–120 mg PO tid
Verapamil (Calan SR)	120–480 mg PO qd
Diltiazem (Cardizem)	360 mg/d PO, divided tid or qid
Diltiazem (Cardizem LA)	180–360 mg PO qd
Other	
Ranolazine (Ranexa)	500 mg twice daily and increase to 1000 mg twice daily as needed, based on clinical symptoms

[1]Not FDA approved for this indication.

Several cardioselective β-blockers, including atenolol (Tenormin) and metoprolol (Lopressor), have been shown to be effective antianginals that are fairly well tolerated in patients with underlying bronchospastic disease. Dosing is important for β-blocker efficacy. A study comparing atenolol with placebo showed that all doses from 25 through 200 mg/day were effective in reducing angina, but only the two highest doses led to an increase in exercise tolerance. Certain β-blockers have intrinsic sympathomimetic activity, including pindolol (Visken)[1] and acebutolol (Sectral).[1] Although they may be effective in reducing angina, they should be used with caution in patients with a prior history of myocardial infarction and in those with left ventricular dysfunction, because they may not reduce heart rate or blood pressure at rest.

When β-blockers are used to treat angina, a goal resting heart rate should be between 55 and 60 beats/min. Caution should be

[1]Not FDA approved for this indication.

used in patients with resting bradycardia and in those with known reactive airway disease. Atenolol is renally excreted and should be used with caution in the elderly and in those with known renal dysfunction.

Calcium Channel Blockers

Calcium channel blockers are classified as either dihydropyridines or nondihydropyridines. The former group includes amlodipine (Norvasc), felodipine (Plendil)[1], nifedipine (Procardia), and nicardipine (Cardene); the latter includes diltiazem (Cardizem) and verapamil (Calan). There are differences among the two subclasses in terms of chronotropic, dromotropic, and inotropic effects.

Calcium channel blockers positively alter myocardial oxygen supply and demand, mainly through direct arterial vasodilatation. The nondihydropyridines also exhibit negative chronotropic and inotropic effects, thus further lowering myocardial oxygen demands.

One of the early quick-release preparations of a dihydropyridine calcium channel blocker, nifedipine, was reported to potentially induce myocardial infarction when used to treat angina. This was most likely due to a rapid drop in afterload leading to reflex adrenergic activation. Sustained-release preparations of nifedipine (Procardia XL), as well as the other dihydropyridines, have been proven safe and effective in patients with cardiovascular disease. Although amlodipine and felodipine are tolerated in patients with left ventricular systolic dysfunction, other calcium channel blockers should be avoided in this patient subset.

Ranolazine (Ranexa)

Ranolazine (Ranexa) is a new and unique antianginal drug approved for the treatment of stable angina. It is a sustained-release preparation that has been approved for patients who remain symptomatic while on standard angina pharmacotherapy. Its mechanism of action may be through reduction of fatty acid oxidation or effects on sodium shifts and intracellular calcium levels. QT prolongation has been reported, but a significant increase in arrhythmias has not been seen. Side effects include dizziness, constipation, and nausea. Dosing is 500 or 1000 mg twice daily, and the major route of metabolism is the cytochrome P 450 system. Ranolazine should be used cautiously in patients who are taking other pharmacologic agents that have the potential to prolong the QT interval, and in patients with liver cirrhosis.

Ivabradine (Corlanor)[1]

Heart rate has a profound effect on diastolic perfusion time and subsequent myocardial oxygen supply. Ninety percent of coronary blood flow occurs in diastole. Therefore, an elevated heart rate may result in myocardial ischemia and angina. Ivabradine (Corlanor) selectively reduces heart rate without affecting inotropic function or coronary vasomotor tone. Ivabradine does not affect central aortic pressure or ventricular repolarization.

Ivabradine is a selective and specific inhibitor of the cardiac pacemaker current (If) that controls the spontaneous diastolic depolarization in the sinus node and regulates heart rate. It is metabolized by both the liver and the gut by oxidation through the cytochrome P450 3A4 (CYP3A4). Although ivabradine has a low affinity for CYP3A4, potent inhibitors and inducers of CYP3A4 may affect its plasma levels. Although nondihydropyridine calcium channel blockers should not be co-administered, other first-line coronary artery disease medications such as β-blockers, renin-angiotensin-aldosterone system inhibitors, aspirin, and HMG-CoA reductase inhibitors can be safely combined. Starting dosage is 5 mg twice daily in patients <75 years old, and 2.5 mg twice daily for patients ≥75 years old. No dosage adjustments are necessary in patients with renal impairment or creatinine clearance >15 mL/min. In patients with moderate hepatic impairment, caution is advised, and ivabradine is contraindicated

in patients with severe liver impairment. The maintenance dose is ≤7.5 mg twice daily, with up titration possible after 4 weeks if initial dose is well tolerated, symptoms persist, and heart rate is >60 bpm. Ivabradine is contraindicated in patients with a pre-treatment resting heart rate <70 bpm.

Heart rate reduction triggered by ivabradine appears to be greatest in those patients with highest pre-treatment baseline heart rates. Borer et al. showed that ivabradine improved exercise stress testing variables in a dose-dependent fashion. In this study, ivabradine improved time to 1 mm ST-segment depression as compared to placebo ($P = .016$). In a pooled analysis of 5 randomized, double blind, parallel-group studies of patients with stable angina, ivabradine ≥5 mg/day (maximum dose 7.5 mg/day) resulted in a 14.5% heart rate reduction, a −59.4% change in the number of angina attacks per week, and a −53.7% change in the consumption of nitrates.

There is mounting clinical evidence that ivabradine improves angina symptoms and quality of life (QOL) regardless of age, gender, and pre-treatment angina class. It also appears to improve prognosis and reduce hospitalizations in angina patients with left ventricular systolic dysfunction.

Medication Combinations

Many patients with chronic stable angina require more than one antianginal medication to control their symptoms. Current guidelines recommend β-blockers or calcium channel blockers as initial therapy unless otherwise contraindicated, with the addition of nitrates as symptoms dictate. Further medications may be added and individualized to each patient based on their degree of angina and overall clinical response.

However, it is important to recognize medication side effects when deciding which agents to combine. β-Blockers block the atrioventricular (AV) node and exert a portion of their effectiveness through this mechanism. The nondihydropyridine calcium channel blockers also have AV-nodal blocking properties and therefore should be used cautiously with β-blockers, especially in patients with preexisting conduction system disease. The dihydropyridine agents do not have AV-nodal blocking effects and may be a safer choice when used in combination with β-blockers. Nitrates do not have a side-effect profile that raises concerns when they are used with β-blockers or with calcium channel blockers.

Antiplatelet Therapy

The common etiology leading to an acute ischemic syndrome is a platelet-rich clot occurring at the site of a significant coronary artery stenosis, often after a plaque rupture. Antiplatelet medications have been shown to consistently decrease morbidity and mortality in a wide array of cardiovascular disease patients. A meta-analysis suggested that for patients with stable cardiovascular disease, low-dose aspirin therapy (50 to 100 mg daily) is as effective as higher doses (>300 mg). In this patient population, aspirin therapy resulted in a 26% reduction in myocardial infarction; the number of patients needed to treat to prevent a myocardial infarction was 83.

The Antiplatelet Trialists' Collaboration study demonstrated a reduction in myocardial infarction, stroke, and death in high-risk cardiovascular patients treated with antiplatelet therapy. Consensus guidelines recommend indefinite oral aspirin for the secondary prevention of cardiovascular events in all angina patients.

Clopidogrel (Plavix)[1] is an effective alternative to aspirin for the treatment of stable cardiovascular disease in those patients with a true aspirin allergy. However, there are no compelling data to indicate that clopidogrel (or newer agents, such as prasugrel [Effient][1] and ticagrelor [Brilinta][1]) are superior to aspirin in this particular patient population. In patients with unstable angina, dual antiplatelet therapy with aspirin and clopidogrel is recommended.

---

[1] Not FDA approved for this indication.

[1] Not FDA approved for this indication.

Oral Anticoagulation

The use of vitamin K antagonists to reduce cardiac events in patients with stable ischemic heart disease has been shown to be beneficial, with results tempered by the cost of a substantial increased risk of bleeding. With the advent of newer antithrombotic agents, also referred to as direct oral anticoagulants (DOACs), there has been renewed interest in further modulating the coagulation cascade to positively affect clinical outcomes.

The recent Rivaroxaban for the Prevention of Major Cardiovascular Events in Coronary or Peripheral Artery Disease (COMPASS) study evaluated the use of a factor Xa inhibitor, rivaroxaban (Xarelto), with or without aspirin vs. aspirin monotherapy in patients with stable atherosclerotic vascular disease. Rivaroxaban (Xarelto) dosing was 5 mg twice daily as monotherapy, 2.5 mg twice daily (referred to as a vascular dose) with 100 mg ASA, or 100mg ASA.

Although the primary combined endpoint revealed positive results in the rivaroxaban plus aspirin group, this was at the cost of a significant increase in overall bleeding events. If these events are separated into fatal or critical organ bleeding only, the findings favor a vascular dose of rivaroxaban plus aspirin for treatment of stable atherosclerotic vascular disease patients. Unfortunately, these results are equivocal when all bleeding events are taken into consideration. Moreover, the positive findings of this trial are driven mainly by a reduction in ischemic stroke and not myocardial infarction (49% RRR for ischemic stroke and 14% RRR for myocardial infarction). Although atrial fibrillation and/or prior use of systemic anticoagulation were exclusion criteria, certainly the percentage of this patient population with subclinical atrial fibrillation cannot be discounted.

Therefore, at this time there is no convincing evidence that adding antithrombotic therapy to aspirin or antithrombotic monotherapy should replace goal directed medical therapy of appropriate antiplatelet medications.

Invasive Assessment

The decision to pursue an invasive treatment approach differs significantly in patients with chronic stable angina and in those with acute coronary syndromes. Within both groups, accurate risk stratification is the key consideration in choosing who will benefit from coronary angiography and subsequent percutaneous coronary intervention. An invasive strategy in unstable angina patients has been shown to reduce recurrent acute coronary syndrome events consistently in many trials. A routine invasive strategy is recommended for patients with non-ST-segment acute ischemic syndromes who have refractory ischemia, elevated cardiac biomarkers suggesting myocardial necrosis, or new ST-segment depression on ECG monitoring.

In patients with unstable angina, there are significant gender differences in outcomes related to the use of invasive therapy. Both men and women with elevated biomarkers from myocardial necrosis have comparable reductions in rates of death, myocardial infarction, and rehospitalization with invasive treatment strategies. However, in the absence of positive biomarkers, women appear to have potentially negative outcomes with an invasive approach. The current American College of Cardiology and American Heart Association guidelines recommend a conservative approach in such women.

Patients diagnosed with stable angina comprise a vast array of clinical presentations. The two most heated debates in this arena concern the initial choice of medical therapy versus an invasive approach, and when to cross over from a medical treatment plan to an invasive one. The Atorvastatin Versus Revascularization Treatment (AVERT) trial studied the effects of intensive lipid-lowering therapy on ischemic events in a relatively low-risk population of patients with single- or two-vessel disease compared with percutaneous transluminal coronary angioplasty. AVERT randomized 341 patients to medical therapy plus atorvastatin 80 mg or to angioplasty followed by usual medical care (which included the option of statin therapy at the choice of the treating physician). The medical treatment group experienced a 36% reduction in the composite endpoint of ischemic events compared with the angioplasty group. This difference was due primarily to repeated angioplasty, coronary artery bypass grafting, or hospitalization for worsening angina. The primary outcome of this trial from a practical standpoint was that high-dose statin therapy was safe in this patient population and did not increase cardiovascular events, compared with an angioplasty-based treatment plan.

One of the keys in interpreting the available data is recognizing that by the time many of these trials are published, the percutaneous treatment choices are often outdated. Early trials used mainly balloon angioplasty; later trials used early-generation bare metal stents. Equally as important is to determine what the background medical treatment plans were for any particular trial on this subject. Often, lipid therapy was not aggressive, hypertension management was not confirmed to be adequate, and intravenous glycoprotein IIb/IIIa antagonists were either not available or not used as a standard protocol when indicated.

The Clinical Outcomes Utilizing Revascularization and Aggressive Drug Evaluation (COURAGE) trial was designed to address the potential advantages of current medical therapy over a percutaneous approach in patients with demonstrable ischemia but stable CAD. Of the 35,000 patients screened, only 2287 met the study inclusion criteria. All participants of the COURAGE trial underwent a coronary angiography, and patients with high-risk anatomic findings such as severe left main coronary artery stenosis were excluded. The biggest difference in this trial compared with previous studies was that strict guideline-based medical therapy was followed in both groups. In the entire cohort, 85% of subjects were taking a β-blocker, 93% were taking a statin, and 85% were taking aspirin. The final interpretation of the COURAGE trial results was not that medical therapy is superior for all patients with CAD, but that in selected cohorts, aggressive medical therapy is an appropriate first step in the treatment of ischemic heart disease.

It is well accepted that a coronary artery lesion ≥70% is clinically significant. Historically, the interventional cardiologist has relied on visually estimating this value during coronary angiography to determine when a percutaneous intervention is appropriate. However, physiology-guided revascularization has become an established practice in the management of patients with coronary artery disease. Both instantaneous wave free ration (iFR) and fractional flow reserve (FFR) are well-studied techniques that allow assessment of the pressure differences across a coronary artery stenosis.

iFR isolates a specific period in diastole where pressure and flow are linearly related, which is referred to as the wave-free period. During this time, competing forces (waves) that affect period diverge; an iFR value below 0.9 suggests flow restriction (normal value is 1.0). iFR is measured at rest, without the need for pharmacologic vasodilators or stressors.

FFR utilizes a guidewire that is passed through a coronary lesion and allows for measurement of both blood flow and pressure. After direct administration of the hyperemic agent adenosine (Adenocard)[1], the pressure difference across a stenosis is determined. An FFR of ≤0.80 is considered clinically significant.

Physiologic assessment of obstructive coronary artery disease adds clarity to the visual angiogram interpretation, thereby leading to more appropriate coronary interventions.

The ORBITA trial was a 200-patient placebo-controlled randomized trial assessing the efficacy of percutaneous coronary intervention (PCI) compared with a placebo sham procedure for the relief of angina in patients with severe (>70%) single-vessel coronary artery disease. Patients were randomized in a 1:1 fashion, and all patients had assessment of their coronary lesion by both FFR and iFR. All patients were assessed by cardiopulmonary exercise testing, symptom questionnaires, and dobutamine stress echocardiography before and six weeks after the procedure.

Compared with placebo, PCI reduced ischemia as assessed by stress echocardiography. However, there was no difference in the primary endpoint of exercise time between the two arms, or

---

[1] Not FDA approved for this indication.

statistically significant differences between the two groups with respect to angina frequency. Changes in the Duke treadmill score and exercise time were both numerically higher in the PCI arm, which poses the question of small sample size effects on these outcomes.

Within the spectrum of stable ischemic heart disease, a portion of patients have coronary arteries that have chronic total occlusions (CTO). Some of these ischemic heart disease patients may suffer from coronary reserve insufficiency and develop recurrent angina.

Since a CTO lesion cannot contribute to collateral blood flow, development of further CAD is often poorly tolerated. CTO lesions are encountered in clinical practice at a frequency of 16%–18%, but only intervened upon in 5%–10% of cases. We suspect this discrepancy in prevalence and treatment is based on the combination of a high rate of technical difficulty coupled with the uncertainty of clinical benefit.

Unfortunately, successful treatment of CTO lesions does not appear to benefit all patients with chronic ischemic heart disease. Patients with underlying diabetes have a reduction in major adverse cardiac events (MACE) when compared to standard medical therapy. This same finding, however, is not seen in non-diabetic patients with CTO lesions.

Novel Therapies
External Counterpulsation
External counterpulsation is a noninvasive method of increasing coronary blood flow through diastolic augmentation. Large blood pressure cuffs are placed on both legs and thighs and are inflated to a pressure of 300 mm Hg in early diastole (triggered by the patient's ECG), promoting venous return to the heart. The mechanism is unclear but may be related to enhanced endothelial function, improved myocardial perfusion, and possibly placebo effect. Several small studies have suggested a clinical reduction in angina episodes, but no positive mortality benefit has yet been published. A meta-analysis that included 13 observational studies and followed 949 patients with stable angina. Using the CCS classification scheme, there was at least a one-class improvement in 86% of the study population. Contraindications to this treatment include certain aortic valvular diseases, aortic aneurysm, and peripheral vascular disease.

Spinal Cord Stimulation
For patients whose angina is refractory to medical therapy and who are not candidates for revascularization, spinal cord stimulation may be considered. Little intermediate or long-term data are available, but many short-term studies suggest reduced angina episodes. Placement of the device and subsequent stimulation at the C7-T1 level suggests that the mechanism of action is reduced pain sensation.

Acupuncture
Acupuncture has been shown to be of benefit for the relief of both acute and chronic pain in various medical conditions. With respect to patients with documented CAD and symptomatic angina, there are only limited data currently available to recommend this modality.

A recently published randomized trial of treating chronic stable angina patients with acupuncture as an adjunct to standard medical therapy was undertaken in China. It was a small study of 398 relatively healthy angina patients. Those with prior myocardial infarction or a history of congestive heart failure were excluded. Patients were randomized to the following groups; disease-affected meridian (DAM), nonaffected meridian (NAM), sham acupuncture group, and a wait-list group. Treatment was 3 times per week for 4 weeks; each session was for 30 minutes. The greatest reduction of angina episodes occurred in the DAM group as compared to each of the other 3 groups.

This is the largest published clinical trial showing evidence that adding acupuncture to goal-directed medical therapy reduces angina frequency. There were some study limitations that are worth mentioning that may soften the results. Namely, the operators were not blinded to their treatment plans, angina episodes were reduced in the sham and wait-list groups (suggesting a strong placebo-associated effect), and the study population was small.

Other Causes of Angina
Syndrome X
The cardiac syndrome X refers to patients who have normal or near-normal epicardial coronary arteries and episodic chest pain. This disorder is much more common in women and is often seen in patients younger than 50 years of age. The chest pain episodes may last longer than 30 minutes and may have a variable response to sublingual nitrates. Patients with syndrome X often describe typical stress-induced angina. Risk factors include hypertension, diabetes, and hyperlipidemia. Female patients are typically postmenopausal and frequently have stress-induced symptoms and ischemia on stress imaging. They often respond to standard angina medications and typically have a better prognosis than patients with significant epicardial plaque.

Vasospastic or Prinzmetal Angina
The classic definition of Prinzmetal angina is chest pain with documented ST-segment elevation during symptoms or during exercise in the face of angiographically normal or near-normal coronary arteries. Over the years, the definition has expanded to include patients who have classic angina symptoms commonly relieved with nitrates or calcium channel blockers and minimal or no CAD. It has been shown that patients with nonobstructive CAD may be prone to focal artery spasm at the stenosis site; therefore, the previous requirement of normal coronary arteries is not an absolute necessity. Other disease states (e.g., Raynaud phenomenon) can increase a patient's development of coronary artery spasm, as can illicit drug usage (e.g., cocaine). Vasospasm is more common in active smokers. β-Blockers should be used cautiously in these patients because they may exacerbate coronary spasm. Patients with angiographically documented intramyocardial bridging may be prone to focal coronary spasm and subsequent angina pectoris.

Newer Imaging Techniques
Calcium Scoring
Coronary artery calcium scoring is a well-studied imaging modality used to assess a patient's pretest probability of CAD. With respect to evaluation for angina, one must remember that electron-beam computed tomographic (CT) scanning does not offer physiologic data and therefore does not allow determination of myocardial ischemia. This study is most useful in the workup of a low-risk patient with an atypical chest pain syndrome. If such a patient has an elevated calcium score, other studies may be reasonable and further assessment of the patient's cholesterol values should be performed.

Computed Tomographic Coronary Angiography
CT coronary angiography is a noninvasive way to image the coronary arteries. Similar to electron-beam CT, it does not provide physiologic data regarding coronary artery perfusion, but it does provide anatomic information such as the presence and percentage of coronary artery stenosis. Although selected patients with stable or unstable angina may be considered candidates for CT angiography, its main utility is to evaluate patients for chest pain who are otherwise at low risk and have a low pretest probability. Because of the volume of intravenous contrast required by CT angiography, the risk of contrast nephropathy must be considered when contemplating this study.

Summary
The approach to the patient with angina should be based on a global assessment and intensive treatment of all identified cardiovascular risk factors. It is recommended that all patients receive the appropriate dose of statin and antiplatelet therapy. Noninvasive testing is helpful for an initial diagnosis and to guide the

decision for a more invasive approach. Familiarity and adherence to current treatment guidelines is of paramount importance. There are important gender differences that should not be overlooked in the clinical presentation of angina and in the approach to optimal therapy.

References

Allan BS, Krumholz HM, SM reviewing The SPRINT Research Group: N Engl J Med 2015 Nov 9 Chobanian AV, *N Engl J Med*, 2015 Nov 9.

Anderson JL, Adams CD, Antman EM: ACC/AHA 2007 guidelines for the management of patients with unstable angina/non-ST-elevation myocardial infarction: A report of the American College of Cardiology/American Heart Association Task Force on Practice Guidelines, *J Am Coll Cardiol* 5067:e1–e157, 2007.

Antithrombotic Trialists Collaboration: Collaborative meta-analysis of randomized trials of antiplatelet therapy for prevention of death, myocardial infarction, and stroke in high risk patients, *BMJ* 324:71–86, 2002.

Berger J, Brown D, Becker R: Low-dose aspirin in patients with stable cardiovascular disease: A meta-analysis, *Am J Med* 121:43–49, 2008.

Bhatt DL, Steg PG, Miller M, et al: Cardiovascular risk reduction with icosapent ethyl for hypertriglyceridemia. *N Engl J Med* 380:11–22, 2019.

Blood Pressure Lowering Treatment Trialists Collaboration: Effects of different blood pressure lowering regimens on major cardiovascular events: Results of prospectively-designed overviews of randomized trials, *Lancet* 362:1527–1545, 2003.

Boden WE, O'Rourke RA, Teo KK: Optimal medical therapy with or without PCI for stable coronary disease, *N Engl J Med* 35:1503–1516, 2007.

Borer JS, Fox K, Jaillon P: Antianginal and antischemic effects of Ivrabidine, a novel I(f) inhibitor, in stable angina:a randomized, double-blind, multicentered, placebo-controlled trial, *Circulation* 107:817–823, 2003.

Cholesterol Treatment Trialists' Collaborators: Efficacy and safety of cholesterol-lowering treatment: Prospective meta-analysis of data from 90,056 participants in 14 trials of statins, *Lancet* 366:1267–1278, 2005.

De Bruyne B, Fearon WF, Pijls NH: Fractional flow reserve-guided PCI for stable coronary artery disease, *N Engl J Med* 371:1208–1217, 2014.

Eikelboom JW, Connolly SJ, Bosch J, et al: COMPASS Investigators. Rivaroxaban with or without aspirin in stable cardiovascular disease, *N Engl J Med* 377:1319–1330, 2017.

Fefer P, Knudtson ML, Cheema AN, et al: Current perspectives on coronary chronic total occlusions: the Canadian multicenter chronic total occlusions registry, *J Am Coll Cardiol* 59:991–997, 2012.

Fihn SD, Gardin JM, Abrams J: 2012 ACCF/AHA/ACP/AATS/PCNA/SCAI/STS guideline for the diagnosis and management of patients with stable ischemic heart disease: A report of the American College of Cardiology Foundation/American Heart Association Task Force on Practice Guidelines, and the American College of Physicians, American Association for Thoracic Surgery, Preventive Cardiovascular Nurses Association, Society for Cardiovascular Angiography and Interventions, and Society of Thoracic Surgeons, *J Am Coll Cardiol* 60:e44–e164, 2012.

Gibbons RJ, Abrams J, Chatterjee K, et al: ACC/AHA 2007 guideline update for the management of patients with chronic stable angina: A report of the American College of Cardiology/American Heart Association Task Force on Practice Guidelines (Committee to Update the 2002 Guidelines for the Management of Patients with Chronic Stable Angina) Reston, VA, American College of Cardiology, American Heart Association Available at: www.acc.org/qualityandscience/cl inical/guidelines/stable/stable_clean.pdf (accessed August 20, 2014).

Grundy SM, Cleeman JI, Merz NB: Implications of recent clinical trials for the National Cholesterol Education Program Adult Treatment Panel III guidelines, *Circulation* 110:227–239, 2004.

Heart Outcomes Prevention Evaluation Study Investigators: Effects of an angiotensin-converting-enzyme inhibitor, ramipril, on cardiovascular events in high-risk patients, *N Engl J Med* 342:145–153, 2000.

James PA, Oparil S, Carter BL: 2014 evidence-based guideline for the management of high blood pressure in adults: Report from the panel members appointed to the eighth Joint National Committee (JNC 8), *JAMA* 311:507–520, 2014.

Mehta SR, Cannon CP, Fox KA: Routine vs selective invasive strategies in patients with acute coronary syndromes: A collaborative meta-analysis of randomized trials, *JAMA* 293:2908–2917, 2005.

Messerli FH, Mancia G, Conti CR: Dogma disrupted: Can aggressively lowering blood pressure in hypertensive patients with coronary artery disease be dangerous? *Ann Intern Med* 144:884–893, 2006.

Montalescot G, Sechtem U, Achenbach S: Editor's choice: 2013 ESC guidelines on the management of stable coronary artery disease: The Task Force on the management of stable coronary artery disease of the European Society of Cardiology, *Eur Heart J* 34:2949–3003, 2013.

Petraco R, Al-Lamee R, Gotberg M: Real-time use of instantaneous wave-free ratio: results of the ADVISE in-practice: an international, multicenter evaluation of instantaneous wave-free ratio in clinical practice, *Am Heart J* 168:739–748, 2014.

Ray K, Cannon C: Optimal goal for statin therapy use in coronary artery disease, *Curr Opin Cardiol* 20:525–529, 2005.

Sabatine MS, Giugliano RP, Keech AC: Evolocumab and clinical outcomes in patients with cardiovascular disease, *N Engl J Med* 376:1713–1722, 2017.

SEARCH Collaborative Group: Intensive lowering of LDL cholesterol with 80mg versus 20mg simvastatin daily in 12,064 survivors of myocardial infarction: A double-blind randomised trial, *Lancet* 376:1658–1669, 2010.

Stone G, Teirstein P, Rubenstein R: A prospective, multicenter, randomized trial of percutaneous transmyocardial laser revascularization in patients with nonrecanalizable chronic total occlusions, *J Am Coll Cardiol* 39:1581–1587, 2002.

Stone NJ, Robinson J, Lichtenstein AH, et al: 2013 ACC/AHA guideline on the treatment of blood cholesterol to reduce atherosclerotic cardiovascular risk in adults: A report of the American College of Cardiology/American Heart Association Task Force on Practice Guidelines, Circulation.

Tendera M, Borer JS, Tardif JC: Efficacy of I(f) inhibition with Ivabradine in different subpopulations with stable angina pectoris, *Cardiology* 114:116–125, 2009.

Weber MA, Schiffrin EL, White WB: Clinical practice guidelines for the management of hypertension in the community, *J Clin Hypertens* 16:14–26, 2014.

Wenger NK: *Cardiac Rehabilitation: A Guide to Practice in the 21st Century*, New York, 1999, Marcel Dekker.

Whooley MA, Jonge P, Vittinghoff E: Depressive symptoms, health behaviors, and risk of cardiovascular events in patients with coronary heart disease, *JAMA* 300:2379–2388, 2008.

Acupuncture as Adjunctive Therapy for Chronic Stable Angina: A Randomized Clinical Trial.

Zhao L, Li D, Zheng H: *JAMA Intern Med*, 2019 Jul 29.

2017 ACC/AHA/AAPA/ABC/ACPM/AGS/APhA/ASH/ASPC/NMA/PCNA Guideline for the Prevention, Detection, Evaluation, and Management of High Blood Pressure in Adults: A Report of the American College of Cardiology/American Heart Association Task Force on Clinical Practice Guidelines.

Zhu Y, Meng S, Chen M, et al: Long-term prognosis of chronic total occlusion treated by successful percutaneous coronary intervention in patients with or without diabetes mellitus: a systematic review and meta-analysis, *Cardiovasc Diabetol* 20:29, 2021.

AORTIC DISEASE: ANEURYSM AND DISSECTION

Method of
David G. Neschis, MD

CURRENT DIAGNOSIS

- Because the majority of patients with abdominal aortic aneurysms are asymptomatic, the majority of abdominal aortic aneurysms are detected on imaging studies performed for other indications.
- Patients older than 50 years who present with abdominal or back pain of unclear etiology should be considered for evaluation of possible abdominal aortic aneurysm.
- Asymptomatic men older than 65 years who have ever smoked are eligible for abdominal aortic aneurysm screening.
- All patients older than 60 years who have a strong family history of abdominal aortic aneurysms should be considered for screening.
- Patients presenting with sudden onset of chest or back pain without clear etiology should be evaluated for dissection.
- Dissection can mimic numerous other conditions.

CURRENT THERAPY

Indications for Repair of Aneurysm
- Fusiform abdominal aortic aneurysms greater than 5.5cm in maximum diameter
- Most saccular aneurysms and pseudoaneurysms
- Thoracic and thoracoabdominal aortic aneurysms of greater than 6cm in maximal diameter
- Aneurysms that are symptomatic or are rapidly enlarging

Indications for Repair of Aortic Dissection
- Dissections involving the ascending aorta
- Dissections involving only the descending aorta are usually managed medically unless complicated by the following: unrelenting pain, end organ ischemia, or significant aneurysmal degeneration to greater than 6cm in maximal diameter

Abdominal Aortic Aneurysms

Epidemiology

A ruptured abdominal aortic aneurysm is a devastating event leading to approximately 15,000 deaths per year, and it is the 13th leading cause of death in the United States. It is the 10th leading cause of death in men. Once rupture occurs, there is an 85% chance of death overall and approximately 50% mortality in the patients who make it to the hospital alive. Clearly, the goal is to identify this life-threatening lesion and repair prior to rupture. Abdominal aortic aneurysms are approximately four times more prevalent in men than in women. The overall incidence in persons older than 60 years is approximately 3% to 4%, with incidence as high as 10% to 12% in an elderly hypertensive population.

Risk Factors

Men are approximately 4 times more likely than women to develop an abdominal aortic aneurysm. Clearly, older persons, particularly those older than 60 years, are at higher risk. Tobacco use is probably the strongest preventable risk factor, with tobacco users being approximately eight times more likely to be affected than nonsmokers. Hypertension is present in approximately 40% of patients with abdominal aortic aneurysms. Family history also plays a significant role. In fact, men who have first-degree female relatives who had aneurysms are approximately 18 times more likely than the general population to develop an abdominal aortic aneurysm. There is also a strong correlation between abdominal aortic aneurysms and other peripheral artery aneurysms. Patients with bilateral popliteal artery aneurysms have an approximately 50% to 60% risk of having an abdominal aortic aneurysm.

Pathophysiology

An aneurysm is a dilatation of a blood vessel that could occur in any blood vessel in the body, even in the veins. Most commonly it is defined as a dilatation of approximately 1.5 to 2 times at that diameter of the adjacent normal vessel.

The definition of a pseudoaneurysm is often misunderstood. The attempt to describe a pseudoaneurysm in terms of the number of layers of the artery wall involved does nothing to help resolve this confusion. A pseudoaneurysm is a walled-off defect in the artery wall. A circular shell of adventitial and surrounding connective tissue contains the blood, preventing free hemorrhage. However, there remains continued flow out and back into the arterial lumen, resulting in a classic to-and-fro pattern on duplex ultrasound. The most common cause of a pseudoaneurysm is iatrogenic, from needle puncture, but it also can be caused by trauma or focal rupture of the artery at the site of an atherosclerotic ulcer.

The etiology of true aneurysms is not clear, although in the past these have been attributed to atherosclerosis. However, it is well known that the majority of patients with abdominal aortic aneurysms do not have associated significant occlusive disease. Biochemical studies have demonstrated decreased quantities of elastin and collagen in the walls of aneurysmal aortas. It is believed that a family of enzymes known as matrix metalloproteinase (MMP), particularly those that have collagenase and elastase activity, are likely involved in development of arterial aneurysms. The propensity for growth and rupture is based on Laplace's law, $T = PR$, where T represents wall tension (or in other words the propensity to rupture), P is the transmitted pressure, and R is the radius. This explains why patients with hypertension and those with larger aneurysms are at higher risk for aortic rupture.

Prevention

Currently the most effective means to prevent aneurysm rupture is early detection and elective repair. Avoidance of smoking and aggressive control of blood pressure would likely be helpful in preventing aneurysmal development and growth. Patients with known abdominal aortic aneurysms that are relatively small and at low risk for rupture are generally serially followed with imaging studies over time. These patients are advised to avoid straining (e.g., heavy lifting), avoid smoking, and keep their blood pressure well controlled.

Investigation is ongoing in efforts to develop a medication that may be helpful in slowing the growth of abdominal aortic aneurysms. It has been known since 1985 that tetracycline antibiotics have activity against MMPs. There had been several animal studies and at least one small human study suggesting that doxycycline (Vibramycin)[1] may be effective at slowing the growth of abdominal aortic aneurysms. Currently, larger human studies are ongoing. At this point, there are no formal recommendations regarding the use of doxycycline for the purpose of slowing aneurysmal growth.

Clinical Manifestations

Approximately 75% of abdominal aortic aneurysms are asymptomatic and discovered incidentally. Unfortunately, physical examination is an unreliable method for detecting aneurysms or determining aneurysm size. In heavier patients it may be simply impossible to adequately palpate the aorta. The majority of aneurysms are incidental findings identified on imaging studies performed for other reasons. Occasionally, an aneurysm is first detected upon operation for another condition.

Unfortunately, when an aneurysm becomes symptomatic, this is usually a sign of impending rupture. Symptoms related to abdominal aortic aneurysms can include abdominal or back pain. The classic triad of findings in the setting of abdominal aortic aneurysm rupture includes abdominal pain, hypotension, and a pulsatile abdominal mass. This triad, however, occurs in only approximately 20% of the patients. Often a high index of suspicion needs to be maintained.

The episode of hypotension associated with aneurysm rupture may be manifested as an episode of syncope or near-syncope before the patient arrives at the hospital. It is quite possible for the patient to have a contained rupture of the abdominal aorta and appear quite stable with a normal blood pressure in the emergency department. Although uncommon, a primary fistula between the aneurysm and gastrointestinal tract can occur and manifest as gastrointestinal bleeding.

Diagnosis

Several imaging modalities are available that can accurately diagnose and measure abdominal aortic aneurysms. Real-time B-mode ultrasound scanning has the advantage of being almost universally available, relatively inexpensive, and essentially risk free. The major disadvantage, however, is that it is technician dependent. Computed tomography (CT) scans can provide a very accurate representation of the aorta in a very short study time (Figures 1 and 2). The use of iodinated contrast is not necessary to obtain a gross size

---

[1] Not FDA approved for this indication.

Figure 1 Large abdominal aortic aneurysm. Notice how the majority of this aneurysm is filled with laminated thrombus. The flow lumen is only mildly dilated, and this aneurysm could be missed on angiography alone.

measurement of the aorta. The contrast, however, helps delineate the flow lumen more clearly, and it is quite valuable in planning repair. Disadvantages include the use of ionizing radiation and the use of iodinated contrast material. MRI is also accurate in determining the size of the aneurysm; however, study times are longer, equipment is less widely available, and the expense is considerable. Angiography, while excellent for evaluating the status of important aortic branches and for evaluating occlusive disease, is not an accurate study for the purpose of determining maximal diameter of the aneurysm. Often aneurysms are filled with laminated thrombus, and the flow lumen, which was seen on aortography, is not representative of the true aneurysm size.

Figure 2 Classic image of a ruptured abdominal aortic aneurysm, which in this case can be seen even without the use of intravascular contrast. Note the lack of symmetry and obliteration of tissue planes in the retroperitoneum on the left.

Treatment

The decision on when to intervene in an abdominal aortic aneurysm is based on a careful analysis of the patient's risk for rupture versus the risk of operative repair. Historically, open repair can be performed with less than 5% in-hospital mortality. Based on historical studies it was estimated that the risk of rupture for an approximately 5-cm aneurysm was about 1% per year, which increased dramatically to 6.6% for aneurysms between 6 and 7 cm. It has been fairly well established for years that aneurysms larger than 5.5 cm are generally recommended for repair and those less than 4 cm are generally observed over time. There remains a gray area for moderate aneurysms in the 4- to 5.5-cm category.

Two large prospective randomized trials were developed to answer this question. These include the United Kingdom Small Aneurysm Trial and the Department of Veterans Affairs Aneurysm Detection and Management (ADAM) trial. Both these studies randomized patients with moderately sized aneurysms to observation versus open repair. Results of both trials were fairly similar. The rupture rate for aneurysms under observation was 0.5% to 1% per year, and neither trial showed a difference in long-term survival. Both studies concluded that it was relatively safe to observe patients with aneurysms less than 5.5 cm in diameter, particularly in men who would be compliant with the follow-up regimen. The diameter of the aneurysm, however, should not be the only data point used for a decision on whether to repair.

Women seem to have a higher rupture rate for a particular aneurysm diameter than men, perhaps because they are starting with smaller aortas to begin with. Patients with COPD may be at higher risk for rupture as well. Saccular or eccentric-shaped aneurysms may also have a higher propensity to rupture and should not be subject to diameter recommendations for fusiform aneurysms (Figures 3 and 4). Additionally, rapidly growing aneurysms—growing at a rate faster than approximately 0.5 cm per year—should be considered for repair.

Figure 3 Axial CT slice and reconstructed images of a saccular abdominal aortic aneurysm. This lesion could also be described as a pseudoaneurysm. For these, treatment is recommended because it is thought that the risk of rupture is higher than for a similarly sized fusiform abdominal aortic aneurysm.

Figure 4 Angiogram of patient in Figure 3, demonstrating aneurysm before and after deployment of an endograft, which successfully excluded the lesion from the circulation.

Once it has been determined that repair is indicated, a number of options are available. Traditional open repair involves a relatively large abdominal incision, cross clamping of the aorta, and replacement of the aneurysmal segment with a graft of polyethylene terephthalate (Dacron) or polytetrafluoroethylene (PTFE; Teflon). Often the iliac arteries are involved, and in these cases a bifurcated graft is placed. Open repair is quite durable and very effective at preventing aneurysm-related deaths. Long-term complications are rare, and patients following open repair generally enjoy 95% freedom from issues related to the repair over the course of their lifetime. Disadvantages, however, include the large incision and an approximate 1-week hospital stay. Recovery to a relatively normal level of function occasionally takes months. In the past, many patients were deemed too old or frail to be expected to undergo open surgery.

Endograft repair has revolutionized the practice of vascular surgery. Using small incisions placed at the groin and performing the procedure under fluoroscopic guidance, devices can now be advanced into the aorta from the femoral artery. Using angiography as a guide, the graft typically is deployed below the renal arteries and effectively excludes the aneurysm from the circulation. Advantages include small incisions and very short hospital stays. Patients are typically discharged on the first or second day after aneurysm repair. Recovery to normal activity is also quite rapid, taking approximately 1 to 2 weeks. Use of this modality has allowed treatment of older and frailer patients who previously were denied treatment due to concerns of operative risk.

Endograft repair, however, is clearly not without its disadvantages. Currently, the durability of endograft repair is unknown, and these patients are subject to frequent serial imaging. Also, there is a higher incidence of graft-related complications, which can occur in up to 35% of patients. These include the development of leaks of blood into the aneurysm sac outside the graft device, issues related to graft failure and migration, and graft limb thrombosis. These grafts are also quite expensive.

Two major prospective randomized trials studying traditional open versus endograft repair are often cited. These include the United Kingdom–based EVAR-1 trial (first Endovascular Aneurysm Repair trail) and the Dutch-based DREAM trial (Diabetes REduction Assessment with ramipril and rosiglitazone Medication trial). Both studies randomized patients who were believed to be good risks for open repair to endograft versus traditional open repair. The results of both of these studies were relatively similar in that both studies demonstrated a clear early survival benefit for patients in the endograft group. However, this came at a cost of an increased incidence of graft-related complications in the endograft group and a higher cost for the endograft group. Additionally, at 2 to 4 years, there was no clear difference in long-term survival in either group.

Ultimately, the decision about whether to proceed with open or endograft repair is a decision between surgeon and patient based on the patient's aortic anatomy, overall health, and the patient's and physician's preference. It would appear, however, that older and frail patients with good anatomy should be strongly considered for endograft repair.

Monitoring

Patients with abdominal aortic aneurysms should be evaluated for the presence of femoral and popliteal aneurysms (particularly in men) and for thoracic aortic aneurysms. After open repair, a follow-up CT scan with contrast should be considered approximately 5 years out to evaluate for the integrity of the graft (i.e., pseudoaneurysms), as well as development of new aneurysms. Patients who have undergone endograft repair require more-intensive monitoring. Typical regimens include a contrast-enhanced CT scan approximately 2 weeks after repair, then 6 months after repair, and then based on the perceived stability of the graft, approximately yearly thereafter. Some centers have used duplex ultrasonography for evaluating patients after endograft repair in efforts to reduce the amount of ionizing radiation the patients receive. However, it should be remembered that duplex ultrasound is highly technician dependent, and follow-up of patients with endograft repairs using only duplex ultrasound should be performed in experienced centers.

Thoracic Aortic Aneurysms

Thoracic aortic aneurysms (TAAs) are limited to the chest cavity. Although they are less common than infrarenal abdominal aortic aneurysms, they share similar risk factors. The male-to-female ratio incidence of the TAA is approximately 1:1.

In the past, the threshold for repair was at a diameter greater than 6 cm. This threshold was chosen due to the higher operative risks associated with repair of the thoracic aorta. Now with the availability of endograft, patients with good anatomy are generally recommended for repair at a diameter similar to those for the infrarenal aorta.

Open repair involves performing a thoracotomy and cross-clamping the aorta. Repair in this location is often performed with the addition of extracorporeal bypass to maintain perfusion to the viscera and spinal cord drain performance of the repair. Although the risk of paraplegia in the treatment of infrarenal aortic is exceedingly low, the risk of paraplegia from a repair of an isolated TAA is approximately 6%. Endograft devices for repair of TAA are now widely available and have reduced the incidence of paraplegia to approximately 3%.

Thoracoabdominal Aortic Aneurysms

By definition, thoracoabdominal aortic aneurysms require entrance to both the thoracic and abdominal cavity to perform repair. These lesions are usually true aneurysms of the aorta and should not be confused with dissection. Repair of thoracoabdominal aortic aneurysms is quite complex and carries risks of death and paraplegia as high as 20% in some settings. These procedures are generally performed at larger institutions with considerable experience with this condition. Unfortunately, endograft devices for the repair of thoracoabdominal aortic aneurysms are limited to a handful of centers in the United States.

Thoracic Aortic Dissection

Thoracic aortic dissection is the most common aortic emergency, even more common than ruptured abdominal aortic aneurysm. This potentially fatal condition is rare in patients younger than 50 years and is approximately two times more common in men than women. Patients at risk include patients with a history of connective tissue disorders and patients with severe, poorly controlled hypertension.

An aortic dissection occurs when there is loss of integrity of the intima and blood dissects into the media. Once in the media, there is a natural plane through which dissection is quite easy.

Although there are various classification systems for aortic dissection, the Stanford classification is perhaps the most widely used and the most useful. In this classification, any dissection that involves the ascending aorta, whether it involves the ascending aorta alone or both the ascending and descending thoracoabdominal aorta, are classified as type A. Dissections that do not involve the ascending aorta are classified as type B. This classification is useful because type A dissections require urgent surgery. Type B dissections are typically managed medically unless they are associated with complications such as unremitting pain, aneurysmal expansion, and end-organ ischemia. By convention, aortic dissections that are evaluated within 14 days after the onset of symptoms are considered acute, and those evaluated beyond 14 days are considered chronic.

Helical CAT scanners with the use of contrast are excellent at defining the location and extent of aortic dissection. However, being alert to the potential for this diagnosis requires a high index of suspicion. Aortic dissection can mimic a variety of common conditions based on the extent of the dissection and the aortic branches involved (Table 1). Uncomplicated type B dissections are typically managed medically. This is usually performed in an intensive care setting with the use of intravenous medications to control contractility and, if necessary, hypertension.

In the past, due to the friability of dissected aortic tissue, the results of operative repair for type B dissections have been particularly poor. Currently, endograft repair with the purpose of excluding the entry point of dissection and reestablishing flow

TABLE 1 Dissection: The Great Mimic

TERRITORY INVOLVED OR AFFECTED BY DISSECTION	MIMICS
Rupture into pericardial sac	Cardiac tamponade
Dissection through aortic valve	Acute aortic insufficiency
Dissection occluding coronary arteries	Myocardial infarction
Involvement of cerebral vessels	Stroke
Involvement of subclavian arteries	Upper extremity ischemia (cold arm)
Dissection running down descending thoracic aorta	Severe back pain and paralysis
Mesenteric artery obstruction	Mesenteric ischemia
Renal artery obstruction	Oliguria and acute renal failure
Iliac artery occlusion	Lower extremity ischemia (cold leg)

to the true lumen is gaining popularity in the treatment of complex dissection. This at times may be supplemented by stenting of affected aortic side branches and fenestration to establish a connection between the true and false lumen to restore perfusion to certain organs. Once the acute phase has passed and medically treated patients are under good hypertensive control, these patients are then converted to an oral medication regimen and transferred out of the intensive care setting. Patients need to be followed up with serial CT imaging after discharge to evaluate for aneurysmal degeneration of the false lumen. This evaluation should occur every 6 months until the patient is stable and then yearly thereafter.

In cases where the total aortic diameter grows to greater than 6 cm, repair for the purpose of preventing rupture is indicated, although this is often technically more complicated than treating a fusiform aneurysm in the absence of a previous dissection. Patients should strictly adhere to their blood pressure medication regimen for life.

References

Blankensteijn JD, de Jong SE, Prinssen M, et al: Two-year outcomes after conventional or endovascular repair of abdominal aortic aneurysms, *N Engl J Med* 352(23):2398–2405, 2005.

Crawford ES, Crawford JL, Safi HJ, et al: Thoracoabdominal aortic aneurysms: Preoperative and intraoperative factors determining immediate and long-term results of operations in 605 patients, *J Vasc Surg* 3(3):389–404, 1986.

Daily PO, Trueblood HW, Stinson EB, et al: Management of acute aortic dissections, *Ann Thorac Surg* 10(3):237–247, 1970.

EVAR Trial Participants: Endovascular aneurysm repair versus open repair in patients with abdominal aortic aneurysm (EVAR trial 1): Randomised controlled trial, *Lancet* 365(9478):2179–2186, 2005.

EVAR Trial Participants: Endovascular aneurysm repair and outcome in patients unfit for open repair of abdominal aortic aneurysm (EVAR trial 2): Randomised controlled trial, *Lancet* 365(9478):2187–2192, 2005.

Lederle FA, Wilson SE, Johnson GR, et al: Immediate repair compared with surveillance of small abdominal aortic aneurysms, *N Engl J Med* 346(19):1437–1444, 2002.

Lee ES, Pickett E, Hedayati N, et al: Implementation of an aortic screening program in clinical practice: Implications for the Screen For Abdominal Aortic Aneurysms Very Efficiently (SAAAVE) Act, *J Vasc Surg* 49(5):1107–1111, 2009.

Nevitt MP, Ballard DJ, Hallett Jr: Prognosis of abdominal aortic aneurysms. A population-based study, *N Engl J Med* 321(15):1009–1014, 1989.

Nienaber CA, Rousseau H, Eggebrecht H, et al: Randomized comparison of strategies for type B aortic dissection: The INvestigation of STEnt Grafts in Aortic Dissection (INSTEAD) trial, *Circulation* 120(25):2519–2528, 2009.

Rentschler M, Baxter BT: Pharmacological approaches to prevent abdominal aortic aneurysm enlargement and rupture, *Ann N Y Acad Sci* 1085:39–46, 2006.

ATRIAL FIBRILLATION

Method of
Lin Yee Chen, MBBS, MS; and Samuel C. Dudley Jr., MD, PhD

CURRENT DIAGNOSIS

- History taking and physical examination for atrial fibrillation (AF) should focus on determining symptom severity (to decide on treatment strategy), risk of thromboembolic stroke, and associated cardiovascular risk factors.
- Symptoms include palpitations, chest discomfort, shortness of breath, and reduced exercise capacity. Some patients have no symptoms.
- Investigations include a 12-lead electrocardiogram (ECG) for confirmation; transthoracic echocardiogram to evaluate left atrial size, left ventricular ejection fraction, and rule out valvular abnormalities; and blood tests for thyroid, renal, and hepatic function.

CURRENT THERAPY

- Rate control: Achieve average ventricular rate of less than 110 beats/min by using atrioventricular node (AVN) blockers or catheter ablation of AVN
- Rhythm control: Prevent AF recurrence by using antiarrhythmic drugs or catheter ablation (pulmonary vein isolation)
- Stroke prophylaxis: Risk stratification and stroke prevention by oral anticoagulation or left atrial appendage closure
- Risk-factor management or lifestyle modification: Prevent AF by weight management, intensive blood pressure lowering, and exercise training

TABLE 1	Risk Factors of Atrial Fibrillation
Cardiovascular risk factors	
Older age	
Male sex	
Diabetes mellitus	
Overweight and obesity	
Hypertension	
Chronic kidney disease	
Structural heart disease	
Valvular heart disease	
Cardiomyopathy (dilated, restrictive, and hypertrophic)	
Congenital heart disease	
Coronary heart disease	
Left ventricular diastolic dysfunction	
Left atrial enlargement	
Family history	
Genetics (polygenic and monogenic inheritance)	
Inflammation	
Low serum magnesium	
Heavy alcohol consumption	
Poor cardiorespiratory fitness	
Low physical activity	
Premature atrial contractions or supraventricular ectopy	

Epidemiology

AF is the most common sustained arrhythmia in the adult general population. Globally, the estimated number of individuals with AF in 2010 was 33.5 million. Between 1990 and 2010, the global estimated age-adjusted prevalence rate of AF increased from 569.5 to 596.2 per 100,000 men and from 359.9 to 373.1 per 100,000 women. This increase in prevalence was accompanied by a substantial increase in health burden: disability-adjusted life-years increased by 18.8% in men and 18.9% in women from 1990 to 2010. Finally, the lifetime risk for development of AF in adults at age 40 is 1 in 4.

Risk Factors and Pathophysiology

Table 1 shows the known risk factors of AF; many of these are also risk factors for atherosclerotic disease. Traditional cardiovascular risk factors such as diabetes, hypertension, and obesity can lead to AF via the following pathway: cardiovascular risk factors → left ventricular diastolic dysfunction → structural and functional alterations in the atria (enlargement, impaired function, fibrosis, etc.) → AF. The aforementioned pathway creates the substrate for AF; premature atrial contractions and supraventricular ectopic beats are the trigger for AF. Other pathophysiologic pathways include inflammation and increased oxidative stress, leading to electrical remodeling and, consequently, AF.

Clinical Manifestations

Common symptoms of AF include palpitations, irregular heartbeat sensation, lightheadedness, dyspnea, chest discomfort, and fatigue. Some patients may have no symptoms at rest but report poor stamina or easy fatigability with physical activity. Other patients, particularly among the elderly, may be asymptomatic.

Diagnosis

The absence of distinct P waves with irregularly irregular RR interval on the ECG are the sine qua non for diagnosing AF. Rhythm documentation can be obtained via the standard 12-lead ECG, Holter monitors that can record up to 48 hours, leadless patch monitors that can record up to 2 weeks, or implantable loop recorders. Newer wearable technologies that can diagnose AF include smartwatches and smartphones with specialized apps.

Paroxysmal AF is defined as AF that terminates spontaneously typically in less than 24 hours and in all cases in less than 7 days. AF that continues for more than 7 days and requires cardioversion for conversion to sinus rhythm is termed persistent AF. Long-standing persistent AF is AF that has been continuous for more than 1 year. Permanent AF exists when both patient and physician have decided not to pursue further attempts to maintain sinus rhythm.

Differential Diagnosis

These include other supraventricular arrhythmias such as atrial tachycardia, atrial flutter, long runs of premature atrial contractions, and multifocal atrial tachycardia.

Treatment

Rate Control

The goal of rate control is to prevent excessive ventricular rate response. This is a reasonable treatment strategy given data from randomized controlled trials (RCTs) that did not show any difference in cardiovascular outcomes between rate-control and rhythm-control strategy.

The AFFIRM (Atrial Fibrillation Follow-up Investigation of Rhythm Management) trial found no difference in mortality or stroke rates between patients assigned to rhythm-control and ventricular rate-control strategies. Similarly, the RACE (Rate Control versus Electrical Cardioversion for Persistent Atrial Fibrillation) trial found that rate control was not inferior to rhythm control for prevention of death.

The RACE II study showed that lenient ventricular rate control targeting a heart rate of lower than 110 beats/min was not inferior to stricter rate control of less than 80 beats/min. Lenient rate control is more convenient and requires fewer outpatient visits and fewer medications.

TABLE 2	Pharmacologic Agents for Rate Control		
DRUG	**INTRAVENOUS ADMINISTRATION**	**USUAL ORAL MAINTENANCE DOSE**	**MAJOR SIDE EFFECTS**
β Blockers			
Metoprolol (Lopressor)[1]	2.5–5 mg IV bolus; up to 3 doses	100–200 mg (long acting) daily	Bradycardia, hypotension, heart block, asthma, heart failure
Atenolol (Tenormin)[1]	N/A	25–100 mg qd	
Esmolol (Brevibloc)	50–200 μg/kg/min IV	N/A	
Propranolol (Inderal)	1–3 mg IV	10–40 mg tid	
Carvedilol (Coreg)[1]	N/A	3.125–25 mg bid	
Nondihydropyridine Calcium Channel Antagonists			
Verapamil (Calan)	5–10 mg bolus	80 mg tid or up to 360 mg (long acting) daily	Hypotension, heart block, heart failure
Diltiazem (Cardizem)	0.25–0.35 mg/kg	60 mg tid or up to 360 mg (long acting) daily	
Digitalis Glycosides			
Digoxin (Lanoxin)	0.25–0.5 mg	0.125–0.25 mg qd	Digitalis toxicity, bradycardia, heart block

[1]Not FDA approved for this indication.
IV, Intravenous.

Other than pharmacologic agents (Table 2), catheter ablation of the AVN is effective in controlling ventricular rate in patients with AF. AVN ablation is indicated if patients fail to achieve adequate ventricular rate control despite maximum doses of AVN blockers.

Rhythm Control

Although AF is associated with an increased risk of stroke and mortality, current evidence indicates that there is no difference in the rates of these cardiovascular outcomes between rhythm- and rate-control strategies. In the CABANA (Catheter Ablation vs Antiarrhythmic Drug Therapy for Atrial Fibrillation) trial, based on intention-to-treat analysis, there was no significant difference between catheter ablation and drug therapy with respect to a primary composite outcome of death, disabling stroke, serious bleeding, or cardiac arrest. However, in selected younger patients with paroxysmal AF, rhythm control may be a better approach. Additionally, catheter ablation to maintain sinus rhythm in selected patients with symptomatic AF and heart failure with reduced left ventricular ejection fraction may reduce mortality rate and hospitalization for heart failure. Finally, in patients who continue to have symptoms despite an adequately controlled ventricular rate, rhythm control is an appropriate next step.

Rhythm control can be achieved by the use of antiarrhythmic drugs (Table 3) or catheter ablation. In patients with paroxysmal and persistent AF who have failed at least one antiarrhythmic drug, catheter ablation by pulmonary vein isolation is indicated to maintain sinus rhythm. In persistent AF, the STAR AF II (Substrate and Trigger Ablation for Reduction of Atrial Fibrillation Trial Part II) showed that performing additional linear ablation or ablation targeting complex fractionated electrograms does not improve rhythm control compared with pulmonary vein isolation alone. The optimal approach to ablate persistent AF remains to be defined.

Stroke Prophylaxis

Stroke prevention is a two-stage process: determination of thromboembolic stroke risk and selection of prevention strategy. The most commonly used risk-stratification scheme for stroke prevention is the CHA_2DS_2-VASc score (https://www.mdcalc.com/cha2ds2-vasc-score-atrial-fibrillation-stroke-risk) (Table 4). Oral anticoagulation is recommended for CHA_2DS_2-VASc score of 2 or greater in men or 3 or greater in women. Aspirin should not be used for stroke prevention in AF.[1]

[1]Not FDA-approved for this indication.

Oral Anticoagulants

These include vitamin K antagonists (warfarin [Coumadin]) and non–vitamin K oral anticoagulants or novel or direct oral anticoagulants (DOAC) (Table 5). Compared with warfarin, DOACs are as effective in preventing thromboembolic stroke in AF. The risk of intracranial hemorrhage from the use of DOACs is 33% to 60% less than that with warfarin. Other advantages of DOACs over warfarin include the facts that there are fewer interactions with food and there is no need for monitoring the international normalized ratio.

Left Atrial Appendage Closure

The Watchman device is approved by the US Food and Drug Administration (FDA) for stroke prevention in AF patients with a contraindication to long-term oral anticoagulation and who are at risk of thromboembolic stroke. Patients, however, must be able to take oral anticoagulants for at least 6 weeks after implantation of the device.

Risk Factor Management and Lifestyle Modification

Recent compelling evidence underscores the importance of a fourth pillar of AF management: risk-factor and lifestyle modifications.

Weight Loss

An RCT has shown that weight reduction with intensive risk-factor management results in a reduction of AF symptom burden and severity and reversal of cardiac remodeling.

Intensive Blood Pressure Lowering

Blood pressure lowering targeting a systolic blood pressure of 120 mm Hg is associated with lower incidence of AF compared with 140 mm Hg.

Exercise Training

A small RCT showed that, compared with nonexercise control patients, high-intensity interval training reduced AF burden and improved atrial contractile function. This time-efficient form of exercise can potentially overcome the lack-of-time problem—an oft-quoted reason for poor compliance with regular aerobic exercise.

Complications

Other than thromboembolic stroke, heart failure, and death, AF is also associated with greater cognitive decline and risk of dementia. More recently, AF has been reported to be

TABLE 3 Pharmacologic Agents for Rhythm Control

DRUG	USUAL ORAL MAINTENANCE DOSE	MAJOR SIDE EFFECTS
Flecainide (Tambocor)	50–200 mg bid	Hypotension, atrial flutter with high ventricular rate
Propafenone (Rythmol)	150–300 mg tid	
Propafenone Extended Release (Rythmol SR)	225–425 mg bid	
Sotalol (Betapace)	80–160 mg bid	Bradycardia, hypotension, QT prolongation, torsades de pointes
Dofetilide (Tikosyn)	125–500 μg bid	QT prolongation, torsades de pointes
Amiodarone (Pacerone)[1]	100–200 mg qd	Hypotension, bradycardia, QT prolongation
Dronedarone (Multaq)	400 mg bid	QT prolongation

[1]Not FDA approved for atrial fibrillation.

TABLE 4 CHA$_2$DS$_2$-VASc Score

RISK FACTOR	SCORE
Congestive heart failure, LV dysfunction	1
Hypertension	1
Age ≥75 years	2
Diabetes mellitus	1
Stroke, TIA, or thromboembolism	2
Vascular disease (MI, PAD, complex aortic plaque)	1
Age 65–74 years	1
Sex category: female	1

MI, Myocardial infarction; LV, left ventricular; PAD, peripheral arterial disease; TIA, transient ischemic attack.

TABLE 5 Non–Vitamin K Oral Anticoagulants

DRUG	USUAL DOSE	COMMENTS
Direct Thrombin Inhibitor		
Dabigatran (Pradaxa)	150 mg bid	Reversal agent (Idarucizumab [Praxbind]) FDA approved; interacts with P-glycoprotein inhibitors and inducers
Factor Xa Inhibitor		
Apixaban (Eliquis)	5 mg bid	Interacts with P-glycoprotein and CYP3A4 inhibitors and inducers
Edoxaban (Savaysa)	60 mg qd	Avoid if CrCl >95 mL/min due to increased rate of stroke
Rivaroxaban (Xarelto)	20 mg qd	Interacts with P-glycoprotein and CYP3A4 inhibitors and inducers; should be taken with evening meal

Special Considerations

Subclinical Atrial Fibrillation

Subclinical AF is commonly detected from interrogation of cardiac implantable electronic devices. Whether subclinical AF poses the same health risks as clinical AF is the subject of much debate and active investigation.

Atrial Fibrillation Burden

A corollary to the problem of subclinical AF is that of AF burden—the amount of AF that a patient has. Studies based on cardiac implantable electronic devices suggest that a higher AF burden is associated with a higher risk of thromboembolic stroke, but it is unclear whether the risk increases continuously or whether a threshold exists.

References

Abed HS, Wittert GA, Leong DP, et al: Effect of weight reduction and cardiometabolic risk factor management on symptom burden and severity in patients with atrial fibrillation a randomized clinical trial, JAMA 310:2050–2060, 2013.

Chen LY, Bigger JT, Hickey KT, et al: Effect of intensive blood pressure lowering on incident atrial fibrillation and p-wave indices in the ACCORD Blood Pressure Trial, Am J Hypertens 29:1276–1282, 2016.

Chen LY, Norby FL, Gottesman RF, et al: Association of atrial fibrillation with cognitive decline and dementia over 20 years: the ARIC-NCS (Atherosclerosis Risk in Communities Neurocognitive Study), J Am Heart Assoc 7(6).

Chen LY, Sotoodehnia N, Bůžková P, et al: Atrial fibrillation and the risk of sudden cardiac death: the Atherosclerosis Risk in Communities (ARIC) Study and Cardiovascular Health Study (CHS), JAMA Intern Med 173:29–35, 2013.

Chugh SS, Havmoeller R, Narayanan K, et al: Worldwide epidemiology of atrial fibrillation: a Global Burden of Disease 2010 Study, Circulation 129:837–847, 2014.

January CT, Wann LS, Calkins H, et al: 2019 AHA/ACC/HRS focused update of the 2014 AHA/ACC/HRS guideline for the management of patients with atrial fibrillation: a report of the American College of Cardiology/American Heart Association Task Force on Clinical Practice Guidelines and the Heart Rhythm Society, Circulation, 2019. https://doi.org/10.1161/CIR.0000000000000665.

Lloyd-Jones DM, Wang TJ, Leip EP, et al: Lifetime risk for development of atrial fibrillation—The Framingham Heart Study, Circulation 110:1042–1046, 2004.

Malmo V, Nes BM, Amundsen BH, et al: Aerobic interval training reduces the burden of atrial fibrillation in the short term a randomized trial, Circulation 133:466–473, 2016.

Marrouche NF, Brachmann J, Andresen D, et al: Catheter ablation for atrial fibrillation with heart failure, N Engl J Med 378:417–427, 2018.

Okin PM, Hille DA, Larstorp ACK, et al: Effect of lower on-treatment systolic blood pressure on the risk of atrial fibrillation in hypertensive patients, Hypertension 66:368–373, 2015.

Packer DL, Mark DB, Robb RA, et al: Effect of catheter ablation vs antiarrhythmic drug therapy on mortality, stroke, bleeding, and cardiac arrest among patients with atrial fibrillation: the cabana randomized clinical trial, JAMA 321:1261–1274, 2019.

Van Gelder IC, Groenveld HF, Crijns HJGM, et al: Lenient versus strict rate control in patients with atrial fibrillation, N Engl J Med 362:1363–1373, 2010.

Van Gelder IC, Hagens VE, Bosker HA, et al: A comparison of rate control and rhythm control in patients with recurrent persistent atrial fibrillation, N Engl J Med 347:1834–1840, 2002.

Verma A, Jiang CY, Betts TR, et al: Approaches to catheter ablation for persistent atrial fibrillation, N Engl J Med 372:1812–1822, 2015.

Wyse DG, Waldo AL, DiMarco JP, et al: A comparison of rate control and rhythm control in patients with atrial fibrillation, N Engl J Med 347:1825–1833, 2002.

associated with a higher risk of sudden cardiac death in the general population. Apart from stroke prevention and rate and rhythm control to prevent heart failure, we currently lack effective prevention strategies for dementia and sudden cardiac death.

CONGENITAL HEART DISEASE

Method of
Richard A. Lange, MD, MBA; and Joaquin E. Cigarroa, MD

CURRENT DIAGNOSIS

- Examine blood pressures in arms and legs, pulse oximetry, mucous membranes and nail beds, respiratory rate, and peripheral pulses.
- In addition to listening over the precordium for heart sounds and murmurs, palpate for thrills and evidence of right or left chamber enlargement.
- Ancillary testing should include chest radiography, electrocardiography, and echocardiography.
- Consult a cardiologist if the physical examination or ancillary tests suggest congenital heart disease.

CURRENT THERAPY

- All congenital heart disease patients should have long-term follow-up for possible complications.
- Endocarditis prophylaxis is recommended for subjects with:
  - Unrepaired cyanotic congenital heart disease
  - Recently repaired congenital heart disease (<6 months after surgical or percutaneous repair)
  - Repaired congenital heart disease with residual defects
- Closure of defects with large left-to-right shunts (i.e., atrial septal defect, ventricular septal defect, atrioventricular canal, or patent ductus arteriosus) is recommended unless pulmonary vascular obstructive disease is far advanced.
- Patients with bicuspid aortic valves should be monitored for aortic root dilation.
- Pregnancy should be avoided in women with cyanotic congenital heart disease because of high maternal and fetal morbidity and mortality rates.

Congenital heart disease affects 0.4% to 0.9% of live births. Nowadays, most survive to adulthood because of improved diagnosis and treatment. Congenital cardiac defects can be categorized according to the presence or absence of cyanosis (due to right-to-left shunting) and the amount of pulmonary blood flow (Box 1).

| **BOX 1** | Categorization of Congenital Heart Disease |

Acyanotic Cardiac Defects
Increased pulmonary blood flow
- Atrial septal defect
- Ventricular septal defect
- Atrioventricular canal defect
- Patent ductus arteriosus
Normal pulmonary blood flow
- Aortic stenosis
- Pulmonic stenosis
- Aortic coarctation

Cyanotic Cardiac Defects
Normal pulmonary blood flow
- Ebstein's anomaly
Decreased pulmonary blood flow
- Tetralogy of Fallot
- Eisenmenger syndrome

Acyanotic Conditions
Atrial Septal Defect

Atrial septal defect (ASD) occurs in female patients two to three times as often as in male patients. Although most result from spontaneous genetic mutations, some are inherited.

The physiological consequences of ASD result from the shunting of blood from one atrium to the other; the direction and magnitude of shunting are determined by the size of the defect and the relative compliances of the ventricles. A small defect (<0.5 cm in diameter) is associated with a small shunt and no hemodynamic sequelae, whereas a sizable defect (>2 cm in diameter) usually is associated with a large shunt and substantial hemodynamic consequences. In most patients with ASD, the right ventricle is more compliant than the left; as a result, left atrial blood is shunted to the right atrium, causing increased pulmonary blood flow and dilation of the atria, right ventricle, and pulmonary arteries (Figure 1). Eventually, if the right ventricle fails or its compliance declines, the magnitude of left-to-right shunting diminishes.

In a patient with a large ASD, a right ventricular or pulmonary arterial impulse may be palpable, and wide, fixed splitting of the second heart sound is present. A systolic ejection murmur, audible in the second left intercostal space, is caused by increased blood flow across the pulmonic valve; flow across the ASD itself does not produce a murmur.

Because ASDs initially produce no symptoms or striking physical examination findings, they are often undetected for years. Small defects with minimal left-to-right shunting cause no symptoms or hemodynamic abnormalities, so they do not require closure. Even patients with moderate or large ASDs (characterized by a ratio of pulmonary to systemic blood flow of 1.5 or more) often have no symptoms until the third or fourth decade of life. Over the years, the increased blood volume flowing through the right heart chambers usually causes right ventricular dilation and failure. Obstructive pulmonary vascular disease (Eisenmenger syndrome) occurs uncommonly in adults with ASD.

The symptomatic patient with an ASD typically reports fatigue or dyspnea on exertion. Alternatively, the development of supraventricular tachyarrhythmias, right heart failure, paradoxical embolism, or recurrent pulmonary infections might prompt the patient to seek medical attention. Although an occasional patient

Figure 1 Atrial septal defect. Blood from the pulmonary veins enters the left atrium, after which some of it crosses the atrial septal defect into the right atrium and ventricle *(longer arrow)*. Thus left-to-right shunting occurs. (Reprinted with permission from Brickner ME, Hillis LD, Lange RA: Congenital heart disease in adults. First of two parts. N Engl J Med 2000;342:256–263.)

with an unrepaired ASD survives to an advanced age, those with sizable shunts often die of right ventricular failure or arrhythmias in their 30s or 40s.

Echocardiography can reveal atrial and right ventricular dilation and identify the ASD's location. The sensitivity of echocardiography may be enhanced by injecting microbubbles in solution into a peripheral vein, after which the movement of some of them across the defect into the left atrium can be visualized.

An ASD with a pulmonary-to-systemic flow ratio of 1.5 or more should be closed (surgically or percutaneously) to prevent worsening right ventricular dysfunction. Prophylaxis against infective endocarditis is not recommended for patients with ASD (repaired or unrepaired) unless a concomitant valvular abnormality is present.

Ventricular Septal Defect

Ventricular septal defect (VSD) is the most common congenital cardiac abnormality, with similar incidence in boys and girls. Approximately 25% to 40% of them close spontaneously by 2 years of age.

The physiological consequences of a VSD are determined by the size of the defect and the relative resistances in the systemic and pulmonary vascular beds. A small defect causes little or no functional disturbance, because pulmonary blood flow is only minimally increased. In contrast, a large defect causes substantial left-to-right shunting, because systemic vascular resistance exceeds pulmonary vascular resistance (Figure 2). Over time, however, the pulmonary vascular resistance usually increases, and the magnitude of left-to-right shunting declines. Eventually, the pulmonary vascular resistance equals or exceeds the systemic resistance; the shunting of blood from left to right ceases; and right-to-left shunting begins (e.g., Eisenmenger physiology).

A small, muscular VSD can produce a high-frequency systolic ejection murmur that terminates before the end of systole (when the defect is occluded by contracting heart muscle). With a moderate or large VSD and substantial left-to-right shunting, a holosystolic murmur, loudest at the left sternal border, is audible and is usually accompanied by a palpable thrill. If pulmonary hypertension develops, the holosystolic murmur and thrill diminish in magnitude and eventually disappear as flow through the defect decreases.

Figure 2 Ventricular septal defect. When the left ventricle contracts, it ejects some blood into the aorta and some across the ventricular septal defect into the right ventricle and pulmonary artery (*arrow*), resulting in left-to-right shunting. (Reprinted with permission from Brickner ME, Hillis LD, Lange RA: Congenital heart disease in adults. First of two parts. N Engl J Med 2000;342:256–263.)

Echocardiography is usually performed to confirm the presence and location of the VSD and to delineate the magnitude and direction of shunting. With catheterization, one can determine the magnitude of shunting and the pulmonary vascular resistance.

The natural history of VSD depends on the size of the defect and the pulmonary vascular resistance. Adults with small defects and normal pulmonary arterial pressure are generally asymptomatic, and pulmonary vascular disease is unlikely to develop. In contrast, patients with large defects who survive to adulthood usually have left ventricular failure or pulmonary hypertension (or both) with associated right ventricular failure.

Closure of VSDs (surgically or percutaneously) is recommended if the pulmonary vascular obstructive disease is not severe. Prophylaxis against infective endocarditis is recommended for patients with unrepaired VSD and those with a residual shunt despite surgical or percutaneous closure.

Atrioventricular Canal Defect

The endocardial cushions normally fuse to form the tricuspid and mitral valves, as well as the atrial and ventricular septa. Atrioventricular (AV) canal defects are caused by incomplete fusion of the endocardial cushions during embryonic development. They are the most common congenital cardiac abnormality in patients with Down syndrome. Such cushion defects include a spectrum of abnormalities, ranging from ASD with a cleft anterior mitral valve leaflet to a common AV canal defect in which a single AV valve in association with a large ASD and VSD is present.

A common AV canal defect permits substantial left-to-right shunting at both the atrial and ventricular levels, which leads to excessive pulmonary blood flow and resultant pulmonary congestion within months of birth. Eventually, the excessive pulmonary blood flow leads to irreversible pulmonary vascular obstruction (e.g., Eisenmenger physiology).

In the patient with an AV canal defect and left-to-right intracardiac shunting, the physical examination reveals a loud holosystolic murmur audible throughout the precordium. As pulmonary vascular resistance increases, the holosystolic murmur diminishes in intensity and duration, eventually disappearing as flow through the defect decreases.

AV canal defects require surgical repair if the magnitude of pulmonary vascular obstructive disease is not prohibitive. Although such patients might initially benefit from medical treatment with diuretics and afterload reduction, the onset of heart failure symptoms is generally the point at which surgery is considered. Prophylaxis against infective endocarditis is recommended for patients with repaired and unrepaired AV canal defects.

Patent Ductus Arteriosus

The ductus arteriosus connects the descending aorta (just distal to the left subclavian artery) and the left pulmonary artery. In the fetus, it permits pulmonary arterial blood to bypass the unexpanded lungs and to enter the descending aorta for oxygenation in the placenta. Although it normally closes spontaneously soon after birth, it fails to do so in some infants, so that continuous flow from the aorta to the pulmonary artery (i.e., left-to-right shunting) occurs (Figure 3). The incidence of patent ductus arteriosus (PDA) is increased in pregnancies complicated by persistent perinatal hypoxemia or maternal rubella infection as well as among infants born prematurely or at high altitude.

A patient with PDA and a moderate or large shunt has bounding peripheral arterial pulses and a widened pulse pressure. A continuous "machinery" murmur, audible in the second left intercostal space, begins shortly after the first heart sound, peaks in intensity at or immediately after the second heart sound (thereby obscuring it), and diminishes in intensity during diastole. If pulmonary vascular obstruction and hypertension develop, the murmur decreases in duration and intensity and eventually disappears.

With echocardiography, the PDA can usually be visualized, and Doppler studies demonstrate continuous flow in the pulmonary trunk. Catheterization and angiography allow one to quantify the

Figure 3 Patent ductus arteriosus. Some of the blood from the aorta crosses the ductus arteriosus into the pulmonary artery *(arrows)*, with resultant left-to-right shunting. (Reprinted with permission from Brickner ME, Hillis LD, Lange RA: Congenital heart disease in adults. First of two parts. N Engl J Med 2000;342:256–263.)

Figure 4 Coarctation of the aorta. Coarctation causes obstruction to blood flow in the descending thoracic aorta; the lower body is perfused by collateral vessels from the axillary and internal thoracic arteries through the intercostal arteries. (Reprinted with permission from Brickner ME, Hillis LD, Lange RA: Congenital heart disease in adults. First of two parts. N Engl J Med 2000;342:256–263.)

magnitude of shunting and the pulmonary vascular resistance and to visualize the PDA.

The subject with a small PDA has no symptoms attributable to it and a normal life expectancy. However, it is associated with an elevated risk of infective endarteritis. A PDA of moderate size might cause no symptoms during infancy; during childhood or adulthood, fatigue, dyspnea, or palpitations can appear. Additionally, the PDA can become aneurysmal and calcified, with subsequent rupture. Larger shunts can precipitate left ventricular failure. Eventually, pulmonary vascular obstruction can develop; when the pulmonary vascular resistance equals or exceeds the systemic vascular resistance, the direction of shunting reverses.

One third of patients with an unrepaired moderate or large PDA die of heart failure, pulmonary hypertension, or endarteritis by 40 years of age, and two thirds die by 60 years of age. Because of the risk of endarteritis associated with unrepaired PDA (about 0.45% annually after the second decade of life) and the safety of surgical ligation (generally accomplished without cardiopulmonary bypass) or percutaneous closure, even a small PDA should be ligated surgically or occluded percutaneously. Once severe pulmonary vascular obstructive disease develops, ligation or closure is contraindicated.

Aortic Stenosis

A bicuspid aortic valve is found in 2% to 3% of the population and is four times more common in males than in females. The bicuspid valve has a single fused commissure and an eccentrically oriented orifice. Although the deformed valve is not typically stenotic at birth, it is subjected to abnormal hemodynamic stress, which can lead to leaflet thickening and calcification. In many patients, an abnormality of the ascending aortic media is present, predisposing the patient to aortic root dilation. Twenty percent of patients with a bicuspid aortic valve have an associated cardiovascular abnormality, such as PDA or aortic coarctation.

In patients with severe aortic stenosis (AS), the carotid upstroke is usually delayed and diminished. The aortic component of the second heart sound is diminished or absent. A systolic crescendo–decrescendo murmur is audible over the aortic area and often radiates to the neck. As the magnitude of AS worsens, the murmur peaks progressively later in systole.

In most patients, echocardiography with Doppler flow permits an assessment of the severity of AS and of left ventricular systolic function. Cardiac catheterization is performed to assess the severity of AS and to determine if concomitant coronary artery disease is present.

The symptoms of AS are angina pectoris, syncope or near syncope, and those of heart failure (dyspnea). Asymptomatic adults with AS have a normal life expectancy. Once symptoms appear, survival is limited. The median survival is 5 years once angina develops, 3 years once syncope occurs, and 2 years once symptoms of heart failure appear. Therefore patients with symptomatic AS should undergo surgical or percutaneous valve replacement.

Pulmonic Stenosis

Pulmonic stenosis (PS) is the second most common congenital cardiac malformation (after VSD). Although typically an isolated abnormality, it can occur in association with VSD.

The patient with PS is usually asymptomatic, and the condition is identified by auscultation of a loud systolic murmur. When it is severe, dyspnea on exertion or fatigue can occur; less often, patients have retrosternal chest pain or syncope with exertion. Eventually, right ventricular failure can develop, with resultant peripheral edema and abdominal swelling.

In patients with moderate or severe PS, the second heart sound is widely split, with its pulmonic component soft and delayed. A crescendo-decrescendo systolic murmur that increases in intensity with inspiration is audible along the left sternal border. If the valve is pliable, an ejection click often precedes the murmur. On echocardiography, right ventricular hypertrophy is evident; the severity of PS can usually be assessed with measurement of Doppler flow.

Adults with mild PS are usually asymptomatic and do not require a corrective procedure. In contrast, patients with moderate or severe PS should undergo percutaneous balloon dilation.

Aortic Coarctation

Aortic coarctation typically consists of a diaphragm-like ridge extending into the aortic lumen just distal to the left subclavian artery (Figure 4), resulting in an elevated arterial pressure in both arms. Less commonly, the coarctation is located immediately proximal to the left subclavian artery, in which case a difference in arterial pressure is noted between the arms. Extensive collateral arterial circulation to the lower body through the internal thoracic, intercostal, subclavian, and scapular arteries often develops in patients with aortic coarctation. Aortic coarctation, which is two to five times as common in males as in females, can occur in conjunction with gonadal dysgenesis (e.g., Turner's syndrome), bicuspid aortic valve, VSD, or PDA.

On physical examination, the arterial pressure is higher in the arms than in the legs, and the femoral arterial pulses are weak and delayed. A harsh systolic ejection murmur may be audible along the left sternal border and in the back, particularly over the coarctation. A systolic murmur, caused by flow through collateral vessels, may be heard in the back.

On chest radiography, increased collateral flow through the intercostal arteries causes notching of the posterior third through eighth ribs. The coarctation may be visible as an indentation of the aorta, and one may see prestenotic and poststenotic aortic dilation, producing the "reversed E" or "3" sign. Computed tomography, magnetic resonance imaging, and contrast aortography provide precise anatomic delineation of the coarctation's location and length.

Most adults with aortic coarctation are asymptomatic. When symptoms are present, they are usually those of hypertension: headache, epistaxis, dizziness, and palpitations. Complications of aortic coarctation include hypertension, left ventricular failure, aortic dissection, premature coronary artery disease, infective endocarditis, and cerebrovascular accidents (due to rupture of an intracerebral aneurysm). Two thirds of patients older than 40 years who have uncorrected aortic coarctation have symptoms of heart failure. Three fourths die by the age of 50 years and 90% by the age of 60 years.

Surgical repair or intraluminal stenting should be considered for patients with a transcoarctation pressure gradient greater than 30 mm Hg, with the choice of procedure influenced by the age of the patient, anatomic considerations of the coarctation, and the presence of concomitant cardiac abnormalities. Persistent hypertension is common despite surgical or percutaneous intervention, and recurrent coarctation or aneurysm formation at the repair site may occur.

Cyanotic Conditions
Ebstein's Anomaly
With Ebstein's anomaly, the tricuspid valve's septal leaflet and often its posterior leaflet are displaced into the right ventricle, and the anterior leaflet is usually malformed and abnormally attached or adherent to the right ventricular free wall. As a result, a portion of the right ventricle is atrialized, in that it is located on the atrial side of the tricuspid valve, and the remaining functional right ventricle is small (Figure 5). The tricuspid valve is usually regurgitant, but it may be stenotic. Eighty percent of patients with Ebstein's anomaly have an interatrial communication (ASD or patent foramen ovale) through which right-to-left shunting of blood can occur.

The severity of the hemodynamic derangements in patients with Ebstein's anomaly depends on the magnitude of displacement and the functional status of the tricuspid valve leaflets. On the one extreme, patients with mild apical displacement of the tricuspid valve leaflets have normal valvular function; on the other extreme, those with severe leaflet displacement or abnormal anterior leaflet attachment, with resultant valvular dysfunction, have an elevated right atrial pressure and right-to-left shunting if an interatrial communication is present.

The clinical presentation of subjects with Ebstein's anomaly ranges from severe right heart failure in the neonate to the absence of symptoms in the adult in whom it is discovered incidentally. Older children with Ebstein's anomaly often come to medical attention because of an incidental murmur, whereas adolescents and adults may be identified because of a supraventricular arrhythmia.

On physical examination, the severity of cyanosis depends on the magnitude of right-to-left shunting. The first and second heart sounds are both widely split, and a third or fourth heart sound is often present, resulting in triple or even quadruple heart sounds. A systolic murmur caused by tricuspid regurgitation is usually present at the left lower sternal border.

Figure 5 Ebstein's anomaly. With Ebstein's anomaly, the tricuspid valve is displaced apically, a portion of the right ventricle is atrialized (i.e., located on the atrial side of the tricuspid valve), and the functional right ventricle is small. (Reprinted with permission from Brickner ME, Hillis LD, Lange RA: Congenital heart disease in adults. Second of two parts. N Engl J Med 2000;342:334–342.)

Echocardiography is used to assess the presence and magnitude of right atrial dilation, anatomic displacement and distortion of the tricuspid valve leaflets, and the severity of tricuspid regurgitation or stenosis.

Prophylaxis against infective endocarditis is recommended. Patients with symptomatic right heart failure should receive diuretics. Tricuspid valve repair or replacement in conjunction with closure of the interatrial communication is recommended for older patients with severe symptoms despite medical therapy and those with less severe symptoms who have cardiac enlargement.

Tetralogy of Fallot
Tetralogy of Fallot is characterized by a large VSD, an aorta that overrides both ventricles, obstruction to right ventricular outflow (subvalvular, valvular, supravalvular, or in the pulmonary arterial branches), and right ventricular hypertrophy (Figure 6).

Most patients with tetralogy of Fallot have substantial right-to-left shunting through the large VSD because of increased resistance to flow in the right ventricular outflow tract; the magnitude of right ventricular outflow tract obstruction determines the magnitude of shunting. Because the resistance to flow across the right ventricular outflow tract is relatively fixed, changes in systemic vascular resistance affect the magnitude of right-to-left shunting: A decrease in systemic vascular resistance increases right-to-left shunting, whereas an increase in systemic resistance decreases it.

Patients with tetralogy of Fallot typically have cyanosis from birth or beginning in the first year of life. In childhood, they might have sudden hypoxic spells, characterized by tachypnea and hyperpnea, followed by worsening cyanosis and, in some cases, loss of consciousness, seizures, cerebrovascular accidents, and even death. Such spells do not occur in adolescents or adults. Without surgical intervention, most patients die in childhood.

On physical examination, patients with tetralogy of Fallot have cyanosis and digital clubbing. A right ventricular lift or tap is palpable. The second heart sound is single, because its pulmonic component is inaudible. A systolic ejection murmur, audible along the left sternal border, is caused by the obstruction to right ventricular outflow. The intensity and duration of the murmur are inversely related to the severity of right ventricular outflow

Figure 6 Tetralogy of Fallot. Tetralogy of Fallot is characterized by a large ventricular septal defect, obstruction of the right ventricular outflow tract, right ventricular hypertrophy, and an aorta that overrides the left and right ventricles. With right ventricular outflow tract obstruction, blood is shunted through the ventricular septal defect from right to left *(arrow)*. (Reprinted with permission from Brickner ME, Hillis LD, Lange RA: Congenital heart disease in adults. Second of two parts. N Engl J Med 2000;342:334–342.)

Figure 7 Eisenmenger syndrome. In response to substantial left-to-right shunting, morphologic alterations occur in the small pulmonary arteries and arterioles *(inset)*, leading to pulmonary hypertension and the resultant reversal of the intracardiac shunt *(arrow)*. In the small pulmonary arteries and arterioles, medial hypertrophy, intimal cellular proliferation, and fibrosis lead to narrowing or closure of the vessel lumina. With sustained pulmonary hypertension, extensive atherosclerosis and calcification often develop in the large pulmonary arteries. (Reprinted with permission from Brickner ME, Hillis LD, Lange RA: Congenital heart disease in adults. Second of two parts. N Engl J Med 2000;342:334–42.)

obstruction; a soft, short murmur suggests that severe obstruction is present.

Laboratory examination reveals arterial oxygen desaturation and compensatory erythrocytosis. Echocardiography can be used to establish the diagnosis and to assess the location and severity of right ventricular outflow tract obstruction.

Complete surgical repair (closure of the VSD and relief of right ventricular outflow tract obstruction) is recommended to relieve symptoms and to improve survival; it should be performed when patients are very young. Those with tetralogy of Fallot (repaired or unrepaired) are at risk for endocarditis and therefore should receive antibiotic prophylaxis before dental or elective surgical procedures.

Patients with repaired tetralogy of Fallot require careful follow-up, because they can subsequently develop atrial or ventricular arrhythmias, pulmonic regurgitation, right ventricular dysfunction, or recurrent obstruction of the right ventricular outflow tract.

Eisenmenger Syndrome
With substantial left-to-right shunting, the pulmonary vasculature is exposed to increased blood flow under increased pressure, often resulting in pulmonary vascular obstructive disease. As the pulmonary vascular resistance approaches or exceeds systemic resistance, the shunt is reversed (right-to-left shunting develops), and cyanosis appears (Figure 7).

Most patients with Eisenmenger syndrome have impaired exercise tolerance and exertional dyspnea. Palpitations are common and most often result from atrial fibrillation or flutter. As erythrocytosis (due to arterial desaturation) develops, symptoms of hyperviscosity (visual disturbances, fatigue, headache, dizziness, and paresthesias) can appear. Patients with Eisenmenger syndrome can experience hemoptysis, bleeding complications, cerebrovascular accidents, brain abscess, syncope, and sudden death.

Eisenmenger syndrome patients typically have digital clubbing and cyanosis, a right parasternal heave (due to right ventricular hypertrophy), and a prominent pulmonic component of the second heart sound. The murmur caused by a VSD, PDA, or ASD disappears when Eisenmenger syndrome develops.

The chest x-ray reveals normal heart size, prominent central pulmonary arteries, and diminished vascular markings (pruning) of the peripheral vessels. On transthoracic echocardiography, evidence of right ventricular pressure overload and pulmonary hypertension is present. The underlying cardiac defect can usually be visualized, although shunting across the defect may be difficult to demonstrate by Doppler because of the low jet velocity.

Even though patients with Eisenmenger syndrome have severe pulmonary hypertension, they have a favorable long-term survival: 80% at 10 years after diagnosis, 77% at 15 years, and 42% at 25 years. Death is usually sudden, presumably caused by arrhythmias, but some patients die of heart failure, hemoptysis, brain abscess, or stroke.

Phlebotomy with isovolumic replacement should be performed in patients with moderate or severe symptoms of hyperviscosity; it should not be performed in asymptomatic or mildly symptomatic patients regardless of the hematocrit. Repeated phlebotomy can result in iron deficiency, which can worsen the symptoms of hyperviscosity, because iron-deficient erythrocytes are less deformable than iron-replete ones. Anticoagulants and antiplatelet agents should be avoided, because they exacerbate the hemorrhagic diathesis.

Patients with Eisenmenger syndrome should avoid intravascular volume depletion, high altitude, and the use of systemic vasodilators. Because of high maternal and fetal morbidity and mortality, pregnancy should be avoided. Patients with Eisenmenger syndrome who are undergoing noncardiac surgery require meticulous management of anesthesia, with attention to maintenance of systemic vascular resistance, minimization of blood loss and intravascular volume depletion, and prevention of iatrogenic paradoxical embolization. In preparation for noncardiac surgery, prophylactic phlebotomy (usually of 1 to 2 units of blood, with isovolumic replacement) is recommended for patients with a hematocrit greater than 65% to reduce the likelihood of perioperative hemorrhagic and thrombotic complications.

Lung transplantation with repair of the cardiac defect or combined heart–lung transplantation are options for patients with Eisenmenger syndrome who are deemed to have a poor prognosis (as reflected by the presence of syncope, refractory right heart failure, a high New York Heart Association [NYHA] functional class, or severe hypoxemia). Because of the somewhat limited success of transplantation and the reasonably good survival among patients treated medically, careful selection of patients for transplantation is imperative. Although pulmonary vasodilators improve exercise capacity, they have not been proved to improve survival.

References

Bhatt AB, Foster E, Kuehl K, et al: on behalf of the American Heart Association Council on Clinical Cardiology: Congenital heart disease in the older adult: a scientific statement from the American Heart Association, *Circulation* 131:1884–1931, 2015.

Brickner ME, Hillis LD, Lange RA: Congenital heart disease in adults. First of two parts, *N Engl J Med* 342:256–263, 2000.

Brickner ME, Hillis LD, Lange RA: Congenital heart disease in adults. Second of two parts, *N Engl J Med* 342:334–342, 2000.

Lange RA, Hillis LD, Vongpatanasin WP, Brickner ME: The Eisenmenger syndrome in adults, *Ann Int Med* 128:745–755, 1998.

Neidenbach R, Niwa K, Oto O, et al: Improving medical care and prevention in adults with congenital heart disease—reflections on a global problem—part II: infective endocarditis, pulmonary hypertension, pulmonary arterial hypertension and aortopathy, *Cardiovasc Diagn Ther* 8(6):716–724, 2018.

Stout KK, Daniels CJ, Aboulhosn JA, et al: 2018 AHA/ACC guideline for the management of adults with congenital heart disease: executive summary: a report of the American College of Cardiology/American Heart Association Task Force on Clinical Practice Guidelines, *Circulation* 139:e637–e697, 2019.

CONGESTIVE HEART FAILURE

Method of
Alex Schevchuck, MD, MS; and Mark E. Garcia, MD

CURRENT DIAGNOSIS

- Recognize clinical symptoms and signs of congestive heart failure (HF).
- Determine left ventricular ejection fraction (EF) using imaging modalities.
- Identify the potential etiologies.
- Evaluate hemodynamic status.

CURRENT THERAPY

- Current therapies differ for heart failure with preserved (HF-pEF) and reduced EF (HFrEF).
- Angiotensin converting enzyme inhibitors (ACEIs), angiotensin-receptor blockers (ARBs), angiotensin receptor-neprilysin inhibitor (ARNI), and mineralocorticoid receptor antagonists (MRAs) play a pivotal role in reducing morbidity and mortality in patients with HFrEF.
- Diuretics are useful in both HFrEF and HFpEF patients to treat congestion and fluid volume removal. A patient with decompensated heart failure may need intravenous diuretic treatment for decongestion caused by intestinal edema and malabsorption of oral diuretics. High-dose IV diuretic is important for treatment of decompensated HF.
- There are limited treatment options for HFpEF. The mainstay of therapy in HFpEF is using diuretics to relieve congestion and treatment of coexisting diseases.
- In advanced heart failure, identification of high-risk features and early referral for consultation with an advanced heart failure specialist are important.

Heart Failure Definition

The definition of heart failure has been variable in part caused by a wide spectrum of etiologies and pathologic processes resulting in this disease.

Heart failure is a clinical syndrome that includes a variety of signs and symptoms of systemic and/or pulmonic congestion from cardiac dysfunction. Specifically, systolic insufficiency and/or elevated ventricular filling pressures result in decreased perfusion and congestion. The symptoms of heart failure commonly include shortness of breath with exertion or at rest, fatigue, limited exercise capacity, and edema. Figure 1 shows the new proposed universal definition of heart failure.

Heart failure can sometimes be confused for a cardiomyopathy and/or a low EF. A cardiomyopathy is a disease state of the myocardium, such as ischemic heart disease or hypertrophic cardiomyopathy. This may lead to the heart failure syndrome but is not necessarily needed to develop heart failure. Thus these terms are not synonymous or interchangeable. Likewise, a low EF does not automatically imply the diagnosis of heart failure in absence of the clinical syndrome.

There are four stages of clinical development and progression of heart failure (Table 1).

Epidemiology

Based on 2013 to 2016 NHANES data, there were 6.2 million adults with congestive heart failure in the United States, and this number has increased from 5.7 million from 2009 to 2012. This represented about 2% of the U.S. population. Projections now show that by the year 2030, the prevalence of HF may increase to nearly 3%, or >8 million adults. The prevalence of HF increases with age, approaching >12% of the population in the age group of 80 and older.

In the ARIC study, the incidence of HF in subjects ≥55 years-old was 1 million cases in 2014 and was slightly higher among women comparatively to men and among African Americans comparatively to whites.

The lifetime risk of developing heart failure is 20% to 45% in subjects ≥45 years of age. HF mortality depends on the type of heart failure, demographics, and history of hospitalizations. Although HF survival has improved with the development of contemporary therapies, 1-year mortality remains substantial, nearing 30%. The overall cost of HF care was ~30 billion dollars in 2012. By 2030, the cost is projected to increase by 127%, to nearly 70 billion a year.

Heart Failure Classification Based on Left Ventricular Ejection Fraction (LVEF)

HF classification based on LVEF has been updated in the 2021 Universal Definition of Heart Failure document and is summarized in Table 2.

EF-based classification further implies prognostic and therapeutic differences. Thus patients with EF ≤40 benefit from specific treatments for heart failure with a reduced LVEF. HF with a mildly reduced ejection fraction has been a controversial topic and generally represents heterogeneous phenotypes that may benefit from treatments for a reduced EF and also may have a worse prognosis than patients with a preserved EF. If a patient has had heart failure with low EF that has improved to ≥40% as

Figure 1 Universal definition of heart failure. BNP: Brain natriuretic peptide

TABLE 1 Stages of Development and Progression of HF

Stage	A AT RISK FOR HF	B PRE-HF	C HF	D ADVANCED HF
Symptoms	No prior or current symptoms of HF	No prior or current symptoms of HF	Prior or current symptoms of HF	Severe symptoms of congestion, dyspnea at rest, recurrent hospitalization despite GDMT
Clinical features	Presence of HTN, CVD, DM, obesity, exposure to cardiotoxins, family history of familial cardiomyopathy	Presence of one of the following: Structural heart disease Abnormal cardiac function Elevated BNP or troponin level in case of cardiotoxins	Symptoms are caused by structural or functional heart abnormality (i.e., systolic dysfunction or elevated filling pressures)	Requires advanced therapies (VAD, transplant) or palliative care

CVD, cardiovascular disease; DM, diabetes mellitus; HTN, hypertension; GDMT: guideline-directed medical therapy; VAD: ventricular assist-device.

TABLE 2 Classification of Heart Failure Based on LVEF

HF CLASS ACCORDING TO LVEF (MUST HAVE SIGNS AND SYMPTOMS)	ACRONYM	LVEF, %
HF with reduced Ejection Fraction	HFrEF	≤40
HF with mildly reduced Ejection Fraction	HFmrEF	41–49
HF with preserved Ejection Fraction	HFpEF	≥50
HF with preserved Ejection Fraction, improved	HFpEF, improved	Prior <40, now ≥40

TABLE 3 NYHA Functional Classification

NYHA FC	FUNCTIONAL CAPACITY
I	No limitations. Can perform high level of activity without symptoms (for example, running, cycling, weightlifting).
II	Slight limitations. Tolerate lower or moderate level activities well, may have limitations with higher level activities (for example, regular walking causes no symptoms, but a run may cause shortness of breath).
III	Significant limitations. Symptoms with low-level activities such as with daily activities such as walking, household chores, etc.
IV	Symptoms at rest, dyspnea with any physical activity.

a result of treatment or a natural cause, the patient is subcategorized into the "HF with preserved Ejection Fraction, improved" class. Clinicians have to keep in mind the limitations of the LV assessment methods. For example, echocardiography may have variability in EF quantification based on a quantification method, reader experience/style, and image quality. An EF decrease from 41% to 39% may not necessarily represent a clinical change or deterioration from HFmrEF to HFrEF but rather be attributed to a measurement variability. Verification tests, such as cardiac magnetic resonance imaging (MRI) or multiple-gated acquisition (MUGA) scan, may be used to validate if the change is true before major therapeutic changes are made.

Functional Capacity

New York Heart Association (NYHA) Functional Class is commonly accepted classification of functional capacity in symptomatic and advanced (stages C and D) heart failure patients. Functional class has prognostic and therapeutic implications. Four NYHA functional classes (FC) are listed in Table 3.

NYFA functional class should be assessed at the time of heart failure diagnosis and then reassessed during subsequent encounters to track progress of heart failure treatment and for monitoring of disease progression.

Left Ventricular Physiology and Hemodynamic Profile

Left ventricular performance depends on three major components: preload, afterload, and contractility. The preload is the maximum amount of myocardial stretch prior to onset of ventricular systole. A clinically accepted measure of preload is the left ventricular end-diastolic pressure (LVEDP), which can be measured directly using cardiac catheterization techniques or indirectly using transthoracic echocardiography. The relationship between cardiac output (CO) and preload is described by Frank-Starling mechanism (Figure 2, Panel A). CO will continue to increase in response to increasing

Figure 2 Effects of preload and afterload on cardiac output.

preload, until the LV stretch reaches the point when actin and myosin fibers lose interlink. Any further increase in preload past this point will result in decrease in CO.

Afterload, on the other hand, has a hyperbolic relationship with the stroke volume (see Figure 2, Panel B). Any reduction in afterload results in an increase in CO and vice versa.

The contractility is a highly debated term in the myocardial physiology world and sometimes is referred to as *inotropy*. This generally implies an intrinsic force or an intensity of a myocardial contraction that is affected by positive and negative inotropic agents. Many conditions that affect the myocardium may also adversely affect the contractility.

The preload-CO relationship determines four hemodynamic profiles (Table 4).

Neurohormone and Sympathetic Nervous System Activation

Heart failure leads to a decreased cardiac output, and in this disease state multiple detrimental physiologic pathways are activated. This includes the renin-angiotensin-aldosterone system (RAAS) and the sympathetic nervous system (SNS). The RAAS is activated in this low perfusion state where the kidney senses the decreased perfusion pressure stimulating the release of renin. Renin is responsible for activating angiotensin-I, which is then further activated to its more potent form angiotensin-II by the angiotensin converting enzyme. Angiotensin-II binds to the AT1 receptor and this process triggers multiple cardiovascular and renal effects including vasoconstriction, triggering of sodium and water absorption in the renal tubules, stimulating aldosterone release, and several direct detrimental myocardium effects including hypertrophy and fibrosis.

Activation of the sympathetic nervous system during heart failure is a complex pathway that is associated with increased catecholamine levels and increased sympathetic tone. Activation of the SNS initially can be considered beneficial in early HF because this has a wide range of effects including increased heart rate and cardiac contractility, but long-term activation has significant detrimental effects leading to further cardiac remodeling and arrhythmias.

Activation of these systems directly contributes to cardiac remodeling and worsening of HF. These pathways allow for multiple different therapeutic interventions that have been proven to improve survival, decrease hospitalizations, decrease symptoms, and potentially improve cardiac function.

Diagnosis

Clinical diagnostic criteria for HF are listed in Box 1. For establishing a definite diagnosis of heart failure in this study, two major or one major and two minor criteria have to be present concurrently.

Echocardiography plays a key role in diagnosis of heart failure. Transthoracic echo (TTE) provides information about the left and right ventricular systolic function, chamber sizes, structural disease such as ventricular hypertrophy, valve structure and function, relaxation function, presence of the intracardiac shunts, and ventricular filling pressures and pulmonary artery pressure. TEE may be helpful to clarify details on cardiac structure, such as anatomy of shunts or mechanism of valve dysfunction.

TABLE 4	Heart Failure Hemodynamic Profiles	
	NORMAL LVEDP	**ELEVATED LVEDP**
Normal CO	A "warm and dry"	B "warm and wet"
Decreased CO	L "lethal, cold, and dry"	C "cold and wet"

BOX 1 — Clinical Criteria for CHF Diagnosis

Major Criteria
- Paroxysmal nocturnal dyspnea or orthopnea
- Neck-vein distention
- Rales
- Cardiomegaly
- Acute pulmonary edema
- S_3 gallop
- Increased venous pressure (≥16 cm of water)
- Circulation time ≥25 sec
- Hepatojugular reflux

Minor Criteria
- Ankle edema
- Night cough
- Dyspnea on exertion
- Hepatomegaly
- Pleural effusion
- Vital capacity ↓ 1/3 from maximum.
- Tachycardia (rate of ≥120/min)

Major or Minor Criterion
- Weight loss ≥4.5 kg in 5 days in response to treatment

Cardiac CT may provide information on cardiac and vascular structure. Cardiac MRI is excellent at the evaluation of cardiac structure, function and chamber size, as well as assessing and diagnosing myocardial disease, such as tumors, fibrosis, thrombi, and inflammatory and infiltrative processes.

Nuclear radiology offers a MUGA scan that is considered a superior EF evaluation method and a myocardial perfusion viability testing, which is an important tool for evaluation of ischemic heart disease.

Left heart catheterization (a percutaneous catheter placement into the left ventricle) allows for a direct measurement of the LVEDP but is rarely performed as a standalone test because of associated risks. This is generally reserved for cases involving other percutaneous cardiac procedures, such as a coronary angiogram. A right heart catheterization (sometimes referred to as a Swan-Ganz catheter or pulmonary artery [PA] catheter) offers a lower complication risk profile and is our favorite method of invasive hemodynamic assessment.

A 12-lead electrocardiography (ECG) is an important test for HF patients. It may diagnose cardiac arrhythmias or ischemic disease, or can be suggestive of other myocardial diseases (i.e., amyloid) providing a clue to the etiology of HF.

Laboratory and Diagnostic Tests

In the newly decompensated HF patient, several laboratory tests should be obtained including serum creatinine, blood urea nitrogen, serum electrolytes, complete blood counts, urinalysis, liver function tests, thyroid stimulating hormone, and fasting lipid panel. In patients with a new HF diagnosis, it is reasonable to screen for hemochromatosis and HIV and to obtain diagnostic tests if there is a clinic concern for systemic disease such as rheumatologic diseases, amyloidosis, or pheochromocytoma.

Natriuretic peptide biomarkers include B-type natriuretic peptide (BNP) and N-terminal pro-B-type natriuretic peptide (NT-proBNP). Natriuretic peptides are released from the heart tissues when stretching (increased intracardiac volume and/or pressure). Circulating natriuretic peptides have a vasodilation and natriuretic response. BNP is the biologically active form and is inactivated by the enzyme neprilysin. Inhibition of the neprilysin enzyme is a target for sacubitril-valsartan. Natriuretic peptide levels can be useful in the ambulatory setting when the evaluation of dyspnea is unclear, assisting with the diagnosis of new onset HF, and in the emergency setting when normal natriuretic peptide levels can help rule out HF. There is no role of serial natriuretic testing in the hospitalized or ambulatory setting but it can be useful when assessing changes in symptoms and upon hospital discharge because the level can help in establishing disease severity and be a predictor of worse outcomes.

Troponin levels can be elevated in decompensated HF. Troponin elevations in HF are not diagnostic to HF but provide information on prognosis in HF and should be obtained on hospital admission.

Therapy for HFrEF
Diuretics (High Dose IV Diuretic Is Important)

Loop diuretics are the mainstay of therapy to relieve congestion in HFrEF and HFpEF. In hospitalized patients already on loop diuretic therapy, the IV dose should exceed the outpatient oral dose and should be given as intermittent boluses or infusion. Consider dosing the IV loop diuretic at 2.5 times the home oral dose. If resistant to initial IV loop diuretic dose, then consider doubling the initial dose. If resistance to IV diuretic continues then consider adding a thiazide diuretic. We prefer IV chlorothiazide, 500 mg × 1, 30 minutes before infusion of a loop diuretic. IV or PO metolazone (2.5–5 mg × 1) or HCTZ 25 mg PO × 1 can also be used. Chronic oral loop diuretics should be adjusted to maintain euvolemia.

Renin-Angiotensin-Aldosterone System Inhibitors
Angiotensin-Converting Enzyme Inhibitor (ACEI)

In patients with HFrEF, ACEIs are indicated and can reduce morbidity and mortality. ACEIs are now considered a class effect in

HFrEF. ACEI block the conversion of angiotensin-I to angiotensin-II, thus avoiding vasoconstriction and other direct myocardial detrimental effects of angiotensin.

Angiotensin Receptor Blocker (ARB)
In similar fashion to ACEIs, ARBs are indicated in HFrEF to reduce morbidity and mortality. ARBs block angiotensin II from binding to the AT1 receptor and avoid the vasoconstriction and other direct myocardial detrimental effects of angiotensin.

Angiotensin Receptor–Neprilysin Inhibitor (ARNI)
ARNI is a combination drug with ARB effect and added neprilysin inhibition (Sacubitril/Valsartan [Entresto]). Neprilysin is an enzyme responsible for the degradation of BNP, and by inhibiting neprilysin circulating BNP is available for further vasodilation and natriuretic effects. ARNI provided further morbidity and mortality benefit compared with ACEI. When possible, patients should be transitioned from an ACEI or ARB to an ANRI. If already on an ACEI, then an ARNI should not be taken within 36 hours of the ACEI to avoid drug interactions. ARNI can cause hypotension, renal insufficiency, and angioedema.

Aldosterone Antagonists
Aldosterone antagonists include spironolactone (Aldactone) or eplerenone (Inspra).[1] They can further reduce morbidity and mortality in HFrEF when added to a background of ACEI/ARB/ANRI and beta blocker. In HFpEF, aldosterone antagonist can be considered to decrease hospitalization. But be aware of the risk of hyperkalemia.

Sympathetic Nervous System
There are three appropriate beta blockers for HFrEF that reduce morbidity and mortality. These include metoprolol succinate (Toprol XL), carvedilol (Coreg), and bisoprolol (Zebeta).[1] When initiating a beta blocker for HFrEF, the patient should have resolution of congestive symptoms and typically will already be on ACEI/ARB/ARNI. Beta blockers are contraindicated in cardiogenic shock.

Hydralazine and Isosorbide Dinitrate Combination
Hydralazine in combination with isosorbide dinitrate is a vasodilator. Hydralazine-isosorbide dinitrate (ISDN) combination (BiDil) or hydralazine and isosorbide dinitrate as a separate combination is indicated for patients self-described as African American and with persistent significant symptoms (NHYA III-IV) while on a background of maximal tolerated ACEI/ARB/ARNI, beta blocker, and aldosterone antagonist. Hydralazine-isosorbide dinitrate combination can also beneficial in those patients that cannot tolerate an ACEI/ARB/ARNI but not as a replacement for those that are able to tolerate.

Sodium-Glucose Cotransporter-2 Inhibitors (SGLT2 Inhibitors)
SGLT2 inhibitors are a newer therapy that is an adjunctive therapy to the existing guideline-directed medical therapy (GDMT). SGLT2 inhibitors can be considered in HFrEF patients with or without diabetes and are associated with reduced cardiovascular events.

Ivabradine
Lower heart rates in HFrEF are associated with better outcomes. Ivabradine (Corlanor, Lancora) is an adjunctive medication to the existing GDMT and can further reduce heart rate. Ivabradine can be considered in HFrEF (LVEF ≤35%) for those in sinus rhythm and on maximal tolerated beta blocker dose when the resting heart rate ≥70 beats per minute.

Digoxin
Digoxin (Lanoxin) can be added as an adjunctive medication in HFrEF and is associated with reduced hospitalizations. Digoxin should be used with caution in the elderly and those with renal dysfunction.

[1]Not FDA approved for this indication.

TABLE 5 Acute Decompensated HF Therapies Based on the Hemodynamic Profile

	NORMAL LVEDP	ELEVATED LVEDP
Normal CO	A "warm and dry" GDMT	B "warm and wet" IV diuretic GDMT
Decreased CO	L "lethal, cold, and dry" Cardiac replacement therapy (circulatory assist devices, cardiac transplant) Palliative care	C "cold and wet" IV inotropes IV diuretics

GDMT, Guideline-Directed Medical Therapy.

Treatment strategies for acute decompensated heart failure based on hemodynamic profile are described in Table 5. Treatment pathways for HFrEF stage C are shown on Figure 3.

Device Therapies
Medicine therapy is the cornerstone of HF treatment, but there are several other therapeutic options that need to be incorporated to further improve survival and decrease symptoms in patients that have demonstrated a lack of response to initial management and through intensification of that therapy. For patients with HFrEF, device therapy including implantable cardioverter-defibrillator (ICD) and cardiac resynchronization therapy (CRT) are proven modalities that further improve survival, and referral to an electrophysiologist and/or heart failure specialist is indicated. ICD can help prevent sudden cardiac death (SCD) in patients with ischemic or nonischemic cardiomyopathies at least 40 days post-MI with LVEF of ≤35% and NYHA II or III symptoms on GDMT or NYHA I with LVEF ≤30%. CRT is indicated in patients with an LVEF of ≤35% and LBBB with persistent symptoms. Transcatheter mitral valve repair (TMVR) using MitraClip™ (Abbott, IL, USA) is another device option in HF patients that decreases mitral regurgitation severity in secondary mitral regurgitation and improves survival in persistent HF.

Therapy for HFpEF
HFpEF is a complex heterogeneous disease where the mortality and morbidity parallel that of HFrEF. Drug therapies have fallen short in being able to significantly impact this disease. A few medical therapies can have impact on this disease including diuretics, which are the mainstay of therapy in relieving congestion; aldosterone antagonists have potential benefit by decreasing hospitalizations, and exercise training can be used to improve symptoms. Treatment of coexisting diseases that drive HFpEF are equally important in the management. This includes addressing coexisting systemic diseases including hypertension, diabetes, obesity, sleep apnea, ischemic heart disease, and chronic kidney disease.

Advanced Heart Failure
Stage D HF or advanced HF are those patients with symptoms at rest or with minimal exertion, recurrent hospitalizations, or refractory symptoms despite appropriate medical therapy. An important key factor in HF management is early identification of high-risk patients for consideration of advanced HF therapies. Early referral to a HF specialist or HF program is key and needs to be considered especially when there is a new onset of HF with unclear etiology, needing assistance with GDMT management, comorbid conditions that increase complexity of management, a persistent reduced LV function despite GDMT, needing referrals for possible device therapies, or having high-risk features (Table 6).

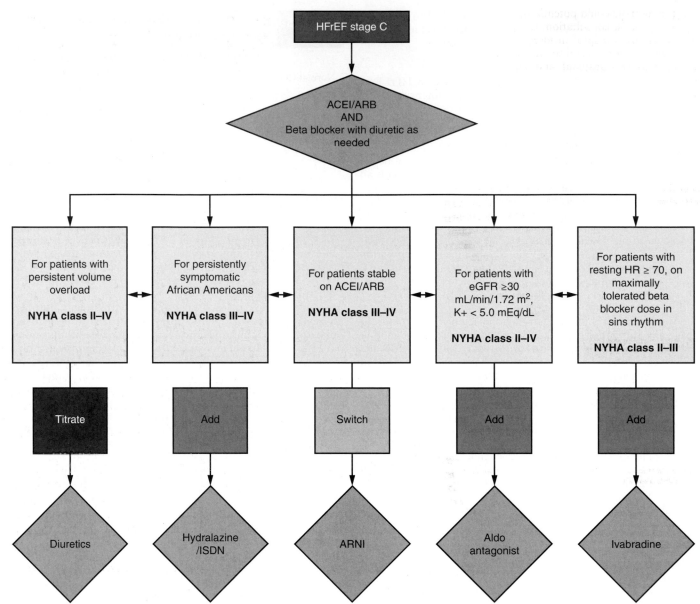

Figure 3 GDMT treatment algorithm for HFrEF stage C. Adapted from 2017 ACC Expert Consensus Decision Pathway for Optimization of Heart Failure Treatment: Answers to 10 Pivotal Issues About Heart Failure With Reduced Ejection Fraction: A Report of the American College of Cardiology Task Force on Expert Consensus Decision Pathways.

TABLE 6	I-NEED-HELP: Identifying Patients Needing Referral to an HF Specialist or an Advanced Therapy
I	Intravenous inotropes
N	New York Heart Association (NYHA) class IIIB/IV or persistently elevated Natriuretic peptides
E	End organ dysfunction
E	EF ≤35%
D	Defibrillator shocks
H	Hospitalizations ≥2
E	Edema despite escalating diuretics
L	Low systolic blood pressure (≤90), tachycardia
P	Prognostic medications; Progressive intolerance or down-titration of guideline-directed medical therapy

From Maddox, Thomas. M., et al. 2021 "Update to the 2017 ACC Expert Consensus Decision Pathway for Optimization of Heart Failure Treatment: Answers to 10 Pivotal Issues About Heart Failure With Reduced Ejection Fraction." Journal of the American College of Cardiology 77.6 (2021): 772-810.

These situations could potentially have a significant benefit from an HF specialist consultation. Using the acronym I NEED HELP (see Table 6) is helpful in identifying those potentially needing consideration for referral to an HF specialist for advanced therapies including transplant and mechanical circulatory support (MCS).

References

Borlaug B: Evaluation and management of heart failure with preserved ejection fraction, *Nat Rev Cardiol* 17(9):559–573, 2020.

Bozkurt B, et al: Universal definition and classification of heart failure: a report of the heart failure Society of America, heart failure association of the European Society of Cardiology, Japanese heart failure Society and Writing Committee of the universal definition of heart failure, *J Card Fail*, 2021.

Felker GM, et al: Diuretic therapy for patients with heart failure, *J Am Coll Cardiol* 75(10):1178–1195, 2020.

Maddox TM, et al: 2021 "Update to the 2017 ACC Expert Consensus Decision pathway for Optimization of heart failure treatment: answers to 10 pivotal Issues about heart failure with reduced ejection fraction," *J Am Coll Cardiol* 77(6):772–810, 2021.

McKee PA, et al: The natural history of congestive heart failure: the Framingham study, *N Engl J Med* 285(26):1441–1446, 1971.

Ponikowski P, et al: 2016 ESC Guidelines for the diagnosis and treatment of acute and chronic heart failure: the Task Force for the diagnosis and treatment of acute and chronic heart failure of the European Society of Cardiology (ESC) Developed with the special contribution of the Heart Failure Association (HFA) of the ESC, *Eur Heart J* 37(27):2129–2200, 2016.

Tsutsui H, et al: JCS 2017/JHFS 2017 guideline on diagnosis and treatment of acute and chronic heart failure—Digest version, *Circ J* 83(10):2084–2184, 2019.

Virani SS, et al: Heart disease and stroke statistics—2020 update: a report from the American Heart Association, *Circulation* 141(9):e139–e596, 2020.

Yancy CW, et al: 2013 ACCF/AHA guideline for the management of heart failure: executive summary: a report of the American College of Cardiology Foundation/American Heart Association Task Force on practice guidelines, *Circulation* 128(16):1810–1852, 2013.

Yancy CW, et al: 2017 ACC/AHA/HFSA focused update of the 2013 ACCF/AHA guideline for the management of heart failure: a report of the American College of Cardiology/American heart association Task force on clinical practice guidelines and the heart failure Society of America, *J Am Coll Cardiol* 70(6):776–803, 2017.

HEART BLOCK

Method of
Kelley P. Anderson, MD

CURRENT DIAGNOSIS

- Assess risk for heart block in the absence of symptoms or heart block on electrocardiogram (ECG).
  - Review cardiac or systemic disorders associated with cardiac conduction disease (CCD), ECG pattern, family history, maternal antibodies, cardiac interventions, and surgery.
- Evaluate documented asystole or bradycardia due to heart block.
  - Classify heart block: transient, recurrent, progressive, permanent.
  - Grade signs and symptoms: none, mild, severe.
- Evaluate signs or symptoms of possible transient heart block with no documentation.
  - Establish temporal pattern: recent versus remote onset, solitary versus recurrent, daily, weekly, monthly, yearly.
  - Grade signs and symptoms: none, mild, severe.
  - Document rhythm during symptoms: telemetry monitoring, Holter monitor, external loop recorder, implantable recorder.

CURRENT THERAPY

- Methods of heart rate support:
  - Immediate: intravenous catecholamines, atropine, or aminophylline[1]; transcutaneous pacing
  - Short term: transvenous temporary pacing
  - Long term: permanent pacemakers
- Pacemaker configuration:
  - Number of leads: 1, 2, 3, 4 or leadless
  - Lead locations: right atrial appendage, Bachman's bundle, right ventricular apex, outflow tract, left ventricle, coronary sinus, His bundle, left bundle branch area
  - Programming to minimize ventricular pacing: manufacturer dependent, biventricular pacing, His bundle pacing, left bundle branch area pacing

[1]Not FDA approved for this indication.

Heart block refers to block or delay of electrical propagation between the atria and ventricles. It is a form of cardiac conduction disease (CCD), which applies more generally to disorders of electrical impulse formation or propagation anywhere along the cardiac conduction system from the sinus node to the ventricular myocardium. Heart block or CCD may present as a syndrome, as an electrocardiographic (ECG) pattern, or as a mechanism of serious signs and symptoms such as sudden death or syncope. Pacemaker therapy is an effective treatment, but it is associated with significant short- and long-term complications. This underscores the importance of recognizing preventable and reversible causes of heart block for accurate targeting of permanent pacing. Risk stratification of patients with heart block, assessment of the benefits and risks of the therapeutic options, and patient education and guidance are largely in the domain of heart rhythm specialists. However, heart block may be encountered unexpectedly in any patient during any clinical encounter. Furthermore, some patients may require evaluation in the absence of known cardiac disease because of increased risk of CCD, or increased risk of CCD in family members or future children. A basic understanding of heart block may be useful to initiate emergency treatment and to recognize patients who warrant further evaluation or specialist referral.

Epidemiology

The prevalence and incidence of heart block are difficult to establish because they are strongly dependent on the demographic and clinical characteristics of the population sample. The prevalence is higher among the elderly and those with cardiovascular disease. First-degree heart block, defined as prolongation of the PR interval >200 ms on ECG, occurs in the population setting with prevalence of 0.7% to 2% in the young and up to 14% in the elderly. Higher degrees of heart block can be expected to be less common but similarly associated with age and underlying cardiovascular disease. In a study of the Framingham population, the prevalence of first-degree heart block was 1.6% and was associated with an incidence of pacemaker implantation of 59 per 10,000 person-years in persons with a PR interval >200 ms compared to 6 per 10,000 person-years in persons with a PR interval <200 ms. Approximately 36% of the pacemakers were for high-grade block.

In 1420 elderly subjects with common risk factors randomized to continuous monitoring by implanted loop recorder (ILR group, mean monitoring duration 39 months) versus 4503 controls in usual care, 4.1% demonstrated first-degree or low-grade second-degree heart block (95.1% asymptomatic) compared with 0.8% in controls. High-grade second-degree block or complete block was observed in 3.1% of the ILR group (28.3% asymptomatic) and in 1.5% of controls. More patients in the ILR group underwent pacemaker implantation with no demonstrable improvements in outcomes. This study suggests that detection of conduction disturbances is increased by longer periods of monitoring, that heart block in elderly patients is infrequent but not rare, that many subjects with incident heart block are asymptomatic, and that pacemaker implantation does not necessary improve outcomes based on the nearly 6 years of observation in the subjects enrolled in this study.

Risk Factors

Patients with genetic or acquired CCD and patients subject to trauma or surgical procedures that can damage the conduction system are at increased risk for developing symptomatic advanced heart block. In the Framingham population, subjects with first-degree AV block had an increased risk of mortality, atrial fibrillation, and pacemaker implantation. However, the vast majority with risk factors never develop symptomatic heart block and have not been shown to benefit from intense monitoring or prophylactic pacemaker placement. The few possible exceptions are discussed below.

Pathophysiology

The function of the cardiac conduction system is to initiate and coordinate cardiac contraction to circulate blood according to physiological needs. Electrical activation is initiated by pacemaker cells of the sinus node regulated by the autonomic nervous system. Unlike conduction in common electrical circuits in which electrons flow along a conductor according to the voltage gradient, electrical activity in cardiac cells propagates from segment to segment of the cell membrane in cardiac myocytes (myocardial cells) and in specialized cardiac conduction cells. Energy-requiring ion pumps maintain an electrochemical gradient across the insulating cell membrane. Electrical activity opens voltage-sensitive ion channels causing regenerative electrical activity as ions shift along their electrochemical gradient. Electrical activity in a single cell excites several adjacent cells via gap junctions. This cascade effect makes it possible for a single cell impulse to spread rapidly throughout the myocardium to enhance synchronous contraction. This also provides a safety mechanism in that each myocardial cell can be activated by many electrical paths. In addition, specialized conduction cells exhibit automaticity (impulse formation). Although normally latent because normal activation inhibits spontaneous discharge, when the normal impulse is blocked, discharges from these subsidiary physiological pacemakers provide vital heart rate support.

Block of electrical activation can occur due to failure of any step in the process, for example, lack of metabolic energy, electrolyte imbalance, inflammatory disruption of the membrane, block of ion channels by drugs, or interference with gap junction function due to infiltration of fibrous tissue (Table 1). Because of the extensive redundancy and interconnectivity and because of the capacity to compensate for injury by electrical and anatomic remodeling, there may be extensive damage before signs or symptoms of heart block occur. Regions of the heart where there are fewer alternative paths for electrical activation, such as proximal portions of the His-Purkinje system where all conducting fibers are confined

to a relatively small area, are more vulnerable to complete block. Subsidiary pacemakers sometimes fail to provide adequate rate support when heart block occurs because of preexisting injury. If the patient survives an episode of heart block, there is a possibility for recovery due to remodeling. However, remodeling can be maladaptive and result in an adverse long-term outcome by further conduction system damage, by left ventricular dysfunction, and by bradycardia-induced ventricular tachyarrhythmias (VTAs). The mechanisms of bradycardia-induced VTAs are not known, but bradyarrhythmias precipitate torsades de pointes, a specific form of VTA, in the presence of drugs that block potassium channels, electrolyte disturbances, certain genetic abnormalities of ion channel function, heart failure, and myocardial hypertrophy. A comprehensive list of drugs that may account for bradyarrhythmia-related ventricular arrhythmias is available at www.torsades.org.

Although there are many potential causes of heart block, the pathophysiology is not known for the vast majority of cases because there are no tests that allow detailed structural or functional examination in patients. By the time of death, morphologic examination may reveal only nonspecific changes such as fibrosis. Instead, most etiologies are inferred by history of recent or past exposures (e.g., trauma or radiation), concomitant disorders (e.g., muscular dystrophy, cardiac sarcoidosis), abnormal test results (e.g., Lyme disease) or family history (e.g., SCN5A sodium channel mutations) (Table 2). Because most etiologies cannot be verified, the clinician must remain open to alternative explanations and accept the likelihood of multiple contributors.

Some patients, usually young, otherwise healthy individuals, present with prolonged asystole due to heart block but have no other detectable abnormalities and have excellent outcomes in the absence of intervention beyond counseling. This suggests that autonomic influences alone can cause prolonged heart block and suppression of subsidiary pacemakers. It is not known whether such responses result from an abnormality or an exaggerated normal reflex. However, the identification of such patients is important because most can be managed without pacemakers.

TABLE 2 Etiologies of Heart Block

- Frequently permanent or progressive (examples)
  - Alcohol septal ablation (acute, delayed)
  - Cardiomyopathies (hypertrophic, idiopathic, mitochondrial)
  - Catheter ablation (atrioventricular nodal reentry, accessory atrioventricular connections)
  - Congenital heart block (neonatal lupus)
  - Congenital heart disease (endocardial cushion defects)
  - Genetic disorders (SCN5A sodium channel mutations, gap junction gene mutations, fatty acid oxidation disorders, PRKAG2 mutations, LMNA gene mutations)
  - Hypertension
  - Idiopathic fibrosis and calcification (Lev's disease, Lenegre's disease)
  - Infectious disorders—destructive (endocarditis)
  - Infiltrative disorders (amyloidosis)
  - Myocardial infarction
  - Neuromyopathic disorders (myotonic dystrophy, Erb's dystrophy, peroneal muscular atrophy)
  - Noninfectious inflammatory disorders (HLA-B27–associated disorder, sarcoidosis)
  - Tumors (mesothelioma, metastatic cancer)
  - Valvular heart disease
- Frequently transient or reversible (examples)
  - Blunt trauma (baseball)
  - Cardiac surgery (valve replacement)
  - Cardiac transplant rejection
  - Central nervous system
  - Drugs (antiarrhythmics, digoxin [Lanoxin], edrophonium [Enlon])
  - Electrolyte disturbances (hyperkalemia)
  - Metabolic disturbances (hypothermia, hypothyroidism)
  - Increased vagal activity
  - Infectious disorders—nondestructive (Lyme disease)
  - Myocardial ischemia
  - Myocarditis (Chagas disease, giant cell myocarditis)
  - Rheumatic fever

TABLE 1 Mechanisms of Conduction Disturbances (Examples)

- Prolonged refractory period (vagal activity, drugs, ischemia)
- Sarcolemmal ion gradient disturbances (hyperkalemia, hypokalemia)
- Sodium channel dysfunction (SCN5A mutations, sodium channel blocking drugs such as lidocaine, procainamide, flecainide [Tambocor], amiodarone [Cordarone], and imipramine [Tofranil])
- Calcium channel dysfunction (verapamil [Isoptin], diltiazem [Cardizem], mutations)
- Energy deprivation (ischemia, cyanide)
- Cell dysfunction (inflammation, barotrauma, thermal injury)
- Cell death (apoptosis, ischemic necrosis, inflammatory necrosis, surgical trauma, ablation)
- Congenital structural defects (endocardial cushion defects)
- Gap junction disturbances (fibrosis, edema, inflammation, genetic defects)
- Genetic defects (SCN5A and NKX2.5 mutations)

Prevention

Prevention of heart block is a challenge for the future. Some instances can be prevented by treatment of inflammatory disorders that cause heart block, such as Lyme disease or cardiac sarcoid. Other individuals who should be identified are those with conditions that place them, their relatives, or their unborn children at risk for heart block. This includes patients and family members with genetic disorders associated with heart block. Genetic testing and counseling may be appropriate in some patients with a family history of CCD. Pacemaker therapy may be indicated in some patients with neuromuscular disorders, in particular myotonic dystrophy or Kearns-Sayre syndrome, in the presence of CCD that would be considered low-grade in other individuals. Neonatal lupus syndrome is a rare disorder with a high mortality rate and risk of permanent complete heart block in survivors. This occurs in pregnant women with anti-Ro/SSA or anti-La/SSB antibodies. Some such women have autoimmune disorders such as systemic lupus erythematosus and Sjögren's syndrome, but many are symptom free. Members of this group may benefit from counseling and anticipatory evaluation and treatment of offspring. Although controversial, fetal monitoring of pregnant women with anti-Ro/SSA and/or anti-La/SSB antibodies and treatment of those with signs of fetal conduction system involvement have been recommended. It should be recognized that with current methods the vast majority of heart block events cannot be predicted or prevented, and the vast majority of persons with risk factors never develop symptomatic heart block.

Clinical Manifestations

Most of the symptoms experienced by patients with heart block are common and nonspecific, including syncope, lightheadedness, fatigue, and dyspnea. Asystole or profound bradycardia may cause syncope, death, or other manifestations of hypoperfusion. Rarely, first-degree AV block results in significant symptoms (e.g., fatigue, palpitations, chest fullness), probably due to atrial contraction against a partially closed mitral valve.

Diagnosis

Because various arrhythmias and other cardiac and noncardiac disorders may be responsible for similar symptoms, it is important to identify the cause. An ECG recording of asystole or bradycardia due to heart block at the time of symptoms strongly suggests a causal relationship, but this is usually difficult to accomplish because the symptoms are often transient and infrequent. Absence of arrhythmias at the time of symptoms is also helpful in excluding heart block as the cause. Asymptomatic heart block is not infrequent. Cardiac conduction disturbances are classified by the pattern of ECG complexes. A normal 12-lead ECG lessens the probability of conduction disturbances due to structural changes but it does not eliminate the possibility of transient third-degree block due to reversible functional effects such as intense vagal activity or ischemia. Significant disease of the His bundle may be electrocardiographically silent, but more often concomitant distal disease is evident in the form of fascicular or bundle branch block or a nonspecific intraventricular conduction delay. In a patient with syncope, the presence of bifascicular block raises the possibility of transient third-degree block as the mechanism and of progression to permanent complete block. Most patients with conduction disorders are not symptomatic and do not progress to complete block. However, the combination of right bundle branch block (RBBB) and left posterior fascicle block has a greater tendency to progress to complete block than the more common RBBB and left anterior fascicle block. Nevertheless, conduction disturbances of the His-Purkinje system should not be assumed to be responsible for syncope or cardiac arrest because they are relatively common in patients with cardiovascular disorders that cause syncope or cardiac arrest due to other mechanisms. Conduction disturbances can cause dyssynchronous contraction and result in adverse remodeling. In addition, they can mask or mimic the ECG signs of myocardial infarction. Alternating bundle branch block refers to a changing ECG pattern in which both RBBB and left bundle branch block are observed or

when the bifascicular block pattern switches between the anterior and posterior fascicle involvement. This pattern is considered a harbinger of complete block and warrants continuous monitoring and evaluation for permanent pacemaker implantation.

Differential Diagnosis

The challenge in second- and transient third-degree AV block is distinguishing between block in the AV node, which is often functional and reversible, and infranodal block, which often progresses to permanent complete heart block. ECG clues that block is in the AV node include normal QRS duration (<100 ms), type I (Wenckebach) pattern, PR prolongation before blocked impulses and PR shortening after pauses, occurrence during enhanced vagal activity (e.g., sleep), narrow QRS escape complexes, and no factors favoring infranodal block. ECG clues for infranodal block include prolonged QRS duration (≥120 ms), type II pattern, and escape QRS complexes broader than intrinsic complexes. Type II second degree AV block is almost always due to block in the His-Purkinje system. Other second-degree AV block ECG patterns have poor sensitivity and specificity for site of block.

Unsustained polymorphic ventricular tachycardia is an ominous sign in any context and may result from a variety of cardiac, metabolic, and autonomic abnormalities. However, in the presence of heart block it suggests that heart rate support may be necessary to prevent sustained VTA. QT prolongation and postpause U-wave accentuation should be sought as other harbingers of bradycardia-related VTA.

The importance and value of ECG documentation of heart block cannot be overemphasized. ECGs are subject to artifact and may be misleading when standards for acquisition and analysis are not followed. Multiple tracings of suspicious events should be obtained in multiple leads when possible. A 12-lead simultaneous rhythm recording mode is available on most modern ECG machines and should be used when continuous recordings are obtained to document arrhythmias.

Clinicians encounter heart block in three general contexts. For the patient with documented heart block, the clinician selects therapy based, in part, on whether the arrhythmia is permanent or likely to recur. There are currently no tests that provide direct information about the pathologic state of the AV conduction system. Instead, these outcomes must be inferred from functional assessment, that is, from the ECG or electrophysiological testing. Other indirect sources such as coronary angiography, magnetic resonance imaging, nuclear imaging, and myocardial biopsy, as well as a large number of specific laboratory tests, are often helpful for identifying disorders that may be causative or associated with heart block and that may affect the choice of treatment.

Another common context is the patient with symptoms for whom the objective is to verify or exclude heart block as the mechanism by correlating the cardiac rhythm with symptoms. Real-time monitoring (e.g., in-patient telemetry) is used for patients who might require immediate access to drugs or pacing devices to prevent or terminate asystole or bradycardia-dependent VTA. Holter monitoring is useful for patients who have very frequent events (at least 1 every 24 hours), and they are useful for capturing asymptomatic rhythm disturbances. External recorders are applied for a month or longer and are very helpful to associate rhythm abnormalities with symptoms and to rule out a rhythm disorder as the cause of symptoms in patients with at least one event per month. Patients with infrequent events may be candidates for implantable loop recorders, which monitor for greater than a year. Modern monitors will provide a permanent record of arrhythmias on activation by the patient or by a detection algorithm.

Electrophysiological studies allow precise measurements of AV node and His-Purkinje system function and can provide definitive information regarding the site of block if the conduction disturbance occurs during the study. Additional tests have been developed that "stress" the AV conduction system, including rapid atrial and ventricular pacing and administration of drugs such as procainamide and disopyramide (Norpace). The provocation of heart block is assumed to indicate a propensity for spontaneous AV block. Unfortunately, the sensitivity is low and a negative test does not imply a low risk of future episodes. Electrophysiological studies have the additional advantage of providing immediate test results, as well as providing the results of programmed stimulation for provocation of supraventricular and VTAs, which may be included in the differential diagnosis.

Therapy

The object of the evaluation and management for heart block is to prevent death and morbidity by (1) heart rate support in patients with poorly tolerated bradycardia; (2) monitoring and standby heart rate support in patients at high risk for asystole or severe bradycardia; (3) identifying and treating reversible causes of heart block; (4) identifying patients at high risk for sudden death, syncope, or recurrent symptoms; and (5) selecting and implanting the appropriate rate support system as soon as safety permits.

Advanced cardiac life-support guidelines apply to the patient who is unresponsive or severely compromised by heart block. However, heart block is rarely the primary problem. Therefore evaluation and treatment of other disorders should continue while efforts to obtain the appropriate heart rate are underway.

The initial evaluation should include a detailed history and physical examination and review of current and previous ECGs and rhythm strips to determine whether heart block is present or occurred in the past and whether there were symptoms or other evidence of hemodynamic compromise. Basic laboratory tests (electrolytes, metabolic panel, cardiac biomarkers, thyroid function, blood count, and coagulation studies) and basic imaging (chest x-ray and echocardiography) are usually appropriate. The patient should then be stratified for the appropriate level of care: (1) the unstable patient who requires ongoing evaluation and treatment in an intensive care setting, (2) the stable patient at high risk for asystole or complications who needs temporary transvenous pacing or other invasive procedures, (3) the patient at moderate risk who requires continuous monitoring and standby noninvasive heart rate support measures, (4) the patient at low risk who requires rapid but not immediate access to heart rate support measures that hospital monitoring provides, and (5) the patient at low risk who can be evaluated and managed as an outpatient. Additional testing and procedures may be necessary to determine the etiology of heart block and to determine whether there is a significant risk of future adverse events.

Determination of the need for long-term heart rate support, as well as other issues that may affect implantable device selection (e.g., risk for VTAs), should be accomplished as soon as possible because the risk of complications and anxiety associated with temporary heart rate support measures increases over time. Major societies have developed guidelines for implantable rhythm management devices (http://www.cardiosource.org/Science-And-Quality/Practice-Guidelines-and-Quality-Standards.aspx; http://www.escardio.org/guidelines-surveys/Pages/GuidelinesList.aspx). The reasons for the selected therapy, including the rationale for any deviation from established guidelines, should be documented and provided to the patient. This will reduce future confusion or misunderstanding about the original rationale for implantation that can affect management of patients with device complications, recalls (safety alerts), and those with a compelling need for device upgrade or explantation.

Patients with acute coronary syndromes require special consideration. The incidence of heart block in patients with myocardial infarction based on creatine phosphokinase as the marker of necrosis is approximately 10%. Although the incidence is probably lower using more sensitive markers such as troponin, heart block is still likely to be associated with increased in-hospital mortality due to larger infarct size. Tachycardia and high blood pressure increase myocardial oxygen consumption. Therefore overcorrection of heart rate and blood pressure should be avoided and ischemia should be relieved by reperfusion as soon as possible. Studies in the prethrombolytic era did not demonstrate a benefit in mortality with prophylactic temporary transvenous pacing, and complications were frequent. The risks of transvenous insertion may be higher in patients requiring administration of thrombolytics and other anticoagulants. Catheter-based revascularization methods should be given strong consideration because of established effectiveness, the possible avoidance of thrombolytic drugs, and because transvenous temporary pacing, if needed, is readily and safely accomplished during the procedure. Suggestions for standby temporary pacing (Table 3) should take into consideration the risks of transvenous pacing based on local circumstances (experience, fluoroscopic guidance, insertion site, use of anticoagulants, etc.). Most conduction disturbances associated with myocardial ischemia or infarction resolve quickly but can persist for days or weeks. The need for permanent pacemaker implantation as a consequence of myocardial infarction is rare, and prophylactic pacemaker implantation in high-risk subsets has not been shown to reduce mortality. Guidelines for temporary and permanent pacing in acute myocardial infarction have been published (http://www.cardiosource.org/Science-And-Quality/Practice-Guidelines-and-Quality-Standards.aspx; http://www.escardio.org/guidelines-surveys/esc-guidelines/Pages/GuidelinesList.aspx).

Selection of the correct therapeutic approach balances the risks and benefits of therapy against the risks of heart block for both immediate and long-term management. Catecholamines (dobutamine, dopamine, epinephrine, isoproterenol [Isuprel]) are useful for emergency, temporary, and standby heart rate support. The standby mode is accomplished by a prepared infusion at the bedside. To avoid underdoses or overdoses at the time of sudden symptomatic heart block, the optimal dose can be established in advance by test doses starting at low infusion rates. Atropine (0.5 mg every 3–5 minutes, with a maximum dose of 0.04 mg/kg or total of 3 mg) may be useful for treatment or pretreatment of patients who develop heart block at the level of the AV node in the context of elevated vagal tone (e.g., in association with nausea or endotracheal tube suction). Atropine should be avoided in patients with infranodal AV block because prolonged asystole sometimes occurs due to more frequent His-Purkinje system depolarization from increased sinus rate. Vagal activity inhibits sympathetic activity; therefore, reduction of vagal tone by atropine disinhibits sympathetic activity and may account for the unpredictable effects of atropine on heart rate. Elevations in heart rate after atropine can persist for hours and cannot be readily reversed. Aminophylline[1] (2.5–6.3 mg/kg IV) is reported to reverse heart block resistant to atropine and epinephrine by antagonizing adenosine. Stimulation of β-adrenergic receptors increases sinus node and subsidiary pacemaker rates, AV node and His-Purkinje system conduction velocities, and myocardial contractility. The effective refractory period shortens in most tissue but this effect varies with dose and specific tissue type. Dobutamine[1] (2–40 μg/kg/min) is a useful β-receptor agonist because it increases cardiac output and lowers filling pressures without

---

[1] Not FDA approved for this indication.

TABLE 3	Suggestions for Temporary Pacing in Acute Myocardial Infarction

- Transvenous pacing
  - Asystole or poorly tolerated bradycardia unresponsive to atropine or aminophylline
  - Persistent third-degree AV block
  - Alternating RBBB and LBBB, or RBBB and alternating LAFB and LPFB
  - Bifascicular block, new
  - Second-degree AV block (any type) and QRS >110 ms
  - Any indication listed below at time of cardiac catheterization if performed
- Standby transcutaneous pacing
  - Any indication listed above until transvenous pacing system inserted
  - Transient asystole or poorly tolerated bradycardia
  - Bifascicular block, uncertain time of onset, or old
  - Second-degree AV block (any type) and QRS <110 ms
  - New first-degree AV block

Abbreviations: AV = atrioventricular; LAFB, LPFB=left anterior, left posterior fascicle block; LBBB, RBBB=left, right bundle branch block.

excessive rise or fall of blood pressure. Dopamine[1] (2–20 µg/kg/min IV) stimulates β_1-adrenergic receptors and increases heart rate by enhancing impulse formation and conduction, as well as myocardial contractility. At higher doses (10–20 µg/kg/min) dopamine causes vasoconstriction by α_1-receptor stimulation. Isoproterenol (0.02–0.06 mg IV bolus, 0.5–10.0 µg/min IV infusion) stimulates β_1- and β_2-adrenergic receptors and enhances vasodilation more than the other catecholamines. This can result in unwanted hypotension in some circumstances but it is also less likely to cause a reflex increase in vagal tone than drugs that cause vasoconstriction. Epinephrine (1 mg IV boluses for cardiac arrest, 0.2–1 mg subcutaneously, 0.5–10 µg/min IV) stimulates both α- and β-adrenergic receptors. It is recommended for asystolic cardiac arrest in part because it increases myocardial and cerebral flow. However, the increase of systemic vascular resistance may be detrimental by augmenting metabolic acidosis and decreasing cardiac performance in patients with poor left ventricular function. The suggested dose ranges are broad because the response to β-adrenergic stimulants such as improved AV conduction varies widely and may be affected by β-adrenergic receptor down-regulation in patients with chronic elevations in sympathetic activity such as patients with long-standing heart failure.

Temporary pacing includes primarily transcutaneous and transvenous approaches. Transthoracic, transesophageal, and transgastric approaches are rarely used. Transcutaneous pacing provides noninvasive heart rate support, as well as immediate access to countershock, but it is often so painful that most patients require sedation. For these reasons its principal uses are for short-term pacing during cardiopulmonary resuscitation and standby pacing in patients at risk for bradyarrhythmias. Capture is not achieved in some patients. Therefore users should be ready to continue mechanical cardiopulmonary support and seek alternative methods. If used in standby applications, ventricular capture should be verified in advance. Capture is often difficult to ascertain because transcutaneous stimuli cause large deflections on the ECG, and pectoral muscle stimulation can be confused with a pulse. Capture should be verified by careful ECG analysis at subthreshold and suprathreshold stimulus amplitudes and confirmed by appropriately timed femoral artery pulses, Korotkoff sounds, or arterial pressure waveforms.

Transvenous insertion of an electrode catheter is the method of choice for most patients who require temporary pacing. This approach is reliable and safe when performed by competent staff with strict aseptic technique, fluoroscopic guidance, and appropriate catheters. Small studies suggest that long-term (>5 days) temporary pacing can be accomplished with active-fixation permanent pacemaker leads attached to an external pulse generator (not approved by the US Food and Drug Administration [FDA]). Tunneling the lead may enhance stability and reduce the risk of infection.

Monitoring

Patients with high-grade or symptomatic heart block require close monitoring until the process is reversed by treatment or a pacemaker is implanted. All patients who receive pacemakers require lifelong follow-up by a trained team of physicians, nurses, and ancillary personnel using standard procedures guided by practice guidelines and manufacturer recommendations.

Complications

Catecholamines used to increase heart rate may precipitate tachyarrhythmias by electrophysiological effects mediated by adrenergic receptors or by myocardial ischemia, and they may worsen hemodynamic status. The adverse effects of catecholamines increase with duration of exposure. Ischemia and receptor-mediated electrophysiologic effects occur immediately after administration; changes in gene expression of ion channels begin as early as several hours; and long-term changes such as myocardial hypertrophy, apoptosis, and fibrosis occur within 24 hours and may progress over much longer periods. This suggests that the duration and dose of catecholamine infusions should be minimized. Complications of temporary transvenous pacing include inadequate pacing or sensing thresholds, vascular complications, pneumothorax, myocardial perforation, infection, and dislodgment. Permanent pacemakers are highly effective, safe, and cost-effective with few contraindications. Although the complications are rarely life threatening, they should be carefully considered and acknowledged. Septicemia or endocarditis has been reported in 0.5% of patients. In patients with pacemaker-related endocarditis, the in-hospital mortality rate is reported to be over 7% with a 20-month mortality rate over 25%. The rate of significant complications has been reported to be 3.5%. About 10% of pacemakers will become infected or develop some other type of failure that may require extraction. In a recent series the rate of major complications associated with extraction was 1.4%. There is a long-term continuous risk of infection, thrombosis, and erosion. In young persons there is a periodic need to replace generators and leads. Abandoned leads block venous access and extractions are associated with significant risks. Perhaps of greater consequence is the constant inconvenience of lifelong follow-up, electromagnetic interference, and false alarms from electronic surveillance devices, as well as exclusion from important procedures, such as magnetic resonance imaging of the thorax. Conventional pacing, that is, from the right ventricular apex, is now known to be detrimental and may cause adverse ventricular remodeling, atrial fibrillation, heart failure, and premature death. Although it has been shown that patients with reduced left ventricular function are at greater risk for adverse effects, it is not known how to identify other patients at risk. Strategies for reducing the adverse effects of conventional pacing are under study, and recommendations are evolving. Because the decision for pacemaker implantation includes selection of lead configuration, lead locations, and pacing mode, patient guidance and education are complex.

Conclusions

Heart block remains a challenge because the cellular mechanisms responsible are poorly understood, prediction of symptomatic heart block (who and when) is unreliable, treatments that restore normal conduction do not exist for most conditions, and pacemaker therapy can have significant long-term adverse consequences. Fortunately, innovations and technological advances such as leadless pacemakers and conduction system pacing have expanded options for personalized therapy, and remote monitoring has enhanced early detection of problems and has reduced the inconvenience of device monitoring. Ongoing clinical trials will provide guidance in pacemaker configurations and programming that will minimize adverse effects. In the future, achievements in molecular biology will elucidate mechanisms and produce treatments that will relegate artificial pacemakers to museum pieces.

References

Diederichsen SZ, Xing LY, Frodi DM. Prevalence and prognostic significance of bradyarrhythmias in patients screened for atrial fibrillation vs usual care: post hoc analysis of the LOOP randomized clinical trial. *JAMA Cardiol.* 8(4):326-334, 2023.

Glikson M, Nielsen JC, Kronborg MB, et al. 2021 ESC Guidelines on cardiac pacing and cardiac resynchronization therapy. *Eur Heart J.* 42:3427, 2021.

Groh WJ, Bhakta D, Tomaselli GF, et al. 2022 HRS expert consensus statement on evaluation and management of arrhythmic risk in neuromuscular disorders. *Heart Rhythm.* 19: e61, 2022.

Kusumoto FM, Schoenfeld MH, Barrett C, et al. 2018 ACC/AHA/HRS guideline on the evaluation and management of patients with bradycardia and cardiac conduction delay. *J Am Coll Cardiol.* 74: 932, 2019.

Priori SG, Wilde AA, Horie M, et al., HRS/EHRA/APHRS expert consensus statement on the diagnosis and management of patients with inherited primary arrhythmia syndromes. *Heart Rhythm.* 10: 1932, 2013.

Shah MJ, Silka MJ, Silva JNA, et al. 2021 PACES expert consensus statement on the indications and management of cardiovascular implantable electronic devices in pediatric patients. *Heart Rhythm.* 18:1888, 2021.

HYPERTENSION

Method of
Timothy P. Graham, MD

CURRENT DIAGNOSIS

- Screening should begin at 18 years of age for the general population per U.S. Preventive Services Task Force (USPSTF) recommendations. The screening interval for those 18 to 39 years of age without other risk factors is every 3 to 5 years. For those older than 40 years of age or those with risk factors, annual screening is recommended.
- Stage 1 hypertension is established at blood pressures of 140 mm Hg systolic and 90 mm Hg diastolic if measured in the office, but 135 mm Hg systolic and 85 mm Hg diastolic if based on ambulatory monitoring per Eighth Joint National Committee (JNC 8) and International Society of Hypertension (ISH) guidelines. The AHA/ACC defines stage I hypertension as at or above 130 mm Hg systolic and at or above 80 mm Hg diastolic.
- Stage 2 hypertension is established at blood pressures of 160 mm Hg systolic and 100 mm Hg diastolic per JNC 8 and ISH guidelines. The American College of Cardiology/American Heart Association (ACC/AHA) defines stage 2 hypertension as at or above 140 mm Hg systolic and at or above 90 diastolic.
- Secondary causes of hypertension should be explored and identified to optimize treatment when there is suboptimal response to treatment, worsening hypertension control, no family history of hypertension, onset of hypertension in patients less than 20 years or older than 50 years.

CURRENT THERAPY

- Initial interventions, regardless of stage, should include lifestyle modifications, including low-sodium diet and exercise.
- Optimal pharmacologic therapy should be tailored to account for age, race, and the presence or absence of chronic kidney disease.
- For individuals 60 years of age and older, consider initiation of pharmacotherapy when systolic blood pressure is 150 mm Hg and diastolic blood pressure is 90 mm Hg.
- For individuals younger than 60 years of age but at least 18 years of age, pharmacotherapy should be initiated when systolic blood pressure is 140 mm Hg and diastolic blood pressure is 90 mm Hg.
- First-line agents for nonblack individuals should include thiazide-type diuretics, calcium channel blockers, angiotensin-converting enzyme inhibitors (ACEIs), or angiotensin receptor blockers (ARBs).
- First-line agents for black individuals should include thiazide-type diuretics or calcium channel blockers.
- Individuals with chronic kidney disease should have therapy that includes ACEIs or ARBs.

Epidemiology

Hypertension is one of the most common conditions encountered in primary care offices. According to the AHA/ACC definition of hypertension, hypertension affects 47% of adults in the United States, which represents approximately 116 million people (cdc.gov). The most commonly affected individuals are black adults, with approximately 56% affected.

In the pediatric population, the prevalence of hypertension in the United States is approximately 2.6% (representing nearly 800,000 children), with nearly one-half of this number being classified as obese (body mass index [BMI] >95%).

Risk Factors

Diet and Sodium Intake

Diet is a clear target for nonpharmacologic management of hypertension. Diets that are high in sodium and fat can put individuals at risk for suboptimal blood pressure control. Limiting sodium to less than 2400 mg per day confers some health benefit to individuals at risk for hypertension. Limiting sodium even further to 1500 mg or less is more ideal and typically results in a significant improvement in both systolic and diastolic blood pressure. Additionally, putting limits on the consumption of sweets, red meat, and soda as well as other sugar-sweetened beverages can help weight reduction and overall health.

Sedentary Lifestyle and Obesity

Lack of physical activity is another important risk factor contributing to poor overall health and obesity. Current recommendations endorse engaging in at least 150 minutes of moderate-intensity activity per week. If patients are unable or unwilling to commit to that level of physical activity, then encouraging any physical activity is prudent, as it will convey at least some health benefit. Participation in physical activity results in absolute reduction in chronic comorbidities including hypertension, stroke, heart disease, diabetes, and metabolic syndrome. Resultant weight loss also results in significant improvement in blood pressure. It is noted that a weight loss of 22 pounds has the potential to reduce systolic blood pressure by 5 to 20 mm Hg.

For children and adolescents, elevated BMI is the greatest risk factor for the development of hypertension.

Alcohol Intake

Although moderate alcohol intake is thought to actually reduce cardiovascular risk, heavier consumption is a risk factor for hypertension. Limiting alcohol intake to no more than two drinks per day (with a *drink* defined as 12 oz. of beer, 5 oz. of wine, or 1 oz. of liquor) for men and no more than one drink per day for women (or lightweight men) is beneficial for overall health.

Smoking

Along with the myriad other reasons that tobacco smoking is not a good choice (e.g., cancer risk, chronic obstructive pulmonary disease, stroke, coronary artery disease), it is also a risk factor for hypertension. This is believed to be at least in part caused by a resultant increase in sympathetic nervous system activity, which leads to an increase in myocardial oxygen demand. Additionally, smoking is the leading modifiable cause of death in the United States.

Of note, the use of marijuana results in an increased risk of hypertension-related death. The magnitude of this increase is estimated to be 3.42-fold higher in marijuana users than in nonusers. Risk also further increases with each year of use.

Sleep Apnea

Obstructive sleep apnea is a well-known secondary cause of and independent risk factor for hypertension. Statistically, at least one-half of individuals with sleep apnea also have hypertension.

Age

Age is a nonmodifiable risk factor for cardiovascular disease. Risk is higher in men 55 years of age or older and women 65 years of age or older.

Gender

Gender is another nonmodifiable risk factor. Men are at greater risk for hypertension before 45 years of age. After 45 years of age and until 64 years of age, the risk for men and women is approximately equivalent. At 65 years of age and older, women have a higher hypertensive risk than men.

Race

Black individuals have a prevalence of hypertension than non-black individuals. Statistics from 2019 demonstrated that approximately 56.8% of black men and 57.6% of black women have hypertension compared with approximately 52.7% of white men and 45.4% of white women. Asians had a lower prevalence, at approximately 49.4% of men and 43.6% of women. Hispanic/Latino individuals had an even lower prevalence than white individuals at 46% of men and 35.4% of women.

Family History
Family history is another nonmodifiable risk factor for cardiovascular disease. Individuals with family history of premature cardiovascular disease (men younger than 45 years of age and women younger than 55 years of age) are at increased risk themselves.

Pathophysiology
The pathophysiology of hypertension is a matter of debate. *Essential hypertension*, which is defined as hypertension without a clear secondary cause, makes up the majority of cases. Two primary mechanisms have been proposed for essential hypertension: neurogenic and renogenic (or nephrogenic). The neurogenic model suggests that hypertension is the result of a chronic increase in sympathetic nervous system activity. This is in contrast with the renogenic model, which attributes blood pressure increase to renal origins either through decreased renal blood flow or through renal parenchymal disease.

Prevention
Prevention of hypertension involves optimization of modifiable risk factors. Maintaining a healthy body weight, avoiding smoking, and moderating alcohol use are all key factors in minimizing risk. Additionally, engaging in regular, moderate-intensity cardiovascular exercise and eating a healthy diet without excessive sodium or fat can help significantly reduce cardiovascular risk and optimize health. These risk factors were discussed in detail in the preceding section.

Clinical Manifestations
Hypertension may have very few symptoms or none at all. If symptoms are present, they can include headaches, visual changes, dizziness, nausea, or chest pain. Oftentimes, however, there are no symptoms, and individuals can function for years without being diagnosed.

Diagnosis
Screening
As noted previously, hypertension is oftentimes an asymptomatic condition. As such, screening plays a critical role in early detection to minimize the end-organ damage that could result from untreated, long-standing hypertension. The U.S. Preventive Services Task Force (USPSTF) recommends screening for hypertension in adults who are 18 years of age or older (grade A recommendation). Adults 40 years of age and older and those with increased risk of hypertension should be screened annually. A review of the existing evidence demonstrated minimal harm in screening and a significant resultant benefit in the form of a reduction in cardiovascular disease–related events. Adults 18 to 39 years of age with no additional risk factors should be screened every 3 to 5 years. Recommended screening techniques include measurement of blood pressure in the office setting with either a manual or automatic cuff and ambulatory or home blood pressure measurement. Office measurement should be done with the patient seated and after at least 5 minutes of the patient arriving in the room. Home measurement may be beneficial after the initial screening for confirmation purposes.

For children and adolescents, the USPSTF indicates that the current evidence is insufficient to assess the risk versus benefit of screening in asymptomatic individuals (grade I evidence). The predictive value of childhood hypertension for adult hypertension is modest, with a risk for false-positive readings.

Clinical Diagnosis
Hypertension is classified into two stages based on degree of elevation. In stage 1 hypertension, systolic blood pressure is greater than or equal to 140 mm Hg to 159 mm Hg, and diastolic blood pressure is greater than or equal to 90 mm Hg to 99 mm Hg. Stage 2 hypertension is reached when systolic blood pressure is 160 mm Hg or greater and diastolic blood pressure is 100 mm Hg or greater. Per the 2021 International Society of Hypertension (ISH) guidelines, the setting where the blood pressure is measured affects the threshold for the diagnosis of hypertension. According to the ISH, the above threshold of 140/90 mm Hg applies to the office setting, whereas for home readings, 135/85 should be used. If relying on 24-hour ambulatory monitoring, the thresholds are 130/80 mm Hg when looking at 24-hour average readings, 135/85 mm Hg for daytime average, and 120/70 mm Hg for nighttime average. Also of note, the AHA released a statement in 2017 recommending a change in definition for stage 1 hypertension to greater than or equal to 130/80 mm Hg. The classification and definition is important as the approach to treatment differs for each category, as will be discussed later.

Primary (Essential) Hypertension
Primary hypertension encompasses persistent blood pressure elevation without a discernible cause (idiopathic or of unknown cause). The majority of cases of hypertension will have no discernible cause and fall into this category.

Secondary Hypertension
Secondary hypertension is persistent blood pressure elevation that is the result of some other underlying cause. About 10% of all cases of hypertension will fall into this category. If another cause can be identified, in many cases it may be correctable.

Looking for Secondary Causes
Identifying these underlying causes can be a challenge. Using a systematic method of investigating potential etiologies can simplify this process and improve the chances of identifying a source that with treatment can improve outcomes. One such approach is the *ABCDE* mnemonic. The letter *A* in this mnemonic stands for *accuracy* (making sure the reading is correct—such as checking the cuff for appropriate sizing and measurement technique—and repeating readings that are obtained on automatic cuffs manually). Readings on home monitors may be different from office-based readings for a variety of reasons, such as the effects of "white coat hypertension," *apnea* (considering the presence of obstructive sleep apnea, which is a known contributor to difficult-to-control hypertension), and *aldosteronism* (investigating for the presence of primary hyperaldosteronism through urinary potassium excretion and an elevation in plasma aldosterone level to plasma renin activity). The letter *B* stands for *bruits* (looking for renovascular sources of hypertension/renal artery stenosis, which often presents with renal bruits upon auscultation) and *bad kidneys* (hypertension resulting from renal parenchymal disease). The letter *C* stands for *catecholamines* (elevation that can contribute to "white coat" hypertension as well as overproduction with pheochromocytoma or associated with other conditions such as obstructive sleep apnea and acute stress reactions), *coarctation* (of the aorta), and *Cushing syndrome* (with mineralocorticoid effects of excess glucocorticoids in this setting). The letter *D* represents both *drugs* (including nonsteroidal antiinflammatory drugs, decongestants, estrogens, immunosuppressive agents, as well as nicotine and alcohol) and *diet* (particularly excess sodium intake). The final letter in the mnemonic, *E*, stands for *erythropoietin* (high endogenous levels—such as in chronic obstructive pulmonary disease—or exogenous levels) and *endocrine disorders* (hypothyroidism or hyperparathyroidism). Utilizing a methodical and organized approach to considering potential causes of hypertension can assist with maximizing the chances of optimally controlling blood pressure.

Differential Diagnosis
The differential diagnosis for hypertension coincides with the array of potential secondary causes that were noted earlier (see the "Looking for Secondary Causes" section earlier in this chapter). It is important to rule out potentially treatable secondary causes in the initial phases of hypertension management.

Treatment Approaches

Approaching treatment of a patient with hypertension can be challenging. Many factors must be considered when making these decisions, including reflection on patient age, race, gender, and comorbidities. Each of these factors can influence what the optimal treatment strategy might be. Figure 1 provides a stepwise strategy to blood pressure management.

Initial treatment should always include lifestyle modification as discussed previously, and this modification must be continued throughout the remainder of any management strategies.

JNC 8 Guidelines

In 2014, the Eighth Joint National Committee (JNC 8) released recommendations regarding the treatment of hypertension. These guidelines were a divergence from the prior JNC 7 recommendations, effectively loosening the goals and the levels at which treatment is initiated. The following is a summary of the eight treatment recommendations from JNC 8. (Please note that the strength of recommendation that is referenced corresponds to the following: grade A—strong recommendation based on evidence; grade B—moderate recommendation based on evidence; grade C—weak recommendation with moderate certainty of a small benefit; grade D—recommendation against; grade E—expert opinion with insufficient or conflicting evidence; grade N—no recommendation for or against).

Recommendation 1

Individuals 60 years of age or older in the general population should have pharmacologic treatment initiated at a systolic blood pressure level of 150 mm Hg or a diastolic blood pressure of 90 mm Hg with treatment goals of less than 150 mm Hg systolic and less than 90 mm Hg diastolic. (Strength of recommendation: grade A.)

An additional aspect of this recommendation is that if the pharmacologic treatment results in adequate blood pressure reduction and there is no adverse effect on quality of life or patient health, then the treatment can be continued without alteration. (Strength of recommendation: grade E.)

Recommendation 2

Individuals younger than 60 years of age in the general population should have pharmacologic treatment initiated at a diastolic blood pressure of 90 mm Hg with a treatment goal of less than 90 mm Hg. (Strength of recommendation: grade A for 30 to 59 years of age, grade E for 18 to 29 years of age.)

Recommendation 3

Individuals younger than 60 years of age in the general population should have pharmacologic treatment initiated at a systolic blood pressure of 140 mm Hg with a treatment goal of less than 140 mm Hg. (Strength of recommendation: grade E.)

Figure 1 Algorithm for management of hypertension. ACE, Angiotensin-converting enzyme; *ARB*, angiotensin receptor blocker; *DASH*, Dietary Approaches to Stop Hypertension. (From Chobanian AV. Shattuck Lecture. The hypertension paradox—More uncontrolled disease despite improved therapy. *N Engl J Med* 2009;361:878–887.

Recommendation 4

Individuals 18 years of age or older with chronic kidney disease should have pharmacologic treatment initiated at a systolic blood pressure of 140 mm Hg or a diastolic blood pressure of 90 mm Hg with a treatment goal of less than 140 mm Hg systolic and less than 90 mm Hg diastolic. (Strength of recommendation: grade E.)

Recommendation 5

Individuals older than 18 years of age with diabetes should have pharmacologic treatment initiated at a systolic blood pressure of 140 mm Hg or a diastolic blood pressure of 90 mm Hg with a treatment goal of less than 140 mm Hg systolic and less than 90 mm Hg diastolic. (Strength of recommendation: grade E.)

Recommendation 6

The treatment of nonblack individuals in the general population (including those with diabetes) who require pharmacologic treatment should include thiazide-type diuretics, calcium channel blockers, angiotensin-converting enzyme inhibitors (ACEIs), or angiotensin receptor blockers (ARBs). (Strength of recommendation: grade B.)

Recommendation 7

The treatment of black individuals (including those with diabetes) should include thiazide-type diuretics or calcium channel blockers. (Strength of recommendation: grade B for the general population, grade C for patients with diabetes.)

Recommendation 8

The treatment of individuals older than 18 years of age with chronic kidney disease should include, either as initial or add-on treatment, ACEIs or ARBs to improve renal outcomes. (Strength of recommendation: grade B.)

Recommendation 9

The goal of hypertension treatment is to reach and maintain blood pressure goals consistent with the previous recommendations. If goals are not reached within 1 month of starting pharmacologic treatment, the dose of the initial agent should be increased, or a second agent from recommendation 6 should be added. Blood pressure should continue to be assessed until the goal blood pressure is achieved. If blood pressure goals are not achieved with two agents, a third agent should be added.

- ACEIs and ARBs should not be used together.
- If necessary, other classes of agents can be used if more than three agents are required or if there are contraindications to the agents in recommendation 6.
- Referral to a hypertension specialist should be considered for patients whose blood pressure goals cannot be met with the previous strategies or patients who are more complicated. (Strength of recommendation: grade E.)

ACC/AHA 2017 Hypertension Guidelines

In late 2017, the ACC/AHA released an updated hypertension guideline. This guideline provided a different approach to hypertension management, particularly around blood pressure goals. Hypertension stages have tighter cut points than under the JNC 8 guidelines. Under the ACC/AHA guidelines, normal blood pressure is defined as less than 120/80 mm Hg. Blood pressure is considered elevated when systolic blood pressure is in the 120 to 129 mm Hg range and when diastolic blood pressure remains under 80 mm Hg. Stage 1 hypertension is defined as systolic blood pressure between 130 and 139 mm Hg and diastolic blood pressure between 80 and 90 mm Hg. Stage 2 hypertension is defined as blood pressures that are greater than 140/90. This classification is a deviation from the set points within the JNC 8 recommendations.

Nonpharmacologic

For stage 1 hypertension (140 to 159 mm Hg systolic/90 to 99 mm Hg diastolic), the first treatment step is aggressive lifestyle modification. This includes targeting both diet and exercise. These nonpharmacologic strategies should continue, even if pharmacologic treatment is found to be necessary. The relative effects of lifestyle modification on systolic blood pressure reduction are noted in Table 1. ACC/AHA guidelines also recommend lifestyle changes as initial intervention for individuals with stage 1 hypertension without other cardiovascular risk factors and with an atherosclerotic cardiovascular disease (ASCVD) risk of less than 10%; however, as noted earlier, the definition of stage 1 hypertension is at a lower blood pressure level (130 to 139 mm Hg systolic/80 to 90 mm Hg diastolic).

Diet. Dietary modifications include salt restriction to a level of less than 2400 mg per day, but ideally less than 1500 mg per day. Suggested dietary interventions also include the use of the DASH (Dietary Approaches to Stop Hypertension) framework. This nutritional framework includes recommendations such as increased consumption of fruits and vegetables, preferential use of complex carbohydrates, and consumption of low-fat dairy products. The DASH diet emphasizes the intake of whole grains, fish, poultry, legumes, nuts, and nontropical vegetable oils. This diet also endorses decreasing higher-fat foods.

Exercise. Current exercise recommendations suggest that engaging in a minimum of 150 minutes of moderate-intensity exercise on a weekly basis confers the greatest health benefits. Exercise at this level of intensity reduces the risk of multiple chronic conditions including cardiovascular disease and type 2 diabetes as well as overall all-cause mortality.

Other Lifestyle Modifications. In addition to diet and exercise, other lifestyle interventions can optimize health. Smoking cessation is an important modifiable risk factor and is the single leading cause of preventable death in the United States. Smoking increases the risk of cardiovascular morbidity and mortality, including myocardial infarction.

Alcohol consumption is another important lifestyle modification that can have a significant impact on overall health. The effects of alcohol consumption, unlike smoking, depend on quantity. It has been shown that at moderate levels of consumption, alcohol can actually decrease blood pressure (defined as no more than two drinks per day for men and no more than one drink per day for women). However, when consumed in greater quantity, alcohol can increase blood pressure, contributing to hypertension. It is emphasized that alcohol consumption should not be promoted in nondrinkers simply for the purpose of decreasing blood pressure.

TABLE 1	Effect of Lifestyle and Diet Modifications on Systolic Blood Pressure		
MODIFICATION	**AMOUNT**	**REDUCTION IN SBP (mm Hg)**
Dietary sodium restriction	< 30–50 mmol/day	2–8
Moderation of daily alcohol intake	150–200 mL	2–4
Increased physical activity	30 min 3 × per week	4–9
Reduction in body weight	10 kg or 22 lb	5–10
Adoption of DASH eating plan (high potassium)		8–14

DASH, Dietary Approaches to Stop Hypertension; *SBP,* systolic blood pressure.

Stress reduction is another lifestyle change that can have effects on blood pressure control. The mechanism of this reduction is not clear, but it is hypothesized that it may be related to decreasing autonomic nervous system output. Studies suggest that activities such as transcendental meditation can lead to modest blood pressure reduction. As such, inclusion of these activities in patient treatment plans may provide additional nonpharmacologic options.

Patients frequently ask about the utility of dietary supplements or other natural alternatives for blood pressure management. There is some evidence for select supplements in the management of hypertension, although such effects appear to be small. Examples of natural substances that may convey a small benefit include garlic and cocoa. Evidence is lacking for other agents including vitamin C, coenzyme Q10, omega-3 fatty acids, and magnesium.

Pharmacologic

In cases in which hypertension is more significant or nonpharmacologic methods have failed to adequately reduce blood pressure, initiation of medications is indicated (Table 2). The selection of an agent or agents is based on a number of factors including race and comorbidities. As noted earlier, the JNC 8 guidelines provide a stepwise, evidence-based approach to blood pressure management including recommended cut points where pharmacologic intervention is appropriate.

One of the points of emphasis of the JNC 8 guidelines is that the point of intervention for individuals 60 years of age or older is higher than for those younger than 60 years of age. One should also balance the side effects or risks of medications with the benefits of intervention in this age group. The cut points for individuals with chronic kidney disease and diabetes do not differ from the general population. The choice of agent according to JNC 8 recommendations does not differ based on the presence or absence of diabetes, but it does differ based on race (see recommendations 6 and 7 earlier in this chapter). Individuals with chronic kidney disease also should have an ACEI or ARB included in their treatment regimen (either as a lone agent or an add-on). In practice, decisions will need to be tailored to individual patient needs and also should consider other factors including whether or not the patient is a reproductive-age female (as ACEIs and ARBs are contraindicated in pregnancy). This is where our role as family physicians becomes increasingly important—embracing our ability to look at the whole patient when making treatment decisions.

The ACC/AHA recommends initiation of pharmacologic therapy in adults with high cardiovascular risk or preexisting cardiovascular disease and stage 1 or greater hypertension. Patients with both diabetes and hypertension are also assumed to fall into the high-risk category. Again, the defined level of blood pressure classified as stage 1 hypertension under the ACC/AHA guidelines (130 to 139 mm Hg systolic/80 to 90 mm Hg diastolic) is lower than the JNC 8 criteria, as noted earlier. The ACC/AHA recommendations also emphasize the need to balance comorbidities as well as preferences, life expectancy, and clinical judgment when making decisions regarding antihypertensive initiation and titration in older adults (65 years of age and older).

A recent trial (Hygia Chronotherapy Trial) published in 2019 investigated whether timing of antihypertensive medication administration affected blood pressure control and overall outcomes. This study demonstrated that for patients on one or more antihypertensive medications, administration of at least one agent at bedtime rather than upon awakening resulted in better ambulatory blood pressure readings as well as an overall decrease in

TABLE 2	Antihypertensive Classes			
DIURETICS				
GENERIC	**BRAND NAME**	**CLASSIFICATION**	**MECHANISM OF ACTION**	**DOSING**
Chlorthalidone	Thalitone	Thiazide	Inhibits sodium and chloride reabsorption in distal tubules	25 mg by mouth once daily. May increase to a maximum of 100 mg once daily.
Hydrochlorothiazide	Microzide	Thiazide	Inhibits sodium and chloride reabsorption in distal tubules	25 mg by mouth once daily to a maximum of 50 mg in single or divided doses.
Metolazone	Zaroxolyn	Thiazide	Inhibits sodium and chloride reabsorption in distal tubules	Individualize. 2.5–5 mg once daily.
Triamterene/ hydrochlorothiazide	Dyazide	Potassium-sparing/ thiazide	Inhibits sodium reabsorption in distal tubules	1–2 capsules by mouth once daily (37.5-/25-mg capsules).
Furosemide	Lasix	Loop	Inhibits sodium and chloride reabsorption in ascending loop of Henle	40 mg twice daily by mouth initially. If adding to another antihypertensive, reduce the other agent's dose by 50%
Torsemide	Demadex	Loop	Inhibits sodium and chloride reabsorption in ascending loop of Henle	5 mg once daily by mouth initially. May increase to 10 mg once daily after 4–6 weeks.

Angiotensin-Converting Enzyme (ACE) Inhibitors

Mechanism of action: Suppress the renin-angiotensin-aldosterone system

GENERIC	**BRAND NAME**	**CLASSIFICATION**	**SPECIAL NOTE**	**DOSING**
Fosinopril	Monopril	ACE inhibitor	Only ACE excreted by both renal and hepatic routes	Initially 10 mg once daily. Usual maintenance is 20–40 mg daily in single or 2 divided doses. Max 80 mg per day. If on a diuretic, suspend diuretic for 2–3 days before starting if possible and resume diuretic if pressure is not controlled with fosinopril alone. If diuretic cannot be discontinued, give 10 mg and monitor carefully.

TABLE 2 Antihypertensive Classes—cont'd

GENERIC	BRAND NAME	CLASSIFICATION	SPECIAL NOTE	DOSING
Captopril	Capoten	ACE inhibitor		Take 1 hour before meals. 25 mg two to three times daily by mouth. May increase to 50 mg two to three times daily by mouth. Maximum 450 mg per day.
Ramipril	Altace	ACE inhibitor		2.5 mg once daily by mouth. May increase to a maximum of 20 mg in 1–2 divided doses by mouth.
Enalapril	Vasotec	ACE inhibitor	If on diuretics or if CrCl <30mL/min: suspend diuretic for 2-3 days if possible. Initially 2.5 mg daily and can titriate to maximum of 40 mg daily in divided doses. If not in above category, start at 5 mg daily. Usual range 10-40 mg in 1-2 divided doses.	2.5 mg daily by mouth initially. Typical dose range is 10–40 mg by mouth daily (may be divided doses).
Lisinopril	Prinivil, Zestril	ACE inhibitor	If renal impairment (CrCl 10-30 mL/min): initially 5 mg once daily. On hemodialysis or CrCl <10mL/min: initially 2.5 mg once daily.	10 mg by mouth daily initial dose. Usual dose range 20–40 mg daily. Doses above 40 mg are not shown to have greater effect. If on diuretics, start 5 mg once daily.
Quinapril	Accupril	ACE inhibitor		10–20 mg daily by mouth initial dose if not on diuretics. Usual maintenance 20–80 mg daily in 1–2 divided doses. If on diuretics, suspend diuretics if possible for 2–3 days before starting and resume if blood pressure not controlled on quinapril alone. Initial dose if on diuretics and CrCl 30–60 mL/min 5 mg. If CrCl 10–30 mL/min, then initially 2.5 mg. If elderly, start 10 mg once daily.

Angiotensin II Receptor Blockers (ARBs)

Mechanism of action: Block binding of angiotensin II to angiotensin I receptors with a resultant inhibition of angiotensin II–mediated vasoconstriction, sodium retention, and release of aldosterone

Losartan	Cozaar	ARB	If mild to moderate hepatic impairment, start at 25 mg once daily.	50 mg daily by mouth initial dose (25 mg initial dose if also on diuretics). May titrate to a maximum dose of 100 mg daily.
Valsartan	Diovan	ARB	Adding a diuretic has greater effect than dose increases over 80 mg daily.	80–160 mg daily by mouth initial dose. May titrate to a maximum dose of 320 mg daily.
Olmesartan	Benicar	ARB		20 mg daily by mouth initial dose. May titrate to a maximum dose of 40 mg daily after 2 weeks. If volume-depleted (on a diuretic), consider lower initial dose.
Azilsartan	Edarbi	ARB		80 mg once daily by mouth. If on diuretics, start at 40 mg once daily.

BETA BLOCKERS

GENERIC	BRAND NAME	CLASSIFICATION	MECHANISM OF ACTION	DOSING
Atenolol	Tenormin	Beta-1 selective		50 mg once daily by mouth. May increase to 100 mg once daily after 1 week. Max dose 200 mg daily. May need to lower dose for elderly or if renal impairment.

Continued

| TABLE 2 | Antihypertensive Classes—cont'd |

BETA BLOCKERS

GENERIC	BRAND NAME	CLASSIFICATION	MECHANISM OF ACTION	DOSING
Metoprolol	Lopressor	Beta-1 selective		Immediate-release formulations: 100 mg in single or divided doses. Maximum 450 mg per day.
	Toprol XL	Beta-1 selective		Extended-release formulations: 25–100 mg daily in a single dose. May increase at 1-week intervals. Maximum 400 mg per day.
Propranolol	Inderal	Beta-1 noncardioselective		Immediate-release formulations: 40 mg by mouth twice daily initial dose. Typical dosing 120–240 mg daily. Maximum 640 mg daily.
	Inderal LA, InnoPran XL	Beta-1 noncardioselective		Extended-release formulations: 80 mg once daily at bedtime initial dose. May increase to 120 mg.
Bisoprolol	Zebeta	Beta-1 selective	More beta-1 specific than other beta blockers	5 mg by mouth once daily initial dose (2.5 mg if patient has bronchospastic disease such as asthma, chronic obstructive pulmonary disease, or renal or hepatic impairment). May titrate to a maximum dose of 20 mg per day.
Timolol		Beta-1 noncardioselective	CAUTION: Avoid abrupt discontinuation as may exacerbate ischemic heart disease	10 mg twice daily by mouth initially. Increase weekly if needed. May titrate to a maximum dose of 60 mg per day in 2 divided doses. Usual maintenance 20–40 mg daily.
Labetalol	Trandate	Alpha and beta antagonist		100 mg twice daily by mouth initially. May titrate in 2–3 days by 100-mg twice-daily increments. Maximum dose 2400 mg per day. Usual maintenance dose 200–400 mg twice daily.

CALCIUM CHANNEL BLOCKERS

GENERIC	BRAND NAME	CLASSIFICATION	MECHANISM OF ACTION	DOSING
Nifedipine, extended release	Adalat CC, Procardia XL	Dihydropyridine	Binds to L-type calcium channels in sinoatrial (SA) and atrioventricular (AV) node, as well as myocardium and vasculature	30–60 mg by mouth once daily initially. Titrate over 7–14 days. Maximum 90 mg daily. Swallow whole.
Diltiazem, extended release	Cardizem CD, Cardizem LA, Cartia XT, Dilacor XR	Nondihydropyridine	Binds to L-type calcium channels in SA and AV node (primarily), as well as myocardium and vasculature	180–240 mg by mouth once daily initially. May titrate at 1–2 week intervals. Maximum dose 360 mg per day.
Verapamil	Calan, Calan SR	Nondihydropyridine	Binds to L-type calcium channels in SA and AV node, as well as myocardium and vasculature	80 mg by mouth every 8 hours initially. Usual max 360 mg/day in divided doses. If elderly or small, start at 40 mg 3 times daily.
Amlodipine	Norvasc	Dihydropyridine	Binds to L-type calcium channels in smooth muscle (vasculature)	5 mg by mouth daily initially. May increase by 2.5 mg every 1–2 weeks. Maximum 10 mg per day. For small, elderly, fragile, or hepatic impaired patients and patients on other antihypertensives, start at 2.5 mg daily.

TABLE 2   Antihypertensive Classes—cont'd

CALCIUM CHANNEL BLOCKERS

GENERIC	BRAND NAME	CLASSIFICATION	MECHANISM OF ACTION	DOSING
Felodipine	Plendil	Dihydropyridine	Binds to *L*-type calcium channels in smooth muscle (vasculature)	5 mg by mouth once daily initially without food or with a light meal. May increase to a maximum dose of 10 mg by mouth once daily. Adjust at 2 week intervals. For elderly patients or hepatic impairment, start at 2.5 mg once daily. Do not crush or chew.

ALDOSTERONE ANTAGONISTS

GENERIC	BRAND NAME	CLASSIFICATION	MECHANISM OF ACTION	DOSING
Spironolactone	Aldactone	Selective aldosterone antagonist	Competes with aldosterone receptor sites. Reduces sodium reabsorption	25–100 mg by mouth once daily or divided twice daily. Titrate at 2 week intervals.
Eplerenone	Inspra	Selective aldosterone antagonist	Competes with aldosterone receptor sites. Reduces sodium reabsorption	50 mg by mouth once daily initially. May increase after 4 weeks to twice daily if needed. (May cause hyperkalemia if doses exceed 100 mg per day.) If on concomitant moderate CYP3A inhibitors such as erythromycin, verapamil, saquinavir, fluconazole, then initially start 25 mg daily with a max of 25 mg twice daily.

Alpha-2 Agonists

Mechanism of action: Stimulate presynaptic aldosterone receptors, decreasing sympathetic nervous activity

GENERIC	BRAND NAME	CLASSIFICATION	MECHANISM OF ACTION	DOSING
Clonidine	Catapres, Catapres-TTS	Centrally acting alpha-2 agonist	Stimulation of alpha-2 adrenoreceptors, reducing sympathetic nervous system output	0.1 mg every 12 hours by mouth. Maximum 2.4 mg per 24 hours. (Usual dose range 0.1–0.3 mg every 12 hours.) If using transdermal formulation, 0.1-mg patch applied once every 7 days. May increase by 0.1 mg/day patch after 1–2 weeks. Maximum 0.6 mg/day.
Methyldopa		Centrally acting alpha-2 agonist	Directly affects peripheral sympathetic nerves through stimulation of central alpha-adrenergic receptors	250 mg by mouth every 8–12 hours initially, then can increase every 2 days. (maximum 3 g per day). Typical maintenance dose is 500–2000 mg/day by mouth divided every 6–12 hours. If also on other antihypertensives (other than thiazides), initial max 500 mg/day.

Alpha Blockers

Mechanism of action: Selectively block postsynaptic alpha-1 adrenergic receptors

GENERIC	BRAND NAME	CLASSIFICATION	MECHANISM OF ACTION	DOSING
Prazosin	Minipress	Alpha-1 blocker	Competitive antagonist, reduces vascular resistance	1 mg by mouth every 8–12 hours initially. Give first dose at bedtime. Increase dose slowly. Maintenance dose typically 6–15 mg divided every 6–8 hours. Typical maximum 20 mg per day in divided doses (although may increase to 40 mg per day in divided doses in some patients). When adding other antihypertensives, reduce dose to 1–2 mg 3 times daily and retitrate.

Continued

		TABLE 2 Antihypertensive Classes—cont'd		
GENERIC	**BRAND NAME**	**CLASSIFICATION**	**MECHANISM OF ACTION**	**DOSING**
Terazosin	Hytrin		Selective competitive inhibitor, decreases vascular resistance	1 mg by mouth at bedtime initially. Typical maintenance 1–5 mg daily or in divided dose every 12 hours. Maximum 20 mg per day.
Doxazosin	Cardura		Selective postsynaptic alpha-1 receptor inhibitor, vasodilation	1 mg once daily initially, titrate gradually at 2 week intervals (based on standing BP at 2–6 hours and 24 hours post-dose) to a maximum of 16 mg/day.

*Exceeds dosage recommended by the manufacturer.
Modified from Medscape. Hypertension Medication. Available at: http://www.emedicine.medscape.com/article/241381-medication.

cardiovascular disease–related events. The results of this study are strongly suggestive that prioritizing bedtime dosing of antihypertensive agents for hypertensive patients leads to greater net benefit.

Monitoring

Clinical practice guidelines vary in their recommendations regarding optimal monitoring. It is clear that monitoring in the early stage or during periods of treatment change should be more frequent than during times of stability, somewhere between monthly and every 6 weeks. Once the patient is stabilized, periodic monitoring can occur either every 3 to 6 months for everyone or in a more risk-stratified manner, with lower-risk patients being seen every 6 months and higher-risk patients every 3 months. Monitoring can also be done through home blood pressure monitoring and through the use of telehealth. This method has become more common and is both convenient and easily accessible to patients. There is evidence to support the use of telehealth for hypertension management, particularly in those individuals with difficult-to-treat hypertension and those with medication compliance issues. Ongoing studies work to support the generalizability to other hypertensive patient populations.

JNC 8 recommendations, as previously discussed, suggest that patients with hypertension be monitored on at least a monthly basis until goal blood pressure is achieved, with any necessary adjustments being made at these visits.

Complications

Hypertension is often referred to as *the silent killer*. This menacing name refers to the fact that this condition often presents without any discernible symptoms, which at times can make treatment compliance challenging. One of the greatest concerns with uncontrolled hypertension is the risk of end-organ damage, which is far-reaching.

Uncontrolled hypertension can lead to serious complications including myocardial infarction, stroke, peripheral artery disease, retinopathy, and renal failure. Given that hypertension is at the same time the most common condition we treat as primary care physicians, the opportunities to circumvent these sources of morbidity and mortality present themselves on a daily basis.

References

Al-Ansary L: A systematic review of recent clinical practice guidelines on the diagnosis, assessment and management of hypertension, *PLOS One* 8(1):1–18, 2013.

Bie P, Evans R: Normotension, hypertension and body fluid regulation: brain and kidney, *Acta Physio* 219:288–304, 2017.

Buelt, et al: Hypertension: New Guidelines from the International Society of Hypertension, *Am Fam Physician* 103(12):763–765, 2021 Jun 15.

Carey: Prevention: detection, evaluation, and management of high blood pressure in adults: synopsis of the 2017 American College of Cardiology/American Heart Association Hypertension Guideline, *Ann Intern Med* 168(5):351–358, 2018.

CDC.gov (Accessed 6/18/2022).

Chobanian AV: Guidelines for the management of hypertension, *Med Clin N Am* 101:219–227, 2017.

Garjon J: First-line combination therapy versus firstline monotherapy for primary hypertension (review), *Cochrane Database Syst Rev* 1, 2017.

Goetsch, et al: New Guidance on Blood Pressure Management in Low-Risk Adults with Stage 1 Hypertension, *ACC.org.*, Jun 21, 2021.

Hermida RC, Crespo JJ, Domínguez-Sardiña M, et al: Hygia Project Investigators: Bedtime hypertension treatment improves cardiovascular risk reduction: the Hygia Chronotherapy Trial, *Eur Heart J*, 2019 Oct 22. ehz754. Online ahead of print.

James P, Oparil S, Carter BL: Evidence-based guideline for the management of high blood pressure in adults: report from the panel members appointed to the Eighth Joint National Committee (JNC 8 h), *JAMA* 311(5):507–520, 2014.

Kallioinen A, Hill A, Horswill MS: Sources of inaccuracy in the measurement of adult patients' resting blood pressure in clinical settings: a systematic review, *J Hypertension* 35:421–441, 2017.

Langan R, Jones K: Common questions about the initial management of hypertension, *Am Fam Physician* 91(3):172–176, 2015.

Leeman L: Hypertensive disorders of pregnancy, *Am Fam Physician* 93(2):121–127, 2016.

Mann S: Redefining beta-blocker use in hypertension: selecting the right beta-blocker and the right patient, *J Am Soc Hypertens*1–12, 2016.

Monthly Prescribing Reference. Available at: www.empr.com. [accessed February 16, 2023].

Omboni S, et al: Telemedicine in Hypertension Management, *Hypertension* 76:1368–1383, 2020.

Onusko E: Diagnosing secondary hypertension, *Am Fam Physician* 67(1):67–74, 2003.

Oza R, Garcellano M: Nonpharmacologic management of hypertension: what works? *Am Fam Physician* 91(11):772–776, 2015.

Prescribers' Digital Reference. Available at: www.pdr.net. [accessed February 16, 2023].

Quyen N: Screening for high blood pressure in adults, *Am Fam Physician* 93(6):511–512, 2016.

Sexton S: Screening for high blood pressure in adults: recommendation statement, *Am Fam Physician* 93(4):300–302, 2016.

Sexton S: Screening for primary hypertension in children and adolescents: recommendation statement, *Am Fam Physician* 91(4), 2015. A–D.

Springer K: Chlorthalidone vs. hydrochlorothiazide for treatment of hypertension, *Am Fam Physician* 92(11):1015–1016, 2015.

Medscape: Hypertension. Available at: http://emedicine.medscape.com/article/241381. [accessed May 9, 2017].

Yankey BA, Rothenberg R, Strasser, et al: Effect of marijuana use on cardiovascular and cerebrovascular mortality: a study using the National Health and Nutrition Examination Survey linked mortality file, *Eur J Prev Cardio*, 2017.

HYPERTROPHIC CARDIOMYOPATHY

Method of
Sandeep Sangodkar, DO

CURRENT DIAGNOSIS

- Echocardiography is a mainstay of clinical diagnosis.
- Cardiac magnetic resonance imaging (MRI) can provide important prognostic information.
- Left ventricular outflow tract pressure and flow measurements have a classic dynamic pattern.
- Left ventricular wall thickness of at least 15 mm.

CURRENT THERAPY

Asymptomatic Disease
- Periodic follow-up to assess symptoms and risk for sudden cardiac death.
- Important to counsel patients regarding potential genetic transmission.
- Patients with concurrent atrial fibrillation should be anticoagulated.

Symptomatic Disease
- β-Blockade or calcium channel blockers are drugs of choice.
- Implantable defibrillator is indicated if the patient has risk factors for sudden cardiac death.
- Surgical myectomy may be undertaken in patients who do not respond to pharmacologic therapy.
- Alcohol ablation may be used in patients who are not candidates for surgery.

Definition

Many names, terms, and acronyms (more than 80) have been used to describe hypertrophic cardiomyopathy (HCM). Common names such as *idiopathic hypertrophic*, *subaortic stenosis*, and *hypertrophic obstructive cardiomyopathy*, popular in the literature in the 1960s and 1970s, imply that left ventricular outflow tract (LVOT) obstruction is a required component of the disease, whereas one-third of patients have no obstruction at rest or exertion. The term *HCM*, first used in 1979, encompasses both the obstructive and nonobstructive hemodynamic variants of this disease and is now considered the formal name.

Epidemiology

Although once thought of as a rare entity, HCM is now recognized as a common inherited cardiovascular disease. Epidemiologic studies from various parts of the world report a similar prevalence, thought of as 1 in 200 to 1 in 500 people, which occurs equally among sexes and ethnic groups. This may, in fact, be underreported because many people with HCM are not clinically diagnosed and achieve normal life expectancy without any HCM-related complications.

Risk Factors

HCM is caused by mutations in genes coding for thin and thick filament proteins of the sarcomere. These mutations are inherited in an autosomal dominant pattern with variable penetrance and expression. At least 11 genes have been identified as responsible for causing HCM, with 70% of successfully genotyped patients found to have mutations in the two most-common genes: β-myosin heavy chain and myosin binding protein C. More than 1500 individual gene variants have been identified, which complicates predicting prognosis for individual patients.

Clinical Manifestations

HCM is seen from pediatric to geriatric populations. A classic description of a murmur suggestive of HCM is a harsh crescendo-decrescendo systolic ejection murmur that increases in intensity with Valsalva or standing from a squatting position. Most patients with HCM are asymptomatic or only mildly symptomatic, with the most common presenting complaints being dyspnea or chest pain. The most worrisome manifestation is sudden cardiac death owing to ventricular tachyarrhythmia, seen more commonly in younger symptom-free patients. Systolic anterior motion of the mitral valve can cause significant mitral regurgitation. Heart failure with preserved ejection fraction is another manifestation of HCM; however, systolic dysfunction can be present owing to myocardial scarring. In addition, atrial fibrillation is associated with an increased risk of thromboembolism in patients with HCM and anticoagulation must be considered. Most patients with HCM have normal life expectancy without a need for major intervention.

Pathogenesis

The pathophysiology of HCM stems from multiple abnormalities, including LVOT obstruction, diastolic dysfunction, mitral regurgitation, myocardial ischemia, and arrhythmias. The peak LV outflow gradient is an important factor in determining treatment options. The obstruction was originally thought to be caused by a hypertrophied basal septum that caused ventricular outflow obstruction during systolic contraction. More recently, it is thought mitral valve systolic anterior motion and mitral-septal contact caused by venturi forces on the mitral leaflets and displacement into the outflow tract cause obstruction of LVOT. The increased LV systolic pressure in turn results in elevated diastolic pressures, mitral regurgitation, and, ultimately, decreased cardiac output.

Diagnosis

Clinically, HCM is defined as maximal end diastolic LV wall thickness of at least 15 mm based on echocardiography or cardiac MRI. Patients should have a comprehensive physical and three-generation family history as part of their initial evaluation. A distinction between HCM and physiologic LV hypertrophy from athletic conditioning must be recognized because the athletic hearts may demonstrate enlargement of the cardiac chambers and thickened septum. The likelihood of clinically significant HCM is determined by identification of sarcomere mutations, marked LV thickness (more than 25 mm), and LVOT obstruction with systolic anterior motion and mitral-septal contact. Provocative testing (exercise or pharmacologic) may elucidate the diagnosis of HCM in symptomatic patients presenting with a normal LVOT gradient at rest. Measurement of outflow gradients by echocardiography and invasive pressures by cardiac catheterization show a characteristic dynamic pattern that can be enhanced by loading conditions.

Imaging

The mainstay of imaging has been held by echocardiography. Transthoracic echocardiography is recommended in the initial evaluation of all patients with suspected HCM and family members of those diagnosed with HCM. Transesophageal echocardiography is used for diagnosis and intraprocedural guidance of surgical myectomy and alcohol septal ablation.

In recent years, cardiac magnetic resonance imaging (MRI; CMR) has proven to be an increasingly useful modality in the diagnosis and treatment of HCM. Contrast-enhanced CMR allows imaging of presumed myocardial fibrosis. Late gadolinium enhancement (LGE) is commonly seen in HCM; an extensive percentage of left ventricular mass involvement is associated with higher risk of sudden cardiac death. Consequently, an absence of LGE is associated with a lower risk of sudden cardiac death and can often provide reassurance.

Treatment

Asymptomatic Disease

Given that a large subset of HCM patients are symptom free and will achieve normal life expectancy, it is important to educate patients about the disease process, screen family members, and advise them to avoid strenuous activity. Coronary artery disease has an impact on survival, and thus aggressive modification of risk factors contributing to atherosclerosis (diabetes, hyperlipidemia, and obesity) is recommended. Low-intensity aerobic exercise is reasonable to allow the patient to maintain fitness. Adequate hydration and avoidance of situations leading to vasodilation are encouraged to minimize exacerbation of an existing LVOT obstruction.

Septal reduction therapy is not indicated in a symptom-free patient with any degree of obstruction.

Symptomatic Disease

Pharmacologic Management

β-Blockade is the mainstay of treatment owing to negative inotropic and negative chronotropic effect. Verapamil (Calan)[1] or diltiazem (Cardizem)[1] are reasonable alternatives to β-blockade. Disopyramide (Norpace)[1] may be added if symptomatic despite these medications (Table 1). An important role in management is to discontinue medications that promote outflow tract obstruction via vasodilatory effects such as dihydropyridine calcium channel blocking agents, angiotensin converting enzyme inhibitors, and angiotensin receptor blockers. Low-dose diuretics may provide symptomatic relief; however, high-dose diuretics should be avoided. Digitalis is potentially harmful in patients without atrial fibrillation. Phenylephrine (Neo-Synephrine)[1] is useful when treating acute hypotension in these patients.

For the treatment of atrial fibrillation in HCM, it is recommended to keep a low threshold for initiating prophylactic anticoagulation with a direct-acting oral anticoagulant or vitamin K antagonist caused by a higher risk of thromboembolic stroke.

Invasive Therapies

The major septal reduction therapies are surgical myectomy and alcohol ablation. These should be performed by experienced operators at comprehensive centers in patients with refractory symptoms.

Surgical septal myectomy is considered the most appropriate therapy for eligible patients unresponsive to optimal medical therapy. The most common procedure is a Morrow procedure in which a rectangular trough is created in the basal septum below the aortic valve, which abolishes or reduces the LVOT gradient. Eligible patients include those with severe dyspnea, chest pain, or exertional syncope despite maximal medical therapy. Hemodynamic considerations that determine eligibility consist of an LVOT gradient of at least 50 mm Hg associated with septal hypertrophy and mitral valve systolic anterior motion. Studies have shown that surgical myectomy can reverse heart failure symptoms owing to the fact it permanently removes LVOT obstruction and can reduce mitral regurgitation.

Alcohol septal ablation can benefit adult patients with HCM and LVOT obstruction. This percutaneous procedure involves injection of ethanol into a major septal perforator coronary artery, with the intent of inducing infarction of the basal septal wall near the anterior leaflet contact point. The effectiveness of alcohol septal ablation is not clear in patients with more than 30 mm of septal hypertrophy, and it should not be performed in patients with disease (coronary artery disease, mitral valve repair) that would need surgical correction regardless. Other downsides of septal ablation include an increased risk of complete heart block requiring pacemaker implantation and an undefined risk of arrhythmogenicity owing to scar tissue.

[1] Not FDA approved for this indication.

TABLE 1	Pharmacologic Management of Patients With Obstructive HCM		
		INITIAL DOSE	TITRATE TO MAX DOSE
Symptoms Attributable to LV Outflow Tract Obstruction			
Non-Vasodilating Beta Blockers	Metoprolol	50 mg/day	400 mg/day
	Atenolol	25 mg/day	100 mg/day
	Propranolol	60 mg/day	240 mg/day
Beta Blocker Ineffective or Not Tolerated			
Nondihydropyridine Calcium Channel Blockers	Verapamil	120 mg/day	480 mg/day
	Diltiazem	120 mg/day	360 mg/day
Severe Symptoms Despite Beta Blocker or Nondihydropyridine CCB			
	Disopyramide	200 mg BID	300 mg BID

Role of Implantable Devices

Determining which patients with HCM should receive an implantable cardiac defibrillator (ICD) is challenging given the unpredictability of the disease. ICDs are the only treatment to have proven to decrease mortality given their ability to reliably abort life-threating arrhythmias. All patients with HCM need comprehensive sudden cardiac death risk stratification, with strong consideration for ICD implantation in those with personal history of ventricular fibrillation, sustained ventricular tachycardia, family history of sudden cardiac death, unexplained syncope, abnormal exercise blood pressure response, LGE >15% of LV mass, massive left ventricular hypertrophy (LVH) (>30 mm), or documented nonsustained ventricular tachycardia on Holter monitor. Device-related complications and issues such as inappropriate shocks and multiple generator changes for patients receiving a device at a young age must also be weighed when considering implantation of ICD. Risk scores can be helpful in the processes of shared decision making.

Participation in Sports

HCM has been reported as one of the most common causes of sudden death among competitive athletes; however, SCD is overall a rare event in young people. In the United States, there have been cardiovascular screening initiatives, including history and physical in addition to 12 lead electrocardiograms (ECGs), with limited success. The American College of Cardiology and American Heart Association do not currently recommend a national mandatory cardiovascular screening program.

It is reasonable for most HCM patients to engage in low-intensity competitive sports (golf, bowling) and recreational sporting activities. Participation in competitive sports is a modifiable risk factor, and it is recommended that HCM patients avoid participation in intense competitive sports regardless of age, sex, LVOT obstruction, prior septal reduction, or ICD. In addition, ICD placement should not be implanted for the sole purpose of participating in competitive athletics. For most HCM patients, mild-moderate intensity

Figure 1 A, Gross anatomy section of heart demonstrating septal hypertrophy and LVOT obstruction. B, Microscopic section demonstrating myocyte hypertrophy and disarray.

Figure 2 Cardiac MRI demonstrating septal hypertrophy (A,B) and late gadolinium enhancement (C).

recreational exercise is beneficial for cardiovascular fitness and overall health.

Monitoring

The unpredictability of HCM disease makes regular surveillance a necessity. Patient age has been seen as a predictor of HCM-related events, with sudden death events more common in young patients. With a family history of sudden cardiac death, periodic screening by transthoracic echocardiography (every 12–18 months) is recommended in children by the age of 12 (or younger if the child has signs of early puberty) or if there are plans for intense sports competition. Repeat transthoracic echocardiography is recommended for any change in clinical status or new cardiovascular event. As recognition of the genetic basis of this disease has improved over time, genetic screening and counseling of all first-degree family members of patients with HCM are now recommended.

Future Research

The perception of HCM has evolved from a rare and deadly condition to a more common and treatable disease. Effective use of ICDs for primary prevention and advances in surgical treatment of obstruction now allow most HCM patients to achieve normal life expectancy. Although significant progress has been made in elucidating the etiology and pathophysiology of HCM,

there is much room for advancement. In addition, the relationship between genetics and environmental influences, as well as the management of family members of genotype positive–phenotype negative patients, is still unclear. Although rapid genetic testing to identify those at risk has become more widespread, further understanding of pathogenic mutations is required. Furthermore, advancement in technology will hopefully lead to therapies that can specifically target these pathways.

References

Cannan CR, Reeder GS, Bailey KR: Natural history of hypertrophic cardiomyopathy. A population based study, 1976 through 1990, *Circulation* 92:2488–2495, 1995.

Elliott PM, Anastasakis A, Borger MA: ESC Guidelines on diagnosis and management of hypertrophic cardiomyopathy, *Eur Heart J* 35:2733–2799, 2014.

Gersh BJ, Maron BJ, Bonow RO: 2011 ACCF/AHA guideline for the diagnosis and treatment of hypertrophic cardiomyopathy, *Circulation* 124:e783–e831, 2011.

Marian AJ: Recent advances in genetics and treatment of hypertrophic cardiomyopathy, *Future Cardiol* 1:341–353, 2005.

Marian AJ: Genetic determinants of cardiac hypertrophy, *Curr Opin Cardiol* 23:199–205, 2008.

Maron B, Ommen S, Semsarian C, et al: State of the art review: hypertrophic cardiomyopathy, *JACC* 64(1).

Maron BJ: Hypertrophic cardiomyopathy: a systematic review, *J Am Med Assoc* 287:1308–1320, 2002.

Robinson AK: Imaging in hypertrophic cardiomyopathy, *JACC* 24, 2018.

Ommen S, Mital S, et al: 2020 AHA/ACC guideline for the diagnosis and treatment of patients with hypertrophic cardiomyopathy, *JACC* 76(25).

INFECTIVE ENDOCARDITIS

Samuel Mathis, MD; and Oyetokunbo Ibidapo-Obe, MD

CURRENT DIAGNOSIS

- Infective endocarditis (IE) should be a diagnostic consideration in patients with fever and heart murmur.
- Healthcare related infections account for 25% to 30% of newly diagnosed cases.
- Positive blood cultures are present in approximately 90% of cases. Multiple sets should be obtained prior to initiating antibiotic therapy to improve diagnostic yield.
- Transesophageal echocardiography has the highest sensitivity and specificity in native heart evaluations while alternative imaging techniques can be used in patients with implanted heart valves.
- Complications of disease include heart failure, valvular incompetence, and structural defects such as abscess, perforation, and fistulas.

CURRENT THERAPY

- Empiric therapy for *Staphylococcus aureus* should be initiated after blood cultures have been drawn and before the results are available.
- Antibiotic choice is complex and dependent on culture results and sensitivities of organisms identified.
- Best practices propose a multidisciplinary approach to care for patients with IE and should include specialties such as cardiology, infectious disease/microbiology, and cardiothoracic surgery in cases of complicated IE or if prosthetic valves or a cardiac device is present.
- Neurology or neurosurgery consults should be accessible as up to 30% of patients will experience symptomatic neurologic events during their disease.
- Increasing numbers of patients with IE will require surgical intervention due to complications from disease such as heart failure, embolism, intracardiac abscess, or failure to control infection.
- Outpatient parenteral antibiotic therapy can be considered in a subset of patients based on their culture results and with close follow-up.

Definition

Infective endocarditis (IE) is a microbial infection of the valves or endocardium of the heart.

Epidemiology and Risk Factors

IE remains a rare disease in Western countries with incidence varying by geographic location, predisposing risk factors, and preexisting conditions.

IE has an annual incidence of 3 to 10/100,000 of the North American population with a mortality of about 30% at 30 days and 40% at 1 year.

Over the years, the epidemiology of IE has shifted with a steady increase in healthcare-associated IE accounting for about 25% to 30% of newly reported cases.

Risk factors include advancing age, prosthetic heart valves, congenital heart disease, intracardiac devices, intravenous/parenteral drug use, indwelling venous access lines, diabetes mellitus, or immunosuppression to name a few.

Developing worlds have rheumatic heart disease as a leading risk factor for IE.

Infection with *Staphylococcus aureus* is presently the most prevalent cause of IE accounting for ~26% and overtaking the Strep group, next is *Streptococcus viridans* group at ~19%, other Streptococci at 17.5% and Enterococci at 10.55. The above listed bacteria jointly account for 80% to 90% of all cases of endocarditis.

Pathophysiology

IE occurs as a result of endothelial damage, which invariably exposes the basement membrane on the valve causing a structural abnormality that allows bacteria present in the bloodstream to colonize the initially sterile vegetation (nonbacterial thrombotic endocarditis).

Bacterial involvement and growth enlarge the vegetation, impede blood flow, and cause inflammation with multiple systemic symptoms/signs.

Progressive valve dysfunction can quickly lead to heart failure, and bacterial colonization of the vegetation causes septic emboli into the bloodstream, causing sepsis, and can lead to a metastatic septic site outside of initial vegetation area on the valve.

Prevention

The mainstay of prevention of IE is antimicrobial therapy prior to procedures, which may cause IE. This has been and remains a topic of debate and varies by geographic location worldwide.

The efficacy of antimicrobial therapy as a prophylaxis depends greatly on multiple factors, which include patient's medical conditions in terms of being high risk for IE, the procedure being done, the probability of sending bacteria into the bloodstream as a result of the said procedure, and the evidence backing antibiotic prophylaxis in the patient scenario.

The guidelines have remained dynamic based on review of published literature, most of which seems to favor less use of antibiotics and better patient selection for prophylaxis if needed. See current guidelines in Box 1.

Clinical Manifestations and Diagnosis

The diagnosis of IE is based on findings of bacteremia from an organism associated with IE along with evidence of endocardial involvement. This allows for highly variable presentations of disease. Due to this variability, it is important to perform a detailed history and physical examination to help lead to the diagnosis. Blood cultures should be obtained as discussed below prior to initiating antibacterial therapy to ensure appropriate management of the causative organism. This is especially important in the setting of predisposing conditions or risk factors for IE, including recent invasive procedures, history of structural heart disease, or injection drug use. Because of the insidious nature of the disease process, many patients will present with symptoms within 2 weeks of the inciting event or infection.

The most common presentation includes fever in up to 90% of patients, though it may not be present in immunocompromised patients or those who have received previous antibiotic therapy. This can be seen in postoperative patients after valve replacement or intracardiac devices. Night sweats, fatigue, weight loss, and appetite changes are other nonspecific signs that can indicate an infection and will be present in up to half of patients with IE.

A new or changing regurgitant murmur will also be present on physical examination along with evidence of endocardial involvement. The presentation of such involvement can range from tachycardia and hypotension to embolization of the vegetations causing embolic symptoms. Approximately 25% of patients with IE will present with evidence of embolization. If left untreated, symptoms of heart failure, valvular dysfunction, and destruction of cardiac structures can occur. Other physical exam findings of IE include petechia, splinter hemorrhages, Janeway lesions, Osler nodes, and Roth spots. As these findings can occur in other conditions and have low incidence in proven cases of IE, their diagnostic use is limited.

BOX 1 — Antibiotic Regimens for High-Risk Patients and Dental Procedures[1] (Taken 30–60 Minutes Prior to Procedure)

Oral: Amoxicillin 2 g (child 50 mg/kg) PO 30–60 minutes before procedure

Penicillin Allergy: Cephalexin 2 g (child 50 mg/kg) PO 30–60 minutes before procedure or clindamycin 600 mg (child 20 mg/kg)

or azithromycin or clarithromycin 500 mg (child 15 mg/kg)

Unable to tolerate oral: Ampicillin 2 g IM/IV (child 50 mg/kg)

Unable to tolerate oral and PCN allergy: Cefazolin or ceftriaxone 1 g IM/IV (child 50 mg/kg) or clindamycin 600 mg IM/IV (child 20 mg/kg)

Patients that would benefit from antibiotics due to high risk:
- Acquired valvular heart disease with stenosis or regurgitation
- Valve replacement
- Structural congenital heart disease
- Previous endocarditis
- Hypertrophic cardiomyopathy
  Dental procedures to consider antibiotic prophylaxis:
- Manipulation of the gingival or periapical region of the teeth
- Perforation of oral mucosa
- Extractions

All these regimens are not approved by the FDA for this indication.

Adapted from Bonow RO, Carabello BA, Kanu C, et al: ACC/AHA 2006 guidelines for the management of patients with valvular heart disease: A report of the American College of Cardiology/American Heart Association Task Force on Practice Guidelines (writing committee to revise the 1998 Guidelines for the Management of Patients with Valvular Heart Disease): Developed in collaboration with the Society of Cardiovascular Anesthesiologists: Endorsed by the Society for Cardiovascular Angiography and Interventions and the Society of Thoracic Surgeons. *Circulation* 114(5):e84–e231, 2006.

Differential Diagnosis

There are several conditions that can mimic the symptoms of IE. Consideration of systemic lupus erythematosus, acute rheumatic fever, atrial myxoma, vasculitis, and renal cell carcinoma should be on the differential. Care must be taken to not confuse the complications of IE as the causative etiology for hospitalization. One study found that up to 50% of patients with IE were initially diagnosed with complications of their disease (pneumonia, CNS infection, septic arthritis, heart failure, stroke) before correctly identifying the causative agent. Misdiagnosis was found to significantly increase the risk of comorbidity and in hospital mortality in these patients.

Laboratory Evaluation and Blood Cultures

Blood cultures are one of the major diagnostic criteria used to diagnose IE. They are of utmost importance due to their use in the treatment of IE by identifying the microorganisms involved as well as their antibiotic sensitivities. The continuous bacteremia present in IE means that fever need not be present before ordering blood cultures. In up to 90% of cases, the etiologic agent is identified in the first two blood cultures. It is recommended that three sets of blood cultures be obtained at least 1 hour apart from separate venipunctures for the most sensitive findings (98% of cases successfully identified). Each vial should have at least 10 mL of blood to increase the chances of obtaining an appropriate amount. Alternatively, two sets of three bottles each (two aerobic, one anaerobic—six bottles total) can be drawn if timing of antibiotic therapy is a concern. Unfortunately, the most common cause of negative culture IE is due to prior administration of antibiotic therapy. This results in prolonged, broad coverage antibiotic therapy and increased uncertainty of the diagnosis.

Other lab findings that may be present in IE but are not specific for the disease include a normocytic, normochromic anemia, thrombocytopenia, leukocytosis, and elevations in erythrocyte sedimentation rate (ERS), C-reactive protein, and procalcitonin.

Imaging

Cardiac imaging should be considered if there is a strong clinical suspicion of IE. The inclusion of cardiac imaging of IE has increased the sensitivity of diagnosis (see modified Duke Criteria [Box 2]). Transthoracic echocardiogram (TTE) should be performed if there is clinical suspicion for IE. The echocardiogram should be specifically looking for any oscillating intracardiac mass on the valve or supporting structure which would indicate vegetations. It can also be used to detect abscesses, dehiscence of prostatic valve, or newly identified valvular regurgitations. The sensitivity of detecting vegetations on native valves is approximately 70% with TTE. This is

BOX 2 — Modified Duke Criteria for Infective Endocarditis

Definite Infective Endocarditis:
- Two major

or
- One major and three minor

or
- Five minor

Possible Infective Endocarditis:
- One major and one minor

or
- Three minor

Major Criteria

Positive blood cultures:
- Typical microorganisms consistent with IE from two separate blood culture: viridans group streptococci, *Streptococcus bovis* group, HACED group, *Staphylococcus aureus*; community acquired enterocci with abscess of primary focus

or
- Microorganisms consistent with IE from persistently positive blood cultures: at least two positive blood cultures drawn more than 12 hours apart; all of three or a majority of positive blood cultures in more than four drawn; or single positive blood culture for *Coxiella burnetii* or phage IgG antibody titer >1:800

Evidence of endocardial involvement:
- Echocardiogram positive for IE showing vegetation, abscess, psuedoaneurysm, intracardiac fistula, valvular perforation or aneurysm, new partial dehiscence of prosthetic valve
- Abnormal activity around site of a prosthetic valve detected by PET/CT assuming >3 months after surgery or radiolabeled leukocyte-SPECT/CT
- Definite paravalvular lesions by cardiac CT

Minor Criteria
- Predisposition: predisposing heart condition or injection drug use
- Fever, temperature >38°C
- Vascular phenomena (including those detected by imaging alone): arterial emboli, septic pulmonary infarcts, myotic aneurysm, intracranial hemorrhage, conjunctival hemorrhage, and Janeway lesions
- Immunologic phenomena: glomerulonephritis, Osler's nodes, Roth's spots, and rheumatoid factor
- Microbiological evidence: positive blood cultures not meeting major criteria above or serologic evidence of infection with organism consistent with IE

CT, Computed tomography; *HACEK*, *Haemophilus* spp, *Aggregatibacter* spp, *Cardiobacterium hominis*, *Eikenella* corrodens, *Kingella* spp; *IE*, infective endocarditis; *IgG*, immunoglobulin G; *PET*, positron emission tomography; *SPECT*, single-photon emission computed tomography.

increased to a sensitivity and specificity around 90% if transesophageal echocardiogram (TEE) is used instead. Due to this increased sensitivity, TEE should be used in high-risk patients with a negative TTE. Transesophageal echocardiogram should also be considered in patients with prosthetic valves, those with *S. aureus* bacteremia, and when IE-related complications have occurred such as heart block, cardiac abscess, embolism, or new/worsening murmurs.

Due to the increased number of patients with prosthetic valves or intracardiac devices, TTE and TEE may prove to be unhelpful due to the artifact from these devices. In these cases, additional imaging with F-labeled fluoro-2-deoxyglucose positron emission tomography/computed tomography (F-FDG-PET/CT) or single-proton emission computed tomography-CT (SPECT-CT) should be considered to assess for inflammation around the prosthetic or intracardiac device. These studies have been found to have a sensitivity of 93% in cases of prosthetic valve endocarditis. They have significantly lower sensitivity in cases of native heart disease (22% sensitivity). Thoracic CT scans have significant value in determining presence of perivalvular abscesses, aneurysms, or pseudoaneurysms.

Cerebral magnetic resonance imaging (MRI) should be considered in patients with evidence of embolic neurologic complications as most of these lesions are ischemic in origin.

Treatment
Treatment should be multidisciplinary and involve cardiology, cardiac surgeon, infectious disease, or microbiology. This approach improves outcomes by optimizing appropriate antibiotic regiments and assessments for surgical interventions. Initiating appropriate antibiotic therapy can improve in-hospital survival by 70% to 80%. Recommended antibiotic regimens against common organisms causing IE are listed in Table 1. These should be adjusted based on the organism and susceptibilities.

TABLE 1	Antimicrobial Regimens Against Typical Infective Endocarditis Organisms			
ORGANISM	**SUSCEPTIBILITY**	**REGIMENT**	**DOSAGE**	**DURATION (WEEK)**
Native Valve				
Streptococcus viridans, Streptococcus bovis	Penicillin	Penicillin G	12–18 MU IV per 24 h continuously or in four to six equally divided doses	4
		or ceftriaxone[1]	2 g IV or IM per 24 h	4
		or vancomycin	30 mg/kg IV per 24 h in two divided doses. Max: 2 g/24 h	4
	Penicillin-relative resistance	Penicillin G	24 MU IV per 24 h continuously or in four to six equally divided doses	4
		or ceftriaxone[1]	2 g IV/IM per 24 h 4	4
		plus gentamicin[1]	3 mg/kg IV/IM per 24 h in one dose	2
		or vancomycin	30 mg/kg IV per 24 h in two divided doses (limit 2 g/24 h)	4
Enterococcus spp	Penicillin	Ampicillin	12 g IV per 24 h in six divided doses	4–6
		or penicillin G[1]	18–30 MU IV per 24 h continuously or in six equally divided doses	4–6
		Plus	gentamicin 3 mg/kg IV or IM per 24 h in three divided doses	2
		or ampicillin	12 g IV per 24 h in six divided doses	6
		plus ceftriaxone[1]	2 g IV every 12 h	6
	Penicillin Resistant	Vancomycin	30 mg/kg IV per 24 h in two divided doses (limit 2 g/24 h)	
Staphylococcus spp	Oxacillin	Nafcillin[1] or oxacillin[1]	12 g IV per 24 h in four to six divided doses	6
		or cefazolin	100 mg/kg IV/IM per 24 h in three equally divided doses	6
			6 g IV per 24 h in three divided doses	6
	Oxacillin resistant	Vancomycin plus gentamicin	30 mg/kg IV per 24 h in two divided doses (goal: 1 h peak concentration 30–45 µg/mL and trough 10–15 µg/mL)	6
Prosthetic Valve				
Staphylococcus spp.	Oxacillin-susceptible	Nafcillin[1] or oxacillin[1]	12 g IV per 24 h in four to six divided doses	6
		plus gentamicin	3 mg/kg IV or IM per 24 h in three divided doses	2
		plus rifampin[1]	900 mg IV or PO per 24 h in three divided doses	6
	Oxacillin-resistant	Vancomycin	30 mg/kg IV per 24 h in two divided doses. Goal: 1 h peak concentration 30–45 µg/mL and trough 10–15 µg/mL	6
		plus gentamicin	3 mg/kg IV or IM per 24 h in three divided doses	2
		plus rifampin[1]	900 mg IV or PO per 24 h in three divided doses	6

[1]Not FDA approved for this indication.
Adapted from Bonow RO, Carabello BA, Kanu C, et al: ACC/AHA 2006 guidelines for the management of patients with valvular heart disease: A report of the American College of Cardiology/American Heart Association Task Force on Practice Guidelines (writing committee to revise the 1998 Guidelines for the Management of Patients with Valvular Heart Disease): Developed in collaboration with the Society of Cardiovascular Anesthesiologists: Endorsed by the Society for Cardiovascular Angiography and Interventions and the Society of Thoracic Surgeons. *Circulation* 114(5):e84–e231, 2006.

Patient with IE will require a prolonged duration of intravenous (IV) antibiotic treatment for up to 6 weeks. This is in order to ensure that all bacteria located in the vegetations are completely eradicated. Blood cultures should be repeated every 24 to 48 hours until resolution of bacteremia is confirmed. If surgery is required, a 4- to 6-week course of antibiotics is still recommended to reduce recurrence of IE.

In addition to IV antibiotic therapy, many patients will also be placed on parenteral therapies. In certain cases, patients may be eligible for transition to oral antibiotic to complete the duration of therapy. The criteria for step down therapy are patients who have no indication for surgery, have completed an initial course of IV antibiotics with no bacteremia, have no concerns for absorption of oral therapy in the gastrointestinal tract, have no psychological or socioeconomic concerns that would cause IV therapy to be preferred for adherence, and the organism is susceptible to the prescribed oral regiment. Oral therapy is preferred over IV due to the decreased potential for harm.

Due to increasing microorganism resistance, parenteral therapy typically consists of a beta-lactam and aminoglycoside. They should be taken close together to increase the bactericidal effect. Care should be maintained with close observation of renal function.

Complications and Surgical Indications
Infective endocarditis carries a high in-hospital mortality of up to 30% due to the development of potential complications either prior or during effective treatment. Heart failure or pulmonary edema is common, occurring in up to half of patients with IE, and is the most common indication for urgent surgery. Destruction of the valvular tissues creates significant regurgitation leading to volume overload. Conversely, severe vegetations can cause significant stenosis and lead to the same outcome. In rare cases, this can lead to cardiogenic shock, which is an immediate indication for surgery (within 24 hours). For those with symptoms of heart failure and worsening hemodynamic response, surgery should be considered within 7 days of identification. Patients with heart failure will typically require surgical intervention as medical therapy alone is insufficient at repairing the damage caused by the infection. It is important to note here that valvular or other surgical interventions for IE may be performed in the acute or active phase of infection as delay can significantly increase the mortality.

Other complications include failure to quickly eradicate infection. This can be due to inability or delays in identifying the causative organism or for severe infections. Severe localized infections can cause paravalvular or aortic root abscesses. These abscess formations usually complicate 30% to 40% of IE cases due to their contiguous spread along the tissue planes. Other risk factors for abscess formation include prosthetic valves or difficult-to-treat organisms such as fungi or multidrug-resistant organisms. For this reason, all IE cases associated with prosthetic valves should have surgical consideration. These cases are typically identified by persistently positive blood cultures despite appropriate antibiotic regiments. Abscesses are identified via TEE or the aforementioned imaging studies in patients with prosthetic valves. Due to the abscess formation and deep infection, surgical debridement or valve replacement is almost always required. Surgical evaluation and debridement is the gold standard of abscess identification.

The third major complication of IE relates to septic emboli from valvular vegetations. While one-third of patients with IE will have signs and symptoms of embolization, another one-third can be found to have silent emboli. Neurologic embolization is the most frequent site (40%), followed by lungs (20%), spleen (20%), peripheral arteries (~15%), and kidneys (10%). Embolization most often occurs prior to the initiation of antibiotic therapy and the risk of embolization is reduced by approximately 65% after 2 weeks of antibiotic therapy. Risk factors include vegetations greater than 10 mm in size and infections associated

with *S. aureus* and *Streptococcus bovis*. These embolic events can further complicate treatment by causing metastatic infection sites. Embolic events are an independent risk factor for in-hospital death in IE and as such require surgical evaluation if the vegetations meet certain criteria. Surgery is indicated in valvular vegetations greater than 10 mm with embolic event while on antibiotics, in vegetations greater than 30 mm, and in those with vegetations greater than 10 mm with severe valvular (native and prosthetic) disease who are low operative risk.

Conclusion
Infective endocarditis continues to maintain a relatively high mortality rate even with the advances in both surgical and antibiotic treatment. Prompt diagnosis and targeted antimicrobial therapy are vital to improving outcomes in patients with IE. Surgical evaluation and treatment should be considered relatively early in the disease course. Even with high rates of surgical intervention, in-hospital mortality continues to remain between 15% and 20% in native valves and up to 25% in prosthetic valves. Complications associated with disease progression (heart failure, uncontrolled infections, embolic events) also increase the mortality risk. Therefore a multidisciplinary team should be involved in patients identified with IE to provide best possible outcomes. Additionally, close follow-up after hospitalization should be conducted as up to 30% of patients with IE may require surgery in the first 12 months after diagnosis.

References
Baddour LM, Wilson WR, Bayer AS, et al: On behalf of the American Heart Association Committee on rheumatic fever, endocarditis, and kawasaki disease of the council on cardiovascular disease in the young, council on clinical cardiology, council on cardiovascular surgery and anesthesia, and stroke council. Infective endocarditis in adults: diagnosis, antimicrobial therapy, and management of complications: a scientific statement for healthcare professionals from the American Heart Association, *Circulation* 132:1435–1486, 2015.

Cahill TJ, et al: Challenges in infective endocarditis, *J Am Coll Cardiol* 69(3):325–344, 2017.

Cahill TJ, Harrison JL, Jewell P, et al: Antibiotic prophylaxis for infective endocarditis: a systematic review and meta-analysis, *Heart* 103:937–944, 2017.

Chu VH, Cabell CH, Benjamin Jr DK, et al: Early predictors of in-hospital death in infective endocarditis, *Circulation* 109(14):1745–1749, 2004.

Fowler Jr VG, Miro JM, Hoen B, et al: Staphylococcus aureus endocarditis: a consequence of medical progress, *J Am Med Assoc* 293(24):3012–3021, 2005.

Gaca JG, Sheng S, Daneshmand MA, et al: Outcomes for endocarditis surgery in North America: a simplified risk scoring system, *J Thorac Cardiovasc Surg* 141:98–106, 2011.

Habib G, Lancellotti P, Antunes MJ, et al: 2015 ESC guidelines for the management of infective endocarditis: the Task Force for the Management of Infective Endocarditis of the European Society of Cardiology (ESC). Endorsed by: European Association for Cardio-Thoracic Surgery (EACTS), the European Association of Nuclear Medicine (EANM), *Eur Heart J* 36(44):3075–3128, 2015.

Kang DH, Kim YJ, Kim SH, et al: Early surgery versus conventional treatment for infective endocarditis, *N Engl J Med* 366:2466–2473, 2012.

Kiefer T, Park L, Tribouilloy C, et al: Association between valvular surgery and mortality among patients with infective endocarditis complicated by heart failure, *J Am Med Assoc* 306:2239–2247, 2011.

Li JS, Sexton DJ, Nettles R, et al: Proposed modifications to the Duke criteria for the diagnosis of infective endocarditis, *Clin Infect Dis* 30(4):633–638, 2000.

Liesman RM, Pritt BS, Maleszewski JJ, Patel R: Laboratory diagnosis of infective endocarditis, *J Clin Microbiol* 55:2599–2608, 2017.

Naderi HR, Sheybani F, Erfani SS: Errors in diagnosis of infective endocarditis, *Epidemiol Infect* 146:394–400, 2018.

Nishimura RA, Otto CM, Bonow RO, et al: 2014 AHA/ ACC guideline for the management of patients with valvular heart disease: a report of the American College of Cardiology/American Heart Association Task Force on Practice Guidelines, *J Am Coll Cardiol* 63:e57–e185, 2014.

Rajani R, Klein JL: Infective endocarditis: a contemporary update, *Clin Med (Lond)* 20(1):31–35, 2020.

Spellberg B, et al: Evaluation of a paradigm shift from intravenous antibiotics to oral step-down therapy for the treatment of infective endocarditis: a narrative review, *JAMA Intern Med*, 2020.

Task Force on the Prevention: Diagnosis, and Treatment of Infective Endocarditis of the European Society of Cardiology; European Society of Clinical Microbiology and Infectious Diseases; International Society of Chemotherapy for Infection and Cancer; ESC Committee for Practice Guidelines: Guidelines on the prevention, diagnosis, and treatment of infective endocarditis (new version 2009): the Task Force on the prevention, diagnosis, and treatment of infective endocarditis of the European Society of Cardiology (ESC), *Eur Heart J* 30(19):2369–2413, 2009.

Thornhill MH, Dayer M, Lockhart PB, Prendergast B: Antibiotic prophylaxis of infective endocarditis, *Curr Infect Dis Rep* 19(2):9, 2017.

MITRAL VALVE PROLAPSE

Method of
Kurt M. Jacobson, MD; Peter S. Rahko, MD; and Shenil Shah, MD

CURRENT DIAGNOSIS

- A midsystolic click with or without a middle- to late-peaking crescendo systolic murmur is the classic auscultatory finding of mitral valve prolapse (MVP).
- Key examination maneuvers can help differentiate MVP from other valvular heart diseases.
- Diagnostic echocardiographic findings of MVP are systolic billowing of the mitral valve leaflets 2 mm above the annulus into the left atrium.
- The presence of significant myxomatous thickening of the valve leaflets (>5 mm) is significant for prognosis.

CURRENT THERAPY

- Patients with physical findings of mitral valve prolapse (MVP) should have an echocardiogram to confirm the diagnosis, determine the severity of prolapse, determine the amount of myxomatous thickening, document the severity (if present) of mitral regurgitation, and determine left ventricular size and function.
- Uncomplicated MVP without significant mitral regurgitation can be evaluated clinically every 3 to 5 years.
- Complicated MVP (associated with significant mitral regurgitation, left ventricular structural changes, pulmonary hypertension, atrial fibrillation, or stroke) should be observed closely with serial clinical evaluation and echocardiography.
- Surgery may be required for complicated MVP associated with severe mitral regurgitation. Repair rather than replacement is the procedure of choice and should be performed at surgical centers experienced with mitral valve repair.
- Recommendations for surgery are the same for MVP as for other forms of chronic severe mitral regurgitation.
- Percutaneous intervention with the MitraClip (Abbott Vascular) is an option in symptomatic patients with moderate to severe or severe mitral regurgitation, prohibitive surgical risk, and acceptable anatomy.

Mitral valve prolapse (MVP) has been known by many names, including floppy valve syndrome, Barlow's syndrome, click/murmur syndrome, myxomatous mitral valve disease, and billowing mitral cusp syndrome. MVP is a common cardiac valvular abnormality characterized by redundant, floppy mitral valve leaflets; it is often detected initially by characteristic nonejection clicks or a middle- to late-peaking crescendo systolic murmur on physical examination.

Prevalence

MVP is the most common congenital cause of mitral regurgitation (MR) in adults and the most common indication for mitral valve surgery in the United States today. Previously, it was one of the most overdiagnosed conditions within cardiology, with suggested prevalence rates ranging from 5% to 15%. With the use of current diagnostic standards, rates are much lower; the overestimation was a consequence of diverse and nonuniformly accepted two-dimensional echocardiographic diagnostic criteria. Freed and colleagues, using the Framingham study population and applying consistent and more stringent echocardiographic diagnostic criteria, demonstrated a much lower prevalence of MVP (approximately 2.4%). The incidence appeared to be similar among men and women. Gender differences do exist, however. Women tend to have a more benign course, whereas men tend to have more advanced myxomatous disease resulting in a greater chance of more severe MR.

Classification

Primary MVP is characterized by idiopathic myxomatous change of the mitral valve leaflets or the chordal structures or both. Secondary MVP is present when underlying conditions such as Marfan's syndrome, Ehlers-Danlos syndrome, osteogenesis imperfecta, or other collagen vascular disorders are evident. Certain congenital cardiac abnormalities, including Ebstein anomaly, aortic coarctation, hypertrophic cardiomyopathy, and ostium secundum atrial septal defects, are also associated with MVP. Familial variants with an autosomal dominant pattern of inheritance have been identified, and work to identify the genes involved is under way. The reported prevalence of MVP in first-degree relatives is between 30% and 50%.

Pathology

Macroscopic and microscopic changes can involve both the anterior and posterior leaflets as well as the chordal structures of the leaflet apparatus. Macroscopically, the surface area of the leaflet is increased, providing the accentuated, billowing appearance of the valve leaflets. Additional notable changes are thickening of the individual leaflets, increased leaflet length, thinning and stretching of the chordae, and increased circumference of the mitral valve annulus. At the microscopic level (Figure 1), normal mitral valves have three well-defined layers, each containing cells and a characteristic composition and configuration of the extracellular matrix: the fibrosa, composed predominantly of collagen fibers densely packed and arranged parallel to the free edge of the leaflet; the centrally located spongiosa, composed of loosely arranged collagen and proteoglycans; and the atrialis, composed of elastic fibers. In myxomatous mitral valves, the spongiosa layer is expanded by loose, amorphous extracellular matrix that has more proteoglycans but less collagen and more fragmented elastic fibers. What collagen is present appears to be disorganized and fragmented, giving the appearance of a haphazard layering of the spongiosa. It is this thickening that produces the classic macroscopic appearance of the myxomatous valve on two-dimensional echocardiography.

Clinical Presentation

Most patients with MVP are asymptomatic and will remain so, testifying to the often benign nature of this disease. Previously, various nonspecific symptoms, including fatigue, dyspnea, palpitations, postural orthostasis, anxiety, and panic attacks, were described as an MVP syndrome when present in association with the characteristic nonejection systolic click or middle- to late-peaking crescendo systolic murmur. Other symptoms, including chest discomfort, near-syncope, and syncope, have also been described by patients with MVP. However, in a community-based study, the prevalence of various clinical complaints including chest pain, dyspnea, and syncope was no higher in patients with MVP than in those without evidence of MVP, making such findings nonspecific. In a controlled study that compared symptomatic MVP patients with first-degree relatives with and without echocardiographic evidence of MVP, there also was no association of MVP with atypical chest pain, dyspnea, panic attacks, or anxiety. There was, however, a significant association of MVP with physical findings of systolic clicks, systolic murmurs, thoracic bony abnormalities, low body weight, and low blood pressure. Congestive heart failure, atrial fibrillation, stroke or transient ischemic attack, hypertension, diabetes, and hypercholesterolemia

Figure 1 Morphologic features of normal mitral valves *(left)* and valves with myxomatous degeneration *(right)*. Myxomatous valves have an abnormal layered architecture: loose collagen in fibrosa, expanded spongiosa strongly positive for proteoglycans, and disrupted elastin in atrialis *(top)*. Movat pentachrome stain (collagen stains yellow, proteoglycans blue-green, and elastin black). Modified from Rabkin E, Aikawa M, Stone JR, et al: Activated interstitial myofibroblasts express catabolic enzymes and mediate matrix remodeling in myxomatous heart valves. *Circulation* 2001;104:2525.)

Figure 2 Auscultative findings with changes in position in patients with mitral valve prolapse (MVP). *Abbreviations*: C = click of MVP; S_1, mitral valve closure; S_2, aortic valve closure. Modified from Devereux RB, Perloff JK, Reichek N, et al: Mitral valve prolapse. *Circulation* 1976;54[1]:3–14.)

are no more likely in patients with MVP than in those without MVP. However, previous retrospective studies suggested a higher incidence of cerebral embolic events, infectious endocarditis, severe MR, and need for mitral valve replacement in patients with classic (complicated) versus nonclassic MVP. Symptoms of poor cardiac reserve, such as reduced exercise tolerance, dyspnea on exertion, and fatigue, may reflect the presence of significant MR and warrant clinical concern.

Diagnosis

Symptoms are not predictive of the presence or absence of MVP. Certain physical and auscultatory characteristics on examination do support the diagnosis of MVP. Patients with MVP more often have a lower body mass index, have a lower waist-to-hip ratio, and are taller. Findings of scoliosis, pectus excavatum, and hyperextensibility are also prevalent among patients with MVP. The classic auscultatory findings include a midsystolic click and a middle- to late-peaking crescendo systolic murmur heard best at the apex. The auscultatory findings are best elicited with the diaphragm of the stethoscope, and they change in relation to the first and second heart sounds (S_1 and S_2) in response to changes in left ventricular (LV) volume. Therefore the patient should be examined in several positions: supine (including lateral decubitus), sitting, standing, and, if possible, squatting. Changes in LV filling and volume affect the degree of prolapse.

The most important and most specific finding on auscultation is the presence of a nonejection midsystolic click or clicks caused by snapping of the valve apparatus as parts of the valve leaflets billow into the atrium during systole. Although these clicks can be heard over the entire precordium, they are best heard at the apex. The click can be misinterpreted as a split S_1, a true S_1 with an S_4, or a true S_1 with an early ejection click from a bicuspid

valve. It can be differentiated from an ejection click heard in bicuspid aortic valves by its timing relative to the beginning of the carotid upstroke. Ejection clicks occur as the aortic valve opens and therefore precede the carotid upstroke, whereas the nonejection clicks of MVP occur afterward. Clicks from atrial septal aneurysms are uncommon but can be difficult to distinguish from those of MVP. Ejection clicks and clicks from atrial septal aneurysms are not altered by changes in loading characteristics, allowing them to be differentiated from clicks of MVP. Often, but not always, a middle- to late-peaking crescendo systolic murmur can be appreciated by itself or after a click. The murmur terminates with closure of the aortic valve (A2). This represents MR, and, in general, the duration of the murmur correlates with the severity of the MR. The earlier in systole the murmur is detected, the more severe the MR. Eventually, with more severe MR, the murmur becomes holosystolic. MVP manifestations on examination vary, and they may not always be reproducible, even in the same patient.

Certain maneuvers can aid in more accurately diagnosing MVP on examination (Figure 2). MVP is very sensitive to LV filling, and subtle changes in auscultatory findings elicited by careful examination maneuvers can be instrumental in separating MVP from other valvular abnormalities. Generally, measures that decrease LV volume or increase contractility produce earlier and more prominent systolic prolapse of the mitral leaflets, causing the systolic click and murmur to move closer to S_1. For example, in the transition from squatting to standing, LV volume is reduced, and the onset of the click and murmur is moved closer to S_1. Conversely, anything that increases LV volume, such as leg-raising, squatting, or slowing the heart rate (increased diastolic filling), delays the onset of the click or murmur and usually diminishes its duration and intensity.

Use of Echocardiography

Two-dimensional echocardiography has proved to be the most accurate noninvasive tool for the diagnosis, assessment, and follow-up of clinically suspected MVP. In fact, physical signs of MVP in an asymptomatic patient are an American College of Cardiology/American Heart Association (ACC/AHA) class I indication for use of echocardiography to make the diagnosis of MVP and assess the severity of MR, leaflet morphology, and ventricular size and function. Once the diagnosis is made, follow-up is determined by the severity of MVP. Routine echocardiographic follow-up of asymptomatic patients with MVP is not recommended unless there are significant findings of MR or LV structural changes. Frequency of follow-up in patients with prolapse and MR is determined by the severity of MR and should be at least annual in patients with severe MR.

Diagnostic criteria for MVP on two-dimensional echocardiography are:

- Billowing of one or both mitral valve leaflets or their prolapse superiorly across the mitral annular plane in the parasternal long-axis view by greater than 2 mm during systole
- The degree of thickening of the leaflets

Combined leaflet prolapse of greater than 2 mm and leaflet thickness greater than 5 mm are supportive of classic MVP, whereas prolapse in the absence of increased thickness is considered nonclassic MVP. In addition to more often being associated with the auscultative findings of the click and murmur, the classic form is more commonly associated with increased risk of endocarditis, stroke, progressive MR, and need for mitral valve repair or replacement.

Because the mitral apparatus is saddle-shaped, certain echocardiographic views are more specific than others for determining leaflet prolapse. Most practitioners agree that the parasternal long-axis and apical two-chamber or apical long-axis views are the most accurate for determining prolapse. A finding of prolapse as determined on other views, particularly the apical four-chamber view, is much less specific and frequently leads to a false-positive diagnosis.

Medical Management

Most patients with MVP remain asymptomatic and require no additional management aside from careful observation over time. It is appropriate to provide reassurance that uncomplicated (non-classic) MVP is a non–life-threatening condition and is unlikely to affect longevity. Periodic clinical evaluation every 3 to 5 years is reasonable. Patients who develop palpitations, lightheadedness, dizziness, or syncope should undergo Holter or event monitoring for detection of arrhythmias. Palpitations are frequently controlled with β-blockers or calcium channel blockers, although the presence of specific arrhythmias may mandate additional therapy. Endocarditis prophylaxis is no longer recommended for patients with MVP unless they have a history of endocarditis or valve replacement. Prophylaxis is recommended for patients who have undergone repair if prosthetic material was used (e.g., in ring repairs). Aspirin or warfarin (Coumadin) therapy may be recommended for certain symptomatic patients with neurologic events who have atrial fibrillation, significant MR, hypertension, or heart failure (Table 1).

Patients with classic (complicated) MVP deserve regular clinical follow-up, particularly if MR is present. These patients are more likely to develop moderate or severe MR over time. Patients with mild to moderate MR and normal LV function should be clinically evaluated at least annually and should undergo echocardiography every second or third year if stable. Patients with severe MR should have an annual echocardiogram and closer clinical follow-up. Those who have severe MR and develop symptoms or impaired LV systolic function require cardiac catheterization and evaluation for mitral valve surgery. Often the valve can be repaired rather than replaced, with a low operative mortality rate and excellent short- and long-term results when performed at experienced centers. Preservation of the native valve allows for lower risks

TABLE 1 ACC/AHA Recommendations for Oral Anticoagulation in Patients With Mitral Valve Prolapse

CLASS	RECOMMENDATION
I	ASA therapy (75–325 mg/d) for cerebral TIAs
	Warfarin (Coumadin) therapy for patients ≥65 years in atrial fibrillation with hypertension, MR, or history of congestive heart failure
	ASA therapy (75–325 mg/d) for patients <65 years in atrial fibrillation with no history of MR, hypertension, or congestive heart failure
	Warfarin therapy after stroke for patients with MR, atrial fibrillation, or left atrial thrombus
IIa	ASA therapy is reasonable in patients after stroke who do not have MR, atrial fibrillation, left atrial thrombus, or echocardiographic evidence of thickening ≥5 mm or redundancy of leaflets
	Warfarin therapy is reasonable after stroke for patients without MR, atrial fibrillation, or left atrial thrombus who have echocardiographic evidence of thickening ≥5 mm or redundancy of leaflets
	Warfarin therapy is reasonable for TIAs that occur despite ASA therapy
	ASA therapy (75–325 mg/d) can be beneficial for patients with a history of stroke who have contraindications to anticoagulants
IIb	ASA therapy (75–325 mg/d) may be considered for patients in sinus rhythm with echocardiographic evidence of complicated MVP

Abbreviations: ACC/AHA = American College of Cardiology/American Heart Association; ASA = aspirin; MR = mitral regurgitation; TIA = transient ischemic attack.
Adapted from Bonow RO, Carabello BA, Chatterjee K, et al: 2008 Focused update incorporated into the ACC/AHA 2006 guidelines for the management of patients with valvular heart disease. *Circulation* 118(15):e523–661, 2008.

of thrombosis and endocarditis than does prosthetic valve replacement.

Surgical Management

MVP is the most common cause of adult MR requiring mitral valve surgery. Symptoms of heart failure, severity of MR, presence or absence of atrial fibrillation, LV systolic function, LV end-diastolic and end-systolic volumes, and pulmonary artery pressure (at rest and with exercise) influence the decision to recommend mitral valve surgery. Indications for surgery in patients with MVP and MR mirror those with other forms of nonischemic severe MR. Patient outcomes after mitral valve repair are typically very good, and the surgical risk is lower than for many other forms of cardiac surgery, including mitral valve replacement.

Based on a Cleveland Clinic review of 1072 patients who underwent primary isolated mitral valve repair for MR due to myxomatous disease, the in-hospital mortality rate was 0.3%. The Mayo Clinic reviewed 1173 patients who underwent mitral valve repair for MVP from 1980 to 1999, observing mortality rates of 0.7%, 11.3%, and 29.4% at 30 days, 5 years, and 10 years, respectively.

Because of the remarkably low mortality rates associated with MVP repair, some experts advocate earlier rather than later repair of MVP in asymptomatic patients with severe MR and no evidence of LV dysfunction, pulmonary hypertension, or atrial fibrillation. AHA/ACC recommendations for surgery in patients with chronic primary mitral valve regurgitation are shown in Table 2.

TABLE 2	ACC/AHA Recommendations for Surgery in Patients With Chronic Primary Mitral Valve Regurgitation

CLASS	RECOMMENDATION
I	Mitral valve (MV) surgery is recommended for symptomatic patients with chronic severe primary MR (stage D) and left ventricular ejection fraction (LVEF) >30%
	MV surgery is recommended for asymptomatic patients with chronic severe primary MR and left ventricular (LV) dysfunction (LVEF 30%-60% and/or left ventricular end-systolic dimension [LVESD] ≥40mm, stage C2)
	MV repair is recommended in preference to mitral valve replacement (MVR) when surgical treatment is indicated for patients with chronic severe primary MR limited to the posterior leaflet
	MV repair is recommended in preference to MVR when surgical treatment is indicated for patients with chronic severe primary MR involving the anterior leaflet or both leaflets when a successful and durable repair can be accomplished
	Concomitant MV repair or replacement is indicated in patients with chronic severe primary MR undergoing cardiac surgery for other indications
IIa	MV repair is reasonable in asymptomatic patients with chronic severe primary MR (stage C1) with preserved LV function (LVEF >60% and LVESD <40mm) in whom the likelihood of a successful and durable repair without residual MR is >95% with an expected mortality rate of <1% when performed at a Heart Valve Center of Excellence
	MV repair is reasonable for asymptomatic patients with chronic severe primary MR (stage C1) and preserved LV function (LVEF >60% and LVESD <40mm) in whom there is a high likelihood of a successful and durable repair with 1) new onset of atrial fibrillation or 2) resting pulmonary hypertension (pulmonary artery systolic arterial pressure >50mm Hg)
	MV repair is reasonable for asymptomatic patients with chronic severe primary MR (stage C1) and preserved LV function (LVEF >60% and LVESD <40mm) with progressive increase in LV size or decrease in ejection fraction on serial imaging studies
	Concomitant MV repair is reasonable in patients with chronic moderate primary MR (stage B) undergoing cardiac surgery for other indications
IIb	MV surgery may be considered in symptomatic patients with chronic severe primary MR and LVEF less than or equal to 30% (stage D)
	MV repair may be considered in patients with rheumatic mitral valve disease when surgical treatment is indicated if a durable and successful repair is likely or if the reliability of long-term anticoagulation management is questionable
	Transcatheter MV repair may be considered for severely symptomatic patients (New York Heart Association class III/IV) with chronic severe primary MR (stage D) who have a reasonable life expectancy but a prohibitive surgical risk because of severe comorbidities and remain symptomatic despite optimal goal directed medical therapy for heart failure
III Harm	MVR should not be performed for treatment of isolated severe primary MR limited to less than one half of the posterior leaflet unless MV repair has been attempted and was unsuccessful

Adapted from 2017 AHA/ACC focused update of the 2014 ACC/AHA guidelines for the management of patients with valvular heart disease. *Circulation* 135(25); e1159–e1195, 2017.

Percutaneous Management

In 2013 the FDA approved the MitraClip (Abbott Vascular) for patients with symptomatic degenerative MR who are deemed high risk for mitral valve surgery. The MitraClip technology is based on the Alfieri edge-to-edge repair in which the middle segments of the anterior and posterior leaflet are sutured together to create a double-orifice. It is approved for use in patients with New York Heart Association Class III or IV heart failure despite medical therapy, chronic moderate to severe or severe primary MR, favorable anatomy typically involving the middle segments of the anterior and posterior leaflets, reasonable life expectancy, and prohibitive surgical risk. This approval is based on the results of the Endovascular Valve Edge-to-Edge Repair Study (EVEREST II), which randomized 279 patients to either percutaneous repair or conventional surgery for repair or replacement of the mitral valve with a primary endpoint of freedom from death, from surgery for mitral valve dysfunction, and from grade 3+ or 4+ MR at 12 months. The rates of the combined primary endpoints were 55% in the percutaneous group and 73% in the surgery group (p=0.007). Rates of death (6% and 6%, respectively) and 3+ or 4+ MR (21% and 20%, respectively) were similar in each group. Major adverse events occurred in 15% of patients in the percutaneous repair group versus 48% in the surgery group at 30 days (p<0.001). Although the MitraClip was less effective at reducing MR, it was approved on the bases of its superior safety and similar clinical outcomes.

References

2008 Focused update incorporated into the ACC/AHA 2006 guidelines for the management of patients with valvular heart disease: a report of the American College of Cardiology/American Heart Association Task Force on Practice Guidelines (Writing Committee to Revise the 1998 Guidelines for the Management of Patients With Valvular Heart Disease): endorsed by the Society of Cardiovascular Anesthesiologists, Society for Cardiovascular Angiography and Interventions, and Society of Thoracic Surgeons, *Circulation* 118(15):e523–e661, 2008.

Devereux RB, Kramer-Fox R, Brown WT, et al: Relation between clinical features of the mitral prolapse syndrome and echocardiographically documented mitral valve prolapse, *J Am Coll Cardiol* 8:763–772, 1986.

Feldman T, Foster E, Glower DD, et al: Percutaneous repair or surgery for mitral regurgitation, *N Engl J Med* 364(15):1395–1406, 2011.

Flack JM, Kvasnicka JH, Gardin JM, et al: Anthropometric and physiologic correlates of mitral valve prolapse in a biethnic cohort of young adults: the CARDIA study, *Am Heart J* 138:486, 1999.

Freed LA, Benjamin EJ, Levy D, et al: Mitral valve prolapse in the general population: the benign nature of echocardiographic features in the Framingham Heart Study, *J Am Coll Cardiol* 40:1298–1304, 2002.

Freed LA, Levy D, Levine RA, et al: Prevalence and clinical outcome of mitral-valve prolapse, *N Engl J Med* 341:1–7, 1999.

Gillinov AM, Cosgrove DM, Blackstone EH, et al: Durability of mitral valve repair for degenerative disease, *J Thorac Cardiovasc Surg* 116(5):734–743, 1998.

Levy D, Savage D: Prevalence and clinical features of mitral valve prolapse, *Am Heart J* 113:1281–1290, 1987.

Marks AR, Choong CY, Sanfilippo AJ, et al: Identification of high-risk and low-risk subgroups of patients with mitral-valve prolapse, *N Engl J Med* 320:1031–1036, 1989.

Rabkin E, Aikawa M, Stone JR, et al: Activated interstitial myofibroblasts express catabolic enzymes and mediate matrix remodeling in myxomatous heart valves, *Circulation* 104:2525–2532, 2001.

Savage DD, Devereux RB, Garrison RJ, et al: Mitral valve prolapse in the general population: 2. Clinical features: The Framingham Study, *Am Heart J* 106:577–581, 1983.

Savage DD, Garrison RJ, Devereux RB, et al: Mitral valve prolapse in the general population: 1. Epidemiologic features: The Framingham Study, *Am Heart J* 106:571–576, 1983.

Suri RM, Schaff HV, Dearani JA, et al: Survival advantage and improved durability of mitral repair for leaflet prolapse subsets in the current era, *Ann Thorac Surg* 82(3):819–826, 2006.

PERICARDITIS

Method of
Amir Azarbal, MD; and Martin M. LeWinter, MD

CURRENT DIAGNOSIS

- Acute pericarditis is an inflammatory syndrome thought to be caused by a viral infection in most cases. It is diagnosed when 2 of the following are present: (1) typical anterior pleuritic chest pain, (2) pericardial friction rub, (3) electrocardiography (ECG) changes (widespread ST segment elevation or PR depression, and (4) new or worsening pericardial effusion.
- Leukocytosis and an elevated high-sensitivity C-reactive protein or erythrocyte sedimentation rate (ESR) are present in most cases.
- Echocardiography is routinely used to detect pericardial effusion. Cardiac magnetic resonance imaging or computed tomography can be used to support the diagnosis.

CURRENT THERAPY

- Limitation of physical activity and high-dose aspirin[1] or other nonsteroidal antiinflammatory drugs such as ibuprofen (Advil)[1] plus colchicine[1] is the treatment of choice for idiopathic (presumed viral) pericarditis.
- Corticosteroids with gradual taper can be added for recurrences.
- Antiinflammatory drugs such as azathioprine (Imuran),[1] anakinra (Kineret),[1] and human intravenous immunoglobulin (Gammagard)[1] have been used in difficult cases of recurrent pericarditis
- Pericardiectomy is reserved for refractory cases and constrictive pericarditis.

[1] Not FDA approved for this indication.

Anatomy and Functions of the Pericardium

The pericardium consists of 2 layers. A visceral monolayer comprised of mesothelial cells is adherent to the epicardium and reflects over the origin of the great vessels, where it is continuous with the inner layer of the parietal pericardium. The latter is approximately 2 mm thick and comprised mainly of collagen and elastin. The pericardial sac is the space between visceral and parietal layers and normally contains up to 50 mL of serous fluid. The pericardium has several functions, including (1) acting as a barrier to infections, (2) providing a mechanism whereby hydrostatic pressure is exerted on the surface of the heart when gravitational or inertial forces are altered, (3) participating in neuro-humoral responses, and (4) limiting short-term distention and displacement of the heart, facilitating interactions between the cardiac chambers and modulating pressure-volume relationships and cardiac output.

Acute Pericarditis

The main inflammatory pericardial syndromes include acute and recurrent pericarditis and constrictive and effusive-constrictive pericarditis. These can be isolated to the pericardium or be a component of a systemic disease.

Acute pericarditis is the most common pericardial syndrome and is responsible for approximately 5% of emergency room visits for chest pain and 2% of patients presenting with ST elevations on ECG. An in-hospital mortality rate of approximately 1% has been reported. Acute pericarditis is more common in males.

Recurrence occurs in 15% to 20% of patients within 18 months after a first episode. Acute pericarditis can also involve the myocardium and cause myopericarditis, with elevated cardiac injury biomarkers (e.g., troponin I).

Etiology

Almost any disease that affects the pericardium can cause acute pericarditis. Acute pericarditis can also cause pericardial effusion; the incidence is highly dependent on etiology. Infectious etiologies are considered to be responsible for the majority of cases. In developed countries 80% to 90% of cases are idiopathic, that is, no specific cause is detected on routine evaluation. These cases are assumed to be viral in etiology. Bacterial and rarely fungal infections account for a small percentage of cases in the developed world. However, *Mycobacterium tuberculosis* is the most common cause of pericarditis in developing countries. Very rarely, parasitic diseases such as echinococcus and toxoplasma species can cause acute pericarditis.

Autoimmune diseases are another common cause of acute pericarditis. These include systemic autoimmune diseases such as lupus erythematosus (SLE), rheumatoid arthritis, Sjögren syndrome, and scleroderma, as well as vasculitic diseases such as eosinophilic granulomatosis with polyangiitis or allergic granulomatosis (previously named *Churg-Strauss syndrome*), Takayasu disease, and Behçet syndrome. Other autoimmune disorders associated with acute pericarditis are sarcoidosis, familial Mediterranean fever, and inflammatory bowel disease.

Malignancies affecting the pericardium also cause acute pericarditis. Almost all neoplastic pericarditis is caused by secondary metastases from extracardiac tumors, especially lung and breast cancer.

Pericarditis can occur after myocardial infarction (MI), both early (i.e., 2 to 4 days after MI) and late (Dressler syndrome, ×1 week to 2 months after MI), and after heart surgery. The incidence of post-MI pericarditis has markedly declined because of reperfusion therapy. Trauma such as penetrating and non-penetrating thoracic injury, esophageal perforation, and procedural complications of cardiac procedures (coronary stenting, pacemaker lead insertion, radiofrequency ablation) are all reported. Although these can cause acute cardiac tamponade, acute pericarditis occurs as a late complication within 1 to 2 weeks to as late as 3 months after the initial event. These causes are collectively termed *post-cardiac injury syndromes* and are believed to have an autoinflammatory basis. Acute pericarditis has also been reported as an immune-mediated response to various drugs.

Presentation

The diagnosis of acute pericarditis is made if two of the following are present: (1) typical anterior chest pain, (2) pericardial friction rub, (3) typical ECG changes (widespread ST segment elevation or PR depression, and (4) new or worsening pericardial effusion. In cases with typical chest pain but no other criteria, additional findings that can establish the diagnosis are elevated cardiac injury biomarkers and evidence of pericardial inflammation or thickening based on advanced imaging modalities (cardiac magnetic resonance imaging [cMRI], computed tomography [CT]). An elevation of either high-sensitivity C reactive protein (hsCRP) or the erythrocyte sedimentation (ESR) rate is supportive but not diagnostic.

Chest pain is the most common symptom of acute pericarditis, present in >90% of cases. The pain is typically sharp, located under the sternum or over the left anterior chest, and almost always pleuritic. The trapezius ridge is a classic radiation. The pain is worst supine and improved by sitting forward. Approximately one-third of patients have a pericardial friction rub (a scratchy or squeaking sound at the left sternal border) because of contact between the layers of the pericardium. The friction rub ordinarily has 3 components. Typical ECG changes include ST elevation in all leads except AVR and

III Cardiovascular System

148

sometimes V1, as well as PR segment depression. Over time, these changes either simply disappear or go through a phase of ST segment normalization and T-wave inversion before disappearing. Both the friction rub and ECG changes are often evanescent. In cases where it is difficult to establish a diagnosis, repeated auscultation and ECGs can be rewarding. A pericardial effusion has been reported in as many as two-thirds of patients with acute pericarditis. The great majority are small. Sinus tachycardia and low-grade fever are also common. If cardiac tamponade is present, elevated jugular venous pressure, muffled heart sounds, hypotension, and pulsus paradoxus are seen. Other diagnoses that can be confused with acute pericarditis include acute MI, pleuritis, pulmonary embolism, costochondritis, and herpes zoster before appearance of vesicles.

Features accompanying acute pericarditis that indicate an elevated risk (mainly for development of cardiac tamponade) include fever >38.5°C, subacute onset of symptoms, moderate to large pericardial effusion, lack of response to aspirin or nonsteroidal antiinflammatory drugs (NSAIDs), immunosuppression, white blood cell count >13,000/mm³, anticoagulant therapy, and suspicion of a non-idiopathic/viral cause such as cancer, SLE, or bacterial infection.

Diagnostic Evaluation
Routine evaluation is directed toward identifying patients with or at elevated risk for cardiac tamponade or patients with a non-idiopathic/viral cause. In addition to a careful history, physical examination, and ECG, routine evaluation should include a chest radiograph, CBC, hs-CRP, routine blood chemistries, and an echocardiogram. Echocardiography should be performed in all patients to detect pericardial effusion, which can be hemodynamically significant despite a normal radiographic cardiac silhouette, and to assess cardiac function in cases with myopericarditis. In the vast majority of cases myopericarditis has no long-term prognostic significance.

Clinical Laboratory Data
Leukocytosis and elevated hs-CRP or ESR are present in most cases. The hs-CRP in particular is increased in about 75% of cases and usually normalizes within 1 to 2 weeks. Failure of normalization within this time frame is associated with higher rates of recurrence. In patients with concomitant myocarditis, markers of cardiac injury such as troponin-I are elevated.

ECG
As discussed earlier, typical ECG changes considered to be hallmarks of acute pericarditis include widespread ST segment elevations or PR segment depression (Figure 1). ECG changes are dynamic, and about 60% of patients have the following evolution over time: stage I (PR depression, ST segment elevation), stage II (ST normalization), stage III (T-wave inversion after ST segment

normalization), and stage IV (ST-T normalization). These evolutionary changes have no known prognostic significance.

Imaging
The chest radiograph is normal in acute pericarditis unless a moderate- to large-size pericardial effusion or associated pulmonary pathology is present. The echocardiogram is usually normal except for the common presence of small pericardial effusions (Figure 2). In cases with associated myopericarditis, the left ventricular ejection fraction is almost always normal.

Cardiac MRI or CT typically shows pericardial thickening and enhanced gadolinium uptake (Figure 3). Advanced imaging modalities can be used to support the diagnosis of pericarditis in difficult cases.

Treatment
Treatment of common pericardial syndromes is summarized in Table 1. Reliable patients without high-risk features need not be hospitalized. For treatment of an initial episode of acute idiopathic pericarditis, avoidance of physical activity greater than walking

Figure 2 Parasternal long-axis view of a transthoracic echocardiogram performed in a patient with acute pericarditis showing small to moderate-sized pericardial effusion (asterisk). Also note a pacemaker lead in the right ventricle (arrow) and associated acoustic shadowing artifact.

Figure 3 Cardiac MRI image in a patient with acute pericarditis after intravenous gadolinium administration. Note late gadolinium enhancement of the pericardium along with pericardial thickening indicating inflammation (asterisk). Other findings are pericardial fat (arrowhead) and trivial pericardial effusion (arrow).

Figure 1 Electrocardiogram demonstrating typical changes of acute pericarditis. Note the widespread ST segment elevations with concomitant PR segment depression.

TABLE 1 Treatment Summary of Common Pericardial Syndromes

PERICARDIAL SYNDROME	TREATMENT OVERVIEW	SPECIFIC CONSIDERATIONS
Acute pericarditis	Physical activity restriction *and* NSAIDs *plus* Colchicine[1]	Restriction of physical activity until resolution of symptoms NSAIDs until symptoms resolve and CRP normalizes Colchicine for 2 to 3 months See text for pregnancy and lactation considerations
Recurrent pericarditis	Acute pericarditis treatment *plus* Corticosteroids (in refractory cases) *or* Immunosuppressive therapy (for multiple recurrences) *or* Pericardiectomy (last resort)	Restriction of physical activity until resolution of symptoms NSAIDs until symptoms resolve and CRP normalizes for 1 to 2 weeks with subsequent taper Colchicine[1] for at least 6 months For multiple recurrences, low to moderate doses of corticosteroids until resolution of symptoms and normalization of CRP followed by slow taper Immunosuppressants (anakinra [Kineret],[1] azathioprine [Imuran],[1] intravenous immunoglobulin[1]) for multiple recurrences Pericardiectomy in refractory cases (last resort)
Constrictive pericarditis	Treatment of underlying condition (ie, tuberculosis, inflammation) *or* Pericardiectomy (if chronic and refractory)	In cases of pericardial inflammation, an empiric antiinflammatory regimen may reverse the disease process and obviate the need for pericardiectomy.

[1]Not FDA approved for this indication.

at a normal pace is recommended until symptoms resolve and CRP has normalized. Athletes should refrain from competitive sports activities for at least 3 months. NSAIDs plus colchicine[1] is a first-line pharmacologic treatment. We recommend ibuprofen (Advil)[1] 600 to 800 mg by mouth 3 times daily or aspirin[1] 2 to 4 g by mouth daily in divided doses and colchicine[1] 0.6 mg twice daily (0.6 mg once daily for patients <70 kg) until symptoms resolve and CRP normalizes. The NSAID should then be tapered over 1 to 2 weeks and colchicine continued for 3 months from onset of symptoms. All patients should receive a proton pump inhibitor while receiving NSAIDs.

In pregnancy ibuprofen, aspirin >100 mg/day by mouth, and colchicine are contraindicated after 20 weeks' gestation. Corticosteroids are preferred in this circumstance. In addition, colchicine is contraindicated during lactation.

In patients in whom a specific cause for acute pericarditis other than idiopathic/viral has been identified, the treatment should be directed at that cause. Thus, in patients with autoimmune diseases, corticosteroids may be more appropriate as the initial treatment.

Recurrent Pericarditis

Recurrent pericarditis is the most common complication of acute pericarditis and is defined as a repeat episode after a symptom-free interval of at least 4 to 6 weeks. The recurrence rate after an initial episode of acute pericarditis is approximately 15% to 20% and may increase to as much as 50% after a first recurrent episode. Patients with recurrent pericarditis can be severely incapacitated. Certain rare conditions such as familial Mediterranean fever, tumor necrosis factor receptor–associated periodic syndrome, and other periodic fever syndromes are often characterized by bouts of recurrent pericarditis. Inadequate treatment of a first episode (e.g., inadequate drug doses, too short a treatment duration or too rapid discontinuation, or tapering of medications) can be responsible for recurrences

Recurrent pericarditis after an initial bout of idiopathic/viral pericarditis is currently considered to be an autoinflammatory process (as opposed to an autoimmune disease such as SLE). It is hypothesized that, after an initial viral infection, immune system cross-reaction between viral particles and host tissue occurs. A similar mechanism is believed to be operative in the periodic fever

syndromes. Of course, pericarditis due to other, specific causes can also recur.

The most feared complication of recurrent pericarditis is constrictive pericarditis. The incidence is high (≤30%) in cases of bacterial pericarditis and low to moderate (<5%) in systemic inflammatory diseases and cancer. In patients with recurrences after an initial bout of viral/idiopathic pericarditis, symptoms almost always eventually resolve, and progression to constrictive pericarditis is very rare (<1%).

The diagnosis of a recurrence is based on the same criteria as for an initial episode (i.e., history, friction rub, ECG findings, and a new or worsening pericardial effusion). Elevated hs-CRP, ESR, and white blood cell count remain useful for monitoring disease activity and response to treatment. More advanced imaging modalities such as CT or cMRI are rarely required to diagnose a recurrence but are useful if there is a concern about development of constriction.

In general, for patients with a recurrence after an index episode of idiopathic/viral pericarditis we recommend that treatment be the same as for the initial episode (i.e., restriction of physical activity, NSAID, and colchicine[1]) until complete resolution of symptoms and normalization of hs-CRP. Some patients are able to manage recurrences by initiating treatment at the very first sign of symptoms. If the response is prompt, the recurrence is converted to a minor illness.

Use of corticosteroids for treatment of recurrent pericarditis should be reserved for cases where the above-mentioned measures have failed, especially if recurrences are frequent and severe and do not respond well to NSAIDs. Unusual patients with an initial episode who do not respond to first-line therapy are also candidates. Corticosteroids usually provide rapid relief of symptoms, and almost all patients respond favorably initially. However, corticosteroids appear to increase the chance of further recurrences, especially when high initial doses are used with rapid tapering. High doses also have a much higher incidence of adverse effects. If a decision is made to use corticosteroids, we recommend low to moderate doses (e.g., prednisone[1] 0.25 to 0.5 mg/kg/day or equivalent) usually for about 4 to 8 weeks, followed by gradual tapering (assuming symptom resolution and normalization of hs-CRP) in conjunction with colchicine. NSAIDs may also be included or added later as corticosteroids are tapered. Colchicine should ordinarily be continued for 6 months. During tapering, recurrences typically occur with doses <10 to 15 mg/day dose of prednisone or equivalent. Patients symptom free at this threshold should be treated with smaller subsequent dose decrements at intervals of

[1] Not FDA approved for this indication.

2 to 6 weeks. If possible, recurrences occurring during tapering should be treated with NSAID optimization rather than increasing corticosteroids. To prevent side effects of long-term corticosteroid use, specifically bone loss, consideration should be given to supplementary calcium and vitamin D. Bisphosphonates are recommended in all men ≥50 years and postmenopausal women in whom long-term treatment with corticosteroids at a dose of 5.0 to 7.5 mg/day of prednisone or equivalent is required.

In patients with multiple recurrences (≥3 episodes) despite the aforementioned strategies, alternative drugs have been suggested based on case reports, case series, and small randomized trials. These include azathioprine (Imuran),[1] methotrexate (Trexall),[1] and intravenous human immunoglobulin.[1] Recently, the interleukin (IL)-1β antagonist anakinra (Kineret)[1] (1 to 2 mg/kg/day up to 100 mg subcutaneously for several months) has shown considerable promise; other IL-1β antagonists are in development. Finally, as a last resort for refractory cases of recurrent pericarditis, pericardiectomy may be effective.

Constrictive Pericarditis
Etiology
Constrictive pericarditis is a consequence of chronic forms of pericarditis, especially bacterial (20% to 30%), immune-mediated, and neoplastic (2% to 5%) disease. Some cases are idiopathic. Other causes include cardiac injury syndromes, postradiation, uremia, and sarcoidosis. Before the availability of effective antimicrobial therapy, tuberculous pericarditis was the most important cause, but this is now rare in the developed world. In the third world, tuberculosis remains an important cause of pericardial disease in general and constrictive pericarditis in particular, often in association with HIV/AIDs. It is very rare (<1%) for idiopathic/viral pericarditis to result in constrictive pericarditis.

When tuberculosis was the major cause of constrictive pericarditis, cases typically presented as a very chronic disease with the features described below. Heavy pericardial calcification was a classic feature. In contemporary practice, most cases of constrictive pericarditis occur in conjunction with the syndrome of effusive-constrictive pericarditis, where pericardial effusion and constriction coexist in varying combinations.

Presentation and Physical Findings
Patients with constrictive pericarditis present with signs and symptoms of right heart failure, with small cardiac volumes and preserved ejection fraction (EF). (In extreme cases EF may be reduced due to severely impaired filling.) Symptoms include fatigue, peripheral edema, dyspnea, hepatomegaly, pleural effusions, and ascites. On physical examination, the venous pressure is markedly elevated, with an M- or W-shaped waveform caused by rapid atrial pressure descents. There is a paradoxical rise in venous pressure with inspiration (Kussmaul's sign), consistent with impaired filling of the right ventricle. A paradoxical pulse is present in as many as one-third of patients. Auscultation may reveal a pericardial knock, an early diastolic, medium-frequency sound (occurring slightly earlier than a usual third heart sound) that reflects abrupt cessation of rapid filling of the ventricles caused by the constricting pericardium. Atrial fibrillation is very common.

By definition, patients with effusive-constrictive pericarditis have pericardial effusions of variable size, which often contain adhesions and fibrous strands and are sometimes large enough to cause cardiac tamponade. In these cases, the diagnosis of constriction is often made after pericardiocentesis, when right heart filling pressures remain elevated and typical hemodynamic features become apparent.

Diagnostic Tests
The ECG often reveals nonspecific repolarization abnormalities, but there are no specific findings. In effusive-constrictive pericarditis, low-voltage and electrical alternans may be apparent if there is a large effusion. The chest X-ray film may reveal pericardial calcification, but its incidence is now low. Pleural effusions are common.

Major echocardiographic-Doppler findings include small cardiac chambers, a septal "bounce" because of exaggerated septal motion related to increased ventricular interdependence, increased mitral and tricuspid respiratory flow variation, and pericardial thickening and calcification. Interdependence is explained on the basis of a fixed intrapericardial volume, as a result of which when the volume of one ventricle changes (e.g., during respiration), the volume of the other must change reciprocally.

Cardiac catheterization reveals rapid atrial pressure descents, equalization of left- and right-sided filling pressures, increased respiratory variation in LV and RV systolic pressure (also due to ventricular interdependence) and a characteristic "dip and plateau" or "square root" sign evident in the ventricular diastolic pressure.

Cardiac CT and MRI are the best methods for imaging the pericardium. These demonstrate variable increases in pericardial thickness and calcification if present, although rare cases without increased thickness have been reported. Pericardial calcifications can be especially well visualized by cardiac CT and increased ventricular interdependence can be appreciated on real-time cine MR images. Modern cases of constrictive and effusive-constrictive pericarditis often have prominent pericardial inflammation, best imaged by gadolinium uptake during cMRI.

Treatment
Medical management of constrictive pericarditis is symptomatic and supportive, primarily consisting of diuretics to manage signs of right heart failure. It is important to avoid drugs that slow the heart rate, as these patients are critically dependent on heart rate to maintain cardiac output. Ultimately, these patients become refractory to diuretics.

Pericardiectomy has been considered the most definitive treatment for constrictive pericarditis. However, these are often difficult surgeries with high morbidity and mortality rates and delayed benefit. A number of patients are deemed too debilitated for surgery. Postradiation constriction has been considered a specific contraindication. Before pericardiectomy is undertaken, consideration should be given to a trial of an antiinflammatory regimen, especially in idiopathic cases, cases due to systemic inflammatory diseases, and cases due to post-cardiac injury syndromes. High-intensity gadolinium uptake on cardiac MRI in association with pericardial thickening is a signal that such a regimen may be successful, and apparent cures have been reported. Patients with evidence of intense inflammation often have a subacute course and belong in the subset with effusive-constrictive pericarditis. There have been no formal trials of specific antiinflammatory regimens. We favor a course of intermediate-dose prednisone[1] followed by a gradual taper similar to that recommended for recurrent pericarditis, along with colchicine[1] for at least 6 months. In cases of effusive-constrictive pericarditis presenting with cardiac tamponade, a few days of higher-dose prednisone initially may be reasonable. If an antiinflammatory regimen is to be attempted, we recommend committing to at least 2 to 3 months of prednisone treatment before tapering is begun. Reimaging the pericardium to ensure that inflammation has resolved before tapering is helpful.

References
Adler Y, Charron P, Imazio M: 2015 ESC Guidelines for the diagnosis and management of pericardial diseases. Task Force for the Diagnosis and Management of Pericardial Diseases of the European Society of Cardiology (ESC), *G Ital Cardiol (Rome)* 16:702–738, 2015.

Azarbal A, LeWinter MM: Pericardial effusion, *Cardiol Clin* 35:515–524, 2017.

Cantarini L, Lucherini OM, Brucato A: Clues to detect tumor necrosis factor receptor-associated periodic syndrome (TRAPS) among patients with idiopathic recurrent acute pericarditis: results of a multicentre study, *Clin Res Cardiol* 101:525–531, 2012.

Hoit BD: Anatomy and physiology of the pericardium, *Cardiol Clin* 35:481–490, 2017.

Imazio M, Battaglia A, Gaido L, Gaita F: Recurrent pericarditis, *Rev Med Interne* 38:307–311, 2017.

Imazio M, Brucato A, Cemin R: A randomized trial of colchicine for acute pericarditis, *N Engl J Med* 369:1522–1528, 2013.

Imazio M, Brucato A, Cumetti D: Corticosteroids for recurrent pericarditis: high versus low doses: a nonrandomized observation, *Circulation* 118:667–671, 2008.

Imazio M, Gaita F, LeWinter M: Evaluation and treatment of pericarditis: a systematic review, *JAMA* 314:1498–1506, 2015.

Kyto V, Sipila J, Rautava P: Clinical profile and influences on outcomes in patients hospitalized for acute pericarditis, *Circulation* 130:1601–1606, 2014.

LeWinter MM: Clinical practice: acute pericarditis, *N Engl J Med* 371:2410–2416, 2014.

PERIPHERAL ARTERY DISEASE

Method of
William Michael, MD

Epidemiology and Risk Factors

Peripheral artery disease (PAD), the third leading cause of atherosclerotic morbidity following coronary artery disease and stroke, is estimated to affect 8.5 million Americans older than 40 years of age and more than 230 million people worldwide. The prevalence ranges from ~5% among individuals 40 to 44 years of age up to ~12% among those 70 to 74 years of age. Although PAD is defined as atherosclerotic disease in any arterial vessel outside of the coronary circulation, the most common sites for the development of PAD are the abdominal aorta and vessels of the lower extremities. Patients at increased risk of PAD are those older than 65 years of age and those with diabetes, a history of smoking, hyperlipidemia, and hypertension. Individuals with a family history of PAD or with known atherosclerotic disease in another vascular bed area are also at increased risk.

Pathophysiology

PAD is related to the development of atherosclerotic plaques of the peripheral arteries that leads to reduction of blood flow to peripheral tissues. Classic claudication involves flow-limiting blockages that present as exertional pain in the lower extremities that is caused by lack of oxygen delivery to the peripheral tissues and improves with rest. More serious manifestations of PAD are termed *critical limb ischemia* (CLI) and involve pain at rest or pain that wakes the patient at night, nonhealing wounds/ulcerations in the distal extremities, or gangrene.

Prevention and Screening Recommendations

Prevention of PAD involves controlling risk factors associated with the development of atherosclerotic disease (e.g., diabetes mellitus, history of smoking, hyperlipidemia, hypertension) and appropriately managing these conditions. The U.S. Preventive Services Task Force (USPSTF) states that the evidence for screening for PAD as part of cardiovascular risk assessment is inconclusive (I rating). However, the American Heart Association (AHA) recommends screening with ankle-brachial index (ABI) in adults at high risk of having PAD (those older than 65 years of age and those 50 to 64 years of age with risk factors for atherosclerotic disease).

Clinical Manifestations

PAD can manifest in a number of different ways, and many individuals are asymptomatic (20% to 50%). Classic intermittent claudication presents with exertional leg pain (often in the calf but also in the buttock, hip, thigh, or foot) that resolves within 10 minutes of rest. However, only 10% to 30% of patients present with classic claudication. The remaining 40% to 50% present with "atypical" leg symptoms that include pain that begins at rest, pain that does not cause the patient to stop walking/activity, or discomfort that does not consistently improve with rest. CLI involves pain at rest, nocturnal pain, nonhealing wounds/ulcers that are located distally (e.g., tips of toes, between toes), and gangrene.

Physical Examination

Physical examination has poor sensitivity in assessing patients with asymptomatic PAD but can be helpful in assessing for and differentiating between claudication and CLI versus presentations that are not related to symptomatic PAD. Lower-extremity pulses should be assessed; pulses are graded on a scale of 0 to 3, with 0 being absent, 1 diminished, 2 normal, and 3 bounding. Absent or diminished pulses are suggestive of PAD and disease at a higher level of the vascular tree than the assessed pulse, making assessment of the dorsal pedal or posterior tibial pulses the most useful. Auscultation for femoral arterial bruit can be helpful but is rare in the primary care setting. Examination of the feet should focus on identification of nonhealing lower-extremity ulceration in a characteristic, well-demarcated, or "punched-out" pattern and lack of granulation tissue at the base, consistent with arterial ulceration. Careful inspection should be paid to the toes, especially between the toes and the webbing of the toes, as these lesions may not be readily noticed by the patient. The anterior lower leg is also a common place for arterial ulcers as they have less collateral circulation. Other examination findings of the lower extremity that suggest a diagnosis of PAD include elevation pallor and dependent rubor.

Diagnosis

The initial diagnostic workup for patients with suspected PAD involves obtaining a resting ABI or ABI (Table 1). If the resting ABI is normal (1.0 to 1.4 is normal; ≤0.9 is abnormal) but there remains a high clinical suspicion for PAD, an exercise ABI can be obtained. The ABI is less accurate and can be falsely elevated in the presence of medial artery calcification that can stiffen arteries in the ankle, an issue most often encountered in patients with diabetes or end-stage kidney disease. This can result in an ABI >1.4, which is an uninterpretable result. In such cases, a toe-brachial index (TBI) can be considered. An abnormal TBI may predict poor outcomes beyond ABI in such patients (TBI ≤0.7 is diagnostic of PAD). Arterial duplex ultrasonography is also readily available, low risk, and inexpensive, but it is limited in its ability to detect infrapopliteal stenosis, stenosis that exists in the pelvic or abdominal cavities, or in patients with significant arterial calcifications. More advanced noninvasive studies, such as computed tomography angiography (CTA) and magnetic resonance angiography (MRA) can provide more anatomic detail and is often ordered for patients with PAD who fail medical management and/or are candidates for more invasive interventions. These studies are expensive and come with the added risk of contrast-related complications in certain patient populations. Catheter-based angiography remains the gold standard for diagnosing PAD but is reserved for patients receiving endovascular revascularization.

Ankle-Brachial Index

The ABI is an inexpensive way to assess for PAD and can be done within 15 minutes in the primary care setting or ordered to be

TABLE 1	Ankle-Brachial Index	
ABI	**MAGNITUDE OF PERIPHERAL ARTERY DISEASE**	**TREATMENT CONSIDERATIONS**
>1.4	Cannot interpret	Consider TBI
1.0–1.4	Normal	None
0.91–0.99	Borderline	If high concern, consider exercise ABI
0.7–0.90	Mild PAD	Treat risk factors, discuss supervised exercise therapy and/or medication management
0.41–0.69	Moderate PAD	Treat risk factors, refer to vascular surgeon
<0.4	Severe PAD	Treat risk factors, refer to vascular surgeon

ABI, Ankle-brachial index; *PAD,* peripheral artery disease; *TBI,* toe-brachial index.

completed in a vascular laboratory. To obtain an ABI in clinic, the patient should be placed in the supine position with the head, hips, and heels fully supported. The ABI averages 0.35 higher in the seated position than in the supine position. A Doppler probe should be used to obtain both the ankle and brachial pressure. After allowing for a 5- to 10-minute rest period, the Doppler probe is used to auscultate flow, and a pneumatic cuff is inflated until flow ceases. The cuff is then slowly deflated until the flow signal reappears, and the corresponding pressure is recorded as the SBP of that limb. The process is then repeated for each limb, and the higher ankle and higher brachial pressures are used for calculation. The ankle pressure is then divided into the brachial pressure to obtain the ABI. A score between 1.0 and 1.4 is considered normal, and a score ≤0.9 is consistent with mild to moderate PAD. An ABI ≤0.4 is considered severe PAD. An ABI between 0.91 and 0.99 is considered borderline low, and PAD cannot be ruled out. In such cases, exercise ABI or other noninvasive imaging studies can be helpful to further evaluate for PAD.

Differential Diagnosis

PAD can present with symptoms that are similar to those for other vascular pathologies, neurologic conditions, and musculoskeletal etiologies. For example, the terms *pseudoclaudication* and *neuroclaudication* are used because of similarities in the presentation of claudication in PAD to conditions such as lumbar spinal stenosis, sciatica, or structural back disease. Venous claudication, popliteal artery entrapment syndrome, and various arthritides should also be considered in the differential diagnosis. The presence or absence of classic PAD risk factors, the specific location and description of the pain, in addition to the effect of exercise and rest (Table 2) can help differentiate PAD from these other conditions.

Treatment

Risk-Factor Control

Control of preexisting risk factors is crucial in the treatment of PAD. Patients with modifiable risk factors such as smoking must be aggressively counseled on the importance of smoking cessation. Patient with diabetes, hypertension, and hyperlipidemia should be treated per the most up-to-date guidelines published by the American College of Endocrinology (ACE) and the American College of Cardiology/American Heart Association (ACC/AHA). The Edinburgh study suggested that a sedentary lifestyle has also been shown to increase the risk for development of PAD by showing that physical activity was inversely proportional to the development of PAD.

Tobacco Cessation

The risk of developing PAD is double for a smoker compared with a nonsmoker. The risk is related to the number of cigarettes smoked and the age at which an individual started smoking. Although it takes 30 years after quitting for a former smoker's risk for development of PAD to return to that of a nonsmoker, the importance of smoking cessation cannot be overstated. Patients who smoke should be counseled on quitting at every office visit and offered appropriate pharmacotherapy, nicotine replacement, and/or referral to tobacco cessation programs. However, only one-third of patients with PAD receive these therapeutic recommendations from their primary care team. Patients who successfully quit have lower rates of progression of atherosclerosis in their limbs as evidenced by decreasing rates of decline in their ABIs and lower rates of CLI, amputation, and death.

Glycemic Control

Diabetic patients also carry about double the risk for the development of PAD than do patients without diabetes. Many studies have been designed to look at the role glycemic control should play in reducing both major adverse limb events (MALE) and major adverse cardiovascular events (MACE) in diabetic patients, but the evidence for improved glycemic control in reduction of macrovascular complications for diabetic patients with PAD is lacking, especially in regard to MALE. Multiple studies have demonstrated benefit with sodium glucose transporter 2 inhibitors (SGLT2i) on MACE, heart failure, and overall mortality but did not show a reduction in MALE. In the Canagliflozin Cardiovascular Study (CANVAS), a subgroup analysis suggested that canagliflozin (Invokana) demonstrated up to a twofold increase in risk of amputation in diabetic patients with PAD compared with older insulin management regimens (sulfonylureas, metformin, insulin). The DECLARE-TIMI 58 trial involving dapagliflozin (Farxiga) redemonstrated the overall positive cardiovascular effects of the SGLT2i medications, but the subgroup analysis also demonstrated an increase in amputation risk in diabetic patients with PAD compared with those without PAD. A subsequent subgroup analysis of a study with canagliflozin, the Canagliflozin and Renal Events in Diabetes with Established Nephropathy Clinical Evaluation (CREDENCE) trial, did not show an increase in amputation risk in diabetic patients with PAD, but the concern remains and would benefit from further direct investigation. Trials looking at glucagon-like protein (GLP)-1 receptor agonists suggest a more direct vascular benefit by their mechanism of action and may provide therapeutic advantage over SGLT2i in diabetic patients with PAD. For example, the Liraglutide Effect and Action in Diabetes: Evaluation of Cardiovascular Outcome Results (LEADER) trial demonstrated benefit for diabetic patients in reduction of MACE and MALE in participants with PAD. It should be noted that the reduction in macrovascular complications related to diabetes, such as MACE, heart failure, and diabetic kidney disease provide distinct overall advantages of both the SGLT2i and GLP-1

TABLE 2	Differential Diagnosis for Symptomatic Peripheral Artery Disease				
CONDITION	LOCATION	CHARACTERISTIC	EFFECT OF EXERCISE	EFFECT OF REST	OTHER CHARACTERISTICS
Venous claudication	Entire leg, worse in calf	Tight, bursting pain	After walking	Subsides slowly	History of iliofemoral deep vein thrombosis; edema; signs of venous stasis
Popliteal artery entrapment syndrome	Calf muscles	Tight, tearing pain	After moderate to vigorous exercise (jogging)	Subsides slowly	Typically heavy muscular athletes
Spinal stenosis	Often bilateral buttocks, posterior leg	Pain and weakness	May mimic claudication	Variable relief, but can take a long time to recover	Worse with standing and extending spine
Nerve root compression	Radiates down leg	Sharp lancinating pain	Induced by sitting, standing, or walking	Often present at rest	History of back problems; worse with sitting; relief when supine or sitting
Arthritis (hip, foot, or ankle)	Lateral hip, thigh, foot arch, ankle	Aching discomfort	After variable degree of exercise	Not quickly relieved	Symptoms variable; may be related to activity or present at rest

receptor agonists over older diabetic medications, even in diabetic patients with PAD, despite the potential for increased amputation risk with SGLT2i. However, for the aforementioned reasons, it may be prudent to start with a GLP-1 receptor agonist before deciding to add an SGLT2i in diabetic patients with PAD.

Antithrombic Therapy

The ACC/AHA recommends treatment with once-daily aspirin[1] (81 mg to 325 mg) for patients with PAD based largely on expert opinion. For patients who cannot tolerate aspirin, clopidogrel (Plavix) 75 mg per day is a reasonable alternative. Dual antiplatelet therapy (clopidogrel plus aspirin) may reduce the risk of nonfatal myocardial infarction in patients with PAD and comorbid CAD, but this link is not well established and not generally recommended. However, per the ACC/AHA guidelines, dual antiplatelet therapy may be reasonable to reduce the risk of limb-related events in patients with symptomatic PAD after lower extremity revascularization.

The COMPASS trial looked at patients with symptomatic PAD treated with rivaroxaban (Xarelto) 2.5 mg twice daily and aspirin daily compared with aspirin monotherapy in 7470 patients, and it demonstrated a 46% risk relative risk reduction in MALE and a 24% relative risk reduction in MACE at the expense of a 70% increase in major bleeding events (mainly gastrointestinal), but not a significant difference in fatal bleeding, intracranial bleeding, or bleeding into a critical organ. The VOYAGER trial looked at rivaroxaban 2.5 mg twice daily and aspirin versus aspirin monotherapy in patients who had undergone revascularization for symptomatic PAD and demonstrated similar findings. Based on these trials, rivaroxaban (Xarelto) 2.5 mg twice daily plus aspirin daily is approved by the U.S. Food and Drug Administration (FDA) for the treatment of PAD.

The Warfarin Antiplatelet Vascular Evaluation (WAVE) trial compared warfarin and aspirin to aspirin monotherapy and found no benefit with the combination therapy and a threefold increase in life-threatening and moderate bleed risk compared with aspirin therapy alone. Warfarin is not recommended as part of a PAD treatment plan.

Lipid-Lowering Therapy

PAD is a coronary artery disease equivalent, and as such, patients should be initiated on a high-intensity statin such as atorvastatin (Lipitor) 80 mg or rosuvastatin (Crestor) 40 mg, per ACC/AHA guidelines. The Reduction of Atherothrombosis for Continued Health (REACH) Registry, an observation investigation for subjects at risk for atherothrombotic events, demonstrated that statin use is associated with a reduction in worsening claudication, new CLI, lower extremity revascularization, or amputation.

In the Further Cardiovascular Outcomes Research with PCSK 9 Inhibition in Subjects with Elevated Risk (FOURIER) trial, patients with atherosclerotic disease (with or without PAD) who were maximized on statin therapy and then treated with the proprotein convertase subtilisin/kexin type 9 (PCSK 9) inhibitor evolocumab (Repatha) versus placebo were found to have reduced MALE and MACE at an average 2.2-year follow-up. Although all patients should receive statin therapy, patients with difficult to control low-density lipoprotein and other less commonly used biomarkers such as lipoprotein (a), may help risk-stratify patients who may benefit from therapies such as evolocumab.

Hypertension Therapy

Hypertension should be treated to a goal of <130/80 per current ACC/AHA guidelines. Systolic blood pressure has more of an impact on the development of PAD than diastolic blood pressure. In the Atherosclerosis Risk in the Community (ARIC) study, an increase in the development of PAD was seen in patients with systolic blood pressure over 140 mm Hg (adjusted hazard ratio of 2.6) and between 120 and 139 mm Hg (adjusted hazard ratio of 1.6). Elevated risk for PAD was only observed in patients with diastolic blood pressure above 90 mm Hg. ACC/AHA guidelines can be

followed in regard to initiation and management of blood pressure in patients with PAD similarly as to those who do not have PAD.

Cilostazol

Cilostazol (Pletal) is a phosphodiesterase III inhibitor that is used to treat intermittent claudication. Cilostazol increases cyclic AMP, which results in vasodilator activity and antiplatelet effects. A 2021 Cochrane review confirmed a 2014 review and found participants taking 100 mg to 300 mg of cilostazol daily had a significant decrease in claudication symptoms and an increase in distance walked compared with those taking a placebo. The main side effects were headache and diarrhea; dizziness and palpitations were also noted, but the medication was generally well tolerated. Of note, there is a black box warning on cilostazol, and it should not be used in patients with congestive heart failure, regardless of class. Although cilostazol did improve symptom-free walking distance in patients with PAD, there is insufficient evidence about the effectiveness on MALE or MACE. The typical dose of cilostazol is 100 mg twice daily, and the medication takes 2 to 4 weeks to have an effect on walking distance. Cilostazol should be discontinued if there is no improvement in intermittent claudication symptoms after 3 months. Thrombocytopenia and/or leukopenia can occur in patients on cilostazol, and this has the potential to progress to agranulocytosis if the medication is not discontinued immediately.

Exercise Rehabilitation

Supervised exercise programs have been shown to provide improvements in functional status and quality of life that are similar to endovascular interventions and superior to optimized medical therapy alone. The Supervised Exercise, Stent Revascularization, or Medical Therapy for Claudication Due to Aortoiliac Peripheral Artery Disease : The CLEVER study highlighted both the short-term (6 months) and long-term (18 months) benefits of supervised exercise therapy. A Cochrane review published in 2018 investigated supervised versus unsupervised exercise for intermittent claudication and concluded that although supervised exercise was more effective than unsupervised or home-based exercise programs at improving maximal walking distance, there was no difference in patient-reported quality of life or functional impairment outcomes. This is important to note as not all communities will have access to supervised exercise programs. The structure of most of the programs studied involve walking 30 to 45 minutes three times per week for 12 weeks. Participants would rest when claudication symptoms occur until they resolve and then begin walking again.

Revascularization/Vascular Interventions

Patients with symptomatic PAD should be considered for revascularization if they have persistent, lifestyle-limiting symptoms despite maximal medical therapy and trial of an exercise rehabilitation program. Patients with CLI should also be considered for urgent revascularization. For patients in whom interventional therapy is indicated, referral to an appropriate specialist, often a vascular surgeon, is warranted, and imaging with CTA or MRA to identify the specific anatomic location of the atherosclerotic lesion should be considered. Endovascular techniques, such as balloon angioplasty and stenting, are often preferred to surgical revascularization. However, patients with challenging anatomy may benefit from surgical revascularization with endarterectomy or surgical bypass.

Critical Limb Ischemia

Patients with findings consistent with CLI (Table 3) should be managed by an interdisciplinary team that involves vascular surgery, interventionalist (radiology, cardiology), and wound care specialists. The BASIL (Bypass versus Angioplasty in Severe Ischemia of the Leg) trial found that there was no difference in amputation-free survival and overall survival in patients managed with endovascular intervention versus open surgery. The goal in management of such patients is to minimize tissue loss and preserve the function of the foot while also balancing their inherent surgical risk. Although the rate of developing CLI in patients with PAD is low (<10% over

---

[1] Not FDA approved for this indication.

TABLE 3	Symptoms Characteristic of Critical Limb Ischemia and Acute Limb Ischemia	
	SYMPTOMS	**VASCULAR SURGERY REFERRAL URGENCY**
Critical limb ischemia	Ischemic pain at rest >2 weeks (especially at night), tissue loss (typically painful "punched out," sharply demarcated arterial ulcers on toes, foot), gangrene	Urgent
Acute limb ischemia	Paresthesia, Pain, Pallor, Pulselessness, Poikilothermia (cool/cold), and Paralysis (the "6 P's")	Emergent

5 years), there is a 20% risk of mortality within 1 year of diagnosis if a patient does develop CLI, and revascularization is generally necessary to avoid amputation.

Acute Limb Ischemia

Acute limb ischemia (ALI) is a medical emergency that requires immediate vascular surgery evaluation. It is characterized by an acute loss of tissue perfusion, as opposed to the more chronically poor limb perfusion characteristic of CLI. Immediate recognition of the signs of ALI (see Table 3) is important as reperfusion may need to occur in <6 hours in some cases to salvage function of the limb and minimize tissue loss. Most commonly, ALI is a result of thromboembolism of a stenotic artery, stent thrombosis, or thrombosis of prior surgical revascularization/bypass graft.

Monitoring

The majority of patients with PAD can be managed with a combination of risk-factor modification and medical management that includes a supervised exercise rehabilitation program. Although it is important to note that disease severity will remain stable over a 5-year period in most patients, up to 20% will progressively worsen in their disease course, and <10% will go on to develop CLI. Patients with PAD should be seen in follow-up at least once per year and potentially more frequently depending on the severity of PAD and other comorbid health conditions.

References

Barraclough JY, Yu J, Figtree GA, et al: Cardiovascular and renal outcomes with canagliflozin in patients with peripheral arterial disease: Data from the CANVAS Program and CREDENCE trial, *Diabetes Obes Metab* 24(6):1072–1083, 2022, https://doi.org/10.1111/dom.14671.

Bhatt DL, Flather MD, Hacke W, et al: Patients with prior myocardial infarction, stroke, or symptomatic peripheral arterial disease in the CHARISMA trial, *J Am Coll Cardiol* 49(19):1982–1988, 2007, https://doi.org/10.1016/j.jacc.2007.03.025.

Bonaca MP, Hamburg NM, Creager MA: Contemporary Medical Management of Peripheral Artery Disease, *Circ Res* 128(12):1868–1884, 2021, https://doi.org/10.1161/CIRCRESAHA.121.318258.

Bonaca MP, Wiviott SD, Zelniker TA, et al: Dapagliflozin and cardiac, kidney, and limb outcomes in patients with and without peripheral artery disease in DECLARE-TIMI 58, *Circulation* 142(8):734–747, 2020, https://doi.org/10.1161/CIRCULATIONAHA.119.044775.

Bradbury AW, Adam DJ, Bell J, et al: Bypass versus Angioplasty in Severe Ischaemia of the Leg (BASIL) trial: An intention-to-treat analysis of amputation-free and overall survival in patients randomized to a bypass surgery-first or a balloon angioplasty-first revascularization strategy [published correction appears in *J Vasc Surg* 2010 Dec;52(6):1751. Bhattachary, V [corrected to Bhattacharya, V]], *J Vasc Surg* 51(5 Suppl):5S–17S, 2010, https://doi.org/10.1016/j.jvs.2010.01.073.

Brown T, Forster RB, Cleanthis M, Mikhailidis DP, Stansby G, Stewart M: Cilostazol for intermittent claudication, *Cochrane Database Syst Rev* 6(6):CD003748, 2021, https://doi.org/10.1002/14651858.CD003748.pub5. Published 2021 Jun 30.

Criqui MH, Matsushita K, Aboyans V, et al: Lower extremity peripheral artery disease: contemporary epidemiology, management gaps, and future directions: a scientific statement from the American Heart Association [published correction appears in *Circulation*. 2021 Aug 31;144(9):e193], *Circulation* 144(9):e171–e191, 2021, https://doi.org/10.1161/CIR.0000000000001005.

Dhatariya K, Bain SC, Buse JB, et al: The impact of liraglutide on diabetes-related foot ulceration and associated complications in patients with type 2 diabetes at high risk for cardiovascular events: results from the LEADER Trial, *Diabetes Care* 41(10):2229–2235, 2018, https://doi.org/10.2337/dc18-1094.

Gerhard-Herman MD, Gornik HL, Barrett C, et al: 2016 AHA/ACC guideline on the management of patients with lower extremity peripheral artery disease: executive summary: a report of the American College of Cardiology/American Heart Association Task Force on Clinical Practice Guidelines [published correction appears in *Circulation*. 2017 Mar 21;135(12):e790], *Circulation* 135(12):e686–e725, 2016, https://doi.org/10.1161/CIR.0000000000000470.

Hageman D, Fokkenrood HJ, Gommans LN, van den Houten MM, Teijink JA: Supervised exercise therapy versus home-based exercise therapy versus walking advice for intermittent claudication, *Cochrane Database Syst Rev* 4(4):CD005263, 2018, https://doi.org/10.1002/14651858.CD005263.pub4. Published 2018 Apr 6.

Huber TS, Commentary Anand, Yusuf Xie, et al: The Warfarin Antiplatelet Vascular Evaluation Trial Investigators. Oral anticoagulation and antiplatelet therapy and peripheral arterial disease, *N Engl J Med* 357:217–227, 2007, https://doi.org/10.1177/1531003508319779. Perspect Vasc Surg Endovasc Ther. 2008;20(4):383-384.

Lu Y, Ballew SH, Tanaka H, et al: 2017 ACC/AHA blood pressure classification and incident peripheral artery disease: The Atherosclerosis Risk in Communities (ARIC) Study, *Eur J Prev Cardiol* 27(1):51–59, 2020, https://doi.org/10.1177/2047487319865378.

Murphy TP, Cutlip DE, Regensteiner JG, et al: Supervised exercise, stent revascularization, or medical therapy for claudication due to aortoiliac peripheral artery disease: the CLEVER study [published correction appears in *J Am Coll Cardiol*. 2015 May 12;65(18):2055], *J Am Coll Cardiol* 65(10):999–1009, 2015, https://doi.org/10.1016/j.jacc.2014.12.043.

PREMATURE BEATS

Method of
Randell Wexler, MD, MPH; and T.M. Ayodele Adesanya, MD, PhD

CURRENT DIAGNOSIS

- The cause of a premature beat may be either atrial (premature atrial contractions or PAC) or ventricular (premature ventricular contractions or PVC) in origin.
- PACs are most often benign but are associated with increased risk of atrial fibrillation.
- PVCs may be benign, but underlying ischemia or structural heart disease is not uncommon and must be ruled out with echocardiography.
- PACs and PVCs are most commonly diagnosed by EKG although Holter or event monitoring may be required.
- A heavier PVC burden is associated with increased development of cardiomyopathy and cardiovascular morbidity and mortality.

CURRENT THERAPY

- PACs are treated if their presence causes the patient symptoms and interferes with daily life.
- Beta blockers are most often used for the treatment of symptomatic PACs.
- In patients with underlying structural heart disease, the treatment of PVCs is directed at the underlying cardiac condition.
- Antiarrhythmics show no benefit in treatment of PVCs in patients with cardiomyopathy and should not be used to suppress their presence post myocardial infarction.
- Patients with a PVC burden of > 15% should see an EPS specialist for evaluation and treatment, as there is an increased risk of a significant cardiac arrhythmia.

It is not uncommon for a patient to present to a primary care physician with the complaint of their "heart pounding," "skipping beats," or having "palpitations." Though often the only symptom, patients may also complain of concomitant dizziness, lightheadedness, or

Epidemiology

Venous thromboembolism (VTE) includes deep venous thrombosis (DVT) and pulmonary embolism (PE). VTE affects up to 900,000 patients per year and results in up to 300,000 deaths per year. The incidence has remained constant and may be increasing since the 1980s and increases with age. The annual VTE rate among persons of European ancestry ranges from 104 to 183 per 100,000 person years. Overall VTE incidence may be higher in Black populations and lower in Asians and Asian- and Native Americans. The increasing prevalence of obesity, cancer, and surgery account in part for the persistent VTE incidence. Treatment of an acute VTE appears to be associated with incremental direct medical costs of $12,000 to $15,000 (2014 US dollars) with subsequent complications to increase cumulative costs up to $18,000 to $23,000 per incident case. Sequelae from VTE including recurrent VTE, postthrombotic syndrome (PTS), ulcers, and varicosities increase the incident cost by an average of 75%. The annual incident cost to the US healthcare system is $7 to $10 billion dollars each year.

Risk Factors

Risk factors for VTE include acquired and genetic factors. Acquired factors include increasing age, malignancy, surgery, immobilization, trauma, oral contraceptives and hormone replacement therapy, pregnancy and the puerperium, neurologic disease, cardiac disease, obesity, sepsis, pneumonia, calf muscle pump dysfunction, and inflammatory bowel disease. Genetic factors include antithrombin deficiency, protein C deficiency and protein S deficiency, factor V Leiden, prothrombin 20210A, blood group non-O, abnormalities in fibrinogen and plasminogen, elevated levels of clotting factors (e.g., factors XI, IX, VII, VIII, X, and II), and elevation in plasminogen activator inhibitor-1. When a patient presents with an unprovoked VTE, family history of thrombosis, recurrent thrombosis, or thrombosis in unusual locations, a workup for hypercoagulability, including testing for the conditions noted in the previous sentence, may be indicated, although even in these situations testing is controversial. Routine testing for hypercoagulable states in the setting of a provoked DVT is generally not indicated. Hematologic diseases associated with VTE include heparin-induced thrombocytopenia and thrombosis syndrome, disseminated intravascular coagulation, antiphospholipid antibody syndrome, myeloproliferative disorders, thrombotic thrombocytopenic purpura, and hemolytic uremic syndrome. There are a number of risk prediction scores that have been advanced, the most widely used being the Caprini risk score (https://www.mdcalc.com/caprini-score-venous-thromboembolism-2005). Using the score, factors that have been found to be associated with VTE are counted and summed, and a score is then calculated, which indicates VTE risk, especially in the context of surgical interventions. Others risk prediction scores include the Roger's score assessing the risk of postoperative VTE among non-cardiac surgery patients, the IMPROVE risk score for hospitalized patients, the Padua score for hospitalized medical patients, and the Khorana score to select ambulatory cancer patients for thromboprophylaxis.

Pathophysiology

Although Virchow's triad of stasis, vein injury, and hypercoagulability has defined the events that predispose to VTE formation since the mid-19th century, the understanding today of events that occur at the level of the vein wall and thrombus, including the inflammatory response on thrombogenesis, thrombus resolution, and the subsequent changes to the vein wall and venous valves, is increasingly becoming apparent and may direct therapy in the future. COVID-19 has also been associated with the development of VTE. Infection with COVID-19 induces overlapping pathways that link the inflammatory response to the coagulation response. The overwhelming inflammatory response in patients with COVID-19 infection leads to a hypercoagulable state, microthrombosis, large vessel thrombosis, and ultimately can lead to death. The endothelium in multiple organs, especially the lungs, appears to play a significant role in the process going from reversible dysfunction to irreversible endothelial dysfunction. In COVID-19 critically ill patients, the rate of VTE has generally been reported between 20% and 40%.

Diagnosis

Deep Venous Thrombosis

The diagnosis of DVT can be ruled out with a clinical scoring system known as the Wells score (https://www.mdcalc.com/wells-criteria-dvt) and a negative D-dimer. Wells has classified patients into a system that emphasizes physical presentation, and the most common physical finding is edema. Characteristics that score points in the Wells system include active cancer, paralysis or paresis, recent plaster/cast immobilization of the lower extremity, being recently bedridden for 3 days or more, localized tenderness along the distribution of the deep venous system, swelling of the entire leg, calf swelling that is at least 3 cm larger on the involved side than on the noninvolved side, pitting edema in the symptomatic leg, collateral superficial veins (nonvaricose), and a history of previous DVT. With extensive proximal iliofemoral DVT there may be significant swelling, cyanosis, and dilated superficial collateral veins. The negative predictive value of a low- or intermediate-risk patient as stratified by Wells score and a negative D-dimer is near 100%. The incidence of DVT over the next 3 months in this patient cohort is 0.0% to 0.6%, suggesting that additional testing is unlikely to improve outcomes.

Duplex ultrasound imaging is the gold standard for ruling in the diagnosis of DVT. Duplex imaging includes both a B-mode image and Doppler flow pattern. Duplex imaging demonstrates sensitivity and specificity rates greater than 95%. According to the grade criteria for the strength of medical evidence, duplex ultrasound is given a 1B level of evidence, depending on the pretest probability for DVT. Even at the level of the calf, duplex imaging is an acceptable technique in symptomatic patients. Duplex imaging is painless, requires no contrast, can be repeated, and is safe during pregnancy. Duplex imaging also identifies other causes of a patient's symptoms. Other tests available for making the diagnosis include magnetic resonance imaging (MRI) (especially good for assessing central pelvic vein and inferior vena cava [IVC] thrombosis) and spiral computed tomography (CT) scanning (especially with chest imaging during examination for PE).

A single complete negative lower extremity duplex scan is accurate enough to withhold anticoagulation with minimal long-term adverse thromboembolic complications. This requires that all venous segments of the leg have been imaged and evaluated. If the duplex scan is indeterminate owing to technical issues or to edema, treatment may be based on factors such as biomarkers, with the duplex repeated in 24 to 72 hours. Combining clinical characteristics with a high-sensitivity D-dimer assay can decrease the number of duplex scans performed in the low-risk patient. Although clinical characteristics and D-dimer levels are useful to rule out thrombosis, the converse is not true, and there is no combination of biomarkers and clinical presentation that can rule in the diagnosis. Work is ongoing to establish new biomarkers based on the inflammatory response to DVT. We have data suggesting that a combination of soluble P-selectin and the Wells score can rule in the diagnosis of DVT, whereas D-dimer plus Wells is still the best combination to rule out the diagnosis of DVT.

Conditions that may be confused with DVT include lymphedema, muscle strain, muscle contusion, and systemic problems such as cardiac, renal, or hepatic abnormalities. These systemic problems usually lead to bilateral edema.

Rarely, massive iliofemoral DVT can result in phlegmasia alba dolens (white swollen leg) or phlegmasia cerulean dolens (blue swollen leg). If phlegmasia is not aggressively treated, it can lead to venous gangrene when the arterial inflow becomes obstructed owing to venous hypertension. Alternatively, arterial emboli or spasm can occur and contribute to the pathophysiology. Venous gangrene is often associated with underlying malignancy and is always preceded by phlegmasia cerulea dolens. Venous gangrene is associated with significant rates of amputation and PE and with mortality.

Pulmonary Embolism

The diagnosis of PE historically has involved ventilation-perfusion scanning and pulmonary angiography. However, the most current techniques include spiral CT scanning and MRI, along with assessments of pretest probability and high-sensitivity D-dimer measurements. Age-adjusted D-dimer measurements may increase the diagnostic usefulness of these measurements. CT scanning demonstrates excellent specificity and sensitivity. Emboli down to the subsegmental level can be identified. The sensitivity for isolated chest CT imaging is increased when clinical analysis is added and when adding lower extremity imaging to the chest scan, although with the introduction of higher resolution multidetector-row CT imaging, the need for lower extremity imaging combined with CT is being questioned. Useful alternate techniques when there are contraindications to CT imaging include MRI and ventilation-perfusion imaging.

In low-risk individuals, a score of 0 on the PE Rule-out Criteria (https://www.mdcalc.com/perc-rule-pulmonary-embolism) gives confidence that further testing (D-dimer and CT) is not necessary. The PE Rule-out Criteria include (1) age older than 50 years, (2) pulse less than 100 beats/min, (3) oxygen saturation greater than 95% on room air, (4) absence of unilateral leg swelling, (5) absence of hemoptysis, (6) no recent trauma or surgery, (7) no prior history of VTE, and (8) no exogenous estrogen use.

Axillary and Subclavian Vein Thrombosis

Thrombosis of the axillary and subclavian veins accounts for less than 5% of all cases of DVT. However, it may be associated with PE in up to 10% to 15% of cases and can be the source of significant disability. Upper extremity DVT may be primary (approximately 20%), such as from thoracic outlet syndrome, effort thrombosis, or idiopathic, or secondary (approximately 80%), such as from catheter-related, cancer-associated, surgery-related, or mediastinal tumors. Primary axillary and subclavian vein thrombosis results from obstruction of the axillary vein in the thoracic outlet from compression by the subclavius muscle and the costoclavicular space, the Paget-Schrötter syndrome, noted especially in muscular athletes. Patients with axillary and subclavian vein thrombosis present with arm pain, edema, and cyanosis. Superficial venous distention may be apparent over the arm, forearm, shoulder, and anterior chest wall.

Upper extremity venous duplex ultrasound scanning is used to make the diagnosis of axillary and subclavian vein thrombosis. A secondary DVT (such as related to a central venous catheter or other risk factor) is treated with anticoagulation alone, with the same recommendation regarding anticoagulant type, dose, and duration. If Paget-Schrötter syndrome is suspected, thrombolysis and phlebography are considered as next interventions. If phlebography is performed, it is important that the patient undergo positional phlebography with the arm abducted to 120 degrees to confirm extrinsic subclavian vein compression at the thoracic outlet once the vein has been cleared of thrombus. Because a cervical rib may be the cause of such obstruction, chest x-ray should be obtained to exclude its presence (although its incidence is quite low). Ultimately, decompression of the thoracic outlet with first rib resection (and cervical rib, if present), is necessary to prevent recurrent DVT.

Treatment

Standard Therapy for Venous Thromboembolism

The traditional treatment of VTE is systemic anticoagulation, which reduces the risk of PE, extension of thrombosis, and thrombus recurrence. Because the recurrence rate for VTE is higher if anticoagulation is not therapeutic in the first 24 hours, immediate anticoagulation should be undertaken. For PE, this usually means anticoagulation followed by testing. For DVT, because duplex imaging is rapidly obtained, usually testing precedes anticoagulation. Recurrent DVT

can still occur in up to one-third of patients over an 8-year period, even with appropriate anticoagulant therapy.

The first line of therapy in the modern-day treatment of VTE is DOACs. Currently four DOACs are approved by the US Food and Drug Administration (FDA) for the treatment of DVT and one for prophylaxis of VTE. These include rivaroxaban (Xarelto) and apixaban (Eliquis) as oral monotherapy (both require a loading dose period followed by a lower dose) and dabigatran (Pradaxa) and edoxaban (Savaysa), which require a LMWH bridge, and betrixaban (Bevyxxa)[2] for prophylaxis. Alternatively, LMWH or unfractionated heparin is given for 5 days, during which time oral anticoagulation with vitamin K antagonists (warfarin) is begun and LMWH is discontinued as soon as anticoagulation is therapeutic. With warfarin, it is recommended that the international normalized ratio be therapeutic for 2 consecutive days before stopping heparin or LMWH.

The new oral anticoagulants are favored over warfarin for acute VTE and no cancer. Dabigatran targets activated factor II (factor IIa), whereas rivaroxaban, apixaban, and edoxaban target activated factor X (factor Xa). Dabigatran etexilate is FDA approved for stroke and systemic embolization prevention in patients with nonvalvular atrial fibrillation, for treatment and reduction of DVT and PE in patients who have been treated with a parenteral anticoagulant for 5 to 10 days, and for reducing the risk of recurrence of DVT and PE in adult patients who have been previously treated. It is approved for DVT prophylaxis after hip replacement. Dabigatran etexilate has also been approved in oral pellet form for the treatment of venous thromboembolic events (VTE) in pediatric patients 8 to younger than 18 years of age who have been treated with a parenteral anticoagulant for at least 5 days, and to reduce the risk of recurrence of VTE in pediatric patients 8 to younger than 18 years of age who have been previously treated.

Rivaroxaban is FDA approved for VTE prophylaxis in patients undergoing hip or knee replacements, for stroke and systemic embolization prevention in patients with nonvalvular atrial fibrillation, for VTE treatment, and for reduction in the risk of recurrence of DVT and PE. Rivaroxaban has also been approved to prevent VTE in certain adult patients hospitalized for an acute illness and for those patients after discharge who are at higher risk of VTE due to the decreased ability to move without a high risk of bleeding. It has also received two pediatric indications: (1) the treatment of VTE and reduction in the risk of recurrent VTE in patients from birth to younger than 18 years of age after at least 5 days of initial parenteral anticoagulant treatment, and (2) thromboprophylaxis in children age 2 years and older with congenital heart disease who have undergone a Fontan procedure. Apixaban is currently FDA approved for the prevention of complications of nonvalvular atrial fibrillation, for prophylaxis of DVT after hip or knee replacement surgery, for the treatment of DVT/PE, and for the reduction in risk of recurrence of DVT/PE. Edoxaban has been approved for prevention of stroke and non–CNS systemic embolism in patients with nonvalvular atrial fibrillation and for treating DVT and PE in patients who have been treated with a parenteral anticoagulant for 5 to 10 days. Betrixaban[2] is indicated for the prophylaxis of VTE in adult patients hospitalized for an acute medical illness who are at risk for thromboembolic complications due to restricted mobility and other risk factors. When an anticoagulant bridge is required, LMWH is the standard for initial treatment. LMWH is preferred because it is administered subcutaneously, it requires no monitoring (except in certain circumstances such as renal insufficiency or morbid obesity), and it is associated with a lower bleeding potential. Additionally, LMWH demonstrates less direct thrombin inhibition, more factor Xa inhibition, and antiinflammatory properties. Compared with standard unfractionated heparin, LMWH has significantly improved bioavailability, less endothelial cell binding and protein binding, and an improved pharmacokinetic profile. The half-life of LMWH is dose independent. LMWH is administered in a weight-based fashion.

---

[2]Not available in the United States.

TABLE 1 Case Scenarios for Treatment and Prevention of Venous Thrombosis

	INITIAL MANAGEMENT		DECISION POINT	
	PRIMARY TREATMENT (3–6 MONTHS)		SECONDARY PREVENTION	
CASE	INITIAL MANAGEMENT	PRIMARY TREATMENT	SECONDARY PREVENTION	
Provoked DVT of right leg following a prolonged car ride in an otherwise healthy 61-year-old man	Apixaban 10 mg BID for 7 days or rivaroxaban 15 mg daily for 21 days	Apixaban 5 mg BID for 3 months or rivaroxaban 20 mg daily for 3 months	None	
PE in 79-year-old man with prostate cancer	Apixaban 10 mg bid for 7 days	Apixaban 5 mg bid	Apixaban 5 mg BID	
Pulmonary emboli in a 48-year-old with ESRD	Intravenous heparin	Vitamin K antagonist (Warfarin)	None (secondary to bleeding risk with ESRD)	
Unprovoked DVT in a 50-year-old male with factor V Leiden	Apixaban 10 mg BID for 7 days or rivaroxaban 15 mg daily for 21 days	Apixaban 5 mg BID for 3 months or rivaroxaban 20 mg daily for minimum of 3–6 months	Apixaban 2.5 mg BID, rivaroxaban 10 mg daily or low-dose aspirin	

BID, Twice daily; *DVT*, deep venous thrombosis; *ESRD*, end-stage renal disease.

Warfarin (Coumadin), when used, should be started after heparinization is therapeutic to prevent warfarin-induced skin necrosis. For standard unfractionated heparin, this requires a therapeutic activated partial thromboplastin time (aPTT); for LMWH, warfarin is administered after an appropriate weight-based dose of LMWH is administered and allowed to circulate. Warfarin causes inhibition of protein C and S before factors II, IX, and X, leading to paradoxical hypercoagulability at the initiation of therapy. The goal for warfarin dosing is an international normalized ratio between 2.0 and 3.0.

Fondaparinux (Arixtra) is also approved for the treatment of VTE. It is a synthetic pentasaccharide that has an antithrombin sequence identical to heparin and targets factor Xa. Fondaparinux has been additionally approved for thrombosis prophylaxis in patients with total hip replacement, total knee replacement, and hip fracture; in extended prophylaxis in patients with hip fracture; and in patients undergoing abdominal surgery. It is administered subcutaneously and has a 17-hour half-life. Dosage is based on body weight. It exhibits no endothelial or protein binding and does not produce thrombocytopenia. However, no antidote is readily available. For the treatment of VTE, fondaparinux was found equal to LMWH for DVT, and for PE, it was found equal to standard heparin.

In patients with acute proximal DVT of the leg or acute PE, the most recent *Chest* guidelines suggest anticoagulation therapy alone over interventional therapy such as thrombolytic, mechanical, or pharmacochemical therapy. Specifically, DOACs are suggested over vitamin K antagonist therapy and LMWH if the patient does not have cancer.

Although LMWH has been the historic standard of care for treating cancer-associated VTE, the DOACS edoxaban[1] and rivaroxaban[1] have been found effective but with a higher risk of bleeding than LMWH. A recent study found that apixaban[1] at therapeutic dose was noninferior to the LMWH dalteparin (Fragmin) with no increased risk of major bleeding for treatment of cancer-associated VTE. Rivaroxaban and edoxaban were associated with higher risk of GI major bleeding when compared with LMWH in cancer-related VTE; so for those patients with luminal GI malignancies, LMWH or apixaban is preferred.

With significant thrombotic complications with COVID-19, there are many studies ongoing evaluating anticoagulant prophylaxis and treatment in these patients, to treat not only diagnosed macrothrombosis but also microthrombosis with the intent to improve mortality. Regarding prophylaxis, the NIH COVID-19 Treatment Guidelines Panel recently updated their recommendations. The panel does not recommend for or against routine VTE screening for COVID-19 patients without symptoms of VTE. They do recommend beginning therapeutic anticoagulation in patients with high clinical suspicion for thromboembolic disease but where

diagnostic imaging may not be possible or available. The guidelines state to approach VTE prophylaxis for COVID-19 patients compared with the usual standard of care for those without COVID-19 and does not recommend ongoing VTE prophylaxis after hospital discharge. Regarding treatment, therapeutic-dose heparin (LMWH preferred) should be used for patients who have a D-dimer above the upper level of normal, require low-flow oxygen, and have no increased bleeding risk (platelet count <50 x 10^9/L, hemoglobin <8g/dL, need for dual antiplatelet medication, known bleeding within the past 30 days, known history of bleeding disorder, or an inherited or active acquired bleeding disorder). Prophylactic dose heparin should be used for those patients who are receiving intensive care unit level of care. Intermediate or therapeutic dose heparin is not recommended in these patients. Several randomized trials have demonstrated that therapeutic anticoagulation does not decrease mortality in these very sick patients but may have a higher risk of bleeding events.

Duration of Treatment

The recommended duration of anticoagulation after a first episode of provoked VTE is 3 months for both proximal and distal thrombi (if symptomatic) (Table 1). After a second episode of VTE, the usual recommendation is prolonged oral anticoagulation indefinitely, unless the patient is at high bleeding risk (two or more risk factors) or the patient is very young at the time of presentation. VTE recurrence is increased with homozygous factor V Leiden and prothrombin 20210A mutation, protein C or protein S deficiency, antithrombin deficiency, antiphospholipid antibodies, and cancer until resolved. Long-term oral anticoagulation is usually recommended in these situations. However, heterozygous factor V Leiden and prothrombin 20210A do not carry the same risk as their homozygous counterparts, and the length of oral anticoagulation is shortened for these conditions.

Regarding unprovoked DVT, in those with a low bleeding risk, the recommended length of treatment is extended therapy for more than 3 months, provided the patient is at low or moderate risk of bleeding. Patients at high risk of bleeding should be treated for 3 months and reevaluated. Predicted risk of VTE recurrence and patient preference can be used to guide decision making on who should continue anticoagulation therapy. In patients with VTE in the setting of a minor risk factor (admission to hospital for less than 3 days, surgery with general anesthesia for less than 30 min, estrogen therapy, pregnancy, leg injury with reduced mobility) or major transient risk factor (confined to bed for at least 3 days, surgery with general anesthesia for greater than 30 min), anticoagulation therapy beyond 3 months is not recommended. In patients diagnosed with unprovoked VTE or provoked with an ongoing persistent risk factor, continued anticoagulation with a DOAC is recommended while a vitamin K antagonist is recommended for those with contraindications to DOACs. Additional

[1]Not FDA approved for this indication.

tools that can aid in the decision making to continue or discontinue anticoagulation include thrombosis risk factors, residual thrombus burden, and coagulation system activation. The HERDOO2 score (https://www.mdcalc.com/herdoo2-rule-discontinuing-anticoagulation-unprovoked-vte) has been suggested as a way for identifying women at low risk of recurrent VTE for whom anticoagulation can be stopped.

Extended therapy is now recommended with low-dose DOACs when the risk-benefit relationship favors continued treatment. Extended rivaroxaban showed a significant decrease in recurrent VTE without a significant increase in major bleeding compared with aspirin for an additional 6 to 12 months of therapy after initial therapy. Apixaban as extended treatment of VTE has also been found to provide long-term protection against recurrent VTE. After initial treatment, an additional 12 months of apixaban therapy has been compared with placebo. There was a significant decrease in the rate of VTE without an increase in bleeding risk. In patients who cannot continue on DOACs after initial therapy for VTE and who do not have a contraindication, aspirin should be administered to prevent recurrent thrombosis. Bridging has been a complicated issue when patients on chronic anticoagulation with vitamin K antagonists (with long 5–7 days' half-lives) must undergo an operative procedure and the anticoagulation must be stopped and restarted. However, in low- to moderate-risk patients, bridging is associated with no decrease in thrombotic events but with a higher bleeding risk. In fact, bridging is only indicated currently in those patients with atrial fibrillation and a recent stroke, atrial fibrillation and a high $CHADS_2$ score (5–6), a recent VTE within the past 3 months, and mechanical cardiac valves, especially mitral valves. The availability of DOACs, with short half-lives, has dramatically decreased the need for LMWH-based bridging. In most circumstances, DOACs need to be held only for 1 day for minor procedures and 2 days for major procedures and can be started back as soon as it is felt safe from the surgical or procedural perspective.

Complications

Bleeding is the most common complication of anticoagulation. Risk factors for bleeding while on anticoagulation include age >65, previous bleeding, cancer, renal or liver failure, thrombocytopenia, previous stroke, diabetes, anemia, concurrent antiplatelet therapy, poor anticoagulant control, recent surgery, frequent falls, alcohol abuse, and nonsteroidal antiinflammatory drug use. Presence of zero risk factors (low risk) confers an absolute risk of major bleeding of 0.8% per year. Patients with one risk factor have a risk of 1.6% per year, and those with two or more have a 6.5% risk or higher per year. With standard heparin, bleeding occurs over the first 5 days in approximately 10% of patients. Warfarin is associated with a major bleeding rate of 1% to 2% per year. Even with the new DOACS, bleeding (major plus minor) may occur in 5% to 10% of cases, although the risk of intracerebral bleeding appears to be less than with warfarin. A recent real-world study of non-valvular atrial fibrillation patients suggested that rates of bleeding may be different between DOACs, with ranges between 11% and 16%. Problems specific to the DOACs include the difficulty to reliably reverse their anticoagulant effects and the difficulty with laboratory monitoring. A monoclonal antibody idarucizumab (Praxbind) for the reversal of dabigatran and a recombinant modified human Factor Xa protein andexanet alfa (Andexxa) for the reversal of Factor Xa inhibitors have been FDA approved; however, expense may limit their use. Aripazine[5] (a Factor Xa inhibitor) is under development for the neutralization of apixaban, rivaroxaban, edoxaban, and dabigatran.

Heparin-induced thrombocytopenia (HIT) occurs in 0.6% to 30% of patients. Although historically morbidity and mortality rates have been high, it has been found that early diagnosis and appropriate treatment have decreased these rates. HIT usually begins 3 to 14 days after unfractionated heparin is begun, although it can occur earlier if the patient has been exposed to heparin in the past. A heparin-dependent antibody binds to platelets, activates them with the release of procoagulant microparticles, leading to an increase in thrombocytopenia, and results in both arterial and venous thrombosis. Both bovine and porcine unfractionated heparin and LMWH have been associated with HIT, although the incidence and severity of the thrombosis is less with LMWH. Even small exposures to heparin, such as heparin coating on indwelling catheters, can cause the syndrome. The diagnosis should be suspected with a 50% or greater drop in platelet count, when the platelet count falls below $100,000/\mu L$, or when thrombosis occurs during heparin or LMWH therapy. The enzyme-linked immunosorbent assay detects the antiheparin antibody in the plasma. This test is highly sensitive but poorly specific. The serotonin release assay is used as a confirmatory test that is more specific but less sensitive than the enzyme-linked immunosorbent assay test.

When the diagnosis is made, heparin must be discontinued. Oral anticoagulation should not be given until an adequate alternative anticoagulant has been established and until the platelet count has normalized. Because LMWHs demonstrate high cross-reactivity with standard heparin antibodies, they cannot be substituted for standard heparin in patients with HIT. Agents that have been FDA approved as alternatives include the direct thrombin inhibitor argatroban. Fondaparinux (Arixtra)[1] has also been found effective for treatment of HIT in most cases, but it is not FDA approved for this indication.

Nonpharmacologic Treatments

The symptoms of swelling and leg fatigue can be controlled after DVT by the use of compression stockings. Additionally, walking with good compression does not increase the risk of PE, whereas it significantly decreases the incidence and severity of the PTS in small nonrandomized studies. A recent multicenter randomized trial has suggested that stockings do not prevent development of PTS after a first proximal DVT, and for that reason, the ACCP guidelines suggest not using compression stockings to prevent PTS. It must be remembered that the use of strong compression and early ambulation after DVT treatment can significantly reduce the symptoms of pain and swelling resulting from the DVT, even if the development of PTS is not prevented, and a recent study suggests that certain surrogate markers for PTS may be lessened by the application of immediate compression, and it also reduced residual vein obstruction, which correlated with PTS. Thus, the story on the use of compression stockings to prevent PTS is still evolving.

Aggressive Therapies for Venous Thromboembolism

The goals of DVT treatment are to prevent extension or recurrence of DVT, prevent PE, and minimize the late sequela of thrombosis, namely chronic venous insufficiency. Standard anticoagulants accomplish the first two goals but not the third goal. The PTS (venous insufficiency related to venous thrombosis) occurs in up to 30% to 50% of patients after DVT and in an even higher percentage of patients with iliofemoral level DVT. It has been hypothesized that reopening the vein will alleviate venous hypertension or prevent PTS. This is known as the "open vein hypothesis." The following evidence suggests more aggressive therapies for extensive thrombosis are indicated: experimentally, prolonged contact of the thrombus with the vein wall increases damage. The thrombus initiates an inflammatory response in the vein wall that can lead to vein wall fibrosis and valvular dysfunction. The longer a thrombus is in contact with a vein valve, the more chance that valve will no longer function.

Venous thrombectomy has proved superior to anticoagulation over 6 months to 10 years as measured by venous patency and prevention of venous reflux. Catheter-directed thrombolysis has been used in many nonrandomized studies and, in small, randomized trials, was more effective than standard therapy. Quality of life was improved with thrombus removal, and results appear to be optimized further by combining catheter-directed thrombolysis with mechanical devices. These devices include but are not limited to the Angiojet rheolytic catheter, the EKOS ultrasound accelerated catheter, and new larger bore extraction devices (Penumbra and angiovac). With these devices, thrombolysis is hastened, the amount of thrombolytic agent is decreased, and bleeding is thus decreased. New devices now can remove thrombus without the need for thrombolysis, including rheolytic, clot-capture, and aspiration devices. Additionally, the use of venous stents for iliac venous obstruction has been shown to decrease the incidence of PTS, decrease chronic venous insufficiency, and improve disease-specific quality of life at 1, 6, and 24 months after the treatment.

To more fully elucidate the role of aggressive therapy in proximal iliofemoral venous thrombosis, the ATTRACT trial randomized 692 patients with acute proximal DVT to either anticoagulation alone or anticoagulation plus pharmacomechanical thrombolysis. This study found that more aggressive therapy did not decrease the incidence of PTS but did result in more major bleeding. The severity of the PTS was lessened by the pharmacomechanical thrombolysis, suggesting that more aggressive therapy should be offered to patients with significant iliofemoral venous thrombosis, who do not respond appropriately to a course of anticoagulation. This result also suggests that other factors need to be addressed to prevent PTS in addition to opening up the thrombosed vein.

For PE, evidence exists that thrombolysis is indicated when there is hemodynamic compromise from the embolism. It is controversial whether thrombolysis should be used in situations in which there is no hemodynamic compromise, but there is evidence of right heart dysfunction or there are positive biomarkers. For PE, PE response teams (PERTs) have become common, and they allow for a multidisciplinary group of providers to treat PE in a rapid and coordinated fashion. These teams include (for example) noninvasive clinicians, emergency physicians, clinical pharmacists, endovascular proceduralists, and cardiac, thoracic, and/or vascular surgeons. The efficacy of these teams for treatment of PE is an area of active investigation.

Inferior Vena Cava Filters

Traditional indications for the use of IVC filters include failure of anticoagulation, a contraindication to anticoagulation, or a complication of anticoagulation. Protection from PE is greater than 95% using cone-shaped, wire-based permanent filters in the IVC. With the success of these filters, indications have expanded to the presence of free-floating thrombus tails, prophylactic use when the risk for anticoagulation is excessive, when the risk of PE is thought to be high, and to allow the use of perioperative epidural anesthesia. IVC filters are not recommended as first-line therapy in patients who are treated with anticoagulants.

IVC filters can be either permanent or retrievable. If a retrievable filter is left, then it becomes a permanent filter; the long-term fate of these filters has yet to be defined adequately in the literature. Thus great efforts need to be made to remove retrievable IVC filters when the risk period is over. Most filters are placed in the infrarenal location in the IVC. However, they may be placed in the suprarenal position or in the superior vena cava.

Indications for suprarenal placement include high-lying thrombi, pregnancy or women of childbearing age, or previous device failure filled with thrombus. Although some have suggested that sepsis is a contraindication to the use of filters, sepsis has not been found to be a contraindication because the trapped material can be sterilized with intravenous antibiotics. Filters may be inserted under x-ray guidance or using ultrasound techniques, either external ultrasound or intravascular ultrasound.

References

Ahmed Z, Hassan S, Salzman GA: Novel oral anticoagulants for venous thromboembolism with special emphasis on risk of hemorrhagic complications and reversal agents, *Curr Drug Ther* 11:3–20, 2016.

Amin EE, Bistervels IM, Meijer K: Reduced incidence of vein occlusion and post-thrombotic syndrome after immediate compression for deep vein thrombosis, *Blood* 132:2298–2304, 2018.

ATTACC Investigators; ACTIV-4a Investigators; REMAP Investigators, et al: Therapeutic anticoagulation with heparin in noncritically ill patients with COVID-19, *N Eng J Med* 385(9):790–802, 2021.

Bruinstroop E, Klok FA, Van De Ree MA: Elevated D-dimer levels predict recurrence in patients with idiopathic venous thromboembolism: a meta-analysis, *J Thromb Haemost* 7:611–618, 2009.

Elsharawy M, Elzayat E: Early results of thrombolysis vs. anticoagulation in iliofemoral venous thrombosis. A randomised clinical trial, *Eur J Vasc Endovasc Surg* 24(3):209–214, 2002.

Freund Y, Cachanado M, Aubry A: Effect of the pulmonary embolism rule-out criteria on subsequent thromboembolic events among low-risk emergency department patients: the PROPER Randomized Clinical Trial, *J Am Med Assoc* 319(6):559–566, 2018.

Gross PL, Weitz JI: New anticoagulants for treatment of venous thromboembolism, *Arterioscler Thromb Vasc Biol* 28:380–386, 2008.

Grosse SD, Nelson RE, Nyarko KA, Richardson LC, Raskob GE: The economic burden of incident venous thromboembolism in the United States: a review of estimated attributable healthcare costs, *Thromb Res* 137:3–10, 2016.

Guyatt GH, Akl EA, Crother M: Executive summary: antithrombotic therapy and prevention of thrombosis: American College of Chest Physicians' evidence based clinical practice guidelines, ed 9, *Chest* 141:7S–47S, 2012.

Heit JA, Spencer FA, White RH: The epidemiology of venous thromboembolism, *J Thromb Thrombolysis* 41:3–14, 2016.

Heit JA, Ashrani AA, Crusan DJ, McBane RD, Petterson TM, Bailey KR: Reasons for the persistent incidence of venous thromboembolism, *Thromb Haemost* 117:390–400, 2017.

Hull RD, Pineo GF, Brant R: Home therapy of venous thrombosis with long-term LMWH versus usual care: patient satisfaction and post-thrombotic syndrome, *Am J Med* 122:762–769, 2009.

Kahn SR, Shapiro S, Wells PS: Compression stockings to prevent post-thrombotic syndrome: a randomized placebo controlled trial, *Lancet* 383:880–888, 2014.

Kahn SR, Julian JA, Kearon C: Quality of life after pharmacomechanical catheter-directed thrombolysis for proximal deep venous thrombosis, *J Vasc Surg Venous Lymphat Disord* 8:8–23, 2020.

Kearon C, Akl EA, Comerota AJ: Antithombotic therapy and VTE disease. Antithombotic therapy and prevention of thrombosis: American College of Chest Physicians Evidence-Based Clinical Practice Guidelines, ed 9, *Chest* 141(Suppl):e419S–e494S, 2012.

Kearon C, Aki EA, Ornelas J: Antithrombotic therapy for VTE disease: chest guideline and Expert Panel Report, *Chest* 149:315–352, 2016.

Knepper J, Horne D, Obi A, Wakefield TW: A systematic update on the state of novel anticoagulants and a primer on reversal and bridging, *J Vasc Surg Venous Lymphat Disord* 1:418–426, 2013. 26.

Kucher N: Deep-vein thrombosis of the upper extremity, *N Engl J Med* 364:861–869, 2011.

Merli G, Spyropoulos AC, Caprini JA: Use of emerging oral anticoagulants in clinical practice: translating results from clinical trials to orthopedic and general surgical patient populations, *Ann Surg* 250:219–228, 2009.

Morillo R, Jimenez D, Aibar MA: DVT management and outcome trends, 2001 to 2014, *Chest* 150:374–383, 2016.

Mismetti P, Laporte S, Pellerin O: Effect of a retrievable inferior vena cava filter plus anticoagulation vs anticoagulation alone on risk of recurrent pulmonary embolism: a randomized clinical trial, *J Am Med Assoc* 313:1627–1635, 2015.

Neglen P, Hollis KC, Olivier J: Stenting of the venous outflow in chronic venous disease: long-term stent-related outcome, clinical, and hemodynamic result, *J Vasc Surg* 46:979–990, 2007.

Palareti G, Cosmi B, Legnani C: D-dimer testing to determine the duration of anticoagulation therapy, *N Engl J Med* 355:1780–1789, 2006.

Piazza G, Campia U, Hurwitz S, et al: Registry of arterial and venous thromboembolic complications in patients with COVID-19, *J Am Coll Cardiol* 76(18):2060–2072, 2020.

REMAP-CAP; ACTIV-4a Investigators; ATTACC Investigators; et al: Therapeutic anticoagulation with heparin in critically ill patients with Covid-19, *N Eng J Med* 385(9):777–789, 2021.

Righini M, Ebadi HR, Gal GL: Diagnosis of acute pulmonary embolism, *J Thromb Haemost* 15:1251–1261, 2017.

Schulman S: Advances in the management of venous thromboembolism, *Best Pract Res Clin Haematol* 25:361–377, 2012.

Schulman S, Kearon C, Kakkar AK: Dabigatran versus warfarin in the treatment of acute venous thromboembolism, *N Engl J Med* 361(24):2342–2352, 2009.

Stein PD, Fowler SE, Goodman LR: Multidetector computed tomography for acute pulmonary embolism, *N Engl J Med* 354(22):2317–2327, 2006.

Stevens S, Woller S, Kreuziger L, Bounameaux H, Doerschug K, Geersing G-J, et al: Executive summary: antithrombotic therapy for VTE disease: second update of the CHEST Guideline and Expert Panel Report, *Chest* 160(6):2247–2259, 2021.

Tepper PG, Mardekian J, Masseria C, et al. PloS One 13(11)e0205989. https://doi.org/10.1371/journal.pone.0205989.

Turpie AG, Bauer KA, Eriksson BI: Fondaparinux vs. enoxaparin for the prevention of venous thromboembolism in major orthopedic surgery: a meta-analysis of 4 randomized double-blind studies, *Arch Intern Med* 162(16):1833–1840, 2002.

Vedantham S, Goldhaber SZ, Julian JA: Pharmacomechanical catheter-directed thrombolysis for deep-vein thrombosis, *N Engl J Med* 377:2240–2252, 2017.

Weitz JI, Jaffer IH, Fredenburgh JC: Recent advances in the treatment of venous thromboembolism in the era of the direct oral anticoagulants, *F1000Res* 6:985, 2017.

Wells PS, Anderson DR, Rodger M: Evaluation of D-dimer in the diagnosis of suspected deep-vein thrombosis, *N Engl J Med* 349(13):1227–1235, 2003.

Digestive System

ACUTE AND CHRONIC PANCREATITIS

Method of
George Van Buren II, MD; and William E. Fisher, MD

CURRENT DIAGNOSIS

- Acute pancreatitis is usually caused by gallstones, and chronic pancreatitis is usually caused by alcohol abuse.
- Other less-common causes of acute and chronic pancreatitis are considered only when gallstones and alcohol are definitively ruled out.
- Pancreatic cancer and chronic pancreatitis can sometimes be difficult to distinguish.

CURRENT THERAPY

- There has been a recent trend toward conservative medical therapy for acute and chronic pancreatitis, reserving surgery for select patients.
- In acute pancreatitis, try to avoid necrosectomy except in the setting of infected necrosis with organ failure.
- Asymptomatic pseudocysts can generally be observed.
- Persistent symptomatic pseudocysts can often be addressed endoscopically.
- Medical therapy for chronic pancreatitis includes pain management, nutrition, diabetes control, and cessation of drinking alcohol and smoking.
- Surgical treatment for chronic pancreatitis currently favors strict patient selection and consideration of various surgical techniques.

Acute Pancreatitis

Acute pancreatitis is an inflammatory disease of the pancreas that is associated with little or no fibrosis of the gland. It can be initiated by several factors including gallstones, alcohol, trauma, and infections, and in some cases it is hereditary (Box 1). Very often, patients with acute pancreatitis develop additional complications such as sepsis, shock, and respiratory and renal failure, resulting in considerable morbidity and mortality.

Epidemiology

The annual incidence of acute pancreatitis is probably about 50 cases per 100,000 population in the United States. Approximately 3000 of these cases are severe enough to lead to death. Studies worldwide have shown a rising but variable incidence of acute pancreatitis, including large increases in incidence in pediatric populations.

Risk Factors

Biliary tract stone disease accounts for 70% to 80% of the cases of acute pancreatitis. Alcoholism accounts for another 10%, and the remaining 10% to 20% is accounted for either by idiopathic disease or by a variety of iatrogenic and miscellaneous causes including trauma, endoscopy, surgery, drugs, heredity, infection, and toxins. Medications appear to cause less than 5% of all cases of acute pancreatitis. The drugs most strongly associated with the disorder are azathioprine (Imuran), 6-mercaptopurine (Purinethol), didanosine (Videx), valproic acid (Depakote), angiotensin-converting–enzyme inhibitors, and mesalamine (Asacol). It is difficult to determine whether the drug is responsible. Tobacco use has also been heavily linked to pancreatitis. Meta-analysis has shown cigarette smoking to be associated with acute pancreatitis development in a dose-response manner.

Pathophysiology

Pancreatitis begins with the activation of digestive zymogens inside acinar cells, which cause acinar cell injury. Digestive zymogens are co-localized with lysosomal hydrolase, and cathepsin-B catalyzed trypsinogen activation occurs, resulting in acinar cell injury and necrosis. This triggers acinar cell inflammatory events with the secretion of inflammatory mediators. Studies suggest that the ultimate severity of the resulting pancreatitis may be determined by the events that occur subsequent to acinar cell injury. These include inflammatory cell recruitment and activation, as well as generation and release of cytokines, reactive oxygen species, and other chemical mediators of inflammation, ultimately leading to ischemia and necrosis. Early mortality in severe acute pancreatitis is caused by a systemic inflammatory response syndrome with multiorgan failure. If the patient survives this critical early period, a septic complication caused by translocated bacteria, mostly gram-negative microbes from the intestine, leads to infected pancreatic necrosis. Late deaths are caused by infected necrosis, leading to septic shock and multiorgan failure.

Prevention

Gallstones are present in about 15% to 20% of patients older than 60 years, but only a fraction become symptomatic. Although gallstone pancreatitis can rarely be the first symptom of gallstones, most patients have symptoms of cholecystitis before developing pancreatitis. Thus it is important to make early and prompt referral of patients with symptomatic cholelithiasis for laparoscopic cholecystectomy to prevent life-threatening complications such as acute pancreatitis.

Clinical Manifestations

All episodes of acute pancreatitis begin with severe pain, generally following a substantial meal. The pain is usually epigastric, but it can occur anywhere in the abdomen or lower chest. It has been described as penetrating through to the back, and it may be relieved by the patient's leaning forward. It precedes the onset of nausea and vomiting, with retching often continuing after the stomach has emptied. Vomiting does not relieve the pain, which is more intense in necrotizing than in edematous pancreatitis.

On examination the patient may show tachycardia, tachypnea, hypotension, and hyperthermia. The temperature is usually only mildly elevated in uncomplicated pancreatitis. Voluntary and involuntary guarding can be seen over the epigastric region. The bowel sounds are decreased or absent. There are usually no

BOX 1 Common Causes of Acute Pancreatitis Gallstones

Alcoholism
Hereditary
Hypertriglyceridemia
Trauma (including iatrogenic: ERCP or surgery)
Drugs: azathioprine (Imuran), furosemide, mercaptopurine
    (Purinethol), opiates, pentamidine (Pentam), steroids,
    sulfasalazine (Azulfidine), sulindac (Clinoril), tetracycline,
    trimethoprim-sulfamethoxazole (Bactrim), valproic acid
    (Depakote)
Tumor
Infection (parasitic and viral)
Idiopathic

ERCP, Endoscopic retrograde cholangiopancreatography.

Figure 1 Computed tomographic scan confirming acute edematous pancreatitis.

palpable masses. The abdomen may be distended with intraperitoneal fluid. There may be pleural effusion, particularly on the left side. With increasing severity of disease, the intravascular fluid loss may become life-threatening as a result of sequestration of edematous fluid in the retroperitoneum. Hemoconcentration then results in an elevated hematocrit. However, there also may be bleeding into the retroperitoneum or the peritoneal cavity. In some patients (about 1%), the blood from necrotizing pancreatitis can dissect through the soft tissues and manifest as a bluish discoloration around the umbilicus (Cullen sign) or in the flanks (Grey Turner sign). The severe fluid loss can lead to prerenal azotemia, with elevated blood urea nitrogen and creatinine levels. There also may be hyperglycemia, hypoalbuminemia, and hypocalcemia sufficient in some cases to produce tetany.

Diagnosis

The definition of acute pancreatitis is based on the fulfillment of two out of three of the following criteria: clinical (upper abdominal pain), laboratory (serum amylase or lipase >3× upper limit of normal) and/or imaging (computed tomographic [CT], magnetic resonance imaging [MRI], ultrasonography) criteria. Although serum amylase is often elevated in acute pancreatitis, there is no significant correlation between the magnitude of serum amylase elevation and severity of pancreatitis. Other pancreatic enzymes also have been evaluated to improve the diagnostic accuracy of serum measurements. Specificity of these markers ranges from 77% to 96%, the highest being for lipase. Measurements of many digestive enzymes have methodologic limitations and cannot be easily adapted for quantitation in emergency laboratory studies. Because serum levels of lipase remain elevated for a longer time than total or pancreatic amylase, it is the serum indicator of highest probability of the disease.

Abdominal ultrasound examination is the best way to confirm the presence of gallstones in suspected biliary pancreatitis. It also can detect extrapancreatic ductal dilations and reveal pancreatic edema, swelling, and peripancreatic fluid collections. However, in about 20% of patients, the ultrasound examination does not provide satisfactory results because of the presence of bowel gas, which can obscure sonographic imaging of the pancreas.

A CT scan of the pancreas is more commonly used to diagnose pancreatitis. CT scanning is used to distinguish milder (nonnecrotic) forms of the disease from more severe necrotizing or infected pancreatitis, in patients whose clinical presentation raises the suspicion of advanced disease (Figures 1 and 2). Pancreatic protocol CT scan of the abdomen and pelvis is recommended when not limited by renal insufficiency: a tri-phasic thin, multislice CT scan with an arterial, venous, and delayed phase in conjunction with sagittal and coronal views; no oral contrast, instead drink 1000 cc water to opacify the stomach. The scan assesses the degree of pancreatic necrosis, peripancreatic fluid collections, and the surrounding vascular structures. This tri-phasic scan can also help to detect underlying mass lesions.

Figure 2 Computed tomographic scan confirming acute necrotizing, emphysematous pancreatitis.

Magnetic resonance cholangiopancreatography (MRCP) is also of value to assess the pancreatic duct and biliary tree. This can often reveal pancreatic ductal disruption.

Differential Diagnosis

The clinical diagnosis of pancreatitis is one of exclusion. Hyperamylasemia can also occur as a result of conditions not involving pancreatitis. The other upper abdominal conditions that can be confused with acute pancreatitis include perforated peptic ulcer and acute cholecystitis, and occasionally a gangrenous small bowel obstruction. Because these conditions often have a fatal outcome without surgery, urgent intervention is indicated in the small number of cases in which doubt persists. A tumor should be considered in a nonalcoholic patient with acute pancreatitis who has no demonstrable biliary tract disease. Approximately 1% to 2% of patients with acute pancreatitis have pancreatic carcinoma, and an episode of acute pancreatitis can be the first clinical manifestation of a periampullary tumor.

Treatment

The severity of acute pancreatitis covers a broad spectrum of illness, ranging from the mild and self-limiting to the life-threatening necrotizing variety. Some cases are so mild they can be treated in an outpatient setting. However, most cases require hospitalization for observation and diagnostic study.

A conservative approach has been advocated in the treatment of acute pancreatitis (Box 2). Severity is assessed with imaging results and clinical parameters and is quantitated with scores such as Ranson criteria (Box 3), the Atlanta classification, and the APACHE II (Acute Physiology and Chronic Health Evaluation) score. Severe acute pancreatitis is defined by associated organ dysfunction. The Atlanta classification is based on an international consensus conference held in Atlanta in 1992 and has been updated. APACHE II was designed to measure the severity of disease for adult patients admitted to intensive care units. Though not specific to pancreatitis, APACHE II can be used in an effort to differentiate patients with mild and severe acute pancreatitis. APACHE II scores of 8 points or more correlate with a mortality rate of 11% to 18%.

Upon confirmation of the diagnosis, patients with severe disease should be transferred to the intensive care unit for observation and maximum support. Adequate fluid resuscitation optimizing organ perfusion and oxygenation is essential. The use of prophylactic intravenous antibiotics in the initial stages of severe acute pancreatitis is not proved to be useful. Two randomized, controlled studies failed to show any benefit from antibiotics. Prophylactic antibiotics did not decrease the incidence of infected pancreatic necrosis or lower mortality. Data from these well-designed trials refute prior data from less-rigorous studies suggesting prophylactic antibiotics were useful. Additional studies are required, but there is increasing concern that the prolonged use of potent antibiotics might result in an increased prevalence of fungal infections and possibly increased mortality. Currently, antibiotic therapy should be reserved for treatment of specific infections such as positive blood, sputum, and urine cultures or percutaneous or operative cultures of necrotic tissue.

Randomized clinical trials have also shown a benefit from early nasojejunal feeding compared to total parenteral nutrition. Gastric decompression with a nasogastric tube is selectively used in patients with severe ileus and vomiting but is not necessary in a majority of cases. A debate remains regarding the optimal nutritional management in the majority of pancreatitis patients. There has been a trend toward oral enteric feeding in the less severe cases.

In biliary pancreatitis, the gallbladder must eventually be removed or recurrent acute pancreatitis will occur in 30% to 60% of cases. The timing of the cholecystectomy depends on the severity of the pancreatitis. Usually laparoscopic cholecystectomy is performed during the index admission as soon as the attack of acute pancreatitis has resolved. In more severe cases, the cholecystectomy is delayed and often combined with interventions for late complications of acute pancreatitis. In cases with severe comorbidity, endoscopic sphincterotomy has been considered as an alternative to cholecystectomy. However, if the patient has a postinflammatory fluid collection, bacteria can be introduced during endoscopic retrograde cholangiopancreatography (ERCP), and sphincterotomy should be delayed.

Currently, there is no role for routine early laparotomy and necrosectomy or resection in the setting of acute necrotizing pancreatitis. If the necrotic pancreas becomes infected and the patient fails to respond to conservative treatment, then necrosectomy may be warranted. Patients with infected necrosis are rarely managed conservatively without eventual surgical intervention. However, even in the setting of infected necrosis, there has been consideration for antibiotic therapy until the acute inflammatory response has subsided, if possible, with the view that surgery that is deferred for several weeks is more easily accomplished with one intervention. Patients who suffer from infected necrosis without having clinical signs of sepsis or other systemic complications might not need immediate surgical necrosectomy.

A nonsurgical alternative for the treatment of infected necrosis is percutaneous catheter drainage. This is considered a temporary measure to allow stabilization of the patient so that a safer surgical necrosectomy can be done at a later time. Multiple large drains are required, and patients frequently undergo repeat CT and revision of the drains. Current recommendations are to postpone surgery for as long as possible, usually beyond the second or third week of the disease or later, when necrotic tissue can be easily distinguished from viable pancreas and débridement without major blood loss can be performed. When surgery is performed, tissue-preserving digital necrosectomy is the usual technique rather than a classic surgical resection of the pancreas (Figure 3).

Necrosectomy can be performed by an open anterior approach with closed lavage or with leaving the abdomen open and packing. The packing is replaced at intervals of 24 to 72 hours. Sometimes a left lateral retroperitoneal approach is helpful. Newer approaches are the video-assisted retroperitoneal débridement (VARD). This procedure is a combination of percutaneous drainage and the open lateral retroperitoneal approach. An anterior laparoscopic approach has also been described and mimics the open anterior approach using laparoscopic ports. Surgical necrosectomy is indicated in patients with sepsis caused by infected necrosis and in selected patients with extended sterile necrosis causing severe systemic organ dysfunction and sepsis without a septic focus.

Figure 3 Necrotic material débrided from the retroperitoneum in a case of acute necrotizing pancreatitis.

In some cases, the acute inflammatory process can lead to erosion into retroperitoneal vessels, and acute hemorrhage occurs. This acute emergent complication is best managed with immediate angiography to determine the exact site of bleeding and can often be treated with embolization rather than surgery (Figure 4).

Although previously frowned upon, there has been a move toward enteric drainage of all necrotic collections (even when infected) when technically feasible. This can be initiated through either an endoscopic or surgical approach.

Monitoring

Despite a conservative operative approach, endocrine and exocrine insufficiency develop in as many as half of the patients and are determined by the extent of pancreatic necrosis. Therefore patients must be monitored with blood glucose measurements, stabilization of body weight, and proper nutrition.

Complications

The most common complication after successful management of acute pancreatitis is a pseudocyst. The term "pseudocyst" is currently used to broadly categorize most pancreatic and peripancreatic fluid collections (including walled-off pancreatic necrosis [WOPN] and acute peripancreatic fluid collection). The Acute Pancreatitis Classification Working Group recently proposed a revised Atlanta classification that refers to collections within 4 weeks of symptom onset as either acute peripancreatic fluid collections (APFC) or postnecrotic pancreatic fluid collections (PNPFC), depending upon the absence or presence of pancreatic/peripancreatic necrosis, respectively. After 4 weeks of the onset of symptoms, persistent collections with discrete walls are referred to as pseudocyst or WOPN, again depending upon the absence or presence of necrosis, respectively. In addition, these collections are further classified as sterile or infected and the term "pancreatic abscess" has been abolished.

The management of pseudocysts has followed a minimally invasive trend. Most pseudocysts resolve spontaneously, even beyond 6 weeks, so asymptomatic pseudocysts are usually observed (70% of pseudocysts will resolve without intervention). Endoscopic cystogastrostomy is the approach of choice for symptomatic fluid-predominant pseudocysts when there is minimal necrosis. If there is significant necrotic debris or a solid-predominant pseudocyst, surgical drainage with laparoscopic cystogastrostomy is preferred (Figure 5). This can also be performed with the traditional open technique. Cystojejunostomy (laparoscopic or open) is used in cases in which the site of the pseudocyst precludes drainage into the posterior aspect of the stomach.

Figure 4 Acute necrotizing pancreatitis. (A) Erosion into the splenic artery as seen on computed tomography. (B) Erosion into the splenic artery as seen on angiogram. (C) This complication of acute pancreatitis is best treated with angiographic embolization.

Figure 5 Computed tomographic scan showing fluid-predominant (A) and solid-predominant (B) pseudocysts. The former can be treated with endoscopic cystogastrostomy, and the latter is best treated with laparoscopic cystogastrostomy.

Chronic Pancreatitis

Chronic pancreatitis is a chronic fibro-inflammatory disease of the pancreas characterized by irreversible morphologic changes that typically are associated with pain or permanent loss of function, or both.

Epidemiology

Population studies suggest a prevalence of chronic pancreatitis that ranges from 5 to 27 persons per 100,000 population, with considerable geographic variation. Autopsy data are difficult to interpret because a number of changes associated with chronic pancreatitis, such as fibrosis, duct ectasia, and acinar atrophy, are also present in asymptomatic elderly patients. Differences in diagnostic criteria, regional nutrition, alcohol consumption, and medical access account for variations in the frequency of the diagnosis, but the overall incidence of the disease has risen progressively since the 1960s. Chronic pancreatitis in the United States currently results in more than 120,000 outpatient visits and more than 50,000 hospitalizations per year.

Risk Factors

Alcohol consumption and alcohol abuse are associated with chronic pancreatitis in up to 70% of cases. Other major causes include tropical (nutritional) and idiopathic disease, as well as hereditary causes. There is a linear relationship between exposure to alcohol and the development of chronic pancreatitis.

The incidence is highest in heavy drinkers (15 drinks/day or 150 g/d). Prolonged alcohol use (four to five drinks daily over a period of more than 5 years) is required for alcohol-associated pancreatitis; the overall lifetime risk of pancreatitis among heavy drinkers is 2% to 5%. The duration of alcohol consumption is definitely associated with the development of pancreatic disease. The onset of disease typically occurs between ages 35 and 40 years, after 16 to 20 years of heavy alcohol consumption. Recurrent episodes of acute pancreatitis are typically followed by chronic symptoms after 4 or 5 years. In most cases, chronic pancreatitis has already developed and the acute clinical presentation represents a flare superimposed on chronic pancreatitis.

Tobacco use has also been heavily linked to pancreatitis. Meta-analysis has shown that both ever and current smokers had higher risks of developing pancreatitis compared with never smokers. This causative relationship was verified by the reduced or eliminated risk after smoking cessation. In comparison with current smokers, the risk of pancreatitis decreased for those who were former smokers.

Pathophysiology

Multiple episodes (or a prolonged course) of pancreatic injury ultimately leading to chronic disease is widely accepted as the pathophysiologic sequence. Abundant data indicate that acute pancreatitis may progress to recurrent acute pancreatitis and then to chronic pancreatitis in a disease continuum. Most investigators believe that alcohol metabolites such as acetaldehyde, combined with oxidant injury, result in local parenchymal injury that is preferentially targeted to the pancreas in predisposed persons. Repeated or severe episodes of toxin-induced injury activate a cascade of cytokines, which in turn induces pancreatic stellate cells to produce collagen and cause fibrosis.

The most common form of chronic pancreatitis is the calcifying type, characterized by the development of intraductal stones; the predominant causative agent is alcohol. Progressive functional impairment can develop from the dilated main pancreatic duct. Furthermore inflammatory enlargement of the pancreatic head may cause local complications such as stenosis of the pancreatic or bile duct, duodenal obstruction, or compression of retropancreatic vessels.

The pain caused by chronic pancreatitis is thought to be due to increased pressure in the pancreatic ducts and tissue, "parenchymal hypertension" from pancreatic ductal obstruction. Neural and perineural inflammation is also thought to be important in pathogenesis of pain in chronic pancreatitis. Neuropeptides released from enteric and afferent neurons and their functional interactions with inflammatory cells might play a key role.

Prevention

Because alcohol is the cause of most cases of chronic pancreatitis, cessation of alcohol consumption is recommended to prevent progression to chronic pancreatitis. Unfortunately, the majority of patients are not able to recover from alcoholism, and relapse is common.

Clinical Manifestations

Symptoms of chronic pancreatitis may be identical to those of acute pancreatitis, typically midepigastric pain penetrating through to the back. Patients with chronic pancreatic pain typically flex their abdomen and either sit or lie with their hips flexed, or lie on their side in a fetal position. Unlike ureteral stone pain or biliary colic, the pain causes the patient to be still. Nausea or vomiting can accompany the pain, but anorexia is the most common associated symptom. Patients with continuous pain can have a complication of chronic pancreatitis, such as an inflammatory mass, a cyst, or even pancreatic cancer. Other patients have intermittent attacks of pain with symptoms similar to those of mild to moderate acute pancreatitis. The pain sometimes is severe and lasts for many hours or several days.

Figure 6 Computed tomographic scan of a patient with autoimmune pancreatitis and an inflammatory mass in the head of the pancreas. Preoperative diagnosis is not always possible, but surgery should be avoided because this disease often responds to steroid therapy.

As chronic pancreatitis progresses, endocrine and exocrine insufficiency begin to appear. Patients describe a bulky, foul-smelling, loose (but not watery) stool that may be pale and float on the surface of toilet water. Patients often describe a greasy or oily appearance to the stool or describe an "oil slick" on the water's surface. In severe steatorrhea, an orange, oily stool is often reported. As exocrine deficiency increases, symptoms of steatorrhea are often accompanied by weight loss. Patients might describe a good appetite despite weight loss, or they might have diminished food intake due to abdominal pain. The combination of decreased food intake and malabsorption of nutrients usually results in chronic weight loss. As a result, many patients with severe chronic pancreatitis are below ideal body weight. Usually islet cells are spared early in the disease process despite being surrounded by fibrosis, but eventually the insulin-secreting beta cells are also destroyed, gradually leading to diabetes.

Diagnosis

The diagnosis of chronic pancreatitis depends on the clinical presentation, a limited number of indirect measurements that correlate with pancreatic function, and selected imaging studies. Diagnosis is usually simple in the late stages of the disease because of the presence of structural and functional alterations of the pancreas. Early in the disease, the diagnosis is more difficult. Various classification systems have been developed. The Cambridge classification uses imaging tests such as ERCP, CT, and ultrasound to grade severity. The Mayo Clinic system is based on functional as well as imaging results. Tests of pancreatic function include the secretin-cerulein test, Lundh test, fecal excretion of pancreatic enzymes, and quantitation of fecal fat.

Chronic pancreatitis can be classified as calcifying (lithogenic), obstructive, inflammatory, autoimmune, tropical (nutritional), hereditary, or idiopathic. Autoimmune and hereditary pancreatitis have recently been better understood and diagnosed more than before. Autoimmune pancreatitis is associated with fibrosis, a mononuclear cell (lymphocyte, plasma cell, or eosinophil) infiltrate, and an increased titer of one or more autoantibodies. It is usually associated with autoimmune diseases such as Sjögren syndrome. Increased levels of serum β-globulin or immunoglobulin (Ig)G$_4$ are often present, however autoimmune pancreatitis can present without these markers. This disease can be mistaken for chronic pancreatitis, with an inflammatory mass in the head of the pancreas suspicious for pancreatic cancer (Figure 6). Diagnosis is important because steroid therapy is uniformly successful in ameliorating the disease, including any associated bile duct compression.

Hereditary pancreatitis first occurs in adolescence with abdominal pain; patients develop progressive pancreatic dysfunction, and the risk of cancer is greatly increased. The disease follows

---

| BOX 4 | Treatment of Chronic Pancreatitis |

Pancreatic enzyme replacement
Proper nutrition and vitamin supplementation
Blood sugar control
Long-acting narcotic analgesics at lowest effective doses
Cessation of alcohol and tobacco
Endotherapy (pancreatic duct stenting and removal of stones)
Parenchymal preserving surgery (Frey, Beger) in carefully selected patients

---

an autosomal dominant pattern of inheritance with 80% penetrance and variable expression. Recent mutational analysis has revealed a missense mutation resulting in an Arg to His substitution at position 117 of the cationic trypsinogen gene, or *PRSS1*, one of the primary sites for proteolysis of trypsin. This mutation prevents trypsin from being inactivated by itself or other proteases, and it results in persistent and uncontrolled proteolytic activity and autodestruction within the pancreas. Similarly, *PSTI*, also known as *SPINK1*, has been found to have a role in hereditary pancreatitis and some cases of sporadic chronic pancreatitis. *SPINK1* specifically inhibits trypsin action by competitively blocking the active site of the enzyme.

It is likely that many of the "idiopathic" forms of chronic pancreatitis, as well as some patients with the more common forms of the disease, will be found to have a genetic linkage or predisposition.

Differential Diagnosis

There are several clinical conditions from which chronic pancreatitis needs to be distinguished. Other causes of upper abdominal pain, such as peptic ulcer disease, biliary tract disease, mesenteric vascular disease, or malignancy must be excluded. The major difficulty in the differential diagnosis of chronic pancreatitis is distinguishing it from pancreatic ductal adenocarcinoma. Chronic pancreatitis can closely mimic pancreatic cancer, both clinically and morphologically. In addition, chronic pancreatitis is a risk factor for the development of pancreatic cancer. Although in pancreatic resection specimens this problem may be finally resolved, distinguishing these two diseases preoperatively in small (needle) biopsy specimens is a formidable challenge for the pathologist. Therefore especially in the setting of an inflammatory mass in the head of the pancreas, consideration of pancreatic cancer and surgical referral is important. Workup of these patients should include a pancreatic protocol CT scan, an MRCP, and an endoscopic ultrasound to evaluate the parenchyma and the ducts of the pancreas.

Treatment

Therapy for chronic pancreatitis is aimed at managing associated digestive dysfunction and relieving pain (Box 4). It is important to first address malabsorption, weight loss, and diabetes. When pancreatic exocrine capacity falls below 10% of normal, diarrhea and steatorrhea develop. Lipase deficiency tends to manifest itself before trypsin deficiency, so the presence of steatorrhea may be the first functional sign of pancreatic insufficiency. As pancreatic exocrine function deteriorates further, the secretion of bicarbonate into the duodenum is reduced, which causes duodenal acidification and further impairs nutrient absorption. Frank diabetes is seen initially in about 20% of patients with chronic pancreatitis, and impaired glucose metabolism can be detected in up to 70% of patients.

The medical treatment of chronic or recurrent pain in chronic pancreatitis requires the use of analgesics, a cessation of alcohol use, oral enzyme therapy, and endoscopic stent therapy. Administration of pancreatic enzyme (e.g., Pancrease MT, Pancrelipase, Creon) serves to reverse the effects of pancreatic exocrine insufficiency and might also reduce or alleviate the pain[1] experienced by patients. Interventional procedures to block visceral afferent nerve conduction or to treat obstructions of the main pancreatic

---

[1]Not FDA approved for this indication

duct are also an adjunct to medical treatment. It has been taught that the pain of chronic pancreatitis decreases with increasing duration of the disease, the so-called burn-out phase, where endocrine and exocrine insufficiency occurs and the pain decreases. However, recent studies have called this concept into question, demonstrating continued pain in patients with chronic pancreatitis despite long-standing disease and pancreatic insufficiency. Cessation of alcohol abuse, if possible, causes the pain to stop in about half of the patients.

Pain relief usually requires the use of narcotics, but these should be titrated to achieve pain relief with the lowest effective dose. Opioid addiction is common, and the use of long-acting analgesics by transdermal patch together with oral agents for pain exacerbations slightly reduces the sedative effects of high-dose oral narcotics. Celiac plexus neurolysis has been an effective form of analgesic treatment in patients with pancreatic carcinoma. However, its use in chronic pancreatitis has been disappointing, with about half of the patients deriving a benefit that lasts 6 months or less.

Pancreatic duct stenting is used for treatment of proximal pancreatic duct stenosis, decompression of a pancreatic duct leak, and drainage of pancreatic pseudocysts that can be catheterized through the main pancreatic duct. Pancreatic duct stones can also be removed endoscopically. Stent therapy in chronic pancreatitis definitely plays a role and can help select patients for successful operative therapy. However, the duration of success with stent therapy for chronic pancreatitis is probably less than with surgical therapy.

There has been significant debate over the years regarding the role and type of surgical therapy in chronic pancreatitis. Progressive functional pancreatic impairment can be delayed by surgical decompression of the dilated main pancreatic duct. Furthermore, inflammatory enlargement of the pancreatic head may cause local complications that require further treatment, such as stenosis of the pancreatic or bile duct, duodenal obstruction, or compression of retropancreatic vessels. Surgery may be superior to conservative or endoscopic treatment in terms of pain relief and preservation of pancreatic function and quality of life. Major pancreatic resections for chronic pancreatitis have a significant complication rate, both early and late. Patients with large duct disease who can have nutrition restored, are working, are not drinking alcohol, and have a supportive family structure fare better with surgical therapies. Failure to carefully select patients for either drainage or resection procedures leads to disappointing results. The surgical management of pancreatic duct stones and stenosis has been shown to be superior to endoscopic treatment in randomized clinical trials. Beger introduced the duodenum-preserving pancreatic head resection (DPPHR) in the early 1980s. Later in the decade, Frey and Smith described the local resection of the pancreatic head with longitudinal pancreaticojejunostomy, which included excavation of the pancreatic head including the ductal structures in continuity with a long ductotomy of the dorsal duct. This operation is basically a hybrid of the Beger and Puestow (Partington-Rochelle modification) procedures and is more popular in the United States (Figures 7 and 8).

Previous randomized prospective studies have compared the Whipple, Beger, and Frey procedures for chronic pancreatitis. Patients who had a Beger procedure had a shorter hospital stay, greater weight gain, less postoperative diabetes, and less exocrine dysfunction than standard Whipple patients over a 3- to 5-year follow-up. Pain control was similar between the two procedures. In a study comparing the pylorus-preserving Whipple to the Frey procedure, there was a lower postoperative complication rate associated with the Frey procedure (19%) compared to the pylorus-preserving Whipple group (53%), and the global quality-of-life scores were better (71% vs. 43%, respectively). Both operations were equally effective in controlling pain over a 2-year follow-up. Operation times, intraoperative blood loss, and transfusion requirements have been shown to be decreased with the Frey and Beger procedures compared to the Whipple

Figure 7 Computed tomographic scan of a patient with chronic calcific pancreatitis and a massively dilated pancreatic duct. (A) Axial view with calcified pancreatic head. (B) Axial view with dilated pancreatic duct.

procedure. In long-term (>8 years) follow-up, there was no difference between the Beger and Frey procedures in pain relief, pancreatic insufficiency, quality of life, and late mortality. Compared to the Whipple procedure, the Beger and Frey procedures may produce a lower incidence of immediate complications and diabetes but no significant differences in pain relief. Although these limited pancreatic procedures have a lower initial rate of endocrine dysfunction, the long-term risk of diabetes is more related to the progression of the underlying disease than to the effects of operation.

Recent multicenter randomized, controlled, double-blinded, trial compared DPPHR to partial pancreatoduodenectomy with a primary endpoint of quality of life within 24 months after surgery. The results showed that DPPHR was not superior to partial pancreatoduodenectomy in terms of the primary endpoint, long-term postoperative quality of life. With both resection and drainage procedures offering viable options for treatment, patient selection becomes critical in assuring there is clinical improvement postoperatively.

Recent refinements in the methods of harvesting and preserving pancreatic islets, and standardization of the methods by which islets are infused into the portal venous circuit for intrahepatic engraftment, have improved the success and rekindled interest in islet autotransplantation for chronic pancreatitis. The ability to recover a sufficient quantity of islets from a sclerotic gland depends on the degree of disease present, so the selection of patients as candidates for autologous islet transplantation is important. As

Figure 8 (A) The pancreatic duct is opened to reveal a preoperatively placed pancreatic duct stent. (B) The residual stones removed from the pancreatic duct. (C) In the Frey procedure, the head of the pancreas is cored out in addition to a longitudinal pancreatic ductotomy. The pancreas is drained with a Roux-en-Y limb of jejunum.

success with autotransplantation increases, patients with nonobstructive, sclerotic pancreatitis may be considered for resection and islet autotransplantation earlier in their course, because end-stage fibrosis bodes poorly for transplant success. Patient selection and surgeon experience play a very large role in the outcomes of autotransplantation.

Monitoring

Chronic pancreatitis is of course a chronic disease, so continued monitoring and maintenance therapy is essential after an acute exacerbation of chronic pancreatitis. Pain control, proper nutrition, and alcohol and smoking cessation must be maintained as an outpatient. The clinician must also be looking for the development of common complications. An annual physical exam and CT or MRI should be considered in this population to assess for the progression of disease.

Complications

Pseudocysts in the setting of chronic pancreatitis are less likely to resolve without intervention. Often, the pancreatic duct and bile duct are compressed, and the compression might need to be addressed at the same time as the pseudocyst. A trend toward minimally invasive management remains appropriate, with endoscopic drainage preferred over laparoscopic cystogastrostomy unless additional procedures are required. Resection of a pseudocyst is sometimes indicated for cysts located in the pancreatic tail, or when a midpancreatic duct disruption has resulted in a distally located pseudocyst. Distal pancreatectomy for removal of a pseudocyst, with or without splenectomy, can be a challenging procedure in the setting of prior pancreatitis. An internal drainage procedure of the communicating duct, or of the pseudocyst itself, should be considered when distal resection is being contemplated.

Pancreatic ascites results from a disrupted pancreatic duct with extravasation of pancreatic fluid that does not become sequestered as a pseudocyst but drains freely into the peritoneal cavity. Occasionally, the pancreatic fluid tracks superiorly into the thorax, causing a pancreatic pleural effusion. Both complications are seen more often in patients with chronic pancreatitis, rather than after acute pancreatitis. Paracentesis or thoracentesis reveals noninfected fluid with a protein level greater than 25 g/L and a markedly elevated amylase level. Paracentesis is critical to differentiate pancreatic from hepatic ascites.

ERCP is most helpful to delineate the location of the pancreatic duct leak and to elucidate the underlying pancreatic ductal anatomy. Pancreatic duct stenting may be considered at the time of ERCP. Paracentesis and antisecretory therapy with the somatostatin analogue octreotide acetate, together with bowel rest and parenteral nutrition, is successful in more than half of patients. Reapposition of serosal surfaces to facilitate closure of the leak is considered a part of therapy, and this is accomplished by complete paracentesis. For pleural effusions, a period of chest tube drainage can facilitate closure of the internal fistula. Surgical therapy is reserved for those who fail to respond to medical treatment.

References

Acute Pancreatitis Classification Working Group: Revision of the Atlanta Classification of Acute Pancreatitis. Available at: http://www.pancreasclub.com/resources/AtlantaClassification.pdf. [accessed 25.08.14].

Beger HG, Matsuno S, Cameron JL: *Diseases of the pancreas: Current surgical therapy*, Berlin, 2008, Springer-Verlag.

Beger HG, Warshaw AL, Buchler MW, et al: *The pancreas: An integrated textbook of basic science, medicine, and surgery*, ed 2nd, Malden, MA, 2008, Blackwell Publishing.

Cunha EF, Rocha Mde S, Pereira FP, et al: Walled-off pancreatic necrosis and other current concepts in the radiological assessment of acute pancreatitis, *Radiol Bras* 47(3):165–175, 2014.

Dellinger EP, Tellado JM, Soto NE, et al: Early antibiotic treatment for severe acute necrotizing pancreatitis: a randomized, double-blind, placebo-controlled study, *Ann Surg* 245:674–683, 2007.

Diener MK, Hüttner FJ, Kieser M, et al: Partial pancreatoduodenectomy versus duodenum-preserving pancreatic head resection in chronic pancreatitis: the multicentre, randomised, controlled, double-blind ChroPac trial, *Lancet* 390(10099):1027–1037, 2017 Sep 9. https://doi.org/10.1016/S0140-6736(17)31960-8.

Fisher WE, Anderson DK, Bell RH, et al: Pancreas. In Brunicardi FC, Andersen DK, Billiar TR, et al: *Schwartz's principles of surgery*, ed 9th, New York, 2010, McGraw-Hill, pp 1167–1243.

Forsmark CE, Vege SS, Wilcox CM: Acute Pancreatitis, *N Engl J Med* 375(20):1972–1981, 2016 Nov 17.

Impact of smoking on the risk of pancreatitis: a systematic review and meta-analysis.

Isenmann R, Runzi M, Kron M, et al: Prophylactic antibiotic treatment in patients with predicted severe acute pancreatitis: a placebo-controlled, double-blind trial, *Gastroenterology* 126:997–1004, 2004.

Working Group IAP/APA Acute Pancreatitis Guidelines: IAP/**APA** evidence-based **guidelines** for the management of acute **pancreatitis**, *Pancreatology* 13(4 Suppl 2):e1–15, 2013 Jul-Aug. https://doi.org/10.1016/j.pan.2013.07.063.

Ye X, Lu G, Huai J, Ding J: *PLoS One* 10(4):e0124075, 2015 Apr 16, https://doi.org/10.1371/journal.pone.0124075. eCollection 2015.

Zaheer A, Singh VK, Qureshi RO, Fishman EK: The revised Atlanta classification for acute pancreatitis: updates in imaging terminology and guidelines, *Abdom Imaging* 38(1):125–136, 2013.

ACUTE DIARRHEA

Method of
Joshua Davis, MD

CURRENT DIAGNOSIS

History
- Onset, duration, frequency, and type of diarrhea
- Associated symptoms (e.g., fever, abdominal pain, vomiting)
- Exposures (sick contacts, contaminated food or water, or antibiotics) or travel
- Medical history and immune status
- Current and new medications or supplements

Examination
- Dehydration assessment
- Abdominal examination

Laboratory Testing
- Not routinely needed
- May include metabolic panel for watery diarrhea with severe dehydration
- Complete blood count and stool testing, preferably by polymerase chain reaction, recommended for bloody diarrhea
- Stool testing also recommended in patients who are immunocompromised or have severe or prolonged (>7 days) illness
- Radiologic imaging and endoscopy are rarely needed

CURRENT THERAPY

Symptomatic Therapy
- Oral rehydration in mild to moderate cases of dehydration
- Parenteral rehydration in severe dehydration
- If no contraindications (e.g., fever, dysentery, possibly *Clostridioides difficile*), loperamide (Imodium) at 4 mg orally, followed by 2 mg orally with each loose stool, up to a maximum of 16 mg per day
- Bismuth subsalicylate (Pepto-Bismol) 524 mg orally four times daily for 3 weeks to prevent traveler's diarrhea[1] or as needed for symptomatic care

Antibiotic Therapy
- Antibiotics should be directed toward detected pathogens identified on testing, when they are indicated.
- Antibiotics are rarely indicated empirically or for patients who are healthy and immunocompetent with mild to moderate illness, regardless of testing results.
- Antibiotic resistance rates worldwide are rising due to overuse of antibiotics leading to resistance, particularly to fluoroquinolones.
- Empiric treatment regimens in adults include azithromycin (Zithromax)[1] 1000 mg orally once (or 500 mg twice daily for 1 to 5 days), ciprofloxacin (Cipro) 500 to 750 mg orally once (or 500 mg twice daily for 1 to 5 days), or levofloxacin (Levaquin)[1] 500 mg orally once (or 500 mg daily for 1 to 5 days).
- Empiric pediatric regimen includes azithromycin[1] 5 to 12 mg/kg orally four times daily for 3 days (max 500 mg/day) or a third-generation cephalosporin for patients younger than 3 months
- Initial *Clostridioides difficile* treatment should be either vancomycin 125 mg orally four times daily for 10 days or fidaxomicin (Dificid) 200 mg orally twice daily for 10 days
- Probiotics[7] have been shown to prevent antibiotic-associated diarrhea and *C. difficile* infections. The exact best dose and type is not known.

[1]Not FDA approved for this indication.
[7]Available as dietary supplement.

Introduction

Gastrointestinal symptoms are a common concern in primary care, leading to up to 18% of primary care visits. Acute diarrhea is the second most commonly reported illness in the United States, next to respiratory infections. Diarrhea is defined as the passage of three or more liquid stools in a day or an increase in baseline for a given patient. Some people consider diarrhea an increase in the number of stools, but stool consistency is really the hallmark. Diarrheal stool will conform to the shape of the container. Acute diarrhea is generally diarrhea lasting less than 14 days, whereas diarrhea lasting more than 14 days is termed *persistent*, and diarrhea lasting more than 30 days is *chronic*. This chapter focuses on acute diarrhea, but it is important to recognize that persistent and chronic diarrhea often start as acute diarrhea. Persistent and chronic diarrhea and recurrent bouts of acute diarrhea require a different evaluation that is outside the scope of this chapter.

Epidemiology

Acute diarrhea is a leading cause of death and disability worldwide. Diarrheal illness is the second leading cause of death for children under the age of 5 years, accounting for 18% of total deaths. This equates to about 5000 deaths per day. In developed countries like the United States, death rates are much lower. But acute diarrhea still accounts for 179 million outpatient visits, about 3% to 18% of all visits, in the United States each year. This leads to about 500,000 hospitalizations and 5000 deaths annually.

Etiology

The two major categorizations of acute diarrhea include watery (i.e., osmotic or secretory) diarrhea and bloody/mucousy diarrhea (i.e., inflammatory).

The more common type of diarrhea encountered in the acute setting in the United States is watery diarrhea. This is further broken down into osmotic and secretory diarrhea. Osmotic diarrhea is caused when a substance prevents normal water reabsorption in the intestine. It is most often seen in causes of chronic diarrhea (e.g., lactose intolerance or celiac disease), but, in the acute setting, is normally caused by medication side effects. Secretory diarrhea, on the other hand, is caused when water and electrolytes are pathologically secreted into the intestine. Secretory diarrhea is normally higher volume (>1 L/day) than osmotic diarrhea. As one would expect, the most common complication from watery diarrhea is dehydration.

Acute bloody or mucousy diarrhea is called inflammatory diarrhea or dysentery. This is normally caused by bacterial pathogens like *Salmonella, Shigella, Campylobacter,* and *Escherichia coli* or by parasites like *Entamoeba histolytica*. Patients with inflammatory diarrhea are at higher risk of infectious complications like sepsis, hemolytic uremic syndrome, seizures, or abscesses. It is important to differentiate bloody or inflammatory diarrhea from anatomic causes of gastrointestinal bleeding. Inflammatory bloody diarrhea is typically bright red and lower volume. Anatomic gastrointestinal bleeding can be bright red, maroon, dark, or tarry and is typically higher volume. Hemorrhoids will cause hematochezia but typically not diarrhea. Inflammatory diarrhea often requires further testing and laboratory workup compared with watery diarrhea.

The cause of acute diarrhea is often not identified. Viruses, namely norovirus, are the most common cause of acute diarrhea in adults. Bacteria, bacterial toxins, ova, and parasites are rarer but important causes of diarrhea as well (Table 1). In addition to the common infectious causes, noninfectious causes must also be considered. This includes medication side effects (Box 1), food intolerances, anatomic gastrointestinal bleeding, and early presentations of other gastrointestinal conditions.

Viruses

Viruses are the most common cause of acute diarrheal illness. In children, the most common pathogen is rotavirus, and, in adults, it is norovirus (also called Norwalk virus). Norovirus is

TABLE 1   Common Infectious Causes of Acute Diarrheal Illness

CAUSES	SYMPTOMS	TREATMENTS	RISK FACTORS
Norovirus and rotavirus	Watery diarrhea, fevers, vomiting	Symptomatic only	Contaminated food or water, close living quarters
Enterotoxigenic *Escherichia coli* (ETEC)	Watery diarrhea	Antibiotics rarely needed. Azithromycin,[1] fluoroquinolones, rifaximin, or trimethoprim-sulfamethoxazole	Contaminated food or water
Enterohemorrhagic *E. coli* (EHEC)	Bloody diarrhea, abdominal cramps, rashes, hemolytic uremic syndrome, seizures	Symptomatic only. Antibiotics not recommended	Unpasteurized dairy, uncooked meat, or contaminated water
Shigella	Bloody diarrhea, high fevers, abdominal cramping, rashes, hemolytic uremic syndrome, seizures	Azithromycin[1] or fluoroquinolones; resistance to both has been reported	Contaminated food or water
Clostridioides difficile	High-volume malodorous diarrhea	Oral vancomycin or fidaxomicin	Antibiotic exposure
Vibrio cholera	High-volume watery diarrhea	Fluoroquinolone[1] or tetracycline	Travel to developing nations
Nontyphoid *Salmonella*	Occasionally diarrhea is sometimes bloody, low fevers, abdominal cramping	Rarely needed. Azithromycin,[1] fluoroquinolone, or third-generation cephalosporin[1]	Unpasteurized milk, undercooked eggs or poultry, reptiles
Salmonella typhi	High fever, myalgias, diarrhea not necessarily prominent	Azithromycin (mild)[1] or carbapenems (severe);[1] fluoroquinolones are not recommended	Travel to Southeast Asia, South Asia
Campylobacter jejuni	Watery or bloody diarrhea, fever, abdominal pain, may mimic appendicitis	Rarely needed. Azithromycin[1] or fluoroquinolones; resistance to fluoroquinolones has been reported	
Yersinia enterocolitica	Bloody diarrhea, fever, abdominal pain, occasionally similar to appendicitis	Rarely needed. Trimethoprim-sulfamethoxazole,[1] aminoglycosides, third-generation cephalosporins, fluoroquinolones, or tetracyclines	Undercooked pork, unpasteurized milk, or contaminated water
Entamoeba histolytica	Watery diarrhea and abdominal cramping, rarely dysentery or liver abscess; incubation up to 1 month	Paromomycin +/- metronidazole	Fecal-oral
Cryptosporidium	Prolonged watery diarrhea	Nitazoxanide for immunocompetent patients	Fecal-oral, swimming, found throughout the United States, immunocompromised status
Giardia	Prolonged steatorrhea with flatulence and bloating	Metronidazole,[1] tinidazole, or nitazoxanide	Fecal-oral, found throughout the United States
Cyclospora and *Cystoisospora*	Watery diarrhea, flatulence, and nausea	Trimethoprim/sulfamethoxazole[1]	Travel to tropical regions
Bacillus cereus toxin	Vomiting, with watery diarrhea and abdominal cramping	Symptomatic only	Reheated rice
Staphylococcus aureus toxin	Vomiting, with watery diarrhea and abdominal cramping	Symptomatic only	Mayonnaise, cream-filled bakery products, ham
Clostridium perfringens toxin	Watery diarrhea with abdominal cramping, rarely vomiting	Symptomatic only	Meats and gravies

[1]Not FDA approved for this indication.

commonly referred to as "cruise ship" diarrhea. Although it can occur in this setting, it also commonly occurs in many other settings. These viruses are typically transmitted via the fecal-oral route. Risk factors include exposure to healthcare settings, close quarters, poor food handling, and daycare centers. It normally occurs 1 to 2 days after exposure and is highly transmissible. It is sometimes associated with fever and vomiting. There is no specific treatment other than supportive care for viral causes of acute diarrhea.

Bacteria

E. coli is the most common worldwide bacterial cause of diarrhea. Although *E. coli* is a part of the normal microbiome, there are many subtypes of *E. coli* that cause diarrheal illness. These include enterotoxigenic *E. coli* (ETEC), enteropathogenic *E. coli* (EPEC), enteroaggregative *E. coli* (EAEC), enteroinvasive *E. coli* (EIEC), and enterohemorrhagic *E. coli* (EHEC or Shiga toxin–producing *E. coli*). The two most well-known types of *E. coli* infection are EHEC and ETEC.

EHEC is a strain of *E. coli* that produces Shiga toxin. Shiga toxin invades the endothelium, leading to bloody diarrhea. It also invades other organs, like the lungs, blood vessels, and kidneys. This invasion of nongastrointestinal sites leads to the many complications of EHEC, including hemolytic uremic syndrome, seizures, and thrombotic thrombocytopenic purpura. The media has focused on EHEC as a cause of diarrheal illness related to meat products caused by the O157:H7 strain of *E. coli*. The infection is spread via consumption of contaminated food, unpasteurized dairy products, and unsanitary water. Symptoms usually appear 3 to 5 days after exposure and last as long as 10 days. EHEC should be reported to local public health authorities. Treatment of EHEC is supportive and directed at rehydration and treating and preventing complications. Antibiotics are not recommended in EHEC as they theoretically increase the release of Shiga toxin and worsen outcomes.

ETEC, on the other hand, produces two types of toxins that cause watery diarrhea. Contaminated food or water is the most common source. It is a common cause of "traveler's diarrhea." Symptoms usually appear 1 to 2 days after exposure and may last from 5 to 7 days. Treatment is generally directed at hydration. Antibiotics have been shown to reduce duration of illness, but they are rarely necessary, carry their own side effects, and risk increasing resistance. Antibiotic choices include azithromycin (Zithromax),[1] fluoroquinolones, rifaximin (Xifaxan), or trimethoprim-sulfamethoxazole (Bactrim). Single doses for both azithromycin (1000 mg)[1] and a fluoroquinolone (ciprofloxacin 500 to 750 mg) have been shown to be equally effective to multiple-day therapy. Given rising resistance patterns of *E. coli* from antibiotic overuse, in the rare instance where antibiotics are needed for severe ETEC, stool culture and sensitivities might be considered.

Shigella is the most common pathogen associated with dysentery and bloody diarrhea. Associated symptoms include high fevers and abdominal cramping. It is a nationally reportable disease. Similar to Shiga toxin–producing *E. coli*, shigellosis can cause bacteremia, hemolytic uremic syndrome, seizures, and other complications. Treatment is usually indicated and has historically been a fluoroquinolone (e.g., ciprofloxacin 500 mg twice daily for

5 to 7 days). Resistance to both azithromycin[1] and fluoroquinolones has been increasing in Asia and Africa. In 2018 the Centers for Disease Control and Prevention (CDC) announced a health alert that *Shigella* isolates in the United States had been identified with at least one resistance mechanism to fluoroquinolones. Since then, multidrug-resistant *Shigella* species have been reported in the United States. Susceptibility testing should be considered, and suspected treatment failures should be reported to the CDC.

Clostridioides difficile has been classically associated with antibiotic-associated diarrhea. However, community-based cases in patients without antibiotic exposure are on the rise. One study in emergency department patients showed that, when they tested all patients presenting with diarrhea, *C. difficile* rates were as high as 10%, and 30% of these patients had no risk factors or antibiotic exposure. *C. difficile* typically produces large-volume malodorous watery diarrhea. It is occasionally associated with toxic megacolon. There are very high rates of recurrence. *C. difficile* is typically diagnosed via a two-step algorithm involving both toxin testing and either polymerase chain reaction (PCR) nucleic acid amplification (NAAT) or glutamate dehydrogenase testing. Rarely, endoscopic testing is needed to confirm the diagnosis. Traditionally, it was taught that bleach and handwashing with soap and water (instead of alcohol-based products) were necessary to prevent the spread of *C. difficile*. The Infectious Diseases Society of America (IDSA) has backed off this guideline slightly, and now handwashing is preferred over alcohol-based hand sanitizer only in hyperendemic areas or when there is direct fecal or perineal contact. If antibiotic use is associated with *C. difficile*, it should be discontinued as soon as possible. Common antibiotics highly associated with *C. difficile* include clindamycin, fluoroquinolones, and β-lactam antibiotics. Treatment recommendations for *C. difficile* have recently been updated. Metronidazole (Flagyl)[1] monotherapy is no longer recommended unless no other options are available. Fidaxomicin (Dificid, 200 mg twice daily for 10 days) or oral vancomycin (125 mg four times daily for 10 days) is recommended as first-line therapy in an initial episode of *C. difficile*. Severe or fulminant *C. difficile* (defined as presence of shock, ileus, or megacolon) is typically treated in an intensive care setting with oral vancomycin and intravenous (IV) metronidazole.[1] Rectal vancomycin[1] may also be used if ileus is present. Recurrent episodes of *C. difficile* require either prolonged, tapered vancomycin; a fidaxomicin regimen; or fecal microbiota transplant.

Vibrio cholera, or simply "cholera," is endemic in developing nations and rare in the United States. It leads to profuse, watery diarrhea (classically called "rice-water stools") that usually occurs 1 to 3 days after exposure. Fever is rare. It is a nationally reported disease. Antibiotics are occasionally needed. Options would include azithromycin,[1] fluoroquinolones,[1] or tetracyclines. An example regimen would be doxycycline (Vibramycin) 300 mg once orally.

Salmonella (nontyphoidal) is the most common bacterial cause of foodborne illness in the United States. It is associated with infected poultry, eggs, and milk. Reptiles, including turtles, are a rare cause of transmission as well. Associated symptoms include fever and abdominal cramping. It is required to report all *Salmonella* infections (both typhoidal and nontyphoidal) to public health authorities in the United States. Rarely, nontyphoidal *Salmonella* can lead to invasive infections like bacteremia or meningitis. *Salmonella* is typically self-limited and requires no treatment. In healthy people with *Salmonella* infection, antibiotics generally do not shorten the duration of illness, diarrhea, or fever. Indications for treatment include immunocompromise, severe disease requiring hospitalization, or extremes of age. Treatment, when needed, is typically either azithromycin, a fluoroquinolone, or a third-generation cephalosporin. An example outpatient regimen would be azithromycin[1] 500 mg once daily for 5 days. An inpatient regimen might consist of ceftriaxone (Rocephin)[1] IV once daily for 5 to 7 days. Antibiotic resistance of

---

[1] Not FDA approved for this indication.

[1] Not FDA approved for this indication.

(nontyphoidal) *Salmonella* in the United States, though less common than *Shigella,* has been reported most recently regarding the multidrug-resistant Newport strain originating in Mexico.

Salmonella typhi and *Salmonella paratyphi* are special cases of severe *Salmonella* infection that lead to the diseases called typhoid fever and paratyphoid fever, respectively. These infections are typically much more severe than nontyphoidal *Salmonella,* and they often require hospitalization and antibiotic therapy. Associated symptoms include high fever, rigors, myalgias, headache, and, occasionally, a rash. Diarrhea may or may not be a prominent symptom. Typhoid fever and paratyphoid fever are almost exclusively associated with travel to endemic regions, most commonly South and Southeast Asia. Cases are rarely not associated with travel. The incubation period for typhoid fever is typically 6 to 30 days and 1 to 10 days for paratyphoid fever. Diagnosis typically can be done via blood culture, but stool is also acceptable. Urine culture or bone marrow may be needed. Antibiotic resistance is common in the United States. Fluoroquinolones are not recommended as empiric therapy. Oral azithromycin[1] may be used for mild disease, and ceftriaxone[1] (2 g IV daily) or carbapenems (e.g., meropenem [Merrem] 1 g IV three times daily)[1] are recommended for severe disease while awaiting antibiotic sensitivity testing results. Multidrug-resistant isolates have been found in people who have recently traveled to Pakistan, Iraq, and Southeast Asia, and a carbapenem for empiric therapy is recommended. Duration of therapy is based on severity of illness but is typically 10 to 14 days. Case recurrences have been reported when patients stop antibiotics early.

Campylobacter jejuni is another common bacterial cause of diarrhea in the United States. Diarrhea can be watery or bloody. It is often spread by undercooked meat and poultry. Symptoms may present 2 to 5 days after exposure and last up to 1 week. Associated symptoms include abdominal pain, fever, nausea, and vomiting. It can sometimes mimic appendicitis. In addition to foodborne transmission, it has been associated with exposure to the feces of young dogs and cats, including stool that is carried on their fur and paws. Delayed complications include reactive arthritis, rheumatoid arthritis, irritable bowel syndrome, and Guillain-Barré syndrome. *Campylobacter* is typically self-limited, and mild disease in otherwise healthy patients does not require treatment. Azithromycin and fluoroquinolones are commonly used for treatment, but resistance to fluoroquinolones is common. Treatment is associated with prolonged shedding of resistant organisms. When antibiotics are indicated, antimicrobial susceptibility testing can help guide appropriate therapy. Azithromycin[1] 500 mg daily for 3 days would be one potential treatment regimen.

Yersinia enterocolitica is a rare cause of bacterial diarrhea and is more common in children. It can be transmitted by undercooked pork, unpasteurized dairy products, animal contact, or contaminated water. It frequently has associated symptoms of fever and abdominal pain and can sometimes mimic appendicitis. Delayed complications of *Y. enterocolitica* infection include reactive arthritis and erythema nodosum. It is typically self-limited and rarely needs antibiotic therapy. *Y. enterocolitica* isolates are usually susceptible to trimethoprim-sulfamethoxazole,[1] aminoglycosides, third-generation cephalosporins, fluoroquinolones, and tetracyclines. Given how rarely it is needed, there is insufficient evidence to recommend an outpatient regimen. Complicated *Yersinia* infections can be treated with ceftriaxone[1] 2 g IV daily for up to 21 days.

Parasites

Entamoeba histolytica is a parasitic amoeba that is common in tropical regions. It can be contracted via fecal-oral transmission or contact with contaminated foods or surfaces contaminated with eggs. Only about 10% to 20% of patients will become symptomatic when infected. Incubation is quite long and can be

up to 1 month. It is known to cause liver abscesses. It is required to be reported to public health authorities. Treatment for asymptomatic individuals is monotherapy with the luminal agent paromomycin monotherapy. For symptomatic carriers, metronidazole is used for the invasive component. Paromomycin (Humatin) can be both nephrotoxic and ototoxic, and its use should be closely monitored. Dose is 25 to 35 mg/kg/day, divided in three daily doses for 5 to 10 days.

Cryptosporidium is a parasitic illness that causes watery diarrhea. It is sometimes associated with fever, nausea, or abdominal cramping. Symptoms of cryptosporidiosis generally begin 2 to 10 days after becoming infected with the parasite and continue 1 to 2 weeks, though symptoms for up to 4 weeks have been reported. It is found throughout the United States. *Cryptosporidium* is typically transmitted via the fecal-oral route, including not only by consuming contaminated foods and water but also by swimming in contaminated locations. It is a nationally reportable disease. It is most well-known for affecting immunocompromised individuals, but it can affect immunocompetent individuals as well. Immunocompetent individuals will often recover without treatment. Nitazoxanide (Alinia, 500 mg twice daily for 3 days) is available and approved for treatment of immunocompetent patients older than 1 year with *Cryptosporidium*. It is not clear if nitazoxanide is effective in immunocompromised individuals.

Giardia is one of the few infectious causes of diarrhea that can cause steatorrhea. It is often associated with flatulence and bloating. Symptoms typically start 1 to 2 weeks after infection and continue 2 to 6 weeks. Other, less common symptoms include fever, itchy skin, hives, and swelling of the eyes and joints. Delayed complications typically occur because of malabsorption, and *Giardia* can lead to lactose intolerance later in life. It is a nationally reportable disease. Like *Cryptosporidium*, it is also spread via the fecal-oral route and found throughout the United States. Treatment options include metronidazole,[1] tinidazole (Tindamax), and nitazoxanide. The simplest regimen is tinidazole 2 g once. Combination therapy may be needed for recurrent infections.

Cyclospora cayetanensis and *Cystoisospora belli* (formerly *Isospora*) are common parasites in tropical regions and are spread by contaminated food and water. Symptoms of *Cyclospora* infection begin an average of 7 days after infection, and untreated disease can last several weeks to months. Associated symptoms include flatulence, nausea, and, rarely, fever. This is a nationally reportable disease. Symptoms in most immunocompetent patients will resolve without treatment, though they may be prolonged or may recur. The mainstay regimen for treatment of both *Cyclospora* and *Cystoisospora* is trimethoprim/sulfamethoxazole[1] 800 mg/160 mg twice daily for 7 to 10 days. No alternative regimen has been shown to be effective for *Cyclospora* infections. Pyrimethamine (Daraprim)[1] or fluoroquinolones may be effective second-line agents for *Cystoisospora* infections. Consultation with an infectious disease specialist is recommended for patients who are immunosuppressed, as dosages and duration of treatment may need to be increased.

Bacterial Toxins

Some forms of diarrhea are caused by preformed bacterial toxins. These are all treated symptomatically. The three most common causes are *Bacillus cereus, Staphylococcus aureus,* and *Clostridium perfringens. B. cereus* is commonly associated with reheated rice, and vomiting occurs much more frequently than diarrhea. Incubation is 1 to 6 hours. *S. aureus* is commonly associated with mayonnaise, eggs, cream-filled bakery products, and ham. It also causes vomiting much more frequently than diarrhea, and its incubation is 1 to 6 hours. *C. perfringens* has a longer incubation of 6 to 12 hours and is associated with poultry, meat, and gravy,

---

[1] Not FDA approved for this indication.

BOX 2 History and Physical Examination for Acute Diarrhea

History
- Description of diarrhea (duration, frequency, onset, type)
- Associated symptoms (fever, nausea/vomiting, pain/cramping, rashes, weight loss)
- Previous episodes with similar symptoms
- Medications (see Box 1)
- Recent dietary history (contaminated food or water, poorly prepared food)
- Animal or reptile contacts
- Travel history (endemic regions)
- Sexual history (anal intercourse)
- Vaccination history
- Contact with institutions (hospitals, nursing homes, daycare facilities)
- Employment history (restaurants)
- Immune status (HIV, use of immunosuppressants, congenital illness)

Physical Examination
- Vital signs
- Weight
- Respiratory (hyperventilation may be a sign of acidosis and dehydration)
- Mucous membranes
- Conjunctival pallor
- Skin tenting
- Abdominal palpation (tenderness, rebound, guarding)
- Rectal
- Lymphadenopathy
- Skin (rashes, pallor)

TABLE 2 Indications for Testing in Acute Diarrhea

FINDING	TESTING
Watery diarrhea	None routinely; consider metabolic panel in severe dehydration
Bloody diarrhea	Blood count and stool testing
Fever	Stool testing
Immunocompromised patients	Stool testing
Prolonged illness >7 days	Stool testing
Severe illness requiring hospitalization	Stool testing, blood counts, and metabolic panel
Suspected *Clostridioides difficile*	Multistep stool testing algorithm for organism and toxin
Fulminant *C. difficile*	Computed tomography imaging for ileus or toxic megacolon
Suspected *Shigella* or enterohemorrhagic *Escherichia coli*	Blood count, metabolic testing, and stool testing
Suspected typhoid or paratyphoid fever	Blood cultures, stool cultures, and blood counts
Symptomatic parasitic infection	HIV testing

particularly when prepared in large batches or stored improperly. Diarrhea and cramping are common, but vomiting is rare.

Diagnosis

As with most illnesses, a thorough history and physical examination are the keys to diagnosis (Box 2). Occasionally, adjunctive testing may be required (Table 2). There is no single diagnostic test that is required in the evaluation of acute diarrhea, and most cases will not require any testing. Patients with examination findings of dehydration may require a metabolic panel to assess for electrolyte derangements or renal dysfunction. Patients with dysentery may also require a complete blood count and stool testing.

Testing stool for identification of specific pathogens is recommended in patients with severe or prolonged illness, with exposures or risk factors for invasive disease, or who are immunocompromised. The IDSA recommends stool testing in patients with fever or bloody diarrhea. Stool testing is not indicated in otherwise healthy patients with less than 7 days of watery diarrhea. This includes traveler's diarrhea, of which the causative agents are described previously. Some would argue that historical guidelines for diagnostic testing are overly restrictive in the current environment that offers new diagnostic methods for specific identification of infectious agents and enhanced ability to target therapy. When stool testing is indicated, it is generally recommended to use multiplex PCR testing as the first-line test to identify causative agents. National guidelines recommend that stool cultures and ova and parasite examinations should be reserved for patients with prolonged or severe courses of illness after PCR testing is negative or for those with specific risk factors for parasitic disease (e.g., known exposure, untreated HIV, transplant recipients, those on chemotherapy). Tests like fecal leukocytes or lactoferrin have little to no role in the diagnosis of acute infectious diarrhea.

Radiologic imaging is almost never needed for the evaluation of acute infectious diarrhea. It may be considered in patients with severe illness, severe pain, peritoneal findings on physical examination, or persistent fevers. Imaging is used in these cases to identify rare complications like toxic megacolon, mycotic aneurysms, or intestinal perforation. Endoscopic evaluation is also rarely needed for acute diarrhea, with the major exception being immunocompromised patients with prolonged symptoms.

Prevention

Preventing acute diarrheal illness is equally as important as treatment. The most common routes of transmission are fecal-oral and foodborne. Therefore the best preventive measures include hand hygiene, access to clean water, and proper food preparation and storage techniques. Public health reporting of suspected outbreaks is paramount to prevent spread. Worldwide, access to clean water is a key intervention to prevent diarrheal illness. Exclusive breastfeeding for the first 6 months of life has also been shown to reduce the risk of diarrheal illness.

Patients who are traveling should have pretravel counseling. Travelers should be mindful to have access to clean water (and ice) and choose their food sources carefully. Bismuth subsalicylate (Pepto-Bismol) may be used to prevent traveler's diarrhea in patients who can adhere to the frequent dosing regimens (524 mg orally four times daily for 3 weeks).[1] It is associated with black stools and tongue. Prophylactic antibiotics are typically unnecessary, but they may be used selectively for short-term use in patients at high risk who travel to endemic areas. Typically, fluoroquinolones are used (e.g., ciprofloxacin 500 mg daily for 1 week),[1] though alternative regimens include rifaximin 400 mg to 1100 mg daily[1] for 1 week; trimethoprim/sulfamethoxazole 160 mg/800 mg daily for 1 week;[1] azithromycin 250 mg daily for 1 week,[1] or 1000 mg in a single dose;[1] or doxycycline 100 mg daily for 1 to 3 weeks.[1]

---

[1] Not FDA approved for this indication.

Over 30 randomized controlled trials suggest that probiotics reduce the risk of antibiotic-associated diarrhea and prevent *C. difficile* infections. Exactly which type or dose of probiotic is best is not known, but probiotics should routinely be recommended to any patient with any antibiotic prescription. This is particularly important for high-risk antibiotics like clindamycin (Cleocin) and fluoroquinolones.

Routine vaccines exist for both rotavirus and hepatitis A, and these vaccines have reduced the incidence of these viral causes of diarrhea in the adult population. There are also vaccines approved in the United States for *S. typhi* and *V. cholera*, but these are reserved for patients at high risk of traveling to endemic areas.

Therapy

The vast majority of acute diarrhea is infectious in nature and self-limited. Thus symptom control and supportive care are the bedrocks of treatment. Medical interventions and treatments are rarely needed and sometimes even harmful.

The foundation for treatment of any acute diarrhea is supportive care with oral rehydration, antidiarrheal agents, and other symptomatic agents. It is important to use some form of solution containing electrolytes when treating diarrhea with oral rehydration. This can include juice, electrolyte-containing sports drinks (e.g., Gatorade, Powerade), prepackaged rehydration solutions (e.g., Pedialyte, the World Health Organization [WHO] oral rehydration salts), or homemade oral rehydration solution. The latter can be made by dissolving 6 teaspoons of sugar and 0.5 teaspoon salt in 1 L of water.

Occasionally, IV hydration may be needed. This can be done on an inpatient or outpatient basis depending on severity of illness. An isotonic solution should almost always be used for simple hydration. There is ongoing debate about whether balanced IV solutions (e.g., lactated Ringer solution, Hartmann solution, Plasma-Lyte) improve outcomes over 0.9% ("normal") saline solutions in general critically ill patients. Some randomized studies have shown no difference, and some have shown a benefit to balanced solutions. No studies have shown improved outcomes with 0.9% saline compared with balanced solutions.

Zinc supplementation[1] has been shown to reduce duration of diarrhea in children, particularly those who are malnourished. It is recommended by the WHO, but it seems to have limited uptake in developed countries like the United States. Most of the data support its role in countries with a high prevalence of zinc deficiency.

Antimotility agents are another important way to control and reduce symptoms of diarrhea and risk for dehydration. Loperamide (Imodium) is the most common agent used in this respect, and it has been shown to reduce symptoms. Loperamide may be used to reduce diarrhea at 4 mg orally, followed by 2 mg orally with each loose stool up to a maximum of 16 mg/day. It is recommended in traveler's diarrhea being treated with antibiotics to reduce duration of illness. It is advised to avoid loperamide in children under 18 years of age. It is also recommended to avoid loperamide in patients with high fever or dysentery. Traditionally, loperamide was thought to be contraindicated in patients with *C. difficile* or other bacterial infections as it might lead to delayed clearance and complications like toxic megacolon. More recently, the IDSA notes that addition of an antimotility agent such as loperamide as an adjunct to specific antibacterial therapy for *C. difficile* may be safe,

although no prospective or randomized studies are available. Bismuth subsalicylate is another agent that may reduce stool passage rates, particularly for traveler's diarrhea. Studies show it is most effective when taking 524 mg orally four times daily for 3 weeks.

Occasionally, antibiotics are needed for the treatment of acute diarrhea. This should not be routine practice. Instances where antibiotic treatment should be considered empirically before testing results are available include in infants younger than 3 months with suspected bacterial source of diarrhea, in patients with high fevers and suspected *Shigella* (but not EHEC), in patients who have recently traveled internationally and are febrile with signs of sepsis, and in immunocompromised patients with bloody diarrhea and severe illness. Recommendations for specific antibiotics for specific pathogens identified by testing are listed in Table 1. Duration of antibiotic therapy is typically driven by severity of illness, with mild illness requiring 1 to 5 days of antibiotics and more severe illness requiring a 7- to 10-day course.

There has been interest in the use of probiotics[7] in treating acute diarrhea. Despite the well-evidenced role of probiotics in preventing antibiotic-associated diarrhea and *C. difficile*, the most recent 2020 Cochrane review, based on large trials with low risk of bias, suggests that, for treatment of acute diarrhea, probiotics probably make little or no difference in the number of people who have diarrhea lasting 48 hours or longer, and it is uncertain whether probiotics reduce the duration of diarrhea. Similarly, probiotics are not recommended as a stand-alone or adjunct treatment for *C. difficile* infections.

---

[7] Available as dietary supplement.

References

Abrahamian FM, Talan DA, Krishnadasan A, EMERGEncy ID NET Study Group, et al: Clostridium difficile infection among US emergency department patients with diarrhea and no vomiting, *Ann Emerg Med* 70(1):19–27.e4, 2017.

Collinson S, Deans A, Padua-Zamora A, et al: Probiotics for treating acute infectious diarrhoea, *Cochrane Database Syst Rev* 12(12):CD003048, 2020.

Liao W, Chen C, Wen T, Zhao Q: Probiotics for the prevention of antibiotic-associated diarrhea in adults: A meta-analysis of randomized placebo-controlled trials, *J Clin Gastroenterol* 55(6):469–480, 2021.

McDonald LC, Gerding DN, Johnson S, et al: Clinical practice guidelines for *Clostridium difficile* infection in adults and children: 2017 Update by the Infectious Diseases Society of America (IDSA) and Society for Healthcare Epidemiology of America (SHEA), *Clin Infect Dis* 66(7):e1–e48, 2018.

Meisenheimer ES, Epstein C, Thiel D: Acute diarrhea in adults, *Am Fam Physician* 106(1):72–80, 2022.

Mussell M, Kroenke K, Spitzer RL, Williams JB, Herzog W, Löwe B: Gastrointestinal symptoms in primary care: prevalence and association with depression and anxiety, *J Psychosom Res* 64(6):605–612, 2008.

Nemeth V, Pfleghaar N. Diarrhea. [Updated 2022 Nov 21]. In: StatPearls [Internet]. Treasure Island (FL): StatPearls Publishing.

Riddle MS, DuPont HL, Connor BA: ACG clinical guideline: Diagnosis, treatment, and prevention of acute diarrheal infections in adults, *Am J Gastroenterol* 111(5):602–622, 2016.

Shane AL, Mody RK, Crump JA, et al: 2017 Infectious Diseases Society of America clinical practice guidelines for the diagnosis and management of infectious diarrhea, *Clin Infect Dis* 65(12):1963–1973, 2017.

United States Centers for Disease Control and Prevention Division of Parasitic Diseases and Malaria: *Parasites*, 2022. Available at: https://www.cdc.gov/parasites/index.html.

World Health Organization: *Diarrhoeal Diseases*, 2017. Available at: https://www.who.int/news-room/fact-sheets/detail/diarrhoeal-disease.

---

[1] Not FDA approved for this indication.

BLEEDING ESOPHAGEAL VARICES

Method of
Cecilio R. Azar, MD; and Ala I. Sharara, MD

CURRENT DIAGNOSIS

- Endoscopic screening for esophageal varices is recommended in patients with liver cirrhosis.
- Noninvasive predictors of the presence of large varices, such as splenomegaly and thrombocytopenia, have limited accuracy.
- A combination of clinical and endoscopic findings including the Child-Pugh class, size of varices, and the presence of red wale markings correlates with the risk of first bleeding in patients with cirrhosis.
- Measurement of hepatic venous pressure gradient may be the best indicator of risk and severity of bleeding in patients with varices. It is an invasive test and is not widely available or used routinely in practice.

CURRENT THERAPY

- Nonselective β-blockers and endoscopic band ligation are both effective first-line therapy in the primary prophylaxis of esophageal varices.
- The management of acute variceal hemorrhage consists of prompt resuscitation and correction of coagulation abnormalities, followed by endoscopic and pharmacologic therapy with vasoactive agents. Antibiotic prophylaxis is given to decrease the risk of infection and of rebleeding. Transjugular intrahepatic portosystemic shunt (TIPS) is reserved for refractory, uncontrolled, acute variceal bleeding.
- Strategies for secondary prophylaxis of variceal bleeding include endoscopic band ligation, pharmacologic therapy with nonselective β-blockers with or without nitrates, TIPS, and surgical shunts.
- Comparative cost-effectiveness of secondary prophylaxis strategies is unknown but should take into consideration the cost of failed therapy (e.g., rebleeding, shunt revision) and that of treatment related-complications (e.g., encephalopathy, esophageal stricture).

Epidemiology

Bleeding of esophageal varices is a major complication of portal hypertension, usually in the setting of liver cirrhosis, accounting for 10% to 30% of all cases of upper gastrointestinal hemorrhage. More than any other cause of gastrointestinal bleeding, this complication results in considerable morbidity and mortality, prolonged hospitalization, and increased affiliated costs. Variceal bleeding develops in 25% to 35% of patients with cirrhosis and accounts for up to 90% of upper gastrointestinal bleeding episodes in these patients. About 10% to 30% of these episodes are fatal, and as many as 70% of survivors rebleed following an index variceal hemorrhage. Following such events, the 1-year survival is 34% to 80%, being inversely related to the severity of the underlying liver disease.

Treatment of patients with esophageal varices includes preventing the initial bleeding episode (primary prophylaxis), controlling active variceal hemorrhage, and preventing recurrent bleeding after a first episode (secondary prophylaxis). Data on the optimal management of gastric varices are much more limited, and this topic is not covered in this article.

Pathophysiology

Chronic liver disease leading to cirrhosis is the most common cause of portal hypertension. The level of increased resistance to flow varies with the level of circulatory breach and can be divided into prehepatic, hepatic or sinusoidal, and posthepatic. In cirrhosis, several organ systems are involved in the pathophysiology of portal hypertension. At the splanchnic vascular bed level there is marked vasodilatation and increase in angiogenesis, leading to increase in portal blood flow and formation of collateral circulation, such as gastroesophageal varices, along with decrease in response to vasoconstrictors. At the systemic circulation level, there is an increase in cardiac output, decrease in vascular resistance, and hypervolemia. This hyperkinetic syndrome leads to an effective hypovolemia, with a resultant increase in vasoactive factors to maintain a normal arterial blood pressure.

Varices represent portosystemic collaterals derived from dilatation of preexisting embryonic vascular channels, such as those between the coronary and short gastric veins and the intercostal, esophageal, and azygous veins. In the distal esophagus, over an area extending 2 to 5 cm from the gastroesophageal junction, veins are found more superficially in the lamina propria rather than the submucosa. This results in reduced support from surrounding tissues owing to the predominant intraluminal location of these varices and might explain the predilection for bleeding at this site. The opening and dilation of portosystemic collaterals appears to depend on a threshold portal pressure gradient (measured as hepatic venous pressure gradient [HVPG]) of 12 mm Hg, below which varices do not form. This pressure gradient is necessary but not sufficient for the development of gastroesophageal varices.

Diagnosis

The current consensus states that every patient with liver cirrhosis should undergo an upper endoscopy to detect gastroesophageal varices. The main aim behind screening for gastroesophageal varices is to identify patients requiring prophylactic treatment or further surveillance. Esophageal varices are present in 52% of screened patients and are more prevalent in more advanced disease (43% for Child–Pugh class A versus 72% in Child–Pugh class B or C). On the other hand, gastric varices are present in up to 33% of patients with portal hypertension, with progression rates for both esophageal and gastric varices from small, medium, to large varices of 10% to 15% per year. Several invasive and noninvasive procedures help in detecting portal hypertension and can, with variable accuracy, predict the presence of gastroesophageal varices. Unfortunately, none are sensitive enough to replace endoscopy. A recent meta-analysis showed that transient elastography may be a useful screening tool for the detection of significant liver fibrosis and associated portal hypertension, but it is not useful at predicting the presence or size of esophageal varices. Smaller trials have evaluated the usefulness of spleen and liver MR elastography in assessing portal hypertension and varices, but this modality has not yet found its way into clinical practice. The combination of an elastography value below 20 kPa together and a platelet count above 150,000 nearly excludes the presence of esophageal varices requiring treatment. Endoscopic videocapsule is a new modality introduced for visualizing the esophagus; it allows correct identification of varices in 80% of cases but can have poor accuracy in identifying the presence of hypertensive gastropathy and gastric varices.

Not all esophageal varices bleed; hemorrhage occurs in only 30% to 35% of patients with cirrhosis. Variceal rupture is directly related to physical factors such as the radius, thickness, and elastic properties of the vessel in addition to intravariceal and intraluminal pressure and tension. Endoscopic findings that predict a higher risk of bleeding include larger size of varices and the presence of endoscopic red signs (described as red wale markings) on the variceal wall, indicating dilated intraepithelial and subepithelial superficial veins. A combination of clinical and endoscopic findings, including the Child-Pugh class, size of varices, and the presence or absence of red wale markings, was found to correlate highly with the risk of first bleeding in patients with cirrhosis. Hemodynamic parameters examined as predictors of bleeding include HVPG, azygous blood flow, and direct measurement of intravariceal pressure.

HVPG, calculated by the gradient of wedged and free hepatic vein pressure (normal value, 5 mm Hg), is used most often and provides reliable measurement of portal pressure in patients with cirrhosis. The extent of elevation of HVPG may be the best indicator of risk of bleeding, severity of bleeding, and survival. A rise in pressure in a patient with known varices increases the risk of bleeding, and the extent of portal pressure elevation has an inverse relationship to prognosis after hemorrhage has occurred. In general, however, a linear relationship between the degree of portal hypertension and the risk of variceal hemorrhage or formation of varices does not exist, so this technique cannot be used routinely to identify individual patients at high risk for bleeding.

Treatment

Primary Prophylaxis

The natural evolution of gastroesophageal varices without treatment is characterized by an increase in size from small to large varices, which eventually rupture and bleed. The progression rate ranges from 5% to 30% per year. The incidence of bleeding from small esophageal varices is estimated to be 4% per year, and it is as high as 15% per year for medium to large varices. In a randomized, controlled trial, the nonselective β-blocker timolol (Blocadren)[1] failed to reduce the development of varices or variceal bleeding in patients without varices. Adverse events were more common in the timolol group. Therefore, it is not recommended to start β-blockers in patients who do not yet have esophageal varices.

Based on prospective studies of cirrhotic patients with varices identified at endoscopy and of untreated groups in randomized controlled trials, the risk of bleeding from esophageal varices has been estimated at 25% to 35% at 1 year. Therapy for primary prophylaxis against variceal bleeding (prevention of a first variceal bleeding) is summarized in Table 1.

Pharmacologic Therapy

The general objective of pharmacologic therapy for variceal bleeding is to reduce portal pressure and consequently intravariceal pressure. Drugs that reduce portocollateral venous flow (vasoconstrictors) or intrahepatic vascular resistance (vasodilators) have been used and include β-blockers, nitrates, β_2-adrenergic blockers, spironolactone (Aldactone), pentoxifylline (Trental),[1] molsidomine (Corvaton),[2] and simvastatin (Zocor).[1] Because varices do not bleed at an HVPG less than 12 mm Hg, reduction to this level is ideal, but substantial reductions in HVPG (i.e., by >20%) are also clinically meaningful.

β-Blockers exert their beneficial effect on portal venous pressure by diminishing splanchnic blood flow and consequently gastroesophageal collateral and azygous blood flow. The effectiveness of β-blockers for primary prophylaxis against variceal bleeding has been demonstrated in several controlled trials. Meta-analyses have revealed a 40% to 50% reduction in bleeding and a trend toward improved survival. The estimated overall response rate is 49%, with bleeding rates of 6% in responders and 32% in nonresponders, with a number needed to treat (NNT) of 10.

The nonselective β-blockers, such as propranolol (Inderal)[1] and nadolol (Corgard),[1] are preferred because of the dual benefit of β_1- and β_2-receptor blockade. In the absence of HVPG determination, β-blockers are titrated to achieve a reduction in resting heart rate to 55 beats/min or 25% of baseline. Propranolol is generally given

[1]Not FDA approved for this indication.

[1]Not FDA approved for this indication.
[2]Not available in the United States.

as a long-acting preparation and titrated to a maximum dose of 320 mg/day. Nadolol is initiated at 80 mg daily up to a maximum daily dose of 240 mg. Carvedilol (Coreg)[1] is initiated at 6.25 mg daily and increased if tolerated to 12.5 mg/day. Carvedilol is superior to propranolol at reducing portal hypertension although available data do not allow a satisfactory comparison of adverse events. The portal pressure–reducing effects of β-blockers are not predictable; the resultant reduction in heart rate or the measurement of drug blood levels are not good indicators of response to therapy. For example, portal venous pressure is reduced in about 60% to 70% of patients who receive propranolol therapy, but only 10% to 30% of these patients show a substantial response (i.e., >20% reduction). Additionally, approximately 20% to 25% of patients have no measurable decline in portal pressure despite increasing dosage of propranolol. Non-selective beta-blockers (NSBB) are effective in preventing first and recurrent variceal hemorrhage both in patients with and without ascites. NSBB-induced reduction in portal pressure is associated with lowering the progression of cirrhosis and even death.

Refractory ascites and spontaneous bacterial peritonitis (SBP) are not absolute contraindications to NSBB as previously thought. However, high-dose NSBB (with resultant decrease in mean arterial pressure) should be used with caution because it can be associated with deleterious outcomes. Hence, careful dosing is necessary in these patients with dose reduction/discontinuation for systolic blood pressure <90 mm Hg.

In addition to β-blockers, a number of vasodilators have been investigated in patients with portal hypertension and in animal models of portal hypertension, most notably isosorbide mononitrate (Imdur).[1] Of note, there is increasing evidence that the use of β-blockers can be deleterious in patients with decompensated liver cirrhosis, refractory ascites, and severe circulatory dysfunction (systolic blood pressure 90 mm Hg, serum sodium <30 meq/fL, or hepatorenal syndrome). The exact mechanism of action of nitrates is unclear but is thought to be mediated primarily by reducing intrahepatic resistance and possibly by splanchnic arterial vasoconstriction induced in response to venous pooling and vasodilation in other regional vascular beds. Monotherapy with nitrates is ineffective in primary prophylaxis and can have detrimental effects, particularly in cirrhotic patients with ascites, and should not be used.

The addition of isosorbide mononitrate to β-blockers, however, has been shown to result in an enhanced reduction in portal pressure in humans. In a randomized, controlled trial involving 42 patients with cirrhosis and esophageal varices, a reduction of greater than 20% in HVPG was documented in only 10% in the propranolol group compared to 50% in the combination therapy group. In patients with Child-Pugh class A and B cirrhosis, the addition of isosorbide mononitrate to nadolol has been shown, in a randomized trial, to result in a greater than 50% additional reduction in variceal bleeding rate when compared with nadolol monotherapy (12% versus 29%). However, a large subsequent double-blind, placebo-controlled study failed to confirm these results. Based on the existing evidence, the combination of β-blockers and isosorbide is not recommended in primary prophylaxis.

Endoscopic Therapy
Endoscopic therapies play a prominent role in treatment of esophageal varices. Endoscopic band ligation (EBL) is the endoscopic procedure of choice in the management of esophageal varices. As of 2010, 16 randomized, controlled trials have compared EBL to β-blockers in the primary prevention of variceal bleeding. These studies suffered from significant heterogeneity, and a large number were published in abstract form. Two meta-analyses of these trials showed a slight advantage of EBL over β-blockers in terms of primary prevention of variceal bleeding, but there were no differences in mortality. A recent Cochrane database systematic review found a beneficial effect of band ligation compared to β-blockers in primary prevention of upper gastrointestinal bleeding in adult patients with esophageal varices. Again, there was no difference in mortality.

β-Blockers are cheaper and much easier to administer but are associated with issues of noncompliance and a higher incidence of adverse events (e.g., hypotension, impotence, insomnia) than EBL. However, most of these side effects are easy to manage and none require hospitalization or result in direct mortality. On the other hand, adverse events related to EBL, such as bleeding from band-related ulcers, albeit infrequent, are more significant, often requiring hospitalization and blood transfusion, and may rarely be associated with death.

According to the Baveno consensus conference, nonselective β-blockers should be considered as a first choice for preventing first variceal bleeding in high-risk patients who have not bled, and EBL should be provided for patients with contraindications or intolerance to β-blockers. The recent guidelines by the American College of Gastroenterology (ACG) and American Association for the Study of Liver Diseases (AASLD) recommend using β-blockers in low-risk patients who have medium to large varices but suggest both EBL and β-blockers for high-risk patients as first-line therapy. The optimal primary prophylaxis in patients with decompensated cirrhosis remains unclear and is arguably expedited liver transplantation. The combination of pharmacologic plus endoscopic therapy has been investigated in such patients with conflicting results. In one study, EBL plus β-blockers offered no benefit in terms of prevention of first bleeding when compared to EBL alone. In a more recent study, combination therapy significantly reduced the occurrence of the first episode of variceal bleeding and improved bleeding-related survival in a group of cirrhotic patients with high-risk esophageal varices awaiting liver transplantation.

Management of Acute Variceal Hemorrhage
Variceal hemorrhage is usually an acute clinical event characterized by rapid gastrointestinal blood loss manifesting as hematemesis (which can be massive), with or without melena or hematochezia. Hemodynamic instability (tachycardia, hypotension) is common. Although variceal bleeding is common in patients with cirrhosis presenting with acute upper gastrointestinal hemorrhage, other causes of bleeding, such as ulcer disease, must be considered. Urgent initiation of empiric pharmacologic therapy with vasoactive agents is indicated in situations where variceal hemorrhage is likely. Subsequently, direct endoscopic examination is critical to establish an accurate diagnosis and to provide the rationale for immediate and subsequent therapies. The immediate steps in the management of acute variceal bleeding include: volume resuscitation, prevention of complications, ensuring hemostasis, and initiating measures to prevent early and delayed rebleeding.

Using a MELD-based analysis, the overall 6-week mortality is estimated at 16% (5%–20%), with mortality rates worsening with more advanced disease. Recurrence rates are up to 60% within 1 to 2 years if untreated, and mortality rates as high as 33%.

Patients with variceal hemorrhage and ascites are at increased risk for bacterial infections, particularly spontaneous bacterial peritonitis. This risk appears to be increased in the setting of uncontrolled hemorrhage or as a result of transient bacteremia following endoscopic sclerotherapy or variceal ligation. Short-term systemic antibiotics (e.g., third-generation cephalosporins or fluoroquinolones for 4–10 days) have been shown to decrease the risk of bacterial infections and to reduce rebleeding as well as mortality in cirrhotic patients with gastrointestinal bleeding.

A restrictive transfusion strategy should be used, aiming for a hemoglobin of 7 to 8 gm/dL to avoid volume overexpansion and perpetuation of bleeding. The role of platelet transfusion or fresh frozen plasma administration has not been assessed appropriately. The routine administration of fresh frozen plasma in patients with active variceal bleeding may in fact be detrimental because of the resultant volume expansion and should be discouraged. Hypofibrinogenemia should be treated with cryoprecipitate aiming for levels >100 mg/dL. The use of recombinant activated coagulation factor VII (rFVIIa [Novoseven]),[1] which corrects

---

[1]Not FDA approved for this indication.

prothrombin time in cirrhotic patients, has been assessed in two randomized, controlled trials. The first trial showed, in a post hoc analysis, that rFVIIa administration might significantly improve the results of conventional therapy in patients with moderate and advanced liver failure (Child-Pugh B and C) without increasing the incidence of adverse events. A more recent trial tested rVIIa in patients with active bleeding at endoscopy and with a Child-Pugh score 8 points or higher. This trial failed to show a benefit of rVIIa in terms of decreasing the risk of 5-day failure, but it did show improved 6-week mortality. In a small prospective study involving cirrhotic patients with acute variceal bleeding and new portal vein thrombosis identified by positive intra-thrombus enhancement on contrast ultrasonography, the use of low molecular weight heparin after hemostasis is achieved by band ligation was shown to be safe, well tolerated, and effective, with complete recanalization of the portal vein within 2 to 11 days and no recurrence of bleeding.

Pharmacologic Therapy

Pharmacologic therapy can be administered early, requires no special technical expertise, and is thus a desirable first-line option for managing acute variceal hemorrhage. Drugs that reduce portocollateral venous flow (vasoconstrictors) or intrahepatic vascular resistance (vasodilators) or both have been used to achieve this effect. Vasoconstrictors work by decreasing splanchnic arterial flow, and vasodilators are used in combination with vasoconstrictors to reduce their systemic side effects, but they can also exert an added beneficial effect on intrahepatic resistance (see Table 1).

Vasopressin and Terlipressin. Vasopressin (Pitressin)[1] is a nonselective vasoconstricting agent that causes a reduction of splanchnic blood flow and thereby a reduced portal pressure. Vasopressin, which is associated with severe vascular complications, has been largely replaced by other vasoconstrictors such as its synthetic analogue, triglycyl-lysine vasopressin (terlipressin [Glypressin]).[2] Terlipressin has fewer side effects and a longer biological half-life, allowing its use as a bolus intravenous injection (2 mg every 4 hours for the initial 24 hours, then 1 mg every 4 hours for the next 24–48 hours). Terlipressin has been shown in numerous placebo-controlled trials to control bleeding in about 80% of cases and is the only pharmacologic therapy proven, as of 2010, to reduce mortality from acute variceal hemorrhage. In patients with esophageal variceal bleeding, a 24-hour course of terlipressin was shown to be as effective as a 72-hour course when used as adjunct therapy to successful variceal band ligation. Terlipressin is not currently available in the United States.

Somatostatin, Octreotide, and Vapreotide. Somatostatin,[2] a naturally occurring peptide, and its analogues, octreotide (Sandostatin)[1] and vapreotide (Sanvar),[1] stop variceal hemorrhage in up to 80% of patients and are generally considered equivalent to vasopressin (Pitressin), terlipressin[2] (Glypressin), and endoscopic therapy for the control of acute variceal bleeding. Their precise mechanism of action is unclear but might result from an effect on the release of vasoactive peptides or from reduction of postprandial hyperemia. Somatostatin is used as a continuous intravenous infusion of 250 μg/hour following a 250-μg bolus injection. Octreotide is used as a continuous infusion of 50 μg/hour and does not require a bolus injection. Side effects are minor, including hyperglycemia and mild abdominal cramps. The addition of octreotide or vapreotide to endoscopic sclerotherapy or banding improves control of bleeding and reduces transfusion requirements, with no change in overall mortality. A continuous infusion of octreotide or vapreotide is therefore recommended for 2 to 5 days following emergency endoscopic therapy.

Endoscopy

Endoscopic sclerotherapy stops variceal hemorrhage in 80% to 90% of cases. Its drawbacks include a significant risk of local complications including ulceration, bleeding, stricture, and perforation. Rare systemic complications have been reported including bacteremia with endocarditis, formation of splenic or brain abscesses, and

portal vein thrombosis. Randomized trials in patients with acute variceal bleeding have shown that EBL is essentially equivalent to endoscopic sclerotherapy in achieving initial hemostasis with lesser complications. These include superficial ulcerations, transient chest discomfort, and, rarely, stricture formation. Erythromycin infusion before endoscopy[1] in patients with acute variceal bleeding has been shown to significantly improve endoscopic visibility and to shorten the duration of the procedure.

Balloon Tamponade/SEMS

The use of the Sengstaken-Blakemore or Minnesota tube for hemostasis of variceal bleeding is based on the principle of the application of direct pressure on the bleeding varix by an inflatable—esophageal or gastric—balloon fitted on a rubber nasogastric tube. When properly applied, balloon tamponade is successful in achieving immediate hemostasis in almost all cases. However, early rebleeding following balloon decompression is high. Complications of balloon tamponade include esophageal perforation or rupture, aspiration, and asphyxiation from upper airway obstruction. Balloon tamponade or use of SEMS is generally not recommended and should largely be reserved for rescue of cases of hemorrhage uncontrolled by pharmacologic and endoscopic methods and as a temporary bridge to more definitive therapy. Self-expandable metal stents (SEMS) have recently been shown to be effective in controlling severe bleeding.

Transjugular Intrahepatic Portosystemic Shunt

Treatment with a transjugular intrahepatic portosystemic shunt (TIPS) consists of the vascular placement of an expandable metal stent across a tract created between a hepatic vein and a major intrahepatic branch of the portal system. TIPS can be successfully performed in 90% to 100% of patients, resulting in hemodynamic changes similar to a partially decompressive side-to-side portocaval shunt while avoiding the morbidity and mortality associated with a major surgical procedure. According to the American Association for the Study of Liver Diseases (AASLD) Practice Guidelines, the indications for TIPS are: (1) as rescue therapy for acute variceal hemorrhage refractory to medical and endoscopic intervention; (2) recurrent variceal hemorrhage despite medical and endoscopic treatment; and (3) an emerging indication is early TIPS within 24 to 72 hours of acute variceal hemorrhage in a select patients (e.g., those with basal HVPG >20 mm Hg). The left gastric vein is frequently embolized (embolotherapy) during TIPS creation. TIPS has been shown to be effective in treating refractory, uncontrolled, acute variceal bleeding. Patients with advanced liver disease and multiorgan failure at the time of TIPS have a 30-day mortality that approaches 100%.

Surgery

Surgery is generally considered in the setting of continued hemorrhage or recurrent early rebleeding—uncontrolled by repeated endoscopic or continued pharmacologic therapy—and when TIPS is not available or is not technically feasible. Surgical options include portosystemic shunting or esophageal staple transection alone or with esophagogastric devascularization and splenectomy (Sugiura procedure). Devascularization procedures may be useful in patients who cannot receive a shunt because of splanchnic venous thrombosis. Regardless of the choice of surgical technique, morbidity is high and the 30-day mortality for emergency surgery approaches 80% in some series. Understandably, rescue liver transplantation is not a practical option in patients with uncontrolled variceal hemorrhage.

Secondary Prophylaxis

Variceal hemorrhage recurs in approximately two thirds of patients, most commonly within the first 6 weeks after the initial episode. Patients with advanced liver disease (MELD [model for end-stage liver disease] score ≥18) have an increased risk of early rebleeding and death. Early rebleeding (within the first 5 days) is

---

[2]Not available in the United States.

[1]Not FDA approved for this indication.

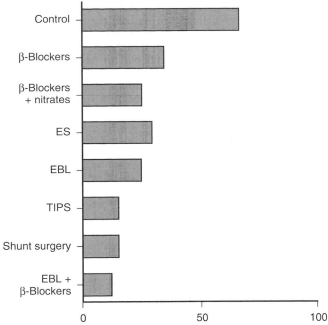

Figure 1 Relative effectiveness of available therapies for preventing recurrent variceal bleeding. The estimates shown are based on the cumulative data available in the literature for recurrent bleeding at 1 year. *Abbreviations:* EBL = endoscopic band ligation; ES = endoscopic sclerotherapy; TIPS = transjugular intrahepatic portosystemic shunt.

reduced by the adjuvant use of octreotide[1] or vapreotide[5]—and possibly terlipressin[2] and somatostatin[2]—after initial endoscopic or pharmacologic control of hemorrhage.

The severity of portal hypertension correlates closely with the severity and risk of rebleeding as well as actuarial probability of survival following an index episode. In a cohort of patients presenting with variceal hemorrhage, those with an initial HVPG greater than 20 mm Hg had a 1-year mortality of 64% compared to 20% for patients with lesser elevations in portal pressure. Given the high risk of recurrent hemorrhage and its associated morbidity and mortality, strategies aimed at prevention should be rapidly instituted following the index episode. The choice of preventive therapy should, therefore, take into consideration the efficacy of therapy, the side effects of the selected treatment, the patient's expected survival, and overall cost. Preventive strategies include pharmacologic, endoscopic, and surgical methods and are listed in Table 1. Relative effectiveness of these strategies is shown in Figure 1.

Pharmacologic Therapy

Reducing the portal pressure by more than 20% from the baseline value pharmacologically results in a reduction in the cumulative probability of recurrent bleeding from 28% at 1 year, 39% at 2 years, and 66% at 3 years to 4%, 9%, and 9%, respectively. Although adjustment of medical therapy based on portal pressure measurement would be ideal, HVPG determination might not be readily available, and treatment must be adjusted using empiric clinical parameters. Several randomized, controlled trials, including a meta-analysis, have demonstrated that β-blockers prevent rebleeding and prolong survival. The addition of isosorbide mononitrate[1] to β-blockers appears to enhance the protective effect of β-blockers alone for preventing recurrent variceal bleeding but offers no survival advantage and reduces the tolerability of therapy. A recent randomized controlled trial showed that carvedilol[1] is as effective as the combination of nadolol (Corgard)[1] plus isosorbide-5 mononitrate in the prevention of gastroesophageal variceal rebleeding, with fewer severe adverse events and similar survival.

Compared with either sclerotherapy or endoscopic band ligation, combination medical therapy is superior in reducing the risk of recurrent bleeding in patients with esophageal variceal hemorrhage, primarily in patients with Child-Pugh class A and B cirrhosis. Notably, in patients who show a significant hemodynamic response to therapy (defined as a reduction in the hepatic venous pressure gradient to <12 mm Hg or >20% of the baseline value), the risk of recurrent bleeding and of death is significantly reduced.

Endoscopy

Endoscopic therapy has been established over the past decade as a therapeutic cornerstone for preventing esophageal variceal rebleeding. Gastric varices, however, are not effectively treated by sclerotherapy or ligation. Patients with recurrent gastric variceal hemorrhage are best treated by *N*-butyl-2-cyanoacrylate injection[1] or by nonendoscopic means such as TIPS. On the other hand, EBL is highly effective at obliterating esophageal varices and is considered the endoscopic therapy of choice for secondary prophylaxis.

Combination modality approaches, usually including an endoscopic and pharmacologic treatment, are pathophysiologically attractive and may be more effective than single therapy. Two randomized, controlled trials have shown that adding β-blockers to EBL reduces the risk of rebleeding and variceal recurrence, suggesting that if EBL is used, it should be used in association with β-blockers. One randomized, controlled trial has evaluated whether EBL could improve the efficacy of the combined administration of nadolol[1] plus isosorbide.[1] In this study, adding band ligation to nadolol plus isosorbide was shown to be superior to nadolol plus isosorbide alone in preventing variceal rebleeding, but there were no significant differences in mortality. The combination of the best endoscopic treatment (EBL) and the best pharmacologic treatment (β-blockers plus isosorbide) may be the best choice in preventing rebleeding but needs further studies for confirmation. Statins improve liver generation of NO and hepatic endothelial dysfunction in experimental models of cirrhosis and may also reduce liver fibrosis. Randomized placebo-controlled trials found that simvastatin[1] decreased HVPG and improved liver perfusion and had an additive effect in patients treated with NSBB, and showed survival benefit in patients with early stages of cirrhosis and variceal bleeding.

Transjugular Intrahepatic Portosystemic Shunt

Transjugular shunting is more effective than endoscopic therapy for preventing variceal rebleeding but offers no survival benefit. The cumulative risk of rebleeding following TIPS placement is 8% to 18% at 1 year. The trade-off, however, is that TIPS is associated with a higher incidence of clinically significant hepatic encephalopathy (new or worsened portosystemic encephalopathy was noted in about 25% of patients after TIPS). Advanced liver disease is the main determinant of poor outcome following TIPS. Consequently, in patients with advanced liver disease, TIPS is best used as a bridge to liver transplantation.

TIPS, using bare stents, has been compared with surgical shunts in two studies (8 mm portocaval H-graft shunt in one and distal splenorenal shunt in the second). Although the first study showed a significantly lower rebleeding rate in the surgical group, the second and larger trial did not find any differences in rebleeding rates, hepatic encephalopathy, or mortality, but it found a significantly higher reintervention rate in the TIPS group. However, the obstruction and reintervention rates are markedly decreased with the recent use of polytetrafluoroethylene (PTFE)-covered stents. According to these data, TIPS using PTFE-covered stents represents the best rescue therapy for failures of medical and endoscopic treatment. In addition to TIPS, balloon-occluded retrograde transvenous obliteration (BRTO) is reserved primarily for prevention of recurrent bleeding, and has recently been included in the AASLD practice guidelines. Typically, it is utilized in patients who are at high risk for TIPS, such as those with elevated MELD (>18), right-sided heart failure, or hepatic encephalopathy. However, a recent prospective study showed that, in patients with

---

[1]Not FDA approved for this indication.
[2]Not available in the United States.
[5]Investigational drug in the United State.

---

[1]Not FDA approved for this indication.

located between the inferior pharyngeal constrictors and the cricopharyngeal muscles. Zenker diverticulum typically presents after age 60 and has a male predominance for reasons that are unclear. It affects only 2 per 100,000 patients per year. Although it can be asymptomatic for years before the development of symptomatology, patients may experience dysphagia, aspiration, and regurgitation of undigested food. The exact cause is unclear, but proposed mechanisms suggest a dysfunction in coordinated swallowing muscle movement and increased intraluminal pressure in the esophagus. There may be an additive component of long-term upper esophageal sphincter irritation from acid reflux.

Diagnosis is primarily made through barium swallow, although small diverticula may be missed (Figure 1). Although endoscopic direct visualization is possible, caution should be exercised owing to the risk of perforation. Small asymptomatic diverticula can be monitored. Zenker diverticulum that are less than 2 cm but symptomatic should be evaluated for possible surgical repair. Zenker diverticulum greater than 2 cm in size, regardless of symptomatology, should be surgically evaluated and repair considered. Methods for closure include endoscopic (flexible and rigid) diverticulostomy and myotomy or traditional surgical resection. Although most patients (>90%) demonstrate symptom improvement, recurrence rates can be as high as 35%. Surgery is associated with much higher morbidity and mortality than endoscopic approaches. Emerging technologies have used different techniques (harmonic scalpel, stapler, etc.) during endoscopic repair. Morbidity and mortality are largely operator dependent.

Traction Diverticulum

Traction diverticula are the only true diverticula of the esophagus. Traction diverticula are rare. Their size tends to stay less than 2 cm. Owing to the proposed mechanism of formation, traction diverticula are isolated to the middle third of the esophagus. It is not fully clear how traction diverticula form. One proposed mechanism is related to a precedent pulmonary infection, most commonly tuberculosis or histoplasmosis, with resultant mediastinal lymph node formation. After the active infection subsides, resultant fibrosis and scarring between the tissues surrounding the mediastinal lymph nodes and esophagus occur. Initially, a small diverticulum develops from this fibrosis, which produces

Figure 1 Zenker diverticulum. (Image courtesy Gastrolab—The Gastrointestinal Site. http://www.gastrolab.net [Accessed August 25, 2014].)

"traction" or a lack of mobility. Diverticular progression results when age-related changes from the dysfunction of coordinated swallowing muscle movement and increased intraluminal pressure in the esophagus develop. Surgical management is rarely needed unless these diverticula become symptomatic or complications, such as fistulas, occur.

Epiphrenic Diverticulum

Epiphrenic diverticula are false diverticula of the distal esophagus affecting only 0.015% of the general population. They are thought to arise secondary to mucosal injury from gastroesophageal reflux and muscle dysmotility. They occur within 10 cm of the gastroesophageal junction, and symptoms include dysphagia, spasmodic chest pain, and gastroesophageal reflux. There does not appear to be a correlation with between diverticular size and symptomatology. With progression of diverticular size, obstruction can become a potential complication. Diagnostic measures start with barium swallow and may be followed with additional tests, including endoscopy, 24-hour pH probe, and esophageal manometry.

Management depends on patient symptoms and size of the diverticulum. If small (<5 cm) and asymptomatic, routine clinical and endoscopic surveillance is permissible. However, any symptomatology necessitates surgical evaluation and repair. Surgical options include open resection and laparoscopy. Partial fundoplication may be indicated, depending on the severity of gastroesophageal reflux present as indicated by ancillary testing of a 24-hour pH probe. Less invasive endoscopic myotomy procedures, successfully used to treat Zenker diverticulum, are judiciously being used to treat epiphrenic diverticulum.

Stomach
Gastric Diverticula

Gastric diverticula are rare, with an endoscopic incidence of 0.01%. Gastric diverticulum may be either true or false in nature. True gastric diverticulae (70% to 75%) are typically congenital and situated along the dorsal wall of the fundus within 2 to 3 cm of the gastroesophageal junction. False diverticulae, which are less common and typically acquired, are located around the antrum of the stomach. Most are asymptomatic and small (<3 cm). Symptoms may include epigastric pain, dyspepsia, and emesis. Rarely, ulcerations, perforations, or bleeding can occur. Diagnosis involves endoscopy, barium swallow, or contrast-aided computed tomography (CT) scan. If symptomatic, typical treatment includes a proton pump inhibitor and monitoring for symptom improvement. Continued symptoms should prompt endoscopic evaluation with biopsies of suspicious lesions with raised or irregular borders. Gastric cancers have been reported in and around gastric diverticulum. Persistent symptoms may necessitate gastrectomy of the diverticulum, especially if concerns about cancer exist.

Small Intestine
Duodenal Diverticula

Diverticula located in the duodenum are relatively common, affecting up to 22% of the general population (Figure 2). Duodenal diverticula may be either true or false diverticula. The most common location is the second portion of the duodenum. Although usually asymptomatic, ulcerative bleeding, perforation, or intermittent obstruction, particularly after eating, may occur. The size and position of the diverticula may lead to complications such as obstruction of the sphincter of Oddi and/or impingement of hepatobiliary tree drainage. This impingement may result in jaundice, right upper quadrant pain, or infection signs/symptoms similar to cholecystitis. Obstruction of the bile duct leading to cholangitis is referred to as Lemmel syndrome.

Duodenal diverticula may be identified on barium swallow, contrast-enhanced CT, magnetic resonance imaging, or endoscopy. Duodenal diverticula found incidentally do not require treatment. If symptoms arise, endoscopic evaluation and surgical resection should be considered. However, intervention should be considered with caution owing to a high risk (30%) of complications, in particular fistula formation and mortality.

Figure 2 Duodenal diverticulum. (Image courtesy Gastrolab—The Gastrointestinal Site. http://www.gastrolab.net [Accessed August 25, 2014].)

Jejunal and Ileal Diverticula

Jejunal and ileal diverticula occur throughout the length of the small intestine in 1% to 2% of the population. There does not appear to be any statistically significant relationship with morbidity or mortality of these types of diverticula with respect to location, gender, size, number, and so forth. These false diverticula are located predominantly where the blood vessels penetrate the muscular wall of the mesenteric side of the bowel. Most are noted incidentally on radiographic studies, but some manifest with symptoms secondary to bleeding, obstruction, or infection. These symptoms are believed to be due to bacterial overgrowth that may occur within the cavity of the diverticulum. Diagnosis can be made with capsule endoscopy or a small bowel barium contrast follow through study, although some may be noted on MRI with intravenous contrast and/or CT with intravenous and oral contrast. Advanced endoscopic procedures such as push enteroscopy and double balloon endoscopy can be used to further evaluate symptomatic diverticula.

Asymptomatic jejunal and ileal diverticula should not be resected. Bacterial overgrowth symptoms may respond to antibiotic treatment and intestinal promotility drug therapy. If diverticulitis is seen radiographically, intravenous antibiotics and bowel rest should be initiated. Surgical intervention with small bowel resection is indicated if symptomatic diverticula persist despite conservative management.

Meckel Diverticulum

Meckel diverticulum is a true diverticulum—a congenital anomaly that occurs owing to incomplete closure of the vitelline duct. This duct typically obliterates during the ninth week of gestational age. Owing to the embryologic origin of the diverticulum, it is almost always located within 2 feet of the ileocecal valve. Meckel diverticulum has a prevalence of 1% to 2% of the population, with a 2:1 male predominance. Approximately 2% of all existing Meckel diverticula will become symptomatic. Symptomatic diverticula most commonly cause nausea, vomiting, and abdominal pain. The sign most commonly associated with Meckel diverticulum is intussusception. This occurs owing to residual fibrous attachments to the umbilicus causing a lead point for the proximal bowel to involute onto the distal bowel. It most commonly presents with bloody mucoid stools, abdominal pain, and vomiting in children younger than 6 years of age, most commonly within the first 2 years of life. However, other symptoms may occur if ectopic tissue exists in the diverticulum. Gastric ectopic tissue may cause abdominal pain and bloody stools from ulceration of the underlying ileal tissue. Duodenal and pancreatic tissues have been identified in Meckel diverticulum but are very rare and do not typically cause symptoms.

Diagnosis in adults requires a high level of suspicion and is aided by the use of a technetium 99m (^{99m}Tc) scan to identify ectopic gastric mucosa in those patients with bleeding and symptoms of ulceration. For children with obstructive signs or symptoms, the diagnosis may be aided by ultrasound and/or computed tomographic scans. Plain film radiographs of the abdomen have low sensitivity and specificity for the diagnosis of intussusception. The sensitivity of the Meckel scan for the pediatric population is 85% to 97% but is much lower in the adult population at 62%. The choice of imaging procedure is dictated by the experience of the radiologic personnel performing the procedure.

Symptomatic Meckel diverticulum should be surgically resected. Up to 90% of intussusception secondary to Meckel diverticulum may be reduced using diagnostic ultrasonography with saline or pneumatic enema. Treatment of Meckel diverticulum largely depends on age and symptomatology because operating on asymptomatic Meckel diverticulum has been shown to have a fivefold increase in complications, such as postoperative bowel obstruction, leaks, ileus, and infection. Many experts have advocated that incidental, asymptomatic Meckel diverticulum should not be resected. Some experts advocate for selective surgical resection of asymptomatic patients with an incidentally noted Meckel diverticulum for the following: healthy young children, healthy adults younger than 50 years of age with palpable abnormalities suggestive of heterotrophic tissue, size longer than 2 cm, or a broad base wider than 2 cm.

Colon

Diverticulosis

The colon is where most diverticula occur in the alimentary tract. Owing to this predominance, this condition is commonly termed *diverticulosis* or *diverticular disease*. Diverticulum of the colon is of the false type. The incidence increases with age. The incidence of left-sided diverticulosis approaches 5% at age 40 and increases to greater than 60% at age 80. Diverticulosis is most commonly located in the sigmoid colon.

The exact pathogenesis of diverticulosis is unclear. The proposed mechanism of colonic diverticular formation places an emphasis on intraluminal pressure buildup. The pressure across the colonic wall increases as the radius of the wall decreases. Accordingly, the radius is the smallest in the sigmoid colon and thus the most likely location of diverticulosis. Normally, pressure is constant throughout the colon. However, as diverticular disease develops, abnormal pressure segmentations occur, resulting in pressure gradient changes in the colon. With increased pressure, the integrity of collagen and elastin in the wall muscle changes, the circular muscles thicken, colonic segments shorten, and the lumen narrows, leading to propagation of the disease. Several risk factors have been associated with the development of diverticular disease: smoking, lack of physical activity, and obesity. By increasing the amount of dietary fiber, it is theorized that the resultant bulking of the stools may decrease the pressure in the colon lumen and prevent diverticular disease progression. Yet, mixed results have been noted on studies of fiber intake and diverticular development and progression of disease. There is no associated risk with the ingestion of caffeine, alcohol, popcorn, seeds, or nuts and the development of diverticulosis, diverticular bleeding, or diverticulitis.

Colonic Diverticular Bleeding

Diverticula tend to develop where an arteriole penetrates the circular muscle layer of the colon. This results in vessels arching over the dome of the diverticulum. This leaves fragile vessels in a vulnerable position of a relatively thin mucosal layer prone to trauma and resultant diverticular bleeding. Bleeding typically manifests as hematochezia—a darkish to bright red bleeding that is typically characterized as brisk and acute in nature. Diverticulosis is attributed to 30% to 50% of all hematochezia. Fifteen percent of patients will experience at least one episode of bleeding in their lifetime, with a recurrent bleeding risk of up to 38%.

Most patients presenting with diverticular bleeding are asymptomatic, but some may experience bloating or cramping.

Selection of the diagnostic modality depends largely on the degree of bleeding and the cardiovascular stability of the patient. Endoscopy is the preferred treatment modality for stable patients owing to its potential for diagnosis and treatment options. Up to 80% of diverticular bleeding can be isolated with direct endoscopic visualization (Figure 3).

Endoscopic failure to identify or control diverticular bleeding may occur in the patient with massive or intermittent bleeding. Depending on the patient's cardiovascular stability and degree of bleeding, the typical evaluative progression if the site of bleeding is not identified is endoscopy, followed by tagged red blood cell scan, and then angiography. Hemodynamically unstable patients may have a high complication risk from the bowel preparation, sedation, or the procedure. Radionuclide imaging can be considered in unstable patients, nondiagnostic endoscopy, or bleeding recurrence. Radionuclide imaging requires that bleeding be active (at least 0.05 to 0.1 mL/min) to accurately isolate the location of the diverticulum. Radionuclide imaging using ^{99m}Tc sulfur colloid (shorter half-life, thus used for acute bleeding) or ^{99m}Tc pertechnetate (longer half-life more useful for intermittent bleeding)-labeled autologous red blood cells can be used to isolate the location of obscure gastrointestinal bleeding. However, numerous studies have produced highly variable sensitivities (26% to 91%). Many advocate for radionuclide imaging to be used as an ancillary test for directing more definitive treatments such as surgery or angiography-directed therapies. Angiography can be used if bleeding is active (at least 0.5 mL/min) and can isolate the bleeding location with a diagnostic yield of 40% to 78%. Angiography can be combined with embolization and/or vasopressin infusion to achieve hemostasis; however, complications may occur, including bowel infarction, rebleeding, and contrast-induced nephrotoxicity.

Diverticulitis

Diverticulosis is largely asymptomatic. Only approximately 4% will develop inflammation and infection known as diverticulitis. The disease severity and complications occur along a spectrum. The proposed mechanism of diverticulitis may be a blocked diverticulum or increased intraluminal pressure inducing. Subsequent vascular compromise and microperforation may occur, leading to localized infection and inflammation. These microperforations are usually sequestered and may lead to small localized abscess formation. This process is generally referred to as uncomplicated diverticulitis. Complicated diverticulitis is classified when a localized abscess or infection infiltrates into adjacent organs or viscera causing macroperforations, fistulas, obstructions, or enlarged abscesses.

The clinical presentation often begins with mild left lower abdominal pain, fever, and leukocytosis. Patients who seek care later in the

disease process may present with sepsis or diffuse peritonitis. Initial diagnosis should be accomplished with history, physical examination, radiographic imaging, and laboratory evaluation. Abdominal radiography has limited utility but may reveal severe complications of diverticulitis such as bowel perforation or bowel obstruction. Ultrasonography and magnetic resonance imaging can be used with high levels of sensitivity and specificity in centers with demonstrated expertise. Ultrasonography has sensitivities and specificities of 92% and 90% for the detection of diverticulitis, respectively. With sensitivities and specificities of 94% and 99%, respectively, CT appears to be the imaging test of choice. This is especially true, as an alternative diagnosis was more likely to be identified with CT than with ultrasonography (50% to 100% vs. 33% to 78%). Those patients with a past medical history of diverticulitis may be empirically treated without imaging, although imaging may be needed if no clinical improvement is noted within 48 hours.

New trials indicate no added benefit with antimicrobial therapy in select patients with uncomplicated diverticulitis. Factors such as pain control, hospitalization rates, and revisits were found to be similar between patients randomized to conservative management and antibiotic administration plus conservative measures. Thus patients may be treated with a liquid diet, analgesics, and close clinical follow-up without antibiotics. Outpatient management is reasonable if the diagnosis is made early in the disease process. Complicated diverticulitis occurs in 25% of all diverticulitis diagnoses, requiring a surgical evaluation and intervention. Optional antibiotic regimens for gram-negative coverage and anaerobic coverage are listed in Table 1. Inpatient management is recommended with any high-risk comorbid conditions, immunosuppression, high-grade fever, leukocytosis, inability to tolerate oral fluids, and/or for elderly patients. Patient improvement should be seen within 48 hours. Those who do not improve should undergo additional evaluation such as repeat imaging or endoscopy. This is done to evaluate for underlying pathology such as cancer or inflammatory bowel disease, which would change the management strategy.

Follow-up scanning should also be considered for cases of slow-resolving diverticulitis. In the past, up to 10% of CT scans in which diverticulitis was the primary diagnosis, cancer could not be fully excluded. As CT scanner resolution has improved, newer studies have demonstrated only a small number of underlying cancers or indeterminate findings. A colonoscopy should be performed to evaluate the extent of diverticular disease and to rule out other comorbid pathology in all patients. Colonoscopy is typically recommended 6 weeks after diverticulitis symptoms have resolved, if one has not been done within the last year. Introduction of stool softeners and a high-fiber diet should begin immediately and continued indefinitely for all patients to help decrease the intraluminal pressure within the colon.

Figure 3 Colonoscopy in a patient with hematochezia from the source isolated to a diverticulum (A) and hemostasis noted after placement of two hemoclips (B). (Courtesy Janak Shah. From Feldman M. *Sleisenger and Fordtran's Gastrointestinal and Liver Disease.* 9th ed. Philadelphia: Elsevier; Figure 117.8.)

TABLE 1	Antibiotic Therapy for Diverticulitis	
OPTIONAL REGIMENS	**DOSAGE (ADULT)**	
Uncomplicated Diverticulitis		
Outpatient (10–14 days)		
Ciprofloxacin (Cipro) and Metronidazole (Flagyl)	500 mg PO bid 500 mg PO tid	
Amoxicillin-clavulanate (Augmentin)[1]	875 mg PO bid	
Moxifloxacin (Avelox)	400 mg PO daily	
Complicated Diverticulitis *Inpatient Transitioning to Outpatient (10–14 Days Total)*		
Piperacillin-tazobactam (Zosyn)[1]	3.375–4.5 g IV every 6 h	
Imipenem-cilastatin (Primaxin)	500 mg IV every 6 h	
Levofloxacin (Levaquin)[1] and Metronidazole	500 mg IV every 24 h 500 mg IV every 8 h	
Ceftriaxone (Rocephin) and Metronidazole	1 g IV every 24 h 500 mg IV every 8 h	

[1]Not FDA approved for this indication.
Clindamycin (Cleocin) may be substituted in metronidazole intolerance/allergy. Antibiotics continued in complicated diverticulitis cases until negative cultures, clinical improvement, or sensitivities obtained on any surgical specimens.
bid, Twice a day; *tid*, three times a day.
Modified from Jacobs DO. Clinical practice: diverticulitis. *N Engl J Med.* 2007;357:2057–2066.

Figure 4 Diverticulitis. (A) Computed tomography (CT) image demonstrates thickened wall of the sigmoid colon *(arrows)* with stranding in the adjacent fat *(*)* indicative of diverticulitis. Fat stranding refers to abnormally increased attenuation of fat from edema and engorgement of lymphatics. (B) CT image slightly more caudal demonstrates an air-filled abscess cavity *(arrows)* with adjacent thickened sigmoid colon wall. (From McNally PR. GI/Liver Secrets Plus, 4th ed. Noninvasive Gastrointestinal Imaging: *Ultrasound, Computed Tomography, Magnetic Resonance Imaging.* Philadelphia: Mosby Elsevier; 2010, Figure 70–16.)

Diverticulitis that is complicated with abscess formation should be evaluated by a surgeon or radiologist for percutaneous drainage using CT or ultrasonography (Figure 4). Depending on location, aspiration or drainage tubes may be used to facilitate drainage. A general recommendation exists for consideration of drainage, preferably with interventional radiology localization, for any abscess measuring greater than 3 to 4 cm.

New research to prevent recurrent diverticulitis with medical management is emerging. Rifaximin (Xifaxan)[1] may help prevent recurrent episodes of diverticulitis. Probiotics[7] have not been shown to prevent recurrence. Fiber may be used as a beneficial supplement for the prevention of recurrent diverticulitis. Debate exists regarding elective segmental colectomy for patients who have experienced recurrent episodes of diverticulitis. Current recommendations suggest surgical consultation with discussion of the benefits and risks of surgery compared with the risks of recurrent diverticulitis. This discussion should take into account the diverticulitis frequency and severity, the impact on the patient's lifestyle, and the patient's other comorbid conditions. This consultation should at a minimum occur after the fourth recurrence of diverticulitis in patients older than age 50. There is insufficient evidence to advise a patient who has experienced fewer than four recurrent cases of diverticulitis or who is younger than age 50 on the benefit of a segmental colectomy.

---

[1]Not FDA approved for this indication.
[7]Available as a dietary supplement.

References

Choi JJ, Ogunjemilusi O, Divino CM: Diagnosis and management of diverticula in the jejunum and ileum, *Am Surg* 79(1):108–110, 2013.

Delavux M: Diverticular disease of the colon in Europe: Epidemiology, impact on citizen health and prevention, *Aliment Pharmacol Ther* 18(Suppl 3):71–74, 2003.

Fry RD, Mahmoud NN, Maron DJ, et al: Colon and rectum. In Townsend Jr CM, Beauchamp D, editors: *Sabiston Textbook of Surgery*, 19th ed, Philadelphia, 2012, Saunders, pp 1309–1314.

Greene CL, McFadden PM, Oh DS, et al: Long-term outcome of the treatment of Zenker's diverticulum, *Ann Thorac Surg* 100:975–978, 2015.

Ishaq S, Sultan H, Siau K, et al: New and emerging techniques for endoscopic treatment of Zenker's Diverticulum: State-of-the-art review, *Digestive Endoscopy* 30:449–460, 2018.

Jacobs DO: Clinical practice, Diverticulitis, *N Engl J Med* 357:2057–2066, 2007.

Janes SE, Meagher A, Frizelle FA: Management of diverticulitis, *BMJ* 332:271–275, 2006.

Kilic A, Schuchert MJ, Awais O, et al: Surgical management of epiphrenic diverticula in the minimally invasive era, *JSLS* 13:160–164, 2009.

Lameris W, van Randen A, Bipat S: Graded compression ultrasonography and computed tomography in acute colonic diverticulitis: Meta-analysis of test accuracy, *Eur Radiol* 18:2498–2511, 2008.

Lin S, Suhocki PV, Ludwig KA, et al: Gastrointestinal bleeding in adult patients with Meckel's diverticulum: The role of technetium 99m pertechnetate scan, *South Med J* 95:1338, 2002.

Maish MS: Esophagus. In Townsend Jr CM, Beauchamp D, editors: *Sabiston Textbook of Surgery*, 19th ed, Philadelphia, 2012, Saunders, pp 1023–1025.

Martinez-Cecilia D, Arjona-Sanchez A, Gomez-Alvarez M, et al: Conservative management of perforated duodenal diverticulum: A case report and review of the literature, *World J Gastroenterol* 14:1949–1951, 2008.

Mohan P, Ananthavadivelu M, Venkataraman J: Gastric diverticulum, *CMAJ* 182:E226, 2010.

Mora-López L, Ruiz-Edo N, Estrada-Ferrer O, et al: Efficacy and safety of nonantibiotic outpatient treatment in mild acute diverticulitis (DINAMO-study): a multicentre, randomised, open-label, noninferiority trial. *Ann Surg.* 274(5):e435, 2021

Morris AM, Rogenbogen SE, Hardiman KM, et al: Sigmoid diverticulitis: A systematic review, *JAMA* 311:287–297, 2014.

Mulder CJ, Costamagna G, Sakai P: Zenker's diverticulum: Treatment using a flexible endoscope, *Endoscopy* 33:991–997, 2001.

Oukachbi N, Brouzes S: Management of complicated duodenal diverticula, *J Visceral Surg* 150:173–179, 2013.

Park JJ, Wolff BG, Tollefson MK, et al: Meckel diverticulum: The Mayo Clinic experience with 1476 patients (1950– 2002), *Ann Surg* 241:529–533, 2005.

Sartelli M, Catena F, Ansaloni L, et al: WSES Guidelines for the management of acute left sided colonic diverticulitis in the emergency setting, *World J Emerg Surg* 11:37, 2016.

Shabanzadeh DM, Wille-Jørgensen P: Antibiotics for uncomplicated diverticulitis, Nov 14, *Cochrane Database Syst Rev* 11, 2012. https://doi.org/10.1002/14651858.

Shah J, Patel K, Sunkara T, et al: Gastric Diverticulum: A Comprehensive Review, *Inflamm Intest Dis* 3:161–166, 2018.

Shahedi K, Fuller G, Bolus R, et al: Long-term risk of acute diverticulitis among patients with incidental diverticulosis found during colonoscopy, *Clin Gastroenterol Hepatol* 11(12):1609–1613, 2013.

Sinha CK, Pallewatte A, Easty Met al, et al: Meckel's scan in children: A review of 183 cases referred to two paediatric surgery specialist centres over 18 years, *Pediatr Surg Int* 29:511–517, 2013.

Strate LL: Lower GI, bleeding: Epidemiology and diagnosis, *Gastroenterol Clin North Am* 34:643–664, 2005.

Verdonck J, Morton RP: Systematic review on treatment of Zenker's diverticulum, *Eur Arch Otorhnolaryngol* 272:3095–3107, 2015.

Weizman AV, Nguyen GC: Diverticular disease: epidemiology and management, *Can J Gastroenterol* 25:385–389, 2011.

Young-Fadok TM: Diverticulitis, *N Engl J Med* 379, 2018. 1635-164.

Zani A, Eaton S, Rees CM: Incidentally detected Meckel diverticulum: To resect or not to resect? *Ann Surg* 247:276–281, 2008.

DYSPHAGIA AND ESOPHAGEAL OBSTRUCTION

Method of
Chrisopher Vélez, MD; John E. Pandolfino, MD; Kumar Krishnan, MD

CURRENT DIAGNOSIS

- The evaluation of dysphagia begins with a careful history, though additional diagnostic testing is often required.
- Oropharyngeal dysphagia is best initially evaluated with a video fluoroscopoic examination, whereas esophageal dysphagia is best evaluated with endoscopy.
- Esophageal dysphagia with negative endoscopy and biopsy should be evaluated next with esophageal physiological testing (esophageal manometry or endoscopic functional lumen imaging probe EndoFLIP).

CURRENT THERAPY

- Underlying neuromuscular conditions such as amyotrophic lateral sclerosis, myasthenia gravis, or Guillain-Barré syndrome should be treated accordingly.
- Endoscopic therapy with dilation (often multiple) is the mainstay of treating fibrotic esophageal strictures regardless of etiology.
- Achalasia can be treated surgically or with dilation, which are equally effective. Minimally invasive endoscopic therapy for achalasia is now a well established alternative treatment approach.

Dysphagia is a symptom generated by the perceived sensation of difficulty or inability to swallow. It ranges in severity from mild difficulty with no associated clinical sequelae, to a complete inability to swallow with aspiration and severe malnutrition. Dysphagia can coexist with and must be distinguished from odynophagia, which is pain when swallowing, with associated swallowing aversion. The etiology of dysphagia is protean and includes two main categories, mechanical obstruction and motor dysfunction.

Epidemiology

Dysphagia is a common condition. In studies of outpatients, 22.6% of patients have reported dysphagia at least several times per month. Only half of these patients had discussed their symptoms with their physician. Elderly patients and women were more likely to note symptoms of dysphagia.

Pathophysiology

Effective swallowing and transfer of food bolus into the stomach requires multiple steps. These steps can be broadly placed into two phases: the oropharyngeal phase and the esophageal phase. The oropharyngeal phase of swallowing ultimately transforms the hypopharynx from a respiratory organ to a digestive organ. It requires five main coordinated steps to occur: (1) elevation of the soft palate and closure of the nasopharynx, (2) relaxation of the upper esophageal sphincter (UES), (3) traction opening of the UES, (4) closure of the laryngeal vestibule and, hence, airway protection, and (5) propulsion of the food bolus by the tongue and pharyngeal constrictors. This process is a carefully coordinated neuromuscular phenomenon with both autonomic and volitional components.

The esophageal phase of swallowing begins when a food bolus passes through the UES. During swallowing, the rapidity of bolus transit into the stomach is accomplished primarily by gravity.

Esophageal peristalsis is a secondary contributor that functions to strip the bolus and clear the esophagus. Primary peristalsis is associated with oropharyngeal swallowing and propagates down through the predominantly striated muscle of the esophagus via a sequential activation pattern originating from the brainstem. This propagation then involves the esophageal smooth muscle where it also engages the intrinsic enteric nervous system to promote peristalsis through a similar but distinct mechanism. Secondary peristalsis is stimulated by distention of the proximal esophagus and will generate a propagating peristaltic contraction similar to primary peristalsis without a swallow-induced trigger. The strength, propagation velocity, and order of peristaltic contractions can be altered, with perturbations potentially leading to motor abnormalities associated with dysphagia.

Diagnosis

Dysphagia is never a normal symptom and always requires additional investigation. The first step in the diagnostic evaluation of dysphagia begins with a careful history to distinguish true dysphagia from other associated conditions such as odynophagia and globus sensation. Odynophagia can coexist with dysphagia; however, the predominant symptom is pain during swallowing. Globus is a sensation of a lump in the throat. It is likely a pharyngeal hypersensitivity that may coexist with other esophageal diseases or occur alone as a functional disorder. Unlike dysphagia, the symptoms in globus persist between swallows and may actually improve during the swallow.

After the above conditions have been ruled out, the next step focuses on distinguishing oropharyngeal dysphagia from esophageal dysphagia. Asking patients if their difficulty swallowing is "above-the-gulp" can differentiate oropharyngeal dysphagia. Unfortunately, patients have a difficult time communicating their symptoms because localization of the point of perceived obstruction is hampered by poor discriminant capacity and may be masked by compensatory mechanisms. Localization of dysphagia to the throat or sternal notch is unreliable because the point of obstruction may be further down in the body. However, localization in the midchest or below is more reliable that the obstruction is esophageal in origin.

As a result, the most useful and underused test for distinguishing oropharyngeal and esophageal dysphagia focuses on observing the patient swallow sips of water in the office. Often this allows the distinction between oropharyngeal and esophageal dysphagia to become apparent. Patients with oropharyngeal dysphagia will have difficulty almost immediately after initiating a swallow, such as coughing, choking, and nasal regurgitation. Patients who can initiate a swallow without difficulty, but note symptoms soon after the swallow, are likely to have esophageal dysphagia. Furthermore, this exercise may be able to elicit associated odynophagia or regurgitation.

Physical examination plays a minor role in evaluating dysphagia outside of assessing the patient's baseline status to rule out malnutrition and dehydration because this will determine whether an expedited evaluation is required. A careful assessment of the oropharynx and a careful neck examination may unmask a mass lesion (i.e. of the thyroid), and a neurologic examination should be performed if oropharyngeal dysphagia is suspected. Additionally, a skin examination and assessment of the oropharyngeal mucosa may be helpful in assessing for potential dermatologic diseases that are associated with esophageal dysphagia. Regardless of findings, most patients will ultimately be referred for diagnostic testing, and this is dependent on the anatomic zone of interest—oropharyngeal versus esophageal (Figure 1).

Diagnostic Testing
Oropharyngeal Dysphagia

Once a distinction is made that the patient is experiencing oropharyngeal dysphagia, the next step in the evaluation should be referral for a video fluoroscopic swallowing examination, also known as a modified barium study. Standard upper endoscopy is of limited value given the general inability to evaluate lesions

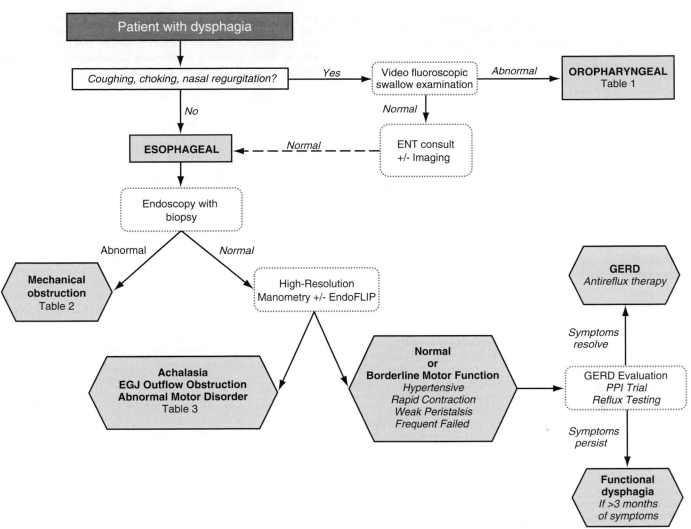

Figure 1 The workup of dysphagia and esophageal obstruction. The first step in the workup of dysphagia focuses on distinguishing oropharyngeal from esophageal dysphagia, which can be done with a history and careful assessment of swallowing during liquid swallows. The workup once this distinction is made is very different. Oropharyngeal dysphagia is typically evaluated by speech pathology and otolaryngology (ENT) based on the results of a video fluoroscopic swallow evaluation. Esophageal dysphagia is evaluated primarily with endoscopy because biopsies and interventions are often required. The primary indication for manometry is to rule out a major motor disorder in patients with a negative endoscopy. Alternatively, the functional lumen imaging probe (FLIP) can be utilized at the time of endoscopy to assess for a primary motor disorder. If a major motor abnormality is not seen on manometry or FLIP, a diagnosis of functional dysphagia should be considered; however, underlying GERD must also be addressed.

in the hypopharynx and the upper esophageal sphincter. Video fluoroscopic swallow examinations have the added benefit of providing functional information in addition to anatomic information. They differ from a standard fluoroscopic examination (i.e., esophogram) by offering the patient various radiopaque food items of different consistency and are often performed by a speech pathologist. They can evaluate delay in initiation of pharyngeal swallowing, aspiration of solids and liquids, retrograde flow of ingested bolus, and residual pharyngeal contents.

If there is a suspicion for a malignancy or mechanical obstruction, a referral to otolaryngology is required. Direct laryngoscopy is used to evaluate for anatomic lesions in the nasopharynx and hypopharynx. In addition to anatomic abnormalities, function can be assessed by having the patient drink liquids with the nasal endoscope positioned in the hypopharynx. Oropharyngeal pooling of liquid indicates ineffective hypopharyngeal clearance and can suggest a high aspiration risk. Cross-sectional imaging is often an adjunct to the functional assessment of videoscopic imaging or direct laryngoscopy when an obstruction is noted without a clear lesion noted on direct examination.

Esophageal Dysphagia

If oropharyngeal dysphagia is excluded on history, the evaluation of dysphagia should proceed to upper endoscopy to rule out a mechanical obstruction. Although an esophogram can be used to assess for obstruction, most patients will eventually require endoscopy to obtain biopsies to rule out malignancy or eosinophilic esophagitis. Additionally, endoscopy has the added benefit of being therapeutic in some circumstances, and thus it is more cost-effective to begin the evaluation with endoscopy. If the endoscopy is negative, the next step is to evaluate for an underlying esophageal motor disorder. This is traditionally done by performing esophageal manometry. Recently, a novel method of assessing esophageal motor function has been developed. The functional lumen imaging probe (FLIP) is a catheter that can be placed at the time of endoscopy. Using a variety of sensors positioned along the length of the probe, it measures diameter and pressure along the esophagus. This information can be used to evaluate for contractility of the esophageal body and esophageal distensibility at the EGJ, thus providing a comprehensive assessment of esophageal motility that is complementary to esophageal manometry and can help resolve borderline cases of motility abnormality prior to the recommendation of potentially invasive surgical or endoscopic therapy. If these studies are negative, a careful evaluation for the presence of gastroesophageal reflux disease (GERD) should be performed and if suspected, the patient may benefit from ambulatory reflux testing or an empiric trial of proton pump inhibitors. Patients with no evidence of obstruction, abnormal esophageal motor function, or evidence of GERD may be classified as having functional dysphagia and they benefit from the use of neuromodulation (with agents used to treat functional gastrointestinal disorders such as tricyclic antidepressants) to improve sensory function.

Oropharyngeal Dysphagia

Differential Diagnosis

The etiology of oropharyngeal dysphagia can be broadly separated based on neuromuscular causes and anatomic causes (Table 1). The most common neurologic cause is cerebrovascular accident (CVA), with an incidence reported between 20% and 80%. CVAs involving the cerebrum, cerebellum, and brainstem can each lead to swallow dysfunction. Cerebral CVA can lead to impairment in mastication and the oral phase of swallowing and can interrupt normal pharyngeal peristalsis. CVA involving the brainstem can lead to disruption of the sensory afferents in the pharynx that help

---

TABLE 1 Oropharyngeal Dysphagia

Iatrogenic

- Medication side effects (chemotherapy, neuroleptics, etc.)
- Postsurgical muscular or neurogenic
- Radiation
- Corrosive (pill injury, intentional)

Infectious

- Diphtheria
- Botulism
- Lyme disease
- Syphilis
- Mucositis (herpes, cytomegalovirus, candida, etc.)

Metabolic

- Amyloidosis
- Cushing's syndrome
- Thyrotoxicosis
- Wilson's disease

Myopathic

- Connective tissue disease (overlap syndrome)
- Dermatomyositis
- Myasthenia gravis
- Myotonic dystrophy
- Oculopharyngeal dystrophy
- Polymyositis
- Sarcoidosis
- Paraneoplastic syndromes

Neurologic

- Brainstem tumors
- Head trauma
- Stroke
- Cerebral palsy
- Guillain-Barré syndrome
- Huntington's disease
- Multiple sclerosis
- Polio
- Postpolio syndrome
- Tardive dyskinesia
- Metabolic encephalopathies
- Amyotrophic lateral sclerosis
- Parkinson's disease
- Dementia

Structural

- Cricopharyngeal bar
- Zenker's diverticulum
- Cervical webs
- Oropharyngeal tumors
- Osteophytes and skeletal abnormalities
- Congenital abnormalities (cleft palate, diverticula, pouches, etc.)

---

trigger pharyngeal swallow, and can also lead to motor dysfunction of laryngeal elevation, glottic closure, and cricopharyngeal relaxation/opening. Tumors in these areas can also produce similar effects. While difficulty swallowing liquids can be associated with oropharyngeal dysphagia, distinguishing between liquid versus solid food dysphagia is not a reliable way to differentiate this type of dysphagia from esophageal dysphagia.

A variety of neuromuscular disease can lead to bulbar symptoms, which manifest as dysphagia. This includes myasthenia gravis, amyotrophic lateral sclerosis (ALS), and Guillain-Barré syndrome (GBS). Clinicians need to be able to identify systemic manifestations of these conditions because dysphagia can often be the first manifestation of neuromuscular disorders.

The most common structural abnormalities of the hypopharynx associated with dysphagia are hypopharyngeal diverticula and cricopharyngeal bars. Acquired hypopharyngeal diverticula are most common in men after age 60 and typically present with symptoms of dysphagia, halitosis, post-swallow regurgitation, or even aspiration of material from the pharyngeal pouch. Hypopharyngeal diverticula are the result of a restrictive myopathy associated with diminished compliance of the cricopharyngeus muscle. The treatment of hypopharyngeal diverticula is cricopharyngeal myotomy with or without a diverticulectomy. Good or excellent results can be expected in 80% to 100% of Zenker's patients treated by transcervical myotomy combined with diverticulectomy or diverticulopexy. Small diverticula may spontaneously disappear following myotomy.

Other anatomic causes associated with oropharyngeal dysphagia that should be considered are cervical osteophytes and head and neck cancers. Cervical osteophytes are associated with cervical spine arthritis and may be confused with a cricopharygeal bar because the dysphagia is structural and localized to the area of the upper esophageal sphincter. It is easily differentiated on contrast studies because the cervical osteophyte can be seen impinging on the upper sphincter. Additionally, head and neck lesions of the larynx, tonsil, tongue, oral cavity, vocal cord, and nasopharynx may also impair bolus transit into the esophagus. Rapid weight loss in a patient with oropharyngeal dysphagia warrants further evaluation for malignancy; however, it is often difficult to distinguish weight loss resulting from malignancy from weight loss secondary to dysphagia. Constitutional symptoms (night sweats, fever, etc.) associated with oropharyngeal dysphagia should raise the suspicion for lymphoma.

Management

The management of oropharyngeal dysphagia is dependent on the underlying cause. Neuromuscular conditions such as stroke may respond to speech therapy and rehabilitation. Systemic neuromuscular dysfunction from conditions such as myasthenia gravis, GBS, or ALS will require treatment of the underlying condition. Patients who cannot safely take oral nutrition may need a temporary enteral feeding tube until swallow function is intact.

Management of dysphagia in patients with head and neck cancers requires a multidisciplinary approach and treatment of the underlying malignancy. Some patients are able to take adequate nutrition with dietary modification (soft or full liquid diet) while undergoing therapy. Patients who are losing weight, are dehydrated, or are unable to meet nutritional requirement by dietary modification alone may require enteral nutrition in the form of a gastrostomy tube. Although endoscopic gastrostomy tube placement is typically safe, and routinely performed in patients with head and neck cancer, there are reports of seeding the gastrostomy tube tract with malignant cells from the pharynx. In such circumstances, a direct gastrostomy tube placed by a radiologist may be preferable.

Esophageal Dysphagia

Esophageal dysphagia can be easily separated into mechanical causes and motor abnormalities after upper endoscopy is performed. Mechanical causes can be further separated into malignant and benign causes of dysphagia, and motor disorders can be conceptualized as primary motor abnormalities versus borderline motor abnormalities. Patients who have symptoms in the context of a normal endoscopy (negative biopsies for eosinophilic esophagitis) and no evidence of a primary motor disorder may also have underlying GERD or functional dysphagia (see Figure 1).

Differential Diagnosis: Mechanical Obstruction (Table 2)

Stricture

Fibrotic esophageal strictures are common and can be caused by erosive esophagitis (peptic stricture), radiation therapy, surgical anastomosis, eosinophilic esophagitis, and desquamating lesions (pemphigus, lichen planus, etc.). Peptic strictures are common and are the result of long-standing erosive esophagitis. They typically occur in the distal esophagus. Such patients often have underlying physiologic derangements that favor aggressive reflux (weak lower esophageal sphincter, hiatal hernia, poor esophageal clearance). Postsurgical anastomotic strictures are an unfortunate consequence of surgical therapy for esophageal disease, but these lesions are often amenable to endoscopic therapy.

Eosinophilic Esophagitis

Eosinophilic esophagitis (EoE) requires some focused discussion because its prevalence in patients presenting with dysphagia is increasing. EoE is a condition characterized by marked eosinophilic infiltrate within the esophageal epithelium. This infiltrate results in characteristic endoscopic findings of esophageal rings, furrows, exudate, and eventually stricture formation. The most common symptom in patients with EoE is dysphagia, which often leads to food bolus impaction. Patients are typically young Caucasians and there is a clear male predominance. Atopic conditions are more prevalent in patients with EoE. Patients should initially be treated with proton pump inhibitor (PPI) therapy because there is an overlap between GERD and EoE. Patients with persistent eosinophilia on PPI therapy can be treated by swallowing inhaled formulations of steroids (fluticasone [Flovent],[1] budesonide [Pulmicort][1]) or a food elimination diet (avoid: soy, nuts, wheat, eggs, dairy, seafood) to reduce the inflammatory component of the disease. Additional therapy with dilation will be required in many patients because histologic improvement does not always result in regression of fibrotic strictures. The esophageal body is more prone to fracture in EoE, and deep mucosal tears are often associated with dilation therapy; thus these lesions may require a more gradual and careful dilation protocol.

---

[1]Not FDA approved for this indication.

TABLE 2	Esophageal Dysphagia (Mechanical)

Mucosal disease
  GERD (peptic stricture)
  Esophageal rings
  Esophageal cancer
  Caustic injury (e.g., lye ingestion, pill esophagitis, sclerotherapy)
  Radiation injury
  Infectious esophagitis
  Eosinophilic esophagitis
  Anastomotic stricture
  Submucosal disease
  Gastrointestinal stromal tumor
  Sarcoidosis
  Invasive carcinoma (primary or secondary)
Mediastinal disease
  Tumors (lymph nodes, lung cancer)
  Infection (histoplasmosis, tuberculosis)
  Vascular compression
  Dysphagia lusoria
  Dysphagia aortica

Rings/Webs

Esophageal webs can exist along the length of the esophagus and lead to dysphagia. The classic triad of proximal esophageal web, iron deficiency anemia, and dysphagia is Plummer-Vinson syndrome. The etiology of this condition is not entirely known; however, it is thought that iron deficiency leads to a decrease in iron-dependent oxidative enzymes, which results in degradation of esophageal tissue, resulting in web formation. Interestingly, iron supplementation alone may result in resolution of symptoms. Whereas Plummer-Vinson syndrome is a rare condition, esophageal webs are relatively common and should prompt an evaluation for caustic pill injury if localized to the transition zone along the aortic impression or distal esophagus. Medications that can be associated with pill esophagitis include NSAIDs, tetracycline, iron, bisphosphonates, potassium, and quinidine.

Malignancy

Dysphagia is often the presenting symptom in a patient with esophageal cancer. There are two subtypes of mucosal cancer in the esophagus, squamous cell and adenocarcinoma. In general, esophageal cancer has a male predominance and is slightly more prevalent among African Americans. The racial disparity is largely due to squamous cell carcinoma, which has noted a sharp decline since the 1960s. Adenocarcinoma tends to be a disease of white men (SEER database). Squamous cell carcinoma typically occurs in the mid esophagus, whereas adenocarcinoma is localized to the distal esophagus where it is associated with intestinal metaplasia (Barrett's esophagus).

Management for Esophageal Obstruction

Endoscopic dilation therapy is the most common therapeutic intervention for patients with nonmalignant mechanical dysphagia. This can be done with a single, large-diameter dilating balloon or semirigid bougie over a guide wire. There has not been any convincing data to demonstrate superiority of balloon dilators over bougie dilators. In cases of membranous webs or Schatzki rings, the goal of endoscopic therapy is to tear the lesion with a single, large-diameter dilation. In the case of a Schatzki ring, postdilation PPI therapy is associated with decreased recurrence rates.

When treating fibrotic strictures (peptic, anastomotic, radiation, EoE), the goal should be gradual stretching of the stricture. The choice of initial dilation size is based on an estimate of the diameter of the stricture. The extent to which a stricture can be dilated is expressed by the endoscopic axiom of the "rule of threes." This refers to the approach whereby the diameter of the stricture is approximated, and no more than three subsequent dilations are performed at 1-mm intervals once resistance is noted. Although there is no controlled trial for support, this approach is used to minimize the most serious risks of dilation therapy, perforation, and bleeding.

In patients with refractory strictures despite dilation therapy, several therapies have been attempted with variable efficacy. Temporary self-expanding stents have been placed to maintain lumen patency. When placed across a stricture, stents serve two purposes. First, they relieve symptoms of dysphagia by maintaining a patent lumen. In addition, the self-expanding nature of the stent provides ongoing radial force, which gradually stretches the lumen. The main disadvantage of stents is their tendency to migrate.

An alternative endoscopic approach is incisional therapy with an electrocautery knife. This is used to make incisions in the mucosa and fibrotic submucosa. This approach has been best studied in the setting of refractory anastomotic strictures; however, no head-to-head comparisons have been made between incisional therapy and other modalities.

Treatment of malignant etiologies for dysphagia will ultimately depend on the tumor type and extent of disease. Benign tumors and early-stage lesions can be treated with endoscopic resection or surgery. Endoscopic therapy using stents is also an

TABLE 3	Esophageal Dysphagia (Abnormal Motor Function)

Achalasia
EGJ outflow obstruction
Absent peristalsis
Spasm
Jackhammer

important component of the treatment of malignancy and may be used during the treatment phase of malignant disorders or as a palliative technique for later-stage disease.

Differential Diagnosis: Motility Disorders (Table 3)

Esophageal motor disorders are defined based on patterns of contractile vigor, propagation, and the presence of deglutitive relaxation. The most common classification scheme is the "Chicago classification," at the time this chapter was written currently in its fourth version. This scheme takes advantage of advanced high- resolution manometry with modifications based on refining disorders into clinically relevant phenotypes compared to earlier classification iterations.

Achalasia

The diagnosis of achalasia is made by esophageal manometry and requires two main manometric criteria: (1) inability of the lower esophageal sphincter to relax and (2) absence of peristalsis. Recently achalasia has been subdivided into three different phenotypes using high-resolution manometry, which are associated with varying clinical outcomes. Patients typically describe both solid and liquid dysphagia. Other common symptoms are regurgitation (especially nocturnal), chest pain, and aspiration. Weight loss and malnutrition may be dominant symptoms as the disease progresses. Given that there is no treatment to reverse absent peristalsis, the treatment is focused on improving esophagogastric junction (EGJ) opening by disrupting the poorly relaxing lower esophageal sphincter. Currently, three modalities exist to treat achalasia: (1) pneumatic dilation with rigid balloons ranging in size from 3 to 4 cm; (2) surgical myotomy paired with or without a fundoplication; (3) per-oral endoscopic myotomy or POEM. It appears that the three treatment approaches are associated with good outcomes with surgery having a more durable single intervention success rate, pneumatic dilation typically requiring multiple sessions and POEM combining the benefit of one treatment session with a non-surgical approach. Botulinum toxin type A (Botox)[1] injected into the lower esophageal sphincter has been shown to reduce EGJ pressure and improve symptoms; however, this treatment only provides temporary relief and should only be reserved for poor surgical candidates or patients unwilling to undergo surgery, dilation, or endoscopic myotomy. Occasionally, esophageal dilatation may progress to a point where EGJ-directed treatment is not adequate and esophagectomy must be performed to prevent severe complications, such as aspiration and severe malnutrition. At times, dysphagia can recur after EGJ-directed therapy; EndoFLIP can help identify patients requiring re-treatment.

Esophagogastric Junction Outflow Obstruction

This pattern of motor disturbance is associated with preserved peristalsis and evidence of high pressures through the EGJ during swallowing. This may be an achalasia variant or could be associated with a subtle obstruction at the distal esophagus not evident on endoscopy. Thus recognition of this pattern should prompt an evaluation for an infiltrating tumor or other potential etiology of obstruction. Treatment is focused on the underlying cause of the obstruction. If distensibility is normal on EndoFLIP, then watchful waiting is appropriate.

[1]Not available in the United States.

Absent Peristalsis

Absent peristalsis is defined as complete absence of contractile activity on all swallows in the context of a normal or low EGJ relaxation pressure. This pattern was previously categorized as scleroderma esophagus if it was found in the context of a hypotensive lower esophageal sphincter; however, this has been abandoned because this pattern may be found in patients with severe GERD without scleroderma. Treatment is focused on aggressive antireflux therapy and lifestyle modifications to reduce dysphagia and caustic injury to the esophagus.

Distal Esophageal Spasm

Distal esophageal spasm is a rare primary motor disorder that can provoke dysphagia and is associated with premature contraction of the esophageal body. Treatment for this disorder is extremely difficult and focuses on medical management with smooth muscle relaxants, such as calcium channel blockers,[1] nitrates,[1] and 5-phosphodiesterase inhibitors.[1]

Jackhammer

Jackhammer esophagus is an extreme form of nutcracker esophagus associated with contractile vigor not encountered in asymptomatic controls or under normal conditions. Previous definitions for hypertensive esophagus had a significant overlap with data from cohorts of asymptomatic controls, and thus the clinical significance of these disorders was unclear. This pattern is associated with dysphagia and chest pain and is typically treated similar to distal esophageal spasm. This motor pattern can also be seen with distal esophageal obstruction, and this should be considered in the differential diagnosis because it would alter management to focus on the obstruction.

Borderline Motor Abnormalities

Borderline motor abnormalities are those associated with ineffective esophageal motility and mild abnormalities of peristaltic propagation (rapid contraction) or hypertensive contraction. These disorders are not considered to be primary motor disorders, and secondary cause for symptoms, such as GERD and visceral sensitivity, should be considered and treated.

Monitoring

Patients with dysphagia or esophageal obstruction should be monitored for three important complications:

- Evidence of aspiration and nocturnal regurgitation because these can be associated with severe complications, such as chemical pneumonitis and aspiration pneumonia.
- Malnutrition and dehydration because this may prompt more aggressive therapy or consideration of non-oral feeding methods.
- Progressive symptoms because this could lead to progression of the disease and early therapy may avoid the above complications.

Acknowledgment

This work was supported by R01 DK079902 (JEP) from the U.S. National Institutes of Health.

[1]Not available in the United States.

References

Bredenoord AJ, Fox M, Kahrilas PJ, et al: Chicago classification criteria of esophageal motility disorders defined in high resolution esophageal pressure topography, *Neurogastroenterol Motil* 24(Suppl. 1):57–65, 2012.

Cook IJ, Kahrilas PJ: AGA technical review on management of oropharyngeal dysphagia, *Gastroenterology* 116:455–478, 1999.

Drossman DA: The functional gastrointestinal disorders and the Rome III process, *Gastroenterology* 130:1377–1390, 2006.

Egan JV, Baron TH, Adler DG, et al: Esophageal dilation, *Gastrointest Endosc* 63:755–760, 2006.

Francis DL, Katzka DA: Achalasia: update on the disease and its treatment, *Gastroenterology* 139:369–374, 2010.

Liacouras CA, Furuta GT, Hirano I, et al: Eosinophilic esophagitis: updated consensus recommendations for children and adults, *J Allergy Clin Immunol* 128:3–20, 2011, e26; quiz 21–2.

Pandolfino JE, Kahrilas PJ: AGA technical review on the clinical use of esophageal manometry, *Gastroenterology* 128:209–224, 2005.

Pandolfino JE, Kwiatek MA, Nealis T, et al: Achalasia: a new clinically relevant classification by high-resolution manometry, *Gastroenterology* 135:1526–1533, 2008.

Spechler SJ: AGA technical review on treatment of patients with dysphagia caused by benign disorders of the distal esophagus, *Gastroenterology* 117:233–254, 1999.

Wilkins T, Gillies RA, Thomas AM, et al: The prevalence of dysphagia in primary care patients: a HamesNet Research Network study, *J Am Board Fam Med* 20:144–150, 2007.

GASTRITIS AND PEPTIC ULCER DISEASE

Method of
Kyle Vincent, MD

CURRENT DIAGNOSIS

- Diagnosis of gastritis and peptic ulcer disease (PUD) is based on history of dyspepsia and elimination of other conditions.
- *Helicobacter pylori* (*H. pylori*) and nonsteroidal anti-inflammatory drugs (NSAIDs) are the most common cause of ulcer disease. Hypersecretory conditions such as Zollinger-Ellison syndrome are rare.
- If testing for *H. pylori* is indicated (test and treat strategy), IgG antibody, urea breath test, and fecal antigen test are available.
- Young patients with no "warning signs" can usually be managed on an outpatient basis without immediate endoscopy.
- Patients older than 55 with bleeding, anemia, loss of more than 10% of body weight, dysphagia, odynophagia, early satiety, history of previous malignancy, lymphadenopathy, abdominal mass, or a previously documented ulcer should undergo upper endoscopy promptly.

CURRENT TREATMENT

- The two principal strategies are empiric treatment or test and treat.
- In areas with an *H. pylori* infection rate of less than 10% a 4–8 week course of proton-pump inhibitors (PPIs) given empirically is appropriate.
- In patients who fail empiric PPI treatment or in areas with an *H. pylori* infection rate of greater than 10%, a test and treat strategy should be employed. A verified noninvasive *H. pylori* test should be used.
- First-line treatment of *H. pylori* consists of a PPI, clarithromycin (Biaxin), and amoxicillin (Amoxil) all taken twice a day for 14 days.
- Test of cure should be undertaken in any patient treated for *H. pylori*.
- NSAIDs should be discontinued or standard dose PPI for ulcer prophylaxis used to treat any dyspepsia.

Epidemiology

An estimated four million Americans have active gastric ulcers with 350,000 new cases diagnosed each year. The lifetime prevalence of this condition is around 10%. The incidence was previously higher in men but is currently equal in men and women. Familial clustering is now believed to result from transmission of *Helicobacter pylori* (*H. pylori*) from person to person or a genetic predisposition to infection with *H. pylori* rather than a genetic predisposition to gastric ulcers.

Risk Factors

Most gastric and duodenal ulcers can be attributed to *H. pylori*, NSAID use, severe physiologic stress, or hypersecretory conditions. In America, 10% of young adults harbor *H. pylori* infections, and this incidence increases with age. Lower socioeconomic status and recent immigration from areas with high rates of infection also increase the incidence of *H. pylori* infection. Hypersecretory conditions such as Zollinger-Ellison syndrome are rare, estimated to be responsible for only 0.1% of all ulcers. These conditions should not be routinely considered except in refractory or recurrent cases or in patients who have multiple ulcers.

Pathophysiology

The low pH of gastric acid is required to kill ingested bacteria and to promote proteolysis and activation of pepsin. Postprandial gastric acid production is stimulated by expression of gastrin from G cells and is inhibited in a negative feedback loop by somatostatin from antral D cells. Contrary to previous beliefs, peptic ulcer disease is not simply due to excessive acid production. Almost all patients with gastric ulcer have normal acid production and only one-third of patients with duodenal ulcer have evidence of increased acid production. The protective mechanisms of the mucosa play an important role in maintaining mucosal integrity.

The gastric and duodenal mucosa forms a gelatinous layer that is impermeable to gastric acid and pepsin. Mucosal blood flow as well as the production of mucus and bicarbonate secretion are largely regulated by E type prostaglandins (PGE). Anything that can disrupt the balance between acid production and the protective barrier has the potential to cause loss of mucosal integrity and tissue exposure to gastric acid and pepsin with subsequent inflammation and potential ulceration.

Two major mechanisms contribute to gastritis and/or ulcer formation. *H. pylori* is a gram-negative curved rod that produces ammonia to control the surrounding pH. Ammonia is toxic to epithelial cells, causing gastritis or duodenitis and damaging mucosal integrity. Many patients with gastritis also have a marked decrease in the number of somatostatin secreting antral D cells, leading to diminished feedback to control acid secretion during gastrin stimulation.

Prevention

The United States Preventative Task Force does not currently recommend routine screening for *H. pylori* in asymptomatic individuals. Prevention is based on avoidance or minimization of risk factors. Long-term NSAID use should be avoided. Prophylactic antisecretory medication should be considered when prolonged NSAID use is necessary. Proton pump inhibitors (PPIs) have better protective efficacy than histamine receptor antagonists (H2RAs) when prolonged NSAID use is necessary. Patients with a previous history of ulcer disease who use steroids or are older than 65 years of age should strongly be considered for prophylaxis with an antisecretory medication. Because of the high risk of gastric ulceration, prophylaxis is recommended for patients experiencing severe physiologic stress such as mechanical ventilation for longer than 48 hours, hypoperfusion, high dose corticosteroids, and large surface area burns (>35% total body surface). Histamine receptor antagonists such as famotidine (Pepcid),[1] cimetidine (Tagamet),[1] and ranitidine (Zantac)[1] or PPIs are recommended. No agent has shown to be clearly

---

[1]Not FDA approved for this indication.

superior for prophylaxis in patients on steroids or undergoing physiologic stress.

No immunization against *H. pylori* is currently available but early stage animal trials are in progress.

Clinical Manifestations

Dyspepsia is defined by the American College of Gastroenterology as chronic or recurrent pain or discomfort centered in the upper abdomen. Discomfort is defined as a subjective negative feeling that is not painful. Discomfort can incorporate a variety of symptoms including early satiety or upper abdominal fullness. A thorough history alone is usually sufficient to establish the diagnosis and to differentiate gastritis and peptic ulcers from other common conditions, though gastritis and peptic ulcer disease are difficult to differentiate from each other. Patients with peptic ulcer disease tend to have symptoms more pronounced with food intake. A patient with a duodenal ulcer usually reports increased pain 2-3 hours after a meal; conversely, a patient with a gastric ulcer tends to have pain precipitated or exacerbated by food intake. However, these classical findings are not reliable diagnostic indicators. Physical examination is important to rule out serious complications from peptic ulcer disease. Patient with a rigid abdomen, rebound tenderness, or guarding should be evaluated with imaging and by a surgeon to rule out perforation. The most common physical finding in peptic ulcer disease is tenderness in the epigastrium.

Differential Diagnosis

The differential diagnosis for gastritis and peptic ulcer disease is broad given its nonspecific nature, but can be narrowed down fairly quickly by a good initial history. The differential diagnosis includes gastroesophageal reflux disease (GERD), cardiac disease, gastric cancer, pancreatitis, pancreatic neoplasm, biliary disease including cholelithiasis or cholecystitis, delayed gastric emptying, or bowel ischemia. Patients presenting with a predominant complaint of heartburn or abdominal pain with heartburn more than once per week should be considered to have GERD until proven otherwise. Any symptoms associated with dyspnea or chest pressure should raise concern for a cardiac etiology. Biliary pain often radiates to the right shoulder and is associated with fatty or greasy foods. Patients with pancreatitis usually describe a severe boring type pain in the epigastrium. They may also get relief from leaning forward.

Diagnosis

While most dyspepsia symptoms can be treated on a nonurgent basis, specific "warning signs" should prompt referral or performance of upper endoscopy. These include age 55 or older, bleeding, anemia, loss of more than 10% of body weight, dysphagia, odynophagia, early satiety, history of previous malignancy, lymphadenopathy, abdominal mass, or a previously documented ulcer.

H. pylori testing is a cornerstone of managing dyspepsia. However, most other laboratory studies are usually not helpful in establishing the diagnosis in uncomplicated peptic ulcer disease or gastritis but may be helpful in eliminating other conditions in the differential diagnosis.

Noninvasive Testing

Antibody Test—Serum IgG antibodies are typically present at 21 days after the onset of *H. pylori* infection but can persist long after active infection. Antibody testing has a sensitivity of 85% and specificity of 79%. The positive predictive value is greatly influenced by the prevalence of the organism in the community and therefore it is less useful in areas with lower rates of *H. pylori* infection. The excellent negative predictive value makes IgG testing a good screening test. However, given that the IgG antibodies can persist for up to a year or longer after infection, it is not as helpful in the acute phase.

Urea Breath Test—This test identifies infection through urease activity. The patient ingests urea labeled with either ^{13}C or ^{14}C. In the presence of *H. pylori*, urease activity produces labeled CO_2 that is expired and can be collected and measured. Sensitivities and specificities of this test exceed 95%. It maintains a strong positive and negative predictive value despite the prevalence of *H. pylori*, but the test is not universally available.

Fecal Antigen Test—This assay uses either polyclonal or monoclonal antibodies to identify *H. pylori* antigens in the stool. The sensitivity and specificity exceed 90% in most studies. Like the breath test, it is unaffected by prevalence, however, both tests are affected by previous exposure to bismuth, antibiotics, and PPIs.

Treatment

The treatment of dyspepsia was revolutionized in the 1990s following the discovery of the role of *H. pylori* in pathogenesis. For patients who present with dyspepsia but no "warning signs," two separate and approximately equivalent treatment strategies are recommended. The "test and treat" option recommends using a validated noninvasive test for *H. pylori* and treatment of positive tests. The "empiric" acid suppression option recommends treating with a PPI for 4-8 weeks without testing for *H. pylori*. The test and treat strategy is recommended for populations where the *H. pylori* infection rate is higher than 10%, in patients with active or past PUD, low-grade gastric mucosa-associated lymphoid tissue (MALT) lymphoma, or history of endoscopic resection of early gastric cancer. As the US prevalence varies from 10% to 40% in different communities, either strategy may be appropriate. The test and treat strategy is more appropriate for most urban areas and in communities with a high immigrant population or known high rates of *H. pylori* infection. In populations with low *H. pylori* prevalence, such as high socioeconomic areas, empiric acid suppression is an appropriate first strategy, followed by *H. pylori* testing in those patients who have continued symptoms (Figure 1).

The recommendations for eradication of *H. pylori* were updated by the American College of Gastroenterology in 2017. Previous regimens had focused on specific PPI medications. This has been replaced with a general recommendation for standard or double dose PPI of choice. There are two key considerations for selection for initial treatment: (1) Is there a penicillin allergy? and (2) Has there been any previous macrolide exposure for any reason? Current first-line treatment is the so-called triple therapy with standard or double dose PPI, clarithromycin (Biaxin), and amoxicillin (Amoxil) for 14 days. This regimen has an eradication rate of 70% to 85%. Studies show no statistical difference between 7- and 10-day treatment regimens; however, there were trends toward higher eradication rates with the longer regimen. In addition, these studies have not been duplicated in the U.S. population where 7-day regimens have shown efficacy rates below 80%. Therefore, regimens less than 10 days are not recommended and 14-day treatment should be considered. In patients who are penicillin allergic, metronidazole (Flagyl)[1] may be substituted for amoxicillin, but resistance rates for metronidazole are more than double those for amoxicillin. Second-line therapy for those with previous macrolide exposure or penicillin allergy is the so-called quadruple therapy. This consists of standard dose PPI, bismuth subcitrate,[2] tetracycline (Sumycin),[1] and metronidazole (Flagyl).[1] Bismuth subcitrate, metronidazole, and tetracycline are available as a combination product, Pylera, which is approved to use with omeprazole for the treatment of patients with *H. pylori* infection and duodenal ulcer disease. There are multiple other regimens with similar eradication rates in European studies that have not been well validated in North America. Nonetheless, they are recommended by the American College of Gastroenterology and can be used for patients who are having difficulty with intolerance to the more common regimens. They are listed in Table 1.

---

[1]Not FDA approved for this indication.
[2]Not available in the United States.

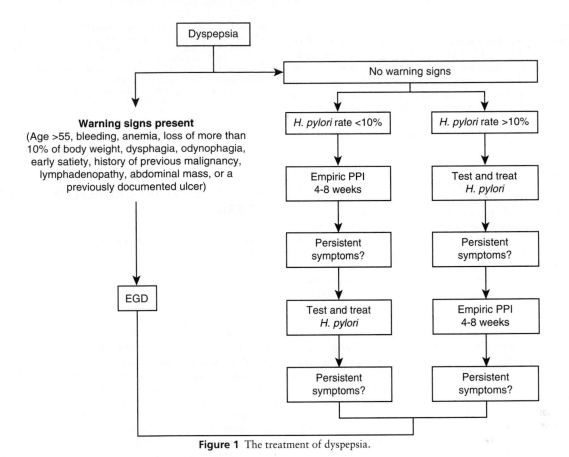

Figure 1 The treatment of dyspepsia.

TABLE 1	*H. pylori* Regimens			
REGIMEN	**ANTIBIOTIC**		**ANTACID**	**DURATION**
Clarithromycin Triple Therapy	Clarithromycin (Biaxin) 500 mg BID	Amoxicillin (Amoxil) 1 g BID[a]	PPI (Standard or double dose)	14 days[b]
Bismuth Quadruple Therapy[c]	Tetracycline (Sumycin)[1] 500 mg QID	Metronidazole (Flagyl)[1] 500 mg QID	Bismuth subcitrate[2] or subsalicylate (Pepto-Bismol) 300 mg QID	PPI (Standard dose)	10-14 days[b]
Concomitant[c]	Clarithromycin (Biaxin) 500 mg BID	Amoxicillin (Amoxil) 1 g BID	Metronidazole (Flagyl)[1] 500 mg BID	PPI (Standard dose)	10-14 days[b]
Sequential[c]	Amoxicillin (Amoxil) 1 g BID and PPI (Standard dose)	Clarithromycin (Biaxin) 500 mg BID and metronidazole (Flagyl) 500 mg BID and PPI (Standard dose)		5-7 days
Hybrid[c]	Amoxicillin (Amoxil) 1 g BID and PPI (Standard dose)	Amoxicillin (Amoxil) 1 g BID, PPI (Standard dose), clarithromycin (Biaxin) 500 mg BID, and metronidazole (Flagyl)[1] 500 mg BID		5-7 days
Levofloxacin triple[c]	Amoxicillin (Amoxil) 1 g BID	Levofloxacin (Levaquin)[1] 500 mg daily	PPI (Standard dose)	10-14 days[b]
Levofloxacin sequential[c]	Amoxicillin (Amoxil) 1 g BID and PPI (Standard dose)	Amoxicillin (Amoxil) 1 g BID, PPI (Standard dose), levofloxacin 500 mg daily, and metronidazole (Flagyl) 500 mg BID	PPI (Standard or double dose)	5-7 days
LOAD[c]	Levofloxacin (Levaquin) 250 mg daily	Doxycycline (Vibramycin)[1] 100 mg daily	Nitazoxanide (Alinia)[1] 500 mg BID	PPI (Double dose)	7-10 days

[a]In patients with penicillin allergy, metronidazole (Flagyl) 500 mg TID can be substituted, although not FDA approved.
[b]14-day courses should be considered secondary to increased eradication rates.
[c]Not FDA approved for this treatment regimen.
[1]Not FDA approved for this indication.
[2]Not available in the United States.

Monitoring

The recommendations for routine testing for eradication of *H. pylori* were updated in 2017. Although strong evidence is lacking, expert consensus supports testing for eradication in most cases. There is clear benefit in testing patients who have persistent symptoms despite the test and treat strategy, any patient with an *H. pylori*–associated ulcer, any patient who has had a resection of any early gastric cancer, or those with an *H. pylori*–associated MALT lymphoma. In these patients, testing should be done no sooner than 4 weeks after the completion of eradication treatment. Patients requiring follow-up endoscopy, such as for an ulcer or MALT lymphoma, should undergo endoscopic testing for eradication. Patients who are not undergoing endoscopy can be tested for eradication with fecal antigen or urea breath testing. The serum antibody test is unreliable for follow-up as it can remain positive for quite some time after successful treatment.

The most common causes of treatment failure are poor compliance with the medications and antibiotic resistance by the organism. Patients should be counseled on the side effects of their regimen and the importance of compliance. About 10% of patients report headaches and diarrhea with PPI use. Clarithromycin (Biaxin) can cause diarrhea, gastrointestinal upset, and altered taste. Similar effects can be seen with amoxicillin and metronidazole. Metronidazole also has disulfiram-like effects if taken with alcohol. Bacterial resistance is relatively rare, with multi-center U.S. data showing resistance rates to be 37% for metronidazole, 10% for clarithromycin, 3.9% for both antibiotics, and 1.4% for amoxicillin. For patients with persistent *H. pylori* infections, a new regimen should be attempted that does not include previously used antibiotics.

Patients who continue to have dyspepsia after successful eradication of *H. pylori* or who have persistent symptoms after a negative test and acid suppression should be considered for upper endoscopy.

Complications

Peptic ulcer disease can have severe complications, almost always requiring hospital admission. The most significant complications are gastric bleeding, perforation, or outlet obstruction.

Gastrointestinal bleeding is the most common cause of death in patients with peptic ulcer disease. Most cases of massive hemorrhage are due to erosion of a posterior ulcer into the gastroduodenal artery. Although the most common site of such hemorrhage is proximal to the ligament of Trietz, profuse bleeding can result in bright red blood from the rectum.

Approximately 5% of peptic ulcers cause perforation. This usually occurs anteriorly through the duodenum or lesser curve of the stomach. These patients often present in extremis with fever, tachycardia, dehydration, and abdominal findings of rigidity and rebound due to chemical peritonitis. Free air is commonly present under the diaphragm. Perforation is almost always requires surgical management.

Gastric outlet obstruction can occur acutely due to inflammation from peptic ulcer disease or more chronically secondary to inflammation and healing that lead to scarring and fibrosis of the duodenum. These patients can present with severe hypochloremic hypokalemic alkalosis due to the loss of hydrogen, potassium, and chloride from gastric secretions. Electrolyte derangements must be corrected prior to any attempted surgery. Initial treatment with balloon dilation can be attempted, especially in cases with newly diagnosed *H. pylori*. If the patient is negative for *H. pylori* or has successfully eradicated the organism, the long-term outcomes of dilation do not compare well to surgery.

References

Chey WD, Leontiadis GI, Howden CW, et al: ACG Clinical Guideline: Treatment of Helicobacter pylori infection, *AM J Gastroenterol* 112:112–238, 2017.

Chey WD, Wong BC: The Practice Parameters Committee of the American College of Gastroenterology: American College of Gastroenterology guideline on the management of *Helicobacter pylori* infection, *AM J Gastroenterol* 102:1808–1825, 2007.

Helicobacter pylori and peptic ulcer disease: FDA approved drug regimens. Available. at. http://www.cdc.gov/ulcer/keytocure.htm. (accessed 30 December 2013).

Mercer DW, Robinson EK: Stomach. In *Sabiston Textbook of Surgery*, ed 18, Philadelphia, 2008, Saunders, pp 1223–1277.

Nordenstedt H, Graham DY, Kramer JR, et al: *Helicobacter pylori*—Negative gastritis prevalence and risk factors, *AM J Gastroenterol* 108:65–71, 2013.

Surgical critical care evidence based-medicine guidelines: Stress ulcer prophylaxis. Available. at. http://www.surgicalcriticalcare.net/Guidelines/stress%20ulcer%20prophylaxis%202011.pdf. (accessed 15 December 2013).

Talley NJ, Vakil NB: The Practice Parameters Committee of the American College of Gastroenterology: Guideline for the management of dyspepsia, *AM J Gastroenterol* 100:2324–2337, 2005.

GASTROESOPHAGEAL REFLUX DISEASE (GERD)

Method of
Mustafa Abdul-Hussein, MD, MSCR

Gastroesophageal reflux disease (GERD) is a motility disorder of the lower esophageal sphincter (LES). The definition of this disease has evolved over time, reflecting better understanding of the roles that transient LES relaxations and acid/pepsin contact with esophageal mucosa play, as well as the ability to identify these events. The diagnosis of GERD has changed from identification of a hiatal hernia, to identification of erosive esophagitis, to the currently accepted patient-centered definition: any symptom or injury to esophageal mucosa resulting from reflux of gastric contents into the esophagus. GERD should not be confused with physiologic gastroesophageal reflux, which is not associated with symptoms or esophageal mucosal injury.

The prevalence of GERD is difficult to ascertain, although several studies have indicated it to be as high as 50% of adults in Western countries, with 10% to 18% experiencing heartburn on a daily basis. Studies using healthcare utilization data may underestimate the prevalence because of self-treatment by individuals in the community, whereas population surveys may overestimate it because of inaccurate assessment of symptoms and absence of objective data. Regardless of the real number, the management of this disease costs more than $10 billion annually in the United States. GERD has been called a disease of White males, although recent data suggest increasing prevalence in Asia and Pacific regions. Recent studies assessing the global prevalence of GERD show that the overall burden of GERD has been worsening, with the prevalent cases increasing by 77.53% from 1990 to 2019.

Pathophysiology

GERD is a motility disorder of the LES characterized by inappropriate or transient relaxations that allow gastric contents to reflux into the esophagus. The LES is a tonically contracted ring of smooth muscle fibers innervated by the vagus nerve. Vagal stimulation during swallowing produces physiologic LES relaxation and is a likely source for transient LES relaxations. Gastroesophageal reflux occurs most frequently during postprandial periods, at a rate of six reflux episodes per hour, but averages two episodes per hour over the entire day. Increasing frequency of reflux in the postprandial period results from gastric distention after a meal and stimulation of tension receptors in the proximal stomach leading to transient LES relaxations (Box 1). A chronically hypotensive LES is not a major mechanism for GERD in most patients but can be seen in cases of severe erosive esophagitis.

Reflux of acidic gastric contents can lead to injury of the esophageal mucosa, including inflammation, ulceration, stricturing, Barrett metaplasia, and adenocarcinoma. Peristaltic clearance, tissue resistance, and salivary bicarbonate make up host defense mechanisms that work by clearing reflux and neutralizing the acid residue on the mucosa. Erosive esophagitis or strictures result in the most severe form of GERD, which includes nocturnal reflux with longer acid contact times, decreased salivary production, and lower frequency of swallowing during sleep.

BOX 1 — Factors That Modulate Transient Lower Esophageal Sphincter Relaxation

Stimulants
- Gastric distention
- Pharyngeal intubation
- Upright orientation
- Foods (fatty foods, caffeine, alcohol)
- Tobacco

Inhibitors
- Recumbency
- Lateral decubitus (left side)
- Anesthesia
- Sleep

BOX 2 — Esophageal Tissue Defense Mechanisms

Preepithelial
- Mucous layer
- Unstirred water layer
- Surface bicarbonate concentration

Epithelial Structures
- Cell membranes
- Intercellular junctional complexes (tight junctions, glycoconjugates/lipid)

Cellular
Epithelial transport (Na^+/H^+ exchanger, Na^+-dependent $Cl^-/HCO3^-$-$HCO3^-$ exchanger)
- Intracellular and extracellular buffers
- Cell restitution
- Cell replication

Postepithelial
- Blood flow
- Tissue acid-base status

BOX 3 — Alarm Symptoms of Gastroesophageal Reflux Disease

Presence of any of the following symptoms requires immediate evaluation:
- Dysphagia
- Odynophagia
- Weight loss
- Spontaneous resolution of symptoms
- Iron deficiency anemia
- Gastrointestinal bleeding

Complications

Acid reflux can lead to significant morbidity if it is not recognized and treated appropriately. Habitual contact of acid and activated pepsin with the stratified squamous epithelium, along with impaired defense mechanisms, results in tissue injury (Box 2). The end result of this process can be ulceration, fibrosis with stricture formation, Barrett esophagus (BE), or adenocarcinoma. These complications can produce alarm symptoms (Box 3). Patients presenting with alarm symptoms should undergo immediate diagnostic evaluation with an esophagogastroduodenoscopy (EGD).

Erosive Esophagitis

The endoscopic finding of erosive esophagitis is seen in fewer than 50% of patients with heartburn. The severity is stratified according to the Los Angeles Classification of Esophagitis. Treatment with a proton pump inhibitor (PPI) for 4 to 12 weeks heals erosive esophagitis in 78% to 95% of cases. The healing effect of antisecretory therapy, and particularly PPIs, demonstrates the important role of acid reflux in causing tissue injury. The recurrence rates for erosive esophagitis are high after discontinuation of PPI maintenance therapy (75%–92%), necessitating continuation of gastric acid suppression.

Strictures

Most strictures caused by GERD are peptic in origin and are located at the squamocolumnar junction. Patients with GERD and strictures, compared with those without strictures, are more likely to have a hypotensive LES, abnormal peristalsis, and prolonged acid clearance time. Stricture formation decreases the luminal diameter, resulting in solid food dysphagia. Dysphagia in these patients is often a combination of decreased luminal diameter and dysmotility of the distal esophageal body with low-amplitude peristalsis. Patients with GERD who develop dysphagia should have immediate barium radiography and an endoscopic evaluation.

Barrett Esophagus

BE is a premalignant condition that may evolve into esophageal adenocarcinoma. The histologic abnormality involves intestinal-like metaplasia of the stratified squamous epithelium. Epidemiologic studies show BE to be more common among Whites, males, and the elderly (mean age, 60 years). The incidence of esophageal adenocarcinoma (EAC) in patients with BE varies based on the degree of dysplasia and, in general, is estimated to have an annual incidence of 0.2 to 0.7. Despite the prevalent use of PPIs in the treatment of GERD, the incidence of adenocarcinoma has been increasing. Current guidelines encourage endoscopic surveillance for patients with BE, yet there are sparse data showing the cost-effectiveness or mortality benefit of this strategy.

Adenocarcinoma

Approximately 50% of esophageal cancers are adenocarcinomas. Since the 1970s, the incidence has been rising for reasons that are still unknown. GERD is a risk factor for EAC, and the risk increases with the duration and severity of GERD symptoms. There is a suggestion that cagA strains of *Helicobacter pylori* are protective against development of BE and adenocarcinoma. The declining incidence of *H. pylori* may be a possible explanation for the rising incidence of adenocarcinoma.

Diagnosis

GERD is largely a clinical diagnosis under the current definition (i.e., any symptom or tissue injury resulting from reflux of gastric contents into the esophagus). Patients with the typical symptoms of heartburn and regurgitation most often associated with meals have a high pretest probability of having GERD. A well-obtained history and symptom questionnaire are usually sufficient to form a presumptive diagnosis and are more cost-effective than ambulatory reflux testing or EGD. An empiric trial of PPI therapy that leads to a significant reduction or resolution of symptoms likely confirms the diagnosis.

The pathophysiology of GERD is much more complex than previously thought. It involves more than acid reflux, because nonacid reflux with a pH greater than 4 can be a common source of symptoms. This entity is unmasked when PPI therapy is found to control gastric acid secretion and impedance-pH testing identifies a temporal relationship between symptoms and episodes of nonacid reflux.

Direct-to-consumer marketing and the availability of over-the-counter PPI medications (e.g., Prilosec OTC) have led to self-treatment of GERD-type symptoms and a consequent change in the type of patients seeking medical care for their symptoms. Patients with typical GERD symptoms that do not completely respond to therapy with PPIs, including over-the-counter and prescription PPIs, warrant a more detailed evaluation of their symptoms. A separate population requiring earlier diagnostic

BOX 4 Clinical Spectrum of Gastroesophageal Reflux Disease–Related Symptoms and Tissue Injury

Esophageal

Symptomatic Syndromes
- Typical reflux syndrome
- Reflux chest pain syndrome

Syndromes With Tissue Injury
- Reflux esophagitis
- Reflux stricture
- Barrett esophagus
- Adenocarcinoma

Extraesophageal

Established Association
- Reflux cough
- Reflux laryngitis
- Reflux dental erosions

Proposed Association
- Sinusitis
- Reflux asthma
- Pulmonary fibrosis
- Pharyngitis
- Recurrent otitis media

---

evaluation includes patients with exclusively atypical GERD symptoms such as cough, hoarseness, throat clearing, asthma attacks, and chest pain. Less commonly, patients presenting with signs or symptoms of tissue injury, such as solid food dysphagia, should also be more rigorously tested for GERD (Box 4).

Patients who have symptoms associated with GERD, whether typical or atypical, are frequently treated empirically with PPI therapy.

Partial responders and nonresponders to PPI therapy should undergo ambulatory reflux testing using combined multichannel intraluminal impedance (MII)-pH or standard pH. MII-pH catheters measure both esophageal pH changes and impedance changes that occur as an ion-rich refluxate passes a pair of ring electrodes, resulting in a drop in the resistance to a low-voltage current between the electrodes. The change in impedance can detect gastroesophageal reflux regardless of the acid content and can distinguish reflux types as liquid, gas, or mixed.

The goals of ambulatory reflux testing are to determine whether the esophageal acid contact time is abnormal, whether there is an abnormal number of reflux episodes, and whether a relationship between reflux and symptoms exists. The advantage of combined MII-pH is its ability to identify both acid and non-acid reflux, so that testing can be done while the patient is on acid-suppression therapy and the artifact of acidic food or beverage ingestion is eliminated; pH-only testing is affected by both of these conditions. The major disadvantage is that MII-pH testing is less available than conventional pH testing.

EGD is specific for detecting reflux-related tissue injury but is not sensitive, because fewer than 50% of patients with GERD-related heartburn have endoscopic findings of reflux. If erosive esophagitis or BE is found on endoscopy, aggressive antisecretory therapy with a PPI is warranted.

A barium esophagram is unlikely to add useful diagnostic information in patients with GERD symptoms without dysphagia. It is a useful tool in distinguishing obstructive from nonobstructive dysphagia and may even be more sensitive than EGD in detecting causes of obstructive dysphagia. Achalasia is often mistaken for GERD during the onset of symptoms, and early use of esophagography may help make this diagnosis.

Management

GERD is predominantly a postprandial event involving transient LES relaxations. The primary focus in management of this disease is to eliminate or improve symptoms, prevent tissue injury, and prevent complications. In most patients with recurrent GERD symptoms, this can be accomplished by controlling gastric acid secretion with antisecretory therapy. PPIs are the most effective pharmacologic therapy for improving symptoms and preventing tissue injury from acid reflux. Individuals with only occasional heartburn may successfully treat symptoms with a combination of lifestyle modifications and over-the-counter antacids, histamine 2 receptor antagonists, or a PPI.

Patients presenting with typical symptoms and a history consistent with GERD should be given a trial of PPI once daily for at least 4 weeks. A validated GERD symptom assessment questionnaire such as the Reflux Disease Questionnaire should be used as an initial screening tool, because symptom response is the primary outcome measure, and subsequent questionnaire responses are useful in comparison with the initial responses for measuring treatment efficacy. If symptoms have not responded or have responded only partially after this trial, then the dosing or frequency of the PPI should be increased over another 4-week period. If the response is still unsatisfactory, diagnostic testing with ambulatory combined MII-pH or pH-only monitoring is indicated.

PPIs are an effective maintenance therapy for most patients with GERD. Both dose and frequency may be adjusted based on clinical response, but GERD is a chronic condition with a high recurrence rate of symptoms without some form of maintenance therapy. This creates a large population of patients on antisecretory therapy for a disease with a low mortality rate, which raises the question of drug safety. There are insufficient data available that would warrant a recommendation against long-term PPI therapy. Clinical judgment in specific patient populations should be used to determine the optimal PPI regimen.

At present, pharmacologic reflux reduction therapy consists solely of the use of baclofen (Lioresal),[1] which has been shown to reduce transient LES relaxations and associated gastroesophageal reflux. The drawback of this medication is its unwanted side effects, which include somnolence and dizziness, limiting its tolerability and clinical utility as a standalone therapy.

Antireflux surgery is another alternative that is effective in limiting GERD symptoms in patients with a positive reflux-symptom relationship. Candidates for surgery include younger patients who do not want to continue chronic PPI therapy and patients with symptomatic nonacid reflux. Today, most antireflux surgery is performed laparoscopically with a 360-degree Nissen fundoplication. The associated mortality rate is small (0.5% to 1%), and this approach is preferred to open laparotomy. Traditional predictors for surgical success have included the presence of typical symptoms (heartburn and regurgitation), symptom response to a trial of PPIs, and an abnormal ambulatory pH study. These criteria exclude the important group of patients with atypical symptoms or symptoms related to nonacid reflux. However, such patients should be considered candidates for antireflux surgery if a positive reflux–symptom relationship can be demonstrated.

In recent years, several endoscopic therapeutic procedures have been developed for the treatment of GERD. Among these procedures, transoral incisionless fundoplication and Stretta are well-studied and viable options. Stretta is the delivery of radiofrequency energy to the gastroesophageal junction (GEJ). Stretta efficacy lies in increasing thickness of LES, decreasing compliance of GEJ without fibrosis, and decreasing transient LES relaxations. Randomized trials showed improvement in GERD symptoms compared with sham procedure, though follow-up periods in these trials were only 6 to 12 months. A metaanalysis of 18 studies and 1441 patients concluded that Stretta is safe, well tolerated, effective in GERD symptom relief, and significantly reduces acid exposure to the esophagus, though it did not consistently normalize pH. In a recent metaanalysis of 28 studies of 2468 patients with mean follow-up time of 25.4 months, Stretta improved

---

[1] Not FDA approved for this indication.

quality-of-life scores and heartburn scores. However, 49% of the patients were still using PPIs at follow-up.

Patients with alarm symptoms and those who are partial responders to PPI therapy should also undergo EGD to aid in determining the cause of the symptoms, such as obstructive dysphagia from peptic strictures, adenocarcinoma, and bleeding esophageal ulcers (which can cause anemia). EGD findings that suggest GERD are a result of acid reflux. However, the incidence of these findings has declined with the use of PPIs.

Nonerosive reflux disease is increasingly common as more patients are converted from acid refluxers to non–acid refluxers with PPI therapy. By definition, these patients have no findings on endoscopy to suggest ongoing GERD. Absence of endoscopic findings does not exclude GERD, however, because tissue injury can occur at the microscopic and macroscopic levels. Patients with either erosive esophagitis or nonerosive reflux disease have dilated intercellular spaces on electron microscopy.

As previously discussed, patients with GERD may develop BE. The metaplastic transformation from normal stratified squamous epithelium to an intestinal-type, columnar-lined epithelium creates a premalignant lesion with a 0.5% per year risk of progression to adenocarcinoma. Screening for BE remains controversial. There is no evidence that screening results in a mortality benefit due to early detection of esophageal adenocarcinoma. Screening of all patients with GERD for BE is clearly not cost-effective, but it is reasonable to target the highest-risk populations, such as White men older than 50 years of age with chronic reflux symptoms. Current American College of Gastroenterology guidelines recommend surveillance endoscopy in patients with known BE at intervals determined by the degree of dysplasia.

References

Bonino J, Sharma P: Barrett's esophagus, *Curr Opin Gastroenterol* 21:461–465, 2005.

Castell DO, Richter JE: *The esophagus*, ed 4, Philadelphia, 2003, Lippincott Williams & Wilkins.

Corley DA, Katz P, Wo JM, et al: Improvement of gastroesophageal reflux symptoms after radiofrequency energy: a randomized, sham-controlled trial, *Gastroenterology* 125:668–676, 2003.

Fass R, Cahn F, Scotti DJ, et al: Systematic review and meta-analysis of controlled and prospective cohort efficacy studies of endoscopic radiofrequency for treatment of gastroesophageal reflux disease, *Surg Endosc* 31(12):4865–4882.

Frye J, Vaezi M: Extraesophageal GERD, *Gastroenterol Clin N Am* 37:845–858, 2008.

Hila A, Agrawal A, Castell D: Combined multichannel intraluminal impedance and pH esophageal testing compared to pH alone for diagnosing both acid and weakly acidic gastroesophageal reflux, *Clin Gastroenterol Hepatol* 5:172–177, 2007.

Hvid-Jensen F, Funch-Jensen P, et al: Incidence of adenocarcinoma among patients with Barrett's esophagus, *N Engl J Med* 365:1375–1383, 2011.

Katz PO, Gerson LB, Vela MF: Guidelines for the diagnosis and management of gastroesophageal reflux disease, *Am J Gastroenterol* 108:308–328, 2013.

Mainie I, Tutuian R, Agrawal A, et al: Combined multichannel intraluminal impedance-pH monitoring to select patients with persistent gastro-oesophageal reflux for laparoscopic Nissen fundoplication, *Br J Surg* 93:1483–1487, 2006.

Mainie I, Tutuian R, Castell D: Comparison between the combined analysis and the DeMeester score to predict response to PPI therapy, *J Clin Gastroenterol* 40:602–605, 2006.

Mainie I, Tutuian R, Shay S, et al: Acid and non-acid reflux in patients with persistent symptoms despite acid suppressive therapy: amulticentre study using combined ambulatory impedance-pH monitoring, *Gut* 55:1398–1402, 2006.

Perry KA, Banerjee A, Melvin WS: Radiofrequency energy delivery to the lower esophageal sphincter reduces esophageal acid exposure and improves GERD symptoms: a systematic review and meta-analysis, *Surg Laparosc Endosc Percutan Tech* 22:283–288, 2012.

Savarino E, Zentilin P, Tutuian R, et al: The role of nonacid reflux in NERD: lessons learned from impedance-pH monitoring in 150 patients off therapy, *Am J Gastroenterol* 103:2685–2693, 2008.

Vakil N: Review article: test and treat or treat and test in reflux disease, *Aliment Pharmacol Ther* 17(Suppl. 2):57–59, 2003.

Vakil N, Van Zanten SV, Kahrilas P, et al: The Montreal definition and classification of gastroesophageal reflux disease: a global evidence-based consensus, *Am J Gastroenterol* 101:1900–1920, 2006.

Verbeek RE, Siersema PD, et al: Surveillance and follow-up strategies in patients with high-grade dysplasia in Barrett's esophagus: a Dutch population-based study, *Am J Gastroenterol* 107:534–542, 2012.

Wang KK, Sampliner RE: Updated guidelines 2008 for the diagnosis, surveillance and therapy of Barrett's esophagus, *Am J Gastroenterol* 103:788–797, 2008.

Zhang D, Liu S, Li Z, Wang R: Global, regional and national burden of gastroesophageal reflux disease, 1990–2019: update from the GBD 2019 study, *Ann Med* 54(1):1372–1384, 2022.

HEMORRHOIDS, ANAL FISSURE, AND ANORECTAL ABSCESS AND FISTULA

Method of
Mary R. Kwaan, MD, MPH

CURRENT DIAGNOSIS

- Although most anorectal complaints are caused by a benign process, it is important to be mindful that the etiology can be a malignancy or other serious medical condition, such as anorectal Crohn's disease.
- A thorough, focused history is often the most helpful diagnostic tool for patients with anorectal complaints.
- In patients in whom no etiology for bleeding is found or there has been a change in bowel movements, a further diagnostic workup should be performed.
- Pain is the predominant symptom with anal fissure, thrombosed external hemorrhoids, and anorectal abscess but is not prominently featured with internal hemorrhoids.

CURRENT THERAPY

- External thrombosed hemorrhoids are treated with evacuation in their early development (<72 hours) but with expectant, supportive management only in their subacute phase.
- Most internal hemorrhoids can be treated with outpatient treatments, including measures to normalize bowel movements and hemorrhoidal banding or injection therapy.
- Anal fissures are treated conservatively with medical therapy but require operative therapy in a minority of cases.
- Anal fistula repair techniques have variable success rates and may require multiple procedures to treat effectively.

A number of conditions cause anorectal symptoms, but the majority of patients present with a complaint of "hemorrhoids." Most anorectal conditions can be diagnosed with a focused history and physical examination. Treatment is aimed at the relief of symptoms, education of the patient, and prevention of further symptoms. Although most anorectal complaints are caused by a benign process, it is important for clinicians to be mindful that in some cases the etiology can be a malignancy or other serious medical condition, such as anorectal Crohn's disease.

History

A thorough, focused history is often the most helpful diagnostic tool for patients with anorectal complaints. Clinicians should inquire about pain, itching, discharge, extra tissue or a lump, and bleeding. It is particularly important to understand the patient's bowel habits with respect to constipation or diarrhea as well as any change in defecatory habits. Other relevant history items include previous anorectal procedures and related medical conditions such as Crohn's disease, malignancy, sexually transmitted diseases, or immunosuppression.

Pain is an important symptom to elicit from patients. In most cases, pain is the predominant symptom with anal fissure, thrombosed external hemorrhoids, and anorectal abscess. Although discomfort from internal hemorrhoids can cause aching, burning, or itching in the setting of tissue prolapse, internal hemorrhoid disease is most often painless. In contrast, external hemorrhoids that are acutely thrombosed cause pain that is severe, constant, and associated with a lump. Fissure pain is often described as a tearing sensation or the feeling of "razor blades" during bowel movements that can continue for more than 1 hour following defecation. Patients with anal fissures might also express a fear of having bowel movements because of pain. Anorectal abscess is often associated with pain, and patients can also present with an acute lump and occasionally a fever. Anal fistula typically is not associated with much pain; rather, patients describe irritation and drainage.

Anal discharge and difficulty with anorectal hygiene are also common complaints. The discharge associated with prolapsing internal hemorrhoids might contain mucus or fecal smearing. In contrast, an anorectal fistula or abscess can spontaneously drain with associated purulent and blood-tinged output.

When a patient has bleeding, specific details to inquire about include color (bright red versus dark blood), amount, frequency, and length of time. When no etiology for bleeding is found, a flexible sigmoidoscopy or colonoscopy should be performed to evaluate for a proximal source. Even if patients are found to have some hemorrhoids, endoscopic evaluation should be strongly considered in patients older than 40 years of age. Although uncommon, the incidence of colorectal malignancy has increased in this age group. Furthermore, patients who are 45 years of age and older should initiate colorectal cancer screening regardless of symptoms based on updated 2021 U.S. Preventive Services Task Force (USPSTF) guidelines. Stool-based screening modalities identify blood in the stool. Therefore patients with anal bleeding should be encouraged to proceed with colonoscopy for screening.

Diagnosis

Although the prone jackknife position allows the greatest exposure, the left lateral decubitus position with the knees up is preferred by patients and usually allows adequate exposure for the anorectal examination. It is critically important to have adequate lighting with a headlight as well as appropriate instrumentation to perform the anoscopy. An adjunctive test that can also be helpful in patients where mucosal (hemorrhoidal) or full-thickness rectal prolapse is suspected is to have patients bear down on the commode and then to examine externally.

The perianal skin is the skin immediately surrounding the anal verge (Figure 1). Perianal inspection includes careful examination of the surrounding skin for excoriation, an external draining orifice in the case of an anorectal fistula, lichenified skin with chronic irritation, other dermatitis, and the presence of perianal lesions. A low-lying anal fistula can be palpated as a fibrotic tract that heads from the external draining site to the anus. The anal verge is the entrance to the anal canal and is defined by the intersphincteric groove. There is frequently a clear demarcation between hair-bearing and non–hair-bearing skin in this location. Careful separation of the anoderm can help visualize an anal fissure located at the anal verge and extending into the anal canal.

A digital rectal examination is helpful for assessing resting and squeeze anorectal tone, palpating the prostate in men, assessing for rectocele in women, detecting any palpable anorectal lesions, and evaluating for tenderness within the anal canal or at the level of the levator ani muscles at the anorectal ring. Internal hemorrhoids, however, are not usually palpable as they readily compress with digital pressure and are not associated with fibrosis. Anoscopy is used to visually examine the anal canal, which is between 4 and 5 cm in length starting at the anal verge and extending to the top of the anorectal ring (top of external sphincter and levator ani muscles). Within the anal canal is the dentate line, which acts as a landmark anatomically and is located approximately 2 cm from the anal verge. The dentate line represents the transition from the squamous epithelial lining of the anus to the columnar epithelial lining of the rectum. Sensation above the dentate line is mediated by autonomic fibers and results in a relative lack of sensation compared with the highly sensitive, somatically innervated tissue below the dentate line. The dentate line is also the location of the crypt anal glands from which anorectal abscesses and fistulas originate.

Hemorrhoids

Hemorrhoids are anal vascular cushions that are present as normal structures in everyone. In the case of internal hemorrhoids, these cushions are arteriovenous channels that have overlying mucosa, submucosal smooth muscle, and supportive fibroelastic connective tissue. It is believed that internal hemorrhoids function by aiding with fine control of fecal continence of liquids and gases. Internal hemorrhoids enlarge and become symptomatic as fixation by submucosal smooth muscle and connective tissue becomes disrupted and loosens. This results in a sliding or prolapsing of the anal canal lining and further engorgement of the internal hemorrhoid tissues. Common exacerbating factors include constipation, diarrhea, aging, and increased abdominal pressure that can occur with chronic straining, pregnancy, heavy lifting, and decreased venous return. Internal hemorrhoids are not palpable on digital rectal examination and instead must be observed on anoscopy. Internal hemorrhoids are typically staged on a scale from I to IV based on the extent of prolapse (Table 1).

Internal hemorrhoids, when symptomatic, most commonly present with painless bright red bleeding or prolapsing tissue (Figure 2). Patients describe bleeding with or after bowel movements. Other symptoms include itching and leakage of mucus in the setting of tissue prolapse. Pain is rarely a prominent symptom except in the case of mixed hemorrhoid disease, when there is a thrombosed external component, or in the case of grade IV incarcerated hemorrhoids.

The central principles for conservative treatment of internal hemorrhoids and for long-term prevention of worsening symptoms are the normalization of bowel habits and avoidance of straining. Ideal bowel habits include having regular, soft, and formed stool resulting in minimal straining with elimination. An ideal diet should have high fiber content along with sufficient fluid intake. A total of at least 30 g of fiber per day is generally recommended. For most patients, this is most easily achieved with the addition of a fiber supplement such as psyllium. Other medical treatment of hemorrhoids includes local anesthetic topical ointments, such as lidocaine gel or ointment, which relieve symptoms but do not improve the hemorrhoids, and steroid ointments, which should only be prescribed for a defined short course

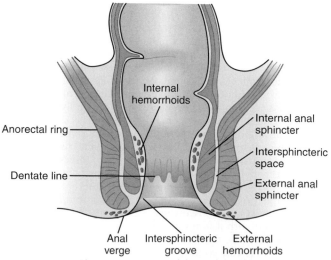

Figure 1 Anatomy of the anal canal.

Anorectal ring
Dentate line
Anal verge
Intersphincteric groove
External hemorrhoids
Internal hemorrhoids
Internal anal sphincter
Intersphincteric space
External anal sphincter

TABLE 1	Staging of Hemorrhoidal Disease
GRADE	DESCRIPTION
I	Protrude only inside the lumen; seen only with an anoscope
II	Protrude during defecation; reduce spontaneously
III	Protrude during defecation; require manual reduction
IV	Permanently prolapsed and irreducible

Figure 2 Prolapsing (grade III) hemorrhoids showing a prominent external component *(right)* and two sites of recent bleeding *(left)*.

for symptoms of itching and irritation. Topical hydrocortisone can thin and atrophy the overlying tissue if used regularly.

Internal hemorrhoids might benefit from further treatment in the setting of persistent prolapse or bleeding. Injection sclerotherapy works through shrinking and scarring the internal hemorrhoid by injecting a sclerosing agent (most commonly 5% phenol in oil [Haemorol]).[1,2] Sodium morrhuate is a sclerosing agent approved only for obliteration of varicosed veins. Alternatively, infrared coagulation may be administered at the apex of the hemorrhoid. Both procedures have moderate effectiveness but are considered less effective than rubber-band ligation, which is widely used in the office setting with favorable results.

Rubber-band ligation, an office procedure, requires the use of a rubber-band ligator (either suction type or a ligator with a clamp) and is performed by placing a rubber band around excess hemorrhoidal tissue at the apex of the hemorrhoid. Rubber-band ligation works by strangulating and cutting off blood flow to the hemorrhoid and by creating a scar that helps fix tissue into place. The band must be placed well above the dentate line to prevent pain. Most patients experience a sensation of pressure with the procedure. Rarely, this procedure can cause significant pain, bleeding, or a vasovagal reaction. In general, only one or two band applications are performed in the same setting to prevent excessive pain or a vasovagal reaction. Multiple rounds of hemorrhoid banding can be used to improve the patient's quality of life and has been shown to be more cost effective than hemorrhoid surgery, which is reserved for more severe prolapse.

Surgical treatment for hemorrhoidal disease should be considered in patients with grade III or IV internal hemorrhoids. Grade IV hemorrhoids, especially associated with dusky prolapsed rectal mucosa, urinary retention, or significant pain should be evaluated urgently by a surgeon, as necrotic tissue requires operative debridement. Surgery is also a consideration in cases in which office procedures and conservative treatment have been ineffective or when internal hemorrhoids are circumferential. In the United States, most hemorrhoidectomies continue to be performed using a closed technique in which the hemorrhoid is excised and the defect sutured closed. Stapled hemorrhoidectomy (also known as a *procedure for prolapsed hemorrhoids* (PPH) or *hemorrhoidopexy*) is used for patients who have more circumferential disease and is performed by excising the rectal mucosa and disrupting blood flow, thereby shrinking hemorrhoidal tissue and lifting the prolapsing tissue into the anal canal. Although stapled hemorrhoidectomy has been demonstrated to be effective and on average less painful, it

does not address external hemorrhoids, costs significantly more, and has been associated with rare but severe complications, including pelvic sepsis, rectal perforation, and rectovaginal fistula.

External hemorrhoids are generally painless, except in the case of thrombosis, and they normally appear as more prominent external perianal tissue or painless skin tags. Thrombosed external hemorrhoids, in contrast, are associated with severe pain and a prominent external lump but not with bleeding or fever. On examination, an external thrombosed hemorrhoid appears as a prominent, blue, and firm perianal lump. Patients who present within 72 hours of onset of symptoms benefit from excision of the hemorrhoid rather than evacuation of the thrombosed clot (Figure 3). In contrast, patients who present after 72 hours should be treated expectantly with conservative supportive care, including sitz baths, normalization of bowel habits with fiber or stool softener, and pain management. The natural history in these cases is for the thrombosed clot to gradually be reabsorbed within several weeks. In many cases, a residual skin tag is noted by the patient and can interfere with anal hygiene.

Anal Fissure

An anal fissure is a tear in the anoderm extending proximally into the anal canal and initially resulting from a traumatic bowel movement. Fissures typically occur in the setting of constipation or diarrhea. Most acute fissures will heal, but some patients have prolonged symptoms, causing them to seek medical attention. The pathophysiology of anal fissures is still not completely understood but is related to local ischemia caused by hypertonia of the internal sphincter. Most anal fissures are located at the posterior midline; some also occur at the anterior midline (Figure 4). Lateral fissures are rare and can be associated with anal malignancy, anorectal Crohn disease, HIV, syphilis, or tuberculosis. In these cases, a biopsy should be strongly considered to confirm the diagnosis.

Patients who present with anal fissure most often have a tearing pain that is associated with bowel movements and continues after defecation along with bright red bleeding with bowel movements. Physical examination demonstrates a tear in the anoderm with an exposed internal sphincter on separation of the anus. Chronic cases also demonstrate a sentinel tag overlying the distal aspect of the fissure.

Conservative treatment for acute anal fissures includes normalization of bowel habits to minimize recurrent trauma to the anoderm and sitz baths for comfort. In cases in which the fissure is chronic or unresponsive to conservative treatment, topical therapy to relax the internal sphincter (i.e., a *chemical sphincterotomy*) is prescribed. Classically, nitroglycerin ointment (0.4% [Rectiv]) has been used but is associated with headaches and lightheadedness. Diltiazem ointment (2%)[1,6] is a commonly used alternative without associated side effects. Either ointment can be applied topically two to three times per day for approximately 8 weeks. Application before bowel movements works best to help with pain on defecation. Reported healing rates are similar and range from 40% to 100%. An alternative agent that can be used for chemical sphincterotomy is botulinum toxin A (Botox)[1], which can be injected in the office or operating room with a single application into the internal sphincter. Although botulinum toxin A appears to be as effective as topical therapy, it is significantly more expensive.

Surgical lateral internal sphincterotomy is the most effective treatment to resolve anal pain associated with fissures and to expedite healing, but it is associated with a small risk of fecal incontinence. This procedure is performed in the outpatient setting and should be considered in cases in which topical medication has failed. This procedure can be performed with an open approach (incising mucosa and exposing muscle) or a closed approach (using landmarks and then dividing muscle by palpation) and can be full thickness (entire internal sphincter) or tailored (partial thickness and length). Most surgeons perform a tailored sphincterotomy from the level of the top of the fissure

[1] Not FDA approved for this indication.
[2] Not available in the United states.

[1] Not FDA approved for this indication.
[6] May be compounded by pharmacists.

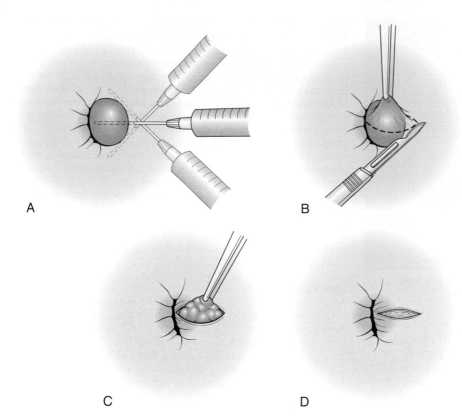

Figure 3 Excision and evacuation of an external thrombosed hemorrhoid. **A,** A local anesthetic is injected into the subcutaneous surrounding tissue and at the base of the hemorrhoid. **B,** The skin over the hemorrhoid is lifted, and a small elliptical excision of skin is made. **C,** The thrombotic clot is evacuated. Additional dissection is sometimes needed in the subcutaneous tissue to extract the clot. **D,** The appearance of the evacuated area. The incision is left open, and the skin heals by secondary intention.

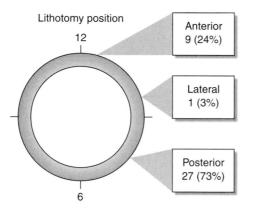

Figure 4 Distribution of the location of anal fissures.

distally, with partial division of the internal sphincter muscle to decrease the risk of postoperative fecal incontinence.

Anorectal Abscess and Fistula

Anorectal abscess is most commonly a self-limiting process thought to result from obstruction and infection of anal glands located in the crypts along the dentate line. Clinicians should be aware that perianal Crohn's disease, trauma, and malignancy can cause an anorectal abscess or fistula. Anorectal abscesses typically manifest with acute pain in the perianal area, acutely painful defecation, an indurated painful area, or fever. Most anorectal abscesses manifest with pain and swelling either superficially at the anal verge or deeper within the ischiorectal fossa. These patients have obvious tenderness, induration, or fluctuance on external and/or digital examination. In contrast, patients with intersphincteric abscesses

have severe pain but minimal findings on external examination and are only suspected on digital rectal examination.

The mainstay of therapy is surgical drainage. Superficial abscesses can be drained using local anesthesia, but more extensive infections typically require general anesthesia. When the abscess is fluctuant and appears easily accessible, an incision and drainage with a local anesthetic can be considered in a motivated patient. Important principles in draining an anorectal abscess include keeping the patient comfortable, using aspiration with a large-bore (14- or 16-gauge) needle to help in the event of difficult localization, using a cruciate incision to ensure adequate drainage, and keeping the incision near the anus to keep any potential fistula tract as short as possible. After the abscess is drained, the area is allowed to heal by secondary intention. Patients are given analgesics and encouraged to take sitz baths. When the abscess is large and extensive, sometimes drainage tubes, débridement, or additional dressing changes are required.

In most patients, drainage of the anorectal abscess is sufficient. However, in one-third of patients, these do not heal and form a fistula with the external opening beyond the anal verge and the internal opening within an infected crypt gland at the dentate line. A recent, small randomized trial suggested that 7 to 10 days of antibiotics after abscess drainage could decrease the risk of fistula formation. Patients developing a fistula can have what appears to be a nearly healed wound but continue to intermittently drain purulent material from the external opening, and some patients continue to have signs and symptoms of infection. Anorectal fistulas are defined by their anatomy and path relative to the sphincter muscles and are classified typically as superficial, intersphincteric, transsphincteric, suprasphincteric, and extrasphincteric, as classically described by Parks (Figure 5). In most cases, patients can proceed directly to the operating room for initial definition of the anatomy and placement of a seton (a length of suture or soft plastic vessel loop that is looped through the fistula), which allows drainage of infection within the tract, prevents recurrent infection, and allows the fistula to mature. Recurrent and complex fistulas may be better defined anatomically with the use of magnetic resonance imaging or endorectal ultrasonography.

Superficial, intersphincteric, or low transsphincteric fistulas can be treated with simple fistulotomy, which opens up the fistula

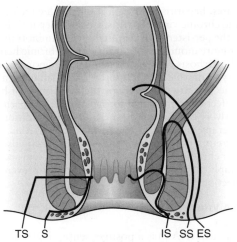

Figure 5 Classification of anal fistulas. *ES,* Extrasphincteric; *IS,* intersphincteric; *S,* superficial; *SS,* suprasphincteric; *TS,* transsphincteric.

tract and allows the tissue to heal by secondary intention. This, however, can result in impaired fecal continence, particularly if the fistula involves a significant amount of sphincter muscle.

If the fistula is too deep for a fistulotomy because of concern about transecting too much sphincter muscle, a variety of methods can be used to repair the fistula. One classic technique is the use of a cutting seton, where a taut seton is progressively tightened over several weeks or months to form a scar in place of the fistula and muscle. A cutting seton may be painful, and the scar is associated with impaired continence in some cases. Fibrin glue and fistula plugs have been proposed as a method to repair a fistula, but the recurrence rate with long-term follow-up is high (>85%). Endorectal advancement flaps are the most well-established method to repair an anal fistula. With this technique, the internal orifice is closed, and healthy tissue is brought down over the internal fistula opening to allow the area to heal. This procedure can be technically difficult: failure most commonly results from ischemia of the flap, and repeat flap procedures are often not anatomically feasible because of scarring and fibrosis. Success rates have been reported between 50% and 80%.

The ligation of intersphincteric fistula tract (LIFT) has been investigated for transsphincteric and suprasphincteric fistulas and shows modest success with the benefit of avoiding any sphincter division. In this procedure, the fistula tract is ligated and partially excised through an intersphincteric approach. Although long-term results are still unknown, reports are favorable (on the order of 60% to 80%) for the short-term success of this technique.

References

Bleier JI, Moloo H, Goldberg SM: Ligation of the intersphincteric fistula tract: An effective new technique for complex fistulas, *Dis Colon Rectum* 53:43–46, 2008.

Coughlin OP, Wright ME, Thorson AG, Ternent CA: Hemorrhoid Banding: A Cost-Effectiveness Analysis, *Dis Colon Rectum* 62:1085–1094, 2019.

Davis BR, Lee-Kong SA, Migaly J, Feingold DL, Steele SR: The American Society of Colon and Rectal Surgeons Clinical Practice Guidelines for the Management of Hemorrhoids, *Dis Colon Rectum* 61:284–292, 2018.

Ghahramani L, Minaie MR, Arasteh P, et al: Antibiotic therapy for prevention of fistula in ano after incision and drainage of simple perianal abscess: A randomized single blind clinical trial, *Surgery* 162:1017–1025, 2017.

Hong KD, Kang S, Kalaskar S, Wexner SD: Ligation of intersphincteric fistula to treat anal fistula: a systematic review and meta-analysis, *Tech Coloproctol* 18:685–691, 2014.

Jayaraman S, Colquhoun PH, Malthaner RA: Stapled versus conventional surgery for hemorrhoids, *Cochrane Database Syst Rev* 4:CD005393, 2006.

Nelson R: Nonsurgical therapy for anal fissure, *Cochrane Database Syst Rev* 4:CD003431, 2006.

Nelson RL: Operative procedures for fissure in ano, *Cochrane Database Syst Rev* 1:CD002199, 2010.

Parks AG, Gordon PH, Hardcastle JD: A classification of fistula-in-ano, *Br J Surg* 63:1–12, 1976.

Shanmugam V, Thaha MA, Rabindranath KS, et al: Rubber band ligation versus excisional haemorrhoidectomy for haemorrhoids, *Cochrane Database Syst Rev* 3:CD005034, 2005.

US Preventive Services Task Force: Screening for Colorectal Cancer, *JAMA* 325(19):1965–1977, 2021.

HEPATITIS A, B, D, AND E

Method of
Varun Takyar, MD; and Marc G. Ghany, MD

CURRENT DIAGNOSIS

Hepatitis A

- Typical prodromal symptoms are nonspecific (e.g., fever, anorexia, nausea, vomiting, diarrhea, abdominal pain, weight loss). In about one-half of patients, prodromal symptoms are followed by icterus (i.e., jaundice, pruritus, and dark urine) lasting 2 weeks.
- Serum aminotransferase levels increase to 10 to 20 times the upper limit of normal during the prodromal phase. Total serum bilirubin increases but rarely exceeds 10 mg/dL during the icteric phase. Biochemical recovery usually occurs within 3 months.
- Acute hepatitis A virus (HAV) infection is diagnosed by the presence of anti-HAV immunoglobulin M (IgM). Anti-HAV IgG appears in the convalescent phase and remains detectable for life. Anti-HAV IgG positivity with the absence of anti-HAV IgM antibodies reflects past exposure or vaccination. The antibody test for HAV usually includes total antibodies (IgM and IgG); thus diagnosis of acute hepatitis A requires specific anti-HAV IgM testing.

Hepatitis B

- Acute hepatitis B virus (HBV) infection may be asymptomatic or present with nonspecific symptoms of anorexia, nausea, and fever with development of icterus, pruritus, right upper quadrant pain, or, rarely, acute liver failure. Globally, it is a major cause of chronic hepatitis.
- Serum alanine aminotransferase (ALT) levels peak with the onset of symptoms.
- Suspected acute HBV infection is diagnosed by the detection of hepatitis B surface antigen (HBsAg), hepatitis B e-antigen (HBeAg), IgM antibody to hepatitis B core antigen, and HBV DNA in serum in the appropriate clinical setting. Anti-HBc IgM is detected during acute HBV infection and may be detected during reactivation of chronic HBV infection.
- Chronic infection is defined as the persistence of serum HBsAg for greater than 6 months. If HBsAg is present, serum HBeAg, antibody to hepatitis B e-antigen, HBV DNA, and serum ALT are used to determine the four phases of chronic infection (immune tolerant, HBeAg-positive and HBeAg-negative immune active, and inactive carrier).

CURRENT THERAPY

Hepatitis A

- Treatment is predominately supportive. Avoid hepatotoxic medications and drugs metabolized by the liver. Acute liver failure with encephalopathy and impaired synthetic function occurs rarely and is more common in patients older than 50 years of age and/or those who have coexisting chronic hepatitis B virus (HBV) or hepatitis C virus (HCV) infections.
- Prevention includes administration of the inactivated or attenuated vaccine for children at 1 year of age and older and for at-risk populations (e.g., intravenous drug users, travelers to regions with high or intermediate hepatitis A virus [HAV] rates, men who have sex with men, patients with chronic liver disease or clotting factor disorders).
- Preexposure passive immunization with pooled human anti-HAV immunoglobulin may be used for those at high or intermediate risk of hepatitis A virus exposure.

- Postexposure passive immunization with pooled human anti-HAV immunoglobulin may be used for close personal contacts of an individual with laboratory-confirmed HAV infection, staff and attendees of childcare centers if one or more children and/or staff are diagnosed with HAV infection, and food handlers during a common-source exposure. Concurrent immunization with inactivated or attenuated vaccines for these at-risk contacts is also warranted.

Hepatitis B

- Acute HBV infection in an adult generally only requires supportive care because of high rates of spontaneous recovery. For people with evidence of acute liver failure, prompt institution of antiviral therapy with a potent nucleos(t)ide analog and referral to a transplant center is recommended. Peginterferon alfa-2a (Pegasys)[1] is contraindicated in persons with acute liver failure.
- Treatment goals of chronic hepatitis B are sustained suppression of HBV DNA to prevent the development of cirrhosis, hepatocellular carcinoma, and liver-related mortality. Cure of chronic HBV infection is currently not possible. Treatment recommendations for chronic HBV differ depending on the phase of infection but are generally indicated for immune-active HBeAg-positive patients with confirmed HBV DNA greater than 2000 to 20,000 IU/mL and serum alanine aminotransferase (ALT) two or more times the upper limit of normal; for immune-active HBeAg-negative patients with HBV DNA greater than or equal to 2000 IU/mL and serum ALT two or more times the upper limit of normal; and patients with liver biopsy–proven moderate to severe inflammation and/or moderate fibrosis. Treatment decisions outside these parameters should be individualized based on the risk for complications (e.g., older age [>40 years], family history of cirrhosis or hepatocellular carcinoma, presence of cirrhosis) and the risk of therapy (e.g., chronic kidney disease, previous treatment history). Four agents are considered first-line—peginterferon alfa-2a (Pegasys), entecavir (Baraclude), tenofovir (Viread), and tenofovir alafenamide (Vemlidy)—based on their safety, effectiveness, and low rates of antiviral resistance. Peginterferon is generally recommended for those who prefer a finite course of treatment and who have clinical and laboratory features predictive of a response to peginterferon (high ALT, low HBV DNA, young age, female gender, and HBV genotype A or B). Peginterferon is contraindicated in persons with decompensated cirrhosis, compensated cirrhosis with clinically significant portal hypertension, autoimmune illnesses, or active psychiatric illness, and during pregnancy. Nucleos(t)ide analogs are more potent inhibitors of HBV DNA replication, generally better tolerated than peginterferon, and usually administered long-term. The ideal endpoint of treatment is loss of HBsAg, though it is rarely observed with any therapy.
- Prevention includes completion of a three-dose HBV vaccination series for all children by 18 months of age, with the first dose administered within 24 hours of birth. Infants whose mothers are HBsAg positive or whose HBsAg status is unknown should receive the last dose by 6 months of age. Vaccination is also recommended for adolescents younger than 19 years of age who have not been vaccinated, all adults ages 19 through 59 years, and adults age 60 years or older with risk factors for hepatitis B infection. A two-dose HBV vaccine is available for adults.
- Hepatitis B immune globulin (HyperHEP B) and HBV vaccination are recommended at birth for infants whose mothers are HBsAg positive. In mothers with viral loads greater than 200,000 IU/mL, antiviral therapy with tenofovir (Viread), telbivudine, or lamivudine (Epivir HBV) in the third trimester of pregnancy (gestation weeks 28–32) can be considered.

[1]Not FDA approved for this indication.

Five viruses, hepatitis A to E, account for the majority of cases of acute and chronic viral hepatitis. Chronic hepatitis is arbitrarily defined as the persistence of elevated serum aminotransferase levels for 6 or more months. Complications of chronic hepatitis (predominantly cirrhosis and hepatocellular carcinoma) account for the majority of morbidity and mortality caused by viral hepatitis. Effective vaccines are available for the prevention of hepatitis A, B, and D infections. A vaccine for hepatitis E has been developed but currently is only available in China. In addition, safe and effective therapy is available for treatment of chronic hepatitis B and C. Therefore it is important to screen individuals who are at high risk for chronic viral hepatitis to provide them access to care, reduce complications, and offer counseling to prevent transmission of infection.

Hepatitis A Virus

Introduction

Hepatitis A virus (HAV) is a positive-sense, single-stranded RNA virus of the *Hepatovirus* genus belonging to the Picornaviridae family. Its genome encodes four structural and seven nonstructural proteins. Four genotypes have been identified, but there is only one serotype. Therefore exposure to one HAV genotype confers immunity to all genotypes.

Natural History

HAV is a cause of acute hepatitis and acute liver failure but not chronic hepatitis (Table 1). In about 5% of cases, a prolonged cholestasis lasting more than 3 months may occur, and, in about 10% of cases, a relapsing hepatitis has been observed up to 6 months after the acute illness with recrudescence of symptoms and flare of hepatitis. Cases of relapsing hepatitis continue to remain infectious with fecal shedding of the virus. These atypical presentations of acute hepatitis A should not be mistaken for evolution to chronic hepatitis, as resolution is the rule. Recovery of HAV is associated with development of lifelong immunity.

HAV replication occurs in hepatocytes, and the virus is shed into the intestine via the biliary system. Viral levels peak during the asymptomatic period, and virus shedding continues until around 2 weeks into the icteric phase. HAV is detectable in the blood, but levels are 1000-fold higher in the feces. Children may shed the virus longer than adults.

The incubation period usually lasts 14 to 28 days. This is followed by the onset of symptoms. The presence and severity of symptoms are variable and age related. Generally, more than 70% of adult patients have a symptomatic illness, compared with only 10% of children younger than the age of 10 years. Typical symptoms are nonspecific and include fever, anorexia, nausea, vomiting, diarrhea, abdominal pain, and weight loss. This prodromal phase is followed by an icteric phase in 40% to 70% of patients with jaundice, pruritus, and dark urine. Physical examination findings are usually unremarkable, but hepatomegaly may be observed. Extrahepatic manifestations are uncommon and may include an evanescent rash and arthralgias.

Laboratory studies during the prodromal phase reveal elevated serum aminotransferase levels greater than 10 to 20 times the upper limit of normal. During the icteric phase, total serum bilirubin increases but generally does not exceed 10 mg/dL. In most patients, jaundice lasts 2 weeks, and a complete clinical and biochemical recovery can be expected in 2 to 3 months.

Epidemiology

Hepatitis A occurs throughout the world (Figure 1), either sporadically or in epidemics. The prevalence of HAV correlates with the level of sanitation and hygiene of a region. In developing countries, more than 90% of children are infected before 10 years of age. In developed countries, including the United States, infection rates are low. Lack of exposure at a young age leads to higher susceptibility in certain high-risk adults, including travelers to endemic areas, injection drug users, and men who have sex with men.

TABLE 1   Hepatitis A, B, D, and E Characteristics

	HEPATITIS A	HEPATITIS B	HEPATITIS D	HEPATITIS E
Classification	Picornavirus, ssRNA(+)	Hepadnavirus, dsDNA	Deltavirus, ssRNA(−)	Hepevirus, ssRNA(+)
Source	Stool	Blood	Blood	Stool
Transmission	Enteric	Percutaneous/permucosal	Percutaneous/permucosal	Enteric
Acute infections (per 1000/year) in the United States	125–200	140–320	6–13	Unknown
Epidemics	Yes	No	No	Yes
Incubation period	15–45 days	30–180 days	30–180 days	15–60 days
Risk of chronic hepatitis	No	Yes	Yes	Yes
Risk of HCC	No	Yes	Yes	No
Acute liver failure	0.10%	0.1%–1%	5%–20%	1%–2%*
Prevention	Pre-/postexposure immunization	Pre-/postexposure immunization	Pre-/postexposure immunization†	Preexposure immunization†

*Higher in pregnancy at 5% to 20%.
†Not available in the United States.
dsDNA, Double-stranded deoxyribonucleic acid; *HCC,* hepatocellular carcinoma; *ssRNA,* single-stranded ribonucleic acid.

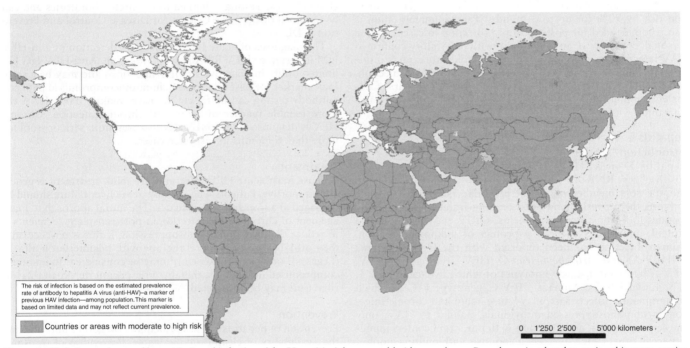

The risk of infection is based on the estimated prevalence rate of antibody to hepatitis A virus (anti-HAV)—a marker of previous HAV infection—among population. This marker is based on limited data and may not reflect current prevalence.

■ Countries or areas with moderate to high risk

0   1'250 2'500   5'000 kilometers

Figure 1 Global prevalence of hepatitis A and infection risk. Hepatitis A has a worldwide prevalence. Prevalence is related to regional income, sanitation, and hygiene. High-income areas (e.g., North America, Western Europe, Australia, New Zealand, Japan, the Republic of Korea, and Singapore) have low levels of hepatitis A virus *(HAV)* endemicity and subsequently a high proportion of susceptible adults. Low-income regions (sub-Saharan Africa and parts of South Asia) have high endemicity levels and very few susceptible adolescents and adults. Middle-income regions have a mix of intermediate and low endemicity levels.

In the United States HAV infection rates have declined by 95% since the introduction of mandatory childhood vaccination in 1995. The overall incidence rate in 2020 was 5 per 100,000 persons, representing a sevenfold increase in cases between 2015 and 2020 due to person-to-person outbreaks in homeless persons and persons who use injection drugs. HAV is spread primarily by the fecal-oral route through the ingestion of contaminated food or water. Humans are the only known reservoir of the virus.

Diagnosis
Serologic testing for antibody to HAV can confirm the diagnosis of acute infection, past exposure, and immunity to the virus. Acute HAV infection is diagnosed by the presence of anti-HAV immunoglobulin M (IgM). Anti-HAV IgG appears in the convalescent phase of infection and remains detectable for life. Past exposure or vaccination confers immunity and is reflected by anti-HAV IgG positivity with the absence of anti-HAV IgM antibodies. The antibody test for HAV usually includes total antibodies (IgM and IgG). Thus to diagnose acute hepatitis A, it is important to order anti-HAV IgM.

Treatment
Given the self-limiting nature of acute hepatitis A, treatment is predominately supportive. Caution should be taken when using hepatotoxic medications or medications metabolized predominately in the liver. Rarely, acute liver failure with encephalopathy and impaired synthetic function can occur. The patients at highest risk for this complication are generally older than 50

years of age and may have coexisting chronic HBV or hepatitis C virus (HCV) infections. Individuals presenting with acute liver failure are more appropriately managed at a liver transplant center.

Prevention

Both inactivated and attenuated vaccines have been licensed against HAV. Inactivated vaccines include HAVRIX (GlaxoSmithKline), VAQTA (Merck), TWINRIX (a combined hepatitis A and B vaccine from GlaxoSmithKline), AVAXIM (Sanofi Pasteur),[2] EPAXAL (Crucell),[2] and HEALIVE (Sinovac).[2] The only live attenuated vaccine is BIOVAC-A (Pukang).[2] The World Health Organization (WHO) recommends routine childhood vaccination for HAV in areas with intermediate infection rates. In the United States the Advisory Committee on Immunization Practices (ACIP) recommends that all children be vaccinated at 1 year of age. Other at-risk populations for whom vaccination is recommended include intravenous drug users, travelers to regions with high or intermediate HAV rates, men who have sex with men, persons in close contact with new adoptees from countries of high or intermediate hepatitis A endemicity, and patients with chronic liver disease or clotting factor disorders.

Passive immunization with immunoglobulin may also be used for preexposure protection among individuals who are at high or intermediate risk of HAV exposure. Pooled human anti-HAV immunoglobulins (GamaSTAN [IGIM]) decrease the HAV infection risk by 90% for up to 3 months. Passive immunization is also recommended for postexposure protection in cases of close personal contacts to an individual with laboratory-confirmed HAV infection, to staff and attendees of child care centers if one or more children and/or staff are diagnosed with HAV infection, and to food handlers during a common-source exposure. Concurrent immunization for HAV in these at-risk contacts is also warranted.

Hepatitis E

Introduction

Hepatitis E virus (HEV) is a nonenveloped, single-stranded, positive-sense RNA virus of approximately 7300 bases in length and the sole member of the Hepeviridae family. Its genome contains three overlapping open reading frames (ORF). ORF1 encodes four nonstructural proteins, ORF2 encodes the capsid protein, and ORF3 encodes a protein of unknown function. Human infection has been reported with the *Orthohepevirus* A (HEV-A) and *Orthohepevirus* C (HEV-C) species of HEV. HEV-A has eight distinct genotypes of which five (genotypes 1, 2, 3, 4, and 7) infect humans. HEV-C, genotype 1 (C-1), which predominantly infects rats, may cause acute and chronic infection in immunosuppressed individuals. Similar to HAV, only one serotype exists, and infection with one strain confers immunity to all others. HEV is likely a zoonosis with multiple nonhuman vectors.

Natural History

HEV is a cause of acute hepatitis and acute liver failure (see Table 1). It can cause chronic hepatitis in immunocompromised individuals. The majority of acute HEV infections are asymptomatic or minimally symptomatic. The incubation period is between 15 and 60 days, and if symptoms arise, they generally consist of anorexia, nausea, vomiting, diarrhea, and abdominal pain. Acute HEV infection rarely causes jaundice, and most symptoms resolve within 6 weeks from onset. A notable exception to the generally favorable outcome is an increased risk of acute liver failure among pregnant women during the second and third trimesters in endemic regions. This leads to a high maternal mortality rate of 15% to 25% and poorer maternofetal outcomes in third-trimester infections. Acute HEV infection may also be associated with a lymphocytic destructive cholangitis.

Chronic HEV infection is defined as the presence of HEV RNA in the serum or stool for more than 6 months. It is uncommon and has been observed in solid-organ transplant recipients, HIV-positive subjects, and other immunocompromised hosts. Chronic HEV infection has only been reported with HEV-A genotype 3 infections. It is unknown if other HEV genotypes can cause chronic HEV infection. Development of cirrhosis has been described as a consequence of chronic infection.

Epidemiology

HEV is found worldwide and can be divided into three distinct geographic patterns: highly endemic, endemic, and nonendemic (sporadic) (Figure 2). Large waterborne epidemics in highly endemic regions are caused by infection with HEV genotypes 1 and 2 in Central America, Africa, and Asia. Sporadic cases of HEV in developed countries (Europe, North America, and Far East Asia) are caused by HEV-A genotypes 3 and 4. The reservoir for autochthonous HEV is unknown but thought to be domestic swine. Sporadic cases may occur in travelers to endemic areas. Interestingly, males are more affected than females in sporadic infections, but this gender bias is not observed during epidemics. HEV is spread by the fecal-oral route, usually through ingestion of contaminated water.

Diagnosis

There are no commercially licensed tests for HEV detection in the United States. Testing is limited to research laboratories and can be obtained through the Centers for Disease Control and Prevention (CDC).

The diagnosis of acute HEV is made by detection of anti-HEV IgM in serum or HEV RNA in stool or serum. Anti-HEV IgG has limited utility in diagnosis of HEV infections and may be a serologic marker for past infection. In immunocompromised patients, antibody testing can be falsely negative, making HEV RNA the more reliable marker of acute and chronic infection. Chronic HEV is diagnosed when HEV RNA is present in sera or stool for more than 6 months in suspected cases.

Treatment

Because most acute HEV infections are mild, treatment is generally supportive. Patients who develop acute liver failure should be managed at a liver transplant center. The initial approach to management of chronic HEV infection in posttransplant recipients is to reduce the level of immunosuppression. If this is unsuccessful, then off-label use of antiviral therapy with peginterferon alfa-2a (Pegasys)[1] or ribavirin (Rebetol)[1] may be considered. In immunocompromised individuals, therapy with peginterferon alfa-2a[1] or ribavirin[1] may be considered.

Prevention

Prevention of hepatitis E relies principally on good sanitation and the availability of clean drinking water. Prevention of transmission in travelers to endemic areas includes avoiding consumption of tap water, street foods, raw vegetables, and raw or undercooked meats such as pork and seafood. A commercially available vaccine for HEV, HECOLIN[2] (Xiamen Innovax Biotech), has been available in China since 2012.

Hepatitis B

Introduction

HBV is a partially double-stranded DNA virus of approximately 3200 bases belonging to the Hepadnaviridae family. HBV consists of an outer lipid shell that surrounds a nucleocapsid consisting of the viral DNA, core protein, and polymerase. HBV has four overlapping reading frames (core, surface, polymerase, and x), which encode for seven viral proteins. Hepatitis B surface antigen (HBsAg) is the marker of infection, and hepatitis B e antigen (HBeAg) is a marker of high viral replication and infectivity. The virus is classified into 10 major genotypes (A to J) that have a

---

[2] Not available in the United States.

[1] Not FDA approved for this indication.
[2] Not available in the United States.

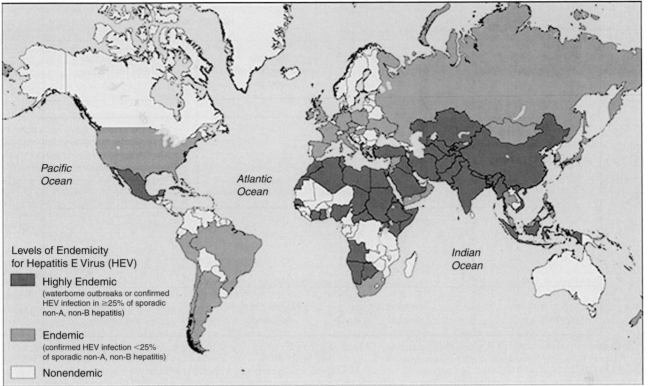

Pacific
Ocean

Atlantic
Ocean

Indian
Ocean

Levels of Endemicity
for Hepatitis E Virus (HEV)

■ Highly Endemic
(waterborne outbreaks or confirmed
HEV infection in ≥25% of sporadic
non-A, non-B hepatitis)

■ Endemic
(confirmed HEV infection <25%
of sporadic non-A, non-B hepatitis)

□ Nonendemic

Figure 2 Global prevalence of hepatitis E virus. Hepatitis E is found worldwide. High endemic areas, defined by greater than or equal to 25% prevalence of sporadic non-A, non-B hepatitis, include parts of Central America and Mexico, Africa, the Middle East, and most of Asia. Endemic areas, defined as less than 25% prevalence of sporadic non-A, non-B hepatitis, include the United States, Europe, Russia, and parts of South America. Remaining regions are regarded as nonendemic.

distinct geographic distribution. Four major serotypes have been described. Humans and Old World primates (e.g., chimpanzees) are the only known hosts.

Natural History

Hepatitis B virus is a cause of acute hepatitis and acute liver failure (see Table 1). Globally, it is a major cause of chronic hepatitis. Infection with HBV is notable for a long incubation period ranging from 1 to 6 months. The majority (two-thirds) of persons with acute HBV infection are asymptomatic, one-third have an icteric presentation, and less than 1% present with acute liver failure. Symptoms of acute HBV are nonspecific and include anorexia, nausea, pruritus, and right upper quadrant pain. Symptoms usually resolve in about 1 to 3 months. Serum alanine aminotransferase (ALT) levels peak with the onset of symptoms. The outcome of acute hepatitis B is strongly influenced by age at exposure. Resolution of acute infection occurs in 95% of persons exposed as adults, but chronic infection ensues in more than 90% of persons exposed as infants.

The natural history of chronic HBV infection depends on a complex interplay between the virus and the host immune response. Chronic HBV infection is often viewed in four phases (as shown in Figure 3) based on HBeAg status and serum HBV DNA and ALT levels. This classification is useful for providing advice on prognosis and need for treatment. Approximately 25% to 40% of persons with chronic infection will be at risk for development of cirrhosis. The 5-year cumulative incidence of cirrhosis in untreated chronic HBV infection is 8% to 20%. Once cirrhosis develops, the 5-year cumulative incidence of decompensated liver disease (ascites, variceal hemorrhage, hepatic encephalopathy) is approximately 20%, and the annual risk of hepatocellular carcinoma is 2% to 5%. Persons who have resolved chronic infection (cleared HBsAg) should be counseled at risk for viral reactivation with use of chemotherapy or other immunosuppressive therapies.

Epidemiology

An estimated 2 billion people worldwide have evidence of past HBV infection, and of these an estimated 296 million have chronic HBV infection. The prevalence of HBV infection is declining worldwide because of the availability of an effective vaccine and implementation of successful vaccination programs. Nevertheless, an estimated 1.5 million new infections occur annually. The prevalence of HBsAg, the serologic marker of chronic infection, is highest (≥8%) in sub-Saharan Africa and Central Asia (Figure 4) and lowest (<2%) in Western Europe, Australia, Canada, and the United States (except Alaska) (see Figure 4). HBV is transmitted vertically, sexually, or through percutaneous routes and is more infectious than human immunodeficiency virus or hepatitis C virus. Individuals considered at high risk for acquiring HBV infection should be screened for chronic hepatitis B by testing for HBsAg (Table 2). In 2023 the CDC recommended that all adults aged 18 years and older should be screened for hepatitis B at least once in their lifetime. The screening panel should include testing for HBsAg, anti-HBs, and antibody to core antigen (anti-HBc).

Diagnosis

A number of serologic markers (viral antigens and antibodies to the viral antigens) and nucleic acid testing are available to diagnose acute and chronic HBV infection. Cases of suspected acute HBV infection are diagnosed by detection of HBsAg, HBeAg, IgM anti-HBc, and HBV DNA in serum in the appropriate clinical setting. Although anti-HBc IgM is detected during acute HBV infection, it is not specific for acute hepatitis B and may be seen during reactivation of chronic HBV infection.

Chronic infection is defined as persistence of HBsAg for greater than 6 months in serum. If HBsAg is present, it is advised to check HBeAg, anti-HBe, HBV DNA, and serum ALT to determine the phase of infection.

HBeAg-positive		HBeAg-negative	
Immune tolerant High replication phase	**Immune active** High replication phase	**Inactive** Low replicative phase	**Immune active** High replicative phase
10^9-10^{10} HBV-DNA (IU/mL) 10^7-10^8		$<10^3$	$>10^5$
ALT			
No treatment indicated	Treatment indicated	No treatment indicated*	Treatment indicated

Figure 3 Phases of chronic hepatitis B virus *(HBV)* infection. Chronic hepatitis B can be viewed in phases defined by hepatitis B e-antigen *(HBeAg)* status and serum HBV DNA and alanine aminotransferase *(ALT)* levels. The initial phase is the immune-tolerant phase, characterized by HBeAg positivity, high HBV DNA level ($>10^7$ IU/mL), and persistently normal ALT levels. This is seen only in persons who acquire the infection at birth or infancy and that persists for two to three decades of life. The next phase is the immune-active phase, defined by continued HBeAg positivity, high HBV viral load ($>10^5$ IU/mL), and elevated ALT levels. The next phase is characterized by loss of HBeAg and development of anti-HBe and heralds a transition from a phase of high viral replication to one of low replication. The viral load is typically less than 10^3 IU/mL, and serum ALT is normal. This phase is termed the *inactive carrier phase*. A proportion of individuals develop raised HBV DNA and ALT levels after HBeAg seroconversion. These persons are said to have transitioned to the immune-escape or HBeAg-negative immune-active phase.

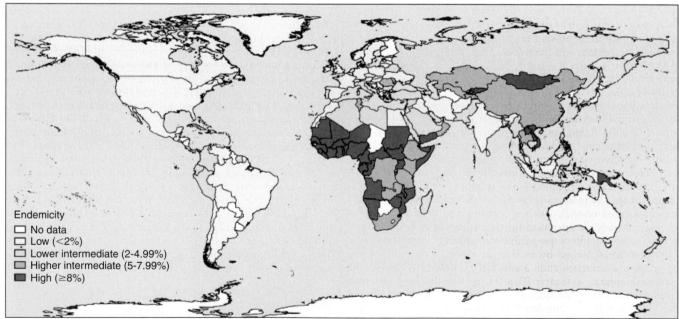

Endemicity
- ☐ No data
- ☐ Low (<2%)
- ☐ Lower intermediate (2-4.99%)
- ☐ Higher intermediate (5-7.99%)
- ■ High (≥8%)

Figure 4 Global prevalence of chronic hepatitis B virus (HBV). Hepatitis B is found worldwide with varying geographic prevalence. High-prevalence areas, defined as a prevalence of hepatitis B surface antigen (HBsAg) greater than or equal to 8%, include western sub-Saharan Africa and Mongolia. Regions of high intermediate prevalence, defined as HBsAg prevalence of 5% to 7%, include China, Southeast Asia, and the remainder of sub-Saharan Africa. Regions of low to intermediate prevalence, defined as HBsAg prevalence of 2% to 4%, include the Mediterranean region, India, the Middle East, Australia, and Japan. Regions with low prevalence, defined as HBsAg prevalence of less than or equal to 2%, include North America and Western Europe. Overall, the prevalence of HBV is declining worldwide.

Treatment

Acute HBV infection in an adult is associated with a high rate of spontaneous recovery, and antiviral treatment is rarely required. Supportive care is advised. For persons with evidence of acute liver failure, prompt institution of antiviral therapy with a potent nucleos(t)ide analog and referral to a transplant center is recommended. Peginterferon alfa-2a (Pegasys)[1] is contraindicated in persons with acute liver failure.

---

[1] Not FDA approved for this indication.

TABLE 2 Centers for Disease Control and Prevention Guidelines for Hepatitis B Virus Screening

Populations recommended or required for routine testing for chronic HBV infections

Persons born in regions of high and intermediate HBV endemicity (HBsAg prevalence >2%)

U.S.-born persons not vaccinated as infants whose parents were born in regions with high HBV endemicity (>8%)

Injection drug users

Men who have sex with men

Persons with elevated alanine aminotransferase/aspartate aminotransferase of unknown etiology

Donors of blood, plasma, organs, tissues, or semen

Hemodialysis patients

All pregnant women

Persons needing immunosuppressive therapy

Infants born to HBsAg-positive mothers

Household, needle-sharing, or sex contacts of persons known to be HBsAg positive

HIV-positive persons

Persons who are the sources of blood or body fluids for exposures that might require postexposure prophylaxis (e.g., needlestick, sexual assault)

HBsAg, Hepatitis B surface antigen; *HBV,* hepatitis B virus.
Modified from Centers for Disease Control and Prevention. Recommendations for identification and public health management of persons with chronic hepatitis B virus infection. *MMWR Morb Mortal Wkly Rep,* 57(RR-8):10–11, 2008

The goals of treatment of chronic HBV are sustained suppression of HBV DNA to prevent the development of cirrhosis, hepatocellular carcinoma, and liver-related mortality. Cure of chronic HBV infection is currently not possible because of persistence of covalently closed circular DNA within the hepatocyte nucleus and integrated HBV DNA. Treatment recommendations differ among regional guidelines, but treatment is generally indicated for HBeAg-positive patients with confirmed HBV DNA greater than 2000 to 20,000 IU/mL and serum ALT two or more times the upper limit of normal, and for HBeAg-negative patients with HBV DNA greater than or equal to 2000 IU/mL and serum ALT two or more times the upper limit of normal and/or liver biopsy–proven moderate to severe inflammation and/or moderate fibrosis. The decision to treat persons outside these parameters should be individualized based on their risk for complications and risk of therapy. Eight agents are approved for the treatment of chronic HBV infection: two interferon preparations (interferon alfa-2b [Intron A has been discontinued by its manufacturer] and peginterferon alfa-2a) and six nucleos(t)ide analogs (lamivudine [Epivir HBV], adefovir [Hepsera], entecavir [Baraclude], telbivudine,[2] tenofovir disoproxil fumarate [Viread], and tenofovir alafenamide [Vemlidy]). Four agents are considered first-line—peginterferon alfa-2a, entecavir, tenofovir, and tenofovir alafenamide—based on their safety, efficacy, and low rates of antiviral resistance. Peginterferon alfa-2a is generally recommended in persons who would prefer a finite course of treatment and who have clinical and laboratory features predictive of a response to peginterferon (high ALT, low HBV DNA, young age, female gender, and HBV genotype A or B). Peginterferon alfa-2a is contraindicated in persons with decompensated cirrhosis, cirrhosis with clinically significant portal hypertension, autoimmune illnesses, or active psychiatric illness and during pregnancy. Nucleos(t)ide analogs are more potent inhibitors of

HBV DNA replication and generally better tolerated than peginterferon alfa-2a. They are usually administered long-term. The ideal endpoint of treatment is HBsAg loss, but this is rarely observed with any therapy (<10% with interferon and after 5 years of therapy with nucleos(t)ide analogs).

Prevention
Vaccination is the primary method of prevention. An effective vaccine against HBV has been available since 1981. In the United States the ACIP has recommended that all infants complete the series of three vaccinations by 18 months of age, with the first dose administered within 24 hours of birth. Infants whose mothers are HBsAg positive or whose HBsAg status is unknown should receive the last dose by 6 months of age. Hepatitis B immune globulin (HyperHEP B) and HBV vaccination is recommended at birth for infants whose mothers are HBsAg positive to prevent maternal-infant transmission of HBV. In mothers with viral loads greater than 200,000 IU/mL, antiviral therapy with tenofovir, telbivudine,[2] or lamivudine in the third trimester of pregnancy (gestation weeks 28–32) can be considered. Vaccination is recommended for all persons younger than 19 years. In 2022 the ACIP recommended vaccination for adults 19 to 59 years of age and adults 60 years or older with risk factors for hepatitis B. Postexposure prophylaxis is recommended for anyone who is exposed to HBV and is considered susceptible to HBV infection and consists of hepatitis B vaccination and/or hepatitis B immune globulin depending on the HBsAg status of the exposure source.

Hepatitis D
Introduction
Hepatitis D virus (HDV) is a viroid that is dependent on HBV for its life cycle. The genome consists of a negative-sense, single-stranded circular RNA virus of approximately 1600 bases, classified as the genus Deltavirus. The virus has an outer lipoprotein envelope HBsAg derived from HBV and is attached to a single structural protein, the HDV antigen (HDAg). There are eight known genotypes. Immunity to HBV prevents HDV infection.

Natural History
Hepatitis D virus is a cause of acute hepatitis, acute liver failure, and chronic hepatitis (see Table 1). Hepatitis D virus infection can occur either simultaneously with HBV (referred to as *coinfection*) or as an infection in a patient with chronic HBV infection (referred to as *superinfection*). The outcome of HBV/HDV coinfection depends on the course of acute hepatitis B infection and is generally self-limiting with a low risk of chronicity (~5%). In contrast, HDV superinfection of a chronic HBV carrier results in chronic HDV infection in more than 90% of cases. Acute liver failure is observed more commonly with coinfection than with superinfection. Chronic HDV infection has a variable course, from an asymptomatic carrier to cirrhosis and decompensated liver disease. In general, HDV infection is associated with more rapid progression to cirrhosis and decompensated liver disease and a higher rate of hepatocellular carcinoma compared with HBV monoinfection.

Epidemiology
In developed countries, the prevalence of HDV has decreased as a consequence of widespread vaccination against hepatitis B. Chronic HDV infection is predominately seen in intravenous drug users or hemophiliacs requiring frequent transfusions. HDV is prevalent in the Amazon basin, Africa, the Mediterranean basin, Central Asia, Mongolia, and Russia (Figure 5). HDV genotype 1 can be found worldwide, but all other genotypes are restricted to specific geographic areas.

HDV is spread by the same routes as HBV infection and is efficiently transmitted by parenteral and sexual exposure. In contrast with HBV, vertical transmission is not a common mode of transmission. Transmission cannot occur in the absence of HBsAg.

---

[2] Not available in the United States.

[2] Not available in the United States.

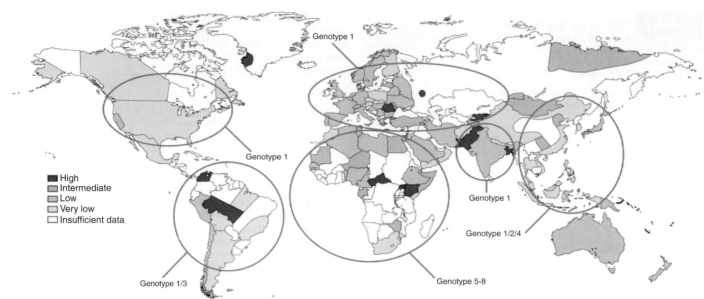

Figure 5 Global prevalence of hepatitis D virus. Hepatitis D is found globally, but prevalence varies among geographic regions. The highest prevalence is observed in Central Africa, Central Asia, and the Amazon. Intermediate-prevalence regions include West Africa and Eastern Europe. Low-prevalence regions include North America, most of Western Europe, and Australia.

Diagnosis

Testing for hepatitis D should be considered in persons presenting with acute hepatitis B who have additional risk factors for HDV, including a history of injection drug use; persons from endemic regions who present with a severe or protracted hepatitis; patients with chronic hepatitis B who develop an acute hepatitis of undetermined origin; and persons with HBsAg-positive chronic hepatitis B from endemic regions. Total anti-HDV (IgM and IgG) and anti-HDV IgM are the only commercially available assays in the United States. Initial testing for HDV should be with total anti-HDV. Chronic infection should be confirmed by a reverse transcriptase polymerase chain reaction assay for HDV RNA.

Treatment

The goals of treatment are long-term suppression of both HDV and HBV to prevent the development of cirrhosis, hepatocellular carcinoma, and liver-related death. There is no effective treatment for HDV. Peginterferon alfa-2a[1] has been used for treatment of HDV. The most effective dose and duration of treatment have not been established. Peginterferon alfa-2a[1] administered for 48 to 72 weeks results in sustained HDV RNA suppression after 6 months of therapy in 17% to 43% of patients. Bulevirtide (Hepcludex),[5] an entry inhibitor, received conditional marketing authorization in 2020 by the European Medicines Agency (the European equivalent of the U.S. Food and Drug Administration). Liver transplantation with the use of hepatitis B immune globulin[1] is an option for patients with decompensated liver disease. Novel agents blocking viral entry and posttranslational prenylation are currently being investigated in clinical studies.

Acknowledgments

This work is supported by the Intramural Research Program of the National Institute of Diabetes and Digestive and Kidney Diseases, National Institutes of Health.

Financial Disclosure

The authors are employees of the U.S. government and have no financial conflicts of interest to disclose.

---

[1] Not FDA approved for this indication.
[5] Investigational drug in the United States.

References

Hoofnagle JH, Nelson KE, Purcell RH: Hepatitis E, N Engl J Med 367(13):1237–1244, 2012.
Hughes SA, Wedemeyer H, Harrison PM: Hepatitis delta virus, Lancet 378(9785):73–85, 2011.
Matheny SC, Kingery JE: Hepatitis A, Am Fam Physician 86(11):1027–1034, 2012.
Trépo C, Chan HL, Lok A: Hepatitis B virus infection, Lancet 384(9959):2053–2063, 2014.

▍HEPATITIS C

Method of
Arthur Y. Kim, MD

CURRENT DIAGNOSIS

- Hepatitis C virus (HCV) is a common infection in the United States, with major morbidity and mortality.
- The incidence of HCV is rising, linked to the opioid epidemic.
- Given the asymptomatic presentation and long period before complications, screening is warranted: one-time routine opt-out testing for adults age 18–79 is recommended, as is periodic repeat testing for increased risk, especially in people who inject drugs (Table 1).
- Diagnosis is made with two-stage testing: initial screening for anti-HCV antibodies followed by HCV RNA testing to confirm the presence of virus.

CURRENT THERAPY

- Novel therapeutic approaches that are safe and highly effective have revolutionized the care of HCV.
- The goal of therapy is cure of virus, which prevents liver-related complications and further transmission.
- Regimens of combination antivirals typically given for 8–12 weeks can cure over 95% of those living with HCV infection.

TABLE 1	Recommendations for One-Time Screening

All adults aged 18–79 years without prior ascertainment of risk

Risk factor–based screening

Risk behaviors

- Injection drug use (current or ever, including those who injected only once)

- Intranasal drug use

Risk exposures

- Persons on long-term hemodialysis (ever)

- Persons with percutaneous/parenteral exposures in an unregulated setting

- Health care, emergency medical, and public safety workers after needlesticks, sharps, or mucosal exposures to HCV-infected blood

- Children born to HCV-infected women

- Prior recipients of transfusions or organ transplants, including

  - Persons who were notified that they received blood from a donor who later tested positive for HCV infection

  - Persons who received a transfusion of blood or blood components or underwent an organ transplant before July 1992

  - Persons who received clotting factor concentrates produced before 1987

- Persons who were ever incarcerated

Other considerations

- HIV infection

- Sexually active persons about to start preexposure prophylaxis for HIV

- Unexplained chronic liver disease and/or chronic hepatitis, including elevated alanine aminotransferase levels

- Solid-organ donors (deceased and living)

- Pregnant women

HCV, Hepatitis C virus.
Modified from http://hcvguidelines.org.

The diagnosis, management, and therapeutic approaches for patients living with HCV have been dramatically transformed in recent years. Most people (over 95%) living with HCV infection can be cured after 8 to 12 weeks of safe oral regimens involving combined antiviral agents. The availability of novel therapies enhances the effectiveness of screening patients for HCV infection who may otherwise be unaware of infection owing to its asymptomatic presentation.

Virology, Pathogenesis, and Natural History
HCV is a single-strand RNA virus whose genome encodes several viral proteins, including nonstructural proteins (NS3/4A, termed protease; NS5A and NS5B, termed polymerase) that may each be specifically targeted by medications. There are seven known families of virus, commonly known as genotypes 1 through 7, many with subtypes (e.g., genotype 1a or 1b).

After acute infection in the majority of individuals, the virus establishes a chronic lifelong infection characterized by high levels of viremia easily detected in plasma; in a minority, the virus is spontaneously cleared. In the latter scenario, HCV is permanently eradicated, as the polymerase is an RNA-RNA polymerase and there is no DNA intermediate to establish latency in the host. Those who achieve clearance of virus, whether spontaneously or via treatment, are susceptible to reinfection if exposed again.

Both the acute and chronic phases of HCV infection are largely asymptomatic. A minority of those with acute infection may present with nonspecific symptoms such as abdominal pain and malaise, with less than 10% presenting with jaundice. Rarely, those with chronic infection may experience extrahepatic manifestations of HCV infection, such as cryoglobulinemic vasculitis, proteinuria or glomerulonephritis, or lymphoma. Otherwise, alanine transaminase (ALT) levels may be persistently or intermittently elevated but may also be within normal range in up to 20% of infected individuals; thus, ALT is considered an imperfect screening test for HCV.

After establishment of chronic HCV infection, fibrosis occurs at a variable rate and may progress to cirrhosis in about 15% to 20% over a 20-year period. Fibrosis may be accelerated by other liver insults, such as alcohol use, nonalcoholic steatohepatitis, and coinfection with HIV or hepatitis B virus (HBV). Those with HCV-related cirrhosis may experience significant morbidity and mortality from various complications; screening for varices and hepatocellular carcinoma is recommended (see chapter on cirrhosis).

Epidemiology
HCV is estimated to infect at least 58 million people worldwide. In the United States, it is the leading bloodborne pathogen and infects over 3 million Americans. The highest-risk groups are those born between 1945 and 1965 (so-called baby boomers), people who inject drugs, and HIV-positive men who have sex with men. In the United States, the incidence reached a peak in the 1970s and 1980s and then steeply declined; in the past decade there has been a resurgence of new incident cases linked to a widespread opioid epidemic.

Owing to the high number of infections that occurred decades ago, a large number of Americans within the baby-boomer cohort are now at risk for unidentified long-standing HCV infection, cirrhosis, and death. HCV-related cirrhosis remains a leading indication for liver transplantation.

Risk Factors
HCV is most efficiently transmitted via exposure to contaminated blood or its components. In the United States, injection drug use (IDU) is the most common mode of transmission. Nosocomial exposure to contaminated blood or blood products and poorly sterilized or reused contaminated medical equipment remains an important risk, especially if strict universal precautions are not instituted. Mother-to-child transmission is not efficient, as only about 5% of children born to HCV-infected women are infected, with higher rates if HIV/HCV coinfection is present. Sexual transmission is considered very rare in the context of heterosexual relationships but does occur at higher rates in men who have sex with men, particularly with HIV and/or practices that result in exposures to blood.

Diagnosis
Two tests are used for the diagnosis of HCV infection: testing for anti-HCV antibodies and measuring HCV RNA. The suggested algorithm is initial serologic testing to assess exposure, followed by HCV RNA testing to determine current or cleared infection. Currently available anti-HCV testing is highly sensitive (>99%) but may be falsely negative in the earliest stages of infection (typically the first 4 to 12 weeks) or in the setting of immunosuppression (such as dialysis or HIV if CD4 cell counts are below 200/mm^3). HCV RNA testing may be utilized to confirm current HCV RNA infection after an initial positive anti-HCV test or in settings when anti-HCV may be falsely negative. There are two types of HCV RNA tests: qualitative HCV RNA tests, which do not quantify the level of viral replication, and quantitative HCV RNA tests. Quantitative testing has improved in recent years and exhibits sensitivity similar to that of qualitative testing; therefore it is preferred in most situations.

GENOTYPE	COMBINATION	USE OF RIBAVIRIN (RBV)	DURATION (WEEKS)	NOTES
1	Elbasvir 50 mg/grazoprevir 100 mg FDC (Zepatier) qd	Add RBV and extend to 16 weeks if baseline NS5A RASs present (genotype 1a only)	12–16	Safe in advanced chronic kidney disease; not recommended in decompensated cirrhosis
	Glecaprevir 300 mg/ pibrentasvir 120 mg FDC (Mavyret) qd	Consider in select re-treatment circumstances	8–16	8 weeks for treatment naive; 12–16 weeks for certain treatment-experienced patients
	Ledipasvir 90 mg/sofosbuvir 400 mg FDC (Harvoni) qd	Add RBV if both interferon-experienced and cirrhosis (12 weeks)	8–24	Antacids reduce absorption; 8 weeks consideration only for naive patients with F0-2 and HCV RNA less than 6M IU/mL
	Sofosbuvir 400 mg/velpatasvir 100 mg FDC (Epclusa) qd	Consider in select re-treatment circumstances	12–24	Antacids reduce absorption
2	Glecaprevir 300 mg/ pibrentasvir 120 mg FDC (Mavyret) qd	Consider in select re-treatment circumstances	8–12	8 weeks for treatment naive; 12 weeks for certain treatment-experienced patients
	Sofosbuvir/velpatasvir FDC (Epclusa) qd	Consider in select re-treatment circumstances	12	Antacids reduce absorption
3	Glecaprevir 300 mg/ pibrentasvir 120 mg FDC (Mavyret) qd	Consider in select re-treatment circumstances	8–16	8 weeks for treatment naive; 12–16 weeks for certain treatment-experienced patients
	Sofosbuvir/velpatasvir FDC (Epclusa) qd	Consider in select circumstances, including cirrhosis + NS5A Y93H mutation	12–24	Antacids reduce absorption
4	Elbasvir/grazoprevir (Zepatier) qd	Consider adding RBV for cirrhosis, prior nonresponder	12–16	
	Ledipasvir/sofosbuvir FDC (Harvoni) qd	Consider for previous SOF failure	12	
	Glecaprevir 300 mg/ pibrentasvir 120 mg FDC (Mavyret) qd	Not proven	8–16	8 weeks for treatment naive; 12–16 weeks for certain treatment-experienced patients
	Sofosbuvir/velpatasvir FDC (Epclusa) qd	Consider in select circumstances	12	Antacids reduce absorption

RBV may be added in select re-treatment situations; refer to https://www.hcvguidelines.org/ for details
FDC, Fixed-dose combination; *NS5A*, nonstructural protein 5A; *RASs*, resistance-associated substitutions; *RBV*, ribavirin; *SOF*, sofosbuvir.

Those with confirmed current HCV infection (positive HCV RNA) should also be tested for HIV and HBV (the latter typically by hepatitis B surface antigen [HBsAg]). Follow-up evaluation includes the HCV genotype, which defines therapeutic options. Discovery of advanced fibrosis or cirrhosis may affect the specifics of recommended antiviral regimens but also has prognostic implications. The likelihood of cirrhosis is dependent on various factors, including advancing patient age, duration of infection, and cofactors such as significant alcohol use or HIV. Noninvasive assessment with serologic testing (such as Fibrosure) or with novel imaging technologies (such as transient elastography) has largely replaced liver biopsies.

Prevention

Prevention of HCV infection should be targeted to the highest-risk groups. For people who inject drugs, clean injecting equipment—including needles, syringes, and other components of drug preparation—is paramount. Risk reduction should also be achieved after viral clearance to prevent reinfection.

Prevention of fibrosis progression includes minimization or abstinence from regular alcohol use, avoidance of fatty liver, and avoidance of primary infection with or control of coexisting viruses (HIV or HBV). For individuals who are not immune, vaccination against hepatitis A virus and HBV is recommended. Patients with coexisting substance use disorder should be referred for appropriate care.

Therapy

Antiviral treatments for hepatitis C have been revolutionized with combination regimens of direct-acting antivirals (DAAs). These new drugs are used in combination with the goal to eradicate HCV. Cure is known as a sustained virologic response (SVR), defined as a negative HCV RNA test 12 or more weeks after cessation of therapy. This definition represents a durable cure in the absence of reinfection. Benefits of SVR include a significant reduction in future liver-related events, especially for those with advanced fibrosis or cirrhosis. Additional benefits include abrogation of further HCV transmission, amelioration of extrahepatic manifestations (if present), and improvement in quality of life. Virtually all patients with current HCV infection are candidates for therapy.

Agents may be classified by the viral protein they target. The following are NS3/4A protease inhibitors: simeprevir, paritaprevir (which requires pharmacologic boosting with ritonavir), glecaprevir, and grazoprevir. NS5A inhibitors include daclatasvir, elbasvir, ledipasvir, ombitasvir, and pibrentasvir; the NS5A nonnucleoside inhibitor dasabuvir; and the NS5B nucleotide polymerase inhibitor sofosbuvir. Simeprevir (Olysio), daclatasvir (Daklinza), and sofosbuvir (Sovaldi) were developed as single agents, but the majority are parts of combination regimens, as described in Table 2. The Infectious Diseases Society of America (IDSA) and American Association for the Study of Liver Diseases (AASLD) maintain guidelines for providers at http://www.hcvguidelines.org, which provides updates with approval of novel agents and as new data become available.

One major consideration in choosing a regimen is the genotype of the virus, although certain regimens such as glecaprevir/pibrentasvir (Mavyret) and sofosbuvir/velpatasvir (Epclusa) are able to treat all genotypes (termed pangenotypic). Other potential influences include presence of cirrhosis, the potential for concomitant drug interactions (including those with HIV coinfection on antiretrovirals), prior treatment experience, and adherence to therapy. Certain regimens such as glecaprevir/pibrentasvir (Mavyret) have been tested for those with advanced renal impairment. Insurance formulary preferences may also dictate the choice. One regimen in particular, elbasvir/grazoprevir (Zepatier), requires testing of genotype 1a virus for resistance-associated substitutions (RASs) associated with decreased response; if these are present, the duration should be increased and ribavirin (Ribasphere) added. In general, almost all patient groups can be offered a regimen with a rate of SVR at or above 95%.

These combinations have favorable safety profiles, with phase III trials reporting very low discontinuation rates. The most common side effects of these regimens are headache and fatigue. At times, ribavirin may be added to the regimen, particularly in the cases of relapse after previous treatment and/or cirrhosis (especially if the patient is decompensated or was previously decompensated).

Drug-drug interactions are also potentially problematic. Sofosbuvir-containing regimens should not be coadministered with amiodarone (Cordarone) owing to reports of symptomatic bradycardia with poor outcomes. Medications may significantly decrease the absorption of HCV antivirals, especially rifampin (Rifadin), carbamazepine (Tegretol), oxcarbazepine (Trileptal), and St. John's wort.[7] For the combinations of ledipasvir/sofosbuvir (Harvoni) and sofosbuvir/velpatasvir (Epclusa), care must be taken if they are coadministered with medications that decrease gastric pH. The involvement of clinical pharmacists may be very useful, along with resources such as the website maintained at the University of Liverpool: http://hep-druginteractions.org.

Monitoring

Compared with previous regimens that were associated with more side effects and complications, current treatments are far more tolerable. Clinical visits or phone calls to monitor for side effects and to promote adherence are optional for patients eligible for simplified therapy (see hcvguidelines.org). Certain regimens may require more intensive monitoring in the presence of cirrhosis, as cases of decompensation have been reported. Those with active HBV replication who are untreated are at risk for reactivation of this virus once HCV is suppressed, with rare cases of liver failure reported; cotreatment of both viruses or very close monitoring is recommended for this subgroup. At this time there are few data for the use of these agents in pregnancy or during breastfeeding.

---

[7]Available as dietary supplement.

References

Edlin BR, Eckhardt BJ, Shu MA, et al: Toward a more accurate estimate of the prevalence of hepatitis C in the United States, *Hepatology* 62(5):1353–1363, 2015.

Ghany MG, Morgan TR; AASLD-IDSA Hepatitis C Guidance Panel: Hepatitis C guidance 2019 update: AASLD-IDSA recommendations for testing, managing, and treating hepatitis C virus infection, *Hepatology* 71(2):686–721, 2020.

Kim A: Hepatitis C virus, *Ann Intern Med* 165(5):ITC33–ITC48, 2016.

Ly KN, Hughes EM, Jiles RB, Holmberg SD: Rising mortality associated with hepatitis C virus in the United States, 2003- 2013, *Clin Infect Dis* 62(10):1287–1288, 2016.

Suryaprasad AG, White JZ, Xu F, et al: Emerging epidemic of hepatitis C virus infections among young nonurban persons who inject drugs in the United States, 2006-2012, *Clin Infect Dis* 59(10):1411–1419, 2014. 2006-2012.

INFLAMMATORY BOWEL DISEASE: CROHN DISEASE AND ULCERATIVE COLITIS

Method of
Mewish Ahmed, MD; Jami A. Kinnucan, MD; and Francis A. Farraye, MD, MS

CURRENT DIAGNOSIS

- Inflammatory bowel disease (IBD) includes Crohn disease (CD) and ulcerative colitis, which are classified as immune-mediated chronic intestinal diseases.
- The pathogenesis of IBD is thought to be related to a dysregulated immune response.
- Clinical features of IBD include chronic diarrhea, abdominal pain, and fatigue. There can also be weight loss, bloody stools, fevers, fistulae (CD), or other extraintestinal manifestations.
- The diagnosis of IBD is made with a combination of symptom history, lab work, stool testing, imaging, endoscopic findings, and histology.

CURRENT THERAPY

- IBD is most optimally managed with a "treat-to-target" strategy.
- Medical therapies for the treatment of IBD are divided into induction therapy and maintenance therapy.
- Classes of medications include 5-aminosalicylates, corticosteroids, biologics, small molecules, and immunomodulators.
- The choice of therapy depends on the type of IBD, disease location, extent of disease, severity of disease, disease prognosis, comorbidities, and patient preference. Special considerations should be given to the aging population and patients who are pregnant.
- Preventive health maintenance should be a routine component of IBD care.

Introduction and Epidemiology

Inflammatory bowel disease (IBD) includes Crohn disease (CD) and ulcerative colitis (UC), which are classified as immune-mediated chronic intestinal diseases. IBD can present at any age, with the most common age at presentation being young adulthood, followed by adults older than age 60 years. The incidence of IBD has been rising over the last few decades. It is more prevalent in Western populations, although the incidence has started to rise throughout the world.

The pathogenesis of IBD is thought to be related to a dysregulated immune response. There is a genetic predisposition, with children and first-degree relatives of patients with IBD having an increased risk. However, only 10% to 20% of patients with IBD have first-degree relatives with the disease. Although genetic loci have been found, they explain a small fraction of the disease risk and phenotype. Environmental factors play a role in disease pathogenesis.

Clinical Manifestations

Clinical features of IBD vary based on disease location and include chronic diarrhea, abdominal pain, and fatigue. Patients can exhibit weight loss, bloody stools, fevers, fistulae (CD), and other extraintestinal manifestations. Extraintestinal manifestations include inflammatory arthritis, skin involvement (erythema nodosum or pyoderma gangrenosum), eye involvement histology, UC appears as chronic inflammation and architectural distortion.

Radiological studies are useful to determine the extent of disease involvement and complications of disease, especially in patients with CD. They do not replace endoscopic evaluation and can be used concomitantly. Computed tomography enterography (CTE) uses oral and intravenous (IV) contrast to identify thickened bowel wall and has a sensitivity of around 90% for CD. Magnetic resonance enterography is an alternative to CTE to avoid cumulative radiation exposure in patients who require frequent disease assessment with imaging. Magnetic resonance imaging is more effective than computed tomography at detecting perianal fistulae. Transabdominal ultrasound with contrast can be helpful in assessing for disease activity in both CD and UC, strictures, bowel wall thickness, and postoperative recurrence of disease. In UC, a plain abdominal film in hospitalized patients may be useful to assess for toxic megacolon; however, imaging does not have as much of a role in evaluation of UC unless patients have severe abdominal pain.

Differential Diagnosis

It is important to consider a differential diagnosis when evaluating patients with acute or chronic GI symptoms. Table 2 lists both infectious and noninfectious IBD mimickers.

Management of Disease

IBD is most optimally managed with a "treat-to-target" strategy. Various targets have been identified by the STRIDE I and II initiatives of the International Organization for the Study of Inflammatory Bowel Diseases. There has been a focus on clinical, endoscopic, histologic, imaging, biomarker, and patient-reported outcomes as potential targets. In Figure 2, from STRIDE II, targets are divided into short-term, intermediate, and long-term for patients with IBD. Table 3 defines these targets. As of 2021, histologic remission and transmural healing do not have enough evidence to support escalating therapy to achieve these parameters but can be helpful adjunctive data to assess the depth of remission.

Medical Management

Medical therapies for the treatment of IBD are divided into *induction therapy* to bring the inflammation under control in the acute setting and *maintenance therapy* to allow for sustained remission. In most situations the medical therapies used for induction can also be used for chronic maintenance therapy. The choice of therapy depends on the type of IBD, disease location, extent of disease, severity of disease, disease prognosis, comorbidities, and patient preference. Table 4 provides a reference for IBD therapies, including formulations, indications, adverse effects, and monitoring.

TABLE 2	Inflammatory Bowel Disease Mimickers
GI infections	*Clostridium difficile*
	Salmonella
	Shigella
	Escherichia coli
	Campylobacter
	Giardia
	Yersinia
	Amebiasis
	Cytomegalovirus colitis (in patients who are immunosuppressed)
	Tuberculosis
Sexually transmitted infections	Chlamydia
	Herpes
	Neisseria gonorrhea
	Treponema pallidum
Noninfectious mimickers	Microscopic colitis
	Diverticulitis
	Segmental colitis associated with diverticulosis
	Ischemic colitis
	Medication associated colitis or enteritis (NSAIDs)
	Solitary rectal ulcer syndrome
	Systemic vasculitis (polyarteritis nodosa, Henoch-Schönlein purpura, Behcet syndrome)
	Celiac disease
	Intestinal lymphoma
	Diversion colitis (in patients with intestinal surgical diversion)

GI, Gastrointestinal; *NSAIDs*, nonsteroidal antiinflammatory drugs.

Figure 2 Stride II treatment targets for UC and CD. *CRP*, C-reactive protein; *IBD*, inflammatory bowel disease; *QoL*, quality of life. (Reprinted with permission from Turner D, Ricciuto A, Lewis A, et al. STRIDE-II: an update on the Selecting Therapeutic Targets in Inflammatory Bowel Disease (STRIDE) initiative of the International Organization for the Study of IBD (IOIBD): determining therapeutic goals for treat-to-target strategies in IBD. *Gastroenterology*. 2021;160:1570-1583.)

TABLE 3　Treatment Targets

IMMEDIATE TREATMENT TARGETS	INTERMEDIATE TARGETS	LONG-TERM TARGETS
Clinical response: 50% decrease in patient reported outcomes 2 (PRO2) CD PRO2: abdominal pain and stool frequency UC PRO2: rectal bleeding and stool frequency	Clinical remission: CD: HBI <5 or CDAI abdominal pain score ≤1 and stool frequency ≤3 UC: PRO2 score 0 (from Mayo score), partial Mayo score <3 with no score >1	Endoscopic healing: CD: SES-CD <3 or absence of ulcerations UC: MES of 0 or UCEIS ≤1
	Normalization of CRP and fecal calprotectin (100–250 mg/g of stool)	QoL measures Absence of disability Normalized health-related QoL

CD, Crohn disease; CDAI, Crohn's Disease Activity Index; CRP, C-reactive protein; HBI, Harvey Bradshaw Index; MES, Mayo Endoscopic Score; QoL, quality of life; SES-CD, Simple Endoscopic Score for Crohn's Disease; UC, ulcerative colitis; UCEIS, Ulcerative Colitis Endoscopic Index of Severity.

TABLE 4　Pharmacologic Therapies for Inflammatory Bowel Disease

MEDICATION CLASS	MEDICATION NAME	INDICATIONS	ADVERSE EFFECTS	MONITORING
5-ASA	Mesalamine rectal suppository (Canasa) Mesalamine enema (Rowasa) Mesalamine extended-release capsule (Pentasa) Mesalamine delayed-release (Apriso, Lialda, Asacol HD) Sulfasalazine (Azulfidine), olsalazine (Dipentum), and balsalazide (Colazal)	Mild to moderate UC (induction and maintenance)	Nausea, vomiting, headache, diarrhea, abdominal pain, interstitial nephritis	Urinalysis and renal function yearly
Corticosteroids	Prednisone Methylprednisolone Budesonide Budesonide-MMX (Uceris extended-release tablet) Rectal hydrocortisone (suppository, foam, or enema) Rectal budesonide foam (Uceris Rectal)	UC and CD (induction and maintenance)	Osteoporosis Adrenal insufficiency Impaired glucose tolerance, infection, fluid retention, hypertension, osteonecrosis, mood and sleep disturbance	DEXA scan if >3 months of systemic use
Biologics				
Anti–TNF-α	Infliximab (Remicade) Adalimumab (Humira) Golimumab (Simponi) (UC only) Certolizumab pegol (CD only)	UC and CD (induction and maintenance)	Infusion reactions, immune-mediated reactions, infections, malignancy (lymphoma, melanoma) Avoid in heart failure, demyelinating disease, or active malignancy	Yearly skin exam TB and hepatitis B
Antiintegrins	Vedolizumab (Entyvio) Natalizumab (Tysabri)	Vedolizumab: UC and CD (induction and maintenance) Natalizumab: CD only (induction and maintenance)	PML (natalizumab), nasopharyngitis	JC virus (natalizumab) TB and hepatitis B
Anti–IL-12/23	Ustekinumab (Stelara)	UC and CD (induction and maintenance)	Nasopharyngitis, other infections, headache, arthralgia	TB and hepatitis B
Anti–IL-23	Risankizumab (Skyrizi)	CD (induction and maintenance)	DILI, nasopharyngitis, headache, arthralgia	Liver enzymes TB and hepatitis B
Small Molecules				
JAK inhibitors	Tofacitinib (Xeljanz) Upadacitinib (Rinvoq)	Tofacitinib: UC (induction and maintenance) Upadacitinib: UC and CD (induction and maintenance)	Hyperlipidemia, lymphopenia, blood clots, infection, herpes zoster, GI perforation	CBC Lipid panel Liver enzymes TB and hepatitis B
S1P receptor modulator	Ozanimod (Zeposia)	UC (induction and maintenance)	Herpes zoster, lymphopenia, bradycardia, HTN, macular edema, elevated liver enzymes	Baseline: ECG CBC Liver enzymes

Continued

MEDICATION CLASS	MEDICATION NAME	INDICATIONS	ADVERSE EFFECTS	MONITORING
Immunomodulators				
Thiopurines	Azathioprine (Imuran) 6-Mercaptopurine (6-MP)	Monotherapy: UC[1] and CD[1] (maintenance) Combination therapy: UC[1] and CD[1] (induction and maintenance)	Hepatotoxicity, leukopenia, lymphoma, pancreatitis, non–melanoma skin cancers, infections	TPMT before initiation CBC and liver enzymes
Methotrexate	Methotrexate (subcutaneous or intramuscular)	Monotherapy: CD[1] (maintenance) Combination therapy: both UC[1] and CD[1] (induction and maintenance)	Myelosuppression, hepatotoxicity, pulmonary fibrosis, teratogen	CBC Liver enzymes
Cyclosporine	Cyclosporine	Induction in acute severe UC[1]	Seizures, nephrotoxicity, neurotoxicity, infections	Not used in maintenance

[1]Not FDA approved for this indication.

5-ASA, 5-Aminosalicylates; *CBC,* complete blood cell count; *CD,* Crohn disease; *DILI,* drug-induced liver injury; *ECG,* electrocardiogram; *GI,* gastrointestinal; *HTN,* hypertension; *IL,* interleukin; *JAK,* janus kinase; *PML,* progressive multifocal leukoencephalopathy; *S1P,* sphingosine-1-phosphate; *TB,* tuberculosis; *TMPT,* thiopurine methyltransferase; *TNF-α,* tumor necrosis factor–α; *UC,* ulcerative colitis.

5-Aminosalicylates

5-Aminosalicylates (5-ASAs) are used as first-line therapy for induction and maintenance of remission of mild to moderate UC. 5-ASA use is limited in CD, although sulfasalazine (Azulfidine)[1] can be considered in mild cases. 5-ASAs work by topical contact, exerting antiinflammatory effects. Rectal formulations are first-line treatment for proctitis (suppositories) and left-sided UC (enemas) up to the splenic flexure. For mild extensive colitis (beyond the splenic flexure), oral 5-ASA is recommended in addition to rectal therapies. For any extent of disease failing to respond to 5-ASA, escalation of therapy is indicated. Once-daily dosing is just as effective as divided dosing. If switching to advanced therapy (biologic or small molecule), there is no indication to continue the 5-ASA to maintain remission.

5-ASA side effects include nausea, vomiting, diarrhea, headache, and abdominal pain. Sulfasalazine may also cause low sperm counts. A small group of patients on 5-ASA may experience worsening of symptoms consistent with a hypersensitivity reaction. Another rare side effect is interstitial nephritis, which occurs in less than 0.3% of patients. To monitor for this, clinicians should monitor renal function several weeks after starting therapy and then yearly.

Corticosteroids

Corticosteroids are antiinflammatory medications that are typically used at the time of diagnosis and during relapses but are not recommended to be used for maintenance of remission because of their extensive adverse side-effect profile with long-term use. Ultimately, the treat-to-target strategy focuses on achieving treatment targets using steroid sparing therapies. Budesonide with controlled-release formulations for either ileum (Entocort EC) or colon (Uceris) disease is an option for clinical relapse with fewer systemic side effects. Topical rectal steroids are available as hydrocortisone suppositories, foam formulations, or enemas. These can be used as initial therapy in mild to moderate left-sided colitis or proctitis, although rectal mesalamine is preferred as the initial agent.

Adverse effects of steroids include mood and sleep disturbances, impaired glucose tolerance, metabolic bone disease, adrenal insufficiency, infections, fluid retention, hypertension, and osteonecrosis of the femoral head. If a patient has required systemic steroids for over 3 months, they should undergo a dual-energy X-ray absorptiometry (DEXA) scan to evaluate for osteopenia.

Biologics

Biologic therapies have transformed the landscape of IBD care. Biologics are recommended to be initiated early in the treatment of patients with moderate to severe UC or CD as they lead to better outcomes, prevention of disease complications, and a higher likelihood of achieving and maintaining remission. Typically, biologics are used both for induction and maintenance of remission.

Anti–Tumor Necrosis Factor–α agents

Anti–tumor necrosis factor-α (TNF-α) therapies block TNF-α, which is a cytokine that mediates inflammation in IBD. They can be used for induction and maintenance for CD and UC. Before initiation of anti–TNF-α agents, screening for latent or active tuberculosis (TB) and hepatitis B must be performed. Infliximab (Remicade or biosimilar) is administered as an IV formulation, whereas adalimumab (Humira or biosimilar) is a subcutaneous formulation. These are both approved for UC and CD. Other formulations include golimumab (Simponi), which is only approved for UC, and certolizumab pegol (Cimzia), which is only approved for CD. Data has also shown that the efficacy of anti–TNF-α agents improves when used in combination with immunomodulators, such as azathioprine (Imuran)[1], 6-mercaptopurine (Purinethol)[1], or methotrexate[1]. This is thought to be due to prevention of anti–drug antibody formation and higher serum drug levels.

Adverse effects of anti–TNF-α agents include infusion reactions (infliximab), which can be acute or delayed, immune-mediated adverse effects, infections, and treatment-related malignancy. Other immune-mediated adverse effects include drug-induced lupus-like reactions and psoriasiform reactions that usually resolve with drug discontinuation.

Those on anti–TNF-α therapy are at increased risk for infection, including opportunistic infections and reactivation of TB and hepatitis B. Although rare, treatment-related malignancy is a risk with anti–TNF-α agents, especially when used in combination with immunomodulators. Although there is no significant risk of development of solid organ tumors, there is an increased risk of non–Hodgkin lymphoma and melanoma. Anti–TNF-α therapies are contraindicated in patients with decompensated heart failure and demyelinating neurologic disease and are relatively contraindicated in patients with active malignancy.

[1]Not FDA approved for this indication.

[1]Not FDA approved for this indication.

Anti-integrins

Anti-integrin agents affect leukocyte trafficking. α4 Integrins are cell adhesion molecules that control the migration of leukocytes across the vascular endothelium and play a significant role in intestinal inflammation.

Natalizumab (Tysabri) is an antibody to α4β1 integrin, and vedolizumab (Entyvio) is a selective α4β7 integrin inhibitor. Because natalizumab is associated with a rare but often fatal disease called progressive multifocal leukoencephalopathy, its use clinically has been limited since the approval of vedolizumab (Entyvio).

Vedolizumab is gut specific and is approved for induction and maintenance of remission in both CD and UC. It has a favorable safety profile with minimal systemic side effects, minimal risk of systemic infections, and no evidence of risk of development of lymphoproliferative disorders.

Anti–IL-12/23

Ustekinumab (Stelara) binds to the p40 subunit of both interleukin (IL)-12 and IL-23 and is approved for induction and maintenance of remission in both CD and UC. The induction dose is a single infusion followed by injections every 8 weeks. Ustekinumab has been shown in the UNITI and UNIFI trials to be efficacious in both CD and UC with a favorable safety profile, rapid onset of action, improvement in fistulizing disease in CD, and efficacy in patients who had previously failed other treatments. The most frequently reported adverse events are nasopharyngitis and upper respiratory tract infections. More serious infections such as diverticulitis, cellulitis, and pneumonia can occur. Ustekinumab has a lower immunogenicity risk relative to other biologics.

Anti–IL-23

Risankizumab (Skyrizi) targets the p19 subunit of IL-23. It has been shown to be effective in the induction and maintenance of remission in patients with moderate to severe CD. It is also being investigated for use in patients with UC. The initial induction dosing with three infusions is followed by maintenance therapy using an on-body subcutaneous injector that can be administered at home every 8 weeks. The most common adverse events include nasopharyngitis, headache, and arthralgia. Serious infections, including herpes zoster and other opportunistic infections, can occur. There is an association with liver injury, therefore it is important to check liver enzymes before initiation and periodically thereafter.

Biosimilars

Biologic agents are large complex molecules of which exact replicas cannot be made. Biosimilars, such as infliximab-dyyb (Inflectra) and infliximab-abda (Renflexis), are very similar in structure to the original molecule but have varying glycosylation patterns that lead to differences in parts of the molecule that are not clinically active. Switching between reference and biosimilar products has not been shown to be inferior to continuing with the original product.

Small Molecules

Small molecule therapies are given orally; have a simple, well-defined structure; and have a favorable pharmacokinetic profile due to lack of immunogenicity.

JAK Inhibitors

Tofacitinib (Xeljanz) and upadacitinib (Rinvoq) are oral medications for IBD that inhibit the janus kinase (JAK) signaling pathway. Tofacitinib targets JAK1, 2, and 3, whereas upadacitinib is a selective JAK1 inhibitor. Both tofacitinib and upadacitinib can be used for induction and maintenance of remission. Tofacitinib has approval for use in moderate to severe UC, and as of June 2023, upadacitinib has approval for use in both moderate to severe UC and CD. JAK inhibitors appear to have a role in the induction of remission in hospitalized patients with acute severe UC as concomitant therapy with IV steroids for those who are at high risk of failure of steroid therapy, such as patients who have previously failed biologics, recently failed IV steroids, or have failed outpatient steroids of 40 mg daily or higher. These therapies are only approved for use in patients with prior exposure to anti–TNF-α therapies.

Adverse effects of this class include an increase in herpes zoster, TB and other infections, blood clots (pulmonary embolism), elevated creatine phosphokinase level, lymphocytopenia, neutropenia and anemia, and elevated lipid levels. Because of the high risk of zoster infections, it is recommended that all patients receive the recombinant herpes zoster vaccination. CBCs and lipid panels should be monitored for patients on JAK inhibitors. GI perforation has also been reported for tofacitinib.

Sphingosine-1-Phosphate Receptor Modulator

Ozanimod (Zeposia) is an oral sphingosine-1-phosphate receptor modulator that promotes sequestration of lymphocytes within lymph nodes, preventing lymphocyte accumulation in the GI tract. It is an oral agent that has been shown to be effective in moderately to severely active UC for induction and maintenance and is currently being studied in phase III clinical trials for moderate to severe CD[1].

Adverse effects include increased risk of infections, including herpes zoster, lymphopenia, bradycardia, elevated liver enzymes, macular edema, and hypertension. Liver enzymes and CBC should be monitored for patients on ozanimod. Because of the risk of bradycardia, patients require an electrocardiogram before initiation.

Immunomodulators
Thiopurines

Thiopurines consist of azathioprine (Imuran)[1] and 6-mercaptopurine (Purinethol)[1]. Because of delayed onset of action, thiopurines are not recommended for induction of remission; however, they can be used for maintenance of remission for both CD and UC as either monotherapy or as combination therapy with anti–TNF-α. Before initiation of a thiopurine, thiopurine methyltransferase enzyme activity or genotype should be checked. Those with low activity may benefit from a lower dose, whereas those with absent activity should not be started on a thiopurine.

Patients on thiopurines are at increased risk of infections, pancreatitis, nonmelanoma skin cancers, and lymphoma (especially non–Hodgkin lymphoma). Hepatosplenic T-cell lymphoma (HSTCL), which is a rare and aggressive form of lymphoma, has been associated with both monotherapy and biologic combination therapy with anti–TNF-α. Often these cases of HSTCL have occurred in younger men. Thiopurines also have risk of hepatotoxicity and leukopenia. A CBC and liver enzymes should be monitored at least every 3 to 4 months.

Methotrexate

Methotrexate works by interfering with DNA synthesis by inhibiting dihydrofolate reductase, a key enzyme in the purine production pathway, thus leading to decreased inflammation. Studies have shown that intramuscular or subcutaneous methotrexate has been effective in the treatment of patients with CD[1], though data have not shown efficacy in patients with UC[1] as monotherapy. Methotrexate may also be used as adjunctive to biologics to reduce immunogenicity. Methotrexate can cause myelosuppression, hepatotoxicity, and pulmonary fibrosis. It is also a teratogen and should be avoided in women of reproductive age unless used with birth control. It is recommended to discontinue methotrexate at least 3 months before planned pregnancy.

Cyclosporine

Cyclosporine is an inhibitor of calcineurin, which is an enzyme that is required for the activation of T cells. Its use in IBD is limited to use as a salvage therapy to induce remission in hospitalized patients with ASUC[1] that is not responsive to

---

[1] Not FDA approved for this indication.

steroids. It is an alternative agent to infliximab, which can also be used in ASUC. Cyclosporine is solely used as induction therapy when there is a plan to transition to an alternative agent for maintenance therapy, such as azathioprine monotherapy or biologic therapy. Side effects include seizures, nephrotoxicity, neurotoxicity, and infections. Cyclosporine requires close monitoring and should not be used unless administered by an experienced clinician.

Surgical Management

The preferred surgical treatment for UC is total proctocolectomy with ileal pouch–anal anastomosis (IPAA). Around 10% to 20% of patients that have UC will require a colectomy by 20 years of diagnosis. Of patients who undergo IPAA, approximately 50% develop an episode of pouchitis. In CD, about 60% of patients will require surgical intervention for active disease or complications. The most common surgery performed for CD is ileocecal resection with primary anastomosis. Other surgical strategies may include small bowel resection, stricturoplasty, segmental colectomy, and total proctocolectomy with end ileostomy. Most patients who undergo surgery for CD will have a recurrence of inflammation and will require postoperative monitoring and, in high-risk individuals, postoperative treatment to prevent recurrence.

Supplemental Therapies

Nutrition and Diet

Patients with IBD are prone to development of micronutrient deficiencies and malnutrition due to malabsorption or because of surgery. Patients with ileal disease or resection of the ileum are more likely to have fat-soluble vitamin and vitamin B12 deficiencies. In patients with known stricturing disease, a low-fiber and low-residue diet is currently recommended. Many special diets have been evaluated for efficacy in IBD with elemental diets proven efficacious in inducing remission of CD in pediatric patients. To improve symptoms, diet modifications are a helpful adjunct to medical therapy. Patients can work with a nutritionist to evaluate which type of diet is best for their quality of life and symptom pattern.

Pain Management

Many patients with IBD struggle with acute and chronic abdominal pain. Pain in IBD can be difficult to treat, especially if the pain is not related to active inflammation. Disease activity should be assessed when patients have worsening abdominal pain, but other etiologies to consider include visceral hypersensitivity, mechanical obstruction due to stricture, fistulae formation, abdominal infection, or abscess.

Chronic use of nonsteroidal antiinflammatory drugs (NSAIDs) has been thought to increase the risk for active inflammation in IBD, though they appear to be safe when used in short courses. Chronic narcotic use has been associated with worse outcomes in patients with IBD. Their use should be minimized and only for acute pain. For chronic pain, neuromodulators and antispasmodics are beneficial. Psychosocial factors play a large role in the pain pathways. Addressing underlying depression, anxiety, and stressors may help pain control. Medication options to consider for acute pain include acetaminophen, tramadol, opiates, NSAIDs, or antispasmodics. For noninflammatory etiologies of pain, tricyclic antidepressants, gabapentin (Neurontin)[1], pregabalin (Lyrica)[1], selective serotonin reuptake inhibitors, serotonin and norepinephrine reuptake inhibitors, and bupropion (Wellbutrin)[1] can be pharmacological options. The use of cannabis[1] has become an area of research interest and has some evidence for use in pain management for patients with IBD. However, its use is limited by current federal illegal status.

Special Populations

Pregnancy

A history of IBD has not been shown to affect fertility rates except for those who have undergone IPAA. In women who have active disease at conception, pregnancy can have varying effects on disease activity, with some patients worsening and others improving. In women who are in remission when they conceive, their disease tends to remain in remission throughout pregnancy but still requires monitoring. It is recommended that female patients with IBD remain on medical therapy during pregnancy to keep disease in remission. There are very few therapies that should be avoided in patients with IBD who are pregnant; these include metronidazole, methotrexate, tofacitinib, upadacitinib, and ozanimod.

Adverse outcomes in pregnancy for women with well-controlled IBD are similar to women without IBD. Active IBD in pregnancy has been associated with small for gestational age, preterm birth, and spontaneous abortion. Venous thromboembolism is increased in patients with IBD, especially in those with active disease. Vaginal delivery is safe in patients with IBD apart from those with active perianal disease.

Aging IBD Population

About 15% of new diagnoses of IBD occur in patients over the age of 60. Patients in this population tend to have more comorbidities and are more prone to infection, venous thromboembolic events, and malignancy. Functional status, frailty, comorbidities, and treatment goals should also be assessed to determine an optimal treatment plan. All routine vaccines should be administered including influenza, pneumococcal, and herpes zoster, especially in this subset of patients. Other comorbidities should be optimally managed to enhance overall health and nutrition and prevent poor outcomes.

Preventive Care

Preventive health maintenance should be a routine component of IBD care. Patients with IBD are at increased risk of infections and regardless of their immunosuppressive status should receive the influenza vaccine yearly and the pneumococcal vaccinations based on guidance from the Centers for Disease Control and Prevention. Subsets of women on immunosuppressive medication for IBD are at increased risk of cervical cancer and therefore should have regular cervical cancer screening. All men and women under the age of 26 should receive the human papilloma virus vaccine. Patients on anti–TNF-α agents, thiopurines, and JAK inhibitors are at increased risk of skin cancer and should have annual skin exams. Those with more than one-third of their colon involved with IBD and who have had IBD for over 8 years should have periodic screening with colonoscopy every 1 to 5 years. Patients with IBD and PSC should begin annual colonoscopy screening at the time of diagnosis with IBD. DEXA scans should be done in patients who have had steroids for over 3 months to assess for osteopenia or osteoporosis. All patients should be screened for tobacco use and counseled on cessation if currently smoking. Depression and anxiety are common in patients with IBD and should be screened annually. Table 5 provides a summary of preventive care in adult IBD patients.

As the prevalence of IBD rises, it has become increasingly important for primary care physicians to be acquainted with the diagnosis, natural history of disease, medication adverse effects, lifestyle recommendations, reproductive counseling, and healthcare maintenance of affected patients.

---

[1] Not FDA approved for this indication.

TABLE 5 Adult Inflammatory Bowel Disease Health Maintenance

	WHO	WHEN
Screening		
Cervical Pap smear	All women (starting at age 21) on systemic immunosuppression	Every 1–3 years*
Dermatologic skin exam	All on systemic immunosuppression	Annually*
Colonoscopy	All with at least one-third colon involved after 8 years of diagnosis	Every 1–2 years
DEXA scan	Steroid use <3 months or other high-risk patients	At least 2 years apart
Depression	All patients	Annually
Smoking	All patients	Annually
Vaccinations		
Influenza (inactivated)	All patients	Annually
Pneumococcal vaccination, either PCV 20 only, or both PCV 13/15 and then PPSV23, 8 weeks apart	If on or considering immunosuppression	Once
Zoster (recombinant vaccine)	Immunocompromised patients aged ≥19 years and patients age 19–49 years at risk for immunosuppression, as well as all aged >50 years	Once
Hepatitis A series	If nonimmune	Once
Hepatitis B series	If nonimmune	Once
Meningococcal	At risk (college students, military recruits) regardless of immunosuppression	Once
HPV vaccine series	All aged 9–26 years regardless of immunosuppression	Once
Tdap	All adults, regardless of immunosuppression	Every 10 years
Varicella (live)	If nonimmune; however, can only be given >4 weeks before starting advanced therapies	Once
MMR (live)	If nonimmune; however, can only be given >4 weeks before starting advanced therapies	Once

*Based on risk factors and with input from gynecology and dermatology.
DEXA, Dual x-ray absorptiometry; *HPV*, human papillomavirus; *MMR*, measles, mumps, and rubella; *PCV*, pneumococcal conjugate vaccine; *PPSV*, pneumococcal polysaccharide vaccine; *Tdap*, tetanus, diphtheria, and acellular pertussis.

References

Abreu MT, Rowbotham DS, Danese S, et al: Efficacy and safety of maintenance ustekinumab for ulcerative colitis through 3 years: UNIFI long-term extension, *J Crohns Colitis* 16:1222–1234, 2022, https://doi.org/10.1093/ecco-jcc/jjac030.

Ananthakrishnan AN, Nguyen GC, Bernstein CN: AGA clinical practice update on management of inflammatory bowel disease in elderly patients: expert review, *Gastroenterology* 160:445–451, 2021, https://doi.org/10.1053/j.gastro.2020.08.060.

Ananthakrishnan AN, Xavier RJ, Podolsky DK: *Inflammatory bowel diseases: a clinician's guide*, Chichester, West Sussex, UK; Hoboken, NJ, 2017, John Wiley & Sons, Inc.

Cohen NA, Rubin DT: New targets in inflammatory bowel disease therapy: 2021, *Curr Opin Gastroenterol* 37:357–363, 2021, https://doi.org/10.1097/MOG.0000000000000740.

Docherty MJ, Jones RCW, Wallace MS: Managing pain in inflammatory bowel disease, *Gastroenterol Hepatol* 7:592–601, 2011.

Drugs for inflammatory bowel disease, *Med Lett Drugs Ther* 60, 107–114, 2018.

Farraye FA, Melmed GY, Lichtenstein GR, Kane SV: ACG clinical guideline: preventive care in inflammatory bowel disease, *Am J Gastroenterol* 112:241–258, 2017, https://doi.org/10.1038/ajg.2016.537.

Ferrante M, Panaccione R, Baert F, et al: Risankizumab as maintenance therapy for moderately to severely active Crohn's disease: results from the multicentre, randomised, double-blind, placebo-controlled, withdrawal phase 3 FORTIFY maintenance trial, *Lancet* 399:2031–2046, 2022, https://doi.org/10.1016/S0140-6736(22)00466-4.

Feuerstein JD, Ho EY, Shmidt E, et al: AGA clinical practice guidelines on the medical management of moderate to severe luminal and perianal fistulizing Crohn's disease, *Gastroenterology* 160:2496–2508, 2021, https://doi.org/10.1053/j.gastro.2021.04.022.

Feuerstein JD, Isaacs KL, Schneider Y, et al: AGA clinical practice guidelines on the management of moderate to severe ulcerative colitis, *Gastroenterology* 158:1450–1461, 2020, https://doi.org/10.1053/j.gastro.2020.01.006.

Ko CW, Singh S, Feuerstein JD, et al: AGA clinical practice guidelines on the management of mild-to-moderate ulcerative colitis, *Gastroenterology* 156:748–764, 2019, https://doi.org/10.1053/j.gastro.2018.12.009.

Lichtenstein GR, Loftus EV, Isaacs KL, Regueiro MD, Gerson LB, Sands BE: ACG clinical guideline: management of Crohn's disease in adults, *Am J Gastroenterol* 113:481–517, 2018, https://doi.org/10.1038/ajg.2018.27.

Mahadevan U, Robinson C, Bernasko N, et al: Inflammatory bowel disease in pregnancy clinical care pathway: a report from the American gastroenterological association IBD parenthood project working group, *Gastroenterology* 156:1508–1524, 2019, https://doi.org/10.1053/j.gastro.2018.12.022.

Rubin DT, Ananthakrishnan AN, Siegel CA, Sauer BG, Long MD: ACG clinical guideline: ulcerative colitis in adults, *Am J Gastroenterol* 114:384–413, 2019, https://doi.org/10.14309/ajg.0000000000000152.

Sandborn WJ, Feagan BG, D'Haens G, et al: Ozanimod as induction and maintenance therapy for ulcerative colitis, *N Engl J Med* 385:1280–1291, 2021, https://doi.org/10.1056/NEJMoa2033617.

Sandborn WJ, Rebuck R, Wang Y, et al: Five-year efficacy and safety of ustekinumab treatment in Crohn's disease: the IM-UNITI trial, *Clin Gastroenterol Hepatol* 20:578–590.e4, 2022, https://doi.org/10.1016/j.cgh.2021.02.025.

Syal G, Serrano M, Jain A, et al: Health maintenance consensus for adults with inflammatory bowel disease, *Inflamm Bowel Dis* 27:1552–1563, 2021, https://doi.org/10.1093/ibd/izab155.

Turner D, Ricciuto A, Lewis A, et al: STRIDE-II: an update on the selecting therapeutic targets in inflammatory bowel disease (STRIDE) initiative of the international organization for the study of IBD (IOIBD): determining therapeutic goals for treat-to-target strategies in IBD, *Gastroenterology* 160:1570–1583, 2021, https://doi.org/10.1053/j.gastro.2020.12.031.

INTESTINAL PARASITES

Method of
Tarvinder Gilotra, MD

CURRENT DIAGNOSIS

Signs and Symptoms
- Watery diarrhea—Most protozoal infections: *Giardia, Blastocystis, Dientamoeba, Cryptosporidium, Cyclospora, Cystoisospora, Microsporidia*
- Dysentery—Most commonly *Entamoeba histolytica;* less commonly *Balantidium coli, Trichuris trichiura* (whipworm)
- Eosinophilia—Throughout chronic infection: *Strongyloides,* schistosomiasis, *Cystoisospora;* usually only in early infection: *Ascaris,* hookworm, whipworm
- Prolonged or severe diarrhea in HIV infection—Spore-forming protozoal infections: *Cryptosporidium, Cyclospora, Cystoisospora, Microsporidia*
- Visible worms passed in stool—*Ascaris,* Taeniasis, *Diphyllobothrium*

Diagnosis of Parasitic Infections
- Stool antigen assay: *Entamoeba histolytica, Giardia, Cryptosporidium*
- Serology*: *Strongyloides,* schistosomiasis
- Stool microscopy for ova and parasites: All intestinal parasites. Sensitivity is increased with repeat examinations if necessary. Concentration, preservation, and staining improve diagnosis of certain pathogens.
- Molecular tests: Traditional polymerase chain reaction (PCR), both nested and multiplexed, real-time PCR, and newer gene amplification technologies including loop-mediated isothermal amplification (LAMP) and Luminex-based assays are gaining popularity in detecting some parasitic infections, especially in low parasite load specimens.
- Proteomics: Mass spectrometry technique. Surface-enhanced laser desorption/ionization–time-of-flight (SELDI-TOF) mass spectrometry, which is based on matrix-assisted laser desorption/ionization time of-flight (MALDI-TOF) mass spectrometry, has been used to identify biomarkers associated with some parasitic diseases such as African trypanosomiasis, Chagas disease, cysticercosis, and fascioliasis.

Note: Key features of intestinal parasitic infection may overlap with other conditions, including nonparasitic infections, and extraintestinal parasites.

*Optimal method of diagnosis in returned travelers and immigrants from endemic to nonendemic areas. Does not distinguish between active and resolved infections.

Intestinal parasites are a diverse group of pathogens with local and global significance. Immigration, international adoption, travel, and the frequency of HIV/AIDS and other immune-compromising conditions (e.g., malignancy, organ transplantation) have all contributed to a need for ongoing or increased awareness of parasitic infections in the United States. Persons who reside in chronic care facilities, children in daycare, and persons whose sexual practices increase the likelihood of fecal–oral contact are also at risk for acquiring intestinal parasitic infection.

Globally, intestinal parasites are responsible for an enormous burden of disease. Although these pathogens are rarely fatal, ongoing exposure to intestinal parasites among persons in endemic areas exacerbates malnutrition, carries multiple morbidities, and causes stunting of growth and development in children, all of which have far-reaching consequences.

Patients who present with diarrheal illness (especially prolonged or travel-associated), unexplained eosinophilia, or expulsion of worms should be evaluated for intestinal parasites. In such cases, a careful history should focus on the patient's country of origin, detailed travel and recreational activities, dietary habits and new or unusual food exposures, occupation, sexual history, sick contacts, and risks for or known immunodeficiency. Some specialists advocate obtaining a complete blood count with differential to assess eosinophil count in all international adoptees and immigrants from areas where parasitic infections are common. If eosinophilia is present, antibody testing for schistosomiasis and strongyloidiasis—two chronic parasitic infections with potentially serious consequences—should be performed, and appropriate therapy should be administered if infection is discovered. For key features of common intestinal parasitic infections, see the Current Diagnosis box.

Diagnosis of intestinal parasites has improved recently with the advent of quick, simple, and accurate stool antigen tests for some major pathogens, such as *Entamoeba, Giardia,* and *Cryptosporidium* species. However, the fecal examination for ova and parasites is still the mainstay of diagnosis in many cases. Whenever possible, stool specimens should be sent to a laboratory with clinical expertise in parasitology, where wet preparation, concentration, or staining can identify most pathogens. Evaluation of fresh specimens and repeated examinations improve diagnostic sensitivity. Key diagnostic points are summarized in the Current Diagnosis box.

This review focuses on basic understanding, recognition, diagnosis, and treatment of common intestinal parasites in the United States and throughout the world. Within each section, parasites are listed in order of relative clinical significance.

Protozoa: Amoebae, Flagellates, and Ciliates
Entamoeba histolytica
Entamoeba histolytica, the cause of amoebic dysentery and amebic liver abscess, is a worldwide pathogen of major clinical significance. Approximately 10% of the world's population and up to 60% of children in highly endemic areas show serologic evidence of infection, and *E. histolytica* is estimated to cause 100,000 deaths per year globally. In the United States, infection is almost exclusively found among returned travelers, immigrants from endemic areas (especially Mexico and Central and South America), men who have sex with men (MSM), and institutionalized persons. *Entamoeba dispar, Entamoeba bangladeshi,* and *Entamoeba moshkovskii* are morphologically indistinguishable from *E. histolytica.* Although these species are usually considered nonpathologic species, there have been increasing reports of *E. moshkovskii* infections associated with gastrointestinal symptoms in humans in endemic areas. Other *Entamoeba,* including *Entamoeba hartmanni, Entamoeba coli, Entamoeba polecki,* and others, can be individually identified on microscopy. Again, these organisms are of uncertain pathogenicity and generally considered as commensal organisms, however *E. polecki, Dientamoeba fragilis,* and *Iodaamopeba bütschlii* have occasionally been associated with diarrheal illness.

E. histolytica exists in two forms: the hardy cyst (infective form) characterized by four nuclei and the trophozoite (responsible for invasive disease), which has a single nucleus and survives poorly outside the human body. *E. histolytica* infection is acquired by ingestion of cysts in contaminated water or food or by sexual transmission through fecal-oral contact. Acquisition of the parasite can result in asymptomatic infection (most common), diarrheal illness, or extraintestinal infection, the latter most commonly manifesting as amebic liver abscess. An appropriately robust layer of colonic mucin may be protective against symptomatic infection, whereas trophozoite attachment to the intestinal epithelium results in penetration of the organism into the submucosal layer, where extensive tissue destruction can take place in the form of apoptosis and lysis of cells, hence the name *histolytica.*

Symptoms of classic amebic dysentery usually begin insidiously over 1 to 3 weeks after infection. Diarrhea is almost universal and typically consists of numerous small-volume stools that can contain mucus, frank blood, or both. Stools are almost always heme positive if not grossly bloody. Abdominal pain and tenesmus are common; fever is present in approximately 30% of cases.

Some patients have a chronic course characterized by weight loss, intermittent loose stools, and abdominal pain. Rare presentations of amebic dysentery include amebomas, which can mimic malignancy, and perianal ulcerations or fistulae. Severe disease can occur in the form of fulminant colitis or toxic megacolon; the latter almost universally requires colectomy. Young age, pregnancy, corticosteroid use, malignancy, malnutrition, and alcoholism predispose to severe infection. Although persons with HIV infection or AIDS can develop invasive disease, E. histolytica does not appear to be a common opportunistic infection, and infection is curable in this population.

Amebic liver abscess is the most common extraintestinal complication of E. histolytica that traffics to the liver via the portal venous system. Cerebral and ocular amebiasis have also been reported. Amebic liver abscess affects children of both sexes equally, but it is up to 7 to 10 times more common in men, indicating that a hormonal milieu likely plays a role. Amebic liver abscess almost always manifests within 3 to 5 months of initial infection, but it can surface years later. Illness is characterized by fever and right upper quadrant abdominal pain that worsens over several days to weeks. Weight loss, jaundice, and cough from diaphragmatic irritation can also occur. Symptoms of dysentery usually are not present, and diarrhea is reported in less than one-third of cases. Hepatomegaly and point tenderness over the liver is present in about 50% of cases. Rupture of the abscess can occur into the abdomen or pleuropulmonary space, manifesting as acute abdomen or empyema. Laboratory abnormalities include leukocytosis without eosinophilia, transaminitis, elevated alkaline phosphatase, and elevated sedimentation rate. Abscess is usually identified as a well-circumscribed hypoechoic mass on ultrasonography, a low-density mass with enhancing borders on computed tomography (CT), and hypointense on T1 and hyperintense on T2-weighted magnetic resonance imaging (MRI). Chest radiograph often demonstrates elevation of the right hemidiaphragm, and pleural effusion may be present. Radionuclide uptake liver scans can help distinguish amebic abscesses as "cold" compared with pyogenic abscesses that are usually "hot."

Diagnosis of intestinal E. histolytica infection has classically relied on stool microscopy, and this remains the only available method in most parts of the world. At least three stool specimens should be examined to improve sensitivity. Cysts visualized in stool cannot differentiate active disease from colonization, and E. dispar, E. moshkovskii, and E. histolytica species. Presence of trophozoites with ingested red blood cells (hematophagous trophozoites) on stool preparation and/or mobile amebae seen on fresh biopsy material stained with iron hematoxylin and/or Wheatley's trichrome are diagnostic of invasive intestinal amebic disease. Contrary to the common belief, presence of hematophagous trophozoites on stool microscopy is not pathognomonic of E. histolytica, as they can be seen with E. dispar infections as well.

Serology can distinguish between E. histolytica (generates antibodies) and E. dispar (does not generate antibodies) infection with good sensitivity in detecting antibodies within 5 to 7 days of infection. Positive serostatus, however, does not discriminate between acute and past infection, but negative serology is quite sensitive in endemic countries. Indirect hemagglutination serology remains the most sensitive test in non-endemic settings.

Diagnosis and species distinction of Entamoeba infection has improved greatly with the advent of antigen tests, now available as enzyme-linked immunosorbent assays (ELISAs), radioimmunoassays, and immunofluorescent probes. The Techlab ELISA E. histolytica stool antigen test is highly sensitive and specific if used on fresh stool specimens. It becomes positive with onset of symptomatic disease and resolves on treatment of infection.

Parasite DNA/RNA PCR, RT-PCR, multiplex PCR (can detect multiple pathogens), and LAMP fecal probes are highly sensitive and can differentiate Entamoeba species.

Aspirate of liver abscess may be necessary to distinguish from pyogenic liver abscess or when empiric therapy fails. Aspirated specimens consist mainly of necrotic hepatocytes ("anchovy paste"), and trophozoites are only seen in less than 20% of cases. Nested multiplex PCR tests on hepatic aspirates might be useful, although sensitivities range from 75% to 100%. As simultaneous colitis and amebic liver abscess are rare, negative stool microscopy and PCR for E. histolytica does not preclude amebic liver abscess. In a patient at high risk for amebic liver abscess (e.g., young male immigrants), an adequate response to a trial of antimicrobial therapy can help confirm the diagnosis as well.

All patients who have confirmed E. histolytica infection and reside in nonendemic areas should be treated regardless of whether they are symptomatic because invasive disease can develop in the future. Asymptomatic cyst passers may be treated with an intraluminal agent alone, such as paromomycin (Humatin) or diiodohydroxyquin (iodoquinol [Yodoxin]).[2] In the United States, the most readily available effective treatment for patients with amebic colitis or liver abscess is metronidazole (Flagyl). It can be given intravenously for patients who are unable to tolerate oral medications. Recommended management is at least a 10-day course of the metronidazole (or tinidazole [Tindamax]) followed by an intraluminal agent (paromomycin for 7 days, or diiodohydroxyquin[2] for 20 days, or diloxanide furoate[2] for 10 days) for all cases of invasive E. histolytica. See Table 1 for medications and doses.

Giardiasis

Giardia duodenalis, previously known as Giardia lamblia or Giardia intestinalis, is the most commonly identified diarrheal parasitic infection in the United States, with an estimated 100,000 to 2.5 million cases per year. It is globally distributed and found in fresh water throughout mountainous regions of the United States and Canada. The organism is a flagellated aerotolerant anaerobe that exists in cyst and trophozoite form. Cysts can survive for several weeks in cold water. Contaminated food and water are the most common sources of infection, but the organism can also be passed by person-to-person contact. In the United States, giardiasis is primarily diagnosed among international travelers, persons with recreational water exposure, institutionalized persons and children in day care, and persons with anal-oral sexual practices.

Illness can result from ingestion of as few as 10 to 25 cysts, which transform into trophozoites in the small intestine and attach to and damage the small bowel wall. Symptomatic disease begins insidiously over approximately 2 weeks in 25% to 50% of persons who ingest Giardia cysts. Others become asymptomatic cyst passers (5% to 15%) or have no signs of infection (35% to 50%). Hallmarks of infection are watery diarrhea, bloating, flatulence, abdominal pain, and weight loss; less commonly, patients have nausea, vomiting, or low-grade fever. Steatorrhea and malabsorption, particularly secondary to Giardia-induced lactase deficiency, is frequently observed. Chronic Giardia infection should be considered in the differential diagnosis for a long-standing diarrheal illness, especially if there is history of exposure to possibly contaminated water. Patients with common variable immune deficiency, X-linked agammaglobulinemia, and IgA deficiency syndromes are at risk for fulminant and sometimes incurable disease, suggesting a significant role for humoral immunity in control of infection. Patients with HIV infection or AIDS usually have a similar presentation as in non-HIV patients, can remain asymptomatic, and can be typically cured of infection with standard therapy. However, profound immunosuppression can be associated with more severe, atypical, disseminated and refractory disease requiring combination therapy with quinacrine[2] and metronidazole.[1]

Diagnosis of giardiasis is made by examination of fresh or preserved stool or by stool antigen assays. Stool microscopy can be specific but has low sensitivity because of intermittent shedding of Giardia cysts. Trophozoites may be directly visualized in fresh liquid stool; semiformed and preserved stool are likely to contain only cysts and should be stained with polyvinyl alcohol and/or formalin

---

[1] Not FDA approved for this indication.
[2] Not available in the United States.

TABLE 1	Pharmacologic Treatment of Major Protozoan Infections.			
CLINICAL SITUATION	**DRUG**	**ADULT DOSE**	**PEDIATRIC DOSE**	**COMMENTS**
Amebiasis				
(Entamoeba histolytica)				
Asymptomatic	Paromomycin* *or*	25–35 mg/kg/d in 3 doses × 7 d	25–35 mg/kg/d in 3 doses × 7 d	
	Iodoquinol[†,2] *or*	650 mg tid × 20 d	30–40 mg/kg/d (max 2 g) in 3 doses × 20 d	
	Diloxanide furoate‡[,2]	500 mg tid × 10 d	20 mg/kg/d in 3 doses × 10 d	
Mild to moderate intestinal disease	Metronidazole *or*	500–750 mg tid × 7–10 d	35–50 mg/kg/d in 3 doses × 7–10 d	Treatment should be followed by a course of iodoquinol or paromomycin in the dosage used to treat asymptomatic amebiasis.
	Tinidazole[1,§]	2 g once daily × 3 d	≥3 y: 50 mg/kg once daily (max 2 g) × 3 d	
Severe intestinal or extraintestinal disease	Metronidazole *or*	750 mg tid × 7–10 d	35–50 mg/kg/d in 3 doses × 7–10 d	Treatment should be followed by a course of iodoquinol or paromomycin in the dosage used to treat asymptomatic amebiasis.
	Tinidazole[§]	2 g once daily × 5 d	≥3 y: 50 mg/kg once daily (max 2 g) × 5 d	
Balantidiasis				
(Balantidium coli)				
Symptomatic and asymptomatic disease	Recommended: Tetracycline[1,‖]	500 mg qid × 10 d	40 mg/kg/d (max 2 g) in 4 doses × 10 d	
	Alternatives: Metronidazole[1] *or*	500–750 mg PO tid × 5 d	35–50 mg/kg/d in 3 doses × 5 d	
	Iodoquinol[2,†]	650 mg tid × 20 d	30–40 mg/kg/d (max 2 g) in 3 doses × 20 d	
Blastocystis hominis				
Symptomatic disease only				Organism's pathogenicity is uncertain.[¶]
Cryptosporidiosis				
(Cryptosporidium)				
Immunocompetent	Nitazoxanide	500 mg bid × 3 d	1–3 y: 100 mg bid × 3 d 4–11 y: 200 mg bid × 3 d ≥12 y: adult dose	FDA approved as a pediatric oral suspension for treating *Cryptosporidium* in immunocompetent children <12 y and for *Giardia*. It might also be effective for mild to moderate amebiasis. Nitazoxanide is available in 500-mg tabs and an oral suspension; it should be taken with food.
Immunocompromised	No optimal therapy available			All HIV-infected patients with cryptosporidiosis should receive HAART whenever possible. Nitazoxanide,[1] paromomycin,[1] or paromomycin + azithromycin[1] may have a role in decreasing diarrhea in chronic cases of HIV-infection.

CLINICAL SITUATION	DRUG	ADULT DOSE	PEDIATRIC DOSE	COMMENTS
Cyclosporiasis				
(Cyclospora cayetanensis)				
	Recommended: TMP-SMX (Bactrim, Septra)[1]	160 mg TMP, 800 mg SMX (1 DS tab) bid × 7–10 d	5 mg/kg TMP, 25 mg/kg SMX bid × 7–10 d	In immunocompetent patients, usually a self-limiting illness. Immunosuppressed patients might need higher doses, longer duration (TMP-SMX qid × 10 d, followed by bid × 3 wk) and long-term maintenance.
	Alternative: Ciprofloxacin[1]	500 mg PO bid × 7 d	(No recommended pediatric dose)[1]	
Dientamoebiasis				
(Dientamoeba fragilis)				
Symptomatic disease only	Iodoquinol[2,†] *or*	650 mg tid × 20 d	30–40 mg/kg/d (max 2 g) in 3 doses × 20 d	
	Paromomycin[1,*] *or*	25–35 mg/kg/d in 3 doses × 7 d	25–35 mg/kg/d in 3 doses × 7 d	
	Metronidazole[1]	500–750 mg tid × 10 d	35–50 mg/kg/d in 3 doses × 10 d	
Giardiasis				
(Giardia lamblia)				
All symptomatic disease and asymptomatic carriage in nonendemic areas	Recommended: Metronidazole[1] *or*	250 mg tid × 5–7 d	15 mg/kg/d in 3 doses × 5 d	
	Nitazoxanide *or*	500 mg bid × 3 d	1–3 y: 100 mg bid × 3 d 4–11 y: 200 mg bid × 3 d	
	Tinidazole[§]	2 g once	50 mg/kg (max 2 g) once	Treatment should be followed by a course of iodoquinol[2] or paromomycin in the dosage used to treat asymptomatic amebiasis.
	Alternatives: Quinacrine[2,**] *or*	100 mg tid × 5 d	6 mg/kg/d (max 300 mg/d) tid × 5 d	Albendazole,[1] 400 mg daily × 5 d alone or in combination with metronidazole[1] may also be effective. Combination treatment with standard doses of metronidazole and quinacrine[2] × 3 wk is effective for a small number of refractory infections. In one study, nitazoxanide was used successfully in high doses to treat a case of *Giardia* resistant to metronidazole and albendazole.
	Furazolidone[2] *or*	100 mg qid × 7–10 d	6 mg/kg/d in 4 doses × 10 d	
	Paromomycin[1]	25–35 mg/kg/d in 3 doses × 7 d	25–35 mg/kg/d in 3 doses × 7 d	Nonabsorbed luminal agent; may be useful for treating giardiasis in pregnancy

Continued

TABLE 1	Pharmacologic Treatment of Major Protozoan Infections.—cont'd				
CLINICAL SITUATION	**DRUG**	**ADULT DOSE**	**PEDIATRIC DOSE**	**COMMENTS**	
Cystoisosporiasis					
(Cystoisospora belli)					
	TMP-SMX[1]	160 mg TMP, 800 mg SMX bid × 7–10 d	5 mg/kg TMP, 25 mg/kg SMX bid × 7–10 d	In immunocompetent patients, usually a self-limiting illness. Immunosuppressed patients might need higher doses, longer duration (TMP-SMX[1] qid × 10 d, followed by bid × 3 wk) and long-term maintenance. For isosporiasis in sulfonamide-sensitive patients, pyrimethamine[1] 50–75 mg qd in divided doses (*plus* leucovorin[1] 10–25 mg/d) is effective.	
Microsporidiosis					
Enterocytozoon bieneusi					
Intestinal disease	Fumagillin[2+]	20 mg PO TID × 14 d		Oral fumagillin (Sanofi Recherche, Gentilly, France) is effective in treating *E. bieneusi* but is associated with thrombocytopenia and neutropenia. HAART can lead to microbiologic and clinical response in HIV-infected patients with microsporidial diarrhea. Octreotide (Sandostatin)[1] has provided symptomatic relief in some patients with large-volume diarrhea.	
	Albendazole[1]	400 mg PO bid × 21 d	15 mg/kg/d in 2 doses (max 400 mg/dose)		
Encephalitozoon intestinalis					
Diarrheal or disseminated disease	Albendazole[1]	400 mg bid × 21 d	15 mg/kg/d in 2 doses (max 400 mg/dose)		

[1]Not FDA approved for this indication.
[2]Not available in the United States.
*Should be taken with meals.
†Should be taken after meals.
‡The drug is not available commercially, but may be available through compounding pharmacies.
§A nitroimidazole similar to metronidazole, tinidazole is FDA approved and appears to be as effective and better tolerated than metronidazole. It should be taken with food to minimize GI adverse effects. For children and patients unable to take tablets, a pharmacist may crush the tablets and mix them with cherry syrup. The syrup suspension is good for 7 d at room temperature and must be shaken before use. Ornidazole, a similar drug, is also used outside the United States. Dosing recommendations are only available for children ≥3 years of age.
ǁContraindicated in pregnant and breastfeeding women and children <8 years of age.
¶Clinical significance of these organisms is controversial; metronidazole 750 mg tid × 10 d, iodoquinol 650 mg tid × 20 d, or TMP-SMX11 double-strength tab bid × 7 d are effective. Metronidazole resistance may be common. Nitazoxanide is effective in children.
**Should be taken with liquids after a meal.
DS, Double strength; *GI*, gastrointestinal; *HAART*, highly active antiretroviral therapy; *max*, maximum; *tab*, tablet; *TMP-SMX*, trimethoprim-sulfamethoxazole.
Modified from World Health Organization. Drugs for parasitic infections, *Med Lett Drug Ther.* 2010;8(Suppl).

preparation. Antigen detection assays including immunochromographic assays, direct immunofluorescence assays, and ELISAs have higher sensitivity with rapid turnaround time. Many assays are commercially available including the ImmunoCard STAT! Cryptosporidium/Giardia Rapid Assay (Meridian Bioscience, Cincinnati, Ohio) that tests for both pathogens simultaneously. Multiplex nucleic acid amplification tests (NAATs) are frequently used to detect various bacterial, viral, and parasitic pathogens as a workup for infectious diarrhea. Although it is rarely necessary, the diagnosis can sometimes be made on duodenal biopsy.

For details of treatment options, see Table 1. Tinidazole (Tindamax) and nitazoxanide (Alinia) are now the preferred agents for initial treatment of giardiasis. Metronidazole[1] is no longer the first-line therapy because of its adverse effects including

[1]Not FDA approved for this indication.

metallic taste, nausea, gastrointestinal discomfort, and headache. Patients who fail first-line therapy might have a persistent source of infection (contaminated water source, close contact with an infected person), immune deficiency predisposing to difficult eradication, or persistence of cysts. Once possible sources of reinfection have been investigated and eliminated, relapsed infections should either be retreated with a longer course of therapy (21 to 28 days) or treated with a different agent. Quinacrine[2] is reserved for refractory cases but is contraindicated in pregnancy. Paromomycin[1] is an alternative in those with contraindications to other agents such as in pregnancy. Patients who fail more than one course of therapy should undergo immunologic workup.

Prevention of *Giardia* infection, as with other parasitic infections, involves primarily close attention to personal hygiene, hand washing, and avoidance of ingestion of fresh unfiltered water. Boiling water or use of a 0.2- to 1-µm water filter offer optimal protection against *Giardia* and other parasitic pathogens, although such filters still might not protect against *Cryptosporidium*.

Blastocystis

Blastocystis, formerly considered a yeast, has now been related to *E. histolytica* and is thought to be an anaerobic protozoan. The pleomorphic nature and karyotype diversity of this organism, its worldwide distribution, and varying diagnostic techniques have led to challenges in its identification and taxonomy. Although it has a worldwide distribution, its prevalence is higher in developing countries and is most commonly isolated in tropical regions. In temperate regions, *Blastocystis (B. hominis)* is detected at a high rate among MSM. It is a commensal of humans and several other animals. It appears to be transmitted via the fecal-oral route, possibly from waterborne sources. *Blastocystis* was long thought to cause only asymptomatic colonization, but there is some evidence to suggest a role in human disease, although this remains controversial. *Blastocystis* has marked morphologic variability and has been known to exist in at least four forms: vacuolated, amoebalike, granular, and cystic, the latter of which is likely to be the infectious form. Ongoing molecular analysis has identified at least 17 subtypes of *B. hominis* (hence now referred to as *Blastocystis* spp., formerly identified as *Blastocystis hominis*) with varying degrees of pathogenicity in humans.

As suggested previously, the majority of infections appear to be entirely asymptomatic, and number of organisms does not appear to accurately predict severity of illness. Symptoms consist mainly of watery diarrhea, bloating, flatulence, abdominal cramps, urticaria, and fatigue. There are typically no pathologic findings on colonoscopy, and there are no reports of invasive disease. Infection is diagnosed by stool microscopy with use of a trichrome or hematoxylin-stained preserved specimen. Fecal leucocytes are generally not found. PCR techniques have also been developed with excellent sensitivity and are available worldwide. The organism is susceptible in vitro to numerous antimicrobials. Asymptomatic detection does not need treatment. Metronidazole[1] and tinidazole[1] are preferred agents for treating symptomatic disease. Trimethoprim-sulfamethoxazole (TMP-SMX, Bactrim)[1] and paromomycin[1] are alternative agents with good efficacy; details are listed in Table 1.

Dientamoeba fragilis

Dientamoeba fragilis was originally classified as an amoeba, but it is more closely related to the flagellates such as *Trichomonas vaginalis*. It is distributed globally, including in the Western nations; however, it is generally more prevalent in areas of the world with limited public sanitation. *D. fragilis* has only recently been recognized as a clinically significant pathogen, possibly because it is difficult to visualize without specific staining techniques. Illness has commonly been found in travelers and MSM,

but it can affect anyone. Some studies suggested a coinfection of *D. fragilis* with *E. vermicularis* as trophozoites were believed to survive in *E. vermicularis* eggs. However, this association has not been consistently demonstrated.

Similar to most other intestinal parasites, *D. fragilis* is now known to exist in both trophozoite and cystic form, although it was known to only have a trophozoite phase for a long time. Despite its genetic relationship to the flagellates such as *Trichomonas*, *D. fragilis* does not have a flagellum and is immotile. Trophozoites range in size from 7 to 20 µm and can be binucleate. Cysts and precystic forms have recently been identified from human fecal specimens, suggesting a fecal-oral mode of transmission.

Most patients are asymptomatic; however, numerous case reports and small series describe patients with no other organisms identified to cause their symptoms who improve significantly after treatment and documented clearance of *D. fragilis* from their stool. Illness is typically subacute to chronic and is characterized by abdominal pain, watery diarrhea, anorexia, fatigue, and malaise. Unlike most other enteric parasites, *D. fragilis* is associated with marked peripheral eosinophilia and can masquerade as allergic colitis. Diagnosis can be challenging because the trophozoites are fragile and usually missed on direct microscopy. If *D. fragilis* is suspected, stool should be preserved with polyvinyl alcohol and quickly stained with iron–hematoxylin and trichrome. PCR-based assays are very sensitive and being increasing used for diagnosis.

Metronidazole[1] remains the drug of choice and has been efficacious in eradication of *D. fragilis* with a 10-day course. Other nitroimidazoles such as tinidazole[1] (better tolerated than metronidazole), secnidazole (Solosec),[1] and ornidazole[2] have been tested with good efficacy, but data are limited. Paromomycin[1] appears to be efficacious but is only backed up by limited data. Iodoquinol (Yodoxin)[2] has been successfully used very commonly in the past; however, its availability has now declined. See Table 1 for medications and doses.

Balantidium coli

Balantidium coli is the largest protozoan that infects humans and is the only ciliate. Balantidiasis is a relatively rare cause of illness and is found primarily in rural agrarian communities in Southeast Asia, Central and South America, and Papua New Guinea. *B. coli* is highly associated with animal farming, in particular, pigs and primates; humans are incidental hosts. The parasite is transmitted by direct contact with animals or on ingestion of water or food contaminated by animal excrement. Persons with malnutrition or immune deficiency are particularly susceptible to infection.

B. coli invades the intestinal mucosa from the terminal ileum to the rectum. About one-half of infections are asymptomatic; the other half result in a subacute or chronic diarrheal illness with abdominal cramping, nausea, vomiting, weight loss, and occasional low-grade fever. Fewer than 5% of patients present with severe or even fulminant dysentery, and rare cases of colonic penetration with peritonitis, mesenteric lymphadenitis, or hepatic infection have been reported.

Diagnosis is made by visualization of trophozoites in fresh stool specimens or preserved and permanently stained samples. The trophozoite is relatively large (40 to 200 microns) and ciliated; cysts are difficult to distinguish. It displays a distinct spiraling motility that can be seen under low power. On stained sample, visualization of *B. coli*'s characteristic bean-shaped macronucleus and spiral micronucleus can help confirm the diagnosis. All patients should be treated regardless of symptoms. Tetracycline[1] (Sumycin and others) is the therapy of choice; alternative agents include metronidazole,[1] tinidazole[1] and paromomycin[1]; see Table 1 for medications and doses.

---

[2] Not available in the United States.
[1] Not FDA approved for this indication.

[1] Not FDA approved for this indication.
[2] Not available in the United States.

Spore-Forming Protozoa and Microsporidia

Cryptosporidium

Cryptosporidium is an intracellular pathogen with worldwide distribution that has been increasingly reported in the United States and other countries including Nordic countries, Denmark, England, and Scotland in the past decade. Humans are most commonly infected by the recently reclassified *Cryptosporidium hominis* (formerly *C. parvum* genotype 1), but *Cryptosporidium parvum* (previously *C. parvum* genotype 2), primarily a bovine pathogen, also causes human disease. *Cryptosporidium* is known to be an important parasitic cause of diarrhea globally; however, it is more frequently associated with overcrowded and poor sanitary environments. In the United States and other developed countries, the incidence is higher in children than in adults. *Cryptosporidium* infections have been reported as sporadic outbreaks of diarrhea and malnutrition syndrome in children from developing countries and as chronic and severe illness in immunocompromised hosts (especially with HIV infection). It is primarily a waterborne illness and has caused multiple outbreaks in the United States secondary to recreational water exposure (e.g., swimming pools, water parks). The best-known outbreak occurred from contamination of the drinking water supply in Wisconsin in 1993 that was thought to be secondary to runoff from the cattle pastures versus contaminated water from melting ice entering water treatment plants through Lake Michigan. It resulted in 403,000 documented cases of cryptosporidiosis and contributed to the deaths of dozens of persons with advanced HIV infection or malignancy.

Cryptosporidium is a coccidian spore-forming protozoa obligate intracellular parasite with a complex life cycle that matures and reproduces both asexually and sexually entirely within human hosts, thereby enabling infection to occur both from environmental sources and by direct person-to-person contact. Its oocysts, the source of infection on ingestion, are markedly hardy; they can withstand heavy chlorination, survive for months in cold water, and are small enough to occasionally evade even the smallest available water filtration systems. As few as 100 oocysts can cause infection, which results when the parasite penetrates small bowel epithelium and replicates just beneath its surface. Villous flattening and small bowel wall edema are seen on pathologic examination from infected persons.

Cryptosporidium infection can be asymptomatic, or it can manifest as mild diarrhea to severe enteritis with or without biliary involvement. Mild illness is usually self-limiting in 10 to 14 days without treatment in immunocompetent patients, although a substantial percentage of patients report a relapse of symptoms after initial improvement. It can have a protracted course with more severe symptoms in immunocompromised hosts. Fulminant and chronic infection has been frequently reported in those with HIV infection (especially those with CD4 <50), malignancy, and in malnourished children. The incubation period ranges from 3 to 28 days following the ingestion of oocysts and appears to be associated with the number of ingested oocysts. The hallmark of infection is explosive watery diarrhea, which can be so voluminous as to resemble cholera and can cause significant dehydration and electrolyte imbalance. Abdominal discomfort, nausea, vomiting, fever, malaise, and myalgia can also be present, and weight loss is common. Extraintestinal manifestations including biliary tract (cholecystitis, cholangitis, pancreatitis) and lung involvement have been reported, particularly in patients with HIV infection.

Diagnosis of *Cryptosporidium* has improved dramatically in recent years with the advent of antigen tests, which are highly sensitive and specific and can be used on a single sample of fresh stool. The ImmunoCard STAT! Cryptosporidium/Giardia Rapid Assay is useful because it can detect both pathogens. PCR is also available, has more sensitivity than direct microscopy, and can differentiate between various genotypes. When such tests are not available, stools submitted for examination should be fixed in formalin and stained for trophozoites or cysts; availability of multiple stool specimens improves the diagnostic sensitivity. Luminal fluid or biopsy specimens obtained during endoscopy can also reveal the organism.

Infection with *Cryptosporidium* is typically a self-limiting illness in otherwise healthy persons, but symptoms can be improved and the course shortened with the antiparasitic nitazoxanide. If nitazoxanide is not available or tolerated, paromomycin can be used, although it is not specifically indicated for this infection. *Cryptosporidium* remains an extremely challenging and potentially devastating infection in immunocompromised patients, especially those with HIV and a low CD4 count (counts <200 increase risk of severe illness, and counts <50 markedly increase risk). Although anticryptosporidial therapies in this population have shown very limited efficacy, restoration of immune function with highly active antiretroviral therapy (HAART) often effects cure. Limited data suggest that a trial of nitazoxanide may be reasonable in this circumstance as well. Appropriate supportive measures are also crucial in all patients with *Cryptosporidium*, including fluid and electrolyte replacement; avoiding lactose products is likely to be beneficial during the first 2 weeks after infection as the brush border regenerates. Appropriate treatment doses for nitazoxanide (Alinia) are listed in Table 1.

Prevention of *Cryptosporidium* infection requires a highly developed public water purification system including flocculation, sedimentation, and filtration. Use of 0.2- to 1-μm personal water filters for campers and hikers greatly reduces but does not eliminate the risk of infection, whereas boiling water before drinking kills oocysts. Close attention to hygiene and avoidance of fecal-oral contact is the mainstay of prevention in the settings of institutional and community outbreaks. Patients should avoid swimming in public pools for 2 weeks after diarrhea resolution.

Cyclospora

Cyclospora cayetanensis is a coccidian with a structure similar to that of *Cryptosporidium*. *C. cayetanensis* is distributed worldwide, most commonly in the tropics and subtropics including Latin America (Guatemala, Peru, Mexico), the Indian subcontinent, and Southeast Asia. Outbreaks in the United States have been associated with import of contaminated produce such as raspberries and snow peas from Guatemala in 1996 and 2004, respectively. Similar outbreaks were attributed to contaminated lettuce and basil from Peru and to cilantro and prepackaged salad from Mexico. It has also become increasingly recognized as a cause of infectious diarrhea in return travelers. Unlike *Cryptosporidium*, *C. cayetanensis* oocysts are shed in the stool as unsporulated oocysts (uninfected) and require a few days of humid environmental conditions to become sporulated infective oocysts, therefore close person-to-person contact as a means of acquiring the infection is unlikely.

All persons are susceptible to infection, but those with HIV are at risk for more severe and prolonged disease, as seen with cryptosporidiosis and isosporiasis. Symptomatic disease appears to be most common in adults who do not have previous exposure to *Cyclospora*, such as travelers or persons who have relocated to endemic areas. Illness begins about 1 week after ingestion of sporulated oocysts and is characterized by watery diarrhea, abdominal cramping, bloating, anorexia, and weight loss. Low-grade fever can occur; marked fatigue is common and can last for weeks or even months, and untreated infections can relapse after apparent resolution. Biliary involvement can occur in patients with HIV coinfection, as with cryptosporidiosis. Cyclosporiasis, similar to infection with other coccidians, causes damage to the small bowel epithelium, with resultant crypt flattening, edema, and inflammatory infiltrate. Lactose deficiency can remain for months after initial infection.

Diagnosis is made by stool examination. As with diagnosis of other parasitic infections, multiple stool specimens improve sensitivity. In the case of *Cyclospora*, concentration of the stool specimen also increases yield. If cyclosporiasis is suspected, specific testing should be requested because the organism exhibits unique properties. Similar to *Cryptosporidium*, organisms can be stained and visualized with Kinyoun acid-fast stain, but they are about two times the size of *Cryptosporidium* (8 to 10 μm in diameter). The cell wall of their oocysts also maintains its autofluorescence under ultraviolet microscopy, and *Cryptosporidium* does not. The commonly used BioFire FilmArray multiplex antigen detection test (BioFire Diagnostics, Salt Lake City, UT) includes *C. cayetanensis.* Various conventional and real-time PCR techniques have been developed with good sensitivity. No serologic tests are available yet.

Cyclosporiasis is best treated with trimethoprim-sulfamethoxazole (Bactrim)[1]; nitazoxanide and ciprofloxacin may be effective for patients who have a sulfa allergy. Patients with HIV infection can require longer courses of treatment or chronic suppressive therapy; appropriate antiretroviral therapy is also important in the treatment of severe or relapsing infections. See Table 1 for details.

Cystoisospora

Cystoisospora belli, formerly *Isospora belli,* is a large coccidian distributed worldwide; however, infections are more frequent in tropical and subtropical areas. In the United States, infections are largely identified in travelers from endemic areas and foreign-born HIV-positive patients. This is the most common parasitic cause of diarrhea in HIV-infected patients in India. Similar to *Cyclospora,* it requires a period of maturation (sporulation) outside the human body and therefore cannot be spread directly from person to person.

It appears to cause largely asymptomatic or mild infection in tropical areas to which it is endemic; the exception is among patients coinfected with HIV and particularly those with AIDS, in whom it is a very common cause of chronic diarrhea in the Caribbean and Central America. Currently in wealthy countries it is found primarily in travelers returning from endemic areas. Illness is typically mild and self-limiting, consisting primarily of watery diarrhea. However, some immunocompetent persons can develop a chronic spruelike syndrome with malabsorption, and those with HIV infection or AIDS often have severe and prolonged diarrhea. *Cystoisospora* can invade to the lamina propria and can cause eosinophilia, which is different from other protozoan infections.

Diagnosis is made by observation of cysts in stool. As with *Cyclospora* and *Cryptosporidia,* they are usually not detected on routine stool ova and parasite examinations, hence acid-fast staining or ultraviolet microscopy techniques should be requested for high suspicion. Stool may also contain Charcot-Leiden crystals. No antigen detection tests are yet available. PCR tests have been developed; however, they are not widely available.

Illness is usually self-limiting in immunocompetent hosts, hence antimicrobial therapy is only indicated when symptoms do not resolve spontaneously in 5 to 7 days. Symptomatic HIV-positive and other immunocompromised patients should always be treated. Trimethoprim-sulfamethoxazole (Bactrim)[1] is the treatment of choice. Ciprofloxacin (Cipro)[1] or pyrimethamine (Daraprim)[1] may be used in cases of sulfa allergy. See Table 1 for medications and doses.

Microsporidia

Microsporidia are eukaryotic organisms that have been recently reclassified as fungi based on molecular genotyping. They are distributed globally, and more than 100 genera have been identified, seven of which contain species known to be pathogenic in humans: *Encephalitozoon, Enterocytozoon, Trachipleistophora, Pleistophora, Nosema, Vittaforma,* and *Microsporidium.* These pathogens cause a wide variety of systemic and focal illness throughout the world.

Many immunocompetent patients in wealthy nations exhibit positive serology for certain types of microsporidial infections without a history of disease or travel. Microsporidia are most commonly associated with systemic infection in immunosuppressed persons, particularly those with HIV and a CD4 count of less than 100 or patients with organ transplants. The mode of transmission is not entirely clear, but the pathogen likely is spread both from water sources and possibly from close household contact.

Encephalitozoon intestinalis and *Enterocytozoon bieneusi* are responsible for intestinal microsporidial infections. *E. bieneusi* has been associated with self-limiting diarrheal illness; *E. intestinalis* is commonly found in stool specimens throughout the developing world, but its pathogenicity is often not certain. Symptomatic infections, most often in patients coinfected with HIV, typically include a gradual onset of watery diarrhea, which may be worse in the morning and after oral intake. Significant volume and electrolyte depletion can occur, as well as fatigue, anorexia, weight loss, and malabsorption. *E. intestinalis* can disseminate and cause acute abdomen with peritonitis, cholangitis, nephritis, and keratoconjunctivitis, and *E. bieneusi* infection can result in cholangitis and nephritis as well as rhinitis, bronchitis, and wheezing. Other microsporidia are implicated in disseminated disease with a wide variety of extraintestinal manifestations including ocular, pulmonary, cerebral, renal, and muscular, both in previously healthy and immunosuppressed hosts.

Diagnosis of microsporidiosis is attained by visualization of spores in stool or in tissue specimens. As suggested by their name, microsporidial spores are much smaller than those produced by spore-forming protozoal infections; most are approximately 1 μm in length and can easily be confused with bacteria or debris on slides. Special staining techniques have been described, but electron microscopy is required for species identification. PCR assays have been increasingly used for highly sensitive identification and speciation. Indirect immunofluorescence assays (IFA) are also available for *Encephalitozoon* spp. and *E. bieneusi.* Albendazole (Albenza)[1] is the treatment of choice for *E. intestinalis.* Treatment of *E. bieneusi* is more challenging. Although some response to albendazole has been reported, oral fumagillin[2] may have more efficacy. Unfortunately, it is not currently commercially available in the United States. Use of appropriate antiretroviral therapy is perhaps the most important treatment for patients with HIV infection or AIDS and chronic microsporidial infections. See Table 1 for medications and doses.

Helminths
Nematodes

Nematodes (roundworms) are cylindrical nonsegmented organisms that are found throughout the world both as free-living species and as human and animal pathogens. Nematodes are the most common type of human parasitic infestation, found in approximately one-fourth of the world's population; often, susceptible hosts carry multiple different pathogenic nematodes. There are at least 60 species that have been shown to infect humans and 10 times that many that cause disease in other animals, but a few pathogens account for the bulk of human infections, in particular *Ascaris,* hookworm, and whipworm. These three organisms all require a period of maturation outside the human body—typically in warm, moist soil—underscoring the fact that repeated contact with fecally contaminated soil or food and water is necessary to sustain the cycle of infestation. *Strongyloides* and *Enterobius* are unique in that they can both complete their life cycle on or within human hosts and therefore can cause chronic infection and be transmitted directly by close person-to-person contact where there is the possibility of fecal-oral contamination.

Ascaris

Ascaris lumbricoides, the most common human helminthic infection, is estimated to affect 20% to 25% of the world's population. Up to 80% of community members are infected in heavily endemic areas, namely in Africa, Asia, and Central and South America. Cases of *Ascaris* infestation are also seen in rural areas in the southeastern United States. *A. lumbricoides* are white to pinkish worms that range from 10 to 40 cm in length. Transmission

[1]Not FDA approved for this indication.

[1]Not FDA approved for this indication.
[2]Not available in the United States.

in humans occurs most commonly by ingestion of infectious human or pig eggs that are oval white bodies with an adherent mucopolysaccharide capsule that clings to multiple surfaces and aids in transmissibility of the parasite. Eggs are also remarkably durable, capable of surviving up to 6 years in moist soil, and able to weather brief droughts and periods of freezing. Another means of transmission is by ingesting uncooked pig or chicken liver containing *Ascaris suum* larvae.

Fecal contamination of water, food, and environmental surfaces such as doorknobs and countertops provides the means of transmission for *Ascaris,* and recurrent infection occurs as long as living conditions that predispose people to infection remain unchanged. Lack of adequate public sanitation, use of human feces as fertilizer (night soil), and frequent contact with soil or shared contaminated surfaces among close household members are risk factors for infection. Persons who move to environments with improved sanitation typically lose their infection within 2 years as all of the adult worms die. Eggs excreted by an infected person must mature outside the human body for approximately 2 weeks. On ingestion by a susceptible host, mature eggs hatch in the small intestine and release larvae, which penetrate the intestinal wall and travel through the venous circulation to the lungs, where they are coughed up and swallowed. They then undergo maturation into adult worms in the intestine and produce eggs by 2 to 3 months after initial infection. The eggs are excreted in the feces and mature outside the body to continue the cycle.

Most persons with *Ascaris* infection are asymptomatic. Approximately 15% of infected people have morbidity, which is associated with young age, large burden of worms, coinfection with other intestinal parasites, and genetic predisposition. In children, infection contributes to malabsorption of protein, fat, and vitamins A and C, and treatment of heavily infected children can improve their nutritional status. *Ascaris* infection can also cause intestinal, pancreatic, or biliary obstruction as a result of worm mass or worm migration. Despite the low incidence of obstructive complications per infected person, the *Ascaris*-related acute abdomen is a significant problem on a global level given the enormous number of people infected. Some patients with intestinal *Ascaris* infection report vague abdominal complaints, such as abdominal discomfort, nausea, vomiting, or diarrhea, but these are relatively rare. Pulmonary migration of a large quantity of worms can produce Loeffler syndrome, or eosinophilic pneumonitis.

Diagnosis is easily attained with standard saline stool preparation, and large numbers of eggs are typically seen. Larvae or worms can also sometimes be seen in sputum or stool samples. In cases of intestinal obstruction, worms may be visualized on upper gastrointestinal series, CT, and even ultrasonography. Multiplex PCR assays are highly sensitive at identification and quantification but are currently not routinely used. Peripheral eosinophilia with *Ascaris* infection is found only during the larval migratory phase, but not at all times. Chronic eosinophilia in an at-risk person suggests another parasitic infection, often *Strongyloides*. Sputum eosinophilia and Charcot-Leyden crystals can be seen, although this is common with many parasitic eosinophilic pulmonary infections.

All persons documented to carry *Ascaris* who have migrated to nonendemic areas should be treated to prevent complications in the future; in endemic areas, adults need only be treated if they are symptomatic. Children have been shown to benefit from intermittent anthelminthic therapy in heavily affected areas of the world. For patients with intestinal obstruction, bowel rest and intravenous hydration are usually sufficient to relieve the obstruction, at which time anthelmintic therapy can be administered. In such cases, gastroenterology consultation should be obtained. In rare cases, surgical intervention is required. Treatment of pulmonary infection is controversial; however, most experts recommend steroid therapy for severe infections followed 2 to 3 weeks later (at the time full-grown worms will have migrated to the intestine) by administration of anthelmintic therapy. *Strongyloides* infection should be ruled out before corticosteroid administration as the latter can induce *Strongyloides* hyperinfection syndrome. The benzimidazoles (mebendazole

[Emverm, Vermox], albendazole [Albenza],[1] levamisole[2]) exhibit excellent activity against *Ascaris*. Ivermectin (Stromectol)[1] and nitazoxanide (Alinia)[1] are suggested as reasonable alternatives. Doses and other options are listed in Table 2. Pregnant women should be treated with pyrantel pamoate (Pin-Away) as albendazole and mebendazole carry a pregnancy class B label. Pyrantel pamoate is a depolarizing neuromuscular blocking agent that causes paralysis in helminths, which prevents them from invading the intestinal wall, eventually resulting in their natural expulsion from the intestinal lumen. Because no consistent teratogenic effects have been demonstrated with albendazole use in late pregnancy, the World Health Organization (WHO) has allowed the use of albendazole to treat mass infections in the second and third trimesters.

Sanitary conditions that allow for proper management of human feces are crucial in control and prevention of *Ascaris* infection; boiling water kills the eggs.

Whipworm (Trichuris)

Trichuris trichiura has become recognized in recent years as a worldwide pathogen and is frequently found as a coinfection with *A. lumbricoides* as they share a similar scope and environmental conditions. Almost 90% of individuals from endemic regions are infected. Sanitary conditions that predispose to ingestion of food and water contaminated with human feces place people at risk for infection.

The adult organism is a small worm about 4 cm in length with a unique whiplike structure that allows its thin tail to become embedded in colonic crypts. Infection is acquired by ingesting *Trichuris* eggs that have undergone embryonation in the soil for 2 to 4 weeks after excretion from a previous host. Larvae emerge from eggs in the intestine and migrate into crypts, where they begin to mature. Egg production begins approximately 3 months later.

Most persons with whipworm carry few worms (approximately 20) and are asymptomatic. As with many other intestinal parasites, children are at greater risk for symptomatic infection, which can cause failure to thrive, anemia, clubbing, inflammatory colitis, and rectal prolapse. Adults with a high worm burden can also experience inflammatory colitis characterized by frequent—often bloody—diarrhea and tenesmus. Infection has been shown to result in production of tumor necrosis factor (TNF)-α by lamina propria cells in the colon, which can contribute to poor appetite and wasting that can be seen with significant infection.

Diagnosis is made by standard stool microscopy without a need to concentrate stool because large numbers of eggs are excreted. Whipworm eggs have a characteristic barrel shape with mucous (hyaline) plugs at either end. Worms can also be seen on colonoscopy, or they can be visualized grossly in cases of rectal prolapse. PCR tests are now available with improved but variable sensitivity for species identification. Peripheral eosinophilia may be seen.

Treatment of symptomatic infections can be accomplished with mebendazole (Emverm, Vermox), albendazole (Albenza),[1] or ivermectin (Stromectol)[1]; see Table 2 for details.

Hookworm

Like other helminthic infections, hookworm affects a substantial portion of the world's population, particularly in rural subtropical and tropical communities where human feces is used as a component of fertilizer. Infection results primarily from parasite penetration into the skin; therefore persons with an agrarian lifestyle and significant soil contact are at greatest risk.

Two species are responsible for the majority of human hookworm: *Necator americanus* and *Ancylostoma duodenale*. *N. americanus* is a smaller and less aggressive pathogen with a longer life span than *A duodenale*. Both parasites are found in warm climates throughout the world; *A. duodenale* exists in smaller pockets in Mediterranean

---

[1] Not FDA approved for this indication.
[2] Not available in the United States.

TABLE 2 Pharmacologic Treatment of Nematode, Trematode, and Cestode Infections

CLINICAL SITUATION	DRUG	ADULT DOSE	PEDIATRIC DOSE	COMMENTS
Anisakiasis				
(Anisakis spp., *Pseudoterranova decipiens)*				
	No recommended medical therapy	—	—	Successful treatment of a patient with anisakiasis with albendazole[1] has been reported.
	Surgical or endoscopic removal of worm			
Ascariasis				
(Ascaris lumbricoides)				
	Albendazole (Albenza)[1,*] *or*	400 mg once	400 mg PO once	
	Mebendazole[†] (Vermox) *or*	100 mg bid × 3 d or 500 mg once	100 mg bid × 3 d or 500 mg once	
	Ivermectin[1,†] (Stromectol)	150–200 µg/kg once	150–200 µg/kg once	In heavy infection, therapy may be given for 3 d.
Enterobiasis				
(Enterobius vermicularis)				
	Mebendazole[†] *or*	100 mg once, repeat in 2 wk	100 mg once, repeat in 2 wk	Because all family members are usually infected, treatment of the entire household is recommended.
	Albendazole[1,*] *or*	400 mg once, repeat in 2 wk	400 mg once, repeat in 2 wk	
	Pyrantel pamoate[‡]	11 mg/kg base (max 1 g) once; repeat in 2 wk	11 mg/kg base (max 1 g) once; repeat in 2 wk	
Hookworm				
(Ancylostoma duodenale, Necator americanus)				
	Albendazole[1,*] *or*	400 mg once	400 mg once	
	Mebendazole *or*	100 mg bid × 3 d or 500 mg once	100 mg bid × 3 d or 500 mg once	
	Pyrantel pamoate[‡,1]	11 mg/kg (max 1 g) × 3 d	11 mg/kg (max 1 g) × 3 d	
Schistosomiasis				
Schistosoma haematobium, Schistosoma mansoni	Praziquantel[§] *or*	40 mg/kg/d in 2 doses × 1 d	40 mg/kg/d in 2 doses × 1 d	
S. mansoni only	Oxamniquine[∥,2]	15 mg/kg once	20 mg/kg/d in 2 doses × 1 d	Praziquantel is first line, but oxamniquine may be effective in some patients in whom praziquantel is less effective.
				Contraindicated in pregnancy
Schistosoma japonicum, Schistosoma mekongi	Praziquantel[§]	60 mg/kg/d in 2 or 3 doses × 1 d	60 mg/kg/d in 3 doses × 1 d	
Strongyloidiasis				
Strongyloides stercoralis	Recommended: Ivermectin[†]	200 µg/kg/d × 2 d	200 µg/kg/d × 2 d	In immunocompromised patients or in patients with disseminated disease, it may be necessary to prolong or repeat therapy or use other agents.

Continued

TABLE 2 Pharmacologic Treatment of Nematode, Trematode, and Cestode Infections—cont'd

CLINICAL SITUATION	DRUG	ADULT DOSE	PEDIATRIC DOSE	COMMENTS
				Veterinary parenteral and enema formulations of ivermectin are used in severely ill patients who are unable to take oral medications.
	Alternative: Albendazole[1],*	400 mg bid × 7 d	400 mg bid × 7 d	
Tapeworm				
(*Diphyllobothrium latum* [fish], *Taenia saginata* [beef], *Taenia solium* [pork], *Dipylidium caninum* [dog])				
	Praziquantel[1] or	5–10 mg/kg PO once	5–10 mg/kg PO once	
	Niclosamide[¶,2]	2 g once	50 mg/kg once	Available in the United States only from the manufacturer
Trichuriasis				
(*Trichuris trichiura*)				
	Recommended: Mebendazole	100 mg bid × 3 d or 500 mg once	100 mg bid × 3 d or 500 mg once	
	Alternatives: Albendazole[1],* or	400 mg daily × 3 d	400 mg daily × 3 d	
	Ivermectin[†,1]	200 μg/kg daily × 3 d	200 μg/kg daily × 3 d	

[1]Not FDA approved for this indication.
[2]Not available in the United States.
*Should be taken with a fatty meal.
[†]Safety of ivermectin in young children (<15 kg) and pregnant women is not yet established. Ivermectin should be taken on an empty stomach with water.
[‡]Limited availability; can be mixed with juice or water to improve palatability.
[§]Should be taken with liquids during a meal.
[‖]Limited or no availability in the United States.
[¶]Available in the United States only from the manufacturer. Must be chewed or crushed thoroughly and swallowed with a small amount of water. Limited or no availability in the United States.
Modified from World Health Organization. Drugs for parasitic infections, *Med Lett Drug Ther.* 2010;8(Suppl).

the tropics in the Americas, Asia, and Africa. *Ancylostoma ceylanicum*, a hookworm of dogs and cats, has been identified as one of the human zoonotic infections in Southeast Asia, tropical Australia, and the Melanesian Pacific Islands. *Ancylostoma braziliense*, a canine intestinal pathogen, causes cutaneous larval migrans in humans because the pathogen cannot penetrate the human dermis.

Hookworms are small helminths, between 0.5 and 1 cm in length. Infection results from larval penetration of the skin on contact with contaminated soil. An intensely pruritic, erythematous, papulovesicular rash called *ground itch* can develop at the site of entry. Parasites then enter the venous or lymphatic circulation and travel to the lungs, at which point an urticarial rash with cough can develop. The larvae are swallowed and migrate to the small intestine, where they attach to the bowel wall with teeth or biting plates and take a continuous blood meal by sucking with strong esophageal muscles. As the larvae lodge in the small intestine, peripheral eosinophilia peaks, and gastrointestinal discomfort with or without diarrhea can result. Large oral ingestion of *A. duodenale* can cause Wakana syndrome, characterized by cough, shortness of breath, nausea, vomiting, and eosinophilia. The most important clinical manifestation of hookworm infection is iron-deficiency anemia, which can be mild or severe and may be accompanied by malabsorption of protein in hosts with heavy burden of disease. Infants and pregnant women can become extremely ill or even die as a result of the anemia.

Hookworm may be difficult to diagnose because light infections often do not produce enough eggs to be readily seen on stool examination; stool should therefore be concentrated if infection is suspected. Eggs do not appear in stool until approximately 2 months after dermal penetration of *N. americanus* and up to 38 weeks from cutaneous entry of *A. duodenale*, hence patients with pulmonary complaints will

higher sensitivity than direct microscopy; however, these are not as widely available yet.

Hookworm infection can be eradicated with benzimidazole anthelmintics; see Table 2 for details. Prevention of hookworm infection, as with other parasites, lies in improved sanitary conditions; wearing shoes is especially important because the majority of infections are acquired through the skin. Mass anthelmintic treatment campaigns have shown some efficacy in reducing disease in children; however, reinfection and concern for development of resistance continue to present significant challenges. Candidate vaccines are currently under investigation.

Toxocara

Human infection is most commonly from the dog ascarid, *Toxocara canis*, and rarely from the cat ascarid, *Toxocara cati*. Humans are infected by embryonated eggs shed by a definitive host (dogs, cats) in contaminated soil or food, and direct contact with a definitive host is usually not a classical mode of transmission. Eggs then hatch into larvae that penetrate the intestinal wall to enter the circulation and embed in various tissues, leading to both visceral larva migrans (VLM), which affects the lungs, liver, heart, muscle, and brain, and ocular larva migrans, which affects the eyes. VLM usually presents as hepatitis (nodular lesions) and pneumonitis (typically with bilateral peribronchial infiltration). Pericarditis, myocarditis, Loeffler endocarditis, heart failure, cardiac tamponade, eosinophilic meningo-encephalitis, cerebral vasculitis, and myelitis have been rarely reported. Ocular larva migrans (OLM) results from a granulomatous inflammatory response to embedded larva that typically presents as a whitish elevated granuloma but red eye from scleritis or uveitis.

Visual impairment leading to blindness from retinal detachment are more serious complications.

ELISA immunoglobulin G (IgG) serology in the appropriate clinical setting is the most commonly used diagnostic modality but cannot differentiate active from past infections. Sensitivity of ELISA for OLM is lower than that for VLM. PCR testing is commercially not available yet. Definite diagnosis is established with biopsy that is rarely indicated.

The treatment of choice is albendazole (Albenza),[1] which is preferred over mebendazole (Emverm, Vermox),[1] especially in neurologic disease and OLM because the latter does not cross the blood-brain barrier. Antiinflammatory corticosteroids are used as adjunctive therapy for cardiac, neurologic, and severe vision-threatening illness.

Strongyloides

Strongyloides stercoralis is a global pathogen that is estimated to affect as many as 100 million people, mostly in tropical regions of the world. In recent years, it has become more commonly recognized in the United States among immigrants as a cause of chronic eosinophilia as well as symptomatic infection.

Strongyloides infection results when filariform larvae dwelling in fecally contaminated soil penetrate the skin or mucous membranes of a susceptible host. Larvae move to the lungs and subsequently to the trachea, where they are coughed up and swallowed. Females, about 2 cm in length, lodge in the lamina propria of the duodenum and proximal jejunum, where they begin to oviposit. Rhabditiform larvae (noninfectious form) emerge from these eggs and either transform into infectious filariform larvae (infectious form) that can repenetrate the intestinal wall (autoinfection; unique to *S. stercoralis* among other helminths) or are passed into the feces, at which point they can begin a free-living cycle and reproduce sexually or can molt directly into an infectious form ready to enter a subsequent susceptible host.

Persons infected with *Strongyloides* are typically asymptomatic. Those who have symptoms might report abdominal discomfort, diarrhea alternating with constipation, or, rarely, blood-tinged stool. Severe intestinal infections can occur and are manifest by chronic watery or mucous diarrhea. In such cases, colonoscopy reveals excessive bowel wall thickening and copious secretions, or edema (catarrhal enteritis or edematous enteritis). Parasite migration through the dermis can manifest as pathognomonic serpiginous, erythematous, and pruritic patches along the buttocks, perineum, and thighs, known as *larvae currens ("running" larvae)*.

Strongyloides appear to attain a balanced state in their host, with similar numbers of adult worms throughout the many years of infection. During periods of host immunocompromise, particularly in patients taking corticosteroids, *Strongyloides* can enter into a state of rapid autoinfection and rampant reproduction called *hyperinfection syndrome,* which results in devastating illness. Persons with HIV infection do not seem to be at particular risk for symptomatic disease or hyperinfection, but hyperinfection has been linked to human T-lymphotropic virus type 1 (HTLV-1) infection. *Strongyloides* has also caused hyperinfection in organ transplant patients whose donor had been infected asymptomatically with the parasite. Although it has long been thought that steroid-induced immune compromise was the major trigger for hyperinfection, growing evidence suggests that steroids themselves may be the culprit by directly inducing the accelerated life cycle in the parasite.

The hyperinfection syndrome is characterized by systemic illness with fever, cough, hypoxia, patchy or diffuse pulmonary infiltrates with alveolar microhemorrhages, and dermatitis; it can include myocarditis, hepatitis, splenic abscess, meningitis and cerebral abscess, and endocrine organ involvement. Larvae migrating out of the intestines can drag bacteria with them, resulting in gram-negative or polymicrobial sepsis. The prognosis of *Strongyloides* hyperinfection syndrome is grave, even with highly effective anthelmintic treatment given the diffuse nature of this disease. However, earlier recognition and intensive supportive care result in cure.

Diagnosis of uncomplicated *Strongyloides* infection in endemic areas can be challenging because few larvae are passed in stool, and numerous examinations may be necessary to detect them. ELISA IgG serologies to filariform larvae are highly sensitive, but positive results cannot distinguish between active and past infections. Moreover, serologies can be falsely negative in immunocompromised hosts. It is, however, the test of choice for persons who have migrated to nonendemic areas, and all persons in this setting should be treated. Ivermectin (Stromectol) is the treatment of choice; albendazole (Albenza)[1] has some activity again *S. stercoralis* and can be tried as an alternative; see Table 2 for medications and doses. During the first days of treatment, patients can experience intense dermal pruritus as parasites die. Eosinophilia and positive ELISA results can persist for months, even after effective therapy.

Enterobius

Human pinworm infection, caused by the threadlike nematode *Enterobius vermicularis*, is found throughout the world and continues to be diagnosed commonly in the United States, especially in children 5 to 10 years of age. It is the most common helminthic infection in the United States and Europe. Its persistence is likely related to the fact that pinworm does not require a period of maturation outside the human body, and autoinfection or transmission by very close contact sustains the parasite within communities. *E. vermicularis* is at maximum 1 cm long with a tapered tail, and it dwells in the cecum, appendix, and adjacent colon. At night, female worms travel to the anus and lay small (25 to 50 μm), double-walled oval eggs in the perianal skin. Within 6 hours, the eggs embryonate within their capsule and are infectious. In scratching the perianal area and subsequently bringing his or her hand to the mouth, the host ingests the embryos, which then hatch in the bowel about 2 months later and continue the cycle of infection. Embryonated eggs can also attach to bedclothes, thereby placing other household members with close contact at risk for infection. In family groups, infection is associated with close living quarters, poor hand washing, and infrequent washing of clothes and sheets. It can also be prevalent among institutionalized persons.

Infection is often asymptomatic, but it can cause perianal itching, which helps facilitate persistent infection by encouraging frequent touching of the perianal area. Rarely, worms migrate into ectopic foci and produce painful genitourinary tract disease with granulomatous inflammation; pinworm infection rarely results in pain that mimics acute appendicitis.

Pinworm infestation is best diagnosed by the classic Scotch tape test, which involves placing and immediately removing a piece of sticky tape firmly across the perianal area early in the morning when the eggs have been deposited. The tape can then be brought into a physician's office or laboratory, where it is placed sticky-side down for microscopic examination to detect the eggs. Sensitivity can be increased by examining at least three specimens. Eggs are small (25 × 50 microns) with a characteristic "bean-shaped" appearance. It is also sometimes possible to see the white small female worms directly on the perianal region, although they are so small (8 to 13 mm in length) that they may easily be mistaken for residual bits of toilet paper. Although *E. vermicularis* is susceptible to standard albendazole[1] or mebendazole (see Table 2), pyrantel pamoate (Pin-Away, OTC) is most frequently used in the United States as it is cheap and effective. All household contacts should be empirically treated with the same regimen to avoid reintroducing infection from family members who may be asymptomatically carrying the parasite. Careful laundering of all bedclothes is recommended as well.

---

[1] Not FDA approved for this indication.

[1] Not FDA approved for this indication.

Anisakiasis

Anisakiasis is a descriptive term for human infection with parasites of two distinct genera: *Anisakis* and *Pseudoterranova*. Humans are incidental hosts for these roundworms that inhabit multiple species of fish and other marine animals (tuna, mackerel, hake, cod, sardines, and cephalopods) as intermediate hosts, and marine mammals such as whales, seals, sea lions, and walruses as final hosts. Humans acquire the parasite in its larval stage by eating undercooked or raw fish (e.g., sushi, ceviche), therefore the condition predominates in cultures in which uncooked fish is consumed. Cases are most commonly reported from Japan but are seen throughout the world in other coastal nations and among restaurateurs.

On consumption of fish with anisakid larvae embedded in its musculature, humans can experience immediate symptoms in the form of itching or burning in the throat, which can provoke coughing that expels the parasite. If the parasite is swallowed, the larva attempts to embed in the gastric musculature at the pylorus. This can produce acute, short-lived epigastric abdominal pain and possibly immediate vomiting, at which point the parasite might again be ejected. If the larva does manage to penetrate gastric tissue, it dies because it is incapable of further tissue invasion in humans. An intense inflammatory response to the dead pathogen can then result, with gastric pain, nausea, and occasionally diarrhea with blood or mucus if a gastric ulcerative lesion has resulted. Eosinophilic enterocolitis, ileitis, appendicitis, and focal peritonitis and abscess formation from penetration of larva into the peritoneum are also rarely reported. Bronchoconstriction, angioedema, and anaphylaxis have been described mimicking seafood allergy. *Pseudoterranova* appears to cause milder symptoms and less tissue invasion, and the worm might simply be vomited several days after initial ingestion and presented to a physician, often by an alarmed patient. Because the vast majority of infections are caused by a single organism, vomiting of the parasite results in a definitive cure, and patients can be reassured. Diagnosis in patients with ongoing symptoms related to an embedded parasite is ultimately endoscopic. Effective cure results on endoscopic or surgical removal of the worm. Albendazole[1] as an effective therapy is reported; however, data are limited.

Trematodes

Schistosoma

Schistosomes are freshwater pathogens that are found in areas of endemicity in Africa, South America, Southeast Asia, and parts of the Middle East. These small trematodes cause varied, often chronic infections that can carry significant morbidity, although some species cannot invade beyond the dermis in humans and result strictly in cercarial dermatitis or swimmer's itch. There are five species of schistosomes known to cause disease in humans: *Schistosoma haematobium*, found through much of Africa and parts of the Middle East; *Schistosoma mansoni*, also native to Africa and the Middle East as well as Latin America; *Schistosoma japonicum*, present in China, Southeast Asia, and the Philippines; *Schistosoma mekongi*, found only in the Mekong River basin in Laos and Cambodia; and *Schistosoma intercalatum*, endemic only in West Africa.

All persons who come in contact with schistosomes are at risk for infection, even with brief exposure to fecally contaminated freshwater in which the intermediate hosts of the pathogen (snails) reside. Frequency and degree of infection tend to be highest in children in endemic areas and then level off in the early teenage years, likely secondary to level of environmental exposure and possibly to host immunity. *S. haematobium* causes disease in the genitourinary system; the others cause intestinal, hepatic, and sometimes pulmonary diseases.

Infection is acquired rapidly on contact with freshwater (including brief swims or by repeated splashing, as can occur during river rafting), when free-living fork-tailed schistosomal larvae (cercariae) penetrate human skin and lose their tail. These schistosomulae can cause intense itching and a papulovesicular, pruritic rash at the site of penetration, swimmer's itch. Invasive schistosomulae then enter the venous bloodstream and reach the liver through portal venules, where they mature into adults. Adult worms then migrate against the portal venous flow to the mesenteric venules of the gut (*S. mansoni, S. japonicum, S. intercalatum, S. mekongi*) and vesical venous plexus *(S. hematobium)*, where male and female forms mate for life. Females begin to oviposit, and the resultant inflammatory response to the eggs can cause either acute illness or chronic fibrosis and granulomatous inflammation of the tissues in which they reside.

Acute illness, called *Katayama fever*, is more common among hosts who have not been previously exposed to the organism and can be quite severe and even fatal. Katayama fever begins 3 to 8 weeks after infection, with acute onset of fever, chills, myalgias, cough, urticaria, angioedema, abdominal pain, hepatomegaly, and lymphadenopathy. Eggs might not yet be present in stool at the time of diagnosis. Chronic schistosomiasis is a slowly progressive illness presenting chiefly with intermittent abdominal pain, diarrhea, and anorexia. Colonic ulceration with gastrointestinal bleeding and iron-deficiency anemia from huge parasitic burden has been described. Hepatosplenic schistosomiasis can be caused by granulomatous inflammation surrounding the eggs, eventually leading to periportal fibrosis (Symmers pipestem fibrosis), portal hypertension, and splenomegaly. Portal hypertension can then lead to portosystemic collateral vessel development along with deposition of eggs in the pulmonary vasculature. Granulomatous inflammation in the pulmonary tissues eventually causes endarteritis, fibrosis, pulmonary hypertension, and cor pulmonale. *S. haematobium* infection can manifest as gross or microscopic hematuria, irritative urinary symptoms, and chronic bacterial urinary tract infections; ultimately ureteral fibrosis, hydronephrosis, and granulomatous genital lesions also can ensue. Neuroschistosomiasis can cause both myelopathy and intracerebral lesions and can have varied presentation including seizures, focal deficits, encephalopathy, and rapidly progressive transverse myelitis.

Diagnosis of schistosomiasis is by observation of eggs in stool (intestinal disease), urine (urinary tract disease), or biopsy specimens, or by serum antibody testing. Concentration of stool may be necessary to detect the pathogen. The eggs of the three most common species of schistosomes can be readily identified microscopically: *S. haematobium* has an inferior spine, *S. mansoni* has an inferolateral spine, and *S. japonicum* lacks a spine. Quantification of eggs is important as the parasitic burden is proportional to the risk of complications and is usually reported as light (up to 100 eggs/gram), moderate (100 to 400 eggs/gram), and severe (>400 eggs/gram) in stool specimens. Eosinophilia is a hallmark of chronic infection and is a common cause of asymptomatic eosinophilia among immigrants from endemic regions of the world. Serology is useful, particularly in return travelers with low parasitic burden; however, it can be negative in early infection as it takes 6 to 12 weeks after exposure to become positive. It is highly specific but cannot distinguish acute, chronic, or cleared infection. Antigen testing targeting specific schistosomal glycoproteins, circulating cathodic antigen (CCA, genus specific) and circulating anodic antigen (CAA, more specific to *S. mansoni*) is more sensitive than microscopy and can lead to rapid diagnosis, particularly in specimens with low parasitic burden. Highly sensitive PCR assays have been developed to be used on blood, stool, and urine specimens; however, these are not as widely available. Histopathology is better than microscopy, particularly in ectopic manifestations, but is usually not required.

---

[1] Not FDA approved for this indication.

All patients with schistosomiasis should be treated, and those with chronic manifestations might experience significant regression of even late-stage organ-specific disease. Treatment of choice is praziquantel (Biltricide); see Table 2 for details.

Prevention of schistosomiasis involves improving access to treated water and exploration of avenues to eliminate the intermediate snail hosts. Host immunity does appear to occur, and efforts are underway to better understand and induce such immunity in the form of a vaccine.

Cestodes
Taenia
Human tapeworm infection has long been implicated in North American oral folklore as a cause of insatiable appetite and excessive weight loss. In reality, despite their impressive size of up to 12 meters, tapeworm infection tends to be minimally symptomatic.

Taenia solium, pork tapeworm, and *Taenia saginata*, beef tapeworm, are the two most common flatworm infections of humans (humans are the only definitive hosts) worldwide and occur in any setting in which raw or undercooked meat is served and cattle and pigs have access to feed contaminated with human feces. *T. saginata* is still found in areas of North America and Europe as well as in Central and South America and Africa; *T. solium* is common throughout Mexico, Central and South America, Africa, China, and the Indian subcontinent. Although humans are the definitive hosts for both parasites, *T. solium* is best known for its pathogenicity in the form of cysticercosis. Cysticercosis is not an intestinal parasitic infection.

Domesticated animals acquire infection on ingestion of eggs or gravid proglottids excreted by humans; the eggs mature in their musculature and develop a scolex. When humans consume infected meat, the scolex attaches to the small intestine, and the adult tapeworm develops over approximately 2 months. Adult tapeworms are made up of hundreds to thousands of gravid proglottids and can live for up to 25 years with intermittent shedding in the stool.

Symptoms tend to be mild or absent but can include nausea, abdominal pain, loose stools, anal pruritus, and occasionally weakness or increased appetite, especially in children. Serious illness rarely results when tapeworm proglottids become lodged in the appendix or the biliary or pancreatic duct or are coughed up and aspirated. Some patients come to medical attention when the worm is noted emerging from the anus or on extrusion of proglottids in the stool.

Diagnosis of taeniasis can be made on visualizing the round eggs with hooks and double wall with characteristic striations, however the species cannot be determined unless their proglottids are examined (*T. saginata* has 12 or more uterine branches, whereas *T. solium* has <10). Because the eggs and proglottids are shed intermittently, the sensitivity of microscopy is poor. Serum antibody and antigen tests as well as stool PCR have been developed for diagnosis but are not widely used in clinical practice. Eosinophilia and elevated immunoglobulin E (IgE) levels may be present. Single-dose praziquantel (Biltricide)[1] (see Table 2) is curative in almost all cases, but infectious eggs can still be released in the feces for some time after worm eradication; ingestion of these could result in subsequent development of cysticercosis, so patients should be counseled to avoid fecal-oral contact.

Proper cooking of meat is the mainstay of prevention; disposal of human waste away from animals would also be effective in interrupting the life cycle.

---

[1] Not FDA approved for this indication.

Diphyllobothrium
Diphyllobothrium latum (fish tapeworm) is the longest parasite known to infect humans (10 to 12 m). It is found in freshwater lakes in areas of the Americas, Northern Europe, Africa, China, and Japan and has a complex life cycle involving two intermediate hosts: crustaceans and small fish. Humans and other fish-eating mammals are the definitive hosts and acquire the infection on ingestion of raw fish or roe.

Eggs and proglottids are intermittently shed in human stool that embryonate in the water. Coracidiae hatch from the eggs and are ingested by small crustaceans, the first intermediate hosts. Coracidiae mature into procercoid larvae in the crustaceans that are then ingested by the small freshwater fish (the second intermediate host). Procercoid larvae develop into plerocercoid larvae (sparganum) that are then passed onto the large predator fish (later intermediate host) that is then consumed by humans (definitive host). Sparganum develops into the adult worm inside the human intestine.

The mature adult tapeworm attaches within the small intestine, and hosts are usually asymptomatic. Infected persons might complain of increased appetite, nausea, or abdominal discomfort. Many patients present after passage of portions of the tapeworm in stool, as with taeniasis. In others, diagnosis is incidental on stool examination performed for other purposes or during screening colonoscopy. As with other worms, the parasite occasionally migrates into biliary ducts or causes intestinal obstruction. Attachment of the parasite higher in the intestine competes the host for vitamin B_{12} absorption and can result in vitamin B_{12} deficiency (pernicious anemia).

Diagnosis is made either by visualizing eggs with an operculum (lidlike opening) in an unconcentrated stool or by encountering the adult worm. Proglottids can be differentiated from those in taeniasis by the presence of a rosette-shaped uterus. Eosinophilia is present in a minority of cases. Treatment with praziquantel[1] is curative; see Table 2. Vitamin B_{12} supplementation is necessary in cases of severe or symptomatic deficiency, but it will not recur once the tapeworm is eliminated. Prevention involves not ingesting undercooked fish.

---

[1] Not FDA approved for this indication.

References
Abubakar I, Aliyu SH, Hunter PR, Usman NK: Prevention and treatment of cryptosporidiosis in immunocompromised patients, *Cochrane Database Syst Rev* (1), CD004932.

Bethony J, Brooker S, Albonico M, et al: Soil-transmitted helminth infections: Ascariasis, trichuriasis, and hookworm, *Lancet* 367(9521):1521–1532, 2006.

Boggild A, Yohanna S, Keystone J, Kain K: Prospective analysis of parasitic infections in Canadian travelers and immigrants, *J Travel Med* 13:138–144, 2006.

Boulware DR, Stauffer WM, Hendel-Paterson RR, et al: Maltreatment of strongyloides infection: Case series and worldwide physicians-in-training survey, *Am J Med* 120:545.e1– 545.e8, 2007.

Concha R, Hartington Jr W, Rogers AI: Intestinal strongyloidiasis: Recognition, management, and determinants of outcome, *J Clin Gastroenterol* 39(3):203–211, 2005.

Drugs for Parasitic Infections: *Treatment Guidelines from the Medical Letter*, 2013, pp e1–e31 (11).

Goodgame RW: Understanding intestinal spore-forming protozoa: Cryptosporidia, microsporidia, isospora, and cyclospora, *Ann Intern Med* 124(4):429–441, 1996.

Guerrant R, Walker D, Weller P, editors: *Tropical infectious diseases: principles, pathogens, and practice*, Philadelphia, 1999, Churchill Livingstone.

Huang DB, White AC: An updated review on Cryptosporidium and Giardia, *Gastroenterol Clin North Am* 35:291–314, 2006.

Mandell G, Bennett J, Dolin R, editors: *Mandell, douglas and bennett's principles and practice of infectious diseases*, 5th ed, Philadelphia, 2005, Churchill Livingstone.

Pardo J, Carranza C, Muro A, et al: Helminth-related eosinophilia in African immigrants, Gran Canaria, *Emerg Infect Dis* 12(10):1587–1589, 2006.

Stark D, Beebe N, Marriott D, et al: Dientamoebiasis: Clinical importance and recent advances, *Trends Parasitol* 22(2):92–96, 2006.

IRRITABLE BOWEL SYNDROME

Method of
Arnold Wald, MD

CURRENT DIAGNOSIS

- Fulfilling diagnostic criteria for irritable bowel syndrome (IBS) using Manning or Rome criteria is mandatory but not sufficient, as some organic diseases may also meet these criteria.
- Against the diagnosis of IBS is new onset in old age, a steady progressive course, frequent awakening by abdominal pain or urge to defecate, and weight loss not attributed to depression.
- The diagnostic approach to patients with IBS symptoms with no "alarm signs" includes a complete blood count; stool testing for occult blood or calprotectin; C-reactive protein and colonoscopy if patient is >50 years of age, has positive stool, or aforementioned blood test results; or if there is a poor response to treatment.
- After a diagnosis of IBS is established with confidence, repeated testing is counterproductive unless there is a distinct change in clinical symptoms or new alarm signs develop.

CURRENT THERAPY

- A robust patient–healthcare provider relationship is perhaps the most important determinant of outcome and reduction of healthcare utilization in patients with IBS.
- There is significant support for the use of a low-FODMAP (fermentable oligosaccharides, disaccharides, monosaccharides, and polyols) diet in patients with IBS. Gluten restriction is part of this diet and will cover those patients who believe that they are gluten intolerant in the absence of celiac disease.
- Pharmacologic agents can be divided into those for IBS-C or IBS-D or in any patient with IBS to ameliorate abdominal pain. The evidence to support these agents varies in quality and strength, and none is effective in the majority of patients who have been tested.
- Cognitive behavioral therapy (CBT) can be very effective in IBS with unrelenting symptoms but may also be effective for any patient with IBS who exhibits poor stress management.

Introduction and Definitions
Irritable bowel syndrome (IBS) is a chronic functional disorder of the gastrointestinal (GI) tract characterized by chronic abdominal pain and altered bowel habits in the absence of an organic disease. In the absence of a biologic disease marker, the diagnosis has traditionally been based on a cluster of symptoms. The earliest was the so-called *Manning criteria*, which was based most stringently on the presence of three or more characteristic symptoms (Table 1).

Subsequently, there have been various iterations of IBS criteria created by the Rome study groups that are currently used for research purposes (see Table 1). When evaluating the relevant literature for IBS, it is important to note that various studies have used different criteria that may result in variable data concerning prevalence and economic costs considerations.

From a clinical standpoint, subtypes of IBS have been defined as follows:
- IBS with predominant constipation (IBS-C): Patient reports that abnormal bowel movements are usually constipation (types 1 and 2 in the Bristol Stool Form Scale [BSFS]).

TABLE 1	Criteria for IBS	
MANNING CRITERIA	**ROME IV CRITERIA***
Looser stools with onset of pain More frequent bowel movements at onset of pain Visible distension Feeling of distension Mucus per rectum Feeling of incomplete emptying (often) Strict criteria >3 of above Less strict criteria >2 of above	Recurrent abdominal pain on average at least 1 day per week in the past 3 months associated with two or more of the following: • Related to defecation • Associated with a change in stool frequency • Associated with change in form of stool (appearance)

*Criterion fulfilled for the past 3 months with onset of symptoms at least 6 months before diagnosis.

- IBS with predominant diarrhea (IBS-D): Patient reports that abnormal bowel movements are usually diarrhea (types 6 and 7 in the BSFS).
- IBS with mixed bowel habits (IBS-M): Patient reports that abnormal bowel movements are usually both constipation and diarrhea (more than one-fourth of all the abnormal bowel movements are constipation, and more than one-fourth are diarrhea) using the BSFS.
- IBS Unclassified (IBS-U): Patients who meet diagnostic criteria for IBS but cannot be accurately categorized into one of the other three subtypes.

Epidemiology
Prevalence
Numerous surveys have reported the prevalence of IBS in the community. The majority of these studies have used accepted diagnostic criteria, and some have used more than one definition within the same population. In one meta-analysis, 23 studies used the Manning criteria, 24 used Rome I criteria, 36 used Rome II criteria, and 5 used Rome III criteria. The prevalence ranged from 5% to 10% (United States, China) to 15% to 20% (Canada, Brazil, Russia). There were little or no data from Africa, Central America, and large parts of South America.

The majority of studies did not report the predominant stool pattern in IBS. Of the nine that included IBS-U subtypes as well, there was an even distribution, ranging from 22% to 24% mean prevalence for each of the four subgroups. In general, the pooled prevalence was higher in women than in men (14%; range 11% to 16% vs. 9%; range 7.3% to 10.5%) with significant heterogeneity between studies. There appeared to be no relationship between socioeconomic status in the four studies that reported it and no strong influence of age as well.

It is important to note that the meta-analysis was restricted to studies based on the general population and excluded those based on convenience samples. This makes the data more generalizable to community individuals with IBS.

Causality: A Biopsychosocial Model of Functional Gastrointestinal Disorders Such as IBS
The ability to study causality in a disorder with no biologic disease markers is fraught with difficulties. This is certainly the case with IBS as a representative of functional GI disorders. Many hypotheses have been advanced and found wanting. The current (and in my opinion most relevant) conceptual model is the biopsychosocial construct, as shown in Figure 1.

Figure 1 indicates that predeterminants such as early life experiences together with psychosocial factors may interact with altered gut physiology via the brain-gut axis. This concept infers that these factors are bidirectional and mutually interactive and therefore influence both the clinical presentation and clinical outcomes of the disorder. Among the physiologic processes that may lead to GI symptoms are abnormal gut motility, visceral hypersensitivity, immune dysregulation, inflammation and barrier dysfunction, the intestinal microbiome, diet, and the brain-gut axis. No one factor

Biopsychosocial Conceptual Model

Figure 1 Predeterminants such as early life experiences, together with psychosocial factors, may interact with altered gut physiology via the brain-gut axis. This concept infers that these factors are bidirectional and mutually interactive and therefore influence both the clinical presentation of the disorder and the clinical outcomes. Among the physiological processes that may lead to GI symptoms are abnormal gut motility, visceral hypersensitivity, immune dysregulation, inflammation and barrier dysfunction, the intestinal microbiome, diet, and the brain-gut axis. No one factor alone accounts for the symptoms of IBS, and all must be considered in the management of affected patients. This becomes apparent when considering treatment approaches. *CNS,* Central nervous system; *ENS,* enteric nervous system; *FGID,* functional gastrointestinal disorder. Reprinted with permission from Drossman DA. Functional gastrointestinal disorders: history, pathophysiology, clinical features and Rome IV. *Gastroenterology* 2016; 150:1262–1279.

alone accounts for the symptoms of IBS, and all must be considered in the management of affected patients. This becomes apparent when considering treatment approaches (see later).

Impact on Population Health
Although there is no mortality associated with IBS, symptoms are long lasting, and there are no curative therapies available. As a chronic illness, the economic impact of this disorder is considerable.

In a 2015 survey conducted by the American Gastroenterological Association (AGA), IBS patients reported that their symptoms interfered with work productivity on an average of 9 days per month and missed work on an average of 2 days per month. Indirect costs (e.g., loss of work and reduced productivity) have been estimated to be up to $20 billion annually in the United States, with an estimated annual cost per patient of $9933 (in 2021 U.S. dollars)

In a recent study of indirect costs, impairment experienced at work (presenteeism) accounted for approximately 75% of the total annual indirect costs for respondents with IBS, far in excess of absenteeism from work. Compared with controls, IBS respondents missed significantly more work (5.1% vs. 2.9%), experienced higher levels of presenteeism (17.9% vs. 11.3%), and had greater overall work productivity loss (20.7% vs. 13.2%) and higher daily activity impairment.

Direct Healthcare Costs
Almost 30 years ago, it was estimated that up to 25% of all visits to gastroenterologists in the United States were for IBS, with additional others for other functional GI disorders. This accounted for 3.5 million visits to healthcare practitioners in 1991 and undoubtedly is much higher today. Earlier studies showed that IBS patients made twice as many health visits per year as did age-matched controls and that 78% of the excess visits were for non-GI complaints. A subsequent analysis of this phenomenon suggests that comorbidity in IBS may be a consequence of the psychological trait for somatization, defined as the tendency to amplify the intensity and overinterpret the significance of any somatic sensation. This excess comorbidity is

the primary determinant of excess healthcare costs associated with IBS, although it does not apply to all patients with IBS.

Recent attempts to identify factors leading to high utilizers with IBS have been made. The investigators used a conceptual framework for accessing healthcare services that holds that a decision to use healthcare is related to (1) predisposition to use services; (2) ability to use services; and (3) need for services. The important conclusion was that decisions to use healthcare are not simply influenced by symptom-specific factors but by a variety of lifestyle and (most importantly) economic factors such as health insurance coverage.

Evaluation of Patients with Suspected Irritable Bowel Syndrome
The diagnosis of IBS should be made based on the clinical history, physical examination, minimal laboratory testing, and colonoscopy or other appropriate tests when clinically indicated. Fulfilling diagnostic criteria is, of course, mandatory but insufficient, as some organic diseases may also meet these criteria. The prevalence of organic disease is lowest in IBS-C and highest in IBS-D, followed by IBS-M; the most common consideration would be Crohn's disease. Against the diagnosis of IBS include new onset in old age, a steady progressive course, frequent awakening by pain or need to defecate, and weight loss not attributed to depression. Additional features that would increase concern about organic disease would include a positive family history of colorectal cancer or inflammatory bowel disease as well as rectal bleeding or anemia associated with iron or vitamin B_{12} deficiency.

In the absence of "alarm signs," a consensus diagnostic approach to patients with IBS symptoms is listed on Table 2 (Rome IV).

Tests of Unproven Value
A high prevalence of small intestinal bacterial overgrowth (SIBO) has been claimed by some centers leading to the frequent utilization of either lactulose or glucose breath tests. This hypothesis is based on poor methodology and erroneous conclusions. The original studies have not been reproduced by other centers using either similar and/or better techniques. This has led to the frequent use of expensive antibiotics that can be effective in some patients with bloating and IBS but not because these patients have SIBO.

Food allergy testing is not routinely recommended. Stool for ova/parasites is not recommended unless the patient has traveled to an undeveloped area. Lastly, after a diagnosis of IBS has been established with confidence, repeated testing is counterproductive unless there is a distinct change in clinical symptoms or new alarm signs develop. This is especially so if endoscopy procedures have already been performed.

TABLE 2	Diagnostic Approach to Patients with IBS Symptoms (No "Alarm Signs")
Complete blood count	
Stool for occult blood	
Routine colon cancer screening at ages >45 years	
C-reactive protein (inflammatory marker)*	
Fecal calprotectin/lactoferrin (indicators of inflammation)*	
Stool for *Giardia**	
Celiac serologies*	
Diagnostic colonoscopy <45 years of age (if poor response to Rx)	

*For IBS with predominant diarrhea (IBS-D).

| TABLE 3 | Low-FODMAP Diet |

AVOID OR REDUCE THESE FOODS

FRUCTOSE	LACTOSE	OLIGOS	POLYOLS
Fruits: Apple, mango, pear, watermelon, juice, dried fruit	Milk: Milk from cows/goats/sheep; custard; ice cream; yogurt; eggnog	Vegetables: Beets, broccoli, brussels sprouts, cabbage, fennel, garlic, onion, chicory root	Fruits: Apricot, avocado, blackberry, cherry, nectarine, peach, plum, prune, fig
Other: Asparagus, honey, high-fructose corn syrup, molasses	Cheese: Soft, unripened cheese	Other: Barley, beans, chickpeas, couscous, inulin, lentils, pistachios, rye, soy milk, wheat (pasta, bread), veggie burgers	Vegetables: Cauliflower, corn, mushroom, sweet potato Sweeteners: Ending in "ol" (e.g., xylitol, sorbitol), isomalt

FODMAP, Fermentable oligosaccharides, disaccharides, monosaccharides, and polyols.

Treatment

A validated standardized algorithm for the treatment of IBS does not exist. Treatment therefore depends on the type and severity of symptoms and the nature of associated psychosocial issues in an individual patient. A strong guiding principle is that a robust patient–healthcare provider relationship is an important determinant of outcome and reduction of healthcare utilization. Treatments may generally be divided into dietary and lifestyle modifications, pharmacologic agents, and behavioral therapies, all of which have been validated by randomized controlled studies.

Dietary Modifications

Although fiber supplements are widely recommended for IBS, a meta-analysis of seven high-quality studies failed to find significant benefit, although some benefits might occur with soluble fiber (psyllium) versus insoluble fiber (bran) in IBS-C. Unfortunately, fiber supplements may exacerbate symptoms such as abdominal bloating and discomfort.

Other dietary interventions such as gluten-free and low FODMAP (fermentable oligosaccharides, disaccharides, monosaccharides, and polyols) diets have become increasingly popular. Several studies support the benefit of gluten-free diets in a subset of IBS patients in the absence of celiac disease. It remains uncertain whether the clinical benefits are a consequence of gluten withdrawal, elimination of other wheat proteins and highly fermentable short-chain fatty acids, or a placebo effect. Adding a gluten-free diet to patients who are already on a low FODMAP diet offers no additional benefits. Monash University has a number of resources including an app that are helpful to patients (https://www.monashfodmap.com/).

There is accumulating evidence from prospective controlled studies that dietary FODMAP restriction is associated with significant symptom improvement in many patients with IBS (Table 3). It appears that restriction of both fructose and fructans is most beneficial. Significant symptom improvement was noted in IBS patients compared with a standard Australian diet and also a National Institute for Health and Care Excellence (NICE; England) diet.

Response to a low FODMAP diet is usually assessed after about 2 weeks. Responders are then asked to engage in a structured reintroduction of restricted foods to allow the individual to tailor his or her diet. It is optimal to involve a properly trained dietitian or nutritionist in the care of these patients.

Pharmacologic Agents

Pharmacologic approaches to IBS may be divided into medications for IBS-C, patients with IBS-D, and for any patient with IBS in order to ameliorate abdominal pain (Table 4).

| TABLE 4 | Pharmacologic Agents for IBS |

INDICATION	DRUG	DOSE
IBS-C	Linaclotide (Linzess) Plecanatide (Trulance) Lubiprostone (Amitiza) PEG-3350 (Miralax)[1] Tenapanor (Ibsrela)	72–290 mcg/d[3] 3 mg/d24 mcg bid[3] 8 mg bid 8.5–17 g/d 50 mg bid
IBS-D	Rifaximin (Xifaxan) Alosetron (Lotronex) Eluxadoline (Viberzi) Loperamide (Imodium)[1]	550 mg tid × 2 weeks 1 mg qd to bid 75–100 mg/d 2–16 mg/d
IBS-All	Dicyclomine (Bentyl) Desipramine (Norpramin)[1]	20–40 mg qid 10–100 mg/d (desipramine)

[1]Not FDA approved for this indication.
[3]Exceeds dosage recommended by the manufacturer. Per Amitiza's manufacturer package insert, the recommended dose for IBS-C is 8 mcg bid.

Most drugs work through different pathophysiologic mechanisms. For example, for patients with IBS-C, linaclotide (Linzess), plecanatide (Trulance), and lubiprostone (Amitiza) increase intestinal chloride and water secretion to combat constipation, whereas PEG (polyethylene glycol 3350 [Miralax])[1] does so through a hyperosmolar effect. Tenapanor (Ibsrela) is a new agent that inhibits sodium absorption to increase water secretion. For IBS-D, rifaximin (Xifaxan) is an antibiotic, loperamide (Imodium)[1] is a peripheral μ-opioid agonist, alosetron (Lotronex) works through the serotonin 3 receptor, and eluxadoline (Viberzi) has effects on all three opioid receptors in the gut (mu, kappa, and delta). Tricyclic antidepressants (TCAs) presumably work via central neurochemical changes, and antispasmodics (dicyclomine [Bentyl], encapsulated oil of peppermint[7]) work largely through peripheral anticholinergic pathways. The large and diverse number of drugs are indicative of the lack of fundamental understanding of IBS. Moreover, few drugs are effective in the majority of IBS patients, and there is no more than a 10% to 15% improvement over placebo in most published studies.

The AGA guidelines published in 2014 incorporated the Grading of Recommendations Assessment, Development and Evaluation (GRADE) methodology and best practices as outlined by the Institute of Medicine. Recommendations are either strong or conditional (weak). The evidence that provides the basis for recommendation is rated high, moderate, or

[1]Not FDA approved for this indication.
[7]Available as dietary supplement.

low quality. A similar grading system was used in the recently published American College of Gastroenterology (ACG) guidelines in 2021.

Of the pharmacologic agents for IBS-C, linaclotide (Linzess) received a strong recommendation with high-quality evidence, lubiprostone (Amitiza) received a conditional recommendation on moderate-quality evidence, and PEG[1] was given a conditional recommendation based on weak evidence. The first two agents showed modest benefit over placebo, whereas there are no data to support the use of PEG. For all three agents, adverse effects were relatively few, and diarrhea is perhaps the major side effect. Both linaclotide and lubiprostone are costly (as are eluxadoline [Viberzi] and plecanatide [Trulance]) and may involve high out-of-pocket expenses for patients.

For IBS-D, both rifaximin (Xifaxan) and alosetron (Lotronex) received conditional recommendations based on moderate-quality evidence. The latter is approved by the U.S. Food and Drug Administration (FDA) only for women who have failed all other treatments. There is a very small risk (approximately 1 case/1000 patient years) for ischemic colitis with alosetron. Although loperamide (Imodium)[1] has very low-quality evidence to support its use, it can be very effective if used in a proactive fashion.

The case for TCAs and antispasmodics is based on low-quality evidence, but both agents can be very effective for abdominal pain and, in the case of TCAs, for reducing diarrhea in IBS patients.

Behavioral Therapy

For patients with unrelenting IBS symptoms, cognitive-behavioral therapy (CBT) and gut-directed hypnosis have been found to be beneficial. Such therapies should be performed by experienced and well-trained behavioral specialists who are an integral part of the medical team that treats patients with functional GI disorders. The most robust data for efficacy are for CBT. One potential drawback is that these treatments are provider-intensive approaches, but recent studies suggest that CBT can be as effective when given in a shortened course as the traditional method.

References

Buono JL, Carson RT, Flores NM: Health-related quality of life, work productivity, and indirect costs among patients with irritable bowel syndrome with diarrhea, *Health Qual Life Outcomes* 15(1):35, 2017.

Drossman DA: Functional gastrointestinal disorders: History, pathophysiology, clinical features and Rome IV, *Gastroenterology* 150:1262–1279, 2016.

Eswaran S, Farida JP, Green J, Miller JD, Chey WD: Nutrition in the management of gastrointestinal diseases and disorders: the evidence for the low FODMAP diet, *Curr Opin Pharmacol* 37:151–157, 2017.

Gudleski GD, Satchidanand N, Dunlap LJ, Tahiliani V, Li X, Keefer L, Lackner JM, IBSOS Outcome Study Research Group: Predictors of medical and mental health care use in patients with irritable bowel syndrome in the United States, *Behav Res Ther* 88:65–67, 2017.

Lacey BL, Pimentel M, Brenner DB, et al: ACG Clinical Guideline: management of irritable bowel syndrome, *Am J Gastroenterol* 116:17–44, 2021.

Lembo A, et al.: AGA clinical practice guidelines on the pharmacologic management of IBS with diarrhea, *Gastroenterology* 163:137–151, 2022.

Lovell RM, Ford AC: Global prevalence and risk factors for irritable bowel syndrome: a meta-analysis, *Clin Gastroenterol Hepatol* 10(7):712–721, 2012.

Massey BT, Wald A: Small intestinal bacterial overgrowth: a guide to the use of breath testing, *Dig Dis Sci* 66:338–347, 2021.

Nellesen D, Yee K, Chawla A, Lewis BE, Carson RT: A systematic review of the economic and humanistic burden of illness in irritable bowel syndrome and chronic constipation, *J Manag Care Pharm* 19(9):755–764, 2013.

Radziwon CD, Lackner JM: Cognitive Behavioral Therapy for IBS: How Useful, How Often, and How Does It Work? *Curr Gastroenterol Rep* 19(10):49, 2017.

Rao SS, Yu S, Fedewa A: Systematic review: dietary fiber and FODMAP restricted diet in the management of constipation and IBS, *Aliment Pharm Ther* 41:1256–1270, 2015.

Skodje GI, Sarna VK, Minelle IH, et al: Fructan, rather than gluten, induces symptoms in patients with self-reported non-celiac gluten sensitivity, *Gastroenterology* 154(3):529–539, 2018.

Weinberg DS, Smalley W, Heidelbaugh JJ, Sultan S: American Gastroenterological Association Institute Guideline on the Pharmacological Management of Irritable Bowel Syndrome, *Gastroenterology* 1146–1148, 2014.

MALABSORPTION

Method of
Lawrence R. Schiller, MD

CURRENT DIAGNOSIS

- Recognize the presence of generalized malabsorption by the combination of typical symptoms: diarrhea, greasy stools, flatulence, weight loss, fatigue, edema.
- Recognize the presence of malabsorption of specific nutrients by associated symptoms and those symptoms particular to deficiency states of the malabsorbed substance: flatus, diarrhea, anemia, dermatitis, glossitis, neuropathy, paresthesias, tetany, ecchymosis.
- Documentation of generalized malabsorption is best done by stool analysis demonstrating steatorrhea and acid stools (reflecting carbohydrate malabsorption). Diagnosis depends on visualization of the small bowel by endoscopy or radiography and small bowel biopsy. Additional tests may be needed.
- Documentation of specific malabsorption is best done by demonstrating low blood levels of the malabsorbed substance or by tests designed to measure absorption of that substance. Diagnosis depends on studies designed to identify the likely diagnosis for a given situation.

CURRENT THERAPY

- Once a diagnosis is reached, therapy can be directed toward that specific problem:
  - Gluten-free diet for celiac disease
  - Antibiotics for bacterial overgrowth
  - Pancreatic enzymes for exocrine pancreatic insufficiency
  - Lactose-free diet for lactase deficiency

Every day the average human being consumes 2000–3000 kcal of food, much of it in the form of polymers or other complex molecules that must be digested and absorbed by the gut. The processes of digestion and absorption are complex and are readily disturbed by pathologic processes. More than 200 conditions have been described that can adversely affect nutrient absorption.

Strictly speaking, *maldigestion* refers to impaired hydrolysis of nutrients, usually due to lack of luminal factors, such as bile acids and pancreatic enzymes, and *malabsorption* refers to impaired mucosal transport. For clinical purposes, "malabsorption" is used to describe both processes.

Malabsorption can be generalized (panmalabsorption) or limited to a specific category of nutrients. Generalized malabsorption is usually due to maldigestion or to extensive mucosal dysfunction. Specific malabsorption occurs when a single transport mechanism is disabled.

The causes of malabsorption can be divided into three categories: impaired luminal hydrolysis, impaired mucosal function (mucosal hydrolysis, uptake, packaging, and excretion), and impaired removal of nutrients from the mucosa (Box 1).

Diagnosis

Symptoms and Signs

Most patients with panmalabsorption have changes in their stools (Box 2). Steatorrhea (excess fat in stools) is characterized by pale color, bulkiness, greasiness, and a tendency to float (probably because of incorporated gas). Occasionally patients with

BOX 1 | Causes of Malabsorption or Maldigestion

- Impaired luminal hydrolysis or solublization
  - Bile acid deficiency
  - Impaired mucosal hydrolysis, uptake, or packaging
  - Pancreatic exocrine insufficiency
  - Postgastrectomy syndrome
  - Rapid intestinal transit
  - Small bowel bacterial overgrowth
  - Zollinger-Ellison syndrome
- Brush border or metabolic disorders
  - Abetalipoproteinemia
  - Glucose-galactose malabsorption
  - Lactase deficiency
  - Sucrase-isomaltase deficiency
- Mucosal diseases
  - Amyloidosis
  - Crohn's disease
  - Celiac sprue
  - Collagenous sprue
  - Eosinophilic gastroenteritis
  - Immunoproliferative small intestinal disease (IPSID)
  - Lymphoma
  - Nongranulomatous ulcerative jejunoileitis
  - Drug-induced enteropathy (e.g., olmesartan enteropathy)
  - Radiation enteritis
  - Systemic mastocytosis
- Infectious diseases
  - AIDS enteropathy
  - *Mycobacterium avium-intracellulare*
  - Parasitic diseases
  - Small bowel bacterial overgrowth
  - Tropical sprue
  - Whipple's disease
- After intestinal resection
- Chronic mesenteric ischemia
- Impaired removal of nutrients
  - Lymphangiectasia

BOX 2 | Symptoms and Signs of Malabsorption or Maldigestion

- Changes in stool characteristics
  - Floating stools
  - Pale, bulky, greasy stools
  - Watery diarrhea
- Increased colonic gas production
  - Abdominal distention
  - Borborygmi, increased flatus
- Vitamin and mineral deficiencies
  - Anemia
  - Cheilosis
  - Glossitis
  - Dermatitis
  - Neuropathy
  - Night blindness
  - Osteomalacia
  - Paresthesia
  - Tetany
- Ecchymosis
- Fatigue, weakness
- Edema
- Weight loss, muscle wasting

malabsorption present with watery stools due to the osmotic effects of unabsorbed carbohydrates and short-chain fatty acids.

Abdominal distention and excess flatus also commonly occur due to fermentation of unabsorbed carbohydrate by colonic bacteria. This can occur not only with panmalabsorption but also with malabsorption of specific carbohydrates (e.g., lactase deficiency).

Weight loss is typical with severe panmalabsorption, but it might not be very prominent with lesser degrees of malabsorption due to compensatory hyperphagia. Weight loss is most prominent early in the course of the illness, but body weight usually stabilizes as calorie absorption and body weight come into balance again. This is in contrast to illnesses like cancer or tuberculosis that produce continuing weight loss. If a patient with malabsorption has continuing weight loss, inflammatory bowel disease or lymphoma should be considered.

Abdominal pain is usually not present with malabsorption, although some cramping may be associated with diarrhea. Severe pain should bring chronic pancreatitis, Zollinger-Ellison syndrome, lymphoma, Crohn's disease, or mesenteric ischemia to mind.

Constitutional symptoms of fatigue and weakness commonly occur, even early in the course. In contrast, appetite is impaired only late in the course of most malabsorption states. Edema is uncommon until late in the course unless protein-losing enteropathy is present.

Vitamin and mineral deficiencies can lead to several symptoms or signs. Glossitis and cheilosis are common in patients with water-soluble vitamin deficiencies. Florid beriberi, pellagra, and scurvy are not commonly seen unless malabsorption has been particularly severe or long-lasting. Fat-soluble vitamin deficiencies also are unlikely to develop except when malabsorption has been long-standing because of substantial body stores.

Miscellaneous findings occasionally seen in patients with malabsorption can provide clues to the diagnosis. Aphthous ulcers in the mouth may be seen with celiac disease, Behçet's syndrome, or Crohn's disease. Hyperpigmentation is seen in Whipple's disease, and dermatitis herpetiformis (pruritic, blistering skin lesions) is seen in celiac disease. Scleroderma can manifest with tight skin, digital ulceration, nail changes, and Raynaud's phenomenon. Chronic sinusitis, bronchitis, and recurrent pneumonia suggest cystic fibrosis or IgA deficiency. Several systemic diseases can be associated with malabsorption syndrome (Box 3).

Tests

Routine Laboratory Tests

Routine laboratory tests (Box 4) commonly are abnormal in patients with established malabsorption syndrome. Anemia is common but not universal. Iron deficiency anemia may be the only finding in some patients with celiac disease. Microcytic anemia may be present in Whipple's disease (due to occult blood loss) and in lymphomas manifesting with malabsorption. Macrocytic anemia due to folate or vitamin B_{12} deficiency can occur in short bowel syndrome,

BOX 3 | Systemic Diseases Associated with Malabsorption or Maldigestion

Endocrine Diseases
- Addison's disease
- Diabetes mellitus
- Hypoparathyroidism
- Hyperthyroidism, hypothyroidism

Collagen-Vascular and Miscellaneous Diseases
- AIDS
- Amyloidosis
- Scleroderma
- Vasculitis (systemic lupus erythematosus, polyarteritis nodosa)

Laboratory Tests for Evaluation of Malabsorption or Maldigestion

Complete Blood Count
- Hemoglobin/hematocrit
- Platelet count
- WBC differential count

Biochemistry Tests
- Blood urea nitrogen
- Prothrombin time
- Serum albumin
- Serum calcium
- Serum creatinine
- Serum Potassium

Blood Levels of Potentially Malabsorbed Substances
- Serum iron, vitamin B_{12}, folate, 25-OH vitamin D, carotene

Fat absorption
- Qualitative fecal fat (Sudan stain)
- Quantitative fecal fat (Timed collection)

Protein Absorption and Protein-Losing Enteropathy
- α_1-Antitrypsin clearance
- Fecal nitrogen excretion

Carbohydrate Absorption
- Osmotic gap in stool water
- Quantitative excretion (anthrone)
- Stool pH <5.5
- Stool reducing substances
- D-Xylose absorption test
- Oral glucose, sucrose, and lactose tolerance tests
- Breath hydrogen tests

Vitamin B_{12} Absorption
- Serum B_{12} level

Bile Acid Malabsorption
- Fecal bile acid excretion
- Serum 7α-hydroxy-4-cholesten-3-one (C4)
- ^{75}SeHCAT retention

Small Bowel Bacterial Overgrowth
- ^{14}C-xylose breath test
- Glucose breath hydrogen test
- Quantitative culture of jejunal aspirate

Exocrine Pancreatic Insufficiency
- Secretin/CCK test
- Stool elastase or chymotrypsin concentration

Serologic Testing for Celiac Disease
- Anti-tissue transglutaminase antibody (IgA)
- Anti-endomysial antibody (IgA)

Abbreviations: CCK = cholecystokinin; SLE = systemic lupus erythematosus; ^{75}SeHCAT = selenium-75-labeled taurohomocholic acid; WBC = white blood cell.

---

small bowel bacterial overgrowth, or ileal disease. Lymphopenia may be present in patients with AIDS or lymphangiectasia.

Electrolyte abnormalities may be due to a combination of poor intake and excess loss in stool. Renal function usually is well maintained in malabsorption syndrome, but blood urea nitrogen may be low due to poor protein absorption, and serum creatinine concentration may be low due to depletion of muscle mass. Serum calcium levels may be low due to malabsorption, vitamin D deficiency, or intraluminal complexing of calcium by fatty acids. Hypomagnesemia can produce hypocalcemia or hypokalemia that is resistant to intravenous repletion. Serum phosphorus, cholesterol, and triglyceride levels may be reduced due to poor intake or malabsorption. Liver tests may be abnormal due to fatty liver. Serum protein and albumin levels are well preserved in patients with malabsorption unless protein-losing enteropathy or an acute illness is present.

Prothrombin time is normal unless vitamin K malabsorption (typically associated with steatorrhea), anticoagulant therapy, antibiotic therapy, or colectomy is present.

Assays are available for several potentially malabsorbed substances, including iron, vitamin B_{12}, folate, 25-hydroxyvitamin D, and β-carotene. Malabsorption tends to lower blood levels, but substantial body stores of many of these can mitigate the reduction in concentration that otherwise might occur. Thus, the sensitivity and specificity of these assays for malabsorption are poor.

Tests for Malabsorption

Fat Malabsorption. The simplest test for fat malabsorption is a qualitative microscopic examination of stool using a fat-soluble stain, such as Sudan III. The finding of more than five stained droplets per high-power field is abnormal and correlates well with quantitative measurement of fecal fat excretion. The test is subject to false-positive results with some drugs and food additives, such as mineral oil, orlistat, and olestra.

A more precise estimate of fat absorption is obtained by a quantitative analysis of a timed stool collection (48 or 72 hours). During the collection, a diary of dietary intake should be maintained so that fat excretion can be assessed as a percentage of intake. Normal fat excretion is <7% of intake when stool weight is normal, but it can be twice as high due to voluminous diarrhea without indicating defective mucosal transport of fat. Thus, fat excretion must be judged against stool weight. Stool fat concentration (grams of fat per 100 grams of stool) also is of value. Pancreatic exocrine insufficiency is associated with high fecal fat concentration (>10 g/100 g stool) because, unlike hydrolyzed fat, unhydrolyzed fat does not stimulate colonic water and electrolyte secretion that would dilute fecal fat concentration.

Protein Malabsorption. Fecal nitrogen excretion can be employed as a marker of protein malabsorption, but is not often used in clinical medicine because it adds little to the evaluation. If protein-losing enteropathy is suspected, an α_1-antitrypsin clearance study can be done. In this study, fecal excretion of α_1-antitrypsin, a serum protein that is relatively resistant to hydrolysis by luminal enzymes, is divided by serum concentration of α_1-antitrypsin, and the volume of serum leaked into the lumen can be calculated. Values of more than 180 mL/day are associated with hypoalbuminemia.

Carbohydrate Malabsorption. Carbohydrate malabsorption is difficult to measure directly because fermentation of malabsorbed carbohydrate by colonic bacteria reduces the amount of intact carbohydrate that can be recovered in stool. Indirect estimates of carbohydrate malabsorption can be made by examining fecal pH (<5.5 with carbohydrate malabsorption) or fecal osmotic gap (> 100 mOsm/kg with osmotic diarrhea) based on chemical analysis of stool water. Oral carbohydrate tolerance tests may be used to evaluate absorption of sugars, such as lactose or fructose. Following an oral load of a given sugar, blood glucose levels are monitored; failure of blood glucose to increase suggests malabsorption.

Another test for carbohydrate malabsorption is the D-xylose absorption test. In this test, a 25-gram dose of D-xylose is given orally; blood xylose levels are measured 1 and 3 hours later, and urinary excretion of xylose is measured for 5 hours. Failure of blood xylose to rise above 20 mg/dL at 1 hour or above 22.5 mg/dL at 3 hours or failure of urinary excretion to exceed 5 g in 5 hours suggests malabsorption. In addition, because xylose does not require pancreatic enzymes or bile acids for absorption, an abnormal D-xylose test suggests a mucosal problem as the cause for malabsorption. The results of this test can be misleading if the patient is dehydrated or has ascites, if renal function is compromised, or if bacterial overgrowth is present in the upper small bowel.

Breath hydrogen testing is another method to assess carbohydrate absorption. If substrates such as lactose or sucrose are not absorbed in the small intestine, they pass into the colon, where bacterial fermentation produces hydrogen gas. The hydrogen is absorbed into the bloodstream and then is exhaled. The concentration of hydrogen in exhaled breath can be measured easily; a rise of more than 10 to 20 ppm after ingestion of a specific substrate is consistent with malabsorption. False-positive results can be seen in patients with small bowel bacterial overgrowth, and false-negative results can be seen in patients who lack hydrogen-producing flora or who have been on antibiotics recently.

Vitamin B$_{12}$ Malabsorption. Although the Schilling test has been used to measure Vitamin B$_{12}$ absorption, commercial testing kits are no longer available in the United States. Instead, serum B$_{12}$ levels are measured: low levels are consistent with enough B$_{12}$ malabsorption, but normal levels do not exclude it because enough B$_{12}$ is stored in the liver to maintain serum levels for several years.

Bile Acid Malabsorption. Direct measurement of fecal bile acid excretion in a timed stool specimen can be used to evaluate bile acid malabsorption in the United States. Retention of a radioactive taurocholic acid analogue (SeHCAT, selenium-75-labeled taurohomocholic acid) is used in Europe to assess bile acid malabsorption. Serum 7α-hydroxy-4-cholesten-3-one (C4) reflects bile acid synthesis; higher levels reflect increased synthesis in patients with bile acid malabsorption.

Small Bowel Bacterial Overgrowth. The gold standard method used to test for small bowel bacterial overgrowth in the upper intestine is quantitative culture of jejunal fluid. The sample can be obtained during endoscopy and sent to the laboratory with instructions to quantitate the aerobic and anaerobic flora. Finding more than 10^5 bacteria per mL confirms bacterial overgrowth. Breath tests using glucose, ^{14}C-xylose, and lactulose also have been described for this purpose.

Pancreatic Exocrine Insufficiency. Tests for pancreatic exocrine insufficiency are not commonly used. The gold standard test is a secretin test. This study requires duodenal intubation, injection of secretin, and measurement of bicarbonate output. Measurement of fecal chymotrypsin or elastase activity is only moderately useful in predicting the presence of exocrine pancreatic insufficiency. For most situations, a therapeutic trial using a high dose of pancreatic enzymes with monitoring of the effect on steatorrhea is the best that can be done.

Evaluation of Suspected Malabsorption

When malabsorption is suspected because of the history, physical findings, and setting, the physician must decide if the malabsorption involves just carbohydrates or represents a generalized process (Figure 1). If the malabsorption seems to be limited to carbohydrates because stool pH is less than 6 and no steatorrhea is present, a diet and symptom diary, breath tests using the presumptively malabsorbed substrate, and stool pH to identify acid stools seen with carbohydrate malabsorption are reasonable diagnostic maneuvers.

Suspected generalized malabsorption requires a more intense evaluation. If steatorrhea is confirmed, serology for celiac disease (IgA anti–tissue transglutaminase, and IgA level to exclude IgA deficiency) should be obtained and the small bowel should be visualized with either capsule endoscopy or radiography (small bowel follow-through examination or computed tomography) and biopsied from above by enteroscopy and from below by colonoscopy. During enteroscopy, an aspirate of small bowel contents can be obtained for quantitative culture to look for small bowel bacterial overgrowth. An alternative method to detect small bowel bacterial overgrowth is breath testing (see earlier). Stool samples also should be examined with microscopy or immunoassay for the presence of parasites that may be associated with malabsorption.

This sequence of evaluation often leads to a specific diagnosis. When it does not, empiric trials of high-dose pancreatic enzyme replacement, low-dose bile acid supplementation, or antibiotics can lead to a presumptive diagnosis of pancreatic exocrine insufficiency, bile acid deficiency, or small intestinal bacterial overgrowth.. Hard endpoints (e.g., reduction in quantitative fat excretion) should be used to assess the effectiveness of these empiric trials.

Specific Disorders Associated With Malabsorption
Malabsorption of Specific Nutrients
Disaccharidase Deficiency

Ingested disaccharides such as lactose and sucrose and starch-digestion products such as maltotriose and α-limit dextrins must be hydrolyzed by brush border enzymes into monosaccharides for abosorption by the mucosa. If these brush border enzymes are not active or if the brush border is damaged, malabsorption of the specific carbohydrate substrate results. This can result in gaseousness or osmotic diarrhea when those substrates are ingested. This rarely occurs on a congenital basis, but it commonly occurs as an acquired disorder.

Figure 1 Flow chart for evaluation of malabsorption or maldigestion. *Abbreviations:* CT = computed tomography; R/O = rule out; SB = small bowel.

Lactase deficiency is the most common acquired disaccharidase deficiency. Infant mammals all rely on lactose as the carbohydrate source in milk, but lactase activity is shut off after weaning in most species. Most human populations lose lactase activity during adolescence as a normal part of maturation. Members of the northern European gene pool typically maintain lactase activity into adult life, but lactase activity declines gradually in many. At some point the amount of lactose ingested might exceed the ability of the remaining enzyme to hydrolyze it, resulting in lactose malabsorption and symptoms. This also can occur with acute conditions such as gastroenteritis that can disturb the mucosa and temporarily reduce lactase activity. Patients might not recognize lactose ingestion as a cause of their problem because they have not had difficulty tolerating lactose in the past. Restriction of lactose in the diet (or use of products that have predigested lactose) mitigates symptoms. Use of exogenous lactase as a tablet may only be partially effective because of incomplete hydrolysis of ingested lactose.

In an analogous way, an acquired lack of sucrase-isomaltase activity might lead to digestive symptoms often interpreted as irritable bowel syndrome. This condition can be diagnosed by breath testing and treated with a restrictive diet and sacrosidase, a yeast enzyme with sucrase activity.

Transport Defects at the Brush Border

Glucose-galactose malabsorption is a rare congenital disorder resulting from an inactive hexose transporter in the brush border. Hydrolysis of lactose is intact, but transport across the apical membrane of the enterocyte fails to occur. Fructose absorption, which is mediated by a different carrier, is unaffected.

In all human beings, the ability to absorb fructose is limited by the availability of carriers in the brush border and may be overwhelmed when excess fructose is ingested. This can occur relatively easily nowadays, because high-fructose corn syrup is used frequently as a sweetener in commercial products such as soda pop. Limiting the amount of fructose ingested will reduce symptoms.

Abetalipoproteinemia is a rare condition that prevents absorption of long-chain fatty acids due to failure to form chylomicrons. Use of medium-chain triglycerides that do not require transport in chylomicrons can bypass this defect.

Pernicious anemia develops when failure to secrete intrinsic factor in the stomach prevents vitamin B_{12} absorption by the ileal mucosa. Parenteral replacement with cyanocobalamin by injection (Cyanoject) or nasal spray (Nascobal) is necessary.

Generalized Malabsorption
Celiac Disease

Celiac disease (also known as celiac sprue) is a disorder in which the mucosa of the small bowel is damaged due to activation of the mucosal immune system by ingestion of gluten, a protein component found in wheat, barley, and rye. People who have HLA-DQ2 or DQ8 are susceptible to this condition because these specific antigen-presenting proteins produce particularly strong reactions by interacting with a unique peptide digestion product of gluten. Tissue transglutaminase, an enzyme produced in the mucosa, is an important cofactor in pathogenesis by amplifying the immunogenicity of gluten peptide fragments and is the target of autoantibodies that are characteristic of this disease. The condition produces generalized malabsorption by destroying the villi of the small intestine, reducing the surface area available for absorption.

In addition to malabsorption syndrome with diarrhea and weight loss, celiac disease can produce a host of nonspecific symptoms, including abdominal pain, fatigue, muscle and joint pains, and headaches and seemingly unrelated problems such as iron deficiency anemia, abnormal liver tests, and osteoporosis. These protean manifestations mean that celiac disease must be considered in the differential diagnosis of many conditions. The clinical course is quite variable, with symptoms coming and going. Symptoms can develop during childhood and produce growth retardation or first become manifest in adulthood.

Testing for celiac disease has been simplified by the development of an assay for anti–tissue transglutaminase antibodies. This test largely supplants measurement of antigluten antibodies, although these remain of some use in evaluating adherence to a gluten-free diet. IgA antibodies are the most useful for diagnosis, but IgA deficiency is common enough that an IgA level should be measured concomitantly.

Although serologic tests have high sensitivity and specificity, the implications of adhering to a gluten-free diet are so extreme that the diagnosis of celiac disease should be confirmed whenever possible by small bowel mucosal biopsy, now obtained routinely by endoscopy. An empiric trial of a gluten-free diet may be difficult to interpret because many persons with gastrointestinal symptoms improve with dietary carbohydrate restriction. Wheat starch is particularly hard to digest; ordinarily 20% of wheat starch is not digested and absorbed by the small bowel, and enters the colon.

Treatment of celiac disease at present involves strict lifetime exclusion of gluten from the diet. This is a difficult regimen that excludes most processed foods. Assistance of a dietitian is most helpful. The prognosis with effective treatment is very good. Symptoms should respond to the diet within weeks; failure to do so should prompt an examination of compliance with the diet or reconsideration of the diagnosis. Failure to respond may be seen when lymphoma or adenocarcinoma complicate the course of celiac disease or in cases of "refractory sprue" or "collagenous sprue," which can have a different autoimmune basis from classic celiac disease and which might respond to immunosuppressive drugs such as corticosteroids or azathioprine (Imuran).[1] Persistent diarrhea may be observed in patients with celiac disease who have concomitant microscopic colitis, another condition that is linked to HLA-DQ2 and HLA-DQ8.

Olmesartan (Benicar) and perhaps other angiotensin II receptor blockers can produce enteropathies resembling celiac disease clinically, but which are not related to gluten ingestion. Diarrhea and malabsorption resolve with discontinuing the medication.

Inflammatory Diseases

Diseases that produce extensive mucosal damage by inflammation cause generalized malabsorption by reduction of mucosal surface area, by promotion of small bowel bacterial overgrowth, by ileal dysfunction, or by development of enteroenteral or enterocolic fistulas. Examples include jejunoileitis due to Crohn's disease, nongranulomatous ulcerative jejunoileitis, radiation enteritis, and chronic mesenteric ischemia. With Crohn's disease, previous resection can add to the problem (see later). Therapy aimed at the underlying process can improve absorption; in some cases (e.g., radiation enteritis), no effective therapy is available for the underlying problem, and symptomatic management is all that is possible. This includes use of antidiarrheal drugs to prolong contact time between luminal contents and the small bowel mucosa, ingestion of a reduced-fat diet to reduce steatorrhea, and use of vitamin and mineral supplements to prevent deficiency states.

Infiltrative Disorders

Several conditions involve infiltration of the intestinal mucosa with cells or extracellular matrix that impede absorption or modify mucosal function by secretion of cytokines and other regulatory substances. These include eosinophilic gastroenteritis, systemic mastocytosis, immunoproliferative small intestinal disease (IPSID), lymphoma, and amyloidosis. These conditions are diagnosed by mucosal biopsy, but special stains might have to be employed to identify the infiltrating cells or matrix accurately.

Treatment of the underlying processes can improve absorption, but it is not uniformly effective. For eosinophilic gastroenteritis, a hypoallergenic (elimination) diet and corticosteroids may be useful. Mild systemic mastocytosis is treated with the mast cell-stabilizer sodium chromoglycate, H_1- and H_2-receptor antagonists, and low-dose aspirin.[1] More advanced disease might respond to interferon or cytotoxic chemotherapy. IPSID initially is treated with antibiotics, because small bowel bacterial overgrowth may be a causative factor. Once malignant change has occurred, it is treated like lymphoma with cytotoxic chemotherapy. Amyloidosis affecting the gut is not amenable to therapy and is usually fatal.

---

[1]Not FDA approved for this indication.

Infectious Diseases

Small Bowel Bacterial Overgrowth. Small bowel overgrowth in the jejunum can produce generalized malabsorption. It can occur whenever the mechanisms that reduce overgrowth are compromised. These situations include achlorhydria or hypochlorhydria, motility disorders of the small intestine (e.g., diabetes mellitus or scleroderma), and anatomic alterations (e.g., diverticulosis, gastrocolic fistula, or blind loops postoperatively). Fat malabsorption is attributed to bacterial deconjugation of bile acid. Bacterial toxins or free fatty acids can produce patchy mucosal damage, leading to less efficient carbohydrate and protein absorption. Bacteria also can compete with the mucosa for uptake of certain nutrients such as vitamin B_{12}.

Diagnosis of small bowel bacterial overgrowth can be difficult (see earlier). Treatment consists of antibiotic therapy unless a surgically correctable anatomic defect is discovered. Tetracycline is no longer uniformly effective; amoxicillin–clavulanic acid (Augmentin), cephalosporins, ciprofloxacin (Cipro), metronidazole (Flagyl), and rifaximin (Xifaxan)[1] may be employed. Therapy should be given for 1 to 2 weeks initially and then discontinued. It should be restarted when symptoms recur. If this occurs quickly, longer treatment periods should be considered. Continuous antibiotic therapy is needed rarely.

Tropical Sprue. Tropical sprue is a progressive, chronic malabsorptive condition occurring in both the indigenous population and in visitors residing in certain tropical countries for extended periods. The prevalence of tropical sprue seems to be decreasing for uncertain reasons. The disease starts as an acute diarrheal disease that becomes a persistent diarrhea associated with substantial weight loss and typically megaloblastic anemia. Villi become shortened and thickened (partial villous atrophy), but the flat mucosa of celiac disease is not usually present. Enterocytes have disrupted brush borders and can have megaloblastic changes; the submucosa has a chronic inflammatory infiltrate. Intestinal biopsy is required for diagnosis.

Currently, tropical sprue is believed to represent a form of bacterial overgrowth with organisms that secrete enterotoxins. Most patients have evidence of excessive gram-negative bacterial colonization of the jejunum. The declining prevalence of tropical sprue may be due to improved nutrition, better sanitation, or prompt treatment of acute diarrhea with antibiotics. Treatment consists of pharmacologic doses of folic acid (folate) (5 mg daily[3]), injection of cyanocobalamin (if deficient), and antibiotic therapy for 1 to 6 months. Tetracycline 250 mg four times a day or sulfonamide is the treatment of choice. Newer antibiotics have not been tested extensively in this condition. Improvement should be noted after a few weeks. The prognosis with treatment is excellent; without treatment, tropical sprue can be fatal. Recurrence can occur.

Whipple's Disease. Whipple's disease is a rare chronic bacterial infection with multisystem involvement. The small bowel typically is heavily infiltrated with foamy macrophages containing periodic acid–Schiff (PAS)-positive material, distorting the villi. Small bowel biopsy with special stains or electron microscopy or a specific polymerase chain reaction (PCR) is diagnostic. Foamy macrophages and bacteria can be found outside the intestine in lymph nodes, spleen, liver, central nervous system, heart, and synovium. Accordingly, symptoms are protean. The bacterium has been identified as *Tropheryma whipplei*, a relative of *Acinetobacter*. It does not appear to be very contagious, and no direct person-to-person transmission has been demonstrated. Presumably, differences in host resistance allow proliferation within macrophages without clearance of the bacteria.

Whipple's disease occurs mainly in older white men, but women and all ethnic groups are susceptible. Patients can present with malabsorption syndrome or with symptoms related to the extraintestinal disease (arthritis, fever, dementia, headache, or muscle weakness). Gross or occult gastrointestinal bleeding can occur. Protein-losing enteropathy may be present.

Treatment with any of several antibiotics (penicillin, erythromycin, ampicillin, tetracycline, chloramphenicol, or trimethoprim-sulfamethoxazole [TMP-SMX]) produces excellent symptomatic

responses within days to weeks, but it should be continued for months to years. Even with protracted courses, relapses are common.

Other Infections. *Mycobacterium avium–intracellulare* is another chronic bacterial infection that can cause malabsorption, particularly in patients with AIDS. Mucosal biopsy with special stains to distinguish it from Whipple's disease is essential. Antibiotic therapy can reduce the intensity of infection; clearance depends on immunologic reconstitution with antiretroviral therapy. Clarithromycin (Biaxin) and ethambutol (Myambutol) are recommended as initial therapy.

Parasitic diseases can produce malabsorption by competing for nutrients and causing mechanical occlusion of the absorptive surface and epithelial damage. Protozoa that may be associated with malabsorption include *Giardia lamblia*, *Cystoisospora belli*, *Cryptosporidium*, and *Enterocytozoon bieneusi*. Tapeworms associated with malabsorption include *Taenia saginata* (beef tapeworm), *Hymenolepis nana* (dwarf tapeworm), and *Diphyllobothrium latum* (fish tapeworm).

Giardia lamblia is a cosmopolitan parasite acquired from contaminated water or from another person by fecal-oral transmission. Cysts are relatively hardy, and ingestion of as few as 10 cysts is sufficient to establish infection. Patients with dysgammaglobulinemia (especially IgA deficiency) are likely to become infected. Diagnosis depends on finding the organism (cysts or trophozoites) in stool by microscopy (sensitivity ~50% for a single specimen), or detection of giardia antigens by immunologic testing of stool (sensitivity >90%), multiplex PCR testing (sensitivity >95%), or discovery of the organism on small bowel biopsy.

Therapy consists of a single dose of tinidazole (Tindamax) (2 g), metronidazole (Flagyl)[1] (250 mg three times a day for a week), nitazoxanide (Alinia) (500 mg twice a day for three days), or quinacrine[2] (100 mg three times a day for a week).

Cystoisospora and *Cryptosporidium* spp. are coccidia, protozoa that disrupt the epithelium by intracellular invasion *(Cystoisospora)* or by attaching to the brush border, destroying microvilli *(Cryptosporidium)*. Stool examination or small bowel biopsy can identify the organism. *Cryptosporidium* can be discovered by antigen immunoassay or multiplex PCR testing on stool with excellent sensitivity. *Cystoisospora* can be treated with trimethoprim/sulfamethoxazole (TMP-SMX)[1] or furazolidone.[2] *Cryptosporidium* can be treated by nitazoxanide.

Microsporidia are intracellular organisms now believed to be most closely related to fungi and are implicated in diarrhea and malabsorption in patients with AIDS and other immunodeficiency states. Small bowel biopsy can show partial villous atrophy, and electron microscopy displays characteristic changes. Stool examination occasionally is helpful. No treatment is of proven value.

Tapeworms compete with their hosts for nutrients in the lumen. *Diphyllobothrium latum* can produce vitamin B_{12} deficiency. The others can result in more extensive nutritional deficiencies. Diagnosis is based on stool examination, and treatment depends on the particular organism identified.

Luminal Problems Causing Malabsorption

Pancreatic Exocrine Insufficiency. Pancreatic exocrine insufficiency is the most common luminal problem that results in maldigestion. Patients develop symptoms of malabsorption when pancreatic enzyme secretion is reduced by >90%. There are several clinical features that distinguish pancreatic exocrine insufficiency from mucosal disorders, such as celiac disease. When fat is not digested, it is transported through the gastrointestinal tract as intact triglyceride, which can appear as oil in the stool. In contrast, if fat is digested but not absorbed, it is in the form of fatty acids that can produce secretory diarrhea in the colon, resulting in more voluminous, even watery stools. This has two important ramifications: Fecal fat concentration is lower with mucosal disease (typically

---

[3]Exceeds dosage recommended by the manufacturer.

[1]Not FDA approved for this indication.
[2]Not available in the United States.

<9% by weight), and hypocalcemia due to formation of soaps (calcium plus 2 fatty acids) is seen with mucosal disease but not with pancreatic exocrine insufficiency. In addition, patients with mucosal disease tend to have more problems with water-soluble vitamin deficiencies than those with pancreatic exocrine insufficiency. In some patients with pancreatic exocrine insufficiency, carbohydrate malabsorption can produce substantial bloating, flatulence, and watery diarrhea.

Tests to document pancreatic exocrine insufficiency are not widely available or are nonspecific (see earlier), and so diagnosis usually hinges on a consistent history, demonstration of anatomic problems in the pancreas (calcification or abnormal ducts), and documentation of a response of steatorrhea to empiric treatment with a large dose of exogenous enzymes.

Bile Acid Deficiency. Bile acid deficiency is a less common cause of maldigestion, and malabsorption in this setting is limited to fat and fat-soluble vitamins. The usual setting is a patient with an extensive ileal resection (see later), but this also occurs in certain cholestatic conditions in which bile acid secretion by the liver is markedly compromised, such as advanced primary biliary cholangitis or complete extrahepatic biliary obstruction. As with pancreatic exocrine insufficiency, stools tend to have high fat concentrations (>9% by weight) when bile acid secretion is limited by hepatic or biliary disorders.

Zollinger-Ellison Syndrome. Zollinger-Ellison syndrome produces several abnormalities that can affect absorption. High rates of gastric acid secretion produce persistently low pH in the duodenum, which precipitates bile acid and inactivates pancreatic enzymes. In addition, excess acid can damage the absorptive cells directly.

Postoperative Malabsorption

Substantial malabsorption can result from bariatric or other gastric surgeries. Weight loss can result from inadequate intake due to early satiety or symptoms of dumping syndrome. Malabsorption can result from impaired mechanical disruption of food, mismatching of chyme delivery and enzyme secretion, rapid transit, or small bowel bacterial overgrowth due to loss of the gastric acid barrier. In addition, gastric surgery sometimes brings out latent celiac disease.

Short intestinal resections are well tolerated, but more extensive resections produce diarrhea and malabsorption of variable severity. When these symptoms are associated with weight loss or dehydrating diarrhea, short bowel syndrome is said to exist. In general, nutrient absorptive needs can be met if at least 100 cm of jejunum are preserved, but fluid absorption will be insufficient and diarrhea may be profuse. The process of intestinal adaptation permits improved absorption with time; it depends on exposure of the absorptive surface to nutrients. Absorption of specific substances, such as bile acids or vitamin B_{12}, is reduced permanently by resection of the terminal ileum.

Malabsorption in short bowel syndrome is not due solely to loss of absorptive surface area. Gastric acid hypersecretion, bile acid deficiency, rapid transit (due to loss of the ileal brake), and bacterial overgrowth may be present. These conditions are amenable to treatment and therapy with antisecretory drugs, exogenous bile acids, opiate antidiarrheals, or antibiotics can produce substantial improvement. Injection of teduglutide (Gattex), a glucagon-like peptide-2 intestinal growth factor, or growth hormone in combination with glutamine and a special diet have been approved as treatments for short bowel syndrome; they can reduce the volume of parenteral fluid or nutrients required. Results with small bowel transplantation are improving with the use of better immunosuppressive regimens, and it remains the only cure for select patients with postresection malabsorption.

Attention to nutrition is vital in any patient with malabsorption. If adequate nutrition cannot be maintained by oral intake, nutritional therapy is needed. Because of impaired bowel function, success with enteral nutrition may be impossible; parenteral nutrition may be needed. It is important to distinguish between the need for supplemental fluid and electrolytes and the need for nutrients; total parenteral nutrition is not a good choice for patients who only require fluids and electrolytes.

References

Benardout M, Le Gresley A, El-Shaer A, Wren SP. Fructose malabsorption: causes, diagnosis and treatment. *Br J Nutr* 127:481–489, 2022.

Boumaza A, Azzouz EB, Arrindell J, et al. Whipple's disease and Tropheryma whipplei infections: from bench to bedside. *Lancet Infect Dis* 22:e280–e291, 2022.

Bushyhead D, Quigley EMM. Small intestinal bacterial overgrowth—pathophysiology and its implications for definition and management. *Gastroenterology* 163:593–607, 2022.

Diéguez-Castillo C, Jiménez-Luna C, Prados J, et al. State of the art in exocrine pancreatic insufficiency. *Medicina (Kaunas)* 56:523, 2020.

Felsenreich DM, Langer FB, Eichelter J, et al. Bariatric surgery—how much malabsorption do we need?—a review of various limb lengths in different gastric bypass procedures. *J Clin Med* 10:674, 2021.

Fernández-Bañares F. Carbohydrate malabsorption and intolerance. *Nutrients* 14:1923, 2022.

Frissora CL, Rao SSC. Sucrose intolerance in adults with common functional gastrointestinal symptoms. Proc *(Bayl Univ Med Cent)* 35:790–793, 2022.

Lebwohl B, Rubio-Tapia A. Epidemiology, presentation, and diagnosis of celiac disease. *Gastroenterology* 160:63–75, 2021.

Massey BT, Wald A. Small intestinal bacterial overgrowth syndrome: a guide for the appropriate use of breath testing. *Dig Dis Sci* 66:338–347, 2021.

Misselwitz B, Butter M, Verbeke K, Fox MR. Update on lactose malabsorption and intolerance: pathogenesis, diagnosis and clinical management. *Gut* 68:2080–2091, 2019.

Montoro-Huguet MA, Belloc B, Domínguez-Cajal M. Small and large intestine (I): malabsorption of nutrients. *Nutrients* 13:1254, 2021.

Silvester JA, Therrien A, Kelly CP. Celiac disease: fallacies and facts. *Am J Gastroenterol* 116:1148–1155, 2021.

NONALCOHOLIC FATTY LIVER DISEASE (NAFLD)

Method of
Nicole Boschuetz, MD; Hiep Phan, MD; and Adnan Said, MD, MS

CURRENT DIAGNOSIS

- Suspected in patients with steatosis noted on imaging or elevated liver enzymes (alanine aminotransferase, aspartate aminotransferase, γ-glutamyl transferase) in the setting of metabolic syndrome, type 2 diabetes or obesity
- Diagnosis of exclusion
  - Quantify alcohol use by history
  - Hepatitis C virus antibody and hepatitis B surface antigen should be negative
  - Review medications that can cause steatosis (methotrexate [Trexall], tamoxifen [Nolvadex], diltiazem [Cardizem], amiodarone [Pacerone], steroids)
  - Check serum ferritin, iron saturation (hemochromatosis)
  - Check serum ceruloplasmin and unbound copper (Wilson disease)
  - Check autoantibodies (antinuclear antibody, antismooth muscle antibody) (autoimmune hepatitis)
- Liver biopsy gold standard
  - Not essential for diagnosis
  - Useful for diagnosis of nonalcoholic steatohepatitis and fibrosis
  - Useful in excluding other conditions (if the preceding tests raise suspicion)
- Noninvasive serum tests (more useful for diagnosis or exclusion of advanced fibrosis and potentially in decision to biopsy or perform elastography)
  - Nonalcoholic Fatty Liver Disease Fibrosis Score
  - FIB-4 Index
- Noninvasive imaging tests for diagnosis of steatosis
  - Transient elastography with controlled attenuation parameter score
  - Right upper quadrant ultrasound
  - Magnetic resonance imaging of liver with proton density fat fraction
- Noninvasive imaging tests for diagnosis of fibrosis
  - Transient elastography with FibroScan
  - Magnetic resonance elastography

CURRENT THERAPY

Lifestyle Modifications Mainstay of Therapeutic Plan
- Goal is to lose 7% to 10% of body weight gradually over 6 to 12 months
- Lose no more than 0.5 to 1 kg/week

Dietary Modification
- Reduce calories by 30% (500 to 1000 kcal/day)
- Reduce sugars, simple carbohydrates, fructose-enriched foods, and sugar-sweetened beverages
- Reduce consumption of processed foods and saturated fat
- Coffee consumption (>3 cups/day, avoid adding sugar, syrups) has been shown to be beneficial

Exercise
- 150 to 200 minutes per week divided over 3 to 5 days
  - Moderate to vigorous intensity (swimming, biking, jogging, playing tennis, weights)

Treatment
- Pioglitazone (Actos)[1] can be used for diabetic or nondiabetic nonalcoholic steatohepatitis (NASH) but causes weight gain and does not treat fibrosis
- Vitamin E (800 IU/day)[7] can be used for nondiabetic NASH but does not treat fibrosis
- Bariatric surgery can be considered if indicated for morbid obesity and complications of metabolic syndrome and may reverse NASH

[1]Not FDA approved for this indication.
[7]Available as dietary supplement.

Note: Discussions regarding the naming of nonalcoholic fatty liver disease (NAFLD) and nonalcoholic steatohepatitis (NASH) have been ongoing over the last few years. This is due, in part, to concerns over the use of stigmatizing language. After this chapter was written, the American Association for the Study of Liver Disease (AASLD) released a multi-society consensus statement on new fatty liver disease nomenclature. Steatotic liver disease (SLD) has been chosen as the overarching term to cover the various causes of hepatic steatosis. NAFLD will now be referred to as metabolic dysfunction-associated steatotic liver disease (MASLD), and metabolic dysfunction-associated steatohepatitis (MASH) has replaced NASH. Further categories have been added to include "MetALD," which covers those with MASLD and increased alcohol intake. Further information about these changes can be found in the AASLD consensus paper. At this time, NAFLD and NASH will be used in this chapter, and nomenclature will be updated in future editions.

Nonalcoholic Fatty Liver Disease

Nonalcoholic fatty liver disease (NAFLD) is defined as the presence of hepatic steatosis (hepatic fat accumulation), on imaging or liver biopsy, in the absence of secondary causes for the fat accumulation (such as excessive alcohol consumption, hepatitis B or C, or certain medications). NAFLD is closely associated with metabolic comorbidities, including obesity, diabetes, dyslipidemia, and hypertension and is the most common cause of chronic liver disease worldwide.

NAFLD comprises a spectrum of disease spanning from isolated steatosis (sometimes called nonalcoholic fatty liver [NAFL]) to more advanced liver disease such as nonalcoholic steatohepatitis (NASH) (Figure 1). NASH signifies steatosis with inflammation and hepatocyte injury and has a higher likelihood of progress to cirrhosis, liver failure, and occasionally liver cancer. Besides liver disease, NAFLD is also closely associated with cardiovascular disease (CVD) and malignancy.

Epidemiology of NAFLD

The global prevalence of NAFLD has been steadily increasing over the past 2 decades with the current overall estimate being 32%. Alarmingly, the prevalence in North America was reported to be 48% with the recent U.S. National Health and Nutrition Examination Survey (NHANES) data from 2017 to 2018 demonstrating a prevalence of up to 59% in the United States. Other notable rates include 32% in Asia and 33% in Europe. There are limited recent studies for South America or Africa though previous rates have been estimated to be 30% and 14%, respectively.

In the United States, the prevalence of NAFLD is highest in Hispanic Americans (22% to 45%), followed by non-Hispanic Whites (15% to 33%) and African Americans (13% to 24%). A significant contribution to this ethnic difference can be explained by genetic differences, particularly a single nucleotide polymorphism (SNP) in a gene (PNPLA3) that is involved in triglyceride (TG) (lipid) hydrolysis in the liver, the ethnic prevalence of which mirrors the ethnic differences in frequency of NAFLD.

NAFLD prevalence increases with age, with a range from 22% to 30% from age 30 to a peak in the sixth decade. Very few studies report on NAFLD prevalence after age 70. Pediatric NAFLD is on the rise paralleling childhood obesity trends, but population data are scant, with estimated population prevalence of 7% to 8% in the United States. An autopsy study of 742 children (ages 2 to 19) who died of unnatural causes used liver histology as the gold standard and demonstrated a NAFLD prevalence of 9.6% adjusted for age, sex, race, and ethnicity. Pediatric obesity clinic studies have shown NAFLD prevalence of 34.2% in a meta-analysis.

Differences in sex prevalence also exist with some studies reporting the prevalence of NAFLD in men significantly higher than women (40% vs. 26%).

Although the prevalence of infectious hepatitis has remained stable and even declined, the prevalence of NAFLD has been rising in the global and U.S. adult and pediatric populations, growing in parallel with the epidemic of obesity and metabolic syndrome. The worldwide prevalence of NAFLD was estimated to have progressively increased from 25% to 32% in the last 2 decades. A study using data from the NHANES found that NAFLD prevalence doubled between the survey periods of 1988 to 1994 and 2005 to 2008 from 5.5% to 11%.

In higher-risk populations, such as patients with diabetes, the prevalence of NAFLD is higher, varying from 33% to 70%. In patients with morbid obesity attending bariatric surgery clinics, the prevalence of NAFLD has been reported at 95%.

Risk Factors for NAFLD

NAFLD is a complex disease that has genetic predispositions and is affected by various environmental factors. The degree of contribution of each of the risk factors requires further study and may vary depending on region of the world.

NAFLD is regarded as the hepatic manifestation of the metabolic syndrome (presence of at least three of the following: abdominal obesity, hypertriglyceridemia, low high-density lipoprotein levels, hypertension and high fasting glucose levels). Obesity (defined as waist circumference > 102 cm in men or > 88 cm in women or simplified to body mass index [BMI] ≥ 30) and type 2 diabetes are two of the primary associated risk factors for NAFLD. Underpinning the rising prevalence of these associated conditions and NAFLD are societal and individual trends in unhealthy eating habits (proliferation of high caloric processed foods and diets with a high content of sugar, high fructose corn syrup, and fat) and decreased physical activity levels. The industrialization of food production, as well as deficiencies in neighborhood planning with poor walkability and public transport system availability, are partly to blame for this epidemic.

Being overweight in childhood and adolescence, especially weight gain during school years, is a significant risk factor for development of NAFLD by late childhood and adulthood.

Figure 1 **Histology of nonalcoholic fatty liver disease.** (A) Hepatic steatosis. The *arrow* points to macrovesicular steatosis in hepatocytes. (B) Nonalcoholic steatohepatitis (NASH). The *arrow* points to ballooned hepatocytes. The *arrowhead* points to lobular inflammation. (C) NASH with cirrhosis. The *arrow* points to fibrosis bands (collagen). Trichrome stain.

Several genetic risk factors have been reported, with non-synonymous SNPs in certain genes in particular, *PNPLA3* (patatin-like phospholipase domain-containing protein 3), *TM6SF2* (transmembrane 6 superfamily member 2), and *MBOAT7* (membrane bound O-acyltransferase domain containing 7) being the most consistently validated. The prevalence of the *PNPLA3* SNP is highest in the Hispanic population and leads to the higher prevalence of NAFLD in this population. The *PNPLA3 I148M* genetic mutation has consistently been shown to be the most common genetic determinant of NAFLD and correlates with hepatic steatosis, as well as severity of liver disease and risk of cirrhosis and liver cancer in NAFLD. More recently, loss of function variants in *HSD17B13* (hydroxysteroid 17-beta dehydrogenase 13) and *CIDEB* have been found to be protective against NAFLD and NASH.

Heavy alcohol intake and obesity have been shown to act synergistically in increasing the risk of liver disease. The effect of more moderate alcohol consumption on NAFLD is unclear currently, though recent data suggest that moderate alcohol use lowers odds of NASH resolution and increases risk of malignancy. Any alcohol use should be avoided completely in those with clinically significant hepatic fibrosis. There are population data suggesting that low levels of alcohol use (1 or fewer drinks per day), wine in particular, may be associated with lower risk of developing NAFLD compared with those who drink more or do not drink at all, although these data are of low quality.

NASH, which has a higher chance of progression to fibrosis and cirrhosis, is independently associated with diabetes, age, BMI, and genetic polymorphisms in *PNPLA3*.

Pathophysiology of NAFLD

The hallmark finding of NAFLD is accumulation of triglyceride (TG) in the cytoplasm of hepatocytes. This is caused by an imbalance between lipid buildup (fatty acid uptake and de novo lipogenesis) and removal (mitochondrial fatty acid oxidation and export as a part of very low-density lipoprotein particles). Further factors contributing to transition from a healthy liver to NAFLD include adipose tissue dysfunction, hepatic insulin resistance (IR), dysbiosis of the gut microbiome, toxic metabolites, and genetic factors (Figure 2).

Along with storage of TGs, adipose tissue is involved in the secretion of hormones, cytokines, and chemokines called adipokines. Overnutrition and/or sedentary lifestyle causes obesity and adipose tissue dysfunction, which likely plays a pivotal role in the development of IR and NAFLD. Obesity results in excess free fatty acids (FFAs) entering the liver through the portal circulation, which can increase lipid synthesis and gluconeogenesis. Increased levels of circulating FFAs also lead to peripheral IR along with inflammation and induction of cytokine production, thereby contributing to NAFLD. In NASH, liver cell injury occurs (ballooning hepatocytes, inflammation) along with steatosis and varying degree of fibrosis.

Clinical Manifestations of NAFLD

NAFLD patients are typically asymptomatic until the condition progresses to cirrhosis. Early in the course of disease, it is often found incidentally on abdominal imaging including ultrasound (US), computed tomography (CT), or magnetic resonance imaging (MRI) (hepatic steatosis). Hepatomegaly may be the presenting symptom is some patients. Vague right upper abdominal discomfort, malaise, and/or fatigue can occur in patients with NASH but is very nonspecific.

The other common presentation of NAFLD is with elevation of liver enzymes with mild to moderate elevations in aspartate aminotransferase (AST) and alanine aminotransferase (ALT). However, even advanced NAFLD can present with normal liver

Figure 2 Pathophysiology of nonalcoholic fatty liver disease. An interaction between intestine, adipose tissue, and hepatocytes. *FFAs,* Free fatty acids; *IL,* interleukin; *TLR,* Toll-like receptor; *TNF,* tumor necrosis factor.

enzyme levels in up to 30% of individuals, and NASH cannot be excluded based on normal liver enzymes alone.

NAFLD patients frequently have comorbidities including hyperlipidemia, obesity, metabolic syndrome, hypertension, and type 2 diabetes mellitus. Associated conditions also include hypothyroidism, obstructive sleep apnea, and less commonly hypopituitarism, hypogonadism, polycystic ovarian syndrome, pancreaticoduodenal resection, and psoriasis.

In a community study following NAFLD patients for over 7 years, there was excessive risk of mortality compared with the general population based age- and sex-matched controls (standardized mortality ratio 1.34, 1.003 to 1.76). Given the commonality of risk factors for NAFLD and CVD, cardiac disease is a leading cause of mortality in these patients. A meta-analysis of observational studies also confirmed the increased risk of CVD in NAFLD (odds ratio [OR] 1.64, 1.26 to 2.13) and NASH (OR 2.58, 1.78 to 3.75). Obesity, diabetes, and metabolic syndrome are also risk factors for carcinogenesis, and a multitude of cancers are increased in patients with NAFLD, including liver cancer, breast cancer, kidney cancer, and colon cancer. Liver disease from cirrhosis and liver cancer is the third most common risk of mortality in these patients.

NAFLD is an increasingly common reason for decompensated cirrhosis and liver cancer. Over their lifetime, 5% to 10% of patients with NAFLD progress to cirrhosis. Isolated hepatic steatosis without evidence of hepatocellular injury (NAFL) carries a minimal risk of progression to cirrhosis (<2%). Patients who are older or have type 2 diabetes are at higher risk for progressing to NASH and fibrosis. On the other hand, NASH has a higher likelihood of progress to cirrhosis (5% to 12%), liver failure, and occasionally liver cancer. Additionally, those with NASH who are identified to have stage 2 fibrosis or higher carry a significantly higher lifetime risk of liver-related mortality and morbidity. In these patients, liver disease mortality predominates the clinical picture. Complications of cirrhosis including variceal hemorrhage, ascites, hepatic encephalopathy, and liver failure can occur.

NAFLD is the second most common indication of liver transplantation in the United States after alcohol-related liver disease and is the most common indication of liver transplantation in women. In the U.S. general population, NAFLD is already one of the most common reasons for developing liver cancer with the risk of developing liver cancer in patients with NAFLD-related cirrhosis being 1% to 2% per year. Hepatocellular cancer (HCC) in NASH, like in most other chronic liver diseases, occurs predominantly in the setting of cirrhosis. Age, obesity, diabetes and

PNPLA3 I148M SNP are risk factors for HCC in these patients. NAFLD-associated HCC is the third most common cause of HCC in the United States, and the incidence of NAFLD-associated HCC is increasing the fastest by a 9% annual incidence rate compared with other causes of HCC.

Diagnosis of NAFLD

The diagnosis of NAFLD (Figure 3) is made by confirming the presence of hepatic steatosis on either imaging or liver biopsy, in the absence of alternative explanations for the steatosis. Diagnosing NAFLD based on elevated liver enzymes alone (without imaging or biopsy) is not recommended. Not only are elevations of liver enzymes nonspecific, but they are also frequently normal in patients with NAFLD, including in those with advanced liver disease.

Alternate causes of steatosis that must be excluded before diagnosing NAFLD include the following:
- Alcohol excess (typically defined as >21 standard drinks of alcohol per week in men and >14 drinks per week in women)
- Hepatitis B/C infection
- Medications that cause steatosis (amiodarone [Pacerone], tamoxifen [Nolvadex], methotrexate [Trexall], diltiazem [Cardizem], prednisone)
- Hemochromatosis
- Wilson disease
- Autoimmune hepatitis

These conditions are easily screened for by history and serologies for these conditions. Excess alcohol use alone may lead to hepatic steatosis and steatohepatitis; however, many patients with NAFLD may also drink low or moderate amounts of alcohol. These two causes of hepatic steatosis may work synergistically and contribute to a faster progression of fibrosis, so a thorough alcohol use history should be obtained. During serologic workup in patients with suspected NAFLD, it is common to find elevated ferritin. This is due to NAFLD itself in the majority of cases. In patients with significantly elevated ferritin and transferrin saturation, serum testing for mutations in the hemochromatosis gene *(HFE)* should be performed, and if there are heterozygous or homozygous mutations in this gene, a liver biopsy should be performed for iron quantification. It is also common to find autoantibodies in NAFLD that are often elevated in autoimmune hepatitis (antinuclear antibody > 1:160, anti–smooth muscle antibody > 1:40). These are often epiphenomena, but if the level of liver enzymes is significantly elevated (greater than fivefold above normal), a liver biopsy can be done to exclude autoimmune hepatitis.

Figure 3 Diagnostic evaluation for suspected nonalcoholic fatty liver disease. *ELF,* Enhanced Liver Fibrosis Score; *FIB-4,* Fibrosis-4 score; *HDL,* high-density lipoprotein; *LFTs,* liver function tests; *MRE,* magnetic resonance elastography; *T2DM,* type 2 diabetes mellitus; *TG,* triglyceride; *VCTE,* vibration-controlled elastography.

NAFLD is usually diagnosed in one of two common scenarios:
1. Patients with unsuspected hepatic steatosis detected on imaging done for other indications (US or CT).
2. Patients with unexplained abnormal liver chemistries (liver enzymes), who should be assessed for associated metabolic risk factors (obesity, diabetes mellitus, or dyslipidemia).

Recent guidelines suggest targeted screening for patients at increased risk for advanced liver disease to identify clinically significant fibrosis (stage 2 or greater) including those with type 2 diabetes and medically complicated obesity. For these patients, it is recommended that noninvasive screening should be considered every 1 to 2 years (discussed later).

It is essential to emphasize that a diagnosis of NAFLD includes the determination of whether progressive liver disease, NASH, and/or fibrosis are present to tailor treatment and monitoring. The state of comorbidities including dyslipidemia, obesity, IR, diabetes, hypothyroidism, polycystic ovary syndrome, and sleep apnea is important to evaluate at the initial evaluation to recommend specific treatment for these associated disorders.

Role of Liver Biopsy in NAFLD

Currently, the gold standard for establishing a diagnosis of NAFLD and staging fibrosis is liver biopsy. In NAFLD, liver histology typically shows steatosis graded as mild (<33% of hepatocytes involved), moderate (33% to 66%) or severe (>66%). Other findings seen in NASH include lobular inflammation and hepatocyte ballooning indicative of hepatocyte injury, as well as varying degrees of fibrosis from none (stage 0 fibrosis) to cirrhosis (stage 4 fibrosis).

Although liver biopsy is not essential for diagnosing hepatic steatosis, liver biopsy should be considered in patients with NAFLD in the following situations:
1. Patients who are at increased risk of having steatohepatitis (NASH) and/or advanced fibrosis because no serum or radiologic marker thus far can reliably differentiate NASH from isolated steatosis. Thus patients who are older (>50 years), have long-standing metabolic syndrome, or have noninvasive evaluations that suggest advanced fibrosis should undergo biopsy for better characterization of their liver disease. Discussed later, these noninvasive studies would include NAFLD fibrosis score, Fibrosis-4 (FIB-4) scores, and liver stiffness measured by imaging techniques such as vibration controlled transient elastography (VCTE) or MRI-based elastography (MRE).
2. Liver biopsy should also be considered when presence and/or severity of coexisting chronic liver diseases cannot be excluded

without a liver biopsy. This may include patients with serum antibodies in whom coexistent autoimmune hepatitis cannot be excluded or patients with significantly elevated ferritin and iron saturation.

Despite the useful information obtained in some patients with NAFLD, liver biopsy has several limitations, including sampling error and intraobserver and interobserver variability in interpretation. It is costly, invasive, and carries risks of mortality (up to 0.1%), pain, intraperitoneal bleeding, bile leaks, and infection. As a result, it is not practical for screening millions of at-risk individuals and for frequent repeated assessments. Noninvasive approaches to diagnosis of NAFLD are thus used widely.

Noninvasive Testing in NAFLD
MRI and Ultrasound
Abnormal hepatic steatosis is defined by a liver fat content of 5% or greater. The most accurate noninvasive method to quantify liver fat content is magnetic resonance spectroscopy. However, this modality requires special expertise, is time-consuming, and is not readily available clinically. A good alternative is MRI that uses proton density fat fraction (MRI-PDFF), which provides an accurate estimate of liver fat content and spatial imaging of the liver. Conventional ultrasonography remains the most commonly used imaging modality to diagnose hepatic steatosis. It is widely available and cheaper than MRI but has limited accuracy, especially in obese individuals. Additionally, it is not sensitive in detecting mild steatosis (<33%) and has lower specificity than MRI for fibrosis.

Elastography
Transient elastography-based techniques are increasingly used to diagnose steatosis and estimate the degree of hepatic fibrosis. Fat and fibrosis affect shear wave propagation through tissue, and this property can be used to measure liver attenuation (steatosis) and velocity (fibrosis) using a specialized US (FibroScan). This machine uses an ultrasonic probe placed over the skin in the right upper quadrant to produce shear waves of 50 MHz that pass through the liver. Measurements of shear wave attenuation called controlled attenuation parameter (CAP) assess for presence and grade of hepatic steatosis. CAP has been shown to be less accurate than MRI-PDFF in diagnosing steatosis but is cheaper and a point-of-care quantitative modality.

Serum Testing
Currently there are many widely available serum-based diagnostic panels for NAFLD that use a mix of serum tests and other demographic/anthropometric measures that are combined in single measurements for diagnosis of NAFLD. Examples include fatty liver index (TGs, BMI, γ-glutamyl transferase, waist circumference) and NAFLD Liver Fat Score (metabolic syndrome, type 2 diabetes mellitus, fasting insulin, ALT, and AST). These panels have been found to have sensitivities and specificities in the 70% range and show reasonable accuracy for predicting steatosis. These tests are not as accurate as imaging or biopsy tests; therefore they are less often used clinically and more often used as research tools in epidemiologic research.

Assessing Fibrosis
Fibrosis is highly correlated with outcomes in liver disease and a marker of worse outcomes. Fibrosis histologically is categorized (staged) as follows on liver biopsy:
- F0: no fibrosis
- F1: portal fibrosis without septa
- F2: portal fibrosis with few septa, extending outside of portal areas
- F3: bridging fibrosis or numerous septa without cirrhosis
- F4: cirrhosis

F3 and F4 are categorized as advanced fibrosis, and F0 and F1 are considered no to minimal fibrosis.

Clinical decision aids such as the NAFLD Fibrosis Score (biomarkers evaluated: age, glucose level, BMI, platelet count,

albumin, and AST/ALT ratio) and Fibrosis-4 Index (FIB-4 biomarkers include age, AST, platelet count, ALT) use a combination of serum and clinical variables to predict the presence of advanced fibrosis or cirrhosis. The Enhanced Liver Fibrosis (ELF) test is a serological test that calculates a score based on serum levels of hyaluronic acid (HA), type III procollagen peptide (PIIINP), and tissue inhibitor of matrix metalloproteinase 1 (TIMP-1). It is approved for prognostication when advanced fibrosis is suspected. When used with the FIB-4 score, the sensitivity and specificity are in the 90% range for predicting advanced fibrosis. These tests are most useful in distinguishing patients who may have advanced fibrosis from those without fibrosis and thus may aid in clinical decision making, including referral to a hepatologist and further workup.

Imaging-based techniques such as VCTE (FibroScan) and MRE can be used to identify those at low or high risk for advanced fibrosis (bridging fibrosis or cirrhosis) with more accuracy than serum-based markers. However, MRE is costly and limited by availability of scanners and reading radiologists. On the other hand, VCTE is increasingly available and can widely be used as point-of-care tests in liver clinics for fibrosis assessment. However, the accuracy of these results are limited in settings of significant obesity, ascites, and acute inflammation. As noted above, the ELF test and FIB-4 score can be used in settings where image-based tests such as the FibroScan are not available.

A suggested algorithm for screening for and diagnosing NAFLD/NASH and advanced fibrosis is shown in Figure 3.

Therapy of NAFLD
Treatment of NAFLD (Table 1) entails treatment of the liver disease and the associated metabolic syndrome (obesity, diabetes, hyperlipidemia, and hypertension).

Lifestyle Modifications in NAFLD
Lifestyle modifications are integral in the treatment of NAFLD at any stage and are the principal intervention for patients with isolated steatosis and NASH without fibrosis. Patients are advised to lose 7% or more of their body weight if overweight or obese (3% to 5% weight loss will improve steatosis; 7% to 10% is needed to improve histopathological features of NASH and fibrosis).

This weight loss is best achieved gradually (losing no more than 0.5 to 1 kg per week) and sustained through a combination of diet and exercise.

Basic principles of diet include reducing calories (by at least 30% or by 750 to 1000 kcal/day for an average U.S. adult) and reducing consumption of simple carbohydrates and saturated fat. Encourage a reduction of sugar-sweetened beverages and of fructose-enriched food and drinks. Fresh fruits and vegetables and lean meats and minimizing processed foods are recommended. Although many different diets have been studied and shown to be beneficial (Mediterranean diet), studies have also shown that any diet that follows these basic principles and results in weight loss achieves the benefits of reversing NASH.

Significant alcohol use can exacerbate steatohepatitis, and limiting consumption of alcohol (≤1 drink/day for women and ≤2 drinks/day for men) is recommended in patients with NASH. For patients with liver fibrosis stage 2 or greater, complete abstinence from alcohol is strongly recommended. There is no safe level of alcohol use at that stage.

A preponderance of epidemiologic data also shows that consumption of coffee (3 or more cups) per day is associated with reduced prevalence of NAFLD. If coffee is consumed, it should be caffeinated with no addition of sweetened syrups, sugar, or large servings of milk or other calories that may negate any beneficial effects.

Recommendations for physical activity include at least 150 to 200 minutes of moderate to vigorous physical activity per week (e.g., moderate jogging, weight training, sports such as tennis, swimming, or biking). For patients who do not exercise at

TABLE 1	Therapy of Nonalcoholic Fatty Liver Disease

Assessment of Steatosis and Fibrosis Staging
Consider pharmacotherapy or investigational agents for more advanced liver disease in addition to lifestyle modifications

Lifestyle Modifications Aimed at Weight Loss
Goals
- Lose 7% to 10% of body weight
- Gradual weight loss, no more than 1 kg/week till at goal

Diet Changes
- Reduce calories by 30% (750 to 1000 kcal/day)
- Reduce simple sugars, saturated fat, and sugar-sweetened beverages and foods including fructose-enriched foods

Exercise
- 150 and 200 minutes per week spaced over 5 days
- Moderate to vigorous intensity (e.g., jogging, playing tennis, swimming laps, biking)

Treatment of Associated Metabolic Factors as per Best Practices
Diabetes
- No particular agent proven beneficial as primary treatment for NAFLD, although pioglitazone (Actos)[1] may benefit histological NASH; be aware of potential weight gain
- Metformin (Glucophage)[1] and DPP-4 inhibitors no proven benefit for NASH
- Insulin can cause weight gain and insulin resistance associated with NASH

Dyslipidemia
- Treat per standard guidelines
- Statins are safe to use if indicated (except in decompensated cirrhosis)

Pharmacotherapy for NASH
Pioglitazone[1]
- Histologic benefits in diabetic and nondiabetic NASH except for fibrosis
- Can cause weight gain

Vitamin E[7]
- Histologic benefits in nondiabetic NASH except for fibrosis
- Concerns for long-term use: small risk in in all-cause mortality, increased risk of prostate cancer

Liraglutide (Victoza, Saxenda)[1], Semaglutide (Ozempic, Wegovy)[1], and Tirzepatide (Mounjaro)[1]
- Improve steatosis, but no specific findings of steatohepatitis or fibrosis improvement

Investigational Trials (Generally for Biopsy-Proven NASH)
Efruxifermin[5]
- Phase 2 trial: reduces hepatic fat fraction and improvement of >1 fibrosis stage

Resmetirom[5]
- Phase 3 trial: improves >1 stage of fibrosis and NASH resolution
- Seeking accelerated FDA approval in 2023

Obeticholic Acid (Ocaliva)[1]
- Phase 3 trial: improvement of fibrosis in 18-month period; further analysis period pending

[1]Not FDA approved for this indication.
[5]Investigational drug in the United States.
[7]Available as dietary supplement.
DPP-4, Dipeptidyl peptidase-4; FDA, U.S. Food and Drug Administration; NAFLD, nonalcoholic fatty liver disease; NASH, nonalcoholic steatohepatitis.

baseline, a gradual buildup to this level is recommended. Limited data suggest that the combination of diet and exercise may be more beneficial than either in isolation.

Bariatric surgery may be considered for patients with BMI greater than 40 kg/m² or greater than 35 kg/m² with comorbidities such as diabetes, hypertension, and hyperlipidemia. NAFLD is increasingly being considered a metabolic comorbidity. Bariatric surgery, malabsorptive procedures in particular, has been shown to resolve NASH, improve fibrosis, and sustain significant weight loss in addition to other health benefits. A 5-year follow up of 180 patients undergoing bariatric surgery with biopsy-proven NASH at the time of surgery found resolution of NASH in 84.4% of patients without worsening of fibrosis and improvement in fibrosis in 70.2%. These improvements were associated with higher amounts of weight loss.

Pharmacotherapeutics in NAFLD

Currently, there are no pharmacologic agents the U.S. Food and Drug Administration (FDA) has indicated specifically for NAFLD or NASH. There are, however, pharmacological treatments aimed at different, components of metabolic syndrome that can be used off-label for NAFLD-related liver disease based on controlled studies and published guidelines. These agents, when used for NAFLD, should generally be limited to those with biopsy-proven NASH and fibrosis.

Pioglitazone (Actos)[1] is an insulin-sensitizing agent used in diabetes (PPARγ agonist) and can be used to treat patients with and without type 2 diabetes with biopsy-proven NASH. It has been shown to improve histologic changes in NASH but not fibrosis.

For nondiabetic adults with biopsy-proven NASH, *Vitamin E*[7] administered at a daily dose of 800 IU/day can be used as well and can cause similar histologic improvements as pioglitazone. It must be noted that trials of these agents in NASH were generally limited to 24 months or less, and longer-term benefits are not known.

Side-effect profiles should also be considered with these therapies. Pioglitazone can cause weight gain, has been associated with osteoporosis, and has been known to exacerbate heart failure in susceptible individuals. Vitamin E has some concerns regarding increased all-cause mortality, a potentially small increased risk of hemorrhagic stroke, and in a large trial, increased risk of prostate cancer. If medications are started for treatment of NASH, ALT should be monitored every 6 to 12 months with medications discontinued if there is less than 20% improvement in ALT from baseline or fibrosis progress.

There are numerous pharmacologic agents in phase 1 and phase 2 trials and a few in phase 3 trials for NAFLD. Some of these agents work on glucose or lipid metabolism in the liver, whereas other are antifibrotic or antioxidant.

Glucagon-like peptide-1 (GLP-1) receptor agonists have been approved for the treatment of diabetes and obesity. Although it is not recommended as a specific treatment for NAFLD, recent small studies have found GLP-1 agonists, specifically liraglutide (Victoza, Saxenda)[1] and semaglutide (Ozempic, Wegovy)[1], are associated with improved steatosis and resolution of NASH, though their effect on fibrosis is less clear. Larger studies on the effects of GLP-1 agonists are ongoing. Tirzepatide (Mounjaro)[1], a GLP-1/glucose-dependent insulinotropic polypeptide receptor agonist, and sodium-glucose cotransporter-2 inhibitors have been shown to decrease hepatic fat content and steatosis in small studies, but the effect on liver histology needs to be better defined.

Efruxifermin[5], a fibroblast growth factor 21 analog, has had promising results in a phase 2 trial, significantly decreasing the MRI hepatic fat fraction (HFF) at 12 weeks compared with placebo with an improvement of greater than 1 stage of fibrosis in 55% of the treatment group whose HFF decreased by greater than 30%.

In a recent phase 3 trial, resmetirom[5], a thyroid hormone receptor beta activator, was found to cause greater than 1 stage improvement in fibrosis without worsening NAS and NASH resolution without worsening fibrosis in 26% and 30% of patients, respectively, at the 100-mg dose; its manufacturer is expected to seek accelerated FDA approval in 2023. Obeticholic acid (Ocaliva)[1] has shown promise in a phase 3 trial, which demonstrated improvement in fibrosis on 18-month interim analysis with further investigation into clinical outcomes ongoing. More safety and efficacy data are needed before these medications can be recommended.

---

[1]Not FDA approved for this indication.
[5]Investigational drug in the United States.
[7]Available as dietary supplement.

Currently, the following drugs are not recommended as specific treatment for NAFLD as they have shown no specific benefit for NASH. Metformin (Glucophage)[1] and dipeptidyl peptidase-4 inhibitors are agents that can be used for diabetes including in patients with NAFLD. However, they have no beneficial effect specifically on NASH. Ursodeoxycholic acid (ursodiol [Actigall])[1] and omega-3 fatty acids[7] can be considered for hypertriglyceridemia concurrent with NAFLD but do not specifically improve NAFLD.

Patients with NAFLD are at high risk for cardiovascular morbidity and mortality, and aggressive modification of CVD risk factors should be considered in all NAFLD patients. Statins can be used to treat dyslipidemia in patients with NAFLD, NASH, and NASH cirrhosis but should be avoided in patients with decompensated cirrhosis.

Prevention of NAFLD

Prevention of NAFLD is imperative and is a societal challenge that should focus on reducing obesity and the metabolic syndrome. Early education and focus on healthy nutrition and childhood physical activity are key initiatives as are neighborhood planning for improving access to healthy foods and healthy spaces.

Monitoring of NAFLD

Patients with NASH, especially those with significant fibrosis, are at the greatest risks for increased progression to cirrhosis and mortality. Patients with NASH and F0 or F1 fibrosis are monitored annually for liver disease progression via blood work (liver enzymes and function tests, platelet counts) and physical examinations. Evaluation of fibrosis progression in these patients can be done via noninvasive serum testing (e.g., FIB-4 score), and if there is evidence of progression of serum fibrosis, further testing through liver biopsy or noninvasive testing such as FibroScan or MRE can be done approximately 5 years after diagnosis; however, with high interindividual variation in fibrosis progression, the timeline of testing is tailored to each individual.

For patients with more advanced fibrosis (F2 or higher) at NASH diagnosis, severity of the fibrosis governs the management. Once F3 or F4 fibrosis occurs, the risk of liver-related illness and death increases significantly, making closer follow-up appropriate.

Patients with NASH cirrhosis should be screened for gastroesophageal varices (upper endoscopy) and considered for HCC screening (American Association for the Study of Liver Diseases guidelines recommend US of the liver and serum alpha-fetoprotein measurements every 6 months). Patients with NASH cirrhosis should be referred to specialty care with a gastroenterologist/hepatologist. All patients with NAFLD/NASH should be screened for immunity to hepatitis A and B and vaccinated if not immune.

---

[7] Available as dietary supplement.

References

Diehl AM, Day C: Cause, pathogenesis, and treatment of nonalcoholic steatohepatitis, N Engl J Med 377(21):2063–2072, 2017.

Lassailly G, Caiazzo R, Ntandja-Wandji LC, et al: Bariatric surgery provides long term-resolution of nonalcoholic steatohepatitis and regression of fibrosis, Gastroenterology, 2020.

Lindenmeyer CC, Mccullough AJ: The natural history of nonalcoholic fatty liver disease-an evolving view, Clin Liver Dis 22(1):11–21, 2018.

Loomba R: Role of imaging-based biomarkers in NAFLD: recent advances in clinical application and future research directions, J Hepatol 68(2):296–304, 2018.

Newsome PN, Buchholtz K, Cusi K, et al. A placebo-controlled trial of subcutaneous semaglutide in nonalcoholic steatohepatitis, N Engl J Med 384(12):1113–1124, 2021.

Riazi K, et al: The prevalence and incidence of NAFLD WORLDWIDE: a systematic review and meta-analysis, Lancet Gastroenterol Hepatol 7(9):851–861, 2022, https://doi.org/10.1016/s2468-1253(22)00165-0.

Rinella ME, Lazarus JV, Ratziu V, et al: A multi-society Delphi consensus statement on new fatty liver disease nomenclature, Ann Hepatol 2023 Jun 20:101133. https://doi.org/10.1016/j.aohep.2023.101133. Online ahead of print.

Said A, Akhter A: Meta-analysis of randomized controlled trials of pharmacologic agents in non-alcoholic steatohepatitis, Ann Hepatol 16(4):538–547, 2017.

Tapper EB, Lok AS: Use of liver imaging and biopsy in clinical practice, N Engl J Med 377(8):756–768, 2017.

Tsai E, Lee TP: Diagnosis and evaluation of nonalcoholic fatty liver disease/nonalcoholic steatohepatitis, including noninvasive biomarkers and transient elastography, Clin Liver Dis 22(1):73–92, 2018.

Younossi Z, Anstee QM, Marietti M, et al: Global burden of NAFLD and NASH: trends, predictions, risk factors and prevention, Nat Rev Gastroenterol Hepatol 15(1):11–20, 2018.

Younossi ZM, Loomba R, Anstee QM, et al: Diagnostic modalities for non-alcoholic fatty liver disease (NAFLD), non-alcoholic steatohepatitis (NASH) and associated fibrosis, Hepatology, 2017.

Younossi ZM, et al: Performance of the enhanced liver fibrosis test to estimate advanced fibrosis among patients with nonalcoholic fatty liver disease, JAMA Netw Open 4(9), 2021, https://doi.org/10.1001/jamanetworkopen.2021.23923.

Younossi ZM, Ratziu V, Loomba R, et al: Obeticholic acid for the treatment of non-alcoholic steatohepatitis: interim analysis from a multicentre randomized, placebo-controlled phase 3 trial, Lancet 394:2184–2196, 2019.

PANCREATIC CANCER

Method of
Joshua S. Jolissaint, MD; and Alice C. Wei, MD, MSc

CURRENT DIAGNOSIS

- Pancreatic cancer remains highly lethal. The majority of patients present with advanced-stage disease, and 5-year survival remains below 10%.
- Patients with pancreatic cancer commonly present with jaundice, malaise, fatigue, weight loss, and abdominal pain.
- Routine screening for pancreatic cancer for patients at average risk is not recommended. For high-risk patients, screening may be considered on a case-by-case basis.
- Diagnostic workup should include a contrast-enhanced, pancreas-protocol computed tomography (CT) scan; serum carbohydrate antigen 19-9 (CA 19-9); and staging CT scans of the chest and pelvis.
- Histologic diagnosis is confirmed with endoscopic ultrasound (EUS)–guided fine-needle aspiration (FNA) or biopsy.

CURRENT THERAPY

- Surgical resection is the only available potentially curative treatment; however, only 20% of patients will have resectable disease at presentation.
- Patients with localized cancer and vascular involvement (borderline resectable [BR] or locally advanced [LA]) may be candidates for neoadjuvant therapy with chemotherapy and/or radiation. If neoadjuvant therapy is effective at stabilizing or downsizing the tumor, these patients may then be eligible for resection.
- Systemic chemotherapy is the mainstay of therapy for unresectable patients.
- Palliation of symptoms may require endoscopic or surgical management for both extrahepatic biliary obstruction and gastric outlet obstruction.

Epidemiology

In 2020 there were an estimated 57,600 new cases of pancreatic cancer in the United States. Although pancreatic cancer comprises only 3.2% of all new cancer diagnoses, it is the fourth leading cause of cancer-related death, contributing to 7.8% of cancer-associated mortality and carrying a 5-year overall survival of only <10%. Survival varies based on stage at presentation, with a 5-year survival for patients with early-stage disease of 39.4%, compared with 2.9% for those with metastatic disease. The incidence of pancreatic cancer has been relatively stable over the last decade, at approximately 12.5 cases per 10,000 person-years.

Incidence increases with age, peaking between 65 and 74 years, with a median age at diagnosis of 70 years; it is higher in men than in women (14.9 vs. 11.6 per 10,000 person-years). African Americans are 12.8% to 22.8% more likely than white Americans to be diagnosed with pancreatic cancer and may have incidence rates 75% higher than patients of other races/ethnicities.

Types of Pancreatic Cancer

Cancer of the exocrine pancreas comprises 93% of pancreatic cancer cases, with pancreatic ductal adenocarcinoma (PDAC) as the most common histologic subtype. Less common subtypes include acinar cell carcinoma, adenosquamous carcinoma, and colloid carcinoma. Tumors of the endocrine pancreas, pancreatic neuroendocrine tumors (PNETs), and islet cell tumors comprise the remaining 7% of pancreatic malignancies.

Risk Factors for Pancreatic Ductal Adenocarcinoma

Multiple genetic and modifiable risk factors for PDAC have been elucidated. Smoking is the strongest risk factor and is associated with approximately one-fourth to one-third of diagnoses. Some studies have demonstrated that smoking may double an individual's risk of developing PDAC. Heavy alcohol use (three or more drinks per day) increases the risk of PDAC in a dose-dependent manner. Obesity and both types 1 and 2 diabetes mellitus are also associated with an increased risk; however, the relationship between these metabolic factors is unclear. Studies have demonstrated an increased risk of PDAC with obesity in early adulthood in addition to a greater risk associated with hyperglycemia, insulin resistance, and low levels of physical activity. Chronic pancreatitis may confer more than a seven-fold increased relative risk of PDAC, and the mechanism can be either modifiable (e.g., alcohol-related pancreatitis) or hereditary.

Approximately 10% of PDAC cases have a hereditary/genetic component (Table 1). The *BRCA1* and *BRCA2* genes encode proteins involved in DNA repair, and germline mutations in these genes are highly penetrant, significantly increasing the risk of breast and ovarian cancer in female carriers. Although the risk of PDAC among patients with *BRCA1* mutations is less well established, *BRCA2* mutations confer an approximately threefold increased relative risk. *BRCA2* mutations are seen with

high frequency among both familial and sporadic PDAC cases. Other hereditary syndromes, such as Lynch syndrome or hereditary nonpolyposis colorectal cancer (HNPCC) (*MLH1, MSH2, MSH6,* or *PMS2* genes), familial adenomatous polyposis (FAP) (*APC* gene), Peutz-Jeghers syndrome (*STK11* gene), and familial atypical multiple mole melanoma (FAMMM) (*CDK2NA* gene) also confer an increased risk of PDAC. Mutations in the *ATM* gene and non-O blood groupings have also been associated with an increased risk of pancreatic cancer. In addition, having a single first-degree relative with PDAC increases a patient's risk of developing PDAC by more than four-fold; however, approximately 80% of patients with a family history of PDAC have no known predisposing genetic mutation or cause.

Lastly, 68% to 80% of hereditary pancreatitis is attributed to germline mutations in the *PRSS1* gene, which are inherited in an autosomal dominant fashion and highly penetrant (approximately 80%). Both the *SPINK1* and *CFTR* genes are also associated with familial pancreatitis. Patients who develop symptoms of pancreatitis in this setting have an increased risk of PDAC that increases with age. By the age of 75 years, patients may have a greater than 50% cumulative incidence of pancreatic cancer.

Screening

Currently there is no role for routine screening for pancreatic cancer for patients at average risk. The US Preventive Services Task Force (USPSTF) has issued a grade D rating (meaning that there is moderate or high certainty that these diagnostic methods have no benefit or that the harm outweighs the risk, thus discouraging the use of this service) for either abdominal ultrasonography, abdominal palpation, or serologic markers. For high-risk patients, those with multiple first-degree relatives with PDAC, or individuals with certain germline mutations (see "Risk Factors," earlier), screening may be considered on a case-by-case basis. Some authors have suggested the use of EUS or magnetic resonance cholangiopancreatography (MRCP), although the efficacy of these modalities as screening tools is still unknown. CA 19-9 is a serum biomarker used to track disease progression or recurrence in PDAC; however, CA 19-9 testing should not be used as a screening tool in otherwise healthy patients.

TABLE 1	Selected Genetic Syndromes With Associated Cancer Risk		
SYNDROME	**GENE**	**ESTIMATED CUMULATIVE RISK OF PANCREATIC CANCER***	**ESTIMATED RISK COMPARED WITH THE GENERAL POPULATION***
Peutz-Jeghers syndrome	*STKI11*	11%–36% by age 65–70 years	132-fold
Familial pancreatitis	*PRSS1, SPINK1, CFTR*	40%–53% by age 70–75 years	26- to 87-fold
Melanoma–pancreatic cancer syndrome	*CDKN2A*	14% by age 70 17% by age 75 years	20- to 47-fold
Lynch syndrome	*MLH1, MSH2*	4% by age 70 years	9- to 11-fold
Hereditary breast-ovarian cancer syndrome	*BRCA1, BRCA2*	1.4%–1.5% (women) and 2.1%–4.1% (men) by age 70	2.4- to 6-fold
Familial pancreatic cancer	Unknown in most families	More than three first-degree relatives with pancreatic cancer: 7%–16% by age 70 Two first-degree relatives with pancreatic cancer: 3% by age 70	Three or more first-degree relatives with pancreatic cancer: 32-fold Two first-degree relatives with pancreatic cancer: 6.4-fold One first-degree relative with pancreatic cancer: 4.6-fold

*See the associated reference for individual sources of data.

Presentation and Diagnosis

The presentation of patients with PDAC is variable. The most common presenting symptoms are jaundice and conjugated hyperbilirubinemia due to biliary tract obstruction, both of which are seen more commonly in tumors of the pancreatic head. Nonspecific complaints can include malaise, fatigue, weight loss, steatorrhea, dyspepsia, and abdominal pain radiating to the back. A new diagnosis of diabetes mellitus in patients 50 years of age or older may also indicate the presence of underlying pancreatic cancer; new-onset diabetes mellitus compared with long-standing diabetes mellitus may convey a greater than twofold increase in risk, particularly in African American and Hispanic patients.

If a diagnosis of PDAC is suspected, the initial diagnostic workup should include a contrast-enhanced dual-phase pancreas protocol CT scan and measurement of serum CA 19-9. Early multidisciplinary consultation is encouraged to optimize symptom management and establish the best treatment. Endoscopic intervention may be both diagnostic and therapeutic; if the patient presents with biliary tract obstruction, endoscopic retrograde cholangiopancreatography (ERCP) may be used to relieve jaundice and to obtain a tissue diagnosis (with ERCP and/or EUS-guided FNA and/or biopsy). Staging should be completed with cross-sectional imaging of the chest and pelvis to evaluate for distant metastases. Magnetic resonance imaging (MRI) and positron emission tomography (PET)/CT may be useful adjuncts in characterizing the tumor or ruling out metastatic disease.

Treatment

Surgical resection is the only potentially curative treatment option. However, only approximately 20% of patients with PDAC will have clearly resectable disease (i.e., without mesenteric or portovascular involvement). For this subset of patients, surgical resection is the preferred initial treatment. Tumors of the pancreatic head may be removed by pancreaticoduodenectomy (i.e., the Whipple procedure), whereas tumors of the pancreatic tail may require a distal pancreatectomy with or without splenectomy. More central or larger tumors may require a central pancreatectomy or total pancreatectomy. Patients with vascular involvement and no evidence of metastases are classified as either borderline resectable (BR) or locally advanced (LA). The current National Comprehensive Cancer Network (NCCN) Pancreatic Adenocarcinoma guidelines recommend neoadjuvant chemotherapy with consideration of resection, depending on the patient's tolerance of chemotherapy, their fitness, and the stage of the disease. Currently accepted systemic neoadjuvant chemotherapy regimens include FOLFIRINOX-based regimens (14-day cycles of 85 mg/m^2 oxaliplatin [Eloxatin][1], 400 mg/m^2 leucovorin[1], 180 mg/m^2 irinotecan [Camptosar][1], and 400 mg/m^2 5-fluorouracil [Adrucil] bolus followed by 2400 mg/m^2 infusion over 46 hours), mFOLFIRINOX (without 5-fluorouracil bolus) or gemcitabine (Gemzar) (1000 mg/m^2) and N-albumin-bound (nab) paclitaxel (Abraxane) (125 mg/m^2) (biweekly for 4 weeks). Some patients may benefit from chemoradiation prior to consideration of resection. The optimal duration of neoadjuvant therapy has not been established; however, most clinicians restage after 2 to 3 months of chemotherapy and reevaluate the potential for resection.

For patients who undergo upfront resection, adjuvant chemotherapy has been demonstrated to improve survival following surgery. The most active regimens include mFOLFIRINOX (85 mg/m^2 oxaliplatin[1], 400 mg/m^2 leucovorin[1], 150 mg/m^2 irinotecan[1], and 2400 mg/m^2 5-fluorouracil infusion over 46 hours every 14 days for 12 cycles), gemcitabine plus capecitabine (Xeloda)[1] (1660 mg/m^2/day on days 1 to 21 every 4 weeks), gemcitabine plus nab-paclitaxel (Abraxane), gemcitabine monotherapy, or 5-fluorouracil plus folinic acid (leucovorin) may also be offered for patients who do not tolerate other regimens due to side effects.

[1]Not FDA-approved for this indication.

Systemic chemotherapy dosing and recommendations for patients who do receive neoadjuvant chemotherapy are varied and dependent on clinical considerations.

Most patients will present with unresectable or metastatic disease. For these patients, FOLFIRINOX or gemcitabine plus nab-paclitaxel are the preferred regimens for those with a good performance status (European Cooperative Oncology Group [ECOG] status 0-1). For patients with ECOG performance status of 2, gemcitabine alone is recommended, whereas for patients with a performance status equal to or greater than 3, emphasis should be placed on palliation, with cancer-directed therapy administered on a case-by-case basis. Routine testing of tumor tissue for deficient mismatch repair (dMMR) or high levels of microsatellite instability (MSI-H) using immunohistochemistry (IHC), polymerase chain reaction (PCR), or next-generation sequencing (NGS) is now recommended. The programmed cell death protein 1 (PD-1) inhibitor pembrolizumab (Keytruda) has been approved as second-line therapy in patients who test positive for dMMR or MSI-H.

Managing Symptoms and Complications

Once a diagnosis of pancreatic cancer has been established, all patients should be evaluated for symptomatology, physical function, and fitness. The active treatment of symptoms and introduction of palliative care services should be considered early. Modern palliative care is not synonymous with hospice, and palliation has been shown to both improve quality of life and decrease the use of aggressive care measures at the end of life.

Pain can be a predominant symptom in patients with pancreatic cancer and may be described as a midepigastric pain radiating to the back. This can be often managed by traditional multimodal analgesia, including opioid/narcotic analgesia; however, consideration can be given to celiac plexus neurolysis or palliative radiation for refractory pain due to local tumor invasion. As described earlier, many patients will also present with **jaundice** due to extrahepatic biliary tract obstruction. Decompression can be achieved with endoscopic, surgical, or percutaneous interventions. Endoscopic stent placement is considered the first line of treatment. Although endoscopically placed stents may be associated with higher rates of readmission for in-stent occlusion or recurrent biliary obstruction, these modalities are generally associated with lower rates of adverse events than percutaneous stent placement. Current guidelines recommend placing a self-expanding metal stent (SEMS) when feasible and only after a histologic diagnosis has been made; however, the decision as to whether to place a plastic, covered metal, or uncovered metal stent is nuanced and should be assessed by a multidisciplinary team, including a surgeon and gastroenterologist when available. For patients receiving neoadjuvant chemotherapy, fully covered SEMS are preferred as they are easily removed/exchanged. If endoscopic or percutaneous interventions are unavailable or if unresectable disease is discovered at the time of surgery, surgical biliary bypass in the form of choledochojejunostomy may be performed. This may be accompanied by a gastrojejunostomy for the treatment or prevention of **gastric outlet obstruction** (also known as a "double bypass") (Figure 1). As many as 20% of patients with PDAC of the pancreatic head will develop symptomatic gastric outlet obstruction. If not discovered intraoperatively or in patients with short prognoses or limited functional status, endoscopically placed duodenal stents can provide adequate relief of obstructive symptoms.

Pancreatic cancer is generally regarded as one of the highest risk states that predispose patients to **venous thromboembolism** (VTE), conferring a four- to sevenfold higher risk than that faced by the general population. All patients should be counseled about signs and symptoms that may indicate the presence of VTE—either deep venous thrombosis or pulmonary embolism. Current guidelines recommend the use of low

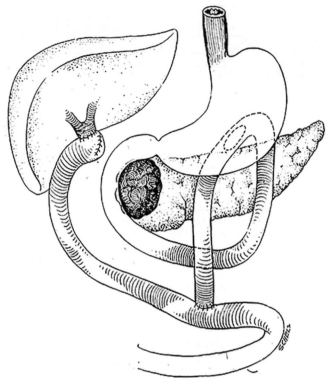

Figure 1 Double bypass showing choledochojejunostomy and gastrojejunostomy with an intact pancreatic head tumor. Reproduced with permission, Scott EN, Garcea G, Doucas H, Steward WP, Dennison AR, Berry DP: Surgical bypass vs. endoscopic stenting for pancreatic ductal adenocarcinoma, *HPB (Oxford)* 11[2]:118–124, 2009.

molecular weight heparin (LWMH) (enoxaparin [Lovenox]) in lieu of warfarin for patients who develop a cancer-related VTE. Routine prophylactic anticoagulation has not been widely adopted due to a lack of survival benefit despite a reduction in VTE events.

Finally, patients with pancreatic cancer may develop **pancreatic exocrine insufficiency** due to pancreatic resection, tumoral destruction of the parenchyma, or blockage of the pancreatic duct. Symptoms include steatorrhea, weight loss, abdominal pain, and malnutrition due to malabsorption of fat-soluble nutrients. Pancreatic enzyme replacement may be started empirically at a dose of 25,000 to 75,000 units of pancrelipase (Creon or Zenpep) per meal with 10,000 to 25,000 units per snack (off-label dosing).

Summary
Pancreatic cancer remains a highly lethal disease. Most patients are not candidates for resection; therefore emphasis should be placed on the palliation of symptoms. However, improvements in chemotherapy over the last decade have increased both survival and rates of resectability.

References
Becker AE, Hernandez YG, Frucht H, Lucas AL: Pancreatic ductal adenocarcinoma: risk factors, screening, and early detection, *World J Gastroenterol* 20(32):11182–11198, 2014.

Heestand GM, Murphy JD, Lowy AM: Approach to patients with pancreatic cancer without detectable metastases, *J Clin Oncol* 33(16):1770–1778, 2015.

Howlader N, Noone AM, Krapcho M, editors: *SEER Cancer Statistics Review*, National Cancer Institute, 1975-2016, Bethesda, MD. (based on November 2019 SEER data submission, posted to the SEER web site, April 2020. https://seer.cancer.gov/csr/1975_2017/.

Khorana AA, Mckernin SE, Berlin J, et al: Potentially curable pancreatic adenocarcinoma: ASCO clinical practice guideline update, *J Clin Oncol* 37(23):2082–2088, 2019.

Kruse EJ: Palliation in pancreatic cancer, *Surg Clin North Am* 90(2):355–364, 2010.

Lee S, Reha JL, Tzeng CW, et al: Race does not impact pancreatic cancer treatment and survival in an equal access federal health care system, *Ann Surg Oncol* 20(13):4073–4079, 2013.

Referenced with permission from the NCCN Clinical Practice Guidelines in Oncology (NCCN Guidelines®) for Pancreatic Adenocarcinoma V.1.2020. © National Comprehensive Cancer Network, Inc. 2020. All rights reserved. Accessed March 23rd, 2020. To view the most recent and complete version of the guideline, go online to NCCN.org.

Rebours V, Lévy P, Ruszniewski P: An overview of hereditary pancreatitis, *Dig Liver Dis* 44(1):8–15, 2012.

Setiawan VW, Stram DO, Porcel J, et al: Pancreatic cancer following incident diabetes in african americans and latinos: the multiethnic cohort, *J Natl Cancer Inst* 111(1):27–33, 2019.

Sohal DPS, Kennedy EB, Khorana A, et al: Metastatic pancreatic cancer: ASCO clinical practice guideline update, *J Clin Oncol* 36(24):2545–2556, 2018.

TUMORS OF THE COLON AND RECTUM

Method of
Richard Huettemann, MD; Colleen A. Donahue, MD; Thomas Curran, MD, MPH; Virgilio V. George, MD; and Pinckney J. Maxwell IV, MD

CURRENT DIAGNOSIS

- Screening of asymptomatic average-risk patients should begin at 45 years of age.
- Colonoscopy should be performed if any screening test results are positive.
- Colonoscopy should be performed on any patient with signs or symptoms of colorectal cancer
- Screening of high-risk patients, those with inflammatory bowel disease (IBD), familial adenomatous polyposis (FAP), hereditary nonpolyposis colorectal cancer (HNPCC), or a significant positive family history, should begin at an earlier age and occur more frequently.

CURRENT THERAPY

- Patients with FAP should undergo early prophylactic colon resection. Patients with HNPCC should be counseled regarding prophylactic total colectomy.
- Colon tumors should be treated with segmental laparoscopic or open resection.
- Chemotherapy is offered for colon cancers with locally advanced, nodal (stage III), or metastatic (stage IV) disease. It may also be considered in stage II patients with high risk features on pathology.
- Rectal tumors that are small (<3 cm), <25% of the rectal circumference, superficial (Tis or T1), lack nodal involvement, and have favorable pathologic characteristics should be removed by transanal techniques.
- Rectal tumors may be treated using open or minimally invasive techniques by performing a total mesorectal excision.
- Combination chemotherapy and radiation therapy is offered for advanced (stage II), nodal (stage III), or metastatic (stage IV) rectal cancer. All rectal cancers should be screened for microsatellite instability prior to initiating treatment.
- Postoperative surveillance includes frequent office evaluations, carcinoembryonic antigen (CEA) levels, endoscopy, and imaging.

Background, Epidemiology, and Etiology
Colorectal cancer is the third most common cancer in men and women, after prostate and lung/bronchus in men and breast and lung/bronchus in women. The American Cancer Society (ACS) expects an estimated 106,970 new diagnoses of colon cancer

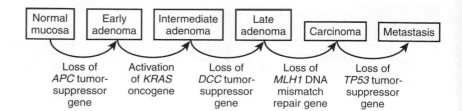

Figure 1 Adenoma to carcinoma sequence.

and an estimated 46,050 new diagnoses of rectal cancer in 2023. The overall incidence of colorectal cancer has been decreasing since the mid-1980s, with a more dramatic decrease in the past decade. This decrease is likely related to an increase in screening with removal of precancerous polyps. However, despite an overall decrease in incidence in colorectal cancer, there has been an increase in incidence of colorectal cancer of those under 50 years of age. The ACS expects an estimated 52,550 deaths from colorectal cancer in 2023, which accounts for 8.6% of all cancer deaths. There has been a similar decrease in mortality since the mid-1980s, again with a sharper decline in the past decade likely related to improved screening as well. Colorectal cancer is a highly treatable and frequently curable malignancy when detected early, with a 91% 5-year survival for localized (stage I and II) disease highlighting the need for better screening.

The development of colorectal cancer is related to a number of factors, including age, diet, activity, environmental exposures, family history, and genetics. Ninety percent of colorectal cancers are diagnosed after 50 years of age, and fewer than 5% of cases are diagnosed before 40 years of age. The peak incidence of diagnosis is in the seventh decade of life. Dietary factors play a role in carcinogenesis as well. Western diets, consisting of high-fat and low-fiber, and the intake of red or processed meats and alcohol have been associated with increased rates of colorectal cancer. It is likely that this low-fiber Western diet slows transit time, leading to increased exposure to carcinogens. Activity level also can play a role in carcinogenesis, as studies have shown an increase in cancer among those with sedentary jobs and a decreased incidence among those with regular exercise. Exposure to cigarette smoke increases the risk of colorectal adenomas and cancers. The ACS Cancer Prevention Study II revealed that 12% of colorectal cancer deaths in the general U.S. population can be attributed to smoking. Family history and genetics also play a significant role in carcinogenesis, as approximately 10% of patients diagnosed have a first-degree relative with colorectal cancer.

Adenomatous Polyps

The progression from normal mucosa to an adenomatous polyp to an invasive colorectal cancer proceeds through a well-defined process, over many years. Aberrant crypt foci develop into micro-adenomas and then into adenomatous polyps. Dysplastic cells develop within the polyp, continue to multiply, become a tumor, and then break through the subepithelial barrier and invade through the layers of the bowel wall, eventually spreading to pericolic tissues or to lymph nodes and distant sites. A number of genes have been implicated in carcinogenesis, including proto-oncogenes *(K-ras, src, c-myc)*, tumor-suppressor genes *(APC, DCC, p53, MCC, DPC4)*, and DNA mismatch repair genes *(MLH1, PMS2, MSH2, MSH6, EPCAM)*. Sporadic colorectal cancers generally develop as a result of several cumulative genetic insults involving these genes (Figure 1).

Familial Colorectal Cancer Syndromes

Familial adenomatous polyposis (FAP) is an inherited, non–sex-linked, Mendelian-dominant disease that accounts for approximately 1% of all colorectal cancers. The high penetrance of FAP means that there is a 50% chance of development within affected families. However, 25% of FAP patients have no family history, likely representing a new, spontaneous mutation. The disorder is caused by mutations in either the tumor-suppressor *APC* gene, which is located on chromosome 5 (5q21–q22), or in the *MUTYH*

gene, which is located on chromosome 1 (1p34.3–p32.1). FAP is characterized by the progressive development of hundreds to thousands of adenomatous polyps located throughout the entire colon. The clinical diagnosis is based on the histologic confirmation of at least 100 adenomas. All patients will eventually develop colorectal cancer. Adenomas generally appear by the mid-20s, and cancers generally appear by the late-30s. An attenuated form of FAP is recognized in which fewer adenomas (12–100) are identified, with cancer developing between 50 and 70 years of age. FAP also exhibits extracolonic manifestations including gastric/duodenal/small bowel polyps, osteomas and desmoid tumors (Gardner syndrome), eye lesions (congenital hypertrophy of retinal pigment epithelium [CHRPE]), papillary thyroid cancer (up to 12% of FAP patients), epidermoid cysts, and brain neoplasms (Turcot syndrome).

Hereditary nonpolyposis colon cancer (HNPCC), also called *Lynch syndrome*, is an inherited, non–sex-linked, Mendelian-dominant disease with virtually complete penetrance. HNPCC is caused by a defect in any of a number of DNA mismatch repair genes *(MLH1, MSH2, MSH6, EPCAM, PMS2)*, which leads to microsatellite instability *(MSI-H)*. A number of criteria have been generated for the diagnosis of HNPCC, including the Amsterdam I and II criteria and the Bethesda guidelines (Box 1). According to the EPICOLON study, the revised Bethesda guidelines are the most discriminating set of clinical parameters for diagnosing HNPCC. However, the use of clinical guidelines alone for Lynch syndrome screening has been shown to underestimate the number of patients with Lynch syndrome. Therefore, in 2009, the NCCN recommended universal Lynch syndrome screening for all colorectal or endometrial cancers.

HNPCC is subdivided into Lynch syndrome types I and II. Lynch type I refers to site-specific nonpolyposis colon cancer, and Lynch type II (formerly called *familial cancer syndrome*) refers to cancers that develop in the colon and related organs such as the endometrium, ovaries, stomach, pancreas, and proximal urinary tract, among others.

Lynch syndrome differs from sporadic colorectal cancer in a number of important ways. It has an autosomal dominant inheritance, a predominance of proximal lesions (75% are found in the right colon), an excess of multiple primary colorectal cancers (18%), an early age of onset averaging 44 years, a significantly improved survival rate of right-sided lesions when compared with family members with distal colorectal cancer (53% vs. 35% 5-year survival), and an increased risk of development of metachronous lesions (24%). Lynch syndrome is the most common hereditary form of colon cancer and affects approximately 1/300 people. Increased surveillance for patients with Lynch syndrome has been shown to reduce cancer-related deaths. Patients and family members of those diagnosed with HNPCC and FAP should undergo genetic testing to aid in future diagnosis and treatment options.

Inflammatory Bowel Disease

Both Crohn's disease (CD) and ulcerative colitis (UC) confer an increased risk of colorectal cancer, with UC approximately double the risk of CD. The duration and severity of CD and the duration and extent (left-sided colitis vs. pancolitis) of UC contribute to cancer risk in inflammatory bowel disease (IBD). Cancer in CD can occur in any segment with inflammation, but is more likely to occur in a stricture or bypass segment given the inability to surveil these areas. Importantly, neoplasia in UC does not follow the adenoma-carcinoma sequence of sporadic colorectal cancer. This change has important screening and treatment implications.

Screening the Average-Risk Patient

Patients with no personal history of colorectal polyps or cancers, no personal history of IBD, no symptoms suspicious for colorectal cancer, no family history of colorectal polyps or cancers, and no evidence of a familial or genetic syndrome can be screened as average risk. Two main categories of screening tests include those that detect adenomatous polyps and cancer (flexible sigmoidoscopy, colonoscopy, double-contrast barium enema, and computed tomography [CT] colonography) and those that primarily detect cancer (fecal occult blood testing [FOBT], fecal immunohistochemical testing [FIT], and stool DNA testing). The goal of screening is to reduce mortality by reducing the incidence of advanced disease. It seems intuitive that tests detecting polyps, the premalignant phase of colorectal cancer, would be preferred to tests detecting only cancers. However, testing for polyps and cancer is generally procedure related, requiring access to care, while testing for cancers can be conducted on stool studies alone and done at home. Screening with simple stool samples has the potential to more easily increase overall screening, but is not preventive without the ability for endoscopic polyp removal.

Regardless of the method employed, testing in the average-risk, asymptomatic patient should begin at 45 years of age based on the most recent updated guidelines because of the increasing disease burden in people younger than 50 years of age. A complete colonoscopy is only required every 10 years, but it requires an oral bowel preparation and carries a small risk of perforation of approximately 1 in 1000. A flexible sigmoidoscopy is required

every 5 years when combined with FOBT annually, and this is the only colorectal cancer screening method that has been studied in a randomized control trial. The testing is more frequent, but it requires only enemas for preparation and carries a lower risk of perforation. Air-contrast barium enemas can be used for screening every 5 years, but they also require an oral bowel preparation and are only diagnostic. CT colonography is an evolving method for screening every 5 years and has the opportunity for more accessible screening; however, there are limitations on the identification of polyps less than 1 cm. It also requires an oral bowel preparation and is only diagnostic; thus it is used in conjunction with flexible sigmoidoscopy and FIT. FOBT and FIT require annual testing. The U.S Food and Drug Administration (FDA) has also approved a FIT-fecal DNA test that is performed at 3-year intervals; however, it is less specific and less cost-effective than FIT, making it unlikely to replace FIT. The most complete screening test, allowing removal of precancerous lesions if identified, remains complete colonoscopy, and importantly, the patient should undergo full endoscopic evaluation if any other screening test is positive.

Screening the High-Risk Patient

High-risk patients include those with a personal history of colorectal polyps or cancers, a family history of colorectal cancer in a first-degree relative, those with Crohn's disease or UC, and those with a personal or family history of FAP or HNPCC. Screening in these patients has been adjusted for changes in incidence and age of onset of neoplasia (Box 2).

Symptoms and Diagnosis

Symptoms of colorectal cancer include bleeding (85%), a change in bowel habits, abdominal pain, malaise, and obstruction. Frequently, anemia may be the only sign a patient exhibits. Patients with symptoms suspicious for colorectal cancer should undergo colonoscopy. An anorectal source of bleeding should not preclude a complete colonic evaluation.

Preoperative Management

Before operative intervention, a complete evaluation should occur, including a careful history and physical examination, routine laboratory testing, and a carcinoembryonic antigen (CEA) level. A complete evaluation of the colon is essential and utilizes colonoscopy with biopsy or barium enema or CT colonography if colonoscopy is incomplete. Bowel preparation with antibiotics is indicated as a routine preoperative measure for colonic surgery per the latest guidelines from the American Society of Colon and Rectal Surgeons (ASCRS).

Preoperative staging should be undertaken for colorectal cancers. This includes CT of the abdomen and pelvis with contrast and CT scan of the thorax to rule out intrathoracic metastatic disease. CT scanning of the abdomen and pelvis are indicated to aid in the evaluation of the extent of localized or metastatic disease and the presence of enlarged lymph nodes. Staging of rectal cancers includes determining the distance from the anal verge (frequently utilizing a rigid proctoscope), the depth of invasion, and the presence of enlarged lymph nodes (utilizing magnetic resonance imaging). Metastatic disease mandates neoadjuvant chemotherapy in the absence of acute symptoms of obstruction or exsanguination. Rectal cancers with locally advanced disease (T3-4, N1-2) or evidence of enlarged metastatic lymph nodes benefit from neoadjuvant chemotherapy and radiation. Preoperative staging allows for the application of neoadjuvant therapy in selected candidates, which can downstage and downsize tumors and can decrease rates of local recurrence in rectal cancer. Neoadjuvant therapy can also allow for sphincter-preserving procedures for previously bulky or very low rectal tumors.

Surgery for Colonic Tumors

The primary therapy for tumors of the colon is operative. The basic principles of surgery for colon cancer include the following:
- Exploration: adequate visual, tactile, and potentially intraoperative hepatic ultrasound staging at the time of primary resec-

BOX 2 | Screening the High Risk Patient for Colorectal Cancer

Risk Category	Age to Begin	Recommendation	Comment
Personal history of <3 adenomas with low- grade dysplasia	5–10 years after the initial polypectomy	Colonoscopy	Examination interval should be based on other clinical factors such as prior examination findings, family history, or preferences of the endoscopist or patient.
Personal history of 3–10 adenomas, or 1 adenoma >1 cm, or any adenoma with villous features or high-grade dysplasia	3 years after the initial polypectomy	Colonoscopy	Adenomas require compete excision. If the follow-up is normal, the next examination should be in 5 years. More than 10 adenomas should raise suspicion of a familial syndrome.
Personal history of colorectal cancer	1 year after resection	Colonoscopy	Patients should undergo high- quality preoperative clearing. Follow-up after normal examinations should be extended to 3 years and then to 5 years
Family history of adenomas or cancer in a first-degree relative <60 years of age or in two first-degree relatives at any age	40 years of age or 10 years before the youngest case	Colonoscopy	Every 5 years
Family history of adenomas or cancer in a first-degree relative >60 years of age or in two second-degree relatives with cancer	40 years of age	Colonoscopy	Screening should be initiated at an earlier age. Intervals based on findings or by the average-risk patient
FAP or suspected FAP	10–12 years of age	Annual FS, counseling for genetic testing if showing polyps	Colectomy should be considered for positive genetic testing/after puberty
HNPCC or risk of HNPCC	20–25 years of age or 10 years before the youngest case	Colonoscopy, counseling for genetic testing	Every 1–2 years. Genetic testing should be offered to first-degree relatives of persons with a known DNA mismatch repair gene, or with one of the first three Bethesda criteria
IBD, Crohn's, or chronic UC	8 years after the onset of pancolitis, or 12–15 years after the onset of left- sided colitis	Colonoscopies with random 4 quad biopsies every 10 cm for dysplasia	Screening should be offered every 1–2 years, and patients are best referred to a center with experience in the surveillance and management of IBD.

FAP, Familial adenomatous polyposis; *FS,* flexible sigmoidoscopy; *HNPCC*, hereditary nonpolyposis colorectal cancer; *IBD,* inflammatory bowel disease.

tion to evaluate for peritoneal, mesenteric, or hepatic disease

- Removal of the entire cancer with enough bowel proximal and distal to encompass the possibility of submucosal lymphatic tumor spread. At least 5-cm margin proximal and distal for colon and upper rectal cancers is recommended. Any negative margin is acceptable in low rectal cancers.
- Removal of regional mesenteric pedicle, including draining lymphatics, based on the predictable lymphatic spread of the disease and the potential for regional mesenteric involvement without concurrent distant involvement
- En bloc resection of involved structures (T4 tumors)
- Segmental colonic resections (right, transverse, left, or sigmoid colectomy) based on the tumor location and blood supply with lymphatic drainage, specifically the ileocolic, middle colic, and left colic arteries. These resections define both a convenient anatomic boundary for standard colonic resection and also provide for adequate regional lymph node clearance because the major draining lymphatics follow these blood vessels in the mesentery. Locally invasive tumors (T4) require en bloc resection of involved structures. Metastatic colonic tumors (M1) may require neoadjuvant chemotherapy before resection or palliation.

Numerous studies have proven that minimally invasive surgery is appropriate and perhaps preferred for colon cancer in experienced hands. There is evidence showing decreased length of stay for minimally invasive surgery without a decrease in oncologic outcomes; reduction in homeostatic insults likely leads to more favorable overall outcomes. The application of minimally invasive techniques for rectal cancer resection is still controversial but is gaining popularity.

Surgery for Rectal Tumors

Two different approaches for rectal tumors include local excision and formal oncologic rectal resection. Local excision is the treatment of choice for a select, small group (3%– 5%) of all patients diagnosed with rectal cancer. Tumors amenable to transanal excision are small (<3 cm), <25% of the rectal circumference, confined to the mucosa or submucosa (Tis or T1), lack nodal involvement by preoperative imaging, and have favorable pathologic characteristics (well or moderately differentiated with no lymphovascular invasion). Tumors in the lower or middle third of the rectum are accessible by simple transanal excision, but tumors of the upper rectum require the use of transanal endoscopic microsurgery (TEMS) or transanal minimally invasive surgery (TAMIS) techniques for resection. Local excision requires a 1-cm normal margin, but the defect generally does not require closure.

Tumors staged at T2 or greater require a formal resection, the type of which depends on the location of the tumor. Upper and middle rectal tumors can generally be managed with a low or very low anterior resection. Lower rectal tumors frequently require a proctectomy with coloanal anastomosis or an abdominoperineal resection (APR) depending on sphincter involvement and patient-related quality-of-life factors. The goal of resection is to obtain a 5-cm distal margin; however, lower tumors can be managed with a 2-cm distal margin. Very low tumors or those involving the sphincter mechanism require an APR. Rectal tumors with a greater depth of rectal wall invasion (T3), evidence of fixation or local invasion (T4), or evidence of lymph nodal (N1–N2) or metastatic (M1) disease mandate neoadjuvant chemoradiation therapy and more recently, total neoadjuvant therapy which includes chemoradiation as well as chemotherapy in the neoadjuvant setting. Proctectomy requires a tumor-specific total mesorectal excision (TME). This involves complete excision of all mesorectal tissue located behind the rectum and no carcinoma at the lateral or circumferential margins. The goal of the TME is to remove all malignant tissue to reduce or eliminate the possibility of locally recurrent disease. Locally advanced rectal tumors may preclude an effective or safe resection. Some indications for likely inoperability include extensive pelvic disease, invasion of ileofemoral vessels, extensive lymphatic involvement or significant lower extremity lymphedema, bony involvement, or life expectancy less than 3 to 6 months.

Minimally invasive surgical techniques are similarly being performed for rectal malignancies. Studies are underway to verify the efficacy and safety of these methods in rectal resection compared with traditional open resection. It has gained widespread popularity and is very commonly used. Given the complexity and constantly evolving management for rectal cancer, we recommend all patients be presented at a multidisciplinary tumor board and referred to a high volume rectal cancer center or rectal cancer center of excellence.

Complicated Disease

Colorectal tumors may present with complications including obstruction, perforation, or significant bleeding. These presentations are generally related to more advanced disease and may preclude a complete staging workup or potential neoadjuvant therapy. Unless patients are unstable or critically ill or the tumor is unresectable, an oncologic resection should be performed. An ostomy is generally performed, whether as an end ostomy or as a proximal loop diversion for a primary anastomosis. Colonic stenting is an attractive option for obstructing lesions as either palliation or as a bridge to resection after medical stabilization and staging for potential neoadjuvant therapy.

Surgery for High-Risk Conditions

High-risk conditions for the development of colorectal malignancies include FAP, HNPCC, and chronic UC. Surgical management may be prophylactic or possibly therapeutic after a malignancy has been diagnosed. The mainstay of operative management in FAP and chronic UC is a total proctocolectomy. Reconstructive options include an ileal pouch-anal anastomosis, a continent ileostomy (Kock pouch), or an end ileostomy. A total abdominal colectomy with ileorectal anastomosis may be performed for temporary preservation of rectal function in selected cases of chronic UC with rectal sparing and FAP with few rectal polyps, but this requires aggressive surveillance of the remaining rectal mucosa's risk of malignancy. Patients with HNPCC should be counseled regarding the increased risk of metachronous cancers and therefore consider subtotal colectomy with ileorectal anastomosis, and a total hysterectomy with bilateral salpingoophorectomy should be offered because of the preponderance of associated gynecologic malignancy at the age of 40 years or after child bearing.

Pathologic Staging and Adjuvant Therapy

Excellent pathologic sampling and review of the operative specimen provides important prognostic and therapeutic information. Current standards recommend at least 12 lymph nodes be removed for adequate staging of colon cancer. The decision for adjuvant chemotherapy and/or radiation therapy is based on pathologic staging. This information also provides prognostic information in terms of survival to the patient and their family.

A number of staging systems have been developed, however the TNM system is most commonly used in the United States (Box 3).

Chemotherapy is offered for colorectal cancers with locally advanced, nodal (stage III), or metastatic (stage IV) disease. There may be a subset of patients with stage II disease and high risk pathologic features who may be recommended for chemotherapy and should be discussed at a multidisciplinary conference. The combination of chemotherapy and radiation therapy for advanced rectal cancer (stages II to IV) has decreased local recurrence and increased survival. The current guidelines recommend total neoadjuvant therapy with both radiation and chemotherapy in the preoperative setting. Additional adjuvant chemotherapy is dependent on the final pathology and extent of chemotherapy received preoperatively. Numerous protocols are available for treatment, with the standard of care being FOLFOX: 5-fluorouracil (5-FU), leucovorin, and oxaliplatin (Eloxatin). Older adult patients or those with multiple comorbidities who may not be able to tolerate full-dose chemotherapy may be candidates for capecitabine (Xeloda) or 5-FU and leucovorin. Numerous study protocols are available at specialized centers evaluating other medications. Newer technologies continue to evolve, such as anti-angiogenesis agents and immunomodulatory agents. The latest development is the use of PDL-1 inhibitors in microsatellite unstable colon and rectal cancers in place of chemotherapy. Therefore, it is highly recommended that all patients are tested for microsatellite instability or mismatch repair deficiency prior to initiating treatment.

Metastatic Disease

Surgical therapy is also available for metastatic disease in certain situations. Metastatic liver lesions amenable to resection can be addressed either at the time of colon resection or after the patient has healed from the colectomy. The lesions could be resected or treated using radiofrequency ablation (RFA), a newer technology allowing in-situ destruction of liver lesions. Similarly, selected pulmonary metastases can be resected, possibly using minimally invasive thoracoscopic techniques. The majority of deaths from colorectal cancer are from metastatic disease; over 20% of patients have widespread disease at diagnosis. A multidisciplinary approach to patients with metastatic disease should be undertaken to discern if it is resectable and what intervention should be pursued.

| BOX 3 | Pathologic Staging Systems for Colorectal Cancer |

Pathologic Features	Stage	TNM	Dukes	Astler-Coller	5-Year Survival
Depth of Invasion					
Lamina propria, muscularis mucosa	0	T0/Tis	A		>90%
Submucosa	I	T1	A	B1	
Muscularis propria	I	T2	A	B1	
Subserosa, pericolic fat	II	T3	B,	B1	70-85%
Adjacent organs, perforation	II	T4	B	B2	55-65%
Lymph Nodal Involvement					
None		N0			
1-3 nodes	III	N1	C	C1, C2	45-55%
>3 nodes	III	N2	C	C1, C2	20-30%
Distant Metastatic Disease					
Absent		M0			
Present	IV	M1	D		<5%

Surveillance

Surveillance for colon and rectal cancer is a lifelong process. Patients are seen and examined in the office every 3 months for 2 years, then every 6 months for 3 years, and then yearly. CEA levels are routinely obtained as a marker for tumor recurrence. Endoscopy should be performed at 1 year postoperatively, given a high-quality preoperative study to clear the entire colon. Normal examinations allow subsequent colonoscopies to occur at 3 years and then every 5 years. Similarly, annual imaging utilizing chest radiography and CT of the abdomen and pelvis are obtained. Patients with increased or rising CEA levels or with evidence of recurrent disease can be evaluated using positron emission tomography (PET). Newer testing for surveillance and treatment response in colorectal cancer is on the horizon, such as circulating tumor DNA; however, these studies are still in process and are not yet part of the national guidelines for surveillance.

References

American Cancer Society: *Cancer facts and figures 2022*, Atlanta, GA, 2022, American Cancer Society. Available at: https://www.cancer.org/content/dam/cancer-org/research/cancer-facts-and-statistics/annual-cancer-facts-and-figures/2022/2022-cancer-facts-and-figures.pdf.

Beart RW, Steele Jr GD, Menck HR, Chmiel JS, Ocwieia KE, Winchester DP: Management and survival of patients with adenocarcinoma of the colon and rectum: a national survey of the commission on cancer, *J Am Coll Surg* 181:225–236, 1995.

Bentrem DJ, Okabe S, Wong WD, et al: T1 adenocarcinoma of the rectum: transanal excision or radical surgery? *Ann Surg* 242:472–479, 2005.

The Clinical Outcomes of Surgical Therapy Study Group: A comparison of laparoscopically assisted and open colectomy for colon cancer, *N Engl J Med* 350:2050–2059, 2004.

Floyd ND, Saclarides TJ: Transanal endoscopic microsurgical resection of pT1 rectal tumors, *Dis Colon Rectum* 49:164–168, 2005.

Lan Y-T, Lin J-K, Li AF-Y, et al: Metachronous colorectal cancer: necessity of postoperative colonoscopic surveillance, *Int J Colorectal Dis* 20:121–125, 2005.

Maetani I, Tada T, Ukita T, et al: Self-expandable metallic stent placement as palliative treatment of obstructed colorectal carcinoma, *J Gastroenterol* 39:334–338, 2004.

Patel SG, May FP, Anderson JC, et al: Updates on age to start and stop colorectal cancer screening: recommendations from the U.S. multi-society task force on colorectal cancer, *Gastroenterology* 162(1):285–299, 2022 Jan, https://doi.org/10.1053/j.gastro.2021.10.007. Epub 2021 Nov 15. PMID: 34794816.

Pinol V, Castells A, Andreu M, et al: Accuracy of revised bethesda guidelines, microsatellite instability, and immunohistochemistry for the identification of patients with hereditary nonpolyposis colorectal cancer, *JAMA* 293:1986–1994, 2005.

Rex DK, Boland CR, Dominitz JA, et al: Colorectal cancer screening: recommendations for physicians and patients from the U.S. multi-society task force on colorectal cancer, *Am J Gastroenterol* 112(7):1016–1030, 2017 Jul, https://doi.org/10.1038/ajg.2017.174. Epub 2017 Jun 6. PMID: 28555630.

Sauer R, Becker H, Hohenberger W, et al: For the german rectal cancer study group. preoperative versus postoperative chemoradiotherapy for rectal cancer, *N Engl J Med* 351:1731–1740, 2004.

Steel SR, Hull TL, Hyman N, Maykel JA, Read TE, Whitlow CB: *The ASCRS textbook of colon and rectal surgery*, ed 4, Springer Nature Switzerland AG, 2022.

Stipa F, Chessin DB, Shia J, et al: A pathologic complete response of rectal cancer to preoperative combined-modality therapy results in improved oncological outcome compared with those who achieve no downstaging on the basis of preoperative endorectal ultrasonography. *Ann Surg Oncol* 13(8): 1047–1053.

TUMORS OF THE STOMACH

Method of
David (Sasha) Mahvi, MD; and Mark Fairweather, MD, PhD

CURRENT DIAGNOSIS

- Screening programs exist in countries with a very high incidence of gastric adenocarcinoma and can be considered elsewhere for individuals at high risk.
- Esophagogastroduodenoscopy with biopsy is the gold standard for diagnosis of stomach tumors.
- Staging workup for adenocarcinoma includes computed tomography (CT) of the chest, abdomen, and pelvis to evaluate for metastatic disease and endoscopic ultrasonography (EUS) to assess T-stage.

CURRENT THERAPY

Adenocarcinoma
- Treatment decisions should be made by multidisciplinary teams.
- Patients with T1a tumors and no further spread can be candidates for endoscopic or surgical resection.
- Patients with T1b tumors without nodal involvement should undergo upfront surgical resection.
- Patients with T2 or higher disease or any nodal involvement should receive perioperative chemotherapy, with the FLOT regimen (5-fluorouracil, leucovorin,[1] oxaliplatin,[1] and docetaxel [Taxotere]) being first-line treatment.
- Surgery consists of either a distal gastrectomy or total gastrectomy depending on tumor location and should include at least 15 lymph nodes for accurate staging.

Gastrointestinal Stromal Tumors
- All tumors greater than 2 cm should be considered for resection.
- No lymphadenectomy is required, and grossly negative margins are sufficient.
- Imatinib (Gleevec), a tyrosine kinase inhibitor, should be offered after surgery to patients with a high-risk of tumor recurrence (either a primary tumor >5 cm or a mitotic rate >5 per 50 high-power field).

Neuroendocrine Tumors
- Type 1 and type 2 tumors can undergo endoscopic resection if they are less than 2 cm in size and are not poorly differentiated or do not invade beyond the submucosa.
- Surgical resection should be performed for all type 3 tumors as well as for type 1 and 2 tumors that have positive margins, recur, or have the worrisome features listed earlier.
- Patients can develop carcinoid syndrome with liver metastases, which can be treated with somatostatin analogues, surgical cytoreduction, or liver-directed therapies.

Gastric Lymphoma
- Mucosa-associated lymphoid tissue (MALT) lymphomas often respond to *Helicobacter pylori* eradication.
- Other lymphomas are treated with chemotherapy, with surgery being reserved for patients with complications such as bleeding or perforation.

[1]Not FDA approved for this indication.

Gastric Adenocarcinoma

Gastric adenocarcinoma is the fourth leading cause of cancer-related death worldwide, accounting for an estimated 768,000 deaths in 2020. Gastric cancer is the fifth most common cancer worldwide, with just over 1 million new cases annually. Although the overall incidence has been downtrending as a result of screening in high-risk populations and the recognition of *H. pylori* as a significant risk factor, the overall crude number of cases has gradually increased because of the aging population. In the United States, gastric cancer is less prevalent, with the 14th highest incidence and 16th highest mortality rate estimated in 2022.

Classification

Historically, gastric adenocarcinomas have been divided into two main subtypes by the Lauren classification system: intestinal and diffuse. Intestinal-type gastric cancers are similar to adenocarcinomas elsewhere in the gastrointestinal tract, appearing in glandular or tubular formations. Intestinal cancers are more likely to occur in male and older adult patients and have a more favorable prognosis. The diffuse subtype lacks cohesive molecules, specifically E-cadherin, and will invade without gland formation.

Risk Factors

There are a number of risk factors for gastric cancer. Although most cancers are sporadic, 1% to 3% are caused by a genetic mutation (most commonly *E-cadherin/CDH-1* mutations). Numerous dietary factors have been linked to subsequent gastric cancer development, including salty or spicy diets, processed meat, smoked fish, refined grains, and lack of adequate fruits and vegetables. Additional lifestyle factors include alcohol and cigarette use. Men are also more likely to develop the disease than women.

A history of *H. pylori* infection or chronic atrophic gastritis also increases a patient's risk of developing subsequent stomach cancer. The International Agency for Research on Cancer estimates that *H. pylori* solely attributes to 36% of gastric cancers in developed countries and 47% in developing countries. Both intestinal and diffuse subtypes of gastric adenocarcinoma are associated with *H. pylori*. *H. pylori* strains with the *cagA* gene have a poorer prognosis. The chronic inflammation and subsequent development of atrophic gastritis can lead to intestinal metaplasia.

There has been an increasing incidence of proximal gastric cancers. Obesity and GERD are risk factors for more proximal lesions.

Screening

National screening programs have been established in Japan and South Korea, both of which have a relatively high incidence of gastric cancer. In Korea, screening is recommended every 2 years starting at 40 years of age. In Japan, screening is performed every 2 to 3 years starting at 50 years of age. Both countries have shown diagnosis at earlier cancer stages improved with utilization of their screening programs. The relative utility and cost-effectiveness of national gastric cancer screening with either upper endoscopy or upper GI series has not been established in countries with a lower relative incidence of gastric cancer. Individualized screening can be considered for those with high-risk genetic syndromes, such as *CDH-1* mutation, Lynch syndrome, Peutz-Jeghers syndrome, and familial adenomatous polyposis. Screening can also be considered in patients with a strong family history of gastric cancer or previously established atrophic gastritis or intestinal metaplasia.

Clinical Manifestations

Patients with gastric adenocarcinoma often have vague symptoms that may not be present until more advanced disease is present. Epigastric abdominal pain (52%) and weight loss (62%) are the most common symptoms, but early satiety, decreased appetite, and nausea can also be present. New-onset heartburn or reflux can be a presenting symptom and warrants further workup, especially in older adults. Melena and anemia can be seen in tumors that are bleeding. A rare subset of patients may have systemic manifestations of gastric cancer. These paraneoplastic syndromes include the Leser-Trelat sign, which is characterized by sudden onset of multiple seborrheic keratoses, and acanthosis nigricans, which appears as dark pigmentation in skin folds. However, these manifestations are not specific to gastric cancer and are benign processes in the majority of patients.

Diagnosis

Esophagogastroduodenoscopy (EGD) with biopsy is the gold standard for gastric cancer diagnosis. This allows for tissue diagnosis as well as anatomic location of the primary tumor. Of note, per the American Joint Committee on Cancer (AJCC) and the Union for International Cancer Control (UICC) TNM classification, 8th edition, esophagogastric junction tumors with an epicenter less than 2 cm into the proximal stomach are classified as esophageal cancers; those more than 2 cm into the stomach are staged as gastric cancers. Gastric adenocarcinomas usually appear as friable ulcerated masses endoscopically. However, it should be noted that the gastric mucosa can appear normal in linitis plastica (an aggressive form of diffuse-type adenocarcinoma), with the only endoscopic finding being poor stomach distensibility.

Deep biopsies beyond the superficial mucosa must be obtained to evaluate for these lesions. Any suspicious lesion should have multiple biopsies taken to improve the diagnostic yield. For example, a single biopsy has a 70% sensitivity for diagnosis compared with 98% with seven biopsies. For this reason, six to eight biopsies are recommended for each suspicious lesion.

For lesions less than 2 cm in size, endoscopic mucosal resection (EMR) or endoscopic submucosal dissection (ESD) can be considered in experienced hands, which can be both diagnostic and therapeutic depending on the pathology of the specimen. The pathology report of the biopsy should include presence of invasion, histologic subtype (intestinal or diffuse), and tumor grade. Unfortunately, in the United States the vast majority of tumors present at later stages of disease.

Staging

Once adenocarcinoma is diagnosed on endoscopic biopsy, patients should undergo CT of the chest, abdomen, and pelvis to evaluate for regional and metastatic disease. For suspicious lesions in the common sites of metastatic disease, such as the liver and lung, a biopsy should be performed for tissue confirmation. Ascitic fluid may be sampled by paracentesis and sent for cytologic and chemical analysis. Involvement of abdominal lymph nodes outside the standard lymphadenectomy resection (i.e., pancreatoduodenal, peripancreatic, middle colic, para-aortic) are classified as distant metastasis.

In patients without evidence of metastatic disease on CT, EUS is recommended to assess the T stage. EUS can also identify enlarged nearby lymph nodes, which can be biopsied using fine-needle aspiration. If there is high clinical suspicion of metastasis but initial CT is unrevealing, integrated positron emission tomography (PET)/CT may be considered. Diagnostic staging laparoscopy may also be useful in detecting occult disease in patients with tumor invasion beyond the submucosa or in whom neoadjuvant therapy is being considered. Staging laparoscopy

TABLE 1	8th Edition AJCC Staging of Gastric Adenocarcinoma		
AJCC Stage	**T-Stage**	**N-Stage**	**M-Stage**
IA	T1	N0	M0
IB	T1	N1	M0
IB	T2	N0	M0
IIA	T1	N2	M0
IIA	T2	N1	M0
IIA	T3	N0	M0
IIB	T1	N3a	M0
IIB	T2	N2	M0
IIB	T3	N1	M0
IIB	T4a	N0	M0
IIIA	T2	N3a	M0
IIIA	T3	N2	M0
IIIA	T4a	N1 or N2	M0
IIIA	T4 b	N0	M0
IIIB	T1 or T2	N3b	M0
IIIB	T3 or T4a	N3a	M0
IIIB	T4b	N1 or N2	M0
IIIC	T3 or T4a	N3b	M0
IIIC	T4b	N3a or N3b	M0
IV	Any T	Any N	M1

is superior to cross-sectional imaging for identifying peritoneal spread and allows for peritoneal fluid sampling for cytologic analysis. A complete blood count and comprehensive metabolic profile should be obtained to evaluate for anemia and electrolyte derangements.

The most recent AJCC/UICC TNM staging classifications were published in 2017. An important update in the new classification system is separate staging for patients with and without neoadjuvant therapy. Early gastric adenocarcinoma is defined as cancers that do not invade past the submucosa (T1); T1a tumors involve the mucosa, and T1b tumors involve the submucosa. T2 tumors involve the muscularis propria, T3 tumors penetrate to the subserosa, and T4 tumors invade beyond the serosa (T4a) or invade adjacent structures (T4b). Regional nodal classification is N1 for 1 to 2 lymph node metastases, N2 for 3 to 6 nodes, N3a for 7 to 15 nodes, and N3b for 16 or more involved nodes. The M1 stage indicates the presence of metastatic disease.

Treatment

It is recommended that treatment decisions for all patients diagnosed with gastric cancer be discussed by a multidisciplinary team including medical oncology, radiation oncology, surgical oncology, gastroenterology, radiology, and pathology. Complete surgical resection of the cancer and adjacent lymph nodes offers the best opportunity for long-term survival when possible. Indicators of surgical unresectability include presence of metastatic disease, involvement of a major vascular structure such as the aorta, or encasement of the celiac axis, hepatic artery, or proximal splenic artery. It should be noted that involvement of the distal splenic artery can still represent resectable disease.

Patients with either Tis or T1a disease (tumor that does not invade past the submucosa) may be candidates for either endoscopic or surgical resection. Patients with T1b cancers (a tumor that invades the submucosa) should undergo upfront surgical resection. Patients with T2 or higher disease or any nodal involvement are recommended to undergo perioperative chemotherapy. Radiation therapy can be considered, especially in cases of locally advanced disease. Patients who are not candidates for curative surgical resection or with metastatic disease should be considered for palliative treatment in addition to systemic chemotherapy.

Surgery

Endoscopic resection with either EMR or ESD can be considered adequate therapy for gastric tumors less than 2 cm in size that (1) are well-differentiated or moderately differentiated, (2) do not penetrate past the submucosa, and (3) do not have evidence of lymphovascular invasion.

Surgical resection typically consists of either a distal/subtotal or total gastrectomy depending on where the tumor is located. Tumors in the proximal third of the stomach typically require total gastrectomy, while a subtotal distal gastrectomy can be performed in the distal two-thirds. There is no survival difference between total and distal gastrectomy for distal tumors, and the quality of life in patients has been shown to be superior with partial gastrectomy when possible oncologically. Patients undergoing surgery should be considered for a diagnostic laparoscopy to detect the possible presence of occult metastatic disease before committing to curative surgery. A 5-cm proximal margin should be obtained with at least a 2-cm distal margin on the duodenum. T4 tumors require en bloc resection of nearby involved organs or structures. Retrieval of at least 15 lymph nodes is necessary for accurate nodal staging.

Minimally invasive gastrectomy, when technically feasible, has been shown to be non-inferior oncologically to open surgery. Additionally, minimally invasive gastrectomy has been shown to have fewer wound complications, decreased postoperative pain, and shorter length of stay.

The appropriate extent of lymphadenectomy for gastric cancer is debated. Although D1 lymphadenectomy involves removal of the perigastric lymph nodes alone, D2 lymphadenectomy involves additional removal of lymph nodes around the left gastric, common hepatic, celiac, and splenic arteries. It is unclear if D2 lymphadenectomy provides an overall survival benefit, with most randomized trials not demonstrating a significant difference between D1 and D2 lymphadenectomy. However, in experienced hands, the additional D2 lymph nodes can provide improved staging information with a minimal increase in morbidity and is now what is typically performed in high-volume cancer centers. D3 lymphadenectomy (para-aortic lymph nodes), however, is associated with increased morbidity and is not presently recommended.

In cases that require reconstruction after a distal gastrectomy, options include Roux-en-Y gastrojejunostomy, Billroth I gastroduodenostomy, and Billroth II gastrojejunostomy. Reconstruction after total gastrectomy is performed with a Roux-en-Y esophagojejunostomy. Placement of a jejunal feeding tube should be considered at the time of operation, especially if a patient is likely to receive adjuvant chemoradiation and/or their nutritional status is poor, though their use is not standardized.

Chemotherapy

The utility of chemotherapy in gastric adenocarcinoma has been established in multiple randomized trials. The first major trial (MAGIC) randomized 503 patients with resectable adenocarcinoma of the stomach, gastroesophageal junction, or lower esophagus to surgery alone versus surgery with perioperative ECF (epirubicin [Ellence],[1] cisplatin,[1] 5-fluorouracil). Chemotherapy consisted of three preoperative and three postoperative cycles. Perioperative ECF resulted in improved 5-year overall survival (36% compared with 23% for patients who received surgery alone). More recently, a randomized phase 2/3 trial of 716 patients with resectable stage II or III gastric or gastroesophageal junction adenocarcinomas was conducted to compare perioperative ECF and perioperative FLOT (fluorouracil, leucovorin,[1] oxaliplatin,[1] and docetaxel [Taxotere]). Survival was significantly improved with FLOT, with a median overall survival of 50 months compared with 35 months with ECF.

In patients who are medically fit and thereby recommended to receive perioperative chemotherapy, the FLOT regimen is recommended. Patients who are unable to tolerate this more aggressive chemotherapy regimen may undergo treatment with a fluoropyrimidine and oxaliplatin[1] or fluorouracil and cisplatin.[1] The ECF regimen is no longer first-line therapy.

For patients who do not receive neoadjuvant therapy, treatment recommendations are guided by the pathologic tumor classification, operative margins, and extent of lymphadenectomy. Those whose final surgical pathology reveals T3, T4, or any N-positive disease should be offered adjuvant chemotherapy. Those with T2N0 disease may be offered either adjuvant chemotherapy or surveillance. All patients with positive operative margins should receive adjuvant chemoradiation. Adjuvant chemotherapy is fluoropyrimidine-based. In patients who received less than a D2 lymphadenectomy, fluorouracil or capecitabine (Xeloda)[1] is recommended before and after fluoropyrimidine-based regimens. For patients who did have a D2 lymphadenectomy, oxaliplatin[1] and fluorouracil or capecitabine[1] is recommended.

Immunotherapy

There are currently ongoing preclinical and early clinical phase trials of various immunotherapy agents in the treatment of gastric adenocarcinoma. However, their use remains investigational at this time.

Radiotherapy

The benefits and indications for radiotherapy are less well-established for noncardia gastric adenocarcinoma. There are currently no randomized trials comparing adjuvant chemoradiotherapy to either surgery alone or surgery and chemotherapy. Preoperative chemoradiotherapy is beneficial in patients with esophageal, gastroesophageal junction, and gastric cardia tumors

---

[1] Not FDA approved for this indication.

as shown in the CROSS trial, but its role specifically in gastric cancer is less clear. Radiotherapy can be considered as an adjunct in multidisciplinary discussions for patients with locally advanced disease.

Palliation

The most common indications for palliative procedures in gastric cancer are gastric outlet obstruction, bleeding, and perforation. Choosing among the various palliative options involves consideration of the risks and benefits specific to each patient's case as well as the patient's goals of care. For patients with an obstructing tumor, especially in the pre-pyloric or antral regions, surgical or endoscopic interventions may be beneficial. For a patient whose life expectancy is greater than 6 months and who is medically fit, surgical gastrojejunostomy may be preferred if technically feasible in either an open or laparoscopic fashion. If the patient is not a surgical candidate, endoscopic stent placement or endoscopic gastrojejunostomy may be considered. Finally, a venting gastrostomy tube is another alternative. However, the patient will no longer be able to eat if this is the only therapy offered, and a feeding jejunostomy tube must be considered for enteral nutrition.

Patients who present with uncontrollable bleeding may initially undergo endoscopic treatment, but this is associated with a high likelihood of recurrent bleeding. Angiographic embolization or radiation therapy are potential alternatives. If these more conservative measures are unsuccessful, palliative resection should be considered. Should a patient pursue operative intervention, lymph node dissection is not required. If patients present with gastric perforation and surgery is within the patient's goals of care, urgent palliative resection may be attempted.

Monitoring

Patients successfully treated with endoscopic resection should undergo a thorough history and physical examination every 3 to 6 months after treatment for the first 1 to 2 years, and then every 6 to 12 months for 3 to 5 years, followed by annual follow-up thereafter. EGD should be performed every 6 months for 1 year and then annually for up to 5 years. CT scans should be performed as clinically indicated by symptoms.

Patients with stage I disease treated by surgery should undergo a history and physical examination every 3 to 6 months after treatment for 1 to 2 years, and then every 6 to 12 months for 3 to 5 years, followed by annual follow-up thereafter. They should have EGD and/or CT scans as clinically indicated by symptoms. These patients must additionally be monitored for nutritional deficiencies, especially involving B_{12} and iron.

Patients with stage II or III disease who received surgery should undergo a history and physical examination every 3 to 6 months after treatment for 1 to 2 years, and then every 6 to 12 months for 3 to 5 years, followed by annual follow-up thereafter. EGD may be performed as clinically indicated. CT of the chest/abdomen/pelvis should be performed every 6 to 12 months for the first 2 years and then annually up to 5 years. PET/CT should be considered as clinically indicated when suspicion for disease recurrence and/or metastasis is high. These patients must also be monitored for nutritional deficiencies.

Complications

In the early postoperative period, patients can develop peritonitis from an anastomotic leak or duodenal stump perforation. Bowel obstructions can also develop. It should be noted that acute afferent limb obstruction in patients who had a Billroth II reconstruction should be treated differently than other small bowel obstructions in that they typically require immediate operative intervention with either surgical revision of the gastrojejunostomy, conversion to a Roux-en-Y anastomosis, or a Braun's enteroenterostomy.

Clinically significant dumping syndrome is seen in approximately 20% of patients after distal gastrectomy. Early dumping, which occurs within 1 hour of eating, is associated with abdominal pain, cramping, nausea, diaphoresis, palpitations, and flushing. Late dumping occurs hours after eating and is caused by hypoglycemia after the postprandial insulin peak. Most patients can be managed conservatively with small, frequent meals and avoidance of exacerbating foods. Octreotide (Sandostatin)[1] can be a useful adjunct in patients with persistent symptoms. Rarely, surgical revision to a Roux-en-Y gastrojejunostomy is required.

Gastrointestinal Stromal Tumors

Gastrointestinal stromal tumors (GISTs) are mesenchymal subepithelial neoplasms. The incidence of GISTs is 7 to 15 cases per 1 million, and the most common tumor location is the stomach. GISTs account for 1% to 3% of stomach neoplasms. GISTs are thought to arise from the interstitial cells of Cajal and are identified histologically by their overexpression of CD117 (KIT). The most common presenting symptom is gastrointestinal bleeding, occurring in approximately 50% of gastric GISTs. Preoperative endoscopic biopsy is not necessary if there is a high suspicion for GIST based on endoscopic submucosal lesion appearance and it is resectable; biopsy should be performed if there is diagnostic uncertainty, if there is concern for metastatic disease, or if neoadjuvant imatinib is being considered. The prognosis for GISTs has greatly improved after the discovery of imatinib, a receptor tyrosine kinase inhibitor that specifically targets c-KIT.

Surgery is the only curative option for patients with gastric GIST. All GISTs >2 cm should be considered for resection. Grossly negative margins are sufficient, and no lymphadenectomy is required given the very low rates of lymph node metastases in these tumors. Care should be taken to preserve the tumor capsule as intraoperative rupture increases the risk of recurrence. Neoadjuvant imatinib can be considered in patients with locally advanced or borderline resectable disease or in whom preoperative tumor shrinkage would potentially reduce surgical morbidity.

Imatinib (Gleevec) is an oral medication taken at a dose of 400 mg daily. Adjuvant imatinib should be offered to patients with a high risk of recurrence, specifically either primary tumor >5 cm in size and/or mitotic rate >5 per 50 high-power field. The phase III ACOSOG Z9001 established the significant improvement in recurrence-free survival with 1 year of adjuvant therapy compared with placebo (98 vs, 83% at 1 year, $P < 0.0001$). Further, the Scandinavian Sarcoma Group XVIII phase III trial showed that 3 years of adjuvant imatinib was superior to 1 year in both recurrence-free survival (65.6 vs. 47.9% at 5 years) and overall survival (92.0 vs. 81.7% at 5 years). However, recurrences are not uncommon after discontinuation of imatinib, and further studies are ongoing to establish if a longer regimen may be more beneficial. For tumors resistant to imatinib, second-line therapy is sunitinib (Sutent), another tyrosine kinase inhibitor. Traditional chemotherapy and hyperthermic intraperitoneal chemotherapy (HIPEC) are not standardly used now after the advent of tyrosine kinase inhibitor therapy.

Neuroendocrine Tumors

Gastric neuroendocrine tumors (gNETs) arise from enterochromaffin-like cells and were previously referred to as *carcinoid tumors*. The incidence of gNETs has increased 15-fold from 1973 to 2012 as a result of increased awareness of the disease, an increased number of upper endoscopies, and possibly increased use of PPIs. There are three distinct subtypes of gNET. Type 1 gNETs are the most common (70% to 80%) and are associated with pernicious anemia and atrophic gastritis. Type 2 gNETs account for 5% to 10% and are associated with Zollinger-Ellison syndrome and multiple endocrine neoplasia type 1. Type 3 gNETs have normal gastrin and stomach acid levels, are solitary lesions, and are more aggressive and tend to metastasize. Neuroendocrine carcinomas are sometimes referred to as type 4 lesions and are poorly differentiated tumors that behave similarly to gastric adenocarcinoma.

---

[1] Not FDA approved for this indication.

Upper endoscopy and biopsy are indicated for diagnosis. The mitotic rate and Ki-67 proliferation index should be measured from the specimen to allow for tumor grading. Patients with type 3 gNETs or with worrisome features (size >2 cm, high grade) should undergo multiphasic abdominal CT or MRI for staging.

Type 1 gNETs less than 1 cm can undergo endoscopic resection or surveillance. If they are greater than 1 cm in size, not high-grade, and EUS shows no invasion beyond the submucosa, endoscopic resection can be performed. If they are poorly differentiated, have invasion beyond the submucosa, or have positive margins after endoscopic resection, surgical resection should be performed. If there is persistent or recurrent disease after surgery, an antrectomy can be considered. For type 2 tumors, gastrinoma resection or high-dose PPI therapy should be initiated. If tumor size is less than 2 cm without worrisome features on biopsy, endoscopic resection can be performed; otherwise surgical resection is recommended. Type 3 tumors, given their more aggressive behavior, should undergo anatomic surgical resection with lymphadenectomy.

If there is metastatic disease to the liver, carcinoid syndrome can occur. Surgical cytoreduction or liver-directed therapies can be offered. The most common systemic therapy utilizes somatostatin analogues (octreotide [Sandostatin] or lanreotide [Somatuline Depot]). If there is disease progression on somatostatin therapy, cytotoxic chemotherapy (i.e., etoposide [Toposar][1] with carboplatin [Paraplatin][1] or cisplatin[1]), everolimus (Afinitor), or interferon-alpha-2b (Intron A)[1] can be given as second-line agents. Peptide receptor radionuclide therapy (PRRT) delivers radiation therapy via binding of the somatostatin receptor by 177-Lu-Dotatate and may be considered in locally advanced or metastatic gNETs.

Gastric Lymphomas

The stomach is the most common extranodal site of lymphoma. Gastric lymphomas account for approximately 3% of gastric malignancies and 10% of lymphomas. The most common presenting symptom is epigastric pain, followed by anorexia, weight loss, nausea, and bleeding. Fever and night sweats are seen in 12% of patients. Diagnosis is established by endoscopic biopsy. The two most common subtypes in the stomach are diffuse large B-cell lymphoma and marginal-zone B-cell lymphoma of mucosa-associated lymphoid tissue (MALT). MALT lymphomas of the stomach often respond to *H. pylori* eradication. Patients with persistent or recurrent disease can undergo radiotherapy or chemotherapy. Surgery is only indicated in patients with complications from their disease such as significant bleeding or perforation.

References

Al-Batran SE, Homann N, Pauligk C, et al: Perioperative chemotherapy with fluorouracil plus leucovorin, oxaliplatin, and docetaxel versus fluorouracil or capecitabine plus cisplatin and epirubicin for locally advanced, resectable gastric or gastro-oesophageal junction adenocarcinoma (FLOT4): a randomised, phase 2/3 trial, *Lancet* 393(10184):1948–1957, 2019.

Corey B, Chen H: Neuroendocrine Tumors of the Stomach, *Surg Clin North Am* 97:333–343, 2017.

Cunningham D, Allum WH, Stenning SP, et al: Perioperative chemotherapy versus surgery alone for resectable gastroesophageal cancer, *N Engl J Med* 355:11–20, 2006.

DeMatteo RP, Ballman KV, Antonescu CR, et al: Placebo-Controlled Randomized Trial of Adjuvant Imatinib Mesylate Following the Resection of Localized, Primary Gastrointestinal Stromal Tumor (GIST), *Lancet* 373(9669):1097–1104, 2009.

Hu Q, Zhang Y, Zhang X, Fu K: Gastric mucosa-associated lymphoid tissue lymphoma and *Helicobacter pylori* infection: a review of current diagnosis and management, *Biomarker Research* 4:15, 2016.

Joensuu H, Eriksson M, Sundby Hall K, et al: One vs Three Years of Adjuvant Imatinib for Operable Gastrointestinal Stromal Tumor: A Randomized Trial, *JAMA* 307(12):1265–1272, 2012.

Noh SH, Park SR, Yang HK, et al: Adjuvant capecitabine plus oxaliplatin for gastric cancer after D2 gastrectomy (CLASSIC): 5-year follow-up of an open-label, randomised phase 3 trial, *Lancet Oncol* 15(12):1389–1396, 2014.

---

[1] Not FDA approved for this indication.

5 Endocrine and Metabolic Disorders

ACROMEGALY

Method of
Moises Mercado, MD

CURRENT DIAGNOSIS

Clinical
- Headaches, visual field defects
- Coarse features, increased size of hands (rings) and feet (shoes)
- Thick, oily skin, skin tags, acanthosis nigricans
- Arthralgias, osteoarthritis
- Paresthesias, carpal tunnel syndrome
- Hypertension, arrhythmia, heart failure
- Glucose intolerance, diabetes, hypertriglyceridemia
- Snoring, sleep apnea
- Risk of colon polyps or colon cancer
- Risk of thyroid cancer

Biochemical
- Glucose-suppressed growth hormone >0.4 ng/mL by ultrasensitive assays or >1 ng/mL by old radioimmunoassays
- Elevated age-adjusted insulin-like growth factor 1

Imaging
- Magnetic resonance imaging

CURRENT THERAPY

- If a pituitary surgeon is available: Transsphenoidal surgery for microadenomas, intrasellar macroadenomas, and debulking or decompressing surgery in invasive macroadenomas
- Depot Somatostatin analogues (SA) (lanreotide autogel [Somatuline Depot] or octreotide LAR [Sandostatin LAR Depot]) as secondary treatment for patients failing surgery or waiting for radiotherapy effect to occur and as a primary treatment for patients with inaccessible lesions, contraindications for surgery, or preference. An effective, orally available octreotide (Mycapssa) has recently been approved by the FDA. The second generation SA pasireotide (Signifor LAR) seems to be somewhat more effective than octreotide or lanreotide.
- Dopamine agonists: Cabergoline (DOSTINEX)[1] is effective alone or in combination with somatostatin analogues in 15% to 30% of patients
- Growth hormone receptor antagonists: Pegvisomant (Somavert) for patients resistant or intolerant to somatostatin analogues and who have tumors >5 mm from the optic chiasm
- Radiotherapy for patients resistant or intolerant to pharmacologic therapy, with clinically and biochemically active disease and a tumor remnant on MRI

[1]Not FDA approved for this indication.

Acromegaly is a disorder resulting from an excessive secretion of growth hormone (GH), with a prevalence of 40 to 60 cases per million and an annual incidence of 3 to 4 per million.

Physiology, Biochemistry, and Regulation of the GH/IGF-1 Axis

GH secretion is regulated at the hypothalamus (Figure 1). The pulsatile secretion of GH-releasing hormone (GHRH) stimulates somatotroph proliferation and GH gene transcription, whereas somatostatin, which is secreted tonically, inhibits GH synthesis. These two hypothalamic signals result in the pulsatile secretion of pituitary GH, with most pulses occurring during the night. GH is also stimulated by ghrelin, a hypothalamic and gastrointestinal orexigenic hormone that binds specific receptors in the somatotroph known as GH-secretagogue receptors. GH exerts its actions through a specific membrane receptor located predominantly in the liver and cartilage, but ubiquitously present in all tissues. One molecule of GH interacts with two molecules of GH receptor, resulting in functional dimerization and conformational changes that lead to the phosphorylation of several kinases and eventually the interaction with target genes such as the insulin-like growth factor (IGF)-1 gene.

IGF-1 is closely related to proinsulin and circulates in plasma bound to six binding proteins (IGFBPs) that are synthesized and released by the liver. IGFBP3 is the most important of these binding proteins and is also GH dependent; it forms a heterotrimeric complex composed of BP3, IGF-1, and the acid-labile subunit (ALS). IGF-1 is responsible for most of the trophic and growth-promoting effects of GH. Blood levels of IGF-1 are increased during puberty, coinciding with the acceleration of somatic growth, and decline with aging. Malnutrition, poorly controlled type 1 diabetes, hypothyroidism, and liver failure all result in diminished IGF-1 concentrations. IGF-1 is the main player in GH negative feedback regulation and it acts at both the pituitary and the hypothalamic levels. Glucose regulates GH release by increasing (hyperglycemia) or decreasing (hypoglycemia) somatostatin synthesis in the hypothalamus. Exercise and amino acids such as arginine also stimulate GH secretion.

Etiopathogenesis of Growth Hormone–Secreting Tumors

The molecular pathogenesis of pituitary tumors includes the inactivation of tumor suppressor genes, the activation of oncogenes, and the trophic effect of factors such as the hypothalamic releasing hormones. Less than 5% of acromegaly cases occur in a syndromic or hereditary context, including type 1 multiple endocrine neoplasia (MEN1), due to inactivating mutations of the gene encoding the tumor suppressor gene menin, MEN4 due to inactivating mutations of CDKN1B (p27), the Carney complex due to mutations of PRKAR1A, the paraganglioma/pheochormocytoma/pituitary adenoma due to a variety of mutations of the genes encoding the different isoforms of succinate dehydrogenase, the familial pituitary adenoma syndrome (FIPA), due to inactivating mutations of the gene encoding the Ary-lhydrocarbion receptor interacting protein (AIP) and X-linked acrogigantism due to duplications of the gene encoding the probable G-protein receptor 101. Patients with isolated familial somatotrophinomas are younger and usually have more aggressive tumors than subjects with sporadic acromegaly. Approximately 40% of GH-producing tumors in whites harbor somatic point mutations of the α subunit stimulatory G protein coupled to the GHRH receptor (GSPα mutations

Figure 1 GH is regulated positively by GHRH and negatively by somatostatin. Fifty percent of circulating GH is bound to the GH binding protein, which represents the extracellular portion of the GH receptor. One molecule of GH dimerizes two molecules of GH receptor, and the ensuing signal transduction results in IGF-1 synthesis and secretion, which exerts negative feedback on GH secretion at the hypothalamic and pituitary levels. *Abbreviations:* ALS = acid-labile subunit; GH = growth hormone; GHRH = growth hormone–releasing hormone; IGF = insulin-like growth factor; IGFBP3 = insulin-like growth factor binding protein 3; IRS = insulin receptor S; JAK2 = Janus kinase 2; SRIH = somatostatin; SSTR = somatostatin receptor.

or GNAS oncogene). This molecular alteration causes constitutive activation of the GHRH receptor, resulting in an increased transcription of the GH gene and the promotion of somatotroph proliferation. Patients with acromegaly whose tumors harbor GNAS mutations usually have a more benign clinical course and appear to be more susceptible to management with somatostatin analogues. Nonwhite acromegalic populations, including persons of Japanese, Korean, and Mexican heritage, have a much lower prevalence of GNAS mutations. *GNAS* mutations occurring in a post-zygotic manner are responsible for the McCune-Albright syndrome, which not infrequently include prolactin (PRL) and to a lesser extent GH-secreting adenomas.

Other molecular events should be present in GSPα-negative somatotrophinomas. Menin is a protein encoded by a tumor suppressor gene located on the short arm of chromosome 11. Inactivating mutations of menin are the molecular basis of type 1 multiple endocrine neoplasia (MEN1); however, GH-secreting tumors occurring out of this context do not have such genetic abnormalities. Inactivating mutations of other putative tumor-suppressor genes located relatively close to the menin locus have been described in several kindreds with familial acromegaly; however, they do not seem to play an important oncogenic role in the sporadic form of the disease. Other genetic alterations such as underexpression of GADD 45γ (growth arrest and DNA damage-inducible protein) and overexpression of the securin molecule PTTG (pituitary tumor transforming gene) have also been shown to be involved in the molecular pathogenesis of acromegaly. Although hereditary acromegaly is rare (less than 2% of the cases), familial somatotrophinomas account for 30% of the tumors seen in the syndrome of familial isolated pituitary adenomas. Patients with isolated familial somatotrophinomas are younger and usually have more aggressive tumors than subjects with sporadic acromegaly. Affected members do not show any molecular alterations in the MEN1 gene. However, 15% of 73 tested families harbor inactivating, germline mutations of the AIP (aryl hydrocarbon interacting protein) gene located on chromosome 11q13.3.

In more than 90% of cases, acromegaly is caused by a sporadic pituitary adenoma. In approximately 70% of these patients, these benign epithelial neoplasms are larger than 1 cm in diameter and are known as *macroadenomas*, whereas one-third of the patients harbor lesions smaller than 1 cm or *microadenomas*. One-third of the patients have tumors that cosecrete GH and prolactin (PRL) (mammosomatoroph cell adenomas). Real pituitary GH-secreting carcinomas, with documented metastasis as the irrefutable malignancy criterion, are exceedingly rare. On rare occasions, acromegaly results from GHRH-secreting neuroendocrine tumors, usually located in the lungs, thymus, or endocrine pancreas. In this scenario, the ectopically produced GHRH leads to hyperplasia of the somatotroph, with the consequent excessive production of GH. Even less common are GH-secreting tumors arising in ectopic pituitary tissue, usually located in the sphenoid sinus. A case of GH-secreting lymphoma has been reported.

Clinical Manifestations

Acromegaly develops insidiously over many years. An 8- to 10-year delay in diagnosis has been estimated from the beginning of the first symptom. Clinical characteristics are often attributed to aging. Symptoms and signs can be divided into those resulting from the compressive effects of the pituitary tumor and those that are a consequence of the GH and IGF-1 excess.

Local Tumor Effects

Headache results from an increase in intracranial pressure and from the effects of GH itself; it is usually described as a dull pain that persists throughout the day. Occasionally, large tumors invading laterally into the cavernous sinuses give rise to cranial nerve syndromes, usually third and sixth. Visual field defects are relatively common with macroadenomas extending superiorly and compressing the optic chiasm. This usually results in different combinations of bitemporal homonymous hemianopia or quadrontopia.

Consequences of the GH/IGF-1 Excess
Skeletal Growth and Skin Changes

A GH excess developing before the pubertal closure of epiphyseal bone leads to an acceleration of linear growth, and this results in gigantism. Once the patient is in adulthood, the GH/IGF-1 excess results in acral enlargement, which is manifested by increases in ring and shoe sizes as well as enlargement of the nose, supracilliary arches, frontal bones, and mandible (Figure 2). There is thickening of soft tissues of the hands and feet; hands are fleshy and bulky and the heel pad is increased. The skin is thickened due to the deposition of glycosaminoglycans and excessive collagen production. Hyperhidrosis and seborrhea occur in 60% of patients; skin tags (previously associated with colon cancer) and acanthosis nigricans are common.

Musculoskeletal System

Generalized arthralgias are present in the majority (80%) of patients. Degenerative osteoarthritis is more common than in

Figure 2 A and B, Skeletal growth and skin changes in acromegaly. (From Salmon JF: *Kanski's Clinical Ophthalmology,* 9th edition. Elsevier, 2020.)

the general population. Paresthesias of the hands and feet and a proximal painful myopathy are often reported. Nerve entrapment syndromes such as the carpal tunnel syndrome occur in nearly half of patients.

Cardiovascular System
Arterial hypertension is found in 30% of patients, and when associated with diabetes, it contributes to the increased mortality rate of the disease. Hyperaldosteronism with low renin levels and the resulting sodium retention play an important role in the pathogenesis of hypertension, but other contributors such as an increased sympathetic tone are also present. Echocardiographic findings include left ventricular and septal hypertrophy with varying degrees of diastolic dysfunction. Symptomatic cardiac disease develops in 15% of patients and is usually due to coronary artery disease, heart failure, and arrhythmias. Although the existence of an acromegalic cardiomyopathy is still controversial, there are patients without hypertension and with angiographically normal coronaries, who develop severe congestive heart failure, in whom histologic evidence of subendocardial, subepicardial, and myocardial fibrosis and necrosis has been documented.

Respiratory Abnormalities
The majority of patients with acromegaly are affected by loud snoring. A significant fraction of these have sleep apnea (with both central and obstructive components) with significant drops in oxygen saturation, which can be complicated by arrhythmias, daytime somnolence, and chronic fatigue.

Abnormalities in Glucose Metabolism
Chronic GH hypersecretion creates a state of insulin resistance, and glucose intolerance has been reported in 30% to 50% of patients with acromegaly; the percentage with fasting hyperglycemia can be close to 30%, depending on the population. Hyperglycemia has correlated with GH concentrations in some studies and with IGF-1 levels in others. Although successful treatment of acromegaly, be it by surgical, pharmacological, or radiotherapeutical interventions, results in significant improvements in metabolic control, the prevalence of diabetes remains higher than in the general population.

Abnormalities in Lipid Metabolism
The classic lipid profile consists of diminished total cholesterol, along with elevated triglyceride concentrations. Intermediate-density lipoprotein (IDL) particles and lipoprotein(a) might also be elevated, and there is a higher percentage of the more atherogenic type II low-density lipoprotein (LDL).

Bone and Calcium Metabolism
Acromegaly is associated with hypercalciuria and hyperphosphatemia. High serum 25-hydroxyvitamin D_3 and urinary levels of hydroxyproline can be found, reflecting a state of increased bone turnover. Cortical bone mineral density is elevated, whereas trabecular bone mass is diminished.

Neoplasia
Retrospective studies suggested that colonic adenomatous polyps and adenocarcinoma were more frequent in acromegalic patients than in the general population. Prospective studies have demonstrated that the risk, albeit smaller than previously thought, is real and probably justifies screening colonoscopy in these patients. Patients with uncontrolled acromegaly have a higher risk of recurrence of premalignant polyps and a higher mortality rate from colon cancer compared with subjects with biochemically controlled disease and the general population. Recently, an increased incidence of well-differentiated thyroid carcinoma has been documented.

Associated Endocrine Abnormalities
A euthyroid goiter is often found but seldom requires specific treatment. Hypopituitarism occurs variably, depending on the size and extension of the tumor and whether the patient has undergone surgery or radiation therapy. Hypogonadotropic hypogonadism is the most common pituitary deficiency, occurring in 20% of patients. A decreased libido is a common presenting complaint in both male and female patients with acromegaly; women often have menstrual and ovulatory disturbances and men complain of impotence.

Although an elevated PRL is common, it does not always reflect cosecretion of this hormone by the somatotrophinoma, but rather an interruption of the descending dopaminergic tone by the tumor compressing the pituitary stalk. Central hypocortisolism and hypothyroidism are less common.

GH-secreting pituitary adenomas are the second, after prolactinomas, pituitary tumor occurring in the context of MEN1 (multiple parathyroid adenomas, pituitary adenoma, and pancreatic islet cell tumors). Acromegaly can also develop in patients with the McCune-Albright syndrome (polyostotic fibrous dysplasia, café au lait spots, and endocrinopathies such as sexual precocity and autonomous thyroid nodules), and occurs in the context of the Carney complex.

Mortality
Life expectancy in patients with acromegaly is decreased by about 10 to 15 years, and the standardized mortality ratio is 1.5 to 2. Most patients die of cardiovascular causes, followed by cerebrovascular

events, respiratory abnormalities, and neoplastic diseases. Hormonal control has a definite impact on survival. Lowering serum GH to less than 2.5 ng/mL results in reduction of the mortality rate to levels comparable with the general population. These safe GH levels were obtained using old radioimmunoassays, and there are no equivalent studies using ultrasensitive GH assays. IGF-1 levels have not been as good as GH as independent predictors of mortality. Other factors associated with an increased mortality include advanced age and the presence of hypertension and diabetes. Mortality rate in acromegaly can be reduced to that seen on the general population when patients are treated using a multidisciplinary approach not only aiming at controlling the GH and IGF-1 levels but also focusing on the management of comorbidities.

Biochemical Diagnosis

Due to the pulsatile nature of GH secretion, random determinations of this hormone are not useful in the diagnosis of acromegaly. The gold standard for the diagnosis is the measurement of GH after an oral glucose load of 75 g; current guidelines state that suppression to less than 0.4 ng/mL (using ultrasensitive assays) reliably excludes the diagnosis. Situations associated with decreased suppression of GH by glucose include puberty, pregnancy, use of oral contraceptives, uncontrolled diabetes, and renal and hepatic insufficiency.

IGF-1 levels reflect the integrated concentrations over 24 hours of GH and correlate well with clinical activity. Blood IGF-1 concentrations decrease with age, reflecting the parallel decline of the somatotropic axis. There is a gender difference in IGF-1 (premenopausal women have lower levels than age-matched male subjects). Other conditions that lower IGF-1 levels include malnutrition, uncontrolled diabetes, and hepatic and renal failure. Normal ranges for IGF-1 should be established in each particular center based on age. The determination of other GH-dependent peptides such as IGFBP3 and ALS has not proved to be superior to IGF-1.

Imaging

Pituitary magnetic resonance imaging (MRI) with gadolinium enhancement allows visualization of lesions as small as 2 or 3 mm in diameter. High-resolution computed tomography (CT) is a reasonable alternative, although it is much less sensitive. An ectopic source of GHRH should be suspected when the MRI is completely normal. In these rare cases, serum GHRH should be measured and the ectopic tumor should be sought, usually with high-resolution CT of the chest and abdomen.

Treatment

The decision as to what therapeutic modality should be used has to take into account medical issues (cardiopulmonary comorbidities, size, and extension of the tumor) as well as the local characteristics of the treating center. The latter refers to the availability of pituitary surgeons and radiotherapeutic technologies as well as the economic feasibility of pharmacologic therapy.

Surgery

Transsphenoidal surgery has been the traditional treatment for acromegaly and achieves biochemical cure (achievement of a post-glucose GH <1 ng/mL and normalization of IGF-1) in 80% to 90% of microadenomas. According to the latest published acromegaly consensus, biochemical cure is defined as a glucose-suppressed GH of 0.4 ng/mL as well as a normal age-adjusted IGF-1. Cure rates for macroadenomas are much lower (40%–50%), and invasive lesions have a very slight chance (<10%) of being cured by surgery. Even though surgery often fails to achieve a full biochemical cure, debulking the pituitary adenoma relieves optic chiasm compression and can result in a sufficient decrement of tumor mass (and therefore of GH production) to allow better results with either pharmacologic or radiotherapeutic regimens.

Pharmacologic Therapy

Somatostatin analogues are the most commonly used medical treatment for acromegaly. Somatostatin inhibits GH secretion and somatotroph cell growth via its interaction with five different somatostatin receptor (SSTR) subtypes. The development of long-acting somatostatin analogues such as octreotide (Sandostatin) and lanreotide (Somatuline) overcame the pharmacologic difficulties of native somatostatin (short half-life, rebound GH secretion, and need for IV administration) and resulted in a more potent inhibition of GH secretion. The most commonly used preparations are intramuscular octreotide LAR (long-acting repeatable) (Sandostatin LAR Depot) and subcutaneous lanreotide autogel (Somatuline Depot), which are administered every 4 weeks. Doses of octreotide-LAR range from 10 to 40 mg and those of lanreotide autogel from 60 to 120 mg, both administered every 4 weeks, although in specific patients the interval of injection can be increased to every 6 or even 8 weeks, thus diminishing the cost of therapy. Octreotide and lanreotide have very high affinities for SSTR-2 and to a lesser extent SSTR-5, which are precisely the most commonly expressed somatostatin receptors in GH-secreting adenomas.

When used after surgery has failed, somatostatin analogues can achieve a safe and a normal IGF-1 in 25% to 35% of patients. Primary treatment with somatostatin analogues is increasingly being used in patients with invasive tumors, when cardiopulmonary contraindications are present, and more recently as a result of the patient's or treating physician's preference. In these settings, biochemical success rates (achievement of a GH <2.5 ng/mL and normalization of IGF-1) have ranged between 30% and 80%, and more than 80% report significant relief of symptoms. More recent trials performed in unselected populations reveal that the real success rate lies between 25% and 35%. Tumor shrinkage occurs in 70% of primarily treated patients. Overall, treatment success is directly related to the abundance of SSTR-2 and SSTR-5 in the tumor. Lower pretreatment GH levels are also associated with a better response to somatostatin analogues. Side effects of somatostatin analogues, including nausea, abdominal pain, alopecia, and biliary sludge, occur in 20% of subjects. The currently recommended biochemical targets when treating patients with somatostatin analogues are the achievement of a GH of 1 ng/mL and an IGF-1 level within the normal age-adjusted range patients with somatostatin analogues is 1 ng/mL.

Pegvisomant (Somavert) is a GH mutant that prevents functional dimerization of the GH receptor, thus acting as an antagonist. Its use results in normalization of IGF-1 in more than 70% of patients, while increasing GH levels. Concern about adenoma growth due to the abolition of IGF-1 negative feedback on the tumoral somatotroph prevents its use in patients with very large lesions in close proximity to the optic chiasm. Transient elevations of liver aminotransferases can occur, although this seldom requires drug discontinuation. Pegvisomant does not compromise insulin secretion, as somatostatin analogues do. GH-receptor antagonists are expensive and should not be used as primary treatment; they are currently indicated in patients who are intolerant or have failed somatostatin analogue therapy.

Few patients respond marginally to difficult-to-tolerate large doses of bromocriptine.[1] Newer dopamine agonists, such as cabergoline,[1] are better tolerated and achieve biochemical control in 20% to 30% of patients. Combination treatment with cabergoline and octreotide appears to be promising in cases resistant to somatostatin analogues.

Radiation Therapy

Both external-beam radiotherapy and radiosurgery are indicated in patients with persistent disease and a demonstrable tumor remnant who are either intolerant or resistant to pharmacologic treatment. Biochemical success occurs in 20% to 60% and requires many years to become apparent. Hypopituitarism, involving at least two axes, develops in more than 50% of patients within 10 years. Serious adverse effects such as brain necrosis and optic nerve damage seldom occur with the currently used techniques that minimize radiation to the normal surrounding tissues. With the currently available radiation techniques, radiotherapy is an effective and safe treatment

---

[1]Not FDA approved for this indication.

alternative. The two major drawbacks of radiotherapy are the time it takes to achieve biochemical control and the almost unavoidable induction of hypopituitarism.

Novel pharmacologic therapies are being developed, some of which will likely become useful particularly in patients who do not respond to current somatostatin analogues. These include the so-called "universal" somatostatin analogue pasireotide (Signifor LAR), which is capable of interacting not only with the SSTRs 2 and 5, but also with subtypes 1 and 3. Pasireotide seems to be slightly more effective than octreotide in achieving GH and IGF-1 targets; however, its major drawback is the worsening of hyperglycemia. Dopastatin[5] is a recently developed chimeric compound that behaves both as an analog and as a dopamine agonist; clinical trials had to be discontinued at early stages due to lack of efficacy. Oral octreotide capsules are a new preparation of octreotide acetate attached to a transient permeability enhancer, which selectively allows the translocation of the somatostatin analog through the paracellular tight junctions. Oral octreotide (Mycapssa Delayed Release capsule), which was granted FDA approval in June 2020, has been shown to be as efficacious as the parenteral preparation in at least three phase III trials, including two open label non-inferiority studies and a more recent placebo-controlled trial.

---

[5]Investigational drug in the United States.

References

Espinosa E, Ramirez C, Mercado M: The multimodal treatment of acromegaly: current status and future perspectives, *Endocr Metab Immune Disord Drug Targets* 14:169–181, 2014.

Espinosa-de-Los-Monteros AL, González B, Vargas G, et al: Clinical and biochemical characteristics of acromegalic patients with different abnormalities of glucose metabolism, *Pituitary* 14:231–235, 2011.

Espinosa de los Monteros AL, Gonzalez B, Vargas G, et al: Octreotide LAR treatment of acromegaly in "real life": long term outcome at a tertiary care center, *Pituitary* 18:290–296, 2015.

Espinosa-de-Los-Monteros AL, Sosa E, Cheng S, et al: Biochemical evaluation of disease activity after pituitary surgery in acromegaly: a critical analysis of patients who spontaneously change disease status, *Clin Endocrinol* 64:245–249, 2006.

Fleseriu M, Deval A, Bondat 1, et al: Maintenance of response to oral octreotide compared with injectable somatostatin receptor ligands in patients with acromegaly: a phase 3, multicenter randomized controlled trial, *Lancet Diabetes Endocrinol* 10:102–111, 2022.

Fleseriu M, Langlois F, Lim DST, et al.: Acromegaly: pathogenesis, diagnosis, and management, *Lancet Diabetes Endocrinol* 10:804–826, 2022.

Gadelha MR, Kasuki L, Lim DST, Fleseriu M: Systemic complications of acromegaly and the impac of the current treatment landscape: an update, *Endocr Rev* 40:268–332, 2019.

Gadhelha M, Gordon MB, Doknic, et al.: ACROBAT Edge. Safety and efficacy of swithcing injected SRL to oral paltusotine in patients with acromegaly. *J Clin Endocrinol Metab* dgac643, 2022.

Garcia Guzman B, Portocarrero Ortiz L, Dorantes Argandar A: Hereditary pituitary tumor syndromes: Genetic and clinical aspects, *Rev Invest Clin* 72:8–18, 2020.

Giustina A, Chanson P, Bronstein MD: A consensus on criteria for cure of acromegaly, *J Clin Endocrinol Metab* 95:3141–3148, 2010.

Giustina A, Chanson P, Kleinberg D, et al: Expert consensus document: a consensus on the medical treatment of acromegaly, *Nat Rev Endocrinol* 10:243–248, 2014.

Gonzalez-Virla B, Vargas-Ortega G, Martinez-Vazquez KB, Espinosa de los Monteros AL, Sosa-Eroza E, López-Felix B, Mendoza-Zubieta V, Mercado M: Efficacy and safety of fractionated conformal radiation therapy in acromegaly: A long-term follow-up study, *Endocrine* 65:386–392, 2019.

Holdaway IM, Rajasoorya RC, Gamble GD: Factors influencing mortality in acromegaly, *J Clin Endocrinol Metab* 89:667–674, 2004.

Kopchick JJ, Parkinson C, Stevens EC, Trainer PJ: Growth hormone receptor antagonists: discovery, development, and use in patients with acromegaly, *Endocr Rev* 23:623–646, 2002.

Mercado M, Abreu C, Vergara-López A, et al: Surgical and pharmacological outcomes in acromegaly: real-life data from the Mexican Acromegaly Registry, *J Clin Endocrinol Metab* 105:dga664, 2020.

Mercado M, Espinosa E, Ramirez C: Current status and future directions of pharmacological therapy for acromegaly, *Minerva Endocrinol* 41:351–365, 2016.

Mercado M, Gonzalez B, Vargas G, et al: Successful mortality reduction and control of comorbidities in patients with acromegaly followed at a highly specialized multidisciplinary clinic, *J Clin Endocrinol Metab* 99:4438–4446, 2014.

Mercado M, Ramirez-Rentería C: Metabolic complications of acromegaly, *Front Horm Res* 49:20–28, 2018.

Portocarrero-Ortiz LA, Vergara-Lopez A, Vidrio-Velazquez M, et al: The Mexican Acromegaly Registry: clinical and biochemical characteristics at diagnosis and therapeutic outcomes, *J Clin Endocrinol Metab* 101:3997–4004, 2016.

Trainer PJ, Newell-Price JDC, Ayuk J, et al.: A randomised, open label, parallel group, phase 2 study of antisense oligonucleotide therapy in acromegaly, *Eur J Endocrinol* 179:97–108, 2018.

ADRENOCORTICAL INSUFFICIENCY

Method of
Fabienne Langlois, MD; Elena V. Varlamov, MD; and Maria Fleseriu, MD

CURRENT DIAGNOSIS

- An initial diagnosis of adrenocortical insufficiency (AI) is based in most cases on an evaluation of morning cortisol level(s), measured at 8 AM in patients who have a normal circadian rhythm.
- A morning cortisol level less than 3 µg/dL to 5 µg/dL supports an AI diagnosis, and a value greater than 15 µg/dL effectively rules out AI.
- To confirm the diagnosis, especially in cases with intermediate cortisol values, a high-dose (250 µg) cosyntropin (Cortrosyn) stimulation test is suggested with a normal cutoff peak cortisol greater than 18 µg/dL to 20 µg/dL at 30 or 60 minutes.
- Primary AI is characterized by elevated endogenous adrenocorticotropic hormone (ACTH) levels and absence of mineralocorticoid hormones in addition to glucocorticoid (GC) deficiency; antibody screening and/or adrenal imaging is indicated.
- Secondary AI is characterized by an inappropriately normal or low endogenous ACTH level and low cortisol with preserved mineralocorticoid hormones. If an exogenous GC source/use is ruled out, pituitary hormone testing and magnetic resonance imaging (MRI) of the pituitary sella is appropriate.

CURRENT THERAPY

- Oral hydrocortisone (Cortef) is the preferred form of steroid to attain physiologic replacement. Doses are usually 15 mg to 20 mg divided into two or three daily doses, with the highest dose in the morning.
- In case of physiologic stress—such as fever, severe infection, or minor surgery—doses should be doubled or tripled (depending on the type of stress or procedure) for the duration of the event.
- In patients with primary AI, fludrocortisone (Florinef), a mineralocorticoid, should be added to the treatment regimen, with a typical dose between 0.05 mg and 0.1 mg daily.
- For adrenal crisis in patients with known AI, administer bolus hydrocortisone injection (Solu-Cortef) 100 mg followed by 50 mg to 100 mg IV every 6 hours to 8 hours or continuous infusion of 200 mg/24 h along with substantial volumes of saline.
- Patients should wear a medical alert bracelet or necklace and have frequent education regarding AI, its treatment, and the prevention of adrenal crisis.

Epidemiology

Primary adrenocortical insufficiency (AI), also known as Addison disease, has a prevalence of 100 to 140 cases per million persons. More than 90% of primary AI in the developed world is secondary to autoimmune adrenalitis, and is more common in women. Secondary AI caused by withdrawal of therapeutic glucocorticoid (GC) administration is the most prevalent; pituitary tumors and surgeries and opioid use are other common etiologies.

Risk Factors
Primary Adrenocortical Insufficiency
A personal or family history of autoimmune disease (e.g., type 1 diabetes, Hashimoto disease, vitiligo, pernicious anemia) is a risk factor for autoimmune adrenalitis. In the context of acute AI in the hospital, thrombosis and secondary adrenal hemorrhage must be

ruled out and the possibility of heparin-induced thrombocytopenia (HIT) elicited if the patient is receiving parenteral anticoagulation. Miliary tuberculosis is the most frequent cause of primary AI in endemic regions. Infiltration in the context of malignancy is often due to a known metastatic cancer; other infiltrative diseases are rare.

Secondary Adrenocortical Insufficiency

The most common risk factor for secondary AI is prolonged use of exogenous GC. In general, patients taking more than 5 mg of prednisone or the equivalent for longer than 3 weeks are at risk for secondary AI. Patients receiving chronic CG will experience adrenal insufficiency symptoms acutely if GC are suddenly stopped. In some patients with GC receptor hypersensitivity, even smaller doses of GC other than oral (topical, injected, or inhaled) can also suppress the hypothalamic-pituitary-adrenal axis. Immunotherapy-related hypophysitis, most often related to inhibition of cytotoxic T-lymphocyte antigen-4 (CTLA-4), but also programmed cell death protein 1 (PD-1), and/or its ligand (PD-L1) induce AI, which is usually irreversible. Chronic opioid use, especially long-acting opioids, can also suppress ACTH and induce secondary AI.

Patients with tumors of the hypothalamic-pituitary region or a history of treatment of such tumors with surgery and/or radiation are at significant risk. Pituitary apoplexy occurs due to hemorrhage or infarction of the pituitary tumor and causes acute secondary AI. Autoimmune lymphocytic hypophysitis is more common in women and usually occurs in the third pregnancy trimester or postpartum. Pituitary ischemia due to severe blood loss postpartum is known as Sheehan syndrome. Patients with traumatic brain injury may experience transient or permanent AI in both the acute and/or recovery phase.

Pathophysiology

Primary AI is characterized by complete destruction of the adrenal cortex, inducing deficits in all hormones: GC, mineralocorticoid, and androgens. With loss of cortisol feedback inhibition, ACTH will be markedly elevated. Secondary AI is characterized by low GC production and reduced adrenal androgens; it is due a defect at the pituitary or hypothalamus level and results in low (or inappropriately normal) ACTH. Mineralocorticoid activity is maintained in secondary AI as it is controlled by the renin-angiotensin-aldosterone system.

Prevention

There is no clinically practicable strategy for preventing primary AI. Opioids and GC-associated secondary AI may be prevented through judicious use of systemic GC and opioids, with efforts made to limit administration to the lowest effective dose for the shortest possible time.

Clinical Manifestations

Primary Adrenocortical Insufficiency

The presentation of primary AI is sometimes dramatic, with a constellation of weakness, fatigue, anorexia, weight loss, nausea, abdominal pain, salt craving, and orthostatic hypotension. Symptoms start as subtle and nonspecific in some patients but may evolve rapidly in adrenal crisis, especially if concomitant stress occurs. The skin and buccal mucosa are often hyperpigmented owing to the effect of excess ACTH on cutaneous melanocortin receptors. Hyponatremia and hyperkalemia (as a result of mineralocorticoid deficiency) are often present.

Secondary Adrenocortical Insufficiency

The presentation of secondary AI is more insidious, with weight loss, fatigue, nausea, and malaise as presenting features. This often leads to a delay in diagnosis. The production of mineralocorticoid is relatively intact in secondary AI, and as such potassium levels are usually normal. Hyponatremia may be present due to an increase in antidiuretic hormone. Hyperpigmentation is not present, reflecting normal or low ACTH levels. Other laboratory abnormalities are less common but hypoglycemia is occasionally observed, especially with concomitant growth hormone deficiency (GHD). Isolated ACTH deficiency in pituitary tumors is rare, and signs and symptoms of other pituitary hormone abnormalities—such as hyperprolactinemia, central hypogonadism, GHD, or central hypothyroidism—may be present.

Diagnosis

Morning cortisol levels (within 2 hours of waking up) of 3 μg/dL to 5 μg/dL or less has a relatively high predictive value for AI; a morning cortisol level greater than 15 μg/dL effectively rules out AI. To confirm the diagnosis of AI, a cortisol stimulation test is performed. Insulin tolerance testing has largely been replaced by stimulation testing with synthetic cosyntropin (ACTH—Cortrosyn, Synacthen). ACTH stimulation testing of cortisol is a reliable method of evaluating adrenal reserve. However, it should not be used in cases of acute secondary AI (less than 6 weeks), such as apoplexy or after recent pituitary surgery, because adrenal atrophy must have occurred for the adrenal response to cosyntropin to be blunted. In high-dose ACTH testing, a cortisol level is checked before and at 30 and 60 minutes after 250 μg of cosyntropin has been administered intravenously. A peak cortisol level greater than 18 μg/dL to 20 μg/dL at 30 or 60 minutes defines a normal response. The low-dose (1 μg) test[1] measures cortisol 20 to 30 minutes after cosyntropin administration and may be more sensitive for the diagnosis of secondary AI. However, the high-dose (250 μg cosyntropin) test remains the standard. The above-mentioned cortisol cutoffs are based on laboratory methods using polyclonal antibody immunoassays. Newer assays (liquid chromatography mass spectrometry [LC-MS/MS]) and some monoclonal antibody immunoassays) have reduced cross-reactivity with cortisol precursors and therefore result in 10% to 20% lower total cortisol levels. For example, lower stimulated cutoffs of 14 μg/dL to 17 μg/dL have been proposed. Additionally, one must consider total serum cortisol level, as this can be affected by diurnal rhythm and binding proteins, which are elevated in hyperestrogenic states and low in hypoalbuminemia. If the clinical picture is not concordant with the investigation, an endocrinology consult should be sought.

Once a diagnosis has been confirmed, a low or normal plasma ACTH level will indicate secondary AI; however, care must be taken with the methodology of the test, as some immunoassays for ACTH can give falsely low results if preanalytic precautions are not respected. An elevated ACTH level (more than twofold the upper limit of normal) typically indicates primary AI, and hyperkalemia, high plasma renin, and simultaneously low aldosterone levels will confirm associated mineralocorticoid deficiency. After the diagnosis of primary versus secondary AI has been established, an etiology should be sought (Boxes 1 and 2). Serology for antiadrenal (anti 21-hydroxylase) antibodies or evidence of other autoimmune diseases is useful in primary AI, given the very large fraction of these patients with autoimmune adrenalitis. In cases with absent antibodies, adrenal computed tomography imaging is indicated. Enlarged adrenal glands with high-density areas or calcification can suggest granulomatous disease or neoplasm. Acute hematoma or fluid collections around the adrenals during an acute adrenal crisis can indicate adrenal hemorrhage. Secondary AI is most often associated with chronic GC therapy but may be caused by a number of other diseases affecting the hypothalamic-pituitary region. If exogenous GC administration has been excluded, pituitary magnetic resonance imaging (MRI) and testing of the other pituitary axes are appropriate.

Differential Diagnosis

Presentation of AI can be subtle (especially in secondary AI), and differential diagnosis is broad and includes a number of illnesses associated with fatigue, weight loss, and malaise as well as occult malignancies, renal or hepatic dysfunction, and electrolyte disturbances. In acute AI crisis, differential diagnosis includes other systemic illnesses associated with orthostatic hypotension and electrolyte abnormalities, including dehydration and distributive and septic shock. Fever can be part of an AI crisis, but an infectious process must be ruled out as the precipitating cause.

Treatment

GC replacement is recommended with oral hydrocortisone two or three times daily for primary AI and once or twice daily for secondary AI. One-half to two-thirds of the daily dose is given upon

---

[1]Not FDA approved for this indication.

BOX 1 | Causes of Primary Adrenocortical Insufficiency

Autoimmune
Isolated
Autoimmune polyglandular syndromes 1 and 2

Infectious
Fungal
    Tuberculosis
    Histoplasmosis
Viral
    Human immunodeficiency virus
    Cytomegalovirus
Parasitic
Syphilis
Rarely bacterial

Bilateral Adrenal Infarction
Hemorrhage
    Anticoagulation
    Sepsis (e.g., meningococcemia)
    Trauma
    COVID-19 infection or vaccination
Thrombosis
    Thrombophilic condition (e.g., antiphospholipid antibody
        syndrome)
    Heparin-induced thrombocytopenia

Neoplastic
Metastatic cancer
    Breast
    Colon
    Melanoma
    Lymphoma
    Non–Small Cell Lung Cancer

Infiltrative Diseases
Hemochromatosis
Primary amyloidosis
Sarcoidosis

Bilateral Adrenalectomy
For bilateral tumors or intractable Cushing syndrome

Familial or Genetic
Classical congenital adrenal hyperplasia
Adrenoleukodystrophy
Familial glucocorticoid deficiency
Adrenocorticotropic hormone insensitivity syndromes
X-linked adrenal hypoplasia (associated with DAX-1 mutation,
    may be of late onset)
Triple-A or Allgrove syndrome (alacrimia, achalasia, adrenal
    insufficiency)

BOX 2 | Etiologies of Secondary Adrenocortical Insufficiency

Iatrogenic/Medication
Chronic steroid therapy, most often oral or parenteral, but
    could also be inhaled, topical, or injected
Chronic opioid therapy
Immunotherapy (CTLA-4 and PD-1/PDL-1 inhibitors)
Drugs used for treatment of Cushing syndrome that can cause
    adrenal insufficiency
    Steroidogenesis inhibitors (ketoconazole, metyrapone,
        osilodrostat, mitotane, etomidate)
    Pituitary tumor directed drugs (pasireotide)
    Glucocorticoid receptor blockers (Mifepristone)

Pituitary Injury
Posttranssphenoidal or transcranial surgery
Radiation to the sella
Infarction/hemorrhage (pituitary apoplexy, Sheehan
    syndrome)
Traumatic brain injury

Tumors of the Sella
Pituitary adenoma
Craniopharyngioma
Meningioma
Rathke cleft cyst
Metastatic cancer

Infiltrative/Inflammatory Diseases
Sarcoidosis, tuberculosis, or other granulomatous diseases
Lymphocytic hypophysitis
Idiopathic adrenocorticotropic hormone deficiency

Congenital
Genetic mutations in transcription factors (PROP-1, PIT-1, etc.)
Midline defect
Septo-optic dysplasia

waking, and the dosage is roughly 15 mg to 20 mg/day (or 10 mg/m^2 to 12 mg/m^2 body surface area per day), typically 10 mg or 15 mg in the morning and 5 mg in the afternoon. Once-daily modified-release hydrocortisone is available in Europe and may better mimic the physiologic circadian rhythm of cortisol, but it is not yet available in the United States. Longer-acting GCs (prednisone, dexamethasone [Decadron]) may be used in patients who remain severely symptomatic in the evenings or early morning hours or who are unable to comply with a multidose hydrocortisone regimen. However, in such cases the risk of overreplacement is much higher.

Patients should be instructed to increase this dosage according to physiologic stress, as doses should be doubled or tripled for the duration of the fever or intercurrent systemic illness. Day-to-day emotional stress does not require an increment in dosing. For surgery, GC parenteral doses should be administered according to the level of surgical stress, such as 25 mg for minor stress (e.g., cataract surgery), 50 mg to 75 mg for moderate stress (e.g., cholecystectomy), and 100 mg to 150 mg daily in divided doses for major stress (e.g., heart surgery).

Patients should wear a medical alert bracelet or necklace and should be dispensed hydrocortisone or dexamethasone injection with instructions for home self-administration in case of vomiting and inability to take oral doses. If symptoms do not improve within hours after injection, patients should seek urgent medical evaluation.

Mineralocorticoid replacement is indicated in most patients with primary AI, and fludrocortisone (Florinef) is the recommended medical therapy, with a typical dose between 0.05 mg and 0.1 mg once daily.

If a patient with known AI presents in adrenal crisis, hydrocortisone (Solu-Cortef) 100 mg bolus followed by 150 mg to 250 mg/day, divided every 6 to 8 hours or as a continuous 200 mg/24 hours intravenous (IV) infusion, is an appropriate initial therapy, with the dose tapered to an appropriate oral dose as the patient's condition improves. Aggressive hydration with a saline solution will help increase the intravascular volume, and high-dose GCs have some mineralocorticoid activity; thus mineralocorticoids are not required in the treatment of acute adrenal crisis.

In critical illness, the treatment of AI should not be delayed if diagnosis cannot be established and the patient is unstable. Baseline cortisol and ACTH levels should preferably be drawn prior to the initiation of treatment and should be interpreted as a stress value (i.e., should be >18 μg/dL). If in doubt, high-dose stress GCs are administered until testing is complete and cosyntropin stimulation testing may be delayed until the patient's condition improves because hydrocortisone has to be suspended at least 24 hours before testing. The controversial entity of suboptimal cortisol response during acute stress may be associated with worse outcomes, but no consensus exists for its diagnosis and treatment. Refer to Table 1 for GC dosage recommendations.

The replacement of dehydroepiandrosterone (DHEA) is controversial and not recommended for all patients by present guidelines. However, a trial may be warranted in selected cases of women with primary AI and persistent symptoms, including low libido and low

TABLE 1 Stress Dose Glucocorticoid Dosage Recommendations for Patients With Adrenal Insufficiency*·†

CLINICAL CONTEXT	MANAGEMENT
Minor surgical or medical stress (for example) Mild fever, colonoscopy, mild gastroenteritis, dental procedures	Hydrocortisone 25 mg/day OR twice the usual maintenance dose on days of stress
Moderate surgical or medical stress (for example) Cholecystectomy, pneumonia, severe gastroenteritis	Hydrocortisone 50–75 mg/day for 1–2 days followed by twice usual dose for 1–2 days, then resume the usual dose
Major surgical or medical stress (for example) Cardiopulmonary bypass, pancreatitis, vaginal delivery	Hydrocortisone 100–150 mg/day for 1–3 days followed by twice to thrice usual dose for 2–7 days, then resume the usual dose
Adrenal crisis Critical illness (for example) Septic shock, hemodynamic instability	Hydrocortisone 100 mg bolus followed by 50–100 mg every 6–8 hours OR continuous infusion of 200 mg/24 h (or 0.18 mg/kg/day)

*For an uncomplicated course, the glucocorticoid dosage should always be individualized according to patient's clinical status.

†Patients with primary adrenal insufficiency may require slightly higher doses compared with patients with secondary adrenal insufficiency and may benefit more from additional intravenous fluids to compensate for the lack of mineralocorticoids.

energy. DHEA is available only as a dietary supplement and has not been approved by the US Food and Drug Administration (FDA).

Monitoring

Patients should be interviewed and examined routinely for indicators of excess GC replacement, such as weight gain, striae, facial plethora, osteoporosis, or glucose intolerance; they should also be checked for under replacement if symptoms of AI persist. Cortisol levels and ACTH are not helpful in monitoring GC doses. Monitoring of mineralocorticoid status should include volume status, electrolytes, blood pressure, and occasionally serum renin levels. The development of hypertension, edema, or hypokalemia could mandate a dose reduction.

Complications

Adrenal crisis is the most severe and life-threatening manifestation of both primary and secondary adrenal insufficiency. In patients with known AI, it occurs at a rate of approximately six cases per 100 patient-years and contributes to approximately 10% deaths; it is more common in primary than secondary AI.

Adrenal crisis is characterized by profound weakness, nausea, vomiting, abdominal pain, and fever and, if not properly treated with GC, can result in cardiovascular collapse resistant to administration of fluids and vasopressors. Precipitating causes of adrenal crisis are mainly gastrointestinal and other infections, acute illness, trauma, surgery, severe emotional distress, and pregnancy. Adrenal crisis usually develops in the setting of lack of GC replacement or failure to administer stress doses of GC during illness or severe physiological stress. Iatrogenic Cushing syndrome can develop if the dose of GC replacement is supraphysiologic long term.

Acknowledgments

The authors thank Shirley McCartney, PhD, for editorial assistance.

References

Annane D, Pastores SM, Rochwerg B, et al: Guidelines for the diagnosis and management of critical illness-related corticosteroid insufficiency (CIRCI) in critically ill patients (Part I): Society of Critical Care Medicine (SCCM) and European Society of Intensive Care Medicine (ESICM) 2017, *Crit Care Med* 45:2078–2088, 2017.

Arlt W, Allolio B: Adrenal insufficiency, *Lancet* 361:1881–1893, 2003.

Husebye ES, Pearce SH, Krone NP, Kämpe O: Adrenal insufficiency, *Lancet* 13 397(10274):613–629, 2021.

Bornstein SR, Allolio B, Arlt W, et al: Diagnosis and treatment of primary adrenal insufficiency: an Endocrine Society clinical practice guideline, *J Clin Endocrinol Metab* 101:364–389, 2016.

Charmandari E, Nicolaides NC, Chrousos GP: Adrenal insufficiency, *Lancet* 383:2152–2167, 2014.

Dillard T, Yedinak CG, Alumkal J, Fleseriu M, et al: Anti-CTLA-4 antibody therapy associated autoimmune hypophysitis: serious immune related adverse events across a spectrum of cancer subtypes, *Pituitary* 13(1):29–38, 2010.

Dorin RI, Qualls CR, Crapo LM: Diagnosis of adrenal insufficiency, *Ann Intern Med* 139:194–204, 2003.

Elhassan YS, Iqbal F, Arlt W, et al.: COVID-19-related adrenal haemorrhage: multicentre UK experience and systematic review of the literature, *Clin Endocrinol (Oxf)* 98(6):766–778, 2023.

Fleseriu M, Hashim IA, Karavitaki N, et al: Hormonal replacement in hypopituitarism in adults: an Endocrine Society clinical practice guideline, *J Clin Endocrinol Metab* 101:3888–3921, 2016.

Husebye ES, Allolio B, Arlt W, et al: Consensus statement on the diagnosis, treatment and follow-up of patients with primary adrenal insufficiency, *J Intern Med* 275:104–115, 2014.

Isidori AM, Venneri MA, Graziadio C, et al: Effect of once-daily, modified-release hydrocortisone versus standard glucocorticoid therapy on metabolism and innate immunity in patients with adrenal insufficiency (DREAM): a single-blind, randomised controlled trial, *The Lancet Diabetes & Endocrinology* 6:173–185, 2018.

Javorsky BR, Raff H, Carroll TB, Algeciras-Schimnich A, Singh RJ, Colón-Franco JM, et al: New cutoffs for the biochemical diagnosis of adrenal insufficiency after ACTH stimulation using specific cortisol assays, *Journal of the Endocrine Society*, 2021. https://doi.org/10.1210/jendso/bvab022. bvab022.

Kazlauskaite R, Evans AT, Villabona CV, et al: Corticotropin tests for hypothalamic-pituitary-adrenal insufficiency: a metaanalysis, *J Clin Endocrinol Metab* 93:4245–4253, 2008.

Ngaosuwan K, Johnston DG, Godsland IF, et al.: Increased mortality risk in patients with primary and secondary adrenal insufficiency, *J Clin Endocrinol Metab*, 106(7):e2759–e2768, 2021.

Rushworth RL, Torpy DJ, Falhammar H: Adrenal crisis, *N Engl J Med* 29(9):852–861, 2019. 381.

Woodcock T, Barker P, Daniel S, et al: Guidelines for the management of glucocorticoids during the peri-operative period for patients with adrenal insufficiency—guidelines from the Association of Anaesthetists, the Royal College of Physicians and the Society for Endocrinology UK, *Anaesthesia* 75(5): 654–663, 2020.

CUSHING'S SYNDROME

Method of
Constantine A. Stratakis, MD, PhD

CURRENT DIAGNOSIS

- Cushing's syndrome remains one of the most challenging diagnoses in endocrine medicine.
- Cushing's disease is caused by corticotropin (ACTH)-producing pituitary adenomas (corticotropinomas) and constitutes the most common cause of endogenous Cushing's syndrome, although its prevalence varies across different age groups.
- Growth failure in children, facial plethora and rounded face, central fat deposition, supraclavicular fat accumulation, buffalo hump, purple striae, thin skin, and proximal myopathy are relatively sensitive clinical features of Cushing's syndrome.
- Ectopic ACTH syndrome occasionally has an unusual presentation of rapid onset, severe weakness, and hypokalemia without classic symptoms of Cushing's syndrome.
- A urinary free cortisol test is the most cost-effective and reliable outpatient screening test.
- A 1-mg overnight dexamethasone screening test is less useful and more expensive than the urinary free cortisol test, but it provides a good alternative for patients in whom urinary collection is impossible or unreliable.
- Midnight salivary cortisol levels greater than 3.6 nmol/L (0.13 μg/dL) have a sensitivity and specificity of approximately 95% for the diagnosis of Cushing's syndrome.
- Undetectable ACTH levels (<1 pmol/L or <5 pg/mL) indicate a primary autonomous adrenocortical disease.
- Postcontrast spoiled gradient-recalled acquisition (SPGR) magnetic resonance imaging (MRI) is superior to conventional MRI for the localization of corticotropinomas in children and adults.
- Computed tomography (CT) is used to investigate adrenal disease in patients with ACTH-independent Cushing's syndrome. Usually, conventional MRI is less useful owing to motion artifacts.

CURRENT THERAPY

- The initial therapy of choice for patients with Cushing's disease is transsphenoidal surgery of the pituitary gland to remove the responsible adenoma.
- Transsphenoidal surgery has a success rate greater than 80% in most experienced centers. Lower success rates and higher incidence of relapse are recorded in less-experienced centers.
- Laparoscopic adrenalectomy has become the treatment of choice for benign adrenal lesions with a diameter of less than 6 cm.
- In stages I to III adrenocortical carcinoma, complete tumor resection offers the best chance for cure.
- Mitotane (Lysodren), an adrenolytic agent, is used in the treatment of metastatic adrenocortical carcinoma and also as an adjuvant for tumors with a high risk of recurrence.
- Medical treatment with ketoconazole[1], metyrapone[1], aminoglutethimide (Cytadren)[2], and mitotane[1] may be used to control hypercortisolism in preparation for surgery; medical adrenalectomy may also be used in cases of cyclic Cushing's syndrome.
- Pasireotide (Signifor) and mifepristone (Korlym) may be used for the treatment of Cushing's disease that cannot be cured by surgery and/or irradiation.
- The most effective treatment option for ectopic ACTH syndrome is resection of the tumor. Somatostatin analogues and various chemotherapeutic regimens have been used in the treatment of metastatic tumors.

[1]Not FDA approved for this indication.
[2]Not available in the United States.

Definition and Epidemiology

Cushing's syndrome remains one of the most difficult diagnoses in endocrinology. By definition, Cushing's syndrome is a multisystem disorder that develops in response to glucocorticoid excess. Iatrogenic Cushing's syndrome is common, but endogenous Cushing's syndrome is a rare condition, with an estimated incidence of 0.7 to 2.4 per million population per year. The etiology of Cushing's syndrome may be excessive adrenocorticotropic hormone (ACTH) production from the pituitary gland, ectopic ACTH secretion by nonpituitary tumors, or autonomous cortisol hypersecretion from adrenal hyperplasia or tumors (Table 1). Cushing's disease refers to the subset of Cushing's syndrome cases caused by an ACTH-producing pituitary adenoma. Cushing's disease is the most common cause of spontaneous Cushing's syndrome in almost all ages, including older children and adolescents. Approximately 20% to 30% (with the exception of very young children) of endogenous Cushing's syndrome is caused by primary adrenocortical diseases that are not ACTH-dependent. Cushing's disease and adrenocortical adenomas occur more commonly in women, with a female-to-male ratio of 3–5:1.

Pathophysiology

Cortisol inhibits the biosynthesis and secretion of corticotropin-releasing hormone (CRH) and ACTH in a negative-feedback loop that is tightly controlled. The hallmark of Cushing's syndrome is the absence of suppression of cortisol levels after low-dose dexamethasone (Decadron) administration owing to autonomous ACTH secretion by a tumor or autonomous glucocorticoid production by a primary adrenocortical disease. It is essential to understand that all diagnostic testing in Cushing's syndrome relies on the disturbance of this feedback mechanism, as revealed by dexamethasone, CRH (corticorelin ovine trifluate [Acthrel]), and all related testing.

ACTH-producing pituitary adenomas are microadenomas (<1 cm in diameter) in 80% to 90% of cases. Macroadenomas are rare and often invasive, with extension outside of the sella turcica. Chronic ACTH hypersecretion commonly leads to secondary adrenocortical hyperplasia.

Ectopic ACTH secretion is most often associated with small cell lung carcinoma, which accounts for half of the cases in adult patients with Cushing's syndrome. The ectopic ACTH syndrome

TABLE 1	Etiology of Cushing's Syndrome in Older Children, Adolescents, and Young Adults*
SYNDROME	**% OF TOTAL**
ACTH-dependent	
Cushing's disease	60–70
Ectopic ACTH syndrome	5–10
Ectopic CRH syndrome	<1
ACTH-independent	
Adrenocortical adenoma	10–15
Adrenocortical carcinoma	5
Bilateral adrenocortical disease	5–10

*In infants and younger children, the distribution is different.
Abbreviations: ACTH = adrenocorticotropic hormone; CRH = corticotropin-releasing hormone.

causes severe hypokalemia and is usually underdiagnosed in patients during advanced stages of neoplasia. Other tumors causing the syndrome are bronchial, thymic, and pancreatic carcinoids; medullary thyroid carcinoma; pheochromocytoma; or other rare neuroendocrine tumors, especially in pediatric patients.

Adrenocortical tumors are more often adenomas that are usually smaller than 5 cm. Adrenocortical carcinomas are rare but very aggressive neoplasms; they most commonly occur as large nonsecreting abdominal masses at diagnosis, and only rarely does Cushing's syndrome develop.

Up to recently, only two types of primary adrenal hyperplasias that are ACTH-independent and cause Cushing's syndrome were known: primary pigmented nodular adrenocortical disease (PPNAD) and ACTH-independent macronodular adrenocortical hyperplasia, also known as massive macronodular adrenocortical disease.

Table 2 lists no fewer than six types of bilateral adrenocortical hyperplasias. They are divided into two groups of disorders, macronodular and micronodular hyperplasias, on the basis of the size of the associated nodules. In macronodular disorders, the greatest diameter of each nodule exceeds 1 cm; in the micronodular group, nodules are less than 1 cm. Although nodules less than 1 cm can occur in macronodular disease (especially the form associated with McCune-Albright syndrome), and single large tumors may be encountered in PPNAD (especially in older patients), the size criterion has biological relevance, because we rarely see a continuum in the same subject: most patients have either macronodular or micronodular hyperplasia. We use two additional basic characteristics in this classification of bilateral adrenocortical hyperplasias: presence of tumor pigment and status (hyperplasia or atrophy) of the surrounding cortex.

Pigment in adrenocortical lesions is rarely melanin; most of the pigmentation in adrenocortical adenomas and bilateral adrenocortical hyperplasias that produce cortisol is lipofuscin. The accumulation of lipofuscin-like material results from the progressive oxidation of unsaturated fatty acids by oxygen-derived free radicals in lysosomes. Lipofuscin pigmentation appears macroscopically as light brown to occasionally dark brown or even black discoloration of the tumor or hyperplastic tissue. Lipofuscin can be seen with a light microscope, but it is better detected by electron microscopy. Massive macronodular adrenocortical disease is a bilateral disease and may be caused by abnormal hormone receptor expression or activating mutations of $G_S\alpha$, which lead to stimulation of steroidogenesis. About 30% to 50% of the cases may be caused by ARMC5 mutations. Another cause of ACTH-independent Cushing's syndrome is primary pigmented nodular adrenocortical disease, usually associated with a syndrome of cardiac myxomas, lentigines, and schwannomas (Carney's complex).

Clinical Manifestations

The clinical presentation of Cushing's syndrome is variable and differs in severity (Table 3). Truncal obesity is the most common

TABLE 2 Bilateral Adrenal Hyperplasias Causing Cushing's Syndrome

LESION	AGE GROUP	HISTOPATHOLOGY	GENETICS	GENE, LOCUS
Macronodular Hyperplasias (Multiple Nodules >1 cm Each)				
Bilateral macroadenomatous hyperplasia	Middle age	Distinct adenomas (usually 2 or 3) with internodular atrophy	MEN1, FAP, MAS, HLRCS; isolated (AD); other	Menin, APC, GNAS, FH, ectopic GPCRs, ARMC5, PRKACA 5
Bilateral macroadenomatous hyperplasia of childhood	Infants, very young children	Distinct adenomas (usually 2 or 3) with internodular atrophy; occasional microadenomas	MAS	GNAS
ACTH-independent macronodular adrenocortical hyperplasia, also known as massive macronodular adrenocortical disease	Middle age	Adenomatous hyperplasia (multiple) with internodular hyperplasia of the zona fasciculata	Isolated, AD	Ectopic GPCRs; WISP2 and Wnt-signaling; 17q22-24, other; ARMC5, PRKACA 5
Micronodular Hyperplasias (Multiple Nodules <1 cm Each)				
Isolated primary pigmented nodular adrenocortical disease	Children; young adults	Microadenomatous hyperplasia with (mostly) internodular atrophy and nodular pigment (lipofuscin)	Isolated, AD	PRKAR1A, PDE11A; PDE8B; 2p16; PRKACA 5 other
Carney complex–associated primary pigmented nodular adrenocortical disease	Children; young and middle aged adults	Microadenomatous hyperplasia with (mostly) internodular atrophy and (mainly nodular) pigment (lipofuscin)	CNC (AD)	PRKAR1A, 2p16; other
Isolated micronodular adrenocortical disease	Mostly children; young adults	Microadenomatous, with hyperplasia of the surrounding zona fasciculata and limited or absent pigment	Isolated, AD; other	PDE11A, PDE8B; other; 2p12-p16, other

Abbreviations: ACTH = adrenocorticotropic hormone; AD = autosomal dominant; APC = adenomatous polyposis coli gene; cAMP = cyclic adenosine monophosphate; CNC = Carney complex; FAP = familial adenomatous polyposis; FH = fumarate hydratase; GNAS = gene coding for the stimulatory subunit alpha of the G-protein (Gsα); GPCR = G-protein-coupled receptor; HLRCS = hereditary leiomyomatosis and renal cancer syndrome; MAS = McCune–Albright syndrome; MEN1 = multiple endocrine neoplasia type 1; PDE8B = phosphodiesterase 8B gene; PDE11A = phosphodiesterase 11A gene; PRKAR1A = protein kinase, cAMP-dependent, regulatory, type I, alpha gene; WISP2 = Wnt1-inducible signaling pathway protein 1; Wnt = wingless-type MMTV integration site family.

clinical sign and is usually the initial manifestation in most patients. Growth failure in children is the most reliable sign of Cushing's syndrome, especially when combined with continuing weight gain. Other symptoms include central fat deposition, supraclavicular fat accumulation, buffalo hump, plethora, rounded face, purple striae, thin skin, proximal muscle weakness, hypertension, impaired glucose metabolism, gonadal dysfunction, and hirsutism (see Table 3). Diabetes mellitus and hypertension also develop. Osteoporosis, mood disorders, emotional lability and cognitive deficits are commonly observed. Proximal myopathy is common, especially in older patients. Ectopic ACTH syndrome caused by small cell lung cancer can have an unusual presentation characterized by rapid onset, severe weakness, and associated hypokalemia without classic symptoms of Cushing's syndrome. In contrast, ACTH-secreting carcinoids manifest with typical clinical manifestations.

Diagnosis
Confirmation of the Diagnosis
The initial evaluation should always include a careful clinical history and physical examination. Reliable symptoms and signs of Cushing's syndrome (see Table 3) should be present in any patient who undergoes evaluation for Cushing's syndrome; patients with no reliable symptoms and signs of Cushing's syndrome should not be investigated, as this often leads to unnecessary, extensive, and expensive testing. It is essential to investigate the use of exogenous glucocorticoids and other conditions that may be associated with mild hypercortisolism, such as alcoholism, anorexia nervosa, severe depression, and morbid obesity; these are pseudo-Cushing's states and are often difficult to exclude, especially in older or chronically ill patients.

The first task in the workup of any patient is documentation of hypercortisolism. On an outpatient basis, this is typically done through the urinary free cortisol test. This is the most cost-effective and reliable outpatient screening test. We typically recommend

TABLE 3 Clinical Manifestations of Cushing's Syndrome

SIGNS AND SYMPTOMS	INCIDENCE (%)
Central obesity	97
Plethora	89
Moon facies	89
Decreased libido	86
Atrophic skin and easy bruising	75
Decreased linear growth	70–80
Menstrual irregularities	80
Hypertension	76
Hirsutism	56
Depression or emotional lability	67
Glucose intolerance/diabetes mellitus	70
Purple striae	60
Buffalo hump	54
Osteoporosis	50
Headache	10

collections over two or three consecutive days so that we avoid errors due to over- or undercollection that are not uncommon with single 24-hour studies. The results of the test need to be corrected for body surface area, as long as total creatinine excretion is normal. A 1-mg overnight dexamethasone test is less useful and more expensive, but it provides a good alternative for patients in whom urinary collection is impossible or unreliable. During these

Figure 1 Algorithm for evaluating patients with Cushing's syndrome. *Abbreviations:* ACTH = adrenocorticotropic hormone; CRH = corticotropin-releasing hormone; CS = Cushing's syndrome; CT = computed tomography; DDAVP = desmopressin; DHPLC = denaturing high-performance liquid chromatography; ICMA = immunochemiluminometric assay; MAD = micronodular disease; MMAD = massive macronodular adrenocortical disease; MRI = magnetic resonance imaging; 17OHS = 17-hydroxysteroids; ON DEX = overnight dexamethasone; PET = positron emission tomography; PPNAD = primary pigmented nodular adrenocortical disease; RIA = radioimmunoassay.

screening tests for hypercortisolism, patients should avoid any activation of the hypothalamic-pituitary-adrenal axis by stress, especially physical. The baseline measurements may be repeated as needed, because cyclic hypercortisolism often precedes overt Cushing's syndrome (Figure 1).

A 24-hour urinary free cortisol excretion of greater than 250 nmol per 24 hours (90 µg/24 hours measured by radioimmunoassay) is highly specific for the diagnosis of hypercortisolism. However, pseudo-Cushing's states are often associated with abnormal levels of 24-hour urinary free cortisol. Administration of 1 mg dexamethasone (15 µg/kg for children) at 11 PM results in suppression of the hypothalamic-pituitary-adrenal axis in normal persons and a fall in plasma and urinary cortisol levels. At 8 AM, serum cortisol should be less than 50 nmol/L (1.8 µg/dL). Unfortunately, dexamethasone is primarily metabolized by the cytochrome P-450 (CYP) system; several drugs, such as phenobarbital, carbamazepine (Tegretol), and rifampicin (Rifadin), that induce the activity of CYP3A4 can lead to false-positive tests. Oral contraceptives also interfere with serum cortisol levels owing to an increase in corticosteroid-binding globulin and by increasing dexamethasone metabolism. The test can only be interpreted if the serum dexamethasone levels reach the expected range; however, this additional requirement can make the test significantly more cumbersome and expensive.

Once hypercortisolism is suspected by the urinary free cortisol or the overnight dexamethasone test, the patient may undergo testing of the cortisol diurnal rhythm. The lack of circadian rhythm of cortisol is the earliest consistent biochemical abnormality of Cushing's syndrome, even in situations of cyclic or other atypical forms of Cushing's syndrome. Serum or salivary cortisol levels at midnight may be used for this test. Normally, the level of serum cortisol begins to rise at 3 to 4 AM and reaches a peak at 7 to 8 AM, falling during the day. A sleeping midnight serum cortisol level lower than 50 nmol/L (1.8 µg/dL) excludes the diagnosis of Cushing's syndrome, whereas a midnight serum cortisol higher than 207 nmol/L (7.5 µg/dL) is highly suggestive of Cushing's syndrome. This test does require inpatient admission. Salivary cortisol levels have an excellent correlation with serum cortisol levels and offer an easy and convenient outpatient way of evaluating circadian rhythm; saliva is also stable at room temperature (for up to 7 days). Midnight salivary cortisol levels greater than 3.6 nmol/L (0.13 µg/dL) have a sensitivity and specificity of approximately 95% for the diagnosis of Cushing's syndrome (see Figure 1).

After the biochemical confirmation of hypercortisolism, the next step is to investigate the source (see Figure 1). Baseline ACTH plasma levels greater than 2 to 5 pmol/L (>20–25 pg/mL) are diagnostic of ACTH-dependent Cushing's syndrome. On the other hand, undetectable ACTH levels (<1 pmol/L or 5 pg/mL) indicate a primary autonomous adrenocortical disease. Values in between should be further investigated with dynamic testing.

High-Dose Dexamethasone Testing
Oral dexamethasone is administrated as 2 mg every 6 hours for 48 hours or as a single 8 mg (120 µg/kg for children) overnight dose. Urinary and serum cortisol levels are suppressed by more than 50% in most patients with Cushing's disease.

Corticotropin-Releasing Hormone Testing
Synthetic ovine CRH (corticorelin ovine trifluate [Acthrel]), an analogue of human CRH is administered intravenously (100 µg), and plasma ACTH and cortisol levels are measured at 15-minute intervals during the next 60 minutes. Patients with Cushing's disease typically have an increase in ACTH or cortisol level of 35% and 22%, respectively. This test has a sensitivity of approximately 85% for the diagnosis of Cushing's disease, but it is often falsely positive in patients with adrenal, ACTH-independent Cushing's syndrome, who do not have a fully suppressed hypothalamic-pituitary-adrenal axis.

Inferior Petrosal Sinus Sampling
None of the noninvasive tests are 100% accurate in distinguishing pituitary (Cushing's disease) from ectopic sources of ACTH. Inferior petrosal sinus sampling (IPSS) is indicated in all cases where an ACTH-dependent source of hypercortisolism is expected but the diagnosis of Cushing's disease versus an ectopic source remains uncertain. Typically, IPSS is done when the ovine CRH and dexamethasone tests are in disagreement or when the pituitary imaging by magnetic resonance imaging (MRI) is negative. An ACTH gradient of central-to-peripheral ACTH levels of 2 or more suggests Cushing's disease. When ovine CRH, human CRH, or desmopressin (DDAVP) testing is performed during IPSS, the diagnostic accuracy of IPSS increases. After ovine CRH stimulation, a central-to-peripheral ratio of ACTH levels of 3 or more suggest the diagnosis of Cushing's disease with specificity and sensitivity greater than 95%. The test is less useful for suggesting the tumor location (right versus left side of the pituitary gland).

Imaging Studies
Pituitary Magnetic Resonance Imaging
Unfortunately, less than 50% of ACTH-producing pituitary adenomas are detectable with MRI, even with the use of contrast enhancement. Typically, we recommend against obtaining an MRI until ACTH dependency is established, because as many as 20% of the patients have an incidental pituitary microadenoma. To avoid false-negative and false-positive imaging, several centers have sought improved methods for MRI detection of ACTH-producing tumors. Our studies demonstrated that postcontrast spoiled gradient-recalled acquisition (SPGR) MRI in addition to the conventional T1-weighted spin echo was superior to conventional MRI for the diagnostic evaluation of corticotropinomas in both children and adults.

Adrenal Imaging
Computed tomography (CT) and MRI are used to investigate adrenal disease in patients with ACTH-independent Cushing's syndrome. Adrenal tumors larger than 6 cm are highly suspicious for adrenocortical carcinomas. The fat content contributes to the differentiation between benign and malignant adrenal tumors. Measurement of Hounsfield units (HU) in unenhanced CT is of great value in differentiating malignant from benign adrenal lesions. Adrenal lesions with an attenuation value of more than 10 HU in unenhanced CT or an enhancement washout of less than 50% and a delayed attenuation of more than 35 HU (on 10- to 15-min delayed enhanced CT) are suspicious for malignancy. MRI with dynamic gadolinium-enhanced and chemical shift technique is as effective as CT in distinguishing malignant from benign lesions. However, MRI is much less useful for detecting adrenal nodularity owing to motion artifacts. Thus, especially for detecting small unilateral adrenocortical adenomas or bilateral micronodular hyperplasia, we recommend a dedicated (thin-sliced) adrenal CT rather than MRI.

Ectopic Adrenocorticotropic Hormone Syndrome
High Resolution Chest-CT 7 and abdominal MRI are the recommended imaging procedures in patients with an IPSS that indicates a nonpituitary ACTH-producing source. Additionally, somatostatin receptor scintigraphy is a useful and complementary tool in the evaluation of patients with ectopic ACTH-dependent Cushing's syndrome. Recent studies have demonstrated a higher sensitivity of somatostatin receptor scintigraphy in comparison to CT or MRI for diagnosing occult ectopic tumors. Additional methods include PET-CT and FDG scans.

Treatment
Untreated chronic hypercortisolism is associated with high morbidity and mortality owing to diabetes mellitus, hypertension, cardiovascular disease, thromboembolism, and suppression of the immune system. Cushing's syndrome should be treated effectively; patients should be closely monitored to rapidly detect recurrent disease.

Treatment of Pituitary Corticotropinomas
Transsphenoidal Pituitary Surgery
The initial therapy of choice for patients with Cushing's disease is transsphenoidal surgery. This procedure is associated with low mortality and morbidity, but complications can include cerebrospinal fluid leaks, meningitis, hypopituitarism, and venous thromboembolism. The success rate for transsphenoidal surgery varies between 60% and 80%, but in experienced centers can be as high as 90% to 95%. Relapses are rare when surgery is performed in an experienced tertiary care center; it can be as high as 30% in less-experienced centers. Postoperative morning serum cortisol levels of less than 50 nmol/L (2 µg/dL) are highly predictive of remission and a low recurrence rate of less than 10% at 10 years.

After successful transsphenoidal surgery, glucocorticoid replacement therapy (hydrocortisone at 12–15 mg/m²/day; 20–30 mg daily in adults) is mandatory until the hypothalamic-pituitary-adrenal axis recovers from the chronic exposure to glucocorticoid excess; this usually takes place within a year after surgery. For recurrent disease, the choice of second-line therapy remains controversial. Repeat surgery can be successful when residual tumor is detectable on MRI imaging, but it carries a high risk of hypopituitarism. Irradiation is recommended in most cases where a tumor is not seen on MRI.

Radiotherapy
Radiotherapy has been used to suppress pituitary secretion of ACTH, but its success rate is variable (50% in some series). It can take as long as 5 years for a full effect; hypopituitarism develops in more than 70% of the patients over a period of 10 to 20 years after the therapy is completed. Stereotactic radiosurgery with gamma knife is associated with a more-rapid effect and a lower risk of hypopituitarism, but it has not been extensively studied.

Medical Treatment to Control Secretion of Adrenocorticotropic Hormone
Cushing's disease responds to the dopamine agonist cabergoline (Dostinex)[1] with a normalization of cortisol production in as many as 40% of the cases. The peroxisome proliferator-activated receptor γ (PPAR-γ) agonist rosiglitazone (Avandia)[1] was demonstrated to be effective in animal models, but it was unsuccessful in controlling ACTH oversecretion in patients with Cushing's disease. A new agent, SOM-230 (pasireotide [Signifor]), blocks both type 2 and type 5 somatostatin receptors and reduces ACTH secretion in vitro. Mifepristone (Korlym), a glucocorticoid receptor antagonist, recently became available for patients who failed surgical or irradiation therapies (see also below).

Bilateral Adrenalectomy
Bilateral adrenalectomy offers a definitive treatment that provides immediate control of hypercortisolism, but this surgery should be reserved for patients with Cushing's disease who have failed all other treatments. Bilateral adrenalectomy in active Cushing's disease often

---

[1] Not FDA approved for this indication.

TABLE 4	Medical Treatment for Hypercortisolism			
MEDICATION	**INITIAL DOSE**	**MAXIMUM DOSE**	**ADVERSE EFFECTS**	
Ketoconazole (Nizoral)[1]	100–200 mg bid/tid	1200 mg	Nausea, vomiting, abdominal pain, weakness, hypothyroidism, gynecomastia, hepatotoxicity, hypertriglyceridemia	
Metyrapone (Metopirone)[1]	250 mg qid	6000 mg	Headache, alopecia, hirsutism, acne, nausea, abdominal discomfort, hypertension, weakness, leucopenia	
Mitotane (Lysodren)[1]	500 mg tid	9000 mg	Nausea, vomiting, anorexia, diarrhea, ataxia, confusion, skin rash, hepatotoxicity	
Aminoglutethimide (Cytadren)[2]	250 mg qid	2000 mg/d	Lethargy, nausea, anorexia, hypothyroidism, somnolence	

[1]Not FDA approved for this indication.
[2]Not available in the United States.

leads to Nelson's syndrome, a condition characterized by unabated progression of a corticotropinoma (owing to the lack of negative feedback by cortisol), very high ACTH levels, and high morbidity.

Treatment of Adrenal Disease

Adrenocortical Tumors

For adrenocortical tumors, the recommended treatment is surgical. Laparoscopic adrenalectomy has become the treatment of choice for benign adrenal lesions with a diameter of less than 6 cm. In stages I to III adrenocortical carcinoma, complete tumor removal by a well-trained surgeon offers by far the best chance for cure. Surgery often needs to be extensive, with en bloc resection of invaded organs, and regularly includes lymphadenectomy. Surgery for local recurrences or metastatic disease is accepted as a valuable therapeutic option and was associated with improved survival in retrospective studies. The overall 5-year survival in different series ranged between 16% and 38%. Median survival for metastatic disease (stage IV) at the time of diagnosis is still consistently less than 12 months.

Radiotherapy has been considered ineffective for treatment of adrenocortical cancer, but it can be indicated to control localized disease not amenable to surgery.

Mitotane (o,p′-DDD [Lysodren]) is the only adrenal-specific agent available for treating adrenocortical cancer. Mitotane is indicated in metastatic adrenocortical carcinoma and can also be used as an adjuvant for tumors with a high risk of recurrence. Mitotane exerts a specific cytotoxic effect on adrenocortical cells, leading to focal degeneration of the fascicular and particularly the reticular zone. In most patients, treatment should be initiated with a dose that does not exceed 1.5 g/day; this is then rapidly increased, depending on gastrointestinal symptoms, to 5 to 6 g/day. This high-dose regimen requires measurement of mitotane blood levels 14 days after initiation of therapy. The dose is then adjusted according to the medicine's plasma concentrations (which should be greater than 14 mg/L) and tolerance of the side effects. Because mitotane treatment induces adrenal insufficiency and increases the metabolic clearance of glucocorticoids, glucocorticoid replacement is indicated, often at higher than normal doses owing to increased clearance.

Cytotoxic Chemotherapy

Cytotoxic chemotherapy includes etoposide (VePesid)[1], doxorubicin (Adriamycin)[1], and cisplatin (Platinol)[1], or streptozocin (Zanosar)[1] plus mitotane. Chemotherapy has limited efficacy for advanced adrenocortical cancer and is associated mainly with partial responses.

Bilateral Adrenal Hyperplasias

The treatment of choice for bilateral adrenal hyperplasias associated with ACTH-independent Cushing's syndrome is bilateral adrenalectomy. Patients require lifelong replacement therapy with glucocorticoids and mineralocorticoids, and they should be adequately educated about the risk of acute adrenal insufficiency.

Treatment of Ectopic Corticotropin Syndrome

The choice of treatment for ectopic ACTH syndrome depends on tumor identification, localization, and classification. The most effective treatment option is surgical resection, although this is not always possible in metastatic disease or in the case of occult tumors. Because the ectopic ACTH syndrome is usually severe and occult tumors can become evident at imaging studies only during the follow-up, medical treatment to control hypercortisolism is often necessary. Bilateral adrenalectomy may be an option to be considered when the hypercortisolism cannot be controlled by other treatment options.

Medical Adrenalectomy

Several drugs that inhibit steroid synthesis are often effective for rapidly controlling hypercortisolism in preparation for surgery, after unsuccessful transsphenoidal surgery or removal of an adrenal tumor such as extensive cancer, or while awaiting the full effect of radiotherapy in recurrent Cushing's disease (Table 4).

Most experience with inhibitors of steroidogenesis has been with metyrapone (Metopirone)[1] and ketoconazole (Nizoral)[1], two medications that appear to be more effective and better tolerated than aminoglutethimide (Cytadren)[2]. Metyrapone reduces cortisol and aldosterone production by inhibiting 11β-hydroxylation in the adrenal cortex. Ketoconazole is a broad-spectrum antifungal drug, which inhibits c17-20 desmolase, cholesterol side-chain cleavage, and 11β-hydroxylation. Ketoconazole is also associated with inhibition of testosterone biosynthesis and gynecomastia.

RU-486, or mifepristone (Korlym), is an antagonist of the progesterone and glucocorticoid receptors. Unexpectedly, the treatment of Cushing's disease with this glucocorticoid antagonist has been associated with increased ACTH secretion and consequent stimulation of cortisol production. RU-486 may be more useful in ectopic ACTH-producing tumors and in adrenal Cushing's syndrome, but its efficacy and potential side effects when administered chronically are currently unknown.

References

Allolio B, Fassnacht M: Clinical review: Adrenocortical carcinoma: clinical update, J Clin Endocrinol Metab 91:2027–2037, 2006.

Assie G, Libe R, Espiard S, et al: ARMC5 mutations in macronodular adrenal hyperplasia with Cushing's syndrome, N Engl J Med 369(22):2105–2114, 2013.

Batista D, Courkoutsakis NA, Oldfield EH, et al: Detection of adrenocorticotropin-secreting pituitary adenomas by magnetic resonance imaging in children and adolescents with Cushing disease, J Clin Endocrinol Metab 90:5134–5140, 2005.

Batista DL, Riar J, Keil M, Stratakis CA: Diagnostic tests for children who are referred for the investigation of Cushing syndrome, Pediatrics 120:e575–e586, 2007.

Bertagna X, Guignat L, Groussin L, Bertherat J: Cushing's disease, Best Pract Res Clin Endocrinol Metab 23:607–623, 2009.

Biller BM, Grossman AB, Stewart PM, et al: Treatment of adrenocorticotropin-dependent Cushing's syndrome: a consensus statement, J Clin Endocrinol Metab 93:2454–2462, 2008.

Boscaro M, Arnaldi G: Approach to the patient with possible Cushing's syndrome, J Clin Endocrinol Metab 94:3121–3131, 2009.

Feelders RA, Hofland LJ: Medical treatment of Cushing's disease, J Clin Endocrinol Metab 98(2):425–438, 2013.

Newell-Price J, Trainer P, Besser M, Grossman A: The diagnosis and differential diagnosis of Cushing's syndrome and pseudo-Cushing's states, Endocr Rev 19:647–672, 1998.

Terzolo M, Angeli A, Fassnacht M, et al: Adjuvant mitotane treatment for adrenocortical carcinoma, N Engl J Med 356:2372–2380, 2007.

[1]Not FDA approved for this indication.　　　　　　　　　　[2]Not available in the United States.

DIABETES INSIPIDUS

Method of
Rami Mortada, MD

CURRENT DIAGNOSIS

- Diabetes insipidus (DI) is a disorder of excess urine production (i.e., "diabetes") that is dilute and tasteless (i.e., "insipidus"). DI contrasts with the concentrated and sweet urine in diabetes mellitus.
- Patients with DI present with polyuria and polydipsia; urine output is usually more than 40 mL/kg/day or more than 3 L/day.
- There are three subtypes of DI:
  - Central DI: due to relative or absolute lack of vasopressin
  - Nephrogenic DI: due to partial or total resistance to the renal antidiuretic effects of vasopressin
  - Dipsogenic DI (also called primary polydipsia): where polyuria is secondary to excessive, inappropriate fluid intake
- Initial labs should include plasma sodium and urine osmolality. Under normal physiologic conditions, the urine osmolality is less than 300 mOsm/L, but if the patient does not have sufficient fluid intake, the urine osmolality can be higher.
- The diagnosis is confirmed by examining urine output and osmolality. It can be followed by an assessment of renal response to the synthetic arginine vasopressin (AVP) analogue desmopressin (DDAVP).
- In primary polydipsia, urine concentration is normal in response to dehydration.
- In central DI, urine concentration does not increase appropriately with dehydration, but does respond to desmopressin (DDAVP). After dehydration in central DI, urine osmolality remains <300 mOsm/kg, and plasma osmolality is >290 mOsm/kg. Urine osmolality rises to >750 mOsm/kg after desmopressin.
- In nephrogenic DI, urine concentration does not increase appropriately with either dehydration or exogenous desmopressin.

CURRENT THERAPY

- The treatment goal is to control polyuria and ensure electrolyte stability.
- In Central DI:
  - The mild form might not require treatment.
  - Significant polyuria can be treated with desmopressin in divided doses: nasal spray 5 to 100 µg/day; tablets 100 to 1000 µg/day; or parenterally 0.1 to 2.0 µg/day.
  - Overtreatment can cause hyponatremia.
- In Nephrogenic DI:
  - Urine output should not be expected to normalize after DDAVP administration.
  - Correct the culprit cause (hypercalcemia or lithium [Eskalith, Lithobid] cessation).
  - Follow a low-sodium, low-protein diet, as tolerated.
  - Hydrochlorothiazide[1] 25 to 50 mg/day may be taken either alone or in combination with indomethacin (Indocin) 25 to 50 mg twice daily.
  - Symptoms may respond partly to high-dose desmopressin (e.g., 4 mcg IM twice daily).
- Primary polydipsia is treated by limiting an excessive fluid intake.

[1]Not FDA approved for this indication.

Physiology of Antidiuretic Hormone

Arginine vasopressin (AVP), also known as antidiuretic hormone (ADH), is a neurohypophysial hormone. It is a peptide hormone that promotes water retention by increasing the permeability of the kidney's collecting duct and distal convoluted tubule to water. It also increases peripheral vascular resistance, which in turn increases arterial blood pressure. In the clinical setting, the terms AVP, ADH, and vasopressin are used interchangeably.

Vasopressin is considered the main hormone involved in the regulation of water homeostasis and osmolality. The regulation and synthesis of vasopressin is under the influence of two systems: osmotic and pressure/volume status. In the case of osmoregulation, a small increase in plasma osmolality produces a parallel increase in vasopressin secretion; a small decrease in plasma osmolality causes a parallel drop in vasopressin.

Vasopressin is one among other hormones and systems that are involved in the regulation of volume and blood pressure. Other factors influence vasopressin production. For example, glucocorticoids inhibit secretion, whereas nausea and vomiting have a stimulatory effect.

Pathophysiology of Diabetes Insipidus

The kidneys exercise one of their urine-concentrating abilities by promoting water retention. If the concentration of vasopressin is decreased, polyuria occurs and diluted urine is excreted. A decrease in total body water results in an increase in the plasma osmolality. If the physiologic response is intact, thirst is stimulated, which leads to an increase in water consumption and the correction of plasma osmolarity. Therefore, unless there is a dysregulation in the thirst mechanisms or water consumption is limited due to a lack of availability (e.g., decreased level of consciousness, immobility, or physical restraints) severe dehydration does not develop.

Clinical Causes

There are three subtypes of diabetes insipidus (DI).

- DI secondary to excess water intake (primary polydipsia)

  Primary polydipsia is a disorder characterized by inappropriate excess fluid intake due to a disordered thirst sensation seen mostly in patients with psychiatric illnesses. A central defect in thirst regulation plays an important role in the pathogenesis of primary polydipsia. Such patients continue drinking even if the plasma osmolality falls below normal. It is not easy to achieve or maintain a low plasma osmolality because vasopressin secretion will normally be suppressed by the fall in plasma osmolality, resulting in rapid excretion of the excess water. If vasopressin regulation is intact, primary polydipsia should not lead to clinically important disturbances in the plasma sodium concentration unless hyposmolar fluid intake overwhelms the kidneys' ability to excrete excess water. Thus the serum sodium concentration is usually normal or slightly reduced in primary polydipsia. These patients may be asymptomatic or present with complaints of polydipsia and polyuria. In rare circumstances where water intake exceeds the kidneys' ability to excrete the water load of about 500 mL/hour, symptomatic severe hyponatremia might result in severe psychosis. Psychosis from hyponatremia in primary polydipsia is most commonly seen in institutionalized patients or in individuals attempting to dilute their urine to avoid a positive urine drug test.

- DI secondary to a decrease in or absence of vasopressin secretion (central DI)

  Central DI may be caused by genetic anomalies of the vasopressin gene (Table 1). Familial neurohypophyseal DI is characterized by the onset of DI with polyuria and polydipsia in childhood or early adulthood. The most common MRI finding in familial neurohypophyseal DI is the progressive disappearance of the posterior pituitary bright spot in children. The normal pituitary bright spot seen on unenhanced T_1-weighted MRI is thought to result from the T_1-shortening effect of the

TABLE 1	Central Diabetes Insipidus (DI) Etiologies
Idiopathic	Unknown etiology
Genetic	Familial neurohypophyseal DI, Wolfram's syndrome (autosomal recessive)
Mass effect	Craniopharyngiomas, primary germ cell tumors, metastatic tumors
Infiltrative diseases	Lymphoma, leukemia, sarcoidosis, amyloidosis
Autoimmune	Lymphocytic infundibuloneurohypophysitis
Trauma	Motor vehicle accident, closed head trauma
Surgical	Surgical intervention at the pituitary region

vasopressin stored in the posterior pituitary. The disappearance of the bright spot corresponds to the disappearance of vasopressin stores in the posterior pituitary. Wolfram's syndrome is a rare autosomal recessive syndrome manifested by DI, diabetes mellitus, optic atrophy, and deafness.

Central DI may be caused by mass lesions of the neurohypophysis, such as craniopharyngiomas, and primary germ cell tumors in childhood. DI can be the initial presentation. MRI often shows a thickened pituitary stalk and may show a hypothalamic mass. Metastasis to the pituitary usually is found with widespread metastatic disease and is twice as likely to involve the posterior pituitary than the anterior pituitary. DI can be associated with pituitary infiltration associated with lymphomas and leukemias.

In granulomatous disease that affects the hypothalamic-pituitary axis, there is usually clear evidence of disease elsewhere in the body. MRI shows an absence of the pituitary bright spot and widening of the hypothalamic-pituitary stalk. Lymphocytic infundibuloneurohypophysitis is a new, well-recognized cause of autoimmune DI, characterized by MRI appearance of a thickened hypothalamic-pituitary stalk and large posterior pituitary gland mimicking a pituitary tumor. Pituitary abscess is a rare cause of pituitary mass and DI. In situations where the cause is not easily diagnosed, an autoimmune process should be suspected. In some patients, the cause is idiopathic.

Central DI may be caused by surgery or trauma to the pituitary region. Vasopressin is normally secreted after any kind of surgical stress, and secretion is more pronounced after surgery to the pituitary region. Only a small percentage of patients undergoing pituitary surgery have permanent DI. A triphasic DI can occur after complete hypothalamic-pituitary stalk transection. The first phase is polyuric and appears within the first 24 hours after surgery. It is thought to be secondary to axonal shock with a resultant inability to release prefabricated vasopressin. The second phase is antidiuretic and starts on about day 6, after stalk injury. It is thought to be secondary to the unregulated release of vasopressin stores. The third phase, also polyuric, starts about day 12, after vasopressin stores have been depleted. It may result in permanent or partial DI or resolve to clinically asymptomatic disease.

The same patterns of DI that occur after pituitary surgery can be seen in patients who experience a closed head trauma. Three-quarters of traumatic induced DI are secondary to motor vehicle accidents. Trauma is usually severe and causes unconsciousness. There is a high association of anterior pituitary deficiency in association with DI induced by head trauma, so the possibility of central hypocortisolism should be considered and treated immediately. DI is reported in 50% to 90% of patients with brain death.

- DI secondary to the lack of renal response to vasopressin (nephrogenic DI)

    Genetic anomalies resulting in a lack of renal response to vasopressin are caused by either a mutation in the V2 receptors or a mutation of the aquaporin 2 water channels gene. The majority of the cases are X-linked recessive disorders in males. Newborns present with polyuria, vomiting, constipation, and failure to thrive. Symptoms usually occur within the first week of life.

Acquired nephrogenic DI can be caused by a kidney disease that distorts the architecture of the kidney and impairs its urine-concentrating ability (e.g., polycystic kidney disease, sickle cell disease). Decreased function of vasopressin or downregulation of aquaporin 2 channels can be caused by hypokalemia, hypercalcemia, and relief of bilateral urinary tract obstruction. Drugs such as lithium (the most common cause of drug-induced nephrogenic DI) and demeclocycline (used clinically to treat a syndrome of inappropriate ADH secretion) may cause nephrogenic DI.

Clinical Manifestations

Patients with central DI typically present with polyuria, nocturia, and polydipsia. The serum sodium concentration in untreated central DI is often in the high normal range, which provides the ongoing stimulation of thirst that replaces urinary water losses. Moderate to severe hypernatremia can develop when thirst is impaired or if there is a lack of access to free water, such as the postoperative period in patients with unrecognized DI or infants with DI. For uncertain pathophysiologic reasons, patients with central DI may develop decreased bone mineral density at the lumbar spine and femoral neck, even if treated with desmopressin.

Nephrogenic DI in its mild form can be asymptomatic. Patients with moderate to severe nephrogenic DI, as with central DI, typically present with polyuria, nocturia, and polydipsia.

Primary polydipsia is the result of an abnormal compulsion to drink water. This disorder is most often seen in middle-aged women and in patients with psychiatric illnesses. The excessive water intake initially drives the excessive urination.

Diagnosis

Polyuria must be distinguished from simple urinary frequency in the absence of excess urine volume. The initial diagnostic approach should be to confirm polyuria, defined as greater than 30 mL/kg or 3 L/day, with a urine osmolality measuring less than 300 mOsm/L. Simple metabolic causes such as hyperglycemia, uremia, and hypercalcemia should be excluded. A definitive diagnosis of DI requires testing of vasopressin production and action in response to osmolar stress. All forms of DI may be partial or complete. In primary polydipsia, the plasma sodium, blood urea nitrogen (BUN), and uric acid are relatively low. In other forms of DI, the plasma sodium and uric acid are relatively high and the BUN is relatively low.

Central DI usually has an abrupt onset resulting from destruction of more than 80% of vasopressin-secreting hypothalamic neurons. The etiology of polyuria is not always evident after history and laboratory tests are completed. In that case, a water restriction test (e.g., dehydration test or water deprivation test) is completed. The water deprivation test is an indirect assessment of the AVP axis, measuring renal concentrating capacity in response to dehydration. It can be followed by assessment of the renal response to the synthetic AVP analogue desmopressin to determine whether any defect identified in urine-concentrating ability can be corrected with AVP-replacement. Office testing is acceptable unless the patient cannot be watched closely. No food or water is allowed. The patient is watched for signs of dehydration and surreptitious water drinking. Baseline measurements include weight, plasma osmolality, sodium, BUN, glucose, and urine volume and osmolality. Weight, plasma osmolality, and urine osmolality are measured hourly. The test is ended if urine osmolality has not increased to more than 300 mOsm/kg for 3 consecutive hours, plasma osmolality has reached 295 to 300 mOsm/kg, or the patient has lost 3% to 5% of body weight. All initial measurements are repeated at the end of the water restriction test. Then, 5 units of aqueous AVP (Pitressin) is administered or 2 µg of desmopressin is given subcutaneously and the plasma osmolality,

TABLE 2	Values Before and After Water Restriction			
	INITIAL PLASMA OSMOLALITY	INITIAL PLASMA SODIUM	POSTTEST URINE/PLASMA OSMOLALITY	POSTTEST URINE/PLASMA OSMOLALITY+ADH
Normal	NL	NL	>1	>1
Central DI	High (high NL)	High (high NL)	<1	>1
Nephrogenic DI	High (high NL)	High (high NL)	<1	<1
Primary polydipsia	Low (low NL)	Low (low NL)	>1	>1

TABLE 3	Treatment Options for Diabetes Insipidus
Central DI	Divide doses of two to three times per day:
	Desmopressin nasal spray 5–100 µg/day
	Desmopressin tablets 0.1–1 mg/day
	Desmopressin injection 0.1–2 µg/day
Nephrogenic DI	Low-salt, low-protein diet
	HCTZ[1] 25 mg one to two times per day
	Indomethacin[1] 25–50 mg bid
	Amiloride[1] 5–10 mg bid
Primary polydipsia	Water restriction to less than 1.5 L/day

[1]Not FDA approved for this indication.

sodium, BUN, glucose, and urine volume and osmolality are measured at 30, 60, and 120 minutes.

In primary polydipsia, urine concentration is normal in response to dehydration (Table 2).

In central DI, urine concentration does not increase appropriately with dehydration, but responds to desmopressin. Urine osmolality remains <300 mOsm/kg, accompanied by plasma osmolality >290 mOsm/kg after dehydration, and urine osmolality rising to >750 mOsm/kg after desmopressin administration.

In nephrogenic DI, urine concentration does not increase appropriately with either dehydration or exogenous desmopressin.

In practice, many results are indeterminate. If central DI is suspected, but the water deprivation test data are inconclusive, a reasonable approach is a therapeutic trial of 10 to 20 µg intranasal desmopressin per day with close monitoring of plasma sodium. If the diagnosis is confirmed, pituitary function testing and cranial MRI should follow.

Treatment

The treatment goal is to improve polyuria and polydipsia symptoms while attempting to treat the etiologic factors (Table 3). This is achieved by appropriate correction of dehydration, if present, and replacing vasopressin or augmenting its effect on the target tissue.

Mild forms of central DI may not require pharmacologic treatment. Desmopressin effectively treats polyuria and polydipsia. Desmopressin comes in different forms, and dosages usually need to be divided.

Hyponatremia from plasma dilution can be avoided by skipping treatment for a short period on a regular basis (e.g., on Sunday). No second dose of desmopressin should be given unless the patient has urine output after the first dose.

Nephrogenic DI may respond to the removal of the offending agent (e.g., lithium) or correction of the underlying electrolyte disturbance (e.g., hypercalcemia or hypokalemia). Drug-induced nephrogenic DI, however, may persist after discontinuation of the drug.

Patients should be instructed to eat a low-sodium, low-protein diet, resulting in a decrease in urine output secondary to the drop in solute excretion. If symptomatic polyuria persists, hydrochlorothiazide[1] can be started. Hydrochlorothiazide presumably acts by inducing mild hypovolemia that induces an increase in proximal sodium and water reabsorption, thereby diminishing water delivery to the vasopressin-sensitive sites in the collecting tubules and reducing the urine output. Indomethacin (Indocin[1]) is an add-on medication if there is not enough response. Given that prostaglandins antagonize the action of vasopressin, indomethacin inhibits renal prostaglandin synthesis and subsequently decreases urine output.

Amiloride (Midamor)[1] might be more effective for lithium-induced nephrogenic DI. This drug closes the sodium channels in the luminal membrane of the collecting tubule cells. These channels constitute the mechanism by which filtered lithium normally enters the collecting tubule cells and interferes with the collecting tubule response to ADH.

The approach to primary polydipsia treatment is reduction in fluid intake. Desmopressin treatment should be avoided due to the risk of hyponatremia.

Monitoring

Primary polydipsia is the most challenging of all types of DI to treat. It requires a multidisciplinary approach that frequently demands medical and psychiatric involvement.

In central DI, patients will require frequent follow-up to adjust desmopressin dosing. Once stable, patients can be seen less frequently to assess symptom control and to check plasma sodium levels to avoid overtreatment resulting in hyponatremia.

In nephrogenic DI, after the precipitating agent has been withdrawn, follow-up is needed to assess the reversibility of polyuria. If acquired nephrogenic DI becomes irreversible, patients might require prolonged pharmacological treatment. In both central and nephrogenic DI, the patient is advised to wear a medical alert bracelet stating the disease and the potential complications.

Acknowledgment
I would like to thank K. James Kallail, PhD, for his contribution to the final editing of this chapter.

[1]Not FDA approved for this indication.

References

Bockenhauer D, Bichet DG: Inherited secondary nephrogenic diabetes insipidus: Concentrating on humans, Am J Physiol Renal Physiol 304:F1037–F1042, 2013.

Crowley RK, Sherlock M, Agha A, et al: Clinical insights into adipsic diabetes insipidus: A large case series, Clin Endocrinol (Oxf) 66:475–482, 2007.

Fujiwara TM, Bichet DG: Molecular biology of hereditary diabetes insipidus, J Am Soc Nephrol 16:2836–2846, 2005.

Hannon MJ, Sherlock M, Thompson CJ: Pituitary dysfunction following traumatic brain injury or subarachnoid haemorrhage, Best Pract Res Clin Endocrinol Metab 25:783–798, 2011.

Monnens L, Jonkman A, Thomas C: Response to indomethacin and hydrochlorothiazide in nephrogenic diabetes insipidus, Clin Sci (Lond) 66:709–715, 1984.

Oiso Y, Robertson GL, Nørgaard JP, Juul KV: Clinical review: Treatment of neurohypophyseal diabetes insipidus, J Clin Endocrinol Metab 98:3958–3967, 2013.

Vande Walle J, Stockner M, Raes A, Nørgaard JP: Desmopressin 30 years in clinical use: A safety review, Curr Drug Saf 2:232–238, 2007.

DIABETES MELLITUS IN ADULTS

Method of

Kristine K. Grdinovac, MD; Candice E. Rose, MD, MS; Ethan Alexander, MD; Daniel R. Tilden, MD; and David C. Robbins, MD, MPH

CURRENT DIAGNOSIS

- Established guidelines define diabetes as a fasting blood sugar ≥126 mg/dL or an HbA1c of ≥6.5% or a blood sugar ≥200 mg/dL 2 hours after a 75-g oral glucose load.
- Prediabetes is defined as a blood sugar of 100 to 125 mg/dL or an HbA1c between 5.7% and 6.4%.
- The diagnostic guidelines are derived from inflection points in the risk of acquiring complications at any given glucose elevation.
- People with prediabetes share a similar risk of cardiovascular disease (CVD) as those with diabetes. Thus, intervention with weight loss, exercise, and metformin[1] is very beneficial in this population.
- Early detection of complications can slow the progression to end-stage disease. Routine surveillance includes annual dilated eye examinations, foot inspection, measurement of microalbuminuria, and measurements of blood lipids and kidney and liver function.

[1]Not FDA approved for this indication.

CURRENT THERAPY

- Treatment should be started early when signs of hyperglycemia appear, including prediabetes. The risks of complications are related to the lifetime duration of hyperglycemia.
- A standard glycemic treatment goal is an A1c below 7%. It is justified, in a few patients, to set a higher goal when factors such as age, desire to lose weight, and catastrophic risk of hypoglycemia (hypoglycemic unawareness), concurrent disease, and/or other barriers are detected. Time in range (TIR), a statistic from continuous glucose monitoring reflecting the time/day capillary glucose is 70 to 180 mg/dL, is an evolving goal. The suggested TIR is 70% or more.
- Because the treatment of diabetes is largely focused on prevention of atherosclerotic disease, aggressive control of blood pressure and lipids is also recommended.
- Treatment of type 2 diabetes mellitus (T2DM) is fundamentally based on diet (weight loss) and exercise with the addition of drugs (or bariatric surgery) when treatment goals are not achieved. No patient should experience uncontrolled hyperglycemia for more than 3 months without the addition of more therapy.
- Metformin is usually the first-line drug. The ADA now considers glucagon-like peptide-1 (GLP-1) receptor agonists and sodium-glucose cotransporter 2 (SGLT2) inhibitors as possible first-line drugs.
- There are now many options for additional medications that may best fit a patient's disease characteristics, financial resources, and lifestyle. Some of the newer (and more expensive) medications are weight-neutral, may promote weight loss, and have shown to reduce the risk of atherosclerotic cardiovascular disease and deterioration in renal function.
- Assessment of glucose control includes periodic measurement of HbA1c, home blood glucose monitoring, and, when appropriate, continuous glucose monitoring.
- Treatment with insulin is an option that can be introduced at any time during the course of T2DM. The goal, ideally, is to normalize the blood sugar without significant or frequent hypoglycemia.

Epidemiology

The increasing prevalence of diabetes in the United States and globally has been described as an epidemic or tsunami that has the potential to overwhelm medical systems worldwide. The number of people who have been diagnosed with diabetes increased from 108 million in 1980 to about 422 million in 2014. The global prevalence has nearly doubled during the same period, from 4.7% to 8.5%. About 34.2 million or 10.5% of Americans are known to have diabetes, and a nearly equal number have the disease but are undiagnosed. The prevalence increases with age, reaching 26.8% of the population 65 years of age or older. Women have a slightly higher prevalence than men, and the disease disproportionately affects people of Hispanic and Asian descent and non-Hispanic Blacks. Not surprisingly, the proportion of people with undiagnosed diabetes is also greatest among those of color and in the lower socioeconomic strata.

In the United States, the yearly incidence of prediabetes (defined as a fasting blood sugar of 100 to 125 mg/dL or HbA1c 5.7% to 6.4%) is estimated to be approximately 35%. On average, 1 in 10 prediabetic patients will become diabetic every year.

The risk factors for diabetes clearly include an interaction of genetic susceptibility and environmental triggers, including obesity. For example, among diabetic patients, 89% are overweight or obese. The U.S. National Health Interview Survey has shown a striking impact of obesity on the risk of acquiring the disease. Among nearly 800,000 respondents, the lifetime risk of diabetes was approximately 7.6% among underweight men and 70.3% for those who were very obese. The effect of increasing weight on the risk of diabetes is linear, with those having a body mass index (BMI) above 30 having at least a fivefold increase in the risk of acquiring diabetes. Central or intraabdominal accumulation of fat has also been shown to be more highly correlated with diabetes than with subcutaneous fat. Thus, individuals of the same body composition who have a predominance of central or intraabdominal fat are much more likely to have insulin resistance, hypertension, diabetes, and dyslipidemia. Intraabdominal fat, in contrast with subcutaneous fat, produces more free fatty acids, inflammatory cytokines, hormones associated with insulin resistance, and reduced amounts of insulin sensitizers such as adiponectin.

The widely used BMI cutoff points for overweight (25 to 30 kg/m^2) and obesity (>30 kg/m^2) are good markers for diabetic risks among non-Hispanic whites and African Americans. However, among Asians and Hispanics, diabetes incidence increases at much lower BMIs, possibly triggered by a more potent impact of central adiposity on insulin resistance and hyperglycemia. In the Diabetes Prevention Program (DPP), a BMI cutoff point of 22 kg/m^2 rather than 25 kg/m^2 was used to identify Asian participants at increased risk for diabetes. These differences should be kept in mind when counseling or treating patients of different ethnicities.

In addition to obesity, a variety of other risk factors include smoking, hypertension, hypercholesterolemia, and, most importantly, physical inactivity. Of these associated risk factors, it is clinically important to recognize that even a modest increase in physical activity and a small reduction in body weight are the only nonpharmacologic interventions prospectively shown to reduce the risk of acquiring or even occasionally reversing diabetes (as shown in the DPP).

The genetics of type 2 diabetes mellitus (T2DM) are complex and incompletely understood despite huge studies seeking the gene variations that increase risk of diabetes. Large population studies have found over 120 gene variants that account for the risk of T2DM, but their contribution is small (about 3% to 10%), and with few exceptions, any given gene variant is practically useless in assessing risk for a particular individual. Thus although weight, waist circumference, and age are clinically useful markers of risk, genetic testing is not yet a clinical tool to predict diabetes. The predominant factors responsible for the diabetes phenotype are environmental rather than genetic. Curiously, identical monozygotic twins show a strong diabetes concordance (76%), even when the twins are raised separately from one another.

Diagnosis and Classification of Diabetes and Prediabetes

The definitions of diabetes and prediabetes are based on standardized and discrete markers of hyperglycemia. On the other hand, the complications of diabetes, most notably atherosclerosis and microvascular disease, are more or less linearly related to the exposure to hyperglycemia over time rather than appearing with any given marker of glycemia. For example, one accepted definition of diabetes is a fasting blood sugar of 126 mg/dL or higher. However, a marked increased risk of CVD is found at lower concentrations of blood glucose. Prediabetic persons, whose fasting blood sugar may range from 100 to 125 mg/dL, have nearly the same incidence of atherosclerotic heart disease as patients assigned a standardized diagnosis of diabetes.

The standard definitions of diabetes are largely based on inflection points in the risk of complications versus a given increment in glycemia. Diabetes then is defined as any of the following abnormalities:

- Hemoglobin A1c 6.5% or higher
- Fasting plasma glucose 126 mg/dL or higher
- A 2-hour glucose of 200 mg/dL or higher after a 75-g oral glucose load (oral glucose tolerance test)

It must be noted that there is some controversy over these values. Not all newly diagnosed individuals will have abnormalities in all three criteria. Furthermore, it is unsettled whether one test better predicts complications than another. Some experts insist that a patient should have at least two abnormal criteria, but this may delay justified clinical intervention and add cost and inconvenience. It is our recommendation to accept any one abnormality as a criterion for a diagnosis of diabetes and justification to begin lifestyle and possibly drug interventions.

The accepted classification of diabetes is, like the laboratory diagnosis, useful but imperfect. *The common phenotype of all types of diabetes is hyperglycemia* and a variety of more subtle abnormalities related to insulin deficiency or insulin resistance such as dyslipidemia, increased tissue oxidation, and macro- and microvascular disease, among others.

Diabetes Is Classified into Four Categories

Type 1 Diabetes

In most cases, type 1 diabetes mellitus (T1DM) is caused by an autoimmune destruction of the insulin-producing beta cells. About 95% of such patients have autoantibodies (glutamic acid decarboxylase-65 [GAD-65], anti–zinc transporter protein, and anti–islet cell antibodies) that mark the gradual (sometimes over many years) or rapid destruction of the beta cells. The result is a complete or near-total loss of endogenous insulin and life-sustaining dependence on insulin therapy. In general, antibody-positive persons who have all three antibodies and those with higher titers become diabetic more quickly than those with low titers of one or two antibodies.

Differentiating T1DM from T2DM can sometimes be a diagnostic challenge. *The age of onset* of T1DM peaks in the mid-teens but is not a reliable diagnostic tool because incident T1DM is seen throughout the human lifespan. Similarly, *thinness* is no longer a reliable phenotype of T1DM since so many individuals are obese. *Ketoacidosis* used to be considered a hallmark of T1DM, but a subset of T2DM patients presents with ketoacidosis, recovers with treatment, and can be successfully treated with oral agents (Flatbush diabetes). The diagnosis can sometimes be even more perplexing because some new-onset T1DM patients will not require insulin for several months after presenting with ketoacidosis. This so-called *honeymoon phase* of diabetes usually lasts less than 6 months.

When the diagnosis is unclear, we occasionally measure C-peptide and glucose simultaneously and the GAD-65 antibody to more clearly differentiate a T1DM patient from the more common T2DM (see definition later in this chapter). Those patients with very low C-peptides in the presence of elevated glucose and the positive anti–GAD-65 antibody are almost always type 1, and insulin treatment is needed from the outset.

Type 2 Diabetes

T2DM accounts for about 95% of the worldwide burden of the disease. The pathophysiology of the disease is fundamentally a simultaneous deficiency in the amount of insulin needed to overcome the insulin resistance, resulting in hyperglycemia, an event that most commonly occurs during midlife. However, the condition is increasingly manifest in childhood or early adolescence in concert with epidemic obesity and inactivity. Adolescent T2DM, now accounting for a significant proportion of diabetes in youth, appears to be a particularly aggressive form of the disease with high risk of late complications.

The cause of the hyperglycemia is complex and multifactorial. There is a progressive nonautoimmune loss of insulin production thought to be caused by aging, loss of beta cells from inflammation and oxidative stress, a genetically programmed loss with age, or, for lack of a better term, *pancreatic exhaustion.* Resistance to insulin is also an essential aspect of the disease that may be detected long before hyperglycemia. The vast majority of patients with T2DM are obese or at least have increased amounts of central fat. Many students of T2DM argue that there are many subtypes or genotypes that share a similar clinical presentation, and future classification schemes may account for those differences. About 5% of the T2DM population are thin, and the cause of their noninsulin-dependent diabetes is not so clear.

Gestational Diabetes

Gestational diabetes (GDM) is typically diagnosed in the second or third trimester of pregnancy on the basis of a 50-g oral glucose tolerance test in women who were not known to be diabetic pre-pregnancy. GDM carries an increased risk of pregnancy complications (hypertension, preeclampsia, large birthweight infants), and treatment with diet, metformin[1], or insulin is commonly used. Importantly, 50% to 80% of women who had GDM will suffer from T2DM within a decade of their pregnancy.

Specific Types of Diabetes Due to Other Causes

This category may account for as much as 5% of clinical diabetes and should not be overlooked. We remind our residents to think of these "other" forms of diabetes on the first visit with every phenotypically type 2 patient. These include cystic fibrosis, glucocorticoid-induced diabetes, Cushing syndrome, hemochromatosis, certain anticancer drugs (e.g., checkpoint inhibitors, alpelisib [Piqray]), HIV protease inhibitors, and monogenic forms of diabetes. The monogenic forms of diabetes can be manifested in the first 3 months of life. Later in life, an autosomal dominant form of non–insulin-dependent diabetes termed maturity-onset diabetes of youth (MODY) is seen. MODY may account for a few percent of the "type 2" diabetic population and is suspected when there is onset of diabetes in the late teens or early adulthood. Genetic testing is commercially available for these polymorphisms and can identify common subtypes that are responsive to high-dose sulfonylurea medication.

Clinical Manifestations

Most patients with T2DM are discovered by elevated glucose on an incidental blood test. Population screening is generally inefficient except among those at very high risk. Otherwise, presenting symptoms include polyuria, polydipsia, nocturia, blurred vision, and/or weight loss resulting from catabolism. Although the peak incidence of T2DM is in midlife, there is an increasing and disturbing increase in the incidence of T2DM in children and adolescents, especially those belonging to racial and ethnic minorities. This is undoubtedly correlated with childhood obesity.

Less frequently, patients can initially present with diabetic keto-acidosis (DKA) or nonketotic hyperosmolar hyperglycemic state (HHS). This typically occurs in combination with some inciting factor, such as infection, stress, or myocardial ischemia. Patients have hyperglycemia, marked dehydration, electrolyte derangements, and altered levels of consciousness and are at increased

---

[1] Not FDA approved for this indication.

risk of death. Other common conditions that are highly correlated with the development of diabetes include polycystic ovarian syndrome, GDM, toxemia of pregnancy, and delivery of infants over 8 lb at birth (large for dates).

Most commonly, T2DM has an insidious onset, and patients can remain asymptomatic for several years, only being diagnosed unexpectedly through routine laboratory workup. Aging, sedentary behaviors, and obesity may tip the balance between insulin action and insulin resistance, resulting in clinical hyperglycemia. At the time of diagnosis, however, asymptomatic patients may already have significant microvascular and/or macrovascular diabetic complications because there is often a long prodrome of hyperglycemia.

Without a doubt, the most common sign of insulin resistance is simply obesity (a large waist or high waist-to-hip ratio) or increased accumulation of central fat, a finding that occurs in 90% to 95% of T2DM patients. Other signs may include acanthosis nigricans, a velvety, hyperpigmented thickening of the skin, typically seen at the nape of the neck and within intertriginous areas such as the axilla (Figure 1). Skin tags around the base of the neck are recognized as a sign of insulin resistance. Necrobiosis lipoidica is a granulomatous skin disorder that is prevalent in up to 65% of patients. It appears as reddish-brown to yellow-brown oval-shaped plaques with central atrophy and telangiectasias that frequently ulcerate (Figure 2).

Long-Term Implications of Glycemic Control

Atherosclerotic cardiovascular disease (ASCVD), stroke, and peripheral vascular disease are the major causes of morbidity and mortality in persons with diabetes. The Framingham study estimated that the relative risk of ASCVD among diabetic patients was three- to fivefold higher than in the nondiabetic cohort, even when accounting for smoking, hypertension, and dyslipidemia. Diabetes itself is an independent risk factor for ASCVD, and multiple studies suggest a correlation between effective glycemic control and risk mitigation of CVD and mortality. Other risk factors for ASCVD include hypertension, dyslipidemia, tobacco use, and family history.

Treatment of hyperglycemia and associated cardiovascular risk factors has clearly been shown to be beneficial in diabetes. Several landmark trials examined the role of intensive glycemic control and ASCVD outcomes. One study, widely quoted and sometimes misinterpreted, seemed to suggest the opposite, that those assigned to very tight control experienced increased risk of death. The Action to Control Cardiovascular Risk in Diabetes (ACCORD) study evaluated the effect of tight glycemic control (HbA1c <6.0% vs. HbA1c of 7% to 7.9%) on the outcomes of nonfatal myocardial infarction (MI), nonfatal stroke, and CVD death. The trial was stopped early because of increased mortality in the intensive therapy group. However, a subset analysis showed that patients with no history of CVD events prior to the study and baseline HbA1c less than 8% had a statistically significant reduction in CVD events. Hypoglycemia did not account for the increased deaths, and the majority of excess deaths were among those who had long-term poor control and were unable to achieve tight control, even when assigned to the aggressive arm of the study.

The Action in Diabetes and Vascular Disease: Preterax and Diamicron MR Controlled Evaluation (ADVANCE) trial aimed to lower HbA1c ≤6.5% in the intensive arm and measured microvascular plus macrovascular (nonfatal MI, nonfatal stroke, CVD death) outcomes. Notably, very few patients were using insulin at the start of this study, but criteria for all participants included having vascular disease or a risk factor for vascular disease. Ultimately, there was no increase in ASCVD mortality or overall mortality between the two arms. The Veteran Affairs Diabetes Trial (VADT) evaluated the value of intensive glycemic control for the primary outcomes of nonfatal MI, nonfatal stroke, CVD death, hospitalization for heart failure, and revascularization. Results of this study showed more CVD deaths in the intensive therapy group than the standard arm, although not statistically significant.

At first glance, these studies suggest that very intensive control of diabetes may lead to increased mortality rather than improved cardiovascular outcomes. It is important to note that in all three trials, ASCVD risk factors were treated aggressively in all participants. All three studies also demonstrated more hypoglycemia in the intensive therapy groups than standard therapy groups. Hypoglycemia, however, did not explain the increased mortality in the intensively treated patients. The studies enrolled many patients who were older (mean age 60 to 66), with a long duration of diabetes (8 to 12 years) and already established CVD or known risk factors. Further subset analyses of each of these trials revealed significant benefits of intensive glycemic control for ASCVD outcomes in those patients with shorter duration of diabetes, lower initial HbA1c at entry, and/or absence of known CVD. We do not see the data from these studies as justification

Figure 2 Necrobiosis lipoidica is a granulomatous skin disorder that is prevalent in up to 65% of patients with diabetes. It appears as reddish-brown to yellow-brown oval-shaped plaques with central atrophy and telangiectasias that frequently ulcerate.

Figure 1 Acanthosis nigricans is a common examination finding of insulin resistance. It presents as a hyperpigmented, velvety, gray-to-brown thickening of the skin folds at the posterior neck and intertriginous folds. From James WD, Elston D, Treat J, Rosenbach M. *Andrews' diseases of the skin: clinical dermatology*, 13th ed., Philadelphia, 2020, Elsevier.

TABLE 1 Treatment Options for Overweight and Obesity in Type 2 Diabetes

TREATMENT*	BMI CATEGORY (KG/M²)		
	25.0–26.9 *(OR 23.0–24.9†)*	27.0–29.9 *(OR 25.0–27.4†)*	≥30.0 *(OR ≥27.5†)*
Diet, exercise, and behavioral therapy	Yes	Yes	Yes†
Pharmacotherapy—weight-loss medications for selected patients	No	Yes	Yes†
Metabolic surgery (vertical gastroplasty or modified Roux-en-Y)	No	No	Yes†*

*Asian Americans in italics.
†For obese patients with comorbidities.
BMI, Body mass index.

for not attempting tight glycemic control in most patients. *Thus intense glycemic control may be more likely to benefit younger patients with shorter duration of diabetes in whom tight control prevents the development of future ASCVD complications.*

Intensive glycemic control also reduces the risk of microvascular complications (retinopathy, nephropathy) in T2DM. As with macrovascular disease, microvascular disease may be present at the time of initial diagnosis of T2DM. Several pivotal trials demonstrated benefits of intensive versus standard blood glucose control on major microvascular outcomes in T2DM. The UK Prospective Diabetes Study (UKPDS) showed the significant impact of early, intensive glycemic control by demonstrating a 25% reduction in the development of microvascular complications in those with newly diagnosed T2DM. At the 10-year follow up, there was continued benefit in reducing microvascular risk as well as risk for MI and death from any cause, demonstrating that early, intensive control of glycemia can provide lasting positive effects on microvascular and macrovascular outcomes.

Prevention and Reversal

Several large, randomized controlled trials have shown that behavior and lifestyle changes are highly effective in preventing T2DM. The strongest evidence comes from the DPP. This trial showed a reduction in incidence of T2DM among prediabetic enrollees by 58% over 3 years. The lifestyle intervention goals of the DPP were to attain and maintain a weight loss of 7% minimum and 150 minutes of physical activity per week, similar in intensity to brisk walking. Few patients actually achieved these modest goals, but the benefit was seen among most patients assigned to lifestyle changes alone. Similarly, modest reduction in weight has a significant protective effect on the progression to diabetes. The DPP study also included a metformin-only arm, and these patients also had a reduction in the incidence of diabetes (about 25%). It has been estimated that prediabetic patients following lifestyle suggestions *and* daily metformin[1] may have the lowest risk of diabetes over time compared with control groups and those receiving intensive lifestyle intervention only or daily metformin only. Outcomes of bariatric surgery and significant weigh loss among T2 DM suggests that reversal of the disease occurs in the majority of patients, especially those whose duration of diabetes is less than 10 yr.

General Medical Management

When caring for the typical T2DM patient, many providers face noncompliant patients with complex problems who show, over time, little progress in overcoming their disease. The treatment of diabetes is perhaps unique in medicine because it relies heavily on changes in patient lifestyle and adherence to complex regimens and imposes heavy economic burdens. The 20-minute clinic visit is unsuited for patients with multiple complaints, and after these visits providers often feel unsuccessful, frustrated with the patients, or worn out from nagging patients to adhere to their regimens.

It is important to find and practice an approach to these patients that focuses on problem solving rather than threatening,

using praise for small changes, setting reasonable goals, and constantly reminding oneself that there are little victories in many patient visits that can be a source of personal reward (Table 1). In our clinic, we rely heavily on the techniques of motivational interviewing, adapted to a short clinic visit, to help the patient identify and solve problems. In addition, we find that motivational interviewing helps the *provider* share in a sense of success, even if that change is small but in the right direction.

General Goals

The treatment of diabetes is goal driven. Although there are discrete goals for average glycemia (HbA1c), blood pressure, and lipid levels, the American Diabetes Association (ADA) recognizes that the goals can be adjusted for a given patient's risks for hypoglycemia, duration of disease, presence of certain comorbidities, established vascular complications, patient preferences, and available resources and system support (Table 2).

Glycemic Goals

Assessment of glycemic control centers around HbA1c and self-monitoring blood glucose (SMBG) values. The average HbA1c correlates well with the SMBG in most instances, although certain situations, such as increased red blood cell turnover, hemoglobinopathies, or recent blood transfusions, may cause discordant results. It is also important to recognize there may be ethnic differences for HbA1c values, as studies have shown higher HbA1c values in African Americans than in Caucasians with the same mean glucose. HbA1c should be measured at least quarterly in patients who are not meeting glycemic goals or twice yearly in those who achieve HbA1c targets.

The ADA recommends an HbA1c target of less than 7% in most nonpregnant adults, suggesting that an even more stringent target HbA1c of less than 6.5% may be appropriate for some patients if it can be achieved without significant hypoglycemia or adverse effects. Conversely, the HbA1c goal may be loosened to less than 8% for patients who are at high risk of hypoglycemia, have limited life expectancy, have advanced complications of diabetes, or have long-standing disease. These guidelines encourage providers to individualize HbA1c goals for each patient, taking patient characteristics as well as risks and benefits into account. Similarly, the Veteran's Affairs/Department of Defense guidelines suggest shared decision making and individualized HbA1c goals, with more aggressive HbA1c goals for patients with a long life expectancy and absent or mild microvascular complications and relaxed HbA1c goals for those with limited life expectancy and significant comorbidities.

In contrast, the American College of Physicians (ACP) recommends that clinicians target an HbA1c of 7% to 8% for most patients with T2DM, with deescalation of pharmacologic therapy for any patients achieving an HbA1c less than 6.5%. The authors of this section do not agree with these guidelines and instead choose to follow the ADA guidelines for HbA1c targets because HbA1c targets closer to 8% put patients at risk for developing more macrovascular and microvascular complications. Although the authors do believe that HbA1c goals should be individualized

TABLE 2 Decision Factors in Selecting Glycemic Goals

DECISION FACTORS	HBA1C <7%	HBA1C >7%–8%
Consequences of hypoglycemia	Low risk of severe hypoglycemia, patient senses hypoglycemia, has access to good support system	High risk, hypoglycemia unawareness, lives alone
Duration of diabetes	Short; tight control early in the disease promotes reduction in complications over time	There is little evidence that tight control late in the disease alters outcome
Life expectancy	Long	Short; reduction in macro- and microvascular diseases seen after years or decades of good glycemic control
Life-shortening comorbidities	Absent	Patients with life-limiting comorbidities may justifiably have glycemic goals that avoid extreme highs and lows
Well-established comorbidities such as retinopathy, nephropathy, neuropathy	Absent. However, improvement in retinopathy and delay in progression of neuropathy are recognized benefits of tight control	Many comorbidities such as end-stage renal disease, moderate-severe ischemic vascular disease, severe peripheral or autonomic nephropathy
Patient preferences	Highly motivated, strong support	Prefers less burdensome therapy, voices resistance to treatment; obstacles potentially modifiable over time
Available resources	Readily available, good health insurance, strong social network	Limited resources, including cost of medication, poor social support, and so on. The provider can choose low-cost medications (human insulins, sulfonylureas, metformin) to attempt to reach glycemic goals

and relaxed when indicated, we target A1c values of less than 7% without hypoglycemia, especially in younger patients with early diagnosis of T2DM, in an attempt to provide the greatest protection against future macrovascular and microvascular complications.

Home SMBG testing remains a mainstay for patients to evaluate and manage blood glucose levels. Patients who are on multiple daily injections (MDIs) of insulin should perform SMBG fasting, before meals, and at bedtime, which is typically three to four checks per day. For patients only on basal insulin, with or without other noninsulin agents, SMBG should be performed at least once daily, ideally fasting. It can be argued that SMBG may not provide added benefit for non–insulin-treated patients, although periodic testing would still be useful to guide treatment and document hypoglycemia. Other studies have found improved glycemic control in patients without insulin therapy who still perform multiple SMBG tests per week. The ADA does not outline specific guidelines for SMBG for patients who are not on MDI.

With advances in technology, continuous glucose monitors (CGMs) are a commonly used tool to assess glucose values (Figure 3). Benefits of CGM include little to no need for SMBG, thus minimizing fingersticks, and continuous data that may alert the patient to glycemic trends and alarm for both high and low blood glucose values. Some CGMs may also be paired with insulin pumps to implement real-time data for basal insulin pump algorithms. Reports can be generated that include multiple data points not achieved with simple SMBG, such as percentage of time CGM is active, glycemic variability, and glycemic patterns over a 24-hour time frame.

A relatively new concept that is included in CGM reports is glycemic "time in range" (TIR), which accounts for the percentage of time a patient is within a desired glucose target. The TIR has a strong correlation with the HbA1c value, and it is typically reported as the *glucose management indicator* (GMI) on CGM reports. In using TIR to assess control, we strive for values of 70% or higher with a coefficient of variation of less than 30%.

The most important principles in the treatment of hyperglycemia can be succinctly summarized as follows:
- Start it early in the disease (arguably even in the prediabetic stages).
- Do not delay additional treatment when glycemic goals are not attained. In our practice, we consider additional interventions every 3 months until the patient's glucose goals are attained.

There is strong empirical evidence supporting these principles. The Epidemiology of Diabetes Interventions and Complications (EDIC) study clearly showed that poor control early in the disease increased the prevalence of complications many years later, even if tight control was implemented at some later, intermediate time point. This delayed risk for complications is called *metabolic memory*. Evidence from practice patterns is that patients with poor glycemic control often stay that way for years as they promise better adherence to weight loss and exercise and negotiate with clinicians who themselves might be fearful of adding medications, especially insulin.

Monitoring

Much like driving a car without a speedometer, a diabetic patient who is unmonitored is at risk of undetected poor control and wide swings in blood sugar. There is little credible evidence that a patient can feel blood sugar highs and lows even when trained in behavioral clinical trials. Before choosing how a patient must be monitored, it is important to determine the frequency needed. The Diamicron MR in NIDDM Assessing Management and Improvement Control (DINAMIC-1) study randomized patients taking a sulfonylurea between no monitoring versus twice-weekly fingerstick testing groups. There was a small but significant difference in A1c between the groups (0.25%). Other studies show that patients doing more frequent testing report a lower score on measures of quality of life while achieving comparable HbA1c levels.

Nevertheless, there are many patients who benefit from frequent monitoring. Those include patients using insulin, those at risk for hypoglycemia, and perhaps a subset who insist on close monitoring as frequent reassurance that they are being properly treated. We have also observed some benefits related to self-learning. Some patients learn which foods produce high excursions in postprandial glucose and self-correct their diet over time based on these data.

Fingerstick Monitoring

The precision and accuracy of available over-the-counter (OTC) monitors are adequate to make safe clinical decisions. In general, the choice of a monitor is based on cost, insurance reimbursement, and features such as memory and the ability to upload stored results for clinical review. We find this latter feature especially useful to detect patterns of diurnal glycemia.

Continuous Glucose Monitoring

CGM offers a tremendous benefit and is extremely useful, if not necessary, in patients treated with insulin. CGM is now recommended for all patients with diabetes on MDIs, continuous

Example of AGP report

AGP Report

Name

MRN

Glucose statistics and targets

26 Feb 2019 - 10 Mar 2019   **13 days**
% Time CGM is active   **99.9%**

Glucose ranges   **Targets** [% of readings (Time/Day)]
Target range 70–180 mg/dL............Greater than 70% (16hr 48min)
Below 70 mg/dL..............................Less than 4% (58min)
Below 54 mg/dL..............................Less than 1% (14min)
Above 250 mg/dL............................Less than 5% (1hr 12min)
Each 5% increase in time in range (70–180 mg/dL) is clinically beneficial.

Average glucose   **173 mg/dL**
Glucose management indicator (GMI)   **7.6%**
Glucose variability   **49.5%**
Defined as percent coefficient of variation (%CV): target ≤36%

Time in ranges

Very high (>250 mg/dL)....................**20%** (4hr 48min)

High...**23%** (5hr 31min)

Target range (70–180 mg/dL)..........**47%** (11hr 17min)

Low...**4%** (58min)
Very low (<54 mg/dL)........................**6%** (1hr 26min)

Ambulatory glucose profile (AGP)

AGP is a summary of glucose values from the report period, with median (50%) and other percentiles shown as if occurring in a single day.

Daily glucose profiles

Each daily profile represents a midnight to midnight period.

Figure 3 The report from a continuous glucose monitor contains valuable information. The time of day is along the x-axis and the blood glucose is along the y-axis. The solid line is the median glucose over 2 weeks and the dark and light shaded areas represent 90% and 95% of the values over the past 2 weeks. On the right, average glucose sensor usage and time and range is documented. The glycemic goals are shown on the graph by two horizontal lines. The glycemic management index (GMI) of 7.6% shows the computer-generated estimate of hemoglobin A1C from the glucose collected over the past ~2 weeks. In this case, the patient suffers from postprandial hyperglycemia after breakfast and the evening meal and a tendency towards hypoglycemia around 3:00 PM and overnight.

subcutaneous insulin infusions, and other forms of insulin therapy. Several devices are available (various Freestyle Libre systems [Abbott, Abbott Park, IL], Dexcom G6/7 [Dexcom Inc., San Diego, CA], and Medtronic Guardian Connect [Medtronic, Minneapolis, MN]). They are all placed on the skin. The Eversense E3 CGM (Ascensia Diabetes Care, Basel, CH) is implanted under the skin and can store glucose data for up to 6 months. Insurance carriers often limit use to patients treated with at least four shots of insulin daily or insulin pumps. The most common devices are small, self-adherent to the skin, shower resistant, easy to apply, and provide continuous readings for 10 to 14 days. Most of the devices have audible low-glucose alarms, a feature useful for patients at risk for hypoglycemia without symptoms (hypoglycemic unawareness). Transmitted data can also alert the patient to trends in blood glucose levels, with directional arrows signaling the rate of increasing or decreasing blood glucose, and notify the patient to act accordingly. The majority of CGMs do not require calibration with fingersticks, and all of them can upload their data to a smartphone or independent reader, which can, in turn, be reviewed both by the patient, a family member, or clinician. "Professional" CGMs are clinic-based and can include blinded or real-time data collection for clinicians. A useful Internet site that accommodates this process with Health Insurance Portability and Accountability Act (HIPAA) compliance is Tidepool (tidepool.org). We consider the availability of continuous glucose monitoring a major advance in patient care.

Frequency of Clinical Visits
The standard frequency of visits for T2DM patients is every 3 to 6 months. We shorten this interval in patients who are in poor control as needed to prevent acute complications. The recommended interval is set, in part, on the duration needed to measure a stable change in HbA1c, which is about 3 months. Other recommendations include the following:
- Actions taken with each visit
  - Blood pressure (orthostatic if indicated)
  - Height, weight, vital signs
  - HbA1c if results are not available within the past 3 months
  - Skin examination
- Annual visits
  - Fundoscopic examination by eye specialist
  - Comprehensive foot examination
  - Laboratory examination to include lipid profile, liver function tests, and spot urine microalbumin/creatinine
  - As indicated: electrolytes, B12, platelet count if considering fatty liver, nonalcoholic steatohepatitis (NASH), or nonalcoholic fatty liver disease (NAFLD)
- Podiatry
  - We generally refer patients to podiatry when there is evidence of reduced blood flow, infection, deformities (claw toes, Charcot foot), heavy calluses, bunions, or neuropathy as determined by errors in sensing the 10-g fiber and loss of vibratory or position sensations. We also use these findings to order custom-fitted shoes that can prevent more serious foot disease.
- Diabetic education/nutrition
  - We find the partnership with a certified diabetes care and education specialist (CDCES, previously known as a *certified diabetes educator* [CDE]) and/or nutritionist invaluable. Even among patients who feel fully informed, an *annual* visit can reinforce good behaviors, inform patients of new treatments, offer inroads to group and formal education, and occasionally assist in management of insulin doses depending on the regulations defining the scope of practice of diabetes educators.
- Cardiology
  - A routine referral to cardiology is not required despite the fact that the majority of T2DM patients will die of ASCVD. Cardiology visits are recommended in patients who plan on starting an intensive exercise program and those with traditional signs of ischemic heart disease (IHD). Keep in mind that diabetic patients are thought to manifest fewer symptoms of IHD, thus the threshold for referral and testing is arguably lower than for many other patients.

Early Detection of Complications
Although the ultimate goal of treatment is prevention of complications, a secondary aim is to find complications and treat them appropriately.

Hypertension
The definition of hypertension for diabetic patients varies between systolic values of less than 130 and 140 mm Hg. Currently, the ADA sets a threshold of less than 130/90 mm Hg for diagnosing hypertension. We recommend three measurements in a seated patient over 15 minutes and using the average of the final two values as the recorded value.

Treatment
Angiotensin-converting enzyme (ACE) inhibitors and angiotensin receptor blockers (ARBs) are usually the drugs of first choice.

Retinopathy
Ophthalmoscopic examination by primary care and diabetes specialists has poor sensitivity and is not considered part of the required examination. A dilated eye examination by a qualified eye specialist is recommended in T2DM patients every year and in T1DM patients annually after 5 years of disease.

Neuropathy
Autonomic neuropathy is common among T2DM patients and is usually first detected by the loss of R-R wave variability on a long-lead electrocardiogram (ECG). Less commonly, it can take the form of gastroparesis, alternating diarrhea and constipation, or orthostatic hypotension. Peripheral neuropathy can take the form of distal, symmetrical dysesthesias, hypesthesia, progressive loss of touch or vibration sensations, and heat-cold insensitivity. These patients are at risk of amputation, foot infection, and bony deformities (Charcot foot).

Treatment
We reserve treatment for patients in whom the symptoms interfere with sleep or daily activities because drugs relieve symptoms but do not alter the course of the disease. Treatment choices for peripheral painful neuropathy include selective serotonin reuptake inhibitors (SSRIs), gabapentin (Neurontin),[1] pregabalin (Lyrica), anticonvulsants, transcutaneous electrical nerve stimulation (TENS), and, ultimately, narcotics. Gastroparesis is treated primarily on the basis of symptoms rather than studies of timed gastric emptying. Small, frequent meals and a vegetarian diet are better tolerated, and there has been some success with erythromycin,[1] metoclopramide (Reglan), or linaclotide (Linzess)[1] to stimulate motility.

Foot Disease
Guidelines suggest a thorough annual foot examination. We include pulses, an estimation of capillary refill, and a 10-point (5 points each foot) 10-g fiber test. Vibration sensitivity using a tuning fork is very hard to judge, although it can be included in the examination, especially if using a 256-cps fork. Patients at risk should be instructed to do a daily foot examination, using a mirror to examine the plantar surface, and should promptly report early signs of infection, sores, or deformities.

Treatment
Prevention is preferable to treatment. Custom shoes should be prescribed to patients with deformities, poor circulation, or neuropathy. Referral to podiatry is needed.

Dyslipidemia/Hyperlipidemia
The development and progression of atherosclerotic cardiovascular disease (ASCVD) is the culprit disease process for the leading cause of morbidity in the United States. For patients with diabetes, the atherosclerotic process is accelerated and morbidity from major adverse cardiovascular events (MACE) is more than double that of the general population without diabetes. The driver of the atherosclerotic process is retention of apolipoprotein B (Apo B) containing lipoproteins in the sub-endothelial space. This drives foam cell development and plaque progression. Therefore, the management of dyslipidemia in the patient with diabetes is of paramount importance.

---

[1] Not FDA approved for this indication.

Pharmacologic intervention for dyslipidemia has progressed substantially, with multiple novel agents coming to market in recent years. While the statin class of medications are the foundational intervention for managing dyslipidemia in diabetes, there are new medications with novel mechanisms that can aid in management. These include the PCSK-9 inhibitors, ezetimibe (Zetia), bempedoic acid (Zetia), and eicosapentaenoic acid ethyl ester (icosapent ethyl [Vascepa]). The impact of newer medications such as inclisiran (Leqvio) remains to be seen.

Overall, the management of lipoproteins in patients with diabetes is key to improving cardiovascular outcomes, and we now have exciting new therapy to help get patients to their goals. Primary prevention utilizing statins should be given to diabetic patients 40-75 years of age. The goal is to reduce LDL by 50% or reaching 70 mg/dl or less. High-intensity statin therapy is recommended for all people with diabetes and ASCVD to target an LDL cholesterol reduction of ≥50% from baseline and an LDL cholesterol goal of <55 mg/dL. Addition of ezetimibe or a PCSK9 inhibitor is recommended if this goal is not achieved on maximum tolerated statin therapy.

Hypertriglyceridemia (and low HDL) are common in diabetes and there is uncertainty about when to treat and if so, with what. When serum triglycerides exceed ~1000 mg/dl, avoidance of pancreatitis is justified by quickly instituting glycemic control, applying short-term starvation, using potent statins (rosuvastatin [Crestor])[1] and fibric acid derivatives. Therapies specifically targeting lower levels of triglycerides in diabetes have not consistently shown cardiovascular benefit (apart from eicosopentanoic acid through the REDUCE-IT Trial). Curiously, fibric acid derivatives, specifically fenofibrate (Tricor, Fenoglide, Trilipix), have significant positive impact on *microvascular* diabetic complications. The fundamental approach to diabetic hypertriglyceridemia is to improve glycemic control which in turn reduces TG production, hastens removal of VLDL, the major TG-containing lipoprotein.

Treatment

Diet and drug treatment follow AHA guidelines. Diabetic dyslipidemia (low HDL, elevated TG) is responsive to improved glycemic control and weight loss. We generally reserve the use of fibrates to those in whom TGs exceed 400 mg/dL. The more potent statins (rosuvastatin [Crestor], atorvastatin [Lipitor]) are favored in patients with hypertriglyceridemia.

Depression

The prevalence of depression among diabetic patients is thought to triple that of the general population. We screen every patient on every visit with a modified Patient Health Questionnaire-9 (PHQ-9). Depression is correlated with poor diabetic control, and ameliorating depression with medication or therapy is associated with an improvement in glycemic control. It has been argued that depression may be both a cause of poor control and a result of it.

Treatment

Ideally, we prefer to combine antidepressant medications with sessions with a skilled therapist. Group diabetic visits have been shown to be helpful and efficient.

Nephropathy

Diabetes is still the most common cause of renal failure in the United States, and it may be largely preventable by tight glycemic control and attainment of normal blood pressure. Screening should include a yearly spot urine test for microalbumin/creatinine. We consider any value above 30 mcg/mg creatine indicative of nephropathy, even in the context of a normal glomerular filtration rate (GFR). Mineralocorticoids (finerenone [Kerendia], possibly eplenerone [Inspra][1]) can be added for additional cardiorenal protection.

Treatment

The presence of microalbuminuria should trigger the prescription of an ACE inhibitor or ARB regardless of the presence of hypertension. These drugs, among others, have been shown to delay end-stage renal disease (ESRD) and slow the decrease in GFR. Sodium-glucose cotransporter 2 (SGLT2) inhibitors are also now recognized to have a benefit in stabilizing or delaying diabetic renal disease. We also carefully follow GFR and refer to nephrology when there is any rapid or otherwise unexplained increase in serum creatinine or a decrease in adjusted GFR to 30 mL/min or less.

Fatty Liver Disease (NASH, NAFLD)

It is estimated that about 60% of patients with T2DM have fatty livers or NAFLD, steatosis unrelated to causes other than the metabolic disturbances of T2DM. Seventeen percent of the T2DM patients will progress to liver fibrosis, a potent risk factor for hepatocellular carcinoma (HCC). HCC is at least two to three times more prevalent among diabetic patients than in the general population. NAFLD is now the leading cause of cryptogenic cirrhosis. Diagnosis of NAFLD is suspected by the presence of elevated serum transaminases, and suspicion is further raised by using one of several scoring systems (FIB4, NAFLD, or *Hepcalc,* a smartphone app) and ordering physiologic tests that measure loss of liver elasticity, such as the Fibroscan. We therefore include a platelet count in our routine annual laboratory tests to calculate the NAFLD or FIB4 and use an *indeterminate* or *likely* score as the basis for referral to hepatology.

Treatment

Weight loss, improved metabolic control, and many diabetic medications such as pioglitazone (Actos),[1] the glucagon-like peptide 1 (GLP-1) receptor agonists, SGLT2 inhibitors, DPP4 inhibitors, and metformin[1] may offer some benefit.

Hypoglycemic Unawareness

It is estimated that about 10% of deaths in T1DM are related to hypoglycemia. A small subgroup of patients loses the adrenergic response to hypoglycemia (usually a blood glucose <60 mg/dL) and are at risk for catastrophic events such as automobile accidents, neurologic decline, and trauma. Such patients must have flexible, elevated glycemic goals. Beta blockers may contribute to the risk, and alternative drugs should be considered in such patients.

Treatment

Later in this chapter we discuss the use of glucagon (GlucaGen, Gvoke, Baqsimi) and the "rule of 15" in the treatment of various degrees of low blood sugar. These patients may derive many benefits from continuous glucose monitoring, especially with devices that have audible alarms when blood sugar trends down sharply. Cognitive behavioral therapy designed to teach at-risk patients to detect early clues to hypoglycemia reduces the frequency of hypoglycemic events. Some studies suggest that adrenergic symptoms reappear in some patients after increasing glycemic goals for a few months.

Erectile and Sexual Dysfunction

Erectile dysfunction (ED) is common among diabetic men, and the clinician should not hesitate to ask if it is a problem during a visit. Surprisingly, unlike other complications, it is not clear if better glycemic control delays or prevents ED. It is also unknown if diabetic women suffer from sexual dysfunction, although some claim that dryness on arousal is more common.

Treatment

Many men respond to tadalafil (Cialis) or sildenafil (Viagra), both of which are now available in generic form. When this fails, we

---

[1] Not FDA approved for this indication.

refer to an experienced urologist who can consider intrapenile injections and prosthetic devices.

Lifestyle

BMI should be calculated at least annually, although it is useful to do at each visit. This can be calculated as weight in kg divided by height in meters squared (kg/m^2) or electronically in the electronic medical record (EMR) or online calculator. BMI should be classified as underweight (<18.5 kg/m^2), normal (18.5 to 24.9 kg/m^2), overweight (25 to 29.9 kg/m^2), or obese (>30 kg/m^2). In general, higher BMIs increase the risk of all-cause mortality and CVD and reduce quality of life. Weight-loss goals and intervention strategies should then be discussed (see Table 1).

Diet

A variety of eating patterns are acceptable for management of T2DM. There is no one preferred eating plan, as it should be individualized for each person. Referral to a registered dietitian nutritionist (RD/RDN) is recommended for all people with diabetes, prediabetes, and GDM to educate and help plan a diet with specific caloric and metabolic goals. Patients with diabetes should have medical nutrition therapy (MNT) with an RD/RDN at the time of diagnosis and as needed throughout their lives.

Reduced overall carbohydrate intake and emphasis on carbohydrates that are high in fiber and minimally processed are recommended. An eating plan emphasizing monounsaturated and polyunsaturated fats and fewer processed foods (Mediterranean-style diet) has been shown to improve glucose metabolism and lower CVD risk. In reality, a diet that is lower in calories and that the patient enjoys enough to continue can cause weight loss.

Exercise

As mentioned previously, 150 minutes per week of moderate to vigorous-intensity exercise improves insulin sensitivity, has been shown to reduce body fat, and is recommended for most patients with T1DM or T2DM. Ideally, this activity is spread over at least 3 days, with no more than 2 days in a row without exercise. Prolonged sitting has negative effects on postprandial blood glucose levels and should be avoided. People with T2DM should decrease the amount of time sitting and other sedentary behaviors. For sedentary activity lasting 30 minutes or longer, a 3-minute (minimum) break of walking, stretching, or isometric exercise is encouraged for improved glycemic control. Resistance training should be done two to three times per week for improved strength as well as improved glycemic control. Even light activities such as housework, gardening, parking farther away, and taking the stairs all have a beneficial impact on weight and blood glucose values. If your patients do not like to "exercise," encourage an increase in normal physical activities.

Weight Loss

Treatment of obesity can delay or prevent the development of T2DM and can be very helpful in the treatment of T2DM. Behavioral therapy, including diet and physical activity, to achieve and maintain weight loss of 5% or more is recommended for patients with T2DM who are obese or overweight. Behavioral therapy should include frequent follow-up with a focus on behavioral strategies, diet changes, and physical activity. For many patients, a calorie deficit of 500 to 750 kcal/day will help achieve this goal. This allows for approximately 1200 to 1500 kcal/day for women and 1500 to 1800 kcal/day for men, although this depends on baseline body weight. Eating plans should be individualized for weight loss while still providing adequate protein, fat, and carbohydrates. Long-term weight maintenance programs are recommended for patients who have achieved their short-term weight loss goal. These programs should include a high level of self-monitoring, including habits, food choices, and portion sizes; they should also continue to encourage a high level of physical activity (at least 200 minutes/week) and at least a weekly body weight check. If a body weight check is done at home, it should be done after using the bathroom first thing in the morning for

consistency. Very-low-calorie diets (800 kcal/day or less) are an option for some people but should be short term (3 months) and prescribed by trained practitioners with close medical follow-up. These patients still need long-term comprehensive weight maintenance counseling.

Drugs That Are Associated with Weight Loss

Medications for treatment of diabetes that are associated with modest weight loss include metformin, SGLT2 inhibitors, amylin mimetics, and alpha-glucosidase inhibitors. GLP-1 receptor agonists such as semaglutide (Ozempic, Rybelsus), dulaglutide (Trulicity), liraglutide (Victoza), and exenatide (Bydureon) produce, on the average, the greatest amounts of weight loss, averaging about 1 lb per month.

Drugs That Are Weight-Neutral or Cause Weight Gain

Dipeptidyl peptidase 4 inhibitors (the "gliptins") are weight-neutral. Sulfonylureas, thiazolidinediones (TZDs), and insulin often cause weight gain, but the amount of weight gain is often overestimated, and the benefit of glucose reduction probably counterbalances the modest weight gain associated with their use.

Drugs Used Specifically for Weight Loss

The U.S. Food and Drug Administration (FDA) has approved a handful of medications to be used in conjunction with diet and exercise for short-term and long-term treatment of obesity. Most of these medications have been shown to improve glycemic control in patients with diabetes and delay progression to diabetes in those at risk. Several of the GLP-1 agonists are formulated in combination with basal insulin in a pen and can be administered in a single injection.

Several medications are FDA approved for long-term weight loss in patients with a BMI 27 kg/m^2 or greater with at least one obesity-associated comorbid condition (T2DM, dyslipidemia, or hypertension). These medications are orlistat (Alli, Xenical), phentermine and topiramate (Qsymia), bupropion and naltrexone (Contrave), liraglutide (Saxenda), and semaglutide (Wegovy). Phentermine (Adipex) is also approved for short-term weight loss. These medications can be helpful for patients in adhering to diet and lifestyle changes. The importance of this adherence cannot be overstated as patients will gain back the lost weight once the medication is stopped if they have not adopted diet and lifestyle changes to continue to promote weight loss or maintenance. Providers should be knowledgeable about the potential risks and benefits of these medications to prescribe appropriately to patients. These medications are contraindicated in women who are pregnant or trying to conceive. We urge our patients to use these in combination with a structured weight-loss program that emphasizes both short-term weight loss and maintenance.

A recent addition to potential medications for weight loss is the dual GLP-1 and glucose-dependent insulinotropic polypeptide (GIP) receptor agonist tirzepatide (Mounjaro).[1] This novel agent has demonstrated substantial and sustained weight loss in trial participants, some with a reduction of over 20% body weight after 72 weeks. However, to date it has not been approved by the FDA for weight loss.

When to Consider Bariatric Surgery

Bariatric surgery, sometimes referred to as *metabolic surgery* because of its weight-loss effects and treatment of T2DM, has been shown in some studies to provide better glycemic control and control of diabetes complications than medical treatment of T2DM. It should be recommended as an option to treat T2DM in patients with a BMI great than or equal to 40 kg/m^2 or those with a BMI 30 to 39.9 kg/m^2 with comorbidities who have tried but not achieved weight loss with other methods. Younger age, shorter duration of diabetes, better glycemic control, and nonuse of insulin are all predictors of reversal of T2DM with bariatric

---

[1] Not FDA approved for this indication.

surgery. Bariatric surgery has been thought of as a "last resort" but should really be considered earlier in the course of the disease. Randomized trials have shown diabetes remission rates of 30% to 60% following Roux-en-Y gastric bypass. However, over 5 to 10 years, diabetes recurrence rates are 35% to 50% but generally with improved glycemic control and less need for medications.

Pharmacologic Therapy

Along with lifestyle modifications, metformin remains the first-line agent for the treatment of T2DM because of its known effectiveness, lack of hypoglycemic effects, low cost, and relatively safe clinical profile. GLP-1 receptor agonists and SGLT2 inhibitors are now also considered reasonable but expensive alternatives. For patients not meeting glycemic targets with metformin alone, the ADA advises an individualized approach in selecting appropriate pharmacologic therapy and escalation of treatment to achieve glycemic goals for patients with T2DM. Many agents now offer added benefits for protection against ASCVD and progression of diabetic kidney disease (DKD) as well as additional weight-loss effects. A patient-centered approach should guide treatment, considering the potential for additional risk factor reduction, mitigating weight gain, hypoglycemia risk, cost, and patient preference (Figure 4). A1c should be checked every 3 months, with escalation of care if targets are not achieved. However, intensification

of care, including initiation of insulin, should not be delayed in patients with markedly uncontrolled glycemia.

After metformin, providers must then consider whether patients are at risk for or have established ASCVD, heart failure, or established DKD. As such, a glucagon-like protein 1 (GLP-1) receptor agonist or SGLT2 inhibitor should be second-line therapy. If a patient does not have high risk or established ASCVD, heart failure, or DKD, second-line agents should be initiated on an individualized basis, accounting for other variables such as weight reduction, hypoglycemia, and cost.

Noninsulin Agents
Metformin
Metformin is a biguanide that inhibits hepatic glycogenolysis and gluconeogenesis. It improves insulin sensitivity in muscle and fat. It can lower A1c by 1.0% to 1.5% on the average, but it occasionally can be very effective, even in new-onset patients with rather high HbA1c levels. Metformin is inexpensive with good efficacy and no risk of hypoglycemia. It is usually weight-neutral and may even provide modest weight loss. Metformin has cardiovascular benefits.

Common adverse effects include gastrointestinal upset, which can be minimized by taking metformin with a meal instead of before a meal or by using the extended-release formula. Gradual

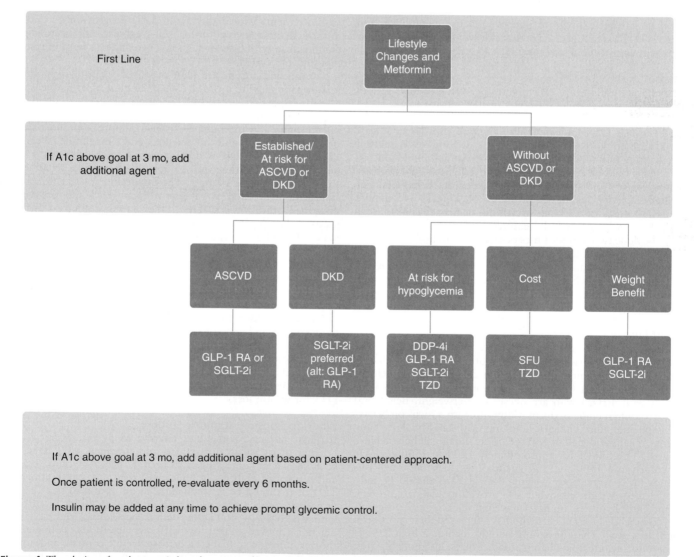

Figure 4 The choice of oral agents is based on many factors including the patient's financial resources and risk or presence of complications. In this figure, we show a decision tree based on the presence or absence of major complications. *ASCVD,* Atherosclerotic cardiovascular disease; *DPP-4i,* dipeptidyl peptidase 4 inhibitor; *DKD,* diabetic kidney disease; *GLP-1 RA,* glucagon-like peptide 1 receptor agonist; *SGLT-2i,* sodium-glucose cotransporter 2 inhibitor; *TZD,* thiazolidinedione. Modified from the ADA Standards of Medical Care in Diabetes, 2020.

titration up to full dose also reduces gastrointestinal side effects, especially when taken with meals. Metformin is associated with a reduction in vitamin B_{12} but rarely with a deficiency. Lactic acidosis is a very rare but catastrophic complication of metformin, usually occurring in patients with significant reduction in GFR.

Metformin has often been inaccurately accused of causing renal damage, and there is little to no evidence to support this belief. The FDA has approved metformin for use in patients with eGFR greater than 30 mL/min/1.73 m^2. The authors typically give a reduced dose of metformin for eGFR less than 60 mL/min/1.73 m^2. As metformin is renally cleared, it should be withheld for 48 hours after iodinated contrast administration to avoid contrast-induced nephropathy. Metformin should be avoided in unstable or hospitalized patients with acute heart failure because of the increased risk of lactic acidosis and worsened myocardial dysfunction. Metformin should be continued as long as it is tolerated and there are no contraindications, even as additional agents including insulin are added. Of note, there is probably little benefit in the use of metformin in T1DM,[1] although it may be beneficial for patients with concomitant insulin resistance caused by overweight/obesity.

Sodium-Glucose Cotransporter 2 Inhibitors

SGLT2 is expressed in the proximal renal tubule and mediates reabsorption of the majority of the glucose load filtered through the kidneys. SGLT2 inhibitors block renal glucose reabsorption, thus promoting excretion of glucose and sodium via glucosuria and lowering blood glucose levels in patients with T2DM. The glucose-lowering effects are independent of insulin, beta-cell function, and insulin sensitivity, thus offering an additional pathway for glucose regulation with low risk of hypoglycemia when used without insulin. These agents lower A1c by 0.5% to 1.0%. Although it is appealing to use these drugs among T1DM patients, the risk of normoglycemic ketoacidosis and lack of FDA approval makes this risky, in our opinion.

Several landmark trials have demonstrated a significant benefit of the SGLT2 inhibitors for both ASCVD risk and DKD. The Cardiovascular Outcome Event Trial in Type 2 Diabetes Mellitus Patients (EMPA-REG OUTCOME) was the first pivotal trial showing reduced composite outcomes for cardiovascular death, nonfatal MI, or nonfatal stroke with the use of empagliflozin (Jardiance). There was a significant relative risk reduction in rates of cardiovascular death by 38%, all-cause mortality by 32%, and hospitalization for heart failure by 35%. As a result of this trial, empagliflozin received FDA approval for reduction of cardiovascular death in adults with T2DM and CVD. The Canagliflozin Cardiovascular Assessment Study (CANVAS) demonstrated reduction in cardiovascular events, but not cardiovascular death, in patients with T2DM at high risk for CVD in the canagliflozin (Invokana) group when compared with the placebo group. Subsequently, the Evaluation of the Effects of Canagliflozin on Renal and Cardiovascular Outcomes in Participants with Diabetic Nephropathy (CREDENCE) trial showed a 30% risk reduction for composite end-stage kidney disease, doubling of serum creatinine level, or death from renal or cardiovascular causes as well as a lower risk of cardiovascular events in patients of the canagliflozin group compared with patients in the placebo group. The Dapagliflozin Effect on Cardiovascular Events randomized double-blind controlled (DECLARE-TIMI 58) trial evaluated time to first event for cardiovascular death, MI, or ischemic stroke, which was reduced in the dapagliflozin (Farxiga) arm when compared with the placebo arm. Although the mechanisms responsible for these clinical outcomes are not well-described, SGLT2-inhibitor–related natriuresis is proposed to account for a favorable effect on blood pressure, while altered myocardial metabolism and weight loss could account for additional benefits to reduction in CVD-related mortality.

Along with the cardiovascular and renal benefits of this drug class, SGLT2 inhibitors also contribute to very modest weight

loss. Unfortunately, they can be expensive, and there is a risk of hypoglycemia if used in combination with insulin or sulfonylureas. Because they are renally cleared, considerations for renal dose adjustment are required. There is also an FDA black-box warning for the risk of amputations with canagliflozin, a finding that has not been uniformly supported in subsequent studies. There is an increased risk of bone fractures with long-term use (canagliflozin), euglycemic DKA, genitourinary and other infections, volume depletion, slight elevation of LDL cholesterol, and Fournier gangrene. The marked benefit in cardiac and renal protection of these drugs must be balanced against the risks of euglycemic DKA, increased urinary tract infections (UTIs) (about 10% in women, >5% in men), and intolerance caused by dehydration. In balance, 90% to 95% of patients prescribed this class of drugs tolerate them well (see Table 2).

Glucagon-Like Peptide 1 Receptor Agonists

The GLP-1 receptor agonists are, with one exception, injectables that act through several mechanisms, including increased insulin secretion in response to hyperglycemia, reduction of gastric emptying, reduction of inappropriate glucagon secretion, and potentially slowing the loss of beta-cell function over time. On the average, they lower HbA1c by 1.0% to 1.5%. This class of medications promotes significant weight loss by enhancing a sense of early satiety and has a low risk of hypoglycemia when used as monotherapy because of its glucose-dependent mechanism of action. These agents have historically been injectable, but recently a new oral GLP-1 receptor agonist (semaglutide [Rybelsus]) was approved.

Like the SGLT2 inhibitors, this class of medications has also demonstrated significant risk reductions in ASCVD and DKD. The Liraglutide Effect and Action in Diabetes: Evaluation of Cardiovascular Outcome Results (LEADER) trial included subjects at risk for CVD and found that liraglutide significantly reduced cardiovascular death, nonfatal MI, or nonfatal stroke, as well as all-cause mortality relative to placebo. Based on the LEADER data, the FDA approved liraglutide (Victoza) for the reduction of major cardiovascular events and cardiovascular deaths in adults with T2DM and CVD. Additional studies have shown benefit of GLP-1 receptor agonists in cardiovascular outcomes. The Trial to Evaluate Cardiovascular and Other Long-Term Outcomes with Semaglutide in Subjects with T2DM (SUSTAIN-6) showed statistically significant reductions in nonfatal MI, nonfatal stroke, or cardiovascular death in the semaglutide (Ozempic) group. An additional meta-analysis of seven GLP-1 receptor agonist cardiovascular outcome trials found that this drug class reduced major adverse cardiovascular events by 12%, all-cause mortality by 12%, and hospitalization for heart failure by 9%. There was also a 17% reduction in a composite of various renal outcomes.

The most common side effects of these agents include mild injection-site reactions, abdominal cramping, and nausea and vomiting, which are typically transient and lessened by gradual dose up-titration. There is a risk of hypoglycemia if used in combination with insulin or sulfonylureas. This class of medications has been found to increase the incidence of benign and malignant C-cell tumors in rodents and is contraindicated in patients with a personal or family history of medullary thyroid carcinoma or multiple endocrine neoplasia 2A or 2B. There have also been postmarketing reports of acute pancreatitis in association with GLP-1 receptor agonists, and they should not be initiated in patients with a history of pancreatitis. Although there are reports of increased incidence of pancreatic cancers and neuroendocrine tumors, a causal relationship has not been established, and the FDA cites insufficient evidence to confirm this risk. Like the SGLT2 inhibitors, these medications may be costly, especially for patients without insurance. The drugs may be poorly tolerated in patients with gastroparesis or previous bariatric surgery. One preparation has been approved for oral use (semaglutide [Rybelsus]) but with a loss of efficacy compared with the injected compound. GLP1 receptor analogs are not labeled for use in T1DM

---

[1] Not FDA approved for this indication.

and are infrequently used to induce weight loss and possibly produce modest improvements in glycemia.

Glucose-Dependent Insulinotropic Polypeptide and Glucagon-Like Peptide-1 Receptor Agonist

Tirzepatide (Mounjaro) is a novel agent that combines both a glucose-dependent insulinotropic polypeptide (GIP) and a glucagon-like peptide-1 (GLP-1) receptor agonist as a once-weekly injection for the treatment of T2DM. The GIP is part of the incretin family of hormones. Its main role is to stimulate insulin secretion, and it also inhibits apoptosis of pancreatic beta cells and promotes proliferation. The combination of GLP-1 and GIP agonists seems to promote greater efficacy in the management of T2DM and significant weight reduction. A multicenter trial demonstrated substantial weight loss in participants over the course of 72 weeks. A 5% weight reduction was achieved by at least 85% of participants. Impressively, at least one-half of the participants achieved a weight loss of 20% body weight with higher doses. Its safety profile is comparable to the GLP-1 receptor agonist class. Tirzepatide was recently approved by the FDA for the treatment of T2DM in adults. Although currently costly, this medication is an exciting advancement in the treatment of T2DM and obesity.

Dipeptidyl Peptidase 4 Inhibitors

The dipeptidyl peptidase 4 (DPP-4) inhibitors work by inhibiting the degradation of incretin hormones (like GLP-1) and thus increasing the half-life to increase insulin secretion in a glucose-dependent manner and decrease glucagon secretion. They lower A1c by 0.5% to 1.0%. They are weight-neutral and do not contribute to hypoglycemia if used as monotherapy. This class of medications is generally well-tolerated, but a few patients complain of upper respiratory symptoms and joint pain. There is a risk of hypoglycemia if used in combination with insulin or sulfonylureas. This class can still be used in renal failure with appropriate dose adjustments. One drug in the class, linagliptin (Tradjenta), is hepatically metabolized, and no dose adjustment is needed in patients with poor renal function. Like the more potent GLP-1 receptor agonists, the DDP-4 inhibitors can be associated with pancreatitis. There is no additive benefit with a DDP-4 inhibitor with GLP-1 receptor agonist, and the combination should be avoided, with preference usually for the GLP-1 receptor agonist. A dose reduction is indicated for patients with renal impairment. Of note, the ADA suggests that DPP-4 inhibitors (except saxagliptin [Onglyza]) may be considered in patients with heart failure[1] because saxagliptin may potentially exacerbate underlying myocardial dysfunction. There is a role for these agents when there is a compelling need to minimize hypoglycemia, when weight neutrality is desired, or in case of significant renal failure.

Thiazolidinediones

TZDs are insulin sensitizers that increase insulin sensitivity in muscle and fat. Pioglitazone (Actos) and rosiglitazone (Avandia) are currently available. They are potent in lowering A1c by 1.0% to 1.5%. They are not associated with hypoglycemia. Pioglitazone may reduce CVD and triglycerides. These medications may cause weight gain in the form of both volume retention and increase in fat mass. There is an FDA black-box warning against the use of these agents in congestive heart failure. They are also associated with an increased risk of bone fractures and small relative risk of bladder cancer with long-term use (pioglitazone). Pioglitazone can also raise LDL cholesterol. There is a role for these agents when patients do not want to use an injectable medication, when cost is an issue, or when there is a need to minimize hypoglycemia. We frequently use them in the uncommon thin type 2 diabetic patient and, anecdotally, seem to have favorable results. Most clinicians avoid the use of TZDs in patients who are already taking insulin because of the risk of edema and congestive heart failure (CHF).

Secretagogues

Sulfonylureas stimulate beta-cell insulin secretion from the pancreas. They can lower HbA1c by 1.0% to 1.5%. These medications are initially effective and inexpensive. However, the authors typically do not prescribe these medications unless cost is an issue. Sulfonylureas lose their efficacy because they result in beta-cell loss over time and also cause weight gain, potentially contributing to further insulin resistance. Newer agents, such as the SGLT2 inhibitors and GLP-1 receptor agonists, preserve islet cell function, maintain their efficacy, and have shown both cardiovascular and renal protective benefits. Sulfonylureas also have a risk of hypoglycemia and should be taken with food. Caution should be used with hepatic or renal impairment.

Other Agents

Other less used agents include amylin agonists (pramlintide [Symlin]), bile acid sequestrants (cholestyramine resin [Questran],[1] colesevelam [Welchol]), and dopamine receptor agonists (bromocriptine [Cycloset]). The authors use these infrequently given their cost, modest impact on glycemia, and relative inconvenience for the patient. See Table 3 for a summary of prescribing noninsulin medications.

Insulin

Insulin is often thought of as the drug of last resort for T2DM. It has a narrow therapeutic window in that the glucose targets are near the threshold for hypoglycemia. Patients have sometimes been preconditioned with fear of insulin, having been threatened by well-intentioned providers saying, for example, "If you don't lose weight, you will need to go on insulin."

Transitioning a patient to insulin requires a fair amount of patient education, a valuable resource especially among small, isolated practices. Patients offer their own resistance seeing the cost, inconvenience, and pain. Insulin injections are sometimes seen as a mark of final deterioration in their disease and associated with catastrophic events: "My uncle lost his leg when he was put on insulin."

Arguably, insulin can be introduced at any stage of diabetes. There is some evidence that early introduction of insulin may preserve islet cell function, but long-term studies have not confirmed or rejected that concept. Conceptually, we see insulin administration as hormone replacement just as giving levothyroxine to a hypothyroid patient. We avoid using insulin as a threat, which may only increase resistance to it when it is finally needed. In practice, insulin is usually prescribed when diet and exercise, oral medications, and perhaps GLP-1 agonists have failed to achieve treatment goals. One should not delay its use when it is needed, keeping in mind the concept of *metabolic memory* discussed earlier in this chapter; the longer patients are hyperglycemic, the more likely they are to have complications in the future.

Conceptual Approach to Insulin Administration in Type 2 Diabetes Mellitus

The primary motivation for using insulin is to achieve the treatment goal. This may go beyond reaching the desired HbA1c threshold because being an average, it does not reflect glucose variability. Evolving concepts suggest that large variations in glucose, even after meals, add to the risk of complications. Thus, TIR (percentage of time that the patient has a blood sugar of 70 to 180 mg/dL) is a concept that will likely move from the domain of the specialist to internal medicine and family practice. Whether the clinician uses a basal-bolus approach (premeal short-acting insulin with a long-acting background insulin) or combinations of regular and neutral protamine Hagedorn (NPH) insulin, the intent is to mimic the postmeal excursions in insulin and to provide a constant background of insulin action. See Table 4 for a summary of insulin preparations.

---

[1] Not FDA approved for this indication.

[1] Not FDA approved for this indication.

TABLE 3 Noninsulin Treatment for Adults with Type 2 Diabetes: Factors to Consider for a Patient-Centered Approach

	EFFICACY	WEIGHT CHANGE	ASCVD BENEFIT	DKD BENEFIT	HYPOGLYCEMIA RISK	COST
Metformin	High	Neutral/modest loss	Benefit	Benefit	None	Low
SGLT2 inhibitor	High	Loss	Benefit	Benefit	Low	High
GLP1-GIP RA	High	Loss+	?	?	None	High
GLP-1 receptor agonist	High	Loss	Benefit	Benefit	Low	High
DPP-4	Low	Neutral	Neutral	Neutral	Low	High
TZD	High	Gain	Potential benefit	Neutral	None	Low
SFU	Intermediate	Gain	Neutral	Neutral	High	Low

ASCVD, Atherosclerotic cardiovascular disease; *DKD*, diabetic kidney disease; *DPP-4*, dipeptidyl peptidase 4; *GLP-1*, glucagon-like peptide 1 receptor; *SFU*, sulfonylurea; *SGLT*, sodium-glucose cotransporter 2; *TZD*, thiazolidinedione.
Modified from the ADA Standards of Medical Care in Diabetes 2021.

TABLE 4 Comparison of Various Types of Insulin

TRADE NAME	GENERIC NAME*	ONSET	PEAK	DURATION	COST
Rapid-Acting					
Admelog	Lispro	15–30 min	30–90 min	3–5 h	$$
Apidra	Glulisine	10–20 min	90–120 min	2–4 h	$$
Fiasp	Aspart + niacinamide	15–20 min	30–90 min	5 h	$$
Humalog	Lispro U100 and U200 formulations	10–20 min	60–180 min	3–5 h	$$
Lyumjev	Lispro-aabc U100 and U200 formulations	15-20 min	60 min	5 h	$$
Novolog	Aspart	10–20 min	2.5–5 h	3–5 h	$$
Short-Acting					
Humulin R, Novolin R	Regular human	16–30 min	4–8 h	4–12 h	$
Humulin R U500	Concentrated regular human	30 min	4–8 h	18–24 h	$$$$
Intermediate-Acting					
Humulin N, Novolin N	NPH (human + protamine)	1–2 h	4–12 h	14–24 h	$
Long-Acting					
Basaglar	Glargine	3–4 h	Flat	11–24 h	$$
Lantus	Glargine	3–4 h	Flat	11–24 h	$$
Levemir	Detemir	3–4 h	Flat	6–23 h	$$
Rezvoglar (Biosimilar glargine)	Glargine-aglr	3–4 h	Flat	11–24 h	$$
Semglee (Biosimilar glargine)	Glargine-yfgn	3–4 h	Flat	11–24 h	$$
Ultra–long-acting					
Toujeo (U-300)	U300 glargine		Flat	24–36 h	$$
Tresiba (U100 and U200)	Degludec		Flat	36–42 h	$$
Combinations†					
Humulin 70/30, Novolin 70/30	NPH 70%/regular 30%	30 min	50 min–2 h and 6–10 h	18–24 h	$
Novolog Mix 70/30	NPH 70%/aspart 30%	15–30 min	50 min–2 h and 6–10 h	18–24 h	$$
Humalog Mix 75/25	NPH 75%/lispro 25%	15–30 min	50 min-2 h and 6–10 h	12–24 h	$$
Humalog Mix 50/50	NPH 50%/lispro 50%	15–30 min	2–4 h and 6–10 h	12–24 h	$$

*Insulins are commonly available in 100 units/mL formulations.
†The fixed combination insulins generally have high inter- and intrapatient variability because of their reliance on NPH as a background or late-peaking insulin. With their use, the practitioner is trading convenience in exchange for flexible dosing. Despite these concerns, some studies have found using these combinations in T2DM produces acceptable control of glucose with slightly more hypoglycemia than multiple daily injections (separate dosing) of basal insulin plus short-acting premeal insulin.
NPH, Neutral protamine Hagedorn.

First Steps

The most common approach to initiation of insulin is to start with a single shot of basal insulin. A conservative approach is to start with 0.2 U/kg and to titrate the dose up until the patient is sleeping without hypoglycemia and waking up with acceptable blood glucose levels (typically 80 to 130 mg/dL). There are a variety of clinically tested titration protocols that allow the patient to adjust to basal insulin without further consulting the provider. These are called *treat-to-target* (TTT). For glargine (Lantus, Basaglar) and detemir (Levemir) insulin, we suggest adding 1 unit per day to the initiating dose until the overnight and fasting targets are reached. Similarly, if the patient experiences overnight hypoglycemia, we reduce the dose by 1 unit. When prescribing ultra–long-acting insulins such as glargine 300 U/mL (Toujeo) and degludec (Tresiba), we modify the TTT by changing the dose by 2 units at 5-day intervals because the pharmacodynamic half-lives of these preparations approach 36 to 40 hours.

Next Steps

A single dose of basal insulin can achieve an HbA1c of less than 7% in at least 50% of T2DM patients. If this target is not reached, we frequently move to a dosing scheme termed *basal-plus-one*. In this case, we add short-acting insulin before the largest meal of the day. Typically, this additional dose can be estimated by dividing the basal insulin dose by one-third and adding that amount as the plus-one premeal dose. The goal of this regimen is to achieve a blood sugar of less than 180 mg/dL 2 hours after the meal. This maneuver will bring HbA1c into the target range in about one-half of patients who fail to be well controlled on a single dose of basal insulin.

Multiple Daily Injections or Basal-Bolus Therapy

MDI is used in many T2DM patients and is the standard of care in T1DM. There are a number of approaches that can be adapted for a given patient's lifestyle and motivation. A helpful statistic is that short-acting insulin in most well-controlled insulin-using patients accounts for 40% to 60% of the total daily dose (TDD).

Fixed Dose Plus Sliding Scale

In this instance, the patient is prescribed a certain number of units of insulin before each meal and given a table to add insulin if the premeal glucose level is above a certain threshold. This might be acceptable in a patient who has regular meals or refuses to learn more complex premeal dose calculations. Endocrinologists frequently dislike the term *sliding scale* because it is often misused to justify giving no premeal insulin when the premeal glucose level is normal. Premeal insulin is given primarily to act on the content of the meal.

Small, Medium, Large

A conceptually simple approach is to assign three premeal doses based on the size of the meal or more specifically the amount of carbohydrate in the meal. Many patients learn to use this dosing scheme with reasonable results.

Carbohydrate Counting with a Correction Factor

This is the gold standard of calculating a premeal dose. It allows for the greatest meal flexibility but at the expense of learning to calculate the grams of carbohydrate in a meal and reliably testing the fingerstick blood glucose before the meal. In addition to working with a nutritionist, a good reference for the carbohydrate content of foods is *Calorie King*, as a paperback or free mobile phone app. Here are the steps needed to calculate carbohydrate ratio (grams of carbohydrate per unit of insulin) and the correction factor (how much insulin to take to correct for premeal hyperglycemia).

- **Estimate the total daily dose (TDD):** Typically, this is about twice the number of units used as basal insulin. Alternatively, a starting TDD for patients with T2DM is approximately 0.5 units/kg.
- **Estimate the carbohydrate ratio:** 500/TDD = grams of carbohydrate requiring a unit of premeal insulin
- **Estimate the correction factor:** 1600/TDD = mg/dL that blood glucose will lower with 1 unit of insulin typically given with

any elevation above 140 mg/dL. Patients will often remember this number as, for example, "1 extra unit for every ___ mg/dL above 140." The 140 mg/dL target can be adjusted up when there is concern about hypoglycemic unawareness or if overall goals are higher than the conventional standards. It can also be expressed as a simple formula:

([blood glucose before the meal] - 140) /correction factor = units needed to treat the premeal hyperglycemia

These formulas provide estimates and give the patient a starting point. Some patients find that they need different insulin dose factors at different meals. In any case, the criteria for success are that patients avoid hypoglycemia between meals and reach their glucose target before the next meal.

Other Factors Affecting Insulin Requirements
Exercise

Exercise can have a marked effect on glucose utilization and insulin sensitivity. The exercising muscle takes in glucose as needed provided that there is *some* insulin in the blood. The glucose transporter on the muscle membrane responds somewhat independently of insulin to local depletion of glucose and glycogen by accelerating glucose transport. In addition, regular exercise reduces insulin requirements both by increasing the efficiency of muscle glucose transport, improving intramuscular energy utilization, reducing insulin resistance, and increasing lean body mass/reducing body fat.

We recommend that patients reduce short-acting insulin in anticipation of exercise. Thus, for example, the premeal short-acting insulin at lunch would be reduced in anticipation of exercise before the evening meal. The amount of the reduction is variable and depends primarily on the duration and intensity of the exercise. We initially suggest decreasing the premeal insulin by one-third, but in long-duration and high-intensity exercise premeal insulin can be reduced drastically or even eliminated in some cases. Patients should have documented education on the impact of exercise on glycemia and must have a source of rapid-acting carbohydrate readily available to them. In the case of children or adolescents, this might mean educating coaches and teachers on the signs and treatment of hypoglycemia.

The window of vulnerability to exercise-induced hypoglycemia extends beyond the time of exercise. During postexercise rest, muscles may continue to take up large amounts of glucose to replete glycogen stores, and hypoglycemic episodes can occur as long as 24 hours after a bout of vigorous exercise.

Sick Days

A common and unfortunate misconception held by some patients is that they do not need insulin if they do not eat. This may be true for some T2DM patients, but many will suffer uncontrolled hyperglycemia and sometimes catastrophic metabolic dysfunction when insulin is withheld for prolonged periods. In some patients, insulin requirements increase during illness because of the stress response. Thus, insulin-using diabetic patients should increase the frequency of blood glucose monitoring, take their basal insulin, and use short-acting insulin. The following are some guidelines:

- Check blood glucose every 4 hours.
- Check urine for ketones, and report moderate or large amounts to the healthcare provider.
- If the blood glucose is less than 200 mg/dL, stay hydrated with Gatorade or a sugar-containing soda.
- If the blood glucose is over 200 mg/dL, drink plenty of sugar-free liquids. In patients who can tolerate a salt load, we recommend broth or soup in a cup (ramen noodle soup).
- Uncontrolled hyperglycemia, nausea and vomiting, or high ketones are indications to alert the provider as soon as possible.

Low Carb or Carbohydrate-free Meals

The popularity of paleo or keto diets confronts healthcare providers with the issue of insulin management with low carbohydrate intake. In most cases, premeal insulin can be reduced and occasionally eliminated based on postprandial blood sugar. We have occasionally observed insulin-using T2DM patients totally eliminate insulin use and return to near-normal glycemia with carefully monitored, hypocaloric ketotic diets.

Types of Insulin

Insulin preparations are categorized by their duration of action. This is referred to as the *pharmacodynamics* (PD) of insulin (duration of action) as opposed to the *pharmacokinetics* (PK) of insulin (circulating half-lives). The distinction between PK and PD is simply because insulin acts on membrane-bound receptors, and subsequent downstream action with most insulins is much longer than the circulating half-lives (PK). All insulins sold in the United States are synthetic, derived from genetically altered yeast or bacteria. All insulins are dosed using "units," a historically interesting measure of bioactivity that was originally derived from the amount of insulin needed to reduce glucose by about 50 mg/dL in a standard laboratory rabbit. The unit now is primarily based on weight (0.0347 mg). Because the molecular weight of some synthetic insulins differs from that of human insulin, the unit is used to ensure that there is equal potency among preparations. That is, 1 unit of any given insulin preparation will be expected to have the same impact on glucose lowering. See Table 4.

The combination insulins generally have high interpatient and intrapatient variability. Despite this, some studies show that twice- or thrice-daily use of these combinations produces acceptable control of glucose with slightly more hypoglycemia than basal insulin plus short premeal insulin.

- *Rapid-acting insulins.* These typically have a duration of action between 3 and 6 hours and are given right before or immediately after meals or used in insulin pumps. Fiasp, an ultra–short-acting aspart insulin, peaks a bit sooner than the short-acting analogues. Some evidence shows a modest decrease in postprandial hypoglycemia and decrease in postprandial glycemia compared with other short-acting analogues.
- *Short-acting insulin (human).* These are the least expensive forms of premeal insulin and are often available without prescription. The reduced cost is offset in part by inconvenience in that they should be taken 30 to 45 minutes before eating (except with premeal hypoglycemia), and they produce slightly more hypoglycemia. We consider them a good option for patients facing high drug costs.
- *Intermediate-acting insulin.* NPH is the only form of this insulin and, like regular human insulin, is much less expensive than the analogue insulins. It is amorphous and thus cloudy. Before use, it should be mixed by rolling the vial or pen rather than vigorously shaking the preparation. Although it can be an adequate lower-cost alternative to analogue insulin, it has relatively high variability in its peak and duration of action. It is associated with slightly more frequent hypoglycemia than the newer basal and ultra–long-acting forms of insulin. Although it theoretically can be given once a day, it is usually given before breakfast and a second dose before the evening meal or bedtime. It can be used in a basal-bolus fashion with one dose at bedtime and regular insulin before each meal. The tendency of an injection of NPH to peak in the afternoon/evening makes it a logical choice in the treatment of glucocorticoid-induced hyperglycemia. A 1 weekly basal insulin is under review by the FDA. An inhaled form of preprandial insulin is available (Afressa), but we do not recommend its use.
- *Basal, or ultra–long-acting, insulin.* These insulin preparations have a duration of action of nearly 24 hours or longer and are often the first insulin used in a treatment regimen. When cost is no object, they are usually the preferred basal preparations, with a few caveats.
  - Detemir (Levemir) has the shortest duration in the class and may not always fill the role as a once-a-day insulin. When used, we prefer to give it at night and sometimes will give it approximately every 12 hours to provide a constant background of insulin.
  - Glargine (Lantus, Basaglar, Toujeo, Semglee) is an acidic insulin that cannot be mixed in the same syringe with other insulins. As such, it sometimes causes minor irritation at the injection site. The primary differences between Basaglar and Lantus, on one hand, and Toujeo on the other, is the concentration of glargine. Toujeo is highly concentrated (300 U/mL), and this increases the duration of action by slowing its absorption from the injection site. Toujeo, then, has a more linear pharmacodynamic profile than its chemical twins and is a bit more forgiving in not requiring a precise dosing time. A new biosimilar insulin approved in the United States for the treatment of diabetes is Semglee (insulin glargine-yfgn). It is considered a generic drug and a more affordable long-acting insulin that is interchangeable with insulin glargine. These insulins do not provide a postmeal peak in insulin. Thus they may be best suited for patients who have some capacity to produce endogenous insulin to act on mealtime calories. Glargine insulin is advertised as a "flat insulin," but it develops peaks if the injected units exceed 0.3 U/kg. Thus it is our practice to split Lantus or Basaglar into two daily shots when the required amount of insulin exceeds approximately 50 U/day. Glargine insulin is usually given at bedtime or with the evening meal, but morning dosing is successful in some patients as well.
  - Degludec (Tresiba) has the longest duration of action of the marketed insulins and has a slight benefit in that its use is associated with a bit less hypoglycemia and more flexible dosing schedules.
- *Pumps.* These devices are infrequently used in general practice, but it is appropriate to be comfortable with suggesting their use to the suitable patients. Pumps are rarely helpful in patients who struggle with compliance and are in poor control. Broadly speaking, pumps fall into two classes: open-loop and semiautonomous pumps. Open-loop pumps must be programmed by the patient or provider to deliver basal doses of insulin as near-constant injections of small amounts of insulin and premeal insulin based on the calculation of the amount of insulin needed to treat premeal hyperglycemia and calorie/carbohydrate content of the meal. Closed-loop pumps (semi-autonomous) are paired through Bluetooth with a continuous subcutaneous glucose monitor and are programmed to vary the amount of basal insulin to maintain a tight range of near-normal glycemia between meals. The patient is still obliged to alert the pump that it is mealtime, and the patient must input the amount of anticipated carbohydrate in the meal. In practice, the pumps are fairly successful at achieving near-normal glycemia with reduced variance.

Hypoglycemia

Hypoglycemia is defined as a glucose concentration of less than 70 mg/dL and is further classified into three levels. Level 1 is a glucose value less than 70 mg/dL but greater than or equal to 54 mg/dL. Level 2 is a glucose value less than 54 mg/dL. Level 3 is any event with severe symptoms that require medical assistance for treatment. Hypoglycemia can present with both neurogenic (autonomic) and neuroglycopenic symptoms. Neurogenic symptoms include adrenergic responses such as tremor, palpitations, and/or anxiety as well as cholinergic responses such diaphoresis, hunger, and paresthesias. Conversely, neuroglycopenic symptoms are those that cause an altered sensorium such as confusion, dizziness, weakness, and drowsiness but can ultimately progress to seizures or coma with severe hypoglycemia. Neuroglycopenic symptoms typically occur with glucose values less than 54 mg/dL.

Studies have suggested significant long-term risks from frequent severe hypoglycemia, including significant cognitive impairment, falls and fractures, and increased mortality. Risk factors for hypoglycemia include advanced age, African American race, longer duration of diabetes, use of sulfonylureas and/or insulin, renal impairment, dementia, alcohol ingestion, and erratic meal timing.

Hypoglycemia is also graded as mild, moderate, or severe. *Mild* is an event in which the patient feels the symptoms and treats the low level on his or her own. *Moderate* events require assistance but do not involve unconsciousness or the need for glucagon. *Severe* hypoglycemia is defined as a seizure, obtundation, need for emergency department visit, or need to call emergency medical technicians

(EMTs). Many patients with well-controlled insulin-treated diabetes experience occasional mild hypoglycemia, and these episodes can be acceptable provided that they are not too frequent or reach moderate-to-severe levels. Moderate and severe events should be addressed with changes in the regimen and a thorough investigation as to why the event occurred, such as skipping a meal or insulin dose error.

Clinicians should be aware that patients with poorly controlled diabetes with frequent episodes of hypoglycemia can often lose their counterregulatory responses to low blood glucose and develop hypoglycemia unawareness in which blood glucose can drop significantly. Thus it is important to ask patients at which glucose threshold they begin to feel symptoms of hypoglycemia. Patients can, occasionally, regain some sensitivity to hypoglycemia by relaxing blood glucose control for several weeks.

Hypoglycemia should be treated with glucose administration if the patient is alert and able to take in food by mouth. The authors educate their patients on the "Rule of 15" for treating hypoglycemia. Patients should ingest 15 g of rapid-acting carbohydrates (such as 4 oz orange juice, 4 oz regular soda, 8 oz skim milk, 3 to 4 glucose tablets, or 15 jellybeans or hard candies) every 15 minutes until fingerstick blood glucose is greater than 70 mg/dL. For prolonged hypoglycemia, we suggest a snack with complex carbohydrates, fats, and protein. It is important to always evaluate the underlying cause of hypoglycemia and adjust the treatment regimen accordingly.

For severe hypoglycemia in which the patient needs the assistance of another person or medical professional, glucagon can be administered. Glucagon is now available in intramuscular (GlucaGen), subcutaneous (GlucaGen, Gvoke), or intranasal (Baqsimi) formulations. The authors always educate patients that use of an emergency glucagon kit warrants evaluation in the emergency department after they have taken it.

Special Populations

Adolescents and young adults with diabetes are a rapidly growing population due to the rising incidences of both type 1 and type 2 diabetes. Among all people with type 1 diabetes, this age group has the highest average HbA1c, is the most likely to experience acute complications such as diabetic ketoacidosis, and presents a unique set of challenges to care systems and providers. Adolescents and young adults with diabetes confront additional challenges as they move from pediatric to adult care and encounter gaps in insurance, pharmacy benefits, and other issues navigating within care systems. In addition, depression and/or diabetes distress are common among these patients, all of which present additional barriers to engagement with diabetes care.

Given these barriers, developing comprehensive programs to prepare and support adolescents before, during, and after their transfer to adult care, including assistance to address health systems barriers to care, is critical. Furthermore, addressing psychological concerns before or alongside glycemic control is needed to improve outcomes in this population. Planning and preparation for transfer to adult care should begin early, starting the process as early as age 14. While there is no established ideal age for transfer to adult care, we suggest a shared decision-making approach that accounts for potential life stressors, systems issues such as changes in insurance coverage, and consideration of local regulations to determine the optimal timing for transfer to adult care. Aside from discussions between patient and provider, a provider-to-provider conversation should occur prior to transfer of care to ensure key clinical details are communicated before the first visit with the new adult-based provider. Resources from the ADA, International Society of Pediatric and Adolescent Diabetes (ISPAD), and the National Alliance to Advance Adolescent Health (gottransition.org) are available to help design and plan transition programs to address the many needs of this growing and vulnerable population.

References

Agarwal R, Filippatos G, Pitt B, et al: FIDELIO-DKD and FIGARO-DKD Investigators: Cardiovascular and kidney outcomes with finerenone in patients with type 2 diabetes and chronic kidney disease: the FIDELITY pooled analysis, *Eur Heart J* 43:474–484, 2022.

Colberg SR, Sigal RJ, Yardley JE, et al: Physical activity/exercise and diabetes: a position statement of the American Diabetes Association, *Diabetes Care* 39(11):2065–2079, 2016.

David M, Nathan DM: for the DCCT/EDIC Research Group: the diabetes control and complications trial/epidemiology of diabetes interventions and complications study at 30 years: overview, *Diabetes Care* Jan 37(1):9–16, 2014, https://doi.org/10.2337/dc13-2112.

Duckworth W, Abraira C, Moritz T, et al: VADT investigators. Glucose control and vascular complications in veterans with type 2 diabetes, *N Engl J Med* 360:129–139, 2009.

El Sayed NA, Aleppo G, Aroda VR, on behalf of the American Diabetes Association, et al: Summary of revisions: standards of care in diabetes—2023, *Diabetes Care* 46(Suppl 1):S5–S9, 2023.

Evert AB, Dennison M, Gardner CD, et al: Nutrition therapy for adults with diabetes or prediabetes: a consensus report, *Diabetes Care* 42:731–754, 2019.

Gerstein HC, Miller ME, Genuth S, et al: ACCORD study group. Long-term effects of intensive glucose lowering on cardiovascular outcomes, *N Engl J Med* 364:818–828, 2011.

Grundy SM, Stone NJ, Bailey AL, et al: 2018 AHA/ACC/AACVPR/AAPA/ABC/ACPM/ADA/AGS/APhA/ASPC/NLA/PCNA guideline on the management of blood cholesterol: a report of the American College of Cardiology/American Heart Association Task Force on Clinical Practice Guidelines, *Circulation* 139(25):e1082–e1143, 2019. Erratum in: *Circulation* 18;139(25):e1182–e1186, 2019.

Heerspink HJL, Stefansson BV, Correa-Rotter R, et al: DAPA-CKD Trial Committees and Investigators: dapagliflozin in patients with chronic kidney disease, *N Engl J Med* 383:1436–1446, 2020.

Holman RR, Paul SK, Bethel MA, et al: 10-year follow-up of intensive glucose control in type 2 diabetes, *N Engl J Med* 359:1577, 2008.

Jardine MJ, Mahaffey KW, Neal B, et al: CREDENCE study investigators. The Canagliflozinand Renal Endpoints in Diabetes with Established Nephropathy Clinical Evaluation (CREDENCE) study rationale, design, and baseline characteristics, *Am J Nephrol* 46:462–472, 2017.

Jastreboff AM, Aronne LJ, Ahmad NN, et al: Tirzepatide Once Weekly for the Treatment of Obesity, *N Engl J Med*, 2022. https://doi.org/10.1056/NEJMoa2206038.

Newman CB, Blaha MJ, Boord JB, et al: Lipid management in patients with endocrine disorders: an Endocrine Society Clinical practice guideline, *J Clin Endocrinol Metab* 105(12):dgaa674, 2020. 2020. Erratum in: *J Clin Endocrinol Metab* 13;106(6):e2465, 2021.

Patel A, MacMahon S, Chalmers J, et al: ADVANCE collaborative group. intensive blood glucose control and vascular outcomes in patients with type 2 diabetes, *N Engl J Med* 358:2560–2572, 2008.

Skyler JS, Bergenstal R, Bonow RO, et al: Intensive glycemic control and the prevention of cardiovascular events: implications of the ACCORD, ADVANCE, and VA diabetes trials, *Diabetes Care* 32(1):187–192, 2009, https://doi.org/10.2337/dc08-9026.

U.S. Department of Veterans Affairs, U.S. Department of Defense: VA/DoD Clinical practice guideline for the management of type 2 diabetes mellitus in primary care, version 5.0. April 2017. Available at: https://www.healthquality.va.gov/guidelines/CD/diabetes/VADoDDMCPGFinal508.pdf.

U.S. Preventive Services Task Force: Screening for abnormal blood glucose and type 2 diabetes mellitus: U.S preventive services task force recommendation statement, *Ann Intern Med* 163(11):861–868, 2015.

Zeitler P, Arslanian S, Fu J, et al: ISPAD clinical practice consensus guidelines 2018: type 2 diabetes mellitus in youth, *Pediatr Diabetes* 19(Suppl 27):28–46, 2018. https://doi-org.proxy.kumc.edu/10.1111/pedi.12719.

DIABETIC KETOACIDOSIS

Method of
Aidar R. Gosmanov, MD, PhD, DMSc

CURRENT DIAGNOSIS

- Initial evaluation includes physical examination and comprehensive metabolic panel, serum osmolality, serum ketones and β-hydroxybutyrate, complete blood count, urinalysis, urine ketones, and arterial blood gases.
- Search for precipitating causes. Omission of insulin, underlying medical illness, cardiovascular events, gastrointestinal disorders, recent surgery, stress, medications, eating disorders, psychological stress, insulin pump malfunction, and infection are potential causes; white blood cell count greater than 25,000 suggests presence of infection.
- β-Hydroxybutyrate of 3.8 mmol/L or greater in adults indicates presence of diabetic ketoacidosis (DKA), even if serum ketones are negative.
- Patients with severe chronic kidney disease (CKD) require careful evaluation of acid-base status.

- Start intravenous fluids early before insulin therapy.
- Potassium level should be more than 3.3 mEq/L before insulin therapy is initiated. Supplement potassium intravenously if needed.
- Initiate continuous insulin infusion at 0.14 U/kg/h and measure bedside glucose every 1 h to adjust the insulin infusion rate.
- Avoid hypoglycemia during the insulin infusion by initiating dextrose-containing fluids and/or reducing the insulin infusion rate until DKA is resolved.
- Transition to subcutaneous insulin only when DKA resolution is established.

Epidemiology

There were 188,965 hospital discharges for diabetic ketoacidosis (DKA) in 2014 in the United States, compared to 140,000 in 2009 and 80,000 in 1988. The in-hospital fatality rates declined consistently from 2009 to 2014 from 1.1% to 0.4%, although mortality remains high in developing countries. In 2014, the direct and indirect annual cost of DKA hospitalization was $5.1 billion.

Risk Factors

Omission of insulin is the most common precipitant of DKA. Infections, acute medical illnesses involving the cardiovascular system (myocardial infarction, stroke) and gastrointestinal tract (bleeding, pancreatitis), diseases of the endocrine axis (acromegaly and Cushing syndrome), and stress from recent surgical procedures can contribute to the development of DKA by causing dehydration, increase in insulin counterregulatory hormones, and worsening of peripheral insulin resistance. Medications such as diuretics, β-blockers, corticosteroids, second-generation antipsychotics, and anticonvulsants can affect carbohydrate metabolism and volume status and can, therefore, precipitate DKA. Other factors that can contribute to DKA include psychological problems, eating disorders, insulin pump malfunction, lower socioeconomic status, and drug abuse. It is now recognized that new-onset type 2 diabetes mellitus can manifest with DKA. These patients are obese, mostly African American or Hispanic, and extremely insulin resistant on presentation. The use of sodium-glucose cotransporter 2 (SGLT-2) inhibitors has been implicated in the development of DKA in patients with both type 1 and type 2 diabetes. Most recently, the immune checkpoint inhibitors (ICI) used in patients with advanced malignancy can cause DKA de novo in patients without a prior history of diabetes. The DKA risk is significantly more common with use of programmed cell death protein 1 inhibitors such as nivolumab (Opdivo) compared to cytotoxic T-lymphocyte associated antigen 4 inhibitors such as ipilimumab (Yervoy). Early evidence suggests that coronavirus disease 2019 (COVID-19) infection can trigger DKA in subjects without or with prior diabetes history.

Pathophysiology

Insulin deficiency, increased insulin counterregulatory hormones (cortisol, glucagon, growth hormone, and catecholamines), and peripheral insulin resistance lead to hyperglycemia, dehydration, ketosis, and electrolyte imbalance, which underlie the pathophysiology of DKA. The hyperglycemia of DKA evolves through accelerated gluconeogenesis, glycogenolysis, and decreased glucose utilization, all due to absolute insulin deficiency. Owing to increased lipolysis and decreased lipogenesis, abundant free fatty acids are converted to ketone bodies: acetoacetate and β-hydroxybutyrate (β-OHB). Hyperglycemia-induced osmotic diuresis, if not accompanied by sufficient oral fluid intake, leads to dehydration, hyperosmolarity, electrolyte loss, and subsequent decrease in glomerular filtration.

With a decline in a renal function, glycosuria diminishes, and hyperglycemia worsens. With impaired insulin action and hyperosmolar hyperglycemia, potassium uptake by skeletal muscle is markedly diminished, which, along with hyperosmolarity-mediated efflux of potassium from cells, results in intracellular potassium depletion. Potassium is lost via osmotic diuresis, causing profound total body potassium deficiency. Therefore DKA patients can present with a broad range of serum potassium concentrations. A "normal" plasma potassium concentration still indicates that potassium stores in the body are severely diminished and the institution of insulin therapy and correction of hyperglycemia will result in hypokalemia.

On average, patients with DKA have the following deficit of water and key electrolytes: water 100 mL/kg, sodium 7 to 10 mEq/kg, potassium 3 to 5 mEq/kg, and phosphorus 1 mmol/kg.

Clinical Manifestations

Polyuria, polydipsia, weight loss, vomiting, and abdominal pain usually are present in patients with DKA. Abdominal pain can be closely associated with acidosis and resolves with treatment. Physical examination findings such as hypotension, tachycardia, poor skin turgor, and weakness support the clinical diagnosis of dehydration in DKA. Mental status changes can occur in DKA and are likely related to the degree of acidosis and hyperosmolarity. A search for symptoms of precipitating causes such as infection, vascular events, or existing drug abuse should be initiated in the emergency department. Patients with hyperglycemic crises can be hypothermic because of peripheral vasodilation and decreased utilization of metabolic substrates.

Diagnosis

Diagnostic criteria for DKA include blood glucose higher than 250 mg/dL, arterial pH 7.30 or less, bicarbonate level 18 mEq/L or less, and adjusted for albumin anion gap greater than 10 to 12. Therefore initial laboratory evaluation should include a comprehensive metabolic panel and arterial blood gases. Positive serum and urine ketones can further support the diagnosis of DKA but are not required. In early DKA, acetoacetate concentration is low, but it is a major substrate for ketone measurement by many laboratories; therefore ketone measurement in serum by usual laboratory techniques has a high specificity but low sensitivity for the diagnosis of DKA. Conversely, β-OHB is an early and abundant ketoacid that can first signal development of DKA, but its measurement requires the use of a specific assay that is different from ketone measurement. β-OHB of 3.8 mmol/L or higher was shown to be highly sensitive and specific for DKA diagnosis.

In patients with chronic kidney disease stage 4 or 5, the diagnosis of DKA is challenging because of the presence of chronic metabolic acidosis and the possibility of mixed acid-base disorders on presentation with DKA. An anion gap greater than 20 supports the diagnosis of DKA in such patients.

Differential Diagnosis

Hyperglycemic hyperosmolar state is usually not associated with ketosis, but mixed hyperglycemic hyperosmolar state and DKA can occur. Clinical scenarios that may be accompanied by acidosis are described in Table 1. Pregnancy, starvation, and alcoholic ketoacidosis are not characterized by hyperglycemia greater than 250 mg/dL. With hypotension or a history of metformin (Glucophage) use, lactic acidosis should be suspected. Ingestion of methanol, isopropyl alcohol, and paraldehyde[2] can also alter the anion gap and/or osmolality but are not associated with hyperglycemia.

Treatment

The therapeutic goals of management include optimization of volume status, hyperglycemia and ketoacidosis, electrolyte abnormalities, and potential precipitating factors. DKA management workflow is presented in Figure 1. The efficiency of

---

[2]Not available in the United States.

TABLE 1 Laboratory Evaluation of Metabolic Causes of Acidosis

LAB VALUE	DKA	STARVATION KETOSIS	LACTIC ACIDOSIS	UREMIC ACIDOSIS	ALCOHOL KETOSIS	SALICYLATE POISONING	METHANOL OR ETHYLENE GLYCOL POISONING
pH	↓	Normal	↓	Mild ↓	↑↓	↑↓*	↓
Plasma glucose	↑	Normal	Normal	Normal	↓ or normal	Normal or ↓	Normal
Plasma ketones†	↑↑	Slight ↑	Normal	Normal	↑	Normal	Normal
Anion gap	↑	Slight ↑	↑	Slight ↑	↑	↑	↑
Osmolality	↑	Normal	Normal	↑ or normal	Normal	Normal	↑↑
Other	—	—	Lactate ↑	BUN ↑	—	Serum level +	Serum level +

*Respiratory alkalosis or metabolic acidosis.
†Acetest and Ketostix (Bayer, Leverkusen, Germany) measure acetoacetic acid only; thus, misleadingly low values may be obtained because the majority of "ketone bodies" are β-hydroxybutyrate.
BUN, Blood urea nitrogen; *DKA*, diabetic ketoacidosis.

early DKA therapy can be improved by clustering key diagnostic and therapeutic steps in one protocol that is easy to understand by both nursing staff and physicians. Table 2 provides one example of such a DKA care bundle. Given the complexity of the condition management, provision of a single care bundle/order set allows the fundamentals of DKA treatment to be delivered safely and efficiently while giving the providers guidance on tackling unanticipated issues during DKA care. Special considerations should be given to patients with congestive heart failure and chronic kidney disease (CKD). These patients tend to retain fluids; therefore caution should be exercised during volume resuscitation in these patient groups.

Bicarbonate therapy is not indicated in mild and moderate forms of DKA because metabolic acidosis should correct with insulin therapy. The use of bicarbonate in severe DKA is controversial owing to a lack of prospective randomized studies. It is thought that the administration of bicarbonate actually results in peripheral hypoxemia, worsened hypokalemia, paradoxical central nervous system acidosis, cerebral edema in children and young adults, and an increase in intracellular acidosis. Because severe acidosis is associated with worse clinical outcomes and can lead to an impairment in sensorium and a deterioration of myocardial contractility, bicarbonate therapy may be indicated if the pH is 6.9 or less. Therefore the infusion of 100 mmol (2 ampoules) of bicarbonate in 400 mL of sterile water mixed with 20 mEq potassium chloride over 2 hours and repeating the infusion until the pH is greater than 7.0 can be recommended pending the results of prospective trials.

A whole-body phosphate deficit in DKA can average 1 mmol/kg. Insulin therapy during DKA will further lower serum phosphate concentration. Prospective randomized studies have failed to show any beneficial effect of phosphate replacement on the clinical outcome in DKA. However, a careful phosphate replacement is sometimes indicated in patients with serum phosphate concentration less than 1.0 mg/dL and in those with cardiac dysfunction, anemia, or respiratory depression who have a serum phosphate level between 1.0 and 2.0 mg/dL. An initial replacement strategy may include infusion of potassium phosphate at the rate of 0.1 to 0.2 mmol/kg over 6 hours, depending on the degree of phosphate deficit (1 mL potassium phosphate solution for intravenous use contains 3 mmol phosphorous and 4.4 mEq potassium). Overzealous phosphate replacement can result in hypocalcemia; therefore close monitoring of phosphorous and calcium levels is recommended. Patients who have renal insufficiency or hypocalcemia might need less-aggressive phosphate replacement.

When DKA is resolved, and independent of the patient's ability to tolerate oral intake, transition to subcutaneous insulin must be initiated. Patients are given intermediate neutral protamine Hagedorn (NPH) or long-acting insulin (detemir [Levemir], glargine [Lantus]) 2 hours before termination of intravenous insulin to allow sufficient time for the injected insulin to start working (Table 3). Once the patient can eat, we recommend the addition of short- or rapid-acting insulin for prandial glycemic coverage (see Table 3). This is the basal-bolus insulin regimen and provides physiologic replacement of insulin. It is common to see transition from intravenous to subcutaneous insulin using sliding-scale insulin only. This strategy as a sole approach should be discouraged because it cannot provide the necessary insulin requirement in patients recovering from hyperglycemic crisis and beta-cell failure.

If the patient used insulin prior to admission, the same dosage can be restarted in the hospital. Insulin-naïve patients require insulin at a total dose of 0.5 to 0.8 U/kg/day divided as 50% basal insulin and 50% as prandial insulin before each meal. Initially, after DKA resolution and given the possibility of fluctuating oral intake, the use of once-daily long-acting insulin such as glargine or detemir to provide basal insulin coverage is encouraged. Long-acting insulin glargine U300 (Toujeo) and insulin degludec (Tresiba), which were approved by the FDA in 2015, as well as biosimilar insulin glargine (Basaglar), which was approved in 2016, have not been studied in hospitalized patients treated for DKA and, therefore, cannot be recommended for subcutaneous administration immediately following DKA resolution. For patients who are not able to adhere to or afford multiple daily insulin injections, conversion of inpatient basal-bolus insulin regimen before discharge to split-mix insulin preparation (Humulin 70/30, Novolin 70/30, Humalog mix 75/25, Novolog mix 70/30) twice a day that contains a mixture of intermediate-acting insulin NPH and short-acting insulin formulations such as regular (Humulin R, Novolin R), aspart (Novolog), or lispro (Humalog) can be considered. Finger-stick glucose measurements before each meal and at night should be taken after discontinuation of intravenous insulin to correct for possible fluctuations in insulin needs while in the hospital.

Monitoring

Serial measurements—every 2 to 4 hours—of metabolic parameters are required to monitor therapy and then confirm the resolution of DKA. DKA is considered resolved when plasma glucose is less than 200 to 250 mg/dL, serum bicarbonate concentration

Figure 1 Diabetic ketoacidosis management protocol. *BG,* Blood glucose.

is 15 mEq/L or higher, venous blood pH is greater than 7.3, and anion gap 12 or less. In general, resolution of hyperglycemia, normalization of bicarbonate level, and closure of the anion gap is sufficient to stop insulin infusion. The anion gap is calculated by subtracting the sum of Cl^- and HCO_3^+ from measured (not corrected) Na^+ concentration and can improve even before the restoration of serum bicarbonate owing to hyperchloremia from normal saline infusion. Venous pH is adequate for assessing the degree of acidosis, with consideration that it is 0.02 to 0.03 lower than arterial blood. If plasma glucose is less than 200 mg/dL but bicarbonate and pH are not normalized, insulin infusion must be continued, and dextrose-containing intravenous fluids started. The latter approach will continue to suppress ketogenesis and prevent hypoglycemia.

Complications
Hypoglycemia is the most common complication and can be prevented by the timely adjustment of insulin dosage and frequent monitoring of blood glucose levels. Hypoglycemia is defined as any blood glucose level below 70 mg/dL. If DKA is not resolved and blood glucose level is below 200 to 250 mg/dL, decreases in insulin infusion rate and/or addition of 5% or 10% dextrose to current intravenous fluids may be implemented (see Figure 1). For patients in whom DKA is resolved, strategies to manage hypoglycemia depend on whether the patient is able to eat or not. For patients who are able to drink or eat, ingestion of 15 to 20 g of carbohydrates—for example, four glucose tablets or 6 oz orange or apple juice or "regular" soft drink—is advised. In patients who are allowed nothing by mouth, are unable to swallow, or have an altered level of consciousness, administer 25 mL 50% dextrose IV or give 1 mg glucagon IM if no IV access is present. Blood glucose should be rechecked in 15

minutes; only if the glucose level is less than 80 mg/dL should these steps be repeated.

Non–anion-gap hyperchloremic acidosis occurs from urinary loss of ketoanions, which are needed for bicarbonate regeneration, and preferential reabsorption of chloride in proximal renal tubules secondary to intensive administration of chloride-containing fluids and low plasma bicarbonate. The acidosis usually resolves and should not affect the treatment course. Cerebral edema has been reported in young adult patients. This condition is manifested by the appearance of headache, lethargy, papillary changes, or seizures. Mortality is up to 70%. Mannitol (Osmitrol) infusion and mechanical ventilation should be used to treat this condition. Rhabdomyolysis is another possible complication resulting from hyperosmolality and hypoperfusion. Pulmonary edema can develop from excessive fluid replacement in patients with CKD or congestive heart failure.

Prevention
Discharge planning should include diabetes education, selection of an appropriate insulin regimen that the patient can understand and afford, and preparation of set of supplies for the initial insulin administration at home. Many cases of DKA can be prevented by better access to medical care, proper education, and effective communication with a healthcare provider during an intercurrent illness.

Sick-day management should be reviewed periodically with all patients. It should include specific information on when to contact the healthcare provider, blood glucose goals and the use of supplemental short- or rapid-acting insulin during illness, insulin use during fever and infection, and initiation of an easily digestible liquid diet containing carbohydrates and

Diabetic Ketoacidosis

TABLE 2 Diabetic Ketoacidosis Order Set

Allergies: □ NKDA or □ **Other (specify):**

Baseline Labs:
□ CBC w/ Diff, CMP, Magnesium, Phosphorus, ABG, Serum Ketones, Fingerstick Blood Glucose, Hemoglobin A1c
□ Urinalysis □ Troponins q6h ×3 □ β-hydroxybutyrate □ Other (specify):

Follow-up Labs:
□ Fingerstick Blood Glucose q1h □ BMP, Magnesium, Phosphorus q2h □ VBG q____h
□ BMP, Magnesium, Phosphorus q4h □ Other (specify):

Consults: □ Endocrinology □ Diabetes Education

Nursing: □ Strict I + O

PHASE I: INITIAL MANAGEMENT

Initial Potassium Replacement for baseline potassium <3.3mmol/L
□ Potassium Chloride_____mEq IVPB (infuse at 10mEq/h)

Initial Fluid Replacement
□ 2 L bolus 0.9% NaCl at 500 mL/h OR □_____L bolus 0.9%NaCl at_____mL/h (specify)

Insulin Therapy:
Do NOT start insulin infusion until K+ > 3.3 mmol/L
□ Regular Human Insulin Continuous Infusion: (specify below)
□ 0.14 units/kg/h (_____units/h)
□ 0.05 units/kg/h (_____units/h) (if end-stage renal disease)

PHASE 2: USE UNTIL BLOOD GLUCOSE <250 mg/dL for the FIRST TIME during insulin therapy

BLOOD GLUCOSE (MG/DL)	INSULIN INFUSION RATE (ROUND UP TO NEAREST WHOLE NUMBER)	FLUID THERAPY
<100	See PHASE 3	
100–250	Decrease current infusion rate by half, MOVE to PHASE 3	D5 ½ NS + KCl 20 mEq/L at 200 mL/h
>250 AND: a) Glucose dropped by less than 50 mg/dL in 1 h b) Glucose dropped by 50–100 mg/dL in 1 h c) Glucose dropped by over 100 mg/dL in 1 h	a) Maintain current infusion rate and CALL MD for additional bolus (0.1 units/kg) b) Maintain current infusion rate c) Decrease current infusion rate by half	½ NS + KCl 20 mEq/L at 200 mL/h

PHASE 3: USE FOR ALL BLOOD GLUCOSE READINGS AFTER PHASE 2, or if blood glucose is <100 mg/dL at any time

BLOOD GLUCOSE (MG/DL)	INSULIN INFUSION RATE (ROUND UP TO NEAREST WHOLE NUMBER)	FLUID THERAPY
<70	1. HOLD insulin infusion and give 1 amp D50W IV 2. NOTIFY MD and check fingerstick blood glucose every 15 min until glucose >70, then every 1 h until glucose >100 3. RESTART insulin at half the previous rate when glucose >100	D5 ½ NS + KCl 20 mEq/L at 200 mL/h
70–100	1. HOLD insulin infusion and give ½ amp D50W IV 2. NOTIFY MD and recheck BG in 15 min 3. RESTART insulin at half the previous rate when glucose >100	D5 ½ NS + KCl 20 mEq/L at 200 mL/h
101–200	• If current rate ≥2 units/h, decrease rate by half • If current rate <2 units/h, continue current rate	D5 ½ NS + KCl 20 mEq/L at 200 mL/h
201–250	Maintain current infusion rate	D5 ½ NS + KCl 20 mEq/L at 200mL/h
> 250	Return to PHASE 2	

ABG, Arterial blood gas; *BMP*, basic metabolic profile; *CBC*, complete blood count; *CMP*, comprehensive metabolic panel; *IVPB*, intravenously per bag; *NKDA*, no known drug allergies; *VBG*, venous blood gas.

salt. Most importantly, the patient should be advised to never discontinue insulin and to seek professional advice early in the course of the illness. The patient or family member must be able to accurately measure and record insulin administered, blood glucose, and blood β-hydroxybutyrate with a point-of-care device when blood glucose is higher than 300 mg/dL. Recent studies demonstrated that β-OHB testing in outpatient setting is more effective than urine acetoacetate testing in preventing

TABLE 3	Pharmacokinetics and Pharmacodynamics of Subcutaneous Insulin Preparations			
INSULIN	**ONSET OF ACTION**	**TIME TO PEAK**	**DURATION**	**TIMING OF DOSE**
Regular (Humulin R, Novolin R)	30–60 min	2–3 h	8–10 h	30–45 min before meal
Aspart (Novolog)	5–15 min	30–90 min	4–6 h	15 min before meal
Ultra-rapid Aspart (Fiasp)	2.5 min	63 min	5–7 h	Within 0–20 min after meal start
Glulisine (Apidra)	15 min	30–90 min	5.3 h	15 min before meal
Lispro (Humalog)	5–15 min	30–90 min	4–6 h	15 min before meal
NPH (Humulin N and Novolin N)	2–4 h	4–10 h	12–18 h	Twice a day
Detemir (Levemir)	2 h	No peak	12–24 h	Once or twice a day
Glargine (Lantus)	2 h	No peak	20–24 h	Once a day
Glargine (Basaglar)	2 h	No peak	20–24 h	Once a day
Glargine U-300 (Toujeo)	6 h	No peak	24–36 h	Once a day
Degludec (Tresiba)	1 h	No peak	42 h	Once a day

DKA, which may reduce the costs of care of patients with insulin-dependent diabetes. COVID-19-positive patients with diabetes outside of a hospital environment should be particularly vigilant in monitoring home blood glucose and/or β-OHB until the resolution of infection. Most recent studies have convincingly demonstrated that the implementation of intermittently scanned continuous glucose monitoring as part of global care of a type 1 diabetes patient can significantly reduce risk of new or recurrent DKA episodes.

Because of the significant cost of repeated admissions for DKA, resources should be directed toward educating primary care providers and school personnel so that they can identify signs and symptoms of uncontrolled diabetes earlier.

References

Benoit SR, Zhang Y, Geiss LS, et al: Trends in diabetic ketoacidosis hospitalizations and in-hospital mortality--United States, 2000-2014, *MMWR Morb Mortal Wkly Rep* 67:362–365, 2018.
Cardoso L, Vicente N, Rodrigues D, et al: Controversies in the management of hyperglycaemic emergencies in adults with diabetes, *Metabolism* 68:43–54, 2017.
Desai D, Mehta D, Mathias P, et al: Health care utilization and burden of diabetic ketoacidosis in the U.S. over the past decade: a nationwide analysis, *Diabetes Care* 41:1631–1638, 2018.
Fadini GP, Bonora BM, Avogaro A: SGLT2 inhibitors and diabetic ketoacidosis: data from the FDA Adverse Event Reporting System, *Diabetologia* 65:1385–1389, 2017.
Hirsch IB: Insulin analogues, *N Engl J Med* 352:174–183, 2005.
Jeyam A, Gibb FW, McKnight JA, et al: Flash monitor initiation is associated with improvements in HbA1c levels and DKA rates among people with type 1 diabetes in Scotland: a retrospective nationwide observational study, *Diabetologia* 60(1):159–172, 2022.
Kamel KS, Halperin ML: Acid-base problems in diabetic ketoacidosis, *N Engl J Med* 372:546–554, 2015.
Kitabchi AE, Umpierrez GE, Miles JM, et al: Hyperglycemic crises in adult patients with diabetes, *Diabetes Care* 32:1335–1343, 2009.
Kitabchi AE, Umpierrez GE, Murphy MB, et al: Hyperglycemic crises in adult patients with diabetes: a consensus statement from the American Diabetes Association, *Diabetes Care* 29:2739–2748, 2006.
Li J, Wang X, Chen X, et al: COVID-19 infection may cause ketosis and ketoacidosis, *Diabetes Obes Metab* 22:1935–1941, 2020.
Sheikh-Ali M, Karon BS, Basu A, et al: Can serum beta-hydroxybutyrate be used to diagnose diabetic ketoacidosis? *Diabetes Care* 31:643–647, 2008.
Stamatouli AM, Quandt Z, Perdigoto AL, et al: Collateral damage: insulin-dependent diabetes induced with checkpoint inhibitors, *Diabetes* 67(8):1471–1480, 2018 Aug.
Tzamaloukas AH, Ing TS, Siamopoulos KC, et al: Pathophysiology and management of fluid and electrolyte disturbances in patients on chronic dialysis with severe hyperglycemia, *Semin Dial* 21:431–439, 2008.
Umpierrez GE, Smiley D, Kitabchi AE: Narrative review: ketosis-prone type 2 diabetes mellitus, *Ann Intern Med* 144:350–357, 2006.
Vellanki P, Umpierrez GE: Increasing hospitalizations for DKA: a need for prevention programs, *Diabetes Care* 41(9):1839–1841, 2018.

GENDER AFFIRMING CARE

Method of
Molly McClain, MD, MPH, MS

CURRENT DIAGNOSIS

- The diagnosis of gender dysphoria can be made by any clinician trained and licensed to manage behavioral health diagnoses. A team approach to care of gender expansive people, particularly youth, is optimal. Linking the expertise of primary care, endocrinology, nursing, and behavioral health is preferred though not always possible.
- Primary care is becoming the most appropriate and accessible venue to receive gender care, similar to endocrinologic diagnoses that are routinely addressed in the primary care setting, such as diabetes or thyroid anomalies.
- The diagnostic terminology has changed over time as the understanding of gender has evolved. Gender identity and expression is most accurately represented as a continuum. Diversity in gender is not a pathology. To reflect this, terms such as "transsexualism" or "gender identity disorder of children" are no longer used.
- The current diagnosis "gender dysphoria" is categorized in the Diagnostic and Statistical Manual of Mental Disorders (DSM-V). When the 11th revision of the International Statistical Classification of Diseases and Related Health Problems (ICD-11) is initiated, the diagnosis will become "gender incongruence," which will be categorized as a sexual health diagnosis. The significance of this shift is that there will no longer be a diagnostic requirement for significant distress or impairment related to one's gender.
- That gender diversity should require a diagnosis is up for debate. However, the World Health Organization included gender incongruence in the ICD-11 to ensure trans and nonbinary people's access to gender affirming care, as well as adequate health insurance coverage for these services.
- There are no current recommendations to screen for gender diversity in childhood or adolescence by primary care physicians or healthcare professionals. This may change given the increasing proportion of youth who identify as gender expansive, the long-term benefits of access to affirming care if desired, and the reticence that youth have in discussing gender identity with their families and providers.
- Box 1 defines commonly used terminology.

CURRENT THERAPY

- There is a paucity of data related to general health and long-term effects of hormone therapy or pubertal blockade for gender diverse people. The most commonly utilized guidelines from the World Professional Association of Transgender Health (WPATH), the Endocrine Society and the University of San Francisco (UCSF) Transgender Center of Excellence are based on available empirical evidence and clinician consensus.
- In addition to the above guidelines, general principles support the creation of an affirming environment for patients. Principles such as informed consent recognize that the medical provider is not a gatekeeper to desired therapies but is an advisor to the patient for their own decision making in the setting of limited empirical data.
- Trauma-informed care, or a healing-centered approach, is based on facilitating a safe environment where patient empowerment and dignity is supported, recognizing people's inherent strengths and capacities.
- Patient-centered care recognizes that everyone's gender journey is different, and there is no "full transition" that has a shared meaning. This requires the provider to follow the lead of the patient in terms of their personal gender goals, which may not include medications or surgery.
- As avoiding harm is an important ethical stance of medical professionals and use of accurate names and pronouns has been shown to dramatically reduce suicidal behavior, using correct names and pronouns are part of the care plan.
- Withholding of gender affirming treatments, or access to a physician who can, is not a neutral option given the well-documented evidence of depression, anxiety, substance use, and suicidality in the setting of lack of access to gender affirming medical therapies.

Epidemiology

The estimates of the number or percentage of those who are gender diverse are based on limited and incomplete data. Per the most recently updated version of the World Professional Association of Transgender Health Standards of Care Version 8 published in 2022, the best estimates or proportions of gender expansive people vary based on the study design. In health systems-based studies the estimates range from 0.02% to 0.1%, whereas in survey based studies the numbers are higher. For adults the range was 0.3% to 0.5%, and for children and adolescents the range was 2.5% to 8.4%. The higher rates in survey-based studies may be accounted for by differences of use of diagnostic codes for health systems studies compared with self-report of most surveys. The dearth of data is largely related to the lack of options to select a gender other than male and female on most surveys, census data collection tools, and health system electronic medical records. In addition, the discrimination faced by gender expansive people results in reduced disclosure of gender in settings when the option to select something other than male or female is available.

Structural Determinants of Health Outcomes

The key determinant of health for gender expansive people is gender affirmation. The depth and breadth of discrimination against gender expansive people in families, education, healthcare, housing, and employment creates severe social and economic exclusion. It is this exclusion, not any biologic determinant, that leads to poorer health outcomes compared with cisgender counterparts. An observational study with nearly 28,000 trans and nonbinary respondents found that nearly 60% reported significant rejection from family because of their gender identity or harassment so severe that almost one-sixth reported leaving school in K-12 or higher education settings. Additionally, 19% were refused medical care because of their gender, and 41% reported attempting suicide (compared with 1.6% of the general population).

On the other hand, data demonstrates that gender affirmation and social/economic inclusion dramatically improves health outcomes. Use of appropriate name and pronouns have been shown to decrease suicide attempts by 56% in one study. Access to medications that suspend puberty or initiate appropriate puberty has been shown to confer lifetime protection against suicide. Even in the face of extensive institutional discrimination, family acceptance has been shown to have the most significant protective effect against homelessness, incarceration, tobacco smoking, drug and alcohol use, anxiety, depression, and suicidal behaviors.

Experts in the neurobiology of trauma describe a lack of gender affirmation as "not being seen or heard." This involves a significantly broader conceptualization of trauma than the diagnostic criteria for posttraumatic stress disorder. Many physical and behavioral health issues that gender expansive people experience stem from chronically not being seen or heard in regard to their gender. The effects of chronic trauma, or stress, on health have been well-documented. The concept of allostatic load might explain the physiologic link between discrimination and ill-health. Short bursts of stress that cause release of cortisol, adrenaline, and other hormones responsible for the "fight or flight" response is adaptive. However chronic, repeated exposures to stress and the chronic release of cortisol is similar to long-term administration of corticosteroids; no system in the human body is left unaffected. As a result, it is common for gender expansive people and anyone who has been exposed to chronic stress to experience depression, anxiety, self-harm, suicidal ideation and attempt, and substance use in addition to autoimmune issues (including mast cell activation), autonomic nervous system dysregulation (such as postural orthostatic tachycardia syndrome), chronic pain, increased rates of metabolic disorders, and increased risk of cardiovascular concerns. Recognizing the wide-ranging effects of trauma (in addition to recognition of people's resilience) can support creation of care plans that validate people's medical concerns while also attending to the likely root cause of trauma. Behavioral health providers who are skilled in the trauma-informed model, and in the many evidence-based modalities of trauma processing, can be very helpful in the care of all people with an extensive history of discrimination and social exclusion.

Evaluation

It is important to create a clinical environment that is affirming, including intake forms with gender neutral language and inclusive options for patient gender selection. All clinic staff should be trained on the importance of correct name and pronoun use and for all clinic employees to use their own pronouns during introductions.

At the initial visit, healthcare professionals might elicit the individual's history including the patient's gender as described by the patient, their gender journey, social support, past medical/surgical/behavioral health history, family history, whether the patient is currently engaged in behavioral health counseling, and the goals of care. Goals of care might include primary care, medical therapy for pubertal suppression or hormone therapy, and/or gender confirmation surgeries. There is no single or "correct" way that people engage in their gender journey, and it is the clinician's role to follow each individual's lead and to provide support and assistance in reaching the stated goals. It is important to use the patient's name, gender (as stated by the patient), and pronouns throughout the visit and consistently in documentation. The identification statement might read "25-year-old male (designated female at birth or DFAB, he/him) here to discuss hypertension."

The diagnosis of gender dysphoria is based on Diagnostic and Statistical Manual of Mental Disorders (DSM)-5 criteria and can be made by any clinician who has been trained and licensed to diagnose and manage behavioral health diagnoses.

The diagnosis supports the consistency (lasting 6 months or greater), and insistence and persistence of one's gender being incongruous with that designated at birth. Commonly, the description of someone's gender journey elicits elements that support the diagnosis. These elements include incongruence of one's experienced gender, their primary and/or secondary sex

BOX 1 | Terminology

Sex: An assignment or designation made at birth (e.g., male, female, or intersex) typically on the basis of external genital anatomy. The appearance of external genital anatomy is the most common method of assigning sex at birth. Other attributes that contribute to sex include sex chromosomes, H-Y antigen, gonadal anatomy, sex hormone levels, and internal and external genitalia. Gender is not based on the appearance of external genitalia. Use of the term "assigned or designated male, female, or intersex at birth" is preferred to "female to male," "male to female," or "transgender man or woman" as these terms are limited to binary gender identities and are less precise. Use of "transgender man or woman" does not clearly indicate true gender nor the gender the individual was assigned at birth.

Gender identity: A person's concept of self as male, female, a blend of both, or neither. One's gender identity can be the same or different from sex assigned at birth. Gender identity results from a complex interaction of biologic traits, environmental factors, self-understanding, and cultural expectations.

Gender expression: The external presentation of one's gender, as expressed through one's name, clothing, behavior, social roles, hairstyle, or voice. This may or may not conform to socially defined behaviors and characteristics typically associated with being masculine or feminine.

Gender diverse/expansive: A term that is used to describe people with gender behaviors, appearances, or identities that do not align with the culturally expected norms assigned to their gender designated at birth. It can be considered an umbrella term for people who identify as transgender, genderqueer, gender fluid, gender creative, gender independent, or agender, as examples.

Transgender: A subset of gender diverse people whose gender identity does not align with their designated gender or sex at birth and is persistent, consistent, and insistent over time.

Cisgender: A term used to describe a person whose gender is congruent with the gender or sex they were assigned at birth.

Agender: A term that people may use when their identity does not align with gender at all.

Nonbinary/gender fluid: A term one might use to describe themselves if their gender does not align exclusively with male or female or if their gender identity is dynamic over time.

Gender affirmation or confirmation surgery: This term is used for both top and bottom surgeries for those interested in surgery as part of their gender journey.

Sexual orientation: This term describes an individual's attraction to other people or lack thereof. Sexual orientation and gender identity develop separately and they are not linked to each other. There are many terms that people of all genders use to describe their sexual orientation including asexual, pansexual, demisexual, bisexual, gay, straight, and aromantic, to name a few.

characteristics, desire to have their primary and secondary sex characteristics be more aligned with their experienced gender, and desire to treated by others as their experienced gender.

It is optimal for gender care to occur in the setting of team-based care consisting of primary care, endocrinology, nursing, behavioral health, and case management. However, expert consensus is consistent with the reality that this type of care is not always accessible. The Endocrine Society recommends that clinicians who diagnose and manage therapies for gender dysphoria be trained in use of the DSM and International Statistical Classification of Diseases and Related Health Problems (ICD), have the ability to determine capacity for consent, be knowledgeable in prescribing and monitoring hormone therapies, and stay abreast of the most current recommendations. Similar to other endocrinologic issues seen in primary care, referral to specialists may be warranted in specific cases but can in large part be addressed by primary care healthcare professionals.

Given the extensive discrimination experienced by gender diverse people, it is helpful for clinicians to have a healing-centered approach in all aspects of care. Healing-centered care orients the care process beyond the effects of trauma that people may have faced and brings focus toward their inherent strength and healing capacity. Creating a therapeutic alliance of safety and respect between the patient and healthcare professional is another foundation of healing-centered care. This concept can be helpful when considering physical examinations.

Many gender expansive people have experienced negative interactions with medical professionals, including inappropriate physical examinations that are incongruent with the presenting issue. To help people feel more comfortable, clinicians can consider making clear that the patient has the right to refuse anything that makes them uncomfortable and that the examination will be based only on the current needs for the visit. It is helpful to ask the patient "Is it ok with you if I listen to your heart and lungs?" and only proceed when consent has been given for each examination. There is little indication for genital examination at the initial visit unless the patient has a stated concern that would warrant it.

Treatment

Preventive Health

While there are very few studies that have addressed preventive health in gender expansive populations, there are general principles that can help the clinician advise the patient in their choices regarding health maintenance and preventive care. If an organ is present, follow the same guidelines as for cisgender patients and use gender affirming or gender-neutral language as much as possible.

Bone health is an important consideration for people who may be status post gonadectomy and who may have had subphysiologic levels of sex hormones secondary to pubertal suppression or initiation of hormone therapy. The recommendation for all trans and nonbinary people is to start bone density screening at age 65, and for people between 50 and 64 to be considered for bone density screening if other risk factors are present.

There are mixed data on whether people on hormone therapy are at higher risk for cardiovascular disease. Therefore screening for cardiovascular disease is the same as current recommendations for all people. When calculating the atherosclerotic cardiovascular disease (ASCVD) risk score, it may be more accurate to use the patient's predominant hormonal milieu when selecting gender on the risk calculator.

There are no data that people on hormone therapy have higher rates of any type of cancer. For cancer screenings, if an individual has a particular body part or organ and meets criteria for screening based on risk factors or symptoms, the patient should be advised on risks and benefits of that screening regardless of hormone use. For breast cancer screening, if tissue is present, the patient should be advised to follow the same guidelines used for ciswomen. Cervical cancer screening is recommended for anyone with a cervix and guidelines used for ciswomen are appropriate regardless of hormone use. Cervical anatomy changes with testosterone use lead to a 10-fold higher incidence of nonsatisfactory cytology results; therefore it is advised to always perform HPV cotesting. Self-swab for HPV alone is an alternative option that can be used by people who find cotesting unacceptable.

Sexually transmitted infection screening is the same for all people as supported by the Centers for Disease Control and Prevention and the U.S. Preventive Services Task Force. Discussion of pre- and post-exposure HIV prophylaxis should be considered for all who meet the criteria. Questions around sexual activity should be limited to the patient's concerns. It is helpful to ask, "What words do you use to describe your genitals?" before discussing anatomy or sexual practices. Attending to sexual health and satisfaction is an important part of whole person care. There is evidence that many people of all genders are reticent to discuss sexual health with clinicians. Inclusion of a question regarding sexual health in one's review of systems for all patients during all visits may facilitate comfort in discussing sexual health. For example, "Are you currently sexually active and do you have any questions or concerns?"

Hormone Therapy

Gender goals may include initiation of hormone therapy. The intent of hormone therapy is to express secondary sex characteristics and to feel more internally aligned with one's affirmed gender. Because gender is a spectrum and goals for hormone therapy might include masculinization, feminization, or nonbinary/gender-fluid goals, it is necessary to ask what an individual's gender and goals for therapy include. Although there is mixed evidence about the safety profile of exogenous hormones compared with endogenous hormones, it can be helpful to consider hormone therapy as initiation of an individual's true puberty and then a lifelong continuation of the hormonal milieu of their accurate gender.

Prior to initiation of hormone therapy, DSM criteria for gender dysphoria must be met and decisional capacity must be established. Any untreated psychiatric issues that affect someone's ability to make safe and informed decisions for themselves is a contraindication to initiation of hormone therapy. The provider should verify absence of hormone-sensitive malignancies and whether the patient has past or current medical issues that may increase the likelihood of side effects from the hormones. It is also imperative that the patient is informed that hormone therapy could irreversibly affect fertility yet does not protect against pregnancy or sexually transmitted illness.

Feminizing regimens consist of an antiandrogen (most commonly spironolactone [Aldactone][1] in the United States or GnRH agonist for suppression of all sex hormones) and bioidentical estradiol (Estrace, generic).[1] Prior to initiation, the medication's effects and possible side effects must be discussed. In addition to the likely effect on fertility, venous thromboembolic events (VTE) can occur while on estradiol, and the patient should have detailed information on signs and symptoms of both deep vein thrombosis and pulmonary embolism. Tobacco use increases this risk, and clinicians can work with their patients on tobacco cessation if indicated. Effects individuals might look forward to are softening of skin, thinning of body hair growth, fat redistribution, decreased muscle mass, decreased sperm production, decreased spontaneous erections, and breast development. Voice timbre is not typically affected by feminizing therapies. The most commonly used formulations are oral tablets (taken daily), patches (switched once or twice weekly), or injectables (once a week). Subcutaneous and intramuscular injections are equally effective. There is no evidence that any formulation has the capacity to cause more feminization than another as they are all the same medication. The effectiveness stems from the consistency of dosing and level of estradiol and testosterone in the serum. Prior to initiation of hormone therapy, baseline labs should be obtained to evaluate for preexisting issues (chemistry panel, hemoglobin A1c, liver function tests, lipid panel, vitamin D, complete blood count (CBC), and differential, and estradiol and testosterone levels). It is advised to start with a lower dose of antiandrogen and estradiol (50 mg spironolactone daily, and 2 mg PO, injectable at 2.5 mg once a week, or 0.05 mg/day once weekly or twice weekly transdermal patch). Per the Endocrine Society, follow-up should occur every 3 months during the first year of hormone therapy, with previsit labs (estradiol and testosterone levels and chemistry panel if on spironolactone). At each visit, doses of both medications can be adjusted based on patient preference and laboratory values. The final goal for estradiol serum level is between 100 to 200 pg per mL, and the goal for serum testosterone, if full suppression is desired, is below 50 ng per dL. Some patients may be interested in progesterone. There have not been high-quality studies performed on the effects of progesterone. Many people who advocate its use feel that it leads to mood stabilization and more rounded, though not larger, breasts. Bioidentical progesterone (Prometrium)[1] at 100

mg daily is a reasonable starting dose. People should be warned that it can decrease estradiol serum levels, so a 3-month follow-up with sex hormone levels may be helpful.

Masculinizing therapy consists of some formulation of testosterone only. The most commonly used formulations are injectable (subcutaneous is equally effective as intramuscular), topical gel (or compounded topicals), and patches. The possible side effects of testosterone must be discussed prior to initiation and include erythrocytosis and possible VTE secondary to chronic untreated erythrocytosis. Large population analyses have not shown increased risk of cardiovascular outcomes compared with cismales. Concern for metabolic effects should be considered but have not been consistently demonstrated in studies. The effects of masculinizing hormones include acne, increased body hair growth, male-pattern baldness, increased libido, clitoromegaly, vaginal atrophy, and more readily achievable fat loss and muscle gain. As with feminizing hormones, it is advised to start with a lower dose and increase based on laboratory values and patient preference. For optimized masculinization, the goal serum testosterone is between 400 and 1000 ng per dL. Prior to initiation of hormone therapy, baseline labs should be obtained to evaluate for preexisting medical problems (chemistry panel, hemoglobin A1c, liver function tests, lipid panel, vitamin D, CBC and differential, and estradiol and testosterone levels). A reasonable starting dose is 30 mg injectable testosterone cypionate (Depo-Testosterone)[1] once weekly. Follow-up during the first year is every 3 months with previsit testosterone, estradiol, and hematocrit/hemoglobin levels. Dose change at these visits can be guided by patient preference and serum levels. An increase or decrease by 10 mg may be a reasonable increment at each quarterly visit.

Gender expansive goals can be achieved by lower doses of hormone therapy or "microdosing." If someone is interested in nonbinary outcomes, whether subtle feminizing or masculinizing changes are desired, all of the above instructions can be applied. However, the goal serum levels differ. For nonbinary masculinization the serum level of testosterone should be as close to 400 ng/dL as possible. This is easier to achieve with either daily topical testosterone at lower doses or low doses of injectable testosterone administered twice weekly to achieve a decreased range of peak and trough levels. If people on feminizing hormones are interested in nonbinary outcomes and/or maintenance of sexual function, the serum goal for estradiol is still between 100 and 200 pg/mL, and people can choose to use an antiandrogen to achieve the desired effect. Lower doses of spironolactone may lead to decreased feminizing effect, and the patient can balance what is most affirming to them in terms of feminization and maintenance of sexual function. As long as either estradiol or testosterone is within physiologic range, bone health is maintained.

Gender Affirming/Confirmation Surgery

As with hormone therapy, not all gender expansive people are interested in gender affirming/confirmation surgeries. The term "sex reassignment surgery" is no longer favored. For those who are interested, access to procedures improves mental health outcomes. Most guidelines suggest that people who undergo gender confirmation surgery be 18 years or older and have been on affirming hormones for at least 12 months. If patients have severe dysphoria and do not meet these criteria, clinicians can still consider supporting the medical necessity of a procedure if they feel it is indicated. "Top surgery" includes chest reduction or breast augmentation. Top surgery requires a letter from a behavioral health provider to verify the diagnosis. The patient need not be engaged in therapy long term to acquire letters for surgery. "Bottom surgery" includes hysterectomy with or without oophorectomy, orchiectomy, vaginoplasty, phalloplasty, and metoidioplasty. For any procedure that may affect fertility, two letters from behavioral health providers should be completed. The choice to undergo hysterectomy is based on patient preference. There is no

[1]Not FDA approved for this indication.

[1]Not FDA approved for this indication.

evidence that hysterectomy is indicated in the setting of long-term masculinizing regimens, nor is there evidence of harms specific to people on testosterone. Those who choose to undergo hysterectomy or orchiectomy should be counseled on the need for lifelong exogenous hormones. Other procedures may include facial feminization, tracheal shave, and gluteal lift.

Insurance coverage differs by insurance carrier and state. There are some states in which the medical and surgical coverage for gender dysphoria must be supplied by insurance carriers; it is helpful for healthcare professionals to have some understanding of the legal context of the state and city they practice in for patient pursuit of surgery. It is also helpful to know what (if any) procedures are available locally and the experience that patients have with local surgeons.

Youth

Affirming care for youth includes provision of developmentally appropriate care focused on recognizing the individual's gender experience, creation of a nonjudgmental partnership with the whole family, and facilitation of discussions regarding risks and benefits of medical treatments if desired. The prevalence of youth who identify as gender diverse may be higher than that of adults. And similar to data for adults, gender expansive youth have dramatically elevated levels of depression, anxiety, disordered eating, self-harm, substance use, suicidal ideation, and attempts compared with cisgender counterparts. Gender affirmation is the key determinant of health for gender expansive youth, as it is for adults. Data has shown that while family rejection does little to change the gender identity of youth, family acceptance has the most powerful impact on decreasing the above health outcomes. The second most impactful intervention is access to medical therapy if desired. The American Academy of Pediatrics encourages families to seek gender-informed therapy and explore legitimate fears, concerns, and confusion regarding how best to support their gender diverse or gender questioning youth. The care of youth is best provided within the context of multidisciplinary care. However, this is not always available.

Providing affirming primary care and gender care during prepubertal stages of childhood is identical to care of all children with regular well-child visits and acute care visits as needed. When youth begin to experience pubertal changes, they may experience worsening dysphoria. If desired, pubertal suppression using GnRH agonist starting at Tanner stage II or III is indicated. Pubertal suppression allows for cessation of pubertal development, which can decrease dysphoria and allow for continued clarification of gender identity. While pubertal suppression is described as reversible, the long-term effects on bone health and fertility are currently unknown and families should be informed of this. The Endocrine Society guidelines and the World Professional Association for Transgender Health (WPATH) delineate adolescent eligibility for GnRH agonist treatment that can be helpful for providers to use during evaluation of patients who desire pubertal suppression. GnRH agonists can be started if the youth has demonstrated consistent gender incongruence, has decisional capacity, and has been informed of effects and side effects and options to preserve fertility. In addition, the patient and guardians must have given consent, a pediatric endocrinologist or other clinician experienced in pubertal assessment must agree with initiation of pubertal suppression, the patient must be in Tanner stage G2/B2, and there must be no medical contraindications. It is encouraged, but not necessary, for the youth to be engaged in behavioral health support. The dosing, monitoring, and laboratory schedules for safe administration of GnRH agonists can be found in the Endocrine Society Guidelines of 2017.

The timing of pubertal induction with hormone therapy while on GnRH analogs should be based on patient and family-centered circumstances. There is no empirical evidence to support a particular age of hormone therapy initiation. The recommendation of initiation at age 16 was based on the age cut-off of certain countries regarding medical decision making and is not consistent with average age of endogenous puberty. This can make the decision of when to initiate hormone therapy more complex.

Other Considerations
Voice Training

Gender diverse individuals may want speech therapy to support their gender affirmation. Masculinizing hormones affect voice tenor permanently, but feminizing regimens do little in this regard. Some speech and language pathologists are specialized in voice feminization or masculinization practices, and for those who find this prohibitively expensive (or if this service is not available locally), there are many smartphone applications that can assist people in voice training.

Fertility Counseling, Gamete Preservation, and Contraception

While pubertal suppression and hormone therapy affect fertility, there is no data regarding the specifics with which to counsel patients and families. In terms of informed consent, it is most appropriate for people to recognize that the likelihood of having biologic children is drastically reduced, if not impossible. Patients should be counseled to seek gamete preservation if desired. If biologic children are desired, it is safest to postpone initiation of all medications until gamete preservation has been completed. At the same time, none of the medications protect against pregnancy or sexually transmitted infections. Condom use is safe and effective for everyone, and for people on masculinizing hormones more acceptable forms of contraception include progesterone-only birth control pills, Nexplanon, and Mirena IUD.

Hair Removal

Hair removal from face and body may be pursued for aesthetic purposes or in preparation for surgery. It is best to suggest a hair removal specialist who provides affirming care and can offer electrolysis and laser hair removal for a tailored approach. The patient should first query their insurance carrier for possible coverage of hair removal. It is more common that insurance will cover hair removal in the setting of preoperative preparation for vaginoplasty as this is a requirement for that procedure.

Legal Considerations

Legal considerations include legal name change, change of gender and/or name on legal documents, providing letters of medical necessity for procedures, and addressing possible insurance denials of medical and/or surgical coverage. The process for legal name change, change of name and gender on birth certificates, and other state-based documents such as driver's licenses differs by state. Many states require that a medical provider write a letter demonstrating that someone meet criteria for gender dysphoria to change any legal documents, but some do not require this form of gatekeeping. Typically, if the state does require provider documentation or signatures, the format for any letter should be readily accessible and easy to create. To change federal documents, such as passports, there is a form letter that is easy to find online (https://transequality.org/know-your-rights/passports) that should be adjusted per patient and clinician as indicated, printed on letterhead, and signed in blue ink.

References

1. World Professional Association for Transgender Health. Standards of Care Version 8. Available at https://www.wpath.org/soc8/chapters. [accessed 1/27/2023].
2. Hembree WC, Cohen-Kettenis PT, Gooren L, et al: Endocrine treatment of gender-dysphoric/gender-incongruent persons: an endocrine society clinical practice guideline, *JCEM* 102:11, 2017. Available at https://academic.oup.com/jcem/article/102/11/3869/4157558. [accessed 24 February 2021].
3. USCF. Guidelines for the Primary and Gender-Affirming Care of Transgender and Gender Nonbinary People. Available at https://transcare.ucsf.edu/guidelines. [accessed 2/24/2021].
4. Rafferty J: Ensuring comprehensive care and support for transgender and gender-diverse children and adolescents, *AAP* 142:4, 2018. Available at https://pediatrics.aappublications.org/content/pediatrics/142/4/e20182162.full.pdf. [accessed 2/24/2021].
5. The Lancet. Series on Transgender Health. Available at https://www.thelancet.com/series/transgender-health. [accessed 2/24/2021].
6. National Center for Transgender Equality. U.S. Transgender Survey. Available at https://transequality.org/issues/us-trans-survey. [accessed 2/24/2021].

GOUT AND HYPERURICEMIA

Method of
Saima Chohan, MD

CURRENT DIAGNOSIS

- Gout is the most common inflammatory arthritis in men and is increasing in prevalence.
- A definitive diagnosis of gout requires the demonstration of monosodium urate crystals in synovial fluid or tophi.
- Gouty arthritis often begins in the joints of the lower extremity.
- Septic arthritis, rheumatoid arthritis, and calcium pyrophosphate disease (pseudogout) can mimic gout and should be ruled out.

CURRENT THERAPY

- The goals of successful gout treatment include terminating the acute attack, preventing intermittent attacks, and undertaking long-term therapy to avoid chronic arthritis.
- Indications for the chronic treatment of gout include frequent attacks, recurrent arthritis, and kidney disease.
- A serum urate level of less than 6.0 mg/dL is the goal when urate-lowering therapy is being used.
- Nonpharmacologic treatment includes lifestyle modification and dietary changes.
- The mainstay of urate-lowering therapies remains xanthine oxidase inhibition.

Epidemiology

Gout, or monosodium urate crystal deposition disease, is the most common inflammatory arthritis of men and is an increasingly common problem among postmenopausal women. It is a chronic disorder, affecting more than 5 million people in the United States and increasing in both prevalence and incidence, especially in persons older than 65 years. Gout is often accompanied by serious comorbid disorders (hypertension, cardiovascular disease, chronic kidney disease, and all of the component features of the metabolic syndrome) and is managed in primary care practice in about 90% of affected persons. Therefore identifying risk factors, optimizing diagnosis, and choosing the appropriate treatment for gout are important skills for a wide array of caregivers.

Pathophysiology and Risk Factors

Uric acid is the end product of purine metabolism in humans. Hyperuricemia, a serum urate concentration exceeding urate solubility (6.8 mg/dL), is an invariable accompaniment of gout, although serum uric acid levels might not be elevated during an acute attack. Hyperuricemia predisposes affected persons to urate crystal formation and deposition, leading to the inflammatory responses underlying the symptoms of gout. Thus treatment of gout is aimed at reducing and maintaining serum urate concentration at subsaturating levels, usually set at less than 6.0 mg/dL.

Hyperuricemia

Risk factors for hyperuricemia include obesity, hypertension, hyperlipidemia, insulin resistance, renal insufficiency, and the use of diuretics. Diets rich in certain foods are also associated with increased risk for gout. Many studies with large patient cohorts have demonstrated a relationship between hyperuricemia and hypertension, cardiovascular and peripheral vascular disease, chronic kidney disease, and diabetes mellitus. The association of hyperuricemia and metabolic syndrome has also been shown in children and adolescents. Interventional trials of asymptomatic patients with hyperuricemia and high cardiovascular risk must be performed before such treatment can be advocated.

Diagnosis

Acute gout is characterized by an abrupt onset of joint pain, erythema, and swelling, usually of one joint but less commonly of more than one. The arthritis most often occurs first in the joint of a lower extremity, especially the first metatarsophalangeal (MTP) joint at the base of the great toe. The predilection for this site is thought to be secondary to cooler acral temperature or repeated trauma and pressure on this joint.

The gold standard for the diagnosis of gout is the demonstration of monosodium urate crystals by polarized light microscopy either in joint fluid aspirated during an acute attack or between attacks or from material aspirated from suspected tophi. To aspirate the first MTP joint, the joint is first identified by palpating the space at the base of the metacarpal on the dorsal aspect while flexing and extending the toe. The needle is then inserted perpendicularly into the joint space to avoid the extensor hallucis tendon. Synovial fluid from affected joints should immediately be examined under polarized microscopy to confirm the diagnosis of needle-shaped crystals with negative birefringence. If polarized microscopy is unavailable, then fluid should be promptly sent in a sterile tube to an appropriate laboratory for crystal confirmation.

Unfortunately the equipment and analytical expertise necessary to make this diagnosis are not widely available to primary care physicians. As a result, the diagnosis of acute gout is commonly made on clinical grounds, using the 2015 classification criteria of the American College of Rheumatology and the European League Against Rheumatism. These diagnostic guidelines use a point system and emphasize the presence of signs of inflammation (redness, tenderness, and loss of joint function), abrupt onset, monoarticular involvement, occurrence in the first MTP joint, presence of tophi, and radiographic findings.

The initial symptoms and signs of gout often arise after many years of asymptomatic hyperuricemia. In untreated or inadequately treated patients, the course of the disease often involves acute attacks at increasing frequency, with shortening of asymptomatic periods (called intercritical gout) and, ultimately, the development of chronic joint disease (gouty arthropathy) and tophi (masses of urate crystals in a chronic inflammatory matrix) in bone, joints, skin, and even solid organs (Figure 1).

Indications for Treatment

Early in gout, patients might have attacks that are separated by years and are manageable over the course of a few days with antiinflammatory medications and adjuncts such as joint rest and the application of ice. Over time, the attacks usually become more frequent, prolonged, and disabling, eventually requiring long-term urate-lowering treatment aimed at preventing the deposition of urate crystals and eventually abolishing acute flares and resolving tophi. Indications for urate-lowering (antihyperuricemic) therapy are listed in Box 1.

Treatment

Acute Gout

Gouty arthritis occurs suddenly, and attacks are often very painful and disabling. Patients describe an acute onset of exquisite pain, swelling, erythema, and inability to bear weight on the afflicted joint. Occasionally patients have constitutional symptoms including fever and chills, with an elevated sedimentation rate and white blood cell count. To terminate an attack, nonsteroidal antiinflammatory drugs (NSAIDs), colchicine (Colcrys), or corticosteroids can be offered. If given at full anti-inflammatory dosage, NSAIDs have a rapid onset and are quite efficacious in relieving pain and shortening the duration of an attack. The utility of this class of drugs may be limited by renal insufficiency, cardiovascular risk factors, and gastrointestinal bleeding. Although indomethacin (Indocin), sulindac (Clinoril), and naproxen (Naprosyn) are all approved by the US Food and Drug Administration (FDA) for

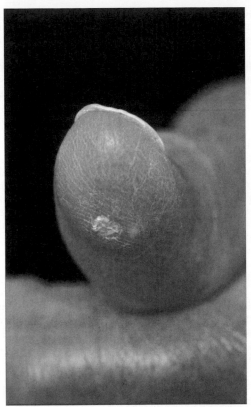

Figure 1 Intradermal urate deposit (tophus). (Reprinted with permission from Mandell BF: Gout and crystal deposition disease. In Weisman MH, Weinblatt ME, Louie JS, Van Vollenhoven R, editors: *Targeted Treatment of the Rheumatic Diseases*, Philadelphia, 2010, Saunders, pp 293–302.)

treating acute attacks of gout, nearly every drug in this class and the selective cyclooxygenase (COX) 2 inhibitors also have considerable efficacy. High-dose salicylate therapy lowers serum uric acid by interfering in renal urate transport; low-dose aspirin[1] has the opposite effect, but it is often continued in gout patients because of its overriding importance in managing coronary artery disease.

Oral colchicine has been used to treat gout for many years as an unproven drug with no FDA dosage recommendations or prescribing information. In July 2009, however, the FDA approved Colcrys, a single-ingredient colchicine product, for the first day of treatment of acute gout attacks at a low-dose regimen of 1.2 mg followed by 0.6 mg in 1 hour (total 1.8 mg). With this regimen, colchicine can be used to abort an attack if it is taken immediately after the development of the first symptom of gout flare. Higher colchicine doses (0.6 mg every hour until symptoms improve or until gastrointestinal symptoms of diarrhea, nausea, or vomiting develop for a total of 4.8 mg over 6 hours)[3] have traditionally been recommended. A randomized placebo-controlled trial comparing the low- and high-dose regimens showed both approaches to have equivalent efficacy in pain relief at 24 hours (compared with placebo). However, adverse gastrointestinal events were significantly less common with the low-dose regimen. In subjects warranting additional flare treatment, continued use of colchicine 0.6 mg twice daily (reducing to once daily as the flare subsides) is appropriate in persons with normal renal and hepatic function. Oral colchicine is now available in generic form and in two branded versions (Colcrys, Mitigare).

Gastrointestinal symptoms are generally the first clinical signs of colchicine toxicity in patients with normal renal and hepatic function. More serious toxicities do occur and include neuromyopathy, aplastic anemia, and worsening renal and hepatic function. Patients with

BOX 1   Indications for Urate-Lowering Therapy

- Frequent and disabling gouty attacks are often defined as two or three flares annually, although this is not evidence based; the decision to treat is based on both number of flares and the disability resulting from flares.
- Chronic gouty disease: clinically or radiographically evident joint erosions.
- Tophaceous deposits: subcutaneous or intraosseous.
- Gout with renal insufficiency.
- Recurrent kidney stones.
- Urate nephropathy.
- Urinary uric acid excretion exceeding 1100 mg/day (6.5 mmol), when determined in men younger than 25 years or in premenopausal women.

renal or hepatic impairment should be treated with caution; because of potentially serious drug-drug interactions, colchicine should be avoided in patients receiving cyclosporine (Neoral), clarithromycin (Biaxin), verapamil (Calan), or amlodipine (Norvasc). Intravenous colchicine is not available in Europe. The FDA has stopped the marketing of unapproved injectable colchicine products in the United States and discourages the compounding of intravenous colchicine because of reports of preparation errors causing deaths.

Corticosteroids provide a safe alternative for patients with contraindications to NSAIDs or colchicine. For isolated mono-articular attacks, especially of medium or large joints, aspiration of joint fluid and intra-articular injection with triamcinolone acetonide (Kenalog) 20 to 40 mg can quickly terminate an attack. For polyarticular attacks or attacks in smaller joints, systemic corticosteroids (oral or intramuscular) may be used. Oral prednisone starting at 20 mg twice daily with a taper over 10 to 14 days is very effective. Patients can have rebound attacks if oral steroids are terminated too quickly; thus methylprednisolone (Medrol) dose packs should be avoided. If intramuscular injection is required, a single dose of triamcinolone 40 mg may be used.

There is interest in agents blocking the action of interleukin 1 (IL-1), a cytokine thought to play a major role in initiating and sustaining acute gouty inflammation. Anakinra (Kineret)[1] and canakinumab (Ilaris) are potent injectable IL-1 inhibitors; studies are ongoing to assess the utility of these agents to mitigate acute attacks. In 2013 canakinumab became the first biologic agent approved for acute gout in Europe. It was approved by the European Medicines Agency for symptomatic treatment of adult patients with frequent gouty arthritis attacks in whom NSAIDs and colchicine are contraindicated, are not tolerated, or do not provide an adequate response and in whom repeated courses of corticosteroids are not appropriate. Rilonacept (Arcalyst),[1] which is also in this class, was declined approval for gout by the FDA in 2012 because of concerns about its long-term safety.

Intercritical Gout

After an attack subsides, management is directed at preventing recurrent attacks. During acute attacks of gout, normal serum urate concentration is reported in up to 40% of affected patients, and thus it is not an accurate reflection of the true urate pool. Confirmation of hyperuricemia is best achieved either before the resolution of an attack or 2 to 4 weeks after it to achieve an accurate serum urate concentration. There is a generalizable correlation between the serum urate level and the risk for a recurrent attack.

Prophylaxis of future attacks during early urate-lowering therapy can consist of colchicine at doses of 0.6 mg once or twice a day (based on renal function) or NSAIDs. If chronic NSAIDs are used, acid-reducing medications such as proton pump inhibitors or histamine-2 blockers may be used for patients at risk for gastrointestinal bleeding.

Long-Term Urate-Lowering (Antihyperuricemic) Therapy

The aim of urate-lowering therapy is to reduce and maintain serum urate at concentrations below those at which extracellular fluids are saturated with monosodium urate. In general an ultimate serum urate concentration of less than 6.0 mg/dL is advised. Urate lowering can be achieved either by increasing urinary excretion or decreasing production of urate.

Nonpharmacologic urate-lowering treatment begins with lifestyle changes. Diet and weight loss must be addressed. Obesity and weight gain are risk factors for gout, and weight loss has been shown to decrease the risk of gout. A purine-restricted diet has often been recommended to patients but is often unpalatable and impractical. Reduction in alcohol intake, namely beer and liquor, can effectively reduce urate levels. Similarly, a reduced intake of red meat and shellfish also lowers the risk of recurrent gouty attacks. Studies have shown an increased frequency of attacks in patients who consume fruit juices and soft drinks containing high-fructose corn syrup, an ingredient not found in diet drinks.

Once the decision is made to institute serum urate–lowering therapy, the duration of treatment is indefinite and must be long-term to be effective. The majority of patients with gout and tophaceous disease will continue to have attacks if therapy is discontinued; thus education is a key part of the treatment plan. Patients should be instructed that, with initiation of any urate-lowering therapy, they will be at increased risk for a flareup and thus must continue regular use of prophylactic agents as outlined earlier. At least 80% to 95% of cases of hyperuricemia and gout are attributable to impaired urate excretion, which is reflected in diminished urate clearance or fractional excretion of uric acid but not usually in low daily urine uric acid excretion. In practice, 24-hour urine collections are rarely performed. Patients are preferentially treated with xanthine oxidase inhibitors because of the easier dosing schedule and many patients have contraindications to uricosurics such as renal insufficiency and kidney stones.

Uricosurics

Relative to medications aimed at urate synthesis, uricosurics are relegated to second-line treatment of patients with elevated urate burden or tophaceous disease. The most commonly used uricosuric agent in the United States is probenecid. This is a very effective drug that concentrates and promotes urinary excretion of urate. Its utility is limited in patients with renal insufficiency, and probenecid is not recommended as first-line therapy in patients with nephrolithiasis or uric acid overexcretion. The maintenance dose of probenecid required to achieve and maintain serum urate concentration at less than 6.0 mg/dL is 0.5 to 3 g/day[3] administered in 2 or 3 daily doses. Once goal serum urate concentration has been achieved with a uricosuric agent, the risk of uric acid calculi is diminished because urinary uric acid excretion becomes normal.

Lesinurad (Zurampic) is another uricosuric agent; it is an inhibitor of renal transport proteins and was approved by the FDA in 2016. It is used at a dose of 200 mg/day in combination with a xanthine oxidase inhibitor, including allopurinol (Zyloprim) or febuxostat (Uloric). In 2017, the FDA approved a combination product of lesinurad 200 mg and allopurinol 300 mg (Duzallo), one tablet in the morning for hyperuricemia. This product is also available as a tablet containing lesinurad 200 mg and allopurinol 200 mg for patients with renal impairment. The drug has a boxed warning regarding the risk of acute renal failure.

Other drugs found to have uricosuric effects include fenofibrate (Tricor),[1] a fibric acid derivative used to treat hyperlipidemia, and the antihypertensives losartan (Cozaar)[1] and amlodipine (Norvasc).[1] These agents have mild uricosuric properties and may be useful adjuncts to urate-lowering therapy. The ingestion of skim milk has been shown to lower serum urate levels through uricosuric effects. Lower urate levels have also been seen in patients who consume coffee, but the mechanism of action is unknown.

Xanthine Oxidase Inhibitors

Allopurinol (Zyloprim) and febuxostat (Uloric) are the only FDA-approved xanthine oxidase inhibitors for the treatment of gout. Allopurinol, introduced in 1966, is approved in doses of 100 to 800 mg/day. More than 90% of patients with gout treated with urate-lowering medication in the United States are given allopurinol, but dosages of more than 300 mg/day are rarely employed and often patients do not achieve serum urate concentrations of 6.0 mg/dL or less. Appropriate use of allopurinol is limited for several reasons. There are genuine concerns about allopurinol drug interactions, gastrointestinal intolerance, rashes (ranging from mild to life threatening), and the rare but sometimes fatal hypersensitivity syndrome. Allopurinol should be avoided with the immunosuppressives azathioprine (Imuran) and 6-mercaptopurine (Purinethol) because it can increase the risk of bone marrow toxicity. That can occur because these medications are partially metabolized by xanthine oxidase. Allopurinol should not be taken with ampicillin owing to an increased risk of rash.

Effective dosing of allopurinol is often not achieved because of compliance with published but disputed recommendations for allopurinol dose reduction in states of renal impairment. Allopurinol should be initiated at 100 mg/day in patients with creatinine clearance of 40 mL/min or greater, and it should be titrated in 100-mg increments every 2 to 4 weeks, with the endpoint of dosing determined by achievement of serum urate concentration of 6.0 mg/dL or less.

The FDA approved febuxostat (Uloric) in 2009. Unlike allopurinol, this is a nonpurine analog and selective xanthine oxidase inhibitor that is not incorporated into purine nucleotides and does not appear to affect pyrimidine metabolism. Febuxostat is primarily metabolized by oxidation and glucuronidation in the liver, with little renal excretion; this contrasts with the renal elimination of oxypurinol, the main allopurinol metabolite. The recommended starting dose of febuxostat is 40 mg/day, with an increase to 80 mg/day if serum urate concentrations do not reach goal urate levels in 2 weeks in patients with normal renal function. In Europe, higher dosages (80–120 mg/day)[3] have received approval, and studies have affirmed the efficacy and safety of dosing in this range. In the FOCUS trial, a 5-year study of efficacy and safety, febuxostat was shown to have durable maintenance of serum urate concentration at 6.0 mg/dL or less, nearly complete elimination of gouty flares, and resolution of baseline tophi in subjects. In 2019, a boxed warning was added by the FDA as studies showed that febuxostat was associated with an increased risk of cardiovascular and all-cause mortality compared with allopurinol. Although an advantage of febuxostat over allopurinol is that it can safely be taken by patients with creatinine clearance greater than 30 mL/min, we recommend allopurinol in patients with elevated cardiovascular risk.

Pegloticase

Pegloticase (pegylated porcine recombinant uricase [Krystexxa]) was granted FDA approval in 2010 for the treatment of refractory gout. Humans lack the enzyme uricase, which converts uric acid to allantoin, a more soluble purine degradation product. Replacement of this missing enzyme allows direct conversion of urate to allantoin with eventual depletion of increased body urate pools and control of disease, including resolution of tophi. Recombinant uricase therapy profoundly lowers serum urate concentration, as was demonstrated in two large trials. Pegloticase is approved at a dosage of 8 mg IV every 2 weeks.

New Therapies

Canakinumab (Ilaris) is a monoclonal antibody that can be used for the treatment of gout flares in adults who have had an inadequate response to treatment or who cannot tolerate NSAIDs, colchicine, or corticosteroids. The dosage is 150 mg in a single subcutaneous injection. Safety concerns include a history of immunosuppression, active or underlying chronic infections such as tuberculosis, pregnancy, breastfeeding, close temporal administration of a live

---

[1]Not FDA approved for this indication.

[3]Exceeds dosage recommended by the manufacturer.

vaccine, and a risk of allergic reactions. A number of other novel agents with new therapeutic targets for the treatment of acute and chronic gout are under investigation.

References

Becker MA, Chohan S: We can make gout management more successful now, *Curr Opin Rheumatol* 20:167–172, 2008.

Dalbeth N, Stamp L: Allopurinol dosing in renal impairment: Walking the tightrope between adequate urate lowering and adverse events, *Semin Dial* 20:391–395, 2007.

Neogi T, Jansen T, Dalbeth N et al, et al: 2015 Gout Classification Criteria: An American College of Rheumatology/European League Against Rheumatism Collaborative Initiative, *Arthr Rheum* 67:2557–2568, 2015.

Schumacher HR, Becker MA, Lloyd E, et al: Febuxostat in the treatment of gout: 5-year findings of the FOCUS efficacy and safety study, *Rheumatology* 48:188–194, 2009.

Stamp L, O'Donnell JL, Zhang Met, et al: Using allopurinol above the dose based on creatinine clearance is effective and safe in patients with chronic gout, including those with renal impairment, *Arthritis Rheum* 63:412–421, 2011.

Sundy JS, Becker MA, Baraf HS, et al: Reduction of plasma urate levels following treatment with multiple doses of pegloticase (polyethylene glycol–conjugated uricase) in patients with treatment-failure gout. Results of a phase II randomized study, *Arthritis Rheum* 58:2882–2891, 2008.

Terkeltaub R, Furst DE, Bennett K, et al: High versus low dosing of oral colchicine for early acute gout flare, *Arthritis Rheum* 62:1060–1068, 2010.

Zhu Y, Pandya BJ, Choi HK: Comorbidities of gout and hyperuricemia in the US general population: NHANES 2007-2008, *Am J Med* 125:679–687, 2012.

Macdonald TM, Ford I, Nuki G, et al: Protocol of the Febuxostat versus Allopurinol Streamlined Trial (FAST): a large prospective, randomised, open, blinded endpoint study comparing the cardiovascular safety of allopurinol and febuxostat in the management of symptomatic hyperuricaemia, *BMJ Open* 4(7):e005354, 2014. Epub 2014 Jul 10.

HYPERALDOSTERONISM

Method of
Ruchi Gaba, MD; and Lawrence Chan, MD

CURRENT DIAGNOSIS

- Hyperaldosteronism may be suspected in patients with severe, resistant, or early-onset hypertension and hypertensive patients with family history, hypokalemia, adrenal mass, and obstructive sleep apnea. Evaluation begins with measurement of morning plasma aldosterone concentration (PAC in ng/dL) and plasma renin activity (PRA in ng/mL/h) in a sodium- and potassium-repleted state and off of significantly interfering medications (spironolactone [Aldactone], eplerenone [Inspra], amiloride [Midamor], triamterene [Dyrenium], potassium-wasting diuretics, and licorice-derived products[7]) for at least 4 weeks.
- Elevated PRA and PAC suggest secondary hyperaldosteronism; suppressed PRA and PAC suggest conditions mimicking hyperaldosteronism; suppressed PRA but elevated PAC suggests primary hyperaldosteronism (screening positive if PAC/PRA ratio > 20 to 40 and PAC > 5 to 10 ng/dL).
- Positive screening of primary hyperaldosteronism should be confirmed with one of the following tests: intravenous saline suppression, oral salt loading, fludrocortisone (Florinef)[1] suppression, or captopril (Capoten)[1] challenge test (may skip if spontaneous hypokalemia, renin below the detection limit, and PAC > 20 ng/dL).
- Once primary hyperaldosteronism is biochemically confirmed, computed tomography of the adrenal glands is recommended to exclude adrenocortical carcinoma and help subtype primary hyperaldosteronism.
- If surgical treatment is considered, adrenal vein sampling is indicated to differentiate unilateral versus bilateral lesions (may skip if the patient is <35 years with spontaneous hypokalemia, PAC > 30 ng/dL, and unilateral adenoma). A cortisol-corrected aldosterone ratio from the high to the low side greater than 4:1 with cosyntropin (Cortrosyn) stimulation confirms unilateral aldosterone excess.

---
[1]Not FDA approved for this indication.
[7]Available as dietary supplement.

CURRENT THERAPY

- Laparoscopic adrenalectomy is recommended for unilateral disease. Otherwise, medical treatment with a mineralocorticoid receptor antagonist (MRA; spironolactone [Aldactone] as the primary agent and eplerenone [Inspra][1] as an alternative) is recommended.
- Spironolactone: 12.5 to 25 mg/day titrated to a maximum dose of 400 mg/day to achieve normal blood pressure (BP) and normokalemia. Side effects include increased serum creatinine, hyperkalemia, gynecomastia, and menstrual irregularities.
- Eplerenone: 25 mg once or twice daily titrated to a maximum dose of 100 mg/day to achieve normal BP and normokalemia. Side effects include increased creatinine, hyperkalemia, hypertriglyceridemia, increased liver enzymes, headache, and fatigue.
- Amiloride (Midamor)[1] or triamterene (Dyrenium)[1] (epithelial sodium channel antagonists) can be used in those who cannot tolerate MRAs or are still hypertensive/hypokalemic while on MRAs. Other antihypertensive agents are also added if necessary to control hypertension.

---
[1]Not FDA approved for this indication.

Introduction

Hyperaldosteronism is a state of excessive aldosterone secretion. Primary hyperaldosteronism occurs due to autonomous hypersecretion of aldosterone that is independent of renin and angiotensin II and is relatively nonsuppressible, whereas secondary hyperaldosteronism occurs due to activation of the renin-angiotensin-aldosterone system (RAAS). The pathophysiology and symptoms of primary hyperaldosteronism can manifest at a broad continuum; thus it is best considered as a syndrome rather than a binary disease. Primary hyperaldosteronism not only contributes to cardiovascular, kidney, and metabolic disease but is also the most common cause of secondary hypertension, and recent reports suggest that 5% to 20% of hypertensive patients have primary hyperaldosteronism (as opposed to less than 1%, as previously reported). Secondary hyperaldosteronism includes two different categories: one is compensatory activation of the RAAS due to decreased effective circulating volume, as in congestive heart failure and liver cirrhosis; the other is overactivity of the RAAS accompanied by hypertension, as in renovascular hypertension. There are also several conditions that mimic aldosterone excess through various mechanisms that present with hypertension and other metabolic perturbations. Except for the compensatory activation of the RAAS, these conditions cause secondary hypertension with or without other metabolic consequences, such as hypokalemia and metabolic alkalosis, which bring them to medical attention. This chapter covers the current approaches to hyperaldosteronism for patients suspected of having hypertension secondary to excess aldosterone production.

Pathophysiology

Aldosterone is a steroid hormone produced by the zona glomerulosa in the adrenal gland and contributes to volume and potassium homeostasis via its action primarily on the principal cells in the collecting tubule of the kidney. The main stimuli of aldosterone secretion are angiotensin II and hyperkalemia, which increase synthesis and activity of aldosterone synthase mediated by calcium signaling. Angiotensin II releases calcium from the endoplasmic reticulum, whereas both angiotensin II and hyperkalemia depolarize membrane potential and open voltage-gated calcium channels. Therefore changes in genes regulating ionic homeostasis and membrane potential can affect aldosterone secretion. Aldosterone and angiotensin II are part of the RAAS; plasma renin from the juxtaglomerular apparatus converts angiotensinogen to

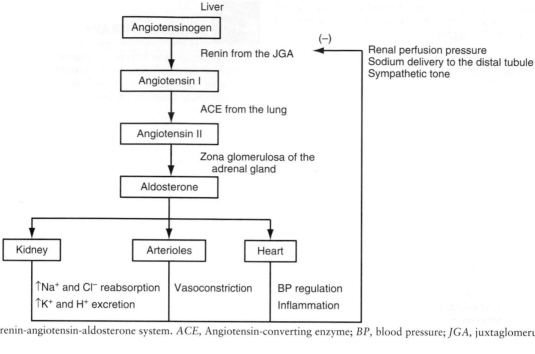

Figure 1 The renin-angiotensin-aldosterone system. *ACE,* Angiotensin-converting enzyme; *BP,* blood pressure; *JGA,* juxtaglomerular apparatus.

angiotensin I, and angiotensin-converting enzyme converts angiotensin I to angiotensin II. Subsequently, angiotensin II stimulates secretion of aldosterone. Renin secretion is controlled by renal artery pressure, sodium delivery to the distal nephron, and sympathetic activation (via β1). Increased effective arterial circulating volume from the action of aldosterone decreases renin secretion by negative feedback (Figure 1). Other minor factors involved in aldosterone secretion are adrenocorticotropic hormone (ACTH) and hyponatremia (which increase aldosterone secretion) and atrial natriuretic peptide (which decreases aldosterone secretion).

Aldosterone binds to the nuclear mineralocorticoid receptors. Activation of the mineralocorticoid receptors upregulates the basolateral Na$^+$/K$^+$ pumps and the epithelial sodium channels (ENaC), leading to increased reabsorption of Na$^+$ and Cl$^-$ and secretion of K$^+$ and H$^+$. The mineralocorticoid receptors can also be activated by other hormones with mineralocorticoid activity. Cortisol is able to bind to the mineralocorticoid receptors with similar affinity as aldosterone but normally is converted to inactive cortisone by 11β hydroxysteroid dehydrogenase 2 (11β HSD2). Mutations/inhibition of 11β HSD2 or very high cortisol levels above the capacity of 11β HSD2, as in Cushing syndrome (particularly ectopic Cushing syndrome), and glucocorticoid resistance can cause activation of the mineralocorticoid receptors. Aldosterone precursors such as deoxycorticosterone have a weak mineralocorticoid effect but can cause features of hyperaldosteronism when they are present at very high levels, as in some forms of congenital adrenal hyperplasias (11β hydroxylase deficiency or 17α hydroxylase deficiency) or deoxycorticosteroid-secreting tumors. In addition, activating mutations of the ENaCs also cause increased sodium absorption and hypertension mimicking hyperaldosteronism (Liddle syndrome).

With the development of specific antibodies against human CYP11B2 (aldosterone synthase) and its application to immunohistochemistry, diverse histopathological and genetic characteristics of primary hyperaldosteronism have been determined. An international consensus for the nomenclature and definition of adrenocortical lesions from patients with unilateral primary hyperaldosteronism was endorsed by the World Health Organization and includes aldosterone-producing adenoma (APA), aldosterone-producing nodule (APN), aldosterone-producing micronodule (APM) (formerly known as "aldosterone-producing cell cluster"), aldosterone-producing diffuse hyperplasia, and, rarely, aldosterone-producing adrenocortical carcinoma.

Multiple aldosterone-producing lesions can occur within a single adrenal gland, and adrenal lesions identified by imaging studies might not necessarily be the source of aldosterone excess. Incidental nonfunctioning adenomas can commonly occur in patients with primary hyperaldosteronism; in these cases, satellite APA or APN/APM in the adjacent or contralateral adrenal tissue may be the source of excess aldosterone production. Multiple APMs appear to be a common histologic feature of idiopathic hyperaldosteronism.

Whereas heritable forms are rare, somatic mutations causing primary hyperaldosteronism are common. Next-generation genetic sequencing has resulted in the identification of somatic mutations in approximately 90% of the APAs, which are a major cause of primary hyperaldosteronism. The mutation occurs in one of the aldosterone-driver genes, which include *KCNJ5, ATP1A1, ATP2B3, CACNA1D, CACNA1H,* and *CLCN2,* causes alteration of intracellular ion homeostasis, and enhances aldosterone production. In a small subset of APAs, somatic activating mutations in the *CTNNB1* gene, which encodes β-catenin, have also been detected. Interestingly, race and sex impact the somatic mutation spectrum of APA. Specifically, somatic mutations in the *KCNJ5* gene, encoding an inwardly rectifying K$^+$ channel, are common in APAs from Asian populations, as well as in women regardless of race.

Clinical Manifestations

The continuum in the pathophysiology of primary hyperaldosteronism translates into a spectrum of symptoms based on severity ranging from mild to overt. Primary hyperaldosteronism usually presents with normokalemic hypertension. Hypokalemia is present only in 9% to 37% of cases and may indicate more severe cases. A few rare patients might present with hypokalemia but have a normal systemic blood pressure (BP). Patients with primary hyperaldosteronism usually do not develop severe volume overload or edema because of aldosterone escape possibly related to atrial natriuretic peptide, pressure natriuresis, or decreased sodium absorption at other nephron segments. Metabolic alkalosis, mild hypernatremia (due to reset osmostat from volume expansion), and hypomagnesemia may be observed. Glomerular filtration rate and urinary albumin excretion can be elevated independent of systemic hypertension. Target organ (heart and kidney) damage and cardiovascular-related morbidity and mortality are higher in primary hyperaldosteronism than in essential hypertension with similar degrees of BP elevation. In fact, milder phenotypes of primary hyperaldosteronism pathophysiology (i.e., renin-independent aldosterone production that lies below the categorical thresholds for overt primary hyperaldosteronism [PA]) are independently associated with the development or progression of cardiovascular and kidney disease. Once hypertension has developed, the magnitude of the pathophysiology is associated with risk for worsening hypertension, incident structural heart disease, adverse cardiovascular events, and death. Thus, even though considered "overt primary hyperaldosteronism," there exists a large and clinically relevant spectrum of milder forms of the disease. Moreover, primary hyperaldosteronism is associated with an increased risk of type 2 diabetes mellitus and metabolic syndrome, which is attributable to both decreased insulin secretion and increased insulin clearance, as well as concurrent cortisol cosecretion. PA frequently co-occurs with obstructive sleep apnea given its association with obesity and its pathophysiology of chronic volume retention with a prevalence of 21% to 34%. Finally, it increases the risk for both osteoporosis and fractures, possibly mediated by hypercalciuria-induced secondary hyperparathyroidism.

Secondary hyperaldosteronism (when it is not from hypovolemia) and other conditions mimicking hyperaldosteronism can present with similar features as primary hyperaldosteronism plus specific manifestations for each disease entity. Depending on the mechanism of disease, more severe volume overload and pulmonary edema may be found (e.g., renovascular hypertension) because aldosterone escape may not work.

Evaluation

Screening

Despite its substantial clinical and public health implications, PA remains highly underdiagnosed. Hyperaldosteronism may be suspected based on severe (BP > 150/100 on three separate occasions) or resistant hypertension (uncontrolled BP despite use of three conventional antihypertensive agents including a diuretic, or well-controlled BP in the presence of four or more antihypertensive agents), early-onset hypertension without known risk factors, and hypertension with other features such as family history of hyperaldosteronism, early-onset hypertension, cerebrovascular accident at a young age, hypokalemia, adrenal mass, and obstructive sleep apnea. Currently there is no evidence-guided screening strategy. Some experts believe that routine screening for primary hyperaldosteronism is warranted in newly diagnosed hypertension considering its high prevalence, whereas others recommend that targeted screening is more appropriate, such as the Endocrine Society guidelines for primary hyperaldosteronism in 2016 (Box 1).

When a decision is made to screen for excessive mineralocorticoid effect, one should first examine the plasma renin and aldosterone levels (i.e., plasma renin activity [PRA, ng/mL/h] and plasma aldosterone concentration [PAC, ng/dL]). It is important to note that several factors can affect PRA and PAC, such as age,

medications, time of day, diet (salt intake), posture, method of blood collection, level of potassium, and level of creatinine (Table 1). Diuretics (both potassium sparing and wasting) and mineralocorticoid antagonists can have a significant effect on PRA and PAC. Angiotensin-converting enzyme inhibitors (ACEIs)/angiotensin receptor blockers (ARBs) and dihydropyridine calcium channel blockers can affect PRA and PAC modestly. Ideally, all medications and other factors that may affect PRA and PAC should be removed; unfortunately, it is not always practical and safe to do this because of the possibility of uncontrolled hypertension. If necessary, antihypertensive agents that affect PRA and PAC only minimally, such as slow-release verapamil (Calan SR), hydralazine (Apresoline), prazosin (Minipress), doxazosin (Cardura), or terazosin (Hytrin), can be used. The Endocrine Society 2016 guidelines recommend certain caveats that optimize the chance for obtaining more easily interpretable PRA and PAC results (Box 2). However, if needed, the screening can occur irrespective of concurrent medications or the time of day to simplify the approach and maximize opportunities to test. If there is renin suppression, defined as a plasma renin activity less than 1.0 ng/mL/h or corresponding plasma renin concentration less than 10 mU/L despite the use of medications that increase renin, it should raise suspicion for presence of nonsuppressible aldosterone.

Patterns of PRA and PAC help differentiate among primary hyperaldosteronism, secondary hyperaldosteronism, and conditions mimicking hyperaldosteronism. Differential diagnoses according to different patterns of PRA and PAC are listed in Box 3. If both PRA and PAC are high, further investigation for causes of secondary hyperaldosteronism should follow. If both PRA and PAC are suppressed, further investigation for conditions that mimic hyperaldosteronism is indicated. Suppressed PRA and elevated PAC suggest primary hyperaldosteronism. The next step is to calculate the aldosterone renin ratio (ARR), and the individual aldosterone and renin values should be individually evaluated. An ARR greater than 20 to 40 is considered screening positive for primary hyperaldosteronism. PAC greater than 15 ng/dL was recommended by some investigators to avoid false-positive ARR from very low renin level, but in many cases PAC can be less than 15 ng/dL, though this occurs more commonly in bilateral adrenal hyperplasia (BAH) than in aldosterone-producing adenoma. More recently, a new approach has been advocated wherein a "high-risk" patient with a suppressed renin should be assumed to have PA until proven otherwise. This approach is distinct from the stepwise approach prescribed by guidelines. By refining the approach to assume PA until proven otherwise in high-risk phenotypes, there is an increase in the probability of making a clinical diagnosis and/or initiating empiric treatment with MRAs for a wider array of PA phenotypes, especially the underrecognized mild ones. Diagnostic flow and subsequent management of hyperaldosteronism are summarized in Figure 2. Of note, there is no consensus on cutoff values for PRA, PAC, or ARR. There exist systematic differences in the calibration of aldosterone assays that have to be taken into account. The measurement of aldosterone by liquid chromatography–tandem mass spectrometry, which is now widespread, is 27% to 87% lower compared with immunoassay-based techniques. Moreover, a single cross-sectional circulating aldosterone level is not a reliable indicator of integrated physiology; an obtained high level can be informative, but a low value is not exclusionary. With aldosterone production and sensitivity being extremely variable and with systematic differences in measurement, screening tests should be repeated if results are inconclusive or if PA is strongly suspected but the initial screening tests are negative. Confirmatory tests should follow to avoid false positives.

Confirmatory Tests of Primary Hyperaldosteronism

The positive screening test should be followed by one or more confirmatory tests to avoid false positives. The confirmatory tests are designed to physiologically suppress aldosterone levels that would normally occur in the absence of primary hyperaldosteronism. However, some experts believe that some aldosterone-producing

---

BOX 1	Groups Indicated for Case Detection With Relatively High Prevalence of Primary Hyperaldosteronism

Sustained blood pressure > 150/100 mm Hg on three different occasions
- Drug-resistant hypertension (>140/90 mm Hg despite three medications, including a diuretic)
- Hypertension and hypokalemia (spontaneous or diuretic-induced)
- Hypertension and family history of early-onset hypertension or cerebrovascular accident at a young age (<40 years)
- Hypertension with adrenal incidentaloma
- Hypertensive first-degree relatives of primary hyperaldosteronism patients
- Hypertension with obstructive sleep apnea

TABLE 1	Medical Factors That May Affect Aldosterone and Renin Measurement		
	EFFECT ON ALDOSTERONE	**EFFECT ON RENIN**	**EFFECT ON ALDOSTERONE–RENIN RATIO**
Medications			
β-Blocker	↓	↓↓	↑
Central α$_2$ agonists (clonidine [Catapres], α-methyldopa [Aldomet])	↓	↓↓	↑
NSAIDs	↓	↓↓	↑
K$^+$ wasting diuretics	→↑	↑↑	↓
K$^+$ sparing diuretics	↑	↑↑	↓
ACE inhibitors	↓	↑↑	↓
Angiotensin II receptor blockers	↓	↑↑	↓
Dihydropyridine Ca^{2+} blockers	→↓	↑	↓
Renin inhibitors	↓	↓ plasma renin activity	↑
		↑ direct renin concentration	↓
Potassium Status			
Hypokalemia	↓	→↑	↓
Potassium loading	↑	→↓	↑
Dietary Sodium			
Sodium restricted	↑	↑↑	↓
Sodium loaded	↓	↓↓	↑
Others			
Advanced age	↓	↓↓	↑
Renal impairment	→	↓	↑
Oral contraceptives*	↑	↑ plasma renin activity	→
		↓ direct renin concentration	↑
Pregnancy	↑	↑↑	↓
Renovascular hypertension	↑	↑↑	↓
Malignant hypertension	↑	↑↑	↓

*Premenopausal women have higher aldosterone level during the luteal phase and lower renin level throughout the cycle than men. False-positive aldosterone renin ratio during the luteal phase was reported when direct renin concentration was used.
ACE, Angiotensin-converting enzyme; *NSAIDs,* nonsteroidal antiinflammatory drugs.

lesions are not completely independent of the RAAS, and confirmatory suppression tests can give false-negative results. Other experts think that confirmatory tests are not necessary for those with obvious clinical/biochemical features. Those with spontaneous hypokalemia, renin level below the detection level plus PAC greater than 20 ng/dL may not need further confirmatory tests. Furthermore, there is no gold standard confirmatory. Therefore factors such as cost, accessibility, feasibility, patient compliance, local expertise, and accuracy of assay should be taken into consideration in selecting confirmatory tests. The Endocrine Society guidelines in 2016 state that any of the following four confirmatory tests can be used: oral salt loading test, saline suppression test, fludrocortisone (Florinef)[1] suppression test, and captopril (Capoten)[1] challenge test (Table 2). Finally, there is increasing evidence that cortisol cosecretion can commonly occur in primary hyperaldosteronism with a prevalence range from 4% to 27%. It usually happens in patients with a visible adrenal mass on cross-sectional imaging, as clinically relevant hypercortisolism usually requires some degree of adrenocortical neoplasia and is associated with increased risk for adverse events. Screening can be conducted by measuring a baseline serum dehydroepiandrosterone sulfate and performing a 1-mg overnight dexamethasone[1] suppression test (DST). Cortisol-producing adenoma-related somatic mutations in unilateral primary aldosteronism with concurrent autonomous cortisol secretion have been noted with a prevalence of approximately 36.7%. The presence of these mutations is associated with higher post-DST cortisol levels and larger adenoma size, though no eventual effect on outcomes after surgery has been noted.

Subtype Classification of Primary Hyperaldosteronism

Once primary hyperaldosteronism is biochemically confirmed, subtype classification follows to guide treatment. Lateralization of the source of excessive aldosterone production is crucial as the next step, as unilateral lesions such as APAs can be treated surgically. In contrast, bilateral lesions, such as BAHs, which account for almost 60% to 70% of the cases and in general are a milder disease, are treated medically. Aldosterone-producing carcinoma is rare but should be ruled out. In this regard, computed tomography (CT) of the adrenal glands should be done first to rule out aldosterone-producing carcinoma and obtain anatomic information. However, imaging studies are usually not reliable enough to lateralize lesions. If surgical treatment is considered, adrenal

[1] Not FDA approved for this indication.

Correct hypokalemia to 4 mmol/L.
- Liberalize sodium intake.
- Withdraw the following agents that markedly affect PRA and PAC for at least 4 weeks: spironolactone (Aldactone), eplerenone (Inspra), amiloride (Midamor), triamterene (Dyrenium), potassium-wasting diuretic, and products made from licorice.[7]
- If not diagnostic and hypertension can be controlled with relatively noninterfering medications, withdraw the following agents for at least 2 weeks: β-blockers, central α2 agonists (clonidine [Catapres], methyldopa [Aldomet]), NSAIDs, ACEIs/ARBs, renin inhibitors, and dihydropyridine calcium channel antagonists.
- If necessary, start other antihypertensive agents that have fewer effects on ARR: slow-release verapamil (Calan-SR), hydralazine (Apresoline) (with verapamil to prevent reflex tachycardia), prazosin (Minipress), doxazosin (Cardura), and terazosin (Hytrin).
- Obtain blood for PRA and PAC midmorning after the patient has been up for at least 2 h and seated for 5 to 15 min.
- Establish use of estrogen products and menstrual cycles. Premenopausal females have higher ARR than men, especially during the luteal phase. False-positive ARR was reported during the luteal phase and from the use of estrogen products when direct renin concentration was used.

[7]Available as dietary supplement.
ACEI, Angiotensin-converting enzyme inhibitor; *ARB,* angiotensin receptor blocker; *ARR,* aldosterone renin ratio; *NSAIDs,* nonsteroidal antiinflammatory drugs; *PAC,* plasma aldosterone concentration; *PRA,* plasma renin activity.

Causes of Primary Hyperaldosteronism: ↓ PRA and ↑ PAC (>5–10 ng/dL); ARR >20–40

Most Common

Aldosterone-producing adenoma
- Bilateral adrenal hyperplasia or idiopathic hyperaldosteronism

Less Common

Unilateral hyperplasia or primary adrenal hyperplasia
- Familial hyperaldosteronism type I or glucocorticoid remediable aldosteronism
- Familial hyperaldosteronism type II
- Aldosterone-producing adrenocortical carcinoma
- Ectopic aldosterone-secreting tumor (ovary, kidney)
- Multiple endocrine neoplasia type 1

Causes of Secondary Hyperaldosteronism: ↑ PRA and ↑ PAC; ARR ≈10

Renovascular hypertension
- Diuretic use
- Renin-secreting tumor
- Malignant hypertension
- Coarctation of the aorta

Causes of Conditions That Mimic Mineralocorticoid Excess: ↓ PRA and ↓ PAC

Congenital adrenal hyperplasia
- Exogenous mineralocorticoid
- Deoxycorticosterone-producing tumor
- Cushing syndrome
- 11β HSD2 deficiency
- Altered aldosterone metabolism
- Liddle syndrome
- Glucocorticoid resistance

ARR, Aldosterone renin ratio; *PAC,* plasma aldosterone concentration; *PRA,* plasma renin activity.

vein sampling (AVS) should be performed. Most cases of primary hyperaldosteronism are sporadic; about 5% are familial, mostly via autosomal dominant inheritance. Young patients (<20 years of age) and those with family history of primary hyperaldosteronism or strokes at young age (<40 years) should have genetic testing for glucocorticoid remediable aldosteronism (GRA) or familial hyperaldosteronism type I, which is caused by the hybrid gene of 11β hydroxylase and aldosterone synthase (increased aldosterone synthesis by ACTH). Patients with GRA are less likely to be hypokalemic than other patients with primary hyperaldosteronism, perhaps because of the circadian nature of ACTH secretion. In very young patients, *KCNJ5* germline mutations, causing familial hyperaldosteronism type III, should be tested. Familial hyperaldosteronism type II is clinically indistinguishable from nonfamilial hyperaldosteronism and can be caused by gain-of-function mutations in the *CLCN2* (chloride voltage-gated channel 2) gene. Familial hyperaldosteronism type IV generally involves patients with early-onset hypertension and primary hyperaldosteronism before the age of 10. Germline mutations in the *CACNA1H* (calcium voltage-gated channel subunit alpha1H) gene occur in type IV patients who also exhibit mental retardation and developmental disorders, as well as seizures and neurologic abnormalities in some patients.

Imaging

CT and magnetic resonance imaging (MRI) scans of the adrenal glands provide one of five conclusions: normal adrenal glands, unilateral macroadenomas (>1 cm), minimal unilateral adrenal limb thickening, unilateral microadenomas (≤1 cm), and bilateral macroadenomas and/or microadenomas. APAs are typically smaller than 2 cm, and BAHs exhibit either normal or nodular changes. Aldosterone-producing adrenal carcinomas are almost always larger than 4 cm in diameter and have imaging characteristics suspicious for malignancy. However, there are limitations: small APAs may be missed, hyperplasia may be misread as adenomas, and nonfunctional tumors are radiologically indistinguishable from APAs. Although several studies suggested imaging criteria for different subtypes, no study has conclusively established specific criteria that differentiate among different subtypes of primary hyperaldosteronism. In fact, CT accurately lateralizes in only about 50% to 70% of cases, and there is no evidence that MRI is superior to CT for subtype classification. Therefore AVS is required to differentiate unilateral from bilateral lesions if surgical resection is being pursued. Patients younger than 35 years with marked hyperaldosteronism with spontaneous hypokalemia and PAC greater than 30 ng/dL and solitary unilateral adenoma may not need AVS, because nonfunctioning tumors are uncommon in this young age group.

Adrenal Vein Sampling

Aldosterone levels are measured from adrenal venous blood samples (Box 4) obtained through adrenal vein cannulation to distinguish between unilateral and bilateral lesions. Unilateral lesions are associated with a marked increase in PAC on the side of the tumor (and suppressed PAC on the other side), whereas bilateral lesions have little difference between the two sides. AVS should be performed only by experienced physicians in part because recognition and successful cannulation of the right adrenal vein especially can be challenging. Complications of AVS include adrenal hemorrhage, adrenal infarction, adrenal vein perforation, and adrenal vein thrombosis, which occur only rarely (<2.5%) in the hands of a physician skilled in the procedure.

The use of cosyntropin stimulation to minimize stress-induced fluctuation in aldosterone level is controversial, and some believe that it has no effect on AVS accuracy. If cosyntropin is not used, then AVS should be done in the morning after overnight

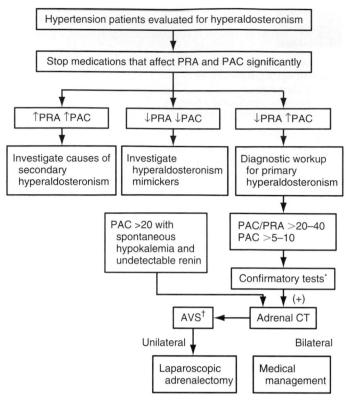

Figure 2 Evaluation of hyperaldosteronism. *AVS,* Adrenal vein sampling; *CT,* computed tomography; *PAC,* plasma aldosterone concentration in ng/dL; *PRA,* plasma renin activity in ng/mL/h. *May skip if spontaneous hypokalemia, renin level below the detection limit, and PAC >20 ng/dL. †If surgical treatment is pursued. May skip if <35 years old, spontaneous hypokalemia, PAC > 30 ng/dL, and unilateral adenoma.

recumbency to avoid postural aldosterone changes and reflect circadian aldosterone secretion.

In reality, different centers use different techniques, protocols, and interpretation criteria. The Endocrine Society guidelines in 2016 provide interpretation criteria with and without cosyntropin use. The first step for interpretation is to determine whether the procedure was done correctly. The adrenal vein–to–inferior vena cava cortisol ratio should be greater than 5:1 with cosyntropin given and greater than 3:1 without cosyntropin. If the ratio is significantly lower than these values, improper cannulation is implied. Next, divide the PAC values for the right and left adrenal veins by their respective cortisol values to correct the dilutional effect of the inferior phrenic vein flow into the left adrenal vein; this is termed the *cortisol-corrected aldosterone* (A/C). If cosyntropin is used, an A/C ratio of the high to the low side of greater than 4:1 indicates unilateral aldosterone hypersecretion, whereas an A/C ratio of less than 3:1 suggests bilateral aldosterone hypersecretion. These cutoffs were reported to have sensitivity of 95% and specificity of 100% for unilateral lesions. If the A/C ratio is between 3:1 and 4:1, the results of AVS should be interpreted in the context of CT, clinical findings, and other tests. Without cosyntropin, an A/C ratio of the high to the low side of greater than 2 or an A/C ratio of the high side to the periphery greater than 2.5 plus an A/C ratio of the low side to the periphery of less than 1 (suppressed contralateral aldosterone secretion) is consistent with unilateral aldosterone excess.

Ancillary Tests

Clinical findings and other ancillary tests may help differentiate unilateral APAs from BAHs. BAHs will respond with increase in plasma aldosterone to postural stimulation, whereas APAs will not. Plasma 18-hydroxycorticosterone level tends to be higher in APAs compared with BAHs. Iodocholesterol scintigraphy may be able to show functional correlation of anatomic abnormalities (but is not available at most centers). APA-specific tracers such

as (11)C-metomidate for positron emission tomography may be useful. Interpretation criteria of these tests are listed in Table 3. Patients with APAs tend to be younger (<40 years), predominantly female, very hypertensive with marked hypokalemia (<3 mmol/L), and tend to have a very high PAC (>25 mg/dL) compared with those with BAHs.

Treatment

Treatment of secondary hyperaldosteronism and conditions mimicking hyperaldosteronism depends on their etiology. Treatment of primary hyperaldosteronism is discussed here. The goals of treatment of primary hyperaldosteronism are (1) normalization of the serum potassium in hypokalemic patients, (2) normalization of the BP, and (3) reversal of the effects of hyperaldosteronism on the cardiovascular system. When a small group of patients were followed after treatment with adrenalectomy or MRAs, left ventricular mass was reduced (faster with adrenalectomy than MRAs), increase in carotid intima-media thickness and arterial stiffness was reversed, glomerular filtration rate and urinary albumin secretion decreased and became similar to that in essential hypertension, and excessive cardiovascular risk compared with essential hypertension disappeared. Cardiovascular complications were rather related to age, duration of hypertension, and smoking. In addition, there was an improvement in the quality of life at 3 months, which was sustained at 6 months. Therefore timely diagnosis and treatment is essential. For unilateral lesions, surgical resection of the affected adrenal gland is recommended mainly to obviate the need for prolonged medical treatment and side effects. Moreover, adrenalectomy in unilateral PA significantly reduces the risk for cardiovascular events, kidney disease, type 2 diabetes mellitus, and mortality while improving quality of life compared with medical therapy. More recently, ablative procedures in the treatment of unilateral AP have been attempted, but future clinical trials of ablation versus adrenalectomy are needed to compare their clinical and cost-effectiveness and further define patient populations that are likely to benefit.

For bilateral lesions, medical treatment is recommended because surgical risk outweighs benefits. BP control per se does not reduce risk of cardiovascular complications unless renin activity is restored to normal (>1 ng/mL/h), which can be accomplished by salt restriction or increasing the dose of the MRA. MRAs are a key component of medical treatment and used as a preoperative measure or maintenance treatment (GRA should be treated with the lowest dose of glucocorticoid that can normalize BP and potassium levels rather than MRAs). A low-sodium diet (sodium <100 mEq/day = 2.3 g/day or salt 6 g/day) is also important, because left ventricular hypertrophy is associated with urine sodium excretion in primary hyperaldosteronism but not in essential hypertension. Other lifestyle changes include aerobic exercise, smoking cessation, and weight loss.

Unilateral Hypersecretion

Adrenalectomy, usually laparoscopic, is recommended. MRAs such as spironolactone (Aldactone) and eplerenone (Inspra)[1] can be used to control BP in patients awaiting adrenalectomy and also to prevent postoperative hypoaldosteronism. Postoperatively, normal saline is given to maintain volume status, MRAs and potassium supplements are discontinued, and antihypertensive medications may be reduced. To confirm biochemical cure, PAC and PRA should be checked shortly after the operation, though renin levels might not change immediately. Risk factors for persistent hypertension after adrenalectomy include older age, duration of hypertension (>5 years), use of two or more antihypertensive agents preoperatively, BP higher than 165/100 mm Hg, low ARR preoperatively, low urine aldosterone, poor response to spironolactone preoperatively, family history of more than one first-degree relative with hypertension, and elevated serum creatinine level. When patients are unwilling or unable to undergo curative adrenalectomy, MRA therapy should be used as the alternative.

---

[1] Not FDA approved for this indication.

TABLE 2	Protocols and Interpretation of Recommended Confirmatory Tests		
	PROTOCOL	**INTERPRETATION**	**REMARKS**
Oral sodium loading test	Place the patient on a high-sodium diet (>200 mmol/day) for 3 days. Replace potassium to compensate for the kaliuresis induced by the high-sodium diet. Collect a 24-h urine on the third day for determination of aldosterone, sodium, and creatinine; adequate if the urine sodium >200 mmol/24 h	Confirmed if the 24-h urine aldosterone is >12 mcg (33.3 nmol) to 14 mcg (38.8 nmol). Ruled out if the 24-h urine aldosterone is <10 mcg (27.7 nmol). The test is equivocal if the value falls in between	Do not perform this test in patients with severe uncontrolled hypertension, renal failure, cardiac failure/ arrhythmias, or severe hypokalemia
IV saline infusion test*	1. Place the patient supine 1 h before drawing blood for morning baseline fasting levels of renin, aldosterone, cortisol, and potassium 2. Infuse 2 L of 0.9% NaCl over 4 h, keeping the patient supine. Monitor blood pressure and heart rate 3. After 4 h, draw blood for measurement of renin, aldosterone, cortisol, and potassium	Confirmed if the PAC is >10 ng/dL (277 pmol/L). Ruled out if the PAC is <5 ng/dL (139 pmol/L). If the PAC falls between these values, the test is equivocal	Do not perform this test in patients with severe uncontrolled hypertension, renal failure, cardiac failure/ arrhythmias, or severe hypokalemia
Fludrocortisone[1] suppression test	Give 0.1 mg fludrocortisone every 6 h for 4 days, with the potassium level checked every 6 h to be sure that it is greater than 4 mmol/L Encourage a liberal sodium diet to keep urinary sodium excretion greater than 3 mmol/kg/day On day 4, draw blood for an upright 7 a.m. plasma cortisol level and 10 a.m. plasma aldosterone, renin, and cortisol levels	Confirmed if the 10 a.m. PAC is >6 ng/dL, as long as PRA is <1 ng/mL/h and the plasma cortisol at 10 a.m. is less than at 7 a.m. (to exclude the ACTH effect)	The test may require hospitalization. Risks include severe hypokalemia, QT changes, worsening of left ventricular function, hypertension, and frequent phlebotomy
Captopril[1] challenge test	Give 25–50 mg captopril after the patient has been sitting or standing for 1 h. The patient remains seated throughout the test. Draw blood for measurement of plasma renin, aldosterone, and cortisol at time 0, at 1 h, and at 2 h	Normally, captopril suppresses PAC by more than 30% from baseline. Confirmed if there is no suppression of PAC and PRA remains suppressed. The false-negative rate for this test is high because suppression occurs in more than 30% of cases. A slight decrease in aldosterone can suggest bilateral adrenal hyperplasia	

*The patient may be seated for 30 minutes before and during the infusion to improve sensitivity, and PAC > 6 ng/dL (170 pmol/L) confirms primary hyperaldosteronism.
[1]Not FDA approved for this indication.
ACTH, Adrenocorticotropic hormone; *IV*, intravenous; *PAC*, plasma aldosterone concentration; *PRA*, plasma renin activity.

BOX 4	Adrenal Vein Sampling

- After both adrenal veins have been cannulated, draw baseline samples for PRA, PAC, ACTH, and cortisol from the peripheral such as cubital or iliac, right adrenal vein, and left adrenal vein.
- Inject 250 mcg of cosyntropin (Cortrosyn) after cannulation, or infuse 50 mcg cosyntropin per hour beginning 30 min before adrenal vein cannulation. This reduces stress-related fluctuations in aldosterone and cortisol values and augments the biochemical gradients. (This step is controversial.)
- Draw blood for aldosterone and cortisol levels at 5, 15, and 30 min from the peripheral site and from each adrenal vein.

ACTH, Adrenocorticotropic hormone; *PAC*, plasma aldosterone concentration; *PRA*, plasma renin activity.

Bilateral Hypersecretion

MRAs and/or ENaC antagonists combined with other antihypertensives are used. One study showed that spironolactone had stronger antihypertensive effect than eplerenone, but there is insufficient evidence to choose one medication over another. When MR antagonist therapy is recommended, patients should be counseled on dietary sodium reduction (<1500 mg per day) as it can result in volume contraction, a rise in renin, and normalization of BP.

Spironolactone is the most widely used MRA. It is very effective in decreasing BP. The medication is initiated at 12.5 to 25 mg/day and can be titrated to 400 mg/day, with most patients requiring at least 200 mg/day. Potassium should be maintained at normal levels without use of potassium supplements. Use of spironolactone can be limited by side effects: antiandrogenic effects can cause gynecomastia in men, and progesterone effect can cause menstrual irregularities in women. There are drug interactions to consider: spironolactone increases the half-life of digoxin (Lanoxin) and salicylates, and other nonsteroidal antiinflammatory drugs may decrease the effectiveness of spironolactone. Serum potassium and creatinine should be closely monitored for the first 4 to 6 weeks, in particular for those with renal insufficiency or diabetes. Spironolactone is not recommended if creatinine clearance is less than 30 mL/min.

Eplerenone[1] is a competitive and selective antagonist of the aldosterone receptors. It has a lower binding affinity to

---

[1]Not FDA approved for this indication.

TABLE 3	Interpretation of Dynamic Testing
TEST	**FINDINGS**
Screening Test	
PAC/PRA ratio	Positive if >20–40 with PAC >5–10 ng/dL
Confirmatory Tests	
Oral sodium loading test	Positive if 24-h urine aldosterone excretion is >12–14 mcg
Saline infusion test	Positive if PAC after infusion is >10 ng/dL
Fludrocortisone[1] suppression test	Positive if upright PAC is >6 ng/dL on day 4 at 10 a.m.
Captopril[1] challenge test	Positive if PAC does not decrease by 30% and PRA remains suppressed
AVS	
With cosyntropin stimulation	A/C ratio (the high to the low side) >4:1 → unilateral aldosterone excess A/C ratio 3:1–4:1 → unclear A/C ratio <3:1 → bilateral aldosterone excess
Without cosyntropin stimulation	A/C ratio from the high to the low side >2:1 → unilateral aldosterone excess A/C ratio from the high side to the periphery >2.5 and A/C ratio from the contralateral side to the periphery <1 → unilateral aldosterone excess
If Equivocal AVS	
Postural stimulation test	PAC falls or fails to rise by 30%: consistent with APAs PAC increases by at least 33%: consistent with BAHs
Recumbent 18-hydroxycorticosterone	>100 ng/dL is consistent with APAs
NP-59 iodocholesterol scintigraphy	Unilateral early uptake (<5 days): consistent with unilateral aldosterone excess Bilateral early uptake (<5 days): consistent with bilateral aldosterone excess Negative scan does not rule out either etiology
(11)C-metomidate positron emission tomography	Preliminary data showed (11)C-metomidate uptake in APA

[1]Not FDA approved for this indication.

A/C ratio, Cortisol-corrected aldosterone ratio; *APA,* aldosterone-producing adenomas; *AVS,* adrenal vein sampling; *BAH,* bilateral adrenal hyperplasia; *PAC,* plasma aldosterone concentration; *PRA,* plasma renin activity.

androgen and progesterone receptors than spironolactone. This leads to fewer side effects. Eplerenone is 25% to 50% less potent in antagonizing the aldosterone receptors than spironolactone. Eplerenone has a short half-life and should be taken twice daily. Dosing is started at 25 mg twice daily, with a maximum dose of 100 mg/day. Again, serum potassium and creatinine should be closely monitored for the first 4 to 6 weeks in particular for those with renal insufficiency or diabetes. Other adverse effects include hypertriglyceridemia, increased liver enzymes, headache, and fatigue. Eplerenone is contraindicated if serum potassium is greater than 5.5 mEq/L at initiation, if creatinine clearance is less than 30 mL/min, or if there is concomitant use of strong CYP3A4 inhibitors such as ketoconazole (Nizoral) and itraconazole (Sporanox).

ENaC antagonists, amiloride (Midamor)[1] and triamterene (Dyrenium),[1] can be used in patients who cannot tolerate MRAs or are still hypertensive/hypokalemic while on MRAs. Amiloride is prescribed at 10 to 20 mg/day in divided doses. Side effects include dizziness, fatigue, and impotence. Triamterene is dosed at 100 to 300 mg/day in divided doses, and its side effects are mainly dizziness and nausea. Addition of thiazide diuretics can help control BP by relieving volume overload. If BP remains uncontrolled, other antihypertensive agents such as ACEIs/ARBs or calcium channel blockers may be used.

---

[1] Not FDA approved for this indication.

References

Adler GK, Murray GR, Turcu AF, et al: Primary aldosteronism decreases insulin secretion and increases insulin clearance in humans, *Hypertension* 75, 2020. 1251–125.

Baudrand R, Guarda FJ, Torrey J, Williams G, Vaidya A: Dietary sodium restriction increases the risk of misinterpreting mild cases of primary aldosteronism, *J Clin Endocrinol Metab* 101:3989–3996, 2016.

Bayomy O, Zaheer S, Williams JS, Curhan G, Vaidya A: Disentangling the relationships between the renin-angiotensin-aldosterone system, calcium physiology, and risk for kidney stones, *J Clin Endocrinol Metab* 105:1937–1946, 2020, https://doi.org/10.1210/clinem/dgaa123.

Born-Frontsberg E, Reincke M, Rump LC, et al: Cardiovascular and cerebrovascular comorbidities of hypokalemic and normokalemic primary aldosteronism: results of the German Conn's registry, *J Clin Endocrinol Metab* 94:1125–1130, 2009.

Bouhanick B, Delchier MC, Lagarde S, et al: Radiofrequency ablation for adenoma in patients with primary aldosteronism and hypertension: ADERADHTA, a pilot study, *J Hypertens* 39:759–765, 2021.

Boulkroun S: Old and new genes in primary aldosteronism, *Best Pract Res Clin Endocrinol Metab* 34, 2020.

Brown JM, Siddiqui M, Calhoun DA, et al: The unrecognized prevalence of primary aldosteronism: a cross-sectional study, *Ann Intern Med* 173(1):10–20, 2020, https://doi.org/10.7326/M20-0065. Epub 2020 May 26. PMID: 32449886; PMCID: PMC7459427.

Catena C, Colussi G, Lapenna R, et al: Long-term cardiac effects of adrenalectomy or mineralocorticoid antagonists in patients with primary aldosteronism, *Hypertension* 50:911–918, 2007.

Catena C, Colussi GL, Nadalini E, et al: Cardiovascular outcomes in patients with primary aldosteronism after treatment, *Arch Intern Med* 168:80–85, 2008.

Cohen JB, Cohen DL, Herman DS, Leppert JT, Byrd JB, Bhalla V: Testing for primary aldosteronism and mineralocorticoid receptor antagonist use among U.S. veterans: a retrospective cohort study, *Ann Intern Med* 174(3):289–297, 2021, https://doi.org/10.7326/M20-4873. Epub 2020 Dec 29. PMID: 33370170; PMCID: PMC7965294.

Fujimoto K, Honjo S, Tatsuoka H, et al: Primary aldosteronism associated with subclinical Cushing syndrome, *J Endocrinol Invest* 36:564–567, 2013.

Funder JW: Primary aldosteronism and cardiovascular risk, before and after treatment, *Lancet Diabetes Endocrinol* 6:5–7, 2018.

Funder JW, Carey RM, Mantero F, et al: The management of primary aldosteronism: case detection, diagnosis, and treatment: an Endocrine Society clinical guideline, *J Clin Endocrinol Metab* 101:1889–1916, 2016.

Gordon RD, Gomez-Sanchez CE, Hamlet SM, et al: Angiotensin-responsive aldosterone-producing adenoma masquerades as idiopathic hyperaldosteronism (IHA: adrenal hyperplasia) or low-renin essential hypertension, *J Hypertens* 5:S103–S106, 1987.

Hundemer GL, Curhan GC, Yozamp N, et al: Cardiometabolic outcomes and mortality in medically treated primary aldosteronism: a retrospective cohort study, *Lancet Diabetes Endocrinol* 6:51–59, 2018.

Hundemer GL, Imsirovic H, Vaidya A, et al: Screening rates for primary aldosteronism among individuals with hypertension plus hypokalemia: a population-based retrospective cohort study, *Hypertension* 79(1):178–186, 2022, https://doi.org/10.1161/HYPERTENSIONAHA.121.18118. Epub 2021 Oct 18. PMID: 34657442; PMCID: PMC8664996.

Hundemer GL, Vaidya A: Primary aldosteronism diagnosis and management: a clinical approach, *Endocrinol Metab Clin North Am* 48(4):681–700, 2019, https://doi.org/10.1016/j.ecl.2019.08.002. PMID: 31655770; PMCID: PMC6824480.

Hundemer Gregory L, Vaidya A: "Management of endocrine disease: the role of surgical adrenalectomy in primary aldosteronism." *Eur J endocrinol* 183(6):R185–R196, 2020. Web.

Kempers MJ, Lenders JW, van Outheusden L, et al: Systematic review: diagnostic procedures to differentiate unilateral from bilateral adrenal abnormality in primary aldosteronism, *Ann Intern Med* 151:329–337, 2009.

Kono T, Ikeda F, Oseko F, Imura H, Tanimura H: Normotensive primary aldosteronism: report of a case, *J Clin Endocrinol Metab* 52(5):1009–1013, 1981, https://doi.org/10.1210/jcem-52-5-1009. PMID: 6262353.

Lechner B, Lechner K, Heinrich D, et al: Therapy of endocrine disease: medical treatment of primary aldosteronism, *Eur J Endocrinol* 181:R147–R153, 2019.

Mete O, Erickson LA, Juhlin CC, et al: Overview of the 2022 WHO classification of adrenal cortical tumors, *Endocr Pathol* 33:155–196, 2022.

Mulatero P, Bertello C, Rossato D, et al: Roles of clinical criteria, computed tomography scan, and adrenal vein sampling in differential diagnosis of primary aldosteronism subtypes, *J Clin Endocrinol Metab* 93:1366–1371, 2008.

Nanba K, Rainey WE: Genetics in endocrinology: impact of race and sex on genetic causes of aldosterone-producing adenomas, *Eur J Endocrinol* 185(1):R1–R11, 2021.

Ng E, Gwini SM, Libianto R, et al: Aldosterone, renin, and aldosterone-to-renin ratio variability in screening for primary aldosteronism, *J Clin Endocrinol Metab* 108(1):33–41, 2022. Erratum in: *J Clin Endocrinol Metab.* 2023;108(5):e206.

O'Toole SM, Sze WC, Chung TT, et al: Lowgrade cortisol cosecretion has limited impact on ACTH-stimulated AVS parameters in primary aldosteronism, *J Clin Endocrinol Metab* 105:e3776–e3784, 2020.

Parthasarathy HK, Menard J, White WB, et al: A double-blind, randomized study comparing the antihypertensive effect of eplerenone and spironolactone in patients with hypertension and evidence of primary aldosteronism, *J Hypertens* 29(5):980–990, 2011.

Pimenta E, Gordon RD, Ahmed AH, et al: Cardiac dimensions are largely determined by dietary salt in patients with primary aldosteronism: results of a case-control study, *J Clin Endocrinol Metab* 96:2813–2820, 2011.

Reincke M, Fischer E, Gerum S, et al: Observational study mortality in treated primary aldosteronism: the German Conn's registry, *Hypertension* 60:618–624, 2012.

Rossi GP, Barisa M, Allolio B, et al: The adrenal vein sampling international study (AVIS) for identifying the major subtypes of primary aldosteronism, *J Clin Endocrinol Metab* 97:1606–1614, 2012.

Rossi GP: A comprehensive review of the clinical aspects of primary aldosteronism, *Nat Rev Endocrinol* 7:485–495, 2011.

Rossi GP, Bernini G, Caliumi C, et al: A prospective study of the prevalence of primary aldosteronism in 1,125 hypertensive patients, *J Am Coll Cardiol* 48:2293–2300, 2006.

Rossi GP, Seccia TM, Pessina AC: Adrenal gland: a diagnostic algorithm—the holy grail of primary aldosteronism, *Nat Rev Endocrinol* 7:697–699, 2011.

Rutherford JC, Taylor WL, Stowasser M, Gordon RD: Success of surgery for primary aldosteronism judged by residual autonomous aldosterone production, *World J Surg* 22(12):1243–1245, 1998.

Sawka AM, Young WF, Thompson GB, et al: Primary aldosteronism: factors associated with normalization of blood pressure after surgery, *Ann Intern Med* 135:258–261, 2001.

Scholl UI: Genetics of primary aldosteronism, *Hypertension* 79:887–897, 2022.

Sechi LA, Novello M, Lapenna R, et al: Long-term renal outcomes in patients with primary aldosteronism, *JAMA* 295:2638–2645, 2006.

Stowasser M: Update in primary aldosteronism, *J Clin Endocrinol Metab* 100:1–10, 2015.

Sukor N, Gordon RD, Ku YK, et al: Role of unilateral adrenalectomy in bilateral primary aldosteronism: a 22-year single center experience, *J Clin Endocrinol Metab* 94:2437–2445, 2009.

Takeda M, Yamamoto K, Akasaka H, et al: Clinical characteristics and postoperative outcomes of primary aldosteronism in the elderly, *J Clin Endocrinol Metab* 103:3620–3629, 2018.

Thuzar M, Young K, Ahmed AH, et al: Diagnosis of primary aldosteronism by seated saline suppression test—variability between immunoassay and HPLC-MS/MS, *J Clin Endocrinol Metab* 105:e477–e483, 2019.

Vaidya A, Brown JM, Carey RM, Siddiqui M, Williams GH: The unrecognized prevalence of primary aldosteronism, *Ann Intern Med* 173(8):683, 2020.

Vaidya A, Carey RM: Evolution of the primary aldosteronism syndrome: updating the approach, *J Clin Endocrinol Metab* 105(12):1–3783, 2020.

Vorselaars WMCM, Nell S, Postma EL, et al: Clinical outcomes after unilateral adrenalectomy for primary aldosteronism, *JAMA Surg* 154:e185842, 2019.

Williams TA, Gomez-Sanchez CE, Rainey WE, et al: International histopathology consensus for unilateral primary aldosteronism, *J Clin Endocrinol Metab* 106(1):42–54, 2021.

Wu WC, Peng KY, Lu JY, et al: Cortisol-producing adenoma-related somatic mutations in unilateral primary aldosteronism with concurrent autonomous cortisol secretion: their prevalence and clinical characteristics, *Eur J Endocrinol* 187(4):519–530, 2022.

Yozamp N, Hundemer GL, Moussa M, et al: Intraindividual variability of aldosterone concentrations in primary aldosteronism: implications for case detection, *Hypertension* 77:891–899, 2021.

Zennaro MC, Boulkroun S, Fernandes-Rosa F: An update on novel mechanisms of primary aldosteronism, *J Endocrinol* 224:R63–R77, 2015.

HYPERLIPIDEMIA

Method of

Ming Li, MD, PhD; Xiaoming Jia, MD; Mandeep Bajaj, MD; and Lawrence Chan, MD

CURRENT DIAGNOSIS

- Hyperlipidemia is diagnosed based on lipid profile in the context of global cardiovascular risk. The exception is when the triglyceride level is greater than 500 mg/dL because of substantial risk of pancreatitis.
- Secondary causes of hyperlipidemia, such as hypothyroidism, alcoholism, uncontrolled diabetes mellitus, kidney disorders, pregnancy, and medications, should be thoroughly investigated and treated if diagnosed.
- Possibility of familial hyperlipidemia based on the lipid profile, family history, and physical examination should be considered because cardiovascular risk can be underestimated and treatment can be challenging.

CURRENT THERAPY

- Therapy should be guided by goals of treatment based on estimated cardiovascular risk unless triglyceride (TG) level is 500 mg/dL or greater, in which case lowering TG to prevent acute pancreatitis is a priority.
- Low-density lipoprotein cholesterol (LDL-C) is a primary target, followed by non–high-density lipoprotein cholesterol (non-HDL-C) as a secondary target, with individualized goals dictated by ASCVD risk assessment (see Table 2). TG has also emerged as a target to further reduce residual cardiovascular risk in select patients with high cardiovascular risk.
- A healthy lifestyle is encouraged for all individuals to reduce risk of atherosclerotic cardiovascular disease (ASCVD). Lifestyle therapy is especially indicated for patients with hyperlipidemia.
- Weight loss is the most effective lifestyle intervention for hypertriglyceridemia and metabolic syndrome. For patients with severe hypertriglyceridemia (TG ≥ 500 mg/dL), a low-fat or very-low-fat diet should be initiated for prevention of pancreatitis.
- Statins are the cornerstone of cholesterol-lowering therapies, with proven efficacy for both primary and secondary prevention of ASCVD; the intensity of statin therapy should be dictated by the degree of cardiovascular risk.
- Nonstatin therapies for LDL-C lowering can be added to maximally tolerated doses of statins to achieve further cholesterol lowering, as indicated by the patient's ASCVD risk.
- Icosapent ethyl (Vascepa) can be added to statin therapy for patients with high TG levels and either established ASCVD or diabetes with additional cardiovascular risks for further reduction of residual ASCVD risk.
- All other cardiovascular risk factors should be treated aggressively at the same time.

Hyperlipidemia is a condition of elevated serum lipids and lipoproteins. Hyperlipidemia is associated with an increased risk of atherosclerotic cardiovascular disease (ASCVD) and, if triglyceride (TG) level is greater than 500 mg/dL, pancreatitis. The primary goals of management of hyperlipidemia are to decrease the risk of ASCVD and pancreatitis. ASCVD, as defined by the *2018 Multisociety Guideline on the Management of Blood Cholesterol*, encompasses acute coronary syndrome; history of myocardial infarction; stable or unstable angina; coronary or other arterial revascularization; stroke; transient ischemic attack; or peripheral arterial disease, including aortic aneurysm; all of atherosclerotic origin. ASCVD is the leading cause of mortality in the United States. Consumption of low-density lipoprotein cholesterol (LDL-C) by vascular macrophages plays a central role in the development of atherosclerosis, and it is well established in epidemiology, genetics, and clinical studies that lower LDL-C levels are closely associated with fewer ASCVD events in a linear relationship, as summarized by the mantra "lower is better." Appropriate treatment of hyperlipidemia is therefore essential in patients with established cardiovascular disease (secondary prevention), whereas detection and treatment of hyperlipidemia are guided by the risk of ASCVD in patients without known clinical ASCVD (primary prevention).

The prevalence of hyperlipidemia varies with the definition of hyperlipidemia and the population studied. The percentage of U.S. adults with a total cholesterol level of 240 mg/dL or higher declined from 19% to 14% in men and from 21% to 15% in women from 1988 to 2008. This may be in part due to increased use of lipid-lowering medications, from 3.4% to 15.5%. However, major risk factors for cardiovascular disease actually have become more common: the prevalence of obesity (body mass index $\geq$ 30 kg/m^2) increased from 19.9% to 31.6% in men and from 25.2% to 34.1% in women, and the prevalence of diabetes increased from 5.5% to 11.1% in men and from 4.6% to 6.3% in women over this period. Therefore optimal treatment of hyperlipidemia to reduce cardiovascular risk is of paramount importance.

Various societies and professional organizations have published clinical guidelines for hyperlipidemia. The *2018 Multisociety Guideline on the Management of Blood Cholesterol* is widely endorsed by physician societies in the United States, whereas in Europe, the *2019 European Society of Cardiology and European Atherosclerosis Society (ESC/EAS) Guidelines for the Management of Dyslipidaemias* is the most influential. The two are largely consistent but with notable differences. We mostly adhere to the 2018 Multisociety guideline and incorporate updates in more recent American guidelines, especially the *2021 ACC Expert Consensus Decision Pathway (ECDP) on the Management of ASCVD Risk Reduction in Patients With Persistent Hypertriglyceridemia,* the *2022 ACC ECDP on the Role of Nonstatin Therapies for LDL-Cholesterol Lowering in the Management of Atherosclerotic Cardiovascular Disease Risk,* and recent results of randomized clinical trials yet to be covered in current guidelines.

Pathophysiology

Lipids have two main points of entry into the circulation: the gut (exogenous pathway) and the liver (endogenous pathway). The exogenous and endogenous pathways are interconnected by intermediate pathways (reverse cholesterol transport pathway and others). These pathways are outlined in Figure 1.

Exogenous Pathway

Lipids in food are emulsified by bile acids and then hydrolyzed into fatty acids and cholesterol by pancreatic lipases in the intestinal lumen. Inside the intestinal cells, fatty acids and cholesterol are reesterified and then packaged with apolipoprotein (Apo) B48 into chylomicrons. Chylomicrons are secreted into the intestinal

lymph and delivered to the systemic circulation. At peripheral tissues, TGs are hydrolyzed by lipoprotein lipase (LPL). Released free fatty acids are then taken up for further metabolism or storage. Chylomicron remnants are taken up by the liver via the chylomicron remnant receptors. LPL plays a central role in clearance of both exogenous and endogenous TGs. A deficiency of LPL is the main cause of familial hyperchylomicronemia. It is regulated by insulin and thyroid hormone. A deficiency of insulin or thyroid hormone in uncontrolled diabetes mellitus and hypothyroidism, respectively, leads to secondary hypertriglyceridemia. Apo CII is an essential cofactor for LPL, while Apo CIII and secreted glycoproteins angiopoietin-like 3 (ANGPLT3) and angiopoietin-like 4 (ANGPLT4) are known inhibitors.

Endogenous Pathway

The endogenous pathway begins in the liver with the synthesis of TG-rich very-low-density lipoproteins (VLDLs). Microsomal triglyceride transfer protein (MTP) facilitates the transfer of lipids onto Apo B100 and stabilizes the protein for secretion as VLDLs. VLDLs, as chylomicrons, undergo lipolysis by LPL, releasing free fatty acids, generating smaller particles called intermediate-density lipoproteins (IDLs, also known as VLDL remnants). IDLs are either removed by the liver or further processed into cholesterol-rich LDLs. LDLs are taken up into the liver or other cells via LDL receptors (LDLRs), a process regulated by cellular cholesterol requirement. Therefore inhibition of cholesterol synthesis leads to increased expression of LDLR at the cell surface and clearance of LDL-C, which is the major mechanism of action of statins and bempedoic acid (Nexletol) for lowering cholesterol. A secreted protease known as proprotein convertase subtilisin/kexin type 9 (PCSK9) binds to cell surface LDLR and promotes the latter's destruction in lysosome by preventing it from recycling to the cell membrane.

Macrophages in the arterial wall can also take up LDLs via the scavenger receptors and become foam cells. Foamy macrophages play a key role in the development of atherosclerosis. Recent research has further suggested that the precursors of macrophages, monocytes, can also uptake lipoprotein particles in circulation and transform into foamy monocytes, which may also play a role in atherogenesis.

Reverse Cholesterol Transport

High-density lipoproteins (HDLs) are the major lipoproteins involved in the transport of cholesterol from peripheral tissues back to the liver. HDLs are synthesized by both the hepatocytes and the enterocytes in the form of small discoidal particles containing Apo AI and phospholipids. HDLs acquire additional lipids and apolipoproteins from TG-depleted chylomicrons and VLDL remnants. HDLs remove free cholesterol from tissues with the help of Apo AI and esterify it with lecithin cholesterol acyltransferase. Cholesteryl esters are then transferred to Apo B 100-containing lipoproteins (VLDLs, IDLs, and LDLs) by cholesteryl ester transfer protein (CETP). HDLs can also be taken up directly by the liver class B type I scavenger receptors.

Plasma Lipids and Atherosclerosis

Multiple studies have shown that total cholesterol and LDL-C levels contribute to cardiovascular disease risk and that lowering of total cholesterol and LDL-C levels reduces the risk. Non–HDL-C (i.e., total cholesterol – HDL-C = VLDL + IDL + LDL-C) reflects total atherogenic lipoprotein burden and may be a better risk indicator than LDL-C, especially in people with combined hyperlipidemia, diabetes, metabolic syndrome, and chronic kidney disease. Table 1 shows the classification of lipid profile.

Recent mendelian randomization studies have suggested that TG-rich lipoproteins, including chylomicrons, VLDLs, and their remnants, also have a causal relationship with ASCVD. Therefore not only does hypertriglyceridemia represent an independent cardiovascular risk marker, but it is also a significant risk factor and a target for therapy. Currently available TG-lowering therapies vary greatly in efficacy for reducing ASCVD. Although there is no

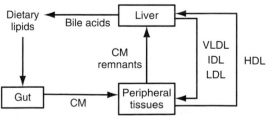

Figure 1 Overview of exogenous and endogenous pathways of lipid metabolism. *CM,* Chylomicrons; *HDL,* high-density lipoproteins; *IDL,* intermediate-density lipoproteins; *LDL,* low-density lipoproteins; *VLDL,* very-low-density lipoproteins.

TABLE 1	Classification of LDL, Total Cholesterol, HDL-C, and Triglycerides (mg/dL)
LDL-C (mg/dL)	
<100	Optimal
100–129	Near optimal/above optimal
130–159	Borderline high
160–189	High
≥190	Very high
Total Cholesterol (mg/dL)	
<200	Desirable
200–239	Borderline high
≥240	High
HDL-C (mg/dL)	
<40	Low
≥60	High
Triglycerides (mg/dL)	
<150	Normal
150–199	Borderline high
200–499	High
≥500	Very high

Based on the National Cholesterol Education Program Adult Treatment Panel III guidelines.

HDL-C, High-density lipoprotein cholesterol; *LCL*, low-density lipoprotein; *LDL-C*, low-density lipoprotein cholesterol.

evidence supporting niacin, fibrates (gemfibrozil and fenofibrate), or regular omega-3 fish oil (eicosapentaenoic acid [EPA] and docosahexaenoic acid [DHA]) in preventing ASCVD, icosapent ethyl (Vascepa), which is an EPA-only omega-3 acid ethyl ester, is able to reduce ASCVD in patients with elevated TG and heightened ASCVD risk; however, the cardioprotective effect is not correlated with the degree of TG lowering. Therefore the exact role of TG in contributing to ASCVD remains to be defined.

It is significant that mendelian randomization studies suggest that HDL-C does not have a causal relationship with ASCVD. Moreover, medications that increase HDL-C (i.e., niacin and CETP inhibitors) have largely failed to show efficacy in ASCVD risk reduction in randomized clinical trials. Therefore although HDL-C was shown to be inversely associated with cardiovascular risk, the mechanism of the relationship between HDL-C and ASCVD is not fully understood. Importantly, ASCVD cannot be viewed as a disease caused solely by a lipid disorder; rather, it is the result of a complex interplay between dyslipidemia, metabolic derangements, inflammation, and endothelial dysfunction. For instance, even mildly elevated TGs (≥150 mg/dL) can suggest metabolic syndrome, an important risk factor for cardiovascular disease. Meanwhile, chronic systemic inflammation was shown to accelerate atherogenesis, and therapies that target inflammation have been demonstrated in clinical trials to reduce the risk for ASCVD.

Additionally, the level of lipoprotein (a) [Lp(a)] is progressively associated with ASCVD risk. A mendelian randomization study suggested that elevation of Lp(a) is an independent causal risk factor. It is considered a risk-enhancing factor for ASCVD if greater than 50 mg/dL. Lp(a) is a special type of LDL, with apoB conjugated with apolipoprotein (a) [apo(a)]. Apo(a) is structurally similar to plasminogen and promotes atherosclerosis and thrombosis. The Lp(a) level is mostly determined genetically (e.g., with polymorphism of the apo[a] gene). Lifetime exposure to severely elevated Lp(a) levels can lead to premature ASCVD.

Pharmacologic treatments (PCSK9 inhibitors and niacin) and lipoprotein apheresis can effectively lower Lp(a), though niacin has no proven cardiovascular benefits. It remains to be determined whether PCSK9 inhibitors and lipoprotein apheresis lower ASCVD risk via lowering Lp(a).

Plasma Lipid and Pancreatitis

Hypertriglyceridemia is the third most common cause of acute pancreatitis. In addition, acute pancreatitis associated with hypertriglyceridemia is often more severe. The risk of acute pancreatitis is progressively increased when the TG level is greater than 500 mg/dL and especially so when it is greater than 1000 mg/dL. The exact mechanism whereby severe hypertriglyceridemia triggers pancreatitis is poorly understood but is thought to be related to proinflammatory effects of fatty acids released by pancreatic lipase.

Evaluation

Global Cardiovascular Risk Assessment

Risk assessment is an integral part in the evaluation of patients with hyperlipidemia. Contemporary guidelines from the United States provide detailed algorithms for risk stratification. The 2013 and 2018 cholesterol guidelines identified four subgroups of patients for whom the benefits of statin therapy outweigh the risk. Secondary prevention patients are automatically considered to be at high risk for recurrent ASCVD events and, thus, would necessitate initiation of lipid-lowering therapy. In the 2018 Multisociety guideline, secondary prevention patients may be further stratified into those at very high risk and those at not very high risk for ASCVD, based on the presence or absence of high-risk features. The value of further delineating risk among secondary prevention patients was, in part, to facilitate the evidence-based use of newer nonstatin therapies (i.e., ezetimibe [Zetia],[1] bempedoic acid [Nexletol], and PCSK9 inhibitors).

Among primary prevention patients, a history of diabetes mellitus or significantly elevated LDL-C (≥190 mg/dL) signifying a likely genetic cause of hypercholesterolemia automatically warrants initiation of lipid-lowering therapy. In primary prevention patients with hyperlipidemia but without these two high-risk features, a global cardiovascular risk score can be used to further stratify a patient. Global risk scores estimate 10-year cardiovascular risk, which combines the effects of well-known risk factors, using one of several risk-calculation tools. Individual tools have been developed based on large epidemiology studies examining a limited number of available risk factors. Traditional risk factors such as age, sex, cigarette smoking, cholesterol, diabetes, and blood pressure are able to predict 80% to 90% of the cardiovascular events in people 40 years or older. However, these tools may not accurately estimate cardiovascular risk in individuals with unaccounted risk factors or those with demographics distinct from the populations used to derive the risk scores. The risk score most commonly used (and endorsed by guidelines) in the United States is the Pooled Cohort Equation (PCE). The PCE is used to estimate a 10-year risk for ASCVD for men and women aged 40 to 79 years of White or Black race, incorporating age, sex, race, HDL and total cholesterol, diabetes, hypertension, and smoking status (https://tools.acc.org/ascvd-risk-estimator-plus/). The 2018 Multisociety guidelines recommend the initiation of statin therapy in patients with intermediate (≥7.5% to <20%) and high (≥20%) 10-year ASCVD risk, with consideration of statins even in select patients with borderline 10-year risk (5% to <7.5%). Of note, the risk stratification system used by the European guidelines, known as the Systematic COronary Risk Evaluation (SCORE) algorithm, considers similar risk factors but gives an estimate of 10-year cardiovascular mortality (www.heartscore.org).

---

[1] Not FDA approved for this indication.

Risk-Enhancing Factors

As the PCE does not consider risk factors with smaller population effect, the 2013 guideline and the 2018 Multisociety guideline recommend that individuals with borderline to intermediate ASCVD risk based on the PCE be assessed for additional risk-enhancing factors (Table 2). These risk enhancers, when present, significantly increase cardiovascular risk in affected individuals. The Endocrine Society's *Clinical Practice Guidelines on Lipid Management for Patients With Endocrine Disorders* describes additional risk-enhancing factors to consider (Table 2). Presence of these factors in patients with borderline and intermediate 10-year ASCVD risks would favor initiating statin therapy. Additionally, some of these risk-enhancing factors are themselves treatable targets (e.g., hypothyroidism and hypertriglyceridemia).

Risk Reclassifying With Coronary Artery Calcium Score

If the decision to initiate LDL-C–lowering therapy remains uncertain after ASCVD risk assessment (e.g., in patients with borderline to intermediate ASCVD risk), measuring a coronary artery calcium (CAC) score is recommended by the 2018 and later

---

TABLE 2 Risk Groups and Treatment Goals (*2018 Multisociety Blood Cholesterol Guidelines, 2021 ACC ECDP on Persistent Hypertriglyceridemia,* and *2022 ACC ECDP on Nonstatin Therapies*)

	RISK CATEGORY	RECOMMENDED STATIN THERAPY TO INITIATE	TREATMENT GOAL	NONSTATIN THERAPY
Secondary Prevention	Very high risk*	High-intensity statin	LDL-C reduction ≥ 50%, LDL-C < 55 mg/dL, non-HDL-C < 85 mg/dL	Ezetimibe PCSK9 mAbs Bempedoic acid Inclisiran Icosapent ethyl[†]
	Not very high risk	High-intensity statin	LDL-C reduction ≥ 50%, LDL-C < 70 mg/dL, non-HDL-C < 100 mg/dL	Ezetimibe PCSK9 mAbs Bempedoic acid Inclisiran Icosapent ethyl[†]
Primary Prevention	LDL-C ≥190 mg/dL	High-intensity statin	LDL-C reduction ≥ 50%, LDL-C < 100 mg/dL, non-HDL-C < 130 mg/dL	Ezetimibe PCSK9 inhibitors Bempedoic acid Inclisiran
	Diabetes mellitus	Moderate-intensity statin if 10-year ASCVD risk‡ < 7.5%	LDL-C reduction ≥ 30–49%, LDL-C < 100 mg/dL, non-HDL-C < 130 mg/dL	Ezetimibe after escalating to high-intensity statin
	Diabetes mellitus	High-intensity statin if 10-year ASCVD risk ≥ 7.5–20%, diabetes specific risk enhancers present§, or subclinical atherosclerosis present	LDL-C reduction ≥ 50%, LDL-C < 100 mg/dL, non-HDL-C < 130 mg/dL	Ezetimibe Icosapent ethyl[†]
	Diabetes mellitus	High-intensity statin if 10-year ASCVD risk ≥ 20%	LDL-C reduction ≥ 50%, LDL-C < 70 mg/dL, non-HDL-C < 100 mg/dL	Ezetimibe Icosapent ethyl[†]
	High risk (10- year ASCVD risk ≥ 20%)	High-intensity statin	LDL-C reduction ≥ 50%, LDL-C < 70 mg/dL, non-HDL-C < 100 mg/dL	Ezetimibe
	Intermediate risk (10-year ASCVD risk ≥ 7.5–20%)	If risk enhancers‖ present or if CAC score elevated, should initiate moderate intensity statin	LDL-C reduction ≥ 30–49%, LDL-C < 100 mg/dL, non-HDL-C < 130 mg/dL	
	Borderline risk (10-year ASCVD risk 5% to <7.5%)	If risk enhancers present, then may consider moderate intensity statin	LDL-C reduction ≥ 30–49%, LDL-C < 100 mg/dL, non-HDL-C < 130 mg/dL	
	Low risk (10-year ASCVD risk <5%)	Statin deferred		

*Very high risk defined by a history of multiple major ASCVD events or at least one major ASCVD event plus multiple high-risk conditions (age ≥65 years, heterozygous familial hypercholesterolemia, history of coronary bypass surgery or percutaneous coronary intervention outside of the major ASCVD events, diabetes mellitus, hypertension, chronic kidney disease, current smoking, persistently elevated LDL-C ≥100 mg/dL despite maximally tolerated statin and ezetimibe, or history of congestive heart failure).

†If persistent fasting TG ≥ 150 mg/dL with history of ASCVD or diabetes mellitus with age ≥ 50 years with additional high-risk features.

‡10-year ASCVD risk as estimated by the Pooled Cohort Equation.

§Diabetes-specific risk enhancers include long duration of disease (type 2 ≥ 10 years; type 1 ≥ 20 years), albuminuria ≥ 30 mcg of albumin/mg creatinine, eGFR < 60 mL/min/1.73 m², retinopathy, neuropathy, and ankle-brachial index <0.9.

‖Risk enhancers include family history of premature ASCVD, chronic kidney disease, metabolic syndrome, inflammatory disease, conditions specific to women (i.e., preeclampsia, premature menopause), ethnicity (i.e., South Asian ancestry), persistently elevated LDL-C ≥160 mg/dL, persistently elevated TGs (≥175 mg/dL), high sensitivity C-reactive protein ≥2.0 mg/L, lipoprotein (a) ≥50 mg/dL or 125 nmol/L, apolipoprotein B ≥130 mg/dL, and ankle-brachial index <0.9. The Endocrine Society recognizes endocrine disorders, including persistent Cushing syndrome and Cushing disease, high-dose chronic glucocorticoid therapy, adult growth hormone deficiency, acromegaly, and hypothyroidism, as additional risk enhancers.

ACC ECDP, American College of Cardiology Expert Consensus Decision Pathway; *ASCVD,* atherosclerotic cardiovascular disease; *CAC,* coronary artery calcium; *eGFR,* estimated glomerular filtration rate; *LDL-C,* low-density lipoprotein cholesterol; *non–HDL-C,* non–high-density lipoprotein cholesterol; *PCSK9,* proprotein convertase subtilisin/kexin type 9.

guidelines to reclassify the patient's risk. A CAC score is an indicator of total burden of calcified plaques in coronary arteries as measured by computed tomography. A CAC score of 0 Agatston unit (AU) can downclassify the patient to low risk and justify deferral of statin therapy. A score of 100 AU or greater or in the 75th percentile or greater up-classifies borderline risk patients to intermediate risk, warranting moderate intensity statins. A score between 1 and 99 AU would justify moderate intensity statin treatment for patients above 55 years old. A score of 300 AU or greater upclassifies patients to the high-risk category, justifying initiation or intensification to high-intensity statins.

Measurement of Lipid Profiles

Lipid profiles should be measured as a part of global risk assessment, and the frequency of checkup is determined by age, sex, and risk factors for cardiovascular disease. In patients on lipid-lowering therapy, a lipid panel should be performed after initiation or dose change in therapy; it should also be performed periodically in patients on stable therapy to assess treatment efficacy and medication adherence.

A fasting lipid profile (fasting for 8 to 12 hours) ensures the most accurate lipid assessment, specifically of TGs (and subsequently LDL-C, if calculated using the Friedewald equation), but is inconvenient for patients. A strict requirement for fasting may become a barrier to timely risk assessments for many patients. Nonfasting lipid profile is accurate for total cholesterol, HDL-C, Apo B, and Apo AI. Recent studies show that differences in TG levels according to fasting time are small; thus calculated LDL-C is often minimally affected in nonfasting samples. Therefore, a nonfasting lipid panel has been accepted by the 2018 Multisociety guideline and other recent guidelines as an option for initial screening or establishing an LDL-C baseline before starting statin treatment, unless a previous lipid panel showed a TG level greater than 400 mg/dL. A fasting lipid profile is still recommended for monitoring adherence to lipid-lowering therapies and identifying cases of metabolic syndrome, severe hypertriglyceridemia, and genetic lipid disorders, including a family history of premature ASCVD.

LDL-C can either be calculated or measured directly. The standard method used to derive LDL-C from other components of the lipid panel is the Friedewald equation (LDL-C = total cholesterol – HDL-C – TG/5), in which TG/5 is used to calculate VLDL cholesterol (VLDL-C). This equation should be used with appropriate caution: it becomes less accurate if TG is 200 mg/dL or greater; it becomes invalid with TG of 400 mg/dL or greater. LDL-C can be underestimated at levels less than 70 mg/dL. A new method, the Martin-Hopkins equation, was found to be more accurate when TGs are between 150 and 400 mg/dL and when non-HDL-C is low. Instead of a fixed factor of 5, as in the Friedewald equation, the Martin-Hopkins method uses an adjustable factor for TG:VLDL-C ratio. When the TG is greater than 400 mg/dL, an enzymatic assay is available to directly measure LDL-C.

Outside the standard lipid profile, the 2018 Multisociety guideline also considered Apo B and Lp(a) as relatively indicated in assessment of ASCVD risk in select populations. The Apo B level reflects the number of atherogenic lipoprotein particles but measurement is limited by expense and test accuracy. Because the Apo B level is strongly associated with the non-HDL-C level in most situations, it does not seem to add to diagnostic value except in patients with elevated TG levels (≥200 mg/dL). In patients with a family history of premature ASCVD or with personal ASCVD not explained by traditional risk factors, testing of Lp(a) may be considered.

Other medical conditions may also affect lipid profiles. Secondary causes include hypothyroidism, nephrotic syndrome, dysgammaglobulinemia, use of progestin (especially those with androgenic activity), cholestasis, use of protease inhibitors, chronic kidney disease, uncontrolled diabetes, obesity, excessive alcohol intake, use of thiazide or β-blockers, use of corticosteroids, use of oral estrogen (not transdermal), and pregnancy. These conditions should be detected and treated, if appropriate, to improve control of hyperlipidemia.

Family history of premature cardiovascular disease and hyperlipidemia and physical findings such as xanthomas, xanthelasmas, and premature arcus cornealis may suggest familial hypercholesterolemia. As the risk for ASCVD associated with very elevated levels of atherogenic lipoproteins begins to accumulate very early in life, patients with familial hypercholesterolemia should be treated aggressively.

Treatment

Overview

Treatment is primarily aimed at lowering LDL-C level, which has been shown to decrease the risk of cardiovascular disease in numerous randomized clinical trials and metaanalyses. Every reduction of LDL-C of 1 mmol/L (~39 mg/dL) is associated with an approximate 22% reduction in cardiovascular risk. The absolute risk reduction by lowering LDL-C is proportional to the global cardiovascular risk; therefore patients with higher baseline LDL-C levels and higher ASCVD risks stand to reap the most benefits in starting lipid-lowering therapy early and adequately. In patients with severe hypertriglyceridemia (i.e., TG ≥ 500 mg/dL and especially ≥ 1000 mg/dL), TG should be treated to less than 500 mg/dL to prevent acute pancreatitis.

Treatment Targets

The 2013 ACC/AHA guideline departed from the traditions of previous lipid guidelines by not setting hard LDL-C targets and, instead, emphasizing percentage reduction of LDL-C as a primary goal and the use of statins of corresponding strength. In short, the desired LDL-C reduction from baseline is 50% or greater, with high-potency statin for secondary prevention, and between 30% and 49% for primary prevention with moderate-intensity statins, except for patients with higher 10-year ASCVD risk.

Since then, additional nonstatin therapies have become available. In particular, cardiovascular outcome trials for PCSK9 inhibitors show that cardiovascular risk progressively decreases as LDL-C levels are reduced to the lowest achievable level (i.e., <25 mg/dL) without any notable harm. As such, the principle of "lower is better" has been validated for all levels of LDL-C. Considering these findings, the 2018 Multisociety guideline introduced LDL-C thresholds for adding nonstatin therapies for secondary prevention patients with or without high-risk features. The 2022 ACC ECDP for Nonstatin Therapies further lowered these thresholds for secondary prevention patients and set LDL-C thresholds for primary prevention patients as well.

The treatment goals and approaches according to the 2018 Multisociety Cholesterol Guidelines, 2021 ACC ECDP on Hypertriglyceridemia, and 2022 ACC ECDP on Nonstatin Therapies are summarized in Table 2. Briefly, these guidelines recognize three separate goals for LDL-C–lowering treatment for different risk groups, including percentage reduction, LDL-C level, and non–HDL-C level. Moderate- and high-intensity statins are the first-line treatment options. Different nonstatin therapies for LDL-C and TG lowering can be added after maximally tolerated statins fail to achieve appropriate goals for the respective risk group.

Lifestyle Therapy

The 2018 Multisociety guideline strongly recommended that all individuals, regardless of lipid status, assume a heart-healthy lifestyle. As accumulative exposure to atherogenic lipoproteins since childhood increases lifetime risk of ASCVD, lifestyle interventions should be initiated as early as possible. Dietary modification to limit intake of lipids is an essential component given that the main source of lipids is dietary fat. Saturated fatty acids and trans unsaturated fatty acids increase LDL-C, whereas dietary fibers and phytosterols decrease LDL-C. Carbohydrates do not affect LDL-C but increase TGs and decrease HDL-C, particularly if they have a high glycemic index. Intake of fructose, a component of sucrose, increases TGs and decreases HDL-C. Body weight reduction, increasing physical activity, and avoidance of a sedentary lifestyle have a small effect on LDL-C, but they reduce TGs, increase HDL-C, and are associated with improved

TABLE 3	Lifestyle Therapy for Persistent Hypertriglyceridemia (2021 ACC ECDP on Persistent Hypertriglyceridemia)		
	TG < 500 mg/dL	TG 500–999 mg/dL	TG ≥ 1000 mg/dL
Added sugars (% calories)	< 6%	< 5%	Eliminate
Total fat (% calories)	30–35%	20–25%	10–15%
Alcohol	Restrict	Eliminate	Eliminate
Aerobic activity	At least 150 minutes of moderate intensity or 75 minutes of vigorous intensity aerobic activity each week, or equivalent combinations of both		
Weight loss (% of body weight)	5%–10% weight loss		

ACC ECDP, American College of Cardiology Expert Consensus Decision Pathway; TG, triglycerides.

cardiovascular outcome. Alcohol intake has an adverse effect on TGs and therefore should be restricted or avoided in patients with hypertriglyceridemia. Moderate alcohol drinking is associated with higher HDL-C levels, but there is no evidence that any amount of alcohol is cardioprotective.

Individual patients will need different approaches based on their cardiovascular risk and lipid profiles. Generally, total dietary fat is recommended to constitute 25% to 35% of the total calorie intake, mainly as mono- or polyunsaturated fat, limiting saturated fats to less than 7% and trans fats to less than 1% of the total calorie intake. Therapeutic lifestyle changes for lowering LDL-C include diets with emphasis on vegetables, fruits, whole grains, low-fat dairy products, poultry, fish, legumes, nontropical vegetable oils, and nuts, as well as limited intake of sweets, sugar-sweetened beverages, and red meats; further reduction of saturated fats (<5% to 6% of the total caloric intake) and avoidance of trans fats; weight reduction; and increased regular physical activity. The amount of cholesterol intake is not well correlated with LDL-C level, and there is no recommended limit for intake. Management of other risk factors, such as smoking cessation and controlling blood pressure in hypertensive patients and blood glucose in diabetics, is also very important.

With severe hypertriglyceridemia (TG ≥ 500 mg/dL), the capacity of plasma LPL becomes saturated; further fat intake would significantly raise TG level even higher and potentially precipitate acute pancreatitis. Therefore it is important to start a low-fat or very-low-fat diet in patients with severe hypertriglyceridemia. Alcohol and added sugars should be avoided as well. Weight loss is considered the single most effective lifestyle therapy for persistent hypertriglyceridemia and metabolic syndrome and may lead to a 50% to 70% reduction of TG level in the long term. The 2021 ACC ECDP on Persistent Hypertriglyceridemia made specific recommendations regarding lifestyle therapies for persistent hypertriglyceridemia based on the TG levels, as outlined in Table 3.

Pharmacologic Agents

The currently available lipid-lowering agents can be classified based on their mechanism of action. Statins (3-hydroxy-3-methylglutaryl coenzyme A [HMG-CoA] reductase inhibitors), ezetimibe, bempedoic acid, PCSK9 inhibitors, bile acid sequestrants, MTP inhibitor, and ANGPLT3 inhibitor are used primarily to reduce LDL-C. Fibrates, niacin, and omega-3 fatty acid prescriptions are used primarily for the treatment of hypertriglyceridemia. These classes of agents differ with regard to degree and type of lipid lowering, and agents within the same group may differ in efficacy and side effects. Conventional dosing regimens and common adverse effects are summarized in Table 4. Expected changes in lipid profiles are shown in Table 5. The choice of drug depends on the specific lipid abnormalities, the patient's tolerability to the medication, and concurrent medical conditions. In general, statins are the most effective drugs to lower cardiovascular risk and are the treatment of choice when medications are indicated based on the global cardiovascular risk. If the treatment goal is not achieved by statins or statins are not tolerated, other validated nonstatin therapies (ezetimibe, bempedoic acid, and PCSK9 inhibitors) may be considered, followed by other agents such as bile acid sequestrants. If the primary goal is to lower TGs, fibrates, omega-3 fatty acids, or niacin may be more effective.

Statins

Statins are usually the first drug of choice in patients with high cholesterol levels to reduce cardiovascular risk and have been validated in multiple randomized controlled trials and their meta-analyses. Furthermore, risk reduction was apparent in a wide range of patients in both primary and secondary prevention; in men and women, smokers, patients with diabetes; and those with hypertension. In general, statins result in a high degree of LDL-C reduction. The approximate equipotent dosages of various statins and their cholesterol-lowering effects are listed in Table 6. The 2013 and 2018 cholesterol guidelines recommend moderate- or high-intensity statins (see Table 6) based on the global risk. Statins inhibit HMG-CoA reductase, the rate-limiting enzyme in cholesterol biosynthesis. By blocking cholesterol biosynthesis, statins upregulate the LDLR on the hepatocytes and increase clearance of IDL and LDL. In addition to their direct effects on lipid metabolism, statins have been reported to have pleiotropic effects (e.g., reduced formation of reactive oxygen species, inhibition of platelet reactivity, and decreased vasoconstriction).

Statins are usually well tolerated. Potential common side effects include myopathy, fatigue, headaches, and nonspecific gastrointestinal symptoms such as dyspepsia. Elevation of liver enzymes occurs in less than 1%. There is also a small but significant association with increase in risk of developing diabetes. Myopathy is one of the most common causes for cessation of statins. Myalgia can occur in about 10% to 20% of patients, which is much more often than reported in the clinical trials. The risk of rhabdomyolysis, however, is very low (0.1 to 0.2 per 1000 person-years). Risk for myopathy is increased in patients with advanced age, female sex, small body habitus, hypothyroidism, alcoholism, vitamin D deficiency, medical conditions (particularly liver or kidney disease), major surgery, excessive physical activity, history of myopathy, family history of myopathy, high-dose statins, and interacting medications or food such as grapefruit juice (>1 L/day). Simvastatin (Zocor), lovastatin (Mevacor), and atorvastatin (Lipitor) are primarily metabolized through CYP3A4, which is inhibited by protease inhibitors, cyclosporine (Neoral, Sandimmune), amiodarone (Cordarone, Pacerone), nondihydropyridine calcium channel blockers, fibrates, and other agents. Pravastatin (Pravachol) is metabolized by the kidney, not by the P450 system. Fluvastatin (Lescol) and rosuvastatin (Crestor) are primarily metabolized through CYP2C9. Pitavastatin (Livalo) is marginally metabolized by CYP2C9 and to a lesser extent by CYP2C8. Simvastatin and lovastatin should be avoided in patients receiving protease inhibitors. Statin dosage should be reduced in patients taking cyclosporine. Because of significant risk of myopathy and rhabdomyolysis related to high-dose simvastatin, the U.S. Food and Drug Administration (FDA) recommends that 80 mg/day should not be used. The FDA further recommends that the dose be limited to 20 mg if the patient is also taking amiodarone,

TABLE 4	Major Drugs for Management of Hyperlipidemia				
AGENT	**STARTING DAILY DOSAGE**	**DOSAGE RANGE**	**MECHANISM**	**SIDE EFFECTS**
Statins				
Lovastatin (Mevacor)	20 mg	10–80 mg	Decreased cholesterol synthesis, increased hepatic LDL receptors, decreased VLDL release	Myalgias, arthralgias, high liver enzymes, dyspepsia
Pravastatin (Pravachol)	40 mg	10–80 mg		
Simvastatin (Zocor)	20–40 mg	5–40 mg		
Fluvastatin (Lescol)	40 mg	20–80 mg		
Atorvastatin (Lipitor)	10–20 mg	10–80 mg		
Rosuvastatin (Crestor)	10 mg	5–40 mg		
Pitavastatin (Livalo)	2 mg	2–4 mg		
Cholesterol Absorption Inhibitors				
Ezetimibe (Zetia)	10 mg	10 mg	Deceased intestinal cholesterol absorption	High liver enzymes
Combination Therapies (Single Pill)				
Ezetimibe/Simvastatin (Vytorin)	10/20 mg	10/10–10/40 mg		
ATP Citrate Lyase Inhibitor				
Bempedoic acid (Nexletol)	180 mg		Inhibit cholesterol synthesis, increase LDLR and cholesterol clearance	Uric acid level increase, gout, tendon rupture
Combination Therapies (Single Pill)				
Bempedoic acid/Ezetimibe (Nexlizet)	180/10 mg			
PCSK9 Inhibiting Monoclonal Antibodies (Subcutaneous)				
Alirocumab (Praluent)	75 mg every 2 weeks	75–150 mg every 2 weeks	Increased hepatic LDL receptors	Injection site reactions, nasopharyngitis, upper respiratory tract infection, influenza, back pain
Evolocumab (Repatha)		140 mg every 2 weeks or 420 mg monthly		
PCSK9 Inhibiting siRNA (Subcutaneous)				
Inclisiran (Leqvio)	284 mg at baseline and 3 months, then every 6 months		Increased hepatic LDL receptors	Injection site reactions, arthralgia, bronchitis
ANGPLT3 Inhibiting Monoclonal Antibody (Intravenous Infusion)				
Evinacumab (Evkeeza)	15 mg/kg every 4 weeks		Inhibiting LPL and endothelial lipase	Nasopharyngitis, dizziness
Bile Acid Sequestrants				
Cholestyramine (Questran)	8–16 g	4–24 g	Increased bile acid excretion, increased LDL receptors	Bloating, constipation, elevated TGs
Colestipol (Colestid)	2 g	2–16 g		
Colesevelam (Welchol)	3.75 g	3.75 g		
Fibrates				
Fenofibrate (Tricor)	48–145 mg	48–145 mg	Increased LPL activity, decreased VLDL synthesis	Dyspepsia, myalgia, gallstones, high liver enzymes
Gemfibrozil (Lopid)	1200 mg	1200 mg		
Fenofibric acid (Trilipix)	45–135 mg	45–135 mg		
Niacin				
Immediate release	250 mg	250–3000 mg	Decreased VLDL synthesis	Flushing, high glucose, uric acid, high liver enzymes
Extended release (Niaspan)	500 mg	500–2000 mg		

Continued

TABLE 4 · Major Drugs for Management of Hyperlipidemia—cont'd

AGENT	STARTING DAILY DOSAGE	DOSAGE RANGE	MECHANISM	SIDE EFFECTS
Omega-3 Fatty Acid Prescriptions				
Icosapent ethyl (Vascepa)	4 g	4 g		Arthralgia, atrial fibrillation, lower extremity edema
Omega-3 fatty acid ethyl esters (Lovaza)	4 g	4 g		Eructation, dyspepsia, and taste perversion

ATP, Adenosine triphosphate; *LDL*, low-density lipoprotein; *LDLR*, low-density lipoprotein receptor; *PCSK9*, proprotein convertase subtilisin/kexin type 9; *TG*, triglycerides; *VLDL*, very-low-density lipoprotein.

TABLE 5 · Metabolic Effects of Each Lipid-Lowering Drug Class

	LDL-C	HDL-C	TGs
Statins	↓ 21%–55%	↑ 2%–10%	↓ 6%–30%
Fibric acids	↓ 20%–25%	↑ 6%–18%	↓ 20%–35%
Niacin	↓ 10%–25%	↑ 10%–35%	↓ 20%–30%
Bile acid sequestrants	↓ 15%–25%		May ↑
Cholesterol absorption inhibitors	↓ 10%–18%		
PCSK9 inhibitors	↓ 39%–62%	↑ 4%–7%	↓ 12%–17%

HDL-C, High-density lipoprotein cholesterol; *LDL-C*, low-density lipoprotein cholesterol; *PCSK9*, proprotein convertase subtilisin/kexin type 9; *TG*, triglycerides.
Adapted from Lipoprotein Management in Patients With Cardiometabolic Risk, Consensus Statement from the American College of Cardiology Foundation and the American Diabetes Association (ACC/ADA) (2008), and American Association of Clinical Endocrinologists' (AACE) Guidelines for Management of Dyslipidemia and Prevention of Atherosclerosis (2012).

TABLE 6 · Equipotency and Percentage Reduction in Total Cholesterol According to the Different Types and Doses of Statins

REDUCTION IN TOTAL CHOLESTEROL (%)	PRAVASTATIN (PRAVACHOL), mg	FLUVASTATIN (LESCOL), mg	SIMVASTATIN (ZOCOR) *, mg	ATORVASTATIN (LIPITOR), mg	ROSUVASTATIN (CRESTOR), mg
6–15	5	10	–	–	–
15–17	10	20	5	2.5	–
22	20	40	10	5	–
27	40†	80†	20†	10†	5†
32	80†	–	40†	20†	10†
37	–	–	(80)	40‡	20‡
42	–	–	–	80‡	40‡

*See the text for the FDA warning.
†Moderate-intensity statins (reduction of LDL-C 30%–49%).
‡High-intensity statins (reduction of LDL-C ≥ 50%).
FDA, U.S. Food and Drug Administration; *LDL-C*, low-density lipoprotein cholesterol.
Modified from Penning-van Beest FJA, Termorshuizen F, Goettsch WG, et al. Adherence to evidence-based statin guidelines reduces the risk of hospitalizations for acute myocardial infarction by 40%: a cohort study. *Eur Heart J*. 2007;28:154–159.

amlodipine (Norvasc), or ranolazine (Ranexa), and to 10 mg/day if taking diltiazem (Cardizem), dronedarone (Multaq), or verapamil (Calan). Addition of fibrates increases the risk of myopathy; in patients on a statin, fenofibrate (Tricor) is preferred, whereas gemfibrozil (Lopid), which has a much higher risk of rhabdomyolysis, is contraindicated. Symptoms of statin myopathy are heaviness, stiffness, cramping associated with weakness during exertion, and tendon-associated pain. Location of symptoms can be at the thighs, at the calves, or generalized. Symptoms can be very nonspecific, and differentiating statin-related myopathy from other causes is not easy. Therefore baseline symptoms, physical examination, and assessment of creatinine kinase level before the initiation of statins can be very helpful. Modifiable risk factors for statin-induced myopathy, such as hypothyroidism and vitamin D deficiency, should be optimally managed. Further decisions regarding stopping, dose reduction, or switching medications can be made based on the severity of symptoms, level of creatinine kinase elevation, and presence of rhabdomyolysis. In patients who develop myopathy while on simvastatin or atorvastatin, if the decision is to continue treatment with a statin, one option is to cautiously switch them to pravastatin, fluvastatin, or rosuvastatin, which are less prone to cause myopathy. Alternatively, lower statin dosing or less frequent dosing may be considered. For instance, rosuvastatin has a long duration of action and can be taken once every other day[1] or weekly,[1] if necessary. For

---

[1] Not FDA approved for this indication.

patients who cannot tolerate statins, other agents should be used, starting with validated nonstatin agents.

Ezetimibe

Ezetimibe is the first in a new class of pharmaceutical agents that primarily targets the cholesterol transport protein Niemann-Pick C1–like 1 protein in the intestine. Ezetimibe is an efficacious and cost-effective add-on agent in people taking a statin, if the LDL-C goal is not achieved or high doses of statin cannot be tolerated. Ezetimibe was shown to modestly decrease LDL-C and cardiovascular events when added to simvastatin in high-risk patients in the Improved Reduction of Outcomes: Vytorin Efficacy International Trial (IMPROVE-IT) study. Moreover, ezetimibe has become a generic prescription in the United States, and its safety profile is well characterized. Elevated liver enzymes have been reported, but the risk of hepatotoxicity seems to be no different from that of placebo.

PCSK9 Inhibitors

The PCSK9 protein plays a major role in regulating the number of LDLRs at the cell surface, including on hepatocytes. Binding of the LDLR by PCSK9 leads to the destruction of the LDLR. Therefore interference with the binding capacity of PCSK9 to LDLR or silencing the expression of the *PCSK9* gene allows more LDLRs to recycle to the cell surface, effecting the removal of more of the circulating plasma LDL. Over a decade ago, individuals with gain-of-function mutations of the *PCSK9* gene were found to underlie a rare form of autosomal dominant hypercholesterolemia. Subsequently, individuals with loss-of-function mutations were found to have very low LDL-C levels and were protected from coronary heart disease. These discoveries led to the development of pharmacologic agents directed against PCSK9 as a novel cholesterol-lowering treatment.

To date, three anti-PCSK9 agents with different mechanisms of action have been approved by the FDA for lowering cholesterol. Two of them are human monoclonal antibodies (alirocumab [Praluent] and evolocumab [Repatha]), whereas the other is small interference ribonucleic acid (siRNA) (inclisiran [Leqvio]). All are administered by subcutaneous injection and have similar efficacy in LDL-C reduction. Both alirocumab and evolocumab have been shown to provide cardiovascular benefit in outcome trials, whereas the cardiovascular outcome trial for inclisiran is expected to close in 2024.

In the Further Cardiovascular Outcomes Research With PCSK9 Inhibition in Subjects With Elevated Risk (FOURIER) trial, evolocumab was found to significantly reduce the risk for ASCVD events in patients with clinical ASCVD and LDL-C of 70 mg/dL or greater or a non–HDL-C level of 100 mg/dL or greater who were receiving optimized lipid lowering using a high-intensity statin or at least atorvastatin 20 mg with or without ezetimibe. Similarly, in the Evaluation of Cardiovascular Outcomes After an Acute Coronary Syndrome During Treatment With Alirocumab (ODYSSEY OUTCOMES) trial, alirocumab was shown to significantly reduce the risk for ASCVD events in patients with recent acute coronary syndrome who had a LDL-C of 70 mg/dL or greater, a non–HDL-C of 100 mg/dL or greater, or an apo B level of 80 mg/dL or greater and who were receiving statin therapy at a high-intensity dose or at the maximum tolerated dose. Taking into account the results, the 2018 Multisociety guidelines and the *2022 ACC ECDP on Nonstatin Therapies* recommended the consideration of PCSK9 inhibitors in secondary prevention patients on maximally tolerated statin and in primary prevention patients with high baseline LDL-C levels of 190 mg/dL or greater not from secondary causes if treatment goals appropriate for the risk are not achieved (Table 2). Both alirocumab and evolocumab are also indicated for heterozygous and homozygous familial hypercholesterolemia (HeFH and HoFH, respectively) as an adjunct to other LDL-C–lowering therapies.

With lack of cardiovascular outcome results, inclisiran, at this time, should be considered as an alternative to the monoclonal antibodies for PCSK9 if the latter fails to achieve appropriate LDL-C goals. Inclisiran is typically administered in clinic twice annually after initial injections at baseline and 3 months; thus it is particularly useful for patients who have difficulty with self-administering the monoclonal antibodies that are required every 2 weeks or monthly.

PCSK9 inhibitors are powerful LDL-C–lowering agents and enable reduction of LDL-C by up to approximately 60% as a single agent or an adjunct therapy. Moreover, the absolute level of LDL-C achieved may be as low as less than 25 mg/dL. There have been concerns regarding the potential adverse effects that may occur at such low LDL-C levels, such as neurocognitive side effects. However, results from these trials and their subanalyses have not shown a significant signal, although more long-term follow-up analysis is needed. Common side effects associated with PCSK9 inhibitors include injection site reactions, nasopharyngitis, upper respiratory tract infection, influenza, and back pain.

A significant hurdle to more widespread use of PCSK9 inhibitors is their high cost. Since their approval in 2015 by the FDA, the cost of evolocumab and alirocumab has consistently decreased and approached the threshold of cost-effectiveness. As a result, the *2022 ACC ECDP on Nonstatin Therapies* dropped the value statement on PCSK9 inhibitors and lowered the threshold for adding them.

Bempedoic Acid

Bempedoic acid (Nexletol) is a new anticholesterol medication that decreases cholesterol synthesis by inhibiting ATP citrate lyase. It is a prodrug, requiring conversion in the liver by very-long-chain acyl-CoA synthetase, which is absent in muscle and is thus expected to have minimal muscle side effects compared with statins. Bempedoic acid added to maximally tolerated statin therapy led to a mean of 18% further reduction in LDL-C. A fixed dose combination of bempedoic and ezetimibe (Nexlizet) added to a maximally tolerated dose of statins led to a 38% reduction of LDL-C. It is well tolerated, with the main side effects being an increase in uric acid level and tendon rupture. It is approved for patients with ASCVD or HeFH who require further LDL-C lowering, and the *2022 ACC ECDP on Nonstatin Therapies* suggested that it be added after ezetimibe and PCSK9 inhibitors if further LDL-C lowering is indicated. In a recently finished CLEAR outcome trial, patients with ASCVD or at high risk for ASCVD who did not tolerate or would not take any statins were given bempedoic acid or placebo; after a median follow-up of 40.6 months, patients treated with bempedoic acid had significantly reduced 4-point major adverse cardiovascular events, the study's primary end point. Although this result has yet to be reflected in any guidelines, it would be reasonable to consider bempedoic acid for both primary[1] and secondary prevention if the desired LDL goal has not been achieved after maximally tolerated statin and ezetimibe. A possible cost-effective algorithm for adding nonstatins could be adding ezetimibe if less than 25% further reduction is needed to reach treatment goal, bempedoic acid/ezetimibe combination (Nexlizet) if 25% to 50% reduction is needed, and PCSK9 inhibitors if 50% or greater reduction is needed.

Bile Acid Sequestrants

Bile acid sequestrants have been in clinical use for many decades. These agents promote fecal excretion of bile acids. The liver responds with increased integration of cholesterol into bile acid synthesis to maintain a stable bile acid pool. The consequent decrease in cholesterol in the liver leads to upregulation of the LDLR and enhanced LDL clearance from the plasma. HMG-CoA synthase activity can increase, so combination therapy with statins would be synergistic, especially in patients with a suboptimal response. Available agents are cholestyramine (Questran), colestipol (Colestid), and colesevelam (Welchol). Most side effects involve the gastrointestinal tract, with constipation and bloating being the most common. These agents may interfere with the absorption of warfarin, phenobarbital, levothyroxine (Synthroid), and digoxin (Lanoxin), among other medications. Patients on multiple medications should be advised to take bile acid sequestrants 1 hour before or 4 hours after taking the other medications. These agents can also cause elevation of TG level

---

[1] Not FDA approved for this indication.

and are contraindicated if TG level is greater than 500 mg/dL. As they are not systemically absorbed, the bile acid sequestrants may be the preferred agents when systemic absorption is to be avoided, such as during pregnancy or lactation.

Fibrates

The effect of fibrates on cardiovascular outcomes is not as favorable as with statins. However, fibrates can be useful in subsets of patients with high TGs and low HDL-C. Recently the Action to Control Cardiovascular Risk in Diabetes (ACCORD) lipid trial showed that addition of fenofibrate to simvastatin in type 2 diabetic patients with cardiovascular risk factors did not improve cardiovascular outcomes, although there was a trend for better outcomes in a subgroup with TGs greater than 204 mg/dL and HDL-C less than 34 mg/dL. Fibrates have multiple favorable metabolic effects, including activation of peroxisome proliferator-activated receptor-α (contributing to the regulation of both lipid and carbohydrate metabolism), stimulation of LPL (increasing TG hydrolysis), and downregulation of Apo CIII (improving lipoprotein remnant clearance as Apo CIII inhibits lipoprotein lipase). An enhanced VLDL-to-LDL conversion may lead to mild LDL-C elevation in some patients. This effect may decrease over weeks as the LDLRs are upregulated. Fibrates are generally well tolerated. The most common side effect is dyspepsia. Other side effects include myopathy and hepatic enzyme elevation, particularly when fibrates are added to statins. The use of gemfibrozil (Lopid) should be avoided in patients on statin therapy due to increased risk for muscle-related adverse events. Fibrates increase the risk of gallstones, and patients on warfarin (Coumadin) may need dose adjustment. Monitoring of liver enzymes is recommended, at baseline and within 3 months and then periodically. Creatinine level can be increased through unclear mechanisms.

Niacin

Niacin or nicotinic acid effectively decreases the hepatic production of VLDL and thus LDL-C levels and raises HDL-C levels by reducing cholesterol transfer from HDL to Apo B–containing lipoproteins and HDL clearance by the liver. Niacin is also the most potent agent currently available to reduce the level of Lp(a); however, this effect on the reduction of cardiovascular events in patients with elevated Lp(a) is not known. Several trials showed the effect of niacin in preventing cardiovascular disease; however, the benefit of adding niacin to statins has not been proved. Niacin did not improve cardiovascular risk when added to simvastatin in patients with high risk for cardiovascular disease in the Atherothrombosis Intervention in Metabolic Syndrome with Low HDL/High TGs: Impact on Global Health Outcomes (AIM-HIGH) study and the Heart Protection Study 2–Treatment of HDL to Reduce the Incidence of Vascular Events (HPS2-Thrive) study. There were excess adverse events and trends toward signs of harm among the niacin groups. The FDA has recently withdrawn the approval for the coadministration of niacin extended-release tablets (Niaspan) with statins. The most common side effect of niacin is flushing. This can be avoided or minimized by initiating therapy with a low dose of niacin, taking an aspirin 1 hour before niacin, avoiding hot foods or beverages at the time the niacin is taken, or switching to extended-release forms (Niaspan). Hepatotoxicity can occur at any time. Immediate-release forms are less likely to cause hepatotoxicity than sustained-release forms (Slo-Niacin). Extended-release forms can minimally elevate transaminases, but significant hepatotoxicity is rare. They can, however, also cause dose-dependent reversible thrombocytopenia, which can be insidious and severe. When switching to different forms, it is recommended that one should start with low doses and titrate up to achieve desired response. Liver function tests should be monitored regularly, at baseline and every 3 months for the first year, and then periodically. Other side effects include pruritus, increased uric acid levels, and hyperglycemia.

Omega-3 Fatty Acid Prescriptions

Highly purified omega-3 fatty acid preparations containing either a mixture of EPA and DHA (Lovaza) or EPA alone (Vascepa) are effective agents used in the treatment of hypertriglyceridemia, the first FDA-approved indication for these agents. Omega-3 fatty acids are polyunsaturated fatty acids and are essential in humans. A significant proportion of omega-3 fatty acids is consumed in the diet. Major dietary sources of omega-3 fatty acids include nuts, vegetable oils, flax seeds, and leafy vegetables, as well as fish and fish oil. EPA and DHA are the two major types of marine-derived omega-3 fatty acids. The mechanism by which omega-3 fatty acids lower TGs is incompletely understood.

Multiple clinical trials have been examining the efficacy of omega-3 fatty acid in improving cardiovascular outcome. Although trials using lower doses of EPA-DHA mixtures (≤1 g total daily) have shown inconsistent results, findings from recent trials assessing higher doses of pure EPA have been more favorable.

Purified EPA was first shown in the Japan Eicosapentaenoic acid Lipid Intervention Study (JELIS) trial to significantly reduce risk for major coronary events in patients with hypercholesterolemia. Subsequently, the Reduction of Cardiovascular Events With Icosapent Ethyl–Intervention Trial (REDUCE-IT) study, a large, randomized controlled trial, assessed the efficacy and safety of purified EPA ethyl ester, icosapent ethyl (Vascepa) in secondary prevention and high-risk primary prevention patients with reasonably controlled LDL-C but elevated TGs. The REDUCE-IT trial showed that treatment with icosapent ethyl was associated with a significant reduction in ASCVD events. In secondary analyses, icosapent ethyl has also been shown to reduce the risk for total ischemic events (first plus subsequent events). Results from REDUCE-IT suggest that high-risk patients with elevated TGs reap additional cardiovascular benefits from icosapent ethyl, when the latter is added to LDL-C lowering therapies. Lastly, the overall rates of adverse events were not significantly different between the treatment and control arms of REDUCE-IT. However, there were increased rates of atrial fibrillation and peripheral edema associated with patients taking icosapent ethyl observed in the trial. On the strength of the REDUCE-IT trial, the FDA has approved icosapent ethyl for reduction of cardiovascular events in high-risk patients with elevated TG levels. Icosapent ethyl has also been incorporated into the *2021 ACC ECDP on Persistent Hypertriglyceridemia,* which recommends icosapent ethyl be added to other cholesterol-lowering medications in patients with clinical ASCVD or in diabetic patients who are more than 50 years old and who have an additional risk factor, if the fasting TG level is 150 mg/dL or greater.

Evinacumab

Evinacumab (Evkeeza) is a human monoclonal antibody against ANGPLT3, a dual inhibitor for LPL and endothelial lipase. Genetic deficiency of ANGPLT3 was associated with a very low level of LDL-C and TGs and significantly reduced ASCVD risk. The mechanism for LDL reduction with ANGPLT3 inactivation is independent from LDLR; thus evinacumab could be effective for patients with HoFH. In the ELIPSE HoFH trial, evinacumab was shown to reduce LDL-C by approximately 50% in HoFH patients on stable therapy with baseline LDL-C of 70 mg/dL or greater. The treatment was well tolerated, with side effects comparable to the placebo group. Currently, evinacumab is approved by the FDA for treating patients with HoFH who need further LDL-C reduction. It is administered via intravenous infusion every 4 weeks.

References

The AIM-HIGH Investigators: Niacin in patients with low HDL cholesterol levels receiving intensive statin therapy, N Engl J Med 365:2255–2267, 2011.

Bhatt DL, Steg PG, Miller M, et al: Effects of icosapent ethyl on total ischemic events: from REDUCE-IT, J Am Coll Cardiol, 2019.

Bhatt DL, Steg PG, Miller M, et al: Cardiovascular risk reduction with icosapent ethyl for hypertriglyceridemia, N Engl J Med 380(1):11–22, 2019.

Brunzell JD, Davidson M, Furberg CD: Lipoprotein management in patients with cardiometabolic risk: consensus conference report from the ADA and the ACC foundation, J Am Coll Cardiol 51:1512–1524, 2008.

IMPROVE-IT Investigators: Ezetimibe added to statin therapy after acute coronary syndromes, N Engl J Med 372:2387–2397, 2015.

Carroll MD, Kit BK, Lacher DA, et al: Trends in lipids and lipoproteins in U.S. adults, 1988–2010, JAMA 308:1545–1554, 2012.

Dullaart RP: PCSK9 Inhibition to reduce cardiovascular events, *N Engl J Med* 376:1713–1722, 2017.

Eckel RH, Jakicic JM, Ard JD, et al: 2013 ACC/AHA guideline on lifestyle management to reduce cardiovascular risk: a report of the American College of Cardiology/American Heart Association task force on practice guidelines, *J Am Coll Cardiol* 63:2960–2984, 2014.

Everett BM, Smith RJ, Hiatt WR: Reducing LDL with PCSK9 inhibitors — the clinical benefit of lipid drugs, *N Engl J Med* 373:1588–1591, 2015.

Ginsberg HN, Elam MB, Lovato LC, et al: Effects of combination lipid therapy in type 2 diabetes mellitus, *N Engl J Med* 362:1563–1574, 2010.

Greenland P, Alpert JS, Beller GA, et al: 2010 ACCF/AHA guideline for assessment of cardiovascular risk in asymptomatic adults: a report of the American College of Cardiology Foundation/American Heart Association Task Force on Practice Guidelines developed in collaboration with the American Society of Echocardiography, American Society of Nuclear Cardiology, Society of Atherosclerosis Imaging and Prevention, Society for Cardiovascular Angiography and Interventions, Society of Cardiovascular Computed Tomography, and Society for Cardiovascular Magnetic Resonance, *J Am Coll Cardiol* 56:e50–e103, 2010.

Grundy SM, Cleeman JI, Merz CNB, et al: Implications of recent clinical trials for the national cholesterol education program adult treatment panel III guidelines, *Circulation* 110:227–239, 2004.

Grundy SM, Stone NJ, Bailey AL, et al: AHA/ACC/AACVPR/AAPA/ABC/ACPM/ADA/AGS/APhA/ASPC/NLA/PCNA guideline on the management of blood cholesterol: executive summary: a report of the American College of Cardiology/American Heart Association Task Force on Clinical Practice Guidelines, *J Am Coll Cardiol* 2018. pii: S0735-1097.

Hlatky MA, Kazi DS: PCSK9 inhibitors: economics and policy, *J Am Coll Cardiol* 70(21):2677–2687, 2017.

Huffman MD, Capewell S, Ning H, et al: Cardiovascular health behavior and health factor changes (1988–2008) and projections to 2020: results from the National Health and Nutrition Examination Surveys (NHANES), *Circulation* 125:2595–2602, 2012.

Jellinger PS, Smith DA, Mehta AE, et al: American Association of Clinical Endocrinologists' guidelines for management of hyperlipidemia and prevention of atherosclerosis, *Endocr Pract* 18:1–78, 2012.

Joy TR, Hegele RA: Narrative review: statin-related myopathy, *Ann Intern Med* 150:858–868, 2009.

Kazi DS, Moran AE, Coxson PG, et al: Cost-effectiveness of PCSK9 inhibitor therapy in patients with heterozygous familial hypercholesterolemia or atherosclerotic cardiovascular disease, *JAMA* 316(7):743–753, 2016.

Keaney JF, Curfman GD, Jarcho JA: A pragmatic view of the new cholesterol treatment guidelines, *N Engl J Med* 370:275–278, 2014.

2019 ESC/EAS guidelines for the management of dyslipidaemias, *Eur Heart J* 41:111–188, 2020.

Musunuru K, Kathiresan S: Surprises from genetic analyses of lipid risk factors for atherosclerosis, *Circ Res* 118(4):579–585, 2016.

Third report of the National Cholesterol Education Program (NCEP) expert panel on detection, evaluation, and treatment of high blood cholesterol in adults (Adult treatment panel III) final report, *Circulation* 106:3143–3421, 2002.

Newman CB, Blaha MJ, Boord JB, et al: Lipid management in patients with endocrine disorders: an Endocrine Society clinical practice guideline, *J Clin Endocrinol Metab* 105:3613–3682, 2020.

Nissen SE, Lincoff AM, Brennan D, et al: CLEAR Outcomes Investigators. Bempedoic acid and cardiovascular outcomes in statin-intolerant patients, *N Engl J Med* 388(15):1353–1364, 2023.

O'Connell C, Horwood K, Nadamuni M: Correction of refractory thrombocytopenia and anemia following withdrawal of extended release niacin, *Am J Hematol* 91(7):E318, 2016.

Orringer CE, Blaha MJ, Blankstein R, et al: The National Lipid Association scientific statement on coronary artery calcium scoring to guide preventive strategies for ASCVD risk reduction, *J Clin Lipidol* 15(1):33–60, 2021.

Otvos JD, Collins D, Freedman DS, et al: Low-density lipoprotein and high-density lipoprotein particle subclasses predict coronary events and are favorably changed by gemfibrozil therapy in the Veterans Affairs High-Density Lipoprotein Intervention Trial, *Circulation* 113:1556–1563, 2006.

Penning-van Beest FJA, Termorshuizen F, Goettsch WG, et al: Adherence to evidence-based statin guidelines reduces the risk of hospitalizations for acute myocardial infarction by 40%: a cohort study, *Eur Heart J* 28:154–159, 2007.

Phan BAP, Dayspring TD, Toth PP: Ezetimibe therapy: mechanism of action and clinical update, *Vasc Health Risk Manag* 8:415–427, 2012.

Reiner Z, Catapano AL, De Backer G, et al: ESC/EAS guidelines for the management of dyslipidaemias: the task force for the management of dyslipidaemias of the European Society of Cardiology (ESC) and the European Atherosclerosis Society (EAS), *Eur Heart J* 32:1769–1818, 2011.

Reyes-Soffer G, Ginsberg HN, Berglund L, et al: American Heart Association Council on Arteriosclerosis, Thrombosis and Vascular Biology; Council on Cardiovascular Radiology and Intervention; and Council on Peripheral Vascular Disease. Lipoprotein(a): a genetically determined, causal, and prevalent risk factor for atherosclerotic cardiovascular disease: a scientific statement from the American Heart Association, *Arterioscler Thromb Vasc Biol* 42(1):e48–e60, 2022.

Ridker PM, Cook NR: Statins: new American guidelines for prevention of cardiovascular disease, *Lancet* 382:1762–1765, 2013.

Robinson JG, Farnier M, Krempf M, et al: Efficacy and safety of alirocumab in reducing lipids and cardiovascular events, *N Engl J Med* 372:1489–1499, 2015.

Robinson JG, Rosenson RS, Farnier M, et al: Safety of very low-density lipoprotein cholesterol levels with alirocumab, *J Am Coll Cardiol* 69(5):471–482, 2017.

Sabatine MS, Giugliano RP, Keech AC, et al: Evolocumab and clinical outcomes in patients with cardiovascular disease, *N Engl J Med* 376(18):1713–1722, 2017.

Sabatine MS, Giugliano RP, Wiviott SD, et al: Efficacy and safety of evolocumab in reducing lipids and cardiovascular events, *N Engl J Med* 372:1500–1509, 2015.

Schwartz GG, Steg PG, Szarek M, et al: Alirocumab and cardiovascular outcomes after acute coronary syndrome, *N Engl J Med* 379(22):2097–2107, 2018.

Stone NJ, Robinson J, Lichtenstein AH, et al: ACC/AHA guideline on the treatment of blood cholesterol to reduce atherosclerotic cardiovascular risk in adults: a report of the American College of Cardiology/American Heart Association task force on practice guidelines, *J Am Coll Cardiol* 63:2889–2934, 2014.

Tall AR, Rader DJ: Trials and tribulations of CETP inhibitors, *Circ Res* 122(1):106–112, 2018.

Tsimikas S: A test in context: lipoprotein(a): diagnosis, prognosis, controversies, and emerging therapies, *J Am Coll Cardiol* 69(6):692–711, 2017.

Virani S, Morris P, Agarwala A, et al: 2021 ACC expert consensus decision pathway on the management of ASCVD risk reduction in patients with persistent hypertriglyceridemia, *J Am Coll Cardiol* 78(9):960–993, 2021.

Writing Committee, Lloyd-Jones DM, Morris PB, Ballantyne CM, et al: 2022 ACC expert consensus decision pathway on the role of nonstatin therapies for LDL-cholesterol lowering in the management of atherosclerotic cardiovascular disease risk: a report of the American College of Cardiology Solution Set Oversight Committee, *J Am Coll Cardiol* 80(14):1366–1418, 2022.

Wu H, Ballantyne CM: Dyslipidaemia: PCSK9 inhibitors and foamy monocytes in familial hypercholesterolaemia, *Nat Rev Cardiol* 14(7):385–386, 2017.

Xu JQ, Murphy SL, Kochanek KD, Arias E: *Mortality in the United States, 2021*. NCHS Data Brief, no 456, National Center for Health Statistics, 2022. Accessed July 13, 2023 https://stacks.cdc.gov/view/cdc/122516.

Xu L, Perrard XD, Perrard JL, et al: Foamy monocytes form early and contribute to nascent atherosclerosis in mice with hypercholesterolemia, *Arterioscler Thromb Vasc Biol* 35:1787–1797, 2015.

Yokoyama M, Origasa H, Matsuzaki M, et al: Effects of eicosapentaenoic acid on major coronary events in hypercholesterolaemic patients (JELIS): a randomised open-label, blinded endpoint analysis, *Lancet* 369(9567):1090–1098, 2007.

HYPERPARATHYROIDISM AND HYPOPARATHYROIDISM

Method of
Claudio Marcocci, MD; and Filomena Cetani, MD

CURRENT DIAGNOSIS

Primary Hyperparathyroidism

- Third most common endocrine disorder and most common cause of hypercalcemia in the general population.
- Diagnosis based on confirmed hypercalcemia (total calcium [albumin corrected] or ionized calcium) associated with elevated or inappropriately normal serum parathyroid hormone (PTH) level.
- Hypercalcemia on routine blood testing or in postmenopausal women investigated for osteoporosis is typically the first clue to the diagnosis.
- Mainly occurs as a solitary disease (90%) but may be part of hereditary syndromes.
- Genetic causes should be searched for in young patients.

Secondary Hyperparathyroidism

- Secondary hyperparathyroidism defines any condition in which the increased PTH secretion occurs as a normal physiologic response, often mediated by a decrease of serum calcium.
- Vitamin D deficiency, as a result of inadequate nutritional intake/sun exposure, malabsorption, liver diseases, or chronic renal failure, is the most common cause.
- At variance with primary hyperparathyroidism, secondary hyperparathyroidism is characterized by low or, more often, low-normal serum calcium and decreased urinary calcium excretion.

Hypoparathyroidism

- Rare disorder.
- Inadvertent removal or damage to the parathyroid gland during thyroid surgery and, much less frequently, autoimmune destruction are the most common causes.
- Diagnosis based on low serum calcium along with undetectable or inappropriately low serum PTH level.

CURRENT THERAPY

Primary Hyperparathyroidism
- Parathyroidectomy is the only definitive therapy.
- Surgery should be considered in all cases and recommended in patients with symptoms and in those who, albeit asymptomatically, meet the surgical criteria.
- Surveillance without surgery can be considered in patients without symptoms who do not meet the surgical criteria.
- Patients not undergoing surgery should be given vitamin D when indicated, and calcium intake should not be restricted.
- Medical treatment can be considered in selected cases: antiresorptive therapy to increase bone mineral density and cinacalcet (Sensipar) to lower serum calcium.

Hypoparathyroidism
- Severe hypocalcemia is a medical emergency and treatment with intravenous calcium should be promptly instituted and maintained for 24 to 48 hours; oral therapy with calcium and active vitamin D metabolites should be started as soon as practical.
- The goal of chronic treatment is to maintain serum calcium in the low-normal range, avoiding hypocalcemic symptoms and long-term complications.
- Chronic conventional therapy is based on adequate calcium intake (calcium supplement needed in most cases) and active vitamin D metabolites.
- Recombinant full-length parathyroid hormone 1 to 84 (Natpara) has been approved by the U.S. Food and Drug Administration and European Medicines Agency for patients not controlled with conventional therapy.
- An individualized approach is necessary to optimize patient care. Lifelong monitoring is needed to decrease the risk of complications.

TABLE 1 Hereditary Forms of PHPT and Related Involved Gene

DISORDER	GENE	PATTERN OF INHERITANCE
Multiple endocrine neoplasia type 1	MEN1	Autosomal dominant
Multiple endocrine neoplasia type 2A	RET	Autosomal dominant
Multiple endocrine neoplasia type 4	CDKN1B	Autosomal dominant
Multiple endocrine neoplasia type 5	MAX	Autosomal dominant
Hyperparathyroidism–jaw tumor syndrome	CDC73	Autosomal dominant
Familial isolated hyperparathyroidism	MEN1, CDC73, CASR, GCM2, CDKN1B	Autosomal dominant
Familial hypocalciuric hypercalcemia type 1	CASR	Autosomal dominant
Familial hypocalciuric hypercalcemia type 2	GNA11	Autosomal dominant
Familial hypocalciuric hypercalcemia type 3	AP2S1	Autosomal dominant
Neonatal severe hyperparathyroidism	CASR	Autosomal recessive

AP2S1, Adaptor-related protein complex 2 sigma 1 subunit; *CASR*, calcium-sensing receptor; *CDC73*, cell division cycle 73; *CDKN1B*, cyclin-dependent kinase inhibitor 1B; *GCM2*, glial cells missing transcription factor 2; *GNA11*, G protein subunit alpha 11; *MAX*, myc-associated factor x; *MEN1*, multiple endocrine neoplasia type 1; *PHPT*, primary hyperparathyroidism; *RET*, rearranged during transfection.

Primary Hyperparathyroidism

Epidemiology
Primary hyperparathyroidism (PHPT) is currently the third most common endocrine disorder and the most frequent cause of hypercalcemia in the general population.

The disease was considered rare until the early 1970s, when its incidence in the United States rose dramatically after the introduction of serum calcium in the multichannel autoanalyzer. The incidence varies according to geographic areas and assessment measures; recent data in the United States indicate an incidence of 79.6 per 100,000 person-years in women and 35.6 per 100,000 person-years in men of all races, with the highest rate among Black people. The incidence peaks in the sixth decade of life. The prevalence ranges between 1 and 7 cases per 1000 adults. Most cases occur in women (with a female-to-male ratio of 3:1), but there is no sex difference before the age of 45 years. PHPT is rare in children and adolescents.

Pathogenesis
PHPT mainly occurs as a solitary disease (90%) but may be part of hereditary syndromes (e.g., multiple endocrine neoplasia [MEN] types 1, 2A, 4, and 5; hyperparathyroidism–jaw tumor syndrome; familial isolated hyperparathyroidism) (Table 1). A single, benign adenoma is found in 80% to 85% of cases, multigland involvement in 15% to 20%, and parathyroid carcinoma in less than 1%. Multigland involvement is more common in hereditary cases, particularly MEN1. In the absence of local infiltration or metastases, the diagnosis of parathyroid carcinoma may be difficult at histology. Genetic studies (*CDC73* gene mutations) and immunohistochemical studies (loss of parafibromin [the protein encoded by the *CDC73* gene] expression) may help in equivocal cases. Predisposing factors are external neck irradiation in childhood and long-term lithium therapy.

PHPT is characterized by excessive parathyroid hormone (PTH) secretion from one or more parathyroid glands, due to the loss of the homeostatic control of PTH synthesis and secretion. Extracellular ionized calcium (Ca^{2+}_o) is the main regulator of PTH secretion. Ca^{2+}_o interacts with the Ca^{2+}-sensing receptor (CaSR) present on the surface of parathyroid cells; there is an inverse sigmoidal relationship between Ca^{2+}_o concentration and PTH release. In adenomas, hypercalcemia is due to the loss of normal sensitivity of the parathyroid cell to the inhibitory action of Ca^{2+}, whereas in parathyroid hyperplasia the increased number of parathyroid cells, which have a normal sensitivity to the inhibitory action of Ca^{2+}, causes hypercalcemia. Serum phosphate, 1,25-dihydroxyvitamin D ($1,25(OH)_2D$), and fibroblast growth factor 23 are also involved in the control of PTH secretion.

Although major progress has been made in the last two decades, the molecular basis of PHPT is still unclear in the majority of cases. The clonality of most parathyroid tumors suggests a defect in the pathways that control parathyroid cell proliferation or the expression of PTH. The genes involved are listed in Table 1. Germline mutations are often found in hereditary forms. On the other hand, somatic mutations may occur in sporadic cases, even though germline mutations have also been described in apparently sporadic cases.

Clinical Presentation
In recent years the clinical presentation of PHPT in Western countries has changed from a symptomatic disease, characterized by hypercalcemia and renal (nephrolithiasis and nephrocalcinosis) and skeletal (osteitis fibrosa cystica, fragility fractures) manifestations, to one with subtle and nonspecific clinical manifestations (asymptomatic PHPT). Nephrolithiasis remains the most common classic clinical manifestation (15% to 20%), and silent stones are frequently detected at ultrasound. Bone mineral

density (BMD) is reduced particularly at sites rich in cortical bone (one-third distal radius). Studies using peripheral high-resolution quantitative computed tomography (CT) have shown involvement of both cortical and trabecular sites, the latter confirmed by the trabecular bone score (TBS) at the lumbar spine. An increased rate of vertebral and nonvertebral fractures has also been documented. Nonclassical manifestations, including subtle cardiovascular abnormalities and psychological and cognitive symptoms, have also been reported.

A new variant of PHPT (normocalcemic PHPT) has recently been identified, namely patients with increased serum PTH levels in the absence of hypercalcemia (also by measurement of ionized calcium) or other causes of secondary hyperparathyroidism (SHPT). This condition, called normocalcemic PHPT, has been typically recognized in persons evaluated for low BMD, in whom PTH was measured even in the absence of hypercalcemia. In some cases, this new phenotype may represent an early phase of classical hypercalcemic PHPT, when PTH elevation precedes the occurrence of hypercalcemia.

Evaluation and Diagnosis

The finding of hypercalcemia on routine blood testing or in postmenopausal women investigated for osteoporosis is typically the first clue to the diagnosis of PHPT. Hypercalcemia should be confirmed in repeated testing, preferably evaluating albumin-corrected total calcium (measured total calcium in mg/dL + [0.8 × (4.0 − serum albumin in g/dL)]) or ionized calcium. The next diagnostic step is the measurement of serum PTH. An elevated (or unexpectedly normal) serum PTH in the face of hypercalcemia is virtually diagnostic of PHPT. Serum phosphate is normal or in the low-normal range in mild PHPT and low in severe cases. A low or undetectable PTH level in a patient with hypercalcemia rules out the diagnosis of PHPT. The most common cause of PTH-independent hypercalcemia is malignancy, where hypercalcemia is due to the secretion by the tumor of PTH-related peptide, a molecule that shares with PTH the amino-terminal active part but does not cross-react in the PTH assay, or osteolytic lytic bone metastases. Urinary calcium should also be measured. If hypercalciuria is greater than 400 mg per day, a more extended evaluation of the stone risk profile should be performed. Urinary calcium measurement is also useful to exclude familial hypocalciuric hypercalcemia, which is suggested by the finding of the calcium-to-creatinine clearance ratio of less than 0.01.

A hereditary form of PHPT, accounting for 5% to 10% of cases, should be sought in patients younger than 30 years at diagnosis, with a family history of hypercalcemia and/or neuroendocrine tumors (see Table 1). In this setting serum calcium should be measured in first-degree relatives and genetic tests performed. Parathyroid cancer should be suspected in individuals, especially males, with marked hypercalcemia, a palpable neck mass, and serum PTH concentration 3 to 10 times the upper normal value. Some ultrasound features may raise the suspicion for cancer, such as a large (i.e., >3 cm) lobulated hypoechoic/heterogeneous parathyroid gland with irregular borders, thick capsule, suspicious vascularity, and calcifications.

Renal ultrasound should be performed in all patients, even in those with no history of nephrolithiasis, because recent studies have shown that silent kidney stones are common in patients with asymptomatic PHPT. Routine BMD testing by dual-energy x-ray absorptiometry (DXA) at the lumbar spine, hip, and distal forearm is also an essential component of the evaluation. BMD is typically low at the one-third distal radius, a site of enriched cortical bone, but a few patients may show predominant cancellous bone involvement, as documented by vertebral osteopenia or osteoporosis. The involvement of the trabecular compartment is also confirmed by the TBS at the lumbar spine. Vertebral imaging by x-ray or DXA (vertebral fracture assessment [VFA]) should also be routinely performed to detect silent vertebral deformities because vertebral fracture risk is increased in asymptomatic patients.

Neck imaging (ultrasound and sestamibi scanning) has no value in the diagnosis of PHPT, but it is a useful tool for localizing the abnormal parathyroid gland in patients selected for parathyroidectomy (PTx). Sestamibi has the advantage of localizing the ectopic parathyroid gland outside the neck. The 4D CT protocol has emerged as a useful tool. Recently 18F-fluorocholine positron emission tomography has proven to be useful in the localization of hyperfunctioning parathyroid glands before surgery.

Treatment

The aim of treatment is to remove all hyperfunctioning parathyroid tissue, resolve biochemical abnormalities, improve BMD, and decrease the risk of nephrolithiasis and fractures.

Surgical Treatment

Parathyroid surgery represents the only definitive cure of PHPT. Successful PTx normalizes serum calcium and PTH, improves BMD, and decreases the risk of nephrolithiasis and fragility fractures. Patients selected for surgery should be referred to an experienced parathyroid surgeon. A focused, minimally invasive approach, guided by imaging studies associated with intraoperative monitoring of serum PTH, is the preferred surgical procedure in sporadic PHPT. In experienced hands the rate of surgical cure reaches 95% to 98% with a negligible rate of surgical complications. In hereditary cases the surgical approach (bilateral neck exploration by classical cervicotomy) may differ because multigland involvement is common. An en bloc resection of the parathyroid lesion together with the ipsilateral thyroid lobe with clear gross margins and the adjacent structures is recommended when parathyroid carcinoma is suspected. Particular attention should be paid to avoid seeding of neoplastic parathyroid cells. Surgery should be considered for any patient with a confirmed diagnosis of PHPT and recommended in those with symptomatic disease.

Patients with mild hypercalcemia (serum calcium < 12 mg/dL [3 mmol/L]) can proceed directly to surgery. When serum calcium is higher, preoperative treatment with saline infusion eventually followed by loop diuretics, intravenous (IV) bisphosphonates, denosumab (Prolia, Xgeva)[1], or cinacalcet (Sensipar) may be considered to reduce serum calcium levels and decrease the risk of complications, particularly cardiac arrhythmias, which are associated with more severe hypercalcemia.

Surgery is also a reasonable option for patients with asymptomatic PHPT. International guidelines provide guidance to select patients who should be referred for surgery or followed without surgery. The most recent revised (2022) guidelines for surgery or monitoring are reported in Table 2. These guidelines are largely consistent with the previous ones and recommend PTx for all patients with symptomatic PHPT and asymptomatic patients who meet one or more of the indicated criteria. The new indications for surgery in asymptomatic patients include a 24-hour urinary calcium excretion greater than 250 mg/day in women and 300 mg/day in men. According to the guidelines, about 60% of patients with asymptomatic PHPT meet the criteria for surgery. As mentioned before, patients with mild PHPT may have subtle cardiovascular abnormalities and complain of psychological and cognitive symptoms. It is unclear whether and to what extent these abnormalities are reversible after successful PTx; for now they are not considered indications for surgery. Nonetheless, surgery could be considered in a middle-aged patient in whom asymptomatic PHPT is associated with increased cardiovascular risk (metabolic syndrome, hypertension, ischemic heart disease) if the surgical risk is low.

Randomized clinical trials have also shown that patients with sporadic asymptomatic PHPT who do not meet the surgical criteria may benefit from surgery, not only because it normalizes serum calcium and PTH, but also because it improves BMD and quality of life (QoL). On the other hand, surgery could be postponed in hereditary cases with mild hypercalcemia, because multigland disease, occasionally with asynchronous involvement of the various parathyroid glands, is not uncommon and carries

---

[1] Not FDA approved for this indication.

TABLE 2	Guidelines for Surgery for Patients With Asymptomatic PHPT and Monitoring for Those Followed Without Surgery	
PARAMETER	**GUIDELINES FOR SURGERY**	**GUIDELINES FOR MONITORING**
Serum calcium	>1 mg/dL (0.25 mmol/L) above the upper normal limit	Annually
Skeletal	BMD by DXA: T-score < –2.5 at lumbar spine, femoral neck, total hip, or distal one-third radius Vertebral fractures by x-ray, CT, MRI, or VFA	BMD by DXA every 1–2 years at lumbar spine, total hip, or distal one-third radius Spine x-ray or VFA or TBS when clinically indicated (e.g., back pain or height loss)
Renal	Creatinine clearance < 60 mL/min Daily urinary calcium excretion > 250 mg in women and >300 mg in men Nephrolithiasis or nephrocalcinosis by x-ray, ultrasound, or CT	Serum creatinine annually If renal stone suspected: 24-hour urinary calcium Renal imaging by x-ray, ultrasound, or CT
Age	<50 years	–

BMD, Bone mineral density; *CT*, computed tomography; *DXA*, dual x-ray absorptiometry; *MRI*, magnetic resonance imaging; *PHPT*, primary hyperparathyroidism; *TBS*, trabecular bone score; *VFA*, vertebral fracture assessment.
Modified from Bilezikian et al. Evaluation and management of primary hyperparathyroidism: summary statement and guidelines from the Fifth International Workshop. *J Bone Miner Res.* 2022;37:2293-2314.

an increased risk of surgical complications and recurrence/persistence of PHPT.

Therefore individual counseling addressing the benefits and risks of PTx is mandatory, and the preference of the patients should be taken into account. It is well-known that parathyroid surgery, when performed by skilled neck surgeons, is safe, cost-effective, and associated with low perioperative morbidity. On the other hand, it is important to recognize that PTx, particularly if performed by inexperienced surgeons, may be associated with complications that could be invalidating and not acceptable for a patient with mild disease and a good QoL. In this regard, the choice of surgery may be reconsidered in a patient with asymptomatic PHPT in whom parathyroid surgery was initially advised or selected by the patient when preoperative imaging studies are negative. Indeed, in this setting the patient may feel uncomfortable undergoing a blind neck exploration, a surgical procedure more extensive than the minimally invasive approach and carrying the greatest risk of complications. Regarding normocalcemic PHPT, because of limited data, no guidelines for surgery have been recommended.

Nonsurgical Management
As mentioned before, many patients with PHPT do not meet the criteria for surgery. These patients, as well as those who decline surgery or have contraindications to surgery, need to be monitored.

Monitoring. Randomized clinical studies have shown stability over a short period of observation (up to 2 years) in patients with asymptomatic PHPT followed without surgery and benefits in those who underwent PTx even if they did not meet the criteria for surgery. The extension up to 5 years of one of these randomized studies has shown a more frequent occurrence of a vertebral fracture in patients belonging to the observation group than in those cured by PTx. However, this difference was not observed in the extension study up to 10 years. Long-term observational

studies indicate that the disease remains stable in the majority for up to 8 to 9 years, but more than one-third of patients show a progression of the disease.

Calcium intake should not be restricted, and an intake appropriate for age and sex as in the general population (preferably with food) should be recommended. Vitamin D–depleted patients should be supplemented with daily doses of 800 to 1000 IU of vitamin D; weekly or monthly doses calculated on this daily dose can also be used. A serum level of 25(OH)D greater than 20 ng/mL should be reached, and the attainment of a higher target (>30 ng/mL) is suggested by some guidelines.

General principles for monitoring are reported in Table 2. Serum calcium and creatinine (creatinine clearance preferred over estimated glomerular filtration rate [eGFR]) should be measured annually, and BMD at the lumbar spine, total hip, and distal forearm should be measured every 1 to 2 years. Vertebral morphometry (by x-ray or VFA) or TBS should be performed when clinically indicated (back pain, height loss). Finally, 24-hour urinary collection for biochemical stone risk profile and renal imaging (x-ray, ultrasound, or CT) should be performed if there is a suspicion of renal stones.

Parathyroid surgery should be recommended in patients who are followed without surgery in the following instances: (1) serum calcium concentration greater than 1 mg/dL above the upper normal limit; (2) significant reduction of creatinine clearance; (3) detection of nephrocalcinosis or kidney stones; (4) BMD T-score at any site less than –2.5 or the finding of a significant (greater than the least significant change as defined by the International Society for Clinical Densitometry) decrease of BMD, even if the T-score is not less than –2.5; and (5) clinical fractures or morphometric vertebral fractures, even if asymptomatic.

Medical Treatment. No medical treatment is currently available to cure PHPT. Therefore when PTx is indicated and there are no contraindications for surgery, medical treatment should not be considered a valuable alternative option. Medical treatment may be considered for patients who have contraindications to surgery or are unwilling to undergo PTx, as well as for those who have failed surgery. Treatment should be guided by the aim of therapy.

Calcimimetics. If the aim of treatment is to reduce serum calcium, the calcimimetic cinacalcet (Sensipar) can be effective. The serum calcium typically declines over a few weeks and may normalize in most patients with moderate hypercalcemia. In addition, cinacalcet increases serum phosphate and only slightly reduces PTH concentration but has no effect on BMD. The beneficial effects are sustained over time as long as the drug is used. Adverse events are dose related: modest and transient when low doses of cinacalcet are used (up to 30 mg twice daily), but rather frequent, particularly gastrointestinal, symptoms, occasionally severe enough to require treatment withdrawal, when higher doses are employed. The use of cinacalcet has been approved by the U.S. Food and Drug Administration (FDA) for the treatment of severe hypercalcemia in patients with PHPT who are unable to undergo PTx, and by the European Medicines Agency (EMA) for the reduction of hypercalcemia in patients with PHPT, for whom PTx would be indicated on the basis of serum calcium levels (as defined by relevant guidelines) but in whom surgery is not clinically appropriate or contraindicated. As clearly stated, the EMA indications leave more room for the use of cinacalcet.

Cinacalcet should not be used as an initial treatment or in patients who do not meet the approved criteria for its prescription. The long-term safety of cinacalcet has not been established. Moreover, the rather high cost is another important limit for its long-term use.

Antiresorptive Therapy. If the aim is to increase BMD, antiresorptive therapy can be considered. Alendronate (Fosamax) is the bisphosphonate that has been more extensively used and shown to be effective in reducing bone turnover markers and increasing BMD. Over a short period of time, its effectiveness in increasing BMD is comparable to that observed after successful PTx. No effect has been shown on serum calcium and PTH levels. BMD also improved in a retrospective study that included 50 elderly women treated with denosumab for 2 years.

Combined Therapy With Cinacalcet and Antiresorptive Therapy. As mentioned before, cinacalcet is effective in the control of hypercalcemia but has no effect on BMD. Conversely, bisphosphonates increase BMD, with no effect on serum calcium. Limited data indicate that combination therapy is associated with both the calcium-lowering effect of cinacalcet and the skeletal advantage of bisphosphonates. Therefore if a patient has a low BMD and serum calcium concentration appropriate for the use of cinacalcet, combined therapy could be of benefit. A recent study has shown that denosumab[1] is effective in increasing BMD and lowering bone turnover irrespective of cinacalcet treatment and might be a valid option for patients in which surgery is undesirable.

Pregnancy and Lactation

PHPT may be diagnosed during pregnancy by the finding of hypercalcemia on routine blood testing. There are some distinctive features that should be considered in the evaluation and management: (1) pregnancy is associated with hemodilution and occasionally hypoalbuminemia, and therefore it would be preferable to measure ionized calcium; (2) the hereditary form should be sought because of the young age of pregnant women; and (3) women with mild elevation of calcium should be managed conservatively, mostly by hydration—in the case of worsening of hypercalcemia PTx in the second trimester and cinacalcet[1] may be considered.

Secondary Hyperparathyroidism

SHPT defines any condition in which the increased PTH secretion occurs as a normal physiologic response, often mediated by a decrease of serum calcium. Vitamin D deficiency, as a result of inadequate nutritional intake/sun exposure, malabsorption, liver diseases, or chronic renal failure, is the most common cause. Other, less common causes include vitamin D resistance (Fanconi syndrome, vitamin D receptor defects), PTH resistance (pseudohypoparathyroidism, hypomagnesemia), drugs (calcium chelators, inhibitors of bone resorption, and drugs that interfere with vitamin D metabolism [phenytoin and ketoconazole]), acute pancreatitis, and osteoblastic metastases (prostate and breast cancer).

SHPT should always be considered and ruled out before making the diagnosis of normocalcemic PHPT. At variance with PHPT, SHPT is characterized by low or, more often, low-normal serum calcium and decreased urinary calcium excretion. An elevation of serum phosphate levels can be a clue to pseudohypoparathyroidism.

A prolonged stimulation of PTH synthesis and secretion, as may occur in end-stage renal failure and severe gastrointestinal diseases, may lead to the emergence of an autonomous clone of parathyroid cells into a single gland, leading to hypercalcemia (tertiary hyperparathyroidism).

Hypoparathyroidism

Hypoparathyroidism (HypoPT) is the clinical spectrum caused by insufficient production of PTH by the parathyroid glands. The major distinguishing feature is hypocalcemia, resulting from inadequate mobilization of calcium from bone and reabsorption of calcium at the distal tubule, and decreased activity of renal 1α-hydroxylase and therefore generation of calcitriol; as a consequence, the intestinal calcium absorption will be reduced.

Epidemiology

HypoPT is a rare condition designated in both the United States and Europe as an orphan disease. The estimated prevalence is 37 and 24 per 100,000 inhabitants in the United States and Europe, respectively.

Pathogenesis

HypoPT can be congenital or acquired (Table 3).

---

[1] Not FDA approved for this indication.
[1] Not FDA approved for this indication.

TABLE 3	Classification of Hypoparathyroidism*

Congenital

Isolated
Defective PTH biosynthesis *(PTH)* ^
- Abnormal development of parathyroid glands *(GCMB, GCM2, GATA3)*
- Autosomal dominant hypocalcemia
- Type 1 *(CASR)*
- Type 2 *(GNA11)*

Associated with additional features or organ defects
- Autoimmune
- Isolated
- Polyglandular syndrome type 1 *(AIRE)*
- Di George syndrome *(TBX1)*
- Sanjad-Sakati/Kenny-Caffey type 2 *(TBCE)*
- Kenny-Caffey type 2 *(FAM111A)*
- Mitochondrial DNA mutations

Defective action of PTH
- Pseudohypoparathyroidism
- Type 1a *(GNAS)*
- Type 1b *(STX16, GNAS;* in sporadic form paternal UPD)
- Type 1c *(GNAS)*
- Type 2 (not yet identified)

Acquired

Destruction or removal of the parathyroid glands
- Postoperative (neck surgery)
- Radiation induced
- Infiltration of the parathyroid glands (metastatic, granulomatous)
- Deposition of heavy metals (iron, copper)

Reversible impairment or PTH secretion or action
- Severe magnesium deficiency
- Hypermagnesemia (e.g., due to tocolytic therapy)
- CaSR-stimulating antibodies

*Mutated genes are indicated in parentheses.
AIRE, Autoimmune regulatory; *CASR,* calcium-sensing receptor; *FAM111A,* family with sequence similarity 111 member A; *GATA3,* GATA-binding protein 3; *GCMB,* glial cell missing gene; *GCM2,* glial cell missing homolog 2; *GNA11,* G protein subunit alpha 11; *GNAS,* GNAS complex locus; *PTH,* parathyroid hormone; *STX16,* syntaxin 16; *TBCE,* tubulin folding cofactor E; *TBX1,* T-Box1; *UPD,* uniparental disomy.

Congenital HypoPT is usually hereditary and may be isolated or combined with organ defects. The autoimmune is the most common form and may be either isolated or part of the autoimmune polyglandular syndrome type 1 (APS1). The other forms are much rarer.

Acquired HypoPT is much more common than the congenital counterpart. Bilateral neck surgery for thyroid or parathyroid disorders is the most common cause. Postoperative HypoPT can be transient (caused by reversible parathyroid ischemia and resolving within a few weeks) or chronic/permanent (caused by irreversible parathyroid damage such as ischemia, electric scalpel damage, or, rarely, inadvertent removal of parathyroid glands). Its rate largely depends on the experience of the surgeon and the extent of the neck surgery.

Clinical Presentation

The clinical manifestations of HypoPT are largely related to the level of serum calcium and the speed of its fall and may range from asymptomatic cases, when hypocalcemia is mild (corrected calcium ≥ 7.0 mg/dL [1.75 mmol/L]), to a severe, life-threatening condition that requires hospital admission and intensive treatment. In mild cases signs related to neuromuscular irritability, namely the Chvostek sign (twitching and/or contracture of the facial muscles produced by tapping on the facial nerve just anterior to the ear and just below the zygomatic bone) and Trousseau sign (carpal spasm evoked by inflating a sphygmomanometer cuff above systolic blood pressure for several minutes), may be present at physical examination. Moderate to severe hypocalcemia (corrected calcium < 7.0 mg/dL [1.75 mmol/L]) is usually

TABLE 4 Calcium Preparation and Vitamin D Metabolites in the Management of Hypocalcemia

CALCIUM		
AGENT	**FORMULATION AND DOSE**	**COMMENTS**
Calcium gluconate	One ampule of 10% calcium gluconate contains 93 mg; preferably diluted in 5% dextrose	Tissue necrosis may be caused by elemental calcium; preferably diluted in 5% dextrose extravasation in the adjacent subcutaneous space
Calcium salts		
Calcium carbonate	40% elemental calcium by weight; 1 g calcium carbonate contains 400 mg elemental calcium	Best absorbed with meals in an acidic environment; constipation is a common side effect
Calcium citrate	21% elemental calcium by weight; 1 g calcium citrate contains 210 mg elemental calcium	Well absorbed independent of meal and acid environment; in patients with atrophic gastritis or taking proton pump inhibitors

VITAMIN D METABOLITES			
MEDICATION	**TYPICAL DAILY DOSE**	**TIME TO ONSET OF ACTION**	**TIME TO OFFSET OF ACTION**
Calcitriol [1,25(OH)$_2$D]$_3$ (Rocaltrol)	0.25–2.0 µg once or twice	1–2 days	2–3 days
Alfacalcidol[1] [1α(OH)D][1]	0.5–4 µg once	1–2 days	5–7 days
Dihydrotachysterol[1,†]	0.3–1.0 mg once	4–7 days	7–21 days
Vitamin D$_2$ (ergocalciferol) (Drisdol)[1] or vitamin D$_3$ (cholecalciferol)[1,†]	25,000–200,000 IU	10–14 days	14–75 days

[1]Not available in the United States.
*This compound is rapidly activated in the liver to 25(OH) dihydrotachysterol.
†These compounds could be used in a setting where active vitamin D metabolites are not available and/or are too expensive.
Modified from Shoback D. Clinical practice. Hypoparathyroidism. *N Engl J Med.* 2008;359:391-403.

symptomatic, even though there is no strict relationship between the severity of symptoms and the degree of hypocalcemia. In patients with postoperative HypoPT, symptoms usually appear on the first postoperative day, but, in some cases, hypocalcemia may become clinically manifest even after 3 to 4 days. Classical manifestations include paresthesias, carpopedal spasm, tetany, seizures, positive Chvostek and Trousseau signs, and prolongation of the QT interval on electrocardiography. Papilledema and subcapsular cataract can be present. Pseudohypoparathyroidism is a group of genetic disorders caused by end-organ resistance to the action of PTH. Patients with the type 1a variant have a typical phenotype (Albright hereditary osteodystrophy), characterized by short stature, shortened fourth and fifth metacarpals, rounded face, and mild intellectual deficiency. Other endocrine glands, including the thyroid and the gonads, may be dysfunctional. This clinical and endocrine phenotype is also typical of patients with type 1c. Patients with type 1b have PTH resistance and in some cases partial resistance to thyroid-stimulating hormone and mild brachydactyly. Patients with the type 2 variant have PTH resistance in the absence of the aforementioned clinical phenotype.

Evaluation and Diagnosis

The finding of low albumin–corrected serum calcium, high serum phosphate, and inappropriately low or undetectable serum PTH confirms the diagnosis of HypoPT. A recent neck surgery strongly suggests the postoperative form. A family history of hypocalcemia suggests a genetic cause. Coexistence of other autoimmune endocrinopathies (e.g., adrenal insufficiency) or candidiasis prompts consideration of APS1. Immunodeficiency and the presence of other congenital organ defects point to DiGeorge syndrome. Genetic testing may be warranted to confirm the diagnosis of this and other genetic forms. Magnesium should also be measured because magnesium deficiency impairs the secretion of PTH and its action in target tissues. Urinary calcium is usually low because of the low filtered calcium. The 24-hour calcium-to-creatinine clearance ratio is increased in patients with the activating mutation of *CaSR*. A biochemical profile of low serum calcium and

high phosphate levels, together with high serum PTH, in the absence of vitamin D deficiency, reflects the PTH-resistant state and suggests a case of pseudohypoparathyroidism.

Treatment

The goal is to control symptoms of hypocalcemia and improve QoL while avoiding side effects and complications. The target serum calcium concentration is in the lower part of the normal range. Treatment relies on the administration of calcium (oral [dietary or supplements] or IV), active vitamin D metabolites, magnesium, and, where available, recombinant human PTH1-84 (Natpara). Thiazide diuretics may help reduce hypercalciuria; a low-phosphate diet and phosphate binders may help control hypophosphatemia and lower the calcium–phosphate product.

Acute Hypoparathyroidism

Acute hypocalcemia typically follows neck surgery and may be favored by a low vitamin D status and magnesium deficiency that, when present, should be corrected before surgery. In patients with high risk (total thyroidectomy, repeated thyroid surgery), perioperative administration of calcitriol (Rocaltrol) decreases the incidence of postoperative hypocalcemia and shortens the hospital stay.

Mild Hypocalcemia. In mild hypocalcemia (corrected calcium ≥ 7.0 mg/dL [1.75 mmol/L]), oral calcium supplements (usually calcium carbonate, 1 to 3 g daily in divided doses) alone or combined with active vitamin D metabolites should be administered. Calcitriol is typically initiated at an initial dose of 0.5 to 1.0 µg twice daily; equivalent doses of 1α-calcifediol[2] (1.0 to 2.0 µg) may also be used (see later [Chronic Hypoparathyroidism, Conventional Therapy] for more details on calcium and active vitamin D therapy) (Table 4). Serum calcium is checked weekly until optimal levels are reached.

Moderate to Severe Hypocalcemia. Patients with moderate to severe hypocalcemia (corrected calcium < 7.0 mg/dL [1.75 mmol/L]) are usually admitted to the hospital and treated with IV

[2]Not available in the United States.

calcium until an oral regimen can be started. One to two ampules of 10% calcium gluconate diluted in 50 to 100 mL of 5% dextrose should be infused over a period of 10 to 20 minutes with electrocardiographic and clinical monitoring. The calcium infusion will raise the serum calcium concentration for no more than 2 to 4 hours; thus this initial treatment should be followed by a continuous infusion (50 to 100 mL/h) of a solution containing 1 mg/mL of elemental calcium (11 ampules of 10% calcium gluconate added to 5% dextrose in a final volume of 1 L). The rate should be adjusted according to corrected serum calcium level, which should be measured initially every 1 to 2 hours and subsequently every 4 to 6 hours and should be maintained at the lower limit of the normal range while the patient is asymptomatic. This calcium infusion protocol maintained for 8 to 10 hours will raise serum calcium by approximately 2 mg/dL. Oral administration of active vitamin D metabolites and calcium should be started as soon as practical. Calcitriol is typically initiated at a dose of 0.5 to 1.0 µg twice daily; oral calcium (1 to 3 g daily in divided doses) is also added.

If hypocalcemia is due to magnesium deficiency, the previous protocol should be applied while magnesium is being replaced by administering IV magnesium sulfate (initial dose 2 g as a 10% solution over 10 to 20 minutes, followed by 1 g/h in 100 mL) until a normal serum level of magnesium is reached. The only administration of magnesium will be unable to correct hypocalcemia because hypomagnesemia inhibits the secretion of PTH and consequently the renal activation of 25(OH)D and induces a peripheral resistance to the action of PTH.

The rate of calcium infusion should be increased if symptoms of hypocalcemia recur. The IV infusion should be slowly tapered and discontinued when an effective regimen of oral calcium and active vitamin D is reached (up to 24 to 48 hours or longer) and stable desired serum calcium levels are obtained.

Chronic Hypoparathyroidism

The goal of therapy is to maintain serum calcium in the low-normal range, avoid hypocalcemic symptoms and long-term complications, and improve QoL. An individualized approach is necessary to optimize patient care. Guidelines for the management of chronic HypoPT have only recently been developed by the European Society of Endocrinology, the American Association of Clinical Endocrinologists, the American College of Endocrinology, and a panel of international experts.

Conventional Therapy. An adequate calcium intake from dietary sources (mainly dairy products) should be recommended, but calcium supplements (1 to 3 g daily in divided doses) are needed in almost all adult patients. Calcium carbonate is generally preferred because fewer pills per day are needed. Calcium carbonate requires an acidic gastric environment to be absorbed and should be taken with meals. Its bioavailability decreases in patients with atrophic gastritis or taking proton pump inhibitors. In these circumstances, calcium citrate, which is well absorbed independent of meal and acid environments, should be preferred. Calcium citrate might also be a preferred option for patients who complain of gastrointestinal side effects using calcium carbonate or who prefer to take calcium supplements outside mealtimes. Calcium carbonate and calcium citrate interfere with levothyroxine absorption; therefore a patient who has had a thyroidectomy should be advised to take levothyroxine well apart from calcium supplements.

Before the availability of synthetic active vitamin D metabolites, supraphysiologic doses (25,000 to 200,000 IU daily) of either cholecalciferol (vitamin D_3) or ergocalciferol (vitamin D_2) were used (Table 4). Nowadays, active 1α-hydroxylated vitamin D metabolites are preferred because patients with HypoPT have impaired renal activation of 25(OH)D. Calcitriol (Rocaltrol) and alfacalcidol (One-Alpha)[2] have a similar time of onset, but the latter has a longer time of offset (5 to 7 days vs. 2 to 3 days). Calcitriol is more potent (about 50%) than alfacalcidol when compared in terms of the calcemic effect. The daily dose of calcitriol

in adults ranges between 0.25 and 2.0 µg, equal to 0.5 to 4 µg of alfacalcidol. Weight-based dosing (0.01 to 0.04 µg/kg per day), eventually associated with calcium supplements (20 to 40 mg/kg per day), should be used in infants and young children. Adult doses should be used in older children. Another active vitamin D analog, dihydrotachysterol,[2] is also available in some countries. Where active vitamin D metabolites are not available or too expensive, large doses of parent vitamin D can still be used, but attention should be paid to the risk of vitamin D toxicity.

A low vitamin D status is not uncommon in patients with HypoPT, and patients with vitamin D deficiency treated with active vitamin D metabolites should be supplemented with vitamin D_2 or D_3, because active vitamin D metabolites do not correct hypovitaminosis D.

Active vitamin D metabolites stimulate intestinal absorption of phosphate, which may cause hyperphosphatemia and an increased calcium–phosphate product, with the risk of soft tissue calcification. In this setting, the intake of phosphate-rich foods should be reduced, and the daily dose of calcium supplements should be increased because calcium binds phosphate.

Hypercalciuria (≥250 mg [6.25 mmol] in women, ≥300 mg [7.5 mmol] in men, or >4 mg [0.1 mmol]/kg body weight in both sexes) is a common feature in patients with chronic HypoPT, because of the lack of PTH-dependent renal tubular reabsorption of calcium. In such instances a low-sodium diet should be advised either alone or combined with the administration of a thiazide diuretic that decreases renal calcium excretion. The combination of thiazide with amiloride[1] may further lower urinary calcium excretion and decrease the risk of hypokalemia. Thiazide diuretics are not advised in autosomal dominant hypocalcemia, a condition caused by mutations of the *CaSR*. Magnesium deficiency, when present, should also be corrected.

Lifelong monitoring is needed in patients with chronic HypoPT. No study has evaluated how to best monitor these patients. The target serum calcium concentration is within the low-normal range, with no symptoms of hypocalcemia. In some patients a higher serum calcium level is needed to be symptom-free. A baseline renal imaging should be obtained. The published guidelines of the European Society of Endocrinology and the recent guidelines of the international experts participating in the Fifth International Workshop on the evaluation and management of primary hyperthyroidism suggest measuring ionized or albumin-corrected total calcium, phosphorus, magnesium, and creatinine (eGFR) every 3 to 12 months; 25(OH)D every 6 to 12 months; and 24-hour urinary calcium excretion every 6 to 24 months. They also suggest performing renal imaging when patients have symptoms of nephrolithiasis or increasing serum levels of creatinine. Biochemical monitoring should be performed weekly or every other week when changing the daily dose of calcium or active vitamin D metabolites or introducing a new drug. It is important to note that serum calcium may fluctuate once the therapeutic regimen has been stabilized. Several comorbidities (e.g., gastrointestinal disease, diarrhea, immobilization) and drugs (loop and thiazide diuretics, systemic glucocorticoids, proton pump inhibitors, antiresorptive drugs, cardiac glycosides, and chemotherapeutics) may interfere with calcium homeostasis, and therefore patients should be periodically asked about their occurrence or use.

Conventional therapy only partially restores calcium homeostasis, and patients with chronic HypoPT have a reduced QoL and an increased risk of comorbidities, which include nephrocalcinosis, nephrolithiasis, impaired renal function, neuropsychiatric diseases, muscle stiffness and pain, infections, and seizures. An increased rate of intracerebral calcifications and cataracts has been documented in nonsurgical HypoPT. Bone mineral content is increased in patients with chronic HypoPT, but cancellous bone microarchitecture is abnormal.

Parathyroid Hormone. Until recently, HypoPT was the only major hormonal insufficiency state not treated with the missing hormone. The development of the recombinant human

---

[2] Not available in the United States.

[1] Not FDA approved for this indication.

N-terminal 1 to 34 fragment (rhPTH$_{1-34}$) and the full-length 1 to 84 (rhPTH$_{1-84}$) molecule has stimulated several studies on its use as replacement therapy, which led to the approval by the FDA of rhPTH$_{1-84}$ for the management of chronic HypoPT.

The official recommendation is to consider rhPTH$_{1-84}$ therapy "only in patients who cannot be well-controlled on calcium and active forms of vitamin D and for whom the potential benefits are considered to outweigh the potential risk." Treatment should be started with subcutaneous administration in the thigh of 50 µg once daily, while reducing by 50% the daily dose of active vitamin D if serum calcium is greater than 7.5 mg/dL (1.875 mmol/L). Serum calcium should be monitored every 3 to 7 days and the daily dose of rhPTH$_{1-84}$ titrated every 4 weeks, aiming to reduce the daily calcium supplements to 500 mg and discontinue active vitamin D therapy while maintaining the serum calcium in the low-normal range. Afterward, serum calcium should be monitored every 3 to 6 months. Hypercalcemia has been reported in some cases, but a careful adjustment of the daily dose may decrease this risk. A "black box" in the official recommendation highlights the potential risk of osteosarcoma (studies in rats have shown that both rhPTH$_{1-34}$ and rhPTH$_{1-84}$ can cause osteosarcoma). However, there is no evidence that individuals treated with either PTH molecules are at increased risk for osteosarcoma. The safety and efficacy of rhPTH$_{1-84}$ in pediatric patients have not been established. The EMA has approved the use of rhPTH$_{1-84}$ as an adjunctive therapy for adults with chronic HypoPT who cannot be adequately controlled with standard therapy alone.

The FDA and the EMA have approved using rhPTH$_{1-84}$ in patients with HypoPT, and that leaves room for decision-making in individual cases. The guidelines recently elaborated by a panel of international experts suggest considering the use of rhPTH$_{1-84}$ therapy, where available, in any patient with chronic HypoPT of any etiology, except in patients with autosomal dominant hypocalcemia. Unfortunately, the manufacturing company (Takeda) will discontinue manufacturing rhPTH$_{1-84}$ globally at the end of 2024 due to unresolved issues that are specific to the product.

TransCon PTH is an investigational prodrug consisting of PTH (1-34) transiently conjugated to a polyethylene glycol carrier molecule providing stable PTH concentrations in the physiologic range for 24 hours a day. TransCon PTH was developed as a therapy for the treatment of HypoPT. After subcutaneous injection with exposure to physiologic pH and temperature, the linker is cleaved, releasing PTH (1-34) in a controlled manner.

A Phase 3 double-blind, placebo-controlled study with TransCon PTH 18 µg daily versus placebo recently evaluated safety and efficacy in 84 patients with chronic HypoPT. At 26 weeks, cessation of active vitamin D was possible in 93% of participants while maintaining normal serum calcium. Statistically significant reductions in 24-hour urine calcium were also observed in comparison to placebo. Improvements in QoL were also observed. The ongoing phase 3 and phase 2 open-label extension studies will provide data on the long-term efficacy and safety of TransCon PTH therapy for HypoPT.

Pregnancy and Lactation

There are limited data to inform treatment strategies in chronic HypoPT in pregnancy and lactation. The guidelines, recently updated, and the expert consensus of the European Society of Endocrinology suggest the use of active vitamin D metabolites and oral calcium as in nonpregnant women. Frequent monitoring (every 2 to 3 weeks) of serum calcium, possibly ionized calcium, is recommended. No studies have addressed the use of rhPTH$_{1-84}$ therapy in pregnant women. The FDA suggests that it should be used "only if the potential benefit justifies the potential risk to the fetus."

References

Arnold A, Levine A: Molecular basis of primary hyperparathyroidism. In Bilezikan JP, et al: *The parathyroids, basic and clinical concept*, London, 2015, Academic Press, pp 279–296.

Bilezikian JP, Bandeira L, Khan A, et al: Hyperparathyrodism, *Lancet* 1:168178, 2018.

Bilezikian JP, Khan A, Silverberg SJ, et al: Evaluation and management of primary hyperparathyroidism: summary statement and guidelines from the fifth international workshop, *J Bone Miner Res* 37:2293–2314, 2022.

Bilezikian JP, Cusano NE, Khan AA, et al: Primary hyperparathyroidism, *Nat Rev Dis Prim* 2:16033, 2016.

Bilezikian JP, Khan A, Potts Jr JT, et al: Hypoparathyroidism in the adult: epidemiology, diagnosis, pathophysiology, target-organ involvement, treatment, and challenges for future research, *J Bone Miner Res* 26:2317–2337, 2011.

Bilezikian JP, Silverberg SJ, Bandeira F, et al: Management of primary hyperparathyroidism, *J Bone Miner Res* 37:2391–2403, 2022.

Bollerslev J, Rejnmark L, Marcocci C, et al: European Society of Endocrinology Clinical Guideline: treatment of chronic hypoparathyroidism in adults, *Eur J Endocrinol* 173:G1–G20, 2015.

Bollerslev J, Rejnmark L, Zahn A, et al: European expert consensus on practical management of specific aspects of parathyroid disorders in adults and in pregnancy: recommendation of the ESE educational program of parathyroid disorders, *Eur J Endocrinol* 186:R33–63, 2021.

Cetani F, Marcocci C: Parathyroid carcinoma. In Bilezikian JP, editor: *The parathyroids, basic and clinical concepts*, London, 2015, Academic Press, pp 409–422.

Cetani F, Pardi E, Aretini P, et al: Whole exome sequencing in familial isolated primary hyperparathyroidism, *J Endocrinol Invest* 43:231–245, 2020.

Cusano NE, Silverberg SJ, Bilezikian JP: Normocalcemic primary hyperparathyroidism, *J Clin Densitom* 16:33–39, 2013.

EMA/CHMP/124164/2017 Media and public relations. http://www.ema.europa.eu/docs/en_GB/document_library/Press_release/2017/02/WC500222215.pdf, 2017.

Khan AA, Koch C, Van Uum SHM, et al: Standards of care for hypoparathyroidism in adults, *Eur J Endocrinol EJE* 18-0609.R1, 2018. https://doi.org/10.1530/EJE-18-0609. [Epub ahead of print].

Khan A, Rejnmark L, Rubin M, et al: PaTH forward: a randomized, double-blind, placebo-controlled phase 2 trial of TransCon PTH in adult hypoparathyroidism, *J Clin Endocrinol Metab* 107(1):e372–e385, 2021.

Khan AA, Bilezikian JP, Brandi ML, et al: Evaluation and management of hypoparathyroidism summary statement and guidelines from the second international workshop, *J Bone Miner Res* 37:2568–2585, 2022.

Khan AA, Rubin MR, Schwarz P, et al: Efficacy and safety of parathyroid hormone replacement with TransCon PTH in hypoparathyroidism: 26-week results from the phase 3 PaTHway trial, *J Bone Miner Res* 38(1):14–25, 2023.

Leere JS, Karmisholt J, Robaczyk M, et al: Denosumab and cinacalcet for primary hyperparathyroidism (DENOCINA): a randomised, double-blind, placebo-controlled, phase 3 trial, *Lancet Diabetes Endocrinol* 8:407–417, 2020.

Lundstam K, Pretorius M, Bollerslev J, et al: Positive effect of parathyroidectomy compared to observation on BMD in a randomized controlled trial of mild primary hyperparathyroidism, *J Bone Miner Res* 38(32–380), 2023.

Mannstadt M, Bilezikian JP, Thakker RV, et al: Hypoparathyroidism, *Nat Rev Dis Prim* 3:17055, 2017. http://www.ema.europa.eu/docs/en_GB/document_library/Press_release/2017/02/WC500222215.pdf.

Mannstadt M, Clarke BL, Vokes T, et al: Efficacy and safety of recombinant human parathyroid hormone (1-84) in hypoparathyroidism (REPLACE): a double-blind, placebo-controlled, randomised, phase 3 study, *Lancet Diabetes Endocrinol* 1:275–283, 2013.

Marcocci C, Bollerslev J, Khan AA, Shoback DM: Medical management of primary hyperparathyroidism: proceedings of the fourth international workshop on the management of asymptomatic primary hyperparathyroidism, *J Clin Endocrinol Metab* 99:3607–3618, 2014.

Marcocci C, Cetani F: Clinical practice, primary hyperparathyroidism, *N Engl J Med* 365:2389–2397, 2011.

NATPARA: *Shire-NPS pharmaceuticals*, Inc, 2015. [package insert] https://www.accessdata.fda.gov/drugsatfda_docs/label/2015/125511s000lbl.pdf.

NATPAR. https://www.ema.europa.eu/en/medicines/human/EPAR/natpar.

Mazoni L, Matrone A, Apicella M, et al: Renal complications and quality of life in postsurgical hypoparathyroidism: a case-control study, *J Endocrinol Invest* 45:573–582, 2022.

Pretorius M, Lundstam K, Hellström M, et al: Effects of parathyroidectomy on quality of life: 10 years data from a prospective randomized controlled trial on primary hyperparathyroidism (the SIPH-study), *J Bone Miner Res* 36(1):3–11, 2021.

Rubin MR, Bilezikian JP, McMahon DJ, et al: The natural history of primary hyperparathyroidism with or without parathyroid surgery after 15 years, *J Clin Endocrinol Metab* 93:3462–3470, 2008.

Seabrook AJ, Harris LE, Velosa SB, et al: Multiple endocrine tumors associated with dermline MAX mutations: multiple endocrine neoplasia type 5? *J Clin Endocrinol Metab* 106:1163–1182, 2021.

Sidhu PS, Talat N, Patel P, et al: Ultrasound features of malignancy in the preoperative diagnosis of parathyroid cancer: a retrospective analysis of parathyroid tumours larger than 15 mm, *Eur Radiol*, 2011.

Shoback D: Clinical practice. Hypoparathyroidism, *N Engl J Med* 359:391–403, 2008.

Shoback DM, Bilezikian JP, Costa AG, et al: Presentation of hypoparathyroidism: etiologies and clinical features, *J Clin Endocrinol Metab* 101:2300–2312, 2016.

Treglia G, Piccardo A, Imperiale A, et al: Diagnostic performance of choline PET for detection of hyperfunctioning parathyroid glands in hyperparathyroidism: a systematic review and meta-analysis, *Eur J Nucl Med Mol Imag* 46:751–765, 2019.

Vignali E, Viccica G, Diacinti D, et al: Morphometric vertebral fractures in postmenopausal women with primary hyperparathyroidism, *J Clin Endocrinol Metab* 94:2306–2312, 2009.

HYPERPROLACTINEMIA

Method of
Ming Li, MD, PhD; and Lawrence Chan, MD

CURRENT DIAGNOSIS

- Hyperprolactinemia is diagnosed by biochemical tests based on two-site immunoassay, which can be confounded by extreme hyperprolactinemia (hook effect) and biologically inactive macroprolactinemia.
- Hyperprolactinemia can be caused by physiologic, pharmacologic, or pathologic conditions; careful clinical, laboratory, and radiology evaluations are required to identify its underlying cause.
- The most common causes of hyperprolactinemia include medications, prolactinoma, and other pituitary and hypothalamic/pituitary stalk diseases.
- Clinical features of hyperprolactinemia include galactorrhea, menstrual abnormalities (in women), impotence (in men), infertility, and osteoporosis.
- Patients with prolactinoma may also have local compression symptoms including headache, visual disturbance, and hypopituitarism.
- Pituitary magnetic resonance imaging (MRI) is the imaging method of choice for diagnosing prolactinoma and other sellar/parasellar lesions.

CURRENT THERAPY

- For secondary hyperprolactinemia, treatment should be directed at correcting underlying causes.
- Treatment goals for prolactinoma are relief of symptoms and the long-term effects of hyperprolactinemia and of tumor mass effects.
- The dopamine agonists cabergoline (Dostinex) and bromocriptine (Parlodel) are effective in normalizing the prolactin level and shrinking the tumor in patients with prolactinoma.
- Surgery and radiotherapy of prolactinoma are reserved for patients resistant to or intolerant of medical therapy.
- Temozolomide (Temodar)[1] monotherapy is the first-line chemotherapy for aggressive or malignant prolactinomas after failing standard treatments.

[1]Not FDA approved for this indication.

Biochemistry and Physiology of Prolactin

Prolactin is a polypeptide hormone produced by pituitary lactotroph cells. It is also produced locally in a variety of extrapituitary tissues such as mammary glands, decidua, gonads, brain, liver, fat, pancreas, and the immune system, along with its receptors. Prolactin is highly pleiotropic in terms of its functions. Many of its actions collectively support puerperal lactation. Prolactin displays considerable sequence homology to growth hormone (GH) and placental lactogen. The prolactin and GH receptors both belong to the class I cytokine/hematopoietic receptor superfamily. Prolactin is responsible for maturation of the mammary glands during pregnancy, but it plays only a minor role in pubertal mammary development, which requires GH instead. It appears not to be an essential hormone for nonchildbearing individuals. Rare patients deficient in either prolactin or its receptor are largely healthy despite difficulty with fertility and lactation.

Prolactin circulates mainly as a 23-kDa 199-aa polypeptide. Several of its cleavage products exist in blood, which may have functions unrelated to lactation; for example, one 16-kDa cleavage product of prolactin displays antiangiogenic and prothrombotic properties and has been implicated in the development of preeclampsia and peripartum cardiomyopathy. Several forms of prolactin aggregate, known as macroprolactins, also exist in circulation at lower levels. They are formed either by covalent bonding of prolactin monomers or by their nucleating around autoimmune immunoglobulin G. These macroprolactins are not biologically active in vivo and have a prolonged half-life. At times they can build up in the circulation to a level high enough to cause diagnostic difficulties.

Among the major pituitary hormones, prolactin is unique for its predominantly negative mode of regulation by the hypothalamus. It does not have a known hypothalamus-derived releasing hormone. Instead, lactotrophs are under tonic inhibition by dopamine secreted from hypothalamic neurons. Increase in prolactin output is mostly mediated by withdrawing dopaminergic control in response to environmental cues, such as physical activity, stress, and nipple stimuli (Figure 1). Under experimental and pathologic conditions, several factors, including thyrotropin-releasing hormone, vasoactive intestinal peptide, oxytocin, and vasopressin, have been shown to increase prolactin secretion, but these peptides appear to play only minor and insignificant roles for the physiologic regulation of prolactin.

Estrogen is the main driver of prolactin secretion during pregnancy. Stimulated by persistently elevated estrogen, lactotrophs grow in number and size. By term the pituitary gland can reach two to three times its normal size, and prolactin levels increase some 20-fold. Along with placental hormones such as estrogen, progesterone, and placental lactogen, prolactin drives the maturation of the mammary glands. Lactation starts after parturition, when estrogen withdraws from the circulation. Frequent infant suckling maintains physiologic hyperprolactinemia, which is important for sustained milk production. In addition, hyperprolactinemia during this critical period provides a natural although unreliable way of contraception. This is achieved by suppression of the hypothalamus-pituitary-gonad axis. Hyperprolactinemic hypogonadism and parathyroid hormone–related peptide (PTHrP) secreted from mammary epithelial cells help mobilize skeletal calcium store in support of milk production. Through its receptors in liver, intestine, fat, and pancreas, prolactin also adjusts maternal nutrient metabolism to meet the nutrition needs of the fetus during pregnancy and breast-feeding newborns. In the brain, prolactin modifies parental behavior toward closer infant attendance (see Figure 1).

Pathophysiology of Hyperprolactinemia

Physiologic hyperprolactinemia as occurs during pregnancy and nursing is essential for child raising through the actions of prolactin in target organs discussed above. Similar changes in these organs under the influence of persistent pathologic hyperprolactinemia in the absence of pregnancy and lactation, however, are inappropriate and could lead to a variety of undesired long-term consequences.

Mammary Glands

One common symptom of persistent hyperprolactinemia is galactorrhea; that is, milk production not associated with childbirth or breast-feeding. Because puerperal lactation normally ends within 6 months after delivery or weaning, any milk production beyond this point is also considered galactorrhea. Because maturation of mammary glands is completed during pregnancy, galactorrhea typically happens in women between 20 to 35 years of age with previous childbirths. It also occurs in nulligravid women, women postmenopause, and men, although less frequently.

Prolactin is a known mitogen for mammary epithelial cells, and concern has been raised regarding its potential role in the pathogenesis of breast cancer. In a large prospective study by the Women's Health Initiative, there was evidence of a significant increase in breast cancer incidence in women postmenopause with high

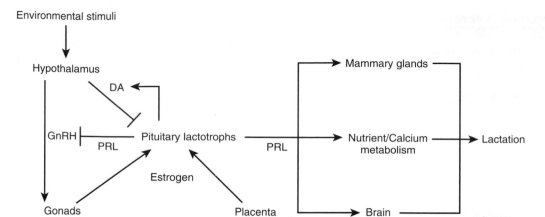

Figure 1 Physiology of prolactin and its regulation. At baseline, prolactin production and secretion are under tonic inhibition by dopamine released from hypothalamic neurons. The hypothalamus controls prolactin production by altering output of dopamine after integrating environmental stimuli and changes in hormonal homeostasis. Prolactin increases hypothalamic dopamine output, providing a negative feedback regulatory loop. Estrogen stimulates prolactin synthesis and secretion during pregnancy. Prolactin supports puerperal lactation via its action on the mammary glands, nutrient/calcium metabolism, and brain. Unlike most other anterior pituitary hormones, feedback regulation of prolactin secretion does not occur via factors produced by a peripheral endocrine target organ. Prolactin also suppresses the hypothalamic-pituitary-gonadal axis by inhibiting GnRH release. *DA,* Dopamine; *PRL,* prolactin.

normal prolactin levels, which is within the highest quartile of the normal range compared with those in the lowest quartile. On the other hand, increased breast cancer risk has not been observed in patients with overt hyperprolactinemia. In fact, early parity and lactation history are strong protective factors against breast cancer. Further research is required to resolve these seemingly discrepant observations.

Female Reproductive System

Persistent hyperprolactinemia significantly diminishes the pulsatile release of gonadotropin-releasing hormone (GnRH). Because GnRH neurons do not themselves express prolactin receptors, prolactin exerts its effects on their afferent neurons instead by suppression of secretion of kisspeptin, a potent secretagogue for GnRH. Prolactin receptors are also found in the gonads, and prolactin has been reported to inhibit folliculogenesis and estrogen production in the ovary directly. However, this likely has only a limited contribution to infertility and hypogonadism associated with hyperprolactinemia, because the hypothalamus-pituitary-gonad axis can be reactivated by administration of GnRH or kisspeptin, with return of ovulation and fertility in subjects with hyperprolactinemia.

Male Reproductive System

As in women, hyperprolactinemia causes secondary hypogonadism and infertility in men by suppression of GnRH pulses and a decrease in luteinizing hormone and follicle-stimulating hormone levels. Patients often have low or low normal testosterone levels, as well as abnormal sperm counts and morphology in semen analysis. Patients usually seek medical attention for diminished libido and impotence. The central nervous system (CNS) actions of prolactin are likely partly responsible for these symptoms, because restoration of testosterone level alone is often inadequate for symptom relief, which occurs only when prolactin levels also return to normal.

Adrenal Glands

Prolactin stimulates the synthesis of androgen in the zona reticularis of the adrenal cortex. Mild elevations in serum levels of adrenal androgens—for example, dehydroepiandrosterone (DHEA) and dehydroepiandrosterone sulfate (DHEA-S)—are seen in approximately 50% of women with hyperprolactinemia. Symptoms of clinical hyperandrogenism such as hirsutism and acne are rare in these patients. When present, they are almost always associated with a concurrent increase in testosterone level.

Elevation of adrenal androgens in hyperprolactinemia may contribute to the suppression of GnRH release in the hypothalamus and secondary hypogonadism.

Skeletal System

Premenopausal women with hyperprolactinemia have lower bone density and approximately a 4.5 times higher risk for osteoporotic fractures. Hypogonadism associated with hyperprolactinemia is the main cause of bone loss, whereas restoration of sex hormones with either hormone replacement or correction of hyperprolactinemia improves bone density. Bone density is preserved in women with hyperprolactinemia who continue to have regular menses. Nonetheless, not all studies showed a clear correlation between the degree of bone loss and duration of amenorrhea or levels of sex hormones, suggesting involvement of additional processes. For example, the levels of PTHrP were found to be significantly higher in patients with hyperprolactinemia and correlated well with bone density measurements. Correction of hyperprolactinemia by dopamine agonists was shown to normalize PTHrP levels.

Metabolic Effects of Hyperprolactinemia

During pregnancy and nursing, physiologic elevation of prolactin, via signaling in fat, small intestine, pancreas, and liver, regulates maternal nutrient metabolism to meet the needs of the fetus and newborn, leading to hyperphagia, weight gain, insulin resistance, and leptin resistance. Similarly, pathologic hyperprolactinemia is strongly correlated with obesity, insulin resistance, hyperlipidemia, diabetes, and all-cause and cardiovascular mortality, although the clinical presentations vary greatly. Medications blocking prolactin release were reported to improve cardiometabolic risk factors. Bromocriptine (Cycloset) is approved by the U.S. Food and Drug Administration (FDA) as a hypoglycemic agent for treating type 2 diabetes. It remains to be determined what level of prolactin is associated with higher cardiovascular risk; high normal and mildly elevated prolactin levels have been reported as cardioprotective. Hyperprolactinemia has not been formally recognized as a risk enhancer for considering lipid-lowering therapies by the Endocrine Society's recent *Clinical Practice Guidelines on Lipid Management in Patients With Endocrine Disorders*. It would be advisable to screen for and treat established cardiovascular risk factors in patients with hyperprolactinemia and consider testing for coronary calcium score in patients with borderline to intermediate cardiovascular risk, if decisions regarding lipid-lowering therapies remain uncertain.

TABLE 1   Causes of Hyperprolactinemia

Physiologic

Pregnancy

Lactation and breast stimulation

Neonatal period

Physical activity

Stress

Sexual intercourse

Pharmacologic

Dopamine antagonists—antipsychotics and antiemetics

Tricyclic antidepressants

Selective serotonin reuptake inhibitors

Antihistamines (H2)

Verapamil (Calan)

Protease inhibitors

Dopamine synthesis inhibitors

Pathologic

Pituitary Diseases

Prolactinoma

Plurihormonal adenomas

Lymphocytic hypophysitis

Empty sella syndrome

Macroadenoma with or without suprasellar extension

Idiopathic hyperprolactinemia

Hypothalamic/Pituitary Stalk Diseases

Tumors: meningioma, craniopharyngioma, germinoma, metastasis, etc.

Granulomas

Infiltrative diseases

Irradiation

Trauma

NEUROGENIC: chest wall lesions, spinal cord lesions, herpes zoster, and epileptic seizure

Paraneoplastic syndrome

Systemic Diseases

End-stage renal disease

Cirrhosis

Adrenal insufficiency

Pseudocyesis

Adapted from Bronstein (2016); Melmed et al. (2016).

Etiology of Hyperprolactinemia

Any conditions that affect production or clearance of prolactin can lead to hyperprolactinemia (Table 1). Physiologic hyperprolactinemia is transient and adaptive, whereas persistent hyperprolactinemia from pharmacologic and pathologic causes is often symptomatic with undesired long-term consequences. Pituitary adenomas overproducing prolactin (prolactinomas) are the most important cause of pathologic hyperprolactinemia. In addition to the elevated prolactin levels, prolactinomas produce pathologic local mass effects. Secondary hyperprolactinemia is most commonly related to disruption of dopaminergic control of lactotrophs, secondary to the use of dopamine antagonists or hypothalamic and pituitary stalk lesions.

Epidemiology and Natural History of Prolactinoma

Prolactinoma is the most common type of pituitary adenoma, contributing to approximately 40% to 50% of pituitary tumor cases. Prolactinomas are categorized according to size into microprolactinomas (<1 cm) and macroprolactinomas (>1 cm). Clinically these two conditions behave very differently and can be considered as separate entities. In general, macroprolactinomas tend to grow progressively and are often locally invasive; they are also generally more resistant to treatment and have a higher risk of recurrence. On the other hand, microprolactinomas rarely progress in size (~7% of cases) and have a good chance (~15% of cases) of going into remission on their own.

The prevalence of prolactinoma has been estimated to be 500 cases per million with an incidence of about 27 cases per million per year based on survey of asymptomatic populations. In autopsy series, however, lactotroph neoplasms staining positive for prolactin are much more common, being found in approximately 5% of the subjects. They are predominantly microadenomas. Only a small fraction of these small lactotroph neoplasms develop overt hyperprolactinemia by escaping tonic dopaminergic suppression from the hypothalamus, presumably via down-regulation of dopamine D2 receptor-mediated signaling pathway and/or bypassing the portal system for blood supply. Microprolactinomas predominantly affect women of childbearing age, with a female-to-male ratio of approximately 20:1. Macroprolactinoma, on the other hand, shows no sex predilection. Neoplastic transformation of lactotroph involves accumulation of genetic and epigenetic events. The best understood candidate genes involved include the pituitary tumor–transforming gene (PTTG) and the heparin-binding secretory transforming (HST) gene. Pituitary tumor–transforming gene expression is positively regulated by estrogen.

Most prolactinomas occur sporadically. Most prolactinomas are benign, although they can be locally invasive. Malignant prolactinomas, as defined by the presence of extrapituitary metastases, are extremely rare. Familial cases, such as those associated with multiple endocrine neoplasia I (MEN I) and familial isolated pituitary adenoma (FIPA), typically occur at a younger age and are more often macroprolactinomas that are locally invasive.

Clinical Manifestations

Clinical manifestations of prolactinomas fall under two categories: systemic effects of hyperprolactinemia and local compression symptoms.

Symptoms of Hyperprolactinemia

Persistent hyperprolactinemia inappropriately recapitulates symptoms associated with normal pregnancy and nursing. In extreme cases, hyperprolactinemia has been associated with delusions of pregnancy in susceptible individuals, for example, some women on psychotropic medications.

Menstrual abnormalities and infertility are the most common symptoms associated with hyperprolactinemia in women of childbearing age. These symptoms may be masked by use of oral contraceptive pills, which often delays diagnosis. The mildest cases include women presenting with infertility caused by shortened luteal phase despite preserved regular menses. As the degree of hypogonadism worsens, patients experience menstrual irregularities ranging from anovulatory cycles to oligomenorrhea and amenorrhea. Patients with amenorrhea may also experience psychological stresses and other menopausal symptoms like vaginal dryness and dyspareunia. Of note, high prolactin levels may sometimes mask vasomotor symptoms of women in menopause and perimenopause with prolactinoma, who may develop hot flashes once they are successfully treated with dopamine agonists.

Galactorrhea occurs in up to 80% of cases of hyperprolactinemia. This will need to be differentiated from nipple discharges of other causes, especially those from breast neoplasms. Further evaluation with breast imaging and cytology is indicated when the discharge is unilateral, bloody, or associated with a breast mass. Galactorrhea is by definition milk-like in appearance, and when in doubt, Sudan Black B staining showing fat globules is confirmatory. Although considered a classic sign and symptom for hyperprolactinemia, galactorrhea per se is a poor predictor for hyperprolactinemia in the absence of additional symptoms, because it can be seen in about 10% of healthy women of childbearing age. If amenorrhea is present at the same time, the patient should be assumed to harbor a prolactinoma unless proven otherwise. The degree of galactorrhea is quite variable, from barely expressible to bothersome bra stain and copious free flow, and does not necessarily reflect the severity of hyperprolactinemia. In fact, most patients with galactorrhea and normal menses have normal prolactin levels. On the other hand, in some patients with extremely high levels of prolactin, galactorrhea could be masked by severe hypogonadism.

Men with hyperprolactinemia mainly present with impotence and diminished libido, which is not always corrected with testosterone replacement. As noted in the section on pathophysiology, these symptoms are not all caused by hypogonadism but may involve the central effects of prolactin. Other symptoms and signs of hypogonadism, such as loss of body hair and muscle bulk, are less common. Infertility could also occur with decrease in sperm count and morphology, although hyperprolactinemia is only present in approximately 5% of male patients seeking treatment for infertility.

For both male and female patients, persistent hypogonadism from hyperprolactinemia leads to osteoporosis and increased risk of fracture. This could be effectively treated with either sex hormone replacement or dopamine agonists.

Mass Effects of Prolactinomas

Headache is the most common neurologic symptom caused by pituitary tumors. It can occur even with microadenomas presumably caused by dural stretch. More severe headache results from larger tumors, especially those with extrasellar invasion, and occasionally from apoplexy.

Visual disturbance typically only happens with macroadenomas with suprasellar extension impinging on the optic chiasm, leading to loss of visual acuity and visual field defects. The typical pattern of visual field defect is bitemporal hemianopsia, which usually starts from the upper field and progresses downward as the tumor impinges upward from below. Ophthalmoparesis typically happens in the setting of apoplexy and only rarely results from parasellar invasion of the cavernous sinus and impingement of cranial nerves III, IV, or VI.

By compressing the rest of the pituitary gland, including the stalk, prolactinoma can cause deficiencies of other anterior pituitary hormones including GH, thyroid-stimulating hormone (TSH), and adrenocorticotropic hormone, in addition to hypogonadism from the hyperprolactinemia. The degree of the risk is proportional to tumor size.

Cerebrospinal fluid (CSF) rhinorrhea occurs when a macroprolactinoma invades inferiorly into the sphenoid sinus. Other rare compressive symptoms from giant prolactinomas include epilepsy (temporal lobe involvement), exophthalmos, and hydrocephalus. Life- and vision-threatening emergencies could arise from apoplexy and CNS infection.

Laboratory Evaluation

Prolactin Assay and Pitfalls

Hyperprolactinemia is diagnosed by individual measurements of serum prolactin levels. Patients should be well rested, because physical activity stimulates prolactin secretion. Fasting is normally not needed but can be justified when the initial reading is only mildly elevated, to rule out meal effects. Dynamic tests such as thyrotropin-releasing hormone stimulation do not appear to add to diagnostic value and are not recommended. The level of prolactin may provide valuable diagnostic clues. Secondary hyperprolactinemia rarely exceeds 150 ng/mL. On the other hand, a prolactin level of greater than 100 ng/mL is highly suggestive, and severe hyperprolactinemia of greater than 500 ng/mL is virtually diagnostic for prolactinoma. On rare occasions, secondary hyperprolactinemia can produce prolactin levels in the prolactinoma range. For example, risperidone (Risperdal)-induced hyperprolactinemia could be as high as 250 to 500 ng/mL, and patients with

end-stage renal disease who are on antipsychotics or antiemetics can have prolactin levels greater than 1000 ng/mL. The size of the prolactinoma shows a rough correlation with the serum prolactin level. Patients with microprolactinomas usually have prolactin levels in the range of 50 to 300 ng/mL, whereas those with macroprolactinomas have levels of 200 to 5000 ng/mL.

Most clinical laboratories measure prolactin using a two-site immunoassay. A capture antibody first affixes prolactin in the sample to a solid matrix. Subsequently, a second signal antibody is attached to the now-immobilized prolactin. The signal antibody is engineered to carry either a radioisotope or a chemiluminescent enzyme to provide a readout. The assay is accurate within its designed linear range, which is typically under 10,000 ng/mL. Beyond this level, both capture and signal antibodies could be saturated, preventing the signal antibody from attaching. As a result, signal outputs will be falsely diminished. This phenomenon, known as the hook effect, produces a falsely low reading that could lead to the misdiagnosis of a macroprolactinoma as a nonfunctioning pituitary tumor. This artifact can be circumvented by repeating the assay with a 100-fold diluted sample. Many laboratories also opt for an additional washout step to eliminate excess prolactin before adding the signal antibody, preempting the artifact.

Macroprolactinemia is another potential diagnostic pitfall masquerading as true hyperprolactinemia. Macroprolactins are biologically inactive prolactin aggregates that could accumulate in blood to a high level. Macroprolactinemia does not cause any morbidities but could contribute to analytical difficulties as the antibodies used in prolactin assays cross-react with macroprolactins. Most laboratories rely on polyethylene glycol (PEG) precipitation to determine the proportion of macroprolactins and the true concentration of monomeric prolactin. Up to 25% of monomeric prolactin can be also precipitated by PEG, potentially masking true hyperprolactinemia. Therefore patients with macroprolactinemia may still need to be further evaluated if clinical suspicion is high for true hyperprolactinemia.

Other Supporting Laboratory Tests

After confirming hyperprolactinemia, a simple chemistry panel may reveal or suggest the underlying cause, such as chronic kidney disease and cirrhosis. A pregnancy test (beta human chorionic gonadotropin level) is essential for women of childbearing age, and hypothyroidism needs to be ruled out with a TSH assay. Both pregnancy and hypothyroidism may have presenting symptoms of sellar mass and hyperprolactinemia and therefore be mistaken for prolactinoma.

For established prolactinoma cases, it is important to also assess other pituitary axes. Up to 20% of GH-secreting tumors co-secrete prolactin, and insulin-like growth factor 1 (IGF-1) level is an essential screening test for these cases. If hypogonadism is suspected, levels of luteinizing hormone, follicle-stimulating hormone, and sex hormones (testosterone or estrogen) should be obtained. Screening for central hypothyroidism and secondary adrenal insufficiency should be done with TSH, free thyroxine (T4), and morning cortisol levels, respectively, for patients with pituitary tumors larger than 6 mm.

Neuroimaging

Pituitary imaging should be considered for all patients with unexplained significant hyperprolactinemia, especially if there are signs or symptoms of local compression. Magnetic resonance imaging (MRI) with and without gadolinium contrast with dedicated pituitary protocol is the test of choice. Compared with other modalities, MRI provides superior soft tissue contrast, revealing the tumor's inner structure and its relationship to surrounding tissues, including cavernous sinus, pituitary stalk, and optic chiasm. Computed tomography scan still has a role for patients with metal implants or other contraindications for MRI and is especially useful for revealing bony erosions and tissue calcification; its use is limited by suboptimal soft tissue contrast and exposure to ionizing radiation.

Visual Field Testing

A formal visual field test with a perimeter is recommended when suprasellar extension of a pituitary adenoma brings it close to the optic chiasm. Improvement or worsening in visual field often precedes imaging evidence of tumor shrinkage or expansion during treatment. Therefore visual field testing is an excellent monitoring tool for patients under treatment for macroadenoma and visual impairment.

Diagnosis

Prolactin testing is usually prompted by suggestive signs and symptoms of hyperprolactinemia such as menstrual abnormalities, infertility, and galactorrhea. A careful history, including medication use, physical examination, and routine laboratory evaluation (see preceding sections), is invaluable for uncovering secondary causes. Pituitary imaging should be performed when no other underlying causes are found, especially if the levels of prolactin are higher than 100 ng/mL. A diagnostic algorithm shown in Figure 2 provides a framework for a structured and cost-effective workup of hyperprolactinemia.

Differential Diagnosis

An exhaustive list of etiologies is provided in Table 1. A few entities deserve additional comments.

Drug-induced hyperprolactinemia is common and at times may produce serum prolactin levels matching those in patients with prolactinoma (see prior section on laboratory evaluation). A more typical range of prolactin level is 25 to 100 ng/mL for drug-induced hyperprolactinemia. It is not always possible to correlate in time the initiation of the culprit drug with the onset of symptoms or rise of prolactin levels. The way to confirm medication-related hyperprolactinemia is to discontinue the putative offending agent(s) for 3 days before repeating a prolactin assay. Some medications may require a longer period of abstinence, and in such cases the level of prolactin can be retested later if the second value is reduced but still elevated. Before discontinuing psychotropic medications, one should consult with the prescribing psychiatrist to prevent worsening of the patient's mental symptoms.

Pseudoprolactinoma refers to a nonfunctioning sellar or suprasellar mass associated with hyperprolactinemia caused by stalk disruption. The prolactin level is seldom >150 ng/mL for pseudoprolactinomas. Accordingly, the Pituitary Society's 2006 guidelines for the diagnosis and management of prolactinomas use 150 ng/mL as a cutoff for diagnosing prolactinoma. Recent literature, however, has revealed significant overlap of prolactin levels in patients with true prolactinoma and secondary hyperprolactinemia <150 ng/mL. Taking into consideration tumor volume in assessing prolactin levels significantly improves diagnostic accuracy. In patients with prolactin levels ≤150 ng/mL, a prolactin level/tumor volume ratio of 0.065 (ng/mL)/mm³ accurately separates patients with nonfunctional pituitary tumors from true prolactinomas without any overlap. Before making a diagnosis of pseudoprolactinoma, one must exclude hook effect with a 100-fold diluted sample. Prolactin levels are typically normalized within several days after initiation of dopamine agonists, because lactotrophs are still sensitive to dopamine, but local compressive symptoms do not improve. In contrast, patients with true macroprolactinoma experience a more gradual decrease in prolactin levels after they are put on dopamine agonists, but they could expect improvement in compressive symptoms within 12 hours to days and imaging evidence of tumor shrinkage in weeks.

Polycystic ovary syndrome (PCOS) and hyperprolactinemia are among the most common causes of menstrual irregularities and infertility and affect women of similar ages. PCOS has also been associated with hyperprolactinemia. However, multiple studies have shown that the prevalence of hyperprolactinemia in women with PCOS is not significantly higher than that of matched populations. Although mild elevations of DHEA-S or DHEA are common in patients with hyperprolactinemia, hirsutism is rare and, when present, is always associated with an increase in testosterone level, likely reflecting possible coexisting PCOS. Therefore the presence of hyperprolactinemia in patients with PCOS or hirsutism warrants additional evaluation.

Management of Secondary Hyperprolactinemia

Treatment of secondary hyperprolactinemia should focus on correcting the underlying conditions; for example, treating hypothyroidism and resection of nonfunctioning pituitary tumors. For drug-induced hyperprolactinemia, the responsible medications should be removed or replaced with alternatives. Newer antipsychotics such as aripiprazole (Abilify) may be used in place of older agents such as risperidone (Risperdal) because they have better metabolic/hormonal profiles. For irreversible conditions such as end-stage renal disease, hyperprolactinemia can be effectively controlled with dopamine agonists. Ectopic prolactin secretion,

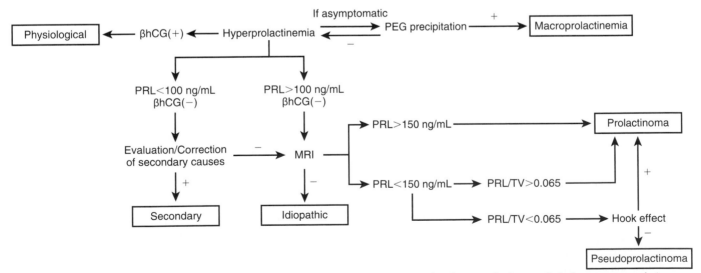

Figure 2 Diagnostic algorithm for hyperprolactinemia. If hyperprolactinemia occurs in the absence of relevant clinical symptoms and signs, one should rule out macroprolactinemia by PEG precipitation. When hyperprolactinemia is confirmed, pregnancy should be ruled out with a βhCG test. In the absence of pregnancy, if the PRL level is higher than 100 ng/dL, the pretest probability for a prolactinoma is high enough to justify a pituitary MRI scan, even if potential secondary causes exist. Regardless of prolactin levels, secondary causes should be carefully evaluated with medication history, physical examination, and laboratory tests such as thyroid function tests and chemistry panel, and appropriately treated. If hyperprolactinemia remains unexplained or persists despite correction of other contributing factors, a pituitary MRI is in order. Patients with negative sellar findings have idiopathic hyperprolactinemia. Patients with sellar mass may have either prolactinoma or pseudoprolactinoma. The latter is suggested by a discordant prolactin level less than 150 ng/mL and prolactin/tumor volume ratio lower than 0.065 (ng/mL)/mm³, after hook effect has been ruled out. *βhCG*, β Human chorionic gonadotropin; *PRL*, prolactin; *PRL/TV*, prolactin level/tumor volume ratio in nanograms per milliliter per cubic millimeter.

HYPERTHYROIDISM

Method of
William J. Hueston, MD

CURRENT DIAGNOSIS

- Hyperthyroidism or thyrotoxicosis is most often caused by Graves' disease, toxic nodular goiter (Plummer's disease), or acute thyroiditis.
- Common symptoms in hyperthyroidism are tachycardia, elevated systolic blood pressure, tremor, and anxiety. Patients with Graves' disease also might exhibit exophthalmos. In contrast, elderly patients can present with apathetic hyperthyroidism, which can be confused with hypothyroidism.
- Hyperthyroidism should be suspected in all patients who present with atrial fibrillation, palpitations, panic disorder, or unexplained tremors.
- Thyroid storm is an acute, life-threatening condition usually occurring in patients with undiagnosed or untreated hyperthyroidism placed under physiologic stress.
- An elevated free T_4, usually with a low thyroid-stimulating hormone is the hallmark of hyperthyroidism, and anti–thyroid-stimulating hormone antibodies can help identify Graves' disease.
- Ultimately, a thyroid scan and uptake are usually necessary to differentiate the cause of hyperthyroidism.
- Subclinical hyperthyroidism is an uncommon finding of uncertain long-term clinical significance but treatment for patients over 65 with cardiac disease or osteoporosis should be considered.

CURRENT THERAPY

- In patients with Graves' disease or autonomous thyroid nodules (toxic nodular goiter), short-term treatment includes thyroid suppression medications (such as methimazole [Tapazole]) and β-blockers (such as propranolol [Inderal][1]). Long-term management with radioiodine thyroid gland ablation is often pursued once symptoms are controlled.
- Patients with acute thyroiditis might need transient β-blockade but can often be managed expectantly until symptoms abate and thyroid hormone levels normalize. A small number of patients (~10%) have persistent hypothyroidism after an episode of illness.
- Thyroid storm is a medical emergency that requires close monitoring along with an antithyroid drug, β-blockers, corticosteroids, and iodine-potassium solution (Lugol's solution).

[1]Not FDA approved for this indication.

Epidemiology

Hyperthyroidism is relatively uncommon and usually caused by three conditions: Graves' disease, toxic nodular goiter, or acute thyroiditis. Graves' disease is the most common cause of hyperthyroidism in the United States and usually affects younger patients from the teens to the 40s. Like other autoimmune diseases, women are at higher risk (seven to eight times) than men. Toxic nodular goiter accounts for 15% to 30% of hyperthyroid diagnoses. It usually occurs after age 50 years, is more common in women, and follows several decades of multinodular thyroid disease. A less-common cause is administration of amiodarone. Amiodarone is about one third iodine and can cause hyperthyroidism either through iodine-induced thyroid damage or from increased thyroxine synthesis owing to excessive iodine.

Subclinical hyperthyroidism, defined as an abnormally low TSH but normal free thyroxine (T_4) and triiodothyronine (T_3) affects 1% to 2% of the population. This condition is most common with mild forms of hyperthyroidism but also can be observed transiently in thyroiditis. Subclinical hyperthyroidism is more common in individuals over age 70 and those with iodine-deficient diets.

Risk Factors

There are no known environmental or reversible risk factors for any of the causes of hyperthyroidism. Graves' disease is associated with a specific human leukocyte antigen (HLA) region on chromosome 6 *(CTLA 4)*.

Pathophysiology

The most common causes of hyperthyroidism are shown in Box 1.

Graves' disease is an autoimmune disorder caused by antibodies against thyroid-stimulating hormone (TSH) receptors on the thyroid gland. Graves' disease is associated with many other autoimmune diseases, including pernicious anemia, vitiligo, type 1 diabetes mellitus, autoimmune adrenal disease, Sjögren's syndrome, rheumatoid arthritis, and lupus. As with these other disorders, the etiology is unknown.

Toxic nodular goiter, also known as Plummer's disease, results from the development of autonomous thyroid adenoma. Patients who develop a toxic nodular goiter usually have a long history of many other nodules that spontaneously burn out over time, but then develop a single large nodule (usually 2.5 cm or greater) that continues to produce thyroid hormone in such large quantities that patients become hyperthyroid. No clear cause is known for the development of the nodules.

Acute thyroiditis can also produce hyperthyroidism. Several different conditions can cause thyroiditis (see Box 1). The inflammation resulting in thyroiditis is thought to be related to subacute viral infections or autoimmune reactions; suppurative thyroiditis is a rare bacterial thyroid infection, usually caused by *Staphylococcus aureus*. During the acute period of thyroid inflammation, damage to the gland leads to the release of stored thyroxine from thyroid lakes, producing hyperthyroidism. However, after the initial release of thyroid hormone from the stored lakes, damage to the gland inhibits production of new thyroxine. After the initial surge in thyroid hormone levels, thyroxine levels drop, often to levels that can result in transient hypothyroidism. Most patients return to the euthyroid state after the thyroid gland heals, but about 10% of patients with acute thyroiditis remain chronically hypothyroid.

Other, less common causes of hyperthyroidism include excessive exogenous administration of thyroid medications. This is most commonly the result of over-replacement of thyroxine (Levoxyl, Synthroid) in patients with hypothyroidism, but it may be intentional for weight loss. Because thyroxine and

---

| **BOX 1** | Conditions Causing Hyperthyroidism |

Graves' disease
Autonomous thyroid nodule (toxic nodular goiter)
  Acute thyroiditis
- Hashimoto's thyroiditis
- Subacute granulomatous thyroiditis (de Quervain's thyroiditis)
- Subacute lymphocytic thyroiditis (silent or painless thyroiditis)
- Suppurative thyroiditis (bacterial infection of thyroid)
  Excessive exogenous thyroid use
- Over-replacement after thyroid ablation or for hypothyroidism
- Thyroxine (Synthroid) abuse for weight loss
  Iodine overconsumption
  Amiodarone administration

triiodothyronine (T_3) are highly protein bound, over-replacement is most common if patients experience hypoproteinemia, such as in nephrotic syndrome, cirrhosis, or malnutrition.

Excessive iodine consumption, referred to as the Jod-Basedow effect, can also lead to thyrotoxicosis. The source of the iodine may include iatrogenic sources such as iodine-containing medications or radiologic contrast agents.

Several other medications, such as amiodarone (Cordarone), lithium, and interferon α (Intron A) also can cause thyrotoxicosis by causing drug-induced thyroiditis.

Prevention

There are no known strategies to prevent hyperthyroidism. For patients with hypothyroidism, annual monitoring of TSH levels is recommended to ensure that patients receive the appropriate replacement dose and not over-replacement.

Clinical Manifestations

Patients with hyperthyroidism complain of a variety of symptoms that can include anxiety, tachycardia, wide-pulse pressure hypertension, palpitations, fine tremor, weight loss, heat intolerance, and, particularly in the elderly, confusion or delirium. Patients with Graves' disease also have ophthalmopathy characterized by lid retraction and exophthalmoses that can lead to optic nerve damage. In contrast, older patients can have few of the classic signs of hyperthyroidism and instead might complain of fatigue or weakness (apathetic hyperthyroidism), unexplained delirium, weight loss, heart failure, or isolated atrial fibrillation.

Some patients have a rapid escalation of symptom severity (thyroid storm) that is life-threatening if not identified and treated promptly. These patients usually have underlying thyrotoxicosis from Graves' disease complicated by a secondary physiological stressor such as infection, surgery, or trauma. This is a medical emergency and needs immediate attention, including hospitalization with close observation.

On physical examination, patients with hyperthyroidism due to Graves' disease or thyroiditis might have a diffusely enlarged and mildly tender thyroid gland. In suppurative thyroiditis, the thyroid gland is red, hot, and very tender and accompanied by a fever and other systemic signs of severe infection. Patients with toxic nodular goiter can have palpable nodules in their thyroid gland and often have a single palpable nodule.

Diagnosis

Hyperthyroidism is diagnosed by finding an elevation in the free thyroxine (T_4) level accompanied by a low TSH level. Patients with Graves' disease often have positive anti–thyroid receptor antibody titers. Only anti-thyroglobulin receptor antibody testing is helpful because it can help differentiate Graves' disease from other causes. No other anti-thyroid tests are clinically indicated. Once the thyroid level abnormalities are found, a definitive diagnosis of the cause for the hyperthyroidism is needed to select the appropriate treatment strategy.

Other conditions can produce a depressed TSH but normal free T_4 levels. These include T_3 toxicosis and subclinical hyperthyroidism. T_3 toxicosis refers to situations where triiodothyronine (T_3) is produced in excess rather than thyroxine (T_4); this can occur in any of the conditions that can cause hyperthyroidism, as well as in surreptitious triiodothyronine (Cytomel) ingestion.

Thyroid scanning and radiolabel uptake are usually necessary to differentiate the causes of hyperthyroidism. Thyroid scanning and uptake rely on the thyroid gland to concentrate radioactive molecules, such as iodine-131 (^{131}I) or technetium. Because of the risk of thyroid storm with iodine administration, patients should be treated with antithyroid drugs for 2 to 8 weeks before a scan and the drugs should be stopped at least 4 days before the test. Patients with Graves' disease show increases in uptake and diffuse distribution of the tracer throughout the thyroid gland. Patients with toxic nodular goiter also have increased uptake, but the isotope is concentrated in a one or a few focal areas, with the remainder of the thyroid gland suppressed. In contrast, patients

TABLE 1	Treatment Strategies for Hyperthyroidism	
TREATMENT	**DRUG**	**DOSAGE**
Graves' Disease and Toxic Nodular Goiter		
Thyroid hormone suppression	Methimazole Propylthiouracil	Initial: 30–40 mg/d Maintenance: 5–15 mg/d Initial: 300–400 mg/d Maintenance: 100–300 mg/d
β-Blockade	Propranolol[1] Metoprolol (Lopressor)[1]	10 mg qid 50–100 mg bid
Thyroid gland removal	Radioactive iodine ablation Thyroidectomy	
Acute Thyroiditis		
β-Blockade transiently May need thyroid replacement long term		
Thyroid Storm		
Thyroid hormone suppression	Propylthiouracil	300–400 mg/d
β-Blockade	Propranolol[1]	1 mg/min IV to max 10 mg[3]
Iodine	Lugol's solution	1–2 gtt mixed in water tid
Cardiac and fluid monitoring	Dexamethasone (Decadron)[1]	2 mg q6h

[1]Not FDA approved for this indication.
[3]Exceeds dosage recommended by the manufacturer.

with thyroiditis have decreased uptake of the radiolabel and a washed-out or mottled distribution on scanning.

Differential Diagnosis

Symptoms of hyperthyroidism also occur in patients with panic disorder and other anxiety conditions. These patients can have sinus tachycardia, tremor, and nervousness that mimic hyperthyroidism.

Treatment

Treatment depends on the cause of the hyperthyroidism (Table 1). In Graves' disease, immediate goals of treatment include reducing thyroid hormone production and blocking the peripheral effects of the excessive thyroid hormone. About 30% to 60% of patients, mostly adolescents, enter remission spontaneously, and the remission may be permanent. Remission rates are highest for those with a small goiter, no ophthalmopathy, thyroglobulin levels less than 50 μg/mL, and thyroxine levels less than 20 μg/dL. Signs of remission include a decreased ratio of T_3 to T_4, lower thyroid-stimulating thyroglobulin levels, and decreased radioactive iodine uptake on rescanning. When remissions do occur, it is usually within a year of starting antithyroid medications.

For those who do not undergo spontaneous remission, which includes most adults, consideration should be given to thyroid gland ablation to permanently treat this condition. Although the dosage can be calculated to attempt to leave patients euthyroid, permanent hypothyroidism occurs in about half of all patients treated with radioactive iodine ablation.

The initial approach to toxic nodular goiter is similar to that for symptom control, but thyroid ablation should be recommended routinely because remissions are very rare.

Thyroid gland production of hormone can be reduced rapidly with either methimazole (Tapazole) or propylthiouracil.

For treatment of Graves' disease, methimazole is the preferred treatment and has the advantage of less frequent dosing, which improves compliance. Propylthiouracil is an alternative that is recommended for women in the first trimester of pregnancy and patients who cannot tolerate methimazole. However, the FDA issued a black box warning about the use of propylthiouracil in 2010 because of liver toxicity; physicians should be aware of this and use propylthiouracil only when methimazole is not suitable. With both drugs, clinicians need to be aware of drug-associated agranulocytosis, which can result in life-threatening bacterial infections. In patients on either of these medications who develop a sore throat, fever, or other signs of infection, a white blood cell count should be done immediately to ensure that they are not neuropenic. Additionally, antithyroid drugs are associated with drug-induced lupus syndromes and other forms of vasculitis.

In addition to reducing production of thyroid hormone, initial therapy for patients with Graves' disease and toxic nodular goiter should include a β-blocker to reduce the tachycardia, tremor, hypertension, and anxiety. A β-blocker that crosses the blood-brain barrier, such as propranalol (Inderal)[1] or metoprolol (Lopressor)[1], is the best choice in this situation because these also reduce the central nervous system effects such as anxiety, as well as the vascular problems caused by thyroid hormones.

Thyroid storm requires immediate attention and should be managed in the hospital setting, especially in older patients where tachycardia and hypertension can lead to cardiac instability. Prompt administration of β-blockers and propylthiouracil along with cardiac monitoring for dysrhythmias and appropriate fluid management are essential for managing this life-threatening condition. Once antithyroid drugs have been administered, iodine-potassium solution (Lugol's solution) at a dose of 1 or 2 drops three times a day should be administered, which will further reduce thyroid hormone production and reduce peripheral conversion of T_4 to T_3. Finally, corticosteroids also have been shown to rapidly reduce thyroid hormone levels in thyroid storm.

For long-term management, thyroid ablation with radioactive iodine (sodium iodide, ^{131}I) can restore patients to a permanent euthyroid state. However, radioactive iodine thyroid ablation often results in destruction of more thyroid than optimal, causing hypothyroidism. Radioactive iodine thyroid ablation is contraindicated in pregnancy. For patients in whom radioactive iodine is either contraindicated or not acceptable, thyroidectomy is an option. Thyroidectomy almost always results in permanent hypothyroidism, as well as having other risks inherent in surgery including hypoparathyroidism and recurrent laryngeal nerve damage.

In patients with hyperthyroidism associated with acute thyroiditis, symptoms often resolve by the time the evaluation is complete. In the interim, symptoms can be managed with β-blockers. β-Blocker therapy can be discontinued fairly rapidly (2 to 3 weeks) after the initial onset of symptoms.

Indications for the treatment of subclinical hyperthyroidism are less clear. Based on recommendations of the American Thyroid Association, patients with a persistently low TSH who are over age 65 or who have underlying cardiac disease or osteoporosis should be considered for treatment. The treatment strategy should be directed at the presumed cause of the condition and may include antithyroid medication for suspected Graves' Disease or thyroid ablation for toxic nodular goiter or a solitary autonomous nodule.

Monitoring

In patients on antithyroid drugs, thyroid hormone levels should be monitored frequently until they reach a stable euthyroid state. Any change in the patient's underlying health, especially changes that could alter protein levels, should prompt reevaluation. In addition, patients who have thyroid ablation need follow-up testing of TSH and free T_4 levels to ensure that sufficient thyroid tissue has been destroyed to reverse their hyperthyroidism but not make them hypothyroid. This should be done 6 to 8 weeks following ablation therapy.

---

[1] Not FDA approved for this indication.

Complications

Complications of hyperthyroidism include acute and chronic conditions. Acutely, the most concerning complications are cardiac dysrhythmias, especially atrial fibrillation. Chronically, excessive thyroxine is associated with cardiomyopathy and osteoporosis. In patients with ophthalmopathy, untreated Graves' disease can lead to progressive vision loss and blindness.

Hyperthyroidism in pregnancy, even when adequately treated, has been shown to be an independent risk factor for cesarean section but not for any additional pregnancy complications. Some patients with existing hyperthyroidism may experience transient increases in free T_4 levels during pregnancy that can be associated with hyperemesis gravidarum. Assessing free T_4 levels in pregnant patients who have hyperthyroidism and develop hyperemesis may be useful.

References

Cooper DS: Antithyroid drugs for the treatment of hyperthyroidism caused by Graves' disease, *Endocrinol Metab Clin North Am* 27:225–247, 1998.
Kharlip J, Cooper DS: Recent developments in hyperthyroidism, *Lancet* 373:1930–1932, 2009.
Lazarus JH: Hyperthyroidism, *Lancet* 349:339–343, 1997.
Nayak B, Hodak SP: Hyperthyroidism, *Endocrinol Metab Clin North Am* 36(3):617–656, 2007.
Zimmerman D, Lteif AN: Thyroxicosis in children, *Endocrinol Metab Clin North Am* 27:109–126, 1998.
Donangelo I, Suh SY: Subclinical hyperthyroidism: When to consider treatment, *Amer Family Phys* 95:710–716, 2017.

HYPOKALEMIA AND HYPERKALEMIA

Method of
Jie Tang, MD

CURRENT DIAGNOSIS

- The "initial approach" to the evaluation of dyskalemia is to determine if it is secondary to transcellular shifts (in vitro or in vivo) of potassium (K) or a result of a true change in total body K.
- A thorough history and physical will provide useful information regarding the causes of hypokalemia and hyperkalemia, especially in cases of low or high intake of K, and transcellular shifts.
- Key steps in the diagnostic approach to hypokalemia include assessments of urinary K excretion and acid-base status.
- Key steps in the diagnostic approach to hyperkalemia include assessments of renal function and aldosterone activity.

CURRENT THERAPY

- For both hypokalemia and hyperkalemia, it is critical to assess the underlying transcellular K shift, given the risk of rebound hyperkalemia after K repletion or hypokalemia after K restriction and removal.
- In cases of severe dyskalemia, close cardiac monitoring is needed.
- The aggressiveness of therapy for dyskalemia is directly related to the rapidity with which the condition has developed, the absolute level of serum K, and the clinical evidence of toxicity.
- In severe or symptomatic cases of hypokalemia, both intravenous and oral K repletion are often needed.
- In severe or symptomatic cases of hyperkalemia, supported by electrocardiogram (ECG) abnormalities, both immediate temporizing measures and definitive therapy for K removal are necessary.

Epidemiology

Hypokalemia is defined as a serum K level of 3.5 mmol/L or lower. It is a common electrolyte disorder encountered in clinical practice. According to one study, serum K less than 3.6 mmol/L was found in up to 20% of hospitalized patients. The majority of these patients had serum K concentrations between 3.0 and 3.5 mmol/L, but as many as 25% had values less than 3.0 mmol/L. Even mild or moderate hypokalemia increases the risks of morbidity and mortality in patients with cardiovascular disease. Hyperkalemia is defined as a serum K of 5.5 mmol/L or higher. The prevalence among hospitalized patients not yet on dialysis was reported to be about 3.3%, and among them, up to 10% had significant hyperkalemia ($\geq$6.0 mmol/L). Hyperkalemia also carries a significantly increased risk of mortality.

Risk Factors

People most at risk for hypokalemia are those who are malnourished, with poor oral intake; those who use certain medications, such as diuretics; and those who have uncontrolled vomiting or diarrhea. People most at risk for hyperkalemia are those with reduced kidney function, those who have a history of diabetes mellitus, or those who take certain medications, such as angiotensin-converting enzyme inhibitors.

Pathophysiology

K is the most abundant cation in the human body. It regulates intracellular enzyme function and helps determine neuromuscular and cardiovascular tissue excitability. The total body store is approximately 55 mmol/kg of body weight. Over 98% of total body K is located in the intracellular fluid (primarily in muscle), and less than 2% in the extracellular fluid. A typical Western diet provides 40 to 120 mmol of K per day. Tight control of the serum K is primarily accomplished by the kidney, where approximately 95% of body K is excreted. Under normal circumstances, K losses in stool and sweat are small. In addition, the interplay of several hormonal systems (insulin, catecholamine), serum tonicity, and the internal acid-base environment contribute to the exchange of K between the extracellular fluid and intracellular fluid, which helps keep the serum K concentration tightly controlled. Hypokalemia occurs when there is a significant intracellular K shift or a reduced total body K store from poor intake, or excessive renal or extrarenal loss, whereas hyperkalemia develops when there is a significant extracellular shift, high body K load, or ineffective K elimination (aldosterone resistance/deficiency or reduced renal function).

Prevention

For patients at risk for hypokalemia, adequate dietary K intake is essential. Additional K supplements may be needed for patients taking high doses of diuretics (especially thiazide diuretics) or experiencing prolonged vomiting or diarrhea. For patients with hyperkalemia and severe kidney dysfunction, dietary K restriction is critical in maintaining body K balance. Sometimes, the empirical use of K exchange resin is needed to prevent hyperkalemia. Lastly, medications that contribute to hypokalemia or hyperkalemia should be avoided if possible.

Clinical Manifestations

Mild hypokalemia (serum K 3.0 to 3.5 mmol/L) is usually well tolerated. Moderate hypokalemia (serum K 2.5 to 3.0 mmol/L) may cause nonspecific symptoms, such as fatigue, weakness, muscle cramps, and constipation. When the serum K drops to less than 2.5 mmol/L, muscle necrosis and flaccid paralysis with eventual respiratory failure may occur. K depletion also causes supraventricular and ventricular arrhythmias, especially in patients on digitalis therapy. Although severe hypokalemia is more likely to cause complications, even minimal decreases in serum or total body K can be arrhythmogenic in patients with underlying heart disease or who are receiving digitalis therapy. Lastly, increases in systolic and diastolic blood pressures can occur in patients with hypokalemia while they are on a liberal salt diet. Overall, the likelihood of symptoms tends to correlate with the rapidity of the decrease in serum K. As with hypokalemia, patients with hyperkalemia may present with nonspecific complaints such as fatigue and malaise. But the predominant manifestations in more severe hyperkalemia are neuromuscular and cardiac. Neuromuscular symptoms range from muscle weakness to paralysis. Cardiac arrhythmias, including asystole, ventricular tachycardia or fibrillation, and pulseless electrical activity, can also occur in severe hyperkalemia.

Diagnosis

Figures 1 and 2 illustrate the diagnostic approaches to hypokalemia and hyperkalemia. It is important to assess for pseudodyskalemia (in vitro shift of K) and dyskalemia from in vivo transcellular shift of K because neither is associated with disturbances in total body K balance. Although cellular shift of K and changes in total body K occur as isolated problems, they frequently coexist. In hypokalemia, the assessment of renal K excretion is a key step in the initial diagnostic evaluation, followed by the assessment of acid-base status. In hyperkalemia, medical history and laboratory testing can help identify altered K distribution, reduced urinary K excretion, or an excessive K load from exogenous intake or transcellular leakage. Under normal circumstances, high K intake alone is not sufficient to lead to significant hyperkalemia unless there are other risk factors present such as reduced aldosterone action or significant loss of kidney function. Measurement of the transtubular potassium gradient (TTKG) has been widely used as a diagnostic tool in both conditions. However, recent evidence suggests that the assumption inherent in the calculation of the TTKG lacks validity. That said, I still find it useful in the initial assessment.

Differential Diagnosis

Figures 1 and 2 outline a diagnostic approach, including differential diagnosis, for hyperkalemia and hypokalemia.

Therapy

The treatment of hypokalemia depends on the underlying cause, the degree of K depletion, and the risk of K depletion to the patient. In general, hypokalemia secondary to cell shift is managed by treating underlying conditions. For example, hypokalemia in the setting of catecholamine increases, as in chest pain syndromes, is managed with appropriate treatments for the pain. However, when cell-shift hypokalemia is associated with life-threatening conditions such as paresis, paralysis, or hypokalemia in the setting of myocardial infarction, the administration of K is indicated. With K depletion, replacement therapy depends on the estimated degree of decreases in total body K. For example, decreases in total body K accompanied by a fall in serum K from 3.5 to 3.0 mmol/L are associated with a K deficit of 150 to 200 mmol. Decreases in serum K from 3 to 2 mmol/L are associated with 200- to 400-mmol additional decreases in total body K. K can be administered intravenously but in limited quantities (10 mEq/h into a peripheral vein; 15 to 20 mEq/h into a central vein). Larger K requirements can only be accomplished by oral therapy or with dialysis.

The acute management of hyperkalemia depends on the presence or absence of ECG and neuromuscular abnormalities. In the absence of symptoms or ECG abnormalities, hyperkalemia is treated conservatively—for example, by decreasing dietary K or withdrawing offending drugs. In the presence of ECG abnormalities or symptoms, the goal of therapy is to stabilize cell membranes. First-line therapy includes calcium gluconate, 10 to 30 mL IV as a 10% solution (onset of action 1 or 2 minutes). Although the mechanism remains undefined, calcium "stabilizes" the cardiac membranes. The dose can be repeated after five minutes if the ECG changes persist or recur. Other therapies include 8.4% IV sodium bicarbonate[1], 50 to 150 mEq (onset 15 to 30

---

[1]Not FDA approved for this indication.

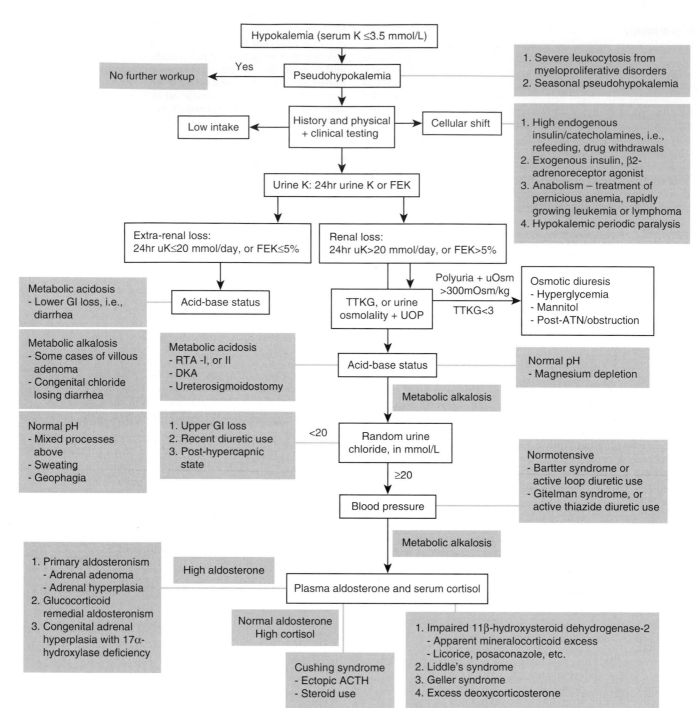

Figure 1 The diagnostic approach to hypokalemia. *ACS,* Acute coronary syndrome; *ATN,* acute tubular necrosis; *DKA,* diabetic ketoacidosis; *FEK,* fractional excretion of K; *GI,* gastrointestinal; *Met,* metabolic; *RTA,* renal tubular acidosis.

minutes), and rapid-acting insulin[1] 5 to 10 units intravenously (onset 5 to 10 minutes). Insulin increases the activity of the Na-K-ATPase pump in skeletal muscle and drives K into cells. Glucose 50%, 25 g intravenously, is given simultaneously with insulin to prevent hypoglycemia. Albuterol given as 0.5 mg in D5W IV or 10–20 mg in 4 mL normal saline by nebulizer (onset 15 to 30 minutes), also activates the Na-K-ATPase and drives K into cells. K driven intracellularly generally begins to move extracellularly again after approximately 6 hours, increasing the serum K concentration. Therefore, therapy to remove K from the body should be started simultaneously. Reductions in total body K may be achieved through a K exchange resin. The primary K resin used is sodium polystyrene sulfonate (Kayexalate). One gram of this medication binds approximately 1 mEq of K and releases 1 to 2 mEq of sodium back into the circulation. This medication may be given orally (onset 2 hours) or by enema with sorbitol to induce diarrhea (onset 30 to 60 minutes).

In 2015, patiromer, a polymer that exchanges calcium for potassium in the gastrointestinal tract, was approved by the Food and Drug Administration (FDA) for the management of hyperkalemia. In 2018, sodium zirconium cyclosilicate (SZC), a novel nonabsorbed, nonpolymer zirconium silicate compound that exchanges hydrogen and sodium for potassium and ammonium was also approved by the FDA for the same indication. Both agents are well tolerated and effective. Patiromer is administered orally at an initial dose of 10 g three times a day for up to 48 hours, followed by a maintenance dose of 10 g daily (maximum daily maintenance dose 15 g/day).

Figure 2 The diagnostic approach to hyperkalemia. *Hyperkalemia may occur with higher GFR if K load is excessive. *ACEI*, Angiotensin-converting enzyme inhibitor; *ARB*, angiotensin receptor blocker; *ENAC*, epithelial sodium channel; *GFR*, glomerular filtration rate; *NSAIDs*, nonsteroidal anti-inflammatory drugs; *RTA*, renal tubular acidosis.

If renal function is adequate, volume expansion with simultaneous diuresis can be attempted. Finally, hemodialysis is very effective in removing excess K.

The chronic management of hyperkalemia starts with dietary K restriction. Other management options include the use of diuretics, cessation or dose reduction of renin-angiotensin-aldosterone system inhibitors, and/or intermittent use of Kayexalate. Both patiromer and SZ are also well tolerated, safe, and effective in the chronic management of hyperkalemia. Just as important, they may allow the optimal use of renin-angiotensin-aldosterone system inhibitors in patients who have been previously untreated, had their dose reduced, or stopped treatment altogether.

Monitoring

Treatment for severe or symptomatic dyskalemia requires close cardiac monitoring and frequent laboratory testing to prevent overcorrection. If insulin and glucose are used in patients with hyperkalemia, blood sugars should be monitored for approximately 6 hours to identify and treat hypoglycemia from the insulin.

Complications

Complications from dyskalemia include cardiac arrhythmias, neuromuscular events, and, rarely, death. There are potential treatment-related complications if pseudodyskalemia or dyskalemia from in vivo transcellular shift is not recognized.

References

Gennari FJ: Hypokalemia, *N Engl J Med* 339:451–458, 1998.
Krishna GG, Kapoor SC: Potassium depletion exacerbates essential hypertension, *Ann Intern Med* 115:77–83, 1991.
Paice BJ, Paterson KR, Onyanga-Omara F, et al: Record linkage study of hypokalaemia in hospitalized patients, *Postgrad Med J* 62:187–191, 1986.
Stevens MS, Dunlay RW: Hyperkalemia in hospitalized patients, *Int Urol Nephrol* 32:177–180, 2000.

HYPONATREMIA

Method of
Beejal Shah, MD; and Susan L. Samson, MD, PhD

CURRENT DIAGNOSIS

- Perform a thorough history and physical examination with focus on the accurate assessment of volume status, neurologic symptoms and signs, current medications, and concurrent illnesses.
- Classify the hyponatremia as hypovolemic, euvolemic, or hypervolemic.
- Determine whether the hyponatremia is acute or chronic, based on the history and the clinical manifestations.
- Order key laboratory tests, including a basic metabolic panel (serum sodium, glucose, blood urea nitrogen, and creatinine), plasma osmolality, urine osmolality, and urine sodium.

CURRENT THERAPY

- Severe and symptomatic hyponatremia should be treated with hypertonic saline (3%) at 1 to 2 mL/kg per hour. Neurologic status and serum sodium should be monitored every 2 to 4 hours. The objective is to raise sodium by 2 mEq/L per hour (or to >125 mEq/L) until deleterious neurologic symptoms improve. After this, the rate of infusion should be titrated to increase the serum sodium by 0.5 to 1.0 mEq/L per hour, with a maximum increase of 6 to 8 mEq/L over 24 hours and no more than 18 mEq/L over 48 hours, to avoid precipitating osmotic demyelination.
- As a general rule, the treatment of hyponatremia should be adjusted for the serum sodium to increase by 0.5 to 1.0 mEq/L per hour with a maximum increase of 6 to 8 mEq/L over 24 hours and no more than 18 mEq/L over 48 hours.
- Acute hyponatremia (<48 hours) with neurologic symptoms should be treated more rapidly than chronic hyponatremia, a 4 to 6 mEq/L increase in serum sodium over 6 hours can reverse severe neurologic symptoms.
- Before a diagnosis of SIADH is made, rule out adrenal insufficiency and hypothyroidism.
- Most cases of euvolemic hyponatremia are caused by the syndrome of inappropriate antidiuretic hormone (SIADH), which usually can be managed with fluid restriction, salt tablets, and vasopressin receptor antagonists ("vaptans") as indicated.
- Discontinue thiazide diuretics in all cases of hypoosmolar hyponatremia.
- Hypovolemic and hypervolemic hyponatremia require therapy to correct the underlying cause (e.g., heart failure) and restore status to euvolemia.
- Vasopressin receptor antagonists (vaptans) are approved for short term management of euvolemic and hypovolemic hyponatremia. The same parameters apply for rate of sodium correction and monitoring as in conventional therapy.
- Overcorrection of hyponatremia should be recorrected in patients at high risk for osmotic dymelination.

Homeostasis maintains the concentration of sodium in the serum between 138 and 142 mEq/L (normal, 135–145 mEq/L) despite variations in water intake. Hyponatremia is defined as a serum sodium concentration of less than 135 mEq/L, although normal range values may differ slightly among laboratories, usually to a minimum normal sodium of 133 mEq/L. It is one of the most common electrolyte abnormalities found in the inpatient setting, occurring in up to 2.5% of patients, and it is a significant marker for mortality, associated with a 60-fold higher risk of death. It is not clear whether hyponatremia

itself is the cause of a more adverse prognosis or whether it echoes the degree of stress caused by illness. In the outpatient setting, chronic hyponatremia is most prevalent among the elderly and nursing home residents. The approach to management of hyponatremia is highly dependent on the underlying process. Establishing the correct etiology is critical, because inappropriate treatment can worsen hyponatremia. Therapy must be administered judiciously because of the risk of severe neurologic sequelae, including central nervous system demyelination. However, with a systematic approach to the differential diagnosis of hyponatremia, the correct diagnosis can be made and therapy initiated.

Clinical Presentation

Acute hyponatremia is defined as hyponatremia of less than 48 hours in duration. Mild symptoms include headache, nausea, vomiting, confusion, and weakness, which usually occur with a sodium level of less than 129 mEq/L. More severe neurologic manifestations—seizure and coma—are seen usually below a threshold of 120 mEq/L, although there currently is no evidence-based critical sodium level above which neurologic sequelae do not occur. The neurologic manifestations of acute or recurrent symptomatic hyponatremia can be delayed, so continued monitoring is important.

In contrast, patients with chronic hyponatremia more often are asymptomatic or have blunted symptoms. In elderly patients with mild chronic hyponatremia, subtle neurocognitive manifestations can occur, with decreased balance, lowered reaction speed, memory loss, and directed gait. Mild hypoosmolar hyponatremia is not independently associated with increased morbidity and mortality. Even so, the underlying etiology needs to be determined because of the potential for other factors (e.g., new medications, dehydration, occult illness) to contribute to the development of more severe hyponatremia with its potential for neurologic injury.

Regulation of Water Balance

Approximately two thirds of total body water is contained in the intracellular fluid (ICF) and one third as extracellular fluid (ECF). Plasma osmolality is tightly regulated between 280 and 290 mOsm/kg and reflects the osmolality of the ECF. A change in plasma osmolality results in a shift of total body water between the ECF and the ICF to maintain their osmolar equivalence. Because sodium is the major osmole in the ECF, hyponatremia most often is a manifestation of decreased osmolality, so-called hypoosmolar or hypotonic hyponatremia.

Renal Handling of Water

The major osmoregulatory hormone is arginine vasopressin, also called antidiuretic hormone, which is synthesized in the paraventricular and supraoptic nuclei of the hypothalamus. It is transported along axons to the posterior pituitary, where it is processed and stored in vesicles. Vasopressin secretion is regulated by osmotic and nonosmotic stimuli. Secretion occurs with a 1% to 2% rise in osmolality (>288 mOsm/kg), as detected by receptors in the anterolateral walls of the hypothalamus adjacent to the third ventricle. Vasopressin secretion is inhibited when the plasma osmolality is lower than 280 mOsm/kg. The major nonosmotic stimulus is a decrease in effective circulating volume, which is detected by baroreceptors in the aortic arch and carotid sinuses. Although this mechanism requires a large drop (10%–15%) in blood pressure, the secretory response is more robust than for increases in osmolality. As such, acutely lowered blood pressure can override the inhibitory signal of low osmolality because of the need to maintain perfusion. Other physiologic nonosmotic stimuli include catecholamines and angiotensin II, but there is a long list of hormones and pharmacologic agents that induce or repress vasopressin secretion (Table 1).

The renal site of action of vasopressin is the V_2 receptors on the basolateral membrane of collecting duct cells in the distal nephron. The hormone-receptor interaction initiates intracellular signaling via cyclic adenosine monophosphate–dependent pathways, resulting in translocation of cytoplasmic aquaporon-2 channels to the surface of the collecting duct luminal membrane. These channels allow movement of water back into the cell for

TABLE 1	Molecules That Regulate Vasopressin Secretion

STIMULATE VASOPRESSIN RELEASE	INHIBIT VASOPRESSIN RELEASE
Hormones and Neurotransmitters	
Acetylcholine (nicotinic)	Atrial natriuretic peptide
Angiotensin II	γ-Aminobutyric acid
Aspartate	Opioids (κ receptors)
Cholecystokinin	
Dopamine (D_1 and D_2)	
Glutamine	
Histamine (H_1)	
Neuropeptide Y	
Prostaglandin	
Substance P	
Vasoactive inhibitory peptide	
Pharmacologic Agents	
Adrenaline (epinephrine)	Butorphanol (Stadol)
Cyclophosphamide (Cytoxan)	Ethanol
High-dose morphine	Fluphenazine (Prolixin) Glucocorticoids
Nicotine	Haloperidol (Haldol)
Selective serotonin reuptake inhibitors	Low-dose morphine
Tricyclic antidepressants	Phenytoin (Dilantin)
Vincristine (Oncovin)	Promethazine (Phenergan)

Figure 1 The differential diagnosis of hypoosmolar hyponatremia. *Abbreviations:* RTA = renal tubular acidosis; SIADH = syndrome of inappropriate antidiuretic hormone.

A rapid rise in plasma osmolality from aggressive treatment causes water to rapidly shift out of the cells, resulting in demyelinosis of neurons. In the past, this was termed pontine demyelinosis, but it has also been reported for extrapontine neurons and is now referred to as osmotic demyelination. The sequelae are permanent and devastating. There is clinical progression from lethargy to a change in affect, to mutism and dysarthria, and finally to spastic quadriparesis and pseudobulbar palsy.

Classification and Differential Diagnosis of Hyponatremia

Initial evaluation of hyponatremia requires a systematic and sequential approach. First, a thorough history and physical examination are required. It is important to identify any history of brain injury, stroke, mental illness, or chronic illness and the patient's current medication usage. On examination, special attention should be paid to mental status and neurologic abnormalities; manifestations of cardiac, hepatic, or renal disease; and signs of adrenal insufficiency or hypothyroidism. From the assessment of volume status, the hyponatremia should be classified as hypervolemic, euvolemic, or hypovolemic; each of these conditions leads in a different direction for diagnosis and treatment of the underlying cause (Figures 1 and 2). Finally, it should be determined whether the hyponatremia is acute (<48 hours) or chronic, because this can determine the time course of treatment.

For the laboratory work-up, essential basic tests are the serum sodium and potassium levels, renal function tests with blood urea nitrogen (BUN) and creatinine, and liver function tests. It is likely that these tests have already been performed, motivating the assessment of hyponatremia. After this, the plasma osmolality (P_{Osm}), urine osmolality (U_{Osm}), and urine sodium concentration are key diagnostic tests. P_{Osm} is directly measured in the laboratory and also can be calculated. Calculated osmolality is the sum of the concentrations of the known major osmoles—sodium and glucose—in the ECF and the BUN:

$$P_{Osm} = (2 \times Na) + (glucose) + (BUN)$$

The calculation is done in SI units. For sodium, mEq/L is the same as the SI unit, mmol/L; if glucose and BUN values were reported in mg/dL, they must be divided by 18 and 2.8, respectively, to convert to SI units (mmol/L). The directly measured osmolality should be within 10 to 12 mOsm/kg of the calculated value; an increased osmolar gap compared with the calculated value points toward the presence of additional osmoles in the plasma that are causing hypertonicity.

later reabsorption into the circulation. This results in a net concentration of urine and decreased plasma osmolality.

Renal Handling of Sodium

In addition to renal water handling, sodium reabsorption and excretion are important for maintenance of water homeostasis. The renin-angiotensin-aldosterone system is activated by reduced arterial perfusion pressure sensed by the juxtaglomerular apparatus of the afferent renal arteriole. Reduced arteriole effective volume (low or perceived) is sensed by the juxtaglomerular apparatus, which secretes renin, activating the renin-angiotensin system. This cascade of events ultimately stimulates aldosterone secretion, which acts at the distal nephron to cause reabsorption of filtered sodium via Na^+, K^+-adenosine triphosphatase (ATPase)–dependent sodium channels.

Central Nervous System Response to Hyponatremia/Hypoosmolality

Osmolar equivalence between the ECF and ICF is closely maintained by shifts in water between the two compartments. The major symptoms and signs of hyponatremia are neurologic in nature and are a clinical manifestation of swelling of the cells in the central nervous system, which results in cerebral edema. The most devastating consequence is herniation due to anatomic limitations on brain volume within the confines of the skull. Premenopausal women are at the highest risk for brain injury from hyponatremia.

A major compensatory mechanism in the central nervous system is the extrusion from the cells of intracellular solutes, which prevents further water influx. In the first few hours, inorganic ions (potassium, sodium, chloride) move out of the cell. After a few days of persistent hypoosmolality, the cells further compensate by extruding organic osmoles (glutamate, taurine, inositol). The clinician must be aware of this protective adaptation, because it necessitates a slower time course of correction during treatment.

Figure 2 Laboratory findings in hypoosmolar hyponatremia. *Abbreviations:* FENa = fractional excretion of sodium; Osm = osmoles; SIADH = syndrome of inappropriate antidiuretic hormone.

Because hyponatremia usually is a reflection of plasma osmolality, most patients also have a low P_{Osm}, and the clinician often can proceed to the differential diagnosis of hypoosmolar (or hypotonic) hyponatremia after excluding pseudohyponatremia (which usually has normal osmolality) and hyperosmolar hyponatremia. Pseudohyponatremia can occur if the plasma lipid or protein content is greatly increased in the plasma (usually to >6%–8% of volume), as in extreme hypertriglyceridemia and paraprotein disorders. These extra components decrease the aqueous portion of the plasma volume and thereby interfere with the laboratory measurement of sodium by dilutional, indirect methods such as flame photometry. Most laboratories now use direct measurement of sodium to avoid this problem.

Hyperosmolar hyponatremia can occur if there are additional osmoles present that cause water movement from the ICF into the ECF, resulting in ECF expansion and dilutional hyponatremia. Overall, the total body water and total body sodium are unchanged in this situation. An important clinical example occurs with hyperglycemia, and the reported sodium value should be corrected for high glucose by the clinician by adding 1.6 mEq/L to the measured Na for every 100 mg/dL rise in glucose above 200 mg/dL. Because glucose is included in the calculation of osmolality, there will be no significant osmolar gap.

Other osmotically active solutes encountered clinically are mannitol, which is used to manage increased intracranial pressure, and glycine, which is used for irrigation in urologic procedures. Mannitol and glycine are retained in the ECF and are not part of the calculated osmolality, so their presence results in an osmolar gap. High levels of alcohol or ethylene glycol also increase the osmolality, but these substances are so quickly metabolized that an osmolar gap may not be apparent by the time testing is performed.

Once pseudohyponatremia and hypertonicity have been ruled out, the diagnosis is narrowed to hypoosmolar hyponatremia. The combined physical examination and laboratory results allow classification of the patient as having hypervolemic hyponatremia with excess total body sodium, hypovolemic hyponatremia with a deficit of total body sodium, or euvolemic hyponatremia with near-normal total body sodium.

Hypovolemic Hyponatremia

The causes of hypovolemic hyponatremia can be classified as extrarenal or renal (see Figure 1). Signs of volume contraction are apparent on examination, including poor skin turgor, skin tenting (forehead), decreased or undetectable jugular venous pressure, dry mucous membranes, and orthostatic changes in blood pressure and pulse rate. If the volume status is not completely clear from the examination, laboratory values can be helpful (see Figure 2), but they need to be interpreted in the context of renal function tests. If the urine osmolality is less than maximally concentrated (<500 mOsm/kg), an infusion of 0.5 to 1 L of isotonic saline over 24 to 48 hours may help with differentiation. With hypovolemia, the sodium will begin to correct and the patient should improve clinically. Conversely, if

the patient is actually euvolemic, such as with syndrome of inappropriate antidiuretic hormone (SIADH), discussed later, the serum sodium level will remain constant or decrease due to retention of free water with a concomitant increase in urinary sodium.

Extrarenal causes of hyponatremia include gastrointestinal losses and third-space losses such as in severe burns and pancreatitis. In the volume-depleted state, with intact renal function, the urine sodium is low (<10 mEq/L), reflecting a normal response by the kidney to maximally reabsorb sodium in response to volume depletion.

The renal causes of hypovolemic hyponatremia involve the inappropriate loss of sodium into the urine, and this is reflected by a urine sodium concentration of greater than 20 mEq/L.

Thiazide diuretics cause renal sodium loss, so the urine sodium is high. However, they also impair the kidney's diluting capacity, decreasing free water excretion and concentrating the urine. Only certain patients may be susceptible to hyponatremia while on thiazides. These patients may have an abnormally sensitive thirst response to the mild hypovolemia induced by the diuretics, causing increased water intake. Elderly women are the most susceptible, and hyponatremia can occur within days after initiation of thiazide therapy. Additional laboratory results reveal hypokalemia and a metabolic alkalosis. It is appropriate to stop the diuretic and restore potassium levels and volume status. Patients often have a recurrence of hyponatremia if rechallenged with thiazides. Loop diuretics, such as furosemide, are a less frequent cause of hyponatremia, which occurs only after long-term therapy.

In the absence of diuretic use, a urine sodium concentration greater than 20 mEq/L with hypovolemia is evidence for underlying renal pathology. Patients with salt-wasting nephropathy, from a number of causes (see Figure 1), usually have significant renal failure, with a creatinine value in the range of 3 to 4 mg/dL. Because of the large net sodium loss, this condition is treated with salt tablets. Renal tubular acidosis causes bicarbonaturia, which requires a compensatory excretion of urinary cations, mainly Na^+ and K^+, to maintain electroneutrality. Similarly, excretion of ketones into the urine also demands additional electrolyte losses in spite of ECF volume depletion, leading to a loss of sodium.

Cerebral salt wasting (CSW), although it could be considered an extrarenal cause, also involves the renal loss of sodium (>20 mEq/L). The biochemical presentation is very similar to that of SIADH, but the diagnosis of CSW is restricted to cases involving extreme central nervous system pathology. CSW is most commonly associated with subarachnoid hemorrhage but also has been reported with stroke, brain trauma, infection, metastases and after neurosurgery. Onset of CSW is usually within the first 10 days after the neurologic event.

CSW may be a protective mechanism against increased intracranial pressure. The proposed pathophysiologic mechanism of CSW is controversial, but one hypothesis is that the initiating event is a primary natriuresis, with renal loss of sodium, caused by the secretion of natriuretic peptides. Clinical studies have found both increased brain natriuretic peptide and increased atrial natriuretic peptide in neurosurgical patients with hyponatremia. Both hormones are vasodilators that increase the glomerular filtration rate while suppressing the renin-angiotensin system. This increases renal sodium losses, as well as water excretion, resulting in volume depletion. Vasopressin levels rise in response to low volume, so that it becomes biochemically difficult to differentiate CSW from SIADH, with a urine sodium level greater than 20 mEq/L, low uric acid, and high urine osmolality. It is helpful if CSW patients have signs of volume depletion in combination with the laboratory results. Also, the hyponatremia of CSW responds to normal saline, whereas SIADH worsens with normal saline. CSW is relatively rare in most case series, and it is important to rule out other causes for natriuresis.

Hypervolemic Hyponatremia

There are a variety of causes of hypervolemic hyponatremia (see Figure 1), all of which are a result of decreased effective circulating volume. To correct this imbalance, the ECF expands, leading to fluid retention and hyponatremia. In spite of the increased total body water and low serum sodium on testing, all of these patients have some degree of total body sodium excess. In many cases, volume overload is clinically evident from the presence of subcutaneous edema, ascites, elevated jugular venous pressure, or pulmonary edema.

In congestive heart failure (CHF), patients can develop hyponatremia with only 2 to 3 L of fluid intake per day despite normal renal function. The decreased filling pressures and cardiac output of CHF are perceived as volume depletion, detected by the baroreceptors. This stimulates vasopressin secretion, overriding the signal of low osmolality detected by the hypothalamic osmoreceptors. This lack of inhibition of vasopressin secretion is believed to be the most important contributing factor to the development of hyponatremia. In addition, decreased right atrial pressures result in inhibition of secretion of atrial natriuretic peptide, contributing to the water and sodium gain. With the low perfusion pressure, there is a decrease in the glomerular filtration rate, which is sensed by the juxtaglomerular apparatus, causing neurohumoral activation of the renin-angiotensin system and sympathetic nervous system. This leads to increased circulating levels of catecholamines, angiotensin II, and aldosterone, further stimulating tubular sodium and water reabsorption. In the absence of diuretics, the urine sodium level is very low (<10 mEq/L) in patients with CHF because of activation of the renin-angiotensin-aldosterone system and maximal tubular reabsorption of sodium. Also, there is less than maximally dilute urine (usually >300 mOsm/kg) in the absence of diuretic therapy. An elevated brain natriuretic peptide concentration helps to confirm the hypervolemia.

A similar mechanism is at work in cirrhotic patients, in whom the incidence of hyponatremia is even higher and is a strong predictor of poor outcome. In cirrhosis, low albumin results in third-spacing and decreased effective circulating volume. In addition, portal hypertension leads to splanchnic vasodilation, which also decreases the effective circulating volume. This serves to activate vasopressin secretion and the renin-angiotensin-aldosterone system.

Hyponatremia is less common in acute and chronic renal failure, but it can occur with a significant decrease in glomerular filtration rate accompanied by severe hypoalbuminemia. Interpretation of the laboratory results may be confounded by a high urine sodium concentration (>20 mEq/L) that reflects the concomitant presence of tubular dysfunction. Hyponatremia can develop in stage IV or V renal failure when fluid intake is in excess of 3 L/day.

Euvolemic Hyponatremia

Euvolemic hyponatremia is caused by impaired excretion of free water by the kidney. The differential diagnosis is more limited (see Figure 1) and the majority of cases are due to SIADH (Table 2). However, this often is a diagnosis of exclusion, and hypothyroidism and adrenal insufficiency must be ruled out clinically or biochemically in patients with euvolemic hyponatremia.

Hypothyroidism leads to reduced glomerular filtration rate and decreased flow to the distal nephron, causing maximal reabsorption of water to maintain arterial volume. Hypothyroidism has to be severe to cause hyponatremia and usually is obvious on

| TABLE 2 | Causes of SIADH |

CNS Disorders

Mass lesions (tumors; CNS abscess; intracranial hemorrhage or hematoma)
Stroke
CNS infections or inflammatory diseases
Spinal cord lesions
Acute psychosis
Pituitary stalk lesions
Hydrocephalus
Dementia
Guillain-Barré syndrome
Head trauma

Pulmonary Disorders

Viral/bacterial pneumonia
Positive-pressure ventilation
Bronchogenic carcinoma (small cell)
Acute respiratory failure
COPD
Tuberculosis
Aspergillosis
Pulmonary abscess

Medications/Drugs

Vasopressin analogues (desmopressin [DDAVP])
NSAIDs
Tricyclic antidepressants
Phenothiazines
Butyrophenones
SSRIs/SNRIs
Morphine
Opiates
Chlorpropamide (Diabinese)
Clofibrate (Atromid-S)[2]
Cyclophosphamide (Cytoxan)
Vincristine (Oncovin)
Nicotine
Tolbutamide (Orinase)
Barbiturates
Acetaminophen (Tylenol)
ACE inhibitors
Carbamazepine (Tegretol)
Omeprazole (Prilosec)
MDMA (Ecstasy)
Lamotrigine (Lamictal)
Sodium valproate (Depakote)
Monomaine oxidase inhibitors
Ifosfamide (Ifex)
Melphalan (Alkeran, Evomela)
Platinum agents

Other

Pain
Nausea
HIV infection/AIDS
Prolonged exercise (e.g., marathon running)
Idiopathic
Acute intermittent porphyria

[2]Not available in the United States.
Abbreviations: ACE = angiotensin-converting enzyme; AIDS = acquired immunodeficiency syndrome; CNS = central nervous system; COPD = chronic obstructive pulmonary disease; DDAVP = 1-deamino, 8-D arginine-vasopressin; MDMA = methylenedioxymethamphetamine; NSAIDs = nonsteroidal antiinflammatory drugs; SSRIs = selective serotonin reuptake inhibitors.

examination. However, in the elderly population, apathetic hypothyroidism may be difficult to diagnose. Hypothyroidism can be confirmed by the presence of a high level of thyroid-stimulating hormone and a low level of free T_4 (thyroxine). Treatment involves thyroid hormone replacement and supportive care.

In primary adrenal insufficiency (Addison's disease), the concomitant aldosterone deficiency results in hyponatremia combined with hyperkalemia, prerenal azotemia, a urine sodium concentration greater than 20 mEq/L, and a urine potassium level lower than

20 mEq/L. In secondary or central adrenal insufficiency, the adrenal zona glomerulosa remains intact for the secretion of aldosterone. However, glucocorticoid deficiency still causes impaired water excretion, which can lead to dilutional hyponatremia. Vasopressin release may be stimulated by the nausea, vomiting, and orthostatic hypotension that occurs with adrenal insufficiency. Finally, corticosteroids normally inhibit vasopressin release, so their deficiency leads to enhanced vasopressin release, causing retention of free water that further contributes to the hyponatremia. The appropriate diagnostic test is a 250-μg ACTH (cosyntropin, Cortrosyn) stimulation test, although an extremely low 8 AM cortisol level (<3 μg/dL) can be diagnostic. Treatment consists of glucocorticoid replacement.

Syndrome of Inappropriate Antidiuretic Hormone

SIADH is the most common cause of euvolemic hypoosmolar hyponatremia. Edema, ascites, and orthostasis are absent, and thyroid, adrenal, and renal functions are normal. Recent diuretic use should be ruled out. The primary event is the release of vasopressin, which results in water retention. The increased intravascular volume stimulates a natriuresis, which actually is appropriate, but the resulting loss of sodium compounds the hyponatremia. There is an extensive list of causes of SIADH, usually involving pulmonary or central nervous system pathology (see Table 2). A number of medications also are known to stimulate vasopressin release or to potentiate its antidiuretic properties at the level of the kidney (see Tables 1 and 2).

The diagnosis of SIADH is suggested by a low P_{Osm} (<280 mOsm/kg) with a high U_{Osm} (>100 mOsm/kg), confirming water retention and an inappropriately concentrated urine. A spot urine sodium level will be greater than 20 mEq/L, and usually greater than 30 mEq/L. Other helpful laboratory findings include low plasma uric acid (<4 mg/dL), which has a positive predictive value of 73% to 100% for SIADH in this setting. In complicated cases confounded by use of diuretics, the fractional excretion of uric acid has a positive predictive value of 100% for SIADH when the calculated excretion is greater than 12%.

Reset osmostat can be considered a form of SIADH, but the hyponatremia is usually chronic, mild, and asymptomatic. Vasopressin release continues to be regulated, but at a lower threshold of plasma osmolality. The thirst threshold may be altered as well. Interventions to raise the sodium usually have short-lived effects, and the sodium resets at its previous value over time. Therefore, treatment is not recommended if the sodium level is stable and the patient is asymptomatic. A physiologic example of reset osmostat is seen in pregnancy, when the normal sodium range is lowered by 5 mEq/L.

Other Causes of Euvolemic Hypoosmolar Hyponatremia

Primary or psychogenic polydipsia should be considered in patients presenting with hyponatremia and a history of psychiatric illness and treatment. Almost 6% to 7% of psychiatric inpatients are at risk for hyponatremia from increased water intake. The polydipsia may be related to a lowered osmolar threshold for thirst, below the threshold of suppression of vasopressin secretion. This can be further complicated by the side effect of dry mouth caused by many psychiatric medications, which compounds the increased thirst and water intake. Because the kidney is capable of excreting up to 15 to 20 L/day of dilute urine, the fact that hyponatremia develops in these patients may point toward an additional and inappropriate increase in vasopressin release or sensitivity. These patients are clinically euvolemic because of renal excretion of the excess water and have otherwise normal laboratory results except for a dilute urine (<100 mOsm/kg), which is caused by vasopressin suppression and helps differentiate primary polydipsia from SIADH. However, some patients have mildly concentrated urine (>100 mOsm/kg), in which case the psychiatric history helps with the diagnosis.

Exercise-induced hyponatremia (e.g., from marathon running) is a form of euvolemic hypoosmolar hyponatremia primarily caused by retention of water relative to fluid lost via sweating or renal excretion. Vasopressin levels are inappropriately increased during exercise-induced hyponatremia. Most importantly, it is an acute hyponatremia, developing in less than 24 hours, and should be treated accordingly.

Vasopressin levels also may be inappropriately high, secondary to pain or the use of NSAIDs, which remove prostaglandin inhibition of vasopressin release. Low solute intake combined with high fluid intake also can cause hyponatremia, as with beer potomania or a low-protein "tea and toast" diet in elderly patients. In both cases, the lack of solute in the urine does not allow retention of water in the filtrate, so the excess water is not excreted.

Hyponatremia also is common after pituitary surgery (transsphenoidal or by craniotomy) and may be a result of damage to the hypothalamic-pituitary tract that causes release of preformed vasopressin from damaged neurons. Often, hyponatremia occurs as the second phase of the classic triphasic response: transient diabetes insipidus, transient SIADH, followed by permanent diabetes insipidus. Hyponatremia can be delayed up to 1 week postoperatively, and sodium should be monitored during the second week as well. Contributions by central adrenal insufficiency and hypothyroidism also are considerations after pituitary surgery, although with these conditions there will be obvious clinical manifestations in addition to the hyponatremia.

Management

The major considerations for choosing the type and time course of treatment for hyponatremia are the duration of hyponatremia (acute or chronic) and the presence of neurologic signs and symptoms, especially severe manifestations such as altered mental status or seizure (see Table 2). Treatment options for hyponatremia include fluid restriction, saline infusion (hypertonic or isotonic), vasopressin receptor antagonists and demeclocycline (Declomycin).[1] Also, treatment of the underlying abnormality, such as CHF or salt wasting, and correction of volume status are important for hypovolemic or hypervolemic patients. Autocorrection may occur after initiation of therapy, especially in cases of hypovolemia, adrenal insufficiency, or thiazide use. Once treatment is started, the contribution of the nonosmotic stimulation of vasopressin secretion is removed, and the patient is able to raise the sodium level by 2 mEq/L per hour over 12 hours.

Acute Severe Symptomatic Hyponatremia

Acute severe hyponatremia is defined as a rapid fall in sodium in less than 48 hours to less than 120 mEq/L. Under these circumstances, most patients develop neurologic symptoms because of the rapid fluid shifts between the ECF and the ICF in the brain. If left untreated, it can result in irreversible neurologic damage and death. Because of the acute drop in sodium, initial rapid correction is acceptable and should not lead to osmotic demyelination. Treatment is aimed at raising the sodium enough to resolve the neurologic signs and symptoms. The goal is to raise the serum sodium by 1 to 2 mEq/L per hour or to greater than 125 mEq/L until symptoms resolve. Hypovolemic patients will respond to infusion of isotonic saline (normal saline 0.9%), especially if the urine sodium concentration is less than 30 mEq/L. If the neurologic findings are severe, hypertonic saline (3%) may be infused at rate of 1 to 2 mL/ kg per hour, or even up to 4 to 6 mL/kg per hour if the imbalance is life-threatening. A loop diuretic can be combined with the saline to enhance solute-free water excretion. In exercise-induced hyponatremia, hypertonic (3%) saline is the preferred treatment to prevent cerebral edema due to water shifting into the brain along the osmotic gradient. A hypertonic (3%) saline 100 mL bolus can be given to promptly decrease the osmotic gradient, which is promoting water entry into cells. Thereafter, in the inpatient setting, hypertonic (3%) saline infusion should be continued to promote correction of hyponatremia. Sodium levels should be monitored every 2 to 4 hours in patients undergoing hypertonic infusion. Once symptoms resolve, the rate of correction should be reduced to 0.5 to 1 mEq/hr, and the total rise in sodium should not exceed 18 mEq in 48 hours. Studies demonstrate a 6 mEq/L increase in serum sodium in 6 to 12 hours can reverse the most severe neurologic symptoms of acute hyponatremia. No benefit has been observed for faster rates of correction of hyponatremia, whether acute or chronic. Useful formulas to determine the rate of infusion

---

[1]Not FDA approved for this indication.

Parameters for acute or chronic hyponatremia:
Do not increase serum Na by more than 9 mEq in 24 hours and 18 mEq in 48 hours

Symptomatic hyponatremia with severe neurologic symptoms (acute <48 hrs or chronic >48 hrs)
1. Correct serum Na at a rate of 1–2 mEq/l per hour (for 2 to 4 hours) until symptoms have resolved
2. Correct Na at a rate of less than 9 mEq/24 h

Acute hyponatremia symptoms
1. Correct at rate of 0.5 to 1 mEq/L per hour to a maximum of 9 mEq/24 h

Chronic hyponatremia with mild symptoms or asymptomatic
1. Correct at a rate of 0.5 mEq/L per hour with fluid restriction
2. Treat underlying etiology

Calculation of the rate of infusion of saline to correct hyponatremia
1. Change in serum sodium per liter infusate

$$(\Delta Na/L) = \frac{Infusate\ [sodium] - Serum\ [sodium]}{TBW + 1}$$

2. Amount of infusate (in L) required in 24 hours

$$L = \frac{desired\ change\ in\ sodium\ (\Delta Na)\ over\ 24\ hrs}{\Delta Na/L\ (from\ 1)}$$

3. Rate of infusate to raise serum Na by desired amount

$$ml/hr = \frac{L\ (from\ 2) \times 1000\ mL/L}{24\ hr}$$

4. (Simplified) Hypertonic saline infused at 1–2 mL/kg per hour

Infusate	Infusate [Na] (mmol/L)
5% sodium chloride in water	855
3% sodium chloride in water	513
Isotonic saline (0.9%)	154
Ringer's lactate solution	130
0.45% sodium chloride in water	77
0.2% sodium chloride in water	34
5% dextrose in water	0

Total Body Water (TBW) is equal to 60% of body weight in young adult men and 50% in young adult women. Older patients have less TBW. In elderly males, TBW is equal to 50% of body weight and in elderly females it is 45%.

Monitoring:
1. Monitor frequently for clinical improvement or worsening of symptoms
2. If on hypertonic saline or severely symptomatic check sodium q2–4 hrs.
3. If undergoing treatment but asymptomatic, check sodium q6–12 h.

Figure 3 Treatment of hyponatremia. *Abbreviation:* TBW = total body water.

for fluids are provided in Figure 3. The formulas can only estimate the rate of correction, and sodium should be measured frequently.

Chronic Hyponatremia

Chronic hyponatremia is defined as a gradual fall in sodium over more than 48 hours. By this time, the brain has begun to compensate for hypoosmolality by extrusion of solutes. However, the patient is at risk of osmotic demyelination if hyponatremia is treated too aggressively. If the duration of hyponatremia is unknown, the recommendation is to assume that it is chronic. However, as with acute hyponatremia, severe neurologic symptoms and signs need to be treated with hypertonic saline until they resolve, after which the rate of correction can be slowed to 0.5 to 1 mEq/L per hour. Most cases of osmotic demyelination occur with correction rates of greater than 12 mEq/L in 24 hours, but there are cases reported with increases of 9 or 10 mEq/day. Asymptomatic hyponatremia can be treated with an infusion of isotonic saline calculated to raise the sodium by 0.5 to 1 mEq/hour. If the patient has a dilute urine (<200 mOsm/kg), water restriction may be sufficient. Data support favorable outcomes for a maximum target rise in serum sodium of 6 to 8 mEq for any 24 hour period.

Syndrome of Inappropriate Antidiuretic Hormone

The mainstays of treatment of SIADH are fluid restriction and treatment of the underlying cause. Mild SIADH usually can be controlled with fluid restriction alone.

In most cases of SIADH, the degree of fluid restriction required can be calculated. It is dependent on three factors: the daily osmolar load, the minimum U_{Osm}, and the patient's maximum urine volume. A typical diet has a daily osmolar load of 10 mOsm/kg of body weight. For a 70-kg person, this would be 700 mOsm/day. With SIADH, the urine osmolality is held constant for that particular patient, as revealed by a spot U_{Osm}. If the U_{Osm} is 500 mOsm/kg and the solute load is 700 mOsm, the fluid load has to be less than 700/500 or 1.4 L/day just to maintain the serum sodium level. Fluid intake above this amount will cause the sodium to decrease.

When needed, salt tablets (sodium chloride tablet 1-3 g taken once to three times daily) can help to make up for renal loss of sodium in SIADH. With symptoms and severe hyponatremia, short-term use of hypertonic saline may also be instituted to restore sodium to the ECF compartment. Loop diuretics (e.g., furosemide [Lasix]) can increase free water clearance when given with solute (e.g., hypertonic saline or salt tablets). In refractory

cases, demeclocycline[1] (300–600 mg PO twice daily)[3] can be used. Demeclocycline (Declomycin) antagonizes the actions of vasopressin by inhibiting formation of cyclic adenosine monophosphate in the collecting duct. Long-term use is limited by the side effect of photosensitivity and by nephrotoxicity in patients with underlying liver disease. Vasopressin receptor antagonists also are important adjunct treatments (see later discussion). A less commonly used treatment is urea (powder or capsules),[1,6] which causes an osmotic diuresis and increased free water excretion. Preclinical data support that urea may decrease osmotic demyelination.

Cerebral Salt Wasting

Management of CSW involves treatment of the underlying neurologic problem, as well as volume replacement. CSW often is difficult to differentiate biochemically from SIADH, but the rise in vasopressin in CSW is secondary to volume depletion. As a result, CSW responds to volume replacement with isotonic saline, suppressing release of vasopressin, whereas SIADH worsens with this therapy. The recommended correction rate is 0.7 to 1.0 mEq/L per hour, with a maximum of 9 mEq per 24 hours. Salt tablets may also be given to replete total body sodium. Fludrocortisone (Florinef 0.05 to 0.1 mg every 12 hours), an aldosterone receptor agonist, is a third-line treatment to encourage volume expansion and sodium retention, but the potassium concentration and blood pressure should be monitored. Fluid restriction is inappropriate for CSW and should be avoided, especially in patients with subarachnoid hemorrhage, because volume depletion can exacerbate cerebral vasospasm and cause infarction. The duration of CSW is usually 3 to 5 weeks.

Vasopressin Receptor Antagonists

Vasopressin receptor antagonists, or vaptans, are a treatment option for clinically significant euvolemic hyponatremia defined as a serum Na <125 mEq/L or if hyponatremia is symptomatic and resistant to correction with standard therapy. Vaptans also can be used for asymptomatic hypervolemic hyponatremia, but the benefit must clearly outweigh the risk, and the patient should be refractory to standard therapy. There are currently two FDA-approved vaptans, conivaptan (Vaprisol) and tolvaptan (Samsca). Conivaptan is a dual V_{1a}/V_2 arginine vasopressin receptor

---

[1]Not FDA approved for this indication.
[3]Exceeds dosage recommended by the manufacturer.
[6]May be compounded by pharmacists.

antagonist and tolvaptan is a selective V_2 arginine vasopressor receptor antagonist with about 29 times the affinity to the V_2 receptor compared to conivaptan. The primary action of both medications is to block the binding of vasopressin to its receptors in the distal nephron which leads to a decrease in translocation of the aquaporin-2 channels to the apical membrane of the collecting duct in the renal tubule. As a result, vaptans cause an increase in excretion of solute-free water resulting in a rise in serum sodium.

Conivaptan is an IV formulation approved for inpatient hospital use for euvolemic and hypervolemic hyponatremia. It is contraindicated for hypovolemic hyponatremia, euvolemic or hypervolemic hyponatremia with moderate to severe central nervous system (CNS) symptoms, and hypervolemic hyponatremia due to cirrhosis. Conivaptan should be used very cautiously in patients with hypervolemic hyponatremia due to heart failure because safety data are limited and efficacy has not been clearly established. Conivaptan is not recommended in those with severe renal impairment CrCl < 30 mL/min. Conivaptan is given intravenously with a bolus of 20 mg over 30 minutes in 100 mL of 5% dextrose in water (D5W) followed by a continuous infusion of 20 mg conivaptan diluted in 250 mL of D5W over 24 hours. After the initial day of treatment, conivaptan can be continued for an additional 1 to 3 days. Sodium is monitored every 2 to 4 hours and the dose may be titrated to 40 mg per 24 hours to obtain an increase in sodium of 0.5 to 1.0 mEq/L per hour. In clinical trials, the average rise in serum Na after 4 days of therapy is about 6 mEq/L. During conivaptan treatment, fluid restriction can be liberal or is not required. Close monitoring of the rate of sodium rise, neurologic status, and hemodynamic stability are required and treatment should be discontinued or resumed at a reduced dose if clinically indicated. The most common side effects of conivaptan are infusion site reactions and to a lesser degree headache, hypotension, nausea, constipation, and postural hypotension.

Tolvaptan is an oral V_2 receptor antagonist that carries the same indications for use as conivaptan. Tolvaptan should be initiated only in the hospital setting for careful monitoring of potassium and the rate of Na rise, and then can be used in the outpatient setting. The starting dose is 15 mg once daily and can be titrated to 60 mg daily after the initial 24 hours. Patients should not be on fluid restriction for the first 24 hours of tolvaptan therapy and be advised to drink based on thirst. Tolvaptan carries a risk of serious liver injury. The FDA recommends that tolvaptan should not be used for durations longer than 30 days or in any patient with underlying liver disease. Monitoring parameters are equivalent to conivaptan the drug should be stopped promptly in patients with abnormal liver tests or symptoms of hepatotoxicity. In clinical studies, the average rise in serum Na after 4 days of therapy is 4.2 mEq/L and 5.5 mEq/L after 30 days of therapy. The vaptans are a substrate and potent inhibitor of cytochrome P-450 3A4 isoenzyme (CYP3A4). Prior to initiation of therapy drug-drug interactions should be reviewed with the pharmacists and vaptans are contraindicated with other CYP3A4 inhibitors.

Overcorrection of Hyponatremia

If the correction of chronic hyponatremia exceeds our therapeutic limits over the course of 6, 12 or 24 hours, the approach to readjust treatment depends on the risk of osmotic demyelination. In acute hyponatremia, the risk of osmotic demyelination due to overcorrection is lower especially if the etiology is due to water intoxication. The risk for cerebral injury is greatest when hyponatremia is both longer in duration and at lower sodium levels (i.e., <120 mEq/L). Risk factors for osmotic demyelination with correction for chronic hyponatremia are serum sodium less than 105 mEq/L, hypokalemia, alcoholism, malnutrition and advanced liver disease. Overcorrection is prevented by careful monitoring of serum sodium and urine output at least every 4 to 6 hours. If the 24 hour increase has exceeded 8 mEq/L, active therapies to raise serum sodium should be held over the next 24 hours. In high risk patients for ODS where serum sodium correction is above 8 mEq/L over 24 hours, therapeutic re-lowering of serum sodium may be justified. In such cases, 2 to 4 µg of desmopressin (DDAVP)[1] in combination with 3 mL/kg infusion of 5% dextrose in water given over 1 hour

has been effective. A serum sodium should be checked after each infusion and therapeutic re-lowering repeated if indicated. In chronic hyponatremic patients not at high risk for ODS, studies have shown 10 to 12 mEq increases over 24 hours were still safe.

Summary

Hyponatremia is a common electrolyte abnormality and is usually caused by decreased plasma osmolality. Accurate assessment of volume status is a key to determining the underlying cause and choosing the correct treatment approach. The biggest risk of hyponatremia and its treatment is the possibility of severe neurologic sequelae, including fatal cerebral edema and osmotic demyelination. Therefore more aggressive initial treatment is needed in patients with neurologic manifestations (hypertonic saline), but a more conservative approach (e.g., fluid restriction) is needed for less symptomatic patients. Vasopressin antagonists are additional tools for the treatment of euvolemic or hypervolemic hyponatremia refractory to more conservative measures. In patients at high risk for ODS, overcorrection of serum sodium should be avoided and recorrected with holding active therapy or treating with desmopressin and D5W.

References

Androgué HJ: Consequences of inadequate management of hyponatremia, *Am J Nephrol* 25:240–249, 2005.

Cerdà-Esteve M, Cuadrado-Godia E, Chillaron JJ, et al: Cerebral salt wasting syndrome: Review, *Eur J Intern Med* 19:249–254, 2008.

Dineen R, Thompson CJ, Sherlock M: Hyponatremia presentations and management, *Clin Med (Lond)* 17:263–269, 2017.

Ellison DH, Berl T: Clinical practice: The syndrome of inappropriate antidiuresis, *N Engl J Med* 356:2064–2072, 2007.

Fenske W, Störk S, Koschker A: Value of fractional uric acid excretion in differential diagnosis of hyponatremia patients on diuretics, *J Clin Endocrinol Metab* 93:2991–2997, 2008.

Gankam Kengne F, Decauz G: Hyponatremia and the Brain, *Kidney Int Rep* 3:24–35, 2018.

Hew-Butler T, Rosner MH, et al: Statement of the Third International Exercise-Induced Hyponatremia Consensus Development Conference, *Clin J Sport Med.* 25:303–320, 2015.

Hoom EJ, Zieste R: Diagnosis and treatment of hyponatremia: Compilation of the guidelines, *J Am Soc Nephrol* 28:1340–1349, 2017.

Jovanovich AJ, Berl T: Where vaptans do and do not fit in the treatment of hyponatremia, *Kidney Int* 83:563–567, 2013.

Sterns RH, Silver AM, Hix JK: Urea for hyponatremia? *Kidney Int* 87:268–270, 2015.

Verbalis J, Goldsmith S, Greenberg, et al: Diagnosis, evaluation, and treatment of hyponatremia: expert panel recommendations, *Am J Med.* 126:S5–S41, 2013.

HYPOPITUITARISM

Method of
Fabienne Langlois, MD; Elena V. Varlamov, MD; and Maria Fleseriu, MD

CURRENT DIAGNOSIS

- Hypopituitarism is rare and occurs most commonly due to sellar tumors and their subsequent treatment (pituitary surgery and radiation); less commonly hypopituitarism is due to infiltrative disease, cancer immunotherapy, traumatic brain injury, congenital and other disorders.
- Heightened awareness is required, as clinical manifestations are often nonspecific and insidious, and patients can deteriorate and experience adrenal crisis if hypopituitarism is not detected and treated.
- Diagnosis is based on a combination of low baseline peripheral gland hormones (cortisol, thyroid hormone, insulin-like growth factor-1 [IGF-1], testosterone, and estrogen) and low or inappropriately normal pituitary hormones as well as complementary dynamic testing for adrenal insufficiency (AI) and growth hormone (GH) deficiency.
- Pituitary imaging should be performed when a biochemical diagnosis is confirmed or pituitary disease is suspected based on neurologic symptoms (headaches and peripheral vision loss).

---

[1]Not FDA approved for this indication.

CURRENT THERAPY

- Glucocorticoid (GC) replacement is the most critical of all replacements for hypopituitarism; in such cases hydrocortisone is the preferred medication.
- Physiologic replacement of each pituitary deficiency is individualized and monitored with clinical assessment and/or laboratory measurements.
- Of note: interactions exist between different hormones, thus changes or replacement in one hormonal axis may affect other axes.

Epidemiology

Hypopituitarism results from a partial or complete pituitary hormone deficiency. Current epidemiology is not well known. A 2001 Spanish population study showed a prevalence of 45.5 cases per 100,000 and an incidence of 4.2 per 100,000 individuals per year. This estimate is likely conservative, as clinical awareness, imaging studies, and overall understanding of hypopituitarism pathophysiology have improved over the last two decades.

Pathophysiology

The pituitary gland is a small endocrine gland (~1 cm in size) located in sella turcica of the sphenoid bone at the base of the brain; its function is closely linked to the hypothalamus and is controlled by various neurohormonal and nonhormonal inputs. The pituitary secretes hypophyseal hormones into the systemic circulation, stimulating target peripheral glands to produce specific hormones, which in turn feed back to the hypothalamic-pituitary system and maintain a highly regulated homeostasis (Figure 1).

The pituitary is composed of two functionally distinct structures that differ in embryologic development and anatomy: the adenohypophysis (anterior pituitary) and the neurohypophysis (posterior pituitary). The anterior pituitary is responsible for GH, prolactin, ACTH, TSH, LH, and FSH. The posterior pituitary has a neural

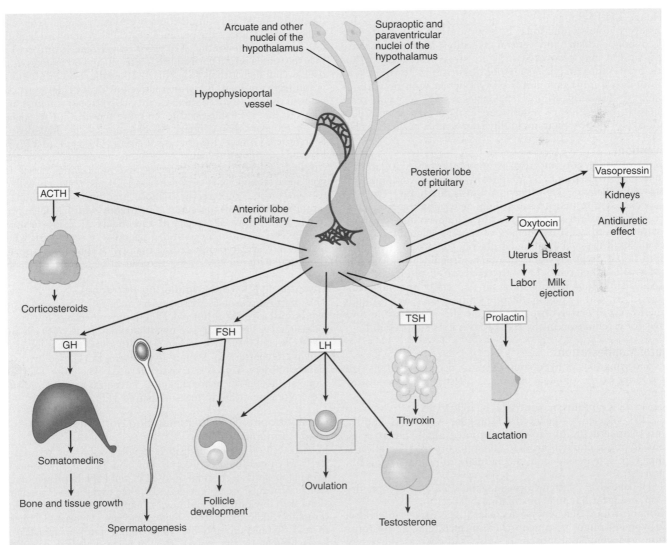

Figure 1 Relationships between hypothalamic hormones, pituitary hormones, and target organs. Numerous hormone-releasing and hormone-inhibiting factors formed in the arcuate and other hypothalamic nuclei are transported to the anterior pituitary by hypophysioportal vessels. In response to hypothalamic hormones, the anterior pituitary secretes the following: corticotropin, which evokes corticosteroid secretion by the adrenal cortex; growth hormone *(GH)*, which elicits production of insulin-like growth factors by the liver; follicle-stimulating hormone *(FSH)*, which stimulates spermatogenesis and facilitates ovarian follicle development; luteinizing hormone *(LH)*, which elicits testosterone secretion by the testes, facilitates ovarian follicle development, and induces ovulation; thyroid-stimulating hormone *(TSH)*, which stimulates thyroxin secretion by the thyroid gland; and prolactin, which induces breast tissue growth and lactation. The posterior pituitary hormones, which are formed in the supraoptic and paraventricular nuclei, are transported by nerve axons to the posterior lobe, where they are released by physiologic stimuli. Oxytocin induces the ejection of milk from the breast and stimulates uterine contractions during labor. Vasopressin increases water reabsorption by the kidneys. *ACTH,* Adrenocorticotropic hormone. From Brenner GM, Stevens CW: *Brenner and Stevens' Pharmacology,* 5th ed., pages 359–365. Elsevier; 2018.

origin and stores vasopressin (or antidiuretic hormone [ADH]) and oxytocin, which are produced in the hypothalamus. Therefore any damage to the hypothalamic-pituitary unit can cause an isolated or combined hormonal deficiency (Table 1).

Different etiologies affect various hormonal patterns. In approximately 70% of cases, the anterior pituitary is affected by a locally expanding tumor, causing mass effect. The most frequent pituitary hormonal deficiency related to sellar tumors is growth hormone (GH) deficiency, followed by gonadal axis hormones (luteinizing and follicle-stimulating hormones [LH/FSH]), and thyroid-stimulating hormone (TSH) deficiencies. However, in other etiologies, the pattern of pituitary deficiency differs. For example, in immunotherapy-related hypophysitis, adrenocorticotropic hormone (ACTH) is the first and most common deficiency noted. Lymphocytic hypophysitis preferentially affects the adrenal and gonadal axes. Infiltrative diseases can also manifest as diabetes insipidus (DI) and/or anterior pituitary dysfunction. Congenital diseases may affect one or more axes and usually present in childhood; for example, an Anosmin-1 (ANOS1) mutation results in isolated hypogonadotropic hypogonadism (Kallmann syndrome) and failure to go through puberty, whereas a PROP-1 mutation presents with low GH, TSH, and LH-FSH.

In severe illness, functional hypopituitarism may cause low GH, hypogonadism, and central hypothyroidism, which are transient and may recover with acute stress resolution. Traumatic brain injury may cause hypopituitarism in up to 30% to 40% of cases, most commonly as GH deficit with or without gonadal dysfunction. Many deficiencies resolve within a year. Surgery in the pituitary region can lead to one or complete pituitary hormone deficit, including transient or permanent DI.

Prevention

In most cases, hypopituitarism is not preventable. Awareness is most important for early diagnosis, as the development of hormonal deficiencies is often insidious and characterized by nonspecific symptoms such as fatigue or weight changes. Pituitary surgery should be performed by a high-volume pituitary neurosurgeon to decrease the risk of surgery-related hypopituitarism. High-dose or prolonged glucocorticoid (GC) therapy suppresses the hypothalamic-pituitary-adrenal (HPA) axis and may also alter the gonadal and thyroid axes. Prolonged opioid use can also induce hypopituitarism, especially adrenal insufficiency (AI) and hypogonadism. Limiting GCs and opioids to the lowest effective dose and for the shortest possible time allows for a reduction in the risk of HPA axis suppression.

Clinical Manifestations

Signs and symptoms of hypopituitarism vary depending on the type and severity of the pituitary hormones affected and also disease duration.

Signs and symptoms may include the following:
- ACTH deficiency—generalized fatigue, weakness, nausea, loss of appetite, failure to thrive, hypotension, hyponatremia, and hypoglycemia (note that mineralocorticoid secretion is intact; thus hyperkalemia, the hallmark of primary AI, is not present).
- TSH deficiency—fatigue, weight gain, cold intolerance, dry skin, bradycardia, and constipation.
- Gonadotropin deficiency—decreased sex drive; infertility; in women, oligo- or amenorrhea; in men, erectile dysfunction; gynecomastia; muscle atrophy; and decreased exercise capacity.
- GH deficiency—failure to thrive and short stature in children; some adults are symptomatic, experiencing fatigue, abdominal fat deposition, weight gain, and decreased concentration, memory, productivity, and quality of life.
- Prolactin—inability to lactate.
- ADH deficiency—polyuria, polydipsia with excessive thirst, hypernatremia if uncompensated.

Detailed Diagnosis

The diagnosis of hypopituitarism is based on a combination of high clinical suspicion, imaging studies, and demonstration of inappropriate pituitary hormone in the setting of low levels of a target peripheral gland hormone.

In most cases, once a single pituitary hormone deficit is confirmed, other axes should be tested and pituitary magnetic resonance imaging (MRI) performed. In cases of peripheral vision deterioration with or without headaches, imaging should not be delayed.

Corticotropin (Adrenocorticotropic Hormone)

AI is confirmed when low cortisol level is measured early in the morning, before 9 a.m. An early-morning serum cortisol level greater than 15 μg/dL in a patient who is not critically ill is usually sufficient to rule out AI, and a level below 3 μg/dL to 5 μg/dL is strongly suggestive of AI. Additionally, serum cortisol testing should be repeated and interpreted in the clinical context (e.g., time of day, acute illness status) and also according to levels of cortisol binding proteins (lower in malnutrition and hypoalbuminemia and higher in hyperestrogenic states). If the serum cortisol level is between 5 μg/dL and 15 μg/dL, an ACTH stimulation test should be performed to confirm diagnosis. An ACTH stimulation test evaluates adrenal reserve that is diminished without the presence of ACTH. A standard high-dose test involves administering 250 μg of cosyntropin (Cortrosyn) and then measuring serum cortisol levels after 30 and 60 minutes. A cortisol level of higher than 18 μg/dL to 20 μg/dL at 30 or 60 minutes is considered normal. In an alternative low-dose (1 μg) test,[1] cortisol is measured 20 to 30 minutes after cosyntropin administration. This test has been suggested to be more sensitive for the diagnosis of secondary than primary AI. Nevertheless, the high-dose test is preferred. Of note, lower cortisol cutoffs (14 μg/dL to 17 μg/dL) have been proposed recently for new, more selective assays (liquid chromatography/mass spectrometry and monoclonal rather than polyclonal immunoassays), which have less cross-reactivity with cortisol precursors; however, these cutoffs need further validation. The serum ACTH level is measured concurrently with baseline cortisol to distinguish between primary and secondary AI. A low or normal ACTH level is consistent with the diagnosis of central AI, while a high ACTH level (typically greater than twice above the upper limit of normal) with primary AI (refer to AI section for further details).

Thyrotropin (Thyroid-Stimulating Hormone)

The key to a diagnosis of secondary (central) hypothyroidism is inappropriately low or normal TSH in the presence of low free T_4. Occasionally, in pituitary or hypothalamic disease, TSH is minimally elevated (usually less than 5 mU/L) and often has lower bioactivity. In contrast, in primary hypothyroidism caused by thyroid gland disorders, TSH is markedly elevated. Therefore TSH levels alone are not sufficient for diagnosis in central hypothyroidism. It is therefore important to measure paired TSH and T_4 levels.

Gonadotropins (Follicle-Stimulating Hormone and Luteinizing Hormone)

In men, central hypogonadism is diagnosed by low testosterone levels when measured between 8 a.m. and 10 a.m. in conjunction with inappropriately normal or low LH and FSH. In premenopausal women, irregular or absent periods (after exclusion of pregnancy) along with low estrogen and low or inappropriately normal gonadotrophins indicate central hypogonadism. Hyperprolactinemia, thyroid dysfunction, and hyperandrogenic states (in females) and hemachromatosis (in males), should be excluded as a cause of gonadal dysfunction. In contrast, in primary hypogonadism and in the postmenopausal state, FSH and LH are markedly elevated.

Growth Hormone

GH secretion is pulsatile, and a single low measurement of GH is not diagnostic of GH deficiency (GHD). Low age- and sex-adjusted IGF-1 in adults is suggestive of GHD; however, normal IGF-1 does

[1]Not FDA approved for this indication.

not rule out GHD. Provocative testing with glucagon (GlucaGen),[1] GH-releasing hormone (GHRH), arginine (R-Gene 10), macimorelin (Macrilen), or insulin tolerance tests are recommended for the diagnosis of GHD in adults. Diagnostic cutoffs differ for different tests and for different body mass indices; therefore careful interpretation is important for accurate diagnosis. When three or more pituitary deficiencies are present along with low IGF-1 levels, confirmatory provocative testing is not required.

Vasopressin (Antidiuretic Hormone)
Hypernatremia in DI may occur due to low ADH, although it is not always present in compensated states if the patient has unlimited access to free water. When hypernatremia is suspected by polyuria and polydipsia, simultaneous measurement of serum and urine osmolality is recommended as an initial test for DI. High serum osmolality (>295 mOsmol/L) and concurrent low urine osmolality (<300 mOsmol/L) are diagnostic of DI. In subtle or unclear cases, a water deprivation test should be performed. Measurement of serum copeptin level at baseline, after water deprivation, hypertonic saline, or with arginine stimulation using specific cutoffs can be helpful in diagnosis. Copeptin is derived from ADH preprohormone and is more stable than ADH; however, copeptin assays may not be available in some countries.

Differential Diagnosis
Hypopituitarism causes secondary endocrine organ failure and should be distinguished from primary failure (primary AI, primary hypothyroidism, and primary hypogonadism), where the corresponding pituitary hormone will be elevated. An ACTH stimulation test can be normal for more than 2 weeks in patients with an acute onset of central AI, such as pituitary apoplexy or after pituitary surgery, because the adrenal cortex is able to respond to stimulation for several weeks until it undergoes atrophy in the presence of low ACTH. Critical illness may result in temporary suppression of TSH, GH, and gonadotrophins and does not require hormonal replacement in the acute period. Obesity can be a cause of male hypogonadotropic hypogonadism. Central DI should be distinguished from nephrogenic DI and primary polydipsia by means of a water deprivation test or other confirmation testing.

Treatment
Glucocorticoid Replacement
Oral hydrocortisone (Cortef) is the preferred GC. A typical replacement regimen is 15 mg/day to 20 mg/day as a single or divided dose (e.g., two-thirds in the morning and one-third in the early afternoon) due to its short half-life. Single doses in the morning can also be used in patients with central AI. A once-daily dual-release hydrocortisone formulation has been designed to mimic physiologic cortisol production; this is available in Europe but not in the United States. Of note, GC replacement at physiologic doses does not require treatment for bone protection or gastric ulcer prophylaxis.

Longer-acting GCs (prednisone, dexamethasone [Decadron]) may be used in patients who remain severely symptomatic in the evenings or early morning hours or who are unable to comply with a multidose hydrocortisone regimen. However, in such cases the risk of overreplacement is much higher.

Patients and families should be educated about the "sick day regimen" (i.e., to double or triple their daily dose for 3 days to 5 days according to the degree of physical stress or illness). In cases of repeated vomiting or deterioration of illness, it is recommended that patients administer injectable GC (hydrocortisone [Solu-Cortef] 100 mg IM or dexamethasone [Decadron] 4 mg IM) and seek immediate medical attention.

Minor surgical stress (e.g., cataract removal) requires additional administration of intravenous (IV) 25 mg hydrocortisone on the day of surgery only. The suggested dose for moderate stress (e.g., cholecystectomy) is 50 mg to 75 mg IV in divided doses on the day of surgery and the first postoperative day. Severe stress (e.g., coronary bypass surgery) requires 100 mg to 150 mg IV in divided doses for 2 days to 3 days with a subsequent rapid taper to the daily maintenance dose in an uncomplicated surgery (refer to the earlier section on adrenal insufficiency for further details).

Adrenal crisis and critical illness in adrenally insufficient patients are managed by administering a 100-mg IV bolus of hydrocortisone followed by 50 mg to 100 mg every 6 hours to 8 hours or continuous infusion of 200 mg/24 hours with the dose gradually decreased as the patient's condition improves. Additionally, it is recommended that patients wear a medical bracelet indicating AI risk.

Thyroid Deficiency
Central hypothyroidism is treated by T_4 replacement (levothyroxine [Euthyrox, Levoxyl, Synthroid]). A standard replacement dose for complete central hypothyroidism is 1.6 μg/kg/day; however, lower doses are needed in cases of partial deficiency. TSH should not be used as a marker of adequacy of replacement. Instead, one should adjust the dose to target free T_4 levels in the mid to upper half of the normal range and consider a lower target in elderly patients and in those with comorbidities in an effort to avoid over replacement.

Thyroid replacement should be administered only after corticosteroids have been replaced or adrenal function has been confirmed to be normal. Thyroid replacement in untreated AI can provoke an adrenal crisis.

Sex Hormone Deficiency
Testosterone replacement in men and estrogen (plus progesterone if the uterus is present) replacement in women is appropriate in symptomatic patients without contraindications after a discussion regarding risks and benefits. Combined oral contraceptive or hormone replacement therapy may be offered to premenopausal women. Premenopausal women not receiving estrogen replacement have an increased risk of cardiovascular disease and osteoporosis. Testosterone improves libido, sexual function, anemia, and bone density in men. Prostate, breast, and uterine cancer are contraindications to sex steroid replacement. Patients at high risk for thrombotic and cardiovascular events, including smokers, are poor candidates for hormone replacement.

Growth Hormone Deficiency
GH replacement (somatropin [Genotropin, Humatrope]) is administered as a daily injection; longer-acting formulations are in clinical trial testing for adults. In GH-deficient adults, GH replacement improves body composition, has a modest effect on the maintenance of bone density, and improves quality of life. Although mortality in patients with hypopituitarism is increased, GH replacement has not been shown to improve mortality. Side effects of treatment include worsening of insulin resistance, joint pain, and peripheral edema. Although GH replacement has not been directly linked to cancer development or tumor regrowth, replacement is contraindicated in cases of active cancer.

Diabetes Insipidus
Desmopressin (DDAVP) therapy is individualized based on the patient's symptoms (severity or persistence of polyuria and polydipsia) and serum sodium levels especially during the initiation phase of therapy due to risk of hyponatremia from overcorrection. Desmopressin may be administered orally, intranasally (in some countries), or via a sublingual route; in a hospital setting it may be given via an IV or subcutaneous route. A low dose is used at initiation to avoid hyponatremia. Some patients with partial DI are only mildly symptomatic and prefer no treatment while keeping sodium levels normal with adequate water intake.

Monitoring
Patients should be periodically assessed for signs of GC overreplacement (weight gain, facial rounding, hyperglycemia, and osteoporosis) or under-replacement (nausea, fatigue, joint pain) and the GC dose adjusted accordingly.

---

[1]Not FDA approved for this indication.

Monitoring for thyroid, GH, and gonadal deficiencies in patients receiving replacement therapy includes periodic clinical assessment and measurement of hormone levels (free T_4, IGF-1, testosterone, and sodium.). Regular follow-up by an endocrinologist is warranted.

Interaction exists between the various hormone replacements. For example, thyroid replacement and GH affect GC metabolism and may cause AI in patients with low adrenal reserve. Higher maintenance hydrocortisone doses may be required in patients who initiate GH or thyroid replacement. Oral estrogen can increase cortisol- and thyroid-binding globulins, resulting in an increase of the total cortisol and thyroxine levels and relative decrease in the bioavailable free hormone; therefore careful interpretation of test results is necessary.

Special Circumstances

Fertility and Pregnancy

New assisted reproductive techniques have led to the increased prevalence of women with hypopituitarism achieving fertility, and birth rates seem to be high in women with hypopituitarism achieving pregnancy. During pregnancy, many continuous adjustments in pituitary hormonal replacement should be considered.

Although GCs, levothyroxine, and desmopressin are safely prescribed during pregnancy, GH treatment regimens vary significantly between countries. GH is not approved for use in pregnancy, but several publications have shown that it can improve outcomes in women pursuing fertility.

In women with hypopituitarism who desire to be pregnant, close monitoring is needed, and such patients will benefit from an evaluation at a pituitary center of excellence.

Complications

Complications arise from a failure to diagnose hypopituitarism, especially in the event of an acute onset or severe illness or trauma, as untreated AI can result in cardiovascular collapse, organ failure, and death. Insufficient chronic replacement can lead to persistent symptoms and poor quality of life, whereas over replacement can result in the development of iatrogenic Cushing syndrome, iatrogenic hyperthyroidism, and other complications.

Conclusion

Early recognition and treatment of hypopituitarism is essential to reduce morbidity and mortality and improve quality of life. Care for patients with multiple pituitary deficiencies is often complex and requires expert management by an endocrinologist in conjunction with a pituitary neurosurgeon when surgical treatment for pituitary lesion is required. Although some pituitary deficiencies except adrenal and thyroid may recover or may not necessitate treatment, most patients require lifelong hormonal replacement and follow-up.

References

Brenner GM, Stevens CW: In *Brenner and Stevens'* pharmacology, ed 5, © 2018, Elsevier.

Carmichael J: Anterior pituitary failure. In Melmed S, editor: *Pituitary*, ed 4, 2007, Elsevier Inc., pp 329–364.

Fleseriu M, Hashim IA, Karavitaki N, et al: Hormonal replacement in hypopituitarism in adults: an endocrine society clinical practice guideline, *J Clin Endocrinol Metab* 101(11):3888–3921, 2016.

Higham CE, Johannsson G, Shalet SM: Hypopituitarism, *Lancet* 388(10058):2403–2415, 2016.

Honegger J, Schlaffer S, Menzel C, et al: Diagnosis of primary hypophysitis in Germany, *J Clin Endocrinol Metab* 100(10):3841–3849, 2015.

Molitch ME, Clemmons DR, Malozowski S: Evaluation and treatment of adult growth hormone deficiency: an Endocrine Society clinical practice guideline, *J Clin Endocrinol Metab* 96(6):1587–1609, 2011.

Regal M, Paramo C, Sierra SM, Garcia-Mayor RV: Prevalence and incidence of hypopituitarism in an adult Caucasian population in northwestern Spain, *Clin Endocrinol (Oxf)* 55(6):735–740, 2001.

Vila G, Fleseriu M: Fertility and pregnancy in women with hypopituitarism: a systematic literature review, *J Clin Endocrinol Metab* 105(3):e53–e65, 2020.

Javorsky BR, Raff H, Carroll TB, Algeciras-Schimnich A, Singh RJ, Colón-Franco JM, et al: New cutoffs for the biomechanical diagnosis of adrenal insufficiency after ACTH stimulation using specific cortisol assays, *J Endocr Soc*, bvab022, 2021. https://doi.org/10.1210/jendso/bvab022.

Ueland GA, Methlie P, Oksnes M, Thordarson HB, Sagen J, Kellmann R, et al: The short cosyntropin test revisited: new normal reference range LC-MS/MS, *J Clin Endocrinol Metab* 103(4):1696–1703, 2018.

HYPOTHYROIDISM

Method of
William J. Hueston, MD

CURRENT DIAGNOSIS

- Hypothyroidism is more common in women as they age.
- The signs and symptoms of hypothyroidism are nonspecific and can mimic other diseases found in the elderly, so clinicians need to have a high index of suspicion.
- The key diagnostic test is to find a low free T_4. The presence of an elevated TSH indicates primary hypothyroidism, and a low TSH indicates secondary hypothyroidism.
- There is insufficient evidence for screening for hypothyroidism in asymptomatic adults.

CURRENT THERAPY

- Thyroxine replacement with L-thyroxine (Synthroid, Levoxyl) is the treatment for hypothyroidism. Medication should be titrated to normalize the thyroid-stimulating hormone (TSH) level, which is usually achieved at an overall dose of 100 to 150 μg.
- Initial dosing for those with potential cardiac disease should be started low (25–50 μg/day) and advanced slowly every 6 to 8 weeks.
- Partial substitution of triiodothyronine (Cytomel) for thyroxine should be reserved for elderly patients with persistent neurocognitive dysfunction despite normalization of their TSH.
- Patients who have subclinical hypothyroidism with a TSH >10.0 should be considered for treatment. Patients with a TSH lower than this do not require therapy.

Epidemiology

Hypothyroidism is second only to diabetes in the prevalence of endocrine disorders in adults in the United States. Hypothyroidism occurs in up to 18/1000 population, with women outnumbering men by approximately 10:1. Rates of hypothyroidism increase dramatically with age, so that about 2% to 3% of all older women have hypothyroidism, and the prevalence is up to 5% in nursing home populations.

The prevalence of subclinical hypothyroidism, defined as an elevated TSH in the presence of normal free thyroxine (T_4) and triiodothyronine (T_3) levels increases with advancing age. Women, individuals over 65, and those from European heritage are at higher risk for subclinical hypothyroidism.

Risk Factors

Thyroid conditions are more common in patients who have a family history of thyroid disorders. In addition, hypothyroidism, as well as thyroid cancers, are more common in patients who had neck irradiation in childhood. However, most cases of hypothyroidism occur in people who have no risk factors.

Pathophysiology

Several conditions can lead to hypothyroidism (Box 1). Two categories, hypothyroidism after thyroiditis and iatrogenic hypothyroidism secondary to treatment of Graves' disease, account for the overwhelming majority of cases of hypothyroidism in the United States.

The most common non-iatrogenic condition causing hypothyroidism in the United States is Hashimoto's thyroiditis. Most idiopathic hypothyroidism also represents Hashimoto's thyroiditis that has followed an indolent course. Hashimoto's thyroiditis, also called chronic lymphocytic thyroiditis, is the most common of the inflammatory thyroid disorders and the most common cause of

| BOX 1 | Conditions Causing Hypothyroidism |

Thyroiditis
Hashimoto's thyroiditis
Subacute granulomatous thyroiditis (de Quervain's thyroiditis)
Subacute lymphocytic thyroiditis (silent or painless thyroiditis)

Iatrogenic Hypothyroidism
Radioactive iodine treatment of Graves' disease
Thyroidectomy

Secondary Hypothyroidism (Pituitary Dysfunction)
Pituitary surgery
Intercranial radiation
Congenital panhypopituitarism

Other Causes
Infiltratative diseases (sarcoidosis, amyloidosis, hemochromatosis)
Drugs (lithium, interferon, amiodarone [Cordarone])
Iodine deficiency

| BOX 2 | Symptoms and Signs of Hypothyroidism |

Common Symptoms
Lethargy
Weight gain
Constipation
Slowed mentation, forgetfulness
Depression
Hair loss
Dry skin
Neck enlargement or goiter

Physical Examination Findings
Goiter
Low blood pressure and slow pulse
Hair thinning or loss
Dry skin
Confusion
Depressed affect
Non-pitting edema

goiter in the United States. The prevalence of Hashimoto's thyroiditis has been increasing dramatically since the 1960s in the United States, but the cause for this rise is unknown. In patients with acute thyroiditis, either subacute granulomatous (also known as de Quervain's) and subacute lymphocytic (also known as silent or painless), transient hypothyroidism is common after an acute attack, and 10% of these patients also develop long-term hypothyroidism.

Another common cause of hypothyroidism is a medical intervention to treat Graves' disease or thyroidectomy for chronic fibrocytic thyroiditis (Riedel's struma). Radioactive iodine ablation of the thyroid for Graves' disease often results in underproduction of thyroxine in the remaining tissue, necessitating thyroid replacement.

A third uncommon cause of hypothyroidism that should not be overlooked is secondary hypothyroidism due to hypothalamic or pituitary dysfunction. These conditions are seen primarily in patients who have received intracranial irradiation or surgical removal of a pituitary adenoma.

Finally, a variety of other conditions including infiltration of the thyroid (amyloidosis, sarcoidosis), iodine deficiency, or medications (such as amiodarone [Cordarone] or interferon) can cause hypothyroidism.

Prevention

There are no known interventions to prevent hypothyroidism. According to their 2015 analysis, the US Preventive Services Task Force found insufficient evidence to support early detection through routine screening of asymptomatic persons.

Clinical Manifestations

Individual who have hypothyroidism can present with a variety of symptoms, many of which are not specific. Consequently, clinicians must have a high index of suspicion for hypothyroidism when patients come in with any one or combination of the symptoms that could signal hypothyroidism.

Symptoms of hypothyroidism include lethargy, weight gain, hair loss, dry skin, constipation, poor concentration, trouble thinking or forgetfulness, and depression (Box 2). In older patients, hypothyroidism easily can be confused with Alzheimer's disease or other conditions that cause dementia. Patients who present with depression also should have their thyroid function assessed.

The thyroid examination in most patients with hypothyroidism is completely normal. Patients might have a painless goiter; tenderness in the thyroid is generally a sign of active inflammation consistent with acute thyroiditis. Once the thyroid inflammation has subsided, thyroid function might return to normal. Other physical findings that can occur with hypothyroidism include low blood pressure, bradycardia, nonpitting edema, generalized hair loss especially along the outer third of the eyebrows, dry skin, and a lag in the relaxation phase of reflexes that can be assessed most easily in the ankle jerk reflexes.

Finally, there is an association between hypothyroidism and obstructive sleep apnea although it is unclear if this is a causal relationship.

Subclinical hypothyroidism usually has no, or very subtle clinical symptoms which could be explained by other conditions. The primary finding in subclinical hypothyroidism is the abnormal laboratory values. Subclinical hypothyroidism in pregnancy is associated with increases in pregnancy loss, premature rupture of membranes, and neonatal death, but limited evidence does not show a reduction in these risks with thyroid supplementation during pregnancy.

Diagnosis

The diagnosis of hypothyroidism is based on finding a low free thyroxine (T_4) level, usually with an elevation in the thyroid stimulating hormone (TSH) levels. For patients with hypothyroidism due to pituitary dysfunction, also called secondary hypothyroidism, both the free T_4 and the TSH levels are low.

One situation where clinicians need to be wary is evaluating thyroid status in patients who are severely ill. During times of acute physiological stress, patients may have mildly elevated TSH levels that suggest hypothyroidism but are, in fact, euthyroid. This condition, called euthyroid sick syndrome, does not require treatment with thyroid replacement and resolves within a few weeks of recovery, but it may be difficult to distinguish from preexisting or new-onset hypothyroidism. Clinicians need to use other clinical symptoms to try to differentiate euthyroid sick syndrome from hypothyroidism. Even though it does not require treatment, the presence of euthyroid sick syndrome in a critically ill patient is a poor prognostic sign.

In contrast to hyperthyroidism, there is no role for thyroid scans or iodine uptake testing in patients with hypothyroidism. The only exception to this is when the clinician identifies a mass on physical examination. In that situation, scanning or other imaging is essential to determine the malignancy potential of the mass.

Differential Diagnosis

The differential diagnosis for hypothyroidism is broad and depends on the primary complaints given by patients. For patients with slowed mentation, depressed affect, or confusion, clinicians should suspect depression. Patients with lethargy and a slow pulse and low blood pressure might have adrenal insufficiency. Patients with constipation need to have colonic obstruction from a mass considered as well. In the elderly, common drugs that can cause depression (such as centrally acting antihypertensive agents), bradycardia (such as β-blockers or calcium channel blockers), constipation (calcium channel blockers), hair loss, or confusion also should be considered.

In patients with pituitary failure, other pituitary hormones are likely to be deficient as well, so clinicians should look for evidence of adrenal and gonadotropic failure.

Treatment

The treatment for hypothyroidism is thyroxine replacement (Synthroid, Levoxyl). The usual dose required to achieve full replacement is between 100 μg and 150 μg, although patients who are treated with radioactive iodine and have some remaining thyroid activity might require lower doses. For patients with known heart disease or at risk for heart problems, doses should be initiated at 25 to 50 μg with increases of 25 μg every 4 to 6 weeks guided by TSH levels. Young patients who are at low risk for cardiac problems can be started at doses of 100 μg.

In choosing an agent to use for thyroid replacement, there is good evidence that generic substitutes are just as effective as brand-name drugs. A detailed study examining the metabolic effectiveness of a variety of generic drugs compared with a brand-name medication demonstrated no clinical or subclinical differences among preparations. So even though clinicians often hear that they should use a brand-name drug to maintain the stability of the replacement dose, this is not supported by the evidence.

One area of uncertainty is whether the addition of triiodothyronine (T_3, Cytomel) adds additional benefit to thyroid replacement with thyroxine. In some studies with elderly patients, subjects with continued neurocognitive dysfunction benefited from the addition of T_3 at a dose of 125 μg, with a concomitant decrease in the T_4 dose of 50 μg. However, subsequent studies of younger patients (aged 29–44 years) failed to find any benefits of partial T_3 substitution. Furthermore, studies of patients on doses of T_4 adequate to restore TSH levels to normal have been found to have normal T_3 levels. At this time, routine use of T_3 cannot be recommended; however, for selected elderly patients who have lingering confusion, depression, or slow mentation on adequate doses of T_4, a trial of T_3 partial substitution might be tried. Both the American Thyroid Association and European Thyroid Association recommend a trial of combination therapy for patients who are using single therapy with thyroxine alone who are persistently dissatisfied with their therapy.

Another situation where there is controversy is the use of thyroid replacement in patients with a mildly elevated TSH and a normal free T_4. This condition, called subacute hypothyroidism or mild hypothyroidism, is more common in white, elderly women. It has been observed that thyrotropin (TSH) levels naturally rise with age, however. In many instances these changes are simply due to aging and do not represent a pathologic process.

While some studies have shown clinical improvement in symptoms when low doses of T_4 are given to these patients, these patient populations tend to be those with preexisting thyroid disease (such as Graves' disease), and studies have had only a small number of patients. Expert panels in the US and Europe have suggested using the TSH level and the presence of anti-thyroid antibodies as guides for therapy, but that most patients with this condition will not require any therapy. Additional evidence against routine treatment is provided by a systematic review, and meta-analysis showed no improvement in quality of life or thyroid-related symptoms in patients with subclinical hypothyroidism who received levothyroxine supplementation.

When considering treatment for subacute thyroiditis, patients with a TSH under 7 generally do not require any therapy unless there are other individual patient risk factors such as existing cardiac disease or cognitive symptoms. Treatment is reasonable in those with a TSH level of 10.0 because these patients may be most symptomatic and have a progression rate of 5% to overt hypothyroidism.

When the TSH is <7, almost half of all patients will revert to normal within 2 years. Patients with a TSH <10 do not require any therapy unless there are other individual patient risk factors such as existing cardiac disease or cognitive symptoms. Treatment is reasonable in those with a TSH level of 10.0 because these patients may be most symptomatic and have a progression to overt hypothyroidism of 5%.

Monitoring

In general, once a patient receives a full replacement dose of T_4 (usually between 100 and 150 μg) and has a TSH consistently in the normal range, there is little likelihood that their thyroid requirement will change over time. Although many advocate annual retesting of TSH to ensure patients are euthyroid, there is no evidence to show this is necessary.

Some conditions do warrant closer monitoring of the TSH level. Because T_4 and T_3 are highly protein bound, any conditions where a patient's serum protein status changes should prompt additional testing. This includes conditions that lower serum protein levels, such as liver disease, nephrotic syndrome, or malnutrition, as well as those where serum proteins are increased, such as pregnancy or initiation of estrogen therapy. Because patients' dietary protein usually decreases with advancing age, older patients whose diet declines can also require monitoring and a lowering of their T_4 dose over time.

Patients with subclinical hypothyroidism also might benefit from annual retesting of their free T_4 levels. Approximately 10% of patients with subacute hypothyroidism progress to hypothyroidism within 3 years of diagnosis. Because of this, yearly testing is recommended. Also, 50% of patients with subacute hypothyroidism have positive anti-thyroid antibodies; however, routine testing for these is not recommended.

Complications

Most of the complications of hypothyroidism are associated with undertreatment or overtreatment. Patients with inadequately treated hypothyroidism are at higher risk for cardiac disease. On the other hand, over-replacement of thyroxine increases the risk of both atrial fibrillation and osteoporosis.

In addition, Hashimoto's thyroiditis is associated with other endocrine autoimmune diseases such as Addison's disease and pernicious anemia. Clinicians should be aware of these associations and not overlook new endocrine disorders that might have clinical features similar to hypothyroidism.

Finally, patients with Hashimoto's hypothyroidism also are at higher risk for the future development of lymphoma. Clinicians should educate patients about the need to have newly enlarged lymph nodes evaluated and be aggressive about evaluating symptoms or signs consistent with the development of a lymphoma.

References

Bekkering GE, Agoritsas T, Lytvyn L, et al: Thyroid hormone treatment for subclinical hypothyroidism: a clinical practice guideline, *BML* 356:I2006, 2019.

Biondi B, Cappola AR, Cooper SA: Subclinical hypothyroidism: A review, *JAMA* 322:153–160, 2019.

Bunevicius R, Kazanavicius G, Zalinkevicius R, Prange AJ: Effects of thyroxine as compared with thyroxine plus triiodothyronine in patients with hypothyroidism, *N Engl J Med* 340:424–429, 1999.

Dong BJ, Hauck WW, Gambertoglio JG, et al: Bioequivalence of generic and brand-name levothyroxine products in the treatment of hypothyroidism, *JAMA* 277:1205–1213, 1997.

Feller M, Snel M, Moutzouri E: Association of thyroid hormone therapy with quality of life and thyroid-related symptoms in patients with subclinical hypothyroidism: A systematic review and meta-analysis, *JAMA* 320:1349–1359, 2018.

Helfand M, Crapo LM: Screening for thyroid disease, *Ann Intern Med* 112:840–849, 1990.

Peeters RP: Subclinical hypothyroidism, *New Engl J Med* 376:2556–2565, 2017.

Sawin CT, Chopra D, Azizi F, et al: The aging thyroid. Increased prevalence of elevated serum thyrotropin levels in the elderly, *JAMA* 242:1386–1388, 1979.

Surks MI, Ortiz E, Daniels GH, et al: Subclinical thyroid disease: Scientific review and guidelines for diagnosis and management, *JAMA* 291(2):228–238, 2004.

U.S. Preventive Services Task Force: Screening for thyroid disease: Available at http://www.ahrq.gov/clinic/uspstf/uspsthyr.htm [accessed July 11, 2015].

OBESITY IN ADULTS

Method of
Meera Shah, MBChB, MRCP (Edin)

CURRENT DIAGNOSIS

- The diagnosis of obesity is based on the patient's body mass index (BMI), which is a ratio of weight to height. However, there are recognized limitations to using BMI alone when defining obesity.
- Waist circumference can aid the identification of patients who are not obese by BMI criteria but who are still at heightened metabolic risk.
- Certain ethnic groups, such as Asians, have a higher body fat content at a lower BMI and are therefore defined as being overweight or obese at lower BMI cutoffs.
- Diagnosing obesity early, and recognizing it as a chronic disease, allows for discussion and formulation of a plan to mitigate health risks associated with this disease.

CURRENT THERAPY

- The cornerstone of any weight management program is lifestyle intervention that focuses on calorie restriction, an increase in physical activity, and behavioral modification. A multidisciplinary team approach offers the greatest benefit.
- The most effective pharmacotherapies for obesity modulate appetite regulation.
- Pharmacotherapy for obesity can be considered as an adjunct to lifestyle modification in the appropriate patient, after having a thorough discussion about benefits and associated risks.
- Weight loss procedures can be considered in patients with medically complicated obesity. This tends to be the most effective way of losing weight but is also associated with the highest risk. Therefore appropriate patient selection is key.

Obesity was recognized as a complex, chronic disease by the American Medical Association in 2013. The designation of obesity as a disease recognizes that obesity develops in response to an aberration in physiology, and its designation as a chronic disease recognizes that obesity is often present for a time period greater than a year and often requires ongoing medical attention and impairs activities of daily living.

Epidemiology

Obesity is a global phenomenon. At the current rate of growth, it is projected that by the year 2030, almost one in two adults in the United States will have a BMI of greater than 30 kg/m². With a higher prevalence of obesity comes a greater burden of obesity-associated chronic disease and comorbidities. Managing obesity is therefore a public health priority.

Obesity and Health Disparity

Obesity disproportionately affects certain racial, ethnic, and socioeconomic groups. Between 2017 and 2018, non-Hispanic Black adults (49.6%) had the highest age-adjusted prevalence of obesity, followed by Hispanic adults (44.8%), non-Hispanic White adults (42.2%) and non-Hispanic Asian adults (17.4%). Within these racial and ethnic differences, prevalence of obesity was lowest in women with college degrees compared with people with lower educational attainment, while in men there was no observable difference in obesity prevalence based on education level.

Among non-Hispanic White and Hispanic men, obesity prevalence was lower in the lowest and highest income groups

TABLE 1	BMI Classification and Weight
CLASSIFICATION	**BODY MASS INDEX, kg/m²**
Underweight	≤18.5
Normal Weight	18.5–24.9
Overweight	25.0–29.9
Obesity, Class I	30.0–34.9
Obesity, Class II	35.0–39.9
Obesity, Class III	≥40

compared with the middle-income group. Conversely, obesity prevalence was higher in the highest income group than in the lowest income group among non-Hispanic Black men. Among non-Hispanic White, non-Hispanic Asian, and Hispanic women, obesity prevalence was lower in the highest income group than in the middle and lowest income groups. Obesity prevalence was not affected by income in non-Hispanic Black women.

The reasons for these health disparities in adults with obesity are complex. However, there is widespread recognition of the fundamental importance of preventing childhood obesity, as children with obesity are more likely to become adults with obesity.

Diagnosis

The current definition of obesity is based on the body mass index (BMI). The BMI is defined as follows:

$$\frac{\text{Weight (kg)}}{\text{Height (m}^2)}$$

BMI is a practical measure of an individual's degree of adiposity and generally correlates well with comorbidities. However, it is well-recognized that BMI has several limitations with regard to body composition and weight distribution and may therefore be misleading if taken as the only measure of obesity, particularly at lower BMI values.

Waist circumference roughly correlates with visceral adiposity and can be an important adjunct when assessing risk associated with obesity in patients with a BMI below 35 kg/m². In adults with a BMI of 25 to 34.9 kg/m², waist circumference of greater than 102 cm (40 in.) for men and 88 cm (35 in.) for women is associated with greater risk of developing hypertension, type 2 diabetes, and coronary heart disease. Waist circumference is measured with the measuring tape situated above the iliac crest and snugged up against the skin. There is significant intraoperator variability, which limits the reproducibility and use of this metric in the longitudinal assessment of patients with obesity.

BMI cutoffs (Table 1) are applicable to the general population in the United States. Certain ethnic group such as Asians have a higher body fat content at a lower BMI and are therefore defined as being overweight or obese at lower BMI cutoffs (23–24.9 kg/m² and greater than 25 kg/m², respectively).

Assessing the Patient With Obesity in the Office

Once the patient has been diagnosed with obesity, effort then should turn toward understanding the etiology of the disease in the individual patient and assessing for comorbidities associated with obesity.

The following components in the patient's history should be elicited:

- Age of onset of weight gain
- Weight loss attempts
- Changes in dietary patterns
- History of exercise and activity in general
- A comprehensive medication history

The dietary assessment should ideally be performed by a registered dietitian.

A comprehensive medication history may identify medications that are associated with weight gain. Chief among these are psychotropic medications, antidepressants, antiepileptics, insulin secretagogues, and glucocorticoids. Progestational hormones and implants, antihistamines, and oral contraceptives may contribute to weight gain in some patients. Wherever possible, the potential for weight gain should be considered when starting patients with obesity on a new medication. If a weight-neutral alternative exists, effort should be made to switch the patient from a medication that could be contributing to weight gain as long as the underlying disease process remains adequately managed on the new medication regimen. This can be difficult to achieve particularly when dealing with psychotropic medications and requires careful coordination with the patient's other prescribers.

The physical examination of the patient should focus on assessing for a pattern of weight distribution that may confer higher risk (i.e. higher waist circumference than BMI alone would confer) as well as physical findings that may elude to a secondary cause of obesity such as glucocorticoid excess, thyroid dysfunction, or dependent edema.

Comorbidities Associated With Obesity

Type 2 Diabetes

It is estimated that about 85% patients with type 2 diabetes are in the overweight or obese category.

The prevalence of diabetes has increased over the years in line with the increase in population-level obesity. The risk of developing type 2 diabetes in people with obesity increases when there is a strong family history of the disease, a prior history of gestational diabetes, or a weight distribution that is metabolically unfavorable (i.e., high waist circumference). Certain high-risk groups, such as South Asians, are 30% to 50% more likely to develop diabetes than their White counterparts despite having a lower BMI.

A fasting plasma glucose concentration of greater than or equal to 126 mg/dL or hemoglobin A1c of greater than or equal to 6.5% on two separate occasions can be used to make a diagnosis of type 2 diabetes.

When considering treatment for patients with type 2 diabetes and obesity, careful attention should be paid to the choice of antihyperglycemic agent. Weight-neutral options or medicines that actively promote weight loss such as GLP-1 receptor agonist or SGLT-2 inhibitors should be prioritized where possible. Conversely, patients on medications that can promote weight gain such as sulfonylureas or insulin should be counseled on alternative regimens. In patients with type 2 diabetes, weight loss of 5% to 10% is associated with hemoglobin A1c reductions of 0.6% to 1.0% and reduced need for diabetes medications.

Prevention of type 2 diabetes is possible with modest weight loss. Participants in the Diabetes Prevention program who were at high risk for developing type 2 diabetes and who were able to lose about 7% body weight through lifestyle intervention delayed development of diabetes by approximately 35%. In overweight and obese adults at risk for type 2 diabetes, average weight loss achieved with lifestyle intervention of 2.5 kg to 5.5 kg over 2 years reduces the risk of developing type 2 diabetes by 30% to 60%.

Thyroid Dysfunction

The 2021 guidelines published by European Society of Endocrinology recommends thyroid function testing in all patients with obesity, even in the absence of a clinical suspicion for hypothyroidism. The guideline is an acknowledgment of a relatively simple diagnostic test, low risk treatment, and potential for untreated hypothyroidism to adversely affect weight loss efforts. Thyroid-stimulating hormone (TSH) is the first thyroid hormone that should be measured. If this is elevated, free thyroxine (free T4) should be measured to accurately classify the disease process.

Reproductive Dysfunction

Obesity in women increases the risk for menstrual dysfunction, infertility, and adverse outcomes in pregnancy. Obesity is an independent risk factor for erectile dysfunction in men. Weight loss has been shown to improve several aspects of reproductive function in both men and women.

Cardiovascular Disease

Obesity increases the risk of coronary heart disease, heart failure, and overall cardiovascular mortality. People with obesity have a higher likelihood of developing risk factors that lead to cardiovascular disease such as hypertension and dyslipidemia.

Hypertension is a common chronic disease. Obesity has been shown to worsen hypertension; conversely there is a dose-response relationship between weight loss and improvements in blood pressure. Hence, even modest weight loss of less than 5% body weight can improve blood pressure in a clinically meaningful way.

Screening for dyslipidemia is best performed with a fasting lipid profile. Treatment guidelines for dyslipidemia are based on underlying comorbidities and calculated risk for developing atherosclerotic cardiovascular disease. Modest weight loss (less than 3 kg) leads to improvement in serum triglycerides and high-density lipoprotein (HDL) and low-density lipoprotein (LDL) cholesterol. In the presence of obesity, other modifiable risk factors such as smoking, hypertension, and sedentary lifestyle should be aggressively targeted.

Obstructive Sleep Apnea

Obstructive sleep apnea is a common but underrecognized complication of obesity. Patients with obesity who present with clinical features suspicious for sleep apnea or a neck circumference of greater than 17 inches in men or 16 inches in women should be screened for sleep apnea. Untreated sleep apnea has numerous health consequences related to the cardiorespiratory system and may also make it difficult for the patient to successfully lose weight. In addition to sleep apnea, obstructive lung disease, apnea-hypopnea syndromes, and restrictive lung disease are common complications of obesity that improve with weight loss.

Fatty Liver Disease

End-stage liver disease from nonalcoholic fatty liver disease is one of the most common reasons for liver transplantation in the world. The prevalence of nonalcoholic fatty liver disease increases as BMI increases, and up to 80% of patients with a BMI of greater than 40 kg/m^2 are estimated to have steatosis. The diagnosis of fatty liver disease is made on imaging, most commonly ultrasound. Weight loss is the first line of treatment for fatty liver disease; 5% to 10% weight loss has been shown to improve liver biochemistries and liver histology.

Mechanical Complications From Weight

Patients with overweight and obesity are at high risk of developing degenerative joint disease in weight-bearing joints. This in turn can promote further weight gain, and a vicious cycle therefore develops. A multidisciplinary approach comprising calorie restriction, behavioral therapy, physical therapy, and pain management is often necessary to achieve successful weight loss in this group of patients.

Gastroesophageal reflux is another mechanical complication from carrying excess weight, resulting from increased intraabdominal pressure from visceral adiposity. Patients who lose weight often see improvements in reflux symptoms.

Risk of Cancer

A number of malignancies are associated with obesity. In 2012 in the United States, about 28,000 new cases of cancer in men (3.5%) and 72,000 in women (9.5%) were due to overweight or obesity. The risk of developing esophageal, stomach, liver, kidney, gallbladder, pancreas, and colorectal cancers is higher in people who are overweight or obese. Endometrial carcinoma, breast cancer (in postmenopausal women), and ovarian cancer occur more commonly in women who are overweight or obese. Obesity also worsens several aspects of cancer survivorship such as quality of life, recurrence, progression, and prognosis.

Psychosocial Functioning

Patients with obesity frequently face stigma in areas such as education, employment, and healthcare, resulting in inequity and loss of opportunity. Patients with obesity often correlate their mental health and well-being with their ability to lose weight, and this can be a challenging situation to navigate. One condition that has been shown to correlate with obesity is seasonal affective disorder. Patients with this diagnosis are prone to gaining weight in the wintertime.

Treatment

Weight loss can only occur with the creation of an energy deficit in an individual. The cornerstone of any weight management program is lifestyle intervention that focuses on calorie restriction, increase in physical activity, and behavioral modification. Other modalities that can help promote weight loss include pharmacotherapy and weight loss procedures. These can be considered adjuncts to lifestyle intervention if lifestyle intervention alone does not produce the desired outcomes.

Successful management of obesity involves a multidisciplinary team working in partnership with the patient. Prior to making specific recommendations, the patient encounter should address the following:

1. Assessing the patient's readiness for change. The clinician can ask, "How prepared are you to make changes in your diet, to be more physically active, and to use behavior change strategies such as recording your weight and food intake?" A patient who is not ready to engage in changes will not be receptive to counseling on lifestyle changes.
2. Identification of barriers. Limitations to activity because of mechanical joint pain or lymphedema are relatively common and specific strategies to manage these may be necessary. Time and financial resources are also common barriers to successful weight loss. Identifying and acknowledging barriers can help build trust and forge a partnership with the patient.
3. Goal-setting. Patients are often overwhelmed by the amount of weight they need to lose. Clarifying that small but meaningful weight loss will improve health can be helpful to the patient. Aiming for 5% to 10% weight loss over 6 months is a reasonable initial goal.

Lifestyle Intervention Program

The key components of a lifestyle intervention prescription are listed in Table 2. An individualized lifestyle intervention program, based on the patient's dietary preferences, physical activity ability, and underlying motivation is most likely to result in successful weight loss.

Pharmacotherapy for Weight Loss

Appetite regulation is a complicated process that involves peripheral gut signaling, central coordination of those signals, and modulation by the environment, emotion, and behavior. Pharmacotherapy for weight loss primarily focuses on central appetite regulation and the most effective weight loss medications are appetite suppressants. Thus they act to reduce caloric intake while simultaneously often reducing cravings.

Current US Food and Drug Administration (FDA)-approved weight loss medications are indicated for individuals with a BMI ≥30 kg/m² or BMI ≥27 kg/m² with at least one obesity-associated comorbid condition who are motivated to lose weight, as an adjunct to comprehensive lifestyle intervention to help achieve targeted weight loss and health goals.

The FDA-approved weight loss medications, their dosing, and their side effect profile are listed in Table 3. All current FDA-approved weight loss medications, with the exception of weekly

TABLE 2	Components of a Lifestyle Intervention Program
COMPONENT	
Diet	*Calorie restriction of 300–500 kcals/day.* Goal for most women: 1200–1500 kcals/day. Goal for most men: 1500–1800 kcals/day. There is no specific dietary macronutrient composition that promotes long-term weight loss. The best predictor of weight loss is dietary adherence; hence patients should be counseled on dietary strategies that are most likely to be sustained.
Physical activity	*Goal: ≥150 minutes a week of moderate-intensity exercise* Patients should be encouraged to increase physical activity wherever able. The first goal may be to decrease sedentary time. Patients can aim for 10 minutes of activity at a time. Self-monitoring of activity, such as using a step-counter, can be helpful. Patients with multiple comorbidities and limitations to activity may benefit from a specific physical activity prescription from a physical therapist.
Behavioral therapy	Behavioral modification is key to ensuring long-term success. Daily monitoring of food and activity can help patients make behavioral changes. Ideally, patients will also be enrolled in a structured behavioral modification curriculum supervised by a behavioral psychologist. Patients benefit from regular feedback and support of their efforts.

Adapted from Heymsfield SB, Wadden TA. Mechanisms, pathophysiology, and management of obesity. *N Engl J Med.* 2017;376(15):1492.

TABLE 3	FDA-Approved Pharmacologic Agents for Weight Loss	
NAME/TRADE NAME	**DOSING**	**COMMON SIDE EFFECTS**
Orlistat/ Xenical™	120 mg TID with meals	Bloating, abdominal cramps, diarrhea, steatorrhea
Phentermine-Topiramate ER/ Qsymia®	3.75/23 mg daily for 2 weeks, then 7.5/46 mg daily thereafter High dose therapy is 11.25–69 mg daily for 2 weeks, then 15–92 mg daily thereafter	Phentermine side effects: Constipation, dry mouth, tachycardia, insomnia, hypertension Topiramate side effects: Paresthesias, dizziness, cognitive dysfunction, kidney stones, glaucoma
Naltrexone-SR/bupropion-SR/ Contrave®	Each tablet contains 8 mg naltrexone and 90 mg bupropion. Titrate by 1 tablet a week until maximal therapeutic dose of 2 tablets twice daily	Nausea, constipation, dry mouth, headache
Liraglutide/Saxenda®	Titrate by 0.6 mg daily every week until maximal therapeutic dose of 3 mg daily subcutaneously	Nausea, abdominal discomfort, constipation, or diarrhea.
Semaglutide/Wegovy®	Start at 0.25 mg subcutaneously weekly for 4 weeks, then 0.5 mg weekly for 4 weeks, then 1 mg weekly for 4 weeks, then 1.7 mg weekly for 4 weeks, then 2.4 mg weekly	Nausea, vomiting, constipation or diarrhea, gallbladder-related symptoms

semaglutide, have an average reported clinical efficacy of 5% to 10% weight loss over 6 months. Because these weight loss medications are relatively similar in efficacy, choice of therapy is typically guided by the principle of minimizing medication interactions and side effects. All current FDA-approved weight loss medications are category X in pregnancy, and patients should be counseled to avoid pregnancy while taking these medications.

Phentermine (Adipex-P) is a short-acting sympathomimetic that has been approved for short-term weight loss (i.e., 12 weeks). However, phentermine is often used off-label for longer periods of time in patients who show a response to the medication in both weight loss and weight maintenance phases. Retrospective analyses of phentermine users demonstrated no increase in cardiovascular morbidity and no increase in addictive potential with phentermine use. If phentermine monotherapy is being considered as a long-term weight loss medication, the risks and benefits of this approach should be thoroughly discussed with the patient and an appropriate monitoring plan instituted.

Topiramate (Topamax) monotherapy is also used off-label to assist with weight management. Topiramate is a carbonic anhydrase inhibitor that has beneficial effects on appetite suppression and satiety. A meta-analysis on the efficacy and safety of topiramate in weight loss showed that patients on topiramate on average were able to lose an additional 5.3 kg over patients on placebo. Most common side effects with topiramate were noted to be paresthesias (tingling of the fingers), changes in taste, and psychomotor impairment.

Semaglutide (Ozempic) is a once-weekly GLP-1 receptor agonist that has been FDA approved for the treatment of obesity and for type 2 diabetes. In early 2021, a number of phase three randomized, placebo-controlled trials using semaglutide at a dose of 2.4 mg once weekly (weight loss dose) were published. The Semaglutide Treatment Effect in People with Obesity (STEP) randomized controlled trials were designed to study the weight loss effect of high-dose semaglutide in patients with and without type 2 diabetes (STEP 1, 2, and 3) and weight maintenance in patients without type 2 diabetes (STEP 4 and 5). On average, participants taking 2.4 mg semaglutide subcutaneously once weekly were able to achieve 15% weight loss compared with patients on placebo who achieved 2% to 5% weight loss. Overall, the gastrointestinal (GI)-related side effect profile was higher in the semaglutide group (nausea, constipation, diarrhea, gallbladder-related conditions), and treatment discontinuation was seen in approximately 3% of participants in that group.

Monitoring Patients on Weight Loss Medications

Patients on weight loss medications should be evaluated early and often to ensure continued efficacy of the drug and to monitor for side effects. The best predictor of overall response to a weight loss medication is weight loss achieved in the first 3 months. In general, 5% weight loss in the first 3 months is indicative of a "responder." If a patient with a previously upward weight trend is able to maintain their weight on the new medication after 3 months of use, then that patient may still be considered a responder. Patients who have had significant changes to their health, overall medication regimen, or physical activity routine may not achieve the goal of 5% weight loss over 3 months; in these situations a longer duration of follow-up might be necessary to determine whether the patient is a responder to the medication.

Except for the scenarios listed above, patients who do not achieve a 5% weight loss over 3 months have several options. If appetite suppression is inadequate per clinical history, then a higher dose of the drug or a different weight loss medication could be considered. Patients could also benefit from meeting with a dietitian to ensure that their dietary plan is adequately calorie-restricted. If a patient has significant side effects from the medication, then an alternative weight loss medication could be considered.

Patients should be seen every 3 to 6 months to assess their weight loss trends and monitor for side effects and the potential for new medication interactions. Patients with a clinically meaningful weight loss can also be retested for improvements in their metabolic profile (e.g., fasting glucose), as this may affect therapeutic decision making.

Weight loss typically slows down after about 6 months of therapy, sometimes referred to as a "weight plateau"; this is a physiologic adaptation to weight loss. Specifically, it is estimated that for each kilogram of lost weight, calorie expenditure decreases by about 20 to 30 kcal/day whereas appetite increases by about 100 kcal/day above the baseline level prior to weight loss. Hence, the default trend is for weight loss followed by weight regain. This is an important phenomenon to highlight with patients who can become frustrated that their efforts are not yielding results. Patients may be more willing to engage in modifications to their dietary intake or energy expenditure to overcome this when they understand how metabolic adaptation occurs with weight loss.

Procedural Interventions for Weight Loss
Endoscopic Interventions

Endoscopic weight loss procedures, such as the endoscopic sleeve gastroplasty (ESG) and endoscopic intragastric balloon, are increasing in popularity because of their efficacy and noninvasive nature.

The ESG is a procedure whereby the patient's stomach capacity is endoscopically reduced, creating a gastric sleeve the size of a small banana. A systematic review and meta-analysis to evaluate the efficacy and safety of ESG in adults showed the average total body weight loss to be approximately 17%. 2.2% of patients in this cohort experienced side effects, most commonly GI-related.

Most patients included in the analysis had a BMI between 30 and 40 kg/m², thus this procedure may not yield similar results in patients with class III obesity (BMI greater than 40 kg/m²). The procedure is also technically challenging and may therefore not be widely available. Patients interested in the ESG should continue to be counseled on making sustainable lifestyle changes following the procedure to ensure long-term weight maintenance.

Intragastric balloon devices are approved to treat obesity in patients with a BMI greater than 30 kg/m². In this procedure, a gastric balloon is endoscopically inserted and filled with saline. It remains in place for 6 months, after which it is removed following endoscopic deflation. The intragastric balloon increases satiety and decreases gastric emptying, thus promoting decreased caloric intake and ultimately weight loss. Total body weight loss at 12 months is approximately 10%; patients who lose weight with the balloon in place often see some degree of weight regain following balloon removal. Adverse effects are most commonly seen in the first week following balloon placement and consist of nausea and constipation. Balloons that are left in place for greater than 6 months run the risk of causing gastric erosion.

Cellulose and Citric Acid (Plenity®)

Plenity is an FDA-cleared, prescription-only aid for weight management. It is made from naturally derived cellulose and citric acid, forming a three-dimensional (3D) matrix in the stomach when ingested with water, and is not absorbed systemically. This product is indicated in overweight and obese adults with a BMI of 25 to 40 kg/m², when used in conjunction with diet and exercise.

It is currently the only FDA-approved weight loss aid that can be used in patients with a BMI as low as 25 kg/m². Access to Plenity is currently only available via a mail-order program.

In a multicenter, double-blind, placebo-controlled 24-week study of 436 patients with a mean BMI 33 to 34 kg/m², patients were randomized to either 3 Gelesis100 (former name of Plenity) capsules taken with 500 mL water 20 to 30 minutes before lunch and dinner or placebo. Participants were prescribed a hypocaloric diet and asked to do 30 minutes of moderate-intensity exercise a day. Mean weight loss achieved was 6.4% in the treatment arm versus 4.4% in the placebo arm. Approximately 60% of participants in the treatment arm achieved at least a 5% weight loss, a threshold that is considered clinically relevant. Adverse GI effects were higher in the treatment arm (38% vs. 28%), but the dropout rate was similar in both groups.

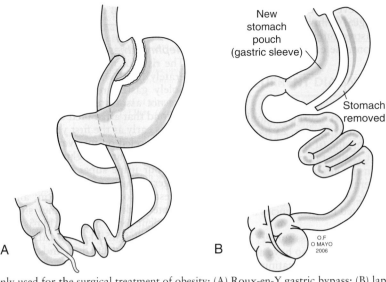

Common bariatric procedures

New stomach pouch (gastric sleeve)

Stomach removed

O.F O MAYO 2006

A   B

Figure 1 Techniques commonly used for the surgical treatment of obesity: (A) Roux-en-Y gastric bypass; (B) laparoscopic sleeve gastrectomy.

Bariatric Surgery

Bariatric (or metabolic) surgery results in significant weight loss leading to remission or resolution of several weight-related comorbidities. Compared with usual obesity care, bariatric surgery has also been shown to prolong life expectancy. Bariatric surgery is indicated in patients with a BMI greater than 40 kg/m^2 or in patients with a BMI greater than 35 kg/m^2 with associated weight-related comorbidities. There are compelling data that patients with diabetes with a BMI as low as 27 kg/m^2 may benefit from bariatric surgery, but this has not been adapted into practice.

Candidacy for bariatric surgery is determined on medical and psychological grounds. Patients interested in bariatric surgery should be motivated and ready for the significant and lifelong changes that occur after surgery. Psychological contraindications to pursuing surgery include untreated major depression or psychosis, other active psychiatric illness including chemical dependency, binge-eating disorders, and the inability to comply with nutritional requirements including lifelong vitamin supplementation.

There are several types of bariatric surgeries. Here we present the two most common, which are the laparoscopic Roux-en-Y gastric bypass (RYGB) and the laparoscopic sleeve gastrectomy (Figure 1).

Roux-en-Y Gastric Bypass

In this surgery, a small "pouch" is formed from the proximal part of the stomach, which is divided and separated from the distal part of the stomach. The pouch has a capacity of approximately 1 tbsp at the time of creation. The small intestine is divided approximately 100 cm distal to the pylorus; one end forms the anastomosis with the pouch and the other and is anastomosed at the jejunum about 75 to 100 cm distal to the pouch. These anatomic alterations result in restriction of food intake and decrease absorption capacity of the small intestine, thus leading to weight loss. The average weight loss seen after gastric bypass surgery is approximately 30% of total body weight.

Patients who undergo gastric bypass surgery often develop an aversion to high sugar content and fatty foods (i.e., calorie-dense foods). This in turn does help decrease total caloric intake. Patients can often develop lactose intolerance as well, which limits their total dairy consumption.

Guidelines for multivitamin supplementation following RYGB is outlined below (Table 4).

Complications from RYGB can be categorized as either surgical complications or nutritional complications. In the immediate

TABLE 4	Guidelines for Standard Multivitamin and Mineral Supplementation After Bariatric Surgery
SUPPLEMENT	**DOSING AND SUPPLY**
200% of recommended daily allowance for vitamins and minerals	Two chewable multivitamins daily Patients with renal impairment may need dose adjustment
Elemental calcium	1500–2000 mg daily with meals, in divided doses. If supplements are required, calcium citrate is better absorbed in a low acid environment such as post-gastric bypass
Vitamin D	3000–5000 units of vitamin D3 daily, total through dietary intake and supplements
B12	1000 mcg deep subcutaneous injection monthly OR 500–1000 mcg orally daily

postoperative period, anastomotic ulcerations and strictures may occur, requiring reintervention. Longer-term surgical complications may include the development of intestinal obstruction from internal hernias or adhesions. Overall, the mortality from bariatric surgery is less than 1%. Nutritional deficiencies after RYGB most commonly involve deficiencies of iron, vitamin D, and calcium. This is partly driven by the exclusion of the proximal duodenum, which is the major side of absorption of these specific nutrients.

Sleeve Gastrectomy

The sleeve gastrectomy is the most widely performed bariatric procedure worldwide. In this surgery, approximately 80% of the body of the stomach is removed, leaving behind a tubular structure that resembles a shirtsleeve. The average weight loss seen with the sleeve gastrectomy is approximately 15% to 25% of total body weight. The sleeve gastrectomy is the preferred bariatric procedure in patients who have a need to be consistent with absorption of specific medications, for example antirejection medications after organ transplantation.

Guidelines for multivitamin supplementation following sleeve gastrectomy is outlined below (Table 4).

patients are at risk for hyperglycemia, hyperlipidemia, and hypercapnia, all of which can be exacerbated by metabolic changes associated with critical illness. As with any critically ill patient, those with obesity will preferentially use protein and carbohydrate for energy and cannot effectively draw upon adipose tissue for energy. These patients require nutrition support to minimize loss of lean body mass.

The concept of "hypocaloric feeding" has emerged as the preferred way to feed critically ill patients with obesity. Energy delivery is restricted to approximately 60% to 70% of estimated energy requirements, and protein delivery is high (typically >2 g/kg ideal body weight [IBW]). This is to avoid hyperglycemia, hyperlipidemia, and hypercapnia while providing the protein required to spare lean body mass and support recovery. Small-scale studies employing this feeding method have demonstrated that patients can achieve positive nitrogen balance. One study found decreased ICU length of stay, decreased antibiotic days, and a trend toward decreased mechanical ventilation days.

Energy and protein delivery for critically ill patients with obesity is guided by BMI. The ASPEN-SCCM guidelines recommend providing 11 to 14 kcal/kg of actual weight for patients with a BMI of 30 to 50 kg/m² or 22 to 25 kcal/kg IBW for patients with a BMI greater than 50 kg/m². For protein delivery, ASPEN and SCCM recommend protein provision of 2 g/kg or greater IBW for patients with class I and class II obesity (BMI of 30–35 kg/m² and 35–40 kg/m², respectively), and, for patients with class III obesity (BMI > 40 kg/m²), protein provision should be 2.5 g/kg or greater IBW.

Other Conditions and Nutritional Treatments

The catabolic response to major surgery, trauma, burn, and sepsis is characterized by a net breakdown of body protein stores to provide substrates for gluconeogenesis and acute-phase protein synthesis. Adequate nutrition can attenuate whole-body catabolism but rarely, if ever, prevents or reverses the loss of lean body mass during the acute phase of injury. Several strategies to prevent the loss of lean body mass have been investigated, including growth hormone, growth factors, and conditionally essential amino acids, such as glutamine.

Growth hormone is a potent anabolic agent, and administration to humans increases the rate of wound healing, decreases rates of wound infection, and decreases the catabolism and muscle wasting of critical illness. However, a large European trial found increased morbidity and mortality in patients with prolonged critical illness who received high doses of growth hormone. Thus the use of growth hormone in patients who are in the acute phase of critical illness is not recommended.

Alternative anabolic agents such as oxandrolone (Oxandrin)[1] and testosterone[1] are being pursued to induce positive nitrogen balance and enhance wound healing in critically ill patients. These anabolic steroid hormones increase protein synthesis and can reduce the rate of protein breakdown. In a study of patients with alcoholic hepatitis, administration of oxandrolone was associated with lower mortality compared with patients receiving placebo. The patients receiving oxandrolone had improvements in the severity of their liver injury and the degree of malnutrition. Several studies have demonstrated a benefit of oxandrolone use in the burn patient population. Other anabolic steroid hormones, such as methandienone[2] and nandrolone decanoate (Deca Durabolin),[2] have been shown to increase protein anabolism and nitrogen balance in hospitalized patients.

Hormone treatment should be reserved for patients with major burns and documented impaired healing, patients who have large wounds or enterocutaneous fistulae who have impaired healing, patients with muscle wasting and weakness associated with AIDS or other failure to thrive conditions, and, in general, patients who have not responded to aggressive nutritional support but whose underlying disease processes are controlled. Growth factors have not been shown to decrease length of time on a respirator in ICU

patients. In fact, such factors can increase ventilator time and worsen outcome.

Glutamine-supplemented PN solutions administered to trauma or critically ill patients can improve overall nitrogen balance, enhance muscle protein synthesis, improve intestinal nutrient absorption, decrease gut permeability, improve immune function, and decrease hospital stays and costs in some patient populations. A review of 14 randomized trials in surgical and critically ill patients found that glutamine supplementation was associated with reduced mortality, lower rates of infectious complications, and a decreased hospital stay. The greatest benefit was in patients receiving high-dose (>0.29 g/kg/day) parenteral glutamine.

However, a recent randomized trial of glutamine and antioxidant micronutrient supplementation in critically ill patients showed a trend toward increased 28-day mortality and significant in-hospital and 6-month mortality in patients receiving glutamine supplementation. There were limitations in this study in that baseline glutamine levels were not checked for all patients; in a subset of 66 patients with plasma glutamine levels evaluated, all had normal levels at baseline. This suggests that glutamine supplementation may not be appropriate for all critically ill patients. In addition, patients received approximately 50% of goal energy requirements and approximately 45% of goal protein delivery from glutamine. The total amount of glutamine given in this study was significantly higher than the dose of glutamine usually recommended. This raises the possibility that there is an optimal "therapeutic window" for glutamine administration: giving too little glutamine may not be efficacious, and giving too much may be toxic. Further investigation is required before a definitive recommendation can be given based on this study alone.

Patients with intestinal dysfunction requiring PN, such as those with short-bowel syndrome or mucosal damage after chemotherapy and/or radiation therapy, might benefit from glutamine-containing PN. Glutamine-containing PN might also be beneficial in patients with immunodeficiency syndromes, including AIDS, immune-system dysfunction associated with critical illness, and bone marrow transplantation; patients with severe catabolic illness; patients with multiple trauma; and patients with other diseases associated with a prolonged ICU stay. Glutamine-supplemented solutions should not yet be considered routine care and should not be used in patients with significant renal insufficiency or in patients with significant hepatic failure. A recent ASPEN position paper summarizes recommendations for use of both enteral and IV glutamine.

Common Complications and Management
Catheter Sepsis

Catheter-related bloodstream infection (CRBSI) is an infection that originates from the catheter itself and is confirmed by culture. Central line–associated bloodstream infection is a bloodstream infection without another identified focus of infection in a patient with a central line in place for at least 48 hours before the development of infection. Central venous CRBSIs range from 3% to 20% in hospitalized patients and are the most common complication of central venous catheters. Colonization of the skin, intraluminal contamination from manipulation of the catheter hub or IV connectors, and seeding of microorganisms from the bloodstream are common sources of infection. Common organisms associated with CRBSIs include *Staphylococcus epidermidis*, *Staphylococcus aureus*, *Enterococcus* spp., *Candida albicans*, *Escherichia coli*, *Klebsiella* spp., *Pseudomonas* spp., and *Enterobacter* spp., as well as resistant strains such as methicillin-resistant *S. aureus* and vancomycin-resistant enterococci.

Management of patients with catheter infection depends on their clinical condition. In extremely ill patients with high fevers who are hypotensive or who have local signs of infection around the catheter site, the catheter should be removed, its tip cultured, and peripheral and central venous blood cultures should be obtained. In CRBSI, the organisms that grow from the catheter

---

[1] Not FDA approved for this indication.
[2] Not available in the United States.

PROBLEM	POSSIBLE ETIOLOGY	TREATMENT
Glucose		
Hyperglycemia, glycosuria, hyperosmolar nonketotic dehydration, or coma	Excessive dose or rate of infusion, inadequate insulin production, concomitant steroid administration, infection	Decrease the amount of glucose given, increase insulin, administer a portion of calories as fat
Diabetic ketoacidosis	Inadequate endogenous insulin production and/or inadequate insulin therapy	Give insulin Decrease glucose intake
Rebound hypoglycemia	Persistent endogenous insulin production by islet cells after long-term high-carbohydrate infusion	Give 5%–10% glucose before parenteral infusion is discontinued
Hypercarbia	Carbohydrate load exceeds the ability to increase minute ventilation and excrete excess CO_2	Limit glucose dose to 5 mg/kg/min Give greater percentage of total caloric needs as fat (up to 30%–40%)
Fat		
Hypertriglyceridemia	Rapid infusion	Decrease rate of PN infusion
	Decreased clearance	Allow clearance (~12 h) before testing blood
Essential fatty acid deficiency	Inadequate essential fatty acid administration	Administer essential fatty acids in doses of 4%–7% of total calories
Amino Acids		
Hyperchloremia metabolic acidosis	Excessive chloride content of amino acid solutions	Administer Na^+ and K^+ as acetate salts
Prerenal azotemia	Excessive amino acids with inadequate caloric supplementation	Reduce amino acids Increase the amount of glucose calories
Miscellaneous		
Hypophosphatemia	Inadequate phosphorus administration with redistribution into tissues	Give 15 mmol phosphate/1000 IV kcal Evaluate antacid and Ca^{2+} administration
Hypomagnesemia	Inadequate administration relative to increased losses (diarrhea, diuresis, medications)	Administer Mg^{2+} (15–20 mEq/1000 kcal)
Hypermagnesemia	Excessive administration; renal failure	Decrease Mg^{2+} supplementation
Hypokalemia	Inadequate K^+ intake relative to increased needs for anabolism; diuresis	Increase K^+ supplementation
Hyperkalemia	Excessive K^+ administration, especially in metabolic acidosis; renal decompensation	Reduce or stop exogenous K^+ If ECG changes are present, treat with calcium gluconate, insulin, diuretics, and/or sodium polystyrene sulfonate (Kayexalate)
Hypocalcemia	Inadequate Ca^{2+} administration; reciprocal response to phosphorus repletion without simultaneous calcium infusion	Increase Ca^{2+} dose
Hypercalcemia	Excessive Ca^{2+} administration; excessive vitamin D administration	Decrease Ca^{2+} and/or vitamin D administration
Elevated liver transaminases or serum alkaline phosphatase and bilirubin	Enzyme induction secondary to amino acid imbalances or overfeeding	Reevaluate nutritional prescription Cycle TPN Avoid overfeeding calories Consider change to a blended lipid rather than 100% soybean oil-lipid Consider administering carnitine

ECG, Electrocardiographic; *IV,* intravenous; *PN,* parenteral nutrition; *TPN,* total parenteral nutrition.

tip are the same those identified in the peripheral blood culture, and typically more than 10^3 organisms are grown from cultures of the catheter tip.

Specific therapy should be initiated against the primary source in patients in whom a source of infection other than the catheter tip is present. Peripheral blood cultures should be obtained. Blood cultures should not be taken from the central venous catheter port dedicated for PN because this increases the risk of contaminating the line. If the infection resolves, central venous feedings can be continued while making sure to maintain euglycemia. If a source is not identified and the symptoms persist, the catheter should be removed, and its tip should be cultured. If the culture of the catheter tip returns positive or if the index of suspicion is high, empiric antibiotic therapy is initiated and later narrowed to target the specific microorganism once culture and susceptibility data become available. If removal of the catheter is indicated and is not possible because of lack of access sites or high risk of bleeding complications, then salvage therapy (systemic antibiotics plus antibiotic lock therapy or ethanol lock therapy) or, as a last resort, exchange of the catheter over a guidewire with systemic antibiotics and antibiotic lock therapy may be considered, with long-term ethanol lock therapy to prevent further infections. Central venous feedings may be continued during this interval if the patient is stable. It is important to note that changing the site of catheter, rather than salvage therapy or guidewire exchange, is preferred in patients in whom infection is suspected.

Other Complications

Common complications, their etiologies, and treatments are outlined in Table 4. Prolonged administration of PN can result in altered hepatic function and can lead to liver failure.

| BOX 3 | Management of Parenteral Nutrition-Related Liver Dysfunction |

Have the patient eat, if possible.

Avoid administering large amounts of glucose or protein calories.

Supply intravenous fat emulsions (up to 30% of total calories).

Consider addition of blended lipid emulsions with lower concentrations of soybean oil.

Cycle the parenteral nutrition, infusing for 10 to 12 hours/day.

Reevaluate energy needs; reduce energy delivery if liver dysfunction persists.

Transaminases may be elevated 1 to 2 weeks after initiating PN, but this often resolves without any change in the composition of PN or rate of administration. However, in patients receiving long-term PN (>20 days), prolonged elevations of alkaline phosphatase followed by elevated levels of serum transaminases can occur, even after therapy is discontinued.

Serum levels of alkaline phosphatase and bilirubin initially remain normal, but they rise in many patients who receive long-term PN. Patients who do not receive lipids in the PN solution have more frequent and severe hepatic abnormalities, most likely due to higher carbohydrate loads. Excess glucose increases insulin secretion, which stimulates hepatic lipogenesis and results in hepatic fat accumulation. Fatty infiltration is the initial histopathologic change; it is readily reversible and might not be accompanied by altered liver function tests.

Longer PN therapy may be associated with cholestasis, cholelithiasis, steatosis, and steatohepatitis and can progress to active chronic hepatitis, fibrosis, and eventual cirrhosis. The management of PN-related liver dysfunction is summarized in Box 3.

Complications are minimized and nutritional therapy maximized when the care of patients who require specialized nutritional support is supervised by a nutrition support team. Ideally, the nutrition support team consists of a pharmacist, dietitian, nurse, and physician.

References

Al-Omran M, Albalawi ZH, Tashkandi MF, Al-Ansary LA: *Enteral versus parenteral nutrition in acute pancreatitis,* Cochrane Database Syst Rev, 2010. http://dx.doi.org/10.1002/14651858.CD002837.pub2. CD002837.

A.S.P.E.N, Ayers P, Adams S, Boullata J, et al: Parenteral nutrition safety consensus recommendations, *JPEN J Parenter Enteral Nutr* 38:296–333, 2014.

A.S.P.E.N. Board of Directors: Guidelines for the use of parenteral and enteral nutrition in adult and pediatric patients, *JPEN J Parenter Enteral Nutr* 26:1SA–138SA, 2002.

Bistrian BR, McCowen KC: Nutritional and metabolic support in the adult intensive care unit: key controversies, *Crit Care Med* 34:1525–1531, 2006.

Boullata JI, Gilbert K, Sacks G, et al: A.S.P.E.N. Clinical guidelines: parenteral nutrition ordering, order review, compounding, labeling, and dispensing, *JPEN J Parenter Enteral Nutr* 38(3):334–377, 2014.

Butler SO, Btaiche IF, Alaniz C: Relationship between hyperglycemia and infection in critically ill patients, *Pharmacotherapy* 25:963–976, 2005.

Evans DC, Corkins MR, Malone A, et al: The use of visceral proteins as nutrition markers: an ASPEN position paper, *Nutr Clin Pract* 36:22–28, 2021.

Heyland DK, Dhaliwal R, Suchner U, Berger MM: Antioxidant nutrients: a systematic review of trace elements and vitamins in the critically ill patient, *Intensive Care Med* 31:327–337, 2005.

Heyland D, Muscedere J, Wischmeyer PE, et al: A randomized trial of glutamine and antioxidants in critically ill patients, *N Engl J Med* 368:1489–1497, 2013.

Li Y, Tang X, Zhang J, Wu T: Nutritional support for acute kidney injury, *Cochrane Database Syst Rev,* 2010. https://doi.org/10.1002/14651858.CD005426.pub3. CD005426.

McClave SA, Chang W-K, Dhaliwal R, Heyland DK: Nutrition support in acute pancreatitis: a systematic review of the literature, *JPEN J Parenter Enteral Nutr* 30:143–156, 2006.

McClave SA, Taylor BE, Martindale RG, et al: , Guidelines for the provision of nutrition support therapy in the adult critically ill patient: Society of Critical Care Medicine (SCCM) and American Society for Parenteral and Enteral Nutrition (A.S.P.E.N.), *JPEN J Parenter Enteral Nutr.* 40:159–211. 40:1200, 2016. Erratum in: JPEN J Parenter Enteral Nutr 2016.

McMahon MM, Nystrom E, Braunschweig C, et al: A.S.P.E.N. Clinical guidelines: nutrition support of adult patients with hyperglycemia, *JPEN J Parenter Enteral Nutr* 37:26–36, 2013.

O'Grady NP, Alexander M, Burns LA, et al: Guidelines for the prevention of intravascular catheter-related infections, *Clin Infect Dis* 52:e162–e193, 2011. Also available at http://www.cdc.gov/hicpac/BSI/BSI-guidelines-2011.html. accessed December 5, 2013.

Vanek VW, Matarese LE, Robinson M, et al: A.S.P.E.N. Position paper: parenteral nutrition glutamine supplementation, *JPEN J Parenter Enteral Nutr* 26:479–494, 2011.

Worthington P, Balint J, Bechtold M, et al: When is parenteral nutrition appropriate? *JPEN J Parenter Enteral Nutr* 41:324–377, 2017.

PHEOCHROMOCYTOMA

Method of

Matthew A. Nazari, MD; Abhishek Jha, MBBS; Katherine Ilona Wolf; and Karel Pacak, MD, PhD, DSc

CURRENT DIAGNOSIS

- The most common clinical sign of a pheochromocytoma/paraganglioma (PPGL) is hypertension; when combined with the triad of headache, palpitations, and diaphoresis, the diagnosis should be suspected.
- A biochemical diagnosis of PPGL should be established with elevated plasma or urinary fractionated metanephrines and plasma methoxytyramine.
- Localize tumors with anatomic imaging (computed tomography [CT] or magnetic resonance), followed by specific functional imaging using positron emission tomography (PET) modalities.
- Following diagnosis, a thorough medical and family history should be obtained to assess for syndromic clinical presentations of PPGL. If available, all patients with confirmed PPGL should undergo genetic testing.
- If a causative pathogenic variant is identified, the patient's first-degree relatives should be appropriately tested. Positive individuals should be presymptomatically screened with plasma or urinary fractionated metanephrines and imaging as described, if appropriate.

CURRENT THERAPY

- Prompt surgical excision remains the primary treatment for PPGL. If feasible, cortical sparing adrenalectomies should be attempted in patients with bilateral or hereditary PPGLs (except succinate dehydrogenase subunit B [*SDHB*]–related disease) to prevent lifelong corticosteroid supplementation.
- One to two weeks prior to the operation, patients with biochemically active tumors should be started on a preoperative α- followed by β-adrenoceptor blockade to avoid unopposed α-adrenoceptor stimulation leading to vasoconstriction and hypertensive crisis. At minimum, a normotensive patient should be maintained on low-dose calcium channel blockers.
- After surgery, scheduled clinical follow-up is necessary, particularly in cases of underlying pathogenic variants or large tumors (>5 cm), which are more likely to metastasize.
- Management of metastatic PPGL requires a multidisciplinary approach involving surgical excision alongside pharmacologic, radio-, and chemotherapies.

The 2022 World Health Organization (WHO) Classification of Tumors of Endocrine Organs defines pheochromocytoma (PHEO)* as a chromaffin cell tumor arising from the adrenal medulla, or an intraadrenal paraganglioma. Lesions smaller than 1 cm within the adrenal gland are called micropheochromocytomas.

---

*From this point forward, PHEO represents pheochromocytoma and paraganglioma unless otherwise specified.

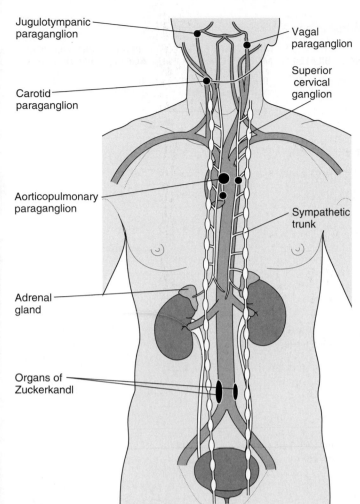

Figure 1 Important anatomic distribution of chromaffin tissue composing paraganglia.

Jugulotympanic paraganglion

Vagal paraganglion

Carotid paraganglion

Superior cervical ganglion

Aorticopulmonary paraganglion

Sympathetic trunk

Adrenal gland

Organs of Zuckerkandl

Paragangliomas (PGLs) are functionally similar tumors that originate along the extra-adrenal ganglia and are further classified as parasympathetic or sympathetic. Predominantly located in the head and neck, parasympathetic PGLs are locally invasive, rarely develop metastases, and secrete dopamine/methoxytyramine, with a minority (approximately 5% or less) producing and releasing norepinephrine/normetanephrine. In contrast to their parasympathetic counterparts, sympathetic PGLs are concentrated primarily in the abdomen and pelvis, with 2% found in the mediastinum and 1% in the neck. Abdominal PGLs often derive from the organ of Zuckerkandl, a collection of neural crest cells above the bifurcation of the aorta at the origin of the inferior mesenteric artery (Figure 1). Biochemically, PHEOs are characterized by the synthesis, metabolism, storage, and almost always the release of metanephrines/methoxytyramine (in approximately 98% of cases) and usually the release of catecholamines (in approximately 70% of cases).

Epidemiology

Previously, PHEOs were primarily diagnosed at autopsy. However, as the sensitivity of biochemical assays and imaging scans increased, the incidence of PHEO likewise swelled. A recent European analysis estimates that the age-standardized incidence rate increased from 0.29 to 0.46 from 1995 to 2015, respectively. While PHEO can occur at any age (including childhood, particularly when associated with germline pathogenic variants), the average age of diagnosis is most commonly in the fifth decade. Although no consistent gender preference has been reported, in the Netherlands, a statistically significant number of PHEOs occurred in females (55%) compared to their male counterparts (45%). The PHEO to PGL ratio

is approximately 0.80 to 0.20, respectively. Approximately 30% to 40% of patients with PHEO carry a germline or somatic pathogenic variant in one of the 25 known PHEO susceptibility genes (see "Genetics" below). The rate of malignancy varies from 0% to 71% depending on genetic background, with succinate dehydrogenase subunit B (*SDHB*)–related disease, the most clinically aggressive.

Genetics

While complete consensus is lacking, 30% to 40% of PHEOs are hereditary, with a significant percentage (upwards of 20%) of apparently sporadic tumors carrying pathogenic variants. Identification of a genetic alteration allows for appropriate treatment algorithms and management of subsequent endocrinopathies or syndromic neoplasias in the proband and at-risk relatives as well.

At present, at least 25 PHEO susceptibility genes have been discovered, which can broadly be categorized into major and minor contributors, with the major genes representing 85% to 90% of all hereditary tumors. Well-known hereditary pathogenic variants include von Hippel-Lindau tumor suppressor (*VHL*), *RET* proto-oncogene resulting in multiple endocrine neoplasia (MEN) types 2A and 2B, neurofibromin 1 (*NF1*) tumor suppressor, and the succinate dehydrogenase (*SDHx*) subunits *SDHB* and *SDHD* genes. The minor susceptibility genes, representing 10% to 15% of hereditary tumors include *SDHA*, *SDHC*, succinate-CoA ligase GDP-forming subunit beta (*SUCLG2*), succinate dehydrogenase assembly factor 2 (*SDHAF2*), fumarate hydratase (*FH*), Myc-associated factor X (*MAX*), hypoxia-inducible factor 2 alpha (*HIF2A*), malate dehydrogenase 2 (*MDH2*), isocitrate dehydrogenase 1 (*IDH1*), isocitrate dehydrogenase 2 (*IDH2*), H-RAS and K-RAS proto-oncogenes, transmembrane protein 127 (*TMEM 127*), cold-shock domain containing E1 (*CSDE1*), mastermind like transcriptional coactivator 3 (*MAML3*) fusion genes, prolyl hydroxylase 1 and 2 (*PHD1/2*), iron regulatory protein 1 (*IRP1*), *MDH2*, kinesin superfamily member (*K1F1B*), dihydrolipoamide S-succinyltransferase (*DLST*), and DNA methyltransferase 3 alpha (*DNMT3A*). Characteristics of the most important hereditary tumor syndromes are described in Table 1.

Several well-established PHEO syndromes (Box 1) exhibit characteristic clinical features. Rare PGL-associated syndromes include Carney triad and Carney-Stratakis syndrome, which are characterized by *SDHB* and *SDHD*-related gastrointestinal stromal tumors (GISTs). The novel recently described Pacak-Zhuang syndrome consists of *HIF2A*-associated PGLs in the setting of polycythemia, duodenal somatostatinomas, and marked, permanent choroidal thickening and tortuous dilated veins in the choroid and retina. Another rare, recently described PHEO syndrome is characterized by pheochromocytomas, paragangliomas, and giant cell tumors of bone associated with a postzygotic *H3F3A* pathogenic variant.

In conjunction with the United States Endocrine Society Clinical Practice Guidelines, recent publications have emphasized genetic counseling and subsequent testing in all patients diagnosed with PHEO, regardless of suggestive family history or age at presentation. Within the United States, several commercially available PHEO gene panels screen patients for the most prevalent hereditary genetic syndromes via DNA sequencing and deletion/duplication analysis. However, broad, comprehensive genetic panels covering 10 to 12 genes are expensive and may not be covered by insurance. In patients with a confirmed PHEO, an algorithm (Figure 2) based on family history, syndromic clinical features, and biochemical phenotype could be used to tailor genetic testing and reduce the financial burden. If genetic testing is positive for hereditary PHEO, all first-degree relatives should undergo genetic evaluation. Asymptomatic carriers should undergo annual biochemical evaluation with plasma metanephrines and whole-body magnetic resonance (MR) imaging every other year for surveillance. Genetic testing in children (Box 2) should be approached on an individual basis following discussion with parents/guardians, geneticists, and psychiatrists due to the ethical and legal ramifications. Children should only be screened if they will be offered regular surveillance.

TABLE 1	Characteristics of Hereditary Pheochromocytoma Syndromes and Pathogenic Variants								
SYN-DROME	PATHOGENIC VARIANT	GENE	PROTEIN FUNCTION	PENETRANCE	BILATERAL	METASTATIC/ MULTIFOCAL	PHEO OR PGL	PEAK AGE (Y)	BIOCHEMICAL PHENOTYPE+
MEN2	10q11.2	*RET*	Receptor tyrosine kinase	50%	50–80%	Rare	PHEO	40	ADR
VHL	3p25-26	*VHL*	VHL protein/ E3 ubiquitin protein ligase	10–30%	50%	5%	PHEO	30	NA
NF-1	17q11	*NF-1*	NF-related protein	1–2%	16%	5–10%	PHEO	50	ADR
PGL1	11q23	*SDHD*	Membrane-spanning subunit; D subunit of SDH	90% if paternally transmitted†	Inconsistent Reports	5–20%#	PHEO/ PGL	35–40	NA and/or DA; some biochemically silent
PGL2 -SDH5	11q12.2	*SDHAF2/*	Assembly factor for SDHA	100% if paternally transmitted	56%	91%	PGL	30–40	Unknown
	3p14.1	*SUCLG2*	Catalytic enzyme: B subunit of succinyl-CoA-synthetase	Likely low		47%	PHEO/ PGL	37	ADR; some NA and DA
PGL3	1q21	*SDHC*	Membrane-spanning protein; C subunit of SDH	Inconsistent Reports	Inconsistent Reports	Rare	PHEO/ PGL	38	NA and/or DA; some biochemically silent
PGL4	1p36	*SDHB*	Catalytic iron-sulfur protein; B subunit of SDH	30-50%	Rare	31–71%	PHEO/ PGL	30	NA and/or DA; some biochemically silent
PGL5	5p15	*SDHA*	Catalytic flavoprotein; A subunit of SDH	10–13%‡	Inconsistent Reports	30-66%	PHEO/ PGL	40	NA and/or DA; some biochemically silent
	2q11.2	*TMEM127*	Transmembrane protein	Inconsistent Reports	33%	<5%	PHEO	43	ADR
	14q23	*MAX*	bHLHLZ transcription factor	Inconsistent Reports*	67%	<25%	PHEO	32	Mixed ADR and NA+
PZS	2p21	*HIF2A (EPAS1)*	Subunit of a hypoxia-inducible transcription factor	None	100	>40%	PHEO/ PGL	17	NA

Abbreviations: Adrenergic (*ADR*), Basic helix-loop-helix leucine zipper (*bHLHLZ*), Dopaminergic (*DA*), Multiple endocrine neoplasia (*MEN*), Noradrenergic (*NA*), Neurofibromatosis (*NF*), Pacak-Zhuang Syndrome (*PZS*), Paraganglioma (*PGL*), Pheochromocytoma (*PHEO*), Succinate dehydrogenase (*SDH*), von Hippel-Lindau (*VHL*)
Adrenergic: Phenotype characterized by increased levels of epinephrine or epinephrine/metanephrine. Noradrenergic: Phenotype characterized by increased levels of norepinephrine or norepinephrine/normetanephrine
†Observations at the National Institutes of Health report lower penetrance
#Excluding head and neck PGLs, where the rate of malignancy is approximately 5–10%
‡Observations at the National Institutes of Health report a much lower penetrance, almost zero percent
*Probable paternal transmission only

Clinical Manifestations

As a result of episodic catecholamine secretion on and stimulation of α- and β-adrenoceptors, the clinical manifestations of PHEO are related to hemodynamic and metabolic instability. While the majority of primary clinical indicators (Box 3) for PHEO are nonspecific, when several symptoms are taken in conjunction, the diagnosis should be considered. Patients with three or more signs and symptoms of catecholamine excess (hyperhidrosis, palpitations, pallor, tremor, and nausea), especially when combined with a body mass index of less than 25 kg/m² and a heart rate greater than 85 beats per minute, are 7.5-fold more likely to have a PPGL. Symptoms may occur spontaneously or as a result of direct tumor manipulation, anesthesia, or ingestion of tyramine-rich foods, which trigger catecholamine release and subsequent crisis. Unfortunately, patients may not exhibit any signs or symptoms of PHEO, thereby delaying a timely diagnosis. Therefore, if biochemistry or imaging suggests PHEO, the diagnosis may not be excluded based on the patient's asymptomatic state.

Differential Diagnosis

Referred to as the "great mimic," PHEO manifests with a myriad of signs and symptoms that are easily misconstrued for more common disorders, which often prevents a timely diagnosis. Consideration should be given to conditions that also result in sympathomedullary activation, including hyperadrenergic and renovascular hypertension, panic disorders, menopausal syndrome, temporal lobe epilepsy, and other neuroendocrine tumors that release vasoactive substances. Patients with a presumptive diagnosis of PHEO should be screened biochemically. If results are unequivocal, a normal response to the clonidine suppression test will effectively rule out PHEO.

BOX 1 — Important Syndromic Pheochromocytoma Presentations

von Hippel-Lindau Syndrome
Type 2A
- Retinal and central nervous system hemangioblastomas
- Pheochromocytoma
- Endolymphatic sac tumors
- Epididymal cystadenomas

Type 2B
- Renal cell cysts/carcinomas
- Retinal and central nervous system hemangioblastomas
- Pancreatic cysts/neoplasms
- Pheochromocytoma
- Endolymphatic sac tumors
- Epididymal cystadenomas

Type 2C
- Pheochromocytoma

Multiple Endocrine Neoplasia
Type 2A
- Medullary thyroid carcinoma
- Pheochromocytoma
- Hyperparathyroidism
- Cutaneous lichen amyloidosis

Type 2B
- Medullary thyroid carcinoma
- Pheochromocytoma
- Marfanoid habitus

FMTC: Familial Medullary Thyroid Carcinoma
Neurofibromatosis Type 1
- Neurofibromas
- Café-au-lait macules
- Lisch nodules
- Scoliosis
- Cognitive impairment
- Pheochromocytoma

Other Pheochromocytoma Syndromes
Carney Triad
- Gastrointestinal stromal tumor
- Pulmonary chondroma
- Paraganglioma

Carney-Stratakis Syndrome
- Gastrointestinal stromal tumor
- Paraganglioma

Pacak-Zhuang Syndrome
- Paraganglioma
- Somatostatinoma
- Polycythemia
- Retinal abnormalities
- Vascular malformations

H3F3A Pathogenic Variant
- Pheochromocytomas
- Bone giant cell tumors
- Periaortic and bladder paragangliomas

Adapted from Lenders JW, Eisenhofer G, Mannelli M, et al: Phaechromocytoma. *Lancet* 366:665–675, 2005.

Biochemical Evaluation

PHEOs are capable of secreting all, none, or any combination of catecholamines—epinephrine, norepinephrine, and dopamine. Plasma metanephrines (the O-methylated metabolites of parent catecholamines) is the current gold-standard diagnostic criteria to detect and exclude a diagnosis of PHEO. Twenty-four-hour urinary metanephrines is a comparable alternative when plasma is not available. Definitive diagnosis is likely when biochemical evaluation is greater than two times the upper reference limit (URL) (Figure 3). Diagnostic accuracy of plasma metanephrines is enhanced with age-specific upper reference limits. To reliably interpret test results, specific conditions (Box 4) should be ensured throughout the blood draw. Additionally, there are a variety of foods and medications (Table 2) that interact either directly or indirectly with catecholamine measurement and should therefore be avoided for 12 hours prior to collection. Patients with acute or chronic kidney disease, particularly those on dialysis, commonly have elevated plasma metanephrines (although likely less than three to four times the URL of normal). If necessary, liquid chromatography with tandem mass spectrometry is a quick and cost-effective means to detect and remove potentially interfering substances.

Confirmatory follow-up testing is necessary in almost all cases of PHEO given the high false-positive rate. Repeat plasma or urinary metanephrines and catecholamines, or the clonidine suppression test, can be used in equivocal cases, as secondary validation or in patients in whom interfering drugs cannot be stopped. Prior to clonidine suppression testing, patients should undergo a complete medication review with consideration to hold antihypertensives given predilection for profound hypotension in response to clonidine. Additionally, diuretics, antidepressants, and β-adrenoceptor blockers have been reported to interfere with test results and should be held when appropriate. The patient should be fasting overnight and resting comfortably supine for 20 minutes prior to baseline blood draw. Clonidine (Catapres)[1] is administered at a dose of 0.3 milligrams (mg) per 70 kg, with appropriate dose adjustments as necessary (upwards of 0.5 mg based on weight), and subsequent repeat blood draw 3 hours after administration.

With an increasing proportion of hereditary PHEO, it is important to distinguish their various catecholamine profiles, which can help guide genetic testing. In the last several years, the O-methylated metabolite of dopamine—methoxytyramine—has been used to confirm head and neck PGLs, which solely secrete dopamine and are therefore missed with standardized biochemical analysis. Furthermore, recent literature points to plasma methoxytyramine as a novel biomarker for metastatic PPGL, which can be used in conjunction with large tumor size, germline pathogenic variants (particularly *SDHx*), and the presence of extra-adrenal PGLs to indicate a higher likelihood of metastatic disease.

Localization of Pheochromocytoma

Imaging should be pursued after clear biochemical evidence is confirmed. In rare instances, biochemically negative disease can be present. For optimal results, initial anatomic scans should consist of whole-body CT or MR imaging. T2-weighted MR imaging is preferred in patients in whom radiation exposure should be limited, those with a CT contrast allergy, and for the detection of skull-based lesions with the presence of known surgical clips. Ultrasound is not recommended for the localization of PHEO but may be utilized in children and during pregnancy if MR imaging is unavailable. Anatomic imaging is only sufficient for PHEO confirmation if the adrenal gland is the sole site of involvement (tumors <5 cm in size) and the metanephrine level is very high—all other patients should proceed with functional imaging, which is also useful in ruling out metastatic disease.

Currently, there are four primary nuclear imaging techniques used to confirm or detect metastatic PPGL (iodine-123 metaiodobenzylguanadine [^{123}I-MIBG], gallium-68 DOTA(0)-Tyr(3)-octreotate [^{68}Ga-DOTATATE], fluorine-18-fluorodihydroxyphenylalanine [^{18}F-FDOPA], and fluorine-18-fluorodeoxyglucose [^{18}F-FDG]). Several algorithms (Figure 4) have been proposed based on tumor location, genetic predisposition, and presence of metastatic disease. While ^{18}F-FDG was previously preferred for comprehensive localization of metastatic disease, recent systematic reviews have reported the superiority of ^{68}Ga-DOTATATE in apparently sporadic and *SDHx*-related metastatic PPGL. However, for other inherited PHEO (*NFI, VHL, RET, MAX*) or apparently sporadic PHEO, ^{18}F-FDOPA is the preferred positron emission tomography (PET) radiopharmaceutical. Recently, copper-64-DOTATATE

Figure 2 Targeted algorithm for genetic analysis in patients with confirmed pheochromocytoma. If both normetanephrine and methoxytyramine are elevated, follow the algorithm for methoxytyramine. If both normetanephrine and metanephrine are elevated, follow the algorithm for metanephrine. *SDHAF2* pathogenic variant screening should be considered in patients who suffer exclusively from head and neck paragangliomas and who have familial antecedents, multiple tumors, or a very young age of onset and in whom *SDHB/C/D* gene pathogenic variants are negative. Only the most common genes are listed. *FMH*, Family medical history; *PHEO*, pheochromocytoma. (Adapted from Karasek D, Shah U, Frysak Z, et al: An update on the genetics of pheochromocytoma. *J Hum Hypertens* 27[3]:141–147, 2013.)

BOX 2	Considerations for Pediatric Genetic Testing

- Parent/Guardian should meet with geneticist and/or psychiatrist in the absence of the child to discuss implications for genetic testing and subsequent screening recommendations if positive.
- Parent/Guardian should be given adequate time to reflect on their consultation and develop a plan to discuss why the child is undergoing the testing and the implications of the results.
- Medical providers should work with the family to avoid testing or revealing results close to or falling on birthdays, religious holidays, or important school activities, as this may negatively impact the memory of these events.
- If possible, avoid simultaneously testing multiple siblings given the potential impact of discordant results.
- If positive, genetic counselors should emphasize the importance of "at risk" vs. "being ill" and provide all parties with the appropriate space to express their immediate reactions, ask questions, and process their emotions.

Adapted from Lahlou-Laforet K, Consoli SM, Jeunemaitre X, et al: Presymptomatic genetic testing in minors at risk of paraganglioma and pheochromocytoma: our experience of oncogenetic multidisciplinary consultation. *Horm Metab Res* 44:354–358, 2012.

BOX 3	Clinical Indications to Screen for Pheochromocytoma

- Patients with a known pheochromocytoma susceptibility pathogenic variant or a positive family history.
- Patients with triad of headaches, sweating, and tachycardia (regardless of blood pressure).
- Patients with recent onset of uncontrolled hypertension on greater than three to four standard oral therapies.
- Patients with previous history of hypertension, tachycardia, or arrhythmia following anesthesia, surgery, or ingestion of medications known to precipitate symptoms of pheochromocytoma.
- Patients with an incidental adrenal mass.

[^{64}Cu-DOTATATE] was FDA approved and has been found to be comparable to ^{68}Ga-DOTATATE in metastatic PPGL per preliminary results. Given the relatively novel status of ^{68}Ga/^{64}Cu-DOTATATE and ^{18}F-FDOPA, these modalities may not be available at a particular institution. In this case, physicians should proceed with traditional ^{18}F-FDG. The use of ^{123}I-MIBG scintigraphy should be limited to patients with known metastatic PHEO in the evaluation and eligibility for targeted radionuclide therapy with ^{131}I-MIBG.

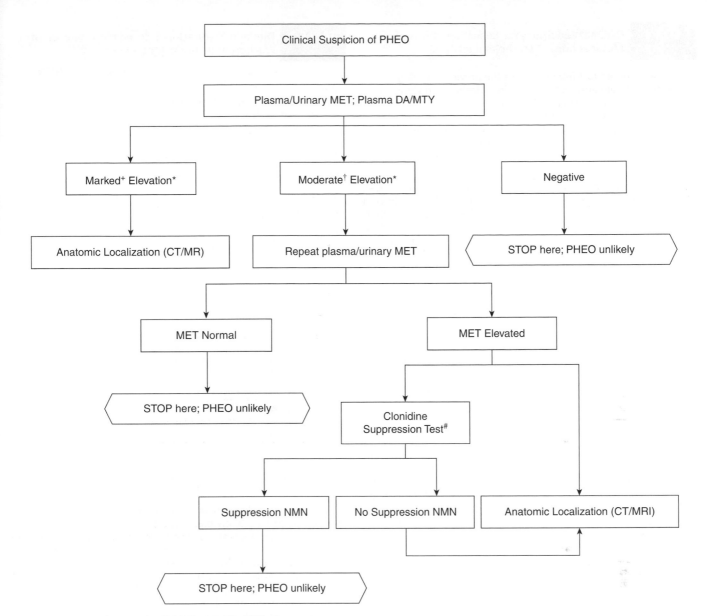

+Marked: greater than 2x the URL of normal
†Moderate; less than 2x the URL of normal
*First rule out any drug-related false elevation of MET/MTY (see Table 2) or renal failure
#If suspicion for PHEO is low or interfering drugs cannot be held
CT: computed tomography; DA: dopamine; MET: metanephrines; MR: magnetic resonance;
MTY: methoxytyramine; NMN: normetanephrine.

Figure 3 Algorithm for biochemical diagnosis of pheochromocytoma. *CT*, Computed tomography; *DA*, dopamine; *MET*, metanephrines; *MR*, magnetic resonance; *MTY*, methoxytyramine; *NMN*, normetanephrine.

Treatment

The preferred, localized treatment for PHEO is surgical resection. Even in patients with metastatic disease or where complete excision is not feasible, debulking procedures are favorable to reduce hormonal secretion and prevent anatomic complications. To ensure patient safety throughout the perioperative period, a multidisciplinary team should include a medical internist/endocrinologist, anesthesiologist, and surgeon, preferably in an experienced center (see "Perioperative Management" for details). For metastatic, systemic treatment options, see "Metastatic Pheochromocytoma."

Preoperative Medical Preparation

Surgical resection bears high perioperative risks and complications, which can be mitigated with an appropriate α- and β-adrenoceptor blockade. Over the past decade, multiple case series have called into question the necessity of such medical management. However, the United States Endocrine Society Clinical Practices guideline recommend an α-adrenoceptor blockade to ensure the protection of patients, secondary to prolonged circulating catecholamines. While patients are most at risk for a catecholamine and subsequent hypertensive crisis during induction of anesthesia and direct tumor manipulation, daily psychological and physical stressors are just as likely to result in a sudden release of catecholamines. Therefore, it is imperative patients be adequately blocked even without a surgical plan.

At minimum, blood pressure should be treated preoperatively for 7–14 days barring extenuating circumstances (Figure 5). The most commonly used nonselective α-adrenoceptor blocker is phenoxybenzamine (Dibenzyline). However, this medication may be expensive, poorly covered by insurance, and is associated with nasal congestion, fatigue, and ejaculatory dysfunction—which may be rate limiting for patients. Selective α1-adrenoceptor

- Patient should fast from midnight the previous evening
- Patient should abstain from nicotine, alcohol, and vigorous exercise for 12 hours prior to collection
- Establish intravenous access
- Patient should lie supine in quiet, dark room without distraction for 15–20 min prior to collection

TABLE 2 | Diet and Medication-Induced* Interference of Fractionated Plasma Metanephrines

	MN	NMN
Diet		
Tomatoes, beans, coffee, cheese, wine, fermented foods	↑	↑
Medications		
TCA	-	↑↑
SNRI#	-	↑↑
MAOi##	↑↑	↑
Phenoxybenzamine	-	↑
Sympathomimetics+	-	↑↑
Labetalol	-	↑
Cocaine	-	↑↑
β-Adrenoceptor Blocker	-	↑
Methyldopa/Carbidopa	-	↑
Buspirone	↑↑	↑↑

*All increases are relative and depend on drug dose, duration of treatment, and quantity of food.
‡Drug interference is not seen with mass spectrometry-based assays. Elevated NE is related to contamination during high-performance liquid chromatography.
#Reported cases of SSRIs potentially leading to elevated norepinephrine level.
##Also elevated MN and MTY.
+Pseudoephedrine, nicotine, amphetamines.
↑Moderate elevation.
↑↑Marked elevation.
MAOi, Monoamine oxidase inhibitor; *MN,* metanephrine; *NE,* norepinephrine; *NMN,* normetanephrine; *SSRI,* selective serotonin reuptake inhibitor; *SNRI,* serotonin norepinephrine reuptake inhibitor; *TCA,* tricyclic antidepressants.

blockers include doxazosin (Cardura), prazosin (Minipress), and terazosin (Hytrin). Selective adrenoceptor blockers have a shorter duration of action and are more likely to result in first-dose orthostatic hypotension, while the long-acting phenoxybenzamine is associated with postoperative hypotension. In low-risk, normotensive patients, calcium channel blockers and metyrosine (Demser) can be utilized if available within the institution.

If tachycardia ensues, cardioselective β1-adrenoceptor blockers, such as atenolol (Tenormin) or metoprolol (Lopressor), can be initiated 2 to 3 days after α-adrenoceptor administration. β-Adrenoceptor blockers *cannot* be given prior to initiation of an α-adrenoceptor blocker as unopposed antagonism can result in severe hypertensive crisis. In patients with persistent tachyarrhythmia, cardioselective calcium channel blockers diltiazem (Cardizem) or verapamil (Isoptin), ivabradine (Corlanor) can be used; however, it is not approved by the FDA for this indication.

Perioperative Management

As stated previously, an appropriate preoperative blockade is a necessity to ensure 24 hours of systolic blood pressure less than 140 mm Hg prior to surgery. Orthostatic hypotension is tolerated, but not below 80/45 mm Hg. Immediately prior to surgical intervention patients should receive 1 to 1.5 L of intravenous crystalloid. Operative approach should be decided on an individual basis by the surgeon. When appropriate and feasible, small, nonmetastatic PHEOs and retroperitoneal PGLs should be surgically excised with a minimally invasive technique. Locoregional invasion is difficult to assess preoperatively; therefore, suspected cases should initially be explored by laparoscopy with conversion to an open procedure in the face of critical adhesions. In non-*SDHB*-related bilateral PHEOs, an adrenocortical sparing procedure is recommended to avoid permanent glucocorticoid deficiency.

Intraoperatively, direct communication between the surgeon and anesthesiologist—particularly during tumor manipulation and excision—is imperative to minimize hemodynamic fluctuations secondary to massive catecholamine release or pharmacotherapy. Careful and continued monitoring of postoperative hemodynamic stability is crucial. Common complications include hypertension, hypotension, arrhythmias, adrenocortical insufficiency, and hypoglycemia. Within the immediate (first 24 hours) postoperative period, transient hypertension is likely attributable to pain, volume overload, or autonomic instability, which should be treated symptomatically. However, persistent hypertension should be concerning for incomplete tumor resection, metastatic disease, excess fluid administration, or underlying essential hypertension. Recommended first-line management is with short-acting, easily titratable agents, such as nicardipine (Cardene) or labetalol (Trandate). Attempts to repeat plasma/urinary metanephrine levels to assess for residual disease burden should be delayed for five to seven days following surgery to ensure resolution of operative catecholamine spikes. In a postoperative hypotensive (SBP <90 mm Hg) patient, hemorrhage should be excluded before deliberating a differential. Alternative etiologies include prolonged adrenoceptor blockade action, abrupt cessation of serum catecholamines, chronically low circulating plasma volume, or blood loss. The primary treatment modality is fluid resuscitation or blood transfusion, if needed. Vasopressors should be used sparingly, especially when metyrosine or long-acting β-adrenoceptor blockers were used preoperatively.

Postoperative tachyarrhythmias (>100 beats/min) may be a reflex response in patients with postoperative hypotension or the result of continued catecholamine release, while bradyarrhythmias (<60 beats/min) are due to a variety of concerns. For persistent abnormal rhythms, expert evaluation is recommended. If adrenal insufficiency is expected postoperatively, patients should receive 50 to 100 mg hydrocortisone (Cortef) prior to induction, followed by 25 to 50 mg every 8 hours thereafter. Barring any postoperative complications, transition to an oral steroid regimen 24 to 48 hours after surgery (glucocorticoid and mineralocorticoid) and provide appropriate education on adrenal crisis, emergency bracelets, and dosage adjustments in times of sickness. In the absence of catecholamine excess, upregulated liver glycogenolysis and inhibition of insulin secretion may cease, leading to postoperative hypoglycemia. Importantly, the classic signs and symptoms may be masked in the immediate postoperative period and should be routinely monitored for the first 24 hours following surgery.

Hypertensive Crisis

The most dangerous PHEO-related complication, a hypertensive crisis, can manifest with a severe headache, visual disturbances, myocardial infarction, congestive heart failure, or a cerebrovascular accident. Immediate treatment with repetitive 5-mg intravenous boluses of phentolamine (Regitine)—a short-acting, reversible, nonselective α-adrenoceptor agonist—should be repeated every 2 minutes until hypertension is adequately controlled (or initiate a continuous infusion). If unavailable, continuous infusions of sodium nitroprusside (Nitropress), labetalol (Trandate), or nicardipine (Cardene) are alternative options, with appropriate dose de-escalation upon the resolution of hypertension and subsequent symptoms related to the crisis.

Metastatic Pheochromocytoma

According to the 2022 WHO report, metastatic PHEO is only established by the presence of chromaffin cells where they are

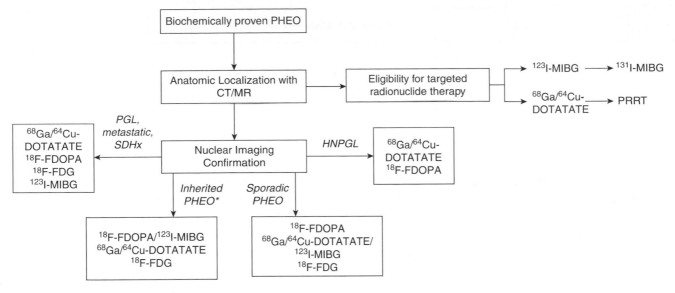

*Non-*SDHx* related

Figure 4 Imaging algorithm for pheochromocytoma localization. (Adopted from Taieb D, Hicks RJ, Hindie E, et al.: European Association of Nuclear Medicine Practice Guidelines/Society of Nuclear Medicine and Molecular Imaging Procedure Standard 2019 for Radionuclide Imaging of Pheochromocytoma and Paraganglioma. *Eur J Nucl Med Mol Imaging* 46:2112–2137, 2019; and Taieb D, Jha A, Treglia G, et al: Molecular imaging and radionuclide therapy of pheochromocytoma and paraganglioma in the era of genomic characterization of disease subgroups. *Endocr Relat Cancer.* 26:R627–R6, 2019.)

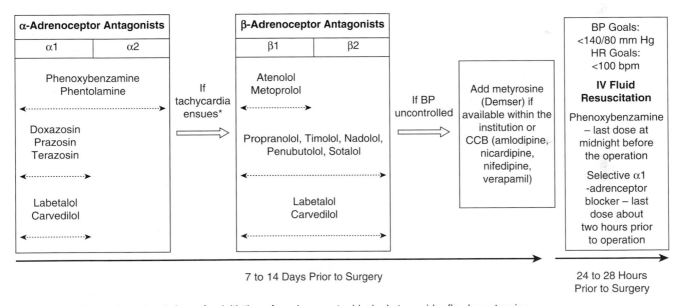

*Must be given at least 2 to 3 days after initiation of α-adrenoceptor blockade to avoid reflex hypertension

Figure 5 Preferred preoperative treatment regimen for pheochromocytoma. (Adapted from Wolf KI, Santos JRU, Pacak K: Why take the risk? We only live once: The dangers associated with neglecting a preoperative alpha adrenoceptor blockade in pheochromocytoma patients. *Endocr Pract.* 25:106–108, 2019.)

normally absent. PHEO metastasizes via a hematogenous or lymphatic route with the bones and lymph nodes considered the only definitive sites of metastasis. While the lungs and liver are also common sites of metastasis, they may also be sites of primary tumor development. Recent data suggest that almost half of patients with metastatic PHEO present within 1 year of initial diagnosis, while greater than 70% of patients will develop metastatic disease within 5 years of their primary diagnosis. At the time of primary tumor resection, over 75% of metastatic PHEO patients have a tumor larger than 5 centimeters (cm), with one study reporting a median tumor diameter of 7.0 cm. From a genetic perspective, around half of all patients with metastatic disease do not express a germline pathogenic variant and are apparently sporadic; however, of the remaining 50%, anywhere from 10% to 42% have been

associated with *SDHB*-related disease. Biochemically, markedly elevated norepinephrine and/or dopamine/methoxytyramine are associated with the presence of metastases, especially in patients with *SDHx*-related disease, and can be utilized to monitor disease progression. Current publications indicate that the 5-year overall survival ranges from 62% to 85%, while the median overall survival varied between 6 and 24 years. Location and type of tumor also indicate a higher likelihood of malignancy, with extra-adrenal PGLs the most worrisome for metastatic disease. Meanwhile, head and neck PGLs were associated with improved prognosis and very rarely reported cases of rapidly progressive disease.

Management of metastatic PPGL (Figure 6) requires a multidisciplinary approach, consisting of targeted pharmacology, radiotherapy, chemotherapy, and surgery. Surgical debulking

Figure 6 Treatment algorithm for metastatic pheochromocytoma/paraganglioma. (Adapted from Nolting S, Ullrich M, Pietzsch J, et al: Current management of pheochromocytoma/paraganglioma: A guide for the practicing clinician in the era of precision medicine. *Cancers* 11:1505, 2019).

procedures continue to be the mainstay of palliative treatment. Delaying any procedures is positively correlated with rapidly progressive metastatic disease and should be avoided whenever possible. Chemotherapy with cyclophosphamide (Cytoxan)[1], vincristine (Oncovin)[1], and dacarbazine (DTIC-Dome)[1], CVD, is the primary therapeutic modality in patients with rapidly progressive (within 3 to 6 months) PHEO. While only 30% of the metastatic PHEO population exhibits clinical benefit, the reported advantages in *SDHB*-related disease is as high as 80%. Temozolomide (TMZ [Temodar])[1] is the only other chemotherapeutic agent with significant experience in PHEO patients. Emerging targeted therapies include adjunctive olaparib (Lynparza)[1] in combination with TMZ, belzutifan (Welireg)[1] in patients with a causative *HIF2A* pathogenic variant tyrosine kinase inhibitors (sunitinib [Sutent][1] or cabozantinib [Cabometyx][1]), and various immunotherapies (including chimeric antigen receptor expressing T cells or CAR-T-cell therapy).

For patients with slow to moderate progression, eligibility for targeted radiolabeled therapy should be considered with ^{131}I-MIBG and peptide receptor radionuclide therapy (PRRT) if they have avid disease on ^{123}I-MIBG and ^{68}Ga/^{64}Cu-DOTATATE, respectively. Targeted radiotherapy with high-specific activity ^{131}I-MIBG (Azedra) is the only FDA-approved treatment for metastatic or inoperable PPGL. In 68 PPGL patients receiving targeted radiotherapy with high-specific activity ^{131}I-MIBG (up to two cycles), 23% had a partial response (PR) and 69% had stable disease (SD) totaling 92% SD and PR as evaluated by the Response Evaluation Criteria in Solid Tumors (RECIST) 1.0. Furthermore, a reduction in baseline antihypertensive medication (lasting 6 months or longer) was achieved in 25% of patients, with 68% of patients showing a complete response (CR) or PR in serum chromogranin levels. The median overall survival (OS) achieved was 36.7 months from the first treatment. In the event Azedra is unavailable, low-specific activity ^{131}I-MIBG may be considered. PRRT with lutetium-177/yttrium-90[1]-DOTATATE/DOTATOC has been used to treat patients with metastatic or inoperable PPGL. In a meta-analysis of 179 pooled patients treated with 1 to 11 cycles of PRRT using various dose regimens and radiopharmaceuticals, 90% of patients had achieved PR or SD. However, currently, lutetium-177 DOTATATE (^{177}Lu-DOTATATE, Lutathera) is not approved by the FDA for metastatic PHEO in the United States; however, the recent National Comprehensive Cancer Network guidelines recommend ^{177}Lu-DOTATATE

---

[1] Not FDA approved for this indication.

along with high-specific activity ^{131}I-MIBG for the treatment of metastatic PPGL, and a clinical trial (NCT03206060) with ^{177}Lu-DOTATATE is currently ongoing.

There are several up-and-coming novel therapeutic agents that will hopefully be approved for treatment of metastatic PPGL after further validation, including HIF-2α, mTOR, and P13K inhibitors, as well as cold somatostatin analogs (octreotide[1] and lanreotide[1]) and immunotherapy.

Prognosis and Monitoring

The long-term survival of patients after surgical excision of a solitary PHEO without evidence of metastsis is the same as age-adjusted normal subjects. A longitudinal follow-up study determined that recurrences are more likely in patients with extra-adrenal PGLs and those with germline pathogenic variant. Following treatment, 25% of patients continue to have well-controlled hypertension on oral medications. Periodic, lifelong biochemical and/or imaging surveillance is required for all patients, but especially for those with an underlying hereditary disorder. Frequency of follow-up depends on the surgical pathology, presentation at diagnosis, and biochemical profile. Patients with metastatic disease should have routine, scheduled observation with a specialist to ensure proper care.

---

[1] Not FDA approved for this indication.

References

Amar L, Pacak K, Steichen O, et al: International consensus on initial screening and follow-up of asymptomatic SDHx mutation carriers, *Nat Rev Endocrinol* 17:435–444, 2021.

Berends AMA, Buitenwerf E, de Krijger RR, et al: Incidence of pheochromocytoma and sympathetic paraganglioma in the Netherlands: a nationwide study and systematic review, *Eur J Intern Med* 51:68–73, 2018.

Bjorklund P, Pacak K, Crona J: Precision medicine in pheochromocytoma and paraganglioma: current and future concepts, *J Intern Med* 280:559–573, 2016.

Carrasquillo JA, Chen CC, Jha A, et al: Imaging of pheochromocytoma and paraganglioma, *J Nucl Med* 62:1033–1042, 2021.

Carrasquillo JA, Chen CC, Jha A, et al: Systemic radiopharmaceutical therapy of pheochromocytoma and paraganglioma, *J Nucl Med* 62:1192–1199, 2021.

Crona J, Taieb D, Pacak K: New perspectives on pheochromocytoma and paraganglioma: toward a molecular classification, *Endocr Rev* 38:489–515, 2017.

Crona J, Lamarca A, Ghosal S, et al: Genotype-phenotype correlations in pheochromocytoma and paraganglioma: a systematic review and individual patient meta-analysis, *Endocr Related Cancer* 26(5):539–550, 2019.

Darr R, Kuhn M, Bode C, et al: Accuracy of recommended sampling and assay methods for the determination of plasma-free and urinary fractionated metanephrines in the diagnosis of pheochromocytoma and paraganglioma: a systematic review, *Endocrine* 56:495–503, 2017.

Dmitriev PM, Wang H, Rosenblum JS, et al: Vascular changes in the retina and choroid of patients with epas1 gain-of-function mutation syndrome, *JAMA Opthalmol*, 138:148–155, 2020.

Eisenhofer G, Goldstein DS, Walther MM, et al: Biochemical diagnosis of pheochromocytoma: how to distinguish true from false-positive test results, *J Clin Endocrinol Metab* 88:2656–2666, 2003.

Eisenhofer G, Lenders JW, Siegert G, et al: Plasma methoxytyramine: a novel biomarker of metastatic pheochromocytoma and paraganglioma in relation to established risk factors of tumour size, location and SDHB mutation status, *Eur J Cancer* 48:1739–1749, 2012.

Else T, Marvin ML, Everett JN, et al: The clinical phenotype of SDHC-associated hereditary paraganglioma syndrome (PGL3), *J Clin Endocrinol Metab* 99:E1482–E1486, 2014.

Geroula A, Deutschbein T, Langton K, et al: Pheochromocytoma and paraganglioma: clinical feature-based disease probability in relation to catecholamine biochemistry and reason for disease suspicion, *Eur J Endocrinol* 181:409–420, 2019.

Gupta G, Pacak K: Precision medicine: an update on genotype/biochemical phenotype relationships in pheochromocytoma/paraganglioma patients, *Endoc Pract* 23:690–704, 2017.

Hadrava Vanova K, Pang Y, et al: Germline SUCLG2 variants in patients with pheochromocytoma and paraganglioma, *J Natl Cancer Inst* 11;114:130–138, 2022.

Hamidi O, Young Jr WR, Iniguez-Ariza NM, et al: Malignant pheochromocytoma and paraganglioma: 272 patients over 55 years, *J Clin Endocrinol Metab* 102:3296–3305, 2017.

Hescot S, Curras-Freixas M, Deutschbein T, et al: Prognosis of malignant pheochromocytoma and paraganglioma (MAPP-Prono Study): a european network for the study of adrenal tumors retrospective study, *J Clin Endocrinol Metab* 104(6):2367–2374, 2019.

Ilanchezhian M, Jha A, Pacak K, et al: Emerging treatments for advanced/metastatic pheochromocytoma and paraganglioma, *Curr Treat Options Oncol* 21(11):85, 2020.

Jha A, Patel M, Carrasquillo JA, et al: Choice is good at times: the emergence of [64Cu]Cu-DOTATATE-based somatostatin receptor imaging in the era of [68Ga]Ga-DOTATATE, *J Nucl Med* 63:1300–1301, 2022.

Jha A, Patel M, Carrasquillo JA, et al: Sporadic primary pheochromocytoma: a prospective intraindividual comparison on six imaging tests (CT, MRI, and PET/CT Using 68Ga-DOTATATE, 18F-FDG, 18F-FDOPA, and 18F-FDA), *AJR Am J Roentgenol* 218:342–350, 2022.

Jha A, Taieb D, Carrasquillo JA, et al: High-specific-activity 131I-MIBG vs 177Lu-DOTATATE therapy: an evolving conundrum in targeted radionuclide therapy of metastatic pheochromocytoma and paraganglioma, *Clin Cancer Res* 27:2989–2995, 2021.

Jha A, de Luna K, Balili Ca, et al: Clinical, diagnostic, and treatment characteristics of SDHA-related metastatic pheochromocytoma and paraganglioma, *Front Oncol* 22(9):53, 2019.

Jochmanova I, Pacak K: Genomic landscape of pheochromocytoma and paraganglioma, *Trends Cancer* 4:6–9, 2018.

Jochmanova I, Wolf KI, King KS, et al: SDHB-related pheochromocytoma and paraganglioma penetrance and genotype-phenotype correlations, *J Cancer Res Clin Oncol* 143(8):1421–1435, 2017.

Kunst HP, Rutten MH, de Mönnink JP, et al: SDHAF2 (PGL2-SDH5) and hereditary head and neck paraganglioma, *Clin Cancer Res* 17:247–254, 2011.

Karasek D, Shah U, Frysak Z, et al: An update on the genetics of pheochromocytoma, *J Hum Hypertens* 27:141–147, 2012. 2013.

Lahlou-Laforet K, Consoli SM, Jeunemaitre X, et al: Presymptomatic genetic testing in minors at risk of paraganglioma and pheochromocytoma: our experience of oncogenetic multidisciplinary consultation, *Horm Metab Res* 44:354–358, 2012.

Lang F, Jha A, Meuter L, et al: Identification of isocitrate dehydrogenase 2 (IDH2) mutation in carotid body paraganglioma, *Front Endocrinol (Lausanne)* 20:731096, 2021.

Lenders JW, Duh QY, Eisenhofer G, et al: Pheochromocytoma and paraganglioma: an endocrine society clinical practice guideline, *J Clin Endocrinol Metab* 99:1915–1942, 2014.

Lenders JW, Eisenhofer G, Mannelli M, Pacak K: Phaeochromocytoma, *Lancet* 366(9486):665–675, 2005.

Mamilla D, Araque KA, Brofferio A, et al: Postoperative management in patients with pheochromocytoma and paraganglioma, *Cancers* 11, 2019.

Muth A, Crona J, Gimm O, et al: Genetic testing and surveillance guidelines in hereditary pheochromocytoma and paraganglioma, *J Intern Med* 285:187–204, 2019.

Nazari MA, Rosenblum JS, Haigney MC, et al: Pathophysiology and acute management of tachyarrhythmias in pheochromocytoma: JACC review topic of the week, *J Am Coll Cardiol* 28;76:451–464, 2020.

Neumann HP, Bausch B, McWhinney SR, et al: Germ-line mutations in nonsyndromic pheochromocytoma, *N Engl J Med* 346:1459–1466, 2002.

Nolting S, Ullrich M, Pierzsch J, et al: Current management of pheochromocytoma/paraganglioma: a guide for the practicing clinician in the era of precision medicine, *Cancers* 11:1505, 2019.

Nölting S, Bechmann N, Taïeb D, et al: Personalized management of pheochromocytoma and paraganglioma, *Endocr Rev*, 43:199–239, 2022.

Pang Y, Liu Y, Pacak K, Yang C: Pheochromocytomas and paragangliomas: from genetic diversity to targeted therapies, *Cancers (Basel)*, 28;11:436, 2019.

Pacak K: New biology of pheochromocytoma and paraganglioma, *Endocr Pract* 28:1253–1269, 2022.

Pacak K: Preoperative management of the pheochromocytoma patient, *J Clin Endocrinol Metab* 92:4069–4079, 2007.

Pacak K, Eisenhofer G, Carrasquillo JA, et al: Diagnostic localization of pheochromocytoma: the coming of age of positron emission tomography, *Ann N Y Acad Sci* 970:170–176, 2002.

Pamporaki C, Prodanov T, Meuter L, et al: Determinants of disease-specific survival in patients with and without metastatic pheochromocytoma and paraganglioma, *Eur J Cancer* 169:32–41, 2022.

Patel M, Jha A, Ling A, et al: Performances of modalities in succinate dehydrogenase A- related metastatic pheochromocytoma and paraganglioma, *Cancers (Basel)* 14:3886, 2022.

Rao D, Peitzsch M, Prejibisz A, et al: Plasma methoxytyramine: clinical utility with metanephrines for diagnosis of pheochromocytoma and paraganglioma, *Eur J Endocrinol* 177:103–113, 2017.

Taieb D, Hicks RJ, Hindie E, et al: European association of nuclear medicine practice guideline/society of nuclear medicine and molecular imaging procedure standard 2019 for radionuclide imaging of pheochromocytoma and paraganglioma, *Eur J Nucl Mol Imaging* 46:2112–2137, 2019.

Taieb D, Jha A, Treglia G, Pacak K: Molecular imaging and radionuclide therapy of pheochromocytoma and paraganglioma in the era of genomic characterization of disease subgroups, *Endocr Related Cancer* 26:R627–R652, 2019.

Tella S, Jha A, Taieb D, et al. A Comprehensive Review of Evaluation and Management of Cardiac Paragangliomas. *Heart* 106:1202–1210, 2020.

Toledo RA, Qin Y, Cheng ZM, et al: Recurrent mutations of chromatin-remodeling genes and kinase receptors in pheochromocytomas and paragangliomas, *Clin Cancer Res* 22:2301–2310, 2016.

van Hulsteijn LT, Dekkers OM, Hes FL, et al: Risk of malignant paraganglioma in SDHB-mutation and SDHD-mutation carriers: a systematic review and meta-analysis, *J Med Genet* 49:768–776, 2012.

Wang K, Crona J, Beuschlein F, et al: Targeted therapies in pheochromocytoma and paraganglioma, *J Clin Endocrinol Metab* 107:2963–2972, 2022.

Wolf KI, Santos JRU, Pacak K: Why take the risk? We only live once: the dangers associated with neglecting a pre-operative alpha adrenoceptor blockade in pheochromocytoma patients, *Endocr Pract* 25:106–108, 2019.

THYROID CANCER

Method of

Michael Holyoak, DO; Teresa Sciortino, MD; and Rudruidee Karnchanasorn, MD

CURRENT DIAGNOSIS

- Most thyroid cancer will present as incidentally discovered thyroid nodules.
- The vast majority of thyroid nodules are benign, and risk of malignancy can be reliably estimated based on sonographic features.
- Thyroid function should always be assessed if a nodule is discovered. If thyroid stimulating hormone is low, a thyroid uptake and scan should be obtained.
- The American Thyroid Association and the American College of Radiology's Thyroid Imaging Reporting and Data System uses ultrasound features to determine risk of malignancy and the need for fine needle aspiration (FNA).
- Approximately 90% to 95% of thyroid nodules are benign and can be monitored with serial ultrasound. FNA is only indicated for nodules equal to or greater than 1 cm.
- Benign nodules can be monitored with ultrasound at intervals based on their risk of malignancy.
- The vast majority of thyroid cancer is classified as differentiated thyroid cancer. Medullary thyroid cancer is less common and somewhat more aggressive. Anaplastic thyroid cancer is a rare and very aggressive thyroid cancer that typically presents at a more advanced stage.

CURRENT THERAPY

- Although thyroid cancer is relatively common, it is responsible for a very small portion of cancer-related mortality.
- Some experts have expressed concern about potentially unnecessary morbidity associated with overtreatment of very low risk differentiated thyroid cancers (DTCs), particularly micropapillary carcinoma.
- Most patients with thyroid cancer should be managed surgically. Smaller, lower risk differentiated cancers can be treated with lobectomy. Larger or higher-risk tumors should be treated with total thyroidectomy and compartment neck dissections based on the presence of lymphadenopathy.
- Radioactive iodine should be used based on the American Thyroid Association (ATA) risk stratification.
- Patients with DTC should be monitored longitudinally using serum thyroglobulin levels and serial ultrasound.
- Thyroid stimulating hormone suppression is indicated for many patients postoperatively, initially based on their ATA risk and later on their response to therapy.
- Patients with medullary thyroid cancer should undergo surgery and be monitored with serial carcinoembryonic antigen and calcitonin levels in addition to imaging studies.
- Patients with anaplastic thyroid cancer typically require aggressive surgery, often including tracheostomy and management by a multidisciplinary team.

Epidemiology

Thyroid nodules are highly prevalent. Data show that approximately 5% to 10% of patients will have palpable nodules, and approximately 34% of patients will have nodules detectable by ultrasound. The prevalence of nodules increases significantly with age, and they are three to four times more common in women. Only a small portion of thyroid nodules (about 5% to 15%) are malignant. From the early 1980s to mid-2010s, the incidence of thyroid cancer rapidly increased before reaching a plateau and subsequent decline beginning in the late 2010s. Despite the near tripling of new diagnoses during this time period, thyroid cancer mortality has remained relatively low, as the upward trend in diagnosis has been primarily driven by small, early-stage differentiated papillary thyroid carcinomas (PTCs). Many of these indolent, slow-growing cancers would otherwise have gone undetected without advances in ultrasonography and other detection modalities. In one study involving patients with low-risk differentiated thyroid cancers (DTCs) who were monitored without surgery, only 10% were found to have disease progression at a median follow-up interval of 6 years. Clinical guidelines have been modified with the increased understanding of the potential harms of overdiagnosis and treatment, resulting in a leveling off and decreased rate of newly diagnosed cases in more recent years.

Risk Factors

The majority of thyroid cancer cannot be attributed to specific risk factors. Nutritional factors including iodine intake have been associated with an increased risk of thyroid nodularity. Childhood exposure to ionizing radiation is one particularly well-documented risk factor for thyroid cancer. In a large retrospective study, individuals treated with radiation for Hodgkin disease were 27 times more likely to have thyroid nodules than those treated without radiation. Family history is an important risk factor, with one study showing a 10-fold increased risk in first-degree relatives of patients with thyroid cancer. An elevated thyroid stimulating hormone (TSH) level in the setting of thyroid nodularity has been associated with an increased risk of thyroid cancer. Cigarette smoking has been negatively correlated with risk of thyroid cancer.

Pathophysiology

Thyroid cancer may arise from two major parenchymal cell types: thyroid follicular cells giving rise to DTC and parafollicular, or C-, cells giving rise to medullary thyroid cancer (MTC). DTCs are responsible for more than 95% of cases of thyroid cancer (Table 1). DTC includes PTC, follicular thyroid carcinoma (FTC), and the follicular variants, including Hurthle cell cancer. Another related variant of thyroid tumor termed noninvasive follicular thyroid neoplasm with papillary-like nuclear features (NIFTP) has an exceptionally low recurrence rate of less than 1% at 15 years. NIFTP is best described as a benign tumor and does not require completion thyroidectomy or radioactive iodine (RAI). PTC metastasizes via the lymphatic system, typically to cervical lymph nodes. FTC and its variants classically spread hematogenously, which contributes to a less favorable prognosis. The *BRAF* mutation is the most frequently encountered mutation in non-MTC and is present in 50% to 70% of patients with PTC. *TERT* mutations are frequently present in high-risk forms of PTC. Mutations in the *RAS* family of oncogenes are also commonly present in FTC.

Poorly differentiated thyroid carcinomas are high-risk cancers that classically spread hematogenously to lung and bone. These cancers are also derived from follicular cells.

MTC originates from parafollicular or calcitonin-producing C cells. Mutations of the *RET* protooncogene are thought to be responsible for the majority of cases. *RET* mutations are classically inherited in an autosomal dominant pattern; however, they can occur sporadically. All patients diagnosed with MTC should be screened for *RET* mutations. If such testing is positive, first-degree relatives should be screened as well. Specific *RET* mutations result in specific phenotypes with varying risks of MTC. Knowledge of the specific *RET* mutation guides the need and timing of prophylactic thyroidectomy; this is of particular importance in the pediatric setting. MTC is part of the classic presentation of patients with multiple endocrine neoplasia type 2 (MEN 2), which also includes a risk of pheochromocytoma and parathyroid adenomas.

Anaplastic thyroid cancer (ATC) is an uncommon (<1%) but aggressive form of cancer. Despite its rarity, ATC is responsible for as much as 50% of thyroid cancer–related mortality. Patients

TABLE 1	Overview of Thyroid Tumor Subtypes				
SUBTYPE	**ORIGIN CELL TYPE**	**% OF THYROID CANCER**	**5-YEAR SURVIVAL**	**COMMON MUTATIONS**	
PTC	Follicular	~80%	~99%	*BRAF, TKR*	
FTC	Follicular	~15%	~98%	*RAS, PAX8-PPARG*	
NIFTP	Follicular	0.4%–2.6%	N/A	*RAS*	
PDTC	Follicular	~1%	~62%	*RAS, P53*	
MTC	Parafollicular/C-cell	~3%	~90%	*RET*	
ATC	Follicular	~1%	~7%	*BRAF, TERT, P53*	

ATC, Anaplastic thyroid cancer; *MTC,* medullary thyroid cancer; *NIFTP,* neoplasm with papillary-like nuclear features; *PDTC,* poorly differentiated thyroid carcinomas.

usually present with advanced disease, commonly with symptoms of hoarseness or dysphasia due to local invasion. Approximately 50% of ATCs arise from a known DTC, with the hypothesis of dedifferentiation changes from preexisting DTC to aggressive ATC.

Clinical Manifestations

Most patients with thyroid cancer, particularly with DTCs, present asymptomatically with incidentally discovered thyroid nodularity on imaging. More aggressive forms of thyroid cancer, including poorly differentiated cancers and ATC, can present with symptoms related to regional invasion, including dysphasia, hoarseness-related recurrent laryngeal nerve injury, and tracheal compression.

Diagnosis

All patients suspected of having thyroid nodules should undergo ultrasound and measurement of their serum TSH levels. A TSH below normal should prompt a scintigraphic evaluation with thyroid uptake and scan to assess for functioning or "hot" nodules. Fine needle aspiration (FNA) is not generally indicated for hyperfunctioning nodules because of a low likelihood of malignancy. Thyroid scintigraphy is not needed when serum TSH is normal or elevated. Serum calcitonin measurement used as a screening test for MTC remains controversial because of its low specificity.

Ultrasound is a critical step in evaluating thyroid nodules. It is not only safe and cost-effective but also reliably determines risk of malignancy and therefore need for FNA. Suspicious sonographic features of nodules associated with increased risk of malignancy include hypoechogenicity (darker than normal thyroid parenchyma), microcalcifications, irregular margins, taller than wide shape, and evidence of extrathyroidal extension. Ultrasound of the central and lateral neck compartments is critical to screen for suspicious lymphadenopathy, which can influence the surgical approach. The American Thyroid Association (ATA) recommends FNA using a risk stratification system based on size and sonographic patterns. FNA is recommended for nodules equal to or greater than 1 cm with intermediate (10% to 20% malignancy risk) or high suspicion patterns (>70% to 90% risk), 1.5 cm for low suspicion (5% to 10% risk), and 2 cm for very low suspicion (<3%). Purely cystic nodules are benign and do not need FNA.

The Thyroid Imaging Reporting and Data System (TIRADS) is another validated clinical tool produced by the American College of Radiology (ACR). It uses a points system based on sonographic features to stratify nodules into one of five TIRADS categories: TR1, benign; TR2, not suspicious; TR3, mildly suspicious; TR4, moderately suspicious; and TR5, highly suspicious, with malignancy risks of 0.3%, 1.5%, 4.8%, 9.1%, and 35%, respectively. TR1 and TR2 nodules do not require FNA. FNA is indicated for TR3 nodules starting at 2.5 cm, TR4 at 1.5 cm, and TR5 at 1 cm. Nodules less than 1 cm are too small for FNA based on both the ATA and ACR-TIRADS owing to the slow-growing nature of micropapillary thyroid cancer. In general, the ACR-TIRADS is more selective than the 2015 ATA guidelines in regard to a decision to pursue FNA. Other considerations governing the need for FNA include specific risk factors of thyroid cancer or syndromes associated with thyroid cancer, such as MEN, Cowden syndrome, familial adenomatous polyposis, and Carney complex. In addition, fluorodeoxyglucose-avid nodules are associated with a malignancy rate of about 35%. However, the recommended FNA size of these nodules remains at least 1 cm or greater.

The 2017 Bethesda system has been the standard method of cytology diagnosis of thyroid nodules, consisting of six categories. Category I, nondiagnostic or unsatisfactory, represents a 5% to 10% malignancy risk; in such cases repeat FNA is required unless the lesion is mostly cystic or ultrasound features of very low suspicion. Category II, benign, represents approximately 70% of specimens and a less than 3% risk of malignancy. Both category III, atypia of undetermined significance/follicular lesion of undetermined significance (AUS/FLUS), and category IV, follicular neoplasm or suspicious for follicular neoplasm (FN/SFN), are associated with a slightly higher malignancy risk: 10% to 30% in AUS/FLUS and 25% to 40% in FN/SFN. The management of both categories III and IV is not straightforward, and various molecular assessments can be used to help with decision making. Currently available molecular tests—including the Afirma GSC, RNA seq panel, and ThyroSeq3 112-gene panel—have high sensitivity and specificity, functioning as rule-out and rule-in tests to decrease the number of unnecessary thyroid surgeries. Category V (suspicious for malignancy [SFN]) and category VI (malignant) carry high rates of malignancy (60% to 75% and 97% to 99%, respectively) and should prompt referral for operative management.

Nodules that do not meet the initial threshold for cytologic assessment require continued sonographic surveillance, the recommended interval of which ranges from 6 to 24 months based on sonographic features. FNA should be performed if there is a 50% increase in the tumor volume or 20% increase in nodule diameter (with a minimum increase in two or more dimensions of at least 2 mm) or once nodules reach the threshold size. A nodule with two negative biopsies should be considered benign.

Therapy

Papillary thyroid microcarcinoma (PTMC) is defined as a small PTC equal to or less than 10 mm in size. PTMCs generally grow very slowly and carry an excellent prognosis. Although many individuals are asymptomatic and do not require treatment, an increased rate of detection has likely resulted in overtreatment. It has been shown that PTMCs in young patients are more likely to progress more than those in elderly patients. Active surveillance for most PTMCs has been shown to be safe, and FNA is not recommended for thyroid nodules smaller than 1 cm. Active surveillance should not be considered in the presence of high-risk features such as nodal metastasis or distant metastasis, vocal cord paralysis due to invasion of the recurrent laryngeal nerve, high-grade malignancy on cytology, or in the case of PTMCs attached to the trachea or located along the path of the recurrent laryngeal nerve. Ultrasound-guided percutaneous ethanol ablation (UPEA) by experienced specialists has been shown to be a safe and well-tolerated definitive minimally invasive alternative for PTMC patients who do not wish to have surgery and are uncomfortable with active surveillance, although UPEA is currently available at only a limited number of centers.

Treatment of thyroid cancer is mainly based on individualized risk stratification, accounting for mortality based on TNM (tumor, node, and metastases) staging, the risk of disease recurrence, and the persistence of structural disease.

Although DTC carries a very low risk of mortality compared with other cancers, the TNM staging system remains an accurate predictor of mortality. Recent changes to the system recommend that patients younger than 55 years of age at the time of diagnosis receive only stage I (no distant metastases) or stage II (distant metastases present) classification. Ten-year disease-specific survival rates for stages I to IV were 99.5%, 94.7%, 94.1%, and 67.6%, respectively.

In addition to TNM staging, an individualized risk stratification outlined by the ATA 2015 guidelines is an important milestone for the assessment of risk of thyroid cancer recurrence and persistence of structural disease. The ATA system uses variables such as histology, extent of the first surgery, and postoperative thyroglobulin (Tg) to guide initial postoperative therapy and treatment in follow-up. Patients with tumor sizes less than 4 cm without clinical lymph node metastases or micrometastases measuring less than 2 mm in five or fewer lymph nodes can be classified as ATA low risk. Intermediate-risk disease is defined as DTC with minimal extrathyroidal extension or aggressive histology. High-risk disease includes patients with gross extension, distant metastases, any lymph node metastases greater than 3 cm, as well as FTC with greater than four foci of vascular invasion. In contrast, minimally invasive FTC is considered low risk.

The ATA recommends either total thyroidectomy or lobectomy for low-risk patients with DTC. The decision to proceed with total thyroidectomy or lobectomy primarily depends on tumor size and patient preference. Low-risk patients are not routinely treated with RAI.

Use of RAI after total thyroidectomy is based on individualized risk stratification accounting for extent of tumor, histology type, age, and presence of distant metastases. Radioiodine is typically delayed several months after surgery to allow for complete recovery and assessment of the biochemical response with Tg. Serum Tg reaches its nadir approximately 4 to 6 weeks postoperatively, and measurement at this point is perhaps the most accurate method of appraising the quality of surgery and probability of cure.

RAI remnant ablation uses a low dose of radioiodine-131 (131-I), around 30 mCi, to destroy any residual thyroid tissue postoperatively. Remnant ablation thus facilitates the interpretation of subsequent serum Tg levels and follow-up RAI whole-body scans to detect any residual or recurrence disease or metastatic foci. Remnant ablation is not routinely recommended in ATA low-risk DTC patients.

Adjuvant treatment uses a higher dose of 131-I (75 to 150 mCi) postoperatively to destroy microscopic thyroid cancer and/or suspected residual disease to potentially decrease recurrence and mortality. RAI adjuvant treatment should be considered in ATA intermediate-risk DTC patients.

Primary treatment with RAI uses 100 to 200 mCi of 131-I to destroy known locoregional and/or distant metastasis with a goal of cure, reduced recurrence and mortality, and/or palliation among high-risk DTC patients.

Serum TSH should be elevated before proceeding with RAI, as TSH potentiates RAI uptake by iodine-avid tissues including normal thyroid tissue and most thyroid cancers. This has historically been accomplished by withdrawing thyroid hormone replacement for approximately 2 weeks until TSH increases to 30 or more. During this time patients should be instructed to consume a low-iodine diet. The use of recombinant human TSH, thyrotropin alfa (Thyrogen), is also a safe and effective alternative to thyroid hormone withdrawal in the detection of recurrent/residual thyroid cancer and facilitation of RAI ablation.

TSH suppression therapy (TST) requires supraphysiologic doses of exogenous thyroid hormone, with the goal of lowering serum TSH. TSH has trophic effects on thyroid tissue, and a subnormal serum TSH may minimize tumor growth and reduce the risk of progression of advanced thyroid cancer. Aggressive TST is not recommended for low-risk patients but may improve survival outcome for those at high risk. Serum TSH levels that were consistently maintained in the subnormal to normal ranges have led to better outcomes in patients at all stages of disease compared with subjects whose serum TSH levels were in the normal to elevated ranges.

Localized treatments with external beam radiation are sometimes needed for gross residual disease or bone metastases. Surgery may be necessary when bone metastases threaten a limb's function.

Systemic treatments for advanced DTC and MTC include tyrosine kinase inhibitors (TKIs). These agents are reserved for patients with progressive or unresectable disease or tumor that is threatening vital structures. TKI-associated adverse effects are common and include hypertension, hand-foot skin reactions, diarrhea, rash, fatigue, and weight loss. The dose of TKI often needs to be titrated based on tolerability.

Most patients with MTC have advanced disease at the time of diagnosis, leading to an unfavorable prognosis. Cure is much more probable if all disease is intrathyroidal at the time of diagnosis. Early identification and complete surgical resection are ideal for the definite treatment of MTC. Calcitonin is a specific serum marker, and its doubling time is the most important prognostic factor for survival and disease progression. Serum carcinoembryonic antigen (CEA) is usually elevated in advanced cases and is often used as a tumor marker in conjunction with calcitonin. The risk of recurrence is low when postoperative calcitonin is undetectable. Patients with low but detectable calcitonin level less than 150 pg/mL likely have persistent or recurrent disease confined to neck lymph nodes and can be followed every 6 to 12 months with physical examination, neck ultrasound, and serial measurement of calcitonin and CEA. If postoperative calcitonin is greater than 150 pg or has a rapid doubling time, additional imaging studies are required to evaluate for distant metastases. If there is concern for disease progression, systemic therapy with vandetanib (Caprelsa) or cabozantinib (Cometriq) should be considered. Before starting this, the possibility of using a local treatment should be evaluated to delay systemic therapy, along with a multidisciplinary team approach.

Patients with ATC usually present with a rapidly enlarging neck mass that can cause compressive neck symptoms and invasion of the adjacent recurrent laryngeal nerve, leading to dysphonia, or compression of the trachea, causing airway obstruction. Ultrasound remains the primary imaging study for ATC, but additional studies, including computed tomography (CT) with contrast of neck, abdomen, and pelvis; positron emission tomography CT, if available; and brain magnetic resonance imaging, can be used. Because of the risk of acute airway compromise, an expeditious diagnosis and management plan by a multidisciplinary team is crucial. Ideally a care team would include a pathologist, head and neck surgeon, medical oncologist, radiation oncologist, and endocrinologist. A palliative care physician should also be involved, given ATC's extremely poor prognosis. Patients with ATC and their families should take part in an in-depth discussion about the natural history of the disease, goals of treatment, treatment toxicities, and expected outcomes. Most untreated patients will die of asphyxiation; therefore, treatment addressing the primary neck disease, even with a goal of only palliation, is a priority. Hospice care could be the best option for patients who do not wish to pursue aggressive therapy. Tracheostomy to prevent airway obstruction as a part of palliative care is controversial but may be appropriate for patients with impending airway compromise. In contrast, patients with limited disease should initially be treated with surgery followed by chemoradiotherapy (intensity-modulated radiotherapy plus taxane-based chemotherapy) as a standard of care when feasible, unless hospice is alternatively elected. Patients with widely metastatic or stage IVC disease should instead be treated with palliative systemic therapy or best supportive care.

Recent studies have indicated improvements in overall survival in early multimodality therapy, especially with recent advancements in systemic therapy including targeted and immunotherapies such as the *BRAF* inhibitor dabrafenib (Tafinlar) and the *MEK* inhibitor trametinib (Mekinist), anti-PD1 monoclonal antibody spartalizumab,[5,8] and newer agents such as the peroxisome proliferator-activated receptor-γ agonist efatutazone,[5] and mammalian target of rapamycin inhibitors, which seem to provide a more efficacious treatment in advanced ATC.

Monitoring

Regardless of the initial risk assessment, patients with DTC should be monitored longitudinally and classified as having either an excellent, indeterminate, or incomplete response, both biochemically and structurally, to therapy. Initial monitoring includes serial neck ultrasounds, TSH, and serum Tg and Tg antibody levels at intervals determined by initial risk assessment. An excellent response (1% to 4% recurrence rate) is defined as no clinical, biochemical, or structural evidence of disease. Serum Tg should be less than 0.2 ng/mL with a suppressed TSH, or less than 1 ng/mL if TSH is stimulated. Patients with an indeterminate response (15% to 20% recurrence rate) will have nonspecific biochemical or structural findings. A biochemical incomplete response (20% recurrence rate) reflects abnormally elevated Tg or Tg antibody levels (serum Tg > 1 ng/mL basal or > 10 ng/mL if TSH is stimulated or increasing Tg antibodies) in the absence of disease. A structural incomplete response (50% to 85% recurrence rate) includes persistent or newly identified locoregional or distant metastasis with or without abnormal Tg or Tg antibodies.

Management of Complications

Immediate surgical complications after thyroidectomy are correlated with low-volume surgeons. High-volume surgeons are also associated with an increased risk of postoperative complications; however, this is likely attributable to overall greater case complexity. Potential complications include injury of the recurrent laryngeal nerve leading to temporary or permanent hoarseness, airway difficulty due to bilateral vocal cord paralysis, and need for tracheostomy. Total thyroidectomy can lead to transient or permanent hypoparathyroidism with resultant hypocalcemia. Adequate preoperative vitamin D replacement can help maintain normocalcemia. Postoperatively the parathyroid hormone (PTH) level should be checked; calcitriol (Rocaltrol) may be needed in addition to calcium supplementation if the PTH level is low or undetectable. Serial calcium levels should be obtained after discharge.

Long-term TST can result in adverse outcomes such as osteoporosis, fracture, and cardiovascular disease, including atrial fibrillation. In general, daily levothyroxine (Levoxyl, Synthroid) doses of 1.6 to 1.8 µg/kg are the initial treatment after thyroidectomy, whereas doses of 2.0 to 2.2 µg/kg are needed to suppress the serum TSH. The dosage requirements of individual patients are highly variable and depend on multiple factors, including body mass index, the concomitant use of other medications, and patient adherence. The ATA recommends maintaining serum TSH levels between 0.5 and 2 mU/L in low-risk and intermediate-risk patients with an excellent response to treatment. Mild TSH suppression (TSH 0.1 to 0.5 mU/L) should be used for high-risk patients who have had an excellent response (negative imaging and undetectable suppressed Tg). Mild TSH suppression is also recommended in patients with a biochemically incomplete response. More significant TSH suppression (i.e., serum TSH <0.1) is recommended in patients with residual structural disease or a biochemically incomplete response if they are young or at low risk for complications from iatrogenic hyperthyroidism.

Adverse effects of RAI—including radiation thyroiditis, sialadenitis, and tumor hemorrhage or edema—occur in 10% to 30% of patients. The possibility of adverse effects is dose dependent. Long-term risk of secondary malignancies has been reported; however, the risk is considerably lower when the total dose is less than 100 mCi. Immediately after patients have been treated with RAI, an appropriate isolation protocol is required to protect household members, especially women who are pregnant and infants, from radiation exposure. The required duration of isolation is predominantly based on RAI dose and rate of clearance.

Conclusion

Thyroid nodules are very common and are often discovered incidentally. The vast majority of nodules, approximately 90% to 95%, are benign. Thyroid sonography should be obtained for all nodules, as this reliably predicts the risk of malignancy and need for FNA. DTCs are indolent; FNA is not indicated for nodules less than 1 cm in size. Thyroid function should be assessed before proceeding with FNA. Patients with a TSH below normal should undergo thyroid uptake and scan to investigate for an autonomously functioning nodule or nodules. Most nodules can be monitored with ultrasound alone. Guidelines produced by either the ATA or ACR can reliably determine the need for FNA. PTC is the most common type of DTC and typically has a very favorable prognosis. Lower-risk patients with DTC can be managed with lobectomy. Patients with larger tumors (>4 cm), extrathyroidal extension, or higher-risk cytology should be treated with total thyroidectomy and central neck dissection. Lateral compartment neck dissections should be completed if there is FNA-positive disease.

Low-risk patients with DTC do not need treatment with RAI, whereas intermediate- and high-risk cases should receive RAI. All patients should be monitored longitudinally after initial therapy, both radiographically and biochemically, using serum Tg. The ATA categorizes patient response as excellent, indeterminate, or incomplete. Patients should receive appropriate levels of TSH suppression, initially based on their ATA risk and subsequently on their response to therapy. TSH suppression poses multiple risks if continued long-term.

MTC should be considered of higher risk than DTC and is managed surgically. MTC is often detected later and is usually more advanced than DTC. Calcitonin and CEA levels can be monitored longitudinally. Calcitonin doubling time is a particularly important prognostic factor for following these patients.

ATC is a rare but extraordinarily aggressive and rapidly growing form of thyroid cancer. Patients should be managed by a multidisciplinary team with consideration for tracheostomy because of the risk of asphyxiation in the setting of rapid tumor growth. Aggressive resection and prompt chemotherapy are suitable treatment options in appropriately selected patients with less advanced disease.

References

Biondi B, Cooper DS: Thyroid hormone suppression therapy, *Endocrinol Metab Clin North Am* 48(1):227–237, 2019. https://doi.org/10.1016/j.ecl.2018.10.008.

Brito JP, Hay ID: Management of papillary thyroid microcarcinoma, *Endocrinol Metab Clin North Am* 48(1):199–213, 2019. https://doi.org/10.1016/j.ecl.2018.10.006.

Cabanillas ME, Mcfadden DG, Durante C: Thyroid cancer, *The Lancet* 388(10061):2783–2795, 2016. Print.

Chintakuntlawar AV, Foote RL, Kasperbauer JL, Bible KC: Diagnosis and management of anaplastic thyroid cancer, *Endocrinol Metab Clin North Am* 48(1):269–284, 2019. https://doi.org/10.1016/j.ecl.2018.10.010.

Cho A, Chang Y, Ahn J, Shin H, Ryu S: Cigarette smoking and thyroid cancer risk: a cohort study, *Br J Cancer* 119(5):638–645, 2018. https://doi.org/10.1038/s41416-018-0224-5.

Du L, Wang Y, Sun X, et al: Thyroid cancer: trends in incidence, mortality and clinical-pathological patterns in Zhejiang Province, Southeast China, *BMC Cancer* 18(1):291, 2018. https://doi.org/10.1186/s12885-018-4081-7.

Haugen BR, Alexander EK, Bible KC, et al: 2015 American Thyroid Association management guidelines for adult patients with thyroid nodules and differentiated thyroid cancer: the American Thyroid Association guidelines task force on thyroid nodules and differentiated thyroid cancer, *Thyroid* 26(1):1–133, 2016. https://doi.org/10.1089/thy.2015.0020.

---

[5] Investigational drug in the United States.

[8] Orphan drug in the United States.

Maxwell C, Sipos JA: Clinical diagnostic evaluation of thyroid nodules, *Endocrinol Metab Clin North Am* 48(1):61–84, 2019.

Mayson SE, Haugen BR: Molecular diagnostic evaluation of thyroid nodules, *Endocrinol Metab Clin North Am* 48(1):85–97, 2019. https://doi.org/10.1016/j.ecl.2018.10.004.

Miyauchi A, Ito Y: Conservative surveillance management of low-risk papillary thyroid microcarcinoma, *Endocrinol Metab Clin North Am* 48(1):215–226, 2019. https://doi.org/10.1016/j.ecl.2018.10.007.

Nikiforov YE, et al: Nomenclature revision for encapsulated follicular variant of papillary thyroid carcinoma: a paradigm shift to reduce overtreatment of indolent tumors, *JAMA Oncol* 2(8):10–1029, 2016.

Pal T, Vogl FD, Chappuis PO, et al: Increased risk for nonmedullary thyroid cancer in the first degree relatives of prevalent cases of nonmedullary thyroid cancer: a hospital-based study, *J Clin Endocrinol Metab* 86(11):5307–5312, 2001.

Powers AE, Marcadis AR, Lee M, Morris LG, Marti JL: Changes in trends in thyroid cancer incidence in the United States, 1992 to 2016, *JAMA* 322(24):2440–2441, 2019.

Viola D, Elisei R: Management of medullary thyroid cancer, *Endocrinol Metab Clin North Am* 48(1):285–301, 2019. https://doi.org/10.1016/j.ecl.2018.11.006.

Xing M: Genetic-guided risk assessment and management of thyroid cancer, *Endocrinol Metab Clin North Am* 48(1):109–124, 2019. https://doi.org/10.1016/j.ecl.2018.11.007.

THYROIDITIS

Method of
Leigh M. Eck, MD

CURRENT DIAGNOSIS

- Thyroiditis is a term used to describe a diverse group of disorders associated with thyroid inflammation.
- Thyroiditis can be associated with a euthyroid state, thyrotoxicosis, or hypothyroidism.
- The clinical presentation of thyroiditis will direct the evaluation with useful testing to include measurement of thyroid hormone levels, thyroid antibody testing, white blood cell count, erythrocyte sedimentation rate, thyroid scintigraphy, and thyroid ultrasound.

CURRENT THERAPY

- Abnormalities of thyroid hormone levels resulting from thyroiditis may be transient and require no or only short-term therapy.
- If symptomatic thyrotoxicosis is present, beta-blocker therapy should be initiated.
- Thyroiditis associated with persistent hypothyroidism is managed with synthetic thyroxine (T4, Levoxyl, Synthroid).
- Thyroid pain associated with subacute thyroiditis is managed with a nonsteroidal antiinflammatory drug or, if ineffective, glucocorticoid therapy.
- Acute suppurative thyroiditis requires immediate parenteral antibiotic therapy as well as surgical drainage, if indicated.

Thyroiditis is a term used to describe a diverse group of disorders characterized by inflammation of the thyroid gland (Table 1). Presentation of thyroiditis is variable depending on the etiology. The most common thyroid disorder in the United States, Hashimoto's thyroiditis, most often presents with hypothyroidism. Other forms of thyroiditis may present with thyrotoxicosis because of inflammation in the thyroid gland resulting in the release of stored hormone. Painful thyroiditis is seen with subacute, suppurative and radiation-induced thyroiditis, while other variants are most often painless.

Epidemiology

The most common cause of hypothyroidism in iodine-sufficient areas of the world is *Hashimoto's thyroiditis,* also known as *chronic autoimmune thyroiditis.* Elevated serum antithyroid

TABLE 1	Causes of Thyroiditis

Autoimmune thyroiditis: Hashimoto's thyroiditis, postpartum thyroiditis, silent thyroiditis

Subacute thyroiditis, also known as de Quervain's thyroiditis or subacute granulomatous thyroiditis

Suppurative thyroiditis, also known as infectious thyroiditis or pyrogenic thyroiditis

Riedel's thyroiditis, also known as fibrous thyroiditis

Therapy induced thyroiditis: amiodarone (Cordarone), interferon-alpha, interleukin-2, lithium, tyrosine kinase inhibitors, radioactive iodine, checkpoint inhibitor immunotherapy

peroxidase antibody concentrations are found in ~ 5% of adults and ~ 15% of older women; overt hypothyroidism is seen in up to 2% of the population. A variant of chronic autoimmune thyroiditis, *postpartum thyroiditis,* is a destructive thyroiditis induced by an autoimmune mechanism that occurs within 1 year of parturition. Postpartum thyroiditis occurs in up to 10% of women in the United States. *Silent thyroiditis* is indistinguishable from postpartum thyroiditis, with the exception of lack of temporal relationship to pregnancy. Silent thyroiditis may account for about 1% of all cases of thyrotoxicosis. Many medications are associated with an alteration in thyroid function testing; however, only a few are known to provoke an autoimmune or destructive inflammatory thyroiditis, including amiodarone (Cordarone), lithium, interferon alfa, interleukin-2, tyrosine kinase inhibitors, and checkpoint inhibitor immunotherapy. *Riedel's thyroiditis* is a progressive fibrosis of the thyroid gland with a prevalence of only 0.05% among patients with thyroid disease requiring surgery. *Subacute thyroiditis* is the most common cause of thyroid pain. It occurs in up to 5% of patients with clinical thyroid disease. *Suppurative thyroiditis,* most commonly caused by bacterial infection, is rare because of the thyroid gland's encapsulation, high iodine content, rich blood supply, and extensive lymphatic drainage. *Radiation-induced thyroiditis* occurs in approximately 1% of patients who receive radioactive iodine therapy for hyperthyroidism.

Risk Factors

Hashimoto's thyroiditis is more common in women, particularly older women. Hashimoto's thyroiditis is associated with several gene polymorphisms, suggesting a role for genetic susceptibility. Subacute thyroiditis frequently follows an upper respiratory tract infection, with its incidence highest in summer. Suppurative thyroiditis is most likely to occur in patients with preexisting thyroid disease, those with congenital anomalies such as pyriform sinus fistula, and those who are immunosuppressed.

Pathophysiology

Hashimoto's thyroiditis, postpartum thyroiditis, and silent thyroiditis all have an autoimmune basis. The antithyroid immune response begins with activation of thyroid antigen-specific helper T cells. Once helper T cells are activated, they induce B cells to secrete thyroid antibodies; thyroid antibodies most frequently measured are those directed against thyroid peroxidase and against thyroglobulin. The mechanism for autoimmune destruction of the thyroid likely involves both cellular immunity and humoral immunity. Riedel's thyroiditis is the local involvement of the thyroid in a systemic disease, multifocal fibrosclerosis; the etiology of Riedel's thyroiditis is not known. Although a viral cause of subacute thyroiditis has been proposed, clear evidence for this proposed etiology is lacking. Suppurative thyroiditis is most often associated with a bacterial pathogen; however, fungal, mycobacterial, or parasitic infections may also be the cause. Although rare, radiation-induced thyroiditis may occur following the treatment of hyperthyroidism with radioactive iodine because of radiation-induced injury and necrosis of thyroid follicular cells and associated inflammation.

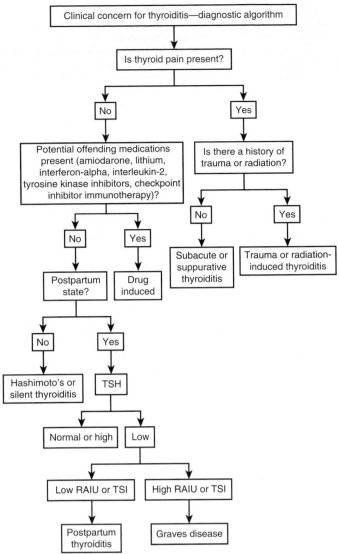

Figure 1 Clinical concern for thyroiditis—diagnostic algorithm. *Abbreviations:* RAIU = radioactive iodine uptake; TSI = thyroid-stimulating immunoglobulins.

Clinical Manifestations

A symmetrical, painless goiter is frequently the initial finding in Hashimoto's thyroiditis. The usual course of Hashimoto's thyroiditis is gradual loss of thyroid function. Among patients with this disorder who have subclinical hypothyroidism, overt hypothyroidism occurs at a rate of about 5% per year. The classic presentation of postpartum thyroiditis occurs in only approximately 30% of afflicted women, with the characteristic sequence of hyperthyroidism, followed by hypothyroidism, and then recovery. Persistent hypothyroidism is seen in up to 30% of women following an episode of postpartum thyroiditis. Silent thyroiditis is marked by a similar characteristic sequence of thyroid hormone dysfunction. However, it is not temporally associated with pregnancy; 20% will have residual hypothyroidism. *Medication-induced thyroiditis* is variable in its presentation. Amiodarone (Cordarone), rich in iodine, is associated with hypothyroidism and hyperthyroidism; type 2 amiodarone-induced thyrotoxicosis is due to a destructive thyroiditis process. Lithium is more commonly associated with hypothyroidism. Interferon-alfa and interleukin-2 can cause both permanent and transient hypothyroidism likely related to the ability of these substances to induce or exacerbate thyroid autoimmune disease. Riedel's thyroiditis presents with neck discomfort or tightness, dysphagia, hoarseness, and a diffuse goiter that is hard, fixed, and often not clearly separable from the adjacent tissues. Generally, patients are euthyroid, and their antithyroid antibody concentrations are often high. Subacute thyroiditis manifests with a prodrome of myalgias, pharyngitis, low-grade fever, and fatigue with subsequent fever and neck pain, and up to 50% of patients have symptoms of thyrotoxicosis. Patients with suppurative thyroiditis are usually acutely ill with fever, dysphagia, dysphonia, anterior neck pain with erythema, and a tender thyroid mass. Radiation-induced thyroiditis presents 5 to 10 days following radioactive iodine treatment with neck pain and tenderness. In addition, there can be a transient exacerbation of hyperthyroidism.

Diagnosis and Differential Diagnosis

The diagnostic approach to suspected thyroiditis can be focused based on an association with thyroid pain and circulating thyroid hormone status (Figure 1). Hashimoto's thyroiditis is diagnosed when a goiter is found on examination with a subsequently noted elevation of thyroid antibodies or when subclinical or overt hypothyroidism is detected with associated elevated thyroid antibodies. Screening for postpartum thyroiditis with a measurement of TSH and free thyroxine should be undertaken in women presenting with symptoms of thyroid dysfunction in the postpartum period. If hyperthyroidism is present, thyroid scintigraphy (if not contraindicated, e.g., breastfeeding) or measurement of thyroid-stimulating immunoglobulins is helpful in the differentiation of postpartum thyroiditis from Graves' disease. The diagnostic approach to silent thyroiditis is similar. The laboratory hallmark of subacute thyroiditis is a markedly elevated erythrocyte sedimentation rate; the leukocyte count is normal or slightly elevated. Thyrotoxicosis may be present; if so, thyroid scintigraphy will reveal a low iodine uptake state. Thyroid antibody testing is typically normal. Thyroid ultrasound reveals a hypoechogenic gland with low to normal vascularity. Suppurative thyroiditis is typically associated with normal thyroid function. Leukocyte counts and erythrocyte sedimentation rates are elevated. Fine-needle aspiration with Gram stain and culture is the diagnostic test of choice. Radiation-induced thyroiditis should be considered if a temporal relationship to radioactive iodine treatment is present. If there is an exacerbation of hyperthyroidism immediately following radiation treatment for the same, consideration of radiation-induced thyroiditis due to the release of preformed thyroid hormone associated with destruction of follicular cells should be considered as an etiology of thyrotoxicosis in addition to the underlying disease process.

Treatment

Once overt hypothyroidism is present in the patient with Hashimoto's thyroiditis, treatment with synthetic L-thyroxine (Levoxyl, Synthroid) therapy is indicated. The average replacement dose of thyroxine in adults is approximately 1.6 mcg/kg body weight per day. Adjustment of dosage is undertaken every 6 weeks until a euthyroid status is achieved. The majority of women with postpartum thyroiditis will not need treatment during either the hyperthyroid or hypothyroid phase. If symptomatic hyperthyroidism is present, beta-blocker therapy can be used; antithyroid medications have no utility in the management of postpartum thyroiditis. Women with symptomatic hypothyroidism should be treated with synthetic thyroxine therapy; in asymptomatic women, initiation of thyroxine therapy should be considered if TSH is >10 mU/L. Management of silent thyroiditis is the same as that for postpartum thyroiditis. Symptoms associated with Riedel's thyroiditis may be relieved with prednisone; a small case series associated improvement and even resolution of the process with tamoxifen (Nolvadex)[1] therapy. Surgery is indicated in Riedel's thyroiditis if compressive symptoms are present. The goal of therapy in subacute thyroiditis is to provide symptom relief. Nonsteroidal antiinflammatory medications

are often adequate to control pain; if insufficient, glucocorticoid therapy should be initiated. Beta-blockade therapy can ameliorate symptoms of thyrotoxicosis if indicated. Suppurative thyroiditis is managed with appropriate antibiotics and drainage of any abscess; the disease may prove fatal if diagnosis and treatment are delayed. Pain associated with radiation-induced thyroiditis can be managed with nonsteroidal antiinflammatory therapy or, if ineffective, a short course of glucocorticoid therapy. Radiation-induced thyroiditis is a self-limited process and will resolve spontaneously within days to weeks.

Monitoring

In the patient with Hashimoto's thyroiditis with a euthyroid state, routine TSH testing should be undertaken given the risk of development of overt hypothyroidism at 5% per year. Any woman who has had postpartum thyroiditis should be monitored very closely for thyroid dysfunction with future pregnancies, as reoccurrence is likely. For women who have fully recovered from postpartum thyroiditis, yearly TSH measurements should be considered because of underlying chronic autoimmune thyroiditis and risk for overt hypothyroidism. Although overall recurrence rates for silent thyroiditis have not been well established, a similar monitoring plan is warranted for this variant of chronic autoimmune thyroiditis. Subacute thyroiditis recurs in only about 2% of patients. Routine monitoring following resolution of process has not been defined.

References

Bogazzi F, Bartalena L, Martino E: Approach to the patient with amiodarone-induced thyrotoxicosis, *J Clin Endocrinol Metab* 95:2529–2535, 2010.

Cooper DS, Ladenson PW: The thyroid gland. 2011. In Gardner DG, Shoback D, editors: *Greenspan's Basic & Clinical Endocrinology*, 9th ed., New York, 2011, McGraw-Hill, Available at. http://accessmedicine.mhmedical.com/content.aspx?bookid¼4380&Sectionid¼39744047. Accessed 23 January 2014.

De Groot L, Abalovich M, Alexander ED, et al: Management of thyroid dysfunction during pregnancy and postpartum: an Endocrine Society clinical practice guideline, *J Clin Endocrinol Metab* 97:2543–2565, 2012.

Pearce EN, Farwell AP, Braverman LE: Thyroiditis, *N Engl J Med* 348:2646–2655, 2003.

Samuels MH: Subacute, silent and postpartum thyroiditis, *Med Clin North Am* 96:223–233, 2012.

---

[1]Not FDA approved for this indication.

Hematology

ACUTE LEUKEMIA IN ADULTS

Method of
Colin Vale, MD; and Anthony Hunter, MD

CURRENT DIAGNOSIS

- Diagnosis of acute leukemia is made based on the presence of myeloid (acute myeloid leukemia [AML]) or lymphoid (T- or B-cell acute lymphoblastic leukemia [ALL]) blasts in blood and/or bone marrow. Acute leukemia may uncommonly have an ambiguous lineage or mixed phenotype.
- Medical history taking should identify risk factors such as prior exposure to chemotherapy for other malignancies (or nonmalignant disorders), antecedent hematologic disorders, familial hematologic disorders, or other inherited genetic disorders (e.g., Down syndrome).
- Clinical examination should identify extramedullary sites of involvement such as meninges/central nervous system (CNS), active infection, hemorrhage, or disseminated intravascular coagulation.
- AML requires the presence of at least 20% blasts in blood or marrow except in selected subsets of disease with specific cytogenetic or molecular aberrations. These include the chromosomal abnormalities t(8;21)(q22;q22), inv(16)(p13q22) or t(16;16)(p13;q22), and t(15;17)(q22;q12), which are associated with more favorable clinical outcomes. Testing for cytogenetic and molecular aberrations is critical for diagnosis, prognosis, and therapy.
- Acute promyelocytic leukemia (APL) is defined by the *PML-RARA* gene fusion, which can be detected by genetic methods or cytogenetics showing t(15;17). APL is a unique entity requiring different therapy and has a favorable prognosis.
- ALL is subcategorized based on B- or T-lymphocyte lineage; cases with less than 20% blasts constitute lymphoblastic lymphoma, which is treated similarly.
- For B-ALL (also in mixed-phenotype acute leukemia), identification of the Philadelphia chromosome, t(9;22)(q34.1;q11.2), or its *BCR-ABL1* gene fusion is essential for proper diagnosis and treatment. As with AML, testing for established chromosomal and molecular aberrations is standard.

CURRENT THERAPY

- Acute myeloid leukemia (AML) is typically treated with intensive initial therapy (induction) followed by repetitive cycles of intensive postremission therapy (consolidation). Induction chemotherapy most commonly consists of anthracycline plus cytarabine (Cytosar). Several acceptable postremission

approaches are used; often, these are repetitive high-dose cytarabine–based regimens.
- Acute promyelocytic leukemia (APL) is uniquely treated with all-*trans*retinoic acid (tretinoin [Vesanoid]) and arsenic trioxide (Trisenox), instead of chemotherapy, although cases with high presenting white blood cell counts may also require chemotherapy or the antibody-drug conjugate gemtuzumab ozogamicin (Mylotarg)[1] for cytoreduction.
- Acute lymphoblastic leukemia (ALL) is treated with multidrug regimens for induction and postremission therapies. Postremission therapies include further intensification cycles and prolonged lower-dose maintenance therapy. Central nervous system–directed therapy is a critical component of treatment, even in patients without clear involvement. Most acute leukemias of ambiguous lineage are treated with ALL-type regimens, although clinical outcomes are poor.
- The use of "pediatric-inspired" ALL regimens for adolescents and young adults has improved outcomes.
- Older patients or those with medical infirmities may require less intensive treatment regimens; because of a greater likelihood of adverse risk disease and higher toxicities, such patients fare worse than younger patients. Novel treatment approaches, such as the combination of a hypomethylating agent and venetoclax (Venclexta) in AML, have led to improved outcomes.
- Because of high relapse risk, allogeneic hematopoietic stem cell transplantation in first remission is an important consideration for all eligible patients with AML except those with favorable-risk disease. High-risk adult patients with ALL are also offered early transplantation. All patients who relapse should be considered for transplantation if remission is again achieved.
- Several subsets of acute leukemia can be treated by effective therapies that target specific aberrant signaling or enzymatic activities or that are directed to unique biologic targets of disease. Most important among these are the tyrosine kinase inhibitors (TKIs), which are used in treating acute leukemia (typically ALL) with *BCR-ABL1*.
- Advances in immunology have rapidly and dramatically improved the options for treatment, especially for those with relapsed B-ALL. Novel antibody constructs and genetically engineered autologous cellular products directed to eliminate B-lymphocytes can induce durable remissions in B-ALL.

[1]Not FDA approved for this indication.

427

Epidemiology

According to data from the National Institutes of Health and American Cancer Society, the incidence of AML in the United States is 4.1 per 100,000 per year, with an estimate of 20,380 new cases for 2023. AML accounts for about 1.0% of all new cancer cases and 33% of all new leukemia cases (but nearly one-half of leukemia deaths). AML is far more common than ALL in adults. Although AML affects all age groups, the incidence increases with advancing age, presenting at a median of 68 years of age. ALL is estimated to occur in 6540 cases in the United States for 2023 and has a bimodal distribution across ages, with a peak in early childhood and a smaller second peak around 70 years of age.

Risk Factors

Most cases of acute leukemia in adults have no established cause. Genetic predisposition, drugs, and radiation have been associated with the development of acute leukemia, particularly AML. Several rare genetic syndromes—including Down syndrome, Fanconi anemia, Bloom syndrome, Li-Fraumeni syndrome, neurofibromatosis type I, short telomere syndromes, Shwachman-Diamond syndrome, and ataxia telangiectasia—are associated with an increased risk for developing acute leukemia. AML with germline predisposition represents an uncommon but important subset of disease. Germline mutations associated with increased risk of developing a myeloid neoplasm include *CEBPA, DDX41, RUNX1, ANKRD26, ETV6,* and *GATA2.* Down syndrome–associated AML and ALL pose an increased risk of toxicity with standard chemotherapy and require dose adjustment (and expert management).

Anticancer drugs are the leading cause of therapy-associated AML. Alkylating agent–associated leukemias typically occur 4 to 6 years after exposure; affected individuals often have multilineage dysplasia and monosomy/aberrations in chromosomes 5 and 7. Topoisomerase II inhibitor–associated leukemias typically occur with shorter latency, 1 to 3 years after exposure; affected individuals often have AML with monocytic features and aberrations involving chromosome 11q23.

Pathophysiology

Acute leukemias are hematologic malignancies arising from hematopoietic progenitor (stem) cells in the bone marrow. Clonal immature cells accumulate in the blood, bone marrow, and occasionally in the extramedullary tissues. These malignant cells divide and proliferate, but they do not differentiate into functional cells. Patients with acute leukemia are immunocompromised and have impaired oxygen-carrying capacity (anemia) and bleeding diathesis (because of thrombocytopenia or disrupted coagulation).

Patients experience complications directly from the accumulation of abnormal immature blasts or indirectly from the reduction in functional hematopoietic cells in the marrow and blood. Leukemic involvement of the bone marrow typically results in cytopenias, which may affect all hematopoietic cell lineages. Patients with acute leukemias typically have evidence of circulating leukemic blasts in the peripheral blood (sometimes with high white blood cell [WBC] counts consisting entirely of blasts), or they may have pancytopenia with no circulating blasts at all. Patients typically require transfusions of red blood cells and platelets and are at risk of life-threatening infectious complications caused by neutropenia. Most patients with acute leukemia die of infection or, less frequently, hemorrhage.

Patients with morphologically similar acute leukemias may experience vastly different clinical outcomes. Increasingly, this is explained by karyotyping or genetic sequencing studies that demonstrate marked heterogeneity in the cytogenetic and gene mutational profiles among patients with acute leukemia. It is clear that morphology and cytochemical staining alone to establish diagnosis does little to explain the pathophysiology and clinical behavior of these varied hematologic cancers. Genetic sequencing studies demonstrate common dysregulation of several critical cellular pathways but also a myriad of genetic alterations that occur only in small subsets. In adults, most cases of AML ultimately arise against the backdrop of a limited number of mutations that accumulate with advancing age. As noted earlier, cases with a clear cause, such as germline predisposition or drug exposure, are rare. The Cancer Genome Atlas (https://cancergenome.nih.gov) and other databases have shown that 5% to 10% of healthy individuals older than 70 years of age have blood cells with potentially "premalignant" mutations that are associated with clonal expansion, referred to as *clonal hematopoiesis of indeterminate potential.* There appear to be a variety of "final insults" that transform these expanded clones to AML, but how these genetic aberrations contribute to leukemic transformation remains incompletely understood. Although the number of mutations per cell in AML is relatively small (median of 13 mutations) compared with other cancers (e.g., melanoma and non–small cell lung cancer may have several hundred mutations per cell), great heterogeneity exists in the mutations identified between individual patients with AML. The same can be said of ALL. Indeed, dramatic differences in mutations/genetic signatures have been observed among patients with childhood, adolescent, young adult, and older adult ALL, respectively, and contribute to dramatic differences in prognosis among these groups.

Great heterogeneity exists not just among patients with different types of acute leukemia, but within each individual patient. Each patient may have several leukemic clones and subclones with slightly different mutational profiles. The presence of genetically different clones and subclones explains why a patient may achieve remission but then experience relapse with more resistant disease. Sensitive clones are eliminated by chemotherapy, whereas surviving clones are likely to be more resistant to subsequent treatment. Furthermore, clones that persist after treatment may emerge with additional novel mutations.

Clinical Manifestations

Patients with acute leukemias often present with similar symptoms. Typically, the onset of illness is no more than 3 months before diagnosis unless the leukemia is associated with an antecedent hematologic disorder. Most have vague symptoms that are consequences of pancytopenia. Fatigue is common, as are anorexia and weight loss. Fever or infection is also common at presentation, and patients may have evidence of abnormal hemostasis (bleeding, easy bruising). Bone pain, lymphadenopathy, nonspecific cough, headache, and diaphoresis (excessive sweating) may also occur. Patients with ALL (compared with AML) are more likely to have lymphadenopathy, splenomegaly, or extramedullary involvement at other sites, such as the testicles or central nervous system (CNS). However, involvement at any of these sites is not exclusive to ALL and can also be observed in AML patients, particularly in cases with monocytic differentiation. Rarely, patients present with primary symptoms caused by extramedullary leukemia. Extramedullary disease in AML is known as a *myeloid sarcoma* (also called a *granulocytic sarcoma* or *chloroma*). This is a tumor mass consisting of myeloid blasts and is most commonly seen in the skin, lymph nodes, gastrointestinal tract, soft tissue, or testis. Patients who present with isolated myeloid sarcoma typically develop blood or marrow involvement quickly thereafter and require systemic treatment akin to that used in patients with systemic disease (not solely surgical resection or local radiation). CNS involvement at initial presentation (headache, cranial nerve palsies) is uncommon; however, patients with ALL have an increased risk of CNS disease and should thus be given intrathecal chemotherapy as prophylaxis even without such symptoms (or detectable CNS involvement).

Severe hemorrhagic complications are relatively infrequent at presentation but are most commonly encountered in acute promyelocytic leukemia (APL). Recognition of this risk at the time of initial presentation is critical, as replacement of fibrinogen or plasma may be lifesaving. Patients with APL often present with disseminated intravascular coagulation (DIC)–associated hemorrhage and may have intracranial hemorrhage or bleeding at other sites. Appropriate therapy for APL such as all-*trans*retinoic-acid (tretinoin [Vesanoid]) should be initiated upon suspicion and not withheld pending genetic confirmation of the classic *t*(15;17) rearrangement. Thrombosis is a less frequent but well-recognized feature of APL. Bleeding associated with coagulopathy may also occur in monocytic AML and with extreme degrees of leukocytosis or thrombocytopenia in other acute leukemias. Retinal hemorrhage caused by thrombocytopenia and extreme leukocytosis is detected in approximately 15% of patients.

Laboratory parameters are quite variable with any type of acute leukemia. The presenting WBC count may be elevated, normal, or low, and a minority of patients present with leukocytosis and high levels of circulating blasts, with hyperleukocytosis defined as WBC count greater than 100,000/μL. Patients with AML and hyperleukocytosis are at increased risk of developing leukostasis, which manifests with CNS and pulmonary symptoms and requires prompt recognition and management. Alternatively, many patients present with low WBC count or even with no circulating blasts. Typically, review of the peripheral blood smear identifies the classic blast—fine, lacy chromatin with one or more nucleoli and a high nucleus-to-cytoplasm ratio, which is characteristic of immature cells. The presence in blasts of abnormal rod-shaped granules called *Auer rods* on light microscopy indicates myeloid lineage.

Anemia is observed at diagnosis in nearly all patients but may not be severe. Decreased erythropoiesis often results in a reduced reticulocyte (immature red blood cell) count; red blood cell survival may be shortened by accelerated destruction. Most patients also present with thrombocytopenia (less than the normal lower limit value of 150,000/μL); severe thrombocytopenia (<10,000/μL) can be life-threatening and requires immediate platelet transfusion.

Diagnosis

When acute leukemia is clinically suspected, in addition to morphologic and flow-cytometric analyses of bone marrow and blood, cytogenetic and genetic tests are mandatory to aid rapid diagnosis, assess prognosis, and inform the best approach to treatment. Clinical features also influence prognosis and treatment selection. These include a history of antecedent hematologic disorder or prior chemotherapy, advanced age, and a strong family history of acute leukemia or related hematologic disorder (all favoring AML); each of these has an adverse prognosis. In ALL, a high WBC count at presentation (>100,000/μL for B-ALL and >30,000/μL for T-ALL) and T-cell phenotype have an adverse prognosis.

Initial assessments should evaluate cardiovascular, pulmonary, hepatic, and renal systems; patients should also be evaluated and treated for infection, tumor lysis syndrome, leukostasis, or DIC. Preparation for transfusion of blood or platelets requires blood type and crossmatch to be determined, and human leukocyte antigen (HLA) testing is required early in the treatment course (before chemotherapy) in consideration of future allogeneic hematopoietic stem cell transplantation (alloHCT). Cytogenetic analysis typically requires bone marrow. Genetic testing (from blood or marrow) continues to evolve and is critical for successful diagnosis, prognosis, and therapy. Younger patients should be counseled regarding fertility preservation at diagnosis.

The diagnosis of AML is based on a finding of at least 20% myeloid blasts by histology, cytochemistry, or flow cytometry in the blood or bone marrow. However, this 20% threshold is not required for diagnosis in cases of myeloid sarcoma or in cases of AML with defining genetic abnormalities; this includes the classic cytogenetic abnormalities *t*(15;17) (diagnostic of APL), *t*(8;21), inv(16), or *t*(16;16). The International Consensus Classification of Myeloid Neoplasms and Acute Leukemias has recently added a new MDS/AML categorization for patients with 10% to 19% blasts to reflect the biologic continuum between MDS and AML. Myeloid blasts stain positive for myeloperoxidase; by flow cytometry, myeloid blasts are typically positive for CD13 and CD33. A prognostic schema developed by the European LeukemiaNet assigns prognostic risk based on cytogenetic and genetic features of disease (Table 1). Some morphologic features are associated with specific cytogenetic or molecular findings such as atypical promyelocytes and *t*(15;17) in APL or dysplastic eosinophils and inv(16) or *t*(16;16). The expression of B-cell markers (CD19, PAX5, cytoplasmic CD79a) is not infrequent in *t*(8;21).

The diagnosis of ALL likewise requires at least 20% lymphoid blasts. Cases with primarily nodal or extranodal involvement and less than 20% blasts in the blood and marrow are classified as lymphoblastic lymphoma. By immunohistochemical methods, lymphoid blasts stain positive for terminal deoxynucleotidyl transferase; by flow cytometry, lymphoid blasts are typically positive for CD10, CD19, CD22, CD79a, and CD20 (variable) for B-ALL and CD3, CD4, CD7, and CD8 for T-ALL.

Patients may uncommonly present with acute leukemia of ambiguous lineage; this classification includes acute undifferentiated leukemias, which express no lineage-defining antigens, and mixed-phenotype acute leukemias, which express antigens defining more than one lineage. However, more common are AML cases that express an aberrant B-cell or T-cell marker (e.g., CD7 on myeloid blasts), referred to as an *aberrant immunophenotype*. Likewise, B-ALL may aberrantly express CD13 or CD33.

Molecular testing is an important component of diagnosis. For AML, molecular testing is performed by next-generation sequencing and/or polymerase chain reaction assays and should, at minimum, include assessment of *FLT3*, *NPM1*, *CEBPA*, *IDH1*, *IDH2*, *RUNX1*, *ASXL1*, *DDX41*, *BCOR*, *EZH2*, *SF3B1*, *SRSF2*, *STAG2*, *U2AF1*, *ZRSR2*, and *TP53*. For ALL, testing is equally complex but is still evolving in terms of commercial availability for important molecular analyses. Critical to the initial assessment of ALL is testing for the *BCR-ABL1* fusion by molecular methods that are widely available; tyrosine kinase inhibitors (TKIs) targeting this lesion are an integral part of treatment of ALL with

TABLE 1	2022 European LeukemiaNet Risk Classification by Genetics at Initial Diagnosis
RISK CATEGORY*	**GENETIC ABNORMALITY**
Favorable	t(8;21)(q22;q22.1)/*RUNX1::RUNX1T1**,† inv(16)(p13.1q22) or t(16;16)(p13.1;q22)/ *CBFB::MYH11**,† Mutated *NPM1**,‡ without *FLT3-ITD* bZIP in-frame mutated CEBPA§
Intermediate	Mutated *NPM1**,‡ with *FLT3-ITD* Wild-type *NPM1* with *FLT3-ITD* (without adverse-risk genetic lesions) t(9;11)(p21.3;q23.3)/*MLLT3::KMT2A**,ǁ Cytogenetic and/or molecular abnormalities not classified as favorable or adverse
Adverse	t(6;9)(p23.3;q34.1)/*DEK::NUP214* t(v;11q23.3); *KMT2A-rearranged*¶ t(9;22)(q34.1;q11.2)/*BCR::ABL1* t(8;16)(p11.2;p13.3)/*KAT6A::CREBBP* inv(3)(q21.3q26.2) or t(3;3)(q21.3;q26.2)/*GATA2, MECOM(EVI1)* t(3q26.2;v)/*MECOM(EVI1)*-rearranged −5 or del(5q); −7; −17/abn(17p)Complex karyotype,# monosomal karyotype** Mutated *ASXL1, BCOR, EZH2, RUNX1, SF3B1, SRSF2, STAG2, U2AF1*, and/or *ZRSR2*†† Mutated TP53§§

*Mainly based on results observed in intensively treated patients. Initial risk assignment may change during the treatment course based on the results from analyses of measurable residual disease.

†Concurrent *KIT* and/or *FLT3* gene mutation does not alter risk categorization.

‡AML with *NPM1* mutation and adverse-risk cytogenetic abnormalities are categorized as adverse-risk.

§Only in-frame mutations affecting the bZIP region of *CEBPA*, irrespective of whether they occur as monoallelic or biallelic mutations, have been associated with favorable outcome.

ǁThe presence of t(9;11)(p21.3;q23.3) takes precedence over rare, concurrent adverse-risk gene mutations.

¶Excluding *KMT2A* PTD.

#Complex karyotype: Three or more unrelated chromosome abnormalities in the absence of other class-defining recurring genetic abnormalities; excludes hyperdiploid karyotypes with three or more trisomies (or polysomies) without structural abnormalities.

**Monosomal karyotype: presence of two or more distinct monosomies (excluding loss of X or Y) or one single autosomal monosomy in combination with at least one structural chromosome abnormality (excluding core-binding factor AML).

††"Myelodysplasia-related gene mutations." For the time being, these markers should not be used as an adverse prognostic marker if they co-occur with favorable-risk AML subtypes.

§§*TP53* mutation at a variant allele fraction of at least 10%, irrespective of the *TP53* allelic status (mono- or biallelic mutation); *TP53* mutations are significantly associated with AML with complex and monosomal karyotype.

AML, Acute myeloid leukemia; *bZIP*, basic leucine zipper region; *PTD*, partial tandem duplication.

Modified from Döhner H, Wei A, Applebaum R, et al. Diagnosis and management of AML in adults: 2022 recommendations from an international expert panel on behalf of the ELN. *Blood*. 2022;140(12):1345-1377.

BCR-ABL1. Likewise, testing by interphase fluorescence in situ hybridization for the major recurrent cytogenetic abnormalities seen in ALL—including ETV6-RUNX1, TCF3-PBX1, and KMT2A rearrangements, among others—is mandatory. Although not yet widely available, testing in B-ALL for the "BCR-ABL1-like" genetic signature identifies a subset of patients with adverse prognosis but potential responsiveness to TKI therapies. BCR-ABL1–like disease has several common genetic features including disruption of B-lymphoid transcription factors including IKZF1, CRLF2, JAK2, and others. Diagnostic testing guidelines for both AML and ALL are delineated and annually updated by the National Comprehensive Cancer Network (https://NCCN.org).

Cytogenetic analysis should be performed on the bone marrow aspirate taken at diagnosis in any patient suspected to have acute leukemia. Prognosis is determined by molecular testing along with the presence of structural or numeric chromosomal abnormalities. Broadly speaking, patients with AML with t(15;17), known as APL as described earlier, have an excellent prognosis, with cure rates greater than 90%. Patients with t(8;21) or inv(16) also have a favorable prognosis. Patients with no cytogenetic abnormalities (cytogenetically normal AML [CN-AML]) have an intermediate prognosis (classification is further dependent on molecular testing; see later discussion), whereas patients with adverse-risk cytogenetic abnormalities (see Table 1) have a poor prognosis with few cures, particularly in older adult patients. At least 20 metaphases are necessary to define a normal karyotype. Molecular testing provides valuable additional information, especially in CN-AML. Favorable genetic risk is observed in those with NPM1 mutations without co-occurring FLT3 internal tandem duplication and also in those with CEBPA in-frame mutations affecting the basic leucine zipper region. Conversely, "myelodysplasia-related gene mutations" (Table 1) and mutations in TP53 (often but not exclusively observed in the setting of complex karyotype) are associated with adverse risk, with TP53-mutated patients demonstrating particularly dismal outcomes. Mutations in genes encoding isocitrate dehydrogenase (IDH) enzymes identify patients who are likely to respond to novel therapies that target these aberrant pathways.

Cytogenetic testing for ALL enables classification into several groups, including, for example, BCR-ABL1 fusion disease. This fusion, known cytogenetically as t(9;22) and colloquially referred to as the Philadelphia (Ph) chromosome (based on the city where it was originally identified), has historically been associated with a poor prognosis. However, the incorporation into multiagent regimens of TKIs that target the aberrantly active kinase has improved clinical outcomes. Other important ALL subsets include KMT2A (formerly MLL) rearrangements at chromosome 11q23 (with various translocation partners but often chromosome 4 in B-ALL), which are associated with an unfavorable prognosis. Many other subsets of ALL exist in the World Health Organization (WHO) classification. Favorable risk is seen in patients with B-ALL with hyperdiploidy (51 to 65 chromosomes) and t(12;21) (p13.2;q22.1), the ETV6-RUNX1 fusion. T-ALL is characterized by activating mutations in NOTCH1 (present in about 60% of cases) and deregulation of a number of transcription factors; immunophenotyping showing an early T-cell precursor phenotype (low expression of CD1a, CD8, CD5) has been associated with an adverse prognosis.

Historically, the diagnosis and classification of acute leukemia was based on the French-American-British morphologic and cytochemical criteria, which assigned patients with AML to one of eight groups designated M0 to M7. Likewise, ALL was classified into L1, L2, and L3 groups. These categories, although still in the vernacular on the clinical wards, are practically obsolete. Diagnosis and classification are based instead on the complex morphologic, flow, cytogenetic, and molecular characterization schemas outlined by the WHO Classification of Haematolymphoid Tumours.

Differential Diagnosis

The differential diagnosis for acute leukemia includes many bone marrow disorders that present with pancytopenia. However, the presence of excess blasts in the blood or marrow limits the diagnosis to AML, ALL, or acute leukemia of ambiguous lineage. For patients without circulating blasts in the blood, highest in the differential diagnosis of pancytopenia are other hematologic cancers with marrow infiltration or bone marrow failure syndromes such as aplastic anemia. Advanced myeloproliferative neoplasms with bone marrow fibrosis and myelodysplastic syndromes can also present similarly, occasionally with rare circulating blasts. Rarely, the pancytopenia caused by the displacement of hematopoietic bone marrow tissue by fibrosis, tumor, or granuloma (called myelophthisis) mimics acute leukemia. Examples include solid organ cancers with extensive marrow involvement and granulomatous disease such as tuberculosis. However, essentially only acute leukemia is the appropriate diagnosis in patients with high-level circulating blasts visualized on light microscopy.

Treatment of Acute Myeloid Leukemia

Treatment of the newly diagnosed adult patient with AML is usually divided into two phases: (1) induction and (2) consolidation (i.e., postremission management). The aim of induction chemotherapy is complete remission (CR), defined as fewer than 5% blasts on a bone marrow aspirate, with recovery of blood counts (absolute neutrophil count >1000/μL and platelet count >100,000/μL). Additional defining criteria of CR include absent circulating blasts and no detectable extramedullary disease. Achievement of CR (or failure to do so) is the best predictor of long-term clinical outcome. The definition of CR is further refined based on the detection of measurable residual disease (MRD) by flow cytometry and/or molecular testing. Marrow response without full blood count recovery meets lesser response definitions (often termed CR with incomplete count recovery); patients with such responses have outcomes inferior to those with CR. Blood count recovery occurs approximately 4 weeks after the initiation of intensive induction chemotherapy. CR is achieved in 60% to 90% of younger patients (depending on molecular risk) and in approximately 2% to 60% of older adult patients (>60 years). Notably, for older adult patients, this estimate is from the subset of patients who are actually offered intensive therapy; many older patients are not treated intensively (or at all) because of medical comorbidities or poor performance status. Long-term survival estimates are approximately 60% for younger patients with favorable-risk disease (see Table 1), 40% for intermediate-risk disease, and 20% for adverse-risk disease. Older adult patients do poorly in each group; indeed, there are very few long-term survivors among older patients with adverse-risk disease.

Induction and consolidation therapies are chosen after considering both patient and disease-specific factors, including overall fitness, comorbidities, and cytogenetic/molecular risk. Intensive induction therapy is the norm in younger patients (<60 years). In older patients, the benefit of intensive therapy is more controversial in all but those with a favorable-risk profile; novel approaches for selecting patients predicted to be responsive to treatment and new therapies remain under investigation. Notably, large data sets have demonstrated that even more infirm older patients with AML benefit from treatment compared with palliative care alone.

Standard induction therapy for AML consists of cytarabine (cytosine arabinoside [AraC, Cytosar]), 100 to 200 mg/m^2/day administered as a continuous infusion for 7 days, and daunorubicin (Cerubidine), 60 to 90 mg/m^2/day for 3 days, commonly known as the 7 + 3 schedule. Idarubicin (Idamycin; 12 mg/m^2/day) is equivalent to daunorubicin. Resistant disease is more frequent in older adult patients and those with prior hematologic disorders, therapy-related AML, or adverse-risk cytogenetic and molecular abnormalities (which are more frequent in older patients). In older adult patients, the long-term outcome is generally poor because of the higher frequency of resistant disease in this group plus an increased rate of treatment-related mortality. As an alternative to intensive induction, unfit or adverse-risk older patients may instead receive lower-intensity therapy with a hypomethylating agent (such as decitabine [Dacogen][1] or azacitidine [Vidaza][1]). For patients older than 75 years of age or those who are not candidates for intensive therapy, the Bcl-2 inhibitor venetoclax (Venclexta) has been approved in combination with hypomethylating agent therapy. A randomized trial demonstrated improved survival and higher remission rates with azacitidine in combination with venetoclax compared with azacitidine alone, and this combination is now considered standard of care in this patient population. All older adult patients should be considered for clinical trials, but those in adverse-risk groups should ideally be offered investigational approaches whenever available.

Induction of first complete remission (CR1) is critical to long-term survival in AML. However, without further therapy, virtually all patients in CR will eventually relapse. Patients are estimated to have 10^{12} leukemic cells at diagnosis, which intensive induction chemotherapy reduces by four to five orders of magnitude. Although this reduces the disease burden by 99.9%, approximately 10^8 residual leukemic cells remain after successful induction therapy. These residual cells may not be measurable at all or may be measurable only by sensitive techniques such as multiparameter flow cytometry or quantitative reverse transcriptase polymerase chain reaction (RT-PCR); they cannot be detected by morphology alone. Thus postremission therapy is designed to eradicate residual (typically undetectable) leukemic cells to prevent relapse and prolong survival. Similar to induction, the type of postremission therapy in AML is selected for each individual patient based on age, fitness, and cytogenetic/molecular risk.

Postremission treatment options include chemotherapy and/or transplantation. The choice between consolidation with chemotherapy alone or transplantation is complex and based on age, risk, and practical considerations. In younger patients receiving chemotherapy, postremission therapy with intermediate/high-dose cytarabine[1] for two to four cycles is standard practice. It is clear that alloHCT is the best relapse-prevention strategy currently available for AML. However, the benefit of alloHCT in reducing relapse risk is offset somewhat by increased morbidity and mortality from transplant-related complications including graft-versus-host disease. Given that relapsed AML is typically resistant to chemotherapy, alloHCT in CR1 is a favored strategy for patients at high risk for relapse. Transplantation is generally recommended for physically fit patients younger than 75 years of age who do not have favorable-risk disease (see Table 1) and have a suitable donor. Donors are typically HLA-matched (related or unrelated) or, increasingly, haploidentical (half-matched sibling, parent, or child). Prognostic factors help in selecting the appropriate postremission therapy in patients in CR1. In general, patients with favorable-risk AML in CR1 are treated with chemotherapy alone, though MRD status may be used to identify patients more likely to benefit from alloHCT. Patients with adverse-risk disease should proceed to alloHCT at CR1 if possible. The decision for alloHCT versus chemotherapy in CR1 for intermediate-risk patients remains in debate, but transplant is typically favored for young, fit patients.

Recent years have seen U.S. Food and Drug Administration (FDA) approval for several targeted drugs. For AML patients with *FLT3* mutation, midostaurin (Rydapt, in combination with induction chemotherapy) and gilteritinib (Xospata, as monotherapy for relapsed AML) have improved outcomes compared with chemotherapy alone. Likewise, agents targeting mutated IDH enzymes 1 or 2 (in AML patients with *IDH1* or *IDH2* mutations) have been shown to be effective in both relapsed and initial therapy settings. Another nontargeted drug, CPX-351 (Vyxeos, a liposomal combination of daunorubicin [an anthracycline] and cytarabine), has been approved in patients with therapy-related AML or AML with myelodysplasia-related changes (including patients with antecedent hematologic disorder). All of these drugs, as well as venetoclax and many other novel agents, are currently in additional clinical trials. Menin inhibition has recently shown particular promise in patients with NPM1 mutations or KMT2A rearrangements.

APL is uniquely treated with all-*trans*retinoic acid (tretinoin) and arsenic trioxide (ATO, Trisenox) rather than chemotherapy, although cases with high presenting WBC counts (>10,000/μL) may require the addition of chemotherapy or the antibody-drug conjugate gemtuzumab ozogamicin (Mylotarg)[1] for cytoreduction. Cases with high WBC counts are at increased risk for fatal hemorrhage and other complications. Low-risk patients (WBC <10,000/μL) have a virtually nonexistent frequency of resistant disease when treated with all-*trans*retinoic acid (tretinoin) and arsenic trioxide. Patients with APL require expert management to address complications of DIC and hemorrhage and the so-called *APL syndrome* (formerly known as *differentiation syndrome* and *retinoic acid syndrome*). APL syndrome is marked by an increasing WBC count, fever, hypoxia, shortness of breath, and fluid accumulation; it occurs up to 3 weeks after treatment initiation. It is common, especially in presentations with higher WBCs, and requires urgent therapy consisting of steroids, diuresis, and possibly cytoreduction.

Treatment of Acute Lymphoblastic Leukemia

Standard chemotherapy treatment of ALL is of much more extended duration and regimen complexity than that of AML. However, the same general principles apply; achievement of CR1 with initial therapy is the critical first step for long-term survival. Postremission therapy in ALL is broken into different segments of various intensity, including consolidation, interim maintenance, delayed intensification, and prolonged (24 to 36 months) maintenance. CNS-directed therapy (systemic chemotherapy with intrathecal chemotherapy, or cranial radiotherapy) is an important and mandatory feature of ALL treatment because of high rates of CNS relapse in patients who do not receive such therapy. Generally, treatment approaches include variations on a five-drug induction combination of cyclophosphamide (Cytoxan), prednisone[1] or dexamethasone (Decadron),[1] anthracycline (doxorubicin [Adriamycin]; or daunorubicin), PEGylated asparaginase (Oncaspar), and vincristine (Oncovin). The principle of therapy for ALL is continuous exposure to multiple chemotherapy agents with non-overlapping resistance mechanisms; all protocols use alternating chemotherapy regimens given over an extended period. Additional agents include methotrexate, cytarabine, 6-mercaptopurine (Purinethol), and others. Examples of common treatment strategies are the Berlin-Frankfurt-Munster (BFM) approach and the hyper-CVAD (hyperfractionated cyclophosphamide, vincristine, doxorubicin, dexamethasone) regimen. Although data are sparse, patients with mixed-phenotype acute leukemias appear to fare better with ALL-like treatment approaches compared with those used in AML.

Unfortunately, although children with B-ALL have favorable long-term survival in the 80% to 90% range, adults fare far worse. Estimated long-term survival rates for adults with ALL are only 30% to 40%. Encouraging data have come from recent cooperative group studies: adolescents and young adults (16 to 40 years of age) treated with "pediatric-inspired" regimens have significantly more favorable outcomes than those treated with "adult" regimens. Pediatric regimens have a greater focus on less myelotoxic therapies such as PEGylated asparaginase, vincristine, and steroids. Unfortunately, older adults (>40 years of age) often have difficulty tolerating such approaches. The addition of nelarabine (Arranon) to first-line therapy has improved outcomes in T-ALL.

As noted previously, the identification of the Ph chromosome ($t(9;22)$) or the *BCR-ABL1* fusion is critical in the initial diagnosis of B-ALL or mixed-phenotype acute leukemia. The introduction of TKIs for Ph-positive patients into multiagent induction and postremission treatment has dramatically improved outcomes and is now standard. AlloHCT in CR1 may not be necessary, especially if a complete molecular remission is rapidly achieved. Imatinib (Gleevec) is a standard TKI; second- or third-generation TKIs such as dasatinib (Sprycel), nilotinib (Tasigna),[1] or ponatinib (Iclusig) are also commonly used for the treatment of Ph-positive acute leukemia.

Additional advances to traditional approaches include the use of CD20 monoclonal antibodies (rituximab [Rituxan][1]) for patients with B-ALL whose lymphoid blasts express this surface marker and nelarabine in T-ALL. Nelarabine is a purine analog with increased activity in T-lymphoid blasts and 30% response

---

[1] Not FDA approved for this indication.

[1] Not FDA approved for this indication.

Figure 1 Structures of the three FDA-approved immune therapies. (From Kegyes D, Jitaru C, Ghiaur G, et al. Switching from salvage chemotherapy to immunotherapy in adult B-cell acute lymphoblastic leukemia. *Blood Rev.* 2023;59:101042.)

rates in the relapsed setting; it is being incorporated into front-line multiagent trials. AlloHCT in adult ALL is more controversial than in AML, although most trials offer alloHCT in CR1 for high-risk disease. MRD status at completion of induction therapy is also increasingly being used to identify patients likely to benefit from alloHCT. The addition of the bispecific antibody blinatumomab (Blincyto; see later) for patients who remain MRD positive after intensive chemotherapy has improved clinical outcomes.

Immune-Based Therapies in Acute Leukemia

Beyond the use of alloHCT, recent years have seen remarkable progress in immunologic therapies for acute leukemia (Figure 1). The FDA recently approved exciting engineered cellular therapies for relapsed malignancies of B-lymphocytes: chimeric antigen receptor (CAR) T cells that target CD19 (in B-ALL and non-Hodgkin lymphoma). Tisagenlecleucel (Kymriah) is approved for relapsed or refractory B-ALL in patients 25 years or younger, and brexucabtagene autoleucel (Tecartus) has been approved for all adult patients. In these cases, autologous B cells are collected by apheresis from the patient, genetically engineered ex vivo to target CD19, and then infused back into the patient to treat CD19+ malignancy (typically after lymphodepleting therapy). In the process, CD19+ normal B cells are also eliminated. High response rates and long-term remissions have been reported in patients with ALL with highly refractory disease using CAR T-cell therapy; complete response rates in the range of 70% to 90% have been observed in CD19+ cancers: ALL, chronic lymphocytic leukemia, diffuse large B-cell lymphoma, and mantle cell lymphoma. Challenges of CAR T cells include issues with uncontrolled immune cell activation (termed *cytokine release syndrome*), neurotoxicity, killing of normal CD19+ B cells, and resistance caused by loss of CD19 expression on leukemic cells (e.g., CD19– relapse). CAR retargeting to other hematologic targets beyond CD19 remains an area of active investigation; CAR T cells targeting the BCMA antigen have recently been approved in multiple myeloma, whereas products targeting CD22 and CD123, among others, appear promising.

Several novel antibodies have also recently been approved. Inotuzumab ozogamicin (Besponsa; targeting CD22 in B-ALL) and gemtuzumab ozogamicin (targeting CD33 in AML) are antibody-drug conjugates that deliver the toxin calicheamicin to lymphoid or myeloid blasts, respectively. Both agents have activity as a monotherapy and may also be incorporated into chemotherapy regimens. Blinatumomab is a CD3-CD19 bispecific T-cell engager; this class of agents functions by linking immune cells to malignant cells resulting in cytotoxicity. Bispecific agents targeting CD7, CD33, CD123, and CD20 are in ongoing clinical trials.

Monitoring

Measurement of residual disease is an important component of management in ALL. Unsurprisingly, initial responsiveness to chemotherapy is a useful predictor for long-term outcome. Persistence of abnormal karyotype after induction among patients in CR is associated with poor clinical outcomes. For patients in morphologic CR, measurement of MRD is an emerging standard in both ALL and AML. More sensitive methods of MRD measurement beyond light microscopy and cytogenetics are increasingly used to aid decision making. Examples of sensitive MRD assessment include immunophenotyping by multiparameter flow cytometry to detect minute populations of blasts or quantitative RT-PCR and other molecular methods to detect leukemia-associated molecular abnormalities. Particularly in B-ALL, early clearance of MRD is favorable. In ALL and in APL, MRD assessment is a very useful and reliable tool to refine prognostication, detect early relapse, and direct the initiation of additional therapy. In AML, MRD identifies high-risk patients, but how to utilize these data to mitigate risk is not yet established in many cases. However, quantitative measurement of mutated *NPM1* transcript levels during first remission provides important and potentially actionable information in that subset of AML.

Management of Complications

The treatment of acute leukemia involves repeated cycles of myelotoxic or immunosuppressive chemotherapy, requiring intensive supportive care. The emergence of infections with multidrug-resistant organisms is a growing concern. In addition, invasive fungal infections are associated with early death. Standard infection precautions include reverse isolation, air filtration, and prophylactic antimicrobials. Recommendations on the latter are best tailored based on institutional antibiograms; in AML patients undergoing intensive induction therapy, antifungal prophylaxis using agents with broad mold coverage is generally recommended.

Transfusion of red blood cells and platelets is a common and necessary part of treatment. Blood products should ideally be leukoreduced (done by the American Red Cross in the United States) to reduce the risk of febrile transfusion reaction and alloimmunization. Particularly in the multicourse induction and postremission therapies in ALL, optimization of supportive care strategies to facilitate the on-time administration of subsequent therapies whenever possible improves outcomes.

References

Arber D, Orazi A, Hasserjian R: International Consensus Classification of Myeloid Neoplasms and Acute Leukemias: integrating morphologic, clinical, and genomic data, *Blood* 140:1200–1228, 2022.

Brown AL, Churpek JE, Malcovati L, et al: Recognition of familial myeloid neoplasia in adults, *Semin Hematol* 54:60–68, 2017.

TCGA Research Network, Ley TJ, Miller C, et al: Genomic and epigenomic landscapes of adult de novo acute myeloid leukemia, *N Engl J Med* 368:2059–2074, 2013.

Döhner H, Wei A, Applebaum F, et al: Diagnosis and management of AML in adults: 2022 recommendations from an international expert panel on behalf of the ELN, *Blood* 140:1345–1377, 2022.

Heuser M, Freeman S, Ossenkoppele G, et al: Update on MRD in acute myeloid leukemia: a consensus document from the European LeukemiaNet MRD Working Party, *Blood* 138:2753–2767, 2021.

Iacobucci I, Mullighan CG: Genetic basis of acute lymphoblastic leukemia, *J Clin Oncol* 35:975–983, 2017.

Khoury JD, Solary E, Abla O, et al: The 5th edition of the World Health Organization classification of haematolymphoid tumours: myeloid and histiocytic/dendritic neoplasms, *Leukemia* 36:1703–1719, 2022.

Lim WA, June CH: The principles of engineering immune cells to treat cancer, *Cell* 168:724–740, 2017.

Maude SL, Frey N, Shaw PA, et al: Chimeric antigen receptor T cells for sustained remissions in leukemia, *N Engl J Med* 371:1507–1517, 2014.

National Comprehensive Cancer Network (NCCN): Clinical practices guidelines in oncology. Available at: https://www.nccn.org/guidelines/category_1. [Accessed March 2023].

Papaemmanuil E, Gerstung M, Bullinger L, et al: Genomic classification and prognosis in acute myeloid leukemia, *N Engl J Med* 374:2209–2221, 2016.

Welch JS, Ley TJ, Link DC, et al: The origin and evolution of mutations in acute myeloid leukemia, *Cell* 150:264–278, 2012.

BLOOD COMPONENT THERAPY AND TRANSFUSION REACTIONS

Method of
Theresa Nester, MD

CURRENT DIAGNOSIS

- Fever greater than 1°C rise during or within 4 hours after transfusion should prompt evaluation of the patient and consideration of a transfusion reaction.
- Fever and pain are the most common manifestations of an acute hemolytic transfusion reaction.
- The point of the transfusion reaction laboratory investigation is to evaluate for hemolysis, either intravascular or extravascular. The majority of reactions are negative for hemolysis.
- The differential diagnosis of a transfusion reaction with respiratory symptoms includes febrile nonhemolytic and circulatory overload (common), allergic or anaphylactic reaction, transfusion-related acute lung injury, acute hemolytic reaction, and bacterial contamination (rare).

CURRENT THERAPY

- The decision to transfuse red blood cells to a patient should depend more on the clinical state of the patient than on an absolute trigger for hemoglobin (Hb) or hematocrit.
- A transfusion trigger of less than 7 g/dL is recommended for hospitalized adult patients who are hemodynamically stable, including critically ill patients. A transfusion trigger of 8 g/dL is recommended for patients undergoing orthopedic or cardiac surgery, as well as those with preexisting cardiovascular disease.
- For severe autoimmune hemolytic anemia, maintenance of Hb at greater than 4 g/dL in younger patients and greater than 6 g/dL in older patients or patients with cardiovascular disease is appropriate.
- Platelets are not typically indicated in thrombotic thrombocytopenic purpura, autoimmune thrombocytopenic purpura, and heparin-induced thrombocytopenia unless the patient has significant bleeding.
- Currently available coagulation tests are not very useful for predicting bleeding in patients with end-stage liver disease. These patients establish a new equilibrium between coagulation, anticoagulation, and fibrinolysis that results in relatively less bleeding than predicted by the international normalized ratio.
- The goal during massive transfusion scenarios should be to prevent marked acidosis, hypothermia, and coagulopathy. The latter is often achieved with replacement of coagulation factors using plasma or cryoprecipitate within the first hour of the resuscitation.
- Cryoprecipitate is useful as a source of concentrated fibrinogen. In a patient who is actively bleeding and has a fibrinogen less than 100 mg/dL, cryoprecipitate is indicated.

Therapeutic Use of Blood Components

The community blood supply depends on two types of donors: whole blood donors and apheresis donors. Units of whole blood are centrifuged and then separated into components within a closed system. Using apheresis techniques, individual components of whole blood can be collected. Citrate is used to keep blood components from clotting.

The decision to transfuse blood to a patient should always include a consideration of the risks versus the benefits. Risks of transfusion-transmitted diseases are small with current testing standards. Transfusion reactions do occur; the most common ones are not life-threatening unless the patient cannot tolerate tachycardia or hypertension. Rarely, a patient experiences a life-threatening reaction. Thus it is important to ensure that the need for the blood component outweighs the risks. Additionally, in a bleeding patient, it is important to check coagulation parameters (platelet count, prothrombin time [PT], international normalized ratio [INR], activated partial thromboplastin time [aPTT], fibrinogen) in addition to hematocrit (Hct) to ensure that the component that will best address the bleeding is being used.

Red Blood Cells
Indications
Red blood cells should be given to increase oxygen-carrying capacity. The hemoglobin (Hb) and Hct levels alone should not be used to determine the need for transfusion; instead, the patient's clinical picture should drive the decision to transfuse. The patient's intravascular volume status, cardiopulmonary function, and baseline vital signs in the presence of anemia should all be considered. When anemia has persisted over weeks and months, large volume transfusion is often not indicated because compensatory mechanisms have had time to work.

Transfusion Triggers
The most recent clinical practice guideline from the Association for the Advancement of Blood and Biotherapies (formerly known as the American Association of Blood Banks) has the following recommendations: in hospitalized adult patients who are hemodynamically stable, including critically ill patients, a transfusion threshold of 7 g/dL is acceptable. In patients undergoing orthopedic or cardiac surgery, and those with preexisting cardiovascular disease, a transfusion threshold of 8 g/dL is recommended. The recommendations do not apply to patients with acute coronary syndrome, severe thrombocytopenia, or chronic transfusion dependent anemia, because of insufficient evidence.

Dosage
One unit of packed red blood cells will increase the Hb by 1 g/dL and Hct by 3% in the patient who is not bleeding or experiencing hemolysis (Table 1).

Autoimmune Hemolytic Anemia
Special Situation
When the autoantibody responsible for autoimmune hemolytic anemia reacts at body temperature, all red blood cell units can appear incompatible. This is because the antibody binds to an epitope common to all red blood cells, such as the band 3 protein. The clinician needs to decide when to transfuse the (apparently) incompatible units. In a patient who has never received a transfusion or been pregnant, there is little possibility of red blood cell alloantibodies in circulation, and the chance of hemolysis (beyond that being caused by the autoantibody) is low. For the patient who has received a transfusion or who has been pregnant in the past, the risk that a circulating red blood cell alloantibody is present and is being masked by the autoantibody is higher; special studies are available to reduce the risk of an alloantibody being overlooked. The transfusion trigger depends on whether the anemia is acute or chronic. For acute severe anemia, maintenance of Hb at greater than 4 g/dL in younger patients and greater than 6 g/dL in older patients or patients with cardiovascular disease is appropriate.

Platelets
Platelets are required as part of normal clotting. The first stage of clot formation is development of a platelet plug over the site of endothelial injury.

Indications
The indications for platelet transfusion may be divided into prevention of bleeding and treatment of bleeding in the setting of thrombocytopenia or platelet dysfunction.

TABLE 1	Component Therapy: Dosage and Expected Increment			
COMPONENT	**DOSE**	**EXPECTED INCREMENT**		**AVERAGE VOLUME**
Red blood cells	1 unit	Hct 3%, Hb 1 g/dL		250 mL
Whole blood platelets	1 unit	Platelet count increased by 5000–10,000/μL		50 mL/unit (1 pool of 6 = 300 mL)
Apheresis platelet	1 unit	Platelet count increased by 20,000–60,000/μL		300 mL/unit
Plasma	10 mL/kg	Factor levels increased by 20%		300 mL/unit
Cryoprecipitate	1 unit	Fibrinogen increased by 5 mg/dL		15 mL/unit
Prepooled cryoprecipitate	1 6-unit pool	Fibrinogen increased by 45 mg/dL		120 mL/pool

Hb, Hemoglobin; *Hct,* hematocrit.

Transfusion Triggers

Prevention of Bleeding. In a stable patient with normal platelet function, transfusion is appropriate if the platelet count is less than 10,000/μL. One randomized, controlled trial has shown that transfusion at platelet counts of 5000/μL to 10,000/μL prevents bleeding in the stable patient. In a stable patient with other hemostatic abnormalities (e.g., on anticoagulation), transfusion is appropriate with a platelet count less than 50,000/μL.

Before a planned invasive procedure such as open lung biopsy, transfusion is appropriate with a platelet count of <50,000/μL. For lumbar puncture, consensus guidelines suggest that a platelet count of 50,000/μL is appropriate, although there are a few large studies suggesting that counts between 20,000 and 50,000/μL may be adequate. A patient undergoing major surgery should receive platelets if the count is less than 50,000 to 100,000/μL. The transfusion should take place as close to the procedure as possible so that the platelets remain in circulation while the procedure is occurring.

Treatment of Bleeding. Platelets may be transfused with a major hemorrhage (e.g., gastrointestinal or genitourinary) and a platelet count less than 30,000 to 50,000/μL. For bleeding with major surgery or trauma, transfusion is appropriate for counts less than 80,000/μL. For bleeding into critical areas (e.g., central nervous system bleeding or diffuse alveolar hemorrhage), platelets may be given for counts less than 100,000/μL.

Dosage

Dosage is determined on the basis of the baseline platelet count, desired platelet count, and estimated blood volume. For a 70-kg patient, 3×10^{11} platelets (4 to 6 units of pooled whole blood platelets or 1 unit of apheresis platelets) increases platelet count by approximately 30,000 to 50,000/μL in the absence of alloimmunization or excessive consumption. For prophylactic therapy, lower dosages have been shown to be as effective as higher dosages in the prevention of bleeding.

Out of ABO Group Platelet Transfusion

Because platelets can only be stored for a maximum of 7 days after collection, and the community platelet supply is collected from volunteer donors, a platelet product that is identical to the patient's ABO type might not be available (Table 2 and Box 1). Thus it may be necessary to infuse a small volume of incompatible plasma (suspending the platelets) to the patient. There is therefore a small risk of hemolysis of the patient's red blood cells if the iso-agglutinin (anti-A or anti-B) titer in the donated plasma is high. Studies of healthy blood donors indicate that these antibody titers are typically low and do not precipitate hemolysis. Transfusion services often have policies that limit the amount of incompatible plasma a patient has received with platelet transfusion. Alternatively, some centers measure the antibody titer in the donated product and give high-titer products only to patients whose red blood cells lack the corresponding ABO antigen.

Unresponsiveness to Platelet Transfusion

A number of clinical factors can result in a patient's less-than-optimal response to platelet transfusion. In addition to

TABLE 2	ABO Compatibility*		
PATIENT'S ABO	**ANTIBODIES IN CIRCULATION**	**COMPATIBLE PACKED RED BLOOD CELLS**	**COMPATIBLE PLASMA**
O	Anti-A, anti-B	O	O, A, B, AB
A	Anti-B	O or A	A or AB
B	Anti-A	O or B	B or AB
AB	None	O, A, B, AB	AB

*For platelet compatibility, see text.

BOX 1	Rh(D) Compatibility

Rh(D) negative patients should receive Rh negative red blood cells and platelet units.*†

Rh(D) positive patients can receive Rh positive or Rh negative red blood cells and platelet units.

Rh compatibility does not apply to acellular components (plasma and cryoprecipitate).

Only 15% of blood donors are Rh negative.

---

*In times of shortage, it becomes necessary to preserve the Rh(D) negative red blood cell inventory for females of childbearing potential (<50 years old).

†Platelet components contain very few red blood cells; Rho(D) immune globulin (RhoGAM) may be administered if prevention of anti-D formation is deemed appropriate. Consult with a transfusion medicine physician if further discussion is needed.

consumption, some of these factors include splenomegaly, fever, and antifungal therapy. Patients who have been sensitized to foreign human leukocyte antigens through prior pregnancy or transfusion can also have a poor response to platelet transfusion. Transfusion medicine consultation regarding the evaluation of refractoriness to platelet transfusion may be indicated.

Special Situations

Uremia. Patients who are dialysis dependent might have an acquired platelet defect as a result of the uremic environment. Transfusion of platelets into this environment will render the transfused platelets dysfunctional. Thus if optimal platelet function is desired, dialysis should be performed frequently. Consider performing dialysis without heparin if the patient is actively bleeding.

Purpura and Thrombocytopenia. In patients with autoimmune thrombocytopenic purpura (ITP), thrombotic thrombocytopenic purpura (TTP), or heparin-induced thrombocytopenia, platelet transfusion is not indicated unless the patient has significant bleeding. Other therapies, such as steroid administration for ITP and plasma exchange for TTP, should be initiated to address the condition.

Plasma

Plasma contains all of the coagulation proteins needed for clot formation, as well as all of the fibrinolytic proteins that prevent systemic thrombosis. There are currently several kinds of plasma, such as fresh frozen, FP24, thawed, and liquid. All contain hemostatic levels of coagulation factors as long as they are stored appropriately. The effect of plasma transfusion on the PT and INR is 4 to 6 hours, owing to the short half-life of coagulation factor VII. Thus other, longer-lasting means of restoring coagulation factors, such as vitamin K administration, should be undertaken if a more durable response is desired.

When replacing coagulation factors with plasma, it is not necessary to have 100% factor replacement as the goal. Hemostasis is typically able to occur if circulating coagulation factor levels are between 40% and 50%. It is important to understand that the relationship between the INR and the percentage factor level is a logarithmic, rather than a linear, relationship (Figure 1). Thus whether the INR is 9 or 1.8, the initial dosage of plasma should be 10 to 20 mL/kg, with recheck of the laboratory values a few minutes after infusion. The more prolonged the INR, the more significant the effect of the dose on the INR.

Transfusion Triggers
For bleeding or imminent surgery that cannot be corrected in a timely manner by vitamin K administration, use plasma to correct an INR greater than 1.8 to 2.0. The exception is patients with end-stage liver disease (see later).

Dosage
At a dosage of 10 mL/kg, each unit has an average of 300 mL (3 to 5 units in a 70-kg adult). This dosage should increase circulating coagulation factors by 20% immediately after infusion.

Special Situations
Liver Disease. The INR is a less useful test in patients with end-stage liver disease. The destruction of liver tissue leads to decreased production of coagulation and fibrinolytic proteins such that a new balance is established. Patients with end-stage liver disease have been shown to have normal levels of circulating thrombin and reduced levels of certain anticoagulant proteins (e.g., protein C), which could explain why they do not bleed as often as predicted with the elevation in INR. Thus the prophylactic use of plasma to correct a mildly prolonged laboratory value in the absence of bleeding is not indicated. It will lead to unnecessary plasma infusion, and the risk of volume overload and transfusion reactions outweighs the benefit in these patients.

Massive Transfusion. In trauma patients, patients with ruptured aortic aneurysms, and patients with other arterial bleeding, massive transfusion may be necessary. The basic principles of such a scenario include taking steps early into the resuscitation to prevent the patient from becoming too cold, acidotic, or coagulopathic to reverse the situation. Some plasma (and cryoprecipitate, if the fibrinogen is very low) should be infused early into the resuscitation to help prevent coagulopathy. Red blood cells and plasma should be infused through a blood warmer, if possible.

Isolated Prolonged aPTT. Other than a deficiency in coagulation factor XI, bear in mind that the differential of an isolated prolonged aPTT includes entities that do not typically require plasma (refer to Figure 2). Hemophilia A, hemophilia B, and von Willebrand disease are no longer treated by plasma but can require factor concentrates to prevent bleeding. Systemic administration of heparin must be reversed by protamine if fast reversal is desired. Note that plasma transfusion will not reverse the effect of heparin. One of the most common causes of a prolonged aPTT is a lupus anticoagulant; this is an antibody directed against phospholipids that typically leads to thrombosis rather than hemorrhage.

Intracranial Hemorrhage or Life-Threatening Bleeding. Reversal of anticoagulation in the setting of intracranial hemorrhage or life-threatening bleeding depends on the anticoagulant. For patients taking warfarin (Coumadin), refer to Box 2.

Prothrombin complex concentrates (PCCs) may be used to replenish factors II, VII, IX, and X rapidly. For reversal of dabigatran (Pradaxa), a direct oral anticoagulant, idarucizumab (Praxbind), is approved by the U.S. Food and Drug Administration (FDA) as a reversal agent. KCentra is a four-factor PCC that has been FDA approved to treat life-threatening hemorrhage in adult patients on warfarin. For reversal of apixaban (Eliquis) and rivaroxaban (Xarelto) in life-threatening bleeding, andexanet alfa (Andexxa) is available.

Cryoprecipitate

Cryoprecipitate contains fibrinogen, coagulation factors VIII and XIII, and von Willebrand factor. The most common current use is as a source of concentrated fibrinogen. It may also be used to treat hemorrhage in the rare patient with factor XIII deficiency.

Indications
Clinical scenarios that increase probability for low fibrinogen include any clinical situation in which disseminated intravascular coagulation (DIC) may be present. These include obstetric bleeding, trauma involving head injury or crush injury, and sepsis. Clinical events that can lead to an isolated decrease in serum fibrinogen concentration include administration of L-asparaginase (Elspar) and surgeries that disrupt bladder or salivary gland endothelium. Fibrinogen concentrates are available for patients who will not accept cryoprecipitate.

Transfusion Triggers
Transfusion is appropriate in patients with low serum fibrinogen, typically less than 100 mg/dL. In cases of massive transfusion, a

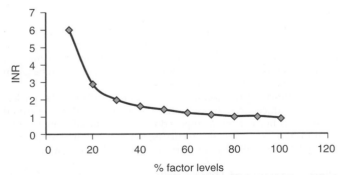

Figure 1 American Association of Blood Banks international normalized ratio compared with percentage factor levels. (Reprinted with permission from Nester T, AuBuchon J. Hemotherapy decisions and their outcomes. In: Roback JD, ed. *AAB Technical Manual*. 17th ed. American Association of Blood Banks; 2011:592.)

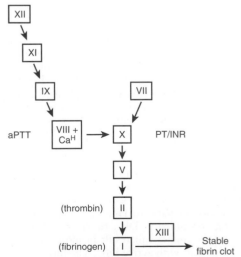

Figure 2 Coagulation cascade.

<table>

| BOX 2 | Guidelines for Correction of Excessive Warfarin Anticoagulation |
</table>

INR Higher Than Therapeutic but <5, No Significant Bleeding
Lower anticoagulant dosage.
Temporarily discontinue drug, if necessary.

INR >5 but <9, No Significant Bleeding
Omit 1 or 2 doses, monitor INR, resume when INR is in therapeutic range.
Alternative if patient is at increased risk of hemorrhage:
- Omit 1 dose.
- Give 1 to 2.5 mg vitamin K orally.
For rapid reversal before urgent surgery:
- Give 2 to 4 mg vitamin K orally.
- Give 1 to 2 mg at 24 hours if INR remains elevated.

INR >9, No Significant Bleeding
Omit warfarin; give 2.5 to 5.0 mg vitamin K orally.
Closely monitor INR; give additional vitamin K, if necessary.
Resume warfarin at lower dose when INR is within therapeutic range.

Serious Bleeding at Any Elevation of INR
Omit warfarin.
Give 10 mg vitamin K by slow IV infusion.
Supplement with plasma or prothrombin complex concentrate depending on urgency of correction.
Vitamin K infusions may be repeated every 12 hours.

Life-Threatening Hemorrhage
Omit warfarin.
Give prothrombin complex concentrate with 10 mg vitamin K by slow IV infusion.
Repeat as necessary, depending on INR.

INR, International normalized ratio.
From Nester T, AuBuchon J. Hemotherapy decisions and their outcomes. In: Roback JD, ed. *AAB Technical Manual.* 17th ed. American Association of Blood Banks; 2011:571–616.

TABLE 3 Transfusion Reactions

MOST COMMON REACTIONS	INCIDENCE
Allergic reaction of mild severity	1:33–1:100
Febrile nonhemolytic reaction	1:100–1:1000 with leukocyte reduction
Transfusion-related circulatory overload	<1:100
MOST DANGEROUS REACTIONS	**INCIDENCE**
Acute hemolytic reaction	1:38,000–1:70,000
Anaphylactic reaction	1:20,000–1:50,000
Transfusion-related acute lung injury	1:1200–1:190,000
Bacterial contamination of red cell unit with gram-negative organisms	1:1,000,000

fibrinogen greater than 100 mg/dL, administration of plasma will replete other coagulation factors being consumed.

Transfusion Reactions
Reactions to transfusion are relatively common; life-threatening reactions are rare (Tables 3 and 4).

Because fever is a feature of both common and dangerous reactions, a transfusion reaction evaluation should be initiated with fever greater than 1°C above patient's baseline temperature at the start of the transfusion. The infusion of product should cease, at least until the laboratory results are known and the patient has responded to treatment. The main point of the laboratory investigation is to evaluate the plasma for abnormal (usually red) color in an effort to detect intravascular hemolysis as quickly as possible. If the clerical check and hemolysis direct antiglobulin tests are negative, one might consider restarting the transfusion with careful surveillance of the patient. A direct antiglobulin test is performed to detect the presence of antibody coating red blood cells in circulation; a positive result could indicate extravascular hemolysis, which is not as dangerous as intravascular hemolysis.

Most Common Reactions
Febrile Nonhemolytic Reaction
Presentation. A febrile nonhemolytic transfusion reaction manifests as a fever greater than a 1°C rise above the patient's baseline, often accompanied by rigors. Hypertension, tachypnea, and transient decrease in oxygen saturation can also occur until the symptoms are treated. Evidence of hemolysis will be absent on laboratory evaluation. These reactions can manifest during or 2 to 3 hours after the transfusion.

Pathophysiology. Cytokines produced by white blood cells present in cellular blood components (red blood cell and platelet units) are responsible for the clinical presentation. Platelets also secrete cytokines; thus leukoreduction of platelet units might not be successful in preventing the reaction.

Acute Management. Administration of an antipyretic is the routine treatment; meperidine (Demerol)[1] may be required to address severe rigors. Slow intravenous (IV) push of 25 mg as a first dose is recommended; an additional 25-mg dose can be given 10 to 15 minutes later if rigors persist.

Prevention of Febrile Nonhemolytic Transfusion Reactions. Ordering leukoreduced red blood cells and platelets (if the hospital inventory is not entirely composed of leukoreduced components) is a preventive measure. For recurring reactions with platelets, volume reduction of the component can reduce the incidence.

Allergic Reaction of Mild Severity
Presentation. Urticaria or flushing occurs during a transfusion. Evidence of hemolysis is absent on laboratory evaluation.

trigger of 150 mg/dL is considered practical, so that the patient becomes less coagulopathic in the time that it takes to draw and review new laboratory values. New evidence indicates that a fibrinogen level of less than 300 mg/dL predicts severe postpartum hemorrhage, as a normal postpartum fibrinogen level is in the 600 mg/dL range. Because component therapy aims to replete coagulation factors to hemostatic (rather than completely normal) levels, consensus guidelines suggest maintaining a fibrinogen level greater than 200 mg/dL during a postpartum hemorrhage.

Dosage
Dosage depends on the type of cryoprecipitate available. If the product requires resuspension in saline before pooling, then 1 unit (average 15 mL volume) will increase fibrinogen by 5 mg/dL. If the product has been pooled in plasma before freezing, then 1 unit will increase fibrinogen by 7 to 8 mg/dL; a 6-unit pool will increase fibrinogen by 45 mg/dL. Check with the transfusion service laboratory regarding which product is available and the expected increment.

Special Situation
DIC is a state where fibrinogen is consumed at a faster rate than other circulating coagulation factors. This is because DIC is typically a thrombin-generating process (thrombin cleaves fibrinogen into fibrin for clot formation). Thus although all coagulation factors are being consumed in DIC, timely repletion of fibrinogen by use of cryoprecipitate can result in more timely cessation of bleeding in a patient with active DIC. The target value is fibrinogen at least 100 mg/dL. If the PT and INR are still prolonged with

---
[1] Not FDA approved for this indication.

TABLE 4 Transfusion Reactions With Respiratory Symptoms

REACTION	CLASSIC SIGNS	RELATIVE FREQUENCY	ACUTE MANAGEMENT (TRANSFUSION STOPPED IN ALL CASES)
Febrile nonhemolytic reaction	Transient tachypnea in the presence of rigors and fever	Common	Antipyretic ± meperidine (Demerol)[1]
Circulatory overload	Hypoxia Crackles in lower lung fields Increased BP Chest radiograph consistent with volume overload	Common	Diuresis
Allergic reaction of moderate severity	Wheezes Possible perioral or periorbital edema Possible hives	Uncommon	IV antihistamines and possibly epinephrine (Adrenalin)
Allergic reaction of marked severity	Wheezes, swollen lips, tongue, uvula Stridor or other signs of airway compromise Very decreased BP	Rare	Epinephrine IV fluids and airway management Bronchodilators and glucagon (GlucaGen)[1] for patient on β-blockers
Transfusion-related acute lung injury	Tachypnea and hypoxia during or within 6 h of transfusion Persisting for several hours Chest radiograph consistent with bilateral white-out	Rare	Respiratory support of noncardiogenic pulmonary edema
Acute hemolytic reaction	Red urine and red serum Hypotension and diffuse oozing may be present Tachypnea (10% of patients)	Rare	Supportive (possibly ICU) care Administration of crystalloid solution Blood component therapy if DIC is present
Bacterial contamination with gram-negative organism	Very decreased BP Fever Nausea, vomiting Possible tachypnea	Rare	Intensive care for support of gram-negative sepsis

[1]Not FDA approved for this indication.
BP, Blood pressure; *DIC*, disseminated intravascular coagulation; *ICU*, intensive care unit; *IV*, intravenous.

Pathophysiology. Allergic reactions are immunoglobulin (Ig) E-mediated reactions against some allergen in the donor plasma. Because all blood components have some amount of plasma, it is possible to experience an allergic reaction with any blood product.

Acute Management. Slowing the infusion rate may be all that is required to alleviate the reaction. Antihistamine administration also addresses the symptoms.

Prevention of Allergic Transfusion Reactions of Mild Severity. A reaction of this type may be a one-time event. For patients with recurrent reactions, transfusing the blood product more slowly (maximum of transfusion over 4 hours) or premedication with antihistamines will reduce the incidence.

Transfusion-Associated Circulatory Overload

Presentation. The patient has respiratory distress, typically during the transfusion, and increase in blood pressure unless cardiac decompensation occurs. Tachycardia, tachypnea, and decrease in oxygen saturation are often present. Jugular venous distension may be seen. Radiographic findings include pleural effusions, perihilar edema, and increased vascular pedicle width.

Pathophysiology. The reaction results in cardiogenic pulmonary edema.

Acute Management. Diuretic should be administered. Supplemental oxygen may be required temporarily to improve oxygen saturation.

Prevention of Transfusion-Associated Circulatory Overload. Slowing the infusion rate with a maximum time of transfusion over 4 hours can prevent the reaction. Diuretic administration may be necessary in patients with poor heart function.

Most Dangerous Reactions
Acute Hemolytic Transfusion Reaction

Presentation. The most common signs include fever with or without rigors and pain. The more commonly reported sites of pain include flank, back, chest, or abdomen. Nausea and vomiting and dyspnea can also occur. In more severe presentations, hemodynamic instability is present, accompanied by oozing from line sites or petechial hemorrhage if DIC is occurring. Red or cola-colored urine is another manifestation of an acute hemolytic transfusion reaction and represents overwhelming of the renal capacity to recirculate free heme.

Pathophysiology. Red blood cells have proteins and carbohydrates on the cell surface that are antigenic. These epitopes are categorized into blood groups based on structure and sharing of a parent protein. A patient who lacks particular epitopes can develop antibodies through pregnancy or transfusion. Such red blood cell alloantibodies then lyse transfused red blood cells that possess the cognate antigen. When time allows for pretransfusion testing, the antibodies are identified, and antigen-negative units are provided. The ABO blood group system is unusual in that almost all patients older than 4 months have naturally occurring antibodies to the A and B antigens that they did not inherit. These antibodies are capable of activating complement and causing intravascular lysis when bound to their cognate antigen. Thus it is of utmost importance to avoid transfusing red blood cells against the ABO antibody in circulation. Refer to the ABO compatibility table (see Table 1).

Acute Management. Management is largely supportive. The end result of intravascular hemolysis and activation of the complement cascade can be shock, uncontrolled bleeding secondary to DIC, and renal failure. Therefore prompt infusion of IV crystalloid solutions are indicated to maintain blood pressure and renal perfusion. The goal for urine flow rate should be more than 1 mL/kg per hour. Coagulation laboratory values should be obtained to determine whether DIC is present; if so, component therapy to reverse the DIC is indicated. If the reaction is severe, intensive care is appropriate, because inotropic agents and mechanical ventilation may be necessary to support the patient.

Prevention of Acute Hemolytic Transfusion Reaction. An acute hemolytic reaction is one of the most feared complications of transfusion. It is also often one of the most preventable. Great care should be given to the pretransfusion blood sample draw, comparing the label to the patient's unique identifiers and labeling the tube at the patient's bedside as soon as the blood is in the tube. Just before transfusion, the unit label attached to the blood product should be compared with the patient's armband to ensure that the product is intended for this particular patient. To prevent intravascular hemolysis from antibodies directed against non-ABO antigens, pretransfusion testing (antibody screen or crossmatch) should be done in advance of the need for red cell transfusion for any patient whose clinical situation indicates a likelihood of needing blood. The exception is a patient who is hemodynamically unstable because of acute red blood cell loss, where uncrossmatched red blood cells are indicated. If the patient's identity is known, a call to the hospital transfusion service in this situation is warranted; explain that the patient needs uncrossmatched red blood cells and ask if there are transfusion records that indicate a need for antigen-negative units.

Allergic Reaction of Marked Severity (Anaphylaxis)

Presentation. Significant drop in blood pressure occurs, typically early into the transfusion. Wheezes, difficulty breathing, and stridor may be present. Tongue or facial edema and hives may be observed.

Pathophysiology. Anaphylaxis is an IgE-mediated reaction against an allergen in the donor plasma. In a patient with absolute IgA deficiency, naturally occurring anti-IgA can precipitate this reaction on binding IgA in the plasma. Antihaptoglobin antibodies can also induce a severe reaction.

Acute Management. Airway and blood pressure support should be provided with the patient recumbent and the lower extremities elevated. The treatment of choice is epinephrine (Adrenalin) 1 mg/mL, also labeled as 1:1000 or 0.1%, using an adult dosage of 0.3 to 0.5 mg per single dose, typically administered intramuscularly to the midquadriceps area. If symptoms persist, the dose may be repeated every 5 to 15 minutes for a maximum of three times, unless palpitations, tremors, or extreme anxiousness occurs. Supplemental oxygen should be administered, and the airway should be maintained. IV fluid administration is also recommended. Bronchodilators such as albuterol can be given as adjunctive treatment for bronchospasm that does not appear to respond to epinephrine. For patients on β-blockers, the addition of IV glucagon (GlucaGen) 1 to 5 mg administered over 5 minutes, followed by infusion of 5 to 15 µg/minute, may be required. The addition of glucocorticoids can help prevent the biphasic reaction that occurs in some patients.

Prevention of Allergic Reaction of Marked Severity (Anaphylaxis). Slow administration with careful observation of any transfusion is required. Premedication with IV antihistamines is appropriate. Steroids may be administered, although their effectiveness has not been confirmed through controlled trials. Epinephrine should be available at the bedside. For severe allergic reactions, a discussion with the transfusion service physician regarding washed components is appropriate.

Transfusion-Related Acute Lung Injury

Presentation. The signs of transfusion-related acute lung injury (TRALI) are difficulty breathing, tachypnea, and hypoxia during or within 6 hours of a transfusion of any blood component. Ideally, signs of underlying lung disease or circulatory overload are absent. Chest radiograph may show diffuse bilateral opacities (white-out). Diuretic administration does not result in improvement. The hypoxemia can progress to the point that the patient requires mechanical ventilation, and thus the patient should be closely monitored while the reaction is occurring.

Pathophysiology. The factors that result in TRALI are not entirely known. In a portion of cases, antibodies against white blood cell antigens are present in donor plasma. These antibodies are believed to bind the cognate antigens on the patient's white blood cells, leading to degranulation and a capillary leak syndrome involving the lungs. Other theories regarding the pathophysiology of TRALI exist. One such theory implicates biologically active substances, such as lipids and cytokines, in the stored blood products. These substances are believed to prime the patient's granulocytes and activate pulmonary endothelium, setting the stage for an additional trigger to cause acute lung injury. Regardless of the cause of TRALI, the end result is an increase in pulmonary vascular permeability and noncardiogenic pulmonary edema. The estimated mortality rate from TRALI is 5% to 8%.

Acute Management. Management consists of supportive care, with particular regard to respiratory support. With adequate supportive care, the process most often reverses over 48 to 96 hours.

Prevention of Transfusion-Related Acute Lung Injury. Marked respiratory compromise is occasionally due to white blood cell antibodies in the patient, which bind cognate antigens in the donated red blood cells or platelet unit ("reverse TRALI"). In these cases, leukoreduction of cellular blood products may reduce the severity of subsequent transfusions, although solid evidence to support this is lacking. For TRALI caused by white blood cell antibodies in the donated product, there are no preventive measures for the clinician to take. The majority of U.S. blood suppliers provide plasma from only male donors, in an effort to reduce the incidence of TRALI caused by multiparous women with white blood cell antibodies.

Bacterial Contamination of a Blood Component

Presentation. The most-common presentation includes fever and rigors, nausea and vomiting, and possible onset of moderate hypotension during or after a platelet transfusion. Rarely, presentation includes signs of overt septic shock, including marked hypotension, typically early into the transfusion of a red blood cell or platelet component. Bacterial contamination of plasma or cryoprecipitate is extremely rare.

Pathophysiology. The most common organisms to contaminate a platelet product are gram-positive organisms such as *Staphylococcus epidermidis*. These organisms are thought to be introduced into the collection bag via a skin plug that results from phlebotomy using a large-gauge needle when sterilization of the phlebotomy site has been ineffective.

The most common organisms to contaminate a red blood cell unit are gram-negative, endotoxin-producing organisms such as *Yersinia enterocolitica*. This organism is introduced into the blood product as a result of asymptomatic bacteremia in the donor, from sources such as the gastrointestinal tract. The donor-screening questionnaire and vital sign assessment at the time of donation help make collection from such a donor a very rare event. Transfusion of a bacterially contaminated red blood cell unit is most often a fatal event. It is important to remember that platelets can also be contaminated by the same gram-negative, endotoxin-producing organisms; in this case, signs of septic shock may manifest.

Acute Management. Blood cultures from the patient should be drawn, and then prompt IV antibiotic administration should begin. Supportive care including inotropic agents and close nursing attention may be required.

Prevention of Bacterial Contamination of a Blood Component. Bacterial contamination is associated with a donor product, and thus preventive measures for the patient do not apply. Blood suppliers perform bacterial detection tests on platelet components or choose to treat platelets with pathogen reduction technology. Transfusion services also have strict policies related to visual inspection of all blood products before they are issued to a patient-care area.

Other Reactions
Delayed Hemolytic Transfusion Reaction

Presentation. The main finding with a delayed hemolytic transfusion reaction is usually an unexplained decrease in Hct within

---

[1] Not FDA approved for this indication.

2 to 7 days after transfusion. The patient often remains symptom free unless the decline in Hb is poorly tolerated. Jaundice can occur, and laboratory values consistent with hemolysis may be positive (elevated indirect bilirubin, elevated lactate dehydrogenase, decreased haptoglobin). Rarely, signs of intravascular hemolysis can occur.

Pathophysiology. The most common source of this reaction is a red blood cell alloantibody that the patient developed with prior transfusion or pregnancy; the antibody titer wanes over time such that pretransfusion testing does not detect the antibody. A unit of red blood cells positive for the cognate antigen is then transfused, and within a few days the patient's memory B cell response produces the antibody again. Transfused cells are then cleared, most often by an extravascular mechanism.

Acute Management. Most transfusion services have a policy to notify the clinician that a serologic delayed hemolytic transfusion reaction is present on testing a new plasma sample from the patient. If the patient's Hct has declined, it may be useful to determine a clinical correlation by obtaining the laboratory values just described. This is of particular importance when the distinction between hemolysis and bleeding will lead to different management strategies for the patient. Although extravascular clearance of Hb is fairly well tolerated by the kidneys, the conservative approach is to increase renal perfusion with IV crystalloid solutions if possible.

Prevention of Delayed Hemolytic Transfusion Reaction. For a patient who routinely receives care through one hospital system, the transfusion service will keep a record of the red blood cell alloantibody and provide antigen-negative cells for transfusion. The prevention, then, is to plan ahead for transfusion when possible, so that fully compatible units can be provided. Uncrossmatched red blood cells may be positive for the cognate antigen.

Allergic Reaction of Moderate Severity

Presentation. The patient has labile blood pressure, either hyper- or hypotension, accompanied by at least one of the following: throat scratchiness, respiratory wheezes, or perioral or periorbital edema. Hives may be present. Gastrointestinal symptoms such as crampy abdominal pain may also be present.

Pathophysiology. This is an IgE-mediated reaction against an allergen in the plasma of the donated product.

Acute Management. Treatment is administration of IV antihistamines. If the respiratory component does not resolve, consider epinephrine administration, and treat similarly to anaphylaxis (see previous section).

Prevention of Allergic Transfusion Reaction of Moderate Severity. Slower infusion of blood products can reduce further episodes of this type of reaction. If the patient is atopic, IV antihistamines may be administered as a premedication. If the patient requires chronic transfusion and experiences this type of reaction on a repeated basis, discussion with the transfusion service regarding washed components may be warranted.

Hypotensive Transfusion Reaction

Presentation. The patient has isolated hypotension (drop in systolic BP greater than 30 but less than 80 mm Hg) that responds quickly to cessation of the transfusion. The reaction classically occurs within the first 15 minutes of infusion of the blood product.

Pathophysiology. Pathophysiology is unclear. Some research indicates that the patient may have slower ability to metabolize bradykinin compared with other individuals.

Acute Management. Stop the transfusion.

Prevention of Hypotensive Transfusion Reaction. Prevention is unclear. In the author's experience, rate of infusion has a role. Slower infusion may help prevent this type of reaction.

Transfusion-Associated Dyspnea

Presentation. Acute respiratory distress that occurs within 24 hours of cessation of transfusion.

Pathophysiology. Pathophysiology is unclear.

Acute Management and Prevention of Transfusion-Associated Dyspnea. Management is supportive and prevention is unclear.

References

Abdel-Wahab OI, Healy B, Dzik WH: Effect of fresh-frozen plasma transfusion on prothrombin time and bleeding in patients with mild coagulation abnormalities, *Transfusion* 46:1279–1285, 2006.

Carson JL, Guyatt G, Heddle NM, et al: Clinical practice guidelines from the AABB: Red cell transfusion thresholds and storage, *JAMA* 316(19):2025–2035, 2016.

Carson JL, Stanworth SJ, Alexander JH, et al: Clinical trials evaluating red blood cell transfusion thresholds: An updated systematic review and with additional focus on patients with cardiovascular disease, *Am Heart J* 200:96–101, 2018.

Cuker A, Burnett A, Triller D: Reversal of direct oral anticoagulants: Guidance from the anticoagulation forum, *Am J Hematol* 94(6):697–709, 2019.

Kaufman RM, et al: Platelet transfusion: A clinical practice guideline from the AABB, *Ann Internal Med* 162(3):205–213, 2015.

Lisman T, Porte RJ: Rebalanced hemostasis in patients with liver disease: Evidence and clinical consequences, *Blood* 116:878–885, 2010.

Patel IJ, Rahim S, Davidson JC, et al: Consensus guidelines for the periprocedural management of thrombotic and bleeding risk in patients undergoing percutaneous image guided interventions—Part II, *Recommendations JVIR* 30(8):1168–1184, 2019.

Savage WJ, Hod EA: Noninfectious complications of blood transfusion. In Fung MK, editor: *AABB Technical Manual*, ed 19, Bethesda, MD, 2017, American Association of Blood Banks, pp 569–599.

Tummula R, et al: Specific antidotes against direct oral anticoagulants: a comprehensive review of clinical trials, *Int J Cardiol* 214:292–298, 2016.

Witt DM, Clark NP, Skov J, Crowther M: *Management of Anticoagulant Therapy: A pocket guide for the clinician*, American Society of Hematology, 2019.

CHRONIC LEUKEMIAS

Method of
Jatin Rana, MD; and Daniel Isaac, DO

CURRENT DIAGNOSIS

Chronic Myelogenous Leukemia
- Clinical symptoms
  - Constitutional symptoms
  - Splenomegaly (abdominal discomfort, early satiety)
- Laboratory parameters
  - Elevated white blood cell count, ~100,000/μL, with differential consisting of various stages of granulocyte maturation from myeloblasts to mature neutrophils
  - Absolute basophilia
- Genetic parameters
  - Presence of *bcr-abl1* by cytogenetics, fluorescence in situ hybridization, or reverse transcriptase polymerase chain reaction

Chronic Lymphocytic Leukemia
- Clinical symptoms
  - B symptoms (fevers, night sweats, weight loss)
  - Lymphadenopathy and/or organomegaly
  - Recurrent infections
- Laboratory parameters
  - Absolute lymphocytosis
  - Anemia
  - Thrombocytopenia
- Immunophenotypic analysis by flow cytometry
  - Monoclonal population of light-chain–restricted mature B cells that express CD19, CD20(dim), and CD23 and coexpress CD5

CURRENT THERAPY

Chronic Myelogenous Leukemia: Chronic Phase
- First-line therapy
  - Imatinib mesylate (Gleevec) 400 mg daily
  - Dasatinib (Sprycel) 100 mg daily
  - Nilotinib (Tasigna) 300 mg twice daily
  - Bosutinib (Bosulif) 400 mg daily
- Later-line therapy
  - Imatinib mesylate (Gleevec)
  - Dasatinib (Sprycel)
  - Nilotinib (Tasigna)
  - Bosutinib (Bosulif)
  - Ponatinib (Iclusig)
  - Omacetaxine mepesuccinate (Synribo)
  - Asciminib (Scemblix)
- High risk for failure
  - Allogeneic stem cell transplantation

Chronic Lymphocytic Leukemia
- Chemotherapy
  - Fludarabine (Fludara)
  - Cyclophosphamide (Cytoxan)
  - Chlorambucil (Leukeran)
  - Bendamustine (Treanda)
- Immunotherapy (monoclonal antibodies)
  - Rituximab (Rituxan)
  - Ofatumumab (Arzerra)
  - Obinutuzumab (Gazyva)
  - Alemtuzumab (Campath)
- Targeted therapy
  - Idelalisib (Zydelig)
  - Duvalisib (Copiktra)
  - Ibrutinib (Imbruvica)
  - Venetoclax (Venclexta)
  - Acalabrutinib (Calquence)

Chronic Myelogenous Leukemia

Chronic myelogenous leukemia (CML) is a myeloproliferative disorder with malignant clonal expansion and pathogenic leukemogenesis. It is defined by a translocation of chromosomes 9 and 22 (the Philadelphia [Ph] chromosome) with the resultant formation of a fusion gene product *bcr-abl* (Figure 1). In 2001, management of the disease changed dramatically with the approval and clinical use of imatinib mesylate (Gleevec), the first tyrosine kinase inhibitor (TKI) targeting the BCR-ABL1 oncoprotein.

Epidemiology and Risk Factors

The worldwide incidence of CML is 1 to 2 cases per 100,000 adults. In the United States, the disorder accounts for approximately 11% to 15% of all new adult cases of leukemia annually. CML is predominately a disorder of adults with a median age at diagnosis of 55 to 60 years. The disease has a slight predominance to males, with a male-to-female ratio of 1.4 to 1.0. The number of patients living with CML is expected to continually increase as a result of successful management of the disorder with TKI therapy. Other than prior radiation exposure, little is known regarding potential risk factors. No specific genetic or familial predisposition to the pathogenesis of CML has been identified.

Pathogenesis

The reciprocal translocation between chromosomes 9 and 22 giving rise to the Ph chromosome is key to the pathogenesis of CML. There is an exchange of genetic material with a portion of the Abelson murine leukemia *(abl1)* gene on the long arm of chromosome 9 relocating next to the breakpoint cluster region *(bcr)* on the long arm of chromosome 22. The presence of the newly formed Ph chromosome (t9;22)(q34;q11.2) is a characteristic

rearrangement seen in approximately 95% of CML cases. This leads to the creation of a hybrid oncogene *bcr-abl1*, which in turn translates into a BCR-ABL1 protein. There are three distinct breakpoint regions in the *BCR* gene, and each one is associated with a unique disease phenotype. The transcript from the most common breakpoint region (major breakpoint cluster region [M-BCR]) is translated into the p210BCR-ABL1 oncoprotein with the molecular consequence of constitutive tyrosine kinase activity. This leads to activation of signal-transduction proteins and upregulation of several key signaling pathways (RAS, JAK/STAT, and PI-3-kinase) with consequential alterations in cellular proliferation, differentiation, adhesion, and survival.

The clinical course of CML can be divided into three distinct phases of the disorder: the chronic phase, in which the vast majority (90% to 95%) of patients are diagnosed, or the more aggressive accelerated and blast phases. The malignant clone acquires additional mutations with time with subsequent progression to the advanced phases of CML. The aberrations most commonly seen at the chromosomal level include trisomy 8, amplification of t(9,22), abnormalities in chromosome 17, trisomy 19, trisomy 21, and monosomy 7, which if present at diagnosis may have a negative prognostic impact on survival. Changes at the molecular level (e.g., *bcr-abl1* kinase domain mutations) are associated with clinical resistance to TKI therapy.

Clinical and Laboratory Characteristics

The malignant disorder of hematopoietic stem cells produces marked myeloid hyperplasia in the bone marrow and resultant uncontrolled proliferation of myeloid cells, erythroid cells, and platelets in the peripheral blood. Up to 50% of CML patients in the United States are asymptomatic at diagnosis and have abnormalities only noted on routine physical examination or with the presence of abnormalities on a complete blood count (CBC). Clinical manifestations seen at presentation include fatigue, weight loss, splenomegaly leading to abdominal fullness and early satiety, malaise, and acute gouty arthritis. Laboratory findings include a markedly elevated white blood cell count (~100,000/μL) with a differential consisting of various stages of granulocyte maturation from myeloblasts to mature neutrophils. There is presence of absolute basophilia and often associated absolute eosinophilia. The findings of an elevated platelet count and anemia can be seen at presentation in approximately 20% to 30% and 50% of patients, respectively. High levels of lactate dehydrogenase (LDH) and uric acid can be seen as a result of increased cellular turnover associated with the disorder.

Without therapy, a patient in the chronic phase of CML will eventually progress to the more aggressive phases in 3 to 5 years. A consensus is lacking on the definition of accelerated phase; however, common features include an increase in the number of peripheral blood myeloblasts and basophils, development of low platelet counts, or discovery of additional clonal cytogenetic abnormalities. The definition of *blast phase* by the International Bone Marrow Transplant Registry (IBMTR) uses criteria of at least 30% blasts in the peripheral blood or bone marrow, or the presence of extramedullary infiltrates of the clonal leukemic cells. The blast phase of CML presents clinically like acute leukemia (30% having a lymphoid morphology, 60% as acute myeloblastic leukemia, and the remainder as megakaryocytic or undifferentiated) with worsening constitutional symptoms, anemia, and bleeding tendencies.

Diagnosis

Clinical suspicion of a CML diagnosis is made from a patient presenting with the typical laboratory abnormalities with or without any physical manifestations (see the Current Diagnosis box earlier in this chapter). Examination of a peripheral blood smear reveals increased neutrophils and immature circulating myeloid cells, increased basophils and eosinophils, a normal to increased number of platelets, and possible normocytic anemia. Obtaining a bone marrow examination with aspirate is essential in the initial workup of a CML patient to appropriately stage the

Figure 1 Schematic of the formation of Philadelphia chromosome (the new chromosome 22) and its physiological consequences. (From Chen, et al. *Protein Kinase Inhibitors as Sensitizing Agents for Chemotherapy*, Fig. 2.1. Elsevier, 2019.)

disorder and to assess for the presence of the Ph chromosome by cytogenetics. The routine cytogenetic study is valuable to evaluate for clonal evolution denoted by the presence of additional karyotypic changes, which may poorly affect prognosis. Utilizing fluorescence in situ hybridization (FISH) or reverse transcriptase polymerase chain reaction (RT-PCR) amplification studies for the detection of the *bcr-abl1* hybrid gene or its transcripts is important both as a baseline confirmatory test for CML and its continued monitoring. FISH analysis has the ability to detect the *bcr-abl1* molecular anomaly using specific probes targeting the chimeric oncogene among interphase nuclei in the peripheral blood. Qualitative RT-PCR can reveal the presence of bcr-abl1 transcripts, whereas continued monitoring of CML patients for the amount of residual disease can be assessed by obtaining quantitative RT-PCR levels. The techniques involving FISH analysis and RT-PCR have both demonstrated high concordance in simultaneous sampling of peripheral blood and bone marrow specimens.

Differential Diagnosis

At presentation, CML can be routinely differentiated from leukemoid reactions, which typically have lower white blood cell counts, absence of basophilia, and presence of Döhle bodies and toxic vacuolation of granulocytes. Temporary extreme neutrophilia and associated left shift can be present after corticosteroid use. The detection of *bcr-abl1* can aid in differentiating CML from other myeloproliferative disorders (essential thrombocytosis, polycythemia vera), chronic neutrophilia leukemia, chronic myelomonocytic leukemia, chronic eosinophilia leukemia, chronic basophilic leukemia, or myelodysplastic syndromes. Rarely, patients can have *bcr-abl1*-negative or atypical CML in which additional mutations *(CSF3R, KRAS/NRAS, SETBP1)* may be present and are associated with a poor outcome.

Prognosis

The introduction of imatinib mesylate and additional TKIs in the 2000s has changed a dismal prognosis of CML into a manageable chronic disorder with a near-normal lifespan. Before the current TKI-based era, the median survival for patients with CML was 5 to 7 years. Oral chemotherapeutics (hydroxyurea [Hydrea] and busulfan [Busulfex, Myleran]) and injectable interferon alfa (interferon alfa-2b [Intron A][1] and peginterferon alfa-2a [Pegasys][1]) were important in achieving hematologic remissions, reducing thrombotic complications, and increasing median survival. Allogeneic stem cell transplantation (allo-SCT) remains a vital option for patients with advanced phases of CML or following failure of multiple TKIs.

CML prognostic scoring systems (Sokal, Euro) have traditionally used basic hematologic data, spleen size, and age to stratify patients into risk groups. Compared with the prior conventional cytotoxic-based scoring systems (Sokal), the new EUTOS Long Term Survival (ELTS) score considers the current TKI treatment era, and age does not hold such a negative impact in the scoring.

The mainstay of managing CML is continuation of long-term TKI therapy to maintain a remission. This has resulted in most patients achieving a normal life expectancy. More recently, there has been a greater acceptance to the concept of TKI therapy discontinuation in carefully chosen patients, for example, chronic phase patients with a minimum TKI therapy duration of 3 years and sustained deep molecular remission of at least 2 years. In such patients, there is an emphasis on more frequent molecular testing and monitoring for adverse events associated with discontinuation (TKI withdrawal syndrome). The recent success of maintaining prolonged treatment-free remission (TFR) is promising. Importantly, in patients who lost a major molecular response (MMR), nearly all were able to regain their response with prompt resumption of TKI treatment.

Monitoring Response to Tyrosine Kinase Inhibitor Therapy

First-line TKI use in CML is aimed at achieving a maximal reduction of leukemia burden with the goal of obtaining a complete cytogenetic response within 12 months of therapy initiation. Peripheral CBCs with differential are frequently ordered until a complete hematologic response is achieved. Quantitative RT-PCR (international scale [IS]) is followed every 3 months to assess for residual *bcr-abl1* transcripts relative to *abl1* transcripts and for the degree of molecular response. Cytogenetics and FISH analysis can be helpful in patients with atypical translocations and atypical *bcr-abl1* transcripts and in those with additional chromosome abnormalities. Milestones of hematologic, cytogenetic, and molecular response to therapy and monitoring recommendations are summarized in Tables 1 and 2. Testing for *bcr-abl1* kinase mutations is recommended in patients who fail to achieve a timely optimal response or display resistance/loss of response to a first-line TKI. Salvage therapy consists of alternative TKI use or consideration of allo-SCT for advanced phases of CML.

Treatment

There are currently four TKIs approved for first-line CML: imatinib (Gleevec), dasatinib (Sprycel), nilotinib (Tasigna), and bosutinib (Bosulif). Each of these TKI therapeutic agents are acceptable options for a patient with newly diagnosed chronic phase CML. The decision of which TKI to choose is dependent on a variety of factors including patient comorbidities, drug toxicity profile, cost, and disease characteristics.

In 2001, the development of imatinib mesylate (Gleevec) changed the treatment landscape for patients with CML. The first-generation TKI was established as the standard of care for first-line patients with chronic phase CML following the International Randomized Study of Interferon Versus STI571 (IRIS) trial. A total of 1106 patients with chronic phase CML were randomized to receive imatinib (400 mg daily) versus interferon alfa (Intron-A)[1] (5 million units/m² daily) plus low-dose cytarabine (Cytosar) (20 mg/m² daily for 10 days per month). At 18 months, the imatinib

TABLE 1	Milestones for Treating Chronic Myelogenous Leukemia Expressed as BCR-ABL1 on the International Scale		
	OPTIMAL*	**WARNING**	**FAILURE**
Baseline	NA	High-risk ACA, high-risk ELTS score	NA
3 months	≤10%	>10%	>10% if confirmed within 1–3 months
6 months	≤1%	>1%–10%	>10%
12 months	≤0.1%	>0.1%–1%	>1%
Any time	≤0.1%	>0.1%–1%, loss of ≤0.1% (MMR)†	>1%, resistance mutations, high-risk ACA

*For patients aiming at treatment-free remission, the optimal response (at any time) is BCR-ABL1 ≤0.01% (MR⁴). A change of treatment may be considered if MMR is not reached by 36 to 48 months.
†Loss of MMR (BCR-ABL1 >0.1%) indicates failure after TFR.
⁴Not yet approved for use in the United States.
ACA, Additional chromosome abnormalities in Ph+ cells; ELTS, EUTOS long-term survival score; MMR, major molecular response; NA, not applicable; TFR, treatment-free remission.
From Hochhaus A, Baccarani M, Silver RT, et al.: European LeukemiaNet 2020 recommendations for treating chronic myeloid leukemia, *Leukemia* 34(4):966–984, 2020.

TABLE 2	European LeukemiaNet Definitions and Monitoring Recommendations	
HEMATOLOGIC RESPONSE	**CYTOGENIC RESPONSE**	**MOLECULAR RESPONSE**
Definitions		
Complete: Platelet count <450 × 10⁹/L WBC count <10 × 10⁹/L Differential without immature granulocytes and with <5% basophils Nonpalpable spleen	Complete: Ph+ 0% Partial: Ph+ <35% Minor: Ph+ 36–65% None: Ph+ >95%	Complete: transcript nonquantifiable and nondetectable Major: ≤0.10
Monitoring		
Check every 2 wk until complete response achieved and confirmed, then every 3 mo unless otherwise required	Check at 3 and 6 mo, then every 6 mo until complete response achieved and confirmed; thereafter every 12 mo if molecular monitoring cannot be ensured; check always for occurrence of treatment failure or unexplained cytopenia	Check every 3 mo until major response is achieved; conduct mutation analysis in case of failure, suboptimal response, or increase in transcript level

Ph, Philadelphia chromosome; *WBC*, white blood cell.
From Baccarani M, Saglio G, Goldman J, et al: Evolving concepts in the management of chronic myeloid leukemia: Recommendations from an expert panel on behalf of the European LeukemiaNet, *Blood* 108(6):1809–1820, 2006; Baccarani M, Cortes J, Pane F, et al.: Chronic myeloid leukemia: an update of concepts and management recommendations of European LeukemiaNet, *J Clin Oncol* 27(35):6041–6051, 2009.

arm was found to have superior outcomes including tolerability, hematologic response, complete cytogenetic response (76.2% vs. 14.5%, P <.001), and freedom from progression to advanced phase (accelerated or blast) CML (96.7% vs. 91.5%, P <.001). Long-term outcomes revealed that the imatinib-assigned group had an overall survival rate of 83.3%, a cumulative complete cytogenetic response rate of 83%, and a 10-year MMR rate of 93%. Because of the high crossover rate from the interferon alfa plus cytarabine arm, no comparative survival benefit was seen with use of the TKI.

The suggested starting dose of imatinib is 400 mg once daily taken with a meal. Higher doses (600 mg daily or 800 mg daily) are associated with increased toxicity without proven overall survival benefit. Although well tolerated by most patients, common side effects include superficial edema, muscle cramps, abdominal pain, nausea, rash, and diarrhea. Patients should be routinely assessed for low blood counts (cytopenias), and those with liver or kidney impairment may require closer monitoring and dose adjustments. Since its introduction, the cost of brand-name imatinib has risen from $30,000 per year to an annual price of $140,000, illustrating the financial toxicity associated with potential long-term TKI-based therapy for CML. Since 2015, the availability of generic imatinib has reduced the annual cost in the United States, albeit the price remains higher compared with other regions of the world.

Second-generation TKIs approved for first-line chronic phase CML include dasatinib (Sprycel), nilotinib (Tasigna), and bosutinib (Bosulif). Compared with the use of imatinib, these agents have demonstrated faster and deeper responses as well as less disease progression to the advanced accelerated and blast phases. Thus second-generation TKIs may be the preferred choice for chronic phase CML patients with high-risk disease.

The phase III Evaluating Nilotinib Efficacy and Safety in Clinical Trials—Newly Diagnosed Patients (ENESTnd) trial evaluated the efficacy and safety of nilotinib versus imatinib in 846 newly diagnosed chronic phase CML patients. Patients in the nilotinib (300 mg twice daily) arm were shown to have improved cumulative rates of MMR (77.7% vs. 62.5%, P <.0001) compared with imatinib 400 mg daily, with no difference in 10-year progression-free survival (86.2% vs. 87.2%). There are increased rates of ischemic heart disease, ischemic cardiovascular events, and peripheral artery disease among those treated with nilotinib, especially at a higher dose (400 mg twice daily). Additional adverse events associated with nilotinib therapy include elevation in blood glucose levels, headaches, rash, QTc prolongation, pancreatitis, and increased liver enzyme levels.

The Dasatinib versus Imatinib Study in Treatment-Naïve Chronic Myeloid Leukemia Patients (DASISON) was a randomized trial of 519 patients with first-line chronic phase CML assigned to dasatinib (100 mg daily) or imatinib (400 mg daily). Treatment with the second-generation TKI demonstrated earlier and more robust MMR rates at 3 months (84% vs. 64%, P <.0001) and deeper molecular response with 4.5-log reduction of *bcr-abl1* transcripts (<0.0032 IS, MR4.5) (42% vs. 33%).

Dasatinib therapy is associated with less nausea, rash, and muscle aches. Patients should be monitored for potential low blood counts and the development of pleural effusions. We await longer follow-up for a recent trial, which has shown effective activity of lower-dose dasatinib (50 mg daily) with a more acceptable safety profile.

In the Bosutinib Versus Imatinib for Newly Diagnosed Chronic Myeloid Leukemia (BFORE) randomized trial, the bosutinib (400 mg daily) arm achieved significantly higher MMR rates (47% vs. 37%, $P = .02$) and complete cytogenetic response rates (77% vs. 66%, $P = .007$) at 12 months compared with imatinib (400 mg daily) therapy. There were similar rates of 2-year survival with both drugs. Patients taking the second-generation TKI are more likely to experience gastrointestinal adverse effects (diarrhea, liver enzyme elevation), which may necessitate dose reductions and temporary holding of the medication.

The preference of using a second-generation TKI as the initial treatment of chronic phase CML should be performed in the context of the available data, understanding the unique side-effect profile of each drug, assessing the cost-effectiveness of long-term treatment, and appropriate patient selection. The ability to achieve response milestones faster and with a deeper response (MR4.5 rates) displays the potential of using second-generation TKIs for patients in whom eventual TKI discontinuation would be considered. The lack of overall survival benefit of these agents compared with imatinib seen in clinical trials could be secondary to effective salvage therapy.

Continuation of long-term therapy with TKIs can be difficult for the patient and provides additional challenges to the treating physician. Routine monitoring for and managing TKI-associated toxicities is as vital as regular assessment of disease response. Despite many short- and long-term toxicities from TKIs graded as mild, they have resulted in poorer patient-reported quality-of-life scores and often can lead to treatment nonadherence. Newly prescribed medications should also be assessed for potential drug-drug interactions with the TKI, which may require dose adjustments.

Other Therapeutic Options

Patients on first-line TKI who fail to meet treatment response milestones, display intolerance to the medication, or have progression/relapse should be assessed for treatment adherence and evaluated for possible drug interaction affecting TKI metabolism. Bone marrow examination should be performed to ensure that the patient has not progressed to an advanced phase of the disease. Often acquisition of novel point mutations in *bcr-abl1* leads to treatment resistance. Determining the type of mutation guides appropriate switching to an alternative TKI. Most of the mutations displaying resistance to imatinib therapy can be overcome by the use of a second-generation TKI. These have the ability to once again achieve high rates of response, especially when compared with increased doses of imatinib (400 mg twice daily). The *T315I* mutation is a unique alteration that confers resistance to all available second-generation TKIs. Ponatinib (Iclusig), a third-generation TKI, is effective in heavily pretreated CML patients and is approved with activity displayed against the *T315I* mutation. However, the drug at the approved dose (45 mg daily) is associated with considerable risk of vascular occlusive disease, thrombotic events, heart failure, and hepatotoxicity. In an attempt to minimize toxicity, it is recommended to reduce the dose upon achieving *bcr-abl1* ≤1%.

In 2012, omacetaxine mepesuccinate (Synribo) subcutaneous injection was approved for patients with resistance or intolerance to two or more prior TKIs. The drug is dosed based on body surface area (1.25 mg/m²) twice daily with an induction and maintenance dosing schedule over 28-day cycles. The approval provided patients with acquired mutations, including *T315I*, an additional treatment option for their difficult-to-control disease. Treated patients should be monitored for cytopenias, bleeding, and hyperglycemia, which may necessitate dose adjustment. In 2021, asciminib (Scemblix) became the latest approved drug for chronic-phase CML patients previously treated with two or more TKIs or for those with the *T315I* mutation. In the ASCEMBL multicenter, randomized clinical trial, asciminib at a dose of 40 mg twice daily was compared with bosutinib 500 mg once daily in the pretreated specified population. The novel agent showed an improvement in MMR rate (25% vs. 13%, $P = 0.029$) compared with bosutinib in addition to a lower discontinuation rate (7% vs. 25%) as a result of adverse reactions. A second trial showed asciminib's ability to be an effective option for chronic phase CMP patients presenting with the *T315I* mutation. The drug was given at 200 mg twice daily and showed an achievement of MMR at 24 weeks in 42% of the patients with the difficult-to-treat mutation status. Dose adjustments may be necessary for hematologic toxicities, hypertension, hypersensitivity reactions, and pancreatic toxicity.

As the only curative option for patients with CML, an evaluation for allo-SCT candidacy is appropriate if optimal response is not achieved after two or more TKIs as a result of resistance, drug intolerance, or inadequate response to newer agents for those harboring the *T315I* mutation. Patients with accelerated phase CML are treated initially with TKI therapy (second or third generation preferred) and early consideration of allo-SCT based on a lack of optimal response. Blast phase CML requires a more aggressive combined approach using the newer-generation TKIs and intensive chemotherapy, followed by immediate allo-SCT in responders. For the advanced phases of the disease, TKI therapy is typically administered at a higher starting dose: imatinib 600 mg daily for accelerated phase and 800 mg daily for blast phase, dasatinib 140 mg daily, nilotinib 400 mg twice daily, bosutinib 500 or 600 mg daily, and ponatinib 45 mg daily. A list of potential palliative options includes hydroxyurea, hypomethylating agents, cytarabine, and busulfan. Unfortunately, survival in endphase CML is measured in months.

Chronic Lymphocytic Leukemia

Chronic lymphocytic leukemia (CLL) is a chronic, mature B-cell neoplasm and is the most common type of leukemia in Western countries. CLL is a heterogeneous disease, and not all patients require treatment at the time of diagnosis, as randomized trials have failed to demonstrate a survival advantage with early treatment strategies. Molecular profiling and whole-exome sequencing have led to improved understanding of the pathogenesis of CLL and significant improvements in our therapeutic approach. Historically, therapy for CLL included alkylating agents, purine analogues, and CD20-directed monoclonal antibodies. However, the treatment approach to CLL has rapidly evolved over the past several years with the advent of targeted agents such as Bruton tyrosine kinase (BTK) inhibitors, B-cell leukemia/lymphoma 2 (BCL2) inhibitors, and phosphoinositide 3-kinase (PI3K) inhibitors. The development of such agents has led to significant improvement in outcomes for these patients including those with high-risk genomic aberrations that had historically been resistant to standard chemotherapies.

Epidemiology and Risk Factors

CLL accounts for approximately 30% of all leukemias in the United States. It is a disease of older adults with a median age at diagnosis of 70 years. CLL occurs more commonly in men than in women, with a male-to-female ratio of approximately 1.7 to 1. The incidence of CLL also varies by race, with a higher incidence in Caucasians. Furthermore, the incidence of CLL in Asian countries is quite low. Although the exact reasons racial disparities exist are not clear, it appears that genetic factors are the most likely explanation. CLL does appear to be seen at a higher frequency among those with a first-degree family member with CLL. There are no clearly identified environmental or occupational risk factors. Most cases of CLL are preceded by development of monoclonal B-cell lymphocytosis (MBL). However, despite the presence of MBL, only a small portion of patients will progress to CLL at a rate of 1% to 2% per year.

Pathogenesis

CLL is a disease of clonal B-cell lymphocytes arrested in B-cell differentiation. The pathogenesis of CLL is complex, and many steps in the developmental pathway have yet to be elucidated. Nevertheless, the development of CLL appears to follow a two-step process in which one first develops MBL due to an unknown event (i.e., gene mutation, epigenetic changes, cytogenetic abnormalities, antigenic stimulation) resulting in proliferation of a clone of B cells. A second event or "hit" occurs (i.e., further cytogenetic changes), leading to accumulation of the malignant clone and subsequent progression to CLL. Malignant cells accumulate as a result of their inability to undergo apoptosis. This is thought to be mediated by overexpression of anti-apoptotic proteins such as BCL2. The exact cell of origin likely differs among cases specifically related to the mutational status of the immunoglobulin variable region genes. FISH detects chromosomal abnormalities in 70% to 80% of patients with CLL, and certain genetic abnormalities are clearly associated with disease prognosis (discussed later in this chapter). Furthermore, it appears that karyotypic abnormalities are acquired throughout the disease course, and such clonal evolution has been associated with progressive disease.

Clinical Manifestations

The clinical manifestations of CLL vary widely, with most patients displaying no clinical symptoms and diagnosis made by routine blood counts showing lymphocytosis. Persistent lymphadenopathy is another common presenting symptom and is present in up to 90% of patients. The spleen is the most commonly enlarged lymphoid organ, and splenomegaly is detected in up to 50% of patients. Splenomegaly can lead to a variety of clinical symptoms including abdominal discomfort or early satiety contributing to poor oral intake and weight loss. Up to 10% of patients may present with "B" symptoms such as unintentional weight loss (10% or more of body weight within previous 6 months), fevers not associated with infection, drenching night sweats, and/or profound fatigue. Importantly, patients with CLL are immunocompromised and can present with recurrent infections. Autoimmune complications of CLL should be considered including hemolytic anemia, immune thrombocytopenia, and pure red cell aplasia, to name a few. Anemia and thrombocytopenia are findings consistent with advanced disease.

Diagnosis

A diagnosis of CLL is suspected when a patient presents with lymphocytosis with an absolute lymphocyte count greater than 5000/μL. Subsequent peripheral blood flow cytometry demonstrates immunophenotypic evidence of a monoclonal B-cell population that coexpresses the T-cell antigen CD5 and B-cell surface antigens CD19, CD20 (usually low/dim expression), and CD23 (Table 3). Typically, there is a low level of surface membrane immunoglobulin (most often IgM) along with a single immunoglobulin light chain, kappa, or lambda, which confirms the clonal nature. The presence of a monoclonal B-cell population with the same immunophenotypic profile but with an absolute lymphocyte count less than 5000/μL is termed *MBL*. Bone marrow aspirate and biopsy are not required for the diagnosis of CLL but may be helpful in certain circumstances.

Differential Diagnosis

Peripheral lymphocytosis can occur in viral or other infectious processes, and immunophenotyping by peripheral flow cytometry is helpful to distinguish between reactive and malignant causes and allows one to establish the diagnosis of CLL. Caution must be taken to differentiate from other low-grade B-cell malignancies (see Table 3). Importantly, one must distinguish mantel cell lymphoma from CLL. As CLL expresses CD23, MCL is typically CD23 negative and is characterized by strong expression of cyclin D1. A lymph node biopsy should be pursued when immunophenotyping of the peripheral blood fails to yield a diagnosis.

Prognosis

Although most patients with CLL are diagnosed with early-stage disease, the prognosis and clinical course is highly heterogeneous. Historically, risk stratification using the Rai or Binet clinical staging systems have been the mainstay of predicting prognosis in clinical practice (Tables 4 and 5). Over the past several years, our understanding of the molecular biology and underlying genetic aberrations in CLL have led to complementary prognostic variables to predict survival, which are widely used in clinical practice today. FISH testing to identify cytogenetic aberrations before treatment has allowed for more robust risk stratification. Specifically, deletion of 13q and trisomy 12 are favorable prognostic abnormalities, whereas deletion of 17p and 11q are higher-risk abnormalities. Deletion of 17p and/or aberrations in *TP53* predict an aggressive disease course and refractoriness to conventional chemoimmunotherapy regimens. The mutational status of immunoglobulin heavy-chain variable genes (IGHV) is also associated with survival. Unmutated *IGHV* genes have a more aggressive clinical course and shorter survival compared with those with mutated

TABLE 3	Differential Diagnosis of Chronic Lymphocytic Leukemia by Immunophenotype					
DISEASE	CD5	CD10	CD20	CD23	SURFACE IMMUNOGLOBULIN	OTHER
Chronic lymphocytic leukemia	+	–	+ (dim)	+	+ (dim)	
B-cell prolymphocytic leukemia	±	–	+	±	+ (bright)	
Mantle cell lymphoma	+	–	+	–	+ (bright)	t(11;14)
Hairy cell leukemia	–	–	+	–	+	CD11c, CD103, CD123 positive
Lymphoplasmacytic lymphoma	– (rarely +)	–	+	±	+	Most have monoclonal IgM paraprotein. Associated with *MYD88* mutations.
Splenic marginal zone lymphoma	±	–	+	±	+ (bright)	

TABLE 4	Rai Staging System for Chronic Lymphocytic Leukemia		
RISK	**STAGE**	**CLINICAL DESCRIPTION**	
Low	0	Lymphocytosis	
Intermediate	I	Lymphocytosis + lymphadenopathy	
	II	Lymphocytosis + hepatomegaly or splenomegaly (± lymphadenopathy)	
High	III	Lymphocytosis + anemia (Hb <11 g/dL)	
	IV	Lymphocytosis + thrombocytopenia (<100,000/µL)	

TABLE 5	Binet Staging System for Chronic Lymphocytic Leukemia	
STAGE	**CLINICAL DESCRIPTION**	
A	Two or less lymphoid areas enlarged	
B	Three or more lymphoid areas enlarged	
C	Anemia (<10 g/dL) or thrombocytopenia (<100,000/µL)	

IGHV genes. Other prognostic factors have also been identified such as lymphocyte doubling time, Beta-2 microglobulin levels, expression of CD38 by flow-cytometry, and ZAP-70 expression in addition to clinical factors (i.e., age, sex, performance status). The CLL-IPI score has been validated by several groups and uses five independent prognostic factors: TP53 deletion and/or mutation, IGHV mutational status, serum B2-microglobulin concentration, clinical stage, and age. This has identified four distinct prognostic subgroups with 5-year overall survival rates ranging from 93% in the low-risk group to 23% in the very-high-risk group. More recently, the International Prognostic Score for Early-stage CLL (IPS-E) scoring system has been developed to predict time to first treatment in early-stage, asymptomatic patients. This system identified three covariates independently correlated with time to first treatment including unmutated IGHV genes, absolute lymphocyte count greater than 1500/µL, and the presence of palpable lymphadenopathy. However, it should be noted that none of these prognostic scoring systems have yet to affect the decision of when to initiate therapy.

Treatment

Not all patients with CLL require treatment at the time of diagnosis. In fact, recent data suggest that although early therapy for high-risk, asymptomatic patients postpones the development of active disease, there is increased toxicity associated with therapy and no clinical data to suggest that such outcomes lead to improved long-term survival. Thus CLL-directed treatment is only indicated for those with active disease as defined by the International Workshop on Chronic Lymphocytic Leukemia Treatment (i.e., progressive marrow failure, symptomatic splenomegaly, bulky lymphadenopathy, rapid lymphocyte doubling time, and/or constitutional symptoms). Therapy for patients with active disease has rapidly evolved over the past several years. It is important to note, however, that patients with advanced CLL are not cured with conventional therapy, thus treatment is directed at alleviating symptoms, improving quality of life, and prolonging survival. With the incorporation of monoclonal antibodies into standard therapy with purine analogues, we began to see significant improvements in patient outcomes, with prolonged remissions in some patients. Additionally, the development of BTK and BCL2 inhibitors has yielded a significant advancement in the treatment of advanced-stage CLL leading to deep remissions, prolonged progression-free survival, and improved overall survival. Importantly, such therapies have yielded marked improvement in outcomes in patients with high-risk disease who historically do not respond or relapse soon after conventional chemoimmunotherapy. Nevertheless, CLL remains an incurable disease, short of allo-SCT.

First-Line Therapy

The choice of first-line therapy in CLL should be made based on patient characteristics and patient preferences/goals as well as on tumor characteristics. Typically, the preferred initial therapy depends on genetic risk stratification and the patient's ability to tolerate therapy. Genetic risk stratification is typically based on IGHV mutational status and the presence of 17p deletion or TP53 mutation. Patients with IGHV-unmutated disease with or without 17p deletion or TP53 mutations are typically treated with targeted agents such as BTK inhibitors or BCL2 inhibitors with or without monoclonal antibodies. For those with IGHV-mutated disease without 17p deletions or TP53 mutations, conventional chemoimmunotherapy and targeted therapy remain treatment options, with no single agreed-upon standard treatment.

First-line therapy with fludarabine (Fludara), cyclophosphamide (Cytoxan), and rituximab (Rituxan) (FCR) has historically been the most commonly used chemoimmunotherapy combination. The addition of rituximab (Rituxan) to fludarabine and cyclophosphamide represented significant progress in the treatment of CLL, with an overall response rate approaching 95% and a complete response rate of 70%. FCR remains an acceptable initial treatment option for younger patients with active disease, specifically those with IGHV-mutated disease who do not harbor 17p deletions or TP53 mutations. For older adult patients (>65 years of age) or those who cannot tolerate FCR, the combination of bendamustine (Treanda) and rituximab (Rituxan) (BR) offers similar efficacy with improved tolerability compared with FCR. Again, BR is a reasonable first-line therapy for those with IGHV-mutated disease without a 17p deletion or TP53 mutation only.

BTK inhibitors such as ibrutinib (Imbruvica) and acalabrutinib (Calquence) and the BCL2 inhibitor venetoclax (Venclexta) are highly effective therapies that have been shown to improve progression-free survival and overall survival. In patients with high-risk disease (17p deletion and/or TP53 mutations or IGHV unmutated), treatment with targeted agents are preferred given improved outcomes demonstrated in multiple clinical trials. In those with standard-risk disease (IGHV-mutated without 17p deletion or TP53 mutation), chemoimmunotherapy and targeted agents appear to be similar in efficacy, and the choice of which agent to use must be individualized. There remains a lack of clinical data directly comparing targeted agents, and the choice of which agent to use must be based on patient preferences and comorbidities. Of note, data from a recent phase III study comparing ibrutinib to acalabrutinib (Calquence) in patients with previously treated disease shows similar efficacy but fewer cardiovascular adverse events with acalabrutinib. Based on this, acalabrutinib is approved by the U.S. Food and Drug Administration (FDA) as initial or subsequent treatment for adults with CLL. Thus options include single-agent ibrutinib (Imbruvica) with or without rituximab (Rituxan) or obinutuzumab (Gazyva) for younger patients or the combination of venetoclax plus obinutuzumab (Gazyva) or acalabrutinib (with or without obinutuzumab). Although the combination of ibrutinib plus venetoclax has shown promise in early studies, this is not yet recommended in routine clinical practice.

Other Therapeutic Options

Treatment of relapsed disease in those who achieve at least a partial remission to first-line therapy requires assessment of time to progression from prior therapy. Early relapse is considered for those who experience disease progression at a shorter interval than the median expected for that treatment (i.e., within 5 to 6 years of targeted therapy and 2 to 3 years of FCR). Targeted therapy with *BTK* inhibitors or *BCL2* inhibitors is the preferred treatment at the time of relapse, with the choice of therapy depending on numerous factors including patient preferences, comorbidities, and first-line therapy received. Additionally, PI3K inhibitors idelalisib (Zydelig) plus rituximab and duvelisib (Copiktra) have gained FDA approval for patients with relapsed CLL after one or two prior lines of therapy, respectively.

Hematopoietic stem cell transplantation remains the only curative therapy for CLL; however, the ideal timing is not clear, and data are limited in nature. Perhaps more important is the associated considerable treatment-related morbidity and mortality. Chimeric antigen receptor T-cell (CAR-T) therapy has been investigated in patients with relapsed or refractory CLL and has shown promising activity in early-phase studies with complete response rates in the largest series of ~28%. Further work is needed to better define the role of CAR-T therapy in patients with relapsed CLL. Patients with relapsed CLL should be encouraged to participate in ongoing clinical trials.

Complications

The most common complications that occur in patients with CLL are related to intrinsic immune dysfunction. Specifically, patients with CLL have abnormal immune responses and thus are at a high risk for infectious complications. Infections are the major cause of mortality in patients with CLL, and patients with recurrent major bacterial infections should be considered for intravenous immunoglobulin therapy (IVIg) (Gammagard S/D). Anemia can be related to direct bone marrow infiltration or hypersplenism. In such circumstances, CLL-directed therapy results in improvement in anemia. Additionally, autoimmune hemolytic anemia and pure red cell aplasia can also occur. Similarly, thrombocytopenia may be related to autoimmune destruction, hypersplenism, or disease burden. CLL transformation to aggressive B-cell lymphomas (most commonly diffuse large B-cell lymphoma), called Richter's transformation, is seen in 5% to 10% of patients. Patients with CLL have a higher risk of secondary malignancies, both hematologic and solid tumors. A retrospective review of the Surveillance, Epidemiology and End Results (SEER) program showed that ~11% of patients with CLL developed a secondary solid tumor. Thus appropriate screening must be undertaken in this population.

References

Condoluci A, Bergamo T, Langereins P, et al: International prognostic score for asymptomatic early-stage chronic lymphocytic leukemia, *Blood*, 2020. https://doi.org/10.1182/blood.2019003453.

Faderl S, et al: The Biology of Chronic Myeloid Leukemia, *N Engl J Med* 341:164–172, 1999.

Hallek M, Shanafelt T, Eichhorst B: Chronic lymphocytic leukemia, *Lancet* 391(10129):14–20, 2018.

Hochhaus A, Baccarani M, et al: European LeukemiaNet 2020 recommendations for treating chronic myeloid leukemia, *Leukemia* 34:966–984, 2020.

Jabbour E, Kantarjian H: Chronic myeloid leukemia: 2020 update on diagnosis, therapy and monitoring, *Am J Hematol* 95:691–709, 2020.

Rawstron AC, Bennett FL, O'Connor SJ, et al: Monoclonal B-cell lymphocytosis and chronic lymphocytic leukemia, *N Engl J Med* 359:575–583, 2008.

Siegel RL, Miller KD, Jemal A: Cancer statistics, CA Cancer, *CA Cancer J Clin* 70(1):7, 2020.

DISSEMINATED INTRAVASCULAR COAGULATION

Method of
Kenneth Byrd, DO

CURRENT DIAGNOSIS

- Disseminated intravascular coagulation (DIC) is an abnormal activation of the coagulation system that is caused by predisposing conditions such as sepsis, malignancy, and trauma.
- Clinical manifestations include organ injury due to microvascular thrombosis and less commonly macrovascular thrombosis. DIC can alternatively present with severe bleeding.
- Laboratory findings include thrombocytopenia, elevated D-dimer, elevated international normalized ratio (INR) and partial thromboplastin time (PTT), and sometimes decreased fibrinogen.
- The International Society on Thrombosis and Haemostasis (ISTH) scoring system predicts overt DIC if score ≥5.

CURRENT TREATMENT

- Aggressive and prompt treatment of the underlying condition causing DIC is paramount.
- If the patient is bleeding or undergoing a procedure, aggressive transfusion support with platelets and fresh frozen plasma (FFP) or cryoprecipitate is often advised.
- Unless the patient is bleeding or undergoing a procedure, FFP or cryoprecipitate is usually not indicated, and platelets are only transfused if less than 20×10⁹/L. The major exception is acute promyelocytic leukemia (APL).
- Prophylactic low-molecular-weight heparin (LMWH) is often indicated in DIC.
- Therapeutic heparin/LMWH is rarely indicated in DIC unless there is clear evidence of a severe prothrombotic state.
- No other treatments are routinely used for DIC, including antithrombin, activated protein C, antifibrinolytics, and thrombomodulin. However, the role of these agents continues to be evaluated.

Introduction

Disseminated intravascular coagulation (DIC) is a complex and often life-threatening manifestation of an acquired disease process. This process is initiated by a strong procoagulant cascade that leads to microthrombi throughout the vasculature. A risk of hemorrhage often follows due to a depletion of platelets, consumption of coagulation factors, and accelerated plasmin formation.

Epidemiology

DIC has been reported in approximately 10% to 20% of critical care admissions. It is an independent predictor of mortality and the risk of death in a patient with sepsis is doubled when accompanied by DIC. Mortality rates vary based on the scoring system used but can be as high as 46%. The mortality rate appears to correlate with the severity of laboratory abnormalities at diagnosis.

Pathophysiology

DIC is primarily a coagulation dysfunction due to excessive procoagulant activity. The overactivation is multifactorial but is mainly due to the generation of excessive thrombin, which is mediated by the extrinsic pathway involving tissue factor and factor VIIa. Thrombin excess leads to increased platelet aggregation and thrombotic occlusion of small and midsize vessels with fibrin. Vascular occlusion leads to the derangement of oxygen supply and tissue demand, which can compromise multiple organs. This effect is compounded by defects in inhibitors of coagulation along with fibrinolytic suppression. Antithrombin activity is diminished due to increased consumption, degradation, and impaired synthesis. Likewise, protein C, tissue factor-pathway inhibitor (TFPI), and thrombomodulin activity are decreased in part due to excess inflammatory cytokines. Fibrinolytic suppression occurs in many instances of DIC due to an increase in plasminogen activator inhibitor-1 (PAI-1), which is the principal inhibitor of the fibrinolytic system.

The excessive activation of the coagulation pathway predictably leads to the depletion of platelets and clotting factors. However, the cause of bleeding in DIC is multifactorial, including consumption of clotting factors, thrombocytopenia, platelet dysfunction, endothelial damage, and excess fibrin degradation products (FDPs) that cause feedback anticoagulant effect.

Clinical Manifestations

The manifestations of DIC are often obscured by the underlying causative etiology. Many times, the diagnosis of DIC is solely laboratory based without any clear clinical manifestations. At other times, DIC may be overtly symptomatic. Recently, it has been suggested that DIC could be divided into clinical subtypes that include asymptomatic, bleeding, and organ failure types. The presentation depends on whether there is a predominance of thrombosis from excessive thrombin activation or bleeding from consumptive coagulopathy.

Overall, the incidence of major bleeding in DIC is 5% to 12%. DIC that presents with acute bleeding is most commonly seen in acute leukemia, obstetric disorders, and trauma. Typical hemorrhagic features of DIC include bleeding from venipuncture sites or indwelling catheters, generalized ecchymosis that develops spontaneously or with minimal trauma, bleeding from mucous membranes, unexpected and major bleeding from around drain sites or tracheostomies, and concealed hemorrhage in serous cavities such as retroperitoneal hemorrhage.

Thrombotic organ failure type of DIC is most commonly seen with sepsis. The incidence of organ involvement secondary to thrombosis is 10% to 40%. This occurs due to thromboses in small and midsize vessels. Many organs can be involved, but it is most commonly seen in the kidneys, lungs, liver, and brain. This can manifest as respiratory distress syndrome, acute kidney injury, confusion, and seizures. The skin can also be involved and present as purpura fulminans or acral ischemia. Macrovascular thrombosis such as venous thromboembolism may present as a later manifestation. COVID-19 frequently presents with a DIC-like coagulopathy. Unlike classic acute DIC, fibrinogen is often elevated and there is excessive thrombotic risk.

Diagnosis

Making the diagnosis of DIC starts with identifying an underlying associated disease state. Table 1 lists the known risk factors for DIC. Once this is established, the diagnosis entails a combination of laboratory values along with an analysis of the clinical presentation. The difficulty with diagnosing DIC is that there is no gold standard and no pathognomonic test. There have been several scoring systems developed for DIC to assist in standardizing the diagnosis. The most commonly utilized is the International Society on Thrombosis and Haemostasis (ISTH) scoring system, which was originally devised in 2001 and has been subsequently validated. The scoring system is outlined in Table 2. A score of ≥5 suggests overt DIC. A score of < 5 indicates a lack of DIC or nonovert DIC (i.e., subtle and compensated hemostatic dysfunction). The ISTH scoring system has a sensitivity of 93% and a specificity of 98%. Most other available scoring systems are more sensitive but less specific for DIC. Importantly, if DIC is suspected but not confirmed, then labs should be repeated to assess trends.

TABLE 1 Risk Factors for Disseminated Intravascular Coagulation (Incidence of Disseminated Intravascular Coagulation Per Etiology)

- Sepsis (35%)
  - Most commonly bacterial
- Severe trauma (up to 50%)
  - Most commonly brain injury or burns
- Malignancy
  - Metastatic cancer (up to 20%)
  - Acute leukemia (15%)
  - Acute promyelocytic leukemia (90%)
  - COVID-19
- Obstetrical
  - Placental abruption
  - Amniotic fluid embolism
  - Postpartum hemorrhage
  - Acute fatty liver of pregnancy
- Vascular malformations
  - Kasabach-Merritt syndrome
  - Large aortic aneurysms
  - Other large vascular malformations
- Severe immunologic reaction
  - Acute hemolytic transfusion reaction
  - Anaphylaxis
- Heat stroke
- Postcardiopulmonary resuscitation

TABLE 2 International Society on Thrombosis and Haemostasis Scoring System

Platelet count × 10^9/L
- ≥100 = 0
- <100 = 1
- <50 = 2

Fibrin marker levels (D-dimer, fibrin degradation products)
- No increase = 0
- Moderate increase (>ULN but <5× ULN) = 2
- Strong increase (≥5× ULN) = 3

Prothrombin time
- <3 s (*INR <1.3) = 0
- ≥3 but <6 s (*INR 1.3–1.5) = 1
- ≥6 s (*INR ≥1.6) = 2

Fibrinogen
- >100 mg/dL = 0
- ≤100 mg/dL = 1

*Assuming the International Survey Index value of the thromboplastin reagents used is close to 1
- A score of ≥5 points is compatible with overt DIC
- The scoring system is only appropriate in patients with an underlying disorder that can be associated with DIC
- If the score if <5 and DIC is still suspected, then consider repeating labs in 1–2 days

DIC, Disseminated intravascular coagulation; *ULN*, upper limits of normal.

The decreased platelet count in DIC is due to excessive thrombin activation and is almost always less than 100 × 10^9/L and often trending down. A normal platelet count without a downward trend would essentially rule out DIC. The INR and PTT are often elevated due to consumption of coagulation factors but can be normal in up to 50% of cases. The vast majority of DIC is also marked by an increase in fibrin-related markers due to increased fibrinolysis. Traditionally, FDPs were used but have largely been replaced by D-dimer. Fibrinogen is traditionally decreased in DIC but is often normal as it frequently surpasses compensated consumption only later in the clinic course. It can also be falsely normal or even elevated as it is an acute phase reactant. It is only rarely severely diminished. A fibrinogen level of <100 mg/dL is seen in <50% of DIC and usually reflects the late, severe, consumptive stage of DIC.

TABLE 3 Differential Diagnosis of Disseminated Intravascular Coagulation

DISEASE	SIMILARITIES	DIFFERENCES	COMMENTS
Liver disease	Low plt; prolonged PT/PTT; low fibrinogen; increased FDP (DIC > Liver disease)	No schistocytes in liver disease; worsening labs in DIC and more stable in liver disease	Factor VIII not very helpful for differentiation. Normal or elevated in liver disease (not synthesized in liver). However, as an acute phase reactant, often normal or elevated in DIC
Thrombotic microangiopathy (TMA)	Low plt; increased FDP (DIC > TMA); decreased ADAMTS13 (TMA lower than DIC)	MAHA in TMA; normal PT/PTT and fibrinogen in TMA; numerous schistocytes common in TMA, but not DIC	Extremely low plt with normal PT/PTT is common in TMA but unusual in DIC; TMA includes TTP, HUS, secondary TMAs
Heparin-induced thrombocytopenia (HIT)	Low plt, increased FDP	Normal PT/PTT in HIT; low fibrinogen unusual in HIT	Plt <20 × 10⁹/L is uncommon in HIT
Catastrophic antiphospholipid syndrome (CAPS)	Low plt; increased FDP; PTT elevation (false elevation of PTT commonly due to LA)	Normal PT in CAPS; lab diagnosis of APLS in CAPS	Normal plt often seen in CAPS and severe thrombocytopenia is rare; microvascular thromboses in both; macrovascular thrombosis is a more common initial presentation of CAPS than DIC
Hemophagocytic lymphohistiocytosis (HLH)	Low plt; prolonged PT/PTT; low fibrinogen; increased FDP	HLH with very high ferritin, TGs, organomegaly, and often hemophagocytosis	

APLS, Antiphospholipid antibody syndrome; *DIC*, disseminated intravascular coagulation; *FDP*, fibrin degradation products; *LA*, lupus anticoagulant; *MAHA*, microangiopathic hemolytic anemia; *plt*, platelet count; *PT*, prothrombin time; *PTT*, partial thromboplastin time; *TG*, triglycerides; *TTP*, thrombotic thrombocytopenic purpura.

Thromboelastography (TEG) and rotational thromboelastometry (ROTEM) testing have been evaluated to assess overall coagulation, including platelet function, and clot dissolving potential. TEG has demonstrated good correlation with clinically important organ dysfunction and survival, although its advantage over usual coagulation assays has not yet been confirmed. The role of these two modalities in DIC is still unclear.

DIC often presents with a small population of schistocytes. If the red blood cell population is > 10% schistocytes, then an alternative diagnosis is more likely (i.e., TMA). Of note, a low ADAMTS13 can be seen in DIC but is usually >30%. There is also frequently a reduction in antithrombin and protein C. These tests are not done routinely and are likely not as sensitive as the ISTH scoring system. Finally, factor VIII can be low in DIC due to consumption, but it can also be elevated at times as it is an acute phase reactant.

The differential diagnosis of DIC is explained in Table 3.

Therapy

The foundation of treatment for DIC is to treat the underlying disorder. If the underlying disorder is reversed, then DIC typically resolves.

During active DIC there may be a need for transfusion support. It is important to note that the following transfusion recommendations are mostly based on low-quality evidence, including expert opinion. In the presence of bleeding, platelet transfusions should be given to keep platelet count greater than 30 to 50 × 10⁹/L. Similarly, in the setting of invasive procedures, platelets should be maintained greater than 20 to 50 × 10⁹/L, depending on the risk of the procedure. Importantly, in the absence of bleeding or procedure, platelets should be transfused only if platelet count is less than 20 × 10⁹/L (a range of 10 to 30 × 10⁹/L has been proposed by various sources). The exception to this threshold would be acute promyelocytic leukemia (APL), in which platelets should be maintained greater than 30 to 50 × 10⁹/L even in the absence of bleeding (less commonly some suggest a 20 × 10⁹/L threshold).

A similar approach to the replacement of factors is indicated. If the patient is bleeding or undergoing a high risk procedure and fibrinogen is less than 150 mg/dL or PT/PTT is greater than 1.5 upper limits of normal (ULN), then fresh frozen plasma (FFP) or cryoprecipitate is recommended. Keep in mind that FFP contains all factors of the soluble coagulation system, while cryoprecipitate contains a concentrated subset of plasma factors including fibrinogen, factor VIII, von Willebrand factor, and factor XIII. The choice between FFP and cryoprecipitate is made on a case-by-case basis and can often be influenced by fluid status. The recommended dose of FFP is 15 to 30 mL/kg and cryoprecipitate is 5 to 10 units. A less frequently used option is 2 g of fibrinogen concentrate. Factor replacement is not indicated in the absence of bleeding or procedure. An exception to this threshold is APL, in which factor replacement could be considered if fibrinogen is less than 100 to 150 mg/dL, even in the absence of bleeding.

In addition to transfusion support and treatment of the underlying etiology, heparin[1] can be considered in a few circumstances. Most importantly, guidelines recommend prophylactic heparin or low-molecular-weight heparin (LMWH)[1] in the absence of bleeding as long as platelet count is greater than 20 to 30 × 10⁹/L, INR greater than 1.5, and fibrinogen greater than 100 mg/dL. This is especially vital in prothrombotic DIC (i.e., sepsis, solid tumor malignancy). An exception to the general use of LMWH prophylaxis is in hyperfibrinolytic DIC (i.e., APL and prostate cancer), in which more caution is advised with heparin use. Therapeutic heparin is uncommonly advised in DIC, but it can be considered in prothrombotic DIC, as evidenced by thromboembolism, purpura fulminans, or acral ischemia. As heparin can partially inhibit activation of the coagulation, it would make sense that it could help offset DIC. In small studies, heparin has shown beneficial effects on coagulation parameters. However, improvement in clinically important outcomes in DIC has not been clearly demonstrated.

---

[1]Not FDA approved for this indication.

Other therapies that have been studied in the treatment of DIC include antithrombin concentrate (AT [Thrombate III]),[1] activated protein C (APC), recombinant thrombomodulin, and antifibrinolytics. Currently, these agents are rarely, if ever, indicated for use. AT and APC have been extensively studied in the setting of sepsis. One of the issues in assessing the benefit of AT and APC is that many clinical trials assess the general sepsis population and do not limit analysis to those specifically with DIC. For AT, there has been no significant reduction in mortality in these studies. However, there is a suggestion that there may be significant benefit in the subset of patients with severe sepsis and DIC. This requires prospective validation. APC has also shown promise at times, including improvement in mortality in an early randomized controlled trial (RCT). However, subsequent studies showed an increased risk of serious bleeding and lack of survival benefit. Therefore, the FDA advised to stop using APC for DIC in 2011.

Caution is advised with the use of antifibrinolytics in DIC. Since the excessive fibrin deposition appears in part to be due to insufficient fibrinolysis, further inhibition of the fibrinolytic system would clearly not be appropriate. This is especially the case in sepsis, but there are a few exceptions to this. Antifibrinolytics can be considered in hyperfibrinolytic DIC (i.e., APL or prostate cancer) only in the setting of life-threatening bleeding. The other exception is in acute trauma. A large RCT showed that early use of antifibrinolytics in trauma was beneficial. However, once the acute phase has passed, further thrombin generation eventually predominates, and the balance is tipped toward thrombosis.

Recombinant soluble thrombomodulin continues to be actively evaluated and shows some potential. While efficacy outcomes have been heterogeneous, a 2020 meta-analysis suggested a 28-day mortality benefit of recombinant thrombomodulin[5] in patients with sepsis and coagulopathy. Results of ongoing studies are pending.

Finally, it is worth mentioning that a Cochrane review evaluated recombinant factor VIIa (NovoSeven)[1] and concluded that it does not have proven efficacy in DIC and that there is an increased risk of arterial thrombotic events. Its use is not advised.

[1]Not FDA approved for this indication
[5]Investigational drug in the United States.

References

Asakura H, Ogawa H: COVID-19-associated coagulopathy and disseminated intravascular coagulation, *Int J Hematol* 113(1):45–57, 2021.

Bakhtiari K, Meijers JC, de Jonge E, Levi M: Prospective validation of the International Society of Thrombosis and Haemostasis scoring system for disseminated intravascular coagulation, *Crit Care Med* 32(12):2416–2421, 2004.

Bernard GR, Vincent JL, Laterre PF, et al: Efficacy and safety of recombinant human activated protein C for severe sepsis, *N Engl J Med* 344(10):699–709, 2001.

Gando S, Levi M, Toh CH: Disseminated intravascular coagulation, *Nat Rev Dis Primers* 2:16037, 2016.

Levi M: Pathogenesis and diagnosis of disseminated intravascular coagulation, *Int J Lab Hematol* 40:15–20, 2018.

Levi M, Scully M: How I treat disseminated intravascular coagulation, *Blood* 131(8):845–854, 2018.

Sanz MA, Grimwade D, Tallman MS, et al: Management of acute promyelocytic leukemia: recommendations from an expert panel on behalf of the European Leukemianet, *Blood* 113(9):1875–1891, 2009.

Squizzato A, Hunt BJ, Kinasewitz GT, et al: Supportive management strategies for disseminated intravascular coagulation, *ThrombHaemost* 116(05):896–904, 2016.

Valeriani E, Squizzato A, Gallo A, et al: Efficacy and safety of recombinant human soluble thrombomodulin in patients with sepsis-associated coagulopathy: A systematic review and meta-analysis, *J Thromb Haemost* 18(7):1618–1625, 2020.

Wada H, Thachil J, Di Nisio M, et al: Guidance for diagnosis and treatment of disseminated intravascular coagulation from harmonization of the recommendations from three guidelines, *J ThrombHaemost* 11(4):761–767, 2013.

Warren BL, Eid A, Singer P, et al: High-dose antithrombin III in severe sepsis: a randomized controlled trial, *JAMA* 286(15):1869–1878, 2001.

HEMOCHROMATOSIS

Method of
Heinz Zoller, MD

CURRENT DIAGNOSIS

- Consider diagnosis in patients with symptoms of iron overload such as fatigue, grayish-brown discoloration of the skin, arthralgias, diabetes, cardiac arrhythmia, or sexual dysfunction.
- High transferrin saturation (TSAT) and a low unbound iron-binding capacity are the clinical biochemical hallmarks of hemochromatosis.
- In patients with high TSAT, homozygosity for the p.Cys282Tyr (C282Y) in the *HFE* gene confirms hemochromatosis genetically.
- Hemochromatosis can be phenotypically diagnosed when transferrin saturation is high, hepatic iron is increased, and spleen iron content is normal.
- Magnetic resonance imaging (MRI) with R2* sequences allows noninvasive quantification of liver and spleen iron.
- Liver biopsy may be required for disease staging or when MRI is not available.
- Genetic testing beyond *HFE* genotyping by multiple gene sequencing can yield alternative genetic hemochromatosis causes but is not necessary for diagnosis because phenotypic diagnosis is sufficient to initiate treatment.

CURRENT TREATMENT

- Management of hemochromatosis requires disease staging and the assessment of hepatic fibrosis, glucose metabolism, heart function, and arthropathy.
- In patients with onset of hemochromatosis before the age of 20 years, left ventricular function, thyroid function, and pituitary function should be assessed.
- Serum ferritin is a surrogate marker for the severity of iron overload but is also increased by inflammation, alcohol intake, and the metabolic syndrome.
- In patients with hemochromatosis with hepatic fibrosis, endocrine, skeletal, and cardiac complications should be recognized and treated accordingly.
- Patients with hemochromatosis with iron overload should be treated by phlebotomy weekly or every other week to achieve a serum ferritin less than 50 ng/mL while avoiding anemia.
- After a ferritin less than 50 ng/mL has been achieved, phlebotomy frequency should be reduced to maintain ferritin less than 100 ng/mL; most patients will require two to six phlebotomies per year.
- Siblings of patients with hemochromatosis should be tested.

Definition and Pathogenesis

Hemochromatosis is defined as a genetic disease caused by deficiency of the hormone hepcidin, which normally controls plasma iron concentrations. The clinical surrogate for hepcidin deficiency is elevated transferrin saturation or low unbound iron-binding capacity (UIBC). Under physiologic conditions, transferrin saturation is maintained in the range of 15% to 45% by hepcidin, which inhibits iron release from cells, mainly the recycling macrophages in the spleen and resorptive duodenal enterocytes. Consequently, hemochromatosis is associated with high intestinal iron absorption, high liver iron concentrations, and low spleen iron. In

Figure 1 Algorithm summarizing the diagnostic path in patients with suspected hemochromatosis.

hemochromatosis, liver iron is increased because elevated transferrin saturation (>65%) results in *nontransferrin-bound iron* in the plasma. The nontransferrin-bound iron is removed from the circulation by hepatocytes. Tissue damage in hemochromatosis has been proposed to result from excess iron in hepatocytes and from redox-active nontransferrin-bound iron in circulation.

Epidemiology

The prevalence of hemochromatosis in populations of European ancestry is about 1 in 1000. The disease is typically diagnosed between 40 and 60 years of age. Hemochromatosis is about four times more common in males than in females. The most common genotype associated with hemochromatosis, present in about 80% to 95% of patients with phenotypic hemochromatosis, is homozygosity for C282Y in the *HFE* gene. This genotype has a prevalence of approximately 1:400 among populations of Northern European ancestry. This means that cumulative lifetime penetrance of hemochromatosis, defined as elevated transferrin saturation and elevated ferritin in C282Y homozygotes, is less than 40%. The prevalence of the C282Y allele in different European populations is variable, ranging from <1% to 12%, with the highest prevalence in Ireland. Disease penetrance among patients homozygous for C282Y increases with age, is higher in males, and is increased by alcohol and a diet high in red meat.

Clinical Features

Fatigue is a typical but nonspecific symptom of hemochromatosis. Signs associated with hemochromatosis include joint pain, bronze discoloration of the skin or porphyria cutanea tarda, diabetes, and hepatomegaly. Advanced hemochromatosis and other coincident risk factors for liver disease, such as viral hepatitis or increased alcohol consumption, can result in progressive fibrosis and cirrhosis, as well as hepatocellular carcinoma. Iron-induced tissue damage is not restricted to the liver and can also affect the endocrine system, heart, bone, and joints. The most common

endocrine manifestation of hemochromatosis in adults is diabetes, which is significantly more common among men with hemochromatosis than in controls. Other common manifestations in adults are osteoporosis and arthropathy, which are often misclassified as rheumatoid arthritis or osteoarthritis. In patients with severe forms of hemochromatosis and early disease onset, cardiomyopathy, hypogonadotropic hypogonadism, and hypothyroidism are more common.

Diagnosis and Disease Staging

In patients with suggestive symptoms or signs of hemochromatosis and siblings of patients with hemochromatosis, the first diagnostic step is determination of transferrin saturation (TSAT) or UIBC and serum ferritin, followed by *HFE* genotyping if TSAT is increased. Iron quantification in the liver and spleen by magnetic resonance imaging (MRI) is recommended in patients with elevated TSAT who are not homozygous for C282Y. Liver biopsy is rarely required because noninvasive methods can be used for fibrosis staging (Figure 1).

Transferrin Saturation or Unbound Iron-Binding Capacity

The pathogenesis and definition of hemochromatosis are based on hepcidin deficiency, which results in elevated TSAT or low UIBC. Studies have shown that TSAT levels are highly variable upon repeat determination. A population-based study has not demonstrated additional value in repeated determination of TSAT, but, in clinical practice, it is recommended to confirm an elevated TSAT in an independent blood sample taken after an overnight fast before further evaluation is pursued in patients with low clinical suspicion of hemochromatosis.

Ferritin

High ferritin is a surrogate marker of iron overload but has limited specificity because alcohol consumption, the metabolic syndrome, and inflammatory and neoplastic diseases can also cause high serum ferritin levels. In patients with hemochromatosis and

Figure 2 Skin discoloration and impaired flexibility of the second metacarpophalangeal (MCP) joint as typical signs in a hemochromatosis patient (left hand). Normal skin color and normal MCP-joint flexibility in a control person.

the absence of any of these conditions, ferritin is correlated with the severity of iron overload. In hemochromatosis, provisional iron overload is defined as the presence of high TSAT and high ferritin levels (males and postmenopausal women >300 ng/mL and women of childbearing potential >200 ng/mL).

Transferrin or Total Iron-Binding Capacity
At physiologic concentrations, iron in circulation is mainly bound to the protein transferrin. Transferrin or total iron-binding capacity is increased in patients with iron deficiency and can be mildly decreased in patients with iron overload. It has limited diagnostic value for the diagnosis of hemochromatosis but is important in the differential diagnosis. In patients with inflammation, alcohol consumption, or end-stage liver disease, the transferrin protein itself can be markedly reduced, resulting in an increased transferrin saturation.

Genetic Testing
Genotyping for the C282Y variant in the *HFE* gene (rs1800562) is recommended in patients with suspected hemochromatosis and repeatedly elevated transferrin saturation. In such patients, homozygosity for the C282Y variant confirms the diagnosis. Because of incomplete penetrance, for patients diagnosed with C282Y homozygosity and with a normal TSAT and normal serum ferritin, a genetic risk for the development of iron overload can be asserted, but the genotype alone is not sufficient for the diagnosis of hemochromatosis. In such individuals, lifestyle modifications (see later) and follow-up are recommended.

A minority of patients with phenotypic hemochromatosis are compound heterozygous for the C282Y and the H63D variant in the *HFE* gene. Because of the high allele frequency of H63D, compound heterozygosity is more common that C282Y homozygosity, though the penetrance of this genotype is much lower than in C282Y homozygotes. Patients with compound heterozygosity with provisional iron overload (elevated TSAT and high ferritin) should be evaluated for the presence of iron overload by MRI and for the coincidence of additional risk factors, including the metabolic syndrome, iron-loading anemias, or alcohol intake. The same applies to patients homozygous for H63D.

Magnetic Resonance Imaging
Quantification of liver and spleen iron can be performed noninvasively by special protocols on MRI. The so-called R2* frequency, expressed in s^{-1} or Hertz (Hz), is directly proportional to tissue iron concentration, where an R2* value of greater than 70 Hz in the liver and greater than 60 Hz in the spleen indicate iron overload in the respective organ. In patients with provisional iron overload (high ferritin and elevated TSAT) who are not homozygous for the C282Y variant, MRI is recommended (Figure 2). The presence of elevated liver iron in the absence of spleen iron overload confirms

the phenotypic diagnosis of hemochromatosis. In patients with elevated liver and spleen iron, other causes of iron overload are typically found, including a history of repeated transfusions, IV iron therapy, or high alcohol intake. A rare genetic cause, important in the differential diagnosis for increased iron concentrations in the liver and spleen, is loss-of-function variants in the cellular iron export pump ferroportin, which is encoded by the SCL40A1 gene. The most common cause of high ferritin with variable TSAT and normal liver iron is the metabolic syndrome. In such patients, hepatic steatosis is present and, in more advanced cases, hepatic and spleen iron can be mildly elevated. An alternative genetic cause for high ferritin with normal liver iron are genetic variants in the 5′ untranslated region of the L-ferritin mRNA.

Fibrosis Assessment
Liver fibrosis is a common complication of hepatic iron overload. In all patients diagnosed with hemochromatosis, the degree of liver fibrosis should be assessed. In the absence of clinically evident cirrhosis, the first step in fibrosis assessment is calculation of the FIB-4 score from patient age, alanine aminotransferase (ALT) level, aspartate aminotransferase (AST) level, and platelet count. A FIB-4 score of less than 1.3 rules out advanced fibrosis, and no further testing is recommended in such patients. As age is an important determinant for the stage of fibrosis, higher cutoff values have been recommended in patients older than 65 years. In patients with hepatomegaly, ferritin greater than 1000 ng/mL and elevated ALT or AST, advanced fibrosis cannot be ruled out. Before elastography became widely available, liver biopsy was recommended. Studies have shown that noninvasive fibrosis assessment by vibration controlled transient elastography has a reasonable predictive value for the diagnosis and exclusion of fibrosis. Hence liver biopsy is now only required for disease staging in hemochromatosis patients with a FIB-4 score of greater than 1.3 and indeterminate results on transient elastography, between 6.5 and 12 kPa.

Liver Biopsy and Hepatocellular Carcinoma Surveillance
Introduction of noninvasive iron quantification by MRI and noninvasive fibrosis assessment by FIB-4 followed by elastography have greatly reduced the need for liver biopsy. Liver biopsy is still recommended in patients with contraindications for MRI, indeterminate readings on elastography, or diagnostic uncertainty. In patients with advanced fibrosis on noninvasive fibrosis assessment or cirrhosis on liver biopsy, surveillance for early detection of hepatocellular carcinoma by biannual abdominal ultrasound should be strongly considered. As treatment can be associated with the regression of cirrhosis, fibrosis stage can be reassessed after excess iron has been removed. In patients with regression of cirrhosis, discontinuation of hepatocellular carcinoma surveillance can be considered.

Family Screening
The majority of patients with hemochromatosis are homozygous for C282Y. The autosomal recessive nature of this *HFE*-associated hemochromatosis renders family screening of siblings cost-effective. In families with three or more children, testing the unaffected spouse before testing the children is also cost-effective. In patients with "non-*HFE* hemochromatosis," genetic testing by sequencing of a gene panel that includes but is not limited to *HFE* can be performed but is not required to initiate treatment because in such patients the diagnosis is based on phenotypic criteria. Rarely, hemochromatosis can be caused by autosomal dominant gain-of-function mutations in SCL40A1, which should be included in the gene panel and also prompt family screening.

Treatment
Phlebotomy
In patients with hemochromatosis and iron overload as indicated by elevated ferritin or on liver MRI, iron removal by phlebotomy is recommended. Phlebotomy can reduce fatigue, prevent progression of fibrosis, and may revert cirrhosis in some patients. Hemochromatosis arthropathy, which can currently only be treated

symptomatically, typically does not respond to phlebotomy. In the initial treatment phase, phlebotomy should be performed weekly or every other week by removing 500 mL of blood after anemia has been excluded by quantifying the hemoglobin concentration. Serum ferritin should be determined every 3 months during the initial treatment phase or when the patient develops anemia, which should ideally be avoided. The treatment goal during the initial phase is a serum ferritin less than 50 ng/mL while avoiding the development of anemia. Once this target has been achieved the patient should enter maintenance treatment with increased time intervals between phlebotomies. As phlebotomy does not correct the genetic cause of hemochromatosis, iron can reaccumulate and maintenance treatment is recommended. The rate of iron reaccumulation is highly variable, and treatment intervals must be individualized. The target ferritin during this treatment phase is serum ferritin in the range of 50 to 100 ng/mL. To achieve this goal, serum ferritin should be checked every 3 months because most patients require two to six phlebotomies per year.

Second-Line Treatment

Erythrocyte apheresis has been shown to be effective in reducing fatigue and achieving target ferritin in clinical trials and has been associated with fewer procedures, milder hemodynamic changes, and shorter treatment duration to achieve treatment targets. Apheresis depends on local availability, local expertise, and reimbursement.

Oral iron chelators are not approved for hemochromatosis, but in patients with needle phobia, limited venous access, or poor tolerance of hemodynamic changes associated with phlebotomy, treatment with oral iron chelators can be considered.

Hepcidin mimetics and drugs that indirectly stimulate hepcidin production are under development and could offer additional benefits in the future, especially in patients with increased transferrin saturation despite having achieved the recommended treatment targets for serum ferritin.

Dietary Recommendations

The most important dietary recommendation in patients with hemochromatosis is to minimize or avoid alcohol consumption. Diets high in bioavailable iron, such as red meat, and high in citrus fruits, which enhance iron absorption, should be reduced. Proton pump inhibitors, low-iron diets, and the intake of coffee or tea can reduce the rate of iron reaccumulation but do not replace phlebotomy. Hemochromatosis patients should avoid handling of raw seafood because of the risk of fulminant infections with *Vibrio vulnificus*.

Summary

Hemochromatosis should be diagnosed before arthropathy, cirrhosis, or heart failure have developed. Early initiation of phlebotomy can prevent these complications and normalize life expectancy. Well-defined diagnostic criteria and the availability of genetic testing can guide physicians and patients to early diagnosis and the prevention of disease complications by phlebotomy.

References

Adams PC, Reboussin DM, Barton JC, et al: Hemochromatosis and iron-overload screening in a racially diverse population, *N Engl J Med* 352:1769–1778, 2005.

Adams PC, Reboussin DM, Press RD, et al: Biological variability of transferrin saturation and unsaturated iron-binding capacity, *Am J Med* 120:999 e1–7, 2007.

Allen KJ, Gurrin LC, Constantine CC, et al: Iron-overload-related disease in HFE hereditary hemochromatosis, *N Engl J Med* 358:221–230, 2008.

Bardou-Jacquet E, Morandeau E, Anderson GJ, et al: Regression of fibrosis stage with treatment reduces long-term risk of liver cancer in patients with hemochromatosis caused by mutation in HFE, *Clin Gastroenterol Hepatol* 18:1851–1857, 2020.

Hagstrom H, Ndegwa N, Jalmeus M, et al: Morbidity, risk of cancer and mortality in 3645 HFE mutations carriers, *Liver Int* 41:545–553, 2021.

Le Lan C, Loreal O, Cohen T, et al: Redox active plasma iron in C282Y/C282Y hemochromatosis, *Blood* 105:4527–4531, 2005.

Legros L, Bardou-Jacquet E, Latournerie M, et al: Non-invasive assessment of liver fibrosis in C282Y homozygous HFE hemochromatosis, *Liver Int* 35:1731–1738, 2015.

Pilling LC, Tamosauskaite J, Jones G, et al: Common conditions associated with hereditary haemochromatosis genetic variants: cohort study in UK Biobank, *BMJ* 364:k5222, 2019.

Rombout-Sestrienkova E, Nieman FH, Essers BA, et al: Erythrocytapheresis versus phlebotomy in the initial treatment of HFE hemochromatosis patients: results from a randomized trial, *Transfusion* 52:470–477, 2012.

Vancloster A, van Deursen C, Jaspers R, et al: Proton pump inhibitors decrease phlebotomy need in HFE hemochromatosis: double-blind randomized placebo-controlled trial, *Gastroenterology* 153:678–680.e2, 2017.

Valenti L, Corradini E, Adams LA, et al. Consensus statement on the definition and classification of metabolic hyperferritinaemia. *Nat Rev Endocrinol* 2023:1-12.

Viveiros A, Schaefer B, Panzer M, et al: MRI-based iron phenotyping and patient selection for next-generation sequencing of non-homeostatic iron regulator hemochromatosis genes, *Hepatology* 74:2424–2435, 2021.

HEMOLYTIC ANEMIAS

Method of
Thomas G. DeLoughery, MD

CURRENT DIAGNOSES

- Suspect hemolysis when anemia is accompanied by signs of red cell breakdown: high low-density lipoprotein (LDH) and indirect bilirubin with a low haptoglobin.
- The reticulocyte count is often high.
- A positive direct antibody test (DAT) confirms the diagnosis of autoimmune hemolytic anemia in the presence of hemolysis.
- In patients with non-immune hemolysis, specific testing is required to make the diagnosis.

At the most basic level, hemolytic anemias are caused by red cell destruction. This destruction can be caused by factors that are either intrinsic or extrinsic to the red blood cell (RBC). The pace of the hemolysis can vary from being only detectable by laboratory abnormalities to fulminant acute severe anemia. A useful way to think about hemolytic anemias is to divide them into hereditary disorders and acquired disorders (Table 1). Defects in any part of the RBC lead to inherited disorders, while acquired disorders are caused by immune-related processes and other etiologies extrinsic to the RBC.

Pathophysiology
Congenital

The major components of the RBC are the membrane, hemoglobin, and enzymes; therefore the three major classes of hereditary hemolytic anemias are caused by defects in any of these three red cell components.

Hereditary spherocytosis is the most common hemolytic anemia caused by membrane defects. This condition is caused by mutation in the proteins that make up the red cell skeleton, which leads to an unstable membrane. The RBCs in hereditary spherocytosis initially have a normal biconcave disc structure, but after repeated passage through the spleen, they gradually lose portions of the membrane and become more spherical as they age (a process known as *splenic conditioning*). These spherocytes are less deformable and because of that are ultimately trapped and destroyed in the spleen. Less common anemias caused by membrane defects are hereditary elliptocytosis and pyropoikilocytosis. The skeletal defects are not as profound in elliptocytosis, so the clinical presentation is usually milder. Most patients with pyropoikilocytosis are homozygous for mutations that cause elliptocytosis and have very unstable red cell membranes; often fragments of RBCs are seen in the circulation.

The most common RBC enzyme defect is glucose-6-phosphate dehydrogenase (G6PD) deficiency. An adequate supply of reduced glutathione (GSH) is necessary to protect the erythrocyte from oxidative damage. G6PD catalyzes the conversion of glucose-6-phosphate to 6-phosphogluconate, in the process reducing NADP to NADPH. NADPH is necessary for the conversion of glutathione (GSSG) to reduced glutathione (GSH). The erythrocyte does not have any other source of NADPH and so is dependent solely

TABLE 1	Hemolytic Anemia: Classification of Common Causes

Congenital

Membrane defects

Hereditary spherocytosis

Hereditary elliptocytosis

Hereditary pyropoikilocytosis

Enzymatic defects

G6PD deficiency

Pyruvate kinase deficiency

Hemoglobin defects

Sickle cell disease

Unstable hemoglobins

Acquired

Autoimmune

Warm antibody IgG

Cold antibody IgM

Drug-induced

Paroxysmal nocturnal hemoglobinuria

Mechanical

Microangiopathic

Toxins

Parasites

on this pathway for reducing power. When G6PD is deficient, this leads to decreased NADPH, which results in decreased GSH. When the RBC undergoes oxidative stress, this lack of reducing power results in damage of red cell proteins, especially hemoglobin. These damaged proteins can aggregate, causing membrane damage and red cell destruction as the crystallized proteins are removed by the spleen.

Pyruvate kinase (PK) deficiency is a hemolytic anemia caused by an enzymatic defect in the glycolytic pathway. Pyruvate kinase catalyzes conversion of phosphoenolpyruvate (PEP) to pyruvate, generating ATP in the same reaction. Deficiency of PK results in decreased levels of erythrocyte ATP. Lack of ATP results in a leaky cell membrane and loss of water and potassium. This leads to cellular dehydration and rigid, nondeformable cells that are susceptible to destruction within the spleen.

By far the most common hereditary hemolytic hemoglobin defect is sickle cell anemia. The abnormal hemoglobin protein forms long polymers that disrupt red cell integrity. There are also very rare defects in hemoglobin that can cause unstable molecules that can crystallize and lead to hemolysis—most often resulting from splenic removal of damaged proteins.

Acquired

Autoimmune hemolytic anemias (AIHAs) can be mediated by either anti–red cell IgG or IgM antibodies. In IgG-mediated disease, the antibody binds to red cell membrane proteins. The antibody-coated RBCs are then phagocytized by macrophages found primarily in the spleen, leading to hemolysis.

In IgM-mediated hemolysis (cold agglutinin disease), the antibody binds to the RBC most often in the periphery of the body. The cold appellation comes from the fact that the antibody binds more strongly when below body temperature. Most commonly, complement is fixed only through C3, and then the C3-coated RBCs are taken up by the macrophages. In rare patients, the IgM can fix complement rapidly, leading to intravascular hemolysis by formation of the end product of complement, the membrane attack complex.

Rare patients can develop immune hemolysis induced by medication. There have been three mechanisms proposed for drug AIHA. The hapten mechanism is most often associated with the use of high-dose penicillin. High doses of penicillin lead to drug incorporation into the red cell membrane by binding to proteins. Another mechanism is the formation of an immune complex of drug, antibody, and red cell membrane which leads to hemolysis. Finally, patients taking certain drugs such as methyldopa will develop a positive direct antibody (DAT) after 6 months of therapy and hemolysis that is indistinguishable from warm antibody AIHA.

In paroxysmal nocturnal hemoglobinuria (PNH), RBCs lack the regulatory membrane proteins that inhibit activated complement proteins. These proteins include membrane inhibitor of reactive lysis (CD59) and decay accelerating factor (CD55). The molecular defect in PNH is a mutation of the phosphatidyl inositol glycan complementation group A (PIG-A) gene located on the X chromosome. This enzyme is required for synthesis of glycosyl phosphatidylinositol (GPI)-linked proteins. Cells derived from the PNH stem cells are deficient in all proteins that are linked to the membrane by a GPI molecule, including those that inactivate complement. Normally there is baseline activation of complement; it is thought that one of the functions of RBCs is inactivation of these active complement proteins. When activated complement binds PNH RBCs instead of being destroyed, the resulting membrane attack complex leads to lysis of the RBC.

Microangiopathic hemolytic anemias (MAHAs) result from destruction of circulating RBCs. Although MAHA is commonly associated with thrombotic microangiopathies such thrombotic thrombocytopenia purpura (TTP) and hemolytic uremic syndrome (HUS), there are many other possible associated disease states. For example, patients with malignant hypertension can have very severe hemolysis resulting from increased shearing of RBCs traversing damaged glomeruli. There may also be associated thrombocytopenia, which can lead to concern that TTP may be present. Hemolysis associated with malignant hypertension resolves rapidly with control of the blood pressure. Scleroderma renal crisis is often accompanied by a MAHA due to both severe hypertension and renal damage.

Cardiac valvular disease can lead to MAHA. This is seen most commonly after mitral valve repair if there is a small defect at the site where the valve ring is sewn in. Ventricular contraction leads to a small resurgent jet that results in a high shear situation in the jet and red cell destruction. In some cases, this can result in severe hemolysis and a transfusion-dependent anemia.

Ventricular-assist devices (VADs) to support heart failure patients can also lead to hemolysis. This is blood flowing through the device being subjected to high shear rates. Most patients have low levels of hemolysis, but with VAD thrombosis there is an abrupt increase in hemolysis because of higher shear forces; an increasing LDH is an indication to look for VAD thrombosis.

Along with MAHA, there are several other syndromes which may cause mechanical damage to RBCs. Clostridium infections can lead to hemolysis by direct damage to red cell membranes. The bacteria secrete an alpha-toxin that has phospholipase activity and leads to the red cell membrane literally dissolving, which causes the hemoglobin to leak out of the cells. In some cases, this can be so severe that the measured hemoglobin may equal the hematocrit. Empty red cell "ghosts" may be seen on the smear.

Wilson disease may cause episodes of hemolysis along with the neurologic and hepatic disease. This is caused by large amounts of hepatic copper entering the circulation and inducing an oxidative hemolysis. The smear can show spherocytes and bite cells (RBCs with defects caused by splenic conditioning). The hemolysis is often transient as it is related to high levels of copper in the serum.

Spur cell anemia is a hemolytic process seen in patients with end-stage liver disease. The lipid metabolism alterations induced

TABLE 2	Drugs That May Precipitate a Hemolytic Crisis with G6PD Deficiency
Acetanilide[4]	
Dapsone	
Furazolidone[2]	
Isobutyl nitrate[4]	
Methylene blue	
Nalidixic acid[2]	
Naphthalene	
Nitrofurantoin (Macrobid)	
Pamaquine[2]	
Phenazopyridine (Pyridium)	
Phenylhydrazine	
Primaquine	
Quinolones	
Sulfacetamide	
Sulfamethoxazole	
Sulfanilamide	
Sulfapyridine	

by severe liver disease lead to cholesterol crystal formation in the red cell membrane. These crystals are removed by the spleen and can lead to both hemolysis and deformed RBCs (spur cells).

Prevention

There are a few supportive steps in patients with hemolysis. Although most food is supplemented with folate, high red cell turnover can increase the need for this vitamin. Patients with hemolysis are often supplemented with folic acid 1 mg daily.[1]

A key preventive measure for those with G6PD deficiency is avoiding agents that can lead to oxidative stress of RBCs. The most complete list of medications found at https://www.g6pd.org/ and common medications are listed in Table 2. Some rarer red cell enzymatic or hemoglobin defects are also sensitive to oxidative stress, so these medications also should be avoided in those diseases.

Clinical Manifestations

Inherited

The severity of congenital hemolytic anemia varies tremendously. Some children are very symptomatic right after birth, while older patients may only present with mild anemia and subtle laboratory findings. A common presentation is a burst of hemolysis with oxidative or other stressors. Hereditary hemolytic anemias are often more severe right after birth, and severity may decrease with age. Patients with congenital anemia can have presentation with extrahematologic problems. Given that the serum bilirubin is increased and more bilirubin is excreted in the bile, they may present with pigmented gallstones. Patients can present with gallbladder disease in their teens or 20s, and this should raise suspicion of a hemolytic anemia. These patients may be more prone to skin ulcers around the ankle that may not heal well.

Classically patients with congenital hemolytic anemias can develop three types of crises. The first is the *hemolytic crisis*. When patients develop fevers or encounter other stressors, the rate of hemolysis may increase, and any inflammation can suppress erythropoiesis, leading to severe anemia. The second type

[1] Not FDA approved for this indication.

of crisis is the *megaloblastic crisis* in which patients become folic acid deficient because of high folate demand associated with increased red cell production. With mass supplementation of folate in the food supply, this incidence has decreased. The final crisis is the *aplastic crisis* in which RBC production is temporarily compromised and the reticulocyte count plummets. This is most commonly found with infections with parvovirus B-19. The infection clears in most patients within 1 week, but patients often require transfusion support during this time.

Hereditary spherocytosis is most prevalent in northern European populations and occurs with a frequency of approximately 1 in 5000. The majority of cases (75%) show an autosomal dominant pattern of inheritance. The remainder result from autosomal recessive inheritance and new mutations. Common clinical features of hereditary spherocytosis include anemia, jaundice, reticulocytosis, splenomegaly, and microspherocytes. Anemia later in life is variable and usually mild. Complications include hemolytic crises, leg ulcers, and gallstones.

With hereditary elliptocytosis, the majority of patients are asymptomatic, and the frequent finding of elliptocytes on the blood smear is of no clinical consequence. However, approximately 10% to 15% of patients have significant hemolysis and may develop anemia. Mild hereditary elliptocytosis is inherited in an autosomal dominant fashion. The incidence is higher in African and Asian populations because of its beneficial impact on malarial infection. Patients with pyropoikilocytosis have severe hemolysis.

G6PD deficiency is the most common enzyme defect in humans and affects an estimated 600 million people worldwide. G6PD deficiency is transmitted as an X-linked recessive condition. There have been hundreds of G6PD variants identified. Enzymatic activity varies from normal with no clinical consequences to severe deficiency resulting in chronic hemolysis and shortened red cell life span, even in the absence of stressors. The two most common variants are the G6PD A- variant that has moderate enzyme deficiency (10% to 15% activity), and the G6PD Mediterranean mutation that has almost no detectable enzyme activity. Despite this, patients with the G6PD Mediterranean mutation have a nearly normal erythrocyte life span except under conditions of metabolic or oxidative stress.

The classic presentation of hemolysis with G6PD deficiency is with oxidative stress. For example, certain medications such as sulfonamides can lead to increased oxidative stress. Patients with G6PD deficiency cannot generate enough reducing power to overcome this stress, which leads to oxidative damage to proteins, especially hemoglobin. The patient presents with fulminant hemolysis that can lead to a severe anemia. As a result of membrane damage, the blood smear can show spherocytes and bite cells. Treatment is removing the offending agent and is otherwise supportive. A unique presentation is *favism*. After eating fava beans, an overwhelming hemolysis develops. This can be idiosyncratic and occur even in patients who have safely eaten the beans in the past.

Pyruvate kinase deficiency is inherited as an autosomal recessive condition. Anemia is variable and may range from a presentation in early infancy requiring transfusions to fully compensated hemolysis presenting with jaundice alone. Many patients have moderate anemia, jaundice, and splenomegaly. Patients with this disorder are also susceptible to the crises identified earlier. Splenectomy may be helpful in severe cases, but response is variable.

Acquired

AIHA patients who have IgG as the offending antibody are said to have *warm antibody AIHA*. The name *warm* comes from the fact that the antibody reacts best at body temperature. The incidence varies by series but is about 1 in 100,000 patients per year, and women are more often affected than men.

Warm AIHA can complicate several diseases. Lupus patients can develop warm AIHA as part of their disease complex. Of the malignancies, the one with the strongest association with AIHA is chronic lymphocytic leukemia (CLL). Series show that 5% to 10% of patients with CLL will have warm AIHA. The disease can appear concurrently with CLL or may develop during the course of the disease.

A rare but important variant of warm AIHA is Evan syndrome. This is the combination of AIHA and immune thrombocytopenia (ITP). One to three percent of AIHA is the Evan variant. The ITP can precede, occur concurrently, or develop after the AIHA. The diagnosis of Evan syndrome should raise concern of underlying disorders. In pediatric and young adult patients, immunodeficiencies such as autoimmune lymphoproliferative disease (ALPS) must be considered. In older patients, Evan syndrome is often associated with T-cell lymphomas.

In rare patients with warm AIHA, IgA or IgM antibodies are implicated. Patients with IgM AIHA often have a severe course with a fatal outcome. Plasma may show spontaneous hemolysis and agglutination. The DAT may not be strongly positive or show C3 reactivity. The clinical clues are C3 reactivity with no cold agglutinins and severe hemolysis, sometimes with intravascular hemolysis.

In cold agglutinin disease, patients often note symptoms related to agglutination of RBCs in the peripheral circulation in addition to hemolysis. For example, acrocyanosis will be noted in cold weather. Rare patients will have abdominal pain when eating cold food resulting from ischemia related to agglutination of RBCs in the viscera. Some patients with cold agglutinins can experience exacerbation of their hemolysis with cold exposure.

In young patients, cold AIHA is often post-infectious (such as from viral and mycoplasma infections), and the course is self-limiting. The hemolysis usually starts 2 to 3 weeks after the illness and will last for 4 to 6 weeks. In older patients, the etiology in over 90% of cases is a B-cell lymphoproliferative disorder, usually with monoclonal kappa B cells. The most commonly seen are marginal zone lymphoma, small lymphocytic lymphoma, and lymphoplasmacytic lymphoma.

A unique cold AIHA is paroxysmal cold hemoglobinuria (PCH). This AIHA is most often postviral and affects children; in the past, it complicated any stage of syphilis. The antibody is IgG directed against the P antigen on the RBC. Binding is best in the "cold," but then complement is activated at body temperature. Because this antibody can fix complement, hemolysis can be rapid and severe, leading to extreme anemia.

Drug-induced AIHA is a rare drug reaction with a lower incidence than drug-related immune thrombocytopenia. The rate of severe drug-related AIHA is estimated at 1 in 1 million individuals, but less severe cases may be missed. Most patients will have positive DAT without signs of hemolysis, though rare patients will have relentless hemolysis resulting in death. With hapten-related AIHA, very few patients will have hemolysis; in these cases, the hemolysis will resolve a few days after discontinuation of the offending drug. With immune complex disease, most often the patient will only have a positive DAT, but rare patients will have life-threatening hemolysis upon exposure or reexposure. The onset of this hemolysis is rapid, with signs of acute illness and intravascular hemolysis. The classic associated drug is quinine, but many other drugs have been implicated.

A virulent form of immune complex hemolysis is associated with both disseminated intravascular coagulation (DIC) and brisk hemolysis. Patients who receive certain second- and third-generation cephalosporins (especially cefotetan and ceftriaxone) have developed this syndrome. The clinical symptoms start 7 to 10 days after receiving the drug. Often the patient has only received the antibiotic for surgical prophylaxis. Warm DAT hemolysis with an acute hematocrit decrease as well as hypotension and DIC develops. Patients are often believed to have sepsis and are then often reexposed to the cephalosporin, resulting in worsening of the clinical status. The outcome is often fatal as a result of massive hemolysis and thrombosis.

Hemolysis caused by methyldopa is indistinguishable from warm AIHA, which is consistent with the notion that methyldopa induces an autoimmune hemolytic anemia. The hemolysis often resolves rapidly after discontinuing the methyldopa, though the Coombs test may remain positive for months. This type of drug-induced hemolytic anemia has been reported with levodopa, procainamide, and chlorpromazine.

In MAHA, the course of the presentation is dictated by the underlying cause. In valvular hemolysis, the onset of hemolysis is soon after the cardiac procedure and may require transfusion support. With VAD hemolysis, most patients have only mild hemolysis, but with pump thrombosis, the hemolysis can be severe. Patients with spur cell anemia have findings of severe liver disease: high INRs and bilirubin (mean of 9.5 mg/dL). Spur cell hemolysis is associated with an ominous prognosis and average survival of a few months.

PNH is characterized by episodes of hemolysis and a propensity for thrombosis and pancytopenia. Often patients can have PNH for years before the diagnosis is made. The hemolysis can range from being well-compensated to transfusion-dependent. Patients with PNH often have a severe thrombophilia; the leading cause of morbidity and mortality (before the release of effective therapy) has been thrombosis. The cause of the hypercoagulable state is unknown, but complement-activated platelets have been implicated.

Diagnosis

There are two steps in the diagnosis of hemolytic anemia. The first step is determining the presence of hemolysis, and the second step is finding the cause. Hemolysis is demonstrated by evidence of both red cell breakdown as well as the compensatory increase in red cell production this stimulates. When RBCs undergo hemolysis, their contents, mostly hemoglobin and also the enzyme LDH, are released. Free hemoglobin is bound by haptoglobin, and the heme moiety is broken down, first to bilirubin and then to urobilinogen, which is excreted in the urine.

The following tests are performed to investigate hemolysis:

LDH: Lactic dehydrogenase is an enzyme found in high concentration in the RBC; hemolysis releases this enzyme into the plasma. Most patients with hemolysis will have an elevated LDH, making this a sensitive test. However, many other processes including liver disease, pneumonia, and so on, will also increase serum LDH.

Serum bilirubin: Heme is broken down to produce bilirubin. Initially unconjugated, the bilirubin is delivered to the liver, where it is conjugated and excreted into the bile. In hemolysis, the unconjugated (indirect bilirubin) is increased as opposed to liver disease, in which the conjugated (direct bilirubin) is increased. If a patient has coexisting liver disease with an elevated direct bilirubin, this test is not reliable.

Serum haptoglobin: Haptoglobin binds free serum hemoglobin and is taken up by the liver. Haptoglobin usually falls to very low levels in hemolysis. It is important to remember that haptoglobin is also an acute-phase reactant that can increase with systemic disease or inflammation. However, patients with advanced liver disease will have low haptoglobin as a result of lack of synthesis, and up to 2% of the population may congenitally lack haptoglobin.

Hemoglobinemia: If the hemolysis is very rapid, the amount of free hemoglobin that is released will overwhelm haptoglobin and lead to the presence of free hemoglobin in the plasma. This can be crudely quantified by examining the plasma. Even minute amounts of free hemoglobin will turn the plasma pink. In fulminant hemolysis, the serum will be cola colored.

Urine hemosiderin: When hemoglobin is excreted by the kidney, the iron is deposited in the tubules. When the tubule cells are sloughed off, they will appear in the urine. The urine can be stained for iron; if positive, this is another sign of hemolysis. This is a later sign as it takes a week for enough iron-laden tubule cells to be excreted in detectable quantities.

Mean corpuscular volume (MCV): The MCV may be larger in hemolysis for several reasons. The size of reticulocytes is larger than normal RBCs, so a brisk reticulocytosis will have a higher MCV. In cold agglutinin disease, the aggregation of RBCs will falsely increase the MCV. Finally, hemolysis can lead to folate deficiency and an increase in MCV.

Reticulocyte count: With hemolysis, the breakdown of RBCs is accompanied by an increase in the reticulocyte count as marrow

TABLE 3 Typical Blood Smear Findings in Hemolysis

Bite Cells

Oxidative hemolytic anemia such as G6PD deficiency

Elliptocytes

Heredity elliptocytosis

Schistocytes

Thrombotic thrombocytopenic purpura, valvular hemolysis

Spherocytes

Hereditary spherocytosis, autoimmune hemolytic anemia, Wilson disease, burns

Spur Cells

Severe liver disease

tries to compensate. The reticulocyte percentage must be adjusted for the hematocrit; a correct value above 1.5% is considered increased. Recently, automated complete blood count machines have taken advantage of the fact that reticulocytes will absorb certain stains, and these machines can directly measure the reticulocyte count via flow cytometry. This results in an "absolute" reticulocyte count. This does not have to be corrected for hematocrit, and levels about 90,000/µL are considered elevated. However, the reticulocyte count can also be increased in blood loss or in patients who have other causes of anemia (such as treated iron deficiency). In addition, as many of 25% of patients with AIHA will never have elevated reticulocyte counts for reasons such as nutritional deficiency, autoimmune destruction of red cell precursors, or lack of erythropoietin.

The blood smear provides vital information (Table 3). The finding of abnormal red cell shapes can be a clue to autoimmune hemolysis or red cell membrane defects. For example, spherocytes are seen in autoimmune hemolytic anemia, heredity spherocytosis, Wilson disease, clostridial sepsis, and severe burns. Schistocytes are a sign of microangiopathic hemolytic anemia and should prompt concerns for such disease processes as thrombotic thrombocytopenia purpura, valvular hemolysis, VAD, march hemoglobinuria, among many others.

In hereditary spherocytosis, the blood smear suggests the diagnosis. Confirmation is by demonstrating an increased osmotic fragility, although direct genetic screening for the molecular defects is becoming more common. The blood smear is also critical for diagnosing hereditary elliptocytosis and hereditary pyropoikilocytosis, although there is an increasing role for genetic diagnosis. Patients with hereditary pyropoikilocytosis are usually homozygous or compound heterozygous for one of the mutations causing mild hereditary elliptocytosis.

Diagnosis of G6PD deficiency is made by measuring enzyme activity. This is best performed after the hemolytic episode is over as reticulocytes have higher G6PD levels and can lead to falsely normal enzyme activity levels.

Increasingly genetic sequencing is being used to screen for inherited disorders, but more experience is required for interpretation of mutations.

AIHAs demonstrate either IgG or complement on the RBC. This is done by the *direct antibody* or *Coombs* test. IgG bound to RBCs will not agglutinate them. However, if IgM that is directed against IgG or C3 is added, the RBCs will agglutinate, proving that there is IgG and/or C3 on the red cell membrane. The finding of a positive DAT in the setting of a hemolytic anemia is diagnostic of AIHA.

There are several pitfalls to the DAT. One is that a positive DAT can be found in 1 in 1000 patients in the normal population and up to several percent of ailing patients, especially those with elevated gamma globulin such as patients with liver disease or HIV. Administration of IVIG can also create a false-positive DAT. Conversely, patients can have AIHA with a negative DAT. Some patients have a low amount of IgG binding the RBC that is below the detection limit of the DAT reagents. Other patients can have IgA or "warm" IgM as the cause of the AIHA. Specialty laboratories can test for these possibilities. The diagnosis of DAT-negative AIHA should be made with caution, and other causes of hemolysis like hereditary spherocytosis or PNH should be excluded.

The DAT in patients with cold AIHA will show cells coated with C3. The blood smear will often show agglutination of the blood, and if the blood cools before being analyzed, the agglutination will interfere with the analysis. Titers of cold agglutinin can range from 1 in 1000 to 1 in over 1 million. The autoantibodies are most often directed against the I/i antigen system, with 90% against I. The I specificity is typical with primary cold agglutinin disease and also following *Mycoplasma* infection. The i-specific antigen is most typical of Epstein-Barr and CMV infections.

In PCH, the DAT is often weakly positive but can be negative. The diagnostic test is the Donath-Landsteiner test. This complex test is performed by incubating samples in three temperature ranges: one set at 0° to 4°C, one set at 37°C, and one incubated first at 0° to 4°C and then 37°C. The diagnosis of PCH is made if only the third tube shows hemolysis.

For many patients, the first clue to drug-associated AIHA is the finding of a positive DAT in a patient taking a suspect drug (Table 4). Specialty laboratories such as Wisconsin Blood Center or the Los Angeles Red Cross can perform in-vitro studies of drug interactions that can produce a certain diagnosis.

For PNH, the diagnosis had been based on an in vitro demonstration of increased sensitivity of RBCs to complement lysis. Currently, flow cytometry is performed to examine cells for the absence of GPI-anchored proteins (CD55 or CD59 on RBCs, other GPI-anchored proteins on white blood cells).

In patients with microangiopathy, the smear will show abundant schistocytes with a marked elevated LDH.

Therapy

Splenectomy is curative for most cases of hereditary spherocytosis but is reserved for patients with severe symptoms. For patients with hereditary pyropoikilocytosis, splenectomy can also be useful.

Most patients with G6PD deficiency require no special management beyond the avoidance of provocative medications and food. Highly symptomatic patients with pyruvate kinase deficiency may respond to splenectomy, and in clinical trials, a small molecule agent that can increase enzyme activity.

Initial management of warm AIHA is prednisone starting at 1 mg/kg daily. It can take up to 3 weeks to see a response. Once the hematocrit is above 30%, the prednisone is slowly tapered. Eighty percent of patients will respond to steroids, but the steroids can be fully tapered off in only 30%. For patients who can be maintained on 10 mg or less of steroids daily, this may be the most reasonable long-term therapy.

Current data show that adding rituximab (Rituxan)[1] to steroids for warm AIHA will improve overall response and should be considered early in most patients. These responses appear to be durable, and for relapses, repeating treatment is effective. It is important to remember that, for most patients, the response to rituximab is a gradual one over months; one should not expect a rapid response. Most studies have used the "traditional" 375 mg/m² dosing weekly for 4 weeks, and another option is 1000 mg repeated once 14 days apart.

Splenectomy is now reserved for patients with warm AIHA who do not respond to steroids or rituximab. Reported response rates in the literature range from 50% to 80%, with 50% to 60% remaining in remission. Timing of the procedure is a balance between allowing time for the steroids to work versus the risk of toxicity of steroids. A patient who is at low risk associated with surgery and has either refractory disease or an inability to be weaned from high doses of steroids should have splenectomy considered early.

---

[1] Not FDA approved for this indication.

TABLE 4	Drugs Implicated in Autoimmune Hemolytic Anemia

Most Common

Cefotetan (Cefotan)

Ceftriaxone (Rocephin)

Piperacillin (Pipracil)

Fludarabine (Fludara)

Other Implicated Drugs

Acetaminophen

Amphotericin B

Beta-lactams (any)

Carboplatin (Paraplatin)

Cephalosporins (any)

Chlorpromazine (Thorazine)

Chlorpropamide (Diabinese)

Cimetidine (Tagamet)

Ciprofloxacin (Cipro)

Diclofenac (Voltaren)

Doxycycline

Enalapril (Vasotec)

Erythromycin

Isoniazid

Levodopa

Melphalan (Alkeran)

Methyldopa

Nonsteroidal antiinflammatory drugs

Omeprazole (Prilosec)

Oxaliplatin (Eloxatin)

Probenciden

Probenecid

Procainamide

Quinidine

Quinine

Rifampin

Sulfa drugs

Teniposide (Vumon)

Tetracycline

Thiazides

Thiopental (Pentothal)

Tolbutamide (Orinase)

Tricyclic antidepressants

For patients who do not respond to either splenectomy or rituximab, therapy is less certain. Although intravenous immune globulin is a standard therapy for immune thrombocytopenia, response rates are low in warm AIHA. Numerous therapies have been reported in small series, but there is no clear approach. Options include the following:

- Azathioprine (Imuran)[1] 75 to 150 mg/day
- Cyclophosphamide (Cytoxan)[1] 1000 mg monthly bolus IV
- Mycophenolate (CellCept)[1] 500 to 1000 mg bid
- Cyclosporine (Neoral)[1] 5 mg/kg daily divided in two doses
- Danazol (Danocrine)[1] 200 mg tid

Our approach has been to use mycophenolate for patients who require high doses of steroids or need transfusions. Patients who need lower doses of steroids may be good candidates for danazol to help wean them from the steroids.

The sparse literature on Evans syndrome suggests that it can be more refractory to standard therapy, with response rates to splenectomy being in the 50% range. In patients with lymphoma, antineoplastic therapy is crucial. Data is accumulating for patients with ALPS: mycophenolate or sirolimus (Rapamune)[1] starting at 2 mg/m², may be effective for splenectomy or rituximab failures.

The importance of diagnosing cold AIHA and differentiating it from warm AIHA is the fact that standard therapy for warm disease steroids is ineffective. C3-coated RBCs are taken up through the reticulo-endothelial system, especially in the liver as well as the spleen, so splenectomy is also an ineffective therapy.

Simple measures to help with cold AIHA should be employed. Patients should be kept in a warm environment and should try to avoid the cold. If transfusions are needed, they should be infused via blood warmers to prevent hemolysis. In rare patients with severe hemolysis, plasma exchange can be considered. Given the culprit antibody is IgM (mostly intravascular), use of plasma exchange can slow the hemolysis to give time for other therapies to take effect.

Therapy of cold AIHA remains difficult. Currently the drug of choice is rituximab.[1] Response can be seen in 45% to 75% of patients but is almost always a partial response; retreatment is often necessary. As with other autoimmune hematologic diseases, there can be a delay in response. There is data to support adding either fludarabine (Fludara)[1] or bendamustine (Treanda)[1] 90 mg/m² to rituximab. The response rates are higher, but so are the complications of therapy. Although more toxic, this combination can be considered in patients with aggressive disease. For acute treatment, the monoclonal antibody sutimlimab (Enjaymo) is available.

For most patients with drug-induced AIHA, discontinuing the offending drug is sufficient. It is doubtful that steroids or other autoimmune-directed therapy is effective. For patients with the DIC-hemolysis syndrome, there are anecdotes that plasma exchange may be helpful. Therapy for patients with positive DAT without signs of hemolysis is uncertain. If the drug is essential, then the patient can be observed. If the patient has hemolysis, the drug must be stopped and the patient observed for signs of end-organ damage.

Transfusions can be very difficult in AIHA. The presence of the autoantibody can interfere with typing of the blood and almost always interferes with the cross-match because this final step consists of mixing the patient's serum with donor RBCs. In most patients with AIHA, the autoantibodies will react with any donor cells, rendering a negative cross-match impossible. Without the cross-match, the concern is that underlying alloantibodies can be missed, which can lead to transfusion reactions.

Some of these concerns may be allayed by remembering that patients who have never been transfused or pregnant will rarely have alloantibodies. Secondly, a patient who has been transfused in the remote past may have an amnestic antibody response but not an immediate hemolytic reaction.

When a patient is first suspected of having AIHA, a generous sample of blood should be given to the transfusion service. This will allow for adequate testing of the sample. Secondly, many centers will test the blood not only for blood groups ABO and D but will also perform full Rh typing and check for Kidd, Duffy, and Kell status. This can allow transfusion of phenotypically matched blood to lessen the risk of alloantibody formation.

One difficult issue is timing of transfusion. Clinicians are often hesitant to transfuse patients with AIHA because of fear of reactions. But in frail patients with severe anemia, especially older adults or those with heart disease, transfusion can be lifesaving. In some cases it can take hours to screen for alloantibodies;

therefore it is often preferable to transfuse patients with severe anemia while carefully observing for reactions.

The treatment for PNH is the complement inhibitor eculizumab (Soliris), a humanized monoclonal antibody that targets complement protein C5, thereby preventing assembly of the terminal complement complex during complement activation. In studies, treatment with eculizumab has been shown to reduce hemolysis as well as improve anemia, fatigue, and quality of life in patients with PNH. In addition, eculizumab has demonstrated efficacy in reducing thrombosis. For patients who experience breakthrough hemolysis with eculizumab, pegcetacoplan (Empaveli) can be of benefit.

Management of Complications

The most concerning complication of splenectomy is overwhelming postsplenectomy infection (OPSI). In adults, the spleen appears to play a minimal role in immunity, except for defense from certain encapsulated organisms. Patients will often present with DIC and will rapidly progress to purpura fulminans. Approximately 40% to 50% of patients will die from sepsis, even when detected early. The overall lifetime risk may be as high as 1 in 500. The organism most commonly found in these cases is *Streptococcus pneumoniae*, which is reported in over 50% of cases. *Neisseria meningitidis* and *Haemophilus influenzae* have also been implicated in many cases.

Patients who have undergone splenectomy must be warned about the risk of OPSI and instructed to report to the emergency department immediately if they develop a fever greater than 101°F or shaking chills. Once in the emergency department, blood cultures should be rapidly obtained and the patient started on antibiotic coverage with agents that cover encapsulated organisms. Patients who are planning to have or are being considered for a splenectomy should be vaccinated for pneumococcal, meningococcal, and *H. influenzae* infections. If patients are planning to be treated with rituximab first, they should also be vaccinated because they will not be able to mount an immune response after receiving rituximab.

The major side effects of rituximab are infusion reactions, and they are often worse with the first dose. These can be controlled with antihistamines, steroids, and, for severe rigors, meperidine (Demerol).[1] Rare patients can develop neutropenia (about 1 in 500) that appears to be autoimmune in nature. Infections appear to be only minimally increased with the use of rituximab. One group at higher risk are patients who are chronic carriers of hepatitis B. These patients may have reactivation of the virus that can be fatal in some cases; patients being considered for rituximab must be screened for hepatitis B. Progressive multifocal leukoencephalopathy is a very rare risk that is more common in cancer patients and heavily immunosuppressed patients. The overall risk is unknown but is less than 1 in 50,000.

Eculizumab is well tolerated except for a risk of meningococcal infection, which is estimated at 1 in 500. All patients receiving this agent should be vaccinated and must report to the emergency department with any sign of infection.

---

[1] Not FDA approved for this indication.

References

Barcellini W, Bruno Fattizzo B: How I treat warm autoimmune hemolytic anemia, *Blood* 137(10):1283–1294, 2021.

Berentsen S: How I treat cold agglutinin disease, *Blood* 137(10):1295–1303, 2021.

Cappellini MD, Fiorelli G: Glucose-6-phosphate dehydrogenase deficiency, *Lancet* 371(9606):64–74, 2008.

Gavriilaki E, Peffault de Latour R, Risitano MA: Advancing therapeutic complement inhibition in hematologic diseases, *PNH and beyond* 139(25):3571–3582, 2022.

Haley K: Congenital Hemolytic Anemia, *Med Clin North Am* 101(2):361–374, 2017.

Hill A, DeZern AE, Kinoshita T, Brodsky RA: Paroxysmal nocturnal haemoglobinuria, *Nat Rev Dis Primers* 3:17028, 2017.

Liebman HA, Weitz IC: Autoimmune Hemolytic Anemia, *Med Clin North Am* 101(2):351–359, 2017.

HEMOPHILIA AND RELATED CONDITIONS

Method of
Bulent Ozgonenel, MD; Roshni Kulkarni, MD; and Meera Chitlur, MD

CURRENT DIAGNOSIS

- The hemophilias and von Willebrand disease (VWD) account for 80% to 85% of inherited bleeding disorders. Hemophilia A and B are X-linked, whereas VWD and rare bleeding disorders (RBDs) are autosomal disorders.
- The diagnosis of hemophilia and other inherited bleeding disorders should be confirmed by specific laboratory assays because screening tests such as prothrombin time (PT) and activated partial thromboplastin time (aPTT) may be normal. Plasma levels of deficient factor determine clinical severity and management.
- Major complications associated with hemophilia are inhibitor development, hemarthrosis, and intracranial hemorrhage. Hemarthrosis is the most common and debilitating complication, and central nervous system (CNS) bleeding is the most common cause of mortality in hemophilia. Mucosal bleeding and menorrhagia are the most common manifestations of VWD. Bleeding manifestations of RBDs are mild, although homozygotes can present with severe disease.
- Newborns have normal levels of factor VIII; therefore the diagnosis of hemophilia A can be established at birth. Vacuum-assisted delivery should be avoided to prevent head bleeds.
- Women and adolescents with menorrhagia and no underlying pathology should be investigated for a bleeding disorder.

CURRENT THERAPY

- Currently there is a paradigm shift in the treatment of hemophilia. In addition to the traditional plasma-derived and recombinant concentrates, the new extended half-life recombinant products have reduced the treatment burden by reducing the frequency of intravenous injections. Novel, subcutaneously administered, nonfactor replacement therapy with prolonged hemostatic efficiency has been a game changer for patients both with and without inhibitors. Gene therapy is on the horizon, offering a promise of cure. Even for von Willebrand disease (VWD) and rare bleeding disorders (RBDs), such as deficiencies of factors VII, XI, XIII, X, and fibrinogen, replacement factor concentrates are currently available. Early and effective treatment and prophylaxis can prevent bleeding episodes, including repeated hemarthrosis and joint destruction in persons with hemophilia. Patients should be tested annually for the presence of inhibitors. Cryoprecipitate is not recommended for the treatment of hemophilia because of concerns regarding transmission of bloodborne pathogens.
- For mild and moderate hemophilia A and VWD, the use of desmopressin (DDAVP) coupled with antifibrinolytics can obviate the use of concentrates. Continued vigilance should be implemented for inhibitory antibodies and new and emerging bloodborne pathogens.
- All patients with inherited bleeding disorders should be immunized against hepatitis A and B and followed in close collaboration with their local hemophilia treatment center (HTC) (https://www.cdc.gov/ncbddd/hemophilia/htc.html). The National Hemophilia Foundation's (https://www.hemophilia.org) Medical and Scientific Advisory Committee (MASAC) guidelines for updated recommendations and product choice should be followed.

Figure 1 Factor VIII protein structure.

TABLE 1	Hemophilia Severity and Clinical Manifestations		
CHARACTERISTICS	**SEVERE (50%–70%)**	**MODERATE (10%)**	**MILD (30%–40%)**
Factor VIII or IX activity (normal 50%–150%)	<1%	1%–5%	>5%
Age of diagnosis	Birth to 2 years	Childhood or adolescence	Adolescence or adulthood
Bleeding patterns	2–4 per month	4–6 per year	Rare
Clinical manifestations	Hemarthroses, muscle, central nervous system, gastrointestinal bleeding, hematuria	Bleeding into joints or muscle following minor trauma, surgical procedure, dental bleeding Rarely spontaneous	Surgical procedures (including dental) and major trauma

Hemophilia A and Hemophilia B

Hemophilia is an X-linked congenital bleeding disorder caused by a deficiency of factor VIII (hemophilia A) or factor IX (hemophilia B). Hemophilia A is the most common severe bleeding disorder and affects 1 in 5000 males in the United States; hemophilia B occurs in 1 in 30,000 males.

Pathophysiology

The *factor VIII* gene is one of the largest genes and spans 186 kb of genomic DNA at Xq28. Intron 22 of the *factor VIII* gene is particularly large and is therefore susceptible to inversion mutations. Inversions of this intron account for 50% of all severe hemophilia A cases, and inversions of other introns, deletions, point mutations, and insertions account for the remainder.

Hepatic and reticuloendothelial cells are presumed sites of factor VIII synthesis. Factor VIII is synthesized as a single-chain polypeptide with three A domains (A1, A2, and A3), a large central B domain, and two C domains (Figure 1). The binding sites for von Willebrand factor (VWF), thrombin, and factor Xa are on the C2 domain, and factor IXa binding sites are on the A2 and A3 domains. The B domain can be deleted without any consequences. VWF protects factor VIII from proteolytic degradation in the plasma and concentrates it at the site of injury.

The *factor IX* gene is 34 kb long and located at Xq26. It is a vitamin K–dependent serine protease composed of 415 amino acids. It is synthesized in the liver, and its plasma concentration is approximately 50 times that of factor VIII. Gene deletions and point mutations result in hemophilia B.

Role of Factors VIII and IX in Coagulation

Factor VIII circulates bound to VWF. It is a cofactor for factor IX and is essential for factor X activation. In the classic coagulation cascade, activation of the intrinsic or extrinsic pathway of coagulation results in sufficient thrombin generation. The fact that bleeding still occurs in hemophilia despite an intact extrinsic pathway has led to the revised cell-based model of coagulation.

The revised pathway incorporates all coagulation factors into a single pathway initiated by factor VII and tissue factor. The contact factors (XI, XII, kallikrein, and high-molecular-weight [HMW] kininogen) are not essential but serve as a backup. Following injury, encrypted tissue factor is exposed and forms a complex with F VIIa. The tissue factor–factor VIIa complex activates factor IX to IXa (which moves to the platelet surface) and factor X to Xa. This generates small amounts of thrombin that activates platelets, converts platelet factor V to Va and factor XI to XIa, and releases factor VIII from VWF and activates it. The factor XIa activates plasma factor IX to IXa on the platelet surface, which together with factor VIIIa forms the tenase complex (factor VIIIa/IXa) that converts large amounts of factor X to Xa. Factor Xa forms a prothrombinase complex with FVa and converts large amounts of prothrombin to thrombin, called *thrombin burst*. This results in the conversion of sufficient fibrinogen to fibrin to form a stable clot. In hemophilia, lack of factor VIII or IX produces a profound abnormality. Factor Xa, generated by FVIIa and tissue factor, is insufficient because this pathway is inhibited by tissue factor pathway inhibitor (TFPI) as part of a negative feedback, and factors VIII and IX, which are required for amplifying the production of Xa, are absent. The primary platelet plug formation and initiation phases of coagulation are normal. Any clot that is formed (from the initiation phase) is friable and porous.

Clinical Features

The diagnosis of hemophilia is often made following a bleeding episode or because of a family history; however, 50% of cases have no family history. Based on the plasma levels of factor VIII or IX (normal levels are 50% to 150%) that correlate with severity and predict bleeding risk, hemophilia is classified as mild (>5%), moderate (1% to 5%), and severe (<1%) (Table 1). Approximately 65% of persons with hemophilia have severe disease, 15% have moderate disease, and 20% have mild disease. Most cases of severe disease manifest by 4 years of age; moderate or mild disease is diagnosed later and often following bleeding secondary to trauma or surgery.

Hemophilia can be diagnosed in the first trimester, using chorionic villus sampling and gene analysis. In the second trimester, fetal blood sampling can be performed. Prenatal diagnosis to determine fetal gender can aid in the management of pregnancy and delivery.

The hallmark of severe hemophilia is hemarthrosis, or bleeding into the joint, that can occur spontaneously or with minimal trauma. The immediate effects of a joint bleed are excruciating pain, swelling, warmth, and muscle spasms, and the long-term effect of recurrent hemarthrosis is the hemophilic arthropathy, which is characterized by synovial thickening and chronic inflammation. Repeated hemorrhage results in a target joint.

Knees, elbows, ankles, hips, and shoulders are commonly affected. Disuse atrophy of surrounding muscles leads to further joint instability. Limitation of joint range of motion resulting from hemarthrosis often correlates positively with older age, non-White race, and increased body mass index, and it adversely affects quality of life.

Muscle hematomas, another characteristic site of bleeding, can lead to compartment syndrome, with eventual fibrosis and peripheral nerve damage. Iliopsoas bleeds manifest with pain and flexion deformity. Gastrointestinal bleeding and hematuria occur less often.

Central nervous system (CNS) hemorrhage is a rare but serious complication with a 10% recurrence rate, and it is the leading cause of mortality in hemophiliacs. Although most newborns with severe hemophilia experience an uneventful course following vaginal delivery, vacuum extraction is associated with an increased CNS bleeding risk. The incidence of intracranial hemorrhage in newborns with hemophilia is 1% to 4%.

Diagnosis

Hemophilia A and B are clinically indistinguishable, and specific factor assays are the only way to differentiate and confirm the diagnosis. Both should be differentiated from VWD. The prothrombin time (PT), platelet function analysis (PFA)-100, and fibrinogen activity are normal. (PFA replaces bleeding time because the bleeding time has low sensitivity and specificity and is operator dependent.) The activated partial thromboplastin time (aPTT) is prolonged when the factor levels are less than 30%. Table 2 shows the characteristics and differences between the hemophilias and VWD.

Female carriers may be asymptomatic except for those with extreme lyonization resulting in low factor VIII or IX levels. Carrier women and girls, whose factor VIII or IX levels are <40%, are therefore also considered to have hemophilia, with the same criteria for severity as boys and men. In fact, the most current terminology reserves the term *carrier* only for women whose factor levels are ≥40%. Carriers are further classified as symptomatic (i.e., with bleeding manifestations) or asymptomatic. It is important to note that carriers may experience bleeding episodes (such as heavy menstrual bleeding, postpartum hemorrhage, or joint bleeding), even with levels of FVIII or IX in the 40% to 60% range. Often with the onset of menarche, asymptomatic girls may become symptomatic as a result of heavy menstrual bleeding. Factor VIII levels increase throughout pregnancy and drop to prepregnancy levels following delivery, but factor IX levels remain constant throughout pregnancy.

Treatment

The treatment for hemophilia consists of replacement therapy with intravenous factor VIII or factor IX concentrates produced by purification of donor plasma (plasma derived) (e.g., factor VIII [human]: Hemofil M, Koate; factor IX [human]: AlphaNine SD, Mononine) or in cell culture bioreactors (recombinant) (e.g., factor VIII [recombinant]: Advate, Afstyla, Kogenate FS, Nuwiq, Xyntha; factor IX [recombinant]: BeneFIX, Ixinity, Rixubis). Careful screening of donors combined with heat treatment and viral inactivation methods have made plasma-derived products safer. Plasma-derived and recombinant products appear to have equivalent clinical efficacy. Cryoprecipitate is no longer recommended because of concerns regarding pathogen safety.

Treatment administered only during bleeding symptoms is known as *episodic therapy,* and periodic administration of factor concentrates to prevent bleeding is known as *prophylactic therapy.* Response to treatment is more effective when it is administered early. Although prophylaxis prevents the development of joint disease, the high cost of factor replacement coupled with the need for venous access makes it expensive, difficult, and out of reach for patients in the developing world.

The goal of treatment is to raise factor levels to approximately 30% or more for minor bleeds (hematomas or joint bleeds) and 100% for major bleeds (CNS or surgery). Administering 1 U/kg of factor concentrate raises plasma factor VIII levels by 2% and factor IX levels by 1.5% (except with the recombinant factor IX product, in which it increases by 0.8%). The half-life of factor VIII is 8 to 12 hours and that of factor IX is up to 24 hours with standard factor products.

Factor concentrates can also be given by continuous infusion (3–4 U/kg/h). The bolus dose varies from 25 to 50 U/kg depending on the severity, site, and type of bleeding and is dosed to the available vial size because of the cost of the products. Table 3 lists the dosing schedule for various types of bleeds.

For prophylaxis, factor VIII 25 to 40 U/kg administered every other day or factor IX 100 U/kg once weekly for BeneFIX and 40 U/kg once weekly for Rebinyn (because of the longer half-life of factor IX) is aimed at preventing joint disease. Prophylaxis may begin at 1 to 2 years of age and is continued lifelong. Self-infusion before any planned strenuous activity is recommended. Because of the complications of central venous catheters (infections, thrombosis, and mechanical), use of a peripheral vein is encouraged.

Extended half-life (EHL) factor products have increased the half-lives by 1.5-fold in the case of factor VIII products and 2.4- to 4.8-fold in the case of factor IX products. EHL factor products have been developed with an aim to decrease the frequency of infusions and improve quality of life for patients with hemophilia, achieved through PEGylation or fusion of the factor protein to the Fc fragment of an immunoglobulin (Ig) or albumin. The first of these EHL products was approved by the U.S. Food and Drug Administration (FDA) in 2014: factor IX (recombinant), Fc fusion protein (Alprolix) for use in patients with hemophilia B, and factor VIII (recombinant), Fc fusion protein (Eloctate) for use in patients with hemophilia A. Subsequently, PEGylated recombinant factor VIII (Adynovate, Takeda Pharmaceuticals, Palo Alto, CA) was approved in 2015, PEGylated recombinant factor IX (Rebinyn, Novo Nordisk, Plainsboro, NJ) was approved in 2017 but not for prophylaxis, and recombinant albumin fusion factor IX (Idelvion, CSL Behring) was approved in 2016 for use in patients with hemophilia. Recently further extension of the half-life of factor VIII was achieved by a novel fusion protein called *BIVV001, now FDA approved and called Altuviiio®,* consisting of a single recombinant FVIII protein fused to a dimeric FC, a D′D3 domain of VWF (FVIII binding domain), and two XTEN polypeptides. The mean half-life of Altuviiio® was three to four times that of recombinant FVIII (37.6 to 42.5 hours vs. 9.1 to 13.2 hours, respectively), thereby allowing weekly dosing.

Novel Therapies for the Treatment of Hemophilia

In recent years, the field of hemophilia treatment has seen dramatic changes. Treatment options that do not target replacement of the missing factor are currently being tested. Factor VIII mimetics such as the bispecific factor IXa– and factor X–directed antibody emicizumab (Hemlibra) (see later) are FDA-approved nonfactor therapy. Rebalancing agents that inhibit endogenous anticoagulants and restore coagulation are in clinical trials and include small interfering RNA (siRNA) targeting antithrombin (Fitusiran; Sanofi Pharmaceuticals, Bridgewater, NJ),[5] anti-TFPI antibody (Concizumab, Novo Nordisk),[5] and products targeting the anticoagulant effect of activated prothrombin complex (APC). The advantages are that these rebalancing agents can be given to patients with either hemophilia A or B, provide the benefits of prophylaxis, and can be given subcutaneously, thereby eliminating the need for intravenous injection. More data are needed regarding the safety and efficacy of these medications.

Gene therapy offers promise of a cure, and trials of gene therapy for both hemophilia A and B are currently in process. This

---

[5] Investigational drug in the United States.

TABLE 2 Hemophilias and von Willebrand Disease: Key Characteristics and Differences

CHARACTERISTIC	HEMOPHILIA A	HEMOPHILIA B	VON WILLEBRAND DISEASE
Incidence	1:5000	1:30,000	1%–3% of U.S. population
Abnormality	Factor VIII deficiency	Factor IX deficiency	VWF (qualitative and quantitative defect)
Inheritance	X-linked, affects males	X-linked, affects males	Autosomal dominant (gene: chromosome 12)
	Gene at the tip of X chromosome	Gene at the tip of X chromosome	Some recessive or compound heterozygotes
Production site	Unknown, liver endothelium	Liver (vitamin K–dependent)	Megakaryocytes and endothelial cells
Function	Cofactor; forms tenase complex with factor IX and activates factor X, leading to a thrombin burst that results in conversion of large amounts of fibrinogen to fibrin	Serine protease (inactive form: zymogen) activated by factor XI or VIIa; forms a tenase complex with factor VIII and activates factor X	Platelet adhesion to site of injury or damaged endothelium
			Protects factor VIII from proteolysis
Classification (normal levels 50%–150%)	Mild (>5%)	Mild (>5%)	Type 1
	Moderate (1%–5%)	Moderate (1%–5%)	Type 2 (2A, 2B, 2M, 2N)
	Severe (<1%)	Severe (<1%)	Type 3
Clinical presentation	Positive family history (30% new mutation) Hemarthroses, hematomas, hematuria, intracranial hemorrhage, gastrointestinal hemorrhage, and so on	Positive family history (30% new mutation) Milder disease, although identical hemorrhage sites as hemophilia A	Positive family history Mucocutaneous bleeding (epistaxis, menorrhagia, postdental bleeding, gastrointestinal bleeding in adults) Can manifest as hemophilia A in Type 3
PFA, bleeding time	Normal	Normal	May be prolonged
PT	Normal	Normal	Normal
aPTT	Prolonged	Prolonged	Prolonged or normal
Factor VIII assay	Decreased or absent	Normal	Decreased or normal (absent type 3)
Factor IX assay	Normal	Decreased or absent	Normal
VWF:Ag	Normal	Normal	Decreased or absent (type 3)
VWF:RCo	Normal	Normal	Decreased or abnormal
VWF multimers	Normal	Normal	Abnormal in types 1, 2A, 2B; absent in type 3
Specific treatment	Recombinant factor VIII (preferred)	Recombinant factor IX	DDAVP (intranasal or intravenous) (FDA approved for type 1)
	Pathogen-safe plasma-derived concentrates	Pathogen-safe plasma-derived concentrates	VWF concentrates (pathogen-safe plasma-derived or recombinant VWF)
	DDAVP for mild cases	DDAVP ineffective	
Inhibitor patients	Immune tolerance, recombinant factor VIIa, APCC	Immune tolerance, recombinant factor VIIa	Inhibitors are rare
Adjunct therapy	Antifibrinolytics	Antifibrinolytics	Hormonal therapy (oral contraceptives), antifibrinolytics

APCC, Activated prothrombin complex concentrates; *aPTT,* activated partial thromboplastin time; *DDAVP,* desmopressin; *FDA,* U.S. Food and Drug Administration; *PFA,* platelet function analyzer; *PT,* prothrombin time; *RCo,* ristocetin cofactor; *VWF,* von Willebrand factor; *VWF:Ag,* von Willebrand factor antigen.

has been a significant breakthrough in the treatment of hemophilia. In December 2011, Nathwani and colleagues reported that a single injection of factor IX–expressing adeno-associated virus (AAV) vector was effective in treating patients with hemophilia B for more than 1 year. Since this breakthrough, more successful gene therapy trials have been currently underway for the treatment of both hemophilia A and B. The trials have incorporated modifications of promoters, transgenes and AAV serotypes, and lentiviral vectors. Results from the initial factor IX gene therapy trials have demonstrated continued factor IX expression at levels shown to decrease bleeding episodes for up to 9 years. In fact, gene therapy for hemophilia B (etranacogene dezaparvovec-drlb [Hemgenix]) was approved by the FDA in November 2022. Gene therapy trials in hemophilia A, although

TABLE 3 Treatment of Bleeding Episodes and Desired Plasma Levels in Hemophilias A and B

TYPE OF BLEEDING	FACTOR DOSE*	DURATION OF TREATMENT	COMMENTS
• Persistent or profuse epistaxis • Oral mucosal bleeding (including tongue and mouth lacerations) • Dental procedures • Acute hemarthrosis • Intramuscular hematomas • Physical therapy	Single dose	1–2 days	• Local pressure, antifibrinolytics, fibrin glue for local control, WoundSeal Powder for epistaxis • Sedation in small children with tongue laceration
• Dental procedures	Single dose	1 hour before procedure	• Antifibrinolytics for 7–10 days
• Acute hemarthrosis, intramuscular hematomas	Single dose	1–3 days	• Lower doses used if treated early • Non–weight bearing on affected joint
• Physical therapy	Single dose	Treat before PT	• Synovectomy (surgical, radioisotope or chemical) considered for target joints
• Gastrointestinal bleeding	Single dose	2–3 days	• May use oral antifibrinolytics
• Persistent painless gross hematuria	Single dose	1–2 days	• PO or IV fluids increased with low-dose antifibrinolytics; risk of clotting in the urinary tract with factor replacement
• Life-threatening bleeding such as intracranial hemorrhage, major surgery, and trauma	Double dose	10–14 days	• Bolus dose followed by continuous infusion (3–4 U/kg/h); may switch to bolus before discharge

*Single dose refers to a factor dose that aims to achieve 40% to 50% factor level and is ~20 to 25 units/kg for factor VIII products and ~50 units/kg for factor IX products. Double dose refers to a factor dose that aims to achieve 80% to 100% factor level and is ~40 to 50 units/kg for factor VIII products and ~80 to 100 units/kg for factor IX products. Factor doses are dosed closest to the vial.
PT, Physical therapy.

still showing benefits in some patients, have shown lower levels of factor VIII expression in the long term compared with hemophilia B. A major limitation to this therapeutic option has been hepatotoxicity typically occurring 1 to 4 months postdelivery of the vector, resulting in transaminitis followed sometimes by loss of gene expression. The long-term outcomes and safety remain to be determined. Table 4 lists novel and current treatments for hemophilia.

Complications of Treatment

One of the most serious complications of hemophilia treatment is the development of inhibitors or neutralizing antibodies (IgG) that inhibit the function of substituted factor VIII and factor IX. Five percent to 10% of all patients with hemophilia and up to 30% of patients with severe hemophilia A develop inhibitors. The incidence of inhibitors in hemophilia B is lower (1% to 3%). Most factor VIII inhibitors arise after a median exposure of 9 to 12 days in patients with severe hemophilia A. They can be transient or permanent and should be suspected if a patient fails to respond to an appropriate dose of clotting factor concentrate. Inhibitors can exacerbate bleeding episodes and hemophilic arthropathy.

Inhibitor levels, measured using Bethesda units (BU), are classified as high titer (>5 BU) or low titer (<5 BU). In patients with low-titer inhibitors, higher-than-normal doses of factor VIII or IX may be used to treat bleeding. For those with high-titer inhibitors, agents that bypass factor VIII or factor IX are used. These include recombinant activated factor VII and, in the case of hemophilia A, activated prothrombin complex concentrates (APCCs) or recombinant porcine factor VIII (currently in prelicensure clinical trials). Immune tolerance induction, a long-term approach designed to eradicate inhibitors, is effective in 70% to 85% of patients with severe hemophilia A; the most important predictor of success of immune tolerance induction is an inhibitor titer of less than 10 BU at the start of immune tolerance induction.

A novel treatment for hemophilia A with inhibitors is emicizumab (Hemlibra), a chimeric humanized antibody that triggers and propagates thrombin generation by binding to both factor IX and factor X. By binding to these coagulation factors, the antibody mimics the function of factor VIII. The medication is given subcutaneously, making it a preferred drug in young children. Emicizumab showed remarkable success in preventing bleeding complications in patients with severe hemophilia A with inhibitors. The FDA initially approved emicizumab in 2017 for routine prophylaxis to prevent or reduce the frequency of bleeding episodes in patients with hemophilia A with inhibitors, but they extended the approval to hemophilia A without inhibitors in 2018 following studies in noninhibitor patients. Emicizumab can be administered subcutaneously once a week, every 2 weeks, or every 4 weeks, and all regimens have been found to be equally effective. In general, emicizumab has been well accepted by patients with hemophilia, especially children and those with difficult venous access, because its treatment regimen does not require intravenous dosing, and the dose frequency is much easier to manage than prophylaxis with conventional factor VIII products. Emicizumab treatment is safe by itself, but thrombotic microangiopathy and thrombotic complications have been observed in hemophilia A, with inhibitor individuals receiving concomitant high doses of APCC for management of breakthrough bleeds while on emicizumab (>100 U/kg of FEIBA for ≥24 hours). Hence it is recommended that recombinant factor VIIa (NovoSeven RT) be used as the first line of treatment for management of breakthrough bleeds in inhibitor patients on emicizumab (MASAC document #255).

Although inhibitors are rare in hemophilia B, they can result in anaphylaxis with exposure to factor IX–containing products. Immune tolerance regimens are associated with nephrotic syndrome and are successful in eradicating the inhibitor only in 40% of cases.

Another important complication of treatment is the transmission of blood-borne pathogens such as hepatitis B and C viruses and human immunodeficiency virus (HIV). In the 1970s, lyophilized plasma factor concentrates of low purity resulted in the transmission of HIV, causing the deaths of many patients with hemophilia. Currently, donor screening for pathogens coupled with viral attenuation by heat or solvent detergent technology

TABLE 4	Treatment Options in Hemophilia*

Factor VIII and factor IX replacement	Standard half-life (SHL) products
	• Plasma-derived
	• Factor VIII: e.g., Alphanate
	• Factor IX: e.g., AlphaNine SD, Bebulin[†]
	Recombinant (many products)
	• Factor VIII: (First, second, third and fourth generation): e.g., Advate
	• Factor IX: e.g., Benefix
	Extended half-life (EHL) products
	First-generation:
	• EHL factor VIII products:
	  • Recombinant, Fc fusion: Eloctate/Elocta[†]
	  • Recombinant, pegylated: Adynovate/Adynovi,[†] Jivi, Esperoct
	• EHL factor IX products:
	  • Recombinant, Fc Fusion: Alprolix
	  • Recombinant, albumin fusion: Idelvion
	  • Recombinant, glycopegylated: Rebinyn/Refixia[†]
	Second-generation
	• Efanesoctocog alfa (Altuviiio): factor VIII–VWF-XTEN fusion protein (hemophilia A only)

Nonreplacement therapy	Bispecific antibody (hemophilia A only) • Emicizumab (Hemlibra) *Rebalancing agents* • *Antithrombin RNA interference molecule* • *Fitusiran[5]* *Anti–tissue factor pathway inhibitor (A-TFPI)* • *Concizumab[5]* • *Marstacimab[5]* *Anti–protein C* • *SerpinPC[5]*
Adjunctive therapy	Antifibrinolytics • ε-Aminocaproic acid (Amicar) • Tranexamic acid (Cyklokapron or Lysteda)[1] • Desmopressin acetate (DDAVP) (Stimate) (hemophilia A only)
Therapy in patients with inhibitors	Recombinant factor VIIa • NovoSeven RT and Sevenfact • Activated prothrombin complex concentrates (e.g., FEIBA) • Recombinant, porcine factor VIII • Obizur (hemophilia A only) • Nonreplacement therapy products
Gene therapy[5]	Hemophilia A • *Valoctocogene roxaparvovec (BMN 270)* • *Dirloctocogene samoparvovec (SPK-8011)* • *BAY 2599023* • *Giroctocogene fitelparvovec (PF-070554480/SB-525)* Hemophilia B • *AMT-060* • Etranacogene dezaparvovec (Hemgenix) • *Fidanacogene elaparvovec (SPK-9001)* • *Verbrinacogene setparvovec (FLT180a)*

*All non–FDA-approved products are italicized.
[†]Brand name available in Europe.
[1]Not FDA approved for this indication.
[5]Investigational drug in the United States.

make these products pathogen safe. However, nonenveloped viruses (parvovirus and hepatitis A) and prions can resist inactivation and can be potentially transmitted.

Patients with bleeding disorders should be encouraged to attend the comprehensive hemophilia treatment centers (HTCs), where they are seen by a multidisciplinary team of hematologists, nurses, social workers, geneticists, physical therapists, dental hygienists, nutritionists, and so on, who educate patients and address issues such as self-care, transitions, and quality of life.

Patients are trained to self-infuse and calculate dosage, maintain treatment logs, and call for serious bleeding episodes. The mortality rate among patients who receive care at HTCs is lower than among those who do not: 28.1% versus 38.3%, respectively. At the HTCs, hemovigilance for bloodborne and emerging pathogens was maintained through participation in the Centers for Disease Control and Prevention (CDC) Universal Data Collection (UDC) project. The grant cycle of the UDC was completed in 2012, and a new surveillance instrument is currently in use (Community Counts) that incorporates collecting information on comorbidities and complications of bleeding disorders in this population. Routine vaccination against hepatitis A and B is recommended.

Von Willebrand Disease

VWD is an inherited (autosomal dominant) bleeding disorder caused by deficiency or dysfunction of VWF, a plasma protein that mediates platelet adhesion at the site of vascular injury and prevents degradation of factor VIII. A defect in VWF results in bleeding by impairing platelet adhesion or by decreasing factor VIII.

VWF is synthesized in endothelial cells and undergoes dimerization and multimerization, forming low, intermediate, and HMW multimers. The HMW multimers are most effective in promoting platelet aggregation and adhesion. Circulating HMW multimers are cleaved by the protease ADAMTS13, which is deficient in patients with thrombotic thrombocytopenic purpura.

VWD is the most common bleeding disorder, affecting 1% or more of the population. It occurs worldwide and affects all races. VWD is classified into three major categories: partial quantitative deficiency (type 1), qualitative deficiency (type 2), and total deficiency (type 3). There are several different variants of type 2 VWD: 2A, 2B, 2N, and 2M based on the phenotype. Approximately 75% of patients have type 1 VWD.

Clinical Presentation

Mucous membrane–type bleeding (e.g., menorrhagia, epistaxis) and excessive bruising are characteristic clinical features in VWD. Bleeding manifestations vary considerably, and in some cases the diagnosis is not suspected until excessive bleeding occurs with a surgical procedure or trauma. Although excessive menstrual bleeding may be the initial manifestation, it takes 16 years for a diagnosis of bleeding disorder. It is for this reason that the American College of Obstetrics and Gynecology recommended screening for hemostatic disorders in all adolescents and women presenting with menorrhagia and no pathology and before hysterectomy for menorrhagia. In infants or small children with type 3 (severe) VWD, excessive bruising and even joint bleeding (caused by very low levels of factor VIII) can mimic hemophilia A.

Diagnosis

Laboratory evaluation for VWD requires several assays to quantitate VWF and characterize its structure and function. Many variables affect VWF assay results, including the patient's ABO blood type. Persons of blood group AB have 60% to 70% higher VWF levels than those of blood group O.

Clinical conditions and disorders with elevated VWF levels include pregnancy (third trimester), collagen vascular disorders, postoperative period, liver disease, and disseminated intravascular coagulation. Low levels are seen in hypothyroidism and the first 4 days of the menstrual cycle.

Symptoms are modified by medications like aspirin or nonsteroidal antiinflammatory drugs (NSAIDs), which can exacerbate the bleeding; oral contraceptives can decrease the bleeding in women with VWD by increasing VWF levels. VWF levels in African American women are 15% higher than in White women. Clinical symptoms and family history are important for establishing the diagnosis of VWD, and a single test is sometimes not sufficient to rule out the diagnosis.

Initial workup should include a complete blood count, aPTT, PT, fibrinogen level, and thrombin time. These tests do not rule out VWD but help rule out thrombocytopenia or factor deficiency

			RISTOCETIN		
TYPE	**FACTOR VIII**	**VWF AG**	**COFACTOR**	**RIPA**	**MULTIMER**
1	↓	↓	↓	↓ or normal	Normal
2A	↓ or normal	↓↓	↓	↓↓	Large and intermediate multimers absent
2B	↓ or normal	↓↓	↓ or normal	↓ to low dose	Large multimers absent
2M	Variably ↓	Variably ↓	↓	Variably ↓	Normal
2N	↓↓	Normal	Normal	Normal	Normal
3	↓↓↓↓	↓↓↓↓	↓↓↓↓	None	Absent
Platelet type	↓ or normal	↓ or normal	↓	↓ to low dose	Large multimers absent

Ag, Antigen; *RIPA*, ristocetin-induced platelet aggregation; *VWF*, von Willebrand factor.

as the cause for bleeding. The closure times on the PFA-100, which has replaced the bleeding time as a screening test in some centers, may be prolonged. The aPTT in VWD is only abnormal when factor VIII is sufficiently reduced.

Specific tests for VWD include ristocetin cofactor assay, a factor VIII activity, and VWF antigen (VWF Ag) assay. The ristocetin cofactor activity measures induced binding of VWF to platelet glycoprotein Ib and is subject to significant intralaboratory and interlaboratory variability, making it an unreliable assay for the diagnosis. In addition, certain mutations in the A1 domain of the VWF, especially the *D1472H* mutation, have been found to attenuate the VWF-ristocetin binding, leading to misdiagnosis of VWD. This has led to the development of the glycoprotein 1bM assay (direct measure of platelet-binding activity of VWF), collagen binding assay (measure of multimeric function), and genotyping (especially for type 2 VWD, which are the new tests available to assist with the diagnosis). Multimer analysis is done by agarose gel electrophoresis using anti-VWF polyclonal antibody and is available at reference laboratories.

In type 1 VWD, the VWF is subnormal in amount, with normal multimer structure. Those with types 2A and 2B VWD lack the HMW multimers. In type 2B, the VWF has a heightened affinity for platelets, often resulting in some degree of thrombocytopenia from platelet aggregation. A useful laboratory test for type 2B is the low-dose ristocetin-induced platelet aggregation (RIPA) assay.

In type 3 (severe) VWD, the affected person has inherited a gene for type 1 VWD from each parent, resulting in very low levels (3%) of VWF (and low factor VIII, because there is no VWF to protect factor VIII from proteolytic degradation). Less commonly, a person with type 3 is doubly heterozygous. Table 5 provides an overview of the laboratory findings in the different variants of VWD.

Treatment

See the "General Hemostatic Agents" section later in this chapter for a discussion on the use of desmopressin (DDAVP) and antifibrinolytic agents.

For patients with type 3 and in patients with type 1 VWD who do not respond adequately to desmopressin, an intermediate-purity plasma-derived concentrate rich in the hemostatically effective HMW multimers of VWF (such as Humate-P) should be used to treat moderately severe or severe bleeding episodes and before surgery. Prophylaxis with VWF concentrates is effective in reducing the bleeding episodes and joint disease in severe VWD. A recombinant VWF concentrate enriched with HMW multimers, Vonvendi (Baxalta, Illinois City, IL) does not contain any factor VIII and is now available and approved for use only in adults.

As in hemophilia, antifibrinolytics are an effective adjunctive treatment for invasive dental procedures or other bleeding in the oropharyngeal cavity. These may be effective even when used alone in some women with VWD with menorrhagia. For epistaxis, Nosebleed QR, a hydrophilic powder (over-the-counter [OTC] product), can help.

Special Situations

Pregnancy

VWF (and factor VIII) levels increase during the third trimester of pregnancy, and women with type 1 VWD have a decrease in bruising or other bleeding symptoms. However, those with type 2 VWD (abnormal VWF) and type 3 (no VWF) have no change in bleeding tendency. Even in type 1 VWD, VWF levels decrease following delivery, so treatment (with intravenous DDAVP or Humate P) may be needed. Antifibrinolytic agents can be used to prevent/treat postpartum hemorrhage.

Acquired von Willebrand Disease

Acquired VWD occurs in persons who do not have a lifelong bleeding disorder. Conditions associated with acquired VWD include underlying autoimmune disease (lymphoproliferative disorders, myeloproliferative disorders, or plasma cell dyscrasias), valvular and congenital heart disease, Wilms tumor, chronic renal failure, and hypothyroidism. The mechanism of acquired VWD is unknown. Medications such as valproic acid can also cause VWD. Removal of the underlying condition often corrects the VWF. DDAVP, Humate P, recombinant factor VIIa (NovoSeven RT),[1] or plasma exchange may be tried, if necessary, to treat bleeding.

Rare Bleeding Disorders

The RBDs account for 3% to 5% of inherited coagulation deficiencies other than factor VIII, factor IX, or VWF deficiencies. They are autosomal recessive and affect both sexes. The prevalence of RBDs ranges from 1 in 500,000 to 1 in 2,000,000. Bleeding manifestations are restricted to persons who are homozygotes or compound heterozygotes. RBDs are common in countries such as Iran, where consanguineous marriages are customary. Ashkenazi Jews are particularly affected by factor XI deficiency. Deficiency of factor XII is a risk factor for thrombosis but not for bleeding. Most cases of RBDs are identified by abnormal screening tests coupled with specific factor assays.

Factor concentrates (recombinant or plasma derived) are available for some of the deficiencies such as FVII, X (Coagadex [human]; Bio Products Laboratory, Durham, NC), XIII (Tretten [recombinant], Novo Nordisk; Corifact [human], CSL Behring, King of Prussia, PA), XI (in Europe), and fibrinogen concentrate (human) (Fibryga, Octapharma, Switzerland; RiaSTAP, CSL Behring). The advantages of concentrates are pathogen safety and small volume. The use of antifibrinolytics and fibrin glue as adjunct therapy for bleeding manifestations is encouraged. Table 6 lists the inheritance, frequency, manifestations, and treatments of the RBDs.

---

[1] Not FDA approved for this indication.

TABLE 6 Rare Bleeding Disorders: Inheritance, Clinical Features, and Treatment

FACTOR	PREVALENCE	TYPE	INHERITANCE	MANIFESTATION AND DIAGNOSIS	TREATMENT	HEMOSTATIC LEVELS	HALF-LIFE
Factor I	1:1,000,000	• Afibrinogenemia • Dysfibrinogenemia • Hypofibrinogenemia	• AR • AD • AD	• Mild bleeding • CNS, umbilical, joint bleeding • Recurrent miscarriage • Prolonged PT, aPTT, TT • Low FI levels • Paradoxical thrombosis	• FFP 15–20 mL/kg • Cryoprecipitate 1 bag/5–10 kg • Fibrinogen concentrate (RiaSTAP) treatment q3–5d	50 mg⁻¹ g/dL	2–5 days
Factor II	1:2,000,000	Type I: hypoprothrombinemia • Type II: dysprothrombinemia	• AR • AR	• Hematomas, hemarthroses, menorrhagia • CNS, umbilical, postpartum hemorrhage • PT abnormal	FFP, PCC 20–30 U/kg for prophylaxis or treatment	20%–30%	3–4 days
Factor V	1:1,000,000	Parahemophilia, labile factor, proaccelerin, Owren disease	AR	• Mucosal bleeding, postpartum hemorrhage CNS bleeding • Platelet factor V deficiency more reflective of bleeding potential • Prolonged PT, aPTT • Normal TT	• FFP • Platelet transfusions • Sometimes antiplatelet antibodies with repeated platelet transfusions	15%–20%	36 h
Factor VII	1:500,000	Proconvertin or stable factor	AR	• Menorrhagia; mucosal, muscle, intracranial bleeds (15%–60%); hemarthrosis • Prolonged PT • Normal aPTT, TT, FI, liver function tests	• Recombinant factor VIIa (NovoSeven), 15–30 μg/kg q2h for major bleeds • FFP, PCC 20–30 U/kg for prophylaxis or treatment • Plasma-derived factor VII concentrates[2],*	15%–20%	4–6 h
Factor X	1:1,000,000		AR	• Menorrhagia; umbilical, joint, mucosal, muscle, intracranial bleeding • Prolonged PT, aPTT	FFP, PCCs 25–40 U/kg Pd FX (Coagadex)	15%–20%	24–48 h
Factor XI (common in Ashkenazi Jews)	1:1,000,000		AR	• Posttraumatic bleeding, menorrhagia • Prolonged aPTT • Normal PT	• Hemoleven*,[5] FFP 15–20 mL/kg • Sometimes inhibitors	15%–20%	
Factor XIII	1:2,000,000		AR	• Intracranial, joint, umbilical bleeding • Delayed wound healing • Recurrent miscarriages • Normal PT, aPTT • ↓ FXIII assay	• Factor XIII concentrate (Corifact) 40 IU/kg q28d to maintain trough level of 5%–20% • FFP 15–20 mL/kg • Tretten, a recombinant factor XIII-A subunit concentrate 35 units/kg/month for prophylaxis; used in patients with factor XIII A subunit deficiency • Cryoprecipitate 1 bag/5–10 kg q3–4 weeks	2%–5%	11–14 days
Combined factor V and VIII	1:2,000,000			• Mucosal bleeding • Prolonged PT, aPTT (disproportionately)	Factor VIII concentrates and FFP	15%–20%	
Vitamin K–dependent multiple deficiencies	1:2,000,000			• Umbilical stump, intracranial, postsurgical bleeding • Skeletal abnormalities • Hearing loss	Oral vitamin K, FFP, PCC	15%–20%	

AD, Autosomal dominant; *aPTT*, activated partial thromboplastin time; *AR*, autosomal recessive; *CNS*, central nervous system; *FFP*, fresh-frozen plasma; *FI*, fibrinogen; *PCC*, prothrombin complex concentrate; *PT*, prothrombin time; *TT*, thrombin time.

*Available in Europe.

[2]Not available in the United States.

[5]Investigational drug in the United States.

Hemophilia and Related Conditions

465

General Hemostatic Agents

For short-term therapy (before dental procedures and minor bleeding episodes), the synthetic vasopressin analog desmopressin acetate (DDAVP injection, Stimate Nasal Spray) is useful both in mild hemophilia A and type 1 VWD and occasionally in type 2A VWD.[1] Some young women with menorrhagia have also benefited from its use at the onset of menses, with a second dose given after 24 hours. The mechanism of action for desmopressin is increase in plasma concentrations of factor VIII and VWF by stimulating release of the endothelial stores of VWF. The levels of both factor VIII and VWF increase threefold to fivefold within 15 to 30 minutes following infusion. A DDAVP trial to determine response is helpful in selecting patients who might benefit from such therapy. For hemostatic purposes, intravenous (0.3 μg/kg in 50 mL of normal saline infused over 15 to 30 minutes) or intranasal dose (150 μg) can be used. The intranasal dose is 15 times larger than that recommended for diabetes insipidus. A multidose intranasal spray formulation (Stimate nasal spray in the United States and Octostim nasal spray in Canada; Ferring Pharmaceuticals, Parsippany, NJ) of 1.5 mg/1 mL delivers 150 μg per spray. The recommended dosage is one spray for patients who weigh less than 50 kg and two sprays (one in each nostril) for those who weigh more than 50 kg. (Note that Ferring Pharmaceuticals issued a voluntary recall of Stimate in July 2020 because of higher-than-specified doses in the sprays. Stimate is not anticipated to be released until 2024. This recall does not affect intravenous doses.) The intravenous route, which was usually used for surgical coverage or for severe bleeding episodes requiring hospitalization, is now the only available route until the intranasal medication is released again.

When necessary, repeat doses may be given at 12- to 24-hour intervals. Tachyphylaxis (diminished response to repeated doses of the medication) occurs as a result of depletion of endothelial VWF stores. Tachyphylaxis is less commonly seen in patients with VWD than in patients with hemophilia. It is important to monitor free water intake following DDAVP administration because it can cause hyponatremia and seizures.

Desmopressin can also be used in the treatment of bleeding in patients with platelet dysfunction secondary to uremia.[1] Desmopressin seems to be effective in reducing blood loss during cardiac surgery in patients who are taking antiplatelet medications.[1] Because desmopressin requires the presence of either factor VIII or VWF to be able to show its effect, it is ineffective in moderate to severe hemophilia A, type 2M VWD, type 2N VWD, and type 3 VWD (there is no VWF to be released from storage sites). Desmopressin should be used with caution in type 2B VWD[1] because it can exacerbate the thrombocytopenia. Some patients with type 2A VWD may respond to desmopressin,[1] and a desmopressin test may be needed to determine benefit. Desmopressin is ineffective in hemophilia B and other coagulation disorders.

Antifibrinolytics such as ε-aminocaproic acid (Amicar; Akorn Inc., Lake Forest, IL) and tranexamic acid (Cyklokapron [Pfizer, New York, NY] or Lysteda [Amring Pharmaceuticals, Berwyn, PA])[1] are used as adjunct therapies in hemophilia, VWD, and other rare bleeding disorders, reducing the need for factor concentrates. The recommended dosage for ε-aminocaproic acid is 50 to 100 mg/kg/dose intravenously or orally (adult dose 4–5 g/dose IV or 5 g/dose PO) every 4 to 8 hours (maximum daily dose 24 g/24 h for children, 30 g/24 h for adults). The recommended dosage for tranexamic acid is 10 mg/kg/dose intravenously three times daily or 25 mg/kg body weight orally three times daily (for adults 1300 mg PO tid for a total of 5 days).

General Measures

Aspirin and aspirin-containing compounds should be avoided in patients with bleeding disorders because they interfere with platelet function and can exacerbate bleeding.

References

Aledort LM: Do hemophilia carriers bleed? Yes, *Blood* 108(1):6, 2006.
Arnold WD, Hilgartner MW: Hemophilic arthropathy. Current concepts of pathogenesis and management, *J Bone Joint Surg Am* 59(3):287–305, 1977.
Bolton-Maggs PH, Pasi KJ: Haemophilias A and B, *Lancet* 361(9371):1801–1809, 2003.
d'Oiron R, O'Brien S, James AH: Women and girls with haemophilia: lessons learned, *Haemophilia* 27(Suppl 3):75–78, 2021.
Flood VH, Gill JC, Morateck PA, et al: Common VWF exon 28 polymorphisms in African Americans affecting the VWF activity assay by ristocetin cofactor, *Blood* 116(2):280–286, 2010.
Franchini M, Mannucci PM: Non-factor replacement therapy for haemophilia: a current update, *Blood Transfus* 14:1–5, 2018.
Gill JC, Wilson AD, Endres-Brooks J, Montgomery RR: Loss of the largest von Willebrand factor multimers from the plasma of patients with congenital cardiac defects, *Blood* 67(3):758–761, 1986.
Hoffman M, Monroe 3rd DM: A cell-based model of hemostasis, *Thromb Haemost* 85(6):958–965, 2001.
Batty P, Lillicrap D: Gene therapy for hemophilia: current status and laboratory consequences, *Int J Lab Hematol* 43(Suppl 1):117–123, 2021.
Miller CH, Dilley AB, Drews C, et al: Changes in von Willebrand factor and factor VIII levels during the menstrual cycle, *Thromb Haemost* 87(6):1082–1083, 2002.
Miller CH, Dilley A, Richardson L, et al: Population differences in von Willebrand factor levels affect the diagnosis of von Willebrand disease in African-American women, *Am J Hematol* 67(2):125–129, 2001.
Nathwani AC, Tuddenham EG, Rangarajan S, et al: Adenovirus-associated virus vector-mediated gene transfer in hemophilia B, *N Engl J Med* 365(25):2357–2365, 2011.
Mulder K, Llinas A: The target joint, *Haemophilia* 10(Suppl 4):152–156, 2004.
National Hemophilia Foundation Medical and Scientific Advisory Council (MASAC): MASAC recommendations concerning the treatment of hemophilia and other bleeding disorders, Available at http://www.hemophilia.org/Researchers-Healthcare-Providers/Medical-and-Scientific-Advisory-Council-MASAC/MASAC-Recommendations.
Pabinger-Fasching I, Pipe S: Innovations in coagulation: improved options for treatment of hemophilia A and B, *Thromb Res* 131(2):S1, 2013.
Pierce GF, Lillicrap D, Pipe SW, Vandendriessche T: Gene therapy, bioengineered clotting factors and novel technologies for hemophilia treatment, *J Thromb Haemost* 5(5):901–906, 2007.
Shapiro A: Development of long-acting recombinant FVIII and FIX Fc fusion proteins for the management of hemophilia, *Expert Opin Biol Ther* 13(9):1287–1297, 2013.
Soucie JM, Nuss R, Evatt B, et al: Mortality among males with hemophilia; relations with source of medical care. The hemophilia surveillance system project investigators, *Blood* 96(2):437–442, 2000.
van Galen KPM, d'Oiron R, James P, et al: A new hemophilia carrier nomenclature to define hemophilia in women and girls: communication from the SSC of the ISTH, *J Thromb Haemost* 19(8):1883–1887, 2021.
Veldman A, Hoffman M, Ehrenforth S: New insights into the coagulation system and implications for new therapeutic options with recombinant factor VIIa, *Curr Med Chem* 10(10):797–811, 2003.
Warrier I, Ewenstein BM, Koerper MA, et al: Factor IX inhibitors and anaphylaxis in hemophilia B, *J Pediatr Hematol Oncol* 19(1):23–27, 1997.
Weyand AC, Pipe SW: New therapies for hemophilia, *Blood* 133(5):389–398, 2019.

HODGKIN LYMPHOMA

Method of
Anusha Vallurupalli, MBBS

CURRENT DIAGNOSIS

- Typically presents as painless cervical or mediastinal lymphadenopathy.
- "B" symptoms (fevers, drenching night sweats, and weight loss >10% of body weight) may be present.
- Tissue diagnosis is made by identifying Reed Sternberg cells on either excisional (preferable) or incisional biopsy. Fine needle aspiration (FNA) is never adequate and should be avoided.

---

[1] Not FDA approved for this indication.

CURRENT THERAPY

- Limited-stage disease (stages I to IIA) with favorable risk factors, termed "early favorable" can be treated with combined modality therapy, (*A*driamycin, *b*leomycin, *v*inblastine, and *d*ubarbazine [ABVD]), for 2 cycles followed by 20 Gy involved-field radiation.
- Limited-stage disease (I to IIA) with unfavorable risk factors, termed "early unfavorable," may be treated with either combined-modality therapy, 4 cycles of ABVD followed by 30 Gy involved-field radiotherapy, or with 6 cycles of ABVD alone. Decisions about therapy should be decided in a multi-disciplinary setting and are usually based on patient age and sex, disease bulk, and area of involved field radiation.
- Advanced-stage disease (IIB to IV) can now be treated with either ABVD or A +AVD for 6 cycles.
- Clinical trials should always be considered for the treatment of disease at any stage, if available.

Epidemiology

There were 8500 estimated new cases of Hodgkin lymphoma (HL) in 2018 with 1050 deaths according to the SEER database. 86.6% patients who underwent treatment were surviving at 5 years between 2008 and 2014. There has been a downward trend in new cases and deaths due to HL over the last 10 years. The median age at diagnosis is 39 years and there is a bimodal age distribution with the highest risk in the age group of 20 to 34 years.

Pathology

HL is classified broadly into classical Hodgkin lymphoma (CHL) and nodular lymphocyte predominant Hodgkin lymphoma (NLPHL) based on the WHO classification system. CHL is the most common type, accounting for 95% of the cases. There are four distinctive histologic subtypes of CHL, Nodular Sclerosis (NS), Mixed Cellularity (MC), Lymphocyte Rich (LR), and Lymphocyte depleted (LD) with NS being the most common subtype.

Pathologically, CHL is characterized by the presence of definitive "Reed Sternberg" (RS) cells, which express CD30 and CD15 on their cell surface. NLPHL, on the other hand, is characterized by "popcorn cells" that express CD20 and CD45 on the cell surface.

Risk Factors

Most cases of CHL are sporadic with no clear risk factors. NS is the most common subtype in United States and developed countries. MC and LR are more common in developing countries and are associated with prior Epstein Barr Virus (EBV) infection. HIV infection is associated with a 5 to 10 times higher risk due to immune suppression and associated EBV infection. The incidence of HL in HIV patients may be increasing in the era of antiretroviral therapy. Increased risk is also seen in other acquired or congenital immunodeficiencies.

There is also increased risk of CHL in families with an index case. According to a Nordic study, there is a threefold increase over the general population risk and the risk is the highest in siblings. Familial risk varies by subtypes and is the highest in the LR subtype.

Clinical Presentation

Painless lymphadenopathy either in the neck (75%) or mediastinal lymph nodes (60%) is the most common presentation for CHL, whereas NLPHL usually presents with painless peripheral lymphadenopathy. "B" symptoms, which include fever higher than 38°C, unintentional weight loss of more than 10% of body weight over 6 months, and drenching night sweats can be present and are often considered unfavorable risk factors. Patients may present with local symptoms from bulky lymphadenopathy such as dyspnea, chest pressure or cough due to mediastinal masses, and neck discomfort and trouble swallowing from cervical lymphadenopathy. Prolonged dyspnea, cough, or chest pressure should be evaluated with appropriate imaging in a young patient when CHL is a consideration in the differential diagnosis. Pruritus can also be seen in some patients and often improves with the treatment of CHL.

Spleen involvement can be seen in 20% of cases and is considered as nodal involvement in CHL. Other extra nodal involvement (e.g., bone marrow, lungs, liver, and bone) is uncommon and is usually associated with advanced unfavorable disease and a poor prognosis. CNS involvement is extremely rare.

Initial lab testing may not show any major abnormalities in early stage and favorable risk patients. The Erythrocyte Sedimentation Rate (ESR) is prognostic in CHL and should be performed at diagnosis in all patients. Anemia, lymphopenia, leukocytosis, and hypoalbuminemia may be seen on labs in advanced and unfavorable risk patients and are a result of cytokine response.

Diagnosis

Adequate tissue sampling is essential in the diagnosis of any lymphoma and is even more indispensable in HL. CHL is characterized by background inflammatory cells, which include polyclonal reactive lymphocytes, neutrophils, and eosinophils with the actual malignant RS cells configuring only 1% to 2% of the total cellularity. As a result, diagnosis is often missed on FNA, which is considered a very insensitive diagnostic methodology. Excisional biopsy is preferable and in cases where it is not possible, multiple core needle biopsies or mediastinoscopic biopsies can be considered, based on the location.

On Haemotoxylin and eosin (H&E) staining of the biopsy, the classic presentation for CHL is a rich inflammatory background interspersed with positive CD15 and CD30 RS cells. RS cells are typically large with bilobed eosinophilic nucleoli and abundant cytoplasm. Mononuclear variants also occur. On immunohistochemistry, RS cells are usually negative for the panlymphoid marker CD45 and the B-cell marker CD20. The presence of RS cells will rule out other conditions in the differential diagnosis, including Non-Hodgkin lymphoma, autoimmune diseases, and infections. The NS subtype also presents with dense bands of fibrosis on H&E staining.

NLPHL is also characterized by atypical malignant cells amidst a polyclonal inflammatory microenvironment composed primarily of small lymphocytes in large nodular meshworks of follicular dendritic cells. The "popcorn" cells characteristic of NLPHL express CD20 and CD45, rather than CD15 an CD30, which is the major pathologic differentiating factor from CHL.

Staging and Risk Prognostication

Staging starts with a thorough history and physical exam. "B" symptoms, pruritus, fatigue, alcohol intolerance, and decrease in performance status may all be noted on the history. Careful palpation and measurements of lymph nodes and spleen as well as documentation of extra nodal involvement are important and can be followed after the initiation of treatment for a clinical response assessment.

The Ann Arbor classification is used for staging. CHL is broadly divided into four stages based on the spread of the lymphoma. Stage I disease is confined to a single lymph-node region, while Stage II is the involvement of multiple lymph-node regions on the same side of the diaphragm, Stage III has involvement of nodal regions on both sides of the diaphragm and Stage IV has extensive involvement of an extranodal site or sites. Each stage is subdivided into "A" and "B" depending on the presence or absence of B symptoms. The Cotswold classification includes an "X" category for bulky disease (Table 1).

Radiographic staging is performed with CT scans in conjunction with PET scanning at diagnosis and repeated after two cycles of chemotherapy and at the end of treatment (EOT). Positron emission tomography–computed tomography (PET-CT) imaging leads to a change in staging in 10% to 30% of patients, more often upstaging. Bone marrow aspirate/biopsy is no longer required for the routine evaluation of patients with HL due to the high sensitivity of PET scan. CNS staging with lumbar puncture (LP) and MRI of the brain is only done if there is a high suspicion based on

TABLE 1	Staging Hodgkin Disease
STAGE	**DEFINITION**
I	Confined to single lymph-node region*
II	Involvement of multiple lymph-node regions on a same side of diaphragm
III	Involvement of nodal regions on both sides of the diaphragm
IV	Extensive involvement of extranodal site(s)
Sub Classification	
A	Absence of "B" symptoms
B	Presence of "B" symptoms
Modifiers	
E	Localized focus of extranodal disease or localized extension of nodal disease into an extranodal site.
S	Splenic involvement (the spleen is considered a nodal site in Hodgkin lymphoma)
X (Cotswold modifier)	Bulky disease (>10 cm or >0.33 of the maximal intrathoracic diameter for mediastinal mass per NCCN guidelines)

*Lymph node regions include: right cervical (including cervical, supraclavicular, occipital, and preauricular lymph nodes), left cervical, right axillary, left axillary, right infraclavicular, left infraclavicular, mediastinal, hilar, periaortic, mesenteric, right pelvic, left pelvic, right inguinal femoral, and left inguinal femoral.
NCCN, National Comprehensive Cancer Network.

symptoms and physical examination. Routine staging laparotomy and bilateral bone marrow biopsies are no longer performed.

Laboratory evaluation includes a complete blood count with differential, complete metabolic profile, including albumin, ESR, and baseline HIV testing. Due to the routine use of anthracyclines, an echocardiogram or multigated acquisition scan (MUGA; also called equilibrium radionuclide angiogram) is necessary prior to initiation of chemotherapy to assess left ventricular ejection fraction. Pulmonary function testing is performed and a detailed tobacco smoking history should be obtained due to the use of bleomycin. A pregnancy test should be performed on all women of childbearing age prior to the initiation of therapy. Fertility counseling is recommended for age appropriate patients even though the infertility risk is low (2% to 10%) with the ABVD regimen. The risk of infertility is higher with other regimens such as bleomycin, etoposide, doxorubicin hydrochloride (Adriamycin), cyclophosphamide, vincristine (Oncovin), procarbazine, and prednisone (BEACOPP).

Regardless of the stage, CHL is highly curable and 86.6% patients were alive at 5 years following treatment. Therefore, it is highly important to diagnose and treat patients appropriately and to monitor for long-term complications in survivors. Staging and risk prognostication are essential in deciding the appropriate treatment regimen. Age greater than 50, bulky disease more than 10 cm, elevated ESR, presence of "B" symptoms, involvement of greater than three nodal groups, and bulky mediastinal mass greater than 0.33 (maximum width of the mass/maximum intrathoracic diameter) are all unfavorable factors in limited stage disease (Stage I to II). In advanced-stage CHL, the international prognostic score is generated using seven adverse risk factors, which include male sex, age greater than 45 years, stage IV disease, serum albumin of less than 4 g per deciliter, a hemoglobin level of less than 10.5 g per deciliter, leukocytosis (a white-cell count of at least 15,000 per cubic millimeter), and lymphocytopenia (a lymphocyte count of less than 600 per cubic millimeter, a count that was less than 8% of the white-cell count, or both). The score predicted the rate of freedom from progression of disease with 42% survival in patients with a score of 5 or higher.

Treatment

Stage I to IIA constitutes limited stage disease and Stage IIB to IV constitutes advanced disease.

Limited Stage Classical Hodgkin Lymphoma

Combined modality treatment using a combination of radiotherapy (RT) and chemotherapy is the treatment of choice for early stage limited disease with favorable risk factors. Various trials over decades have established the role of combined modality treatment with RT alone or chemotherapy alone being the comparator arms.

The HD 10 trial investigated the reduction of number of cycles of doxorubicin (Adriamycin,[1] bleomycin, vinblastine, and dubarbazine [ABVD]) and the dose of involved field radiation (IFRT) in patients with no unfavorable risk factors. One thousand three hundred and seventy patients were randomized into four different groups. Early stage favorable risk factor patients who received 2 cycles of ABVD followed by 20 Gy IFRT had similar 5 year overall survival (OS) as the patients who received 4 cycles of ABVD followed by 30 Gy IFRT. ABVD for 2 cycles followed by 20 Gy IFRT is now the standard of care for Stage IA to IIA disease with favorable risk patients. Four cycles of ABVD followed by 30 Gy of IFRT or 6 cycles of ABVD is recommended for limited stage (stage I to IIA) disease with unfavorable risk factors or bulky disease. Stanford V and BEACOPP (bleomycin, etoposide [Toposar],[1] Adriamycin,[1] cyclophosphamide, vincristine [Oncovin], procarbazine [Matulane], and prednisone) regimens are considered alternate treatment options and generally yield similar excellent results with 5 year OS rates of 90% to 95%. ABVD is the most commonly used regimen due to greater tolerability and less cumulative dosage of anthracyclines.

Advanced-Stage Classical Hodgkin Lymphoma

Advanced-stage CHL (Ann Arbor stages IIB to IV) used to be a fatal disease until the development of the MOPP (mechlorethamine, vincristine [Oncovin], procarbazine, and prednisone) regimen in the 1960s. ABVD for 6 to 8 months was compared to MOPP in a randomized landmark clinical trial and ABVD was found to be equally or more effective and was associated with less toxicity. ABVD is administered on days 1 and 15 of a 28-day cycle for 6 total cycles. Modern outcomes with ABVD for advanced-stage disease produced 5-year freedom from progression and OS of 78% and 90%, respectively. Combined modality treatment with IFRT is considered in patients with bulky disease for tumor consolidation or in patients with an incomplete response to chemotherapy.

Alternative regimens include escalated BEACOPP and Stanford V. Neither of these regimens improved OS when compared to ABVD and were associated with increased treatment-related toxicity. Most recently, brentuximab vedotin (BV) (Adcetris) in combination with an Adriamycin, vinblastine, and dacarbazine (A+AVD) regimen has been approved in the United States for advanced stage CHL based on the phase III randomized ECHELON-1 study. This regimen had a 4.9 percentage-point lower combined risk of progression, death, or noncomplete response when compared with the use of subsequent anticancer therapy at 2 years in comparison to ABVD with a tolerable safety profile. The modified end point is considered a caveat for this study and long-term survival data for this study is still pending. Both ABVD and A+AVD are reasonable first line options in patients with Stage III and IV disease and should be chosen based on the patient's age, financial status, and preference and comorbidities. There are not enough data at this time to recommend A+AVD over ABVD. There are ongoing clinical trials evaluating the efficacy and tolerability of combination regimens with BV and checkpoint blockade (nivolumab [Opdivo]) in front line settings. As of now, ABVD is still the preferred regimen in United States with ongoing debate in regard to alternative regimens.

[1]Not FDA approved for this indication

Relapsed/Refractory Classical Hodgkin Lymphoma

CHL carries an overall excellent prognosis and approximately 85% of patients are cured. However, approximately 15% of patients do relapse or have primary refractory disease and will require salvage treatment. Prognosis, especially in patients with refractory disease or who relapse within 12 months of treatment, has historically been poor with conventional salvage chemotherapy. However, with the advent of targeted therapy and checkpoint blockade, response rates and OS rates for this group have improved significantly. Currently, conventional salvage chemotherapy followed by autologous stem cell transplant, which offers a 50% cure rate, remains the second line option.

BV maintenance is offered starting 30 to 45 days after stem cell transplant for a total of 16 cycles, 3 weeks apart based on phase III randomized AETHERA trial data. Patients randomized to receive brentuximab consolidation had significantly improved progression-free survival of 43 months, compared with 24 months in placebo-treated patients. There are ongoing clinical trials evaluating newer agents in second-line settings and enrollment in clinical trials is preferable for these patients. Patients who relapse after autologous stem cell transplant are usually considered for allogeneic stem cell transplant after they have demonstrated a response with next line options.

BV is a monoclonal antibody that is active against CD30 bound to the microtubule toxin monomethyl auristatin E (MMAE). BV has been FDA approved for third-line treatment after a pivotal phase II study resulted in an ORR of 75% and CR of 34% compared to single agent treatment. BV is administered every 3 weeks by intravenous infusion at a dose of 1.8 mg/kg. BV is now also used in combination with Bendamustine (Bendeka)[1], which, in multiple single institutional retrospective data, showed improved response rates of around 92% compared to BV alone.

Mostly recently, immunotherapy with checkpoint blockade has been studied in CHL after identification of 9p24.1 amplification, which results in universal overexpression of programmed death-1(PD-1) ligands. Nivolumab and pembrolizumab (Keytruda), which are both PD-1 inhibitors, have been studied in phase II studies and have shown overall response rates of around 69% and 67%, respectively. Nivolumab is FDA approved for patients who have relapsed after autologous stem cell transplant and have failed BV. Pembrolizumab is approved for patients who have failed BV. Further studies are evaluating the role of combination treatments with these agents. There are also ongoing clinical trials evaluating newer treatment options such as CD30 engineered CAR T cells.

Treatment of Nodular Lymphocyte-Predominant Hodgkin Lymphoma

Nodular lymphocyte-predominant Hodgkin lymphoma (NLPHL) is typically an indolent disease and presents with early stage disease in peripheral nodal locations. Early stage patients are treated with IFRT alone with excellent response rates. Ten year OS is 95% in these patients. Advanced-stage NLPHL is relatively uncommon and can be treated with either single agent rituximab (Rituxan),[1] due to CD20 positivity on malignant cells, or combination chemotherapeutic regimens such as ABVD and RCHOP (rituximab, cyclophosphamide, hydroxydaunomycin [doxorubicin], Oncovin, and prednisone), depending on the extent of disease and patient comorbidities.

Response Assessment

End-of-treatment (EOT) assessment is more accurate with PET-CT imaging. The Deauville score, which is a 5-point scoring system, is used to assess responses with PET scan imaging. A score of 1, 2, or 3 is considered a complete metabolic response. There is no indication for routine surveillance scans after the EOT assessment. A score of 4 or 5 is considered a suboptimal response and

---

[1]Not FDA approved for this indication

may require a change of treatment plan. Interim PET scanning after two cycles of ABVD therapy has prognostic significance. However, the significance of interim PET scanning with newer combination regimens has not been validated.

Complications and Long-Term Monitoring

CHL is a curable cancer. Short- and long-term complications from treatment require close monitoring, especially given the young age of presentation in most patients. Most short-term side effects are fatigue, nausea, emesis, constipation, increased risk of infections, and peripheral neuropathy. Patients need long-term cardiac monitoring due to the risk of congestive heart failure with anthracyclines and combination IFRT, and the risk of coronary artery disease with IFRT. Bleomycin can cause long-term pulmonary toxicity and patients should be monitored while on active treatment. Prompt discontinuation of bleomycin is warranted if there is any suspicion of pulmonary complications. There is a long-term risk of secondary malignancies and myelodysplastic syndrome in patients treated for HL.

Patients should undergo regular cancer screenings. Yearly complete blood count is warranted. Thyroid evaluation once a year is recommended for patients who have received neck or superior mediastinal IFRT. Mammography is recommended for women starting 8 years after IFRT to mediastinum.

References

Advani RH, Hoppe RT, Baer D, et al: Efficacy of abbreviated Stanford V chemotherapy and involved-field radiotherapy in early-stage Hodgkin lymphoma: mature results of the G4 trial, Ann Oncol 34:1044–1048, 2013.

Armand P, Engert A, Younes A, et al: Nivolumab for relapsed/refractory classic hodgkin lymphoma after failure of autologous hematopoietic cell transplantation: extended follow-up of the multicohort single-arm Phase II CheckMate 205 Trial, J Clin Oncol 36(14):1428–1439, 2018 May 10.

Canellos GP, Anderson JR, et al: Chemotherapy of advanced Hodgkin's Disease with MOPP, ABVD, or MOPP alternating with ABVD, N Engl J Med 327:1478–1484, 1992.

Chen RC, Chin MS, Ng AK, et al: Early-stage, lymphocyte-predominant Hodgkin's lymphoma: patient outcomes from a large, single-institution series with long follow-up, J Clin Oncol 28:136–141, 2010.

Cheson BD, Fisher RI, Barrington SF, et al: Recommendations for initial evaluation, staging, and response assessment of hodgkin and non-Hodgkin lymphoma: the Lugano classification, J Clin Oncol 32(27):3059–3067, 2014 Sep 20.

Connors JM, Jurczak W, Straus DJ, et al: Brentuximab vedotin with chemotherapy for stage III or IV Hodgkin's lymphoma, N Engl J Med 378:331–344, 2018.

Eichenauer DA, Fuchs M, Pluetschow A, et al: Phase 2 study of rituximab in newly diagnosed stage IA nodular lymphocyte-predominant Hodgkin lymphoma: a report from the German Hodgkin Study Group, Blood 118:4363–4365, 2011.

Engert A, Plutschow A, Eich HT, et al: Reduced treatment intensity in patients with early-stage Hodgkin's lymphoma, N Engl J Med 363:640–652, 2010.

Gallamini A, Hutchings M, Rigacci L, et al: Early interim 2-[18 F]fluoro-2-deoxy-Dglucose positron emission tomography is prognostically superior to international prognostic score in advanced-stage Hodgkin's lymphoma: a report from a joint Italian-Danish study, J Clin Oncol 25:3746–3752, 2007.

Hasenclever D, Diehl V: A prognostic score for advanced Hodgkin's disease. International Prognostic Factors Project on Advanced Hodgkin's Disease, N Engl J Med 339(21):1506–1514, 1998 Nov 19.

Jacobson CA, Abramson JS: HIV-associated Hodgkin's lymphoma: prognosis and therapy in the era of cART, Adv Hematol 2012:507257, 2012.

Kharazmi E, Fallah M, Pukkala E, et al: Risk of familial classical Hodgkin lymphoma by relationship, histology, age, and sex: a joint study from five Nordic countries, Blood 126(17):1990–1995, 2015 Oct 22.

LaCasce AS, Bociek RG, Sawas A, et al: Brentuximab vedotin plus bendamustine: a highly active first salvage regimen for relapsed or refractory Hodgkin lymphoma, Blood 11:815183, 2018.

Meyer RM, Gospodarowicz MK, Connors JM, et al: ABVD alone versus radiation-based therapy in limited-stage Hodgkin's lymphoma, N Engl J Med 366:399–408, 2012.

Moskowitz CH, Nademanee A, et al: Brentuximab vedotin as consolidation therapy after autologous stem-cell transplantation in patients with Hodgkin's lymphoma at risk of relapse or progression (AETHERA): a randomised, double-blind, placebo-controlled, phase 3 trial, Lancet 385(9980):1853–1862, 2015 May 9.

Moskowitz CH, Zinzani PL, Fanale MA, et al: Pembrolizumab in relapsed/refractory classical Hodgkin lymphoma: primary end point analysis of the Phase 2 Keynote-087 Study, Blood 128:1107, 2016.

Younes A, Gopal AK, Smith SE, et al: Results of a pivotal phase II study of brentuximab vedotin for patients with relapsed or refractory Hodgkin's lymphoma, J Clin Oncol 30(18):2183–2189, 2012 Jun 20.Olorepera eium, quamendisit quidessin nem faces aped estio endes doluptatiis modio tem isto blaborum invernam, aut est optur maioreh enduntorero dolles dolo dusam esteseq uaest, omniminit, qui dolorum, tem rem eictur archit eium expelit voluptat atiatem harum ium si unt exerum event, apedio eosti blat.

IRON DEFICIENCY ANEMIA

Method of
Susan Evans, MD

CURRENT DIAGNOSIS

- The presence of symptoms and signs depends on the degree of iron deficiency, the time course of the development of iron deficiency, and the overall physiologic state of the patient. Patients may be asymptomatic. Signs and symptoms are more likely if anemia and/or hemodynamic instability are present.
- Symptoms include fatigue, poor exercise tolerance, weakness, headache, pica, dyspnea, dizziness, vertigo, and angina pectoris.
- Signs include pallor, dry and rough skin, brittle nails, defects of the nail bed (koilonychias), atrophy of the lingual papillae, and cheilosis.
- Systolic heart murmur if anemia is present
- Neonates: delayed growth and development
- Adolescents: learning and behavior problems
- Blood loss is the most common cause of iron deficiency
- Iron deficiency is the most common cause of anemia

Laboratory Findings
- Decreased iron on bone marrow aspirate is the gold standard but is rarely used
- Low serum hemoglobin to diagnose anemia
- Low mean corpuscular hemoglobin: late finding
- Low mean corpuscular volume: late finding
- Low serum iron
- High serum iron-binding capacity
- Low percent transferrin saturation (TSAT)
- Low serum ferritin, but may be normal in the presence of inflammation

CURRENT THERAPY

Oral Replacement
- Ferrous sulfate (or another equivalent iron preparation) 325 mg (65 mg elemental iron) once daily or once daily on alternating days if that is better tolerated.
- Avoid taking with meals to increase absorption.

Parenteral Replacement
- Recommended when blood loss exceeds the ability to replace orally, in the context of malabsorption and if oral iron is not tolerated
  - Ferric carboxymaltose (Ferinject and Injectafer)
  - Ferric gluconate (Ferrlecit)
  - Ferumoxytol (Feraheme)
  - Iron sucrose (Venofer)

Unstable Patient
- If the patient is hemodynamically unstable due to anemia, consider blood transfusion

Treatment Endpoint
- Continue iron replacement for 3 months after anemia is resolved and iron replaced.

Epidemiology

Anemia affects more than one-third of the world's population, or 2 billion people. Iron deficiency continues to be the most common cause of anemia. Iron deficiency is the only micronutrient deficiency that remains a significant problem in both developing and developed countries. Iron deficiency refers to a decrease in iron stores below a normal level and can cause fatigue and decreased exercise intolerance even without anemia. In the case of iron deficiency without anemia, iron stores are still adequate for erythropoiesis. Iron deficiency anemia is a more serious condition in which there is not enough erythroid iron available, leading to anemia. Worldwide levels of iron deficiency are estimated to be twice that of iron deficiency anemia.

Risk Factors

Risk factors for iron deficiency anemia include age, socioeconomic status, female gender, race and ethnicity, diet low in iron, disease, and medical treatment. Several groups of people are at an increased risk of iron deficiency based on age or their stage in life. Infants and children ages 0 to 5 years old are at risk for iron deficiency because of their rapid rate of growth, which necessitates increased iron stores. Based on 2019 World Health Organization information, 39.8% of children aged 6 to 59 months were anemic. Adolescent girls and women of child bearing age are also at risk due to iron loss through menstruation. In 2019, 29.9% of women aged 15 to 49 were anemic. In the United States, Black women of childbearing age are 4 to 7 times more likely to have anemia than White women, and for Hispanic women the prevalence is 2 to 3 times that seen in White women. During pregnancy, a woman's iron needs triple because of the expansion of red cell mass, the placenta, and the growth of the fetus. Worldwide, anemia affects 36.5% of pregnant women and is known to increase the risk of cesarean section and maternal mortality. Elderly people are also at risk for iron deficiency for a number of reasons, including inadequate diet, poor absorption due to disease or antacid medicines, or as a complication of chronic disease. The 2025 Global Nutrition Targets aim to decrease the prevalence by 50%.

Dietary causes of iron deficiency anemia include lack of access to or preference against eating a diet including iron rich foods. While 90% of iron in the body is recycled every day, dietary iron is essential for replacing lost iron, which is mainly excreted in bile. Iron supplementation of common foods such as breads and rice in the United States decreases the risk of dietary iron deficiency. Iron is found naturally in both animal products such as meat and in plant based foods such as green leafy vegetables, sweet potatoes, and legumes. As long as they eat a healthy and well-balanced diet, vegetarians and vegans have not been shown to be at an increased risk for iron deficiency; such diets have many other health benefits.

Any illness or therapy that leads to decreased iron absorption or blood loss may cause iron deficiency. Common causes of blood loss include gastrointestinal diseases such as cancer, inflammatory bowel disease, and ulcer disease. Taking aspirin, nonsteroidal anti-inflammatory drugs (NSAIDs), or anticoagulants also increases the risk of gastrointestinal blood loss. Iron absorption is decreased in the context of celiac disease, post gastric bypass surgery, and *Helicobacter pylori* infection. Chronic diseases associated with iron deficiency include chronic kidney disease, rheumatoid arthritis, cancer, obesity, and chronic heart failure. There are also medical treatments that may cause iron deficiency such as antacid medicines, which decrease iron absorption, dialysis that causes blood loss, and erythropoietin therapy that depletes iron stores through increased erythropoiesis. Frequent phlebotomy, including repetitive blood donation or treatment for polycythemia or hemochromatosis, decrease iron stores. Rarely, there may be a genetic cause for iron deficiency anemia such as iron-refractory iron deficiency anemia.

Pathophysiology

Iron in the body can be broken down into two main types: functional iron and storage iron. Functional iron plays many essential roles in the human body. It is found in hemoglobin, which carries oxygen from the lungs to body tissues, and in muscles as myoglobin, which helps with oxygen use and storage. Iron plays a role in enzymatic reactions, DNA synthesis, mitochondrial energy generation, and cell proliferation. Storage iron is found in ferritin, hemosiderin, and transferrin. Iron homeostasis is very important to the body and is regulated through the diet, gastrointestinal absorption, and the recycling of the iron in red blood cells. Total body iron stores are about 3.5 g for men and 2.5 g for women. Approximately 20 to 25 mg of iron is needed daily for red cell production and body processes. Dietary absorption of iron is limited to about 1 to 2 mg/day; the daily requirement is produced through the recycling of iron in used red blood cells by macrophages.

Dietary iron is found in two forms. Heme iron (Fe^{2+}) is found in animal products such as meat, poultry and seafood and is more easily absorbed than plant-based iron. Nonheme iron (Fe^{3+}) is found in plant sources such as beans and lentils, baked potatoes, dark green leafy vegetables, tofu, and cashews. Dietary iron is also found in iron fortified breakfast cereals and enriched breads. Adding foods high in vitamin C to a meal with nonheme iron can increase iron absorption. There are other foods that inhibit the absorption of iron, including polyphenols found in some vegetables, tannins found in tea, and calcium found in dairy products. Dietary iron absorption takes place almost exclusively in the duodenum and upper jejunum.

The recycling of iron from used red blood cells provides about 90% of body iron and is essential for maintaining normal iron levels in the body. Hepcidin, a peptide hormone mainly synthesized in the liver, controls the process of iron absorption and recycling. When serum iron levels are high, hepcidin levels increase in response, which leads to breakdown of the iron transporter called ferroportin. A decrease in ferroportin leaves more iron inside macrophages, enterocytes, and hepatocytes, and the serum iron level decreases. When serum iron levels drop, expression of hepcidin should decrease as well. However, inflammation and infection can cause hepcidin to increase inappropriately; this is one of the ways in which chronic disease contributes to iron deficiency.

Prevention

Prevention plays a large role in the treatment of iron deficiency anemia worldwide and includes both dietary interventions and supplementation. A food-based approach to prevention would include encouraging patients to eat more iron rich foods such as meats and dark green leafy vegetables. A list of iron rich foods is found in Table 1. Heme iron, found in animal sources, is easily absorbed; however, the absorption of nonheme iron from plant sources is affected by the foods with which they are eaten. Foods that can inhibit the absorption of iron include the tannins in tea and coffee and the calcium found in milk. It is best to eat these foods separately from iron rich foods to increase iron absorption. Certain foods increase the absorption of non-heme iron when they are eaten at the same time, including foods that

contain heme (such as meat) or foods that contain vitamin C (such as fruit, orange juice, or broccoli). Encouraging iron fortified foods, which in the United States include cereals, rice, pasta, and bread, is another effective way to prevent deficiency. There are some cases when the risk of developing iron deficiency is so high that supplementation with an oral iron supplement is recommended. The World Health Organization recommends universal supplementation for low-birth-weight infants with 2 mg/kg daily from age 2 months to 23 months. They also recommend universal supplementation for pregnant women with 60 mg iron per day. While supplementation for pregnant women is common practice in the United States, the US Preventive Services Task Force states that there is insufficient evidence to show that these practices help prevent adverse maternal health and birth outcomes. According to the US Preventive Services Task Force, evidence is also insufficient to recommend screening children age 6 months to 2 years of age for iron deficiency anemia in the United States.

Clinical Manifestations

Patients with iron deficiency may be asymptomatic. The presence of symptoms and signs of iron deficiency depend on the degree of deficiency, the time course of the development of iron deficiency, and the overall physiologic state of the patient. Common symptoms of iron deficiency include fatigue, weakness, irritability, poor concentration, decreased exercise intolerance, dry mouth, headache, and restless leg syndrome. Severe iron deficiency can cause pica, a craving to eat substances such as ice, dirt, clay, or paint. Signs of iron deficiency include pallor and a systolic heart murmur if anemia is present, hair loss, atrophy of lingual papillae, and nail changes such as koilonychias.

Diagnosis

Normal hemoglobin levels depend on age, gender, pregnancy status, altitude, and smoking, but in general, an adult male is considered anemic with a hemoglobin level less than 13 g/dL and an adult female at less than 12 g/dL. Iron deficiency may be present with or without anemia; therefore, measuring hemoglobin level is neither a sensitive nor a specific test for iron deficiency. Absolute iron deficiency occurs when the amount of total body iron is low. Functional iron deficiency occurs when there is not enough iron available to meet the demand of body tissues and processes because iron is sequestered either in macrophages or the reticuloendothelial system.

Diagnosing iron deficiency is not straightforward because serum ferritin level, which is often used as a screening test, is affected by gender, age, inflammation, infection, and chronic diseases such as liver disease and cancer. While a serum ferritin concentration less than 12 µg/L makes iron deficiency very likely, a person with inflammation or chronic disease may have iron deficiency at much higher ferritin levels. Increasing the cutoff for normal ferritin concentration to 30 µg/L has been shown to increase sensitivity for iron deficiency, and an even higher cutoff of 100 µg is recommended by some specialty societies. For this reason, utilizing more than one iron status indicator to make the diagnosis is important. A low iron level (<50 µg/dL) and an elevated total iron binding capacity (TIBC >450 µg/dL) also support the diagnosis of iron deficiency. Other supporting labs include a drop in transferrin saturation (TSAT) to less than 16% or less than 20% if inflammation or disease is present. Low mean corpuscular volume (MCV) may be another sign of iron deficiency, but this is generally a late finding, so MCV may be in the normal range. Low MCV can also be seen in thalassemia. Low mean corpuscular hemoglobin concentration (MCHC) is another late finding in iron deficiency. Decreased iron seen on bone marrow aspiration is still considered the gold standard for diagnosing iron deficiency, but it is rarely done due to both cost and patient discomfort.

TABLE 1	Iron Rich Foods
IRON TYPE	**DIETARY SOURCES**
Heme Iron	Beef
	Chicken
	Fish
	Organ Meats
	Oysters
Nonheme Iron	Dark Green Leafy Vegetables
	Beans
	Lentils
	Tofu
	Baked Potato
	Cashews
	Fortified Cereals, Breads and Pasta

Differential Diagnosis

The differential diagnosis of iron deficiency includes causes of fatigue and exercise intolerance such as hypothyroidism, electrolyte disturbances due to diuretic therapy, left ventricular dysfunction, chronic lung disease, malignancies, or liver disease.

Anemia of chronic disease can mimic iron deficiency anemia and may be found concurrently in the same patient. The differential diagnosis for iron deficiency also includes thalassemia, sideroblasitc anemias, and lead poisoning

Treatment

The goal of treatment is to replace iron so that hemoglobin levels normalize, and iron stores are replenished. Treatment of iron deficiency must take into consideration the type of patient being treated and the source and amount of iron deficit or blood loss. Patients who are severely anemic and hemodynamically unstable may be candidates for blood transfusion. For people in groups that are at high risk for iron deficiency, such as infants, toddlers, adolescents, and menstruating women, it is reasonable to start with oral supplementation with iron and only proceed with further work up if that is unsuccessful. However, in patients at low risk for iron deficiency, such as men and post-menopausal women, it is important to determine the underlying cause of iron deficiency. Blood loss is the most common cause of iron deficiency, so this work-up includes evaluation for a source of bleeding. Urinalysis and heme-occult testing are preliminary tests, and upper and lower endoscopy is needed to evaluate for gastrointestinal pathology including cancer, colitis, or celiac disease. If those tests are inconclusive, consider proceeding to video capsule endoscopy to further evaluate the small intestine. Heavy gynecologic bleeding may require further evaluation and treatment. Persistent blood noted on urinalysis would warrant referral to urology for further testing.

Oral iron supplementation continues to be the first line treatment for iron deficiency anemia. Common forms include ferrous sulfate (Feosol), ferrous gluconate (Fergon), and ferrous fumarate (Ferro-Sequels). A typical dose of ferrous sulfate is 325 mg (65 mg elemental iron) daily. However, there is now evidence that a dose of oral iron increases serum hepcidin, which then decreases iron absorption. Based on these findings, an alternate recommendation would be to give a single dose of iron on alternate days. This dosing schedule may increase iron absorption and adherence to treatment due to simpler regimen with decreased side effects. Iron is best absorbed when taken between meals; however, this can also worsen side effects. It is best to take iron separate from acid reducing medicines and foods that inhibit iron absorption. Common side effects of oral iron include diarrhea, nausea, epigastric discomfort, and constipation. Side effects can be lessened by taking iron with food and taking smaller doses such as ferrous gluconate 325 mg (38 mg elemental iron).

Parenteral iron may be indicated when oral therapy is unsuccessful due to malabsorption, when oral iron is not tolerated, or when the rate of absorption with oral supplementation is insufficient due to the rate of blood loss. New forms of parenteral iron are safer, less likely to cause hypersensitivity reactions, and their use is increasing. The dose of IV iron needed can be calculated with the following formula: body weight in kilograms x 2.3 x hemoglobin deficiency (target hemoglobin level—patient hemoglobin level). Add another 500 to 1000 mg iron to replace low iron stores. Parenteral iron preparations licensed for use in the United States include iron sucrose (Venofer), ferumoxytol (Feraheme), ferric carboxymaltose (Ferinject and Injectafer), and ferric gluconate (Ferrlecit). A common dose for iron sucrose is 200 mg IV over 2 to 5 minutes, which is often repeated 5 times or until the target dose of iron is reached. Ferumoxytol has a usual dose of 510 mg IV infusion over at least 15 minutes which can be repeated 3 to 5 days after the initial dose. For patients who weigh ≥50 kg, the dose of ferric carboxymaltose is 750 mg IV over 15 to 30 minutes, and this can be repeated 7 days after the first dose. Ferric gluconate is generally used for patients on dialysis, and the typical dose is 125 mg IV over 10 minutes or IV infusion over 60 minutes per dialysis session.

Monitoring

The earliest marker for successful iron replacement is an increase in the reticulocyte count, which occurs within 5 to 10 days of initiation of iron replacement. Darkening of stools after 2 or 3 days of starting oral iron replacement is a reliable marker of compliance. A hemoglobin increase of 2 g/dL is considered an appropriate response to oral iron replacement. Reaching a serum ferritin level of 100 µg/L will ensure good iron stores in nearly all patients. Once iron deficiency has been corrected, a complete blood count and labs to evaluate iron stores should be checked monthly for 3 months and then every 3 months for a year. If iron levels are not maintained, then further work up is indicated to discover the cause.

Management of Complications

If properly treated, iron deficiency has few complications in adults. Untreated iron deficiency in infants and small children can lead to cognitive development and growth deficits. Treating iron deficiency without identifying the source and cause of blood loss could result in a delay or failure to diagnose gastrointestinal malignancies or other serious clinical problems.

Plummer–Vinson syndrome is a rare clinical condition characterized by a triad of iron deficiency anemia, postcricoid esophageal webs, and dysphagia. The pathogenesis of Plummer-Vinson syndrome remains unclear, though iron and other nutritional deficiencies, genetic predisposition, and autoimmunity have all been implicated in the formation of the webs. Treatment includes the correction of iron deficiency and endoscopic dilation of the esophageal webs to relieve dysphagia.

References

Auerbach M, Adamson JW: How we diagnose and treat iron deficiency anemia, *Am J Hematol* 91(1):31–38, 2016 Jan.

Camaschella C: Iron-deficiency anemia, *N Engl J Med* 372(19):1832–1843, 2015 May 7.

Camaschella C, Girelli D: The changing landscape of iron deficiency, *Mol Aspects Med* 2020 Oct;75:100861. https://www.doi.org/10.1016/j.mam.2020.100861. Epub 2020 May 14. PMID: 32418671

Centers for Disease Control. Recommendation to Prevent and Control Iron Deficiency in the United States. Available at https://www.cdc.gov/MMWR/preview/mmwrhtml/00051880.htm. [Accessed April 16, 2019].

Craig WJ, Mangels AR, American Dietetic Association: Position of the American Dietetic Association: vegetarian diets, *J Am Diet Assoc* 109(7):1266–1282, 2009 Jul.

Engebretsen KV, Blom-Hogestol IK, Hewitt S, et al: Anemia following Roux-en-Y gastric bypass for morbid obesity; a 5-year follow-up study, *Scand J Gastroenterol* 53(8):917–922, 2018 Aug.

Le CHH. The Prevalence of Anemia and Moderate-Severe Anemia in the US Population (NHANES 2003-2012). *PLoS ONE* 11(11):e0166635, 2016.

Lopez A, Cacoub P, Macdougall IC, Peyrin-Biroulet L: Iron deficiency anaemia, *Lancet* 387(10021):907–916, 2016 Feb 27.

Parrott J, Frank L, Rabena R, Craggs-Dino L, Isom KA, Greiman L: American Society for Metabolic and Bariatric Surgery Integrated Health Nutritional Guidelines for the Surgical Weight Loss Patient 2016 Update: Micronutrients, *Surg Obes Relat Dis* 13(5):727–741, 2017 May.

Peyrin-Biroulet L, Williet N, Cacoub P: Guidelines on the diagnosis and treatment of iron deficiency across indications: a systematic review, *Am J Clin Nutr* 102(6):1585–1594, 2015 Dec.

Stoffel NU, Cercamondi CI, Brittenham G, et al: Iron absorption from oral iron supplements given on consecutive versus alternate days and as single morning doses versus twice–daily split dosing in iron–depleted women: two open-label, randomised controlled trials, *Lancet Haematol* 4(11):e524–33, 2017.

World Health Organization: Anaemia in women and children. Available at https://www.who.int/ data/gho/data/themes/topics/anaemia_in_women_and_children. [Accessed 30 March 2022].

World Health Organization/UNICEF/UNU: Iron Deficiency Anaemia: Assessment, Prevention, and Control. A guide for Programme Managers, Geneva, Switzerland, 2001, World Health Organization. Available at https://www.who.int/nutrition/publications/en/ida_assessment_prevention_control.pdf. [Accessed 17 April 2019].

MULTIPLE MYELOMA

Method of
S. Vincent Rajkumar, MD; and Robert A. Kyle, MD

CURRENT DIAGNOSIS

- Malignant clonal plasma cell disorder
- Characterized by presence of a monoclonal immunoglobulin in the serum or urine in most patients
- Typical manifestations include anemia, osteolytic bone lesions, and renal failure
- Initial work-up should include a bone marrow aspiration and biopsy with fluorescent in situ hybridization studies to determine molecular cytogenetic typ0065
- Standard risk: trisomies (hyperdiploidy), t(11;14), and t(6;14)
- High risk: del(17p), gain 1q, t(4;14), (t14;16) or t(14;20)

CURRENT THERAPY

- Do not begin treatment until symptomatic multiple myeloma develops (CRAB: *c*alcium elevated, *r*enal failure, *a*nemia, *b*one lesions) or other myeloma defining events are present. Patients with high risk smoldering multiple myeloma are candidates for preventive therapy with lenalidomide (Revimid) or lenalidomide plus dexamethasone (Decadron)[1] (Rd)
- Decide whether an autologous stem cell transplant is feasible. If it is, one must avoid melphalan (Alkeran) therapy as initial treatment.
- Initial therapy typically consists of a triplet regimen such as lenalidomide (Revlimid), bortezomib (Velcade), dexamethasone (VRd), daratumumab (Darzalex), lenalidomide, and dexamethasone (DRd).
- Patients who are candidates for autologous stem cell transplantation should collect stem cells after 3 to 4 cycles of induction. After collection, patients proceed to either early transplantation, or resume initial therapy and postpone transplant until relapse. After transplant, and after initial therapy in patients who delay transplant, patients should receive maintenance therapy.
- Patients who are not stem cell transplant candidates who are treated with VRd receive about 8 to 9 cycles of triplet therapy followed by maintenance. If DRd is used as initial therapy, the triplet is continued at maintenance doses. Frail patients can be treated with the doublet regimen of Rd, in which case therapy is continued until progression if tolerated.
- Relapsed or refractory myeloma should be treated with one of the active drugs given alone or in combination. Active agents include thalidomide, lenalidomide, bortezomib, carfilzomib (Kyprolis), pomalidomide (Pomalyst), daratumumab (Darzalex), ixazomib (Ninlaro), elotuzumab (Empliciti), isatuximab (Sarclisa), belantamab mafodotin (Blenrep), selinexor (Xpovio), ide-cel (Abecma), cilta-cel (Carvykti), corticosteroids, anthracyclines, and alkylators.

Multiple myeloma is characterized by the neoplastic proliferation of clonal plasma cells. It is typically associated with a monoclonal (M) protein in the serum and/or urine.

Epidemiology

In the United States, multiple myeloma constitutes 1% of all malignant diseases and slightly more than 10% of hematologic malignancies. The annual incidence is 4 to 5 per 100,000; the incidence in African Americans is twice that in whites. The apparent recent increase in rates is probably caused by increased availability and use of medical facilities and improved diagnostic techniques, particularly in the older population. The median age at diagnosis is approximately 70 years.

Risk Factors

The cause of multiple myeloma is unclear. Exposure to radiation might play a role. Persons in agricultural occupations who are exposed to pesticides, herbicides, or fungicides have an increased risk of multiple myeloma. Benzene and petroleum products, hair dyes, engine exhaust, furniture worker products, obesity, and chronic immune stimulation have also been reported as risk factors. The risk of developing multiple myeloma is higher for patients with a first-degree relative with the disease. Clusters of two or more first-degree relatives or identical twins have been recognized.

Clinical Manifestations

Weakness, fatigue, bone pain, recurrent infections, and symptoms of hypercalcemia or renal insufficiency should alert the physician to the possibility of multiple myeloma. Anemia is present in 70% of patients at the time of diagnosis. An M protein is found in the serum or urine in more than 97% of patients with multiple myeloma by immunofixation studies and the serum free light chain (FLC) assay. Lytic lesions, osteoporosis, or fractures are present at diagnosis in 80% of patients and are best detected by whole body low-dose computed tomography (CT) or positron emission tomography (PET)/CT. Magnetic resonance imaging (MRI) and PET/CT are also helpful in patients who have skeletal pain but no abnormality on radiographs or when there are other clinical concerns about the extent of the disease. Conventional radiography is less sensitive and is no longer recommended. Hypercalcemia is present in 15% of patients, and the serum creatinine value is 2 mg/dL or greater in almost 20% of patients at diagnosis.

Diagnosis

If multiple myeloma is suspected, the patient should have, in addition to a complete history and physical examination:

- Determination of values for hemoglobin, leukocytes with differential count, platelets, serum creatinine, calcium, and uric acid
- A radiographic survey of bones, including humeri and femurs using low-dose whole body CT or PET-CT.
- Serum protein electrophoresis with immunofixation
- Quantitation of immunoglobulins (Igs), serum FLC assay
- Bone marrow aspirate and biopsy
- Routine urinalysis
- Electrophoresis and immunofixation of an adequately concentrated aliquot from a 24-hour urine specimen
- Fluorescence in situ hybridization (FISH)
- Measurement of β_2-microglobulin, C-reactive protein, and lactate dehydrogenase

Box 1 lists the International Myeloma Working Group updated criteria for diagnosis of myeloma and related disorders. Metastatic carcinoma, lymphoma, leukemia, and connective tissue disorders can resemble multiple myeloma and must be considered in the differential diagnosis. Patients with multiple myeloma must be differentiated from those with monoclonal gammopathy of undetermined significance (MGUS) and smoldering (asymptomatic) multiple myeloma (SMM). Patients with MGUS and low-risk SMM may remain stable for long periods and not require treatment (see Box 1). Patients with high-risk SMM (any two or more of the following: >20% bone marrow plasma cells, >2g/dL serum M protein, >20 serum FLC ratio) should be considered for lenalidomide (Revlimid)[1] or lenalidomide plus dexamethasone (Decadron)[1] as preventive therapy.

---

[1]Not FDA approved for this indication.

BOX 1 International Myeloma Working Group Diagnostic Criteria.

Monoclonal Gammopathy of Undetermined Significance
- Serum M protein <3 g/dL
- Clonal bone marrow–plasma cells <10%
- Absence of end-organ damage (CRAB) attributable to a plasma cell proliferative disorder

Smoldering Multiple Myeloma
- Serum M protein ≥3 g/dL and/or clonal bone marrow–plasma cells 10%–60%
- Absence of myeloma defining events or amyloidosis

Multiple Myeloma
- Presence of clonal bone marrow plasma cells 10% or greater or biopsy-proven plasmacytoma
- Presence of end-organ damage (CRAB) thought to be related to a plasma cell proliferative disorder or other myeloma defining event (clonal bone marrow plasma cells 60% or higher, serum free light chain ratio 100 or more provided involved free light chain level is 100 mg/L or more, more than one focal lesion on magnetic resonance imaging)

CRAB, Calcium elevated, renal failure, anemia, bone lesions; *M*, monoclonal.
Derived from Rajkumar SV, Dimopoulos MA, Palumbo A, et al. International Myeloma Working Group updated criteria for the diagnosis of multiple myeloma. *Lancet Oncol.* 2014;15:e538–e548.

Treatment

Patients with symptomatic multiple myeloma may be classified as having high-risk or standard-risk disease. High-risk disease is defined as the presence of del(17p), gain 1q, t(4;14), t(14;16), or t(14;20) with FISH. Detection of p53 mutations by sequencing is also considered a cytogenetic high-risk factor. The presence of two high-risk cytogenetic abnormalities is considered "double-hit" myeloma; and the presence of three high-risk abnormalities is considered triple-hit myeloma. Lactate dehydrogenase, circulating plasma cells, and β_2-microglobulin levels are additional important risk factors. Approximately 15% to 20% of patients with symptomatic multiple myeloma have high-risk disease.

Initially, patients are classified into those eligible for an autologous stem cell transplant (SCT) versus those not eligible. An autologous SCT adds approximately 1 year of survival on average when compared with patients treated with conventional-dose chemotherapy alone.

Eligibility for autologous SCT in multiple myeloma varies from country to country. In the United States, decisions are made on a patient-by-patient basis depending on the physiologic age rather than the chronologic age. In most institutions, patients older than 70 years or with serum creatinine greater than 2.5 mg/dL, Eastern Cooperative Oncology Group (ECOG) performance status of 3 or 4, or New York Heart Association (NYHA) functional status class III or IV are considered ineligible for autologous SCT. Although patients with kidney failure may have an autologous SCT, the morbidity and mortality are higher.

Initial Therapy for Transplant-Eligible Patients

The approach to treatment of newly diagnosed myeloma in patients eligible for stem cell transplantation is summarized in Figure 1A. Bortezomib (Velcade), lenalidomide (Revlimid), dexamethasone (Decadon) (VRD)$_1$ is the preferred standard initial therapy for multiple myeloma. In a randomized trial conducted by the Southwest Oncology Group, VRD was superior to lenalidomide plus dexamethasone (Rd) in terms of progression-free survival (PFS) and overall survival (OS). Bortezomib and dexamethasone are typically administered once weekly. In the VRD regimen lenalidomide is given at a dose of 25 mg daily on days 1 to 14 of a 21-day cycle. Bortezomib should be given using the once-weekly schedule to reduce the risk of peripheral neuropathy.

It is also preferable to administer bortezomib subcutaneously to diminish the risk of neuropathy. An alternative to VRD is daratumumab (Darzalex), lenalidomide, dexamethasone (DRD). For patients who are initiated on DRD, all three drugs are continued until progression, with daratumumab administered once-monthly after the first 6 months of therapy. The addition of daratumumab (Darzalex) to VTD (Velcade, thalidomide, dexamethasone) has shown better response rates and PFS compared with VTD, but more data on OS are needed before this approach can be recommended. Similar results are also available with the addition of daratumumab to the current standard of VRD. Daratumumab plus VRD can be considered as pre-trasnplant induction therapy instead of VRD in young patients with high-risk disease. Bortezomib plus cyclophosphamide (Cytoxan) 300 mg/m^2 orally once weekly plus dexamethasone 40 mg once weekly (VCD) is an option for patients presenting with acute renal failure. If lenalidomide is not available, an alternative for initial therapy is bortezomib, thalidomide (Thalomid), and dexamethasone (VTD). For high-risk patients less than 65 years of age, daratumumab plus VRD can be considered as an alternative. In all regimens, it is preferable to administer dexamethasone at a dose no greater than 40 mg per week unless there is need for urgent cytoreduction as in patients with acute renal failure and cast nephropathy.

Autologous Stem Cell Transplantation

Following 3 to 4 months of induction therapy with one of the initial regimens, one must collect the stem cells in patients eligible for transplantation. The stem cells must be collected before the patient is exposed to prolonged therapy, especially melphalan (Alkeran). Granulocyte colony-stimulating factor (G-CSF, Neupogen) with or without cyclophosphamide (Cytoxan) is used for mobilizing stem cells. G-CSF plus cyclophosphamide is preferred in patients who are treated with lenalidomide plus dexamethasone induction, who are older than 65 years, or who have received such therapy for over 4 months. Plerixafor (Mozobil) may also be used for mobilization of hematopoietic stem cells. It is advisable to collect 6×10^6 CD34$^+$ cells/kg, which is sufficient for two transplants in patients below 65 years of age.

The timing of autologous SCT takes into account the patient's wishes, and it may be done early (when the patient recovers from stem cell collection) or delayed until relapse. There is no difference in OS even at 8 years of follow up among patients who receive an autologous SCT immediately following collection of stem cells and those who receive it at first relapse. In general, we prefer an early transplant because this provides a better quality of life and time without therapy.

Melphalan 200 mg/m^2 is the preferred conditioning regimen for autologous SCT. Tandem transplantation is not recommended for most patients. An exception would be young patients (below 65 years of age) with high-risk multiple myeloma, in whom such an approach can be considered on a case-by-case basis.

The mortality rate with autologous SCT is approximately 1%. Unfortunately, multiple myeloma is not eradicated, and the autologous peripheral stem cells are contaminated by myeloma cells or their precursors.

Bone marrow transplantation from an identical twin donor (syngeneic) is the treatment of choice if such a donor is available. Results are superior to allogeneic transplantation.

Maintenance Therapy Following Autologous Stem Cell Transplantation

Randomized trials have tested the value of lenalidomide as maintenance therapy following stem cell transplantation. An OS benefit has been observed in a meta-analysis of three trials. This benefit appears to be mainly restricted to standard-risk patients. An increased risk of second cancers has been noted with lenalidomide maintenance and further follow-up is needed. In another randomized trial improved OS with bortezomib maintenance has been reported, but it is not clear whether the benefit is due to the maintenance therapy or differences in induction therapy between the two groups. We recommend lenalidomide maintenance for

Figure 1 Approach to the treatment of newly diagnosed myeloma in patients eligible for stem cell transplantation (A) and approach to the treatment of newly diagnosed myeloma in patients not eligible for stem cell transplantation (B). *ASCT*, Autologous stem cell transplantation; *DRD*, daratumumab, lenalidomide, dexamethasone; *Dara*, daratumumab; *VRD*, bortezomib, lenalidomide, dexamethasone. Modified from Rajkumar SV. Multiple myeloma: 2020 update on diagnosis, risk-stratification, and management. *Am J Hematol.* 95(5):548–567, 2020.

standard-risk patients following autologous SCT, and following approximately 12 months of initial therapy in patients not eligible for SCT and in patients who delay SCT. In high-risk patients, we recommend bortezomib plus lenalidomide maintenance.

Allogeneic Transplantation
Allogeneic bone marrow transplantation (myeloablative and nonmyeloablative) has been tested in myeloma, but treatment-related mortality is high and graft-versus-host disease is a troublesome problem. Furthermore, only a small proportion of patients with multiple myeloma are eligible. Allogeneic transplantation is currently not recommended for routine use outside of a clinical trial. An exception to this are young patients with high-risk disease in first relapse after autologous transplantation who are willing to assume the high treatment-related mortality associated with allogeneic SCT.

Initial Therapy for Patients Who Are Ineligible for Autologous Stem Cell Transplantation
The initial therapy for patients not eligible for transplantation now resembles that of transplant-eligible patients. The current approach to treatment of newly diagnosed myeloma in patients not eligible for stem cell transplantation is summarized in Figure 1B. Currently, we prefer VRD as initial therapy. An alternative that has been recently approved for initial therapy in the United States is DRD. Other options include VCD and VTD. For frail patients, the doublet regimen of Rd can be used.

When using VRD, we continue the initial chemotherapy regimen for approximately 6 to 9 cycles followed usually by lenalidomide maintenance in standard-risk patients and bortezomib plus lenalidomide maintenance in high-risk patients.

Relapsed or Refractory Multiple Myeloma
Almost all patients with multiple myeloma who survive eventually relapse. If relapse occurs more than 6 months after treatment is discontinued, the initial chemotherapy regimen should be reinstituted. Most patients respond again, but the duration and quality of response are usually inferior to the initial response. Recently, several new drugs have been approved for the treatment of multiple myeloma including pomalidomide (Pomalyst), carfilzomib (Kyprolis), daratumumab (Darzalex), elotuzumab (Empliciti), ixazomib (Ninlaro), selinexor (Xpovio), isatuximab (Sarclisa), belantamab mafodotin (Blenrep), idecabtagene vicleucel (ide-cel [Abecma]), and ciltacabtagene autoleucel (ciltacel [Carvykti]).

Thalidomide
Thalidomide (Thalomid) is usually instituted in a dose of 50 to 100 mg daily and, if necessary, escalated to 200 mg daily if tolerated. It is most often used in combinations such as VTD. Side effects include sedation, fatigue, constipation, rash, deep venous thrombosis (DVT), edema, bradycardia, and hypothyroidism. Virtually all patients develop a sensorimotor peripheral neuropathy. The use of thalidomide in pregnancy is contraindicated, and the System for Thalidomide Education and Prescribing Safety (STEPS) program must be followed to prevent teratogenic effects.

Bortezomib
Bortezomib (Velcade) is a proteasome inhibitor that produces a response rate of approximately 35% in patients with relapsed or refractory myeloma. It is most often used in combinations such as VRD, VCD, or VTD to maximize response rates. The most troublesome side effect is peripheral neuropathy, which can occur in 35% to 40% of patients. The neuropathy is often painful but does improve in most patients after discontinuing bortezomib. The risk of neuropathy can be greatly reduced by using bortezomib in a once-weekly subcutaneous schedule.

Lenalidomide
Lenalidomide (Revlimid) as a single-agent produces an objective response in approximately 30% of patients with relapsed or refractory multiple myeloma. The major side effects are cytopenias, and the dose needs to be modified accordingly. The combination of lenalidomide plus low-dose dexamethasone (Rd) is the backbone of several myeloma treatment regimens.

Carfilzomib
Carfilzomib (Kyprolis) is a new proteasome inhibitor approved for the therapy of patients with multiple myeloma who have received at least two prior therapies, including both an immunomodulatory agent and bortezomib, and have disease progression on or within 60 days of the completion of the last therapy. Carfilzomib needs to be administered intravenously twice weekly. In a recent randomized trial, the combination of carfilzomib, lenalidomide, and dexamethasone (KRD) was found to have superior response rate, PFS, and OS compared with Rd.

Pomalidomide
Pomalidomide (Pomalyst) is an analog of lenalidomide and thalidomide. It has shown significant clinical activity in patients who are refractory to both bortezomib and lenalidomide (dual refractory). It is approved for patients with multiple myeloma who received at least two prior therapies, including both lenalidomide and bortezomib, and have disease progression on or within 60 days of the completion of the last therapy. It is administered orally at a dose of 2 to 4 mg daily for 21 days every 28 days. The major side effects are cytopenias and fatigue.

Elotuzumab

Elotuzumab (Empliciti) is a monoclonal antibody that is approved for the treatment of relapsed myeloma. It targets the signaling lymphocytic activation molecule F7 (SLAMF7). In a randomized trial of 646 patients, elotuzumab plus Rd was superior to Rd, median PFS 19.4 months versus 14.9 months, respectively ($P < .001$).

Daratumumab

Daratumumab (Darzalex) is a monoclonal antibody that is approved for the treatment of relapsed myeloma. It targets CD38, a molecule universally expressed on myeloma cells. Daratumumab has a response rate of approximately 30% in heavily pretreated patients. Two randomized trials have found improvement in PFS with the addition of daratumumab to Rd and bortezomib-dexamethasone, respectively.

Ixazomib

Ixazomib (Ninlaro) is an oral proteasome inhibitor approved for the treatment of relapsed myeloma. It is a boronic acid derivative similar to bortezomib. It is administered once weekly orally. Compared with bortezomib, it has a lower risk of peripheral neuropathy.

Selinexor

Selinexor (Xpovio) is an oral drug that acts by binding to nuclear export protein 1 (XPO1) and selectively blocking the transport of various proteins within the cell. It has been approved in combination with low dose dexamethasone for patients with relapsed or refractory multiple myeloma who have received at least 4 prior therapies, and whose disease is refractory to at least 2 proteasome inhibitors, at least 2 immunomodulatory agents, and an anti-CD38 monoclonal antibody. It is administered orally at a dose of 80 mg twice a week. However, due to toxicities, a once weekly regimen is likely more preferable.

Belantamab mafodotin

Belantamab mafodotin (Blenrep) is an antibody drug conjugate targeting B-cell maturation antigen (BCMA) that is expressed on plasma cells. Belantamab mafodotin has been approved as a single agent in patients with relapsed or refractory multiple myeloma who have received at least 4 prior therapies, including an anti-CD38 monoclonal antibody, a proteasome inhibitor, and an immunomodulatory agent. It has a response rate of approximately 30%. The main adverse effect of concern is grade 3 to 4 keratopathy, which can be seen in approximately 40% of patients, necessitating ophthalmologic evaluation prior to starting therapy and periodically during therapy.

Chimeric Antigen Receptor T (CAR-T) Cell Therapy

Idecabtagene vicleucel (ide-cel; Abecma) and ciltacabtagene autoleucel (cilta-cel; Carvykti) are CAR-Ts targeting BCMA. They have been approved for patients with relapsed refractory myeloma after 4 or more prior therapies, including an immunomodulatory drug, a proteasome inhibitor, and an anti-CD38 antibody. Ide-cel is well tolerated, with less than 5% of patients experiencing severe cytokine release syndrome or neurological toxicity. It has a response rate of 73%, with a response duration of approximately 9 months. Cilta-cel is also well tolerated and has a 2-year progression free survival rate of approximately 60%.

Isatuximab

Isatuximab (Sarclisa) is a monoclonal antibody targeting CD38 and is an alternative to daratumumab. It has been approved in combination with pomalidomide and dexamethasone, as well as in combination with carfilzomib and dexamethasone. In certain patients, isatuximab may be significantly less expensive than daratumumab, which may be a consideration.

Other New Drugs

New drugs that are in clinical trials include new bi-specific antibodies such as teclistamab[5] and AMG-701[5] (targeting BCMA and CD3), talquetamab[5] (targeting GPRC5D and CD3), and cevostamab[5] (targeting FcRH5 and CD3). Venetoclax (Venclexta)[1] has shown promise against t11;14 subtype of multiple myeloma. Iberdomide[5] is a new cereblon targeting agent that has also shown promise.

Supportive Therapy

Radiotherapy

Palliative radiation in a dose of 20 to 30 Gy should be limited to patients who have disabling pain and a well-defined focal process that has not responded to chemotherapy. Analgesics in combination with chemotherapy usually can control the pain. This approach is preferred to local radiation because pain often occurs at another site, and local radiation does not benefit the patient with systemic disease. In addition, the myelosuppressive effects of radiotherapy and chemotherapy are cumulative and can restrict future therapy. Radiation is required for spinal cord compression from plasmacytoma. Postsurgical radiation after stabilization of fractures or impending fractures is rarely needed.

Hypercalcemia

Hypercalcemia must be suspected if the patient has anorexia, nausea, vomiting, polyuria, increased constipation, weakness, confusion, stupor, or coma. If it is untreated, renal insufficiency usually develops. Hydration, preferably with isotonic saline and prednisone (25 mg orally four times daily), is effective in many patients with mild to moderate hypercalcemia (calcium < 13 mg/dL). If more-severe hypercalcemia occurs, zoledronic acid (Zometa) at a dose of 4 mg intravenously over 15 minutes or pamidronate (Aredia) 90 mg given intravenously over at least 2 hours is indicated. Calcitonin (Miacalcin) may be used if rapid reduction of calcium levels is needed. Hemodialysis may be necessary for extremely severe hypercalcemia. The dosage of prednisone must be reduced and discontinued as soon as possible.

Renal Insufficiency

Approximately 20% of patients with multiple myeloma have a serum creatinine level of 2.0 mg/dL or more at diagnosis. Myeloma kidney (cast nephropathy) and hypercalcemia are the two major causes. Myeloma kidney is characterized by the presence of large, waxy, laminated casts in the distal and collecting tubules. Some light chains are very nephrotoxic, but no specific amino acid sequence of the nephrotoxic light chain has been identified.

Dehydration, infection, nonsteroidal antiinflammatory agents, and radiographic contrast media can contribute to acute kidney failure. Hyperuricemia or amyloid deposition can produce renal insufficiency. Nephrotic syndrome rarely occurs in multiple myeloma unless amyloidosis is present.

Maintenance of a high fluid intake producing 3 L of urine per 24 hours is important for preventing kidney failure in patients with Bence Jones proteinuria. If hyperuricemia occurs, allopurinol (Zyloprim) in doses of 300 mg daily provides effective therapy.

Acute kidney failure should be treated promptly with appropriate fluid and electrolyte replacement. Patients with kidney failure should be treated with either VCD or VTD to reduce the tumor mass as quickly as possible. A trial of plasmapheresis is reasonable in an attempt to prevent chronic dialysis. Hemodialysis and peritoneal dialysis are equally effective and are necessary for patients with symptomatic azotemia.

Anemia

Almost every patient with multiple myeloma eventually becomes anemic. Increased plasma volume from the osmotic effect of the

VI Hematology

---

[1]Not FDA approved for this indication.
[5]Investigational drug in the United States.

M protein can produce hypervolemia and can spuriously lower the hemoglobin and hematocrit values. Patients with significant symptoms should be considered for red blood cell transfusion. If a transfusion is indicated, irradiated leukocyte-reduced red cells are preferred.

In patients with newly diagnosed myeloma, induction chemotherapy is often associated with a prompt improvement in hemoglobin levels, so it is better to avoid the use of erythropoietin. Erythropoietin (Epogen) should be seriously considered in relapsed patients receiving chemotherapy who have a persistent, symptomatic hemoglobin level of 10 g/dL or less.

Erythropoietin reduces the transfusion requirement and increases hemoglobin concentration in more than half of patients. Those with low serum erythropoietin values are more likely to respond. Most physicians proceed with a trial of erythropoietin 150 U/kg three times weekly or 40,000 U once a week. Darbepoetin, a long-lasting erythropoietin (Aranesp), may be given weekly or biweekly. Erythropoietin should be discontinued when the hemoglobin reaches 11 g/dL.

Skeletal Lesions

Bone lesions manifested by pain and fractures are a major problem. A skeletal radiographic survey should be repeated at 6-month intervals or sooner if pain develops. Patients should be encouraged to be as active as possible because confinement to bed increases demineralization of the skeleton. Trauma must be avoided because even mild stress can result in a fracture. Fixation of long bone fractures or impending fractures with an intramedullary rod and methyl methacrylate gives excellent results.

All patients with multiple myeloma who have lytic lesions, pathologic fractures, or severe osteopenia should receive an intravenous bisphosphonate. Pamidronate (Aredia) 90 mg intravenously over 2 hours every 4 weeks or zoledronic acid (Zometa) 4 mg intravenously over 15 minutes every 4 weeks are equally efficacious. The dosage of bisphosphonates should be reduced with renal insufficiency. Because renal insufficiency or nephrotic-range proteinuria can occur, serum creatinine and 24-hour urine protein monitoring is necessary. One should seriously consider stopping the intravenous bisphosphonate in patients who have responsive or stable disease after 2 years of therapy. In other patients, we recommend reducing the dose to once every 3 months. A randomized trial has found that denosumab (Xgeva), a monoclonal antibody targeting RANKL, may be as effective in reducing skeletal events as zoledronic acid and may be an option for selected patients with significant renal impairment.

Bisphosphonates should be resumed upon relapse with new-onset skeletal-related events. Osteonecrosis of the jaw can occur in patients receiving bisphosphonates. Although the relationship is unclear, it is essential to obtain a complete dental evaluation and perform preventive dental treatment before beginning bisphosphonates. The patient should practice good oral hygiene during therapy. Invasive procedures (especially dental extractions) should be avoided during bisphosphonate therapy. Osteonecrosis of the jaw should be managed conservatively.

Vertebroplasty or kyphoplasty may be helpful for patients with an acute compression fracture of the spine. Both have been associated with pain relief. Results appear to be better when the procedure is performed shortly after the compression fracture. Leakage of the methyl methacrylate is a potential adverse event. A choice between vertebroplasty and kyphoplasty depends on the expertise of the physician performing the procedure.

Infections

Bacterial infections are more common in patients with myeloma than in the general population. All patients should receive pneumococcal and influenza immunizations despite their suboptimal antibody response. Substantial fever is an indication for appropriate cultures, chest radiography, and consideration of antibiotic therapy. The greatest risk for infection is during the first 3 months after chemotherapy is initiated, and prophylactic antibiotics (levofloxacin [Levaquin] or cotrimoxazole [Bactrim]) should be considered during this period. Antiviral prophylaxis (acyclovir [Zovirax] 400 mg twice daily or valacyclovir [Valtrex] 500 mg once daily) should be given to all patients receiving bortezomib because of the increased risk of herpes zoster. Intravenous immunoglobulin (IVIg, Gammagard)[1] may be helpful in selected patients who have recurrent serious infections despite the use of prophylactic antibiotics. It is inconvenient, associated with side effects, and very expensive. Consequently, few of our patients receive IVIg.

Hyperviscosity Syndrome

Symptoms of hyperviscosity can include oronasal bleeding, gastrointestinal bleeding, blurred vision, neurologic symptoms, or congestive heart failure. Most patients have symptoms when the serum viscosity measurement is more than 4 cP, but the relationship between serum viscosity and clinical manifestations is not precise. The decision to perform plasmapheresis, which promptly relieves the symptoms of hyperviscosity, should be made on clinical grounds rather than serum viscosity levels. Hyperviscosity is more common in IgA myeloma than in IgG myeloma.

Extradural Myeloma (Cord Compression)

The possibility of cord compression must be considered if weakness of the legs or difficulty in voiding or defecating occurs. The sudden onset of severe radicular pain or severe back pain with neurologic symptoms suggests compression of the spinal cord. MRI or CT of the entire spine must be performed immediately. Radiation therapy in a dose of approximately 30 Gy is beneficial in about one half of patients. Dexamethasone (Decadron)[1] should be administered in addition to radiation therapy. Surgical decompression is necessary only if the neurologic deficit does not improve.

Venous Thromboembolism

Patients with multiple myeloma have an increased risk of venous thromboembolism. This is due to the malignancy itself, as well as therapy with lenalidomide, thalidomide, or pomalidomide. All patients receiving lenalidomide (or thalidomide or pomalidomide) need DVT prophylaxis with aspirin[1] (81 mg or 325 mg daily) or full-dose warfarin (Coumadin)[1] or low-molecular-weight heparin.[1]

Emotional Support

All patients with multiple myeloma need substantial and continuing emotional support. The physician's approach must be positive in emphasizing the potential benefits of therapy. It is reassuring for patients to know that some survive for 10 years or more. It is vital that the physician caring for patients with multiple myeloma has the interest and capacity for dealing with incurable disease over the span of years with assurance, sympathy, and resourcefulness.

---

[1]Not FDA approved for this indication.

References

Anderson K, Ismaila N, Flynn PJ, et al: Role of bone-modifying agents in multiple myeloma: American Society of Clinical Oncology Clinical Practice Guideline Update, *J Clin Oncol*, 2018 Jan 17, JCO2017766402. Available at: 10.1200/JCO.2017.76.6402 [Epub ahead of print].

Attal M, Lauwers-Cances V, Marit G, et al: Lenalidomide maintenance after stem-cell transplantation for multiple myeloma, *N Engl J Med* 366:1782–1791, 2012.

Chari A, Vogl DT, Gavriatopoulou M, et al: Oral selinexor–dexamethasone for triple-class refractory multiple myeloma, *N Engl J Med* 372(381):727–738, 2019.

Dimopoulos MA, Oriol A, Nahi H, et al: Daratumumab, lenalidomide, and dexamethasone for multiple myeloma, *N Engl J Med* 375(14):1319–1331, 2016.

Durie BGM, et al: Bortezomib with lenalidomide and dexamethasone versus lenalidomide and dexamethasone alone in patients with newly diagnosed myeloma without intent for immediate autologous stem-cell transplant (SWOG S0777): a randomised, open-label, phase 3 trial, *Lancet* 389(10068):519–527, 2017.

Facon T, Kumar S, Piesner T, et al: Daratumumab plus lenalidomide and dexamethasone for untreated myeloma, *N Engl J Med* 380(22):2104–2115, 2019.

Krishnan A, Pasquini MC, Logan B, et al: Autologous haemopoietic stem-cell transplantation followed by allogeneic or autologous haemopoietic stem-cell transplantation in patients with multiple myeloma (BMT CTN 0102): a phase 3 biological assignment trial, *Lancet Oncol* 12:1195–1203, 2011.

Kyle RA, Rajkumar SV: Epidemiology of the plasma-cell disorders, *Best Pract Res Clin Haematol* 20:637–664, 2007.

Lonial S, Dimopoulos M, Palumbo A, et al: Elotuzumab therapy for relapsed or refractory multiple myeloma, *N Engl J Med* 373:621–631, 2015.

Lonial S, Lee HC, Badros A, et al: Belantamab mafodotin for relapsed or refractory multiple myeloma (DREAMM-2): a two-arm, randomised, open-label, phase 2 study, *Lancet Oncol* 21:207–221, 2020.

McCarthy PL, Owzar K, Hofmeister CC, et al: Lenalidomide after stem-cell transplantation for multiple myeloma, *N Engl J Med* 366:1770–1781, 2012.

Moreau P, Attal MA, Hulin C, et al: Bortezomib, thalidomide, and dexamethasone with or without daratumumab before and after autologous stem-cell transplantation for newly diagnosed multiple myeloma (CASSIOPEIA): a randomised, open-label, phase 3 study, *Lancet* 394(10192):29–38, 2019.

Moreau P, Masszi T, Grzasko N, et al: Oral ixazomib, lenalidomide, and dexamethasone for multiple myeloma, *N Engl J Med* 374(17):1621–1634, 2016.

Munshi NC, Anderson LD, Shah N, et al: Idecabtagene vicleucel in relapsed and refractory myeloma, *N Engl J Med* 384:705–716, 2021.

Palumbo A, Chanan-Khan A, Weisel K, et al: Daratumumab, bortezomib, and dexamethasone for multiple myeloma, *N Engl J Med* 375(8):754–766, 2016.

Raje N, Terpos E, Willenbacher W, et al: Denosumab versus zoledronic acid in bone disease treatment of newly diagnosed multiple myeloma: an international, double-blind, double-dummy, randomised, controlled, phase 3 study, *Lancet Oncol* Feb 8. pii: S1470-2045(18)30072-X. Available at: https://doi.org/10.1016/S1470-2045(18)30072-X.

Rajkumar SV, Jacobus S, Callander NS, et al: Lenalidomide plus high-dose dexamethasone versus lenalidomide plus low- dose dexamethasone as initial therapy for newly diagnosed multiple myeloma: an open-label randomised controlled trial, *Lancet Oncol* 11:29–37, 2010.

Rajkumar SV, et al: International Myeloma Working Group updated criteria for the diagnosis of multiple myeloma, *Lancet Oncol* 15:e538–e548, 2014.

San Miguel J, Weisel K, Moreau P, et al: Pomalidomide plus low-dose dexamethasone versus high-dose dexamethasone alone for patients with relapsed and refractory multiple myeloma (MM-003): a randomised, open-label, phase 3 trial, *Lancet Oncol* 14:1055–1066, 2013.

Sonneveld P, Schmidt-Wolf IGH, van der Holt B, et al: Bortezomib induction and maintenance treatment in patients with newly diagnosed multiple myeloma: results of the randomized phase III HOVON-65/ GMMG-HD4 trial, *J Clin Oncol* 30:2946–2955, 2012.

Stewart AK, et al: Carfilzomib, lenalidomide, and dexamethasone for relapsed multiple myeloma, *N Engl J Med* 372(2):142–152, 2015.

MYELODYSPLASTIC SYNDROMES

Method of
Wafik George Sedhom, MD; and Jamile M. Shammo, MD

CURRENT DIAGNOSIS

- Myelodysplastic syndromes (MDSs) are diseases of the elderly.
- Chronic unexplained cytopenias should be evaluated to rule out MDSs.
- Bone marrow biopsy with cytogenetic testing is necessary for diagnosis.
- The International Prognostic Scoring System, Revised IPSS, and Molecular IPSS are important tools for risk stratification and choice of therapy.

CURRENT THERAPY

- Myelodysplastic syndromes are broadly divided into two therapeutic categories per the International Prognostic Scoring System (IPSS): low-risk disease (encompassing low and intermediate-1 risk groups), and high-risk disease (encompassing intermediate-2 and high-risk groups).
- The Revised IPSS defines five prognostic groups (very low, low, intermediate, high, and very high risk). Treatment options are also dependent on risk category.
- Patients with low-risk disease should receive supportive care and hematopoietic growth factors or luspatercept (Reblozyl); those with the deletion 5q abnormality should be treated with lenalidomide (Revlimid).
- Patients with high-risk disease should be treated with a hypomethylating agent and should be considered for allogeneic stem cell transplantation.

Epidemiology

Myelodysplastic syndrome (MDS) has an annual incidence of approximately 4 in 100,000 people in the United States. Disease incidence increases with age, with a median age of diagnosis of 76 years. Disease in patients younger than 50 years is rare except in the case of therapy-related MDS (t-MDS). Whites are the most affected at 4.2 cases per 100,000 person-years. Men are nearly twice as likely to be affected as women (5.8 vs. 3.3 per 100,000 per year), except in the case of MDS with isolated del(5q), which is more common in women.

Risk Factors

MDS can be classified as primary or secondary. Primary (or de novo) MDS indicates disease where no inciting exposure can be identified. Secondary MDS occurs from exposure to various substances. t-MDS occurs in patients exposed to certain chemotherapeutics, radiotherapy, or both. The onset of t-MDS varies from 2 to 10 years depending on the agent implicated. Tobacco use and occupational exposure to solvents and agricultural chemicals have also been associated with MDS development. A minority of MDS cases might have evolved from an antecedent hematologic disorder such as aplastic anemia or paroxysmal nocturnal hemoglobinuria (PNH). Several rare and inherited genetic "bone marrow failure syndromes"—such as Fanconi anemia, dyskeratosis congenita, Diamond-Blackfan anemia, and Shwachman-Diamond syndrome—have been associated with a higher risk of developing MDS.

Pathophysiology

Ineffective hematopoiesis and resulting cytopenias are major features of the disease. The first step in MDS development arises from a driver mutation in a hematopoietic stem cell that gives growth and survival advantage over wild type cells in the bone marrow. Over time, this mutated stem cell uses hematogenous spread to reach other bone marrow sites (clonal hematopoiesis of indeterminate potential [CHIP]). Additional mutations that increase proliferation are acquired over time until this clone becomes dominant in the bone marrow. Excessive apoptosis of myeloid progenitors, abnormal responses to cytokines and growth factors, epigenetic aberrations resulting in gene silencing, chromosomal abnormalities, and a defective bone marrow microenvironment have all been described in association with MDS. Our understanding of CHIP and clonal cytopenia of undetermined significance in the development of MDS is evolving.

Clinical Manifestations

Some patients with MDS are asymptomatic, but the majority present with cytopenias. Anemia is the most common cytopenia (usually macrocytic), and patients can develop fatigue, pallor, and dyspnea. If presenting with neutropenia or thrombocytopenia, they can develop infections or bleeding/bruising, respectively. Infection is the cause of death in approximately 20% to 35% of cases. Organomegaly and lymphadenopathy are uncommon. Systemic symptoms, like fevers, chills, or weight loss, are uncommon and may be initial signs of progression to leukemia. MDS can transform to acute myeloid leukemia (AML) in 25% to 30% of cases.

Diagnosis

The diagnosis of MDS can be challenging because of its similarity in clinical manifestations and pathology to disorders such as aplastic anemia, myeloproliferative neoplasms, and acute leukemia. The evaluation for MDS begins with a thorough history of potential exposures, family history of bone marrow failure syndromes, and full physical examination. Complete blood cell count may show cytopenias. Iron studies, vitamin B12, and folate levels should be obtained to identify other causes of cytopenias. Peripheral blood smear may show a pseudo–Pelger-Huet anomaly, blasts, or macrocytic red blood cells (RBCs). Patients with unexplained cytopenia(s) should be referred to a hematologist for further evaluation. The gold standard test is bone marrow biopsy and aspirate to identify myeloid dysplasia. Iron stains on the marrow are needed to identify ring sideroblasts, and cytogenetic analysis will identify chromosomal abnormalities driving the disease (observed in 50%

TABLE 1 The WHO 5th Edition Classification of MDS

CLASSIFICATION	BLASTS	CYTOGENETICS	MUTATIONS
MDS With Defining Genetic Abnormalities			
MDS with low blasts and isolated 5q deletion (MDS-5q)	<5% BM and <2% PB	5q deletion alone, or with 1 other abnormality other than monosomy 7 or 7q deletion	
MDS with low blasts and SF3B1 mutation (MDS-SF3B1)		Absence of 5q deletion, monosomy 7, or complex karyotype	*SF3B1*
MDS with biallelic TP53 inactivation (MDS-biTP53)	<20% BM and PB	Usually complex	Two or more *TP53* mutations, or 1 mutation with evidence of *TP53* copy number loss or cnLOH
MDS, Morphologically Defined			
MDS with low blasts (MDS-LB)	<5% BM and <2% PB		
MDS, hypoplastic (MDS-h)			
MDS with increased blasts (MDS-IB)			
MDS-IB1	5–9% BM or 2–4% PB		
MDS-IB2	10-19% BM or 5–19% PB or Auer rods		
MDS with fibrosis (MDS-f)	5–19% BM; 2–19% PB		

BM, Bone marrow; *IB*, increased blasts; *MDS*, myelodysplastic syndrome; *PB*, peripheral blood.
Adapted from Alaggio R, et al.: The World Health Organization Classification of Haematolymphoid Tumours: Lymphoid Neoplasms, ed 5. *Leukemia* 36:1720–1748, 2022.

to 60% of patients). Bone marrow dysplasia involving at least 10% of the cells of a specific myeloid lineage is the hallmark of MDS. The marrow is usually hypercellular. Next-generation sequencing is a highly sensitive test that identifies mutated genes encoding for splicing factors, epigenetic modifiers, and transcription factors, among others. Examples include *SF3B1, TET2, ASXL1, TP53,* and *RUNX1*. These genes can assist in prognostication (*TP53* in del[5q] MDS) or confirming the diagnosis (*SF3B1* in MDS with ringed sideroblasts [MDS-RS]).

Differential Diagnosis
The differential diagnosis of MDS includes other causes of dysplasia. Nutritional deficiencies of vitamin B12, folate, and copper should be ruled out. Drugs such as ganciclovir (Cytovene), valproic acid (Valproic), zinc, and mycophenolate mofetil (CellCept) have also been implicated in dysplastic marrow. These changes are reversible with discontinuation of the drug. Infections of HIV and parvovirus B19 can contribute to cytopenia and dysplasia as well. Hematopoietic disorders such as large granular lymphocytic leukemia and aplastic anemia also should be ruled out. All these reactive causes of dysplasia should be thoroughly evaluated before the diagnosis of MDS is confirmed.

Classification and Risk Stratification
Beginning in 1982, there have been efforts to classify subtypes of MDS to risk-stratify and guide management. The French-American-British (FAB) classification was the first. Currently, two classification schemes are used most widely: the World Health Organization (WHO) and the International Consensus Classification (ICC).

The WHO fifth edition classification (2022) builds upon the principles made with the fourth edition and further separates distinct clinical entities based on genetics or morphology, reflecting the increasing understanding genetics play in the development, prognosis, and therapy for this disease. Genetic categories include MDS with low blasts and del(5q), MDS with low blasts and *SF3B1* mutation (replacing MDS-RS), and MDS with biallelic *TP53* inactivation (a newly defined subtype). Morphologic categories include MDS with low blasts, hypoplastic MDS, and MDS with increased blasts, which is further divided based on blast percentage (Table 1). The 20% blast cutoff that defines AML is retained.

The ICC classification divides MDS into subtypes based on either cytogenetics, the percentage of blasts, or on the amount of dysplasia present. Cytogenetic categories include MDS with mutated *SF3B1* and MDS with deletion of chromosome 5q. MDS with *TP53* mutation is classified into a separate category of *TP53*-mutated myeloid neoplasms (given the clinical similarities of this mutation). Categories of dysplasia include MDS, not otherwise specified without dysplasia, MDS with single lineage dysplasia, and MDS with multiple lineage dysplasia. MDS with excess blasts defines 5% to 9% blasts in bone marrow, whereas the category MDS/AML encompasses blast counts of 10% to 19% (Table 2).

The International Prognostic Scoring System (IPSS) was introduced in 1997 to address the variability in prognosis within FAB subtypes. It predicts survival and risk of evolution to acute leukemia. The IPSS is calculated by adding scores assigned to three variables: blast cell count, cytogenetics, and number of cytopenias. The IPSS was revised in 2012 (IPSS-R) to incorporate five cytogenetic categories and account for the depth of cytopenias in MDS (Tables 3 to 5). IPSS-M is the latest prognostic scoring system that incorporates molecular data. It has the advantages of being personalized to the molecular profile, easy to interpret (an increase of 1 is equal to doubling of risk), and more accurate than the IPSS-R in prognosticating overall survival and transformation to AML. Although the IPSS-M is emerging as a new predictive model, the IPSS and IPSS-R are still widely used to predict the prognosis and clinical behavior of MDS patients and to guide choice of therapy.

Treatment
The treatment of MDS varies from supportive care to allogeneic stem cell transplantation. The objectives of treatment may be improving quality of life, delaying morbidity, extending overall survival, or cure. The treating physician should determine which of these objectives is right for each patient—a decision made by looking at a patient's age, comorbidities, risk (based on IPSS-R/IPSS-M), and incorporation of patient's goals. Stratification into lower-risk and higher-risk MDS is key to guiding management. There are several medications approved by the U.S. Food and Drug Administration (FDA) for MDS treatment, including recent advances that are sure to change the treatment landscape for years to come.

Supportive Care
Supportive care has been the cornerstone of MDS therapy for decades; it includes RBC transfusion for symptomatic anemia, platelet transfusion to reduce the risk of bleeding or to

TABLE 2 ICC Classification of MDS

CLASSIFICATION	DYSPLASTIC LINEAGES	CYTOPENIAS	CYTOSES*	BM AND PB BLASTS	CYTOGENETICS	MUTATIONS
MDS with mutated SF3B1 (MDS-SF3B1)	Typically ≥1	≥1	0	<5% BM; <2% PB	Any, except isolated del(5q), –7/del(7q), abn3q26.2, or complex	SF3B1 (≥ 10% VAF), without multi-hit TP53, or RUNX1
MDS with del(5q)	Typically ≥1	≥1	Thrombocytosis allowed	<5% BM; <2% PB	del(5q), with up to 1 additional, except –7/del(7q)	Any, except multi-hit TP53
MDS, NOS without dysplasia	0	≥1	0	<5% BM; <2% PB	–7/del(7q) or complex	Any, except multi-hit TP53 or SF3B1 (≥ 10% VAF)
MDS, NOS with single lineage dysplasia	1	≥1	0	<5% BM; <2% PB	Any, except not meeting criteria for MDS-del(5q)	Any, except multi-hit TP53; not meeting criteria for MDS-SF3B1
MDS, NOS with multilineage dysplasia	≥2	≥1	0	<5% BM; <2% PB	Any, except not meeting criteria for MDS-del(5q)	Any, except multi-hit TP53; not meeting criteria for MDS-SF3B1
MDS with excess blasts (MDS-EB)	Typically ≥1	≥1	0	5-9% BM; 2-9% PB	Any	Any, except multi-hit TP53
MDS/AML	Typically ≥1	≥1	0	10-19% BM or PB	Any, except AML-defining	Any, except NPM1, bZIP CEBPA or TP53

*Cytoses: Sustained white blood count ≥ 13 × 10⁹/L, monocytosis (≥0.5 × 10⁹/L and ≥10% of leukocytes) or platelets ≥450 × 10⁹/L; thrombocytosis is allowed in MDS-del(5q) or in any MDS case with inv(3) or t(3;3) cytogenetic abnormality.
AML, Acute myeloid leukemia; *BM*, bone marrow; *MDS*, myelodysplastic syndrome; *NOS*, not otherwise specified; *PB*, peripheral blood; *VAF*, variable allele frequency.
Adapted from Arber DA, et al.: International consensus classification of myeloid neoplasms and acute leukemias: integrating morphologic, clinical, and genomic data, *Blood* 140,11: 1200–1228, 2022.

TABLE 3 IPSS-R Prognostic Score Values

PROGNOSTIC VARIABLE	0	0.5	1	1.5	2	3	4
Cytogenetics	Very Good	-	Good	-	Intermediate	Poor	Very Poor
BM Blast %	≤2	-	>2-<5%	-	5-10%	>10%	-
Hemoglobin	≥10	-	8-<10	<8	-	-	-
Platelets	≥100	50-<100	<50	-	-	-	-
ANC	≥0.8	<0.8	-	-	-	-	-

ANC, Absolute neutrophil count; *BM*, bone marrow.

TABLE 4 IPSS-R Prognostic Risk Categories/Scores

RISK CATEGORY	RISK SCORE
Very Low	≤1.5
Low	>1.5–3
Intermediate	>3–4.5
High	>4.5–6
Very High	>6

TABLE 5 IPSS-R Cytogenetic Groups

CYTOGENETIC PROGNOSTIC SUBGROUPS	CYTOGENETIC ABNORMALITIES
Very good	-Y, del(11q)
Good	Normal, del(5q), del(12p), del(20q), double including del(5q)
Intermediate	del(7q), +8, +19, i(17q), any other single or double independent clones
Poor	-7, inv(3)/t(3q)/del(3q), double including -7/del(7q), Complex: 3 abnormalities
Very poor	Complex: >3 abnormalities

From Greenberg PL, Tuechler H, Schanz J, et al. Revised International Prognostic Scoring System (IPSS-R) for myelodysplastic syndromes, *Blood* 120:2454–2465, 2012.

treat bleeding, and use of hematopoietic growth factors such as erythropoiesis-stimulating agents (ESAs) and colony-stimulating factors such as granulocyte colony-stimulating factor filgrastim (Neupogen)[1] and granulocyte-macrophage colony stimulating factor sargramostim (Leukine)[1]. The last two cytokines have

---
[1] Not FDA approved for this indication.

limited efficacy and are not routinely recommended for the treatment of MDS-related neutropenia.

ESAs are generally indicated for symptomatic anemia, transfusion-dependence, or Hgb less than 10 g/dL. Two ESAs are currently available: a recombinant human erythropoietin (rhu-EPO; epoetin alfa [Epogen, Procrit])[1] and a supersialylated form of EPO (darbepoetin alfa [Aranesp])[1]. These are considered the standard of care for the treatment of anemia in patients with low-risk MDS. A predictive model for response to such treatment has been developed by the Nordic MDS study group to guide patient selection. In general, patients with a serum EPO level less than 500 mU/mL and low transfusion burden (<2 units pRBC/month) are likely to respond by improving their hemoglobin level and reducing their need for transfusions.

Thrombopoietin agonists such as romiplostim (N-Plate)[1] and eltrombopag (Promacta)[1] are not yet FDA approved but are sometimes used to alleviate symptomatic thrombocytopenia. Although they have been shown to reduce thrombocytopenia and bleeding rates, they can increase the blast count in some patients. Trials are being conducted to evaluate the efficacy and safety of this intervention.

Immunomodulatory Drugs

The novel class of immunomodulatory drugs includes thalidomide (Thalomid)[1] and lenalidomide (Revlimid). Thalidomide was investigated initially with some success in patients with low-risk disease. However, its use was compromised because of poor tolerability. Lenalidomide has been approved for the treatment of patients with low-risk MDS with deletion 5q because it was shown in clinical trials to result in transfusion independence in about two-thirds of such patients.

Luspatercept (Reblozyl)

A recombinant fusion protein that acts as a ligand trap for transforming growth factor beta superfamily has shown positive results in early phase trials in ameliorating anemia in transfusion-dependent MDS patients. The pivotal MEDALIST trial was a randomized, double-blind, placebo-controlled trial that evaluated the efficacy of luspatercept as defined by the proportion of patients who achieved RBC transfusion independence during any consecutive 8-week period between weeks 1 and 24 of therapy and enrolled 229 transfusion dependent patients with low-risk MDS-RS who were randomized at 2:1 to either luspatercept or placebo. The trial demonstrated that 37.9% of those who were randomized to luspatercept achieved the primary efficacy endpoint compared with 13.2% who received placebo ($P < 0.0001$). Subsequently, the drug was approved by the FDA in 2020 for the treatment of anemia in transfusion-dependent patients with MDS-RS and MDS with ringed sideroblasts and thrombocytosis (MDS-RS-T). The phase III, randomized COMMANDS trial published in 2023 looked to study luspatercept frontline in ESA naïve low-risk MDS. Its primary endpoint was RBC transfusion independence for at least 12 weeks with a Hgb increase of 1.5 g/dL. Results demonstrated a 59% response with luspatercept versus 31% with ESA alone. This data is likely to push luspatercept as frontline therapy for lower-risk MDS in the near future.

Imetelstat

Imetelstat[5] is a telomerase inhibitor that has shown impressive results in the IMerge trial. This double-blind, placebo-controlled trial randomized patients who were refractory or ineligible for ESAs to imetelstat or placebo. For patients reaching the primary endpoint of 8-week transfusion independence, Hgb increased on average 3.6 g/dL with imetelstat compared with placebo, which offers significant improvement in quality of life. Although not yet approved for MDS, it is an exciting new treatment possibility.

---

[1] Not FDA approved for this indication.
[5] Investigational drug in the United States.

Hypomethylating Agents

Two parenteral hypomethylating agents are currently approved for the treatment of MDS: 5-azacitidine (Vidaza) and decitabine (Dacogen). These agents are cytosine analogs known to inhibit and deplete DNA methyltransferase, which adds a methyl group to cytosine residues in newly formed DNA, resulting in the formation of hypomethylated DNA in vitro. The exact mechanism of action in vivo has not yet been identified. Results of randomized clinical trials comparing these agents to best supportive care in patients with MDS have demonstrated a statistically significant improvement in response rate and hematologic improvement. It has been shown for the first time that treatment with 5-azacitidine was reported to result in prolongation of survival in patients with Int-2 and high-risk disease. Both drugs have myelosuppressive properties and comparable response rates. In 2020 an oral hypomethylating agent combining decitabine and cedazuridine (Inqovi) was approved by the FDA for MDS.

Immunosuppressive Therapy

Immunosuppressive therapy with antithymocyte globulin (Thymoglobulin)[1] or cyclosporine (Neoral)[1] or both was evaluated in several clinical trials and was shown to result in durable hematologic responses in a subset of MDS patients—specifically, younger patients with low-risk disease, hypocellular marrows, PNH clone, human leukocyte antigen (HLA)-DR 15 phenotype, and low transfusion need.

Hematopoietic Stem Cell Transplantation

Allogeneic stem cell transplantation is the only curative therapy for MDS patients; this option is feasible for a small subset: typically younger patients with good performance status and an available HLA-matched donor. Approximately 40% of patients can be cured with this modality. The recent introduction of reduced intensity conditioning regimens and nonmyeloablative transplants has resulted in expanding the age limit for performing the procedure, thus reducing transplant-related complications and mortality. However, it has been associated with a higher risk of relapse. Because stem cell transplantation is associated with a high rate of treatment-related death (estimated at 39% at 1 year) and the development of acute and chronic graft-versus-host disease, such treatment is recommended only to patients with high-risk disease. Patients with low-risk MDS may be considered for transplant at disease progression.

Conclusion and Future Direction

MDS is a chronic disease characterized by bone marrow dysplasia with a variable propensity for leukemic evolution. It is curable only by allogeneic stem cell transplantation, which is feasible in only a small subset of patients. For all others, the treatment goal is aimed at improving quality of life and prolonging survival. New drugs are being studied to improve quality of life for patients with MDS, with several exciting changes on the horizon. Meanwhile, a great deal of research is focused on understanding the molecular underpinning of this heterogeneous disorder to enhance our understanding of its biology.

---

[1] Not FDA approved for this indication.

References

Arber DA, Orazi A, Hasserjian RP, Borowitz MJ, Calvo KR, Kvasnicka HM, et al: International consensus classification of myeloid neoplasms and acute leukemias: integrating morphologic, clinical, and genomic data, *Blood* 140(11):1200–1228, 2022.

Bejar R, Stevenson K, Abdel-Wahab O, Galili N, Nilsson B, Garcia-Manero G, et al: Clinical effect of point mutations in myelodysplastic syndromes, *N Engl J Med* 364(26):2496–2506, 2011.

Cazzola M: Myelodysplastic syndromes, *N Engl J Med* 383(14):1358–1374, 2020.

de Swart L, Smith A, Johnston TW, Haase D, Droste J, Fenaux P, et al: Validation of the revised international prognostic scoring system (IPSS-R) in patients with lower-risk myelodysplastic syndromes: a report from the prospective European LeukaemiaNet MDS (EUMDS) registry, *Br J Haematol* 170(3):372–383, 2015.

Fenaux P, Platzbecker U, Mufti GJ, Garcia-Manero G, Buckstein R, Santini V, et al: Luspatercept in patients with lower-risk myelodysplastic syndromes, *N Engl J Med* 382(2):140–151, 2020.

Godley LA, Larson RA: Therapy-related myeloid leukemia, *Semin Oncol* 35(4):418–429, 2008.

Greenberg P, Cox C, LeBeau MM, Fenaux P, Morel P, Sanz G, et al: International scoring system for evaluating prognosis in myelodysplastic syndromes, *Blood* 89(6):2079–2088, 1997.

Hellstrom-Lindberg E, Negrin R, Stein R, Krantz S, Lindberg G, Vardiman J, et al: Erythroid response to treatment with G-CSF plus erythropoietin for the anaemia of patients with myelodysplastic syndromes: proposal for a predictive model, *Br J Haematol* 99(2):344–351, 1997.

Kantarjian H, Issa JP, Rosenfeld CS, Bennett JM, Albitar M, DiPersio J, et al: Decitabine improves patient outcomes in myelodysplastic syndromes: results of a phase III randomized study, *Cancer* 106(8):1794–1803, 2006.

Khoury JD, Solary E, Abla O, Akkari Y, Alaggio R, Apperley JF, et al: The 5th edition of the world health organization classification of haematolymphoid tumours: myeloid and histiocytic/dendritic neoplasms, *Leukemia* 36(7):1703–1719, 2022.

List A, Dewald G, Bennett J, Giagounidis A, Raza A, Feldman E, et al: Lenalidomide in the myelodysplastic syndrome with chromosome 5q deletion, *N Engl J Med* 355(14):1456–1465, 2006.

Ma X, Does M, Raza A, Mayne ST: Myelodysplastic syndromes: incidence and survival in the United States, *Cancer* 109(8):1536–1542, 2007.

Malcovati L, Hellstrom-Lindberg E, Bowen D, Ades L, Cermak J, Del Canizo C, et al: Diagnosis and treatment of primary myelodysplastic syndromes in adults: recommendations from the European LeukemiaNet, *Blood* 122(17):2943–2964, 2013.

Martino R, Iacobelli S, Brand R, Jansen T, van Biezen A, Finke J, et al: Retrospective comparison of reduced-intensity conditioning and conventional high-dose conditioning for allogeneic hematopoietic stem cell transplantation using HLA-identical sibling donors in myelodysplastic syndromes, *Blood* 108(3):836–846, 2006.

Platzbecker U, Della Porta MG, Santini V, Zeidan AM, Komrokji RS, Shortt J, et al: Efficacy and safety of luspatercept versus epoetin alfa in erythropoiesis-stimulating agent-naive, transfusion-dependent, lower-risk myelodysplastic syndromes (COMMANDS): interim analysis of a phase 3, open-label, randomised controlled trial, *Lancet* 402(10399):373–385, 2023.

Rotter LK, Shimony S, Ling K, Chen E, Shallis RM, Zeidan AM, et al: Epidemiology and pathogenesis of myelodysplastic syndrome, *Cancer J* 29(3):111–121, 2023.

Silverman LR, Demakos EP, Peterson BL, Kornblith AB, Holland JC, Odchimar-Reissig R, et al: Randomized controlled trial of azacitidine in patients with the myelodysplastic syndrome: a study of the cancer and leukemia group B, *J Clin Oncol* 20(10):2429–2440, 2002.

Tefferi A, Vardiman JW: Myelodysplastic syndromes, *N Engl J Med* 361(19):1872–1885, 2009.

Zeidan AP U, et al: IMerge: results from a phase 3, randomized, double-blind, placebo-controlled study of imetelstat in patients (pts) with heavily transfusion dependent (TD) non-del(5q) lower-risk myelodysplastic syndromes (LR-MDS) relapsed/refractory (R/R) to erythropoiesis stimulating agents (ESA), *J Clin Oncol* 41(16):7004, 2023.

Zhang Y, Wu J, Qin T, Xu Z, Qu S, Pan L, et al: Comparison of the revised 4th (2016) and 5th (2022) editions of the world health organization classification of myelodysplastic neoplasms, *Leukemia* 36(12):2875–2882, 2022.

NON-HODGKIN LYMPHOMA

Method of
Kevin A. David, MD; and Andrew M. Evens, DO, MBA, MSc

CURRENT DIAGNOSIS

- The etiology of non-Hodgkin lymphoma (NHL) is not known, although several risk factors and conditions are associated with an increased risk of developing lymphoma, including congenital immunosuppression conditions (ataxia-telangiectasia, Wiskott-Aldrich syndrome, and X-linked lymphoproliferative syndrome), acquired immunodeficiency states (e.g., human immunodeficiency virus [HIV] and after solid organ transplantation), viruses (e.g., human T-lymphotropic virus [HTLV]-1 and hepatitis C virus [HCV]), and autoimmune disorders (e.g., Sjögren syndrome, celiac sprue, and systemic lupus erythematosus).
- Patients most commonly present clinically with enlarged, painless lymph nodes, splenomegaly, and bone marrow involvement, but they may also present with other extranodal disease sites (e.g., stomach, skin, liver, bone, brain).
- NHL has many different clinicopathologic subtypes—more than 65 types are included in the World Health Organization (WHO) classification of lymphoid neoplasms. The natural history and prognosis of these vary greatly from indolent and slow-growing types (over many years) to highly aggressive (within weeks) types.
- Excisional lymph node biopsy is the gold standard procedure in establishing the precise NHL histology. Expert hematopathology review incorporating morphologic, immunophenotypic, and genetic features is essential for an accurate diagnosis.

CURRENT THERAPY

- Indolent lymphomas are low-grade and represent slow-growing NHL that may remain stable with low tumor burden, not warranting therapy for several years. The disease is highly responsive to a variety of treatment options (remission rates exceeding 90% with combined rituximab (Rituxan)/chemotherapy), although the clinical course is characterized by repetitive relapses. Outside of early-stage disease and therapy with allogeneic stem cell transplantation, low-grade NHLs are not curable.
- Transformation of follicular lymphoma to a high-grade NHL occurs in 2% to 3% of patients each year; it is less common in other indolent subtypes. Transformation is typically heralded by an aggressive change in the patient's clinical condition.
- Diffuse large B-cell lymphoma (DLBCL), the most common aggressive NHL, is curable in all stages in a majority of patients with rituximab (Rituxan)-based chemotherapy. A variety of primary extranodal DLBCL clinical subtypes warrant specialized therapy, such as primary central nervous system (CNS) lymphoma and testicular lymphoma.
- Long-term survivors are at increased risk for second cancers. The highest relative risk of developing a secondary malignancy occurs more than 21 to 30 years after original diagnosis. Patients who received an anthracycline (e.g., doxorubicin [Adriamycin]) as part of therapy are at a long-term increased risk for cardiovascular disease.

The term *malignant lymphoma* was originally introduced by Billroth in 1871 to describe neoplasms of lymphoid tissue. Generally speaking, lymphomas are neoplasms of the immune system. Traditionally, lymphomas are divided into Hodgkin lymphoma (HL) and non-Hodgkin lymphoma (NHL).

There are many different clinicopathologic subtypes of NHL (>60). By cell of origin, the majority of NHLs are of B-cell origin (85%–90%); T-cell NHLs account for 10% to 15% of lymphomas in the United States, whereas natural killer cell or histiocytic lymphomas are rare (<1%). The NHL subtypes for lymphoid, histiocytic, and dendritic neoplasms as classified by the World Health Organization (WHO) were updated in 2022.

NHLs manifest most commonly clinically with involvement of lymph nodes, spleen, and bone marrow, but they can involve other extranodal sites (stomach, skin, liver, bone, brain, etc.). Peripheral blood involvement uncommonly occurs (leukemic phase of lymphoma). The natural history and prognosis vary greatly among the different subtypes of NHL, from indolent subtypes that are often slow-growing (i.e., therapy not warranted for years) to very aggressive and rapidly fatal types (within weeks) if not treated. Most NHL subtypes are highly treatable, with initial remission rates greater than 90% using combined rituximab (Rituxan)/chemotherapy; however, indolent NHLs are generally incurable, whereas the goal of treating most aggressive NHLs is cure.

Epidemiology

Currently, NHL represents approximately 5% of all cancer diagnoses, being the seventh most common cancer in women and men. Estimates from the American Cancer Society indicate that, in 2023, approximately 80,000 new cases of NHL will be diagnosed in the United States and approximately 20,000 people will die of the disease. In addition, there are approximately 900,000 people living with NHL in the United States.

Geographic Distribution

The incidence of NHL varies throughout the world, in general being more common in developed countries, with rates in the United States of more than 15 per 100,000 compared with 1.2 per 100,000 in China. In the United States the incidence rates of NHL

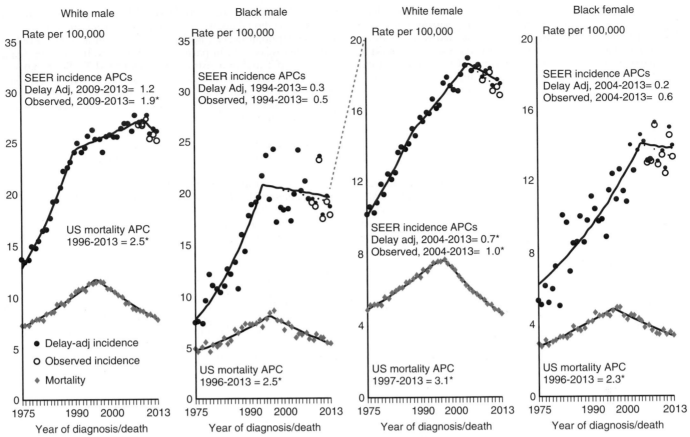

Source: SEER 9 areas and US mortality files (National Center for Health Statistics, CDC).
[a]Rates are age-adjusted to the 2000 US Std population (19 age groups - census P25-1103).
Regression lines and APCs are calculated using the joinpoint regression program version 4.3.0.0. April 2016, National Cancer Institute.
The APC is the annual percent change for the regression line segments. The APC shown on the graph is for the most recent trend.
*The APC is significantly different from zero $P < .05$.

Figure 1 Surveillance, epidemiology, and end results (SEER) observed incidence, SEER delay adjusted incidence, and U.S. death rates for non-Hodgkin lymphoma, by race and sex.

more than doubled between 1975 and 1995, representing one of the largest increases of any cancer. The increases have been more pronounced in White populations, males, older adults, and those with NHL diagnosed at extranodal sites. Similar findings have been reported in other developed countries. The incidence rates of NHL began to stabilize in the late 1990s, although the temporal trends vary by histologic subtype, as well as by race and sex (Figure 1). Some of the increase may be related to improved diagnostic techniques and access to medical care and the increased risk of NHL attributable to human immunodeficiency virus (HIV) infection. However, additional factors are likely responsible for this unexpected increase in incidence.

Age
Overall, NHL incidence rises exponentially with increasing age. In persons older than 65 years, the incidence is 90.9 per 100,000 population compared with 7.1 per 100,000 population for persons aged 20 to 49 years. Except for high-grade lymphoblastic and Burkitt lymphomas (the most common types of NHL seen in children and young adults), the median age at presentation for most subtypes of NHL exceeds 60 years.

Race and Ethnicity
Incidence varies by race and ethnicity, with White people overall having a higher risk than Black people and Asians (incidence rates increased 50%–60% in White people compared with Black people). Most NHL subtypes are more common in White people than in Black people; however, peripheral T-cell lymphoma (PTCL), mycosis fungoides, and Sézary syndrome occur more often in Black people than in White people.

Etiology and Risk Factors
Chromosomal Translocations and Molecular Rearrangements
Nonrandom chromosomal and molecular rearrangements play an important role in the pathogenesis of many lymphomas and often correlate with histology and immunophenotype. These chromosomal changes often result in oncogenic gene products; for example, t(11;14)(q13;q32) translocation results in overexpression of *bcl-1* (cyclin D1) in mantle cell lymphoma (MCL), whereas translocation with 8q24 leads to c-*myc* overexpression in nearly all Burkitt lymphomas and in 10% to 15% of patients with diffuse large B-cell lymphoma (DLBCL). Research to discover more information regarding the prognostic and pathogenic importance of these oncogenes continues, although they are currently used primarily in clinical practice for diagnostic purposes. In addition, these genes serve as potential targets for novel therapeutics.

Environmental Factors
Environmental factors may also play a role in the development of NHL, including particular occupations (e.g., chemists, painters, mechanics, machinists) and chemicals (solvents and pesticides). Patients who receive chemotherapy or radiation therapy for any indication are also at increased risk for developing NHL as a secondary cancer, as discussed later.

Viruses
Several viruses have been implicated in the pathogenesis of NHL, including Epstein-Barr virus, human T-lymphotropic virus (HTLV-1), Kaposi sarcoma–associated herpesvirus (KSHV, also known as human herpesvirus 8 [HHV-8]), and hepatitis C virus

(HCV). Meta-analyses have shown 13% to 15% seroprevalence of HCV in certain geographic regions among persons with B-cell NHL. Furthermore, HCV infection is associated with the development of clonal B-cell expansions and certain subtypes of NHL, particularly in the setting of essential (type II) mixed cryoglobulinemia. HTLV-1 is a human retrovirus that establishes a latent infection through reverse transcription in activated T-helper cells. A minority (5%) of carriers will develop adult T-cell leukemia lymphoma. KSHV-like DNA sequences are often detected in primary effusion lymphomas in patients with HIV infection and in those with multicentric (plasma cell variant) Castleman disease.

Bacterial Infections

Gastric mucosa-associated lymphoid tissue (MALT) lymphoma is seen most often, but not exclusively, in association with *Helicobacter pylori* infection. Infection with *Borrelia burgdorferi* has been detected in approximately 35% of patients with primary cutaneous B-cell lymphoma in Scotland. Studies indicate that *Campylobacter jejuni* and immunoproliferative small intestinal disease are related. European reports have noted an association between infection with *Chlamydia psittaci* and ocular adnexal lymphoma. The infection was found to be highly specific and does not reflect a subclinical infection among the general population. Furthermore, remission of NHL to antibiotics has been reported. Attempts to confirm this association in the Western Hemisphere have been unsuccessful.

Immunodeficiency

Patients with congenital conditions of immunosuppression are at increased risk of NHL. These conditions include ataxia-telangiectasia; Wiskott-Aldrich syndrome; X-linked lymphoproliferative syndrome; severe combined immunodeficiency; acquired immunodeficiency states, such as HIV infection; and iatrogenic immunosuppression. Relative risk of NHL is increased 150- to 250-fold among patients with acquired immunodeficiency syndrome (AIDS); patients usually develop high-grade NHLs, such as Burkitt lymphoma or DLBCL. The incidence of posttransplantation lymphoproliferative disorders (PTLDs) after solid organ transplantation ranges from 1% to 3% in kidney transplant recipients to 10% to 12% in heart and multiorgan transplant recipients, the latter of whom require more potent immunosuppressive therapy.

Autoimmunity

An increased incidence of gastrointestinal lymphomas is seen in patients with celiac (nontropical) sprue and inflammatory bowel disease, particularly Crohn disease. An aberrant clonal intraepithelial T-cell population can be found in up to 75% of patients with refractory celiac sprue before overt T-cell lymphoma develops. Sjögren disease is associated with a sixfold increased risk of NHL overall, with risk varying in part on severity of disease (5–200 times); moreover, the risk specifically of parotid marginal zone lymphoma is increased 1000-fold. In addition, systemic lupus erythematosus and rheumatoid arthritis have been associated with a slightly increased risk of B-cell lymphoma.

Genetic Susceptibility

Several studies have implicated a role for genetic variants in the risk of NHL, including genes that influence DNA integrity and methylation, genes that alter B-cell survival and growth, and genes that involve innate immunity, oxidative stress, and xenobiotic metabolism.

Signs and Symptoms

Fever, weight loss, and night sweats, referred to as B symptoms, are more common in advanced and aggressive subtype NHLs, but they may be present at all stages and in any histologic subtype.

Low-Grade or Indolent Lymphomas

Painless, slowly progressive peripheral adenopathy is the most common clinical presentation in patients with low-grade lymphomas. Patients sometimes report a history of waxing and waning adenopathy before seeking medical attention. Spontaneous regression of enlarged lymph nodes can occur, which may cause a low-grade lymphoma to be confused with an infectious condition. Primary extranodal involvement and B symptoms are uncommon at presentation; however, both are more common in advanced or end-stage disease and in particular indolent NHL subtypes (e.g., gastric MALT and nongastric extranodal MALT). Bone marrow is frequently involved, sometimes in association with cytopenias. Splenomegaly is seen in approximately 40% of patients, but the spleen is rarely the only involved site besides the specific subtype of splenic marginal zone lymphoma.

High-Grade or Aggressive Lymphomas

The clinical presentation of high-grade lymphomas is more varied. Although the majority of patients present with adenopathy, more than one-third present with extranodal involvement alone or with adenopathy, the most common sites being the gastrointestinal tract (including Waldeyer ring), skin, bone marrow, sinuses, genitourinary tract, bone, and central nervous system (CNS). B symptoms are more common, occurring in approximately 30% to 40% of patients. Lymphoblastic lymphoma often manifests with an anterior mediastinal mass, superior vena cava syndrome, and leptomeningeal disease. American patients with Burkitt lymphoma often present with a large abdominal mass and symptoms of bowel obstruction. In addition, certain histologic NHL subtypes manifest with symptoms unique to that particular lymphoma subtype; for example, angioimmunoblastic T-cell lymphoma (AITL) in addition to lymphadenopathy presents with disease features including organomegaly, skin rash, pleural effusions, arthritis, eosinophilia, and varied immunologic abnormalities such as positive Coombs test, cold agglutinins, hemolytic anemia, antinuclear antibodies, and polyclonal hypergammaglobulinemia.

Screening

No effective methods are currently available for screening patients or populations for NHL.

Diagnosis

A definitive diagnosis can be made only by biopsy of pathologic lymph nodes or tumor tissue. It is critical in most cases to perform an *excisional* lymph node resection to avoid false-negative results and inaccurate histologic classification; fine-needle aspirations or core biopsies are often insufficient for diagnostic purposes. When clinical circumstances make surgical biopsy of involved lymph nodes or extranodal sites prohibitive, a core biopsy obtained under computed tomography (CT) or ultrasonographic guidance may suffice, but it often requires the integration of histologic examination and immunophenotypic and molecular studies for accurate diagnosis. A formal review by an expert hematopathologist is mandatory. In addition to morphologic review and immunostaining of tissue, other studies such as detailed cellular immunophenotyping and genotyping for relevant oncogenes are often needed to complete the diagnosis.

In addition to a detailed history and physical examination, baseline staging studies are warranted. These consist of blood tests (complete blood count with differential, complete metabolic panel including liver function tests, and lactate dehydrogenase [LDH]); CT of chest, abdomen, and pelvis; and bone marrow biopsy and aspirate, in some cases (Box 1). For aggressive NHL histologies, functional imaging is advocated (i.e., fluorodeoxyglucose [^{18}F] positron emission tomography [FDG-PET]), as is assessment of ejection fraction in anticipation of anthracycline-based chemotherapy. Testing for history of hepatitis B virus (HBV) is recommended, especially before starting anti-CD20 antibody therapy; evidence suggests that anti-CD20 antibody therapy (e.g., rituximab [Rituxan]) increases the risk of HBV reactivation above the known rate of chemotherapy-associated reactivation. HIV serology should be obtained in patients with relevant risk factors, especially for DLBCL and Burkitt lymphoma. HTLV-1 serology is recommended in patients who present with cutaneous T-cell lymphoma lesions, especially if they have hypercalcemia.

Examination of cerebrospinal fluid and consideration of intrathecal chemotherapy prophylaxis or integration of intravenous high-dose methotrexate are applicable for patients with DLBCL with bone marrow, epidural, testicular, paranasal sinus, breast,

- Excisional tissue biopsy
- Detailed history and physical examination
- CBC with differential, metabolic panel (including liver function), and LDH
- CT scans (chest, abdomen, pelvis)
- Nuclear functional imaging (i.e., FDG-PET)
- Bone marrow biopsy and aspirate
- Heart function (e.g., echocardiogram) if anthracycline therapy anticipated
- Upper endoscopy, colonoscopy, or both
- HIV and HBV testing (with risk factors and/or if monoclonal antibody therapy planned)
- Consider tuberculosis testing (i.e., purified protein derivative with anergy panel) with history of exposure
- Assessment of CSF (when applicable or with risk factors)
- Consider early institution of TLS prophylaxis (e.g., intravenous fluids, allopurinol [Zyloprim])

TABLE 1	Clinical Prognostic Classification of Adult Immunocompetent Non-Hodgkin Lymphomas

LYMPHOMA TYPE	PERCENTAGE OF ALL NON-HODGKIN LYMPHOMAS
Indolent or Low-Grade Non-Hodgkin Lymphomas	
Follicular lymphoma	20–25
Small lymphocytic lymphoma	7
MALT-type marginal zone lymphoma	7
Nodal-type marginal zone lymphoma	<2
Lymphoplasmacytic lymphoma	<2
Aggressive or High-Grade Non-Hodgkin Lymphomas	
Diffuse large B-cell lymphoma	30–35
T-cell lymphomas: peripheral or systemic (multiple subtypes)	10–12
Mantle cell lymphoma	6
Lymphoblastic lymphoma	<2
Burkitt lymphoma	<1

Subtypes are listed in order of most to least common.
MALT, Mucosa-associated lymphoid tissue.

or multiple extranodal sites (especially when in conjunction with elevated LDH). Testing is mandatory for high-grade lymphoblastic lymphoma and Burkitt lymphoma and its variants and primary CNS lymphoma if there is no evidence of increased intracranial pressure. Upper gastrointestinal endoscopy or gastrointestinal series with small bowel follow-through is recommended in some patients with head and neck involvement (tonsil, base of tongue, nasopharynx) and those with primary gastrointestinal disease. MCL is associated with a high incidence of occult gastrointestinal involvement. In addition, magnetic resonance imaging (MRI) of the complete craniospinal axis and ocular examination is advocated with any brain or leptomeningeal disease involvement to rule out multifocal disease.

Classification

The 1965 Rappaport Classification of malignant lymphomas was based solely on architecture and cytology. Since then, with the help of advanced cellular and genetic technologies, numerous new unique NHL entities have emerged. The WHO classification, which continues to emphasize immunophenotyping, genotyping, and clinical features, was revised in 2022. Another way to group the many different lymphoma histologies is by clinical presentation and prognosis (Table 1).

Prognosis

International Prognostic Index

The International Prognostic Index (IPI) was developed as a prognostic factor model for aggressive NHLs treated with doxorubicin (Adriamycin)-containing regimens (Box 2). In the prerituximab (Rituxan) era, persons with no risk factors or one risk factor had a predicted 5-year overall survival (OS) rate of 73%, compared with 26% for high-risk patients with four or five risk factors. In the postrituximab era, the survival rates have improved (see Box 2). A variant of the IPI is also useful in predicting outcome in patients with follicular low-grade lymphoma (FLIPI), MCL (MIPI), and, most recently, Burkitt lymphoma (BLIPI, Box 3).

Molecular Profiling

DNA microarray technology for gene expression profiling has identified distinct prognostic subgroups in many NHL subtypes, including DLBCL and follicular NHL. Patients with germinal center B-like DLBCL have an improved OS compared with other molecular profiles. Additional pivotal work has found that gene expression signatures incorporating mutations in MYD88 (L265P), CD79B, NOTCH1, NOTCH2, and EZH2 and translocations in BCL6 and BCL2 predicted responses to immunochemotherapy and survival. Favorable outcomes were seen in cases with simultaneous BCL6 fusions and NOTCH2 mutations and simultaneous

BOX 2	Enhanced International Prognostic Index Risk Factors and Associated Approximate Cure Rates for Diffuse Large B-Cell Lymphoma

Factors/scoring
- Age, years
- >40 to ≤60: 1
- >60 to ≤75: 2
- >75: 3
- Lactate dehydrogenase (LDH), normalized
- >1 to ≤3: 1
- >3: 2
- Ann Arbor stage III–IV: 1
- Extranodal disease: 1
- Performance status ≥2: 1
- Five-year progression-free survival rates based on score at diagnosis
- Score 0 to 1: 91%
- Score 2 to 3: 74%
- Score 4 to 5: 51%
- Score ≥6: 30%

BOX 3	Burkitt Lymphoma International Prognostic Index

One point assigned for each of the following:
- Age ≥40 years
- ECOG performance status ≥2
- Serum LDH greater than three times ULN
- CNS involvement
  Risk categories and 3-year PFS and 3-year OS:
- Low risk: 0 risk factors; 92% PFS, 96% OS
- Intermediate risk: 1 factor; 72% PFS, 76% OS
- High risk: ≥ 2 factors; 53% PFS, 59% OS

ECOG, Eastern Cooperative Oncology Group; *ULN,* upper limit of normal.

BCL2 translocations and EZH2 mutations. Inferior outcomes were seen in cases with the co-occurrence of MYD88 and CD79B mutations, as well as isolated NOTCH1 mutations. Studies in follicular NHL have identified gene expression signatures that also predicted survival. Interestingly, the genes that defined the prognostic signatures were not expressed in the tumor cells but were expressed by the nonmalignant tumor-infiltrating cells—primarily T cells, macrophages, and dendritic cells.

Treatment

The therapeutic approach for NHL differs for each clinicopathologic subtype. Chemotherapy remains an important modality. However, in some instances, radiation therapy or, rarely, surgical resection plays a role. Biologic approaches, including monoclonal antibodies and antibody-drug conjugates, have shown significant activity and are currently incorporated into many treatment paradigms. In addition, other novel therapeutics targeting the cell surface of lymphoma cells or varied transcription factors continue to be incorporated into treatment paradigms. Autologous and allogeneic stem cell transplantation are mostly reserved for patients with recurrent or refractory disease, although there are some subtypes in which consolidative autologous transplantation after frontline therapy is considered (e.g., MCL and PTCLs).

Indolent B-Cell Non-Hodgkin Lymphomas

Indolent lymphomas are low-grade and represent slow-growing NHLs that may be stable with low tumor burden that may not warrant therapy for several years. The disease is responsive to treatment (remission rates greater than 90% with combined rituximab/chemotherapy), although the clinical course is characterized by repetitive relapses. Outside of early-stage disease and therapy with an allogeneic stem cell transplant, low-grade NHLs are not curable. The median survival of patients with advanced-stage follicular lymphoma in the prerituximab era was 9 to 10 years, although that is currently significantly longer ($\approx$16–18 years). Transformation to a high-grade NHL occurs in 2% to 3% of patients each year with follicular lymphoma (less common in other indolent subtypes) and is typically heralded by an aggressive change in the patient's clinical condition (e.g., B symptoms, rapidly rising LDH).

General Principles

Only a minority of patients present with early-stage disease (i.e., stage I or II). Low-dose involved field radiotherapy is a valid treatment option for these patients (especially stage I without central sites of disease), and associated 20-year disease-free survival rates are greater than 50%. Treatment for patients with advanced-stage disease ranges from observation (i.e., watchful waiting) to anti-CD20 monoclonal antibody therapy (rituximab [Rituxan] or obinutuzumab [Gazyva]) with or without chemotherapy. Treatment choice depends in part on tumor burden and the patient's individual disease characteristics and baseline functional status. Treatment with frontline anti-CD20 monoclonal antibody with chemotherapy (outpatient therapy given once every 3–4 weeks typically for six to eight cycles), followed possibly by 2 years of maintenance therapy with anti-CD20 monoclonal antibody for patients with high tumor burden, is associated with median progression-free survival (PFS) rates of approximately 9 to 10 years.

Treatment options for relapsed indolent lymphoma include repeating rituximab with or without a different chemotherapy regimen, radioimmunotherapy, oral lenalidomide (Revlimid) immunomodulatory therapy, CART therapy, bispecific T-cell engager (BITE) therapy, or stem cell transplantation. There is a small subset of patients with follicular lymphoma who experience early progression to first-line therapy (i.e., within 2 years), and survival rates are significantly inferior with conventional therapies. Autologous stem cell transplantation is an option for patients with relapsed disease, especially early progressors, although an improvement in OS is debated. Allogeneic stem cell transplantation is a potential curative modality for patients with relapsed or refractory disease, although patient selection is critical owing to potential morbidity and mortality related to this therapeutic option.

Special Considerations

Localized gastric MALT lymphoma cases often may be managed with therapy for *H. pylori* infection; radiation is typically reserved for failure to eradicate *H. pylori*. Patients with lymphoplasmacytic

lymphoma (Waldenström macroglobulinemia) can present clinically with hyperviscosity or cryoglobulinemia, which may be managed acutely with plasmapheresis, but ultimately systemic therapy similar to that for other indolent NHLs is warranted. More recently, the Bruton tyrosine kinase (BTK) inhibitor ibrutinib (Imbruvica) was approved by the U.S. Food and Drug Administration (FDA) for the treatment of patients with relapsed or refractory marginal zone lymphoma who require systemic therapy after at least one anti-CD20–based therapy, as well as for frontline treatment for Waldenström's macroglobulinemia.

Aggressive or High-Grade Non-Hodgkin Lymphomas

High-grade B- and T-cell NHLs are typically aggressive lymphomas that are fatal in weeks to a few months if not treated. However, many of these NHLs are curable with multiagent chemotherapy.

General Principles

DLBCL, the most common aggressive NHL, is curable in all stages in the majority of patients (60%–70%). A common treatment is anti-CD20 monoclonal antibody combined with anthracycline-based chemotherapy: rituximab–cyclophosphamide, doxorubicin (hydroxydaunorubicin), vincristine (Oncovin), and prednisone (R-CHOP) or polatuzumab-rituximab-cyclophosphamide-doxorubicin-prednisone (Pola-R-CHP). The number of treatment cycles depends on stage of disease and response to treatment. Standard therapy for advanced-stage disease is six R-CHOP cycles, whereas patients with early-stage disease may receive three or four cycles with or without involved field radiation. There are emerging data regarding the prognostic importance of *MYC* rearrangement (from tumor testing) as a single finding and especially in conjunction with *BCL-2* and/or *BCL6* (i.e., double or triple hit) by molecular studies as well as with immunohistochemical staining. Outcomes with R-CHOP for DLBCL patients with a molecular double hit (e.g., presence of MYC and *BCL-2* rearrangements) are modest; more intensive and novel therapeutic options should be considered. Therapy for relapsed DLBCL typically includes abbreviated salvage non–cross-resistant chemotherapy followed by autologous stem cell transplantation for patients who have chemotherapy-sensitive disease, which is curative in approximately 35% to 45% of patients. However, recent studies have highlighted the efficacy of CART therapy in patients with relapsed/refractory DLBCL, including in cases relapsing within 1 year of first-line therapy or in patients not eligible for autologous stem cell transplantation.

MCL is a B-cell NHL with initial high remission rates (>90%–95%), but it has more modest long-term outcomes, and it is difficult to cure. With standard chemotherapy regimens (e.g., R-CHOP), the median PFS rates are only 18 to 20 months. With more-intensive chemotherapy regimens, especially ones incorporating high-dose cytarabine as a component of induction therapy, 5-year PFS rates are near 70%. Some groups advocate induction therapy with aggressive high-dose cytarabine (Cytosar)[1]-based chemotherapy followed by consolidative autologous stem cell transplantation in first remission. As noted later, there has been the integration of several novel therapeutic agents into the treatment paradigm of MCL. Bendamustine (Bendeka, Treanda) in combination with rituximab has also become a widely used and more tolerable induction regimen, especially in older patients with MCL. Recent studies have also shown a benefit with adding ibrutinib to initial chemotherapy with or without use as part of maintenance therapy.

Burkitt lymphoma and related high-grade NHLs (e.g., lymphoblastic lymphomas) are often rapidly growing malignancies with a doubling time of 24 hours. Prompt initiation of therapy, including aggressive supportive care measures, is often warranted. With aggressive chemotherapy regimens, including prophylactic intrathecal chemotherapy, the majority of Burkitt patients younger than age 40 years are cured (>70%–80%). In addition, there are data showing high efficacy using lower-intensity treatment

[1]Not FDA approved for this indication.

consisting of infused etoposide (Toposar),[1] doxorubicin, and cyclophosphamide with vincristine, prednisone, and rituximab (EPOCH-R), especially for patients with untreated Burkitt lymphoma without CNS involvement, including HIV related.

Systemic (i.e., noncutaneous) PTCLs are mostly aggressive malignancies. They are treatable; however, cure rates are lower compared with most aggressive B-cell NHLs. Standard therapy had consisted of CHOP-based chemotherapy with or without autologous stem cell transplantation in first remission as consolidation. Recently published data from the ECHELON-2 trial combining the antibody–drug conjugate brentuximab vedotin (Adcetris) with cyclophosphamide, doxorubicin, and prednisone (CHP) chemotherapy versus standard CHOP for untreated CD30[+] PTCLs was associated with significantly improved PFS and OS. This regimen (i.e., brentuximab vedotin + CHP) was subsequently FDA approved for this indication. Several additional novel targeted agents have also been FDA approved over the past several years for the treatment of T-cell NHL (see later).

Special Considerations

There are several clinical subtypes of DLBCL that present as primary extranodal manifestations such as primary testicular DLBCL and primary gastric DLBCL. If these lymphomas are localized, treatment typically consists of abbreviated cycles (three to four) of R-CHOP followed by involved field radiation. In addition, CNS prophylaxis with either intrathecal chemotherapy or agents such as intravenous high-dose methotrexate[1] is warranted for testicular DLBCL given the relatively high risk of CNS involvement or relapse.

Primary CNS lymphoma is typically DLBCL; high-dose methotrexate chemotherapy is a key component of therapy with consideration for a consolidative autologous transplantation for younger fit patients.

A long-standing therapeutic maneuver for solid organ transplant–related PTLDs has been reduction of immunosuppression, although, using this approach alone, mortality rates have ranged from 50% to 60% in most series. Evidence with use of initial rituximab-based therapy together with reduction in immunosuppression suggests improved outcomes in the modern era.

The majority of AIDS-related NHLs are aggressive or high-grade types: DLBCL or Burkitt lymphoma. Similar therapy as immunocompetent NHL is often recommended. Response to therapy, including cure rate, has improved significantly with better control of opportunistic infections and highly active antiretroviral therapy (HAART).

Mycosis fungoides and Sézary syndrome are cutaneous T-cell lymphomas that initially might show eczematous lesions. It is often difficult to establish the diagnosis, but eventually the lesions develop into plaques and tumors. Lymph nodes, spleen, and visceral organs may be involved. Sézary syndrome is a variant of mycosis fungoides and shows peripheral blood involvement; patients usually have diffuse erythroderma. Skin-targeted modalities for treatment of early-stage mycosis fungoides include psoralens with ultraviolet A (PUVA) light; narrowband ultraviolet light; skin electron beam radiation; and topical steroids, retinoids, carmustine (BCNU), and nitrogen mustard (Mustargen).[1] Treatment goals in advanced stages are to reduce tumor burden and to relieve symptoms. Treatment options also include monochemotherapy or polychemotherapy, including CHOP; extracorporeal photopheresis; interferons; retinoids; liposomal doxorubicin (Doxil);[1] monoclonal antibodies; recombinant toxins; histone deacetylase inhibitors; and, most recently, the antibody–drug conjugate brentuximab vedotin (Adcetris) and humanized antibody against CCR4, mogamulizumab (Poteligeo).

During therapy for aggressive/high-grade NHLs, attention should be paid to preventing tumor lysis syndrome. Measures to prevent this complication include aggressive hydration, allopurinol (Zyloprim), and frequent monitoring of electrolytes, uric acid,

and creatinine. Rasburicase (Elitek), a recombinant urate oxidase enzyme, is an expensive but potent agent for treating hyperuricemia.

Novel Treatment Options and Modalities

Many new agents targeting specific molecular targets have become available for the treatment of lymphoma (Tables 2 and 3). Novel agents in lymphoma include bortezomib (Velcade) and lenalidomide (Revlimid), which are FDA approved for relapsed or refractory MCL (and lenalidomide also for relapsed follicular and marginal zone lymphoma), and histone deacetylase inhibitors, which are approved for cutaneous T-cell lymphoma and peripheral T-cell NHLs as well. In addition, bortezomib is FDA approved for untreated patients with MCL in combination with immunochemotherapy. Other newer agents that are FDA approved for the treatment of patients with chronic lymphocytic leukemia (CLL), including in higher-risk patient populations (e.g., p53 mutated), are the BTK inhibitors (ibrutinib [Imbruvica], acalabrutinib [Calquence] and zanubrutinib [Brukinsa]) and venetoclax (Venclexta), a BH3 mimetic acting as an inhibitor of BCL2. A 2023 study found that zanubrutinib therapy resulted in longer progression-free survival with fewer toxicities compared with ibrutinib. There are several recently published and a number of ongoing clinical studies to evaluate the optimal sequence and varied combinations for patients with CLL, especially vis-à-vis harnessing frontline targeted therapeutics. A novel class of drugs, EZH2 inhibitors, has also shown promise in relapsed lymphomas through modulation of epigenetic pathways. One of these, tazemetostat (Tazverik), has been approved for use in relapsed follicular lymphoma, with higher response rates in patients harboring EZH2 mutations compared with those without.

The BTK inhibitor acalabrutinib (Calquence) is FDA approved for patients with relapsed or refractory MCL who have received at least one prior therapy. The PI3K inhibitor copanlisib (Aliqopa) is approved for adult patients with relapsed or refractory follicular lymphoma. New anti-CD20 antibodies have also been approved for the treatment of CLL (e.g., obinutuzumab [Gazyva]) as well as antibody–drug conjugates, which contain potent drugs that are conjugated to an antibody. These include brentuximab vedotin (Adcetris), which is FDA approved for newly diagnosed CD30-positive T-cell lymphomas and relapsed anaplastic (T-cell) large-cell lymphoma, and the anti-CD79b monoclonal antibody–drug complex polatuzumab vedotin (Polivy), which the FDA approved in combination with rituximab and bendamustine for relapsed/refractory DLBCL. As noted above, polatuzumab was approved in 2023 as part of combination chemotherapy for newly diagnosed DLBCL in patients with an IPI score of 2 or higher.

These novel therapeutic agents are mostly FDA approved for patients with relapsed or refractory disease; however, there are a multitude of ongoing studies in the frontline/untreated setting and in varied sequences and combinations.

There is also great excitement in the continued application of new immunotherapy approaches in NHL such as checkpoint inhibitors (e.g., programmed death-1 [PD-1] inhibitors) as well as chimeric antigen receptor (CAR) T-cell therapy, which involves removal of T cells from patients followed by bioengineered CARs (e.g., CD19) that facilitate T-cell expansion and antigen/tumor recognition when reinfused into the patient. Axicabtagene ciloleucel (Yescarta), tisagenlecleucel (Kymriah), and lisocabtagene maraleucel (Breyanzi) are anti-CD19 CAR T-cell therapies the FDA approved for patients with relapsed or refractory DLBCL. Overall response rates range from 50% to 72%, with complete remission rates of 32% to 51%. Furthermore, 25% to 35% of patients appear to experience longer-term disease remission. In particular, lisocabtagene maraleucel is specifically approved for patients with DLBCL relapsed within 12 months of initial therapy or not eligible for autologous stem cell transplant. Tisagenlecleucel (Kymriah) and axicabtagene ciloleucel (Yescarta) are also approved for patients with relapsed/refractory follicular lymphoma. There are a multitude of other CAR T-cell and natural killer-based constructs being studied across several lymphoma subtypes.

Whereas CART therapy uses ex vivo manipulation of T cells to facilitate lymphoma-directed cytotoxicity, a novel class of

---

[1] Not FDA approved for this indication.

TABLE 2	Targeted Therapeutics FDA Approved for the Treatment of B-Cell Non-Hodgkin Lymphoma

BTK inhibitors

Mechanism: Bruton tyrosine kinase (BTK) bound by and downstream signaling pathways initiated by B-cell receptor inhibited by small molecule
Notable toxicities: atrial fibrillation, myelosuppression, rash, arthralgias, headache, bleeding, and impaired wound healing (should be held perioperatively and prior to other invasive procedures)

Drug Name	Indication and Year Approved
Ibrutinib (Imbruvica)	Mantle cell lymphoma (2013) CLL/SLL (2014) Waldenström macroglobulinemia (2015) Marginal zone lymphoma (2017)
Acalabrutinib (Calquence)	Mantle cell lymphoma (2017) CLL/SLL (2019)
Zanubrutinib (Brukinsa)	Mantle cell lymphoma (2019) CLL/SLL Marginal zone lymphoma Waldenstrom's macroglobulinemia
Pirtobrutinib (Jaypirca)	Mantle cell lymphoma (2023)

Anti-CD20 monoclonal antibodies

Mechanism: bind to CD20 molecule on B lymphocytes and induce a variety of responses, including antibody-mediated cytotoxicity, complement-mediated cytotoxicity, and apoptosis
Notable toxicities: infusion reactions, hypogammaglobulinemia, hepatitis B virus reactivation, progressive multifocal leukoencephalopathy (rare)

Drug Name	Indication and Year Approved
Rituximab (Rituxan)	Relapsed indolent B-cell lymphomas (1997) Untreated DLBCL with CHOP (2006) CLL (2010) Follicular lymphoma maintenance (2011) Waldenström macroglobulinemia,[1] with ibrutinib (2018)
Obinutuzumab (Gazyva)	Untreated CLL with chlorambucil (Leukeran) (2013) Relapsed rituximab refractory follicular lymphoma with bendamustine (Bendeka) (2016) Untreated follicular lymphoma with bendamustine (2017) Untreated CLL with ibrutinib (2019)
Ofatumumab (Arzerra)	Relapsed CLL (2016)

Anti-CD79b monoclonal antibody

Mechanism: binds to CD79b molecule on B lymphocytes; conjugated monomethyl auristatin E (MMAE) then internalized by lymphocyte; tubulin bound by MMAE, resulting in cell cycle arrest
Notable toxicities: neuropathy, immunosuppression, fatigue, diarrhea

Drug Name	Indication and Year Approved
Polatuzumab vedotin (Polivy)	Relapsed DLBCL with bendamustine and rituximab (2019) Untreated DLBCL in combination with rituximab, cyclophosphamide, doxorubicin, prednisone in patients with IPI of 2 or higher (2023)

Bispecific T-cell engager

Mechanism: CD20 on B cells and CD3 on cytotoxic T cells bound by anti-CD20/CD3 bispecific antibody
Notable toxicities: cytokine release syndrome (CRS): fever, hypotension, hypoxia, tachycardia; neurotoxicity (encephalopathy, headache)

Drug Name	Indication and Year Approved
Mosunetuzumab-axgb (Lunsumio)	Follicular lymphoma (2022)
Epcoritamab (Epkinly)	Relapsed/refractory DLBCL (2023)
Glofitamab (Columvi)	Relapsed/refractory DLBCL (2023)

Immunomodulators

Mechanism: affect T-cell stimulatory pathways, angiogenesis, and cell proliferation
Notable toxicities: myelosuppression, fatigue, rash, thrombosis (prophylactic aspirin or anticoagulants typically advised)

Drug Name	Indication and Year Approved
Lenalidomide (Revlimid)	Relapsed mantle cell lymphoma (2013) Relapsed follicular lymphoma and marginal zone lymphoma (2019)

Anti-CD19 monoclonal antibody

Mechanism: binds to CD19 antigen and mediates B-cell lysis through apoptosis and immune effector mechanisms, including antibody-dependent cellular cytotoxicity (ADCC) and antibody-dependent cellular phagocytosis
Notable toxicities: neutropenia, fatigue, anemia, diarrhea, thrombocytopenia, cough, pyrexia, peripheral edema, and pleural effusions (loncastuximab)

Drug Name	Indication and Year Approved
Tafasitamab-cxix (Monjuvi) in combination with lenalidomide	Relapsed DLBCL (2020)
Loncastuximab tesirine-lpyl (Zynlonta)	Relapsed DLBCL (2021)

TABLE 2 Targeted Therapeutics FDA Approved for the Treatment of B-Cell Non-Hodgkin Lymphoma—cont'd

EZH2 inhibitors	**Mechanism:** inhibit enhancer of zeste homolog 2 (EZH2), a histone methyltransferase responsible for repression of tumor suppressor genes. **Notable toxicities:** fatigue, infection	
	Drug Name	*Indication and Year Approved*
	Tazemetostat (Tazverik)	Follicular lymphoma (2020)
Phosphatidylinositol-3-kinase (PI3Kδ) inhibitors	**Mechanism:** are small molecule inhibitors of PI3 kinase, resulting in inhibition of various cellular processes, such as cellular growth, proliferation, and intracellular trafficking **Notable toxicities:** pneumonitis, colitis, transaminitis, hypertension, hyperglycemia (copanlisib)	
	Drug Name	*Indication and Year Approved*
	Idelalisib (Zydelig)	Relapsed CLL (2014)
	Copanlisib (Aliqopa)	Relapsed follicular lymphoma (2017)
PD-1 (programmed cell death-1) inhibitors	**Mechanism:** block PD-1 on cellular surface, facilitating T-cell–mediated immune killing **Notable toxicities:** pneumonitis, colitis, dermatitis, endocrinopathies (hypothyroidism)	
	Drug Name	*Indication and Year First Approved*
	Pembrolizumab (Keytruda)	Relapsed primary mediastinal large B-cell lymphoma (2018)
Chimeric antigen receptor (CAR) T-cell therapy	**Mechanism:** CD19-expressing lymphoma cells targeted by CD19 directed genetically modified autologous T cells **Notable toxicities:** cytokine release syndrome (fever, hypotension, organ dysfunction), neurotoxicity (mental status changes, confusion, seizures), cytopenias	
	Drug Name	*Indication and Year Approved*
	Axicabtagene ciloleucel (Yescarta)	Relapsed DLBCL (2017) Relapsed follicular lymphoma (2021)
	Tisagenlecleucel (Kymriah)	Relapsed DLBCL (2018) Relapsed follicular lymphoma (2022)
	Brexucabtagene autoleucel (Tecartus)	Relapsed mantle cell lymphoma (2020)
	Lisocabtagene maraleucel (Breyanzi)	Relapsed DLBCL (2021)
BCL-2 inhibitors	**Mechanism:** antiapoptotic activities of protein BCL2 inhibited by small molecule **Notable toxicities:** tumor lysis syndrome, myelosuppression, fever, diarrhea	
	Drug Name	*Indication and Year Approved*
	Venetoclax (Venclexta)	Relapsed CLL/SLL (2016) Untreated CLL/SLL in combination with obinutuzumab (2019)
Proteasome inhibitors	**Mechanism:** inhibit proteasomal clearance of multiple molecules, including proapoptotic molecules **Notable toxicities:** peripheral neuropathy, fatigue, diarrhea	
	Drug Name	*Indication and Year Approved*
	Bortezomib (Velcade)	Relapsed mantle cell lymphoma (2006) Untreated mantle cell lymphoma with chemotherapy (2014)
Nuclear export inhibitor	**Mechanism:** actively binds to export protein 1 (XPO1 or CRM1), inhibiting the nuclear export of tumor suppressors, growth regulators, and antiinflammatory proteins **Notable toxicities:** fatigue, nausea, diarrhea, appetite decrease, weight decrease, constipation, vomiting, pyrexia; dizziness and mental status changes; thrombocytopenia, neutropenia, anemia, and hyponatremia	
	Drug Name	*Indication and Year Approved*
	Selinexor (Xpovio)	Relapsed DLBCL
Radioimmunotherapy	**Mechanism:** targeted radiation to lymphoma cells delivered by monoclonal antibodies **Notable toxicities:** cytopenias (delayed), fatigue, MDS	
	Drug Name	*Indication and Year Approved*
	Ibritumomab tiuxetan (Zevalin)	Relapsed follicular lymphoma (2002) Consolidation for follicular lymphoma after initial chemotherapy (2009)

[1]Not FDA approved for this indication.
CHOP, Cyclophosphamide, doxorubicin, Oncovin, prednisone; *CLL/SLL,* chronic lymphocytic leukemia/small lymphocytic lymphoma; *DLBCL,* diffuse large B-cell lymphoma; *MDS,* myelodysplastic syndrome.

monoclonal antibodies known as bispecific T-cell engagers (BITEs) directs cytotoxic T cells to target tumor-specific molecules. Mosunetuzumab (Lunsumio) is a bispecific CD20-directed CD3 T-cell engager approved for use in patients with relapsed or refractory follicular lymphoma after two or more lines of prior therapy. Epcoritamab (Epkinly) and glofitamab (Columvi) also target CD3 and CD20 and have been approved for relapsed or refractory DLBCL. The investigational agent odronextamab has a similar mechanism of action and has also shown encouraging results in a variety of B-cell lymphoma subtypes.

TABLE 3 Targeted Therapeutics FDA Approved for the Treatment of T-Cell Non-Hodgkin Lymphoma

Histone deacetylase inhibitors	**Mechanism:** modulates acetylation of key targets, including genes involved in cancer-related cellular pathways **Notable toxicities:** QT prolongation, electrolyte abnormalities, cytopenias (especially thrombocytopenia), nausea, fatigue	
	Drug Name	*Indication and Year Approved*
	Romidepsin (Istodax)	Relapsed CTCL (2009)
	Vorinostat (Zolinza)	Relapsed CTCL (2006)
	Belinostat (Beleodaq)	Relapsed PTCL (2014)
Anti-CD30 monoclonal antibody	**Mechanism:** binds to CD30 molecule on T lymphocytes; conjugated monomethyl auristatin E (MMAE) then internalized by lymphocyte; tubulin bound by MMAE, resulting in cell cycle arrest. **Notable toxicities:** peripheral neuropathy, diarrhea, cytopenias, fatigue, pancreatitis	
	Drug Name	*Indication and Year Approved*
	Brentuximab vedotin (Adcetris)	CD30-positive mycosis fungoides and cutaneous anaplastic large cell lymphoma (2017) Untreated CD30-expressing PTCL in combination with CHP chemotherapy (2018)
Anti-CCR4 monoclonal antibody	**Mechanism:** binds CCR4 (CC chemokine receptor type 4) and inhibits downstream signal transduction pathways and chemokine-mediated cellular migration and T-cell proliferation **Notable toxicities:** infusion reactions, infection, rash, fever, edema, nausea, headache, cytopenias	
	Drug Name	*Indication and Year Approved*
	Mogamulizumab (Poteligeo)	Mycosis fungoides (2018) Approved outside United States for adult T-cell leukemia/lymphoma
Folate antagonists	**Mechanism:** are a folate analog that accumulates in lymphoma cells and impairs DNA synthesis **Notable toxicities:** mucositis, myelosuppression, nausea, fatigue	
	Drug Name	*Indication and Year Approved*
	Pralatrexate (Folotyn)	Relapsed PTCL (2009)

[1]Not FDA approved for this indication.
CTCL, Cutaneous T-cell lymphoma; *PTCL*, peripheral T-cell lymphoma.

Follow-Up of Long-Term Survivors

Relapse

Among patients with aggressive lymphomas, such as DLBCL, most recurrences are seen within the first 2 years after the completion of therapy, although later relapses occur uncommonly. Physical examination and laboratory testing at 2- to 3-month intervals and follow-up CT scans at 6-month intervals for the first 2 years after diagnosis are recommended; however, there is ongoing debate regarding the effect that postsurveillance scans have on disease outcomes. Detection of recurrent disease is important in part because these patients may be candidates for potentially curative therapy (e.g., stem cell transplantation). Patients with advanced low-grade NHL are at a constant risk for relapse, as discussed before.

Secondary Malignancies

Long-term NHL survivors are at an increased risk for second cancers. In general, the risk is increased with history of radiation use, but it is also seen with chemotherapy. In a survey of 28,131 Dutch registry patients with NHL who survived 2 years or longer, significant excesses of second cancers were seen for nearly all solid tumors as well as acute myelogenous leukemia (AML) and HL. The standardized incidence ratio (SIR) for solid tumors after NHL was 1.65. The SIRs for solid tumors are increased for up to 30 years after NHL diagnosis, with the highest relative risk of developing a secondary malignancy occurring more than 21 to 30 years after original diagnosis.

Late Treatment Complications

There has been more selective use of radiation as part of therapy for NHL. Thus the risk of certain radiation-induced complications has been reduced in patients treated more recently. Nevertheless, the risk still exists. Transplant recipients are at increased risk for secondary myelodysplasia and AML, regardless of whether they received radiation. All chemotherapy agents may cause long-term morbidity; in particular, patients who received an anthracycline (e.g., doxorubicin [Adriamycin]) are at a long-term increased risk

of cardiovascular disease. Among Dutch and Belgian patients with NHL treated with at least six cycles of doxorubicin-based chemotherapy, cumulative incidence of cardiovascular disease was 12% at 5 years and 22% at 10 years. Risk of coronary artery disease matched that of the general population; however, risk of chronic heart failure was significantly increased (SIR, 5.4), as was stroke (SIR, 1.8). Risk factors associated with excess risk included younger age at start of NHL treatment (<55 years), preexisting hypertension, any salvage treatment, and use of radiotherapy; risk relating to radiotherapy was dose dependent. Continued studies are needed to develop optimal secondary prevention strategies.

References

Bishop MR, Dickinson M, Purtill D, et al: Second-line tisagenlecleucel or standard care in aggressive B cell lymphoma, *N Engl J Med* 386:629–639, 2022.

Brown JR, Eichhorst B, Hillmen P, et al: Zanubrutinib or ibrutinib in relapsed or refractory chronic lymphocytic leukemia, *N Engl J Med* 388(4):319–332, 2023.

Budde LE, Sehn LH, Matasar M, et al: Safety and efficacy of mosunetuzumab, a bispecific antibody, in patients with relapsed or refractory follicular lymphoma: a single-arm, multicentre, phase 2 study, *Lancet Oncol* 23(80):1055–1065, 2022.

Burger JA, et al: Ibrutinib as initial therapy for patients with chronic lymphocytic leukemia, *N Engl J Med* 373(25):2425–2437, 2015.

Chapuy B, Stewart C, Dunford AJ, et al: Molecular subtypes of diffuse large B cell lymphoma are associated with distinct pathogenic mechanisms and outcomes, *Nat Med* 24:679–690, 2018.

Dickinson MJ, Carlo-Stella C, Morschhauser F, et al: Glofitamab for relpased or refractory diffuse large B cell lymphoma, *N Engl J Med* 387:2220–2231, 2022.

Dunleavy K, Pittaluga S, Shovlin M, et al: Low-intensity therapy in adults with Burkitt's lymphoma, *N Engl J Med* 369(20):1915–1925, 2013.

Evens AM, Danilov AV, Jagadeesh D, et al: Burkitt lymphoma in the modern era: real world outcomes and prognostication across 30 US cancer centers, *Blood* 137:374–386, 2021.

Fischer K, Al-Sawaf O, Bahlo J, et al: Venetoclax and obinutuzumab in patients with CLL and coexisting conditions, *N Engl J Med* 380(23):2225–2236, 2019.

Fowler NH, Dickinson M, Dreyling M et al. Tisagenlecleucel in adult relapsed or refractory follicular lymphoma: the phase 2 ELARA trial. 28:325–332, 2022.

Gopal AK, Kahl BS, de Vos S, et al: PI3Kδ inhibition by idelalisib in patients with relapsed indolent lymphoma, *N Engl J Med* 370(11):1008–1018, 2014.

Hemminki K, Lenner P, Sundquist J, Bermejo JL: Risk of subsequent solid tumors after non-Hodgkin's lymphoma: effect of diagnostic age and time since diagnosis, *J Clin Oncol* 26(11):1850–1857, 2008.

Horwitz S, O'Connor OA, Pro B, et al: Brentuximab vedotin with chemotherapy for CD30-positive peripheral T-cell lymphoma (ECHELON-2): a global, double-blind, randomised, phase 3 trial, *Lancet* 393(10168):229–240, 2019.

Jacobson CA, Chavez JC, Sehgal AR, et al: Axicabtagene ciloleucel in relapsed or refractory indolent non-Hodgkin lymphoma (ZUMA-5): a single-arm, multicentre, phase 2 trial, *Lancet Oncol* 23(1):91–103, 2022.

Marcus R, Davies A, Ando K, et al: Obinutuzumab for the first-line treatment of follicular lymphoma, *N Engl J Med* 377(14):1331–1344, 2017.

Morschhauser F, Tilly H, Chaidos A, et al: Tazemetostat for patients with relapsed or refractory follicular lymphoma: an open-label, single-arm, multicentre, phase 2 trial, *Lancet Oncol* 21(11):1433–1442, 2020.

Morton LM, Curtis RE, Linet MS, et al: Second malignancy risks after non-Hodgkin's lymphoma and chronic lymphocytic leukemia: differences by lymphoma subtype, *J Clin Oncol* 28:4935–4944, 2010.

Moser EC, Noordijk EM, van Leeuwen FE, et al: Long-term risk of cardiovascular disease after treatment for aggressive non-Hodgkin lymphoma, *Blood* 107:2912–2919, 2006.

Neelapu SS, Locke FL, Bartlett NL, et al: Axicabtagene ciloleucel CAR T-cell therapy in refractory large B-cell lymphoma, *N Engl J Med* 377(26):2531–2544, 2017.

Olszewski AJ, Jakobsen LH, Collins GP, et al: Burkitt lymphoma international prognostic index, *J Clin Oncol* 39(10):1129–1138, 2021.

Prince HM, Kim YH, Horwitz SM, et al: Brentuximab vedotin or physician's choice in CD30-positive cutaneous T-cell lymphoma (ALCANZA): an international, open-label, randomised, phase 3, multicentre trial, *Lancet* 390(10094):555–566, 2017.

Roberts AW, et al: Targeting BCL2 with Venetoclax in relapsed chronic lymphocytic leukemia, *N Engl J Med* 374(4):311–322, 2016.

Schmitz R, Wright GW, Huang DW, et al: Genetics and pathogenesis of diffuse large B cell lymphoma, *N Engl J Med* 378(1396–1407), 2018.

Schuster SJ, Bishop MR, Tam CS: Tisagenlecleucel in adult relapsed or refractory diffuse large B-cell lymphoma, *N Engl J Med* 380(1):45–56, 2019.

Seghal A, Hoda D, Riedell PA, et al: Lisocabtagene maraleucel as second-line therapy in adults with relapsed or refractory large B-cell lymphoma who were not intended for haematopoietic stem cell transplantation (PILOT): an open-label phase 2 study, *Lancet Oncol* 23(8):1066–1077, 2022.

Shanafelt TD, Wang XV, Kay NE, et al: Ibrutinib-rituximab or chemoimmuno-therapy for chronic lymphocytic leukemia, *N Engl J Med* 381(5):432–443, 2019.

Siegel RL, Miller KD, Fuchs HE, et al: Cancer statistics, 2021, *CA Cancer J Clin* 71(1):7–33, 2021.

Swerdlow SH, Campo E, Pileri SA, et al: The 2016 revision of the World Health Organization classification of lymphoid neoplasms, *Blood* 127(20):2375–2390, 2016.

Trappe RU, Dierickx D, Zimmermann H, et al: Response to rituximab induction is a predictive marker in B-cell post-transplant lymphoproliferative disorder and allows successful stratification into rituximab or R-CHOP consolidation in an international, prospective, multicenter phase II trial, *J Clin Oncol* 35(5):536–543, 2017.

Wang ML, Rule S, Martin P, et al: Targeting BTK with ibrutinib in relapsed or refractory mantle-cell lymphoma, *N Engl J Med* 369(6):507–516, 2013.

Woyach JA, Ruppert AS, Heerema NA, et al: Ibrutinib regimens versus chemoimmunotherapy in older patients with untreated CLL, *N Engl J Med* 379(26):2517–2528, 2018.

Zhou Z, Sehn LH, Rademaker AW, et al: An enhanced International Prognostic Index (NCCN-IPI) for patients with diffuse large B-cell lymphoma treated in the rituximab era, *Blood* 123(6):837–842, 2014.

PERNICIOUS ANEMIA/MEGALOBLASTIC ANEMIA

Method of
Anusha Vallurupalli, MBBS

CURRENT DIAGNOSIS

- Megaloblastic anemia is defined as macrocytic anemia with large, structurally and functionally abnormal red blood cells in the bone marrow and peripheral blood and is most commonly associated with folate or B12 deficiencies.
- In adults, folate deficiency is most commonly due to inadequate dietary intake. Vitamin B12 deficiency is mainly due to cobalamin malabsorption from food due to pernicious anemia, an autoimmune disorder, and gastrointestinal malabsorption.
- Megaloblastic anemia often presents with macrocytosis and hypersegmented neutrophils on peripheral smear.

CURRENT TREATMENT

- Prompt recognition and diagnosis are essential to prevent both short-term and long-term complications.
- Recognition of the underlying etiology for megaloblastic anemia is essential for a long-term treatment plan.
- Vitamin B12 deficiency can be treated with both oral and parenteral therapy and the route and duration of treatment is usually based on underlying etiology.
- If vitamin B12 deficiency is untreated, folate repletion will correct the megaloblastic anemia but not the associated neuropathic changes that occur with B12 deficiency.
- Folate replacement is generally accomplished through the oral route.
- Preventive B12 and folate dosing is warranted in certain high risk patients.
- Both B12 and folate replacements are generally well tolerated.

Introduction

Anemia is one of the most common hematologic disorders encountered on a regular basis in various clinical settings. In 2010, the global prevalence of anemia was 32.9%; that is, more than 2.2 billion people were affected. The World Health Organization (WHO) defines anemia as a hemoglobin (Hb) count of less than 13 g/L in men, less than 12 g/L in nonpregnant women, and less than 11 g/L in pregnant women and the elderly. A Hb of less than 10 g/L in any patient should trigger an evaluation. The etiology of anemia is oftentimes multifactorial, especially in elderly patients. In elderly patients, anemia can exacerbate comorbid cardiac complications such as cardiac ischemia and congestive heart failure. Most of the causes of anemia, especially nutritional causes, can usually be treated efficiently. Therefore, the cause of anemia should be identified and treated promptly to decrease the risk of complications.

Megaloblastic anemia, in general, is defined as macrocytic anemia with large, structurally and functionally abnormal red blood cells in the bone marrow and peripheral blood. Hypersegmented neutrophils are also commonly seen on the peripheral smear. The mean corpuscular volume (MCV) is elevated. Megaloblastic anemia is most commonly associated with nutritional deficiencies, specifically B12 and folate. In most cases, diagnosis is made by blood testing.

Epidemiology

The incidence and prevalence of anemia is highly variable and depends on age, sex, ethnicity, country of origin, socioeconomic status, and multifactorial comorbid conditions.

A retrospective study of 1784 randomly selected older adults living at home found macrocytosis in 6.3% of men and 3.3% of women. Folate and B12 deficiencies are the most common causes of megaloblastic anemia. Folate and B12 nutritional deficiencies are often easily treated.

Etiology
Folate Deficiency

Deficiency of folate is the most common cause of megaloblastic anemia. Folate is abundant in green leafy vegetables and approximately 60% of dietary folate is absorbed in the small intestine. However, folate is not stored in the body for a long duration and needs to be constantly replaced. Body stores of folate only last for approximately 6 months. Other causes include malabsorption and factors affecting folate metabolism (Table 1).

Vitamin B12 Deficiency

Deficiency of vitamin B12 can occur due to insufficient capture of the vitamin B12 from dietary sources because of inadequate intake, as seen in vegetarians and vegans or in patients who are malnourished. Malabsorption, as seen in patients with pernicious anemia, atrophic gastritis, or following gastric surgery, is another major cause (Table 2).

TABLE 1 Causes of Folate Deficiency

Dietary Deficiency

Malabsorption due to abnormalities of the jejunum
- Celiac disease
- Jejunal resection
- Tropical sprue

Drug-induced malabsorption
- Sulfasalazine (Azulfidine)

Increased requirement
- Pregnancy
- Prematurity
- Chronic hemolytic anemias (sickle cell anemia and autoimmune hemolytic anemias)
- Malignant diseases
- Chronic inflammatory disease

Increased loss
- Some skin diseases
- Long-term dialysis

Acquired abnormality of folate metabolism: dihydrofolate reductase inhibitors (methotrexate and sulfamethoxazole/trimethoprim [Bactrim])

Complex or uncertain mechanism
- Ethanol abuse (some cases)
- Anticonvulsant drugs (some cases)
- Oral contraceptive drugs, glutethimide, and cycloserine

Inherited abnormalities of folate absorption and metabolism
- Hereditary folate malabsorption
- Glutamate formiminotransferase-cyclodeaminase deficiency

Adapted from Wickramasinghe SN. Diagnosis of megaloblastic anemias. *Blood Rev.* 2006;20(6):299–318.

TABLE 2 Causes of B12 Deficiency

Dietary Deficiency

Impaired release of B_{12} from food—food cobalamin malabsorption

Inadequate secretion of intrinsic factor
- Pernicious anemia
- Total or partial gastrectomy
- Congenital intrinsic factor deficiency
- Congenitally abnormal intrinsic factor

Impaired release of B_{12} from B_{12}–R binder complex
- Pancreatic insufficiency
- Zollinger-Ellison syndrome

Diversion of dietary B_{12}
- Abnormal intestinal bacterial flora—jejunal diverticula, small intestinal strictures, and stagnant intestinal loops (blind loop syndrome)
- Fish tapeworm infestation

Malabsorption due to abnormalities in the terminal ileum
- Ileal resection
- Crohn disease
- Chronic tropical sprue
- Other acquired diseases
- Imerslund-Gräsbeck syndrome (selective malabsorption with proteinuria)

Drug-induced malabsorption (amino salicylic acid, neomycin, colchicine, slow-release potassium chloride, metformin, phenformin, biguanides, and cholestyramine)

Inactivation of methyl cobalamin by nitrous oxide

Inherited abnormalities of B_{12} transport or intracellular B_{12} metabolism
- Deficiency or abnormality of transcobalamin II
- Defective methyl cobalamin synthesis (hyper homocysteinemia)
- Defective synthesis of both methyl cobalamin and adenosyl cobalamin (hyper homocysteinemia and methylmalonic acidemia)

Adapted from Wickramasinghe SN. Diagnosis of megaloblastic anemias. *Blood Rev.* 2006;20(6):299–318.

TABLE 3 Laboratory Findings in Megaloblastic Anemia

Common for both B12 and folate deficiencies:
- Macrocytosis with elevated MCV, often greater than 100
- Megaloblasts and hypersegmented neutrophils on peripheral smear
- Anemia
- Elevated homocysteine levels

Specific for B12 deficiency:
- Elevated MMA levels
- Elevated LDH, indirect bilirubin, and low haptoglobin in the setting of intravascular hemolysis, which can be seen in severe B12 deficiency.
- Positive intrinsic factor antibodies in patients with pernicious anemia.

LDH, Lactate dehydrogenase; *MCV,* mean corpuscular volume; *MMA,* methylmalonic acid.

TABLE 4 Signs and Symptoms of B12 Deficiency

Neurological Symptoms/Signs	Gastrointestinal Symptoms/Signs
• Dysesthesia and hypoesthesia • Subacute combined degeneration presenting with ataxia, decreased proprioception, and vibratory sensation • Extrapyramidal signs (e.g., dystonia, dysarthria, and rigidity) • Abnormal deep tendon reflexes • Ataxia or positive Romberg test	• Glossitis • Abdominal pain • Dyspepsia likely related to atrophic gastritis or *H. pylori* infection

Psychiatric Symptoms	Rare Manifestations
• Depression or mood impairment • Psychosis • Dementia	• Skin hyperpigmentation • Grey hair

Anemia Symptoms
- Fatigue
- Palpitations
- Exertional dyspnea
- Chest pain
- lightheadedness

Pernicious Anemia

Pernicious anemia is characterized by malabsorption of B12 due to a deficiency of intrinsic factor. It is often associated with other co-existing autoimmune disorders such as celiac disease, Hashimoto thyroiditis, and Sjögren syndrome. Pernicious anemia is usually diagnosed by checking for intrinsic factor antibodies in the blood or by biopsy-proven immune atrophic gastritis. Intrinsic factor neutralizing antibodies are found in the setting of atrophic immune gastritis. *Helicobacter pylori*-related atrophic gastritis is in the differential and, if there is a clinical suspicion, should be evaluated by gastric biopsy. Intrinsic factor antibodies should not be checked after parenteral B12 administration for at least 2 weeks, as it will result in a false negative result.

Clinical Manifestations

Symptoms of anemia and laboratory findings (Table 3) from folate deficiency and B12 deficiency are essentially indistinguishable. B12 deficiency can manifest without anemia and is also characterized by neuropsychiatric symptoms (Table 4). The cause of neurological symptoms is thought to be secondary to the role that vitamin B12 plays in neuronal myelination, although the exact mechanism is not known.

Diagnosis

The diagnosis of pernicious anemia is based on laboratory testing (see Table 3). Complete blood count with differential, peripheral

TABLE 5	Differential Diagnosis of Macrocytic Anemia

- Chronic alcohol abuse
- Myelodysplastic syndromes
- Hypothyroidism
- Chronic lung disease with hypoxia
- Heavy smoking
- Chronic liver disease
- Chronic hemolytic anemia
- Therapy with certain anticonvulsant drugs
- Myeloma (some cases)
- Hypoplastic and aplastic anemia
- Physiologic
- Normal neonates
- Normal pregnancy (some cases)

Adapted from Wickramasinghe SN. Diagnosis of megaloblastic anemias. *Blood Rev.* 2006;20(6):299–318.

blood smear, complete metabolic profile including total and indirect bilirubin, lactate dehydrogenase, and serum folate and B12 levels are all included in the initial diagnostic testing. Methylmalonic acid (MMA) and homocysteine levels in indeterminate situations where the B12 or folate serum levels are borderline low may be helpful. MMA levels are increased in B12 deficiency, whereas MMA levels are normal in folate deficiency. Homocysteine levels are increased in both folate and B12 deficiencies. There may be fluctuations in MMA and homocysteine levels due to underlying concurrent conditions such as renal insufficiency (increased MMA levels), methylmalonic aciduria (increased MMA levels) and hereditary homocystinemia (increased homocysteine levels), and additional bacterial overgrowth in the small intestine (increased MMA levels), in addition to other rare conditions. Intrinsic factor antibody testing should be ordered prior to initiation of parenteral B12 replacement in patients with pernicious anemia.

Bone marrow aspiration and biopsy are not routinely recommended and should be reserved for cases in which there is persistent anemia despite replacement of both B12 and folate with resultant normalized levels. Patients with pernicious anemia should be evaluated for underlying gastric cancer with esophagogastroduodenoscopy. A systematic meta-analysis of 27 studies revealed a pooled gastric cancer incidence rate in patients with pernicious anemia of 0.3/100 person-years and an estimated sevenfold relative risk of gastric cancer.

Differential Diagnosis

The differential diagnosis for macrocytic anemia includes anemia related to chronic alcohol use (with or without liver disease), thyroid failure, and myelodysplastic syndromes (Table 5). Symptoms of copper deficiency can mimic B12 deficiency, can occasionally present with macrocytosis and should be ruled out with serum copper level testing if the patient does not respond to B12 supplementation.

Prevention

Providing food sources with nutrients rich in folic acid and/or B12 is best for preventing megaloblastic anemia. Therapeutic supplementation may be necessary, especially for the very old. The Institute of Medicine (United States) Standing Committee on the Scientific Evaluation of Dietary Reference Intakes has recommended fortification of cereals with multiple B vitamins, including B12. Prophylactic folate treatment should be administered to patients with increased requirements such as those with chronic hemolytic anemias and women who are pregnant. Preventive therapeutic replacement should be offered to all patients who have undergone bariatric gastric surgery or patients with compromised small intestine absorption due to various causes.

Treatment
General Principles

All patients who are identified as having B12 deficiency and/or folate deficiency should be treated. Replacement of the nutrients usually corrects the anemia. Blood transfusions are generally reserved for emergency situations such as severe symptomatic anemia and in patients with cardiac complications (i.e., chest pain, heart failure) associated with anemia. Oral replacement is generally well tolerated and is the first line treatment of choice. Parenteral replacement, especially for B12 deficiency, should be considered in patients with severe B12 deficiency who present with symptomatic anemia, severe neurologic symptoms, pernicious anemia, as well as in patients who are at risk for malabsorption and in women who are pregnant. Replacement with oral folate in a patient with undiagnosed B12 deficiency will improve the anemia but will not reverse the neurological symptoms.

The underlying cause for B12 deficiency and/or folate deficiency should be identified and treated. The duration of therapy depends on the underlying cause of the deficiency. Lifelong replacement is recommended for patients with irreversible causes (e.g., gastric bypass surgery and pernicious anemia). Short term treatment is recommended for patients with reversible causes (e.g., drug induced, reversible causes of malabsorption, inadequate dietary intake, and alcoholism). Both B12 and folate are water soluble vitamins and do not generally cause any major adverse effects.

Treatment of B12 Deficiency

Vitamin B12 is available in oral, sublingual, intramuscular (IM), subcutaneous (SC), and intranasal formulations. Cyanocobalamin is the most available formulation in United States. The oral formulation is generally effective in patients with a reversible cause and is administered at a dosage of 1000 μg daily for at least 1 month followed by either continuation of the same dose for maintenance or the dose can be decreased to 100 to 500 μg daily in patients with mild reversible deficiencies. The parenteral formulation is preferably administered IM at a dose of 1000 μg daily for 1 week followed by 1000 μg once a week for 1 month. The maintenance dose for IM or parenteral deep SC injection is 1000 μg monthly and indefinitely, depending on the etiology. Patients are usually taught to self-administer the injections to minimize the inconvenience of travel, improve compliance, and decrease costs.

Treatment of Folate Deficiency

The replacement dose for folic acid varies between 1 and 5 mg/day. Usually, therapy is continued for at least 3 to 6 months, provided that the underlying causes of the deficiency have been corrected.

Complications and Long-Term Monitoring

Patients with undiagnosed megaloblastic anemia can develop severe anemia and cardiac comorbidities. Neuropsychiatric changes can become irreversible if the B12 deficiency is not treated promptly. Patients may also develop long-term complications from undiagnosed underlying etiologies.

There is no need for frequent monitoring of B12 and folate levels once the underlying cause of the deficiency has been identified and appropriate treatment has been started.

References

Carmel R, Agrawal YP: Failures of cobalamin assays in pernicious anemia, *N Engl J Med* 367:385–386, 2012.

Green R: Vitamin B$_{12}$ deficiency from the perspective of a practicing hematologist, *Blood* 129:2603–2611, 2017.

Inelmen EM, D'Alessio M, Gatto MR, et al: Descriptive analysis of the prevalence of anemia in a randomly selected sample of elderly people living at home: some results of the Italian multicentric study, *Aging (Milano)* 6:81–89, 1994.

Kassebaum NJ, Jasrasaria R, Naghavi M, et al: A systematic analysis of global anemia burden from 1990 to 2000, *Blood* 123:615–624, 2014.

Lahner E, Capasso M, et al: Incidence of cancer (other than gastric cancer) in pernicious anemia: a systematic review with meta-analysis, *Digestive and Liver Disease* 50(8):780–786, 2018.

Wazir SM: Ghobrial I: Copper deficiency, a new triad: anemia, leucopenia, and myeloneuropathy, *J Community Hosp Intern Med Perspect* 7(4):265–268, 2017 Oct.

Wang H, Li L, Qin LL, et al: Oral vitamin B12 versus intramuscular vitamin B12 for vitamin B12 deficiency, *Cochrane Database Syst Rev* 3:CD004655, 2018.

Wickramasinghe SN: Diagnosis of megaloblastic anemias, *Blood Reviews* 20(6):299–318, 2006.

PLATELET-MEDIATED BLEEDING DISORDERS

Eric H. Kraut, MD

CURRENT DIAGNOSIS

- Platelet-mediated bleeding disorders commonly present with bleeding from mucosal surfaces or skin. Bleeding caused by reduced platelet counts may present with petechiae or purpura, whereas abnormalities of function are more likely to present with bleeding after injury or menstruation.
- Evaluation of platelet function used to be measured by the bleeding time. However, it is now more commonly evaluated by the platelet function analysis (PFA)-100 or platelet aggregation studies.
- Thrombocytopenia is most commonly caused by deficient production of platelets from the bone marrow, decreased platelet survival in the circulation, or sequestration of platelets by an enlarged spleen.
- Patients may bleed after trauma at platelet counts less than 50,000/µL and develop petechiae or purpura at platelet counts less than 20,000/µL, but they usually do not have severe bleeding unless platelet counts drop to less than 10,000/µL.
- The most common causes of new thrombocytopenia in the hospitalized patient are drugs or infection, whereas the usual cause of new platelet function abnormalities are medications.
- Patients in the hospital and placed on heparin should have their platelet counts monitored, and a reduction of 50% should be evaluated for heparin-induced thrombocytopenia (HIT).
- Immune thrombocytopenic purpura (ITP) usually presents in outpatients as new-onset mucocutaneous bleeding associated with only a reduced platelet count or unexplained asymptomatic isolated thrombocytopenia.
- Drugs that inhibit platelet activation and aggregation, such as aspirin, clopidogrel (Plavix), and dipyridamole (Persantine) can lead to significant bleeding, especially after surgery or procedures. This effect may last for 7 to 10 days.
- Patients presenting with a lifetime history of easy bruising and or heavy menses should have careful evaluation of their bleeding history and family history of bleeding. If positive, studies to rule out von Willebrand disease or hereditary disorders of platelet granules such as storage pool disorder should be done.

CURRENT THERAPY

- Patients with severe thrombocytopenia (platelet counts <10,000/µL) that is due to impaired production are at risk of severe bleeding and should be considered for platelet transfusions. The benefit of transfusing platelets when the platelet count reaches this level and the patient is not bleeding has been demonstrated as reducing bleeding in some patients in a recent study.
- Standard practice for platelet transfusions is to maintain platelet counts greater than 50,000/µL for patients with gastrointestinal bleeding and 75,000 to 100,000/µL for neurosurgical procedures. Platelet transfusions should be considered for certain other invasive procedures.
- Patients with immune thrombocytopenia should not receive platelet transfusions unless they are having significant bleeding because response to platelet transfusion occurs in less than 10% of patients and is short lasting.
- Patients with immune thrombocytopenic purpura (ITP) who have no bleeding and platelet counts greater than 30,000/µL can be followed without treatment because the risk of bleeding is low.

- In patients with ITP and thrombocytopenia less than 10,000/µL, initial treatment with high doses of corticosteroids in combination with intravenous immunoglobulin (IVIG; Gamunex) induces a rapid rise in platelets, usually within 24 hours.
- Current treatment for patients with ITP who fail prednisone treatment include splenectomy, rituximab (Rituxan),[1] or thrombopoietin agonists (romiplostim [Nplate] or eltrombopag [Promacta]).
- Patients with chronic renal failure can develop severe bleeding diathesis, which appears to be multifactorial including platelet dysfunction. Dialysis can reduce bleeding but not completely correct it. Other treatment that may help to include desmopressin (DDAVP),[1] tranexamic acid (Lysteda),[1] and synthetic erythropoietin (Epogen)[1].
- Patients with drug induced platelet dysfunction who may need to undergo surgery or who are bleeding may require platelet transfusions.
- Patients with inherited platelet disorders and mild bleeding can be treated with DDAVP but, if severe, may require platelet transfusions.

[1]Not FDA approved for this indication.

Platelets are small nonnucleated blood cells that are derived from bone marrow megakaryocytes. Their production is controlled by the hormone thrombopoietin produced in the liver, and they survive in the circulation for 8 to 10 days. On blood vessel injury, they form a seal or plug at the site of injury to limit bleeding. This initial event, termed *primary hemostasis*, occurs after endothelial injury when the subendothelial surface is exposed to circulating blood. Platelets are drawn to the site via von Willebrand factor (VWF), which, in combination with other proteins including fibrillar collagen, fibronectin, and laminin, leads to platelet adhesion. After platelets adhere to the vessel wall, they are activated, undergo a shape change, and release products from their granules. These platelet granule products, including adenosine diphosphate (ADP) and thromboxane A_2, further potentiate this process. Fibrinogen then binds to platelets via GPIIb/IIIa on the platelet surface causing firm platelet aggregation. The platelet secretory release reaction and aggregation recruits other platelets forming a firm hemostatic plug. Platelets also support the coagulation phase by interacting with circulating clotting factors and providing a surface for generation of thrombin. Secondary hemostasis occurs and thrombin-mediated fibrin mesh stabilizes the platelet plug.

Clinical Manifestations

The hallmark of platelet-mediated bleeding disorders is mucocutaneous bleeding such as nose bleeds, prolonged bleeding after tooth extractions, and heavy menstrual bleeding. When the platelet count drops to less than 30,000/µL, one may also see petechiae or purpuric lesions, especially on lower extremities.

Quantitative Platelet Disorders (Thrombocytopenia)

Primary hemostasis depends on an adequate number of platelets to prevent bleeding. A significant reduction in platelets or thrombocytopenia is usually defined as less than 100,000/µL. However, bleeding usually does not occur until the platelet count drops much lower. For example, spontaneous bleeding may only occur when the platelet count is less than 20,000/µL and severe life-threatening bleeding occurs only less than 10,000/µL. Thrombocytopenia can develop due to inadequate platelet production from the bone marrow, reduced platelet survival in the circulation, or sequestration of platelets in the spleen. Differentiating the cause requires evaluation of the patient's associated medical problems, physical findings, drug history, blood chemistry analysis, and possibly bone-marrow sampling.

Decreased platelet production is often the result of chemotherapeutic drugs for cancer, some antibiotics and antivirals (Table 1),

TABLE 1	Drugs Commonly Implicated as Causes of Drug-Induced Thrombocytopenia
CATEGORY	**IMPLICATED IN SEVERAL REPORTS**
Heparin	Unfractionated and low-molecular-weight heparin
Cinchona alkaloids	Quinidine, quinine
Platelet inhibitors	Abciximab (RepPro), eptifibatide (Integrilin), tirofiban (Aggrastat)
Antirheumatic agents	Gold salts
Antimicrobial agents	Linezolid (Zyvox), rifampin, sulfonamides, vancomycin
Sedatives and anticonvulsants	Valproic acid, phenytoin, carbamazepine
Histamine receptor antagonists	Cimetidine
Diuretic agents	Chlorothiazide
Analgesic agents	Acetaminophen, naproxen, diclofenac
Chemotherapy agents	Oxaliplatin (Eloxatin), fludarabine (Fludara), and others

or radiation therapy. These drugs may cause bone marrow injury, including damage to the megakaryocytes. Complete recovery may occur after stopping the offending agent. One common agent that can induce thrombocytopenia is alcohol. Thrombocytopenia associated with reduction in the white blood cell count and or red blood cell count should alert physicians to the possibility of a bone marrow disorder such as forms of leukemia or aplastic anemia. In cases where the cause is not evident, a bone marrow biopsy may be necessary to demonstrate whether there is a malignancy that may require urgent treatment.

Patients with reduced platelet production can often be observed without intervention depending on the severity of the thrombocytopenia, presence of bleeding, or the need to perform invasive procedures. Guidelines for transfusion of platelets to prevent bleeding (prophylactic transfusion) have changed in the last few years. With evidence that severe bleeding may not occur in most patients until the platelet count is less than 10,000/μL, limited platelet resources, and potential for development of alloimmunization to platelets, transfusions are not usually given unless sustained platelet counts are less than 10,000/μL. When platelets are transfused, it is appropriate to measure the response with a platelet count 1 hour post transfusion. The platelet count should rise 30,000 to 40,000/μL for the usual four-pack of platelet transfusion. Patients requiring frequent transfusions may require single-donor apheresis or human leukocyte antigen–matched platelets to obtain a good response.

Thrombocytopenia Resulting from Increased Platelet Destruction

Normally, platelets live in the circulation for 10 days, and the bone marrow replenishes them at the same rate that they are destroyed. Platelet survival may be altered by both nonimmune and immune processes. Severe infections will often lead to increased platelet destruction, and the platelet count returns to normal when the infection is adequately treated. Consumption of platelets also can occur in association with microangiopathic hemolytic anemia, as seen in disseminated intravascular coagulation (DIC) and thrombotic thrombocytopenic purpura and hemolytic uremic syndrome (TTP/HUS). It is important to review the blood smear to document fragmented red blood cells and evaluate coagulation parameters to help differentiate DIC from TTP/HUS and other causes of consumption. TTP/HUS may require specific and urgent treatment to prevent life-threatening complications.

Platelet transfusions are not usually given for TTP because there are reports of patients deteriorating after transfusions.

Immune-mediated platelet destruction is seen in response to several common drugs, including the sulfonamides and vancomycin. The characteristic pattern of immune-mediated platelet destruction is a sharp drop in the platelet count 7 to 10 days after starting the drug. The platelet count may drop to 5000/μL or less. Recognition is important because significant bleeding may occur, and the platelet count will only improve after discontinuation of the drug. Glycoprotein IIa/IIIb inhibitors, which are often used after cardiac stent placement, may cause a dramatic drop in the platelet count to as low as 1000/μL within hours of administration. This is important to recognize because this is one case where platelet transfusions may be necessary to prevent severe bleeding and it can be easily confused with other causes of low platelet counts.

Heparin-induced thrombocytopenia (HIT) is a unique drug reaction for several reasons. First, although thrombocytopenia is the initial sign of this entity, the major and feared complication is arterial and venous thromboses. It appears to affect 4% to 5% of patients exposed to unfractionated heparin and approximately 0.5% of patients exposed to low-molecular-weight heparin. Those at highest risk are female surgical patients who receive a minimum of 4 days of either type of heparin. The classic pattern is exposure to heparin at any dose with development of antibodies to heparin at day 4 and a 50% reduction in platelet count by day 6. The antibodies responsible are to the heparin–platelet factor 4 complex (IgG-PF4). A suspicious clinical pattern and a high antibody titer measured by an enzyme-linked immunosorbent assay are often diagnostic. Patients suspected of having HIT are at a high risk of thromboembolic disease within the first 24 hours of the drop in platelet count, and the heparin should be immediately stopped. However, despite the reduced platelet count, bleeding is unusual. Patients should be placed on an alternative anticoagulant, usually a direct thrombin inhibitor. The platelet count takes approximately 2 weeks to return to normal, and warfarin (Coumadin) should not be started until the platelet count returns to normal to avoid warfarin-associated necrosis. By reducing protein C and protein S, warfarin creates a temporary hypercoagulable state and places the patient at risk for warfarin-associated necrosis during the time when patients are most susceptible to thrombosis from HIT.

Immune thrombocytopenic purpura (ITP), previously termed *idiopathic thrombocytopenic purpura* affects 1 to 3 people per 100,000 but is probably the most common cause of severe isolated thrombocytopenia seen in the outpatient setting. It affects all ages, although ITP in childhood has a unique natural history. Childhood ITP is often associated with viral illness, is commonly transient, and may not need treatment. In adults, 40% of patients may have protracted or recurrent episodes of ITP, and the majority of patients need treatment. It was demonstrated in the 1950s that ITP is caused by circulating antiplatelet antibodies, and, like many autoimmune diseases, it is more common in women. When ITP presents in association with other diseases such as systemic lupus erythematosus or chronic lymphatic leukemia, or in patients with HIV, management of the underlying disease is important. The clinical presentation of ITP depends on the degree of thrombocytopenia. Mild thrombocytopenia of 20,000 to 80,000/μL is often asymptomatic, whereas platelet counts less than 20,000/μL may present with mucocutaneous bleeding and diffuse petechiae and purpura. Thrombocytopenia, an otherwise normal blood count, and peripheral blood smear without evidence of splenomegaly in a patient with no other illness helps to make a tentative diagnosis. A bone marrow biopsy is no longer considered necessary to confirm the diagnosis.

Treatment of ITP has changed over the past several years, and initial treatment after the diagnosis requires evaluation of the platelet count, whether it is increasing or decreasing, and the presence or absence of bleeding. Patients who have counts greater than 20,000/μL without bleeding and who are not in need of an invasive procedure can be observed without intervention. Patients with counts between 10,000 and 20,000/μL may be started on oral prednisone at 1 mg/kg. Patients with severe thrombocytopenia less than 10,000/μL and those who are bleeding can receive high-dose dexamethasone (Decadron) at 40 mg daily for 4 days and intravenous immunoglobulin (IVIG; Gamunex). There is usually a response to treatment within 24 hours. Although usually not helpful or required, approximately 10% of patients will have a response to platelet transfusion, and this can be considered for patients presenting with low platelet counts and bleeding. Refractory or recurrent ITP is a common problem in these patients, and recommendations for treatment include splenectomy, rituximab (Rituxan)[1], or thrombopoietin agonists. The choice of which to use depends on the patient and his or her clinical condition.

Thrombocytopenia Due to Hypersplenism
The platelet mass is distributed 70% in the circulation and 30% in the spleen. Enlargement of the spleen and/or alteration of blood flow in portal hypertension may increase platelet sequestration in the spleen and reduce the platelet count in the peripheral blood circulation. Patients' counts rarely drop to less than 20,000/μL. Thus thrombocytopenia caused by hypersplenism does not usually need any intervention. Patients with hepatitis C and cirrhosis may present with low platelet counts, and this may represent both hypersplenism and secondary immune thrombocytopenia. A trial of steroids may be used if these patients' clinical situation requires therapy.

Qualitative Platelet Function Disorders
Acquired Qualitative Platelet Function Disorders
Acquired disorders of platelet function are commonly seen, because platelets are the target of medications used to prevent arterial and cardiac stent thrombosis. Spontaneous bleeding is not common, but bleeding resulting from trauma or surgery can be a significant clinical problem. Because many patients may be on multiple antiplatelet agents or anticoagulants at the same time, the risk of bleeding needs to be recognized. Acquired qualitative disorders of platelet function may be due to drugs, hematologic diseases, or medical illnesses.

Drugs are the most common cause of acquired platelet dysfunction with differing risks of bleeding due to different targets. Aspirin causes irreversible acetylation of cyclooxygenase I (COX-1) and inhibits generation of prostaglandin A2. Although it is considered a weak antiplatelet agent with up to 25% resistance, aspirin increases the risk of bleeding in otherwise normal patients. Major bleeding was seen in up to 3.7% of patients and, when aspirin is used in combination with other antiplatelet agents or in patients with underlying bleeding disorders, the bleeding risk is higher. Clopidogrel (Plavix) is a thienopyridine prodrug, and the active metabolite irreversibly inhibits the surface receptor $P2Y_{12}$ on platelets. In clinical trials the risk of major bleeding in patients taking clopidogrel was similar to what is described with aspirin. Clopidogrel may significantly increase bleeding after surgery. GPIIb/IIIa receptor antagonists used after cardiac stent placement inhibit platelet aggregation and can induce severe thrombocytopenia.

Malignancies of the bone marrow may produce abnormally functioning platelets or alter platelet function by affecting VWF. The myeloproliferative and myelodysplastic disorders may produce platelets with reduced numbers of granules and may have associated increased risk of gastrointestinal bleeding and bleeding after invasive procedures. Acquired von Willebrand disease, an infrequent cause of abnormal bleeding, can be seen in patients with lymphoproliferative disease, multiple myeloma, and Waldenström macroglobulinemia.

Systemic illness can alter platelets and increase the bleeding risk. Acute and chronic renal failure are common causes of platelet-function abnormalities. In uremia, hemorrhagic complications include upper gastrointestinal bleeding, pericardial bleeding, and intracranial bleeding. Bleeding in renal failure is believed to be multifactorial and includes impaired release of platelet granules, decreased prostaglandin formation, VWF dysfunction, and presence of severe anemia. Effective treatment includes improvement of the anemia with erythropoietin (Epogen)[1] or DDAVP[1] or conjugated estrogens (Premarin).[1]

Hereditary Qualitative Platelet Function Disorders
Inherited abnormalities of platelet function are infrequent disorders that give rise to bleeding of varying severity. Inherited abnormalities of platelet function are often classified according to the type of genetic defect. Bernard-Soulier syndrome (BSS) is a severe bleeding disorder with autosomal recessive inheritance characterized by thrombocytopenia, decreased platelet adhesion, reduced platelet survival, and giant platelets on blood smear. Patients with BSS have defects in the GPIb-IX-V complex leading to reduced binding to VWF. Glanzmann thrombasthenia is an autosomal recessive disorder with defects of integrin αIIbβ3, a receptor on activated platelets that normally binds platelets during aggregation. Platelet aggregation to ADP and thrombin is abnormal. Patients with BSS and Glanzmann thrombasthenia who need treatment require platelet transfusions.

Hereditary disorders of platelet secretion are common reasons patients present to clinicians for evaluation of mucocutaneous bleeding. Defects in platelet dense granules (δ storage pool disease) are suspected in patients with bleeding and a negative work-up for von Willebrand disease. Diagnosis is made by platelet electron microscopy and or platelet aggregation studies. Granule deficiency associated with abnormalities of other lysosome-related organelles may lead to specific phenotypes such as Hermansky-Pudlak and Chediak-Higashi disease. Gray platelet syndrome (GPS), or alpha granule deficiency, is an autosomal recessive disorder with mild bleeding. GPS patients may also be thrombocytopenic. Treatment for bleeding or in preparation for surgery includes DDAVP[1] or platelet transfusions.

---

[1]Not FDA approved for this indication.

References
Aster RH, Curtis BR, McFarland JG, Bougie DW: Drug-induced immune thrombocytopenia: pathogenesis, diagnosis, and management, *J Thromb Haemost* 7:911–918, 2009.

Barbour T, Johnson S, Cohney S, Hughes P: Thrombotic microangiopathy and associated renal disorders, *Nephrol Dial Transplant* 27:2673–2685, 2012.

Estcourt L, Stanworth S, Doree C, et al: Prophylactic platelet transfusion in prevention of bleeding in patients with hematologic disorders and stem cell transplantation, *Cochrane Database Syst Rev* 5:CD004269, 2012. 10.1002/14651858.CD004269.pub.

Hedges SJ, Dehoney SB, Hooper JS, et al: Evidence-based treatment recommendations for uremic bleeding, *Nat Clin Pract Nephrol* 3:138–153, 2007.

Jackson S: Arterial thrombosis: insidious, unpredictable, and deadly, *Nat Med* 17:1423–1436, 2011.

Kam T, Alexander M: *Drug induced immune thrombocytopenia, J Parm Practice* 27:430–439, 2014.

Neunert C, Tenell D, Arnold DM: American Society of Hematology 2019 guidelines for immune thrombocytopenia, *Blood Adv* 10:3829–3866, 2019.

Nurden A, Nurden P: Advances in our understanding of the molecular basis of disorders of platelet function, *J Thromb Haemost Suppl* 1:76–91, 2011.

Parvod S, Myers B: Bleeding and thrombotic complications of renal disease. *Blood Rev.* 25:271–278, 2011.

Raschke RA, Gallo T, Cunz SC, et al: Clinical effectiveness of a Bayesian algorithm for the diagnosis and management of heparin induced thrombocytopenia, *J Thromb Haemost* 15:1640–1645, 2017.

Stanworth SJ, et al: Risk of bleeding and use of platelet transfusions in patients with hematologic malignancies: recurrent event analysis, *Haemostol* 100(6):740–747, 2015.

Tsantes AE, Nikolopoulos GK, Tsirigotis P, et al: Direct evidence for normalization of platelet function resulting from platelet count reduction in essential thrombocytosis, *Blood Coagul Fibrinolysis* 22:457–462, 2011.

Warkentin AE, Donadni MP, Spencer FA, et al: Bleeding risk in randomized controlled trials comparing warfarin and aspirin: a systemic review and meta-analysis, *J Thromb Haemost* 10:512–520, 2012.

Zucker ML, Hagedorn CH, Murphy CA, et al: Mechanism of thrombocytopenia in chronic hepatitis C as evaluated by the immature platelet fraction, *Int J Lab Hematol* 34:525–532, 2012.

POLYCYTHEMIA VERA

Method of
Peter R. Duggan, MD; and Sonia Cerquozzi, MD

CURRENT DIAGNOSIS

- Polycythemia vera (PV) should be considered when there is persistent elevation of hemoglobin (>165 g/L in men and >160 g/L in women) or hematocrit (>49% in men and >48% in women).
- *JAK2V617F* mutation testing and erythropoietin levels should be performed when PV is suspected.
- Bone marrow biopsy and aspiration may be necessary in some cases to confirm the diagnosis of PV and to distinguish PV from other myeloproliferative neoplasms (MPNs).
- PV is highly likely when *JAK2V617F* mutation is present and erythropoietin level is subnormal. When *JAK2V617F* mutation is seen with normal erythropoietin level, PV is possible; bone marrow biopsy is recommended to differentiate PV from other MPNs. When *JAK2V617F* is normal and erythropoietin is low, consider *JAK2* exon 12 mutational analysis or alternative diagnosis of congenital polycythemia. Wildtype *JAK2V617F* with normal or high erythropoietin level makes PV very unlikely, and patients should be investigated for secondary causes of polycythemia.
- Investigations for secondary polycythemia that may be indicated include:
  - Chest x-ray
  - Pulse oximetry
  - Arterial blood gas including carboxyhemoglobin and methemoglobin levels
  - Kidney and liver function tests
  - Abdominal imaging studies (ultrasound or computed tomography scan)
  - Oxyhemoglobin dissociation curve
  - Nocturnal polysomnography

CURRENT THERAPY

- All patients should be treated with phlebotomy and/or cytoreductive therapy to target hematocrit less than 45%.
- Low-dose aspirin[1] (acetylsalicylic acid [ASA]) should be used in *all patients* without a contraindication.
- In *high-risk* patients with polycythemia vera (age ≥ 60 years and/or history of thrombosis), cytoreductive therapy should be used in combination with low-dose ASA.
- Alkylating agents should be avoided as cytoreductive therapy owing to the risk of acute leukemia.
- Conventional cardiovascular risk factors (diabetes, hypertension, hyperlipidemia) should be aggressively managed, and cigarette smoking should be discouraged.
- Thromboembolic events should be managed according to accepted management guidelines. Thromboprophylaxis should be used after surgery and in other high-risk situations.

[1] Not FDA approved for this indication.

Polycythemia vera (PV) is a clonal stem cell disorder characterized by an increase in red blood cell production independent of the stimulation by erythropoietin. PV is the most common of the chronic myeloproliferative neoplasms (MPNs), occurring in approximately 2 to 3 people per 100,000 annually. The median age at diagnosis is 70 years, and it is rare in patients younger than 40 years.

A mutation of the tyrosine kinase Janus kinase 2 (*JAK2*) is consistently found in PV. This sheds some light on the pathogenesis of the disease and is useful in the diagnosis of PV and other MPNs. A single acquired mutation (*V617F*) of the gene for the JH-2 domain of *JAK2* can be found in 90% to 95% of patients with PV. The JH-2 domain functions to inhibit *JAK2* activity. In normal erythropoiesis, binding of erythropoietin to its receptor lifts this inhibition and allows *JAK2* stimulation of cell division and differentiation. In mutated *JAK2*, this inhibitory function is absent, leading to constitutive activity of the tyrosine kinase. This mutation is also present in about half of patients with essential thrombocytosis and primary myelofibrosis. The small number of patients with PV who are negative for the common *JAK2V617F* mutation have another functionally similar mutation within *exon 12*.

Presentation

Many patients with PV are asymptomatic, and PV is diagnosed after the incidental finding of an elevated hemoglobin or hematocrit on routine complete blood cell count. Splenomegaly is present in 30% to 40% of patients. Up to half of patients experience nonspecific symptoms such as weight loss, sweating, headache, fatigue, epigastric discomfort, visual disturbances, and dizziness. Many of these symptoms are likely caused by decreased blood flow due to an increased blood viscosity from polycythemia.

Generalized pruritus is often described, often after a warm bath or shower (aquagenic pruritus). Although the cause of this is unknown, it is thought to be due to the degranulation of increased numbers of mast cells in the skin of patients, releasing histamine and other inflammatory mediators. However, the symptom responds poorly to antihistamines, and it does not always resolve with treatment of PV.

Venous and arterial thromboembolic events are a major cause of morbidity and mortality in PV. Thrombosis at presentation occurs in up to 40% of patients. Ischemic stroke, transient ischemic attack, and myocardial infarction are common, especially among elderly patients. These, along with deep venous thrombosis and pulmonary embolus, are the most common thrombotic events and often result in serious morbidity, disability, and even death. Thrombotic events that are considered unusual in the general population, such as Budd-Chiari syndrome; portal, mesenteric, and other abdominal vein thrombosis; and cerebral venous thrombosis, occur more commonly among patients with PV. The possibility of an underlying MPN should be considered when a patient presents with such an event.

PV can manifest with symptoms of peripheral vascular disease. Patients with erythromelalgia describe a painful burning sensation of the hands and feet; pallor, erythema, or cyanosis of the extremities; and sometimes cutaneous ulceration. Erythromelalgia results from microvascular thrombosis and ischemia due to platelet activation and aggregation and responds well to platelet reduction and antiplatelet agents such as aspirin (ASA).[1]

Almost all patients with PV are iron deficient at diagnosis, even before the onset of therapeutic phlebotomy. Other manifestations of PV include acute gouty arthritis, peptic ulcer disease, erosive gastritis, and hypertension.

Diagnosis and Differential Diagnosis

The 2016 World Health Organization (WHO) diagnostic criteria incorporating recent International Consensus Classification changes for PV are shown in Box 1. The *JAK2V617F* mutation is present in about 95% of cases of PV. Erythropoietin level is decreased in more than 90% and is rarely elevated. Few patients with PV carry a mutation of exon 12 (~ 4%) of the *JAK2* gene instead of the more common *JAK2V617F* mutation. A *JAK2* mutation can also be found in about half of patients with essential thrombocytosis and primary myelofibrosis.

[1] Not FDA approved for this indication.

Diagnostic Criteria for Polycythemia Vera

Diagnosis requires three major criteria or first two major criteria and minor criterion.

Major Criteria
- Hemoglobin > 165 g/L in men, > 160 g/L in women or hematocrit > 49% in men, > 48% in women
- Bone marrow biopsy: hypercellular for age with trilineage growth (panmyelosis)
- Presence of *JAK2V617F* or *JAK2* exon 12 mutation

Minor Criterion
- Subnormal serum erythropoietin level

Differential Diagnosis of Polycythemia

Normal Red Cell Mass
- Relative polycythemia
- Gaisböck syndrome

Elevated Red Cell Mass
Primary Polycythemia
- Polycythemia vera

Secondary Polycythemia
- Congenital EPO receptor mutations
- Chuvash polycythemia
- High-affinity hemoglobin

Appropriately elevated EPO (hypoxia driven)
- Chronic hypoxic lung disease
- Cardiac shunts or cyanotic heart disease
- Sleep apnea
- Methemoglobinemia
- High altitude
- Chronic carbon monoxide poisoning
- Cigarette smoking
- Renal artery stenosis

Inappropriately elevated EPO
- Renal cell carcinoma
- Hepatocellular carcinoma
- Hemangioblastoma
- Uterine fibroids

Other causes
- Erythropoietin-stimulating agents (ESA)
- Androgens (testosterone)
- Kidney transplant

EPO, Erythropoietin.

Thrombotic Risk in Polycythemia Vera

Low Risk
- Age < 60 years and no history of thrombosis

High Risk
- Age ≥ 60 years and/or history of thrombosis

Leukocytosis and thrombocytosis are present in the majority of cases of PV. Red blood cell mass is increased. A nuclear medicine study measuring red blood cell mass and plasma volume is rarely required with the availability of *JAK2* testing, but it may be useful when relative polycythemia is suspected. Bone marrow biopsy and aspiration are not often needed for a diagnosis of PV but have been included as a major criterion within the revised WHO classification. Bone marrow examination can be important for diagnosing PV in the rare cases where *JAK2* is negative and to differentiate PV from other *JAK2*-positive MPNs when the distinction cannot be made based on peripheral blood cell counts.

Erythrocytosis can occur as a result of a number of other conditions in the absence of PV (Box 2). A careful history and physical examination with selected investigations can usually distinguish PV from secondary polycythemia and relative polycythemia (see Current Diagnosis). In relative (apparent, spurious) polycythemia, there is usually only a modest increase in the hematocrit, because of a decrease in plasma volume rather than a true increase in red blood cell mass. Thrombocytosis, leukocytosis, and splenomegaly should be absent. Causes include smoking, dehydration, and use of diuretics, and it is also described in middle-aged, obese, hypertensive men (Gaisböck syndrome).

Red blood cell mass can be elevated owing to increased stimulation of erythropoiesis by high levels of erythropoietin. Erythropoietin can be increased as an appropriate response to chronic hypoxia (sleep apnea, right-to-left cardiac shunts, chronic lung disease, high altitude, smoking, methemoglobinemia), and it can be inappropriately elevated owing to erythropoietin-secreting tumors (renal cell carcinoma, hepatocellular carcinoma, cerebellar hemangioma, uterine fibroids) or decreased kidney perfusion (renal artery stenosis). Familial causes of polycythemia include high-affinity hemoglobins, erythropoietin receptor mutations, and Chuvash polycythemia. Polycythemia occurs in 10% to 15% of patients after kidney transplantation, and this may be due to erythropoietin secretion by the native kidneys or increased sensitivity to erythropoietin. Polycythemia can be drug induced, such as with the use of performance-enhancing drugs (erythropoietin [Epogen], androgens) in athletes and testosterone replacement in men.

Prognosis

Patients with PV have a reduced life expectancy compared with the general population, with a median survival of approximately 14 years or, if younger than 60 years at diagnosis, 24 years.

Despite therapy, thrombosis remains an important cause of mortality. Cardiac disease, ischemic stroke, pulmonary embolus, and other thrombotic events account for 40% of deaths among patients with PV. Nonfatal thrombosis is common, occurring in almost 4% of patients annually. Age and a history of prior thromboembolic events are independent risk factors for thrombosis and can be used to predict a patient's risk of future events (Box 3). Low-risk patients are younger than 60 years and have no history of thrombosis. They experience new events at a rate of 2% per year. For patients older than 60 years or with a past history of thrombosis, this rate is 5% annually, but it can be as high as 11% when both risk factors are present.

The contribution of other cardiovascular risk factors (smoking, diabetes, hypertension, hyperlipidemia) to thrombotic risk in PV has been studied, with inconclusive results. However, because these are major contributors to the development of cardiovascular disease in the general population, they should also be considered when assessing risk in patients with PV. Leukocytosis (white blood cell count > 15 × 10^9/L) has been associated with a higher risk of arterial thrombosis.

Conversely, the risk of major hemorrhage is low, with fatal bleeding responsible for less than 5% of all deaths. However, there is considerable excess mortality from malignancy, in particular transformation to a myelodysplastic syndrome, myelofibrosis, or acute leukemia. The rate of leukemic transformation is less than 10% at 20 years. Risk factors for leukemic transformation include advanced age, leukocytosis, and abnormal karyotype. Approximately 10% of patients transform to myelofibrosis (post-PV myelofibrosis). Risk factors for post-PV myelofibrosis include leukocytosis and *JAK2V617F* allele burden of greater than 50%.

Treatment

The goals of treatment in PV are to lower the risk of thrombosis while minimizing toxicity. This is achieved by a combination of phlebotomy, ASA,[1] and cytoreductive therapy, such as hydroxyurea (Hydrea)[1] or pegylated interferon (PEG-IFN)-based therapy. The use of these therapies can be individualized based on a patient's risk of developing future thromboembolic events. Risk stratification (Box 3) aims at identifying patients with PV at higher risk of thrombotic events who require cytoreductive therapy. Because cerebrovascular and cardiovascular disease are among the main causes of morbidity and mortality for these patients, careful attention should be paid to the management of conventional cardiovascular risk factors. Hypertension, diabetes, and hyperlipidemia should be controlled with standard measures based on current guidelines, and patients should be encouraged to stop smoking. As the hematocrit increases in PV, there is a dramatic increase in blood viscosity. Phlebotomy is the fastest, most effective way to normalize a patient's hematocrit, and it should be initiated immediately in those with newly diagnosed PV. Blood volume should be reduced as rapidly as possible. Usually, 500 mL of blood is removed every 1 or 2 days until the hematocrit is less than 45%. The frequency of phlebotomy or the volume of blood removed can be decreased in elderly patients, those with cardiovascular disease, or others who do not tolerate this schedule. The optimal target in patients with PV is to maintain a hematocrit less than 45% to lower the risk of major thrombotic events and death from cardiovascular causes. Regular phlebotomy eventually results in iron deficiency, at which point most patients' phlebotomy needs to decrease dramatically. Iron replacement should be avoided.

Aspirin

Previous studies did not support the routine use of ASA to prevent thrombosis in PV. However, high doses of ASA were used in these early studies, resulting in excess bleeding in the treatment arm. The results of a recent large randomized trial show that low-dose ASA (100 mg/day) reduces major thrombotic events (nonfatal myocardial infarction, nonfatal stroke, pulmonary embolism, major venous thrombosis). This was accomplished without an increase in bleeding risk. Although there was a trend suggesting more minor bleeding events in those receiving ASA, the rates of major bleeding were identical for those receiving ASA or placebo. The benefit from ASA was seen, even though this study included many low-risk patients without a prior history of thromboembolism. Low-dose ASA (75 to 100 mg daily)[1] should be started in all patients without a contraindication to the drug (history of bleeding or intolerance). Because of the risk of bleeding from acquired von Willebrand disease that can occur with extreme thrombocytosis, ASA should be held when platelets are more than 1500×10^9/L until the count can be lowered by cytoreduction.

Cytoreductive Therapy

Cytoreductive therapy is recommended for high-risk patients with PV (Box 3). Hydroxyurea (HU)[1] or PEG-IFN are the first-line cytoreductive agents most commonly used to treat PV. Aims of cytoreduction are to safely lower blood cell counts, which HU does more so than PEG-IFN. Cytoreduction also decreases spleen size. Randomized data are limited, but HU also appears to reduce thrombotic complications. A starting dosage of 15 to 20 mg/kg daily (1000 to 1500 mg daily) is used. Occasional phlebotomy is still required to maintain hematocrit less than 45%, but the frequency usually decreases with time due to development of iron deficiency and/or if concomitant cytoreduction is used. Myelosuppression is the main toxicity of HU. The lowest dosage that provides therapeutic effect should be used, and excess myelosuppression should be avoided. The dosage can be titrated to ensure that the white blood cell count remains higher than 3.0×10^9/L, neutrophils are higher than 2.0×10^9/L, and platelets are in the normal range.

HU has been associated with leg ulcers and other skin changes, especially after long-term use. There is growing evidence that HU does not contribute to the excess rates of acute leukemia seen in PV; rates are no different than in those treated with phlebotomy alone. However, transformation is clearly associated with the use of other chemotherapeutic agents such as chlorambucil (Leukeran),[1] busulfan (Myleran),[1] and pipobroman (Vercyte),[2] accounting for one-third of the deaths among patients with PV treated with these agents. The use of these agents should be avoided. HU resistance can occur in up to 11% of patients and is associated with increased risk of death. Both HU resistance and intolerance are defined according to the European Leukemia Net criteria.

IFN-α2b (Intron A)[1] has been an alternative first-line therapy and is now only available in controlled-release (pegylated) formulation. It is more common to use PEG-IFN for younger patients (< 60 years), and it is required that patients of childbearing age take PEG-IFN instead of HU due to the teratogenic effects of HU. PEG-IFN-α2a (Pegasys)[1] is the most widely available and is given at 45 to 90 μg weekly, up to a dose of 180 μg weekly. Studies have shown its efficacy in controlling blood cell counts in addition to achieving complete hematologic and molecular responses. The inconvenience of its administration and its side effects, including mood disturbance and flu-like illness, have made it a less desirable first-line option. However, newer formulations of PEG-IFN include ropeginterferon alfa-2b (Besremi; Ropeg [Europe]), which has been studied most recently in comparison with HU for various MPNs and which is a monopegylated, long-acting interferon administered once every 2 weeks or longer. It was FDA approved for PV at the end of 2021 based on results from the phase 3 PROUD/CONTINUATION-PV clinical trials. In the CONTINUATION-PV trial, which included 171 patients, 61% of patients on ropeginterferon alfa-2b met complete hematologic response (CHR) (defined as hematocrit < 45% without phlebotomy for at least 2 months after last phlebotomy, platelets $\leq 400 \times 10^9$/L, leukocytes $\leq 10 \times 10^9$/L, normal spleen size with improved disease burden markers). A total of 71% of patients had a CHR compared with 58% on the standard of care. Ropeginterferon alfa-2b was well tolerated, with serious adverse reactions (incidence > 4%) being urinary tract infection, transient ischemic attack, and depression.

JAK Inhibitors

Ruxolitinib (Jakafi), a JAK1/2 inhibitor, was originally approved in patients with myelofibrosis, including myelofibrosis evolving from PV. There was a significant reduction in spleen size and constitutional symptoms in almost half of these patients. In the phase III RESPONSE trial, ruxolitinib illustrated its effectiveness in controlling hematocrit (<45%), reducing spleen size (≥35%), and improving symptoms in patients with PV who had HU intolerance or resistance, resulting in its approval as a second-line cytoreductive agent in PV. The most common side effects are anemia, thrombocytopenia, and atypical infection risk.

Other Treatment Issues

Hyperuricemia is common in MPNs and occasionally results in kidney stones or gout. Allopurinol (Zyloprim) can be used to reduce uric acid levels in patients with these complications. For those with intractable pruritus, several agents have been used with variable success. Some patients respond to ASA,[1] hydroxyurea,[1] cimetidine (Tagamet),[1] cyproheptadine (Periactin),[1] and/or paroxetine (Paxil)[1] 20 mg daily. Both IFN-α2b[1] and ruxolitinib have been successful in the majority of cases.

---

[1] Not FDA approved for this indication.

[1] Not FDA approved for this indication.
[2] Not available in the United States.

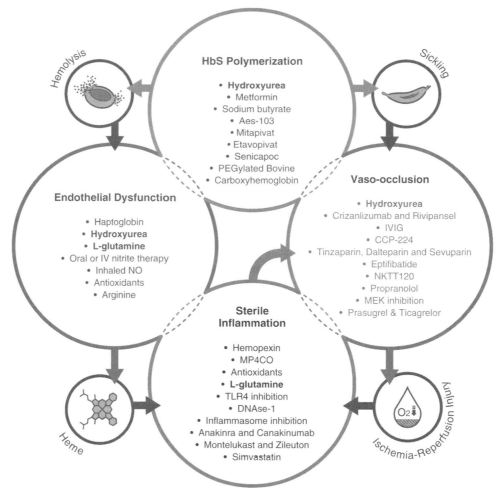

Figure 2 FDA approved and experimental therapies targeting the molecular pathobiology of sickle cell disease. The FDA approved drugs are in bold. (Modified from the Annual Review of Pathology: Mechanisms of Disease, Volume 14 © 2019 by Annual Reviews, http://www.annualreviews.org.)

TABLE 1 Severity of the Main Sickle Cell Syndromes

GENOTYPE	CLINICAL SEVERITY	HEMOGLOBIN (G/DL)
HbSS	Usually marked	6–10
HbS-β⁰-thalassemia	Moderate to marked	6–10
HbS-β⁺-thalassemia	Mild to moderate	9–12
HbSC	Mild to moderate	10–15
HbSS-HPFH	Mild	

HbSC, Heterozygous phenotype; *HbSS*, homozygous phenotype; *HPFH*, hereditary persistence of fetal hemoglobin.

to display the most severe manifestations. On the other end of the spectrum, HPFH, particularly common in Saudi Arabia, or coinheritance of β-thalassemia mitigates the phenotype. Although the net effect of high HbF levels on the phenotype of SCD is beneficial, coinheritance of one or two α-thalassemia alleles has a more complex effect. α-Thalassemia is present in approximately 30% of patients with SCD and is associated with higher hemoglobin, lower mean corpuscular volume (MCV), and decreased rate of hemolysis. These effects are protective toward stroke and leg ulcers but lead to increased rates of vasoocclusive episodes, osteonecrosis, and acute chest syndrome because of increased blood viscosity related to the higher hemoglobin level. Patients with HbSC and HbS/β⁺-thalassemia have an intermediate severity phenotype (Table 1). Haplotypes

of polymorphic sites in the β-globin gene cluster in chromosome 11 have been associated with different disease severity and rates of complications. Other yet unidentified genetic factors predispose certain patients to develop a particularly severe hemolysis with brisk reticulocytosis and a high rate of specific complications that include leg ulcers, priapism, and PH.

Hematology

This section describes the main clinical manifestations of SCD in each organ system (Figure 3 and Table 2).

Baseline or Steady-State Hematologic Abnormalities

Chronic intravascular and extravascular hemolysis causes a chronic anemia of moderate to severe intensity in HbSS and HbS/β⁰-thalassemia, with a hemoglobin range of 6 to 9 g/dL. In HbSC and HbS/β⁺-thalassemia, the anemia may be mild or absent. The anemia of SCD is usually normocytic in HbSS, with anisocytosis and poikilocytosis and a population of small dehydrated dense cells, irreversibly sickled cells, numerous reticulocytes, and schistocytes. Reticulocytosis is common but not compensatory, and nucleated RBCs are seen in acute exacerbations of the anemia such as in splenic or hepatic sequestration. Baseline leukocytosis with neutrophilia is also common and is a poor prognostic sign associated with acute chest syndrome in adults and frequent vaso-occlusive episodes in children. Preclinical studies have shown that leukocytes are not simply a marker of disease activity and acute phase but also have a direct pathogenic role in cellular adhesion and vaso-occlusion. The platelet count is commonly elevated in SCD, particularly in patients who are autosplenectomized as

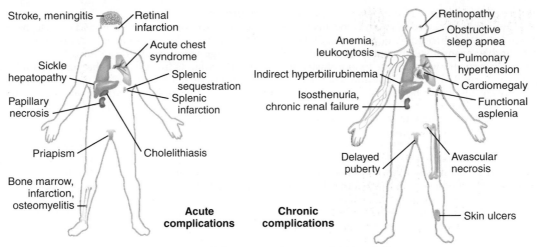

Figure 3 Acute and chronic complications of sickle cell disease.

TABLE 2	Landmark Randomized Clinical Trials in Sickle Cell Disease	
YEAR OF PUBLICATION	**TITLE**	**MAIN FINDINGS**
1986	Prophylaxis with oral penicillin in children with sickle cell anemia: A randomized trial	84% reduction in incidence of infection and no deaths from pneumococcal septicemia in the penicillin group
1995	Multicenter Study of Hydroxyurea in Sickle Cell Anemia (MSH)	Reduced incidence of painful crises, ACS, and transfusion in the hydroxyurea group Survival benefit in follow-up study
1995	Preoperative Transfusion in Sickle Cell Disease Study	A conservative transfusion regimen was as effective as an aggressive regimen in preventing perioperative complications in patients with sickle cell anemia
1996	Multicenter investigation of bone marrow transplantation for sickle cell disease	HCT is safe in SCD with survival and event-free survival at 4 years of 91% and 73% and can lead to cure
1998	Stroke Prevention Trial in Sickle Cell Anemia (STOP)	Transfusion reduces the risk of a first stroke by 92% in children with sickle cell anemia who have abnormal results on transcranial Doppler ultrasonography
2005	Optimizing Primary Stroke Prevention in Sickle Cell Anemia (STOP 2)	Discontinuation of transfusion for the prevention of stroke in children with sickle cell disease results in a high rate of reversion to abnormal blood-flow velocities on Doppler studies and stroke
2009	Improving the Results of Bone Marrow Transplantation for Patients with Severe Congenital Anemias	Nine of 10 adults who received nonmyeloablative allogeneic hematopoietic stem cell transplantation for severe sickle cell disease achieved stable, mixed donor–recipient chimerism and reversal of the sickle cell phenotype, without acute or chronic GVHD.
2011	Pediatric Hydroxyurea Phase III Clinical Trial (BABY HUG)	Children ages 9–18 months randomized to receive hydroxyurea irrespective of disease severity for 2 y had decreased pain episodes, dactylitis, ACS, hospitalization, leukocyte count, and transfusion and increased hemoglobin as compared with children receiving placebo.
2014	Silent Infarct Trial (SIT)	Children with silent cerebral infarcts and normal TCD velocity who were randomized to chronic transfusion therapy had a 58% relative risk reduction in the recurrence of silent cerebral infarct or stroke as compared to those in the observation arm.
2017	Sustain Study	Crizanlizumab, a monoclonal antibody that targets P-selectin, reduced the rate of VOE to a median/year of 1.63 compared to 2.98 with placebo and increased the median time to the first and second crisis.
2019	Realizing Effectiveness Across Continents With Hydroxyurea (REACH)	Children 1 to 10 years of age with sickle cell anemia in four sub-Saharan countries had lower rates of vaso-occlusive pain, malaria, transfusion and death on hydroxyurea (Tshilolo, 2019).

ACS, Acute chest syndrome; *GVHD*, graft-versus-host disease; *HCT*, hematopoietic cell transplantation; *SCD*, sickle cell disease; *TCD*, transcranial Doppler; *VOE*, vaso-occlusive crisis.

a result of repeated splenic infarction, and platelet activation is increased. In the subset of patients with HbSC and HbS/β+-thalassemia who retain a functional spleen and develop splenomegaly, features of hypersplenism may instead be observed with resulting mild pancytopenia.

Hematologic Indices During Vaso-occlusive Episodes
In acute vaso-occlusive episodes the total Hb decreases as a result of hemolysis (by 1.6 g/dL in acute chest syndrome). The lactate dehydrogenase (LDH), reticulocyte count, and other markers of hemolysis such as aspartate transaminase (AST) and

indirect bilirubin are elevated in steady state, and in many—but not all—patients are further increased during vasoocclusive episodes. Haptoglobin levels are chronically depressed in SCD and typically not measurable, even in steady state, in patients with HbS homozygosity. In patients with HbSC, vasoocclusive episodes may be due to increased blood viscosity and RBC sickling, and worsening hemolysis might not be readily appreciated.

Splenic sequestration crises occur mostly in childhood and are characterized by anemia disproportionate to the degree of hemolysis, reticulocytosis, and acute splenomegaly. Splenic sequestration and repeated episodes of splenic infarction eventually lead to autosplenectomy, although some patients develop splenomegaly. Splenic infarction usually manifests with left upper-quadrant pain and may be massive, involving more than 50% of the splenic tissue.

In severe vasoocclusive episodes, massive bone marrow infarction can also occur. In these instances, the peripheral blood smear reveals a leukoerythroblastic picture with immature neutrophilic forms, nucleated RBCs, and teardrop cells. Fat emboli syndrome, a life-threatening complication of vasoocclusive episodes, can then develop as bone marrow fat embolizes to peripheral capillary beds, leading to multiorgan failure.

Red Blood Cell Alloimmunization

RBC alloimmunization is a common complication of transfusional therapy in SCD and occurs in approximately 30% of patients. It is primarily due to the disparate expression of RBC antigens in African Americans as compared with the donor pool, which is mostly composed of whites. Alloimmunization complicates RBC matching and leads to delayed hemolytic transfusion reactions. Alloantigens that become undetectable by indirect Coombs test 2 months after exposure to mismatched blood have the potential to result in future false-negative cross-matching results. A subset of heavily alloimmunized patients with SCD undergoes life-threatening hemolytic reactions upon exposure to mismatched RBC units. In these hyperhemolytic crises, there is intense hemolysis of transfused and non-transfused RBCs and acute anemia. Treatment of hyperhemolytic crises is empirical and includes erythropoietin-stimulating agents (ESAs), parenteral steroids, and intravenous immunoglobulins (Gammagard).[1]

Iron Overload

Hemosiderosis is the other major complication of transfusional therapy in SCD and is characterized by iron deposition in the heart, liver, and endocrine glands, leading to organ failure and significant morbidity and mortality. It commonly occurs in patients who have received more than 10 lifetime transfusions or more than 20 packed RBC units. Liver biopsy is the "gold standard" for diagnosis, but it is an invasive and uncomfortable procedure. Hepatic and myocardial iron quantitation by MRI has supplanted liver biopsy as the preferred test to diagnose iron overload and monitor therapy with iron chelators, although when this is not available diagnosis often rests on the finding of an elevated ferritin and transferrin saturation in the appropriate clinical setting.

Hemostatic Activation and Thrombosis

Numerous studies have shown that arterial and venous thrombosis are common in SCD and include pulmonary embolism, in situ pulmonary thrombosis, and stroke. In SCD, alterations at all levels of the hemostatic system have been described: patients with SCD exhibit increased basal and stimulated platelet activation, increased markers of thrombin generation and fibrinolysis, increased tissue factor activity, and increased von Willebrand factor (vWF) antigen and thrombogenic ultralarge vWF multimers with depressed ADAMTS13 activity. Interestingly, hemostatic activation is amplified during vaso-occlusive episodes, as shown by increases in multiple markers of thrombosis as compared with steady state, suggesting a link between hemolysis and thrombosis.

Neurology

Ischemic stroke is common in SCD, with the highest incidence between 2 and 5 years of age. Patients may develop overt stroke from large vessel occlusion (5% to 8% of patients with HbSS) or silent infarcts from focal ischemia detectable by MRI without symptoms of acute stroke (20% to 35% of patients with HbSS). The pathophysiology of stroke in SCD is unclear, although genetic factors and an unbalance between oxygen demand and supply have been postulated. Multiple epidemiologic studies have shown that the risk factors for ischemic stroke in adult patients include HbSS genotype, severity of anemia, systolic hypertension, male gender, and increasing age. Patients with repeated strokes are at risk for development of anatomic abnormalities and Moyamoya pattern of vascularization, which predisposes to both ischemic and hemorrhagic stroke later in life. The highest incidence of intracerebral hemorrhages occurs in patients older than 20 years.

Both overt and silent strokes have a negative impact on IQ and cause cognitive impairment measurable by psychometric testing. Children and adults with SCD can develop cognitive impairment and subtle signs of accelerated brain aging and vascular dementia even in the absence of focal ischemia by MRI, with a low hematocrit being a predictor of neuropsychological dysfunction. These abnormalities are probably due to chronic and diffuse, as opposed to focal, cerebral anoxia and may be unmasked by psychometric testing.

Ophthalmology

Retinal abnormalities are common in SCD and are often asymptomatic until the occurrence of ophthalmologic emergencies. Retinal disease is due to arteriolar occlusion, with subsequent vascular proliferation, neovascularization, retinal hemorrhage (stage IV), and detachment (stage V). Patients with HbSC are more prone to retinal complications, possibly as a result of increased blood viscosity.

Nephrology

Renal abnormalities are common in SCD and manifest primarily as hematuria, proteinuria, and renal tubular acidosis. Hematuria is usually due to papillary necrosis and is an acute finding that requires supportive care and carries a good prognosis. Rarely, gross hematuria requires urologic consultation. Tubular functional defects include an inability to concentrate the urine (hyposthenuria) and renal tubular acidosis. Hyposthenuria often manifests with enuresis in childhood, and it is clinically relevant because it predisposes patients to an increased risk of dehydration. Renal tubular acidosis similar to type IV renal tubular acidosis is a common finding in SCD and may lead to hyperkalemia, an important consideration in patients already predisposed to hyperkalemia with intravascular hemolysis and whenever therapy with angiotensin-converting enzyme inhibitors is entertained.

Hyperphosphatemia and hyperuricemia are also often observed in SCD. Microalbuminuria may be detected in early adulthood and tends to progress to nephrotic range proteinuria. Focal segmental glomerulosclerosis is the most common glomerular abnormality and it is probably due to glomerular sickling and infarction. There are currently no approved therapies to prevent progression to end-stage renal disease, which occurs in up to 20% of patients and at a median age of 37 years. Renal replacement therapy is often needed in older adults with SCD. Serum creatinine and 24-hour creatinine clearance are not adequate for screening and monitoring of progression of kidney disease, because tubular secretion of creatinine is preserved and glomerular hyperfiltration is common in SCD, leading to a relatively low creatinine and a high glomerular filtration rate even in patients with underlying kidney impairment. Testing for microalbuminuria, plasma cystatin C levels, and hemoglobinuria may instead be used as screening tools for chronic kidney disease.

Leg Ulcers

Leg ulcers occur in 10% to 20% of patients with HbSS and have been associated with a chronically high hemolytic rate. They are

---

[1]Not FDA approved for this indication.

usually located over the malleolar areas and are exquisitely painful, debilitating, disfiguring, and nonhealing. Vascular and plastic surgery consultations are recommended and aim at excluding local vascular problems that can complicate management of the ulcers and at providing prompt débridement and skin grafting. Although hydroxyurea is associated with development of leg ulcers in patients with myeloproliferative disorders, there is no such link with leg ulcers in SCD. Although wound healing may be impaired with hydroxyurea use, patients who develop an increase in fetal hemoglobin and have reduced sickling as a result of hydroxyurea therapy might have a net benefit in terms of tissue oxygenation and perfusion. Transfusional therapy, including exchange transfusional therapy, topical nitrates[1], and nutritional zinc[7] or L-arginine[7] supplementation, have shown benefit in anecdotal reports, but the evidence is inconclusive.

Gastroenterology

Nausea, vomiting, and dyspepsia in SCD are related to delayed gastric emptying and gastrointestinal motility disorders, autonomic neuropathy, or medical therapy. Opiates are often responsible for acute nausea and vomiting, whereas other medications such as hydroxyurea and deferasirox (Exjade) are occasionally responsible for chronic symptoms. Gastroparesis may be due to damage of the microvasculature of autonomic nerves (vasa vasorum) from repeated episodes of sickling.

The liver may be episodically affected by hepatic sequestration crises, heralded by direct hyperbilirubinemia, right upper quadrant pain from distention of the hepatic capsule, acute anemia, and reticulocytosis or by sinusoidal vaso-occlusion leading to severe episodes of intrahepatic cholestasis. Supportive therapy and transfusions are indicated for hepatic vaso-occlusive complications. Exchange transfusion may be the preferred modality for hepatic sequestration with the goal of preventing erythrocytosis once the pooled RBCs are released back into the circulation. Elevation of liver injury tests may be drug induced (hydroxyurea, deferasirox) but also related to hepatic sickling, particularly if it occurs during a vaso-occlusive episode.

Infectious Disease

Patients homozygous for HbSS develop functional asplenia during childhood. This is due to repeated episodes of splenic infarction leading to fibrosis and autosplenectomy. As a result, children are susceptible to overwhelming bacterial sepsis from encapsulated organisms such as *Streptococcus pneumoniae, H. influenzae,* and *N. meningitidis.* High pediatric mortality from sepsis was therefore common before a landmark study published in 1986 demonstrated the benefit of penicillin prophylaxis instituted at birth. Vaccination for encapsulated organisms is also standard of care in children and adults. In spite of preventive measures, the incidence of life-threatening bacterial infections is increased in SCD, and high fever should be treated empirically as in splenectomized patients, with coverage for penicillin-resistant *S. pneumoniae* pending blood culture results. Patients with indwelling venous catheters are at risk of catheter-related bacteremia.

Viral infections with bone marrow–tropic viruses such as Epstein-Barr virus, cytomegalovirus, and predominantly parvovirus B19 place patients at risk for myelosuppression, which can further worsen chronic anemia. In children, infections with parvovirus B19 are responsible for transient red cell aplasia and severe aplastic crises, characterized by acute anemia and reticulocytopenia due to intramarrow destruction of erythroid precursors. Treatment of these episodes includes transfusion and intravenous immunoglobulins[1], besides supportive measures.

Individuals with SCD are known to be particularly vulnerable to H1N1 influenza, which has raised concerns about the outcomes of SARS-CoV-2 infection and COVID-19 in SCD. Epidemiological data show that African Americans have been disproportionately affected during the COVID-19 pandemic, but large studies on the outcomes of COVID-19 in SCD have not yet been published.

Pulmonology

A subset of patients with vaso-occlusive episodes develop acute chest syndrome, the major pulmonary complication of SCD. Acute chest syndrome is a lung injury syndrome defined by fever, pleuritic chest pain, oxygen desaturation, and multilobar radiographic infiltrates associated with severe vaso-occlusive episodes, infection, and bone marrow fat embolization (Figure 4). It usually develops 2 to 3 days after hospitalization for vaso-occlusive episodes and is often misdiagnosed as nosocomial pneumonia or aspiration pneumonia, particularly because it displays a predilection for the lower lobe of the lungs. Although pneumonia often accompanies acute chest syndrome, proper diagnosis is important because acute chest syndrome warrants simple or exchange transfusion in addition to antibiotic therapy and supportive measures. Common infectious pathogens identified in cases of acute chest syndrome include *Chlamydia pneumoniae, Mycoplasma pneumoniae,* and *Legionella pneumophila,* thus dictating inclusion of a macrolide in the antibiotic cocktail. Pulmonary embolism with resulting infarct is also in the differential diagnosis of acute chest syndrome and may occur concurrently in 17% of patients. If not recognized and treated promptly, acute chest syndrome leads to pulmonary failure and carries a high mortality.

Airway hyperreactivity is common in children with SCD and needs to be actively diagnosed and aggressively treated because it is associated with worse SCD outcomes. Children with chronic respiratory symptoms should be tested for bronchial hyperresponsiveness.

Chronic complications of SCD include pulmonary fibrosis and PH. PH is an emergent complication of SCD and is associated with a high morbidity and mortality. Multiple epidemiologic studies have shown that a high baseline hemolysis rate, low hemoglobin, increasing age, a history of leg ulcers, liver dysfunction, iron overload, and kidney failure are risk factors for the development of PH. Three epidemiologic studies and a randomized clinical trial have shown that an elevated tricuspid regurgitant jet velocity (TRV) measured by Doppler echocardiography is a common occurrence in SCD with 30% of the patients having a TRV of 2.5 m/s (2 standard deviations [SDs] above the normal mean) or higher, and 10% of the patients having a TRV of 3.0 m/s (3 SDs above the normal mean) or higher. These have proven to be valuable cutoff values, as a TRV of less than 2.5 m/s, when combined with an N-terminal pro B-type natriuretic peptide (NT-proBNP) value less than 160 has a high negative predictive value for PH. A TRV of 3.0 m/s or higher confers a positive predictive value for having PH by right heart catheterization (RHC) of 60% to 75% and a relative risk for death of 10.6. Controversy exists on the significance of an intermediate TRV value of 2.5 to 2.9 m/s, because it is unclear how accurately it predicts RHC-diagnosed PH. In three subsequent studies, patients with intermediate or high TRV values had a prevalence of PH by RHC ranging from 25% to 65% depending on what specific cutoff value was used as the criteria to perform an RHC (2.5 vs. 2.8) and on whether patients with evidence of end-organ damage were included or excluded. However, it is worrisome that regardless of the prevalence of PH, patients with an intermediate TRV are as a whole at increased risk of death (relative risk 4.4). One screening approach is to consider RHC in all patients with TRV of 3.0 or higher and in patients with intermediate TRV values of 2.5 to 2.9 m/s if the NT-proBNP is greater than 160 pg/mL or the 6-minute walk is less than 333 m or there is a high clinical pretest probability of having PH (mosaic perfusion pattern on computed tomography [CT] scan, low diffusing capacity of the lung for carbon monoxide (DLCO), significant dyspnea on exertion, etc.). It is likely that intermediate TRV values will need to be combined with other measures of right ventricular function and functional capacity such as NT-proBNP, and 6-minute walk to derive a highly predictive composite biomarker of PH. All studies have been concordant on the high risk of death conferred by PH in SCD whether

Sickle Cell Disease

---

[1]Not FDA approved for this indication.
[7]Available as dietary supplement.

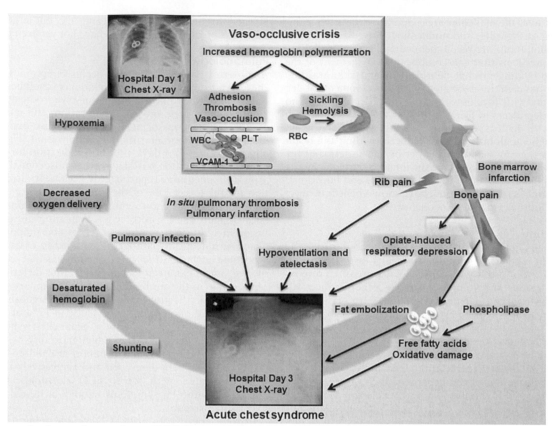

Figure 4 Vicious cycle of acute chest syndrome (ACS). Vaso-occlusive crises are characterized by increased intraerythrocytic polymerization of deoxygenated hemoglobin S, leading to red blood cell sickling, cellular hyperadhesion, hemolysis, and vaso-occlusion in the microvasculature. These processes are responsible for acute pain (pain crisis) and bone marrow necrosis. ACS typically occurs in a subset of patients 2 to 3 days after hospitalization for a vaso-occlusive episode, and radiographically may present as new multilobar, basilar infiltrates on a chest x-ray. Fat embolization from the necrotic marrow is a recognized cause of ACS and is diagnosed by identifying lipid-laden macrophages in the bronchoalveolar lavage. However, pulmonary infection is the most common trigger of ACS and may be superimposed over existing pulmonary infarction. Hypoventilation and molecular pathogens such as reactive oxygen species from ischemia-reperfusion injury and by-products of hemolysis may also play a role in inducing or exacerbating lung injury. Finally, in situ pulmonary thrombosis has been frequently identified as a comorbid condition in patients with ACS and may be caused by endothelial and hemostatic activation. As a result of lung injury, ventilation-perfusion mismatches and shunting ensues, with subsequent hemoglobin desaturation and hypoxemia. Tissue hypoxia in turn triggers further hemoglobin S polymerization and sickling in a vicious cycle.

measured by echocardiography, NT-proBNP, or RHC. Noninvasive transthoracic Doppler echocardiography is recommended by the American Thoracic Society as a screening test in homozygous SCD due to its safety, low cost, and availability. However, the definitive diagnosis of PH requires a confirmatory RHC.

RHC studies of patients with SCD and PH reveal a hyperdynamic state similar to the hemodynamics characteristic of portopulmonary hypertension. It is increasingly clear that pulmonary pressures rise acutely in vaso-occlusive episodes and even more during acute chest syndrome. This suggests that acute PH and right heart dysfunction represent a major comorbidity during acute chest syndrome, and right heart failure should be considered in patients presenting with acute chest syndrome.

Cardiology

Similar to other conditions with chronic anemia, SCD is associated with a hyperdynamic state, low peripheral vascular resistance, and normal blood pressure or hypotension. In this setting, even mild elevation of the blood pressure can indicate relative hypertension and represent a risk factor for stroke. Because there are no studies on the treatment of hypertension in SCD, general guidelines on antihypertensive therapy are applied.

Coronary artery disease is rarely observed in SCD, although many patients complain of chest pain during vaso-occlusive episodes. In these instances, the usual work-up for acute coronary syndrome is recommended. It is possible that myocardial microvascular occlusions are the predominant ischemic event in SCD.

Left-sided heart disease in SCD is primarily due to diastolic dysfunction (present in approximately 13% of patients), although

systolic dysfunction and mitral or aortic valvular disease (2% of patients) can also occur. The presence of diastolic dysfunction alone in SCD patients is an independent risk factor for mortality. Patients with both pulmonary vascular disease and echocardiographic evidence of diastolic dysfunction are at a particularly high risk for death (odds ratio, 12.0; 95% confidence interval [CI], 3.8 to 38.1; $P < .001$).

Cardiac dysfunction is a late complication and the major cause of death in patients with iron overload. Heart failure and conduction defects are the most common abnormalities and warrant emergent iron chelation treatment. Among the iron chelators, deferiprone (Ferriprox) appears to be particularly apt at reducing cardiac iron content. Chelators may be used in combination for cases of severe cardiac decompensation from hemosiderosis.

Methadone (Dolophine) is associated with a risk of QTc prolongation, which carries a risk of arrhythmias and sudden death, particularly in the setting of PH and iron overload. Frequent electrocardiographic (ECG) monitoring, as well as dosage reduction or discontinuation, are warranted in this group, particularly if the QTc is greater than 500 ms.

Endocrinology

Iron overload is a common cause of endocrinopathy in SCD and thalassemia, with the hypophysis, gonads, and thyroid glands being particularly affected. Patients with iron overload should therefore undergo screening for endocrine dysfunction as it is mandated in thalassemia.

However, patients with SCD are at risk for specific endocrine problems regardless of their iron status. Delayed growth and puberty are relatively common, presenting in females with delayed age of menarche by 2 to 3 years and in males with small testicular size and hypospermia. Likely pathogenic factors include increased catabolism, chronic hypoxemia, hospitalizations with prolonged immobility, ischemic insults during vaso-oclusive episodes, and chronic use of opiates.

Priapism

Priapism is the most common urogenital complication in patients with the HbSS genotype. It is a sustained, painful erection in the absence of sexual stimulation from occlusion of the penile blood return. It is defined as stuttering if it lasts from minutes to less than 3 hours and as prolonged if it lasts more than 3 hours. The latter is considered a urologic emergency because of the risk of permanent fibrosis and impotence and requires a urologic consultation. Pseudoephedrine (Sudafed)[1] may lead to detumescence in nonemergency settings, whereas aspiration of the corpus cavernosum is required in the emergency setting and is performed under conscious sedation and local anesthesia. This is usually accompanied by instillation of epinephrine. Other supportive measures, such as intravenous fluids and parenteral opiates, are usually indicated.

Penile shunts are used as a last resort to prevent further episodes of priapism by increasing the cavernous blood flow using native vessels or by creating an arteriovenous shunt. They invariably result in erectile dysfunction, which can be ameliorated by implantation of an inflatable penile prosthesis. There are data showing that sildenafil (Viagra)[1] therapy can prevent priapism by altering vascular smooth muscle tone through inhibition of phosphodiesterase 2 activity.

Diagnosis

The diagnosis of SCD rests on the hemoglobin electrophoresis or high-performance liquid chromatography (HPLC), which allows detection of most hemoglobin variants. In patients with microcytosis α-globin gene sequencing may reveal coinheritance of an α-thalassemia trait.

---

[1]Not FDA approved for this indication.

Neonatal Screening

Children with SCD have an increased susceptibility to bacteremia due to *S. pneumoniae*, which can occur as early as 4 months of age and carries a case fatality rate as high as 30%. Acute splenic sequestration crises also contribute to mortality in infancy. Diagnosis by newborn screening and immediate entry into programs of comprehensive care, including the provision of effective pneumococcal prophylaxis, can reach infants who might otherwise be lost to the healthcare system and has been demonstrated to decrease morbidity and improve survival. Currently, newborn screening and follow-up of SCD are carried out in all 50 states in the United States, as well as in most developed countries, and initiatives are under way to introduce universal newborn screening in most sub-Saharan African countries.

Late Diagnoses and Misdiagnoses

Rarely, patients who were born before the adoption of universal screening or who were lost at the time of follow-up of positive neonatal screening results are only diagnosed late in life. This occasionally occurs in patients with HbSC who might have normal hemoglobin and hematocrit and a mild disease phenotype. Alternatively, the disease may be misdiagnosed as iron deficiency in patients with HbS/β[+]-thalassemia on account of their microcytosis, which places them at risk of futile and potentially harmful prolonged trials of iron supplementation. Patients who have a low HbS level (< 40%) due to recent transfusion or who have only mildly decreased hemoglobin (HbSC or HbS/β[+]-thalassemia) may receive an erroneous diagnosis of sickle cell trait (carrier state).

Treatment

From the original description of SCD in 1910 to the 1970s, there was no efficacious therapy for SCD, and most patients died within the first 2 decades of life, with infectious complications being responsible for the majority of pediatric fatalities. Several preventive and pharmacologic milestones since then, and the realization that care has to occur in a multidisciplinary setting, have profoundly affected the natural history of the disease (Table 3). Median age at death in resource-rich countries was 42 years in male patients and 48 years in female patients

TABLE 3	Manifestations of Sickle Cell Disease With Key Prevention and Treatment Strategies	
MANIFESTATION	**PREVENTION**	**TREATMENT**
Pneumococcal sepsis	Penicillin, Prevnar/Pneumovax vaccination	Antibiotic therapy for penicillin-resistant *Streptococcus pneumoniae*
Splenic or liver sequestration	—	Exchange transfusion
Painful vaso-occlusive episode	Hydroxyurea (Droxia), prevention of exposure to triggers	Intravenous fluids, parenteral opiates, supplemental oxygen
Acute chest syndrome	Incentive spirometry during VOE, hydroxyurea	Transfusion, broad-spectrum antibiotics with atypical coverage
Iron overload	Optimization of transfusion therapy	Iron chelation with deferasirox (Exjade) or deferoxamine (Desferal)
RBC alloimmunization	Transfusion with leukoreduced RBCs	—
CVA	Chronic transfusion in children with high transcranial Doppler velocity	Exchange transfusion and thrombolytics in selected cases
Pulmonary hypertension	Hydroxyurea?, treatment of predisposing conditions such as obstructive sleep apnea, hypoxemia, thromboembolism	Hydroxyurea, chronic transfusion therapy, specific therapy
Kidney disease	Antihypertensive therapy?, hydroxyurea?, ACE inhibitors?	ACE inhibitors?, renal replacement therapy, kidney transplant
Priapism	Hydroxyurea?	Pseudoephedrine (Sudafed)[1], aspiration of corpus cavernosum, sildenafil (Viagra)[1]
Leg ulcers	Hydroxyurea?, topical sodium nitrite?, voxelotor?	Surgical débridement, surgical grafting

ACE, Angiotensin-converting enzyme; *CVA,* cerebrovascular accident; *RBCs,* red blood cells; *TCD,* transcranial Doppler; *VOE,* vaso-occlusive episode (crisis).
[1]Not FDA approved for this indication.

with HbSS, according to data from the Cooperative Study of Sickle Cell Disease in the 1980s (a prehydroxyurea setting), thereby still lagging approximately 2 to 3 decades behind that of the general African-American population. The following sections summarize the therapeutic approach to the most important complications of SCD.

Vaso-occlusive Episodes

Acute pain from vaso-occlusive episodes in SCD is extremely intense, affects both children and adults, and is due to ischemia or necrosis of the vascular beds. Most patients report severe pain in the bones and joints of the extremities, as well as lower back, although acute ischemia and pain can affect unusual sites such as the mandibular area. Infants and young children may experience dactylitis, a painful swelling of the hands from bone marrow infarct in the small bones of the digits. Occasionally, adults may also experience the typical signs of inflammation, such as edema, warmth, and erythema in an affected limb, but a paucity or absence of signs is the norm. Imaging studies such as MRI, positron emission tomography (PET), and bone scan can reveal signs of acute bone marrow infarction in a painful bony area, but they are not routinely used in the work-up of a pain episode, unless osteomyelitis or septic arthritis are suspected.

Intravenous opiates are the mainstay of treatment of a pain episode. Even in opiate-naïve patients with SCD, opioid dosages often exceed those required for other indications. For instance, doses of intravenous hydromorphone (Dilaudid) of 1 to 2 mg are typical in adult patients. However, most patients, are on an oral pain regimen at home and have a history of multiple admissions for vaso-occlusive episodes. In these cases, individualized care based on prior effective regimens and the patient's own perception of the intensity of pain are recommended. After an attempt at controlling the pain with three or four closely spaced opiate boluses is made, patients who are in persistent discomfort or have evidence of underlying complications triggering the vaso-occlusive episode should be admitted and ideally placed on patient controlled analgesia. Nonsteroidal antiinflammatory drugs such as ketorolac (Toradol) have fallen out of favor due to their risks in patients with renal disease and their questionable efficacy. The American Pain Society, the National Heart, Lung and Blood Institute (NHLBI), and the American Society of Hematology have published guidelines for the treatment of acute and chronic pain in SCD.

Common obstacles to prompt and effective care in SCD are the health professional's fear of overdosing the patient, as well as misconceptions about addiction and pseudoaddiction. In general, healthcare professionals tend to overestimate the prevalence of opioid use disorder in SCD and tend to undertreat patients significantly, leading to patients' frustration and anger when their pain demands are not met (pseudoaddiction).

Nonpharmacologic therapies such as biofeedback, relaxation, and localized heat may be effective and should be incorporated into the management of pain episodes whenever possible. Care for vaso-occlusive episodes should also include management of possible precipitating factors: dehydration and hypovolemia should be corrected with hypotonic crystalloids, and an infection work-up should be initiated in patients with fever, hypoxemia, or leukocytosis above baseline. Antiemetics and antipruritus therapy are also usually required.

Prior experiences in multiple institutions have shown that a dedicated facility for effective and rapid management of uncomplicated vaso-occlusive episodes reduces hospitalizations and length of stay and facilitates integration of care—psychological, socioeconomic, and nutritional—in a multidisciplinary approach. This experience is the basis of the concept of the day hospital in SCD and relies on the need to provide prompt assessment and treatment of pain, safe dose titration to relief, monitoring of adverse effects, and adequate disposition (emergency department, inpatient admission, home) in a clinical environment familiar with SCD and the individual patient.

Chronic Pain

Chronic pain is common, and a study using pain diaries compiled by patients shows that most patients with SCD experience pain on an almost daily basis (PiSCES study). Orthopedic problems such as avascular necrosis (AVN) are common and tend to develop early in patients with HbSS disease, thus exposing patients to a lifetime of pain. There is an increasing realization that central sensitization and opiate-induced hyperalgesia also play a significant role in chronic pain in SCD. Unfortunately, there is a dearth of safe and effective strategies to manage chronic pain in SCD. At times, short-acting and long-acting opiates are required to empower the patient to manage pain at home and minimize use of the emergency department. Drugs for neuropathic pain, such as gabapentin (Neurontin)[1], may also be used in combination with opiates because neuropathic pain may develop as a result of tissue ischemia and necrosis.

Patients who have successfully transitioned from pediatric to adult care, have a good support system, and are distracted by their work or school schedules tend to cope better and require less pharmacologic support.

Because analgesic care is life-long, consultation with pain specialists is often valuable, particularly in patients for whom more-sophisticated pain regimens are needed. For instance, the mu-opioid receptor partial agonist buprenorphine (Buprenex, Butrans), opioid rotation, and methadone used as analgesic can help to reduce the total opiate requirements. Several States in the United States have approved the use of marijuana for medical purposes for several conditions including SCD. Although controlled studies on the benefits and risks of medical marijuana in SCD are lacking, studies in sickle mice and anecdotal reports hold promise. Urine toxicology screens and written "opiate agreements" are indicated in patients receiving opiates to ensure adherence with the therapy and to minimize the risk of use of illicit substances, particularly at a time of heightened surveillance for opiate abuse in the United States. The ASH guidelines published in 2020 emphasized an individualized approach in the management of chronic pain in SCD due to the lack of extensive evidence on the benefits of opioids for chronic pain in this population. In addition, they recommended "against the initiation of chronic opiate therapy unless pain is refractory to multiple other treatment modalities" in children and adults with chronic pain from SCD. All recommendations on opioids for chronic pain were "conditional" based on very low certainty in the evidence about effects, and reflect a more guarded stance on opioids due to the deeper appreciation of the risks of chronic opioids for noncancer pain that has emerged in the past few years.

Transfusional Therapy

In SCD, the benefits of transfusion in terms of improved hemodynamics and oxygenation need to be balanced with the risks of iron overload, alloimmunization, transfusion reactions, and viral transmission of infectious agents. Leuko-reduced, sickle-negative RBCs with extended phenotypic matching for Rh Cc, Ee, and Kell, which account for 80% of detected antibodies, are required. By using extended phenotypic matching, the rate of alloimmunization decreased from 3% to 0.5% per unit, and the rate of delayed hemolytic transfusion reactions decreased by 90% in the STOP study. In previously immunized patients, a full RBC match also inclusive of matching for the Duffy, Kidd, and S antigens is recommended. Indications for transfusion include hemoglobin less than 5 g/dL or less than 6 g/dL with symptoms and any severe complication such as stroke, aplastic anemia, splenic or hepatic sequestration, or acute chest syndrome.

Prophylactic transfusions have been considered standard of care before surgery (with the exclusion of minor procedures such as intravenous port placement); the benefit of preoperative transfusions in preventing SCD-related complications in HbSS patients has also been confirmed in a small randomized clinical trial (the TAPS study).

---

[1]Not FDA approved for this indication.

BOX 1 Indications for Transfusion

No Indication
Chronic steady-state anemia
Uncomplicated painful episode
Infections
Minor surgery without general anesthesia
Aseptic necrosis of hip or shoulder
Uncomplicated pregnancy

Unclear Indication
Intractable or frequent painful episodes
Leg ulcers
Before receiving intravenous contrast dye
Complicated pregnancy
Cerebrovascular accident in adults
Chronic organ failure

Simple Transfusion
Symptomatic anemia
- High output cardiac failure
- Dyspnea
- Angina
- Central nervous system dysfunction

Sudden decrease in hemoglobin
- Aplastic crisis
- Acute splenic sequestration

Severe anemia (hemoglobin ~5 g/dL) with fatigue or dyspnea
Preparation for surgery with general anesthesia

Exchange Transfusion
Acute cerebrovascular accident
Multiple organ system failure
Acute chest syndrome
Hepatic sequestration
Retinal surgery

As to the type of transfusion strategy to be used, a clinical trial published in 1995 showed that a conservative prophylactic transfusion regimen to achieve a target hemoglobin of 10 g/dL and any HbS value was as effective as an aggressive regimen to achieve a hemoglobin of 10 g/dL and a target HbS value of less than 30% in preventing postsurgical complications such as acute chest syndrome.

Exchange transfusion (erythrocytapheresis with RBC exchange) is usually reserved for the most severe complications, which include acute chest syndrome with impending pulmonary failure, acute stroke and its prevention in children, multiorgan failure, and sepsis. Box 1 summarizes the main indications for simple and exchange transfusion in SCD, as well as the areas of uncertainty.

Iron Chelation

Patients who have received more than 10 transfusions or 20 units of packed RBCs should be screened for iron overload. Most authorities recommend initiation of iron chelation based on a ferritin level consistently greater than 1000 ng/mL, based on data from the thalassemia literature, although liver iron quantitation by MRI or biopsy should be obtained, when available, prior to therapy and to monitor its effectiveness. In the United States, the oral chelating agents deferasirox (Exjade) and deferiprone (Ferriprox) and the parenteral deferoxamine (Desferal) are available and should be administered until the ferritin level is less than 500 ng/mL for three consecutive measurements. Patients on iron chelation with deferasirox and deferoxamine require monitoring of hepatic, renal, auditory, and visual toxicity, and particular caution has to be exercised in the setting of renal disease, because transient, reversible increases in serum creatinine and rare instances of irreversible acute kidney injury have been reported in patients with underlying renal insufficiency. Deferiprone has been associated with agranulocytosis and neutropenia, mandating close monitoring of the absolute neutrophil count during therapy.

Erythropoietic Stimulating Agents

Although a brisk reticulocytic response is common in SCD, patients who develop renal failure or aplastic crises or who receive therapy with hydroxyurea may experience a relative or absolute reticulocytopenia (<100,000 reticulocytes/mL) and a worsening of their baseline anemia. In these situations, therapy with ESAs may be beneficial.

Because of bone marrow expansion in patients with HbSS, higher starting doses of erythropoietin (Epogen, (Epogen, Procrit)[1] than in patients without SCD may be considered. For darbepoetin (Aranesp)[1], a reasonable starting dose is 100 to 200 µg/weekly or every 2 weeks. ESAs can be titrated by 20% to 25% increases in dose per week in patients who do not respond adequately. Weekly monitoring of hematocrit is essential to avoid overdosage and relative erythrocytosis, which can lead to hyperviscosity and vaso-occlusive episodes.

Nutritional Considerations

Malnutrition, growth retardation, and stunting with findings of low lean and fat body mass are highly prevalent in children and adolescents with SCD, due to their increased caloric demands and a hypermetabolic state. Macronutrient and micronutrient deficiencies are common, and nutritional counseling is warranted. Hypovitaminosis D and low bone mineral density are also prevalent in children and adults. Folic acid[1] is indicated at the dose of 1 mg daily as in other hemolytic diseases, particularly where folate nutritional supplementation programs are absent. Strategies aimed at decreasing iron intake and absorption should be implemented early. There is also growing interest in antioxidant nutraceuticals, particularly in light of the clinical trial showing beneficial effects with L-glutamine (Endari) in SCD; however, evidence on other substances remains limited. The small subset of patients who are overweight or obese is at risk for exacerbating or precipitating common orthopedic problems in SCD such as AVN of the femoral head and its resulting disability. These patients should also receive targeted nutritional counseling.

Hydroxyurea

Since the pediatric hematologist Janet Watson suggested in 1948 that the paucity of sickle cells in the peripheral blood of newborns was due to the presence of increased HbF, there has been interest in developing therapies to modulate the hemoglobin switch from fetal to newborn life and prolong HbF production. Several antineoplastic agents, including 5-azacytidine (Vidaza)[1] and hydroxyurea, became the focus of attention after they were found to increase HbF levels in nonhuman primates and individuals with SCD.

The landmark Multicenter Study of Hydroxyurea in Sickle Cell Disease (MSH) showed that the incidence of painful crises was reduced from a median of 4.5 per year to 2.5 per year in hydroxyurea-treated patients with SCD. The rates of acute chest syndrome and blood transfusion were also reduced significantly. A follow-up for up to 9 years of 233 of the original 299 subjects showed a 40% reduction in mortality among those who received hydroxyurea. This study led to the approval of hydroxyurea (Droxia, Siklos) as the first disease-modifying therapy in adults with SCD. More recent studies showed that hydroxyurea is safe and effective in children and adults with SCD. The recently concluded BABY HUG study showed that children 9 to 18 months with HbSS disease randomized to receive 2 years of hydroxyurea therapy, irrespective of the disease severity, had less dactylitis and fewer pain episodes, hospitalizations, and transfusions than children receiving placebo.

On the molecular and cellular levels, the benefits of hydroxyurea are mostly related to increased intracellular HbF, which prevents the formation of HbS polymers and sickling. In addition to this mechanism, some patients on hydroxyurea who do not adequately increase their HbF levels also display clinical benefits,

[1]Not FDA approved for this indication.

Start therapy if one or more of the following conditions are present:
- frequent pain episodes
- history of acute chest syndrome
- other severe VOE
- severe symptomatic anemia

Starting dose: 15 mg/kg or 7.5 mg/kg if the patient has kidney disease

Endpoints:
- less pain
- increase in HbF to 15%–20%
- increased hemoglobin level to 7–9 g/dL
- improved well-being
- acceptable myelotoxicity

Dose escalation: increase dose by 500 mg every other day every 8 weeks if no toxicity encountered to a maximum of 35 mg/kg

Lab monitoring:
- At time of initiation or escalation: check CBC/differential/reticulocyte count every 2 weeks; serum chemistries every 2–4 weeks, percent HbF every 6–8 weeks
- During maintenance: check CBC/differential/reticulocyte count chemistries monthly, percent HbF every 3 months

Criteria to hold:
- ANC <2000
- Hb <9.0 g/dL and reticulocyte count <80,000 (alternatively start Epo)
- Platelet count <80,000
- Raising creatinine
- 2-fold elevation of AST or ALT over baseline
- 2 months prior to planned conception/pregnancy

Figure 5 Protocol for hydroxyurea treatment.

suggesting that hydroxyurea might have other beneficial rheologic properties.

Although the MSH study only included patients with HbSS, its findings traditionally have been extrapolated to other sickle cell syndromes such as HbSC and HbS/β-thalassemia. A report from Greece, where S/β-thalassemia is highly prevalent, has confirmed that hydroxyurea similarly reduces complications and mortality in patients with HbS/β⁰-thalassemia, with a nonsignificant benefit also observed in HbS/β⁺ thalassemia. Existing guidelines also recommend hydroxyurea in patients with HbSC disease, but there is still no high-level evidence to support this practice.

Hydroxyurea has been indicated at a dosage of 15 mg/kg (7.5 mg/kg in patients with renal disease) in patients with frequent pain episodes, history of acute chest syndrome, other severe vaso-occlusive episodes, or severe symptomatic anemia, although another sensible approach is to prescribe it to all patients with HbSS regardless of their phenotype. End points are less pain, increase in HbF to 15% to 20%, increased hemoglobin level to 7 to 9 g/dL in severely anemic patients, improved well-being, and acceptable myelotoxicity. The dosage can be increased by 500 mg every other day every 8 weeks to a maximum of 35 mg/kg if no toxicity is encountered. Considering the potential myelotoxicity, hepatotoxicity, and nephrotoxicity of this medication, laboratory monitoring needs to be performed every 2 weeks at the time of initiation or escalation and monthly during maintenance therapy. Laboratory studies should include a complete blood cell (CBC) count, differential and reticulocyte count, and serum chemistries. Measurements of HbF can be performed every 3 months. An elevated MCV is a marker of adherence to the therapy.

Criteria for holding hydroxyurea are listed in Figure 5. Patients need to be counseled on the teratogenic potential, as demonstrated in animal studies, as well as the risks of infertility and leukemogenesis, although a growing body of evidence shows that these risks may have been overestimated in patients with SCD.

Other side effects that can affect compliance include, but are not limited to, weight gain, alopecia, skin and nail hyperpigmentation (melanonychia), nausea and vomiting, and mucosal ulcerations. Because of the toxicity concerns, as well as factors intrinsic to long-term preventive therapy, hydroxyurea therapy has had low effectiveness in spite of high efficacy, with underprescribing by healthcare professionals and poor patient compliance being major obstacles to its widespread adoption.

Therapy of Pulmonary Hypertension

Because evidence-based guidelines for managing PH in patients with SCD are not available, recommendations are based upon the pulmonary arterial hypertension literature, case reports, small open-label studies, and expert opinion. For patients with mild PH (tricuspid regurgitant velocity [TRV], 2.5 to 2.9 m/s), it is important to identify and treat risk factors associated with PH such as rest, exercise or nocturnal hypoxemia, sleep apnea, pulmonary thromboembolic disease, restrictive lung disease or fibrosis, left ventricular systolic and diastolic dysfunction, severe anemia, and iron overload. These patients may benefit from aggressive SCD management, including optimization of hydroxyurea dosage and initiation of a chronic transfusion program in those who do not tolerate or respond poorly to hydroxyurea. Consultation with a pulmonologist or cardiologist experienced in PH is also recommended.

For patients with TRV 3 m/s or more, we recommend following the guidelines for TRV 2.5 to 2.9 m/s. In addition, RHC is necessary to confirm diagnosis and to directly assess left ventricular diastolic and systolic function. We would consider specific therapy with selective pulmonary vasodilator and remodeling drugs if the patient has pulmonary arterial hypertension defined by RHC and exercise limitation defined by a low 6-minute walk distance.

US Food and Drug Administration (FDA)-approved drugs for primary pulmonary arterial hypertension include the endothelin receptor antagonists (bosentan [Tracleer] and ambrisentan [Letairis]), prostaglandin-based therapy (epoprostenol [Flolan], treprostinil [Remodulin, Tyvaso, Orenitram], and iloprost [Ventavis]), the phosphodiesterase-5 inhibitors (sildenafil [Revatio]), and riociguat (Adempas), the first member of a new class of drugs, the soluble guanylate cyclase (sGC) stimulators. No published randomized studies in the SCD population exist for any of these agents, although a multicenter placebo-controlled trial of sildenafil for PH of SCD was stopped early because of an unexpected increase in hospitalizations for vaso-occlusive crisis in the treatment group receiving sildenafil.

Anticoagulation is indicated in patients who have evidence of pulmonary thromboembolic complications and is supported by evidence of benefit in other populations with PH.

Hematopoietic Stem Cell Transplantation

Despite improvement of supportive care in SCD, life expectancy remains lower than for those not affected. In addition, quality of life for patients with SCD is usually significantly impaired. Although hydroxyurea can decrease acute complications of SCD such as vaso-occlusive episodes and acute chest syndrome, no satisfactory measures exist to prevent the development of irreversible organ damage in adults. Furthermore, therapy with hydroxyurea is lifelong, and only 20% to 30% of eligible patients are prescribed or actually take the drug.

Currently, allogeneic hematopoietic stem cell transplantation (HCT) remains the only curative treatment. Indications for HCT have been empirically determined from prognostic factors derived from studies of the natural history of SCD. The most common indications for which patients with SCD have undergone HCT are a history of stroke, recurrent acute chest syndrome, or frequent vaso-occlusive episodes.

Allogeneic HCT after myeloablative therapy has been performed in hundreds of pediatric and numerous adult patients with SCD. The backbone of the preparative regimens have consisted of busulfan (Busulfex)[1] 14 to 16 mg/kg and cyclophosphamide (Cytoxan)[1] 200 mg/kg. Additional immunosuppressive

---

[1]Not FDA approved for this indication.

Figure 6 Spectrum of immunosuppression and myelosuppression in preparative regimens in hematopoietic stem cell transplantation (HCT) in sickle cell disease (SCD). Most preparative regimens for HCT in SCD have used a backbone of busulfan (BU) (Busulfex)[1] and cyclophosphamide (CY) (Cytoxan)[1]. Additional immunosuppressive agents include equine antithymocyte globulin (Atgam)[1] or leporine antithymocyte globulin (Thymoglobulin) (ATG)[1], antilymphocyte globulin, total lymphoid irradiation (TLI) or total body irradiation (TBI), fludarabine (Flu) (Fludara)[1], and alemtuzumab (Campath)[1]. Attempts to reduce the intensity of preparative regimens for patients with SCD have been based on one of two approaches. The first is the use of reduced-intensity conditioning regimens to produce less myeloablation. These require donor marrow infusion for hematopoietic recovery. The second is the use of nonmyeloablative regimens, which do not eradicate host hematopoiesis and allow hematopoietic recovery even without donor stem cell infusion. [1]Not FDA approved for this indication. Adapted with permission from Krishnamurti L. Hematopoietic cell transplantation: a curative option for sickle cell disease. *Pediatr Hematol Oncol.* 2007;24:569–575.

agents used have included antithymocyte globulin (Atgam)[1], rabbit antithymocyte globulin (Thymoglobulin)[1], antilymphocyte globulin, or total lymphoid irradiation (Figure 6). Cyclosporine A (Neoral)[1], alone or with mercaptopurine (Purinethol)[1] or methotrexate[1], has been used for posttransplant graft-versus-host disease prophylaxis.

The outcome of HCT for patients with SCD from matched siblings is excellent. Of 1000 recipients of human leukocyte antigen (HLA)-identical sibling transplants performed between 1986 and 2013 and reported to the European Blood and Marrow Transplant, Eurocord, and the Center for International Blood and Marrow Transplant Research, the 5-year event-free and overall survival were 91.4% (95% CI 89.6% to 93.3%) and 92.9% (95% CI 91.1% to 94.6%), respectively. Event-free survival was lower with increasing age at transplantation (hazard ratio [HR] 1.09; $P < .001$) and higher for transplantations performed after 2006 (HR 0.95, $P = .013$). Twenty-three patients experienced graft failure; 70 patients (7%) died, the most common cause of death being infection. Stabilization or reversal of organ damage from SCD has been documented after HCT. In patients who have stable donor engraftment, complications related to SCD resolve, and there are no further episodes of pain, stroke, or acute chest syndrome. Patients who successfully receive allografts do not experience sickle-related central nervous system complications and have evidence of stabilization of central nervous system disease by cerebral MRI. However, the impact of successful HCT on reversal of cerebral vasculopathy has been variable. Current research is focused on improving the applicability of HCT to a greater proportion of patients with SCD by the development of novel conditioning regimens minimizing myeloablation (see Figure 6), the use of novel sources of hematopoietic stem cells such as umbilical cord blood, extending HCT to adult recipients and alternate donors such as matched unrelated donors and haploidentical donors. The aim of these studies is to develop safe and effective alternatives for patients without matched sibling donors, thus increasing the applicability of curative therapy for SCD.

New and Experimental Therapies

The last few years have witnessed a flourishing of new therapeutic approaches for SCD. Three new drugs have received FDA approval and have been incorporated in the clinical practice across the United States, and several are in the pipeline or being reviewed in accelerated approval pathways by the FDA. Several decades of preclinical research in sickle mouse models are finally bearing fruit with pathologic pathways identified in sickle mice being harnessed for the development of molecular targeted biologicals. Finally, gene therapy is currently on the horizon with several gene therapy and gene editing approaches being developed simultaneously.

Antioxidant Strategies

In 2018, pharmacologic L-glutamine (Endari) received FDA approval as the second disease-modifying drug in SCD. A randomized, phase III multicenter trial showed that patients in the L-glutamine group had significantly fewer pain crises and hospitalizations than those in the placebo group. Of note, two-thirds of the patients in both arms received concomitant hydroxyurea. Reassuringly, the drug had relatively mild side effects including nausea and fatigue. L-glutamine presumably acts by reducing oxidant stress in the sickle RBCs, although its effects on major disease parameters such as hemolysis are unclear.

Modulation of Cellular Adhesion

Adhesive interactions between RBCs, white blood cells, and platelets, and between cells and endothelium are implicated in the pathogenesis of vaso-occlusive episodes. Recently, several compounds have been developed to target specific adhesion molecules such as E-selectin and P-selectin. This is a particularly promising area of research that has yielded two compounds in advanced phases of development. The P-selectin inhibitor crizanlizumab has shown significant reduction of the rate of crises per year and longer median time to the first crisis and second crisis when given as intravenous prophylaxis in a double-blind, randomized, phase II clinical trial. The FDA approved crizanlizumab (Adakveo) for the prevention of vaso-occlusive episodes in SCD in November 2019. As in the case of L-glutamine, crizanlizumab can be used with and without concurrent hydroxyurea therapy. The pan-selectin inhibitor rivipansel[5] had shown promising results in a phase II trial of treatment of vaso-occlusive episodes but failed to meet the

---

[5]Investigational drug in the United States.

primary end point of time to readiness for discharge and other key secondary endpoints in a phase III trial.

Modulation of Hemoglobin Oxygen Affinity

Deoxygenation of HbS leads to polymerization, sickling, and hemolysis. Thus strategies aimed at increasing the oxygen affinity of HbS may be beneficial. Clinical trials in adults and children have shown reduced hemolysis and improved hemoglobin with voxelotor, a once daily oral drug that increases the oxygen affinity of hemoglobin maintaining it in the oxygenated state and reducing polymerization and sickling. Unfortunately, these changes were not accompanied by a statistically significant reduction in vaso-occlusive episodes. Voxelotor (Oxbryta) was also approved by the FDA for the treatment of SCD in November 2019.

Another promising strategy to reduce HbS polymerization by modulating oxygen affinity involves the use of pyruvate kinase activators. Both mitapivat (Pyrukynd)[1] and etavopivat[5] are promising pyruvate kinase activators that ameliorate the sickling of SCD RBCs by reduction of 2,3-diphosphoglycerate (2,3-DPG), which in turn increases hemoglobin oxygen affinity.

Modulation of Nitric Oxide

NO is an active biogas and a free radical species that mediates arterial relaxation, cellular adhesion to endothelium, hemostasis, and blood viscosity. In SCD, NO bioactivity is reduced as a result of decreased production due to endothelial perturbation and NO scavenging by cell-free hemoglobin generated during intravascular hemolysis. Dietary supplementation with L-arginine, a precursor of NO, and delivery of exogenous NO or NO bioactivity to the microvasculature in SCD, should promote dilatation of the terminal arterioles where obstruction to flow and tissue damage occurs, improvement of lung ventilation and perfusion is matching, decrease in pulmonary artery pressures, and inhibition of platelet aggregation and cellular adhesion. Although two recent clinical trials on L-arginine supplementation and inhaled NO (DeNOVO trial) for vaso-occlusive episodes failed to show a clinical benefit, optimization of timing and dosing and novel strategies to target the NO pathway might lead to valuable NO therapeutics in the future.

Gene Therapy

The ultimate cure for SCD, gene therapy, is finally on the horizon. A French group first reported that a patient had been successfully treated with lentiviral-mediated insertion of an anti-sickling β-globin gene into autologous stem cells. The transduced cells were then transplanted into the patient who has since experienced long-term remission from SCD. Subsequently, in a clinical trial at the National Institutes of Health (NIH), several patients were treated with autologous hematopoietic stem cells transduced with a lentiviral vector that encodes for a nonsickling hemoglobin with very promising results. Other gene therapy approaches have targeted fetal hemoglobin induction and have harnessed the CRISPR-Cas9 gene editing technology.

Several hurdles need to be overcome before gene therapy will become a viable, large scale therapeutic option for SCD, including technical limitations (e.g., the need for *ex vivo* gene transduction or editing, with the potential loss of stem cell viability), toxicity concerns (e.g., the need for myeloablative chemotherapy to accommodate the auto transplant), cost considerations, and ethical concerns. It is also important to note that gene therapy approaches may not necessarily lead to a cure if they do not result in permanent and high-level suppression of HbS polymerization. Further compounding these concerns, in early 2021 a company performing clinical trials of a lentiviral gene therapy approach for SCD has halted its studies after one gene therapy recipient developed acute myeloid leukemia and others

a myelodysplastic syndrome. The causes of this serious setback are currently being investigated.

Surgical Issues

Preoperative patient optimization includes prophylactic transfusion, close monitoring of pulse oximetry, adequate analgesia based on the patient's opiate tolerance, and monitoring for sickle cell–related complications.

AVN of the femoral heads, and more rarely of the humeral heads, is the most common orthopedic problem in SCD. Surgery is usually deferred until the pain and disability from AVN become intolerable and usually involves total hip or shoulder arthroplasty. This is usually a more involved procedure than in the general population on account of the altered bone anatomy in SCD. Patients with bone marrow expansion may experience thinning of the cortical bone and prosthetic instability, whereas some may suffer from the opposite problem of obliteration of the medullary shaft by sclerotic bone in response to multiple necrotic events.

Patients with SCD tend to develop pigmented gallstones and cholelithiasis. Cholecystectomy is performed in patients with SCD with cholelithiasis, right upper quadrant pain, and a positive hepatobiliary iminodiacetic acid (HIDA) scan. In SCD, the rate of intraoperative complications is higher and so is the rate of reversion from laparoscopic to open cholecystectomy.

Splenectomy has been reserved for patients with massive splenic infarction (>50% of the spleen volume); intractable, recurrent splenic pain; and splenic abscess in the setting of splenic infarction. It is important to limit splenectomy to these few specific circumstances, because overwhelming sepsis and acute PH have been reported in the postsplenectomy period in SCD.

Kidney transplantation has been successfully performed in patients with SCD on chronic renal replacement therapy, although survival at 7 years is lower than in African Americans without SCD (67% vs. 83%). This difference is mostly due to vaso-occlusive complications in the transplanted kidney, possibly exacerbated by the higher hematocrit in the postoperative period from resumption of endogenous erythropoietin production and increased blood viscosity. It is therefore critical to closely monitor ESA therapy in the posttransplantation period to prevent overdosing and relative erythrocytosis. A chronic transfusion program to prevent intrarenal sickling and maximization of hydroxyurea therapy should also be entertained, although its benefits need to be balanced against the risk of HLA alloimmunization and rejection. Combined solid organ and HCT protocols are being developed to overcome these complications. Recently, lung transplantation has been successfully performed in a SCD patient with severe pulmonary arterial hypertension and pulmonary venoocclusive disease.

References

Adams RJ, Brambilla D: Discontinuing prophylactic transfusions used to prevent stroke in sickle cell disease, *N Engl J Med* 353:2769–2778, 2005.

Adams RJ, Brambilla DJ, Granger S, et al: Stroke and conversion to high risk in children screened with transcranial Doppler ultrasound during the STOP study, *Blood* 103:3689–3694, 2004.

Ataga KI, et al: Crizanlizumab for the prevention of pain crises in sickle cell disease, *N Engl J Med* 376:429–439, 2017.

Bunn HF: Pathogenesis and treatment of sickle cell disease, *N Engl J Med* 337:762–769, 1997.

Charache S, Terrin ML, Moore RD, et al: Effect of hydroxyurea on the frequency of painful crises in sickle cell anemia. Investigators of the Multicenter Study of Hydroxyurea in Sickle Cell Anemia, *N Engl J Med* 332:1317–1322, 1995.

DeBaun MR, et al: Controlled trial of transfusions for silent cerebral infarcts in sickle cell anemia, *N Engl J Med* 371(8):699–710, 2014.

Falletta JM, Woods GM, Verter JI, et al: Discontinuing penicillin prophylaxis in children with sickle cell anemia. Prophylactic Penicillin Study II, *J Pediatr* 127:685–690, 1995.

Gaston MH, Verter JI, Woods G, et al: Prophylaxis with oral penicillin in children with sickle cell anemia. A randomized trial, *N Engl J Med* 314:1593–1599, 1986.

Gladwin MT, Sachdev V: Cardiovascular abnormalities in sickle cell disease, *J Am Coll Cardiol* 59:1123–1133, 2012.

---

[1]Not FDA approved for this indication.
[5]Investigational drug in the United States.

Gladwin MT, Sachdev V, Jison ML, et al: Pulmonary hypertension as a risk factor for death in patients with sickle cell disease, *N Engl J Med* 350:886–895, 2004.

Gladwin MT, Vichinsky E: Pulmonary complications of sickle cell disease, *N Engl J Med* 359:2254–2265, 2008.

Gluckman E, Cappelli B, Bernaudin F, et al: Sickle cell disease: An international survey of results of HLA-identical sibling hematopoietic stem cell transplantation, *Blood* 129(11):1548–1556, 2017.

Hoppe CC, Inati AC, Brown C, et al: Initial results from a cohort in a phase 2a study (GBT440- 007) evaluating adolescents with sickle cell disease treated with multiple doses of GBT440, a HbS polymerization inhibitor, *Blood* 130.

Howard J, Malfroy M, Llewelyn C, et al: The Transfusion Alternatives Preoperatively in Sickle Cell Disease (TAPS) study: A randomised, controlled, multicentre clinical trial, *Lancet* 381:930–938, 2013.

Hsieh MM, Fitzhugh CD, Weitzel RP, et al: Nonmyeloablative HLA-matched sibling allogeneic hematopoietic stem cell transplantation for severe sickle cell phenotype, *JAMA* 312(1):48–56, 2014.

Jeong GK, Ruchelsman DE, Jazrawi LM, Jaffe WL: Total hip arthroplasty in sickle cell hemoglobinopathies, *J Am Acad Orthop Surg* 13:208–217, 2005.

Krishnamurti L, Kharbanda S, Biernacki MA, et al: Stable long-term donor engraftment following reduced-intensity hematopoietic cell transplantation for sickle cell disease, *Biol Blood Marrow Transplant* 14:1270–1278, 2008.

Lee MT, Piomelli S, Granger S, et al: Stroke Prevention Trial in Sickle Cell Anemia (STOP): Extended follow-up and final results, *Blood* 108:847–852, 2006.

Little JA, McGowan VR, Kato GJ, et al: Combination erythropoietin-hydroxyurea therapy in sickle cell disease: Experience from the National Institutes of Health and a literature review, *Haematologica* 91:1076–1083, 2006.

Mehari A, Alam S, Tian X, et al: Hemodynamic predictors of mortality in adults with sickle cell disease, *Am J Respir Crit Care Med* 187:840–847, 2013.

Merkel KH, Ginsberg PL, Parker JC, Post MJ: Cerebrovascular disease in sickle cell anemia: A clinical, pathological and radiological correlation, *Stroke* 9:45–52, 1978.

Morris CR, Kato GJ, Poljakovic M, et al: Dysregulated arginine metabolism, hemolysis-associated pulmonary hypertension, and mortality in sickle cell disease, *JAMA* 294:81–90, 2005.

Noguchi CT, Rodgers GP, Serjeant G, Schechter AN: Levels of fetal hemoglobin necessary for treatment of sickle cell disease, *N Engl J Med* 318:96–99, 1988.

Novelli EM, Huynh C, Gladwin MT, et al: Pulmonary embolism in sickle cell disease: A case-control study, *J Thrombosis and Hemostasis* 10:760–766, 2012.

Ohene-Frempong K, Weiner SJ, Sleeper LA, et al: Cerebrovascular accidents in sickle cell disease: Rates and risk factors, *Blood* 91:288–294, 1998.

Niihara Y, et al: A phase 3 trial of l-glutamine in sickle cell disease, *N Engl J Med* 379:226–235, 2018.

Platt OS: The acute chest syndrome of sickle cell disease, *N Engl J Med* 342:1904–1907, 2000.

Platt OS, Brambilla DJ, Rosse WF, et al: Mortality in sickle cell disease. Life expectancy and risk factors for early death, *N Engl J Med* 330:1639–1644, 1994.

Platt OS, Thorington BD, Brambilla DJ, et al: Pain in sickle cell disease. Rates and risk factors, *N Engl J Med* 325:11–16, 1991.

Reiter CD, Wang X, Tanus-Santos JE, et al: Cell-free hemoglobin limits nitric oxide bioavailability in sickle-cell disease, *Nat Med* 8:1383–1389, 2002.

Ribeil J, et al: Gene therapy in a patient with sickle cell disease, *N Engl J Med* 376:848–855, 2017.

Scheinman JI: Sickle cell disease and the kidney, *Nat Clin Pract Nephrol* 5:78–88, 2009.

Smiley D, Dagogo-Jack S, Umpierrez G: Therapy insight: Metabolic and endocrine disorders in sickle cell disease, *Nat Clin Pract Endocrinol Metab* 4:102–109, 2008.

Steinberg MH: Management of sickle cell disease, *N Engl J Med* 340:1021–1030, 1999.

Steinberg MH, Barton F, Castro O, et al: Effect of hydroxyurea on mortality and morbidity in adult sickle cell anemia: Risks and benefits up to 9 years of treatment, *JAMA* 289:1645–1651, 2003.

Telen MJ, Wun T, McCavit TL, et al: Randomized phase 2 study of GMI-1070 in SCD: Reduction in time to resolution of vaso-occlusive events and decreased opioid use, *Blood* 125:2656–2664, 2015.

Tshilolo L, Tomlinson G, Williams TN, et al: Hydroxyurea for children with sickle cell anemia in sub-Saharan Africa, *N Engl J Med* 380:121–131, 2019.

Vichinsky EP, Neumayr LD, Earles AN, et al: Causes and outcomes of the acute chest syndrome in sickle cell disease, *N Engl J Med* 342:1855–1865, 2000.

Vichinsky E, Hoppe CC, Ataga KI, et al: A phase 3 randomized trial of voxelotor in sickle cell disease, *N Engl J Med* 381(6):509–519, 2019.

Walters MC, Patience M, Leisenring W, et al: Bone marrow transplantation for sickle cell disease, *N Engl J Med* 335:369–376, 1996.

Walters MC, Storb R, Patience M, et al: Impact of bone marrow transplantation for symptomatic sickle cell disease: An interim report. Multicenter investigation of bone marrow transplantation for sickle cell disease, *Blood* 95:1918–1924, 2000.

Yawn BP, et al: Management of sickle cell disease: Summary of the 2014 evidence-based report by expert panel members, *JAMA* 312(10):1033–1048, 2014.

THALASSEMIA

Sarah A. Holstein, MD, PhD; and Raymond J. Hohl, MD, PhD

CURRENT DIAGNOSIS

- Complete blood count: anemia (very severe in β-thalassemia major, mild in β-thalassemia minor and α-thalassemia trait), low mean corpuscular volume, variable leukocytosis, thrombocytopenia (secondary to splenomegaly) or thrombocythemia (after splenectomy)
- Peripheral blood smear: hypochromia, microcytosis, anisocytosis, poikilocytosis, target cells, Heinz bodies, nucleated red blood cells
- Evidence of hemolytic anemia: indirect hyperbilirubinemia, elevated lactate dehydrogenase, decreased haptoglobin
- Hemoglobin electrophoresis pattern:
  - β-Thalassemia minor: elevated HbA2 ($\alpha_2\delta_2$)
  - β-Thalassemia intermedia: elevated HbA2, elevated HbF ($\alpha_2\gamma_2$), and decreased HbA ($\alpha_2\beta_2$)
  - β-Thalassemia major: absence of HbA, markedly elevated HbF, and elevated HbA2
  - α-Thalassemia trait: normal
  - Hemoglobin H disease: decreased HbA, presence of HbH (β_4) and HbBart (γ_4)
  - Hemoglobin Barts hydrops fetalis: HbBart, absence of HbA, HbA2, and HbF
- Timing of symptomatic disease:
  - β-Thalassemia minor: asymptomatic
  - β-Thalassemia intermedia: variable
  - β-Thalassemia major: within first year of life
  - α-Thalassemia trait: asymptomatic
  - Hemoglobin H disease: symptomatic at time of birth
  - Hemoglobin Barts hydrops fetalis: death during gestation

CURRENT THERAPY

- Chronic packed red blood cell transfusions for β-thalassemia major (1 to 3 units of packed leukoreduced erythrocytes every 3 to 5 weeks) with a target hemoglobin concentration of 9 to 10.5 g/dL; variable transfusion needs for β-thalassemia intermedia and hemoglobin H disease
- Splenectomy with antibiotic prophylaxis and vaccination
- Iron chelation: deferoxamine (Desferal) or deferasirox (Exjade); deferiprone (Ferriprox)
- Osteoporosis management: calcium with vitamin D supplementation; bisphosphonates
- Allogeneic hematopoietic cell transplantation for β-thalassemia major
- Luspatercept (Reblozyl) for transfusion-dependent adults with β-thalassemia
- Betibeglogene autotemcel (Zynteglo) for children and adults with transfusion-dependent β-thalassemia

Globin Gene Arrangements

Thalassemia syndromes encompass a spectrum of hemoglobin disorders that arise from impaired production of globin chains. The genes that encode globins are located in two clusters: the β gene cluster on chromosome 11 and the α gene cluster on chromosome 16 (Figure 1). The β gene cluster includes the adult globin genes (β and δ) as well as the fetal Aγ and Gγ genes and the embryonic ε gene. The arrangement of the 5′ to 3′ sequence of these genes parallels the order of their developmental expression. Functional hemoglobin is a tetramer that includes two α and two β globin units. The α gene cluster includes two fetal/adult α genes (α_1 and α_2) and the embryonic ζ genes. In the embryo, three hemoglobins are found ($\zeta_2\varepsilon_2$, $\alpha_2\varepsilon_2$, and $\zeta_2\gamma_2$). Fetal hemoglobin (HbF) is composed of two α chains and two γ chains ($\alpha_2\gamma_2$). In adults, the predominant hemoglobin is hemoglobin A (HbA), consisting of two α chains and two β chains ($\alpha_2\beta_2$) (see Figure 1). Hemoglobin A2, consisting of two α chains and two δ chains ($\alpha_2\delta_2$), is a normal variant in adults and typically represents less than 3% of the total hemoglobin (see Figure 1).

In β-thalassemia, there is diminished production of β globin genes, resulting in an excess of α globin chains. Conversely, in α-thalassemia there is impaired production of α globin genes, resulting in an excess of β globin chains. This imbalance of globin production is variable, and the degree of accumulation of unpaired globin chains is directly related to the severity of the disease phenotype. The genetic basis of thalassemia is heterogeneous, and several hundred mutations have been identified. These mutations may affect any level of globin gene expression, including arrangement of the globin gene complex, gene deletion, splicing, transcription, translation, and protein stability. In general, β-thalassemia occurs as a result of mutations, whereas α-thalassemia occurs as a result of gene deletion.

It has been estimated that there are 270 million carriers of thalassemia in the world, including 80 million β-thalassemia carriers. The frequency of β-thalassemia carriers is highest in the malarial tropical and subtropical regions of Asia, the Mediterranean, and the Middle East. The term *thalassemia*, derived from Greek, refers to the Mediterranean Sea. This distribution is secondary to the selective advantage of heterozygotes against malaria. β-Thalassemia is subdivided into major, intermedia, and minor types (Table 1). α-Thalassemia is classified into four syndromes: α-thalassemia trait 2 (loss of one α globin gene [αα/α–]); α-thalassemia trait 1, also referred to as *α-thalassemia minor* (loss of two α globin genes [αα/– – or α–/α–]); hemoglobin H (HbH) disease (loss of three alleles [α–/– –]); and hemoglobin Barts hydrops fetalis (loss of all four α globin loci [– –/– –]).

Pathophysiology

The clinical manifestations of thalassemia and their severity are a consequence of the relative excess of unpaired globin chains. In particular, excess α globin chains are unstable and insoluble and therefore precipitate inside the red blood cell (RBC). These inclusions (precipitated hemoglobin) may be visualized as Heinz bodies. The accumulation of α globin chains leads to a variety of insults to the erythrocyte, including changes in membrane deformability and increased fragility. Free β chains are more soluble than free α chains and are able to form a homotetramer (HbH). The hallmark of thalassemia is an anemia that is a consequence of both increased destruction (i.e., hemolysis) and decreased production (i.e., ineffective erythropoiesis). The bone marrow typically displays erythroid hyperplasia.

Oxidant injury is closely linked with the pathology of thalassemia. Under normal conditions, a small amount of methemoglobin (Fe^{3+}) is formed via oxidation and can then be reduced back to hemoglobin (Fe^{2+}). However, isolated globin chains can be oxidized to hemichromes, some forms of which are irreversibly oxidized. The hemichromes can then generate reactive oxygen species, which can oxidize membrane components, leading to cell injury. There is an increase in membrane rigidity in β-thalassemia, and this appears to be secondary to the binding of partially oxidized α globin chains to components of the membrane skeleton. Increased membrane rigidity in turn leads to decreased membrane deformability and increased destruction. In α-thalassemia, HbH has a left-shifted oxygen disassociation curve and therefore does not readily transport oxygen. HbH erythrocytes have increased rigidity, which is thought to be secondary to interactions between excess β globin chains and the membrane. Unlike with β-thalassemia, HbH erythrocytes have increased membrane stability. Inclusion bodies have been identified in HbH cells, and

Chromosome 11: Beta globin gene cluster

Chromosome 16: Alpha globin gene cluster

Figure 1 Representation of the β and α globin gene clusters. Also shown are the globin tetramers produced during embryonic development. (Reproduced with permission from the Annual Review of Pathology: Mechanisms of Disease, Volume 14 © 2019 by Annual Reviews, http://www.annualreviews.org.)

TABLE 1 Summary of Hematologic and Clinical Features of the Thalassemias

TYPE	HEMATOLOGIC FINDINGS	HEMOGLOBIN ELECTROPHORESIS PATTERN	CLINICAL FEATURES
β-Thalassemia major	Severe anemia, microcytosis, hypochromia, target cells, nucleated RBCs	Absence of HbA, markedly elevated HbF, elevated HbA2	Splenomegaly, jaundice, skeletal abnormalities, abnormal facies; transfusion dependent
β-Thalassemia intermedia	Mild to moderate anemia, microcytosis, hypochromia	Elevated HbA2, elevated HbF, decreased HbA	Splenomegaly; variable transfusion dependence
β-Thalassemia minor	Mild anemia, microcytosis, target cells	Elevated HbA2	None
Hemoglobin Barts hydrops fetalis	Severe anemia, anisopoikilocytosis, hypochromia, nucleated RBCs	HbBart; absence of HbA, HbA2, and HbF	Death during gestation; fetus with massive hepatosplenomegaly, generalized edema
Hemoglobin H disease	Moderately severe anemia, anisopoikilocytosis, microcytosis, Heinz bodies	Decreased HbA; HbH and HbBart present	Splenomegaly, jaundice; generally transfusion dependent
α-Thalassemia trait 1	Mild anemia, hypochromia, microcytosis, target cells	Normal	None
α-Thalassemia trait 2	Normal	Normal	None

HbA, Hemoglobin A; *HbF*, fetal hemoglobin; *HbH*, hemoglobin H; *RBCs*, red blood cells.

there appears to be a correlation between RBC age and solubility of HbH. As cells age, the amount of soluble HbH decreases, and the level of inclusions increases.

It has also been recognized that there is increased phagocytosis of thalassemia RBCs compared with normal controls. The etiology is not completely understood, but it may be a consequence of reduction in surface levels of sialic acid, increase in surface immunoglobulin G binding, and changes in phosphatidylserine localization.

Despite the pronounced hemolysis and marrow erythroid hyperplasia, patients with thalassemia generally do not display the compensatory reticulocytosis that is indicative of the other basis for anemia, ineffective erythropoiesis. Accumulation of α-chain aggregates is thought to lead to death of erythrocyte precursors. Furthermore, abnormal assembly of membrane proteins in erythroid precursors has been demonstrated.

Iron overload is one of the primary causes of morbidity. Even without transfusion, the long-standing anemia, however mild, leads to increased iron absorption in the gut and eventual chronic iron overload. Excessive iron deposition causes devastating damage to multiple organs, particularly affecting the heart, liver, and endocrine organs.

β-Thalassemia Major

Symptoms of β-thalassemia major are not present at birth, because HbF ($\alpha_2\gamma_2$) is present. However, as HbF levels decline over the first year, the signs and symptoms of severe hemolytic anemia begin to manifest. Affected individuals display hepatosplenomegaly from expansion of the reticuloendothelial system as well as extramedullary hematopoiesis, pallor, growth retardation, and abnormal skeletal development. If left untreated, 80% of children with β-thalassemia major will die before 5 years of age.

Laboratory Features

Thalassemia major is characterized by a severe microcytic anemia. Hemoglobin levels may be as low as 3 to 4 g/dL. The peripheral blood smear is markedly abnormal and is notable for hypochromia, microcytosis, anisocytosis, poikilocytosis, target cells, and teardrop cells. Routine stains show the presence of precipitated α globin chains as Heinz bodies. The reticulocyte count is often low. The white blood cell count is often high but may be artifactually elevated as a consequence of automated inclusion of high numbers of circulating nucleated RBCs. The platelet count is typically normal, but progressive hypersplenism can result in decreased platelet counts. Patients who have undergone splenectomy often have increased white blood cell and platelet counts. Iron studies reveal elevated serum iron, transferrin saturation, and ferritin. Consistent with hemolysis and ineffective erythropoiesis, indirect bilirubin and lactate dehydrogenase levels are increased, and haptoglobin levels are low.

Clinical Features

Unique to β-thalassemia major is the development of extramedullary erythropoiesis. This may be so severe that the masses of bone marrow lead to broken bones and spinal cord compression. Sites of involvement include the sinuses and the thoracic and pelvic cavities. The expansion of the erythroid bone marrow can lead to a number of skeletal changes. In particular, characteristic changes in the facial bones and skull result in frontal bossing, overgrowth of the maxillae, and malocclusion. This has sometimes been referred to as *chipmunk facies*. Other bones are also affected, and premature fusion of the epiphyses results in shortened limbs. Compression fractures of the spine may occur. Even if the disease is managed appropriately with transfusions and iron chelation, patients will still suffer from osteopenia and osteoporosis. Possible mechanisms include changes secondary to hypogonadism or increased bone resorption secondary to vitamin D deficiency.

Hepatomegaly and splenomegaly, secondary to extramedullary erythropoiesis and RBC destruction, are prominent. Injury to Kupffer cells and hepatocytes from chronic overload leads to fibrosis and end-stage liver disease. Hepatic iron overload is probably caused in part by comparatively high levels of transferrin receptors. Iron overload and perhaps other factors increase susceptibility to viral hepatitis. Laboratory studies show indirect hyperbilirubinemia, hypergammaglobulinemia, and elevated liver markers. The chronic hemolysis leads to formation of bilirubin gallstones, although cholecystitis or cholangitis is not common. Splenic dysfunction results in immune dysfunction. The shortened erythrocyte survival time leaves patients susceptible to aplastic crisis induced by parvovirus B19 infection. Extramedullary hematopoiesis may also affect the kidneys, and patients often have large kidneys. Rapid cell turnover leads to hyperuricemia, and children may develop gouty nephropathy.

A number of endocrine abnormalities are commonly seen in β-thalassemia major, including hypogonadism, growth failure, diabetes, and hypothyroidism. These abnormalities occur even in chronically transfused patients and may be in part related to iron overload. Endocrine glands, such as the liver and heart, have high levels of transferrin receptor and therefore are more susceptible to iron overload. The typical growth pattern for a child with β-thalassemia major is relatively normal until 9 to 10 years of age. After that time, the growth velocity slows, and the pubertal growth spurt is either absent or reduced. Although secretion of growth hormone does not appear to be altered in thalassemic patients, a reduction in peak amplitude and nocturnal levels of growth hormone has been observed. Amenorrhea is quite common, with 50% of girls presenting with primary amenorrhea. Secondary amenorrhea also develops, particularly in patients who do not receive regular chelation therapy. In males, impotence and azoospermia are common. Primary hypothyroidism typically appears during the second decade of life. The prevalence of diabetes mellitus and impaired glucose intolerance has been estimated at 4% to 20%. Unlike type 1 diabetes mellitus, diabetes associated with thalassemia is rarely complicated by diabetic ketoacidosis. The risk of diabetic retinopathy is lower, but the risk of diabetic nephropathy is higher. Patients with a high ferritin level (>1800 μg/L) experience faster progression to hypothyroidism, hypogonadism, and other endocrinopathies.

Thalassemic patients suffer from extensive cardiac abnormalities. Chronic anemia causes cardiac dilation. Although long-term transfusion can help prevent cardiac dilation, the resulting iron overload leads to cardiac hemosiderosis. Pericarditis, ventricular and supraventricular arrhythmias, and end-stage cardiomyopathy can develop. Ventricular arrhythmia is a common cause of death. Patients may also develop pulmonary hypertension. The degree of iron overload in the heart has traditionally been assessed by cardiac biopsy, but cardiac magnetic resonance imaging (MRI) is increasingly being used.

Vitamin and mineral deficiencies may occur. Folic acid deficiency may develop in patients, presumably as a consequence of increased cell turnover. Although the cause is unknown, patients with β-thalassemia major often have very low serum zinc levels. Serum levels of vitamin E and vitamin C may also be low.

Management of β-Thalassemia Major
Transfusion

The key intervention for the management of β-thalassemia major is chronic transfusion therapy. In particular, during the first decade of life, regular transfusion results in improvements in hepatosplenomegaly, skeletal abnormalities, and cardiac dilation. Patients typically require 1 to 3 units of packed RBCs every 3 to 5 weeks. The optimal target total hemoglobin level has yet to be determined. Alloimmunization does occur, and some blood centers try to leukodeplete their products, match donors by ethnicity, and limit the donor pool for any particular patient. Although the risk of bloodborne infections is currently quite small, regular transfusion of blood products still carries a risk for infections such as human immunodeficiency virus and hepatitis C.

Splenectomy

The general indication for splenectomy is an increase of more than 50% in the RBC transfusion requirement over a period of 1 year. Splenectomy may initially yield a decrease in the RBC transfusion requirement. It has been noted that thalassemia patients are at higher risk for infection after splenectomy than patients who are splenectomized for other reasons. The bacteria that most frequently cause infections in these patients include *Streptococcus pneumoniae, Haemophilus influenzae, Neisseria meningitidis, Klebsiella, Escherichia coli*, and *Staphylococcus aureus*. The increased susceptibility to infection compared with other splenectomized patients is thought to be a result of greater immune dysfunction secondary to iron overload. In particular, it has been reported that iron-overloaded macrophages lose the ability to kill intracellular pathogens. Antibiotic prophylaxis with penicillin, amoxicillin, or erythromycin is recommended for children up to 16 years of age. In addition, patients should receive immunizations, including the pneumococcal, influenza, and *H. influenzae* vaccines.

Iron Chelation Therapy

Because of increased iron absorption and long-term transfusion therapy, iron overload develops. As noted earlier, iron overload causes damage to multiple organs. Because iron is poorly excreted, removal must be accomplished by phlebotomy (not an option in thalassemic patients) or by chelation therapy. Historically, deferoxamine (Desferal) has been the most widely used chelator. This agent may be administered subcutaneously (SQ), intramuscularly (IM), or intravenously (IV). The dosing for chronic iron overload is 1000 to 2000 mg/day (or 20 to 40 mg/kg/day) SQ or 500 to 1000 mg/day IM or 40 to 50 mg/kg/day IV. The IV-only route is indicated for patients with cardiovascular collapse. Multiple studies have shown that deferoxamine therapy improves long-term survival. In addition, intensive therapy with deferoxamine has been shown to improve cardiac function in patients with severe iron overload. However, compliance with daily injections has been a particular problem, and unless regular therapy is given, iron will reaccumulate.

Deferiprone (Ferriprox) was the first orally active chelator to be introduced. It is given three times daily (total of 75 mg/kg/day). Studies have indicated that deferiprone may be as effective as deferoxamine in lowering iron levels. A recent Cochrane review concluded that deferiprone is indicated in the treatment of iron overload in thalassemia major if deferoxamine therapy is contraindicated or inadequate. Agranulocytosis associated with deferiprone has been reported, and because of this risk, the drug has a black box warning on its label. The U.S. Food and Drug Administration (FDA) also requires that medication guides be issued to patient when the drug is dispensed. Deferiprone is currently available at selected specialty pharmacies. Deferiprone is available in Europe and Asia. There has also been interest in combined therapy with deferiprone and deferoxamine, and one study showed that the combination was more effective in removing cardiac and hepatic iron but did not further improve cardiac function.

Deferasirox (Exjade) is the first orally active agent approved for use in the United States. Its longer half-life in comparison with deferiprone allows this drug to be given once daily (total of 20 to 40 mg/kg/day). A phase III trial comparing deferasirox to deferoxamine in patients with thalassemia revealed similar decreases in liver iron concentrations. Side effects include gastrointestinal complaints (abdominal pain, nausea, vomiting, diarrhea) and skin rash. There have been postmarketing reports of acute renal failure, hepatic failure, and cytopenias. It is recommended that serum creatinine, ferritin, and alanine aminotransferase be monitored monthly during therapy. A prospective, randomized study comparing deferiprone and deferoxamine versus deferiprone and deferasirox in 96 patients with β-thalassemia major demonstrated that both regimens reduced iron overload. However, the latter regimen was found to be superior with respect to improving cardiac iron, patient compliance, and patient satisfaction.

The "gold standard" for measurement of liver iron concentration has been liver biopsy with iron measurement by atomic absorption spectrometry. More recently, there has been increasing use of MRI technology to measure liver iron levels. In general, iron content determined by MRI methodology correlates with liver iron concentration determined by biopsy. However, the precision of liver MRI measurement appears to be dependent on iron levels, liver fibrosis, and calibration. Hepatic iron concentration has also been measured using a superconducting quantum interference device, although reported consistency has varied and widespread use of this technique has been limited by expense and complexity.

Novel Agents Targeting Iron Homeostasis

A variety of agents that modulate hepcidin activity are being explored as potential therapies for β-thalassemia. Preclinical data demonstrated that minihepcidins restrict iron absorption. A synthetic hepcidin, LJPC-401, was studied in a phase II trial involving patients with transfusion-dependent thalassemia. However, the study was stopped early as a result of lack of efficacy at an interim analysis. Another phase II study of MTG-300, a hepcidin mimetic, was also stopped. Studies are underway evaluating VIT-2763, an oral ferroportin inhibitor. Finally, approaches that increase hepatic synthesis of hepcidin by suppressing the gene transmembrane protease serine 6 (either via siRNA or antisense oligonucleotides) are currently being evaluated in early-phase trials.

Management of Osteoporosis

Even with calcium and vitamin D supplementation, iron chelation, transfusion therapy, and hormonal therapy, bone loss continues to be a significant problem for thalassemia patients. Recently there has been interest in the use of bisphosphonates. This class of drugs, which includes clodronate (Bonefos)[2], alendronate (Fosamax), pamidronate (Aredia), zoledronate (Zometa), and neridronate (Nerixia)[2], inhibit osteoclastic bone resorption and have found extensive use in the management of Paget disease, osteoporosis, and skeletal metastases. Small studies performed in thalassemia patients have failed to show benefit with clodronate 100 mg IM every 10 days or 300 mg IV every 3 weeks. A very small study using alendronate (Fosamax)[1] 10 mg orally daily revealed an increase in bone mineral density only at the femoral level. Conversely, in a study involving pamidronate (Aredia)[1] 30 or 60 mg IV every month, there was an increase in bone density only at the lumbar level. The most promising results have been achieved with the most potent member of the class, zoledronate. Several trials demonstrated that zoledronate (Zometa)[1] 4 mg IV every 3 or 4 months results in significant improvement in femoral and lumbar bone mineral density and reduces bony pain. The largest randomized trial involved 118 β-thalassemia patients who received calcium plus vitamin D with or without neridronate[2] (given every 90 days). At 6 and 12 months, there was increased bone mineral density as well as decreased back pain and analgesic use in the neridronate arm. Larger long-term trials are necessary before this agent finds widespread use in the management of thalassemia-induced osteoporosis.

Hematopoietic Cell Transplantation

Hematopoietic cell transplantation is the only curative strategy for patients with hemoglobinopathies. Patients are assigned to a risk class (Pesaro class) based on adherence to regular iron chelation therapy, presence or absence of hepatomegaly, and presence or absence of portal fibrosis. Those children with no or little hepatomegaly, no portal fibrosis, and regular iron chelation therapy (class I) have a better than 90% chance of cure, whereas those with both hepatomegaly and portal fibrosis (class III) have long-term survival rates of approximately 60% in older studies.

---

[1] Not FDA approved for this indication.
[2] Not available in the United States.

More recent reports indicate that class III survival has improved to 90%.

The use of human leukocyte antigen (HLA)-identical sibling donors has been preferred, because the use of HLA-mismatched donors has produced inferior results and is associated with increased graft rejection, graft-versus-host disease, and infection. However, it is estimated that only one-third of patients will have a matched donor. The use of unrelated donors has been explored, and initial studies showed poorer outcomes. However, more recent data suggest that matched unrelated donors might be a viable option if a suitable sibling donor is lacking, thanks to improved donor selection and transplantation techniques. The use of partially HLA-matched unrelated cord blood has been reported, although 4 of 9 children did not engraft.

Another emerging technique is the use of reduced-intensity conditioning regimens, although long-term success has yet to be achieved. However, no randomized controlled studies have been performed evaluating the role of transplant in thalassemia patients.

Gene Therapy

Globin gene therapy, achieved through manipulation of autologous stem cells, is an attractive alternative to allogeneic transplantation. There are three major scientific hurdles that must be overcome: design of vectors that yield therapeutic levels of globin gene expression, ability to isolate and transduce autologous stem cells, and development of transplantation conditions that will permit host repopulation. In addition, the safety of viral and nonviral transfections is an issue. Initial studies involved ex vivo transduction of autologous hematopoietic stem cells with a lentiviral vector carrying the transgene. This gene therapy has been administered intravenously or via intrabone injection after a myeloablative conditioning regimen. Many of the patients treated to date have achieved transfusion independence, and thus far no unusual toxicities have been observed.

The first gene therapy to obtain regulatory approval is betibeglogene autotemcel (Zynteglo), which was granted conditional approval by the European Commission for patients with transfusion-dependent non-β_0/β_0-thalassemia who are 12 years of age and older. Subsequently the FDA granted approval of Zynteglo for children and adults with transfusion-dependent β-thalassemia. Zynteglo therapy involves the ex vivo transduction of autologous CD34+ cells with the gene-encoding βA-T87Q-globin via a BB305 lentiviral vector. After a myeloablative conditioning regimen with busulfan (Busulfex)[1], the transduced CD34+ cells are administered (single dose of 5.0×10^6 CD34+ cells/kg). Two ongoing phase III, open-label, single-arm studies of this product enrolled 41 patients aged 4 to 34 years. In the first study, 20 of 22 evaluable patients with a non-β_0/β_0 genotype achieved transfusion independence, and 13 out of the 20 patients were not on iron chelation therapy as of last follow-up. In the second ongoing study, 12 of 14 evaluable patients with a β_0/β_0 or non-β_0/β_0 genotype achieved transfusion independence, and 7 out of the 12 patients were not on iron chelation therapy as of last follow-up. Both studies were 24 months in length and then rolled over into a long-term follow-up study.

Pharmacologic Induction of Fetal Hemoglobin

Induction of HbF expression has been proposed as a therapeutic strategy. For β-thalassemia, induced γ globin gene expression would be predicted to decrease globin chain imbalance by complexing with free α chains. Hydroxyurea (Hydrea)[1] is an antimetabolite thought to interfere with DNA synthesis. It is well established in the management of sickle cell disease, where it has been shown to increase levels of HbF. The use of hydroxyurea in β-thalassemia is much less well established. In the United States, hydroxyurea has been approved for use in sickle cell disease but not for thalassemia. Studies published elsewhere in the world have generally shown improvements in hemoglobin levels in thalassemia intermedia patients, with some patients becoming transfusion independent. A recent metaanalysis on the use of hydroxyurea in patients with transfusion-dependent β-thalassemia concluded that this agent might offer some benefit but that double-blinded placebo-controlled studies are lacking.

5-Azacytidine (azacitidine [Vidaza])[1], an inhibitor of DNA methyltransferase, has been shown to induce HbF. However, concerns regarding long-term use have prevented further evaluation in thalassemia. Decitabine (Dacogen)[1], an analog of 5-azacytidine, has been shown to increase HbF levels in patients with sickle cell disease refractory to hydroxyurea. A small pilot study of low-dose decitabine in β-thalassemia intermedia patients demonstrated an increase in total hemoglobin and hemoglobin F levels. Butyrate,[5] an inhibitor of histone deacetylases, is another agent capable of inducing HbF. However, butyrate and its derivatives (arginine butyrate[5], sodium isobutyramide[5], and sodium phenylbutyrate [Buphenyl][1]) have failed to show significant clinical benefit in thalassemia patients. Therefore no agent has been approved for use in thalassemia patients at this time.

IMR-687 (tovinontrine),[5] a small molecule inhibitor of phosphodiesterase 9, increases intracellular cGMP levels and leads to reactivation of HbF. An interim analysis of a randomized, double blind, placebo-controlled phase IIb study of this agent in adults with β-thalassemia (transfusion-dependent and nontransfusion-dependent cohorts) reported no meaningful benefits in either transfusion burden or hemoglobin, and the sponsor has discontinued further development of this agent for β-thalassemia.

Novel Agents Targeting Ineffective Erythropoiesis

An alternative strategy that is being investigated involves the targeting of ineffective erythropoiesis. Luspatercept-aamt (Reblozyl) and sotatercept (ACE-011)[5] are activin receptor trap ligands that were developed to treat postmenopausal osteoporosis but were noted to increase Hb levels. Initial phase II studies with these agents in thalassemia patients revealed reductions in transfusion burden, increase in Hb, and reduction in liver iron levels. A phase III study comparing luspatercept plus best supportive care to placebo plus best supportive care revealed that 21.4% of patients receiving luspatercept achieved a reduction in transfusion burden compared with 4.5% in the placebo group. Luspatercept (1 mg/kg SQ every 3 weeks) is approved by the FDA for the treatment of anemia in adult patients with β-thalassemia who require regular RBC transfusions.

Janus kinase 2 (JAK2) plays a key role in erythropoiesis, and there is interest in the potential use of JAK2 inhibitors in thalassemia. A phase II study with ruxolitinib (Jakafi)[1] showed a reduction in spleen size. However, there was no clinically relevant improvement in pretransfusion hemoglobin, and subsequent phase III studies are not planned.

The pyruvate kinase activator AG-348 (mitapivat) increased ATP levels, reduced markers of ineffective erythropoiesis, and improved anemia in mouse models of β-thalassemia. Initial results from a phase II study of mitapivat (Pyrukynd)[1] reported an increase an increase in hemoglobin in patients with non–transfusion-dependent thalassemia. Two randomized, placebo-controlled phase III studies evaluating mitapivat in patients with thalassemia are underway.

Antioxidants

Oxidative damage is believed to be an important cause of tissue damage, and there has been interest in the use of antioxidants in thalassemia patients. A variety of substances have been investigated, including ascorbate[1], vitamin E[1], N-acetylcysteine (Mucomyst)[1], flavonoids, and indicaxanthin.[5] A variety of antioxidant effects have been observed in vitro with these agents, but none have been shown to improve anemia in patients with thalassemia.

---

[1] Not FDA approved for this indication.

[1] Not FDA approved for this indication.
[5] Investigational drug in the United States.

β-Thalassemia Intermedia

Given the underlying genetic heterogeneity, it is not surprising that the clinical manifestations of β-thalassemia intermedia are also quite varied. Some patients with more mild forms of β-thalassemia intermedia do not require long-term transfusion therapy. There is no clear consensus about when long-term transfusion should be initiated. Factors that are considered for children include growth patterns, spleen size, and bone development. Transfusion may be necessary during infection-induced aplastic crises. In some instances, transfusions are begun in childhood to help with growth and then discontinued after puberty. Some adults gradually become more anemic and eventually require transfusion. Some authors have argued that starting transfusions early in life is advantageous because the prevalence of alloimmunization appears to increase if transfusion is started after the first few years of life.

Splenomegaly usually develops in all patients, including those who do not require transfusion. With progression of splenomegaly and the accompanying sequestration and hemolysis, there is usually worsening of anemia to the point at which transfusions may be required. Most patients achieve transfusion independence after splenectomy. Gallstones may develop, and a prophylactic cholecystectomy is sometimes performed at the same time as the splenectomy. As with β-thalassemia major patients, thalassemia intermedia patients are at increased risk for infection and should be appropriately vaccinated.

For reasons that are not entirely clear, there is an increased risk of thromboembolic complications in thalassemia intermedia patients compared with thalassemia major patients. An Italian study reported that 10% of thalassemia intermedia and 4% of thalassemia major patients experienced a thromboembolic event. Another study reported that thromboembolism occurred four times more frequently in patients with intermedia versus major disease. This report noted that venous events were more common in the thalassemia intermedia population, whereas arterial events were more common in the thalassemia major population. An even higher rate of venous thrombotic events (29%) was reported in a population of splenectomized patients with thalassemia intermedia. It has been suggested that exposed anionic phospholipids on the surface of damaged RBCs may induce a procoagulant effect. There is no consensus regarding the prophylactic use of antiplatelet agents or anticoagulants in this population.

Patients with thalassemia intermedia may develop iron overload, although it is less severe than in patients with thalassemia major. Even those who are not regularly transfused may develop a degree of iron overload as a result of increased iron absorption. Iron overload may be managed with the iron chelating agents described earlier. Cardiac toxicity, including congestive heart failure, valvular problems, and pulmonary hypertension (leading to secondary right-sided heart failure) resulting from iron overload is not infrequent in the thalassemia intermedia population.

Bone abnormalities and osteoporosis may develop in thalassemia intermedia patients. In a North American study, the prevalence of fractures in these patients was 12%. Leg ulcers involving the medial malleolus are common and are often difficult to treat. Hypogonadism, hypothyroidism, and diabetes may occur, with frequency related to the severity of anemia and iron overload. Pseudoxanthoma elasticum, a syndrome consisting of skin lesions, angioid streaks in the retina, calcified retinal walls, and aortic valve disease, is more common in thalassemia intermedia than in thalassemia major. Currently, no effective therapy exists, although it has been reported that aluminum hydroxide (Alternagel)[1] reduces skin calcification.

β-Thalassemia Minor

Most patients with β-thalassemia minor are asymptomatic. However, they have an abnormal complete blood cell count that may sometimes lead to the misdiagnosis of iron deficiency. Although these patients have a microcytic anemia, it is much less severe than in patients with β-thalassemia major. In general, the hematocrit is greater than 30%. The mean corpuscular volume is typically less than 75 fL, and the RBC distribution width index is normal, in contrast with iron deficiency in which the degree of microcytosis is less and the distribution width index is usually increased. The peripheral blood smear shows the presence of target cells. Hemoglobin electrophoresis typically reveals an increase in HbA2. The normal anemia experienced during pregnancy may sometimes be exacerbated in patients with β-thalassemia minor, necessitating transfusion. Otherwise, no long-term effects of β-thalassemia minor have been described, and no interventions are required.

α-Thalassemia

Laboratory and Clinical Features

Patients with α-thalassemia trait 2 are symptom free and have normal laboratory values, including complete blood count, peripheral smear, and hemoglobin electrophoresis. Individuals with α-thalassemia trait 1 are symptom free, and the disease resembles β-thalassemia minor. The peripheral smear shows a hypochromic microcytic anemia with the presence of target cells. Hemoglobin electrophoresis is normal.

HbH disease does produce symptoms. Unlike β-thalassemia major, in which HbF production protects the fetus, individuals with HbH disease develop hemolytic anemia during gestation and are symptomatic at birth. This is because α globin production is required for HbF ($\alpha_2\gamma_2$). As with β-thalassemia major, patients with HbH disease suffer from the consequences of chronic hemolytic anemia, although the severity is somewhat less. The transfusion requirements for HbH patients resemble those for patients with β-thalassemia intermedia, with transfusion support initiated in the second and third decades of life. These patients also develop iron overload, necessitating treatment with chelation therapy.

Hydrops fetalis with hemoglobin Barts is usually fatal in utero. The utter lack of α globin chain production results in absence of HbF. Hemoglobin Barts, a homotetramer consisting of four γ globin genes, is unable to deliver oxygen to tissues. Severe tissue hypoxia develops, leading to widespread tissue ischemia. High cardiac output failure leads to massive edema (hydrops). In most cases, death occurs in the third trimester or late second trimester. There have been reports of live births after intrauterine transfusion, but survival beyond the perinatal period is exceedingly rare. Prenatal diagnosis of hemoglobin Barts hydrops fetalis may be achieved through DNA-based testing using amniocytes from amniocentesis or chorionic villi sampling. Noninvasive testing is under development, including methods that isolate circulating fetal DNA in maternal peripheral blood.

Management

Patients with α-thalassemia 1 and 2 traits do not require treatment. The management of HbH disease is similar to that described for β-thalassemia.

References

Algiraigri A, Wright N, Paolucci EO, et al: Hydroxyurea for lifelong transfusion-dependent β-thalassemia: a meta-analysis, *Pediatr Hematol Oncol* 34(8):435–448, 2017.

Arab-Zozani M, Kheyrandish S, Rastgar A, et al: A systematic review and meta-analysis of stature growth complications in β-thalassemia major patients, *Ann Glob Health* 87(1):1–17, 2021. 48.

Bhardawj A, Swe KM, Sinha NK, Treatment for osteoporosis in people with β-thalassemia, *Cochrane Database Syst Rev* 5(5):CD010429, 2023.

Bou-Fakhredin R, Motto I, Cappellini MD: Advancing the care of β-thalassaemia patients with novel therapies, *Blood Transfus* 20(1):78–88, 2022.

Kattamis A, Kwiatkowski JL, Aydinok Y: Thalassaemia, *Lancet* 399(10343):2310–2324, 2022.

Langer AL, Esrick EB: β-Thalassemia: evolving treatment options beyond transfusion and iron chelation, *Hematology Am Soc Hematol Educ Program* 2021(1):600–606, 2021.

Porter JB, Garbowski MW: Interaction of transfusion and iron chelation in thalassemias, *Hematol Oncol Clin North Am* 32(2):247–259, 2018.

Sharma A, Jagannath VA, Puri L: Hematopoietic stem cell transplantation for people with β-thalassaemia major, *Cochrane Database Syst Rev* 4(4):CD008708, 2021.

---

[1] Not FDA approved for this indication.

THROMBOTIC THROMBOCYTOPENIC PURPURA

Method of
Ravi Sarode, MD

CURRENT DIAGNOSIS

- A provisional diagnosis based on unexplained microangiopathic hemolytic anemia and thrombocytopenia in the absence of oliguric renal failure is sufficient to initiate emergent plasma exchange (PLEX) for a suspected diagnosis of autoimmune acquired thrombotic thrombocytopenic purpura (TTP).
- The final diagnosis is usually established by the documentation of a severe deficiency (<10% activity) of ADAMTS13 (*a disintegrin and metalloproteinase with thrombospondin 1 motif, 13th member of the family*).
- These laboratory tests are recommended for patient evaluation:
  - Complete blood count (shows anemia and decreased platelet count, usually <30,000/uL)
  - Peripheral blood smear (shows "schistocytes/fragmented red blood cells," a hallmark of thrombotic microangiopathy)
  - Reticulocyte count (elevated)
  - Haptoglobin (usually undetectable in TTP)
  - Lactate dehydrogenase (usually more than twice the upper limit of normal in TTP)
  - Blood urea nitrogen, serum creatinine (determine nonoliguric renal insufficiency, serum creatinine < 2.5 mg/dL)
  - Liver function tests, including direct and indirect bilirubin
  - Troponin (many patients have an ischemic cardiac injury)
  - Plasma ADAMTS13 activity (<10% is diagnostic of TTP) and inhibitor level (usually detected in 90% of cases of acquired TTP) or ADAMTS 13 antibodies by enzyme-linked immunosorbent assays (almost all acquired TTP)
  - Prothrombin time, partial thromboplastin time, fibrinogen, and D-dimers (to rule out disseminated intravascular coagulopathy)
  - Direct antiglobulin test (to rule out autoimmune hemolytic anemia)
  - Urinalysis

CURRENT THERAPY

- The goal is to normalize ADAMTS 13 levels (>50%).
- Daily plasma exchange (PLEX) uses plasma as a replacement fluid (1.0–1.5 total body plasma volume) until the platelet count is greater than 150,000/μL for 2 days. Thereafter, the frequency of PLEX may be guided more judiciously if ADAMTS13 levels are obtained once or twice a week during hospitalization.
- Caplacizumab (Cablivi, 11 mg intravenous loading dose followed by daily 11 mg subcutaneously), a potent disease modifying agent, is a nanobody that interferes with the binding of von Willebrand factor to the GPIb domain on platelets and disrupts the pathophysiology of the disease; thus, it may prevent deaths and reduce the number of PLEXs needed. It is given daily until ADAMTS13 levels are greater than 10% to 20%.
- Prednisone 1 mg/kg/day is tapered gradually as platelet count remains greater than 150,000/uL.
- Rituximab (Rituxan)[1] (either 100 mg fixed dose or 375 mg/m^2 weekly for 4 weeks) is given upfront as soon as the diagnosis of autoimmune thrombotic thrombocytopenic purpura (TTP) is confirmed (reduces length of stay, number of PLEXs, and exacerbations and relapses, and thus overall cost).

- Plasma (10–15 mL/kg) or cryoprecipitate (one dose = 10 units of pooled cryoprecipitate) infusion is used if PLEX will be delayed more than 6 hours on day 1.
- ADAMTS13 testing is done during follow-up to detect early biologic relapse and preemptive rituximab to avoid clinical relapse and hospitalization.
- For exacerbation or relapsing of TTP, the following therapies are used:
  - Rituximab (Rituxan)[1] (100 mg fixed dose or 375 mg/m^2 once a week for 2 to 4 weeks).
  - Cyclosporine (Neoral)[1] (2–3 mg/kg/day up to 6 months).
  - Vincristine (Oncovin)[1] (1.4 mg/m^2 once a week for 4 weeks).
  - Bortezomib (Velcade)[1] (1.3 mg/m^2 one to two cycles or 1 mg fixed dose once a week for 4 weeks).
- Splenectomy as a last resort.

---

[1]Not FDA approved for this indication.

Thrombotic thrombocytopenic purpura (TTP) is a rare (1 to 2 cases per million) but life-threatening thrombotic microangiopathy (TMA) disorder characterized by the presence of microthrombi in the microcirculation of various organs, including the brain, kidneys, heart, and abdominal viscera. Microthrombi consist of platelets and von Willebrand factor (vWF), resulting in microangiopathic hemolytic anemia (MAHA) and thrombocytopenia. MAHA refers to the fragmentation of red blood cells (schistocytes) during their passage through partially occluded arterioles and capillaries by microthrombi. TTP diagnosis requires a high degree of suspicion because a delay in initiating plasma exchange (PLEX), the current standard of care, could result in a poor response or fatal outcome. In the past, diagnosis of TTP was made based on a pentad that included MAHA, thrombocytopenia, neurologic involvement, renal affection, and fever. This pentad was found in patients who had died of TTP, indicating advanced disease; therefore one should not wait for the development of a pentad, which could delay TTP diagnosis and lead to a potentially fatal outcome. Currently, unexplained MAHA and thrombocytopenia in the absence of oliguric renal failure are sufficient to make a working diagnosis of TTP and initiate emergent PLEX. Patients may present with only severe thrombocytopenia and/or with warm autoimmune hemolytic anemia and be managed as nonresponding immune thrombocytopenia/Evans syndrome. However, after a few days, such patients may develop MAHA, establishing a TTP diagnosis. Therefore such patients not responding to standard therapy should have high suspicion of TTP. Similarly, but rarely, a young patient may present with unexplained ischemic stroke without hematologic features and later develop hematologic features.

Pathophysiology

In congenital TTP (Upshaw-Shulman syndrome), ultralarge (UL) multimers of vWF were detected during remission but were absent during relapse. Later, an ADAMTS13 (*a disintegrin and metalloproteinase with thrombospondin 1 motif, 13th member of the family*), vWF-cleaving protease was identified that was responsible for cleaving UL multimers secreted from endothelium into normal-sized vWF multimers seen in normal plasma. This cleavage occurs under high-shear-rate flow conditions in smaller blood vessels where the UL-vWF undergoes unfolding, exposing the cleavage site for ADAMTS13. ADAMTS13 is severely deficient (<10%) in patients with both congenital and acquired (autoimmune) TTP. Persistence of UL-vWF multimers in the microcirculation results in unfolding of the molecule, enabling it to bind to platelets at GPIb, thus producing platelet-vWF microthrombi in capillaries and arterioles that cause end organ ischemic damage (Figure 1). Elevated lactate dehydrogenase (LDH) reflects not only MAHA but also organ damage; hence very high LDH reflects more severe disease.

Figure 1 During normal hemostasis, *ADAMTS13* enzyme cleaves ultralarge multimers of von Willebrand factor (vWF) in normal sizes and prevents the formation of platelet-vWF aggregates under high shear rates. However, in the absence of *ADAMTS13* (a disintegrin and metalloproteinase with thrombospondin 1 motif, 13th member of the family) due to congenital deficiency or autoantibodies, vWF persist as ultralarge multimers that unfold under high shear rates in small blood vessels and induce vWF-platelet microthrombi in various organs, causing ischemic damage.

Classification

TTP can be divided into (1) a congenital form resulting from a genetic defect in the *ADAMTS13* gene and (2) an acquired form due to an autoantibody against the ADAMTS13 enzyme (Figure 2). Congenital TTP can present in the neonatal period, early childhood, or later in life, when it is usually associated with an inciting trigger in the form of pregnancy, severe infection, surgery, or other stress. Acquired TTP is usually idiopathic without an underlying disorder or secondary when associated with an underlying autoimmune disorder, such as systemic lupus erythematosus, HIV, or use of ticlopidine (Ticlid).[2] Other clinical conditions that present with MAHA and thrombocytopenia with nonsevere ADAMTS13 deficiency are grouped under the broader term TMA.

Clinical Presentation

Autoimmune TTP is a disease of young adults (20–50 years of age, female-to-male ratio 2:1), with the majority being African American. Most patients present in the emergency department with an acute onset of vague, anemia-like symptoms (malaise, fatigue, weakness) and thrombocytopenia (petechiae, bleeding gums). Detailed evaluation reveals that these symptoms had their onset several days before presentation. Up to 70% to 80% of patients have some neurologic features, including severe headaches, visual disturbances, focal neurologic deficits, transient ischemic attacks, memory deficits, unusual behavior, confusion, seizures, paraparesis, stupor, and coma. Mild renal insufficiency is seen in less than 50% and fever in less than 15%. Because of the generalized nature of the disease, any organ system can be affected, and ischemic insult to the heart is common.

Diagnosis

Unexplained MAHA and thrombocytopenia constitute the diagnostic features and are associated with elevated LDH, reticulocytosis, undetectable haptoglobin, elevated bilirubin, and nonoliguric renal insufficiency in some patients. A severe deficiency of ADAMTS13 (<10% activity with a detectable inhibitor in up to 90% of patients and antibodies by enzyme-linked immunosorbent assays in almost all) confirms the diagnosis. Because this test is usually sent to a reference laboratory, this level is unavailable in most hospitals at the time of clinical diagnosis. Therefore based on the initial clinical and laboratory features, PLEX should be initiated emergently because a delay can increase not only morbidity but also mortality. A sample for ADAMTS13 must be drawn before initiating PLEX or plasma/cryoprecipitate infusion to avoid measuring enzyme from transfused products. ADAMTS13 is a stable enzyme; if a sample for ADAMTS13 could not be drawn before plasma therapy, a routine coagulation test sample may be used. In congenital TTP, a persistent severe deficiency of ADAMTS13 (without an inhibitor) is associated with *ADAMTS13* gene defect. However, this diagnosis is sometimes made difficult because many patients, especially children and young adults, are often misdiagnosed as having immune thrombocytopenia or anemia of unknown origin or the hemolysis elevated liver enzymes and low platelets (HELLP) syndrome in pregnancy.

Differential Diagnosis

The differential diagnosis of TTP includes clinical conditions that present with MAHA and thrombocytopenia but without severe ADAMTS13 deficiency (i.e., TMA). These conditions include hematopoietic stem cell transplantation, drug toxicities (e.g., mitomycin, clopidogrel [Plavix], cyclosporine A [Neoral]), malignant hypertension (usually mild to moderate thrombocytopenia),

---

[2] Not available in the United States.

Figure 2 Classification of TTP. *Ab,* Antibody; *ADAMTS13,* a disintegrin and metalloproteinase with thrombospondin motif 1, 13th member of the family; *HUS,* hemolytic uremic syndrome; *MAHA,* microangiopathic hemolytic anemia; *PLEX,* plasma exchange; *TMA,* thrombotic microangiopathy; *TTP,* thrombotic thrombocytopenic purpura.

HELLP syndrome with severe preeclampsia, mechanical cardiac devices (e.g., left ventricular assist devices, intraaortic balloon pumps, mechanical heart valves), disseminated intravascular coagulation, vasculitis, and both diarrhea-associated and atypical hemolytic uremic syndrome.

Treatment

PLEX is the standard of care therapy. Its use has reduced mortality from more than 90% to less than 20%. Ideally it should be initiated within 4 to 6 hours of suspected diagnosis. The patient's plasma (which contains autoantibody) is selectively removed during PLEX (1.0–1.5 plasma volume processed) and replaced with donor plasma containing ADAMTS13. Neurologic symptoms usually disappear within 24 to 48 hours. The platelet count is the most useful laboratory parameter in the assessment of initial response. Complete clinical response, defined as normalization of platelet count for at least 2 days with near normal LDH, is generally achieved in most patients with seven to nine daily PLEXs. Thereafter, a gradual taper—that is, PLEX every other day in the first week, twice in the next week, and once in the third week—may be performed. However, the number of PLEXs can be guided by frequent ADAMTS13 measurements to avoid unnecessary PLEXs and reduce exposure to hundreds of plasma donors, thus reducing the risk of transmitting known and unknown pathogens. Another option is to use pathogen-inactivated plasma, such as Octaplas (Octapharma Plasma Centers), which is approved by the U.S. Food and Drug Administration (FDA) for the treatment of TTP. Given the autoimmune nature of the disease, glucocorticoid therapy is often given from the beginning. Approximately 30% to 50% of patients will have an exacerbation of the disease (worsening of clinical or laboratory features after initial response) or relapses (recurrence of the disease 30 days after discontinuation of PLEX). Such patients require additional PLEXs and other immunomodulatory therapies (e.g., rituximab [Rituxan],[1]

cyclosporine [Neoral],[1] vincristine [Oncovin],[1] bortezomib [Velcade],[1] or splenectomy as a last resort). Early rituximab use, within the first week, has recently been shown to reduce number of PLEXs, length of stay, and exacerbation/relapse. Preliminary data also suggest that a lower dosage of rituximab (100 mg weekly for 4 weeks) elicits a similar clinical response as a higher dosage (375 mg/m² weekly for 4 weeks). However, the former offers the benefits of reduced cost, lower infusion time, and fewer side effects. A dialysis-type catheter is required for PLEX and can be placed with ultrasound guidance in patients with platelet counts as low as 5000/μL. With the exception of a life-threatening bleed, platelet transfusion is contraindicated in TTP because it is a thrombotic disorder of platelet consumption and transfused platelets may worsen the condition (with the appearance of new neurologic symptoms, myocardial infarction, etc.). Most fatalities occur during the first few days of diagnosis, probably because of the severity of the disease or delay in the initiation of PLEX. If initiation of PLEX is likely to be delayed, either plasma or cryoprecipitate can be infused temporarily to supplement ADAMTS13.

Caplacizumab (Cablivi), a nanobody that binds to the A1 domain of vWF and blocks its interaction with GPIb/IX/V receptors on platelets, was FDA approved for the treatment of TTP. This is a very potent disease-modifying agent; therefore it should be used in all cases of TTP. A randomized clinical trial showed that caplacizumab given once as an intravenous (IV) bolus (of 11 mg) followed by daily subcutaneous injections (of 11 mg) up to 30 days post-PLEX led to normalization of the platelet count slightly faster and reduced the numbers of PLEXs, disease exacerbations, and possibly deaths but also led to more relapses compared with placebo. It seems that the use of caplacizumab can definitely benefit severe and refractory TTP and may be tailored based on frequent ADAMTS13 testing during the treatment course. Once ADAMTS13 levels are greater than 10% to 20%, caplacizumab should be discontinued to prevent a bleeding tendency due to development of a severe acquired von Willebrand syndrome. Congenital TTP is treated with plasma infusions (10–15 mL/

[1] Not FDA approved for this indication.

kg); however, cryoprecipitate and intermediate purity Factor VIII concentrate that contain adequate ADAMTS13 have been used successfully to avoid volume overload in susceptible patients. In congenital TTP, a recombinant ADAMTS13 has recently been shown to produce very promising results in a phase I clinical trial.

Monitoring

Considering the relatively high frequency of cardiac involvement, cardiac monitoring should be performed initially. Although PLEX is an otherwise safe procedure, complications related to catheter infection and line thrombosis are not uncommon and should be identified as soon as possible to avoid exacerbation of the disease. Exacerbation of TTP is often related to an infection. There is increasing awareness of delayed long-term psychological and psychosocial effects in up to 50% patients; these are probably related to silent cerebral infarct often documented on imaging in these patients. Therefore a careful follow-up is recommended to identify and manage these issues. Because of recent awareness of silent cerebral infarcts in many patients, use of caplacizumab in all cases seems prudent.

Prognosis

Although PLEX has reduced TTP mortality in the last two decades, most deaths occur within 24 to 48 hours of presentation and are due to delay in the administration of PLEX for a variety of reasons, including a delay in diagnosis or line placement or nonavailability of PLEX at the institution. After one PLEX, survival rates can increase to greater than 90%. Importantly, no clinical or laboratory parameter exists to predict outcome or relapse. Frequent ADAMTS13 monitoring is now used during follow-up to detect early biologic relapse (decrease in activity <30%–50%); preemptive rituximab[1] has been used to prevent overt hematologic and clinical relapse and avoid hospitalization.

---

[1] Not FDA approved for this indication.

References

Fujimura Y, Matsumoto M, Isonishi A, et al: Natural history of Upshaw-Schulman syndrome based on ADAMTS13 gene analysis in Japan, *J Thromb Haemost* 9(Suppl 1):283–301, 2011.

Peyvandi F, Rock GA, Shumak KH, Buskard NA, et al: Comparison of plasma exchange with plasma infusion in the treatment of thrombotic thrombocytopenic purpura. Canadian Apheresis Study Group, *N Engl J Med* 325:393–397, 1991.

Sarode R, Bandarenko N, Brecher ME, et al: Thrombotic thrombocytopenic purpura: 2012 American Society for Apheresis (ASFA) consensus conference on classification, diagnosis, management, and future research, *J Clin Apher,* https://doi.org/10.1002/jca.21302.

Sarode R. Thrombotic thrombocytopenic purpura in caplacizumab era – An individualized approach. *Transfs Apher Sci,* https://doi.org/10.1016/j.transci.2023.103682

Shah N, Rutherford C, Matevosyan K, et al: Role of ADAMTS13 in the management of thrombotic microangiopathies including thrombotic thrombocytopenic purpura (TTP), *Br J Haematol* 163:514–519, 2013.

Tsai HM: Thrombotic thrombocytopenic purpura and atypical hemolytic uremic syndrome—An update, *Hematol Oncol Clin North Am* 27:565–584, 2013.

7

Head and Neck

DRY EYE SYNDROME

Method of
Lauren A. Jeang, MD

CURRENT DIAGNOSIS

- Dry eye disease can manifest as a multitude of symptoms, including dryness, burning, irritation, foreign body sensation, and fluctuating vision.
- Patients of older age are more commonly affected.
- Patients can have a combination of contributing factors that culminate in reduced aqueous tear production and increased tear evaporation.
- Environmental causes include fans, air conditioning, low humidity, and electronic screen use.
- Ocular risk factors include contact lens use, blepharitis, and eyelid malposition.
- Systemic diseases such as Sjögren syndrome, thyroid eye disease, graft-versus-host disease, and mucous membrane pemphigoid should be considered in the differential diagnosis, especially if there are other suggestive signs or symptoms.
- Slit-lamp examination and ocular surface staining provide the most helpful clinical findings. Corneal esthesiometry, Schirmer tests, and tear composition assays are useful as adjunct testing.

CURRENT THERAPY

- Patients should be educated on the chronic nature of dry eye disease.
- Treatment depends on the contributing factors and severity of disease. Multiple simultaneous therapies may be required.
- For mild and moderate disease, initial treatment includes environmental modification and artificial tear lubrication.
- If artificial tears are required more than four times a day, preservative-free artificial tears are recommended to avoid ocular surface irritation from preservatives.
- Other treatment options include prescription anti-inflammatory topical medication, punctal plugs, oral medications, autologous serum tears, and scleral contact lenses. Management of blepharitis should also be considered.
- Cases of eyelid malposition or dysfunction may require surgical intervention.
- Extreme disease can lead to sight- or eye-threatening complications and require more aggressive treatment.

Epidemiology

Dry eye syndrome is a multifactorial disease with a wide range of findings including eye discomfort, burning, irritation, blurry vision, altered tear film, and ocular surface damage. The prevalence of dry eye is unclear because of the broad disease definition and lack of universal diagnostic criteria. It is estimated that 20 million people in the United States suffer from dry eye. Signs and symptoms of dry eye increase by every decade of age. Among older age groups, higher rates of dry eye have been reported in women than in men. Additional terms associated with dry eye include dry eye disease, dry eye syndrome, dysfunctional tear syndrome, and keratoconjunctivitis sicca.

Risk Factors

Multiple risk factors have been associated with dry eye disease. Demographic risk factors include older age (>65 years), female sex, and Asian race. Ocular risk factors include blepharitis, meibomian gland dysfunction, ocular rosacea, contact lens wear, and eyelid malposition such as entropion and ectropion. Systemic diseases strongly associated with dry eye include mixed connective tissue disorders, Sjogrens disease, androgen deficiency, and hematopoietic stem cell transplantation. Thyroid orbitopathy increases ocular exposure and tear evaporation, while Parkinson disease decreases blink rate. A wide range of medications including antihistamines, antidepressants, anxiolytics, and isotretinoin can induce eye dryness. Environmental risk factors such as prolonged electronic screen time, low humidity, and fan use can increase tear evaporation from the ocular surface.

Blepharitis and meibomian gland dysfunction are often diagnosed in conjunction with dry eye disease. Blepharitis is a chronic inflammation of the eyelid margins, including the eyelashes and meibomian glands. Meibomian gland dysfunction, which is considered a subcategory of blepharitis, is defined by duct obstruction/atrophy or altered glandular secretions. Both blepharitis and meibomian gland disease can cause eye irritation, inflammatory tear film state, and ocular surface changes.

527

Pathophysiology

Healthy tears are important in maintaining a lubricated ocular surface. The precorneal tear film is classically described as having an inner mucin layer, middle aqueous layer, and outer lipid layer. More recent studies suggest that the tear film may be a complex gel substance containing soluble mucus, water, electrolytes, proteins, and lipids. Mucus from goblet cells protects and hydrates the eye through formation of a glycocalyx on the surface epithelium. Aqueous fluid, protein, and electrolytes are produced by the lacrimal gland. The outer lipid layer is secreted by meibomian glands and prevents rapid tear evaporation of the aqueous layer to the air.

Adequate tear production, maintenance, and clearance is the responsibility of the lacrimal functional unit, which includes the lacrimal glands, cornea, conjunctiva, meibomian glands, eyelids, and their associated sensory and motor nerves. Cranial nerve V1 sensory input from the ocular surface stimulates eyelid blinking, which allows for even distribution of tears across the eye surface and directs excess tears down through the eyelid punctum. Blinking also allows for expression of lipid material into the tear film from the meibomian glands.

Dry eye disease is the result of any condition that affects a component of the tear film or the lacrimal functional unit. Lacrimal gland secretion inhibition may be caused by lacrimal duct obstruction in sclerosing diseases such as mucous membrane pemphigoid, graft-versus-host disease, ocular burns, or by inflammation of the ductal and acinar epithelial cells in Sjögren syndrome. Systemic medications can reduce tear secretion. Corneal hypoesthesia caused by previous herpes simplex or herpes zoster keratitis, prior laser-assisted in-situ keratomileusis (LASIK) surgery, or trigeminal nerve damage can lead to decreased tear production and decreased blinking. Poor eyelid movement from Parkinson disease, Bell's palsy, or increased ocular surface exposure from thyroid eye disease and electronic screen use prevent formation of an even and adequate tear film. Blepharitis and meibomian gland dysfunction prevent adequate meibum secretion and increase inflammatory factors on the ocular surface.

The combination of poor aqueous secretion by the lacrimal gland and increased tear evaporation leads to tear film hyperosmolality, which in turn triggers an inflammatory cascade in the junction between ocular surface epithelial cells. This in turn leads to a loss of epithelial and goblet cells and T-cell recruitment. The resulting loss of corneal epithelium and unstable tear film then propagates this cycle.

Clinical Manifestations

Dry eye can be classified as mild, moderate, or severe. Patients with mild dry eye may have a multitude of complaints including dryness, discomfort, irritation, burning, foreign body sensation, and fluctuating or blurry vision. Vision may improve with blinking or with use of lubricating drops. Worsening vision may be reported with prolonged screen use, upon awakening, or toward the evening. Moderate disease manifests as increasing symptoms and more persistent visual changes. Severe dry eye, especially when caused by an underlying inflammatory condition, may cause sight- or eye-threatening problems such as corneal scarring, thinning, sterile or infectious ulcers, and perforation.

Diagnosis

The diagnosis of dry eye is made clinically. A gross external examination may reveal proptosis, excessive eyelid laxity, trichiasis, entropion, or ectropion. Patients may demonstrate incomplete blinking or lagophthalmos. The skin may demonstrate changes consistent with blepharitis and rosacea, including rhinophyma, erythema, and telangiectasias. Eyelid changes consistent with blepharitis include debris at the eyelash bases, lid margin telangiectasias, and poor meibum flow from the meibomian glands. Slit lamp examination with the aid of fluorescein staining may show evidence of poor tear production and distribution. A drop of saline applied to a fluorescein strip, or a drop of premade 1% or 2% solution is placed on the lower tarsal conjunctiva. Using the cobalt blue filter on the slit lamp, fluorescein may highlight a low tear lake over the lower eyelid (normal is 1 mm), irregular or rapid breakup of the tear film (normal is 10 seconds), and punctate changes representing epithelial cell loss over the cornea. Lissamine Green is another type of stain used to reflect areas of mucin or glycocalyx loss on the conjunctiva. The pattern of staining may suggest the underlying cause. Corneal hypoesthesia is evaluated before the use of any eyedrops. Sensation is evaluated by using a cotton-tip applicator with the fibers twisted to a point or using a Cochet-Bonnet aesthesiometer device.

Schirmer's testing is useful in assessing decreased aqueous tear production. The test can be performed with or without topical anesthesia. A thin strip of filter paper is placed along the lateral one-third of the lower eyelid. The amount of aqueous absorbed after 5 minutes is measured. If topical anesthesia is not used, a value less than 10 mm is considered abnormal. However, there is no established cutoff, and results are poorly reproducible. Therefore the use of Schirmer's testing as a sole diagnostic test is not recommended.

Multiple tear composition assays are available that examine different markers of dry eye including elevated tear osmolality, decreased lactoferrin and lysozyme, and increased matrix metalloproteinase-9 (MMP-9). However, there are conflicting studies on whether or not these markers strongly correlate with symptoms and other examination findings. There is some suggestion that multiple measurements over time may be more useful.

Additionally, the workup should include a careful review of medications and systemic symptoms. Patients with severe or intractable dry eye should raise questions of concurrent dry mouth, arthritis, or history of inflammatory or autoimmune disease. These patients may benefit from evaluation for Sjögren syndrome or another autoimmune condition. Similarly, patients with significant proptosis and lagophthalmos should be examined for possible thyroid disease.

Differential Diagnosis

The differential diagnosis for dry eye disease can be broad because of overlapping signs and symptoms with other ocular diseases. Burning and irritation may be caused by blepharitis or meibomian gland dysfunction without dry eye. Patients presenting with severe dry eye may have another underlying ocular condition such as a thermal or chemical ocular burn, Stevens-Johnson syndrome, graft-versus-host disease, or mucous membrane pemphigoid.

Additional history may elucidate other conditions in the differential diagnoses. Patients with ocular irritation after initiating eye drops may be suffering from topical drug toxicity. Redness, itching, and mucoid discharge can be suggestive of allergic or viral conjunctivitis. Foreign body sensation or eye pain in the setting of recent ocular trauma may be due to a corneal abrasion. Infectious corneal ulceration should also be considered if there is redness, tearing, or decreased vision in a patient with prior ocular trauma or poor contact lens hygiene.

Therapy

Treatment of dry eye disease begins with addressing the underlying cause and educating patients on the nature of this disease. Potential environmental factors should be eliminated first. Air conditioners, heaters, and fans should be avoided or diverted away from the eyes. Patients should be reminded to take short breaks every 20 minutes or consciously blink during prolonged digital screen use. Moisture chamber goggles and humidifiers may help improve periocular humidity. Discontinuation of an offending systemic drug should be considered if medically appropriate.

Basic treatment includes the use of eye lubricants to enhance aqueous volume. Over-the-counter artificial tears dosed two to six times a day is often the first treatment modality. If patients need lubricants more than four times a day, preservative-free artificial tears are recommended over non–preservative-free products. Artificial tear ointments are also available over the counter and are best used at nighttime to avoid blurred vision. Introductory blepharitis management includes warm compresses over the eyelids to soften meibomian gland secretions and eyelid scrubs twice a day to loosen adherent eyelash debris.

Medications can be added in cases of moderate or severe disease. Topical anti-inflammatory medications include cyclosporine 0.05% and 0.09% and lifitegrast 5% which are dosed BID. Patients should be educated on the side effects of these medications, which include burning and, in the case of lifitegrast, a bitter taste. Topical steroids such as prednisolone, fluorometholone, and loteprednol (0.25% suspension) dosed QD to QID are useful in inflammatory dry eye, but should be limited to a few weeks as they can elevate intraocular pressure and promote cataract formation. Topical erythromycin or bacitracin ointment applied to the eyelids multiple times a day or at bedtime for a few weeks has been used for treatment of blepharitis. Oral medications such as doxycycline[1] (20 to 100 mg QOD to BID), minocycline[1] (50 mg QD to BID) and azithromycin[1] (500 mg per day for 3 days in three cycles with 7-day intervals) can been used for their anti-inflammatory properties. Clinicians should keep in mind that tetracyclines are contraindicated in children younger than 8 years of age and in pregnant and nursing patients. Side effects include photosensitivity, gastrointestinal upset, and vaginitis. Azithromycin may cause arrythmias. Initiation of omega-3 and omega-6 supplementation[7] has been suggested to enhance tear film quality, although more studies are required to confirm their efficacy. Patients with Sjögren syndrome or other autoimmune disorders may need more aggressive management of their underlying disorder through oral steroids or disease-modifying antirheumatic drugs (DMARDs).

Punctal occlusion is another option to improve tear volume on the ocular surface once ocular surface inflammation has been controlled. Occlusion can be achieved with dissolvable polymer plugs or more durable silicone plugs. Polymer plugs are positioned deep into the

---

[1]Not FDA approved for this indication.
[7]Available as dietary supplement.

canaliculus to allow for patient comfort, but they require replacement every few months. Silicone plugs are placed over the punctum opening. These are advantageous in that they can last years and be removed at any time. However, if incorrectly sized, they can self-extrude or cause ocular irritation. The largest-diameter plug should be used to avoid dislocation. Permanent punctum occlusion by thermal cautery is reserved for patients who show consistent improvement with plugs or those with severe disease. The biggest side effect of punctal occlusion is epiphora. Therefore it is highly recommended to perform a trial with silicone plugs before performing cautery because of the irreversibility of the procedure.

Various in-office procedures that warm and express the meibomian glands are available. Many involve devices that apply localized heat and massage to the eyelids. Other options include intense pulsed light (IPL) followed by manual gland expression, direct intraductal probing, and microblepharoexfoliation. These procedures can be costly, and data on long-term success are limited. Additional studies are required to confirm their efficacy.

Severe disease states may need "third-tier" treatments. Patients with Sjögren syndrome–associated dry eye disease may benefit from oral secretagogues. Although neither are approved by the U.S. Food and Drug Administration (FDA) for the treatment of dry eye, studies suggest that pilocarpine (Salagen)[1] dosed at 10 to 30 mg a day or cevimeline (Evoxac)[1] may improve symptoms, although perhaps not tear production. Side effects include excessive salivation and sweating.

Another option is autologous serum drops, which are thought to contain anti-inflammatory mediators. They have shown the most benefit in patients with Sjögren syndrome, graft-versus-host-disease, and other dry eye–related ocular surface conditions. Serum drawn from the patient is diluted to various concentrations and is dosed anywhere from four to eight times a day. The need for repeated blood draws, medication refrigeration, and out-of-pocket cost to patients are the biggest drawbacks. This treatment is not formally FDA approved, and more studies are necessary to confirm their general utility.

Scleral contact lenses have been shown to help in refractory or severe cases of dry eye. Scleral lenses are rigid and vaulted over the globe to create a chamber of fluid. This technology protects the corneal surface from eyelid trauma and exposure while constantly hydrating the eye. These lenses require consultation with a specialty-trained optometrist.

Patients with poor eyelid positioning caused by entropion and ectropion may require surgical repair. Patients with severe corneal exposure from poor eyelid closure may need eyelid reconstruction, upper-lid weight placement, tarsorrhaphy (placement of a suture through the eyelids to promote eye closure), or placement of retained amniotic membranes.

Dry eye treatment continues to evolve. There are many promising medications and devices in the pipeline that may expand options for patients in the future.

Monitoring
Patient follow-up depends on the severity of disease and the treatments initiated. Severe disease may require weeks or months of follow-up visits. Patients should be monitored for medication side effects.

Complications
Complications are usually limited to cases of severe dry eye. Persistent corneal epithelial defects may form and cause significant decreased vision. Such compromised corneal epithelium places the eyes at risk for microbial keratitis. Additionally, corneal stromal thinning can occur as a result of prolonged dehydration and uncontrolled inflammation. In some cases, thinning progresses and may result in corneal perforation. Both sterile and infectious keratitis may lead to loss of vision or loss of the eye itself. Therefore urgent ophthalmology referral is warranted in these cases to initiate aggressive dry eye treatment, frequent topical antibiotics, placement of corneal glue, and/or surgical rehabilitation.

[1] Not FDA approved for this indication.

References
Akpek EK, Amescua G, Farid M, Garcia-Ferrer FJ, Lin A, Rhee MK, Varu DM, Musch DC, Dunn SP, Mah FS: American Academy of Ophthalmology Preferred Practice Pattern Cornea and External Disease Panel. Dry Eye Syndrome Preferred Practice Pattern®. *Ophthalmology*. 126(1):P286–P334, 2019.

Amescua G, Akpek EK, Farid M, Garcia-Ferrer FJ, Lin A, Rhee MK, Varu DM, Musch DC, Dunn SP, Mah FS: American Academy of Ophthalmology Preferred Practice Pattern Cornea and External Disease Panel. Blepharitis Preferred Practice Pattern®. *Ophthalmology*. 126(1):P56–P93, 2019.

Craig JP, Nelson JD, Azar DT, Belmonte C, Bron AJ, Chauhan SK, de Paiva CS, Gomes JAP, Hammitt KM, Jones L, Nichols JJ, Nichols KK, Novack GD, Stapleton FJ, Willcox MDP, Wolffsohn JS, Sullivan DA: TFOS DEWS II Report Executive Summary, *Ocul Surf* 15(4):802–812, 2017.

Foulks GN, Forstot SL, Donshik PC, Forstot JZ, Goldstein MH, Lemp MA, Nelson JD, Nichols KK, Pflugfelder SC, Tanzer JM, Asbell P, Hammitt K, Jacobs DS: Clinical guidelines for management of dry eye associated with Sjögren disease, *Ocul Surf* 13(2):118–132, 2015.

Jones L, Downie LE, Korb D, Benitez-Del-Castillo JM, et al: TFOS DEWS II Management and Therapy Report, *Ocul Surf* 15(3):575–628, 2017.

Pflugfelder SC, Stern ME: Biological functions of tear film, *Exp Eye Res* 197:108115, 2020.

GLAUCOMA

Method of
Albert P. Lin, MD; and Kristin Schmid Biggerstaff, MD

CURRENT DIAGNOSIS

Primary Open Angle Glaucoma
- Primary open angle glaucoma is an irreversible optic neuropathy typically associated with elevated intraocular pressure.
- Primary open angle glaucoma is the most common form of glaucoma, affecting more than 68 million people worldwide. There are more than 36 million Asians with the condition, accounting for over 50% of all those affected. The disease has the highest prevalence in Africans, affecting more than 4% of the population, while prevalence in other ethnicities ranges from 1% to 2%. It is more common in older adults: 1 to 2% in 50-year-olds compared with 6% to 12% in 80-year-olds.
- Primary open angle glaucoma is diagnosed by a complete ophthalmic examination, including dilated stereoscopic optic nerve examination and formal visual field.
- Untreated primary open angle glaucoma can lead to slow irreversible loss of vision and blindness. Other common causes of slow and progressive vision loss in older adults include cataracts, macular degeneration, and diabetic retinopathy.

Acute Angle Closure Glaucoma
- Pupillary block in susceptible patients leads to block of aqueous drainage and sudden and extreme rise of intraocular pressure. Acute angle closure can damage the optic nerve, resulting in acute angle closure glaucoma.
- About 0.6% of the global population, or 70 million people, are at risk for acute angle closure. It is more common in Inuits and Asians and rare in African Americans. The risk of acute angle closure increases with age. It is also more common in hyperopes.
- Patients can present with blurry vision, red eye, pain, headache, nausea, or vomiting. Acute angle closure is sometimes misdiagnosed as migraines or gastrointestinal illnesses. Patients with conjunctivitis, keratitis, uveitis, and corneal abrasion can also present with the same symptoms.
- Peripheral iridotomy prevents acute angle closure in susceptible patients. High intraocular pressure can result in irreversible damage of the optic nerve within hours, making acute angle closure one of the true ophthalmic emergencies.

Primary Open Angle Glaucoma

- Topical eye drops, including β-blockers, selective α_2 agonists, carbonic anhydrase inhibitors, prostaglandin analogues, and rho kinase inhibitors, can be used to reduce intraocular pressure.
- Oral carbonic anhydrase inhibitors are typically used in recalcitrant cases until surgery can be performed.
- Laser trabeculoplasty may be used as first-line or adjunct therapy.
- Glaucoma surgery, including trabeculectomy, tube shunt, and cyclodestruction, may be performed if goal intraocular pressure cannot be reached with medical therapy or in nonadherent patients.

Acute Angle Glaucoma

- All glaucoma eye drops are used to reduce intraocular pressure.
- Oral and intravenous medications are added sequentially to reduce intraocular pressure as needed.
- Laser iridotomy can be performed as prophylactic treatment or acutely to break the pupillary block if the patient is unresponsive to medical intervention.
- Emergency glaucoma incisional surgery is performed if the patient is unresponsive to all other treatments.

Glaucoma is an optic neuropathy with characteristic optic nerve head appearance: narrowing of the neuroretinal rim. The optic nerve is a collection of more than 1 million axons from the retinal ganglion cells. The anterior 1-mm portion of the optic nerve within the globe is referred to as the *optic disk* or simply the disk. When the disk is examined with direct or indirect ophthalmoscopy, a cup, or a physiologic empty space, is observed centrally. The remainder of the disk, which has a yellow-orange appearance, contains the axons and is referred to as the *neuroretinal rim*. The area of the cup compared to the entire disk is the cup-to-disk ratio, which is normally less than 0.4 (Figure 1A). When patients develop glaucoma, axons are lost from the neuroretinal rim and the size of the cup increases in relation to the disk. Narrowing of the neuroretinal rim and increased cup-to-disk ratio are the hallmarks of glaucomatous optic neuropathy (see Figure 1B).

Glaucoma can result in significant and irreversible loss of vision and is one of the leading causes of blindness in the world. Early in the disease state, glaucoma is asymptomatic; it is sometimes called "the sneak thief of sight." As the disease progresses, the patient develops decreased peripheral vision and eventually loss of the central vision.

Glaucoma is typically associated with increased intraocular pressure (IOP), but it is possible to have normal-tension or low-tension glaucoma. Glaucoma treatment is focused on the reduction of IOP to prevent or slow optic nerve damage and preserve visual function.

Glaucoma is classified in many ways, and it is most useful to approach it clinically based on the status of the angle, the area between the cornea and iris where aqueous humor exits the globe through the trabecular network. We further discuss primary open angle glaucoma, the most common form of glaucoma, and the management of acute angle closure, one of the true ophthalmic emergencies.

Primary Open Angle Glaucoma

Glaucoma is one of the leading causes of blindness in older adults, especially in patients of African descent. Vision loss from glaucoma is irreversible, and the treatment goal is to reduce IOP, slow disease progression, and preserve visual function during the patient's lifetime. Glaucoma is a slowly progressive disease, and progression to blindness often takes more than 10 years, even in untreated patients. Given its slow progression and the fact that central vision loss occurs in late disease, most patients do well with early diagnosis and treatment. Treatment is more difficult in late disease because the rate of disease progression and visual deterioration is accelerated, sometimes despite good control of IOP.

Due to the early asymptomatic nature of the disease, the patient's adherence to and persistence with treatment is often less than optimal. Studies have shown patients who obtain glaucoma information from physicians in addition to their ophthalmologists have a higher rate of medication adherence. Ophthalmologists have the options to use treatment modalities such as laser and surgery to obtain pressure control and decrease or eliminate the need for medication use.

The American Academy of Ophthalmology recommends asymptomatic patients older than 40 years be referred for ophthalmic evaluation once every several years for early detection of glaucoma and other chronic eye diseases. However, the US Preventive Services Task Force found insufficient evidence to recommend for or against screening for glaucoma in adults. Risks, benefits, and cost effectiveness of screening are beyond the scope of this chapter, but symptomatic patients or patients at high risk for glaucoma (African descent and family history) might benefit from ophthalmology consultation. It is possible to diagnose glaucoma by direct ophthalmoscopy, but this is not a substitute for binocular assessment of the disk through dilated pupils and formal visual field testing. If glaucoma is suspected or diagnosed, primary care visits should include inquiries regarding glaucoma medication use, medication side effects, and the time of last eye examination. Primary care physicians can improve glaucoma outcome by promoting adherence to medication and follow-up. Glaucoma patients need to follow up with their ophthalmologists at least annually, and in severe cases every 3 months, for intraocular pressure checks.

Treatment

Topical Glaucoma Medications

Topical glaucoma medications are administered once or twice daily. Patients should look up, pull down their lower eye lid, drop the

Figure 1 Disk appearance. (A) Normal disk. Cup-to-disk ratio is less than 0.4. (B) Glaucoma. Increased cup-to-disk ratio and narrow neuroretinal rim superiorly and inferiorly (*arrows*).

TABLE 1 Topical Glaucoma Medications: Carbonic Anhydrase Inhibitors

CLASS	β-BLOCKER	SELECTIVE α_2 AGONIST	CARBONIC ANHYDRASE INHIBITOR	PROSTAGLANDIN ANALOGUE	RHO KINASE INHIBITOR	COMBINATION
Medication	Timolol (Timoptic) Betaxolol (Betoptic) Levobunolol (Betagan)	Brimonidine (Alphagan)	Dorzolamide (Trusopt) Brinzolamide (Azopt)	Latanoprost (Xalatan) Travoprost (Travatan) Bimatoprost (Lumigan) Latanoprostene bunod (Vyzulta)	Netarsudil (Rhopressa)	Timolol/Dorzolamide (Cosopt) Timolol/Brimonidine (Combigan) Brimonidine/Brinzolamide (Simbrinza) Netarsudil/latanoprost (Rocklatan)
Dosing	qd or bid	bid	bid	qhs	qd	bid or qd (Rocklatan)
Cap color	Yellow	Purple	Orange	Teal	White	Blue (Cosopt, Combigan), light green (Simbrinza), white (Rocklatan)
Side effects	Bradycardia, COPD, and asthma exacerbation	Allergic conjunctivitis, dry mouth, and fatigue in elderly	Stinging and bitter taste	Hyperemia, lash growth, and increased pigmentation	Hyperemia	See individual components

COPD, Chronic obstructive pulmonary disease.

medication on the inferior conjunctival cul-de-sac, and keep their eyes closed for 5 minutes. Applying gentle pressure next to the bridge of the nose to occlude the puncta can improve absorption of the medication. Medication bottle caps are color-coded by their class, and patients can usually identify their eye drops by color. Glaucoma medications are not subject to first-pass effect through the liver and can sometimes have significant systemic side effects, especially the β-blockers. Topical glaucoma medications are described later and summarized in Table 1.

Prostaglandin Analogues. Latanoprost (Xalatan), travoprost (Travatan), and bimatoprost (Lumigan) are prostaglandin analogues and are color-coded by teal caps. They are administered once at bedtime but may be administered once at any time during the day to promote adherence. They decrease IOP by increasing uveoscleral outflow. Latanoprostene bunod (Vyzulta) is converted into latanoprost and nitric oxide inside the eye and decreases IOP by promoting aqueous outflow through both the uveoscleral and trabecular meshwork pathways. It is considered a prostaglandin analogue with an additional mechanism of action. Side effects are primarily local and include increased conjunctival hyperemia, increased lash growth, and possible irreversible increase in periocular and iris pigmentation.

β-Blockers. Timolol (Betimol, Istalol, Timoptic), levobunolol (Betagan), and betaxolol (Betoptic) are color-coded by yellow caps. They are administered once or twice daily and decrease IOP by decreasing aqueous production. Side effects include bradycardia, exacerbation of chronic obstructive pulmonary disease (COPD) and asthma, impotence, and decreased serum high-density lipoprotein (HDL) cholesterol. Physicians need to be aware that a topical β-blocker is a potential cause of acute changes in cardiovascular or pulmonary status. There are several reported incidents of death following the use of topical β-blockers mostly due to exacerbation of asthma.

Selective α_2 Agonists. Brimonidine (Alphagan) and is a selective α_2 receptor agonist. It decreases IOP by decreasing aqueous production. Allergic conjunctivitis has been reported in up to 10% of patients. Rarely, it causes dry mouth and chronic fatigue and drowsiness in the elderly.

Carbonic Anhydrase Inhibitors. Dorzolamide (Trusopt) and brinzolamide (Azopt) are color-coded by orange caps and are sulfa-based medications. They are administered twice daily and decrease IOP by decreasing aqueous production. This class of medication has minimal systemic side effects. However, some patients complain about transient stinging and a bitter taste in the mouth after administration. These side effects, if tolerable, are not indications for discontinuing therapy.

Rho Kinase Inhibitors. Netarsudil (Rhopressa) affects actin and myosin contraction and decreases IOP by increasing aqueous outflow through the trabecular meshwork. It is color coded white and administered once daily. Conjunctival hyperemia is reported in up to 50% of the patients. Ophthalmologists have also observed pinpoint conjunctival hemorrhages and corneal verticillata (lipid deposits on the corneal epithelium) because these observations are asymptomatic and generally not reported by the patients. Compared to other medications, rho kinase inhibitor has a unique mechanism of action and is considered to be an excellent adjunct medication to lower IOP when other medications are already in use.

Combined Topical Medications. Timolol and dorzolamide (Cosopt) and timolol and brimonidine (Combigan) are color-coded by blue caps. Brimonidine and brinzolamide (Simbrinza) are color-coded by a light green cap. Netarsudil and latanoprost (Rocklatan) are color-coded by white caps. Combined medications decrease exposure to preservatives and can decrease irritation and problems with dry eyes. Adherence might also be improved.

Oral Carbonic Anhydrase Inhibitors
Oral carbonic anhydrase inhibitors include acetazolamide (Diamox), 250 mg or 500 mg given twice daily, and methazolamide (Neptazane), 25 mg or 50 mg given twice daily. They are sulfa-based medications and decrease IOP by decreasing aqueous production. Oral carbonic anhydrase inhibitors are not commonly used today because effective topical medications are available. They are typically used on a short-term basis to achieve IOP control in acute or refractory cases. Side effects can include aplastic anemia, kidney stones, bitter taste, indigestion, paresthesia of the extremities, tinnitus, and polyuria. Clinicians need to consider the possibility of hypokalemia when patients take other diuretics to control blood pressure (Table 2). Acetazolamide may also be given intravenously.

Laser Trabeculoplasty
Argon or selective laser trabeculoplasty can be used to increase aqueous outflow. Laser trabeculoplasty is noninvasive and safe, and it can be performed in the office in less than 10 minutes. Compared to surgery, IOP reduction is limited, up to 25% as primary treatment, but less as an adjunct modality. It is ineffective or less effective in some patients with light trabecular meshwork pigmentation. The effect of laser decreases over time but may be repeated in the case of selective laser trabeculoplasty.

Surgery
The most commonly performed conventional glaucoma surgeries are trabeculectomy, tube shunt, and cyclodestruction. Trabeculectomy (with or without Xen gel stent) and tube shunt are procedures that create an opening in the sclera to increase

TABLE 2	Oral and Intravenous Glaucoma Medications			
	ACETAZOLAMIDE (DIAMOX)	**METHAZOLAMIDE (NEPTA-ZANE)**	**MANNITOL (OSMITROL)**	**GLYCERIN 50%**[1]
Class	CAI	CAI	Hyperosmotic	Hyperosmotic
Dosage	250 or 500 mg bid	25 mg or 50 mg bid	1 g/kg in 30 min	1 g/kg once
Route	PO or IV	PO	IV	PO
Side effects	Bitter taste, indigestion, paresthesia, tinnitus, polyuria, kidney stones, hypokalemia, aplastic anemia, and sulfa allergy		Polyuria, dehydration Exacerbate CHF and diabetes (glycerin)	

CAI, Carbonic anhydrase inhibitor; *CHF*, congestive heart failure
[1]Not FDA approved for this indication.

aqueous outflow. Cyclodestruction destroys the ciliary body and decreases aqueous production. The procedure can be transscleral or endoscopic; the endoscopic method is typically done at the time of cataract surgery. Alternative surgical methods such as deep sclerectomy, Trabectome, canaloplasty, iStent, Kahook dual blade, Hydrus, and trabecolotmy (GATT, Trab 360, OMNI) are performed at the time of cataract surgery to minimize the invasiveness and potential complications associated with traditional glaucoma surgery. However, these minimally invasive glaucoma surgeries (MIGS) are not as effective at lowering the IOP.

Visual Impairment and Blindness

Patients who are visually impaired (Snellen vision of <20/40) or legally blind (Snellen vision of <20/200 or visual field of <20 degrees) may have significantly decreased mobility and ability to function. Continued glaucoma treatment is still important in these patients because even maintenance of count-finger vision can allow the patients some degree of independence. Low-vision devices and services, including high-contrast video magnifiers, audiobooks, eccentric viewers, and mobility training, can allow patients maximal use of their residual vision and improve their confidence and quality of life.

Acute Angle Closure Glaucoma

Pupillary block in susceptible patients blocks aqueous drainage and leads to sudden and extreme rise of intraocular pressure. Acute angle closure can damage the optic nerve, resulting in acute angle closure glaucoma.

About 0.6% of people worldwide are at risk for acute angle closure. It is more common in Inuits and Asians and rare in African Americans. The risk of acute angle closure increases with age. It is also more common in hyperopes (farsightedness).

Mechanism of Acute Angle Closure: Pupillary Block

After aqueous is produced in the ciliary body in the posterior chamber, it travels through the pupil and exits the anterior chamber through the trabecular meshwork located between the iris and the cornea. Pupillary block occurs when the iris contacts the lens and obstructs the flow of aqueous through the pupil. Increased posterior chamber pressure displaces the iris anteriorly against the trabecular meshwork and stops aqueous outflow.

Patients at risk for acute angle closure have narrow occludable angles. These patients have smaller eyes, allowing the lens to contact the iris to initiate papillary block. The distance between the iris and the lens is the shortest when the pupil is mid-dilated. Therefore, patients who present with acute angle closure might have a history of dim light exposure (movies) or use of medications with anticholinergic properties (antihistamines, decongestants, antispasmodics). High IOP causes iris and corneal endothelial cell dysfunction, resulting in nonreactive pupil and hazy cornea, respectively. High IOP also results in inflammation and red eye, as well as severe pain, nausea, and vomiting (Figure 2). Elevated IOP can damage the optic nerve within hours, and acute angle closure needs to be treated on an emergent basis to prevent permanent loss of vision.

Figure 2 Acute angle closure patient with red eye and mid-dilated and nonreactive pupil.

Diagnosis

Patients with acute angle closure can present with blurry vision, red eye, pain, headache, nausea, or vomiting. History can include hyperopia, onset after exposure to a dim environment, or taking anticholinergic medications. Examination findings include decreased vision, conjunctival hyperemia, mid-dilated, nonreactive pupil with or without an afferent papillary defect, and increased IOP (by palpation or tonometry). Acute angle closure is sometimes misdiagnosed as migraines or gastrointestinal illness. Patients with conjunctivitis, keratitis, uveitis, and corneal abrasion can also present with the same symptoms.

Treatment

If acute angle closure is suspected, an emergent referral to ophthalmology is indicated. If an ophthalmologist is not immediately available, the goal will be to medically control the IOP as soon as possible. One drop of topical aqueous suppressant—β-blocker, selective α2 agonist, or carbonic anhydrase inhibitor—should be administered (timolol, brimonidine, and dorzolamide) (see Table 1). The maximum dose of oral or intravenous carbonic anhydrase inhibitor is given: acetazolamide 500 mg or methazolamide 50 mg (see Table 2). The patient is placed in the supine position to allow the lens and iris to fall posteriorly. The patient is reassessed in 30 minutes, and if the condition is not improved, topical drops are repeated. If there is no improvement after another 30 minutes, a hyperosmotic, oral glycerin[1] 1 g/kg or intravenous mannitol (Osmitrol) 1 g/kg over 30 minutes, is administered. Hyperosmotics may be contraindicated in patients with congestive heart failure, and glycerin can cause severe hyperglycemia in diabetic patients.

An ophthalmologist can break the pupillary block by medically lowering the IOP or by performing anterior chamber paracentesis, compression gonioscopy, laser peripheral iridotomy, and, in recalcitrant cases, emergent trabeculectomy. Once the pressure is controlled, it is important to perform an iridotomy in both eyes to prevent future episodes. Patients with patent iridotomies may safely take anticholinergic medications.

[1]Not FDA approved for this indication.

References

Allingham RR, Damji KF, Freedman S, et al: *Shield's Textbook of Glaucoma*, ed 7, Philadelphia, 2020, Lippincott Walters Kluwer.

American Academy of Ophthalmology: Available at: Practice guidelines. Preferred practice patterns. Primary angle-closure disease. November 2020. http://www.aao.org/preferred-practice-pattern/primary-angle-closure-ppp. [Accessed April 30, 2023].

American Academy of Ophthalmology: Practice guidelines. Preferred practice patterns. Primary open-angle glaucoma, November 2020. Available at: http://www.aao.org/preferred-practice-pattern/primary-openangle-glaucoma-ppp [accessed April 30, 2023].

Lin AP, Orengo-Nania S, Braun UK: PCP's role in chronic open-angle glaucoma, *Geriatrics* 64:20–28, 2009.

Nordstrom BL, Friedman DS, Mozaffari E, et al: Persistence and adherence with topical glaucoma therapy, *Am J Ophthalmol* 140:598–606, 2005.

Schwartz GF, Quigley HA: Adherence and persistence with glaucoma therapy, *Surv Ophthalmol* 54:S57–S68, 2008.

Tham YC, Li X, Wong TY, et al: Global prevalence of glaucoma and projections of glaucoma burden through 2040, *Ophthalmology* 121(11):2081–2090, 2014.

US Preventive Services Task Force: Screening for glaucoma, Available at: http://www.uspreventiveservicestaskforce.org/uspstf/recommendation/primary-open-angle-glaucoma-screening; May, 2022. [accessed April 30, 2023].

Zhang N, Wang J, Chen B, et al: Prevalence of primary angle closure glaucoma in the last 20 years: a metaanalysis and systemic review, *Front Med (Lausanne)* 7:624179, 2021.

Zhang N, Wang J, Li Y, et al: Prevalence of primary open angle glaucoma in the last 20 years: a meta-analysis and sysetmic review, *Sci Rep* 2;11(1):13762, 2021.

MÉNIÈRE'S DISEASE

Method of
Terry D. Fife, MD

CURRENT DIAGNOSIS

- Ménière's disease is characterized by recurrent attacks of severe vertigo, nausea, and vomiting typically lasting 1 to 6 hours.
- Ménière's disease causes tinnitus on the side of the affected ear; the tinnitus can change in pitch and loudness during attacks of vertigo.
- Attacks of vertigo are associated with reduced or muffled hearing on the side of the affected ear.
- Fluctuating unilateral hearing loss and low-frequency hearing loss on the side of the affected ear is characteristic.

CURRENT THERAPY

- Initial therapy includes a sodium-restricted diet (preferably <1500 mg of sodium daily) and a diuretic agent (e.g., thiazide diuretics).
- Betahistine,[1] a medication widely used in Europe that may be obtained at compounding pharmacies in the United States, may be helpful in selected patients at a dosage 16 to 48 mg three times daily though some authors have recommended even higher dosages.
- Transtympanic infusion of gentamicin[1] or corticosteroids and endolymphatic sac surgery may be considered as minimally invasive options in patients with serviceable hearing. Gentamicin poses a moderate risk of inducing hearing loss.
- Vestibular nerve sectioning is highly effective in stopping vertigo attacks with a reasonably low risk of causing further hearing loss, but it is a more invasive procedure.
- Labyrinthectomy is highly effective in stopping vertigo attacks but causes complete hearing loss, so it is only an option for patients who have already lost all useful hearing.

Patients who have undergone procedures that cause acute loss of vestibular function often have vertigo for a while after the surgery; the vertigo improves more quickly with vestibular rehabilitative therapy.

[1]Not FDA approved for this indication.

Ménière's disease is a disorder of the inner ear that results in recurrent, spontaneous episodes of vertigo, hearing loss, ear fullness, and tinnitus affecting the same ear. The hearing loss often fluctuates early in Ménière's disease, but fluctuating hearing is not always present. Eventually permanent hearing loss occurs, affecting the low frequencies initially but ultimately affecting all frequencies.

Epidemiology

The reported prevalence of Ménière's disease varies from about 50 to 200 per 100,000. Females are somewhat more prone to Meniere's disease than males, with a female/male ratio of about 1.9:1.

Risk Factors

Possible risk factors for later development of Ménière's syndrome include autoimmune disorders, migraine, syphilitic otitis and viral infection of the inner ear, head trauma, and a family history of Ménière's disease. Despite the emergence of COVID-19, no correlation with Ménière's is evident with infection or following vaccination (Wachova, 2021).

Pathophysiology

The underlying mechanism is generally thought to be due to endolymphatic hydrops, a type of swelling of the endolymphatic compartment that ultimately leads to permanent damage of the inner ear structures. Possible reasons for this periodic swelling of the endolymph compartment include mechanical obstruction of endolymph flow or at least dysregulation of the electrochemical membrane potential between endolymph and perilymph compartments.

Endolymphatic hydrops appears to be the mechanism for a number of conditions that can lead to Ménière's syndrome. When no primary cause is identified, the idiopathic form of the syndrome is called Ménière's disease. When an underlying cause is found, it is referred to as Ménière's syndrome or secondary Ménière's or secondary endolymphatic hydrops. Secondary Ménière's syndrome can result from delayed endolymphatic hydrops in which symptoms come on years after a prior disorder or viral injury of the labyrinth, syphilitic otitis, autoimmune inner ear disease, and trauma.

Prevention

There is no known way of preventing the development of Ménière's disease because it occurs in many people with no risk factors.

Clinical Manifestations

Ménière's disease can manifest with periodic unilateral (or, less commonly, bilateral) hearing loss or isolated attacks of vertigo. Not uncommonly, Ménière's disease has both elements present at its onset, but the vertigo is usually the symptom that gets the most attention. Vertigo usually lasts 1 to 6 hours but can last as little as 30 minutes or as long as all day. Patients prone to motion sickness often report that their dizziness lasts longer because the aftereffect of vertigo lingers longer in those who are motion sensitive. Vertigo attacks in Ménière's disease are often quite severe and generally render patients unable to move around owing to the vertigo, nausea, and recurrent vomiting.

The hearing loss is usually unilateral, and patients might notice fluctuation in hearing accompanied by ear fullness and a low-pitched roaring tinnitus either before or coincident with the vertigo. If audiometry can be performed during this time, low-frequency (250–1000 Hz) hearing loss may be documented and might improve after the attack ceases. This signature fluctuating low-frequency sensorineural hearing loss is very helpful (Figure 1) when found, but getting patients with vertigo attacks in for testing while they are in the acute stage of vertigo is usually not feasible.

Occasionally, patients with Ménière's have sudden random drop attacks in which they abruptly fall without loss of consciousness. These spells, referred to as otolithic crises of Tumarkin, can lead to serious injury and should prompt aggressive treatment. The mechanism is presumed to be related to sudden mechanical deformation or sudden neural discharges related to the otolith structures of the inner ear. Because there is no specific treatment for Tumarkin crises, treatment entails the standard treatments for Ménière's disease in general.

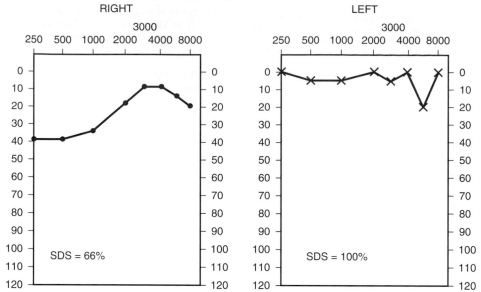

Figure 1 Audiogram showing typical low-frequency hearing trough of Ménière's disease affecting the right ear.

As Ménière's disease progresses, usually over months to years, permanent low-frequency hearing loss develops that gives way to hearing loss at all frequencies. Eventually, the patient can lose all or most hearing on the affected side. Meanwhile, with each vertigo attack, some vestibular function is lost, and so as vertigo attacks continue, vestibular loss ensues, often paralleling the hearing loss. Ménière's occasionally burns out, meaning that enough vestibular function has been lost that acute hydrops no longer produces vertigo. Patients might report less severe dizziness or just a vague feeling of unsteadiness. This usually indicates advanced Ménière's, and unilateral hearing and vestibular loss should be expected.

Bilateral Ménière's disease is present at the time of initial diagnosis in about 10% of cases and by 10 years of symptoms, about 35% have bilateral involvement. Bilateral Ménière's disease has treatment implications because treating one side alone will be unlikely to stop the vertigo attacks, which could be emanating from the untreated side. Surgical treatment of both sides is also problematic because it could leave the patient with bilateral hearing loss, vestibular loss, or both.

Diagnosis

The diagnosis of Ménière's disease is made clinically based on unilateral hearing loss, tinnitus, ear fullness, and episodic vertigo typically lasting 1 to 6 hours. The criteria for definite, probable, and possible Ménière's disease are listed in Box 1. Recent studies using three-dimensional fluid-attenuated inversion recovery (3D-FLAIR) 24 hours after administration of bilateral intratympanic gadolinium (Gd) injection and similar techniques have demonstrated abnormalities consistent with endolymphatic hydrops. MRI at this point, however, is not yet established as useful in affirming the diagnosis of Ménière's disease.

Differential Diagnosis

Vestibular neuritis causes a single attack of vertigo, sometimes with acute hearing loss (labyrinthitis), but it can usually be distinguished from Ménière's disease because vestibular neuritis has a lifetime recurrence rate of only 2%, whereas Ménière's vertigo attacks recur multiple times and cause fluctuating and gradual decline in hearing.

When a patient reports episodic vertigo attacks in the absence of unilateral tinnitus, ear fullness, and hearing loss, one must be cautious in diagnosing Ménière's disease because vestibular migraine

---

BOX 1   Diagnostic Criteria for Ménière's Disease

Definite Ménière's Disease
1. Two or more spontaneous attacks of vertigo, each lasting 20 minutes to 12 hours
2. Audiometrically documented low- to mid-frequency SNHL in the affected ear on at least 1 occasion before, during, or after 1 of the episodes of vertigo
3. Fluctuating aural symptoms (hearing loss, tinnitus, or ear fullness) in the affected ear
4. Other causes excluded by other tests

Probable Ménière's Disease
1. At least 2 episodes of vertigo or dizziness lasting 20 minutes to 24 hours
2. Fluctuating aural symptoms (hearing loss, tinnitus, or fullness) in the affected ear
3. Other causes excluded by other tests

Basura GJ, Adams ME, Monfared A, et al: Clinical practice guideline: Ménière's disease, *Otolaryngol Head Neck Surg* 162:415–434, 2020.

(basilar-type migraine) can produce a similar pattern. Diagnostic criteria have been published for vestibular migraine.

Benign paroxysmal positional vertigo causes brief recurrent spells of spinning without hearing loss, so it is rarely confused with Ménière's disease.

Vertebrobasilar insufficiency can cause isolated vertigo, but the duration is usually only several minutes and without hearing loss, whereas Ménière's attacks last hours and are associated with unilateral auditory symptoms.

Acoustic neuroma (vestibular schwannoma) typically leads to slowly progressive unilateral sensorineural hearing loss, but vertigo is infrequently a prominent feature because patients compensate gradually as their vestibular function wanes due to compressive effects of the tumor.

Fluctuating unilateral hearing loss, ear fullness, and tinnitus can occur without vertigo and is referred to as cochlear hydrops. Such symptoms can precede the development of vertigo but may be treated as Ménière's nonetheless. Lermoyez's syndrome refers to transiently improved hearing and tinnitus during attacks of vertigo. More commonly, however, hearing declines around and during vertigo spells.

Treatment
Medical Management
Treatment of Ménière's disease is mainly aimed at preventing the vertigo attacks, but no treatments are known that reliably restore or arrest hearing loss or tinnitus. It is presumed that if attacks of vertigo, ear fullness, fluctuating hearing, and tinnitus are all stopped, hearing should stabilize, but this is still a supposition. The management of Ménière's is hierarchical, starting with a low-sodium diet and a diuretic and proceeding to more-invasive or destructive surgical procedures only when initial medical treatment fails. When a patient has very frequent vertigo attacks and is disabled, more-aggressive treatment may be considered sooner.

Dietary sodium should be restricted to 1000 to 1500 mg daily. The average person consumes about 4000 mg daily, and the maximum recommended daily intake of sodium is 2300 mg. Because more than 70% of the daily sodium comes from processed foods, this dietary restriction generally requires more than simply stopping the use of table salt, which generally accounts for only about 10% of daily sodium intake for most people.

A diuretic is usually added to the sodium restriction. The most commonly prescribed diuretic is hydrochlorothiazide 25 mg combined with triamterene 37.5 mg (Dyazide)[1] because this combination usually obviates the need for potassium supplementation. Acetazolamide (Diamox)[1] 125 to 250 mg bid or furosemide (Lasix)[1] 10 to 20 mg daily are also options. Patients with severe sulfa allergy can use low-dose ethacrynic acid (Edecrin)[1] 12.5 to 25 mg daily.

An acute attack of vertigo from Ménière's disease can be managed with vestibular suppressants such as dimenhydrinate (Dramamine)[1] 50 mg, meclizine (Antivert) 25 to 50 mg, diazepam (Valium)[1] 2 to 5 mg, or promethazine (Phenergen)[1] 12.5 to 50 mg. Scopolamine in patch form (Transderm-Scōp)[1] is too slow to be useful because it takes hours to be absorbed transdermally. Scopace (oral scopolamine) has been discontinued and is no longer being manufactured in the United States. Scopolamine tablets[1] may be available in certain compounding pharmacies. Nausea can additionally be managed with prochlorperazine (Compazine) 10 mg orally or 25 mg by suppository, with oral or sublingual ondansetron (Zofran)[1] 4 to 8 mg, or with other antiemetics. Generally, the vertigo attacks subside in several hours even without treatment.

Betahistine hydrochloride or dihydrochloride[2] may also be helpful in Ménière's, although it is not commonly used in the United States. The role of betahistine is not firmly established, although it is widely prescribed for vertigo throughout the world. Betahistine may be helpful when successful medical management with diet and diuretics has helped but is inadequate to stop attacks. Betahistine is a vasodilator, a modest H_1 histamine agonist, and a powerful H_3 histamine receptor antagonist. Its method of action in Ménière's is unknown, though it may influence perfusion of the stria vascularis to reduce pressure in the endolymphatic space. Doses of betahistine may start at 8 mg PO three times daily and may be increased to 48 mg three times daily. It is available outside the United States in the form of Serc®, Vertin®, Vertipress®, Betavert® and many other trademarks throughout the world. Betahistine may be made within the United States at compounding pharmacies with a physician prescription[1] and may also be imported from outside the United States for personal use. This is often done using an encapsulated powder form of betahistine dihydrochloride USP (from manufacturers such as Fagron, Inc., St. Paul, MN USA) by weight in capsules with or without filler. Side effects are few, although occasionally patients report some gastrointestinal upset or mild headache. Betahistine is not histamine, and has not been found to cause or aggravate urticaria.

Oral corticosteroids are often used but rarely seem effective except in cases of bilateral Ménière's resulting from autoimmune inner ear disease (AIED). Oral corticosteroids rarely seem to be effective in typical Ménière's disease.

Ménière's attacks have been said to be triggered by caffeine, chocolate, stress, visual stimuli, and dropping barometric pressure. Such triggers should be avoided when possible, but strong associations with these triggers can also occur in migrainous vertigo. Vestibular rehabilitative therapy is not generally helpful in Ménière's because most vertigo attacks remit and the patients have few vestibular symptoms between attacks. However, when vestibular loss has occurred and the patient appears to have not compensated well for it, vestibular rehabilitation can be helpful.

Bilateral Ménière's Disease
The estimated incidence of bilateral Ménière's disease varies in the literature but is estimated to occur in about 15% of cases and bilateral involvement increases over time. The possibility of bilateral involvement weighs on the decision-making for any procedures that sacrifice hearing or vestibular function because it leaves the patient with only one functioning labyrinth.

Serviceability of Hearing
Serviceable hearing is residual hearing that can be useful to the patient by wearing hearing aids. In general, because hearing loss is permanent, one should avoid sacrificing any serviceable hearing.

Injections and Surgical Treatments
Patients who continue to have disabling vertigo despite a low-salt diet, diuretics, and possibly betahistine are considered to have failed conservative medical therapy. The next step in treatment depends on the age, health status, and residual hearing and vestibular function of the patient and also on the surgeon's opinion and experience with the various options. If spells are infrequent, symptomatic management of vertigo attacks may be the best option. Table 1 outlines some of the additional interventional options.

Intratympanic Gentamicin
Transtympanic gentamicin (Garamycin)[1] administration has become increasingly used as an effective treatment of Ménière's disease. This is partly due to the ease of administration of gentamicin and its relative safety. Gentamicin is a commonly used aminoglycoside antimicrobial agent with activity against gram-negative bacteria that also happens to be ototoxic. It damages hair cells of the labyrinth and preferentially affects hair cells of the vestibular neuroepithelium over that of the cochlea. Even so, transtympanic administration still has some risk of causing hearing loss. Gentamicin is administered by injecting a small amount (usually about 0.5 mL) of gentamicin sulfate (80 mg/2 mL) solution through the tympanic membrane into the middle ear space. To avoid rapid drainage through the eustachian tube, the injection is done with the patient supine and kept in that position for an hour or so to allow the gentamicin to absorb through the round window into the inner ear. There are many protocols, but commonly an injection is given once, and additional injections can be considered every 3 to 4 weeks until improvement in vertigo attacks is realized. Studies suggest that intratympanic gentamicin is an effective treatment for vertigo complaints in Ménière's disease but there is some risk of hearing loss.

---

[1]Not FDA approved for this indication.
[2]Not available in the United States.

---

[1]Not FDA approved for this indication.

TABLE 1   Procedures Used in the Management of Ménière's Disease

METHOD	TECHNIQUE	ADVANTAGES	DISADVANTAGES
Procedures Intended to Spare Serviceable Hearing			
Intratympanic corticosteroids	Injection of steroid through the tympanic membrane to the middle ear to be absorbed in the inner ear	Minimally invasive, few side effects	Effectiveness unclear when compared to placebo
Intratympanic gentamicin (Garamycin)[1]	Injection of gentamicin through the tympanic membrane to the middle ear to be absorbed in the inner ear	Simple office-based procedure, low risk profile	Number of injections is unpredictable; some risk of hearing loss
Endolymphatic mastoid shunt	Placing a shunt from the endolymphatic sac to the mastoid air cells	Effective in 50%–75% of cases; low risk of hearing loss; day procedure	Vertigo can recur; effectiveness depends on surgical experience and technique
Vestibular neurectomy	Surgical sectioning of the vestibular part of cranial nerve VIII, sparing the auditory part of the nerve	Highly effective in eliminating vertigo attacks	Requires general anesthesia; risk of facial weakness, hearing loss
Procedures Expected to Eliminate Residual Hearing			
Labyrinthectomy or cochleosacculotomy	Several methods of removing all or part of the labyrinth	Highly effective in stopping vertigo attacks	Inevitable complete hearing loss

[1]Not FDA approved for this indication.

Endolymphatic Sac Surgery

Another option for patients with residual functional hearing is endolymphatic sac shunt or decompression. This procedure eliminates vertigo in 50% to 75% of those treated. Nevertheless, its effectiveness compared with placebo has remained a point of contention based on a number of studies. It has been suggested that the procedure's effectiveness depends on the operative technique and experience of the surgeon.

Intratympanic Steroids

Sometimes, a trial of intratympanic corticosteroids may be offered (Basura, 2020), although its effectiveness in controlled trials is still not compelling. Even so, a trial of corticosteroids administered in this manner poses little risk.

Vestibular Neurectomy

The most definitive procedure for stopping vertigo attacks in Ménière's when the goal is to preserve hearing is vestibular neurectomy. This procedure involves craniotomy and severing the vestibular nerve while preserving the cochlear nerve. This procedure requires overnight hospitalization and general anesthesia, and it does pose some risk to facial nerve function and hearing on the affected side.

Labyrinthectomy

For patients who have unilateral Ménière's disease and no serviceable hearing, labyrinthectomy is a commonly used procedure. This procedure entails the removal of the membranous labyrinth and is highly effective in stopping recurrent vertigo attacks from that ear. In elderly patients or those who are poor surgical candidates, a more limited transtympanic cochleosacculotomy may be performed.

Meniett Treatment

The Meniett device is a portable, low-frequency, pressure-wave delivery system that administers a wave of pressure of about 12 cm H_2O to the middle ear via a tympanostomy tube for about 0.6 seconds pulsed at 6 Hz for 5 minutes about three to five times daily. Quality randomized trials demonstrating effectiveness of this treatment are lacking, and it is recommended by a recent evidence-based guideline that this treatment should NOT be prescribed (Basura, 2020).

Monitoring

Following patients with Ménière's disease should include monitoring of the frequency and severity of vertigo spells and the fluctuation in hearing, ear fullness, and tinnitus. Periodic audiometry is probably the most sensitive measure of stabilization of the condition. Vestibular testing may be considered when changes might alter the treatment strategy. Brain imaging is only helpful in excluding other disorders, but does not yet have an established role in the management of Ménière's disease.

Complications

Known complications include the progression of unilateral and occasionally bilateral hearing and vestibular function. There may also be complications associated with some of the treatments as described earlier. Owing to the unpredictability of the vertigo attacks, many patients avoid certain activities and might even develop agoraphobic features because the attacks are so severe and disruptive. In most cases, these avoidance behaviors improve if Ménière's disease can be controlled.

Conclusion

The management of Ménière's disease is still part art and part science. Treatment options are many, but patients should be reassured that, in most cases, something can be offered to help improve their vertigo and quality of life.

References

Basura GJ, Adams ME, Monfared A, et al: Clinical practice guideline: Ménière's disease, *Otolaryngol Head Neck Surg* 162:415–434, 2020.

Hoskin JL. Ménière's disease: new guidelines, subtypes, imaging, and more, *Curr Opin Neurol* 35:90–97, 2022.

Luca P, Ralli M, Cassandro C, et al: Surgical Management of intractable Meniere's disease. *Int Tinnitus J* 26(1):50–56, 2022.

Nevoux J, Franco-Vidal V, Bouccara D, et al: Diagnostic and therapeutic strategy in Ménière's disease. Guidelines of the French Otorhinolaryngology-Head and Neck Surgery Society (SFORL), *Eur Ann Otorhinolaryngol Head Neck Dis*, 134(6):441–444, 2017.

Pullens B, van Benthem PP: Intratympanic gentamicin for Ménière's disease or syndrome, *Cochrane Database Syst Rev*(3), 2011. https://doi.org/10.1002/14651858.CD008234.pub2. CD008234.

Rizk HG, Mehta NK; Qureshi U. et al. Pathogenesis and etiology of Meniere's disease: a scoping review of a century of evidence. *JAMA Otolryngal Head Neck Surg* 148(4):360–368, 2022.

Wichova H, Miller ME, Derebery MJ: Otologic manifestations after COVID-19 vaccination: the House Ear Clinic experience, *Otol Neurotol* 42:e1213–e1218, 2021.

Yaz F, Ziylan F, Smeeing DPJ, Thomeer HGXM: Intratympanic treatment in Meniere's disease, efficacy of aminoglycosides versus corticosteroids in comparison studies. A systemic review, *Otology and Neurotology* 41(1):1–10, 2020.

OTITIS EXTERNA

Method of
Kimberly Williams, MD

CURRENT DIAGNOSIS

- Pain, itching, or fullness of the ear
- Tenderness of tragus, pinna, or both
- Onset <48 h
- Physical examination findings of erythema, edema, ± drainage and debris

CURRENT THERAPY

- Aural toilet
- Topical antimicrobials
- Analgesic treatment

Otitis externa is an inflammation of the ear canal and can be either acute or chronic. It is often called swimmer's ear.

Epidemiology
Acute otitis externa is a common problem seen in the primary care office. The annual incidence falls between 1:100 and 1:250 with a lifetime incidence approaching 10%. Peak incidence is in children 7 to 12 years old. It does appear to have a genetic link, because it occurs more often in people with blood group type A. Chronic otitis externa affects 3% to 5% of the population.

Risk Factors
Otitis externa is more common in warmer climates with high humidity. Increased water exposure, especially from swimming, places a person at higher risk. Other risk factors include debris from dermatologic conditions such as psoriasis, trauma due to use of hearing aids and ear plugs and abrasions from cleaning of the ear canal. Cerumen helps prevent microbial growth by providing an acidic pH; when cerumen is removed in cleaning, an environment ready for microbial growth is set up.

Pathophysiology
Approximately 95% of acute otitis externa is due to bacterial infection (Figure 1). The other 5% can be attributed to fungal infections or, less commonly, herpes zoster. Fungal infection is more common in chronic otitis externa. Of the bacterial infections, 20% to 60% are due to *Pseudomonas aeruginosa*. *Staphylococcus aureus* is the next major causative organism. Gram-negative organisms account for 2% to 3% of bacterial infections.

Prevention
Prevention is aimed at avoiding water accumulation and retention in the ear canal. Using ear plugs while swimming and using a hair dryer to dry the ear canal after water exposure can be beneficial. The use of acidifying eardrops, such as acetic acid 2% (Vosol), before and after swimming can also help prevent otitis externa. Other preventive measures include stopping the removal of cerumen and avoiding trauma to the ear canal. Finally, proper treatment of dermatologic conditions such as eczema and psoriasis can help reduce debris that can be a risk factor for infection.

Clinical Manifestations
Otitis externa usually develops rapidly over 1 to 2 days. Most patients complain of a feeling of ear pain, fullness, or itching. Hearing loss may be another symptom. Key physical examination findings include tenderness on palpation of the tragus, discomfort with traction on the pinna, edema of the ear canal, and erythema of the canal. Pain may be out of proportion to examination findings.

Figure 1 Acute otitis externa with the canal somewhat narrowed from edema and obstructed by desquamating epithelium, soft cerumen, and purulent discharge; this must be removed to visualize the tympanic membrane and to allow ototopical therapy to penetrate to all the superficially infected areas of the canal skin. Reprinted with permission from Osguthorpe JD, Nielsen DR. Otitis externa: review and clinical update. *Am Family Physician.* 2006;74(9):1510–1516.

Regional lymphadenitis and cellulitis of the pinna and adjacent skin can also be present.

Diagnosis
The diagnosis of otitis externa is made clinically by history and physical examination. The history should be positive for otalgia, itching, or sense of fullness. The exam should be positive for tenderness if the tragus is palpated or if the pinna is pulled up and out. If the cause is bacterial, purulent drainage is usually present. Otoscopy will show diffuse canal edema, usually present with erythema. Often there will be copious amounts of debris. Debris should be cleared to visualize the tympanic membrane. There should be good mobility of the tympanic membrane and the tympanometry curve will be normal unless there is concomitant acute otitis media.

Differential Diagnosis
Middle ear disease should be distinguished from external disease by ensuring that the tympanic membrane is normal. Acute otitis media with perforation of the tympanic membrane may result in purulent middle ear secretions into the external ear canal. Contact dermatitis of the ear canal can mimic otitis externa, and a thorough history of exposure to metals such as nickel and copper, chemicals such as new soaps, topical antibiotics, detergents, cosmetics, and other irritants should be obtained. Fungal infection of the ear canal can mimic bacterial otitis externa. Fungus tends to infect the medial portion of the ear canal and has spores and filaments that can be seen both macroscopically and microscopically. Also in the differential are carcinoma of the external auditory canal, which mimics chronic infection; herpes, which is rare and forms vesicles on the outer ear canal; and radiation therapy.

Therapy
Topical therapy is the treatment of choice in mild to moderate disease in healthy patients. The choice of topical agent is based on cost, ease of administration, and risk of side effects (Table 1). Topical aminoglycoside and fluoroquinolone antibiotics have a response rate of more than 70%. If there is a perforation of the tympanic membrane, ciprofloxacin topical solutions are preferred because of the risk of ototoxicity from aminoglycosides and neomycin. Using a topical steroid in conjunction with topical antibiotic therapy has been shown to shorten duration of ear pain. Duration of topical therapy should be 7 to 10 days. Clotrimazole 1%[1] may be used for superficial fungal infections of the ear canal.

---

[1]Not US Food and Drug Administration approved for this indication.

TABLE 1	Topical Otic Preparations for Treatment of Otitis Externa.		
ACTIVE DRUGE	**BRAND NAME**	**DOSING**	**COMMENTS**
Acetic acid 2% solution with steroid	Vosol HC, Acetasol HC	q4–6h	Can sting/local irritation
Ciprofloxacin/ hydrocortisone	Cipro HC	q12h	Approved if tympanic membrane is perforated
Ciprofloxacin/ dexamethasone	Ciprodex	q12h	Approved if tympanic membrane is perforated
Neomycin, polymyxin B, hydrocortisone	Cortisporin Otic	q6h	Neomycin can cause local irritation, ototoxic potential
Ofloxacin	Floxin Otic	q24h	Can cause local irritation
Tobramycin[1]	Tobrex	q6h	Minimally irritating, ophthalmic preparation, ototoxic potential
Gentamycin[1]	Garamycin	q6h	Ophthalmic preparation, ototoxic potential

[1]Not FDA approved for this indication.

For the topical therapy to be effective, it must be delivered to the tissue of the ear canal. First, the canal must be cleared of debris. This can be done in the physician's office under direct visualization or with lavage of the ear canal using saline or hydrogen peroxide warmed to body temperature. The patient should then be instructed on the proper delivery of the eardrops. Eardrops are administered more effectively if another person delivers the drops. The patient should lie on his or her side with the affected ear up, and drops should be placed in the ear canal until it is filled. The patient should remain on his or her side for 3 to 5 minutes. If greater than 50% of the canal is edematous, a wick made of cellulose material should be placed to facilitate delivery of the drops. The wick may fall out or can be removed by either patient or clinician once the edema has resolved.

Systemic therapy should be used in patients who are immune compromised, including those with diabetes, and in patients with surrounding cellulitis. The systemic therapy chosen should be effective against pseudomonas.

Adequate pain control is another important factor in the treatment of otitis externa. Often this can be achieved with nonsteroidal antiinflammatory medications, but opioid analgesics may be necessary, especially to remove debris. Analgesics should be used early in treatment of the disease.

Monitoring

Patients should respond to therapy in 48 to 72 hours. If therapy fails, the clinician should evaluate adherence to therapy and ability of the drug to be delivered properly. Alternative diagnoses should be considered, including fungal infections, dermatitis, foreign bodies, and middle ear disease with perforation of the tympanic membrane. If the infection has spread outside of the ear canal, systemic therapy should be started.

Complications

One complication of simple otitis externa is malignant otitis externa, an invasive infection of the external auditory canal causing osteomyelitis of the temporal bone. It most commonly occurs in elderly diabetic patients or the immunocompromised. Complications include meningitis, dural sinus thrombosis, cranial abscess, and cranial nerve neuropathy including facial nerve paralysis. Diagnosis may require computed tomography and cultures. Treatment includes systemic antipseudomonal antibiotics and surgical débridement. Contact dermatitis from the topical antimicrobials prescribed for otitis externa may also complicate treatment. This is due to a delayed-type hypersensitivity reaction to one or more of the components of the topical therapy. Neomycin is the most common cause, but hypersensitivity reactions can also occur from other agents including preservatives and fragrances. The reaction is characterized by pruritus, edema, and inflammation of the skin in the auditory canal. It can spread beyond the canal to the pinna and even the skin of the neck. This is treated with topical steroids and by stopping the offending agent.

References

Kaushik V, Malik T, Saeed SR: Interventions for acute otitis externa. *Cochrane Database of Systematic Reviews* 2010, Issue 1. Art. No.: CD004740. https://doi: 10.1002/14651858.CD004740.pub2.

Long M. Otitis externa. *Pediatrics in Review* 2013; 34 (3):133–134.

Rosenfeld RM, Brown L, Cannon CR, et al: Clinical practice guideline: acute otitis externa. *Otolaryngology—Head Neck Surg* 2006; 134:S4.

Schaefer P, Baugh R: Acute Otitis Externa: An update. *Am Fam Physician* 2012; 86(11):1055–1061, 2012.

OTITIS MEDIA

Method of
Gretchen Irwin, MD, MBA

CURRENT DIAGNOSIS

- History of acute onset of symptoms
- Middle ear effusion
  - Bulging tympanic membrane
  - Limited mobility of tympanic membrane or air fluid level visible behind tympanic membrane
- Middle ear inflammation
  - Erythema of tympanic membrane or distinct otalgia

CURRENT THERAPY

- Watchful waiting—appropriate for children:
  - Older than 2 years of age with nonsevere illness
  - Older than 6 months of age with uncertain diagnosis and nonsevere illness
  - Older than 2 years of age with severe illness, but uncertain diagnosis
    - Need close follow-up in 48 hours
    - Consider delayed prescription
- Antibiotics
  - First-line therapy should be amoxicillin (Amoxil) 80 to 90 mg/kg/day[3]
  - Treat 10 days if child younger than 6 years of age, 5 to 7 days if older than 6 years of age
  - Follow up if not improving in 48 hours
- Analgesia
  - Acetaminophen (Tylenol), ibuprofen (Motrin, Advil)
  - Antihistamines and decongestants are of no benefit

- Surgery—consider tympanostomy tubes when:
  - First acute otitis media (AOM) episode at younger than 6 months of age and child with two or more episodes in 6 months or three episodes in 24 months
  - First AOM episode at older than 12 months of age and child with three episodes in 6 months, five episodes in 12 months, or seven episodes in 24 months

[3]Exceeds dosage recommended by the manufacturer.

Epidemiology

Acute otitis media (AOM) is a common condition of childhood, with 1 in 4 children having at least one episode of AOM by 10 years of age. In fact, 86% of children will have at least one episode of AOM within the first year of life. Younger children are more likely to be affected, with a peak incidence noted between 6 and 20 months of age, likely because of the relative immaturity of the immune system and eustachian tube function. On average, $5 billion are spent per year on office visits, lost productivity, and diminished parental quality of life as a result of AOM infections. As a result, research has focused on effective strategies both to prevent episodes of AOM and also to efficiently treat episodes that do occur.

Risk Factors

Identifying children at risk for AOM has been an important strategy to attempt to limit instances of AOM. Unfortunately, many of the risk factors associated with AOM are not modifiable, including male sex, Native American ethnicity, presence of siblings within the home, and a family history of recurrent AOM. Additional risk factors include low socioeconomic status, premature birth, attendance at out-of-home daycare, lack of breastfeeding, and history of poor maternal health during pregnancy. Limited studies have suggested that interventions such as avoiding supine feeding or bottle propping, reducing pacifier use after the first 6 months of life, and eliminating passive tobacco exposure can help reduce the incidence; however, the evidence in which these interventions demonstrate clear impact is limited. Public health programs that encourage breastfeeding and optimal maternal health during pregnancy as well as those focused on reducing tobacco use have perhaps the best opportunity to affect AOM incidence rates. Not only are these identified risk factors for any episode of AOM, but children with these characteristics are also more likely to have recurrent AOM. Although many children will be affected in their lifetimes, those with recurrent disease are most at risk of complications leading to morbidity or mortality.

Other risk factors specifically for recurrent AOM include an early onset of the first episode and low parental education. Pathophysiology AOM has classically been associated with three bacteria, namely, *Streptococcus pneumoniae, Moraxella catarrhalis,* and *Haemophilus influenzae.* The introduction of pneumococcal vaccines has led to a shifting in the frequency with which each pathogen causes disease. In 1999, *S. pneumoniae* was responsible for 40% to 45% of acute otitis media, while *H. influenzae* was responsible for 25% to 30%. In 2017, the bacteria were responsible for 15% to 25% and 50% to 60% of infections, respectively. The frequency of *M. catarrhalis* infections has remained consistent at 12% to 15%. The bacteria responsible for AOM become pathogenic in the setting of eustachian tube dysfunction. A relative obstruction of the eustachian tube develops most commonly secondary to secretions from an antecedent viral upper respiratory infection or allergies, but it may result from neuromuscular conditions or abnormal anatomy. Such relative obstruction creates a negative pressure within the middle ear leading to serous effusion and secondary infection of this collection of interstitial fluid. Thus prevention of AOM is aimed at both reducing the presence of pathogenic bacteria and preventing upper respiratory infections that may create eustachian tube dysfunction. Interestingly,

during the COVID-19 pandemic, cases of otitis media in children decreased. This may be a result of infection control measures such as widespread use of masks or avoidance of healthcare as a strategy to avoid contracting COVID-19.

Prevention

The successes of immunization programs in virtually eliminating childhood illnesses such as measles, polio, and varicella have led to great interest in the development of vaccines capable of eradicating the causative agents of AOM. Immunizations targeting the specific bacteria most commonly associated with AOM have had mixed success, however. For example, although the serotypes contained in the 7-valent pneumococcal conjugate vaccine (PCV, Prevnar) are responsible for approximately 66% of pneumococcal-related AOM, only moderate effectiveness has been noted in reducing AOM incidence among vaccinated children. After the introduction of the 7-valent PCV into practice in February 2000, the incidence of AOM decreased only 6% to 7% among vaccinated children. The 9-valent and 11-valent PCVs2 have been shown to result in a risk reduction of *S. pneumoniae* isolates in children with AOM of 17% and 34%, respectively. An increase in serotype 19A has been noted that is not covered in the 7-, 9-, or 11-valent PCVs2 but is included in the new 13-valent PCV (Prevnar 13). The 13-valent PCV was incorporated into the recommended childhood immunization schedule in February 2010. Since 2010, there has been a steady decline in otitis media attributable to *S. pneumoniae*. Similar vaccines are in development for *H. influenzae* and *M. catarrhalis* as causative agents of AOM. The current *H. influenzae* b vaccine (Hib) has had little impact on AOM because less than 5% of episodes are caused by the type b strain of *Haemophilus*. Instead, nontypeable *H. influenzae* is a much more common cause of AOM. Although the vaccines targeting specific bacteria that have been shown to cause AOM have been successful, so too has the influenza vaccine been shown to affect the course of AOM. In several studies, children who received seasonal influenza vaccine (Fluzone) were found to have fewer episodes of AOM than unvaccinated children. Furthermore, those who did have an AOM episode were found to use fewer antibiotics and have shorter duration of middle-ear effusion compared with unvaccinated counterparts.

With evidence that reducing the incidence of viral influenza may reduce the occurrence of secondary AOM, several other interventions aimed at reducing viral upper respiratory infection incidence have been studied for their impact on AOM rates. The use of zinc[7] and propolis[7] as agents to prevent viral upper respiratory infections, for instance, has been shown to have mixed benefit in reducing AOM in children. In multiple studies, zinc has been well tolerated with no contraindications to use identified. Zinc as a single agent has been shown to prevent AOM only when used in children younger than 5 years of age who are also malnourished. However, when combined with propolis, zinc was shown to be effective at reducing AOM episodes for children with a history of recurrent AOM. Of note, in several trials zinc did not reduce upper respiratory infection rates; rather, rates of secondary AOM alone were decreased. Although not necessarily effective as a preventive measure for all children, zinc and propolis may be an option for children with recurrent infections.

Similarly, probiotics[7] added to infant formula have been shown to be beneficial for some children. Although breastfeeding has been shown to be most beneficial in preventing AOM compared with formula supplementation, infant formulas supplemented with *Lactobacillus rhamnosus* GG and *Bifidobacterium lactis* Bb-12 (Enfamil Premium, Nestlé Good Start) were shown to reduce the incidence of AOM over the first 7 months and the first year. Children who received placebo formula had an incidence of AOM of 50% in the first 7 months, whereas children who received the probiotic-supplemented formula had an incidence of only 22%.

---

[7] Available as a dietary supplement.

Dietary supplementation to limit AOM is not limited to infant formulas, however. Xylitol,[7] a polyol sugar alcohol found in birch plants, plums, strawberries, and raspberries, has been demonstrated in several studies to be effective at preventing both dental caries and AOM, although its dosage forms make administration difficult. Xylitol is available as a chewing gum, which raises concern as a choking hazard in young children. Similarly, in its oral syrup form, xylitol must be administered five times daily to be effective. Studies of thrice-daily dosing have not been able to demonstrate the same preventive effect as dosing five times daily despite a consistent total daily dose of 10 grams per day. Furthermore, emerging evidence suggests that xylitol must be given daily to remain effective at reducing AOM episodes because prophylaxis only during winter months or use only during upper respiratory tract infections is ineffective. Of note, children who have already received tympanostomy tubes receive no prevention benefit from xylitol administration. Research is ongoing to increase physician awareness of xylitol as a possible prophylactic measure because current studies suggest less than one-half of U.S. physicians are aware of xylitol, and less than one-fourth discuss or recommend its use to patients.

Echinacea[7] and osteopathic manipulation have also been cited as potential prophylactic treatments, particularly for children at high risk of recurrence. However, little evidence exists that either are effective. In fact, one large study demonstrated an increased risk of AOM with echinacea use during an upper respiratory tract infection episode and no benefit to manipulation treatment. Ongoing studies are examining the use of these modalities.

Clinical Manifestations

AOM presents with a rapid onset of symptoms that may include fever, chills, ear pain, or ear pulling. In fact, ear pulling and ear rubbing have been demonstrated to be quite sensitive for the diagnosis of AOM in the setting of a history consistent with AOM and middle ear effusion. Often, symptoms may be preceded by upper respiratory symptoms such as rhinorrhea, cough, or congestion. Children who have had tympanostomy tubes placed will likely have a far different presentation, with fever and pain being quite unlikely; rather, a thin, yellow or milky discharge may be the only sign that AOM is present.

Diagnosis

The 2013 update of the guidelines of the American Academy of Pediatrics (AAP) for the diagnosis and treatment of AOM acknowledged that no gold standard exists for the clinical diagnosis of AOM. History and physical examination should be consistent with rapid onset of inflammation in the middle ear. Both pneumatic otoscopy and tympanometry may be useful in the diagnosis of AOM. Tympanic membranes should be evaluated for position, mobility, color, and degree of translucency using pneumatic otoscopy to assess for presence of middle ear effusion or inflammation. Moderate to severe bulging of the tympanic membrane, new onset of otorrhea without other cause, or mild bulging of the tympanic membrane with intense erythema or ear pain should prompt diagnosis of AOM. Furthermore, tympanometry may be useful in determining whether an effusion is present if the diagnosis is otherwise unclear.

One concern of physicians has been accurately diagnosing middle ear inflammation after a child has been vigorously crying. A study of 125 healthy children, age younger than 30 months, assessed the impact of crying on tympanic membrane color by performing otoscopy both before and after administering at least two immunizations. Although crying can cause a pinkening of the tympanic membrane, it should disappear when the child quiets and should be less intense than what is observed with inflammation. True middle ear inflammation results in an angry, red eardrum, not the milder, pink flush seen with vigorous crying. The presence of effusion should also help support a diagnosis of inflammation.

Differential Diagnosis

Otitis media with effusion (OME) is often misdiagnosed as an episode of AOM. Like AOM, OME is common, with 2.2 million episodes annually, representing an estimated cost of $4 billion. OME can also occur with a viral upper respiratory infection and may follow or precede an episode of AOM. OME differs from AOM, however, because fluid may be present in the middle ear with OME, but there are no signs of acute infection. Although OME is not associated with acute infection, it is nonetheless critical to diagnose because research has demonstrated that chronic OME is associated with hearing loss and subsequent developmental delay. In fact, OME in infancy has been shown to be associated with, on average, a 7-point reduction in IQ at 7 years of age. The cornerstone of treatment for OME is observation for 2 to 3 months to allow the effusion to clear. Avoidance of allergens and tobacco exposure that may worsen eustachian tube dysfunction is also important. Decongestants and antihistamines are not effective. If an effusion does not clear within 2 months, a single course of amoxicillin (Amoxil) or penicillin may be given.

Audiometry should be performed in all children with OME for longer than 3 months or, in the setting of language delay, learning problems or suspected hearing loss in a child with OME. If the effusion persists or if a child has multiple episodes of OME or has hearing or learning difficulties as a result of OME, surgical intervention should be considered. Initial surgical intervention for children with persistent OME should be myringotomy with placement of tympanostomy tubes. Tonsillectomy and myringotomy alone are not indicated for treatment of OME. However, adenoidectomy may have a role, particularly in children 4 to 8 years of age. Current recommendations include adenoidectomy only if repeat surgery for OME is needed. However, emerging evidence suggests that adenoidectomy may decrease the need for surgical retreatment, reduce ongoing hearing loss, and be of benefit during initial surgery for older children.

Treatment

The treatment of AOM has been controversial in recent years. Because it is the most common childhood bacterial infection for which antibiotics are prescribed worldwide, debate continues about both the most effective regimen and appropriate time to treat AOM. On average, $2.8 billion are spent per year on antibiotics for episodes of AOM, yet emerging evidence suggests that watchful waiting is appropriate for some children. However, schema that involve watchful waiting have not been fully embraced by U.S. physicians. Judicious use of antibiotic therapy remains key in the prevention of morbidity and mortality associated with otitis media but is not an appropriate therapy for every child. All children require analgesia of some type as well as close, scheduled follow-up, but use of observation or an antibiotic varies with severity of illness and age of the child. Treatment options are summarized in Table 1.

Treatment Options

Observation

For some children with AOM, observation has been shown to be an appropriate therapy that avoids the possible side effects of antibiotics, with low risk of complications developing from an untreated otitis media. Evidence suggests that 78% of AOM episodes will spontaneously resolve within the first few days of infection. In fact, for every 100 otherwise healthy at-risk children with AOM, 80 will improve within 3 days without antibiotic therapy. If the same 100 children were all treated with amoxicillin or ampicillin, 92 would improve, although 3 to 10 would develop a rash and 5 to 10 would develop diarrhea. Thus, in a typical family medicine practice, 16 children with AOM would need to be treated with antibiotics to prevent 1 child from experiencing ongoing otalgia, whereas 1 of every 24 children treated will experience harm related to therapy. Hence, the use of antibiotics is not without risk. Multiple studies have demonstrated that even in children as young as 2 months of age, many will improve

TABLE 1	Treatment Options for Acute Otitis Media					
	AOM WITH OTORRHEA		**AOM WITHOUT OTORRHEA**		**AOM WITH SEVERE SYMPTOMS***	
AGE OF CHILD	UNILATERAL	BILATERAL	UNILATERAL	BILATERAL	UNILATERAL	BILATERAL
6 months to 2 years	Antibiotics	Antibiotics	Antibiotics or observation	Antibiotics	Antibiotics	Antibiotics
>2 years	Antibiotics	Antibiotics	Antibiotics or observation	Antibiotics or observation	Antibiotics	Antibiotics

*Severe symptoms include toxic-appearing child, persistent otalgia for >48 hours, temperature >39°C in the past 48 hours, or uncertain access to follow-up.
AOM, Acute otitis media.

without antibiotic therapy, and delaying antibiotics may prevent undesirable side effects without exposing the child to undue risk. No studies have demonstrated a resurgence of either mastoiditis or meningitis with implementation of watchful waiting for AOM. If observation is chosen as a management strategy for AOM, it is important to reevaluate the child in 48 to 72 hours to ensure that they are improving and that a rescue antibiotic is prescribed if symptoms are not resolving.

Delayed prescriptions are one strategy that has been effective at reducing antibiotic use, maintaining parental satisfaction, and improving healthcare efficiency. Physicians are often concerned that parental satisfaction will decrease if watchful waiting for an episode of AOM is recommended. Interestingly, satisfaction has been tied to the receipt of an antibiotic prescription, though not necessarily the administration of antibiotics to the child. Declines in satisfaction are noted when parents are advised to return to care in 2 to 3 days if the child is not improving while undergoing watchful waiting. By offering a delayed prescription, the parent can avoid the difficulties associated with needing to be seen again if the child fails to improve, and parental satisfaction is maintained even if the child never receives any medication. Parents should be educated that up to one-third of children who initially are treated with observation will eventually need antibiotic therapy. Although this suggests that up to two-thirds of children can avoid unnecessary antibiotics, parents should be aware that many children will go on to need antibiotic therapy. Clearly, however, not every child is a candidate for observation therapy.

Antibiotic Therapy

Antibiotic therapy may be associated with less duration of pain, less analgesic use, and less absence for both children and parents from school and work, respectively. The AAP and the American Academy of Family Physicians in a joint position statement have recommended that, when a decision is made to use antibiotics, amoxicillin (Amoxil) be given as a first-line agent at a dose of 80 to 90 mg/kg/day.[3] For penicillin-allergic children, cefdinir (Omnicef), cefpodoxime (Vantin), or cefuroxime (Ceftin) may be used. Although the cross-reactivity of cephalosporins and penicillins is likely lower than previously believed, if concern exists about treating a child with a cephalosporin, clindamycin[1] (30 to 40mg/kg/day)[3] may be used. Macrolide antibiotics may have limited efficacy. Ceftriaxone (Rocephin) may be used as a single dose for a child who is unable to tolerate oral medications. Although amoxicillin continues to be the preferred first-line agent, 30% to 70% of *S. pneumoniae* strains have become penicillin and macrolide resistant, whereas 20% to 40% of *H. influenzae* has beta-lactamase–producing capabilities. Given the various resistance patterns of organisms, a child who fails to improve on amoxicillin should receive amoxicillin with clavulanate (Augmentin) or ceftriaxone as second-line therapy. Clindamycin (Cleocin) or tympanocentesis to identify a causative organism may also be

considered. Current evidence continues to suggest that a 10-day course is optimal for children younger than 2 years of age. Less benefit to longer-duration therapy is noted in older children, and therefore a shorter 5- to 7-day course is recommended for those older than 2 years of age. If a child has a perforation of the tympanic membrane, treatment considerations may be slightly different. Oral antibiotics continue to be recommended if perforation is a result of the AOM episode; however, if a child has an episode of AOM with tympanostomy tubes in place, topical 0.3% ciprofloxacin/0.1% dexamethasone (Ciprodex Otic) should be added to oral amoxicillin. Table 2 provides antibiotic dosing recommendations. Regardless of the decision to implement watchful waiting or antibiotic therapy, any child with AOM should be expected to improve within 48 to 72 hours. If improvement is not occurring, the child should be reevaluated.

Surgery

For some children, AOM will not be an isolated event. Instead, the child will have recurrent infections and require multiple antibiotic courses throughout a year, prompting consideration of tympanostomy tube placement. Currently, referral for evaluation for tympanostomy tubes is recommended when a child has had three or more episodes of AOM within a 6-month period or more than four episodes within a 12-month period. Some have argued, however, that this recommendation should be considered within the context of the child's age at first presentation. A child who has the first episode of AOM before 6 months of age is likely to go on to have many more episodes. Ultimately, they will likely meet the criteria for myringotomy and thus may warrant a more aggressive approach from the outset. Conversely, a child who presents with a first episode of AOM as an older child is less likely to have recurrent episodes and can therefore be treated in a more conservative manner. Using an age-stratified approach, children who experience a first episode of AOM before 6 months of age should receive tympanostomy tubes if they have two episodes in a 6- or 12-month time period or three episodes in 24 months. Similarly, children who have a first episode of AOM after 1 year of age should receive tympanostomy tubes only if they have three episodes within 6 months, five within 12 months, or seven within 24 months. Referral may also occur if a child has a history of AOM associated with meningitis, facial nerve paralysis, coalescent mastoiditis, or brain abscess. Tympanostomy tubes are also often placed because of prolonged OME resulting in hearing loss and language delay. Myringotomy without tube placement may be considered for either diagnosis of an infection that has not responded to numerous antibiotics or for relief of severe otalgia. AOM episodes will continue to occur despite tympanostomy tube placement. However, episodes will likely be less severe, of shorter duration, and less frequent. In addition to ongoing AOM episodes, tympanostomy tubes can be problematic if they become clogged. New studies in animal models suggest that applying colchicine[1] in the external ear may prevent this complication.

---

[1] Not FDA approved for this indication.
[3] Exceeds dosage recommended by the manufacturer.

[1] Not FDA approved for this indication.

TABLE 2	Antibiotic Selection for Specific Patient Populations			
	ANTIBIOTIC OF CHOICE	**DOSE (MG/KG/DAY)**	**ROUTE**	**DURATION OF THERAPY**
AOM in child older than 2 years	Amoxicillin (Amoxil)	80–90[3]	PO	5–7 days
AOM in child younger than 2 years	Amoxicillin	80–90[3]	PO	10 days
AOM in child with allergy to penicillin	Cefdinir (Omnicef)	14	PO	10 days
	Cefpodoxime (Vantin)	10	PO	5 days
	Cefuroxime (Ceftin)	30	PO	10 days
AOM with inability to tolerate oral medications	Ceftriaxone (Rocephin)	50	IV/IM	1 day
AOM with amoxicillin failure	Amoxicillin with clavulanate (Augmentin)	90 of amoxicillin and 6.4 of clavulanate[3]	PO	10 days
	Ceftriaxone (Rocephin)	50	IV/IM	3 days[3]
AOM with amoxicillin/clavulanate failure	Ceftriaxone (Rocephin)	50	IV/IM	3 days[3]
AOM with ceftriaxone failure and tympanocentesis not available	Clindamycin (Cleocin)[1]	30–40[3]	PO	10 days
Perforated tympanic membrane	Amoxicillin	80–90[3]	PO	10 days
Tympanostomy tube in place	Amoxicillin and topical 0.3% ciprofloxacin/0.1% dexamethasone (Ciprodex Otic)	80–90 8 drops	PO Topical bid	10 days 7 days

AOM, Acute otitis media; *IM,* intramuscular; *IV,* intravenous; *PO,* by mouth.
[1]Not FDA approved for this indication.
[3]Exceeds dosage recommended by the manufacturer.

Analgesia

Regardless of a decision to pursue watchful waiting or antibiotics, analgesics are an important component in the treatment of AOM. Multiple homeopathic interventions and home remedies including application of heat, ice, or mineral oil (Min-O-Ear)[1] have been used for pain control, although no studies exist to verify their effectiveness. Acetaminophen (Tylenol), ibuprofen (Motrin), narcotics, and tympanostomy have all been demonstrated to be effective at reducing pain. However, the side effects of altered mental status, gastrointestinal upset, and respiratory depression with narcotics as well as the skill needed to perform tympanostomy limit the usefulness of these interventions in primary care practice. Antihistamines and decongestants have often been prescribed in an attempt to reduce the fluid volume in the middle ear and hence provide relief. Unfortunately, use of antihistamines and decongestants has been shown to result in a fivefold to eightfold increase in the risk of side effects with no benefits, including no decreased time to cure, no prevention of surgery or complications, and no increased symptom resolution. Therefore antihistamines and decongestants have not been routinely recommended.

Conclusion

AOM continues to be one of the most costly and common childhood illnesses in developed nations throughout the world. Successful management of this condition requires much more than choosing amoxicillin at an appropriate dose and duration or appropriately timing a surgical referral. Vigilant attention to modifying risk factors when possible, promoting immunization, and limiting the spread of viral illnesses has been shown to prevent AOM instances. Furthermore, adhering to diagnostic criteria to attempt to accurately distinguish between AOM and OME as well as implementing observation when appropriate can significantly reduce antibiotic usage, thereby minimizing side effects for patients and the opportunity to develop resistance in pathogens.

RED EYE

Lynn Fisher, MD; and John N. Dorsch, MD

CURRENT DIAGNOSIS

- Bacterial, viral, and allergic conjunctivitis can often be distinguished by the course of spread in the eye, the type of ocular discharge present, and associated symptoms.
- Subconjunctival hemorrhage can occur from trauma, increased intrathoracic pressure, anticoagulants, or idiopathically.
- Physicians should consider referring to an ophthalmologist patients with traumatic injury to the eye, loss of vision, extreme pain not explained by pathology, keratitis, suspected uveitis or glaucoma, chemical injury, or nonhealing corneal abrasion.

CURRENT THERAPY

- Do not use eye patches in patients with corneal abrasions.
- Do not use topical anesthetics for the eye outside a clinic or hospital setting because corneal toxicity can occur.
- Patients with corneal abrasions should be reexamined the following day.
- Patients with corneal abrasions from extended-wear contact lenses often become colonized with *Pseudomonas aeruginosa* and should be treated with appropriate antibiotics (quinolones).

In the primary care office, the most common causes of red eye are conjunctivitis, subconjunctival hemorrhage, and corneal abrasions due to a foreign body. Other common causes of red eye include blepharitis and hordeolum. Less common but serious causes of red eye include viral keratitis, uveitis, scleritis, and angle-closure glaucoma. Other usually less serious causes of red eye include episcleritis, pinguéculum, and pterygium. All primary care physicians should have expertise in recognizing and treating the common causes of red eye and should recognize and refer patients with higher-stakes diagnoses (Boxes 1 and 2).

BOX 1 | Approach to the Patient with Red Eye

The following questions are often helpful in making the diagnosis in patients with red eyes.

- *Is one eye or are both eyes involved?* Infections, allergy, and systemic illness are more likely to cause bilateral eye involvement.
- *Does the patient have intense eye pain?* If yes, likely diagnoses include acute angle closure glaucoma, uveitis, scleritis, keratitis, foreign body, or corneal abrasion.
- *Does the patient have a foreign body sensation?* If so, consider corneal abrasion, trauma, dry eye, keratitis, and other corneal disorders.
- *Is there a discharge?* If it is very copious and purulent, consider gonococcal conjunctivitis. If it is discolored and purulent, consider bacterial conjunctivitis. Copious watery discharge is typical of viral conjunctivitis. Stringy, mucoid discharge is typical of allergic or chlamydial conjunctivitis.
- *Do the eyes itch?* If so, consider blepharitis or allergy in the differential.
- *Are the eyelids swollen?* Consider allergy or infection.
- *Do the eyelids have lumps?* Hordeolum and chalazion should be considered.
- *Do the eyes burn?* Consider blepharitis or dry eye.
- *Is the eye redness recurrent?* Consider herpes keratitis, uveitis, and allergic conjunctivitis.
- *Does the patient have photophobia?* Corneal problems (abrasions, keratitis) and uveitis should be considered.
- *Is there loss of vision?* Consider corneal ulcer, uveitis, and angle closure glaucoma.
- *Is the patient using ocular medications?* Prolonged use of neomycin and sulfa ophthalmic medications can cause sensitization and redness of the eyes.

BOX 2 | Red Eye

Common Causes
- Conjunctivitis: bacterial, viral, allergic
- Subconjunctival hemorrhage
- Corneal abrasion
- Blepharitis

Less Common Causes
Less Serious
- Episcleritis
- Pinguéculum
- Pterygium

More Serious
- Viral keratitis
- Uveitis
- Scleritis
- Angle closure glaucoma

Physical Examination

Always check visual acuity in any patient with an eye complaint. Fluorescein strips (Flu-Glo, Fluorets), topical anesthetic drops, and cobalt blue light are used to examine the cornea for abrasions, keratitis, and ulceration. Cotton-tipped applicators are used to evert the upper eyelid and look for a foreign body.

Pupillary reaction is often affected by angle closure glaucoma and uveitis, but it is rarely affected by conjunctivitis, blepharitis, and corneal disorders. The pupil may be irregular in the patient with uveitis.

Patients with uveitis often have pain in the closed affected eye when a bright light is shined in the normal eye or with convergence of the eyes. This is due to consensual reflex of the pupils to light and accommodation.

Examine the conjunctiva by pulling the lower eyelid down with the examiner's finger. If the bulbar or palpebral conjunctivae are inflamed (i.e., hyperemic, edematous, discharge), conjunctivitis is present. Palpable preauricular nodes may be present with viral conjunctivitis and chlamydial conjunctivitis.

Conjunctivitis

Conjunctivitis is the most common cause of red eye encountered by primary care clinicians. Among the etiologies of conjunctivitis, viral conjunctivitis is the most common. Although patients with conjunctivitis might have some minor irritation of the eyes, they usually do not complain of pain in the eye or loss of vision. Ocular discharge is generally considered to be an important diagnostic feature of conjunctivitis (Table 1). Although much has been written about characterizing conjunctivitis by the nature of the discharge, one meta-analysis failed to find evidence of the diagnostic usefulness of clinical signs or symptoms in distinguishing bacterial conjunctivitis from viral conjunctivitis.

Viral Conjunctivitis

Viral conjunctivitis is often seen in epidemics and is most commonly caused by members of the Adenovirus family. Typically, viral conjunctivitis starts in one eye and spreads to the other eye a few days later. The conjunctivae appear red and swollen, with copious watery discharge (Figure 1). The natural course of viral conjunctivitis is self-limiting, lasting 10 to 14 days. Tender preauricular lymph nodes, when present, indicate the presence of viral or chlamydial conjunctivitis. Management should be directed at scrupulous hygiene. Patients must be informed that their infection is highly contagious. They should avoid close contact with other persons (e.g., towels, direct contact, swimming pools) for 2 weeks and wash hands or use hand sanitizer frequently to prevent the spread of their infection. Topical antibiotics have been prescribed to try to prevent bacterial superinfection, but there is no good evidence that they have any significant impact. Symptomatic treatment with cold compresses and topical vasoconstrictors may be helpful. Conjunctivitis has been reported in patients with coronavirus. If a patient has a red eye with burning and watery discharge that is also associated with fever, cough, shortness of breath, fatigue, or loss of taste/smell, coronavirus should be considered as a potential cause. Clinically significant conjunctivitis was observed in less than 4% of inpatients and 2% of outpatients with confirmed mild to moderate coronavirus from one 2020 study in a training and research hospital in Istanbul, Turkey. There is no specific treatment for conjunctivitis caused by coronavirus.

Bacterial Conjunctivitis

Bacterial conjunctivitis typically starts abruptly in one eye and spreads to the other eye in 1 to 2 days. Usually a purulent discharge is present that persists throughout the day. A variety of gram-positive and gram-negative organisms cause bacterial conjunctivitis, but the most common causes are *Staphylococcus aureus*, *Streptococcus pneumoniae*, and *Haemophilus pneumoniae*. Treatment of bacterial conjunctivitis is usually empiric, but conjunctival scraping for smears and cultures should be done in infants, immunocompromised patients, and patients

TABLE 1	Conjunctivitis		
TYPE	COURSE	CHARACTERISTICS	DISCHARGE
Bacterial	Starts in one eye, often spreads to other eye		Purulent
Allergic	Accompanies allergic rhinitis	Itchy eyes	Mucus
Viral	Usually bilateral	Very red eyes	Watery

Figure 1 Viral conjunctivitis. Reproduced with permission from the University of Michigan Kellogg Eye Center, https://www.kellogg.umich.edu.

with hyperacute conjunctivitis in which *Neisseria gonorrhoeae* or *Chlamydia trachomatis* infection is suspected. Treatment of bacterial conjunctivitis (excluding gonococcal or chlamydial conjunctivitis) usually consists of a topical antibiotic used four times a day (Table 2). Topical antibiotics are usually prescribed for 5 to 7 days, and resolution of conjunctivitis is expected within that time.

Hyperacute bacterial conjunctivitis has an abrupt onset, copious purulent discharge, and rapid progression, and it is usually associated with gonococcal infection in a sexually active patient. Chemosis (edema of the conjunctivae) may be present.

Chlamydial conjunctivitis is acquired through exposure to infected secretions from the genital tract, either direct or indirect. The infection is usually unilateral (at least initially), and often there is involvement of the preauricular node on the ipsilateral side. Gonococcal and chlamydial infections are treated systemically (Box 3).

Conjunctivitis of the Newborn

Chlamydial conjunctivitis is the most common cause of infectious conjunctivitis of the newborn in the United States. Onset of conjunctivitis is 3 to 10 days after birth, but it has been reported as late as 2 months after birth. Erythromycin ointment (Ilotycin 0.5%) or tetracycline ointment[2] given shortly after delivery is effective in preventing chlamydial conjunctivitis but not systemic chlamydial infections. *Chlamydia trachomatis* infections, causing pneumonia and otitis media, can be treated either with ethylsuccinate (EryPed Drops) orally 50 mg/kg/day in four divided doses for 14 days or azithromycin (Zithromycin)[1] 20 mg/kg/day orally up to 1 g daily for 3 days. Chlamydial infections of rectal and urogenital sites can only be treated with erythromycin ethylsuccinate orally 50 mg/kg/day in four divided doses for 14 days.

Gonococcal conjunctivitis of the newborn is a hyperacute infection that occurs 2 to 4 days after birth. It can cause corneal ulceration and loss of vision. Gonococcal conjunctivitis can be prevented with silver nitrate drops[2] or erythromycin (Ilotycin) or tetracycline ointment[2] administered shortly after delivery. Silver nitrate commonly causes a self-limited chemical conjunctivitis, which can delay visual bonding of the infant to the parents in the

---

[1]Not FDA approved for this indication.
[2]Not available in the United States.

TABLE 2	Topical Antibiotics Used to Treat Bacterial Conjunctivitis	
DRUG	DOSAGE	
Bacitracin (Ak-Tracin, Bacticin) ointment	Apply 0.5 inch in eye q3–4 h	
Ciprofloxacin (Ciloxan) 0.3% ophthalmic solution	1–2 gtt in eye q15 min × 6 h, then q30 min × 18 h, then q1 h × 1 d, then q4 h × 12 d[3]	
Gatifloxacin (Zymaxid) 0.5% ophthalmic solution	1 gtt in eye q2 h up to 8 ×/d on day 1, then 1 gtt 2–4 ×/day on day 2–7	
Gentamicin (Gentak, Gentasol) 0.3% ophthalmic solution or ointment	Ointment: 0.5 inch applied to eye 2–3 times per day Solution: 1–2 gtt in eye q4 h	
Levofloxacin (Quixin) 0.5% ophthalmic solution	1–2 gtt in eye q2 h × 2 d while awake, then q4 h while awake × 5 d	
Moxifloxacin (Vigamox) 0.5% ophthalmic solution	1 gtt in eye tid × 7 d	
Neomycin/polymyxin B/ gramicidin (Neosporin) ophthalmic solution	1–2 gtt in eye q4 h × 7–10 d	
Ofloxacin (Ocuflox) 0.3% ophthalmic solution	1–2 gtt in eye q2–4 h × 2 d, then 1–2 gtt in eye qid × 5 d	
Polymyxin B and trimethoprim (Polytrim) ophthalmic solution	1 gtt in eye q3 h × 7–10 d	
Sulfacetamide (Isopto Cetamide, Ocusulf-10, Sodium Sulamyd, Sulf-10, AK-Sulf) 10% ophthalmic solution, ointment	Ointment: 0.5-inch ribbon in eye q3–4 h and q h × 7 d Solution: 1–2 gtt in eye q2–3 h × 7–10 d	
Tobramycin (AK-Tob, Tobrex) 0.3% ophthalmic solution	1–2 gtt in eye q4 h	

[3]Exceeds dosage recommended by the manufacturer.

BOX 3	Treatment of Chlamydial and Gonococcal Conjunctivitis

Chlamydial Conjunctivitis
- Doxycycline (Vibramycin) 100 mg PO bid × 7 days
- Or
- Azithromycin (Zithromax) 1 g PO X 1
- Treat partners

Gonococcal Conjunctivitis
- Ceftriaxone (Rocephin 1 g IM x 1 in patients ≥150 kg, or 500 mg IM x 1 in patients <150 kg)
- Azithromycin (Zithromax) 1 g PO x 1

first few hours of life. Gonococcal conjunctivitis of the newborn is treated with Ceftriaxone (Rocephin) 25 to 50 mg/kg up to 125 mg IM/IV.

Conjunctivitis–Otitis Media Syndrome

Conjunctivitis–otitis media syndrome is a common condition in which children with otitis media also have purulent bilateral ocular discharge. It responds to treatment of otitis media; no topical treatment of conjunctivitis is required.

Methicillin-Resistant *Staphylococcus Aureus* Conjunctivitis

Increasing numbers of cases of bacterial conjunctivitis are caused by methicillin-resistant *S. aureus* (MRSA). MRSA conjunctivitis manifests as bacterial conjunctivitis resistant to conventional therapy and is treated with the same drugs used to treat MRSA in other parts of the body (Doxycycline [Vibramycin],[1] vancomycin [Vancocin], sulfamethoxazole-trimethoprim [Bactrim][1]). Cultures should be obtained when MRSA is suspected.

Allergic Conjunctivitis

Allergic conjunctivitis is an immunoglobulin E (IgE)-mediated condition characterized by bilateral eye involvement, itchy eyes, and mucoid discharge. *Seasonal* conjunctivitis is caused by exposure to common allergens (e.g., pollens, dander) and usually accompanies allergic rhinitis. *Perennial* allergic conjunctivitis is similar to seasonal allergic conjunctivitis, but the symptoms are usually less severe. Patients are usually treated with a systemic antihistamine. Ophthalmic (topical) medications include antihistamine or decongestants, mast cell inhibitors, nonsteroidal antiinflammatory drugs (NSAIDs), H[1]-antagonists, and various combinations of these (Table 3). Milder cases can be treated with a decongestant-antihistamine combination for about 2 weeks. Moderate to more severe cases can require longer use of these medications or the addition of systemic antihistamines or mast cell inhibitors. Some patients require topical corticosteroids or cyclosporine (Restasis)[1] for severe allergic conjunctivitis, but these should be evaluated by an ophthalmologist because of potential complications of therapy.

Subconjunctival Hemorrhage

In subconjunctival hemorrhage, the redness of the eye is localized and sharply circumscribed, and the underlying sclera is not visible (Figure 2). Conjunctivitis is not present, and there is no discharge. There is typically no pain or visual change. Subconjunctival hemorrhage may be spontaneous, but it can also result from trauma, hypertension, bleeding disorders, or increased intrathoracic pressure (e.g., straining, coughing, retching). No treatment is necessary, but investigation may be warranted if the etiology is in question or the hemorrhage is recurrent. Referral to an ophthalmologist should be considered if the subconjunctival hemorrhage is from trauma or has not resolved within 2 to 3 weeks.

Corneal Abrasion

Corneal abrasions typically result from scratching of the corneal epithelium due to trauma, but they can also occur from extended-wear contact lenses. Patients with corneal abrasions present with pain, excessive tearing from the involved eye, photophobia, a foreign-body sensation (like having sand in the eye), and blurry vision.

Corneal abrasions are identified by staining the cornea with fluorescein and examining under cobalt blue light (Figure 3). The eye should also be examined carefully to check for foreign bodies. Topical anesthetic is administered to make the patient comfortable during the examination, but continued use can cause corneal damage.

Management of corneal abrasions consists of pain relief and prevention of infection. Pain can be relieved with topical NSAIDs such as ketorolac (Acular)[1] and diclofenac (Voltaren),[1] oral over-the-counter analgesics, and occasionally oral narcotics. Topical antibiotics are usually prescribed to prevent infection. Antibiotic ointments are lubricating and soothing to the eye, making them

---

BOX 4	Patient Hygiene Measures for Conjunctivitis

- Do not wear contact lens until the conjunctivitis has cleared and resume wear with a new set. Wear and clean your contact lens as recommended by your eye doctor.
- Avoid touching the eyes and if you do, immediately wash your hands. Use a clean towel or tissue each time you wipe your face and eyes.
- Wash your hands or use hand sanitizer frequently. Always wash them before and after eating, after using bathroom, and after sneezing/coughing.
- Do not use eye makeup while an eye is infected with conjunctivitis. Replace eye makeup if the eye becomes infected and never share makeup.

---

[1]Not FDA approved for this indication.

545

TABLE 3	Topical Medications for Allergic Conjunctivitis

GENERIC NAME	BRAND NAME(S)	DOSING	MODE OF ACTION
Azelastine 0.05% solution	Optivar	1 gtt in eye(s) bid	H[1]-antagonist, mast cell inhibitor
Cromolyn 4% solution	Crolom, generic	1–2 gtt in eye(s) 4–6 times per day	Mast cell inhibitor
Emedastine 0.05% solution	Emadine	1 gtt in eye(s) qid	H[1]-antagonist
Epinastine 0.05% solution	Elestat	1 gtt in eye(s) bid	H[1]- and H[2]-antagonist, mast cell inhibitor
Ketorolac 0.5% solution	Acular	1 gtt in eye(s) qid up to 1 week	NSAID
Diclofenac 0.1% solution[1]	Voltaren ophthalmic	1 gtt in eye(s) qid × 2 weeks	NSAID
Lodoxamide 0.1% solution	Alomide	1–2 gtt in eye(s) qid up to 3 months	Mast cell inhibitor
Loteprednol 0.2% susp.	Alrex	1 gtt in eye(s) qd	Corticosteroid
Naphazoline/pheniramine (solution)	• Naphcon-A (OTC) • Opcon-A (OTC) • Visine-A (OTC)	1–2 gtt in eye(s) qd-qid prn	Antihistamine, decongestant
Nedrocomil 2% solution	Alocril	1–2 gtt in eye(s) bid	H[1]-antagonist, mast cell inhibitor
Olopatadine 0.1% solution	Patanol	1 gtt in eye(s) bid	H[1]-antagonist, mast cell inhibitor
Olopatadine 0.2% solution	Pataday	1 gtt in eye(s) qd	Mast cell inhibitor

[1]Not FDA approved for this indication.
NSAID, Nonsteroidal antiinflammatory drug.

a good option for traumatic corneal abrasions. Topical ophthalmic antibiotic ointments commonly used are bacitracin (Bacticin), erythromycin (Ilotycin), and gentamicin (Gentak).

In patients who have corneal abrasions from contact lens overwear, eyes are commonly colonized with *Pseudomonas aeruginosa*. These patients should be treated with topical antibiotics such as ciprofloxacin (Ciloxan) or ofloxacin (Ocuflux) solutions.

Patching of the eye, though a common practice of the past, has not shown evidence of benefit in recent studies. It was found that eye patching can actually cause harm, so this practice is no longer recommended.

Infrequently, patients have traumatic uveitis accompanying corneal abrasion. Traumatic uveitis usually causes significantly more pain than a corneal abrasion, and, if uveitis is suspected, the clinician should consider referral to an ophthalmologist.

Patients with corneal abrasions should be reexamined in 24 hours. Corneal abrasions typically should be healed or greatly improved in 24 hours. If the abrasion is not completely healed after 24 hours, the patient should be examined again in 2 or 3 days. Referral should be considered if any worsening occurs or if the abrasion does not heal within 5 days. Corneal abrasions can be prevented by using protective eyewear.

Other Causes of Red Eye

Other causes of red eye are somewhat less common.

Blepharitis

Blepharitides are inflammatory conditions of the eyelid caused by infection or obstruction of eyelid glands (Table 4). Blepharitis may be accompanied by conjunctivitis. Staphylococcal blepharitis arises from the accessory glands to the eyelashes and causes discharge from the eyelid, often associated with erythema, induration, loss of eyelashes, and crusting of the eyelid (Figure 4). This is treated with hot, moist packs to the eyes, baby shampoo scrubs (3 oz. water and 3 drops baby shampoo used on a washcloth bid), and erythromycin ointment (Ilotycin) at bedtime. Seborrheic blepharitis, a more chronic form of blepharitis, arises from the meibomian glands and causes scaling of the eyelids (Figure 5). Seborrheic blepharitis is often associated with skin disorders such as rosacea, eczema, and seborrheic dermatitis. This is treated with hot, moist packs and baby shampoo scrubs. Resistant cases are treated with oral tetracycline (Sumycin) (or one of its derivatives).

Hordeolum (Stye)

A hordeolum is an acute, painful mass of the eyelid that is caused by inflammation of the glands (Figure 6). It does not usually cause the eye to become red as well. Warm compresses to the eyelid four times a day for 3 to 5 minutes typically causes resolution within 1 week. Because they arise from the same glands, hordeola and blepharitis commonly occur together.

Episcleritis

Episcleritis is a self-limited inflammation of the episcleral vessels and is believed to be autoimmune. It has a rapid onset and usually minimal discomfort. Redness is most often confined to a sector of the eye. Episcleritis usually resolves in 7 to 10 days. Recurrence is not uncommon. Oral NSAID drugs may be prescribed, but treatment is usually not necessary.

Scleritis

Scleritis is, fortunately, much less common than episcleritis. Patients with scleritis experience intense inflammation and deep eye pain. Scleritis is commonly associated with rheumatoid arthritis and inflammatory bowel disease. The patient should be promptly referred to an ophthalmologist if scleritis is suspected.

Figure 2 Subconjunctival hemorrhage. Reprinted with permission from American Academy of Ophthalmology: Managing the red eye. eye care skills for the primary care physician series. San Francisco: American Academy of Ophthalmology, 2001.

Figure 3 Corneal abrasion with fluorescein stain with cobalt blue light. Reprinted with permission from American Academy of Ophthalmology: Managing the red eye. eye care skills for the primary care physician series. San Francisco: American Academy of Ophthalmology, 2001.

TABLE 4	Blepharitis		
TYPE	**SITE OF ORIGIN**	**CLINICAL CHARACTERISTICS**	**TREATMENT**
Staphylococcal	Accessory glands of eyelids	Erythema and induration of eyelid; crusting; discharge; loss of eyelashes	• Warm compresses • Baby shampoo scrubs • Erythromycin ointment (Ilotycin)
Seborrheic	Meibomian glands	More chronic, scaling	1. Warm compresses 2. Baby shampoo scrubs 3. Oral tetracycline for resistant cases

Figure 4 Staphylococcal blepharitis. Reprinted with permission from American Academy of Ophthalmology: Managing the red eye. eye care skills for the primary care physician series. San Francisco: American Academy of Ophthalmology, 2001.

Figure 5 Seborrheic blepharitis. Reprinted with permission from American Academy of Ophthalmology: Managing the red eye. eye care skills for the primary care physician series. San Francisco: American Academy of Ophthalmology, 2001.

Figure 6 Hordeolum. Reprinted with permission from American Academy of Ophthalmology: Managing the red eye. eye care skills for the primary care physician series. San Francisco: American Academy of Ophthalmology, 2001.

Acute Angle Closure Glaucoma

Acute angle closure glaucoma is characterized by acute ocular pain and is often accompanied by vomiting, blurred vision, acute photophobia, pupils unreactive to light, and circumcorneal redness (ciliary flush). Treatment of glaucoma with pilocarpine (Isopto Carpine), topical timolol (Timoptic), and acetazolamide (Diamox) should be started, and the patient should be given an urgent referral to an ophthalmologist.

Anterior Uveitis

Uveitis is the inflammation of the iris and ciliary muscle, often associated with autoimmune disease. Trauma can also cause uveitis. Signs of uveitis include ocular pain, ciliary flush, and occasionally irregularity of the pupil. Prompt referral should be arranged for a patient in whom uveitis is suspected.

In general, referral to an ophthalmologist should be considered for the following:

- Traumatic injury to the eye
- Loss of vision
- Extreme eye pain not explained by pathology
- Keratitis
- Suspected uveitis or glaucoma
- Chemical injury (especially alkali)
- Corneal abrasion not healing

References

Ackay B, Kardes E, Kiray G, et al: Evaluation of ocular symptoms in COVID-19 subjects in inpatient and outpatient settings, *International Ophthalmology* 41:1541–1548, 2021.

American Optometric Association: *Optometric clinical practice guideline: Care of the patient with anterior uveitis*, June 23, 1994. Revised March 1999. PDF available at www.aoa.org/documents/CPG-7.pdf. June 23, 1994 [accessed July 10, 2015].

Arbour JD, Brunette I, Boisjoly HM, et al: Should we patch corneal abrasions? *Arch Ophthalmol* 115(3):313–317, 1997.

Au YK, Henkind P: Pain elicited by consensual pupillary reflex: a diagnostic test for acute iritis, *Lancet* 2:1254–1255, 1981.

Avdic E, Cosgrove SE: Management and control strategies for community-associated methicillin-resistant *Staphylococcus aureus, Expert Opin Pharmacother* 9(9):1463–1479, 2008.

Boder F, Marchant C, et al: Bacterial etiology of conjunctivitis-otitis media syndrome, *Pediatrics* 76:26–28, 1985.

Bradford CA: *Basic Ophthalmology* San Francisco, ed 8, 2004, American Academy of Ophthalmology.

Centers for Disease Control and Prevention. Zika Virus. Symptoms, diagnosis, and treatment. Available at www.cdc.gov/zika/symptoms. Accessed Feb. 3, 2016.

Centers for Disease Control and Prevention: *Sexually Transmitted Diseases Treatment Guidelines*, 2015. Available at www.cdc.gov/std/tg2015/default.htm. Accessed May 25, 2021.

De Toledo AR, Chandler JW: Conjunctivitis of the newborn, *Infect Dis Clin North Am* 6(4):807–813, 1992.

Frith P, Gray R, MacLennan S, et al: *The Eye in Clinical Practice*, Oxford, 1994, Blackwell Scientific.

Jackson WB: Blepharitis: Current strategies for diagnosis and treatment, *Can J Ophthalmol* 43(2):170–179, 2008.

Khan J, Mack H: Management of conjunctivitis and other causes of red eye during the COVID-19 Pandemic, *AJGP* 49(10):656–661, 2020.

Kimberlin D, Brady M, Jackson M: *Red Book. Report of the Committee on Infectious Diseases*, ed 31, AAP Committee on Infectious Diseases, 2018.

Liebowitz HM: The red eye, *N Engl J Med* 343(5):345–351, 2000.

Patterson J, Fetzer D, Krall J, et al: Eye patch treatment for the pain of corneal abrasion, *South Med J* 89(2):227–229, 1996.

Prochazka AV: Diagnosis and treatment of red eye, *Primary Care Case Reviews* 4:23–31, 2001.

Rietveld RP, van Weert H, Riet G, Bindels P: Diagnostic impact of signs and symptoms in acute infectious conjunctivitis: systematic literature search, *BMJ* 327(4):789, 2003.

Tarabishy A: Jeng B: Bacterial conjunctivitis: A review for internists, *Cleve Clin J Med* 75(7):507–512, 2008.

Talbot EM: A simple test to diagnose iritis, *BMJ* 295:812–813, 1987.

Trobe JD: *The Physician's Guide to Eye Care*, ed 2, San Francisco, 2001, Foundation of the American Academy of Ophthalmology.

Wilson SA, Last A: Management of corneal abrasion, *Am Fam Physician* 70:123–130, 2004.

Wong AH, Barg SS, Leung AK: Seasonal and perennial allergic conjunctivitis, *Recent Pat Inflamm Allergy Drug Disc* 3(2):118–127, 2009.

RHINOSINUSITIS

Method of
Ann M. Aring, MD

CURRENT DIAGNOSIS

- Because inflammation of the sinuses rarely occurs without concurrent inflammation of the nasal mucosa, rhinosinusitis is a more accurate term for what is commonly called sinusitis.
- Most cases of sinusitis are caused by viral infections associated with the common cold. Viral rhinosinusitis improves in 7 to 10 days.
- Four signs and symptoms with a high likelihood ratio for acute bacterial sinusitis are double sickening, purulent rhinorrhea, erythrocyte sedimentation rate (ESR) >10mm, and purulent secretion in the nasal cavity. A combination of at least three of these four symptoms and signs has a specificity of 0.81 and sensitivity of 0.66 for acute bacterial rhinosinusitis.
- Acute rhinosinusitis lasts up to 4 weeks, subacute rhinosinusitis lasts from 4 to 12 weeks, and chronic rhinosinusitis lasts 12 weeks or longer. Recurrent acute rhinosinusitis is defined as four or more episodes per year with complete resolution between episodes.
- Radiographic imaging in a patient with acute rhinosinusitis is not recommended unless a complication or an alternative diagnosis is suspected. Computed tomography of the sinuses without contrast media is the imaging method of choice.

CURRENT THERAPY

- Mild rhinosinusitis symptoms of less than 7 days' duration can be managed with supportive care including analgesics, saline nasal irrigation, and intranasal corticosteroids.
- Antibiotic therapy is recommended for patients with sinusitis symptoms that do not improve within 7 to 10 days or that worsen at any time.
- First-line antibiotics include amoxicillin with or without clavulanate.
- Macrolides and trimethoprim sulfamethoxazole (Bactrim) are not recommended for empiric therapy owing to high rates of resistance among *Streptococcus pneumoniae* and *Haemophilus influenzae*.
- For adults allergic to penicillin, doxycycline may be used as an alternative regimen for initial empiric therapy for bacterial rhinosinusitis. According to a recent US Food and Drug Administration (FDA) safety alert, fluoroquinolones such as levofloxacin (Levaquin) and moxifloxacin (Avelox) should be reserved for patients who do not have other treatment options.
- In adults with confirmed acute rhinosinusitis, more than 70% will clinically improve after 2 weeks with or without antibiotic therapy.
- Antibiotic use increases the absolute cure rate by 5% compared with placebo at 7 to 15 days.

Epidemiology of Acute Rhinosinusitis and Predisposing Factors

Each year in the United States, rhinosinusitis affects one in seven adults and is diagnosed in 31 million patients. Rhinosinusitis is the fifth most common diagnosis for which antibiotics are prescribed. Rhinosinusitis has a higher frequency in the winter months and lower frequency in the summer and autumn months.

Predisposing Factors

Predisposing factors for acute rhinosinusitis include viral upper respiratory infections and allergic rhinitis. Anatomic malformations including polyps, deviated nasal septum, foreign bodies, and tumors can also predispose to acute rhinosinusitis.

Pathogenesis and Etiology of Rhinosinusitis

Most cases of acute rhinosinusitis are caused by viral infections associated with the common cold. The most common viruses in acute viral rhinosinusitis are rhinovirus, adenovirus, influenza virus, and parainfluenza virus. Mucosal edema occurs with the viral infection with subsequent obstruction of the sinus ostia. In addition, viral and bacterial infections impair the cilia, which help transport the mucus. The ostia obstruction and slowed mucus transport cause stagnation of secretions and lowered oxygen tension within the sinuses. This environment is an excellent culture medium for both viruses and bacteria and the infectious particles grow rapidly. The body responds with an inflammatory reaction. Polymorphonuclear leukocytes are mobilized, which results in pus formation. The most common bacteria found in acute community-acquired bacterial rhinosinusitis are *S pneumoniae*, *H influenzae*, *Staphylococcus aureus*, and *Moraxella catarrhalis*. Acute adult rhinosinusitis most commonly involves the maxillary and ethmoid sinuses. More than one of the paranasal sinuses can be affected.

Diagnosis of Acute Rhinosinusitis

Diagnosis of acute bacterial rhinosinusitis requires that symptoms persist for longer than 10 days or worsen after 5 to 7 days. Four signs and symptoms with a high likelihood ratio for acute bacterial sinusitis are double sickening, purulent rhinorrhea, ESR >10mm, and purulent secretion in the nasal cavity. A combination of at least three of these four symptoms and signs has a specificity of 0.81 and sensitivity of 0.66 for acute bacterial rhinosinusitis. Table 1 lists the sensitivity, specificity, likelihood ratio, and odds ratio of criteria used to diagnose acute rhinosinusitis. If resistant pathogens are suspected or if the patient's immune system is compromised, bacterial culture of the secretions may be used for diagnosis and to direct therapy.

TABLE 1	Signs and Symptoms of Acute Bacterial Rhinosinusitis		
SIGN/SYMPTOM	**SENSITIVITY (%)**	**SPECIFICITY (%)**	**LR +**	**ODDS RATIO**
Symptoms after upper respiratory tract infection	99	8	1.1	2.1
Facial pain on bending forward	90	22	1.2	0.9
Nasal congestion	90	14	1.0	1.1
Purulent rhinorrhea	89	42	1.5	1.6
Bilateral facial pain, pressure, or fullness	78	32	1.2	1.4
Double sickening	72	65	2.1	*
Previous sinusitis	57	38	0.9	0.4
Upper teeth pain	50	50	1.0	1.2
Unilateral facial pain, pressure, or fullness	46	73	1.7	1.9

Abbreviation: LR = Likelihood ratio.
*No data given in reference.

Imaging

For uncomplicated acute rhinosinusitis, radiographic imaging is not recommended. Plain sinus radiography shows air–fluid levels in patients with both viral and bacterial rhinosinusitis. Sinus computed tomography should not be used for routine evaluation of acute bacterial rhinosinusitis. However, sinus computed tomography without contrast media can be used to identify suspected complications and define anatomic abnormalities.

Differential Diagnosis

The signs and symptoms of acute bacterial rhinosinusitis and prolonged viral upper respiratory infection are similar, which can lead to overdiagnosis of acute bacterial rhinosinusitis. Other conditions that mimic bacterial rhinosinusitis are migraine headache, tension headache, trigeminal neuralgia, and temporomandibular joint disorders.

Treatment of Acute Rhinosinusitis
Symptomatic Treatment

Mild rhinosinusitis symptoms less than 7 days in duration can be managed with supportive care including analgesics, saline nasal irrigation, and intranasal corticosteroids. There are no randomized controlled trials that evaluate the effectiveness of decongestants in patients with sinusitis. Nasal saline is used to soften viscous secretions and improve mucociliary clearance. The mechanical cleansing of the nasal cavity with saline has been shown to benefit patients with rhinosinusitis. Most studies of intranasal corticosteroids are industry sponsored. A 2013 Cochrane review found that patients receiving intranasal corticosteroids were more likely to experience symptom improvement after 15 to 21 days compared with those receiving placebo (73% vs. 66.4%; $p<.05$; number needed to treat [NNT]=15). Antihistamines should not be used for symptomatic relief of acute rhinosinusitis, except in patients with a history of allergic rhinitis.

Antibiotic Treatment

Antibiotic therapy is recommended for patients with sinusitis symptoms that do not improve within 7 to 10 days or that worsen at any time. Amoxicillin with or without clavulanate is recommended as the first-line antibiotic in adults with acute bacterial rhinosinusitis. "High-dose" amoxicillin-clavulanate (Augmentin XR) is recommended for patients with high risk of *S pneumoniae* resistance, recent antibiotic use, or treatment failure. Macrolides and trimethoprim sulfamethoxazole are not recommended for empiric therapy owing to high rates of resistance among *S pneumoniae* and *H influenzae*. Fluoroquinolones are not recommended as first-line antibiotics because they do not demonstrate benefit over beta-lactam antibiotics and are associated with a variety of adverse effects. According to a recent FDA safety alert, fluoroquinolones should be reserved for patients who do not have other treatment options.

Complications and Referral

Complications of acute bacterial rhinosinusitis are estimated to occur in 1 in 1000 cases. Patients with acute bacterial rhinosinusitis who present with visual symptoms (diplopia, decreased visual acuity, disconjugate gaze, difficulty opening the eye), severe headache, somnolence, or high fever should be evaluated with emergency computed tomography with contrast. Sinonasal cancers are uncommon in the United States, with an annual incidence of less than 1 in 100,000 patients. However, cancer should be included in the differential diagnosis. Referral to an otolaryngologist is needed if symptoms persist or progress after maximal medical therapy when computed tomography shows evidence of sinus disease. Table 2 summarizes indications for subspecialist referral in a patient with acute bacterial rhinosinusitis.

TABLE 2	Indications for Subspecialist Referral for Acute Bacterial Rhinosinusitis
Anatomic defects causing obstruction	
Complications such as orbital involvement, altered mental status, meningitis, cavernous sinus thrombosis, intracranial abscess, Pott's puffy tumor (osteomyelitis of front bone)	
Evaluation of immunotherapy for allergic rhinitis	
Frequent recurrences (3–4 episodes per year)	
Fungal sinusitis, granulomatous disease, or possible neoplasm	
Immunocompromised host	
Nosocomial infection	
Severe infection with persistent fever >102°F or 39°C	
Treatment failure after extended antibiotic courses	
Unusual or resistant bacteria	

From Aring AM, Chan MM. Current concepts in adult acute rhinosinusitis. Am Fam Physician 2016;94[2]:97–105.

References

Aring AM, Chan MM: Current concepts in adult acute rhinosinusitis, *Am Fam Physician* 94(2):97–105, 2016.

Chow AW, Benninger MS, Brook I, et al: IDSA clinical practice guideline for acute bacterial rhinosinusitis in children and adults, *Clin Infect Dis* 54(8):e72–112, 2012. Epub 2012 Mar 20.

Cornelius RS, Martin J: Wippold, FJ 2nd, et al. ACR appropriateness criteria sinonasal disease, *J Am Coll Radiol* 10(4):241–246, 2013.

DeSutter AI, Lemiengre M, Campbell H: Antihistamines for the common cold, *Cochrane Database Syst Rev* CD009345, 2015.

Hayward G, Heneghan C, Perera R, Thompson M: Intranasal corticosteroids in management of acute sinusitis: A systematic review and meta-analysis, *Ann Fam Med* 10:241–249, 2012, https://doi.org/10.1370/afm.1338.

King D, Mitchell B, Williams CP, Spurling GKP: Saline nasal irrigation for acute upper respiratory tract infections, *Cochrane Database of Syst Rev* 4, 2015, https://doi.org/10.1002/14651858.CD006821.pub3.

Lemiengre MB, van Driel ML, Merenstein D, et al: Antibiotics for acute rhinosinusitis in adults, *Cochrane Database Syst Rev* 9:CD006089, 2018.

Lindbaek M, Hjortdahl P, Johnsen U: Use of symptoms, signs, and blood tests to diagnose acute sinus infections in primary care: Comparison with computer tomography, *Fam Med* 23:183–188, 1996.

Rosenfeld RM, Piccirillo JF, Chadrasekhar SS, et al: Clinical practice guideline (update): Adult sinusitis, *Otolaryngol Head Neck Surg* 152(2S):S1–39, 2015.

U.S. Food and Drug Administration. FDA Drug Safety Communication: FDA updates warnings for oral and injectable fluoroquinolone antibiotics due to disabling side effects. Available at http://www.fda.gov/Drugs/DrugSafety/ucm511530.htm [accessed January 28, 2017].

Zalmanovici Trestioreanu A, Yaphe J: Intranasal steroids for acute sinusitis, *Cochrane Database Syst Rev* 12, 2013.

TEMPOROMANDIBULAR DISORDERS

Method of
Jeffrey P. Okeson, DMD

Temporomandibular disorder (TMD) is a collective term that includes a number of clinical complaints involving the muscles of mastication, the temporomandibular joints (TMJs) and associated orofacial structures. Other commonly used terms are Costen's syndrome, TMJ dysfunction, and craniomandibular disorders. TMDs are a major cause of nondental pain in the orofacial region and are considered a subclassification of musculoskeletal disorders. In many TMD patients the most common complaint is not with the TMJs but rather the muscles of mastication. Therefore the terms *TMJ dysfunction* or *TMJ disorder* are actually inappropriate for many of these complaints. It is for this reason that the American Dental Association adopted the term *temporomandibular disorder.*

Signs and symptoms associated with TMDs are a common source of pain complaints in the head and orofacial structures. These complaints can be associated with general joint problems and somatization. Approximately 50% of patients suffering with TMDs do not first consult with a dentist but seek advice for the problem from a physician. The family physician should be able to appropriately diagnose many TMDs. In many instances the physician can provide valuable information and simple therapies that will reduce the patient's TMD symptoms. In other instances, it is appropriate to refer the patient to a dentist for additional evaluation and treatment.

Epidemiology

Cross-sectional population-based studies reveal that 40% to 75% of adult populations have at least one sign of TMJ dysfunction (e.g., jaw movement abnormalities, joint noise, tenderness on palpation), and approximately 33% have at least one symptom (e.g., face pain, joint pain). Many of these signs and symptoms are not troublesome for the patient, and only 3% to 7% of the population seeks any advice or care. Although in the general population women seem to have only a slightly greater incidence of TMD symptoms, women seek care for TMD more often than men at a ratio ranging from 3:1 to 9:1. For many patients TMDs are self-limiting or are associated with symptoms that fluctuate over time without evidence of progression. Even though many of these disorders are self-limiting, the health care provider can provide conservative therapies that will minimize the patient's painful experience.

Signs and Symptoms

The primary signs and symptoms associated with TMD originate from the masticatory structures and are associated with jaw function (Box 1). Pain during opening of the mouth or during chewing is common. Some persons even report difficulty speaking or singing. Patients often report pain in the preauricular areas, face, or temples. TMJ sounds are often described as clicking, popping, grating, or crepitus and can produce locking of the jaw during opening or closing. Patients commonly report painful jaw muscles, and, on occasion, they even report a sudden change in their bite coincident with the onset of the painful condition.

It is important to appreciate that pain associated with most TMDs is increased with jaw function. Because this is a condition of the musculoskeletal structures, function of these structures generally increases the pain. When a patient's pain complaint is not influenced by jaw function, other sources of orofacial pain should be suspected.

The spectrum of TMD often includes commonly associated complaints such as headache, neckache, or earache. These associated complaints are often referred pains and must be differentiated from primary pains. As a general rule, referred pains associated with TMDs are increased with any activity that provokes the TMD pain. Therefore, if the patient reports that the headache is aggravated by jaw function, it could very well represent a secondary pain related to the TMD. Likewise, if the secondary symptom is unaffected by jaw use, one should question its relationship to the TMD and suspect two separate pain conditions. Pain or dysfunction due to non-musculoskeletal causes such as otolaryngologic, neurologic, vascular, neoplastic, or infectious disease in the orofacial region is not considered a primary TMD even though musculoskeletal pain may be present. However, TMDs often coexist with other craniofacial and orofacial pain disorders.

Anatomy and Pathophysiology

The TMJ is formed by the mandibular condyle fitting into the mandibular fossa of the temporal bone. The movement of this joint is quite complex as it allows hinging movement in one plane and at the same time allows gliding movements in another plane.

Separating these two bones from direct articulation is the articular disk. The articular disk is composed of dense fibrous connective tissue devoid of any blood vessels or nerve fibers. The articular disk is attached posteriorly to a region of loose connective tissue that is highly vascularized and well innervated, known as the retrodiscal tissue. The anterior region of the disk is attached to the superior lateral pterygoid muscle.

The movement of the mandible is accomplished by four pairs of muscles called the muscles of mastication: the masseter, temporalis, medial pterygoid, and lateral pterygoid. Although not considered to be muscles of mastication, the digastric muscles also play an important role in mandibular function. The masseter, temporalis, and medial pterygoid muscles elevate the mandible and therefore provide the major forces used for chewing and other jaw functions. The inferior lateral pterygoid muscles provide protrusive movement of the mandible, and the digastric muscles serve to depress the mandible (open the mouth).

When discussing the pathophysiology of TMD, one needs to consider two main categories: joint pathophysiology and muscle pathophysiology. Because etiologic considerations and treatment strategies are different for these conditions, they are presented separately.

Pathophysiology of Intracapsular TMJ Pain Disorders

Several common arthritic conditions such as rheumatoid arthritis, traumatic arthritis, hyperuricemia, and psoriatic arthritis can affect the TMJ. These conditions, however, are not nearly as common as local osteoarthritis. As with most other joints, osteoarthritis results from overloading the articular surface of the joint, thus breaking down the dense fibrocartilage articular surface and ultimately affecting the subarticular bone. In the TMJ, this overloading commonly occurs as a result of an alteration in the morphology and position of the articular disc. In the healthy TMJ, the disc maintains its position on the condyle during movement because of its morphology (i.e., the thicker anterior and posterior borders) and interarticular pressure maintained by the elevator muscles. If, however, the morphology of the disc is altered and the discal ligaments become elongated, the disk can be displaced from its normal position between the condyle and fossa. If the disc is displaced, normal opening and closing of the mouth can result in an unusual translatory movement between the condyle and the disc, which is felt as a click or pop. Disc displacements that result in joint sounds might or might not be painful. When pain is present it is believed to be related to either loading forces applied to the highly vascularized retrodiscal tissues or a general inflammatory response of the surrounding soft tissues (capsulitis or synovitis).

Pathophysiology of Masticatory Muscle Pain Disorders

The muscles of mastication are a very common source of TMD pain. Understanding the pathophysiology of muscle pain, however, is very complex and still not well understood. The simple explanation of muscle spasm does not account for most TMD

BOX 1	Common Primary and Secondary Symptoms Associated with Temporomandibular Disorders

Primary Symptoms
Facial muscle pain
Preauricular (TMJ) pain
TMJ sounds: jaw clicking, popping, catching, locking
Limited mouth opening
Increased pain associated with chewing

Secondary Symptoms
Earache
Headache
Neckache

Abbreviation: TMJ = temporomandibular joint.

muscle pain complaints. It appears that a better explanation would include a central nervous system effect on the muscle that results in an increase in peripheral nociceptive activity originating from the muscle tissue itself. This explanation more accurately accounts for the high levels of emotional stress that are commonly associated with TMD muscle pain complaints. In other words, an increase in emotional stress activates the autonomic nervous system, which in turn seems to be associated with changes in muscle nociception.

These masticatory muscle pain conditions are further complicated when one considers the unique masticatory muscle activity known as bruxism. Bruxism is the subconscious, often rhythmic, grinding or gnashing of the teeth. This type of muscle activity is considered to be parafunctional and can also occur as a simple static loading of the teeth known as clenching. This activity commonly occurs while sleeping but can also be present during the day. These parafunctional activities alone can represent a significant source of masticatory muscle pain, and certainly bruxism in the presence of central nervous system–induced muscle pain can further accentuate the patient's muscle pain complaints.

Etiology

Because TMD represents a group of disorders, any of several etiologies may be associated. Problems arising from intracapsular conditions (clicking, popping, catching, locking) may be associated with various types of trauma. Gross trauma, such as a blow to the chin, can immediately alter ligamentous structures of the joint, leading to joint sounds. Trauma can also be associated with a subtler injury such as stretching, twisting or compressing forces during eating, yawning, yelling, or prolonged mouth opening.

When the patient's chief complaint is muscle pain, etiologic factors other than trauma should be considered. Masticatory muscle pain disorders have etiologic considerations similar to other muscle pain disorders of the neck and back. Emotional stress seems to play a significant role for many patients. This can explain why patients often report that their painful symptoms fluctuate greatly over time.

Although most TMD patients do not have a major psychiatric disorder, psychological factors can certainly enhance the pain condition. The clinician needs to consider such factors as anxiety, depression, secondary gain, somatization, and hypochondriasis. Psychosocial factors can predispose certain people to TMD and can also perpetuate TMD once symptoms have become established. A careful consideration of psychosocial factors is therefore important in the evaluation and treatment of every TMD patient.

TMDs have a few unique etiologic factors that differentiate them from other musculoskeletal disorders. One such factor is the occlusal relationship of the teeth. Traditionally it was thought that malocclusion was the primary etiologic factor responsible for TMD. Recent investigations, however, do not support this concept. Still, in certain instances occlusal instability of the teeth can contribute to a TMD. This may be true in patients with or without teeth. Poorly fitting dental prostheses can also contribute to occlusal instability. The occlusal condition should especially be suspected if the pain problem began with a change in the patient's occlusion (e.g., following a dental appointment).

History and Examination

All patients reporting pain in the orofacial structures should be screened for TMD. This can be accomplished with a brief history and physical examination. The screening questions and examination are performed to rule in or out the possibility of a TMD. If a positive response is found, a more extensive history and examination is indicated. Box 2 lists questions that should be asked during a screening assessment for TMD. Any positive response should be followed by additional clarifying questions.

Patients experiencing orofacial pain should also be briefly examined for any clinical signs associated with TMD. The clinician can easily palpate a few sites to assess tenderness or pain, as well as assess for jaw mobility. The masseter muscles can be palpated bilaterally while asking the patient to report any pain

---

BOX 2 Recommended Screening Questionnaire for Temporomandibular Disorder

All patients reporting pain in the orofacial region should be screened for TMD with a questionnaire that includes these questions. The decision to complete a comprehensive history and clinical examination depends on the number of positive responses and the apparent seriousness of the problem for the patient. A positive response to any question may be sufficient to warrant a comprehensive examination if it is of concern to the patient or viewed as clinically significant by the physician.

1. Do you have difficulty, pain, or both when opening your mouth, for instance when yawning?
2. Does your jaw get stuck or locked or go out?
3. Do you have difficulty, pain, or both when chewing, talking, or using your jaws?
4. Are you aware of noises in the jaw joints?
5. Do your jaws regularly feel stiff, tight, or tired?
6. Do you have pain in or about the ears, temples, or cheeks?
7. Do you have frequent headaches, neckaches, or toothaches?
8. Have you had a recent injury to your head, neck, or jaw?
9. Have you been aware of any recent changes in your bite?
10. Have you been previously treated for unexplained facial pain or a jaw joint problem?

Abbreviation: TMD = temporomandibular disorder.

---

or tenderness. The same assessment should be made for the temporal regions, as well as the preauricular (TMJ) areas. While the examiner's hands are over the preauricular areas, the patient should repeatedly open and close the mouth. The presence of joint sounds should be noted along with whether these sounds are associated with joint pain.

A simple measurement of mouth opening should be made. This can be accomplished by placing a millimeter ruler on the lower anterior teeth and asking the patient to open as wide as possible. The distance should be measured between the maxillary and mandibular anterior teeth. It is generally accepted that less than 40 mm is a restricted mouth opening.

It is also helpful to inspect the teeth for significant wear, mobility, or decay that may be related to the pain condition. The clinician should examine the buccal mucosa for ridging and the lateral aspect of the tongue for scalloping. These are often signs of clenching and bruxism. A general inspection for symmetry and alignment of the face, jaws, and dental arches may also be helpful. A summary of this screening examination is shown in Box 3.

Treatment

Most recent studies suggest that TMDs are generally self-limiting, and symptoms often fluctuate over time. Understanding this natural course does not mean these conditions should be ignored. TMD can be a very painful condition leading to a significant decrease in the patient's quality of life. Understanding the natural course of TMD does suggest, however, that therapy might not need to be very aggressive. In general, initial therapy should begin very conservatively and only escalate when therapy fails to relieve the symptoms.

When the physician identifies a patient with a TMD, he or she has two options. The physician can elect to treat the patient or refer the patient to a dentist who specializes in TMD for further evaluation and treatment. The decision to refer the patient should be based on whether the patient needs any unique care provided only in a dental office. The following are some indications for referral to a dentist:

- History of trauma to the face related to the onset of the pain condition
- The presence of significant TMJ sounds during function
- A feeling of jaw catching or locking during mouth opening

All patients with face pain should be briefly screened for TMD using this or a similar cursory clinical examination. The need for a comprehensive history and clinical examination depends on the number of positive findings and the clinical significance of each finding.

1. Palpate for pain or tenderness in the masseter and temporalis muscles.
2. Palpate for pain or tenderness in the preauricular (TMJ) areas.
3. Measure the range of mouth opening. Note any incoordination in the movements.
4. Auscultate and palpate for TMJ sounds (i.e., clicking or crepitus).
5. Note excessive occlusal wear, excessive tooth mobility, buccal mucosal ridging, or lateral tongue scalloping.
6. Inspect symmetry and alignment of the face, jaws, and dental arches.

Abbreviation: TMJ = temporomandibular joint.

- The report of a sudden change in the occlusal contacts of the teeth
- The presence of significant occlusal instability
- Significant findings related to the teeth (e.g., tooth mobility, tooth sensitivity, tooth decay, tooth wear)
- Significant pain in the jaws or masticatory muscles upon awakening
- The presence of an orofacial pain condition that is aggravated by jaw function and has been present for more than several months

The specific therapy for a TMD varies according to the precise type of disorder identified. In other words, masticatory muscle pain is managed somewhat differently than intracapsular pain. Generally, however, the initial therapy for any type of TMD should be directed toward the relief of pain and the improvement of function. This initial conservative therapy can be divided into three general types: patient education, pharmacologic therapy, and physical therapy.

Patient Education

It is very important that patients have an appreciation for the factors that may be associated with their disorder, as well as the natural course of the disorder. Patients should be reassured and if necessary, convinced by appropriate tests, that they are not suffering from a malignancy. Properly educated patients can contribute greatly to their own treatment. For example, knowing that emotional stress is an influencing factor in many TMDs can help the patient understand the reason for daily fluctuations of pain intensity. Attention should be directed toward changing the patient's response to stress or, when possible, reducing exposure to stressful conditions. Patients with pain during chewing should be told to begin a softer diet, chew slower, and eat smaller bites. As a general rule the patient should be told "if it hurts, don't do it." Continued pain can contribute to the cycling of pain and should always be avoided. The patient should be instructed to let the jaw muscles relax, maintaining the teeth apart. This will discourage clenching activities and minimize loading of the teeth and joints.

When pain is associated with a clicking TM joint, the patient should be informed of the biomechanics of the joint. This information often allows the patient to select functional activities that are less traumatic to the joint structures. For example, some patients may report that the pain and clicking are less when they chew on a particular side of the mouth. When this occurs, they should be encouraged to continue this type of chewing.

Pharmacologic Therapy

Pharmacologic therapy can be an effective adjunct in managing symptoms associated with TMDs. Patients should be aware that medication alone will not likely solve or cure the problem. Medication, however, in conjunction with appropriate physical therapy and definitive treatment, does offer the most complete approach to many TMD problems. Mild analgesics are often helpful for many TMDs. Control of pain is not only appreciated by the patient but also reduces the likelihood of other complicating pain disorders such as muscle co-contraction, referred pain, and central sensitization.

Nonsteroidal antiinflammatory drugs (NSAIDs) are very helpful with many TMDs. Included in this category are aspirin, acetaminophen (Tylenol), and ibuprofen. Ibuprofen (Motrin, Advil, Nuprin) is often very effective in reducing musculoskeletal pains. A dosage of 600 to 800mg three times a day for 3 to 5 days commonly reduces pain and stops the cyclic effects of the deep pain input. For patients with gastrointestinal issues, short-term use of a cyclooxygenase-2 (COX-2) inhibitor such as celecoxib (Celebrex) can also be useful.

Physical Therapy

In many patients with TMD, symptoms are relieved with very simple physical therapy methods. Simple instructions for the use of moist heat or cold can be very helpful. Surface heat can be applied by laying a hot, moist towel over the symptomatic area. A hot water bottle wrapped inside the towel will help maintain the heat. This combination should remain in place for 10 to 15 minutes, not to exceed 30 minutes. An electric heating pad may be used, but care should be taken not to leave it on the face too long. Patients should be discouraged from using the heating pad while sleeping because prolonged use is likely.

Like thermotherapy, coolant therapy can provide a simple and often effective method of reducing pain. Ice should be applied directly to the symptomatic joint or muscles and moved in a circular motion without pressure to the tissues. The patient will initially experience an uncomfortable feeling that will quickly turn into a burning sensation. Continued icing will result in a mild aching and then numbness. When numbness begins the ice should be removed. The ice should not be left on the tissues for longer than 5 minutes. After a period of warming a second cold application may be desirable.

The physician should be aware that many TMDs respond to the use of orthopedic appliances such as occlusal appliances, bite guards, and splints. These appliances are made by the dentist and are custom fabricated for each patient. Several types of appliances are available. Each is specific for the type of TMD present. The dentist should be consulted for this type of therapy.

Other Therapeutic Considerations

Sometimes TMDs become chronic and, as with other chronic pain conditions, might then be best managed by a multidisciplinary approach. If the patient reports a long history of TMD complaints, the physician should consider referring the patient to a dentist associated with a team of therapists, such as a psychologist, a physical therapist, and even a chronic pain physician. Generally, patients with chronic TMD are not managed well by the simple initial therapies discussed in this chapter. Often other factors, such as mechanical conditions within the TMJs or psychological factors, need to be addressed. The physician who attempts to manage these conditions in the private practice setting can become very frustrated with the results. It is therefore recommended that if the patient's history suggests chronicity or if initial therapy fails to reduce the patient's symptoms, referral is indicated.

References

de Leeuw RE: Orofacial Pain: Guidelines for Assessment, Diagnosis, and Management, ed 5, Chicago 2013, Quintessence.

Okeson JP: Management of Temporomandibular Disorders and Occlusion, ed 8, St. Louis, 2019, Elsevier.

Okeson JP: Bell's Orofacial Pains, ed 7, Chicago, 2014, Quintessence.

Scrivani SJ, Keith DA, Kaban LB: Temporomandibular disorders, N Engl J Med 359(25):2693–2705, 2008.

UVEITIS

Method of
Curtis E. Margo, MD, MPH; and Grace Levy-Clarke, MD

CURRENT DIAGNOSIS

- Uveitis is classified by anatomic location and etiology.
- Most forms of uveitis are due to infectious or immune-mediated disease.
- Drug-induced uveitis and masquerade disorders (neoplasms) must be excluded in diagnostic evaluations.
- Patients with first-time uveitis should have a medical history, physical examination, and targeted laboratory studies, with the possible exception of adults who have a single episode of mild anterior uveitis that responds to therapy and who have no systemic signs or symptoms.
- Diagnostic evaluation must differentiate infectious from noninfectious uveitis.
- Patients who are immunosuppressed are at higher risk of infectious uveitis and their clinical presentations may be atypical.
- Uveitis in children is uncommon and deserves a thorough medical evaluation at initial presentation.
- Uveitis is managed optimally through a collaborative multidisciplinary approach.

CURRENT THERAPY

- Eradication of infection is the primary objective in infectious uveitis but may require judicious use of local antiinflammatory agents to mitigate structural and functional damage to intraocular tissues.
- The goal of therapy in noninfectious uveitis is to suppress and eliminate inflammation, achieving lasting remission through the stepwise implementation of therapy.
- First-time anterior uveitis in adults with negative medical history and review of systems can be treated with topical corticosteroids and cycloplegic agents and careful clinical monitoring.
- Corticosteroids can be delivered topically, through periocular and intravitreal injection, via sustained release devices implanted in the eye, and systemically.
- Immunomodulating therapy using alkylating agents, antimetabolites, biologic response modulators, or inhibitors of T-lymphocyte signaling are indicated for uveitis not responsive to systemic corticosteroids.
- A thorough history, physical examination, and select laboratory studies are required before initiating immunomodulating therapy. Subspecialty evaluations, when clinically indicated, may also be needed, such as rheumatology, neurology, or infectious disease specialists.

Current Diagnosis

Uveitis describes a heterogeneous group of disorders that have in common inflammation of the uveal tract (i.e., iris, ciliary body, and choroid). Symptoms are nonspecific, usually involving various combinations of blurred vision, ocular discomfort, intolerance to light, and floaters. Onset may be sudden or insidious. Children may have no symptoms. The essential signs of uveitis are the presence of inflammatory cells in the aqueous humor and/or vitreous gel. Sufficient magnification with a slit lamp is required to confidently detect these inflammatory cells and avoid confusion with suspended red blood cells or pigment epithelial cells. Although the uveal tract is the conceptual epicenter of uveal inflammation, there is spillover inflammation in the aqueous humor and vitreous gel, the two anatomic locations used to quantify the severity of inflammation and to monitor response to therapy. Grading schemes for recording the severity of anterior chamber and vitreous inflammatory cell density and protein content (flare) have been published by the Standardization of Uveitis Nomenclature (SUN) Classification Working Group.

Clinical Features and Diagnosis

The anatomic classification of intraocular inflammation into anterior, intermediate, and posterior uveitis and panuveitis guides the diagnostic workup toward the determination of etiology. When the anterior chamber is the principal site of inflammation, the terms iritis or iridocyclitis are often used. When the vitreous is the primary focus of inflammation, the term intermediate uveitis is preferred, but posterior cyclitis or vitritis are commonly used synonyms. Pars planitis is a clinical subtype of intermediate uveitis and is characterized by clumping or a layering of inflammatory cells over the pars plana and anterior retina called "snowballs" or a "snowbank lesion." These characteristic cells may also be seen in sarcoidosis. Posterior uveitis refers to diseases limited to the posterior segment of the eye. Comprehensive anatomical characterization includes retinitis, choroiditis, or neuroretinitis, and is clinically described as focal or multifocal. This classification is informative in developing an appropriate differential diagnosis.

Most cases of uveitis are caused by infection or immune-mediated disease. A substantial proportion of immune-mediated disease is a manifestation of systemic disease. Arriving at a diagnosis of infectious or noninfectious uveitis requires exclusion of drug-induced uveitis and so-called masquerade disorders (usually neoplasms) that mimic uveal inflammation. Most undifferentiated idiopathic forms of uveitis are localized immune-mediated disease whose pathogenesis is not yet understood. Immune-mediated and infectious uveitides may have overlapping clinical features. This is important as some diseases are diagnosed based on clinical features with supporting laboratory findings. The diagnostic evaluation for persons with noninfectious uveitis and no known systemic disorders involves a complete history, review of systems, physical examination, and select laboratory tests. There is limited consensus in the uveitis community regarding appropriate laboratory testing for specific uveitic entities; however, the general recommendation is to make case-specific determinations.

The anatomic categories of posterior uveitis and panuveitis have vastly expanded the number of potential diagnoses. The pattern and distribution of inflammatory lesions of the choroid, retina, and optic nerve, along with a host of other clinical findings (e.g., vascular or perivascular involvement, severity of overlying inflammation, color and shape of choroidal and retinal lesions, etc.) are critical to narrowing the differential diagnosis. The importance of pattern recognition in the diagnosis of posterior uveitis and panuveitis cannot be overstated. Toxoplasma chorioretinitis, the most common form of posterior uveitis, can usually be confidently diagnosed by clinical ophthalmoscopic appearance of a yellow-white retina with overlying vitreal inflammation adjacent to a hyperpigmented chorioretinal scar. On the other hand, the disorders belonging to the so-called white dot syndromes (acute posterior multifocal placoid pigment epitheliopathy, multifocal chorioretinitis with panuveitis, punctate inner choroidopathy, multiple evanescent white dot syndrome, and birdshot chorioretinopathy) require diagnostic studies such as fluorescein angiography, indocyanine green angiography, optic coherence tomography (OCT), and OCT angiography to elucidate. Most of these disorders, and a few others such as Vogt-Koyanagi-Harada disease and sympathetic ophthalmia, are clinically defined syndromes. Laboratory studies in the context of a clinically defined syndrome are used to exclude conditions that could possibly mimic their appearance.

Uveitis occurs in children substantially less often than adults. Although a majority of the same infectious and noninfectious etiologies that occur in adults also affect children, juvenile idiopathic arthritis has a relatively unique clinical presentation in young patients. All four subtypes of juvenile idiopathic arthritis are associated with anterior uveitis, but the pauciarticular category may present with anterior chamber inflammation and advanced band keratopathy with few or no symptoms. This degree of incongruity between symptoms and clinical findings on slit-lamp examination is unusual in adults.

Current Therapy

The heterogeneous nature of uveitis limits the generalizability of a universal therapeutic algorithm. When the cause of uveitis is infection, the goal of therapy is to eradicate the infectious organism while controlling inflammation during the process. For noninfectious uveitis, the goal of therapy is to suppress and eliminate inflammation and to achieve lasting remission. We know from published retrospective studies that early effective treatment minimizes the disease burden, so the current paradigm is the one utilized by rheumatologists, which is a treat to target approach. The severity and pattern of inflammation at presentation and the perceived risk to vision and ocular integrity guide the initial selection of therapy. Timing of treatment escalation and transition to noncorticosteroid therapy are decisions based on multiple factors, including but not limited to ocular and systemic comorbidities. Simultaneous therapies, particularly local and systemic antiinflammatory agents, are commonly used. Multidisciplinary management is ideally suited to combine the expertise needed to track the ocular response to treatment and to prescribe and monitor many of the systemic mediations.

Anterior Uveitis

Anterior uveitis, the most common subset of uveitis, is usually noninfectious. A minority of cases are attributed to viruses, most often herpes simplex virus (HSV), varicella zoster virus (VZV), and cytomegalovirus (CMV). Acute anterior uveitis associated with an underlying viral etiology is typically associated with increased intraocular pressure and iris atrophy. The diagnosis of viral anterior uveitis is typically a clinical one; when a diagnostic dilemma exists, then an anterior chamber tap with PCR analysis is recommended. In general, prompt empiric oral therapy will shorten the course, and tailored maintenance therapy may be indicated to decrease recurrences. For HSV or VZV, therapy with oral acyclovir (Zovirax),[1] valacyclovir (Valtrex),[1] or famciclovir (Famvir)[1] is started. Following clinical resolution of inflammation, maintenance therapy with an oral antiviral drug is recommended. The optimal treatment for anterior uveitis due to CMV is still being evaluated, with current recommendations for systemic therapy (with oral ganciclovir[2] or intravenous foscarnet [Foscavir][1] or intravenous ganciclovir [Cytovene]).[1] Maintenance therapy with topical ganciclovir (Zirgan)[1] or oral valganciclovir (Valcyte)[1] should be considered. The antiviral therapy is used with concomitant topical therapy discussed in the next section. Duration of maintenance therapies for viral anterior uveitis is a clinical decision and should be individualized.

The vast majority of anterior uveitis is noninfectious, for which the mainstay of treatment is topical corticosteroids with cycloplegics (Table 1). There are nearly 20 different preparations of topical corticosteroid (e.g., dexamethasone sodium phosphate 0.1% solution; prednisolone acetate 1.0% suspension [Pred Forte]) that come in suspension or solution (and some as ointment) and in different concentrations. Dose and duration of use is tailored to the clinical setting.

Topical nonsteroidal antiinflammatory agents (e.g., diclofenac 0.1% [Voltaren][1]; ketorolac 0.4% [Acular][1]; flurbiprofen 0.03% [Ocufen][1]) are less effective than topical corticosteroids in controlling the inflammation of anterior uveitis. Their use in combination with topical corticosteroids may be additive.[1]

Topical cycloplegics provide pain relief, and the mydriasis they produce reduces the risk of iridolenticular scarring. The selection of a long-acting (e.g., atropine sulfate 1% [Isopto Atropine] twice daily) versus short-acting cycloplegic agent (e.g., cyclopentolate hydrochloride 0.5%–1.0% [Cyclogyl][1] two or three times a day) is based on clinical features such as severity of inflammation, presence of synechial scarring, age of patient, ability to take topical medications, and so on. Duration of action varies from 1 to 2 weeks for topical atropine to approximately half a day for cyclopentolate.

[1]Not FDA approved for this indication.
[2]Not available in the United States.

TABLE 1	Topical Medications for Anterior Uveitis		
DRUG NAME (TRADE NAMES)	**FORMULATION**	**STARTING DOSE SCHEDULE***
Topical Corticosteroids		
Dexamethasone (Decadron phosphate [Maxidex])	0.1% suspension; 0.1% solution; 0.05% ointment[2]	4 times per day
Difluprednate (Durezol)	0.05% emulsion	4 times per day
Fluorometholine alcohol (Flarex, FML)	0.1 and 0.25% suspensions; 0.1% ointment	2–4 times per day; 1–3 times per day
Loteprednol etabonate (Lotemax)	0.5% suspension	4 times per day
Leteprednol etabonate (Alrex)	0.2% suspension[1]	3 times per day
Prednisolone acetate (Pred Forte, Econopred Plus; AK-Tate)	1.0% suspension	4 times per day
Prednisolone sodium phosphate (Inflamase Forte; AK-Pred)	1.0% solution	4 times per day
Prednisolone acetate (Pred Mild; Econopred)	0.12% suspension	4 times per day
Topical Cycloplegic Agents		
Atropine sulfate (Isopto Atropine)	1.0%	Once or twice a day
Cyclopentolate hydrochloride (Cyclogyl)[1]	0.5% and 1.0%	Twice a day
Homatropine hydrobromide (Isopto homatropine)	2.0%–5.0%	Once or twice a day
Scopolamine hydrobromide (Isopto hyoscine)	0.25%	Once or twice a day
Tropicamide (Mydriacyl)[1]	0.5% and 1.0%	2–3 times a day
Topical Nonsteroidal Antiinflammatory Medications		
Bromfenac (BromSite; Prolensa; Xibrom)[1]	0.075%–0.09% solution	Once or twice daily
Diclofenac (Voltaren)[1]	0.1% solution	2 times per day
Flurbiprofen (Ocufen)[1]	0.03% solution	2 times per day
Ketorolac (Acular LS; Acular)[1]	0.4%–0.5%	3 times per day
Nepafenac (Ilevro; Nevanac)[1]	0.1%–0.3% suspension	1–3 times a day, based on formulation

*More frequent use of corticosteroids dictated by severity of inflammation then tapered based on clinical response.
[1]Not FDA approved for this indication.
[2]Not available in the United States.

Noninfectious anterior uveitis is commonly associated with surgical trauma and accidental blunt trauma (concussive injury). They are usually effectively managed with tapering regimens of topical corticosteroids and cycloplegics.

Oral prednisone (1 mg/kg/day) may be needed for severe or recalcitrant anterior uveitis. Strategies for therapeutic escalation beyond oral corticosteroids parallel that of intermediate or posterior uveitis.

Although topical corticosteroids and cycloplegics do not play a primary role in intermediate and posterior uveitis, they are used as adjuvant therapies for comfort and to minimize the formation of peripheral and posterior synechiae due to associated anterior inflammation/iridocyclitis.

Intermediate Uveitis

Intermediate uveitis, characterized by inflammatory cells in vitreous, peripheral retina, and pars plana, can be associated with systemic disorders such as multiple sclerosis, sarcoidosis, syphilis, toxocariasis (in children), the HLA-B27 spondyloarthropathies and Lyme disease. Vitritis is also a presenting sign of endogenous endophthalmitis and can be mimicked by primary vitreoretinal lymphoma. Once infection, drug-related uveitis, and masquerading conditions are excluded, the approach to therapy for noninfectious forms of intermediate uveitis is similar to the stepladder approach (described later) that typically begins with oral corticosteroids A treat to target approach should be taken, tailored based on disease severity, ocular and systemic comorbidities, and the presence/absence of an underlying systemic rheumatologic disorder. Additionally, known chronic/progressive ocular disorders that historically requires early aggressive systemic therapy such as serpiginuous or birdshot will require special considerations. (Table 2). For pars planitis recalcitrant to medical therapy, options include peripheral ablation of the snowbank lesion with indirect laser photocoagulation and pars plana vitrectomy. Their effectiveness has not been rigorously tested in clinical trials.

Adjunct periocular or intravitreal therapy (i.e., regional therapy) may be an option for noninfectious intermediate, posterior, and panuveitis. Regional therapy delivers medications closer to the site of inflammation. The currently available regional therapeutic options include periocular injections of depot corticosteroids (40 mg triamcinolone acetonide [1 mL of 40 mg/mL Kenalog-40[1]); intravitreal corticosteroid injection through the pars plana (4 mg triamcinolone acetonide suspension [0.1 mL 40 mg/mL Kenalog-40[1]; Triesence]); and a sustained-release corticosteroid implant embedded to either a biodegradable or nonbiodegradable vehicle to achieve sustained release. The implants are injected into the vitreous or surgically fixed to the sclera. Dexamethasone (Ozurdex, 0.7 mg) has a delivery span of 6 months, and fluocinolone acetonide (Iluvien 0.19 mg[1]; Retisert 0.59 mg; Yutiq 0.18 mg) 18 to 36 months. Approved in 2021, a suprachoroidal route, XIPERE™ is 4 mg (0.1 mL of the 40 mg/mL triamcinolone injectable suspension), specifically approved for retinal edema associated with uveitis. In the appropriate clinical setting these options may be tried before moving to oral prednisone or other systemic immune modulator therapy. The risk of endophthalmitis and the need for repeat injections need to be considered.

Posterior Uveitis and Panuveitis

The general diagnostic approach to posterior uveitis and panuveitis begins by excluding infection and drug-induced uveitis and not overlooking the possibility of a masquerade condition. The optimal strategy for laboratory testing to identify a culpable systemic disorder responsible for noninfectious uveitis is a matter of debate. Many posterior and pan uveitides are clinically defined syndromes. For example, Behçet disease, multifocal choroiditis with panuveitis, acute posterior multifocal placoid pigment epitheliopathy, serpiginous choroiditis, punctate inner choroidopathy, multiple evanescent white dot syndrome, Vogt-Koyanagi-Harada disease, and sympathetic ophthalmia are diagnoses based on clinical findings (e.g., ophthalmoscopy, fluorescein angiography, optical coherence tomography, etc.). These syndromes have no confirmatory laboratory tests, other than several with strong human leukocyte antigen (HLA) haplotype associations (e.g., Behçet disease [HLA-B51] and birdshot chorioretinpathy [HLS-A29]).

Management of inflammation associated with noninfectious posterior uveitis requires systemic medications. Most clinicians initiate oral corticosteroids, understanding that high-dose long-term use is associated with serious and predictable side effects. The risk of systemic side effects may be reduced with judicious use of periocular or intravitreal corticosteroid injections, but those routes of administration also have their own potential adverse effects and complications. These range from elevated intraocular pressure and glaucoma to infectious endophthalmitis.

The optimal time to transition to corticosteroid-sparing immunomodulatory therapy is a clinical decision-making process, focused on limiting the long-term systemic side-effects of oral corticosteroids, treating inflammation recalcitrant to oral corticosteroids, and for management of specific diseases expected to fare poorly with less aggressive therapies. The guidelines for treatment escalation should be based on a treat to target approach, to minimize disease burden and improve clinical outcomes. A frequently cited reference is the SITE (Systemic Immunosuppressive Therapy for Eye diseases) Cohort Study series, a retrospective cohort study with multiple publications detailing the use of antimetabolites, T-cell inhibitors, alkylating agents, and other immunosuppressives ascertained from medical records of approximately 9250 patients with ocular inflammation. Data are collected with up to 30 years of follow-up from five U.S. tertiary centers and analyzed by fellowship-trained ocular immunologists. Immunomodulatory therapy for the treatment of uveitis falls into four drug categories: antimetabolites, inhibitors of T-lymphocyte signaling, biologic response modifiers, and alkylating agents (Table 3). Their judicious use has been shown to reduce or eliminate the need for systemic corticosteroids, improve long-term visual prognosis, and reduce ocular complications from inflammation. Meaningful clinical responses should occur within 3 months of initiating therapy. Following achieved clinical end points, patients should be monitored and the decision to taper based on input from patients and disease-specific criteria. A thorough history, physical examination, and select laboratory tests and imaging studies should be completed prior to initiation of therapy, in conjunction with appropriate subspecialty consultation.

The most commonly used antimetabolites for the treatment of noninfectious uveitis are methotrexate (Rheumatrex),[1] azathioprine (Imuran),[1] and mycophenolate mofetil (Cellcept).[1] Oral methotrexate, 7.5 to 15 mg once per week with daily folic acid[1] 1 mg, can be increased to 20 to 25 mg/week based on clinical response. Appropriately adjusted intravenous dose can be tried for persons with gastrointestinal intolerance. Intravitreal injection of 400 µg/0.1 mL has been used for refractory inflammation. Oral azathioprine is begun at 1 mg/kg/day. Depending on clinical response, it can be incrementally increased to 2.5 mg/kg/day. Mycophenolate mofetil is started at 1 to 2 g orally per day in divided doses up to 3 g/day. The manifold side effects of antimetabolites necessitate close clinical monitoring.

Most experience in treating noninfectious uveitis with inhibitors of T-lymphocyte signaling, or calcineurin inhibitors, is with cyclosporine (Sandimmune).[1] Given 2.5 to 5 mg/kg/day in divided doses, cyclosporine can cause nephrotoxicity, bone marrow suppression, and hypertension.

Alkylating agents used to treat noninfectious uveitis include cyclophosphamide (Cytoxan)[1] and chlorambucil (Leukeran).[1] These immunomodulating drugs are titrated to keep white blood cell counts in the range of 3000 to 4500 cells per cubic millimeter. Chlorambucil is started at 0.15 mg/kg/day and cyclophosphamide at 1 to 3 mg/kg/day. Regular monitoring for bone marrow suppression and opportunistic infection is needed for both drugs. Risks of hemorrhagic cystitis with cyclophosphamide may be reduced by consuming generous amounts of water daily.

Biologic response modifiers, or "biologics," have expanded the therapeutic arsenal for treating advanced or severe noninfectious uveitis. This family of medications consists of antibodies directed against key cytokines in the immune response pathway. Most experience in treating noninfectious uveitis has been with tumor necrosis factor-α (TNF-α) inhibitors (infliximab [Remicade][1] and adalimumab [Humira]). Although other biologics have been used to treat advanced or severe

---

[1]Not FDA approved for this indication.

TABLE 2 Treatment of Infectious Uveitis

DIAGNOSIS	INFECTIOUS ORGANISM(S)	TREATMENT	COMMENT
Acute retinal necrosis	Herpes zoster virus (HZV) Herpes simplex virus (HSV) I and II	Acyclovir (Zovirax)[1] 13 mg/kg/dose divided every 8 h IV for 7 days, followed by 800 mg PO 5 times/day for 3–4 months or Famciclovir (Famvir)[1] 500 mg PO q8h or Valacyclovir (Valtrex)[1] 1000–2000 mg PO q8h for induction Ganciclovir (Cytovene)[1] 500 mg IV q12h; maintenance: (duration varies with response) Valganciclovir (Valcyte)[1] 900 mg PO BID for 3 weeks then 450 mg PO BID Ganciclovir[2] 1000 mg PO TID	Adjuvant intravitreal injection options: Ganciclovir (200–2000 μg/0.1 mL)[6] Foscarnet (Foscavir)1 (1.2–2.4 mg/0.1 mL)[6]; Possible role for prednisone (0.5–2.0 mg/kg/day po for up to 6–8 weeks)
Anterior uveitis, viral	HSV	Valacyclovir[1] 1000 mg PO TID Acyclovir[1] 400 mg PO × 5/day 4 weeks Famciclovir[1] 250 mg PO TID	Topical corticosteroids and cycloplegic recommended. Alternative options include an intravitreal ganciclovir (2 mg/0.05 mL).[6] After active infection eradicated, consider maintenance therapy for HSV and CMV
	HZV	Valacyclovir[1] 1 g PO TID Acyclovir[1] 800 mg PO × 5/day 5–6 weeks Famciclovir[1] 500 mg PO TID 5–6 weeks	
	Cytomegalovirus (CMV)	Ganciclovir[1] 5 mg/kg IV BID 2–3 weeks Valganciclovir[1] 900 mg PO BID × 6 weeks, then 450 mg PO BID × 6 weeks	Gancyclovir ophthalmic gel (Zirgan)[1] 0.15% × 5/day (optional)
Cat-scratch disease	Bartonella henselae	Doxycycline (Vibramycin)[1] 100 mg PO BID 2–4 weeks	Children: antibiotic selection based on age, dental maturity.
Cytomegalovirus retinitis	Cytomegalovirus	Ganciclovir 5 mg/kg IV BID for 2–3 weeks followed by maintenance 5 mg/kg/day PO Cidofovir (Vistide)[1] 5 mg/kg/week IV for 2 weeks then 5 mg/kg every 2 weeks Valganciclovir 900 mg BID PO, then PO qd for maintenance. Foscarnet 90 mg/kg IV BID × 2 wks; maintenance 90–120 mg/kg IV daily	Immune reconstitution targets cause of immune compromise.
Diffuse unilateral subacute neuroretinitis (DUSN)	Possible larva of Baylisascaris procyonis, Toxocara canis	Photocoagulation of intraretinal nematode	Destruction of intraretinal larva may preserve vision.
Lyme disease	Borrelia burgdorferi	Doxycycline[1] 100 mg PO BID × 21 days (adults) Amoxicillin[1] 500 mg PO BID (adult); 50 mg/kg PO in divided doses × 14–21 days (children)	Alternative: cefuroxime axetil (Ceftin) 500 mg PO BID × 14–21 days (adult); 30 mg/kg/day PO (children)
Metastatic endophthalmitis (endogenous)	Numerous bloodborne bacteria and fungi	Sepsis treatment protocol; antibiotic selections based on cultures and sensitivities	Role and timing of intravitreal antibiotics and of vitrectomy less well defined
Onchocerciasis	Onchocerca volvulus	Ivermectin (Stromectol) 150 μg/kg single oral dose; repeat at 6 months for the lifespan of adult worm	Corticosteroids to control ocular inflammation; route of administration depends of site of inflammation
Syphilis	Treponema pallidum	Aqueous penicillin G 18–24 million units, IV qd divided doses for 10–14 days	Ocular syphilis is considered a subset of neurosyphilis
Toxocariasis	Toxocara canis or Toxocara catis	Prednisone 1 mg/kg/day PO; timing of antihelminthic therapy unresolved.	Laser ablation and vitrectomy depending on stage of disease. Intraocular larval death incites considerable inflammation
Toxoplasmosis	Toxoplasma gondii	Pyrimethamine (Daraprim): loading dose 50–100 mg PO; treatment dose 25–50 mg/day PO; and sulfadiazine: loading dose 2–4 g PO; treatment dose 1.0 g PO QID, and prednisone (0.5–1.0 mg/kg/day PO) Trimethoprim-sulfamethoxazole (Bactrim DS)[1] 160 mg/80 mg PO BID, plus above regimen of prednisone	Modify doses if pregnant or immune compromised. Some recommend adding clindamycin[1] or azithromycin.[1]
Tuberculosis	Mycobacterium tuberculosis	For first-line therapy for active tuberculosis, follow recommendations on CDC website.	

BID, Twice a day; IV, intravenous; PO, by mouth; TID, three times a day.
[1] Not FDA approved for this indication.
[2] Not available in the United States.
[6] May be compounded by pharmacists.

TABLE 3   Immune Modulator Therapy for Uveitis

GENERIC (TRADE) NAME	DOSE (ROUTE)*	COMMENT/INDICATIONS[†]
Alkylating Agents		
Chlorambucil (Leukeran)[1]	0.15 mg/kg/day (oral)	Behçet disease; juvenile idiopathic arthritis; pars planitis; sympathetic ophthalmia
Cyclophosphamide (Cytoxan)[1]	1 mg/kg/day (oral)	Sclerouveitis; sympathetic ophthalmia
Antimetabolites		
Azathioprine (Imuran)[1]	1–1.5 mg/kg/day (oral) can increase to 2.5 mg/kg/day	Severe anterior uveitis; panuveitis, juvenile idiopathic arthritis; pars planitis, sarcoidosis; sympathetic uveitis; Vogt-Koyanagi-Harada disease (VKH)
Methotrexate (Otrexup, Rasuvo, Rheumatrex, Trexall)[1]	7.5–15 mg/week (oral)	Anterior, intermediate, and posterior uveitis; juvenile idiopathic arthritis; sympathetic uveitis
Mycophenolate mofetil (Cellcept)[1]; Mycophenolate sodium (Myfortic)[1]	Mofetil: 1 g (oral) divided dose/day; Sodium: 360 mg (oral)/day	Anterior, intermediate, and posterior uveitis
Calcinernin Inhibitors		
Cyclosporine (Gengraf, Neoral, Sandimmune)[1]	2.5–5 mg/kg/day (oral) divided dose	Often given with prednisone 10–20 mg/day; Behçet disease; birdshot chorioretinopathy; pan uveitis; posterior uveitis; sarcoidosis; sclerouveitis; sympathetic uveitis; VKH
Tacrolimus (Prograf, Astagraf XL, Envasus XR)[1]	0.15–0.3 mg/kg/day (oral)	Behçet disease; birdshot chorioretinopathy; posterior uveitis
Biologic Response Modifier Tumor Necrosis Factor (TNF)-α Inhibitor		
Adalimumab (Humira)	40 mg every other week subcutaneous injection	Anterior, intermediate and posterior uveitis; juvenile idiopathic arthritis; sarcoidosis
Infliximab (Remicade)[1]	3 mg/kg/day (intravenous) weeks 0, 2, and 6	Behçet disease; anterior uveitis; juvenile idiopathic arthritis; sarcoidosis
Certolizumab pegol (Cimzia)[1]	400 mg subcutaneous induction 1–3 doses; 200 mg every 2 weeks	Refractory uveitis
Golimumab (Simponi)[1]	50 mg subcutaneous every 4 weeks	Juvenile idiopathic arthritis; Behçet disease
Biologic Response Modifier Interluekin-1 Inhibitor		
Anakinra (Kineret)[1]	100 mg subcutaneous daily	Behçet disease
Canakinumab (Ilaris)[1]	150–300 mg subcutaneous every 4–8 weeks	Behçet disease; juvenile idiopathic arthritis
Biologic Response Modifier Anti-Interleukin 6 Receptor		
Tocilizumab (Actemra)[1]	4–8 mg/kg (intravenous) every 2–4 weeks	Juvenile idiopathic arthritis; Behçet disease; persistent macular edema
Biologic Response Modifier Anti-Cd20		
Rituximab (Rituxan)[1]	375 mg/m² intravenous weekly, modify accordingly	Refractory uveitis; juvenile idiopathic arthritis; refractory VKH;

*Therapeutic doses and schedules in clinical trials have differed in loading doses and maintenance doses. Cited doses reflect lower ranges.
[†]Refers to reported success at controlling or eliminating inflammation as a single or as a steroid-sparing agent. Strength of recommendations will vary by level of evidence.
[1]Not FDA approved for this indication.

noninfectious uveitis, their equivalence or superiority to the drugs already mentioned are under study. Etanercept (Embrel)[1] may increase the risk of anterior uveitis in persons with ankylosing spondylitis.

Infliximab (Remicade) is given intravenously beginning with two loading doses of 3 to 5 mg/kg each given 2 weeks apart. Injections are then continued at 4-week intervals. Based on clinical response, dose can be gradually increased to 10 mg/kg. Side effects include infection from activation of latent tuberculosis or hepatitis, drug-induced autoimmune disease, and demyelinating disease. If non-melanoma skin cancer is excluded, current published data indicate that TNF-inhibitors do not increase the risk for solid malignancies. Adalimumab (Humira) is given subcutaneously starting at 40 mg/kg every 2 weeks. Children are started at a reduced dose. Its adverse risk profile is similar to that of infliximab.

Other biologics used to treat noninfectious uveitis such as anti-CD20 monoclonal antibody (Rituximab [Rituxan][1]) have clinically established utility in the treatment of specific disease entities such as severe scleritis, peripheral ulcerative keratitis, ocular mucous membrane pemphigoid, and retinal vasculitis. In these cases the rheumatoid arthritis approved dosing regimen is used: two 1000 mg intravenous infusions separated by 2 weeks (cycle 1) then every 24 weeks or based on clinical evaluation, but not sooner than every 16 weeks. Interferon alfa-2a is associated with flu-like symptoms and depression, which may limit patient acceptance.

Complications of Uveitis

Chronic uveitis gives rise to a variety of ocular complications such as secondary glaucoma; macular edema; corneal dysfunction; neovascularization of the iris, angle, and retina; retinal tears

Uveitis

and detachments; cyclitic membrane formation; and uveal effusion, as well as other conditions. These ocular complications are typically approached by controlling or eliminating ocular inflammation and managing the structural/functional problems according to standards guidelines.

Disease-Specific Recommendations

Strength of recommendations for disease-specific noncorticosteroid immunomodulatory therapy is constrained by the relative lack of prospective clinical trials, drug-to-drug comparison trials, studies that have included patients with diverse forms of uveitis, and the small size of studies. Given these limitations, the strength of recommendations is tempered by a level of evidence for most drugs of 2B or lower on the Oxford Centre for Evidence-Based Medicine level of evidence scale. Mycophenolate preparations,[1] azathioprine,[1] methotrexate,[1] cyclophosphamide,[1] cyclosporine,[1] sirolimus (Rapamune),[1] infliximab,[1] adalimumab, and etanercept[1] have demonstrated varying degrees of success in controlling inflammation, improving visual outcome, and reducing corticosteroid use in severe anterior, intermediate, and posterior uveitis and in panuveitis. Control of inflammation and improved visual acuity in Vogt-Koyanagi-Harada disease have been achieved with systemic methotrexate,[1] azathioprine,[1] mycophenolate preparations,[1] infliximab,[1] adalimumab,[1] and interferon alfa-2a.[1] The uveitis of Beçhet disease, juvenile idiopathic arthritis, pars planitis, and sympathetic ophthalmia responds to chlorambucil.[1] Mycophenolate preparations[1] have had success in various forms of anterior, intermediate, and posterior uveitis. The inflammation of Beçhet disease has been controlled with azathioprine,[1] infliximab,[1] adalimumab,[1] rituximab,[1] and interferon alfa-2a.[1] Sarcoid uveitis has responded to infliximab,[1] and adalimumab.[1] The systemic disease of juvenile idiopathic arthritis has been successfully managed with methotrexate, cyclosporine,[1] mycophenolate mofetil,[1] azathioprine,[1] and TNF-α inhibitors adalimumab and infliximab.[1] Therapeutic vitrectomy and/or laser ablation has been used in different forms of noninfectious uveitis, but evidence of long-term effectiveness is sparse.

Systemic Drug Use in Pregnancy and in Children

Because the teratogenic potential of many immunosuppressive drugs is incompletely understood, it may be prudent to discuss contraception when they are administered to women. The largely unknown teratogenic effects of immunosuppressive agents in men should also be considered. Although prednisone is well tolerated during pregnancy, its use should be carefully comanaged with an obstetrician.

The effects of immunosuppressive drugs are less well studied in children than in adults. Children on immunosuppressive agents should not receive live virus vaccine for 3 months after immunosuppressive use has ended. This would include high-dose corticosteroids. The impact of immunosuppressive drugs and systemic corticosteroids on growth and their collateral effects on social development are not inconsequential. Osteoporosis, adrenal suppression, and heightened susceptibility to infections related to cell-mediated immunity are among the side effects that require monitoring in children. Calcium supplements and vitamin D may be beneficial in some circumstances.

[1]Not FDA approved for this indication.

References

Dick AD, Rosenbaum JT, Al-Dhibi HA, et al: Guidance on noncorticosteroid systemic immunomodulatory therapy in noninfectious uveitis. Fundamentals of Care for UveitiS (FOCUS) Initiative, *Ophthalmology* 125:757–773, 2018.
Foster CS, Kothari S, Anesi SD, et al: The Ocular Immunology and Uveitis Foundation preferred practice patterns of uveitis management, *Surv Ophthalmol* 61:1–17, 2016.
Jabs DA, Nussenblatt RB, Rosenbaum JT: Standardization of Uveitis Nomenclature (SUN) Work Group. standardization of uveitis nomenclature for reporting clinical data. results of the first international workshop, *Am J Ophthalmol* 140:509–516, 2005.

Jap A, Soon-Phaik C: Viral anterior uveitis. diagnosis and management, *Focal Points* 34(5):1–18, 2016. Available at https://store.aao.org/clinical-education/product-line/focal-points.html.
Kempen JH, Daniel E, Gangaputra S, Dreger K, et al: Methods for identifying long-term adverse effects of treatment in patients with eye diseases: the Systemic Immunosuppressive Therapy for Eye Diseases (SITE) Cohort Study, *Ophthalmic Epidemiol* 15(1):47–55, 2008.
Levy-Clarke G, Jabs DA, Read RW, et al: Expert panel recommendations for the use of anti-tumor necrosis factor biologic agents in patients with ocular inflammatory disorders, *Ophthalmology* 121:785–796, 2014. e783.
London NJS, Garg SJ, Moorthy MS, et al: Drug-induced uveitis, *Focal Points* 33(5):1–10, 2015. Available at https://store.aao.org/clinical-education/product-line/focal-points.html.
Lower CY, Lima BR: Pediatric uveitis, *Focal Points* 32(3):1–11, 2014. Available at https://store.aao.org/clinical-education/product-line/focal-points.html.
Schwartzman S: Advancements in the management of uveitis, *Best Prac Res Clin Rheumatol* 30:304–316, 2016.
Wakefield D, McCluskey P, Wildner G, et al: Inflammatory eye disease: pretreatment assessment of patients prior to commencing immunosuppressive and biologic therapy: recommendations from an expert committee, *Autoimmun Rev* 16:213–222, 2017.
Yeh S, Suhler ER, Moorly RS, et al: Biologic response modifiers in uveitis, *Focal Points* 30(3):1–16, 2012. Available at https://store.aao.org/clinical-education/product-line/focal-points.html.

VISION REHABILITATION

Method of
August Colenbrander, MD; and Donald C. Fletcher, MD

CURRENT DIAGNOSIS

- The need for vision rehabilitation needs to be considered whenever patients indicate that they have difficulty performing visual tasks.
- Sometimes, however, patients do not recognize the visual causes of their complaints, therefore:
  - Vision rehabilitation needs to be considered whenever visual acuity is reported as 20/50 or less.
  - Vision rehabilitation also needs to be considered for all patients with reported visual disorders, such as visual field deficits or contrast vision deficits, who have not received this service yet,

CURRENT THERAPY

- Simple cases of reduced visual acuity can be addressed with a variety of magnifying devices, ranging from stronger glasses to electronic devices.
- Improved task lighting can often be helpful.
- Orientation and mobility training can be indicated for patients with visual field loss, even if their visual acuity is still adequate.
- As for any other specialized service, referral to a dedicated low vision service may be indicated.

Vision rehabilitation refers to the multidisciplinary effort of assisting those with various degrees of vision loss in coping with the *consequences* of that loss. To describe vision rehabilitation, the nature of vision itself must be understood. Vision is the major source of information about our environment. The eyes alone contribute as much information to the brain as all other organs combined. It is not surprising therefore that many people fear loss of vision almost as much as loss of life.

Most people will state that "we see with our eyes." On closer examination, this is not true. An isolated eyeball cannot produce any vision; our brain, however, can produce exquisite visual imagery in our dreams, without any input from the eyes.

The ultimate goal of vision is to facilitate interaction with the environment, not just to read letters on a letter chart. To achieve this goal, the visual process goes through three distinct stages. Each stage comes with its own specific problems.

- First is the *optical stage*, where the refractive media of the eye deliver an image to the retina. Familiar problems in this area include refractive errors and cataracts.
- Second is the *receptor stage*, where the optical image is translated into neural impulses. Age-related macular degeneration (AMD) is a significant problem of the receptor stage, which is becoming increasingly common as the population ages.
- Third are various stages of *neural processing*, initially in the inner retina (glaucoma), then in the visual cortex, and finally in higher cortical centers, where the visual input gives rise to visual perception and to visually guided behaviors, actions, and interactions.

The most common visual problems vary for different ages. Today, brain-damage-related vision problems (cerebral visual impairment [CVI]) are the single most prevalent cause of visual impairment in *infants and young children*. Given that vision is so important for normal development, vision loss in infants constitutes a developmental emergency and should be detected and addressed as early as possible. When a child does not smile back at the mother, the mother may be inclined to leave the baby in its crib, instead of holding him or her to provide extra tactile stimulation to compensate for missing visual stimulation.

At *school age* and later, visual health is critical because reading becomes important for academic development. For *adults*, vision is important for maintaining independence in activities of daily living (ADL) and development of vocational skills. For *seniors*, vision loss may exacerbate other age-related dysfunctions. Studies of the elderly have shown correlations between visual impairment and depression, falls, and reduced longevity. In all of these instances, early detection and early intervention are essential; the primary care physician plays a crucial role in this respect.

Four Aspects of Vision Loss

Vision is a complex phenomenon.

A convenient framework for discussing the various impacts of vision loss is to consider four aspects of visual functioning (Figure 1). At a basic level, we may consider how various external causes may result in *structural changes* to the eyes and the visual pathways. For this aspect, the focus is on the tissue; an ocular pathologist is needed to describe the pathologic condition. However, structural changes alone do not determine how well the eyes actually function. Clinicians need to measure various *organ functions*, such as visual acuity, visual field, and contrast sensitivity.

Yet even knowing how the eyes function does not tell us how the person functions. In other words, the *abilities* of the person to perform tasks, such as reading, mobility, face recognition, and ADL, must be considered. Occupational therapists (OTs) and other rehabilitation professionals work with patients to teach them how residual vision can be used most effectively. OTs also assess the person in a societal context. For example, do the visual changes have an impact on the person's *participation* in society, on his or her ability to perform necessary tasks, and on general satisfaction with one's quality of life? It is clear that to cover all aspects of vision rehabilitation, a team approach is necessary and that the patient must be part of that team.

A single ADL may cover several of the above aspects. When reading, the aspect of minimum print size falls under organ function (retinal resolution). Reading speed (words/minute) and reading endurance (hours/day) define abilities of the person; reading endurance may be poor, even if reading acuity is adequate. Reading enjoyment, finally, falls under the aspect of quality of life.

It is helpful to draw a line between the organ side of Figure 1 on the left and the person side on the right. On the left side of the diagram, we discuss *visual functions*, which describe how each eye functions. On the right side, we speak of *functional vision*, which describes how the person functions in vision-related activities. Medical specialists are well versed in dealing with the left side of the diagram. Yet the ultimate goal of all interventions is to improve the patient's quality of life. It is the function of vision rehabilitation to make sure that "eye" doctors become "people" doctors by extending their interest to the right side of the diagram as well.

Comprehensive Vision Rehabilitation

Considering all of these aspects, comprehensive vision rehabilitation involves much more than the patient's performance on a letter chart and requires teamwork by different professionals who specialize in different aspects of vision loss. All vision loss starts with some medical condition, so primary care physicians are well positioned to coordinate team activities. Primary care physicians need to be aware of what other team members can contribute and should know where to locate vision rehabilitation resources and to make appropriate referrals.

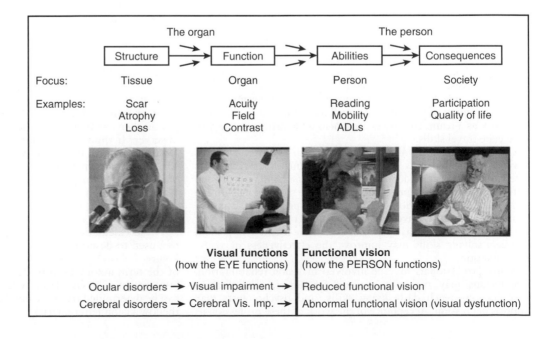

Figure 1 Aspects of vision loss.

Figure 2 Comprehensive vision rehabilitation.

Figure 2 illustrates that comprehensive vision rehabilitation involves much more than the traditional optical low vision care offered in the past, and is still relevant today.

Low vision is a term used to describe individuals whose vision (with appropriate optical correction) is less than normal (low) but who are not blind (vision). Unfortunately, many people in this category do not yet receive the services they need. Such services should include adequate refractive, medical, and surgical care as well as rehabilitative care. The latter may include vision enhancement, vision substitution, and vision assistance as well as the honing of coping skills.

Vision enhancement, which is the traditional focus of low vision care, is primarily oriented at improving residual visual function through visual aids, including a wide range of magnification devices. Additionally, enhancement of contrast, illumination, and filters need to be explored.

Low vision is distinct from blindness (i.e., no vision). For blindness, the emphasis of rehabilitation is entirely on vision substitution. Patients with severe or profound low vision may combine the use of low vision rehabilitation skills with some blindness rehabilitation skills.

Vision substitution expands the options for rehabilitation by optimizing the use of other senses. This can range from using simple tactile markings to sense the position of a stove dial to devices such as talking books, a long cane for travel, and braille for reading. Vision enhancement and vision substitution are not mutually exclusive. A patient may use a magnifier to read price tags and may prefer talking books for recreational reading. A patient with retinitis pigmentosa, which causes reduced night vision, may have normal mobility in the daytime and need a cane at night. Digital audio books may have braille labels.

Vision assistance. A special form of vision substitution involves using the eyes of others. Family members, caregivers, and office personnel should be familiar with *sighted guide* techniques to effectively assist visually impaired patients with minimal embarrassment. *Guide dogs* are also a possibility. Using a guide dog requires training of the patient as well as of the dog so that they can work as a team. Dog users must also demonstrate mastery of long cane travel skills.

Coping skills. How different patients will accept visual aids may differ greatly. It is important to recognize that vision loss often causes a reactive depression. On the one hand, a depressed patient will be less receptive to rehabilitative suggestions. On the other hand, demonstration of rehabilitative success can be a powerful tool to lift a reactive depression and to motivate the patient for further success. It has been shown that the teaching of general problem-solving skills may improve the effectiveness of vision rehabilitation.

Many professionals may be involved in vision rehabilitation. Technicians may prescribe various magnifiers, rehabilitation workers may teach daily living skills, and psychologists may address depression. Acceptance of the work of these professionals will be improved if the trusted primary care physician is credited with making the referrals.

Beyond the factors that directly involve the patient, the environment must also be considered.

The *human environment* is important. As patients go through the stages of adaptation, a supportive home environment is essential. As patients are counseled, it is important to include spouses, children, or significant others to make sure that they understand the condition, know what can be expected, and know how to support the patient. Answering family and caregiver questions directly is often better than leaving this to the patient, who initially may not have absorbed everything that was said. An overprotective environment, which deprives patients of opportunities to do things for themselves, can be as detrimental as an overdemanding one that puts too much emphasis on the patient's shortcomings. The same holds true for the work or school environment and for social groups.

Initially, patients often feel isolated and believe that they are the only ones experiencing these problems. *Peer support groups* can be helpful; in these groups, patients can experience how others are dealing with similar problems.

Finally, the *physical environment* needs to be considered. An uncluttered environment, where things have a defined, fixed place is helpful because it reduces the need for searching. Good general illumination and task lighting often help, because at higher illumination levels retinal cells that are damaged but not dead can still contribute to vision. Good contrast is important: Do not serve milk in a white Styrofoam cup; mark the edges of steps and stairs. The triangles and circles on men's and women's bathrooms are designed to be visible for those with very low vision; braille labels in elevators are useful for people who are totally blind.

How Blind Is Blind?

The most common visual function test is the letter chart, developed by Snellen in 1862. That test determines how large a letter, or other symbol, must be to be recognized by the patient. That size is then compared with the size recognized by a standard observer. If the magnification requirement is 2×, visual acuity is said to be 1/2; if it is 5×, visual acuity is said to be 1/5, etc. That fraction can be recorded in different ways; in the United States, it is customary to use 20 as the numerator (1/2 = 20/40, 1/5 = 20/100); in the British Commonwealth, 6 is used as the numerator (6/12, 6/30); in Europe, decimal fractions are common (0.5, 0.2).

Those calculations are simple; unfortunately, the terminology used to describe various ranges of vision loss is confusing. Figure 3 shows progressively degraded pictures with examples of the terminology used to describe different degrees of visual impairment. The visual acuity level represented by each picture can be determined from the number of lines that are readable on the low vision letter chart.

| Low vision (WHO) | <20/60 | Statutory blindness (SSA) | <20/100 |
| Legal blindness (USA) | <20/200 | Blindness (WHO) | <20/400 |

Figure 3 Ranges of vision loss.

The first picture shows the visual acuity level that is labeled as "low vision" by the World Health Organization (WHO). Although the bottom lines of the letter chart cannot be read, the appearance of the room is near normal. The next picture shows what the US Social Security Administration considers "statutory blindness" for its programs. Although reading regular print is not possible without magnification devices, it is clear that this is far from actual blindness. Other US programs use a different definition for "legal blindness," and the WHO does not consider a person "blind" until he or she has reached the status of the last picture. At that level, reading even the special letter chart is not possible, but one can still navigate the room. Even this level of visual impairment does not constitute actual blindness.

The widespread use of the word "blindness" is unfortunate because it cannot be used with modifiers. One is either blind or sighted; one cannot be "a little bit blind." This black-and-white thinking has hampered the acceptance of vision rehabilitation. Terms such as *vision loss* or *visual impairment* are preferred because they can be used with modifiers, including mild, moderate, severe, profound, and total vision loss. Although "legal blindness" and "severe vision loss" (ICD-9-CM) have the same definition, there is a big difference between telling a patient "you *are* legally blind" and "you *have* a severe visual impairment." The first statement might be followed by "I am sorry, there is nothing more we can do for your eyes"; the second statement leads to the question, "What can we do to help you cope with this problem?"

Vision Rehabilitation Techniques and Devices

Having considered the general outlines of vision rehabilitation, some details of rehabilitative interventions can be discussed. Primary care physicians should know what vision rehabilitation techniques are available so that they can make appropriate referrals.

Optical Problems

The most commonly encountered visual problems are those involving the optical system of the eye.

Refractive errors are the easiest visual problems to deal with. Refractive errors can be corrected with glasses or contact lenses, and for those who hate glasses, by refractive surgery. Even if there are other causes of vision loss, determining the best refractive correction is still important.

Uncorrected refractive error accounts for about half of all visual impairment worldwide. In developed countries, the question may be why people do not avail themselves of the solutions that are available. In developing countries, availability and accessibility of eye care and of the means for correcting refractive errors often do not exist. Providing these services is a matter of infrastructure, not of individual healthcare.

Opacities disrupt visual image formation. Cataracts are the most familiar opacity; they can be removed by surgery. Other opacities of a temporary or permanent nature may occur in the cornea, in the anterior chamber, or in the vitreous cavity. Corneal and conjunctival infections may cause corneal scarring, as is the case in trachoma, a condition that does not exist in the developed world anymore but is still a major cause of vision loss worldwide.

Letter chart acuity is a good way to measure optical problems. It should be understood, however, that letter chart acuity only measures the function of the retinal area where the letter read is projected. Even for a patient with 20/200 acuity, this area is less than 1 degree in diameter. For optical problems this does not matter because foveal defocus predicts equal defocus in all other areas of the retina. For retinal problems, however, visual acuity alone is not sufficient to characterize the visual status.

Magnification is the primary way to compensate for reduced acuity. One way to provide magnification is to bring print closer to the eye. For older adults, this requires reading glasses with extra power. Alternatively, large print may be helpful. Larger print on medicine labels, as required in several states, can reduce medication errors by older adults, who often take several medications. Handheld magnifiers are another option; today, many have built-in LED illumination to provide more light. Video-magnifiers with a table-mounted large screen are ideal for prolonged reading; they can also enhance contrast and brightness, while some devices can even read the text out loud. Tablets, smartphone apps, and dedicated devices can provide similar advantages in a portable form. Today, these electronic means of magnification are increasingly popular because they can provide not only magnification but also contrast enhancement. They also have a larger field of view and allow a more comfortable reading distance with binocular viewing.

Retinal Problems

While primitive forms of cataract surgery have existed for centuries, the study of retinal disorders has only been possible since the invention of the ophthalmoscope in 1851. The ability to

Penicillin or amoxicillin[1] may be used if the isolate is found to be sensitive in vitro. It is important to give an adequate dose because resistance may develop when underdosed.

Antitoxins

There are three antitoxins in the Centers for Disease Control and Prevention (CDC) Strategic National stockpile: raxibacumab, obiltoxaximab, and anthrax immune globulin intravenous (AIGIV). These agents are not readily available to the public. They inhibit binding of protective antigen to the anthrax toxin receptor and translocation of lethal factor and edema factor into cells. There are human and animal data from the pre-antibiotic era that suggest that there is lower mortality in those who received the antitoxin in cutaneous anthrax compared with those who did not. Whether this agent should be given for systemic anthrax is controversial owing to lack of data. Because the mortality rate with systemic anthrax is high whereas the complication of antitoxin treatment is low, the potential benefit from antitoxins outweighs the potential risk from the antitoxins in systemic anthrax. This agent should be given in addition to appropriate antibiotics when systemic anthrax is suspected.

Pregnancy

Overall management is similar to that in the nonpregnant patient. In pregnancy, ciprofloxacin is preferred over doxycycline for both treatment and prevention. Newer fluoroquinolones such as levofloxacin and moxifloxacin[1] are not preferred because embryo toxicity has been observed in animal studies. This was not seen with ciprofloxacin. Transplacental transmission of anthrax is known to occur. Ciprofloxacin, levofloxacin, meropenem,[1] ampicillin,[1] penicillin, clindamycin,[1] and rifampin[1] are known to have adequate concentration in the placenta and at least one agent should be used with treatment.

Prognosis

Uncomplicated cutaneous anthrax has a mortality rate of less than 2% with treatment. Injection anthrax has a mortality rate of 28%, and gastrointestinal anthrax has a mortality rate of 40%. Inhalational anthrax has mortality of 45% despite antibiotics and modern intensive care. Meningitis from anthrax is almost always fatal.

Prevention

Postexposure prophylaxis should be started as soon as possible after exposure. Sixty days of antibiotics for immediate protection and a three-dose series of Anthrax Vaccine Adsorbed (AVA, BioThrax) for long-term protection are recommended by the United States Advisory Committee on Immunization Practices. Ciprofloxacin and doxycycline are recommended as first-line antibiotic therapy for postexposure prophylaxis and are FDA-approved for this indication. Alternative agents include levofloxacin, moxifloxacin, amoxicillin, or penicillin VK (if sensitive); and clindamycin. AVA should be administered at diagnosis and at 2 and 4 weeks. AVA is not FDA-approved for postexposure prophylaxis. Raxibacumab and obiltoxaximab, which are two monoclonal antibodies held in the United States Strategic National Stockpile, have been approved for prevention of inhalation anthrax when alternative preventive therapies are not available or not appropriate.

---

[1]Not FDA approved for this indication.

References

Anthrax. Available at http://www.cdc.gov/anthrax/ [accessed 3.1.2023].

Hendricks KA, Wright ME, Shadomy SV, et al: Centers for disease control and prevention expert panel meetings on prevention and treatment of anthrax in adults, *Emerg Infect Dis* 20, 2014. https://doi.org/10.3201/eid2002.130687.

Knox D, Murray G, Millar M, et al: Subcutaneous anthrax in three intravenous drug users, *J Bone Joint Surg* 93:414–417, 2011.

Logan NA, Hoffmaster AR, Shadomy SV, Stauffer KE: In Versalovic J, editor: *Manual of clinical microbiology*, 10th ed., Washington DC, 2011, ASM Press, pp 381–402.

Meaney-Delman D, Zotti ME, Creanga AA, et al: Special considerations for prophylaxis for and treatment of anthrax in pregnant and postpartum women, *Emerg Infect Dis* 20, 2014. https://doi.org/10.3201/eid2002.130611.

Ruoff KL, Clarridge J, Bernard K: In Garcia LS, editor: *Clinical microbiology procedures handbook*, ed 3rd, Washington DC, 2010, ASM Press. 3.18.1.

Singh K: Laboratory-acquired infections, *Clin Infect Dis* 49:142–147, 2009.

BABESIOSIS

Method of
Cheston B. Cunha, MD; and Burke A. Cunha, MD

CURRENT DIAGNOSIS

- Suspect babesiosis in patients from Ixodes tick-endemic areas who present with a malaria-like illness (MLI) with fever, chills, headache, fatigue, and malaise.
- Clinically, babesiosis usually presents as an acute febrile illness with high fevers (>102 °F), relative bradycardia, and shaking chills accompanied by fatigue and myalgias.
- Myalgias may suggest an influenza-like illness (ILI).
- Severe headaches may suggest an alternate diagnosis (e.g., meningitis).
- Some patients with babesiosis may be short of breath and may go on to develop acute respiratory distress syndrome (ARDS).
- Consider babesiosis for unexplained fevers following blood transfusion.
- In prolonged fevers that meet the definition of fever of unknown origin (FUO), consider babesiosis in patients from endemic areas.
- With babesiosis, there are usually no localizing signs except for splenomegaly. Importantly, no rash is present. If rash is present, consider an alternate diagnosis.
- In babesiosis, nonspecific laboratory test results, considered together, are helpful in excluding or narrowing diagnostic possibilities.
- Common nonspecific laboratory findings of babesiosis include a normal/slightly decreased white blood cell count, relative lymphopenia, atypical lymphocytes, thrombocytopenia, elevated total bilirubin, and high lactate dehydrogenase levels. Sera are mildly elevated.
- The erythrocyte sedimentation rate is usually highly elevated (>90 mm/h) as are serum ferritin levels.
- Definitive babesiosis diagnosis is by peripheral blood smears (thick and thin); thick smears are best for the detection of babesia and thin smears are best to assess the degree of parasitemia.
- In normal hosts, the degree of parasitemia is usually low (1%–5%), but high in compromised hosts (>10%). Severe babesiosis may occur in asplenic individuals (Howell-Jolly bodies reflect the degree of splenic dysfunction), the immunosuppressed, the elderly, and those with coinfections (e.g., ehrlichiosis, Lyme disease).
- If present, babesiosis is diagnosed by peripheral stained blood smears demonstrating the characteristic (but uncommon) "Maltese cross" in tetrads (four merozoites).
- In nonmalarious areas, babesiosis may be diagnosed by demonstrating intraerythrocytic ring forms on the peripheral smear.
- Babesiosis, like malaria, has intracellular ring forms, but babesiosis, unlike malaria, has no intracellular pigment (hemozoin).
- Alternatively, *Babesia microti* serology in the Northeastern United States is diagnostic if IgM titers are highly elevated (>1:64).
- Polymerase chain reaction to detect Babesia is more sensitive than blood smear review. It is particularly useful in patients with a low level of parasitemia.

- Preferred therapy is atovaquone (Mepron)[1] plus azithromycin (Zithromax).[1]
- Alternatively, clindamycin (Cleocin)[1] plus quinine[1] may be used.
- In addition to antibabesia therapy, exchange transfusion may be lifesaving in severe cases.
- For severe cases, continue therapy until degree of parasitemia is <5%.
- Recurrent or persistent babesiosis should be treated for >2 weeks after resolution of parasitemia.
- Doxycycline is not effective in babesiosis.
- Coinfection with other tick-borne pathogens is rare, but possible.

[1]Not FDA approved for this indication.

TABLE 1	Babesiosis	
PREFERRED THERAPY	**ALTERNATE THERAPY**
Azithromycin (Zithromax)[1] 500 mg PO×1, then 250 mg PO q24h×7 days **plus** Atovaquone suspension (Mepron)[1] 750 mg PO q12h×7 days	Clindamycin (Cleocin)[1] 600 mg PO q8h×7 days **plus** Quinine[1] 650 mg PO q8h×7 days

From Cunha CB, Cunha, BA, editors: *Antibiotic Essentials.* 17th ed. New Delhi: Jaypee Brothers Medical Publishers; 2020, p. 271.
[1]Not FDA approved for this indication.

Epidemiology

Babesiosis is a tick-borne zoonosis that clinically presents as a malaria-like illness (MLI). There are many *Babesia* species, but only five are pathogenic in humans. The geographic distribution of babesiosis mimics that of hard-bodied *Ixodes dammini* (*I. scapularis*) ticks and their vertebrate hosts (e.g., dogs, cats, cattle, and rodents). The primary reservoir for babesiosis in the Northeastern United States is the white-footed mouse (*I. dammini* nymphs) and the white-tailed deer (*I. dammini* adults). Sporadic cases of babesiosis also occur in states with the tick vector/vertebrate hosts. Babesiosis may also be acquired by blood/blood product transfusions.

Clinical Features

In the Northeastern United States, babesiosis is usually *B. microti* and clinically manifests as an MLI. Babesiosis may be asymptomatic (IgG seropositive) or a mild, self-limited influenza-like illness (ILI). The incubation period for naturally acquired babesiosis is 1 to 6 weeks and 6 to 9 weeks for transfusion-acquired babesiosis. Clinical presentations in normal hosts are subacute with fever, fatigue, headache, malaise, and anorexia often mimicking Epstein-Barr virus infectious mononucleosis (with false-positive Monospot test results). Babesiosis presenting in patients with prolonged fevers of unknown origins (FUOs) and anorexia/weight loss may mimic a lymphoreticular malignancy. Presentation may be acute in those with impaired splenic function, those on immunosuppressives, or the elderly. Babesiosis may be viewed clinically as the "malaria of Long Island/Nantucket" as it presents with many malarial features, e.g., fever, chills, headache, sweats, myalgias. Excluding epidemiologic considerations, babesiosis differs in geographic distribution from malaria. Clinically, babesiosis differs from malaria in two important aspects. The clinical hallmarks of malaria are acute onset, intermittent fevers, and the classic "malaria paroxysm." Babesia reproduce by asynchronous asexual budding, which is clinically manifest as constant/nonintermittent fever. With malaria, fevers are intermittent with fever periodicity related to the *Plasmodium* species. Only *P. falciparum* has no fever periodicity and like babesiosis has no hepatic phase. Malaria and babesiosis both have extraerythrocytic ring forms, but babesiosis has two distinct morphologic features: extracellular merozoites (tetrads), known as "Maltese crosses," and no extraerythrocytic pigment, which malaria does have.

Unless the liver or spleen is enlarged, the physical features in babesiosis are limited to the fever. The fever curve of babesiosis is remittent without periodicity; fever is between 102 °F and 105 °F and accompanied by relative bradycardia. Rash is not a feature. When babesiosis is suspected, the presence of a rash is either indicative of coinfection, e.g., Lyme disease, or an alternative cause, e.g., viral or drug exanthem. Babesiosis should not be in the differential diagnosis of Rocky Mountain spotted fever with rash on the wrists/ankles. Babesiosis may clinically resemble ehrlichiosis. Peripheral blood smears are the best way to differentiate babesiosis from ehrlichiosis. Nonspecific laboratory abnormalities in babesiosis include normal/decreased white blood cell (WBC) count (leukopenia). Relative lymphopenia is usually present. Atypical lymphocytes are frequently present in the peripheral smear. Thrombocytopenia is a constant finding. The erythrocyte sedimentation rate (ESR) is highly elevated (usually >90 mm/h and often >100 mm/h) as is C-reactive protein (CRP). Since the pathophysiology of babesiosis is that of an acute hemolytic anemia, like malaria, intravascular hemolysis in babesiosis is manifested by increased lactate dehydrogenase (LDH)/total bilirubin. Increased LDH and total bilirubin are the most sensitive indicators of the degree of intravascular hemolysis in babesiosis. The hemoglobin/hematocrit is decreased later in more severe cases. Ferritin levels are highly elevated and prolonged (higher/longer) than would occur with acute-phase ferritin elevations. Since babesiosis impairs T cell function, as in malaria, serum protein electrophoresis often shows polyclonal gammopathy reflecting compensatory B cell hyperactivity. Serum transaminases are mildly elevated, but alkaline phosphatase is unelevated. Cold agglutinins are not a feature of babesiosis. In patients with decreased/absent splenic function, Howell-Jolly bodies are present in the peripheral smear. The number of Howell-Jolly bodies present is inversely proportional to the degree of splenic dysfunction.

Diagnosis of babesiosis is microscopic or serologic. Like malaria, babesiosis may be diagnosed on Giemsa stained blood smears. If malaria is not a diagnostic consideration (geographic distribution, blood transfusion), the presence of intraerythrocytic ring forms is diagnostic. Less common, but more specific, are pathognomonic tetrads (Maltese crosses) of babesiosis in peripheral smears. Also, unlike malaria, there is no extraerythrocytic pigment in babesiosis. Alternatively, elevated IgM *Babesia* species titers are diagnostic.

Therapy

The preferred therapy of babesiosis consists of 7 days combination therapy of azithromycin (Zithromax)[1] plus atovaquone (Mepron).[1] Alternatively, clindamycin (Cleocin)[1] plus quinine[1] for 7 days may be used (Table 1).

Treatment failure may occur in those with impaired T cell function, e.g., patients with HIV or with decreased splenic function. In such cases, exchange transfusion may be lifesaving.

[1]Not FDA approved for this indication.

References

Bonoan JT, Johnson DH, Cunha BA: Life-threatening babesiosis in an asplenic patient treated with exchange transfusion, azithromycin and atovaquone, *Heart Lung* 27:424–428, 1998.

Cunha BA, Raza M, Schmidt A: Highly elevated serum ferritin levels are a diagnostic marker in babesiosis, *Clin Infect Dis* 60:827–829, 2015.

Cunha BA, Mickail N, Laguerre M: Babesiosis mimicking Epstein Barr Virus (EBV) infectious mononucleosis: another cause of false positive Monospot test, *J Infect* 62:531–532, 2012.

Cunha BA, Cohen YZ, McDermott B: Fever of unknown origin (FUO) due to babesiosis in an immunocompetent host, *Heart Lung* 37:481–484, 2008.

Cunha BA, Nausheen S, Szalsa D: Pulmonary complications of Babesiosis: case report and literature review, *Eur J Clin Microbiol Infect Dis* 26:505–508, 2007.

Cunha BA, Crean J, Rosenbaum G: Lipid abnormalities in babesiosis, *Am J Med* 15:758–759, 2000.

Cunha CB: Infectious diseases differential diagnosis. In Cunha BA, editor: *Antibiotic Essentials*, ed 12th, Sudbury, MA, 2013, Jones & Bartlett, pp 474–506.

Hildebrandt A, Gray JS, Hunfeld KP: Human babesiosis in Europe: what clinicians need to know, *Infection* 41:1057–1072, 2013.

Kim N, Rosenbaum GS, Cunha BA: Relative bradycardia and lymphopenia in patients with babesiosis, *Clin Infect Dis* 26:1218–1219, 1998.

Krause PJ, Daily J, Telford SR, et al: Shared features in the pathology of babesiosis and malaria, *Trends Parasitol* 23:605–610, 2007.

Larkin JM: Ticks and tick-related illness, *Med Health RI* 91:209–211, 2008.

Leiby DA: Transfusion-transmitted Babesia spp: bull's-eye on Babesia microti, *Clin Microbiol Rev* 24:14–28, 2011.

Merch K, Holmaas G, Frolander PS, et al: Severe human Babesia divergens infection in Norway, *Int J Infect Dis* 23:37–38, 2014.

Nathavitharana RR, Mitty JA: Diseases from North America: focus on tick-borne infections, *Clin Med* 15:74–77, 2015.

Panduranga V, Kumar A: Severe babesiosis presenting as acute respiratory distress syndrome in an immunocompetent patient, *Conn Med* 78:289–291, 2014.

Rosenbaum GS, Johnson DH, Cunha BA: Atypical lymphocytosis in babesiosis, *Clin Infect Dis* 20:203–204, 1995.

Sharon KP, Krause PJ: Babesiosis. In Cunha BA, editor: *Tickborne infectious diseases diagnosis and management*, New York, 2007, Information Healthcare, pp 111–120.

Usmani-Brown S, Halperin JJ, Krause PJ: Neurological manifestations of human babesiosis, *Handb Clin Neurol* 114:199–203, 2013.

Wudhikarn K, Perry EH, Kemperman M, et al: Transfusion-transmitted babesiosis in an immunocompromised patient: a case report and review, *Am J Med* 124:800–805, 2011.

BACTERIAL MENINGITIS

Method of
Martha Muller, MD

CURRENT DIAGNOSIS

Patient Age Often Determines Clinical Presentation:
- Neonates: nonspecific symptoms
- Classic features: Fever, headache, neck stiffness, altered mental status
- Cerebrospinal fluid (CSF) evaluation
- Elevated opening pressure
- Elevated white blood cell count
- Decreased glucose: CSF–to–blood glucose ratio less than 0.60
- Elevated protein

CURRENT THERAPY

Neonates Younger Than 2 Months
- Most common organisms: *Streptococcus agalactiae, Escherichia coli* or other gram-negative enteric organism, occasional *Listeria monocytogenes*
- Empiric therapy: ampicillin, cefotaxime, or ceftriaxone (should be discussed with a pharmacist to determine risk factors for use)

Infants and Children Older Than 2 Months
- Most common organisms: *Streptococcus pneumoniae, Neisseria meningitidis, Haemophilus influenzae* type B
- Empiric therapy: ceftriaxone and vancomycin (used for potential penicillin-resistant *S. pneumoniae*)

Adults
- Most common organisms: *S. pneumoniae, N. meningitidis*
- Empiric therapy: ceftriaxone and vancomycin

Adults Older Than 50 Years
- Most common organisms: *S. pneumoniae, N. meningitidis, L. monocytogenes*
- Empiric therapy: ceftriaxone, vancomycin, and ampicillin

Bacterial meningitis is a serious, life-threatening infection of the central nervous system. This inflammation of the meninges and subarachnoid space, including the cerebrospinal fluid (CSF), may potentially affect the brain cortex and parenchyma. Bacterial meningitis can occur via several pathophysiologic mechanisms (Table 1). In the neonatal period, most of the offending organisms have colonized mucosal surfaces after contact and aspiration of maternal intestinal and genital tract secretions during the delivery process. The most common mechanism noted outside of the neonatal period involves nasopharyngeal colonization, penetration of the nasopharyngeal mucous membrane barrier with entrance to the interstitial space, and entrance into the capillary bloodstream with subsequent delivery to the meninges or choroid plexus. Once organisms penetrate the CSF, an advantage in their favor exists. In a usual physiologic state, there is essentially an absence of capsule-specific immunoglobulins, complement factors, polymorphonuclear lymphocytes, and other plasma cells within the CSF, making the environment conducive to bacterial proliferation. Available host defenses are apparently ineffectual against encapsulated organisms. The cerebral vasculature is the primary mark for inflammation. Inflammatory changes result in blood-brain barrier disruption, edema, vasospasm and potential arterial thrombosis, as well as cerebral vein occlusions.

Additionally, bacterial and neutrophil-associated inflammatory products may traverse the pial barrier, potentially resulting in neuronal necrosis or cranial nerve compression.

The majority of bacterial meningitis cases occur sporadically. Globally, reported cases of bacterial meningitis increased between 2006 and 2016, with poverty strongly correlated to incidence. Incidence reported in higher-resourced countries has decreased to 0.5 to 1.5 per 100,000 population. Africa continues to bear a significant burden of bacterial meningitis, with incidence reaching 1000 per 100,000 population. Worldwide, bacterial meningitis is linked with significant morbidity and mortality, evidenced by approximately 16 million reported cases in 2013, associated with 1.6 million years lived with disability annually. Although dependent on many factors, including etiologic agent, age, risk factors, and so on, case fatality rates for bacterial meningitis have been reported to be between 17% and 40%.

A disease formerly dominated by *Haemophilus influenzae* in infants has now transitioned to one caused by *Streptococcus pneumoniae*, largely affecting older adult patients. On the whole, *S. pneumoniae* meningitis causes meningitis in children older than 5 years of age and in adults older than 65 years of age. Contrastingly, *Neisseria meningitidis* tends to cause meningitis in older children and young adults. *Streptococcus agalactiae* dominates as the most common organism implicated in bacterial meningitis in neonates and young infants.

Many intrinsic and extrinsic factors increase the risk for developing bacterial meningitis and also affect the potential offending bacteria (Table 1). Additionally, general factors such as poor living conditions and crowded daycare centers influence the potential development of bacterial meningitis.

TABLE 1	Pathophysiologic Mechanisms Associated With the Development of Bacterial Meningitis	
MECHANISM	**EXAMPLES**
Hematologic	Nasopharyngeal colonization with penetration
Traumatic	Skull fractures
Iatrogenic	Cochlear implantation; ventriculoperitoneal shunt placement
Congenital	Dermal sinus
Contiguous infection	Sinuses; middle ear

Diagnosis

The clinical presentation of bacterial meningitis is greatly influenced by patient age. Neonates and infants generally present with nonspecific signs and symptoms, including poor feeding, respiratory distress, fussiness, general weakness, and irritability. Although not universal in babies with bacterial meningitis, fever may also be present in less than 40% and seizures may be present in 15% to 34%. Similarly, hypothermia may be a presenting symptom. In general, patients with bacterial meningitis beyond the neonatal period present with more classic symptoms, including fever, neck stiffness, photophobia, significant headache, nausea, and vomiting. Those patients with associated systemic compromise have higher potential for poor disease outcome.

Physical examination findings are also associated with age, generally displaying more characteristic findings with increasing age. Meningeal irritation may be demonstrated by neck stiffness, the Brudzinski sign (hips and knees flex reflexively when the neck is flexed), and the Kernig sign (flexion of the thigh with the hip and knee at 90-degree angles results in pain on knee extension), with reported sensitivity as low as 9% for Brudzinsky sign and 5% for Kernig sign. A high degree of suspicion for bacterial meningitis in the appropriate clinical setting should be maintained despite physical examination findings as they are not always indicative of the disease. An adult prospective study demonstrated that the classic signs of meningeal irritation demonstrated a sensitivity of only 5% to 30%. Adult patients older than 65 years may present without typical symptoms. Additionally, patients with bacterial meningitis in this population may frequently present with nonspecific confusion. These older adult patients may also have nuchal rigidity that is not associated with bacterial meningitis.

In general, lumbar puncture should be sought without delay, with few contraindications to suggest otherwise. Contraindications include shock, respiratory compromise, and coagulopathy. Indications for obtaining neuroimaging before conducting a lumbar puncture include the presence of focal neurologic findings in children and immunocompromised condition, previous history of central nervous system disease, new-onset seizure, and focal neurologic findings in adults. CSF examination is crucial to the diagnosis of bacterial meningitis. CSF obtained for suspected bacterial meningitis should routinely be evaluated for cell count (red blood cells; white blood cells, with differential as appropriate), glucose, protein, Gram stain, and culture (Table 2). CSF culture serves as

the gold standard for diagnosis, with reported positivity in 50% to 90% of patients. CSF should be evaluated as soon as possible after obtaining it as white blood cells deteriorate within 30 minutes, and elevated white blood cell counts have the potential to metabolize CSF glucose. In general, characteristic CSF findings include elevated white blood cells, low glucose, and elevated protein values (Table 2). It is important to note that the CSF white blood cell count may infrequently be normal, especially very early in the course of illness. Blood cultures should also be obtained for patients with concerns for bacterial meningitis, with reported positivity in 50% to 80% of cases.

The receipt of antibiotics before CSF evaluation may lend to decreased organism recovery via culture. Effective antibiotic therapy can result in sterile cultures within 2 hours for *N. meningitidis* and begin the sterilization process within 4 hours for *S. pneumoniae*. Additional factors that may adversely affect CSF diagnostic utility include the potential for 24 to 48 hours or longer before obtaining culture results, inadequate CSF specimen volumes, fastidious organisms requiring special growth parameters, and inappropriate specimen attainment and transportation to the laboratory. Although CSF glucose and protein values in children may rarely be affected (in general, irregular values tend to persist for many days despite appropriate therapy), a diagnosis of bacterial meningitis may often still be made based on the CSF analyses in the setting of antibiotic pretreatment. Polymerase chain reaction (PCR) is a promising tool in the arsenal for diagnosis of bacterial meningitis, especially in the setting of antibiotic pretreatment, and its evaluation and clinical use are expanding. Notably, the World Health Organization endorses the use of real-time PCR when considering *S. pneumoniae*, *N. meningitidis*, and *H. influenzae* type B for patients with potential meningitis. The diagnostic precision of PCR has been most widely evaluated for *S. pneumoniae*, *N. meningitidis*, and *H. influenzae* and has been reported to be as high as 95% to 100% in cases of culture-proven bacterial meningitis. A prospective study from Sweden reviewing CSF from repeat lumbar puncture demonstrated PCR positivity in 89% of samples taken on days 1 to 3; 70% of samples taken on days 4 to 6; and 33% of samples taken on days 7 to 10. In contrast, all CSF cultures taken from the same samples were negative. With its increasing utilization, PCR sensitivity has been reported as 61% to 100%, 88% to 94%, and 72% to 92% for *S. pneumoniae*, *N. meningitidis*, and *H. influenzae*, respectively. Additionally, false-negative PCR results are rare, occurring in approximately 5% of cases. Latex agglutination and coagglutination techniques, best for detection of bacteria that are actively proliferating and shedding polysaccharide, are infrequently used for the diagnosis of bacterial meningitis.

Complications of bacterial meningitis may occur any time during the course of the illness and include circulatory collapse, disseminated intravascular coagulation, gangrenous digits, focal neurologic findings, seizures, and subdural effusions.

The differential diagnosis of bacterial meningitis in infants and young children includes otitis media, pharyngitis, pneumonia, retropharyngeal abscess, and lymphadenopathy. Additional diagnoses include brain abscess, tuberculous meningitis, aseptic meningitis, meningitis caused by atypical organisms, and sinusitis.

Antibiotic Management

Successful treatment is characterized by a delicate balance between prompt antibiotic administration and host inflammatory response regulation. Underscored by an almost 100% mortality noted for untreated bacterial meningitis, prompt, appropriate antibiotic administration is paramount, generally increasing the chances of survival. This is particularly notable for infants and children in whom case fatality rates are decreased to less than 10% and less than 5%, respectively, for meningococcal meningitis in the setting of appropriate therapy.

Empiric antibiotic therapy should be chosen based on a variety of factors, including most likely bacterial etiology (local antibiograms and resistance patterns should be considered) (Tables 3 and 4), ability to penetrate the blood-brain barrier and achieve

TABLE 2	Anticipated Cerebrospinal Fluid Findings in Bacterial Meningitis
CSF PARAMETER	**TYPICAL FINDINGS**
White blood cell count	>1000 cells/mm³ (may be affected by immunosuppression, neutropenia, atypical pathogens)
Glucose	<40 mg/dL (CSF–to–blood glucose ratio <0.60)
Total protein	>100 mg/dL (increased above normal values for age)
Gram stain	Positivity depends on bacterial burden. Stains positive 97% of the time when cultures grow >10⁵ CFU Specific yield of 70%–90% for *Streptococcus pneumoniae* Specific yield of 30%–90% for *Neisseria meningitidis* Sensitivity low for *Listeria monocytogenes* as few organisms are generally present in CSF
CSF opening pressure	>200 mm H₂O (may be >300 mm H₂O; continued elevation for first 24–48 hours before decrease)

CFU, Colony-forming units; *CSF*, cerebrospinal fluid.

TABLE 3 Empiric Antibiotic Therapy Based on Contributing Factors*

CONTRIBUTING FACTOR	POTENTIAL ORGANISMS	ANTIBIOTIC THERAPY
Age		
<1 month	*Streptococcus agalactiae, Escherichia coli* (gram-negative enteric organisms), *Listeria monocytogenes*	Ampicillin and cefotaxime or ceftriaxone (discuss use in this population with pharmacist)
1–2 years	*Streptococcus pneumoniae, Neisseria meningitidis, Haemophilus influenzae* type B, *S. agalactiae, E. coli*	Ceftriaxone or cefotaxime and vancomycin[1]
2–50 years	*S. pneumoniae, N. meningitidis*	Ceftriaxone or cefotaxime and vancomycin[1]
>50 years	*S. pneumoniae, N. meningitidis, L. monocytogenes*	Ceftriaxone or cefotaxime, ampicillin and vancomycin[1]
Head trauma Penetrating trauma	*Staphylococcus aureus,* coagulase-negative staphylococci, aerobic gram-negative organisms (including *Pseudomonas aeruginosa*)	Vancomycin with either cefepime[1] or meropenem
Neurosurgery	*S. aureus,* coagulase-negative staphylococci, aerobic gram-negative organisms (including *P. aeruginosa*)	Vancomycin with either cefepime[1] or meropenem
CNS shunt placement	*S. aureus,* coagulase-negative staphylococci, aerobic gram-negative organisms (including *P. aeruginosa*)	Vancomycin with either cefepime[1] or meropenem

*Modified from Tunkel AR, Hartman BJ, Kaplan SL, et al: Practice guidelines for the management of bacterial meningitis, *Clin Infect Dis* 39:126–1284, 2004.
[1]Not FDA approved for this indication.

TABLE 4 Special Patient Characteristics Associated With Specific Organisms

BACTERIA	PATIENT CHARACTERISTICS
Streptococcus pneumoniae	Immunocompromised status
Neisseria meningitidis	Complement deficiencies, asplenia, smoking, antibody deficiency
Haemophilus influenzae type B	Native American children; Alaskan Native children
Listeria monocytogenes	Immunocompromised status
Staphylococcus aureus	Neurosurgical procedures, shunt device placement, trauma, underlying disease (e.g., diabetes mellitus), HIV, cardiovascular disease, intravenous drug use

TABLE 5 Antibiotics Commonly Used to Treat Bacterial Meningitis

ANTIBIOTIC	ADULT DOSING	PEDIATRIC DOSING
Ampicillin	2 g every 4 hours	300–400 mg/kg/day divided every 4–6 hours; maximum daily dose: 12 g/day
Cefotaxime[2]	2 g every 4–6 hours	225–300 mg/kg/day divided every 6–8 hours
Ceftriaxone	2 g every 12 hours	50 mg/kg/dose every 12 hours
Cefepime[1]	2 g every 8 hours	50 mg/kg/dose every 8 hours
Meropenem	2 g every 8 hours	40 mg/kg/dose every 8 hours
Vancomycin*[1]	15–20 mg/kg/dose every 8–12 hours	15 mg/kg/dose every 6 hours

*Appropriate loading and level monitoring should be performed by a pharmacist.
[1]Not FDA approved for this indication.
[2]Not available in the United States.

adequate CSF levels, and bactericidal mechanism of action. Beta-lactam antibiotics are frequently used to treat bacterial meningitis and are generally effective against the most commonly associated bacteria. CSF concentrations of these antibiotics, even in the setting of minimal meningeal inflammation, are generally adequate for the minimal inhibitory concentrations for susceptible bacteria. Bacterial resistance patterns also greatly influence empiric antibiotic therapy. Worldwide, penicillin resistance in *S. pneumoniae* has affected recommendations to use vancomycin as part of the empiric antibiotic regimen. Antibiotics should be provided parenterally at maximal clinically indicated doses (Table 5). Antibiotic therapy should not be delayed by the need to obtain neuroimaging. Once a specific organism is isolated, antibiotic therapy should be tailored to treat the organism, completing an appropriate duration of therapy (Table 6).

Adjunctive Therapy

With a goal of decreasing inflammation leading to neuronal death and brain damage, dexamethasone (Decadron)[1] administration is the cornerstone of adjunctive therapy for bacterial meningitis. Data from studies evaluating the effect of steroids on outcomes of infants and children with bacterial meningitis have demonstrated improved meningeal inflammatory indices and decreased audiologic and neurologic sequelae compared with those receiving

[1]Not FDA approved for this indication.

TABLE 6 Duration of Antibiotic Therapy for Uncomplicated Infections Caused by Specific Organisms

PATHOGEN	DURATION OF THERAPY
Streptococcus agalactiae (group B streptococcus)	14 days
Escherichia coli (gram-negative enteric organisms)	21 days
Listeria monocytogenes	21 days
Streptococcus pneumoniae	10–14 days
Neisseria meningitidis	7 days
Haemophilus influenzae type B	7–10 days

placebo; this benefit is most notable for *H. influenzae* meningitis. The data for dexamethasone use to treat *S. pneumoniae* meningitis in children are less vigorous. Additionally, animal models of bacterial meningitis demonstrated decreased vancomycin concentrations and penetration rates in the CSF for those animals receiving dexamethasone. This is important given the potential need to use vancomycin in the treatment of penicillin-resistant *S. pneumoniae* bacterial meningitis.

The American Academy of Pediatrics Committee on Infectious Diseases does endorse the use of dexamethasone for *H. influenzae* type B meningitis. However, the committee does not make a recommendation for routine dexamethasone use in *S. pneumoniae* meningitis. They do provide a consideration of its use in children older than 6 weeks after risks and benefits have been reviewed. There are inadequate data to make a recommendation for dexamethasone use during the neonatal period. The available data demonstrating decreased unfavorable outcomes in adults when using dexamethasone have prompted the Infectious Diseases Society of America to routinely recommend dexamethasone for adults with suspected or proven pneumococcal meningitis. When given, dexamethasone should be provided at a dose of 0.15 mg/kg every 6 hours for 2 to 4 days. It should be given 10 to 20 minutes before or concurrent with the first dose of antibiotic therapy.

Vaccination Prevention

Between 1990 and 2013, global mortality caused by *S. pneumoniae, N. meningitis,* and *H. influenzae* type B decreased by 29%, 25%, and 45%, respectively. Conjugate vaccination strategies have played an important role in improving that landscape. The introduction of *H. influenzae* type B and *S. pneumoniae* conjugate vaccines during the 1990s and 2000s contributed to reports of a decrease in bacterial meningitis in both vaccinated and nonvaccinated populations. The additional benefit of whole-population herd immunity was also described with the introduction of pneumococcal conjugate vaccines. The introduction of conjugated *H. influenzae* type B vaccination programs provided a significant contribution to reducing bacterial meningitis, wherein bacterial meningitis caused by this organism has decreased by almost 100%. Interestingly, initiation of the 7-valent pneumococcal conjugate vaccine (Prevnar 7) in the United States was accompanied by a noted decrease in meningitis caused by vaccine serotypes, initially in children followed by a decrease in adults. However, a concurrent increase in nonvaccine serotypes was noted in response. Likewise, the introduction of the 13-valent pneumococcal conjugate vaccine (Prevnar 13) has also been met with an increased prevalence of nonvaccine serotypes causing bacterial meningitis. Since 2015 there has been a brisk increase in incidence of invasive pneumococcal disease, including meningitis, secondary to non-PCV13 serotypes. Despite the concerns regarding serotype replacement, receipt of several pneumococcal conjugate vaccines in the United States led to a 66% and 33% decrease in rates of pneumococcal meningitis for children younger than 2 years and adults older than 65 years, respectively. Vaccination against *N. meningitidis* has also resulted in a decrease in bacterial meningitis, demonstrating a rate decrease from 13.5 per 100,000 in 1968 to 1985 to 5.2 per 100,000 in 1989 to 2011. Many higher-resourced countries have seen a significant decrease in the incidence of serogroup-C meningitis related to vaccination. Serogroup-B meningitis rose with the decline of serogroup-C meningitis in higher-resourced countries. In 2015 the United Kingdom introduced serogroup-B vaccine 4CMenB (Bexsero), reporting an overall 75% decline in invasive disease.

Immunization against *H. influenzae* type B, *S. pneumoniae,* and *N. meningitidis* has been incorporated into the routine childhood vaccination schedule in the United States. The Advisory Committee on Immunization Practices provides specific vaccine recommendations.

Outcomes/Sequelae

The consideration of patient outcomes is multifactorial, including patient age; time to antibiotic administration, especially as it relates to symptom onset; host factors such as immune response to infection; and time to CSF sterilization. In general, the greatest morbidity and mortality are seen at the extremes of ages (i.e., neonates and older adults). Mortality associated with bacterial meningitis has been 20% to 25% for numerous decades.

Pneumococcal meningitis is associated with the highest case fatality rates, reported as 20% to 37% in high-income countries and as high as 51% in low-income countries. This is in contrast with case fatality rates reported as 3% to 10% worldwide for meningococcal meningitis. A study reported that risk factors implicated in the development of neurologic complications in the pediatric population include age less than 12 months; bacterial etiology, especially *S. pneumoniae;* altered level of consciousness on presentation; delayed presentation; and delayed antibiotic administration.

An important immediate complication related to bacterial meningitis in pediatric patients is the development of subdural effusions. Subdural effusions are described in 20% to 39% of pediatric patients with bacterial meningitis and are notably more common in infants younger than 1 year compared with their older peers. Importantly, although there is the potential for infection, most subdural effusions in this clinical scenario are asymptomatic, demonstrating spontaneous resolution.

Neurologic difficulties have been reported in 20% to 30% of bacterial meningitis events. Similarly, long-standing neuropsychological sequelae have been reported in as many as 50% of those who survive bacterial meningitis. Compared with their well siblings who did not have bacterial meningitis, infants and children with bacterial meningitis are more likely to experience seizures, hearing loss, cognitive disturbances, and behavioral concerns. Similarly, there have been reports of disturbed executive functioning, memory, and intelligence in adults who have recovered from bacterial meningitis.

Seizures, hearing loss, and cognitive impairment are the most commonly reported disabilities after a diagnosis of bacterial meningitis. Seizures complicate bacterial meningitis and have an individual link to increased morbidity. In children, the development of long-standing neurologic complications is less concerning when associated seizures that occur early during the course of illness are easily controlled. In contrast, prolonged or difficult-to-control seizures and seizures developing 72 hours after admission are more likely to be associated with neurologic sequelae and are often indicative of a cerebrovascular event. Neurologic complications have been reported in as many as 50% of those who survive bacterial meningitis. Hearing loss is a common complication of bacterial meningitis. In fact, sensorineural hearing loss has been described as the most broadly reported neurologic sequelae of bacterial meningitis. Hearing loss has the potential to be transient or permanent and is often associated with *S. pneumoniae* meningitis. Sustained hearing loss is generally sensorineural, with incidence reported as 14% for mild hearing loss and 5% for severe hearing loss. The hearing loss typically occurs during the initial days of the infection and can be transient or permanent, underscoring the need for formal hearing evaluation to occur in all patients diagnosed with bacterial meningitis.

References

American Academy of Pediatrics: *Red book report of the committee on infectious diseases 2018-2021,* ed 31.

Brouwe MC, van de Beek D: Epidemiology of community-acquired bacterial meningitis, *Curr Opin Infect Dis* 31:78–84, 2018.

Bystritsky RJ, Chow FC: Infectious meningitis and encephalitis, *Neurol Clin* 40:77–91, 2022.

Costerus JM, et al: Community-acquired bacterial meningitis, *Curr Opin Infect Dis* 30:135–141, 2017.

Davis LE: Acute bacterial meningitis, *Continuum (Minneap Minn)* 24:1264–1283, 2018.

Diallo K, et al: Molecular diagnostic assays for the detection of common bacterial meningitis pathogens: a narrative review, *EBioMedicine* 65:103274103274, 2021.

Figueiredo AHA, et al: Acute community-acquired bacterial meningitis, *Neurol Clin* 809–820, 2018.

Hasbun R: Progress and challenges in bacterial meningitis, *JAMA* 328:2147–2154, 2022.

Kim KS: Acute bacterial meningitis in infants and children, *Lancet Infect Dis* 10:32–42, 2010.

Lexicomp Online: *Adult Lexi-Drugs Online,* Hudson, Ohio, 2021, UpToDate, Inc.

Lexicomp Online: *Pediatric and Neonatal Lexi-Drugs Online,* Hudson, Ohio, 2021, UpToDate, Inc.

Liechti FD, et al: Bacterial meningitis: insights into pathogenesis and evaluation of new treatment options: a perspective from experimental studies, *Future Microbiol* 10:1195–2213, 2015.

McGill F, et al: Acute bacterial meningitis in adults, *Lancet* 388:3036–3047, 2016.

Obaro S: Updating the diagnosis of bacterial meningitis, *Lancet Infect Dis* 19:1160–1161, 2019.

Oordts-Speets AM, et al: Global etiology of bacterial meningitis: a systematic review and meta-analysis, *PLOS One* 13, 2018. https://doi.org/10.1371/journal.pone.0198772. e0198772.

Pajor MJ, et al: High risk and low prevalence diseases: Adult bacterial meningitis, *Am J Emerg Med* 65:76–83, 2023.

Posadas E, et al: Pediatric bacterial meningitis: An update on early identification and management, *EB Medicine* 15:1–20, 2018.

Saez-Llorens X, McCracken GH Jr: Bacterial meningitis in children, *Lancet* 361:2139–2148, 2003.

Syrogiannopoulos GA, et al: Global epidemiology of vaccine-preventable bacterial meningitis, *PIDJ* 41:e525–e529, 2022.

Tunkel AR, et al: Practice guidelines for the management of bacterial meningitis, *CID* 39:1267–1284, 2004.

Van de beek D, et al: Community-acquired bacterial meningitis, *Lancet* 398:1171–1183, 2021.

van de Beek D, et al: Community-acquired bacterial meningitis, *Nat Rev Dis Primers* 2(1–20), 2016.

Wall EC, et al: Acute bacterial meningitis, *Curr Opin Neurol* 34:386–395, 2021.

Zainel A, Mitchell H, Sadarangani M: Bacterial meningitis in children: Neurological complications, associated risk factors, and prevention, *Microorganisms* 9:535, 2021.

Young S and Saguil A: Bacterial meningitis in children. *Am Fam Physician* 105(3):311-312.

BRUCELLOSIS

Method of
Patrick L. Allen, MD

CURRENT DIAGNOSIS

- Brucellosis presents with a variety of nonspecific clinical syndromes, most commonly an unusually persistent, undulating fever often accompanied by musculoskeletal pains. Rare complications include meningitis and endocarditis.
- The key to the diagnosis of brucellosis is maintaining a high degree of clinical suspicion in patients with a suggestive clinical history, such as travel to an endemic area, consumption of unpasteurized dairy products, close contact with potentially infected mammals, or inadvertent laboratory exposure.
- There is no gold standard for the diagnosis of *Brucella* infection. Multiple blood cultures should be drawn but have variable yield. Serologic tests may be helpful but require cautious interpretation, especially in endemic areas. Polymerase chain reaction (PCR) is promising but will require more standardization before widespread acceptance.

CURRENT THERAPY

- Combination therapy with multiple antibiotics is needed to successfully treat and to prevent recurrence.
- Doxycycline (Vibramycin) for 6 weeks plus either rifampin (Rifadin)[1] for 6 weeks or a parenteral aminoglycoside for 1 to 3 weeks are the most commonly recommended regimens.
- Longer therapy, often with three antibiotics in combination, is needed for localized and complicated disease.

[1]Not FDA approved for this indication.

History

Brucellosis, also called Malta fever, Mediterranean fever, and Undulant fever, has plagued humanity for millennia and was described by Sir David Bruce, a Scottish physician serving in the Royal Army Medical Corps. In 1887 he linked it with the causal pathogen, a bacteria later given the doubly eponymous name *Brucella melitensis* (from Malta). Later, additional species were identified, some of which also cause human disease.

As a public health interest, brucellosis is a disease reportable to the Centers for Disease Control (CDC). *Brucella* spp. can be easily cultured, grown, stored, and aerosolized in laboratories. This, together with the high infectivity of aerosolized specimens and a very low infectious dose, explains why brucellosis is recognized as a potential bioterrorism agent. Though its low case fatality rate (about 1%) and long incubation period make it an unlikely modern bioterrorism weapon (and is therefore listed by the CDC as a category B, "second highest priority," bioterrorism agent), the potential morbidity and economic ramifications of a widespread attack should not be underestimated. Fortunately, to date, *Brucella* has never successfully been used as a bioterrorism agent against humans.

Epidemiology

Brucellosis is now rare in the United States but is the world's most widespread zoonosis, found in animals as divergent as alpine ibex, African lions, and Antarctic seals. In humans it is noted as a top neglected disease by the World Health Organization (WHO). Though 500,000 human cases are reported worldwide each year, experts estimate the true incidence is substantially, perhaps 10-fold, higher. Much of the world is endemic, particularly the Middle East and Mediterranean Europe. The control of brucellosis requires well-functioning veterinary and animal husbandry systems; thus it is not surprising that the highest incidence rates of brucellosis are often found in the least developed nations of the world or after times of political instability. For example, when the Syrian conflict starting in 2011 devastated local animal care infrastructure, human brucellosis cases surged in the following years. The United States successfully eradicated *Brucella melitensis* in the 1970s and has nearly eliminated other zoonotic species in livestock; however, *Brucella* continues to be identified in certain populations of bison and elk (in the greater Yellowstone area), as well as in some deer and boar populations. These wild animals do occasionally interact with and infect neighboring domestic animals. Table 1 lists a variety of species of brucellosis, their usual hosts and whether they are considered zoonotic.

In infected ruminants such as cattle and goats, spontaneous abortions are the hallmark clinical presentation, and consumption of infected aborted tissue is the primary means of transmission from animal to animal for *B. melitensis* (causing caprine brucellosis) and *B. abortus* (causing bovine brucellosis, also called contagious abortion). *B. suis* (causing swine brucellosis) also causes abortions and is sexually transmitted in pigs and wild swine. *B. canis*, primarily infecting domestic and wild dogs, is rarely transmitted to humans and requires substantial direct contact, such as assisting with birthing. Other species of *Brucella*, such as *B. ovis* (causing ovine brucellosis, infertility in male sheep), are not considered zoonotic, though rare cases of human transmission have been reported with some species (see Table 1).

The most common cause of human infection is the consumption of unpasteurized dairy products, because the bacteria concentrate in the mammary glands of cattle, goats, and camels. Of the approximately 100 cases of brucellosis diagnosed each year in the United States, most are owing to the consumption of illegally imported soft cheeses from Mexico. Other causes include direct contact with infected animals such as hunters who field-dress animals or meat industry workers who slaughter animals or clean animal products. Brucellosis is the most common laboratory-acquired infection, and this mode of transmission comprises 2% of all human brucellosis cases globally. Laboratory workers can be infected by inadvertent direct contact of infected specimens to mucosal or nonintact skin or through inhalation while sniffing open cultures. Fortunately, when humans are infected with

TABLE 1	Characteristics of *Brucella* Species		
SPECIES	**PRIMARY HOST**	**OTHER HOSTS**	**ZOONOTIC SPREAD**
Brucella melitensis	Goats and sheep	Camels, cattle, yaks, alpacas, ibex	Yes
Brucella abortus	Cattle	Elk, bison, camels, moose	Yes
Brucella suis	Pigs, wild hogs	Hares, horses, reindeer, armadillo	Yes
Brucella canis	Dogs	Foxes, coyotes, cats, racoons	Less common
Brucella ovis	Sheep	Deer, goats, cattle	Not reported
Brucella ceti	Whales, dolphins, porpoises	Narwhals	Rare
Brucella pinnipediae	Seals	Whales, dolphins, porpoises	Rare
Brucella inopinata	Unknown		Rare
Brucella neotomae	Wood rats	Mice, guinea pigs	Rare
Brucella microti	Vole	Foxes	Not reported
Brucella papionis	Nonhuman primates		Not reported

Brucella, they are an accidental, dead-end host; human-to-human transmission is exceptionally rare.

Pathophysiology

Brucella spp. are gram-negative, aerobic, nonmotile, facultative intracellular coccobacilli of the family *Brucellaceae*. They are slow-growing, taking several hours to double. The three most virulent species (see Table 1) have a unique smooth lipopolysaccharide (LPS) that induces an unusually tame immune response in humans. After invading the host's mucosa, brucellae are ingested by macrophages and dendritic cells. There the bacteria employ a variety of sophisticated mechanisms to survive in specialized vacuoles and continue to replicate inside of the endoplasmic reticulum without affecting host-cell integrity. Programmed cell death is initially inhibited by the bacteria until sufficient replication has occurred. Brucellae then induce cell necrosis and release new pathogens, which travel through the bloodstream to regional lymph nodes and eventually to macrophage-rich tissues such as the liver, spleen, and bone marrow where chronic infection is established. Granuloma formation occurs in the lungs, liver, and other organs. Brucellae inhibit tumor necrosis factor-alpha, subsequently inhibiting macrophages and natural killer cells. Humoral immunity plays a limited role in controlling this mostly intracellular infection, though the production of antibrucellae antibodies are useful diagnostically. On the other hand, interferon-γ, causing the classic fevers associated with the disease, is a very important and effective host response against brucellae.

Clinical Manifestations

Brucellosis can affect any organ in the body. Its incubation period is usually 3 to 4 weeks but can be anywhere from 5 to 60 days. Asymptomatic and mild, self-limited infections do occur, but the rate remains unclear. In those with clinical brucellosis, fever is the invariable presentation, though it can be acute, relapsing, or prolonged over days to weeks. Other constitutional symptoms such as rigors, chills, sweats, generalized weakness, and fatigue are common. Skeletal complications such as arthralgias, peripheral arthritis, sacroiliitis, and lumbar spondylitis are the most common complications (40%) and are more difficult to treat, with three times the therapeutic failure rates of nonosteoarticular disease. Brucellosis can cause orchitis and epididymitis in men and spontaneous abortions in women. Other complications include hepatitis, liver granulomas, hepatosplenomegaly, lymphadenopathy, and pneumonia. Neurobrucellosis is rare (5%) and can consist of meningitis, meningoencephalitis, brain or epidural abscesses, and/or demyelination disorders. Endocarditis is also rare, occurring in about 2% of cases but responsible for about 80% of brucellosis deaths. Lab findings may include anemia, mild leukopenia, relative lymphocytosis, elevated transaminases, and elevated inflammatory markers. Children can be affected by brucellosis but are more likely than adults to have a mild course of illness.

Diagnosis

Any prolonged, recurrent, or unexplained fever should evoke a detailed clinical history. If that history reveals travel to an endemic area, consumption of any unpasteurized dairy product, close contact with a potentially infected animal, or potential accidental laboratory exposure, this should prompt a thorough diagnostic evaluation for brucellosis.

Unfortunately, there is no single reliable laboratory test as the gold standard for the diagnosis of brucellosis. The definitive diagnosis relies on isolation of the organism by culture. Blood cultures are of variable sensitivity (10%–90%), and yields improve with multiple blood draws over time, especially if drawn while febrile. Bacteremia is more persistent and therefore more easily diagnosed in early infection; with longer duration of illness, successful culture becomes increasingly elusive. Cerebrospinal fluid should be cultured in patients with any neurologic signs or symptoms, though this also has a low sensitivity (15%–30%). Bone marrow cultures have a higher sensitivity than blood cultures in many, but not all, studies and may slightly increase diagnostic yield. However, most recommend against routine bone marrow cultures, because blood cultures are much more easily obtained and may reveal brucellae, even in patients in whom the diagnosis is not initially being considered. In cases of suspected brucellosis, cultures should be incubated for 4 weeks owing to slow bacterial doubling time; the routine practice of discarding samples after 5 to 7 days increases the chances for a missed diagnosis.

Several techniques may be employed to improve the diagnostic yield of blood cultures. Lysis of white blood cells releases intracellular bacteria, and several experts recommend lysis-centrifugation as the method of choice for brucellae cultures. However, newer automated blood culture detection systems perform with even better sensitivity and faster time to detection of positive cultures. Laboratory personnel must be notified of any clinical suspicion for *Brucella* so that they can take appropriate protective precautions and avoid accidental exposure to the highly infectious bacteria.

In the absence of a positive culture, serologic tests are well established and indispensable diagnostic tools, though they do require cautious interpretation. Numerous serologic assays are available, each with its own unique limitations. Furthermore, individual immune responses to *Brucella* are highly variable, further complicating the interpretation of serologic assays. The standard agglutination test (SAT), developed in 1897, remains the most widely used diagnostic test worldwide, reliably detecting antibodies to the smooth LPS found in the three most common species infecting humans. If coupled with compatible symptoms of brucellosis, a titer of >1:160 (or 1:320 in endemic areas) confirms the diagnosis. A fourfold increase in titers over time is also diagnostic, though usually impractical. The prozone phenomenon, in which antibodies are so abundant that they interfere with expected agglutination, may cause false negative results. In that case, a true positive test will emerge with retesting after serial dilutions. False negatives can also be seen in long-standing chronic infection, as agglutinating antibodies wane over time and are replaced by nonagglutinating antibodies later in infection. False positives can occur owing to cross-reaction of antibodies with several other pathogens that share the smooth LPS, including *Francisella tularensis*, *Escherichia coli* O116 and O157, *Salmonella urbana*, *Yersinia enterocolitica* O:9, *Vibrio cholerae*, *Stenotrophomonas maltophilia*, and *Afipia clevelandensis*. Titers tend to decrease with successful treatment in most patients, but 3% to 5% have immunoglobulin M (IgM) persistence after 2 years, so following SAT titers after treatment is not recommended.

The 2-mercaptoethanol test (2-ME) is a microagglutination assay, similar to SAT but more specific to IgG; it does not react during early disease but can be used to monitor serologic response to treatment. Immunocapture agglutination tests such as Brucellacapt are useful for their sensitivity and single-step simplicity and can also be monitored to assess treatment success. Enzyme-linked immunosorbent assay testing has improved sensitivity over SAT and is recommended for suspected neurobrucellosis or when other serologic tests are negative in suspected brucellosis but is less specific than SAT. The serum dipstick assay offers rapid detection of IgM antibodies, most useful in recently acquired disease. The rose Bengal test (RBT) is a widely used buffered plate agglutination assay, using a suspension of *Brucella abortus* in an acid buffer. The RBT has several advantages over the SAT. It does not have the drawback of the prozone phenomenon. It is more sensitive in chronic infections, because it detects both agglutinating and nonagglutinating antibodies. The RBT is also technically simple, rapid, and cheap, making it an ideal screening test. However, test positivity tends to endure, limiting its usefulness in highly endemic areas where repeated exposure to *Brucella* is likely. A positive RBT should be followed up by a more specific agglutination test, especially in endemic areas. Another alternative is to perform serial dilution of a positive RBT serum specimen; persistent positivity at a >1:8 dilution is more suggestive of true clinical disease.

Nucleic acid amplification assays such as PCR offer striking sensitivity, rapid results, and early detection in as little as 10 days after exposure. First developed in 1990, various genomic targets have since been used to develop several assays. However, much of the developing world lacks the needed infrastructure to implement its use. Further, high interlaboratory variability and a lack of standardization have precluded widespread implementation efforts.

Treatment

Antibiotic therapy is indicated in all diagnosed cases of brucellosis and must be able to penetrate macrophages and act in the acidic intracellular environment. Monotherapy is associated with unacceptably high relapse rates, as are short treatment courses. Therefore WHO guidelines recommend 6 weeks of doxycycline (Vibramycin) plus either streptomycin for 2 to 3 weeks or rifampin (Rifadin)[1] for 6 weeks—both are popular worldwide. Seven days of gentamicin may be used as a substitute for streptomycin.[1] oxycycline plus an aminoglycoside is associated with lower relapse rates than doxycycline plus rifampin (5% vs 12%), but gentamicin requires parenteral, usually intramuscular, administration. Thus doxycycline plus rifampin is an easier and more popular choice, despite slightly higher relapse rates and a potential to increase rifampin resistance in areas coendemic with

---

[1] Not FDA approved for this indication.

TABLE 2	Treatment of Brucellosis Syndromes
CLINICAL SYNDROME	**MANAGEMENT**
Nonlocalized disease	Doxycycline (Vibramycin) 100 mg po bid × 6 weeks + streptomycin 1 g IM daily × 2–3 weeks Doxycycline 100 mg po bid × 6 weeks +gentamicin[1] 5 mg/kg IV daily × 7 days Doxycycline 100 mg po bid × 6 weeks + rifampin (Rifadin)[1] 600–900 mg po daily × 6 weeks
Pregnancy (<36 weeks gestation)	Trimethoprim-sulfamethoxazole (Bactrim DS)[1] 5 mg/kg of TMP component po bid + rifampin[1] 600–900 mg po daily × 4 weeks
Localized disease:	
Osteoarticular (spondylitis, sacroileitis, peripheral arthritis)	Triple therapy: Doxycycline 100 mg po bid × 3 months + rifampin[1] 600–900 mg po daily × 3 months + aminoglycoside as above
Neurobrucellosis	Triple therapy: Doxycycline 100 mg IV or po bid + rifampin[1] 600–900 mg po daily + ceftriaxone[1] 2 g IV q12h until CSF studies normalize
Endocarditis	Surgical valve replacement + aminoglycoside × 4 weeks + doxycycline 100 mg po bid × 6 weeks to 6 months + trimethoprim-sulfamethoxazole[1] × 6 weeks to 6 months

[1] Not FDA approved for this indication.

tuberculosis. In vitro resistance testing is often discrepant with in vivo activity and should not be a therapeutic consideration for brucellosis.

Localized disease is more difficult to treat in terms of likelihood of relapse; treatment often involves a combination of three antibiotics for an even more lengthy treatment course (Table 2). In addition to medical therapy, patients with endocarditis almost always benefit from valve replacement, because this has been shown to reduce mortality.

Monitoring

Patients should be expected to defervesce after an average of 4 to 5 days after initiation of appropriate therapy. Fevers lasting longer than 1 week should prompt consideration for treatment failure or an alternative diagnosis. Clinical relapse is defined as the reappearance of signs or symptoms of brucellosis and is ideally confirmed with positive blood cultures or increasing serology titers. Relapse with brucellosis may occur at a rate of around 5% to 10%, even with good adherence to recommended treatment regimens. Relapses typically present within 12 months after treatment and have a milder clinical course than the incident illness. Risk factors for relapse include male gender, bacteremia, duration of illness <10 days, and thrombocytopenia. Reinfection is also common in endemic areas. Relapses and reinfections are successfully treated with a repeated course of the previously mentioned combination treatment regimens.

Prevention

For individuals, the single most important measure to prevent *Brucella* infection is to avoid any consumption of unpasteurized dairy products, especially when sourced from endemic areas. Even in well-developed nations, brucellae persist in wild animal reservoirs and can easily pass into neighboring domestic animals.

Unpasteurized products at risk include raw milk, soft cheeses, and ice cream. Fermented dairy products such as yogurt, hard cheeses, and sour milk may carry lower infectious risks but should still be avoided if unpasteurized. On a population level, the implementation of routine pasteurization has been shown to markedly reduce human brucellosis cases, and resources should be leveraged to improve consistent access to pasteurization worldwide. Unfortunately, many developing countries currently lack this infrastructure; in these areas, brucellae are found at alarming rates in dairy products.

Hunters and slaughterhouse workers should use rubber gloves while dressing animals and practice meticulous hand hygiene after any contact with killed animals or animal products. It should be noted that infected animals often appear healthy. Veterinarians and park rangers should take similar precautions.

Laboratories must be notified of specimens that have any suspicion for brucellosis. Labs must be meticulously compliant with established laboratory biosafety standards, such as avoiding splashes and aerosolizing procedures, and sniffing culture media. Adequate ventilation should be maintained, and protective barriers should be used where appropriate. In endemic areas, every positive blood culture vial should be initially processed in safety cabinets until brucellae is ruled out, because unanticipated infections are common.

Healthcare personnel caring for patients infected with *Brucella* should adhere to universal precautions, but no additional isolation measures or precautions are recommended, because human-to-human transmission is exceptionally rare. Currently there is no available vaccine to protect humans from brucellosis, though the WHO considers its development a high priority.

Ultimately, eradication among domesticated and wild animals is the only way to reliably prevent zoonotic disease. In domesticated animals, culling (selective slaughtering) of infected animals based on serologic screening is an important surveillance measure in developed countries but is not feasible in most developing nations. Vaccines are available for some animals, including cattle, sheep, goats, and camels. The most commonly used vaccines, S19 and RB-51, are live attenuated vaccines that can infect humans. Veterinarians can be exposed by accidental needle stick or by accidental spray onto mucosa while vaccinating animals. Humans potentially exposed to infectious vaccine products should take prophylactic antibiotics for 3 weeks (doxycycline and rifampin for S19 or doxycycline alone for RB-51) and should undergo serial diagnostic testing.

To add to the challenges of eliminating brucellosis from domesticated animals, we still have much to learn about the complete extent of *Brucella* in the wild. With animal reservoirs well established in so many species throughout the world, complete eradication of brucellosis is likely an unattainable goal.

References

Centers for Disease Control and Prevention: *Bioterrorism agents/diseases*. Available at https://emergency.cdc.gov/agent/agentlist-category.asp, 2018. Accessed 4.13.23.
Centers for Disease Control and Prevention: *Brucellosis*. Available at https://www.cdc.gov/brucellosis/clinicians/, 2021. Accessed 04.13.23.
Corbel MJ: *Brucellosis in humans and animals*, Geneva, 2006, World Health Organization.
"Etymologia: *Brucella* [broo-sel′ə]." *Emerg Infect Dis* 14(8):1337, 2008. https://doi.org/10.3201/eid1408.089999.
Gilbert D, Brucella sp: *The sanford guide to antimicrobial therapy web edition*, Dallas, TX, 2019, Antimicrobial Therapy, Inc.. Available at https://webedition.sanfordguide.com/en/sanford-guide-online/disease-clinical-condition/brucella-sp. Accessed 4.13.23.
Gilbert D, Brucellosis: *The sanford guide to antimicrobial therapy web edition*, Dallas, TX, 2023, Antimicrobial Therapy, Inc. Available at https://webedition.sanfordguide.com/en/sanford-guide-online/disease-clinical-condition/brucellosis. Accessed 4.13.23.
Lalsiamthara J, Lee JH: Development and trial of vaccines against Brucella, *J Vet Sci* 18(S1):281–290, 2017.
Hull NC, Schumaker BA: Comparisons of brucellosis between human and veterinary medicine, *Infect Ecol Epidemiol* 8(1):1500846, 2018.
Pappas G, Akritidis N, Bosilkovski M, Tsianos E: Brucellosis, *N Eng J Med* 352:2325–2336, 2005.
Yagupsky P, Morata P, Colmenero JD: Laboratory diagnosis of human brucellosis, *Clin Microbiol Rev* 33(1):e00073-19, 2020.

CLOSTRIDIOIDES DIFFICILE COLITIS

Method of
Jeffery D. Semel, MD

CURRENT DIAGNOSIS

- *Clostridium difficile* (renamed *Clostridioides difficile*) infection is diagnosed by a combination of clinical and laboratory-findings.
- Diagnosis requires a positive test for the presence of *C. difficile* toxins.
- GDH, or glutamate dehydrogenase, produced by *C. difficile*, can be detected in stool. However, it is not specific and can be produced by non-toxigenic *C. difficile*.
- Enzyme immunoassay testing for toxin A and or B has a variable sensitivity and specificity and a turnaround time of about 24 hours and correlates well with disease activity.
- Polymerase chain reaction testing has a high sensitivity and specificity and a turnaround time of less than 4 hours; correlates less with disease activity, thus identifying patients with colonization as well as active infection. Increasingly, combination testing is being employed to imrove diagnostic accuracy.
- Laboratory testing for *C. difficile* toxins should only be performed on patients with ≥3 unformed stools per 24 hours, who are not on laxatives and is not useful as a test of cure.
- Pathologic findings can help to confirm diagnosis.
- Consider GDH and immunoassay testing for toxin A and or B. If results are discordant, follow with PCR.

CURRENT THERAPY

- If possible, the clinician should first consider discontinuing concurrent antibacterial therapy.
- Treatment should be initiated only after a positive test result for *C. difficile* toxin unless the patient is at high risk for *C. difficile* infection or is severely ill, in which case empirical therapy is justified.
- Treatment recommendations depend on the severity of the disease and whether the patient has a first-time diagnosis or recurrence.
- Clinical parameters that guide treatment include increasing age, leukocytosis, elevation of serum creatinine, and presence of hypotension, shock, ileus, or megacolon.
- Taken orally, fidaxomicin (Dificid) is preferred for initial therapy and recurrences, although it is much more costly than vancomycin, which remains an acceptable choice. Metronidazole (Flagyl)[1] oral, can be used for non-severe disease if these are not available.
- Intravenous metronidazole and or rectal vancomycin (enema)[1],[6] can be added for severe disease.
- FMT (fecal microbiota therapy) is a safe and effective option for recurrent disease that does not respond to oral therapies, and has shown promise in studies of severe or fulminant *C. difficile* infection.
- Antimicrobial stewardship programs are a safe and cost-effective method of reducing the burden of *C. difficile* infections.

[1]Not FDA approved for this indication.
[6]May be compounded by pharmacists.

Pseudomembranous colitis is an inflammatory disease of the colon that is almost always associated with the toxin-producing bacteria *Clostridioides difficile*. In very rare cases, other organisms can be responsible. In this article I discuss *C. difficile* as an important cause of pseudomembranous colitis.

References

Feurstadt, P Louie, TJ, Lashner B: SER-109, an oral microbiome therapy for recurrent Clostridioides difficile infection, *NEJM* 386:220–229, 2022.

Fisbein SRS, Hink T, Reske KA, et al: Randomized controlled trial of oral vancomycin treatment in *Clostridioides difficile* colonized patients, *mSphere* 6: e00936–20, 2021.

Fischer M, Sipe B, Cheng Y, et al: Fecal microbiota transplant in severe and severe-complicated *Clostridium difficile*: A promising treatment approach, *Gut Microbes* 8(3):289–302, 2017.

Goldenberg JZ, Yap C, Lytvyn L, et al: Probiotics for the prevention of Clostridium difficile-associated diarrhea in adults and children, *Cochrane Database Syst Rev* 12:CD006095, 2017.

Jiang ZD, Ajami NJ, Petrosino JF, et al: Randomised clinical trial: faecal microbiota transplantation for recurrent Clostrium difficile infection - fresh, or frozen, or lyophilised microbiota from a small pool of healthy donors delivered by colonoscopy, *Aliment Pharmacol Ther* 45(7):899–908, 2017.

Johnson SW, Brown SV, Priest DH: Effectiveness of oral vancomycin for prevention of healthcare facility-onset *Clostridioides difficile* infection in targeted patients during systemic antibiotic exposure, *Clin Infect Dis* 27:ciz966, 2019, https://doi.org/10.1093/cid/ciz966. {epub ahead of print}.

Johnson S, Lavergne V, Skinner AM et al: Clinical practice guideline by the Infectious Diseases Society of America (IDSA) and Society for Healthcare Epidemiology of America (SHEA): 2021 focused update guidelines on management of *Clostridioides difficile* infection in adults, *Clin Infect Dis* 73(5):e1029–e1044, 2021.

Kyne L, Warny M, Qamar A, et al: Asymptomatic carriage of *Clostridium difficile* and serum levels of IGG antibody against toxin A, *N Engl J Med* 342:390–397, 2000.

Magill SS, O'Leary SJ, Janelle DL, et al: Changes in prevalence of health - care associated infections in U.S. hospitals, *N Engl J Med* 379:1732–1744, 2018.

McDonald LC, Gerding DN, Johnson S, et al: Practice Guidelines for Clostridium difficile Infection in Adults and Children: 2017, *Clin Infect Dis* 66:987–994, 2018.

Song YN, Yang DY, van Zanten SV, et al: Fecal microbiota transplantation for severe or fulminant Clostridioides difficile infection: systematic review and meta-analysis, *J Can Assoc Gastro* 5:e1–e11, 2022.

Oksi J, Aalto A, Sailla P, et al: Real-world efficacy of bezlotoxumab for prevention of recurrent *Clostridium difficile* infection: a retrospective study of 46 patients in five university hospitals in Finland, *Eur J Clin Microbiol Infect Dis* 38:1947–1952, 2019.

Shim JK, Johnson S, Samore MH, et al: Primary symptomless colonisation by *Clostridium difficile* and decreased risk of subsequent diarrhea, *Lancet* 351:633, 1998.

Song YN, Yang DY, van Zanten SV, et al: Fecal microbiota transplantation for severe or fulminant *Clostridioides difficile* infection: systematic review and meta-analysis, *J Can Assoc Gastro* 5:e1–e11, 2022.

CAT SCRATCH DISEASE

Method of
Ronen M. Ben-Ami, MD

CURRENT DIAGNOSIS

- The combination of a compatible clinical syndrome of regional lymphadenopathy with a primary inoculation lesion and cat contact is highly suggestive of cat scratch disease.
- Results of *Bartonella henselae* serology are helpful in confirming the diagnosis; however, up to 20% of patients remain seronegative throughout their disease.
- Detection of *B. henselae* DNA by polymerase chain reaction from pus obtained by needle aspiration or lymph node biopsy is a highly sensitive diagnostic modality and may be particularly useful in seronegative patients.

CURRENT THERAPY

- Typical cat scratch disease is a self-limiting disease; therefore systemic antimicrobials are not routinely indicated in immunocompetent patients with uncomplicated cat scratch disease.
- Indications for antimicrobial therapy include an immunocompromised host, endocarditis, retinitis, and other atypical syndromes.
- Treatment may also be considered for patients who have typical cat scratch disease and who have extensive or bulky lymphadenopathy and are highly symptomatic.
- Suppurative lymph nodes should be drained by large-bore needle aspiration.

Cat scratch disease is a worldwide zoonotic infection caused by *Bartonella henselae*, an intracellular, pleomorphic, gram-negative bacillus. Other *Bartonella* species have rarely been implicated. The disease typically manifests as benign regional lymphadenopathy, but atypical disease can involve almost any organ system and is associated with significant morbidity.

Epidemiology

Bartonella henselae infection is widespread among domestic cats and other felids worldwide, and serologic studies indicate a higher prevalence in warm, humid climates. Transmission among cats occurs via an arthropod vector, the cat flea *Ctenocephalides felis*. *B. henselae* bacteremia is detected at higher rates in feral cats than in domesticated cats and in kittens compared with adult cats, explaining the higher infectivity of these animals. Cats infected with *B. henselae* are asymptomatic. Transmission to humans occurs via a scratch, bite, or lick; contamination of cat scratches by flea feces may enhance *Bartonella* transmission.

Cat scratch disease has been estimated to occur in the United States at a rate approaching 10 per 100,000 population. There is some seasonality, with incidence peaking between September and January. Although traditionally considered a disease of childhood, epidemiologic surveys have found a similar incidence of cat scratch disease in adults, and 6% of patients are 60 years of age or older. Cat contact is the most important risk factor: Almost all patients are cat owners or were otherwise exposed to cats, and about one-half can recall a recent bite or scratch, most commonly by a kitten.

Clinical Manifestations

Cat scratch disease is divided into two clinical syndromes. Typical cat scratch disease is a subacute, self-limiting regional lymphadenopathy and constitutes 80% to 90% of cases. Atypical cat scratch disease encompasses Parinaud oculoglandular syndrome and other clinical entities with systemic extranodal involvement. Bacillary angiomatosis and bacillary peliosis are manifestations of *B. henselae* infection in immunocompromised persons and are not discussed here.

Typical Cat Scratch Disease

A primary skin lesion, usually a papule or pustule, appears at the site of inoculation 3 to 10 days after cat contact and persists for 1 to 3 weeks. Regional lymphadenopathy develops within 1 to 7 weeks and resolves spontaneously after 2 to 4 months. The primary lesion is still present in about two-thirds of patients when they present for evaluation of lymphadenopathy. The most commonly involved lymph nodes are, in descending order of frequency, axillary and epitrochlear nodes, head and neck nodes, and femoral and inguinal nodes. One-third of patients develop lymphadenopathy at multiple sites. Lymph nodes are often painful and red; suppuration occurs in 10% of nodes. Mild constitutional symptoms, including low-grade fever and malaise, are noted in about one-half of the cases. Rash, night sweats, anorexia, and weight loss are uncommon. Infection results in lifelong immunity.

Atypical Cat Scratch Disease

Parinaud oculoglandular syndrome, the most common form of atypical cat scratch disease, is a specific type of regional lymphadenopathy that occurs following conjunctival inoculation of *B. henselae*. The syndrome includes granulomatous conjunctivitis and preauricular lymphadenopathy. Endocarditis and encephalitis represent severe forms of *B. henselae* infection and are more common in older adult patients. Encephalitis manifests with various degrees of altered mental status, agitation, headache, and seizures. Cerebrospinal fluid lymphocytic pleocytosis occurs in only one-third of cases, and brain imaging studies usually fail to show any abnormalities. Neuroretinitis manifests as sudden unilateral loss of visual acuity. The diagnosis is suspected on the basis of typical findings on fundoscopic examination: papilledema and macular exudates in a starlike configuration. However, these findings are not pathognomonic of cat scratch disease. Other ocular findings include uveitis, optic neuropathy, and

TABLE 1 Antibiotic Treatment Regimens for Cat Scratch Disease

CLINICAL SYNDROME	FIRST CHOICE	SECOND CHOICE	COMMENTS
Typical cat scratch disease	Not indicated*	Azithromycin (Zithromax)[1] 500 mg PO on day 1, then 250 mg PO × 4 days	Drain suppurative nodes using large-bore aspiration
Endocarditis	Gentamicin[1] 1 mg/kg IV q8h × >14 days plus doxycycline 100 mg IV/PO bid × 6 weeks	Doxycycline 100 mg PO bid plus rifampicin (Rifadin)[1] 300 mg PO bid × 6 weeks	Some experts recommend extending oral doxycycline treatment × 3–6 months. Surgical valve excision may be required
Neuroretinitis	Doxycycline 100 mg PO bid plus rifampicin[1] 300 mg PO bid × 4–6 weeks	NA	Spontaneous resolution is the rule; the utility of treatment remains unproven
Other atypical cat scratch disease	As for neuroretinitis	NA	Treatment duration should be individualized

[1]Not FDA approved for this indication.
*Treatment may be considered for patients with bulky or extensive lymphadenopathy and for immunocompromised patients.
NA, Not available.

retinal vessel occlusion. Infrequent manifestations are self-limiting granulomatous hepatitis and splenitis and osteoarticular disease. Prolonged fever of unknown origin has been described in children and adolescents, taking the form of relapsing fever in one-half of the cases.

Diagnosis

A compatible clinical syndrome in a person with a positive history of cat exposure suggests cat scratch disease. The diagnosis is most commonly confirmed with specific serologic assays. The immunofluorescence assay and the enzyme-linked immunsorbent assay are comparably sensitive, although cross-reactivity can occur with other organisms such as *Chlamydia* species, *Coxiella burnetii,* and non-*henselae Bartonella* species. A single elevated titer of immunoglobulin (Ig)M or IgG in the acute phase or a fourfold increase of IgG in convalescent serum supports the diagnosis.

Biopsy and histopathologic examination of lymph nodes are usually only performed when malignancy is suspected. Necrotizing granulomas are typically observed. The pleomorphic gram-negative bacilli are best visualized with the Warthin-Starry stain; however, the sensitivity of this method is too low to be clinically useful. Similarly, culture lacks sensitivity and requires prolonged incubation, making it impractical for routine use.

Polymerase chain reaction assays for the detection of *B. henselae* in pus aspirated from suppurative lymph nodes or primary skin lesions are highly sensitive and specific, and they can be performed with a rapid turnaround time. However, these assays are not widely available in most clinical microbiology laboratories.

Differential Diagnosis

Cat scratch disease should be differentiated from other infectious and noninfectious causes of regional lymphadenopathy. Importantly, lymphoma and solid tumors with metastases to lymph nodes may be confused with cat scratch disease. Malignancy should be suspected in patients who have marked constitutional symptoms, who are seronegative, or whose lymphadenopathy fails to resolve spontaneously after more than 6 months. Unlike cat scratch disease, pyogenic lymphadenitis manifests with rapid progression, high-grade fever, and a septic-appearing patient. Mycobacterial infection, syphilis, bubonic plague, tularemia, histoplasmosis, and sporotrichosis should be considered based on the presence of specific risk factors and endemic exposures. *Bartonella* endocarditis must be differentiated from other causes of culture-negative endocarditis, specifically Q fever and brucellosis.

Treatment

Because of the self-limiting course of typical cat scratch disease, patients usually only require observation and reassurance of its benign nature. The goals of therapy are alleviation of symptoms in patients with bulky lymphadenopathy and drainage of suppurating lymph nodes to prevent spontaneous formation of chronic sinus tracts. If drug treatment is initiated, azithromycin (Zithromax)[1] is the agent of choice based on a small randomized placebo-controlled study that showed more-rapid resolution of lymphadenopathy in the azithromycin arm as determined by ultrasonography. Suppurative nodes should be drained by large-bore needle aspiration. Incisional drainage is best avoided because it can promote sinus tract formation.

Atypical cat scratch disease syndromes usually require treatment, but there are scant data to support specific regimens, and treatment duration is not well defined. For patients with endocarditis, treatment with an aminoglycoside for at least 14 days is associated with a higher likelihood of recovery and survival. Uncontrolled data suggest that, for patients with neuroretinitis, treatment with antibiotics and corticosteroids is associated with better visual outcomes than treatment with antibiotics alone (Table 1).

Prevention

Flea control in domestic cats can reduce the likelihood of *Bartonella* bacteremia and transmission to humans. Bites and scratches should be promptly rinsed. HIV-infected patients and other immunocompromised persons should be cautioned about the risks of cat exposure because they are susceptible to disseminated visceral *B. henselae* infection as well as other zoonotic infections such as toxoplasmosis.

[1] Not FDA approved for this indication.

References

Ben-Ami R, Ephros M, Avidor B, et al: Cat-scratch disease in elderly patients, *Clin Infect Dis* 41:969–974, 2005.

Giladi M, Kletter Y, Avidor B, et al: Enzyme immunoassay for the diagnosis of cat-scratch disease defined by polymerase chain reaction, *Clin Infect Dis* 33:1852–1858, 2001.

Goaz S, Rasis M, Binsky Ehrenreich I, et al: Molecular diagnosis of cat scratch disease: a 25-year retrospective comparative analysis of various clinical specimens and different PCR assays, *Microbial Spectr* 10, 2022:e0259621.

Habot-Wilner Z, Trivizki O, Goldstein M, et al: Cat-scratch disease: ocular manifestations and treatment outcome, *Acta Ophthalmol* 96(4):e524–e532, 2018.

Hansmann Y, DeMartino S, Piemont Y, et al: Diagnosis of cat scratch disease with detection of *Bartonella henselae* by PCR: A study of patients with lymph node enlargement, *J Clin Microbiol* 43:3800–3806, 2005.

Jackson LA, Perkins BA, Wenger JD: Cat scratch disease in the United States: An analysis of three national databases, *Am J Public Health* 83:1707–1711, 1993.

Jacobs RF, Schutze GE: *Bartonella henselae* as a cause of prolonged fever and fever of unknown origin in children, *Clin Infect Dis* 26:80–84, 1998.

Raoult D, Fournier PE, Vandenesch F, et al: Outcome and treatment of *Bartonella* endocarditis, *Arch Intern Med* 163:226–230, 2003.

Rolain JM, Brouqui P, Koehler JE, et al: Recommendations for treatment of human infections caused by *Bartonella* species, *Antimicrob Agents Chemother* 48:1921–1933, 2004.

Zangwill KM, Hamilton DH, Perkins BA, et al: Cat scratch disease in Connecticut. Epidemiology, risk factors, and evaluation of a new diagnostic test, *N Engl J Med* 329:8–13, 1993.

CHIKUNGUNYA

Method of
Scott Kellermann, MD, MPH; and Rick D. Kellerman, MD

CURRENT DIAGNOSIS

- Clinically, chikungunya is a diagnosis of exclusion, particularly when laboratory testing is not available. Accurate diagnosis depends on the patient's clinical symptoms and the epidemiology of endemic disease.
- Acute symptoms include incapacitating relapsing bilateral symmetrical polyarthralgia accompanied by high fever, headache, backache, and fatigue. Some may have a pruritic maculopapular rash at onset.
- Chronic symptoms include episodic incapacitating symmetrical polyarthralgia. Many have long-term asthenia and depression.
- From 0 to 7 days of infection, chikungunya virus can be detected via real-time reverse-transcription polymerase chain reaction (RT-PCR).
- For individuals presenting 8 or more days following onset of symptoms, chikungunya virus serologic testing via enzyme-linked immunoassay (ELISA) or indirect fluorescent antibody (IFA) should be performed.
- Immunoglobulin (Ig)M anti–chikungunya virus antibodies are detectable starting about 5 days (range 1–12 days) and persist for several weeks to 3 months.
- Immunoglobulin M antibody levels peak 3 to 5 weeks after the onset of illness and persist for approximately 2 months.
- IgG antibodies begin to appear about 2 weeks following onset of symptoms and persist for years.
- A positive IgG antibody indicates prior chikungunya infection; it does not delineate whether arthritic symptoms are a consequence of prior infection.

CURRENT THERAPY

- Medical treatment is primarily supportive.

The word *chikungunya* is a derivation of the Kimakonde (a Mozambique dialect) word *kungunyala,* meaning "to become desiccated or contorted." In the Democratic Republic of the Congo, it is called *buka-buka,* translated as "broken-broken," reflecting the incapacitating arthralgias that are common manifestations of chikungunya fever.

Epidemiology

Chikungunya, first diagnosed in Tanganyika in 1952, is found in a large percentage of countries in Africa, Asia, and Southeast Asia and is prevalent in India. Chikungunya virus often causes large outbreaks with high attack rates, affecting one-third to three-quarters of the population. Dense human populations and lack of herd immunity likely contribute to the volatile nature of chikungunya epidemics in many regions. In India during 2006, more than 1,250,000 cases of chikungunya were reported, with *Aedes aegypti* implicated as the vector. In late 2013, the first locally acquired cases were reported on Caribbean islands. By the end of 2017, more than 2.6 million suspected cases had been chronicled in the Americas. From 2010 through 2013, 110 cases of chikungunya were documented among U.S. travelers. Following the outbreak in the Americas, there were >4000 cases reported in U.S. travelers from 2014 to 2017, 13 of which were locally acquired in the continental United States. In 2021 there were 36 travel-associated cases of chikungunya; no cases were acquired in the continental United States or its territories.

A 2014 study, undertaken by the Puerto Rico Department of Health and the Centers for Disease Control and Prevention (CDC), demonstrated that chikungunya cases are vastly underreported in Puerto Rico. In passive surveillance of 250 participants, 70 tested positive for past or current chikungunya virus infection (28%). However, only 2 of 25 participants with chikungunya infection who sought care had been reported to health authorities (8%).

It is believed that chikungunya virus originated in Africa and migrated to Asia 200 years ago. Evidence derived from molecular genetics suggests it evolved around 1700; the first recorded outbreak of this disease was probably in 1779.

Interestingly, some medical historians believe that a pandemic of chikungunya occurred in the Western Hemisphere in the 1800s but was diagnosed as dengue fever. The 21st-century researchers who have examined the accounts of this pandemic now speculate that it was caused by chikungunya because the cases exhibited severe joint arthritis, which is more indicative of chikungunya than dengue. The virus then disappeared from the Americas until it reemerged during the last decade. Chikungunya epidemics appear suddenly and unpredictably and proceed explosively.

Risk Factors

Individuals at the highest risk of contracting chikungunya and experiencing more severe symptoms are those who have chronic arthritis, have underlying chronic medical conditions, are over the age of 65 years, or are pregnant. Travelers who spend extended periods of time in endemic areas are at greater risk. These include missionaries, humanitarian aid workers, and those who frequently work outdoors.

Pathophysiology

Chikungunya is an arthropod-transmitted disease caused by a single-stranded RNA arbovirus. Patients develop viremia within a few days of infection. The virus invades and replicates within the joints. Animal models of chikungunya virus pathogenesis suggest the virus directly infects the synovium, tenosynovium, and muscle, leading to production of proinflammatory cytokines and chemokines and recruitment of leukocytes. Typically, infectious virus is cleared from the circulation within days and from joints within a couple of weeks.

There is a wide range of frequency and severity of protracted disease, with chronic musculoskeletal symptomology occurring in 25% to 75% of patients. Why some patients develop chronic joint pain whereas others do not is not well understood. Three hypotheses have been proposed to explain chronic arthritis: persistent viral replication, persistent viral RNA driving an inflammatory response, and autoimmunity. Persistent T-cell activation has been reported in chronic arthritis due to chikungunya virus, but rheumatoid factor and anticyclic citrullinated peptide testing are typically negative.

As with dengue fever and yellow fever, chikungunya cycles from mosquito to human to mosquito. The mosquito *A. aegypti* is the usual vector for transmission of chikungunya. *A. aegypti* is well adapted to urban settings and is widely distributed in the tropics and subtropics worldwide. It prefers the human host. *A. aegypti* breeding sites are associated with elements of human habitation that are seemingly innocuous (i.e., flower vases, water storage vessels, tires, and birdbaths). Eggs, which hatch when submerged, are laid on the walls of these artificial water containers. *A. aegypti* enters homes and will feed indoors and outdoors. A single *A. aegypti* mosquito can infect more than one human because this species may feed on another host if its blood meal is interrupted.

A. albopictus, the Asian tiger mosquito, is also a vector. Both species are found in the Southeastern United States and limited parts of the Southwest. The risk of person-to-mosquito transmission is highest during the viremic first week of illness. Human and nonhuman primates are the main amplifying reservoirs for the virus. Transmission is possible through a needle stick, handling of blood, and aerosol laboratory exposure. No transfusion-related cases have been identified. Previous infection will convey permanent immunity.

Prevention

Currently, no vaccine or preventive drug is available. Several candidate vaccines, including mRNA vaccines, are in Phase III clinical trials. The best preventive measures are wearing permethrin-treated, bite-proof long sleeves and trousers and using a mosquito repellant such as 30% DEET, 20% oil of lemon eucalyptus, or 30% picaridin. Travelers to endemic areas should choose a hotel or lodging with air conditioning or with screens on windows and doors; however, this has only a limited effect because most contacts between the *Aedes* mosquitoes and humans occur outside. Travelers with underlying medical conditions and women late in their pregnancy (because their fetuses are at increased risk) might consider avoiding visiting areas with ongoing chikungunya outbreaks. The CDC's website has excellent information regarding preventive measures: https://www.cdc.gov/chikungunya/prevention/index.html. Standing water, a breeding ground for mosquitoes, should be drained. Customary blood handling procedures are recommended.

If a chikungunya epidemic were to occur in the United States, the standard public health measures of avoidance and mosquito control would be major lines of defense. To prevent local spread, the patient diagnosed with chikungunya should use mosquito repellent for 1 week after the onset of fever.

Clinical Manifestations

Chikungunya virus infection should be considered in patients with acute onset of fever and polyarthralgia, especially in travelers who have recently returned from areas with endemic chikungunya. Joint pain may precede fever; in one outbreak in 2017 among more than 1300 patients in Dhaka, Bangladesh, joint pain preceded fever in 90% of cases.

The incubation period of the chikungunya virus ranges from 1 to 12 days, most typically 3 to 7 days. Chikungunya infection may be divided into an acute phase (<3 months) and chronic phase (>3 months). The acute phase may be further subdivided into viremic (1–3 weeks) and subacute postviremic (4–12 weeks) phases.

The viremic phase is characterized by sudden onset of high-grade fever (often >39°C); severe, incapacitating polyarthralgia/polyarthritis; myalgias; conjunctivitis; and exanthema. Polyarthralgia is reported in 87% to 98% of cases and represents the most characteristic symptom. The joint pain is mostly polyarticular, bilateral, and symmetric and occurs mainly in peripheral joints (wrists, ankles, and phalanges) and some large joints (shoulders, elbows, and knees). Joint swelling is less frequent, occurring in 25% to 42% of cases. Typically, the fever lasts for 2 days and then will defervesce abruptly. Headache and an extreme degree of prostration may persist for a variable period, usually about 5 to 7 days. Symptoms typically resolve in 7 to 10 days. Rare complications include uveitis, retinitis, myocarditis, hepatitis, nephritis, hemorrhage, and neurologic problems such as myelitis, meningoencephalitis, Guillain-Barré syndrome, and cranial nerve palsies. In 40% to 50% of cases, skin involvement is present, consisting of a pruritic maculopapular rash, predominantly on the thorax, localized petechia, and facial edema.

In the subacute phase, fever settles but articular symptoms and fatigue persist. Polyarthritis is usually symmetric and involves small and large joints. Tenosynovitis and bursitis can also occur, which are usually very painful. Patients who have concomitant comorbidities such as osteoarthritis, heart failure, respiratory disease, renal disease, and diabetes are likely to have more severe manifestations of acute infection. Chikungunya infection may also exacerbate underlying rheumatic diseases and relapses of autoimmune arthritis in patients who were in remission prior to infection.

The chronic phase of the disease may follow a pattern similar to rheumatoid arthritis, peripheral spondylarthritis, undifferentiated arthritis, and fibromyalgia. The ankles, knees, hips, wrists, elbows, and metacarpal-phalangeal joints are mainly involved.

Factors such as an age older than 45 years, high viral load ($\geq 10^9$ copies/mL) during the acute phase, and severe immunologic response in postviremic phase are predictors of the development of chronic symptoms.

Approximately 20% of patients with chronic chikungunya infection may have chronic pain with neuropathic features including paresthesia, tingling, numbness, and itching.

A study of pregnant women conducted on the island of Réunion during the 2005 to 2006 epidemic showed that the mother-to-child (vertical) transmission rate was approximately 50% when chikungunya infection occurred in the intrapartum (2 days either side of delivery) period. Delivery by cesarean section did not prevent the transmission of virus. The babies were born healthy; however, they developed fever, weakness, and thrombocytopenia between 3 to 7 days. Neurocognitive outcome was poor in children with perinatal transmission from infected mothers. Chikungunya virus has not been detected in breast milk, and there are no reported cases transmitted though breast milk. Even in endemic areas, women are encouraged to breastfeed.

In a study of 4000 patients with travel-acquired chikungunya in the United States, 18% were hospitalized, and 4 patients died. Hospitalization rates were highest among patients <10 years old (31%) and patients ≥70 years old (33%) and were higher among males than females (23% versus 17%).

Diagnosis

Chikungunya virus infection should be considered in patients presenting with an acute onset of fever and polyarthralgia and relevant epidemiologic exposure where mosquito-borne transmission of chikungunya virus infection has been reported. In humans, chikungunya viremia may exceed 10^9 RNA copies/mL plasma; in addition, viremia may be present prior to onset of symptoms. In the setting of symptomatic infection, viremia usually disappears after 6 to 7 days of illness; however, the virus has been isolated after 8 days, and chikungunya genomic products can be detected as late as day 17 of illness. Instructions for serum diagnostic testing are found on the Centers for Disease Control and Prevention's website: https://www.cdc.gov/chikungunya/hc/diagnostic.html.

Chikungunya virus RNA can be detected by RT-PCR during the first 5 days following onset of symptoms with excellent sensitivity and specificity (100% and 98%, respectively). For individuals presenting 8 or more days following onset of symptoms, chikungunya virus serologic testing via ELISA or IFA should be performed. A positive result establishes a diagnosis of chikungunya virus infection.

Immunoglobulin (Ig)M anti–chikungunya virus antibodies (detected by direct ELISA) are present starting about 5 days (range 1–12 days) following onset of symptoms and persist for several weeks to 3 months. IgG antibodies begin to appear about 2 weeks after onset of symptoms and persist for years. A positive IgG antibody test result indicates prior chikungunya infection; it does not delineate whether arthritic symptoms are a consequence of prior infection. The time between possible exposure and clinical history should be evaluated carefully when making a diagnosis of chronic chikungunya viral arthritis in a patient with a positive IgG test. Chikungunya virus antibodies normally develop toward the end of the first week of illness; therefore to definitively rule out the diagnosis, convalescent-phase samples should be obtained from patients whose acute-phase samples test negative.

Viral culture is mainly a research tool and should be handled under biosafety level (BSL) 3 conditions.

A complete blood count may show lymphopenia and thrombocytopenia. Liver enzymes may elevate, and the serum creatinine might also increase. There are no pathognomonic radiologic findings, and biologic markers of inflammation are normal or modestly elevated.

In many parts of the world, chikungunya is a clinical diagnosis of exclusion, particularly when laboratory testing is not readily available. The probability of accurate clinical diagnosis is predicated on the epidemiology of endemic diseases and the patient's clinical symptoms.

Differential Diagnosis

Prominent arthralgia, high fever, diffuse rash, and absence of respiratory symptoms can help distinguish chikungunya from other illnesses. The differential diagnosis for chikungunya includes influenza, malaria, rickettsia, and a multitude of viruses, especially dengue fever. Zika, dengue, and chikungunya viruses are transmitted by the same mosquitoes, may have similar clinical features, and can occasionally coinfect the same individual. Typically, the signs and symptoms of Zika virus are mild, though Zika infection in pregnancy can result in serious congenital malformations. Clinically differentiating chikungunya from dengue may be difficult; however, in chikungunya, the onset of fever is typically more abrupt and shorter lived, with severe arthralgia, rash, and lymphopenia more prevalent, whereas infection with dengue is more likely to present with neutropenia, thrombocytopenia, and the potential of hemorrhage, shock, and death. The accurate diagnosis of dengue virus infection is essential because proper clinical management of dengue can improve outcomes. Seasonally, chikungunya is more likely to be seen in the summer months when *Aedes* mosquitos proliferate. A single RT-PCR test to evaluate for the presence of all three infections is available through the United States Centers for Disease Control and Prevention and other qualified laboratories: https://www.cdc.gov/zika/pdfs/fact-sheet-for-hcp-eua-trioplex-rt-pcr-zika.pdf

Treatment

Most chikungunya infections are self-limiting and will improve with supportive care, hydration, and analgesia. There is no specific antiviral therapy for acute chikungunya virus infection.

In the acute viremic phase (1–3 weeks), acetaminophen (up to 500 to 1000 mg three times daily) is useful. If acetaminophen is inadequate for symptom relief and once dengue is excluded, any nonsteroidal antiinflammatory drug (NSAID) may be used.

In the subacute phase (4-12 weeks), if there is evidence of severe synovitis and joint swelling, prednisone 10 to 20 mg daily for 5 days tapered over 10 days can be efficacious. The lowest effective glucocorticoid dose possible with a short trial is usually sufficient; however, the individual response to therapy varies substantially. More severely affected patients may require higher doses (0.5 mg/kg daily), and some patients require up to 1 to 2 months of glucocorticoid therapy. Adding oral steroids to NSAIDs will aid in ameliorating symptomology. Weak opioids like codeine or tramadol may be also considered at the lowest dose for the shortest duration necessary.

In the chronic phase (>3 months) of chikungunya arthritis with ongoing synovitis or tenosynovitis, disease-modifying antirheumatic drugs (DMARDs) can be used. The most commonly used DMARD is methotrexate[1] as a single dose at 7.5 to 15 mg/wk, along with folic acid[1] 1 mg/day. Renal function should be assessed. There is limited experience using sulfasalazine.[1] In patients with a complete response for at least 6 months, discontinuation of DMARD therapy should be attempted. In patients who are nonresponsive to methotrexate,[1] a tumor necrosis factor (TNF)-alpha inhibitor[1] is an appropriate consideration.

---

[1] Not FDA approved for this indication.

Monitoring

Chikungunya is a nationally notifiable disease. Cases should be immediately reported to state or local health department officials to facilitate diagnosis and mitigate the risk of local transmission.

Complications

In a 2018 meta-analysis of studies in the Americas, 52% of chikungunya-infected patients in the American continent developed protracted articular symptoms. Because of its potential for chronicity, chikungunya is properly considered a major world health problem. Healthcare professionals should be prepared to address the physical, psychological, and social demands of the lingering sequelae of chikungunya.

Chikungunya is one of the agents researched as a potential biologic weapon.

References

Adams LE, Martin SW, Lindsey NP: Epidemiology of dengue, chikungunya, and Zika virus disease in the US states and territories, *Am J Trop Med Hygiene* 101(4):884–890, 2017. 2019.

Amaral JK, Sutaria R, Schoen RT: Treatment of chronic chikungunya arthritis with methotrexate: a systematic review, *Arthritis Care Res (Hoboken)* 70(10):1501–1508, 2018.

August A, Attarwala H, Himansu S: A phase 1 trial of lipid-encapsulated mRNA encoding a monoclonal antibody with neutralizing activity against Chikungunya virus, *Nat Med* 27(12):2224–2233, 2021.

Cerny T, Schwarz M, Schwarz U: The range of neurological complications in Chikungunya fever, *Neurocrit Care* 27:447–457, 2017.

Edington F, Varjão D, Melo P: Incidence of articular pain and arthritis after chikungunya fever in the Americas: a systematic review of the literature and meta-analysis, *Joint Bone Spine* 85:669, 2018.

Gérardin P, Sampériz S, Ramful D: Neurocognitive outcome of children exposed to perinatal mother-to-child Chikungunya virus infection: the CHIMERE cohort study on Reunion Island, *PLoS Negl Trop Dis* 8(7):e2996, 2014.

Lindsey NP, Staples JE, Fischer M: Chikungunya virus disease among travelers-United States, 2014-2016, *Am J Trop Med Hyg* 98:192, 2018.

O'Driscoll M, Salje H, Chang AY, Watson H: Arthralgia resolution rate following chikungunya virus infection, *Int J Infect Dis* 112(1–7), 2021.

Pathak H, Mohan MC, Ravindran V: Chikungunya arthritis, *Clin Med (Lond)* 19(5):381–385, 2019.

Schilte C, Staikovsky F, Couderc T: Chikungunya virus-associated long-term arthralgia: a 36-month prospective longitudinal study, *PLoS Negl Trop Dis* 7(3):e2137, 2013.

Taksandel A, Vilhekar KY: Neonatal Chikungunya infection, *J Prevent Infect Control* 1(8), 2015.

Zeller H, Van Bortel W, Sudre B: Chikungunya: its history in Africa and Asia and its spread to new regions in 2013–2014, *J Infect Dis* 214(suppl 5):S436–S44, 2016.

CHOLERA

Method of
Mark Pietroni, MD, MBA

Cholera affects about 3 million people per year and kills approximately 100,000. It can kill within hours of the onset of symptoms, and even today the impact of an outbreak of cholera can be catastrophic in locations in which the water and sanitation infrastructure is weak, especially in crisis or war situations. The 21st century has already seen large-scale cholera epidemics in Haiti, Zimbabwe, Pakistan and Yemen, as well as many smaller outbreaks in countries and areas in which cholera is endemic. When cholera is untreated, mortality can be as high as 60% to 70%, but even in epidemics, with appropriate management and well-run diarrhea treatment centers, mortality can be reduced to well below 1%.

Oral rehydration therapy (ORT) is now the mainstay of treatment (Table 1). Developed in the 1960s in Dhaka, Bangladesh, ORT was used to great effect during the Bangladesh Liberation War of 1971. Cholera broke out in the refugee camps outside Calcutta, and the medical services ran out of intravenous fluid. ORT was not accepted as routine therapy by the medical profession at that time. The courageous decision to treat people with ORT saved thousands of lives and convinced

TABLE 1	Composition (mEq/L) of Common Solutions Used for Rehydration						
SOLUTION	NA+	K+	CL-	HCO3-	CITRATE	CA2+	GLUCOSE OR CARBOHYDRATE
Intravenous Solution							
Normal saline	154	—	154	—	—	—	—
Ringer's lactate	130	4	109	28	—	3	—
Ringer's lactate + D5	130	4	109	28	—	3	278
Cholera saline (Dhaka solution)	133	13	98	48	—	—	140
Oral Solution							
Standard ORS	90	20	80	—	10	—	111
Hypo-osmolar ORS	75	20	65	—	10	—	75
ReSoMal*	45	40	76	—	7	—	125

Abbreviations: D_5 = 5% dextrose; ORS = oral rehydration solution; ReSoMal = reduced osmolarity ORS for malnourished children.
Reprinted with permission from Harris JB, Pietroni M: Approach to the child with acute diarrhea in developing countries. UpToDate. Available at http://www.uptodate.com/contents/approach-to-the-child-with-acute-diarrhea-in-developing-countries (accessed August 11, 2016).
*Also contains Mg 6 mmol/L, Zn 300 μmol/L, Cu 45 μmol/L.

the world of the effectiveness of ORT in the management of cholera.

Pathophysiology

Cholera is caused by a gram-negative, comma-shaped bacterium called *Vibrio cholerae*. Clinical disease is caused by two serogroups: *V. cholerae* O1 (which has two biotypes: classical and El Tor) and *V. cholerae* O139. Humans are the only known natural host, and asymptomatic human carriage is rare. *V. cholerae* is rapidly killed by boiling water, but it can lie dormant for months in blue-green algae, crustaceans, and copepods in brackish water, especially in estuaries. The Ganges delta provides an ideal habitat and is believed to be the place cholera first emerged.

Human infection is caused by ingestion of contaminated food or drink or from poor hand hygiene in epidemic situations. Relative or absolute achlorhydria facilitates passage through the stomach. Proliferation occurs in the small intestine, where a number of toxins are released. This results in massive secretion of isotonic fluid into the gut. The fluid passes out of the anus full of vibrios to perpetuate the cycle of transmission. Killing the host does not appear to interrupt this cycle!

The cholera toxin is secreted only by the O1 and O139 serogroups. It has two subunits: A (active) and B (binding). Subunit B binds to receptors in the small intestine and subunit A activates adenylate cyclase. This causes the active secretion of a number of ions into the gut, which drags water by osmosis and also blocks the reabsorption of sodium from the gut. The net result is a massive loss of water, sodium chloride, and bicarbonate. This cannot be replaced by drinking a sodium solution because sodium reabsorption is blocked. However, the addition of glucose to a solution of sodium activates a sodium–glucose co-transporter; sodium is absorbed and water follows by osmosis. This is the basis of oral rehydration therapy for diarrhea today.

Clinical Presentation and Diagnosis

Cholera manifests as an acute watery diarrhea without blood in the stool or (usually) abdominal cramps. The majority of cases are clinically indistinguishable from other causes of watery diarrhea. About 10%-20% will develop dehydration but most require only oral rehydration fluid as treatment. However, some will progress to classic or severe cholera.

The classic picture is of the rapid onset of profuse watery diarrhea (rice-water stool) and vomiting, which is painless and can result in circulatory collapse within hours without effective treatment. The history is usually less than 24 hours, although it

may be longer if the patient is taking oral rehydration solution. Abdominal cramps can occur. Fever is absent. Patients usually remain alert, but severe electrolyte abnormalities such as hypoglycemia and hyponatremia can cause a reduced level of consciousness or convulsions, especially in children. Acidosis is often severe and results in tachypnea, which is commonly misdiagnosed as pneumonia. Patients should be reassessed for the presence or absence of pneumonia 1 to 2 hours after adequate rehydration. The diagnosis of cholera can be confirmed by the presence of rapidly motile vibrios detected by dark-field microscopy or by stool or rectal swab culture. However, the classic history, appearance of the stool, and rapid presentation mean that the diagnosis is usually clinical.

Treatment

A clinical syndrome of acute watery diarrhea (three or more watery stools in the last 24 hours) of short duration (24–48 hours) with or without vomiting associated with dehydration in anyone older than 2 years in an endemic or epidemic situation should be treated as cholera. Children younger than 2 years may be managed in the same way, but other diagnoses such as rotavirus should be considered. The mainstay of management (whatever the causative organism) is appropriate early rehydration, and time should not be wasted worrying about investigations or which antibiotic to use (Figure 1).

The initial assessment should be brief but must:
- Confirm the diagnosis of acute watery diarrhea
- Assess the level of dehydration
- Assess the presence or absence of malnutrition
- Recognize any other comorbidities

Accurate assessment and rapid, appropriate treatment of dehydration is critical to the management of cholera. A simple scoring system based on five clinical signs is sufficient and can accurately predict patients with 5% to 10% (some) dehydration and greater than 10% (severe) dehydration. Common mistakes include overreliance on individual clinical signs and giving too little intravenous fluid during the initial phase and too much during the recovery phase. Patients with less than 5% (no) dehydration and 5% to 10% (some) dehydration can be managed with oral rehydration alone (Box 1) unless there is a reduced level of consciousness or inability to take fluids by mouth. Those with 5% to 10% (some) dehydration must be reassessed every 1 to 2 hours to make sure that hydration is improving.

Patients with severe dehydration require an immediate intravenous fluid bolus of 100 mL/kg given over 3 hours with one

COVID-19

Method of

Thomas E. Dobbs, MD, MPH; and Lucius M. Lampton, MD

CURRENT DIAGNOSIS

- Coronavirus disease 2019 (COVID-19), the illness caused by severe acute respiratory syndrome coronavirus 2 (SARS-CoV-2), presents with a broad spectrum of multisystem clinical manifestations, including fever, dry cough, dyspnea, fatigue, sore throat, gastrointestinal symptoms, headache, chills, myalgias, anosmia, and ageusia, that can lead to severe illness and death in a minority of cases.
- Transmission of SARS-CoV-2 occurs most commonly through droplet and aerosol contact and less commonly by surface contamination.
- Diagnosis is based on detection of SARS-CoV-2 by viral testing of a respiratory sample, usually a nasopharyngeal swab. Serologic tests can detect antibodies from past infection or vaccination.
- Other factors critical for diagnosis and treatment include exposure history, computed tomography findings, laboratory tests, and clinical manifestations of SARS-CoV-2 infection.
- Different variants have demonstrated different clinical presentations, severity of illness, and incubation periods.

CURRENT THERAPY

- Prevention and protection via use of a SARS-CoV-2 vaccine are paramount and offer the best possibility of containing COVID-19 worldwide.
- Other pragmatic recommendations focus on prevention of person-to-person transmission and infection control, which are accomplished by social distancing, handwashing, source control measures, screening, quarantine, contact tracing, and personal protective equipment for healthcare workers.
- For nonhospitalized adults with mild to moderate COVID-19 at high risk of disease progression, several effective therapeutic options should be used, including oral antiviral therapy, intravenous antiviral treatment, and monoclonal antibody (mAb) therapy.
- Patients with moderate or severe disease may require hospitalization, respiratory support, and intensive care. Treatment in hospitalized patients includes supportive care and directed treatment to moderate the inflammatory response.
- Older adults and individuals with underlying chronic medical conditions are at higher risk for morbidity and mortality from COVID-19.
- Efficacy of specific mAbs has been dependent on the infecting variant.

Epidemiology

A novel coronavirus, severe acute respiratory syndrome coronavirus 2 (SARS-CoV-2) was first recognized in December 2019 as the etiologic agent of a serious respiratory illness soon designated *coronavirus disease 2019* (COVID-19). This potentially fatal disease has led to enormous human casualties and a considerable worldwide economic impact. Since COVID-19 was first reported in Wuhan, the capital of Hubei, China, it has reached a pandemic level, spreading over the world and multiplying more hurriedly than any infectious disease in recent memory, with more than 768 million confirmed cases and more 6,952,522 deaths, according to the latest figures (July 26, 2023) as reported to the World Health Organization (WHO). The outbreak has spread throughout the world, and in the United States there have been more than 103 million confirmed cases and over 1.1 million deaths as of July 2023.

This new, highly contagious coronavirus causes a respiratory illness with such symptoms as fever, cough, shortness of breath, and, in some cases, a deadly acute respiratory syndrome that can lead to pneumonia, respiratory failure, or septic shock. Infected persons have shown a range of symptoms from mild to severe illness and death. Symptoms may appear in as few as a couple of days to as long as 14 days after exposure, with variation depending on the variant. Genetic analysis of the virus indicates that it originated in bats, although it is still unclear whether it jumped directly from bats or an intermediary host existed. It appears similar to other zoonotic coronaviruses, like SARS-CoV, which emerged in 2002. Although there is a near-consensus view that the causative agent of COVID-19 has a natural zoonotic origin, several of its characteristics are not easily explained by this hypothesis and suggest the possibility of an alternate hypothesis of a laboratory leak origin. There remains much to be learned about the possible source and evolutionary path of this emerging disease.

In many countries, healthcare facilities have been stressed by a surge in recurrent cases, especially by patients requiring ventilatory support and intensive care. To slow disease spread and allow more time for public health and hospitals to become better prepared, public health efforts initially focused on flattening the epidemic curve with recommendations for physical distancing (referred to by some as *social distancing*) to minimize person-to-person transmission. Closure of schools and workplaces occurred, especially early in the pandemic, as well as cancellation of public events and services such as public transport. Classic public health strategies, including isolation and quarantine, were also implemented as effective countermeasures. However, limited data exist on the comparative effectiveness of these varied policy interventions. The brisk emergence of this devastating pandemic caused by a previously unknown pathogen underscores the perpetual challenges facing modern public health of emerging infectious diseases and the necessity of sustained preparedness.

The availability of safe and effective SARS-CoV-2 vaccines has saved numerous lives and assisted the control of COVID-19 both in the United States and worldwide. However, the emergence of several new variants of the original virus have been recognized that appear to cause significant changes in the way the pathogen behaves, including alterations to its transmissibility. The current vaccines have a limited duration of maximal efficacy, necessitating booster doses to maintain maximal protection. The evolution of variants has rendered vaccines less effective at preventing viral replication, but the protective effects of preventing severe illness have remained robust. Infection with SARS-CoV-2 yields immunity roughly on par with vaccine-induced immunity.

Risk Factors

Exposure history to individuals with COVID-19 is the essential risk factor. Individuals who have had close contact with a known positive patient or who have traveled to or live in an area with high community transmission should be screened if they are symptomatic. Individuals with known exposure should be tested for SARS-CoV-2 at least 5 days from initial exposure. Employment as a healthcare worker engaged in the direct care of patients is also a risk factor. Individuals at higher risk of morbidity and mortality if infected are adults older than 65 years of age, especially those in long-term care facilities and those with chronic illnesses such as hypertension, diabetes, obesity, chronic kidney disease, chronic obstructive pulmonary disease (COPD), asthma, immunocompromised conditions, pregnancy, heart failure, and sickle cell disease. Studies have also revealed that a disproportionate percentage of COVID-19 hospitalizations and deaths occurs in minority and lower-income populations. Disease in children is typically mild, but severe disease from COVID-19 and multisystem inflammatory syndrome in children (MIS-C) occurs, causing over 1400 deaths among children in the United States.

Pathophysiology

Coronaviruses are enveloped, positive-sense single-stranded RNA viruses, which are characterized by clublike glycoprotein spikes on their surface that mediate receptor binding and cell entry during infection. These spikes on the envelope give coronaviruses a *crownlike* appearance under an electron microscope, which is the source of its name, *corona* being the Latin term for "crown." They are the largest group of viruses belonging to the Nidovirales order, which includes the Coronaviridae, Arteriviridae, Mesoniviridae, and Roniviridae families. The Coronavirinae are one of two subfamilies in the Coronaviridae family. Coronaviruses possess an unusually large RNA genome and cause a wide spectrum of multisystem diseases in birds and mammals ranging from upper respiratory infections in chickens to enteritis in pigs and cows to potentially fatal human respiratory disease. To date, only seven human coronaviruses have been identified. Several cause common colds and self-limiting upper respiratory infections. However, at least three have caused widespread deadly outbreaks, including the highly pathogenic severe acute respiratory syndrome coronavirus, Middle East respiratory syndrome coronavirus, and most recently SARS-CoV-2.

Genomic analyses indicate that SARS-CoV-2 probably originated and evolved from a strain found in bats. Most researchers suggest that there probably was an amplifying mammalian host, intermediate between bats and humans. However, it is not certain whether an intermediary exists, as the original strain's mutation could have directly jumped from bats to humans. Although animal-to-human transmission was first presumed, the main exposure mechanism appears to be human-to-human transmission, with symptomatic individuals the most frequent source of spread, although presymptomatic and asymptomatic individuals also contribute to this spread. Transmission is believed to occur primarily through respiratory droplets spread by coughing, sneezing, or talking and via aerosol transmission, especially in closed spaces. Studies also reveal that SARS-CoV-2 can contaminate objects and surfaces for hours and days.

Like other coronaviruses, SARS-CoV-2 is sensitive to ultraviolet rays and heat. These viruses can be effectively inactivated by lipid solvents including ether, ethanol, chlorine-containing disinfectants, and peroxyacetic acid.

Prevention

Vaccination against COVID-19 is the most effective way to prevent SARS-CoV-2 infection and severe illness and over the first 2 years of use, saving an estimated three million lives in the United States alone.* Vaccination is available for everyone 6 months of age and older. Bivalent vaccine products, based on the antigenic characteristics of the initial COVID-19 strain and more recent omicron variants, were recently available for ages 6 months through adulthood. For those without underlying immune compromising conditions, a single dose of bivalent vaccine has been recommended for ages 6 years through adulthood. For children ages 6 month through 5 years of age, dosing recommendations vary by product selected and prior vaccination history.** For patients with moderate to severe underlying immune compromising conditions, including those with a history of transplantation, advanced HIV, active cancer treatment or taking immune suppressive drugs, additional doses have been recommended.** A second bivalent dose, 4 months after an initial bivalent dose, was approved for those over 65 years of age. Monoclonal antibody products for treatment or prophylaxis of COVID-19 are not currently recommended for use as they are unlikely to be effective against actively circulating subvariants.

Given the ever-evolving nature of COVID-19, the FDA's Vaccines and Related Biological Products Advisory Committee recommended the development of a monovalent vaccine, directed at the omicron variant XBB.1.5, for use in the fall of 2023. Pfizer and Moderna have developed monovalent mRNA vaccine products based on this recommendation. Novavax, using a protein subunit vaccine approach, has also developed a vaccine targeting the XBB.1.5 sublineage. On September 12, 2023, the CDC recommended the updated COVID-19 vaccine for everyone 6 months of age and older. Evidence supports the efficacy of the updated vaccine products against the currently circulating strains of the omicron variant. Older individuals and those with higher risk conditions are likely to achieve the greatest benefit from the updated vaccine product. Serious reactions after COVID-19 vaccination are rare, and the risk to benefit ratio strongly favors the vaccination for all recommended age groups. Myocarditis in males 12 to 17 years old has been described following vaccination, but the risk of myocarditis following COVID-19 infection is considerably higher.***

Other Mitigation Measures

Other preventive strategies should focus on isolation of patients and rigid infection control, which includes appropriate measures to provide clinical care for infected patients. Transmission of SARS-CoV-2 is believed to occur usually through respiratory droplets spread from an infectious person to others within 6 feet and through airborne transmission of small droplets over larger distances. In rare instances, an individual just passing through a room that was previously occupied by an infected individual may become infected. For the general public, the primary preventive action is physical distancing (maintaining 6 feet between people) and isolation when ill to minimize transmission. Other general recommendations include avoiding close contact with individuals suffering from acute respiratory infections and washing hands frequently, especially after contact with infected individuals and their environment; individuals with acute airway infections or symptoms should keep their distance from others and follow cough and hand hygiene. Avoiding indoor public gatherings is important during periods of increased transmission, especially for high-risk or immunocompromised individuals.

Studies indicate that the combination of isolation and contract tracing with physical distancing can effectively reduce disease transmission in communities. A variety of public health interventions have been implemented worldwide during the pandemic to reduce transmission. Among the more effective interventions associated with reduced rates of transmission are the use of home isolation after infection, the restriction of mass gatherings, travel restrictions, and social distancing. Studies assert that risk of resurgence follows when these interventions are lifted. A key priority is identifying optimal protective measures that result in the least economic and societal disruption while adequately controlling transmission and infection.

Source control is an important prevention strategy and refers to use of cloth face coverings or face masks to shield an individual's mouth and nose to prevent spread of respiratory secretions when talking, sneezing, or coughing. Because of the potential for asymptomatic and presymptomatic spread, source control measures appear to be an effective prevention tool. The regular use of masks can help protect individuals from contracting COVID-19, with N95 masks more effective than surgical masks, which in turn are more effective than cloth masks. This measure is important to consider during periods of increased transmission, especially for those at greater risk for adverse clinical outcomes.

Patient Isolation and Quarantine

Patients diagnosed with COVID-19 should maintain strict home isolation for at least 5 days from symptom onset or positive test if asymptomatic. If symptoms are absent or improved after 5 days, increased activity with universal mask use may occur through day 10, at which time all restrictions can be lifted. No travel through

---

*https://www.commonwealthfund.org/blog/2022/two-years-covid-vaccines-prevented-millions-deaths-hospitalizations
**https://www.cdc.gov/vaccines/covid-19/clinical-considerations/index.html (Accessed 9/13/2023)

***https://www.cdc.gov/respiratory-viruses/whats-new/covid-vaccine-recommendations-9-12-2023.html a public conveyance should occur within 10 days. Patients with more severe illness or immune compromise should home isolate for at least 10 days.

Quarantine is a term used for persons who are at risk of developing a contagious illness but are not yet ill, for the purpose of preventing future transmission. Close contacts to a case of COVID-19, defined as exposure of 15 minutes or more to an infectious case within 6 feet in a 24-hour period, should quarantine themselves based on vaccination status or history of recent infection.

Infection Control in Healthcare Settings

Infection control measures are critically important in inpatient and outpatient settings to minimize transmission to patients and staff. These recommended measures currently include source control (i.e., use of masks); screening of patients for COVID-19 infection or risk; environmental control; and isolation, quarantine, and testing of healthcare staff as indicated.

Before engaging the healthcare system, patients should be pre-screened for known COVID-19 illness, symptoms of COVID-19, or recent exposure. Patients with potential COVID-19 should be quickly isolated in an area that minimizes the risk of transmission. Healthcare workers should use medically appropriate masks (i.e., N95) and eye protection when caring for potential COVID-19 patients. The Centers for Disease Control and Prevention (CDC) continues to recommend universal mask use in healthcare settings. This is especially important for patients with possible COVID-19 infection.

Environmental cleaning and proper air filtration are important measures to mitigate transmission. Thorough cleaning of the environment and equipment should be performed between patient encounters with an appropriate disinfectant. In the inpatient setting, dedicated equipment should be used when practicable. Proper air filtration is important and should be reviewed with physical maintenance staff. Detailed guidance is available through the American Society of Heating, Refrigerating and Air-Conditioning Engineers resources for healthcare facilities.

Isolation and quarantine of healthcare personnel are critical measures to limit transmission and protect the workforce. Healthcare workers diagnosed with COVID-19 may return to work in 10 days or as early as 7 days if symptoms have improved or are absent, the patient has a negative COVID-19 test within the previous 48 hours (antigen test or nucleic acid amplification test [NAAT]), and the patient is at least 24 hours free from fever. Employees with more severe illness or immune compromise should remain isolated for at least 10 days. Employees who are contacts to a case (without appropriate personal protective equipment) and have an up-to-date vaccination status do not have to discontinue working, but they should test on days 5 to 7. Employees who are not up to date on vaccination should home quarantine for 10 days (or 7 days with a negative test on days 5 to 7). The CDC has alternative recommendations for shortened durations of quarantine for circumstances when healthcare systems are operating in contingency or crisis modes.

Clinical Manifestations

COVID-19 patients can manifest a wide variety of symptoms, with pulmonary inflammation its main pathologic manifestation. The estimated incubation period for COVID-19 is up to 14 days from exposure, with a median incubation time of 4 to 5 days. This varies depending on the infecting variant. The spectrum of illness can range from asymptomatic infection to severe pneumonia with acute respiratory distress syndrome (ARDS) and death. Patients usually report fever; dry cough; shortness of breath; gastrointestinal symptoms such as abdominal pain, diarrhea, anorexia, and vomiting; myalgias; headaches; dizziness; anosmia; dysgeusia; sore throat; fatigue; and chills. Mild pneumonia can occur, but in more severe cases tachypnea, dyspnea, and significant pneumonia can be seen, which can develop into a critical stage with respiratory failure, septic shock, and multiorgan failure. Older adult patients occasionally present with delirium or altered mental status. Adults with severe disease usually present during the second

week of illness, a period that coincides with decreasing viral loads but increasing markers of inflammation, which suggests that host tissue damage is mediated by hyperinflammatory and maladaptive immune responses.

As found in many other viral infections, there appears to be a two-phase immune response in COVID-19. The first is the body's response directly to the viral infection. This is followed by a second reactive-stage infection that precipitates a cytokine release syndrome, a consequence of the host's reaction to the infection and the resulting cytokine activation cascade, which causes autoimmune-induced damage to the lungs, vascular endothelium, gastric mucosa, and other structures. This is mediated by non–T leukocytes and is found to be associated with lymphocytopenia, increased ferritin levels, decreased platelet count, and elevated erythrocyte sedimentation rate. This cytokine storm and its extensive tissue damage and dysfunctional coagulation are thought to result from an overactive immune response mediated in part by interleukin (IL)-6 and other cytokine pathways.

Thrombotic aberration in COVID-19 patients is common and appears to contribute to organ failure and death. Platelet hyperreactivity, which is recognized in COVID-19, also contributes to morbidity through increased platelet-platelet and platelet-leukocyte interactions. Hemostatic alterations that mimic disseminated intravascular coagulopathy associated with sepsis often present with severe COVID-19 illness, with elevated risk of thrombosis rather than bleeding.

Most children with COVID-19 present either without symptoms or with milder symptoms than in adults. Symptoms resemble routine acute chest infections, with pyrexia, dry cough, sore throat, sneezing, myalgia, and lethargy. Less commonly, wheezing, diarrhea, and vomiting have also been noted. An uncommon disorder, MIS-C has also been associated with SARS-CoV-2. MIS-C can result in severe illness in previously healthy children and adolescents. Although it is less common in children, death can result from either complications from infection or MIS-C. A similar syndrome to MIS-C can also occur in adults.

Long COVID or Post-COVID Conditions

A substantial proportion of COVID-19 patients develop a prolonged syndrome of various symptoms that is commonly referred to as *long COVID*. This likely represents a constellation of different pathologic processes, and there is no consensus terminology currently in place. Common symptoms include fatigue, malaise, fever, cough, difficulty concentrating, muscle pain, rash, intestinal disorders, and others. Loss or change of taste and/or smell are common after infection with SARS-CoV-2 but usually resolves over several weeks, though persistent aberrations may occur. Long COVID is more common in those with more severe illness, prolonged hospitalization, need for the intensive care unit (ICU), and unvaccinated status before COVID-19 infection. More than 1 in 10 COVID-19 patients have symptoms 1 month or more after infection. The pathophysiology for these symptoms is not defined, and there is no effective treatment identified. Precluding COVID-19 infection via vaccination and preventive safety measures is the best way to avoid long COVID. Prior vaccination is associated with a substantially lower risk of developing long COVID symptoms. Numerous medical centers are operating specialized clinics that focus on patients with this ill-defined syndrome.

Diagnosis

The diagnosis of COVID-19 is established by a suggestive clinical history including exposure history and clinical manifestations of SARS-CoV-2 infection, confirmed by detection of SARS-CoV-2 nucleic acid (via NAAT) or antigen from an upper respiratory sample (i.e., a nasopharyngeal, nasal, or oropharyngeal specimen). Numerous platforms are currently available for both diagnostic approaches. NAAT has superior sensitivity compared with antigen testing, which is typically faster and more convenient. Home antigen tests are widely available for use, presenting the possibility of patients self-diagnosing before presentation. Lower respiratory tract specimens have a higher viral load and are recommended for intubated or mechanically ventilated patients with clinical signs and symptoms of COVID-19. If the initial viral test results are positive for SARS-CoV-2, the patient should be considered to have COVID-19 and additional testing pursued (i.e., NAAT confirmation), regardless of whether other findings are also present. Because of false-negative test result rates of SARS-CoV-2 viral testing, other data such as imaging and laboratory tests are often helpful in making a presumptive diagnosis. Many cases of COVID-19 are asymptomatic or minimally symptomatic and will test positive by antigen or NAAT. Serologic testing is not recommended for the diagnosis of acute COVID-19. Repeat NAAT for SARS-CoV-2 is not recommended as results may remain positive in the absence of active infection.

Because pulmonary inflammation is the major pathologic manifestation of COVID-19, chest radiography should be the initial imaging study. A plain chest radiograph in COVID-19 may reveal peribronchial thickening (which is typical in viral infections), pneumonia, nonspecific findings, or even negative findings. A chest computed tomography (CT) scan is usually more helpful in providing a definitive diagnosis. Multiple studies reveal that COVID-19 pneumonia is more likely to have a peripheral distribution, ground-glass opacity, fine reticular opacity, bilateral consolidations, and vascular thickening. These studies also reveal that COVID-19 is less likely to have a central plus peripheral distribution, pleural effusion, and lymphadenopathy. However, differentiating radiographic findings of COVID-19 pneumonia, influenza virus pneumonia, and other viral pneumonias in clinical practice remains difficult.

Despite its diagnostic benefits, a chest CT is not recommended as a first-line screening test for those with suspected COVID-19 infection. As well, a chest CT should be used sparingly and reserved for hospitalized patients with clinical indications for CT. If a patient medically declines, a chest CT may be indicated to better assess pulmonary status and disease progression. In the first 2 weeks after symptom onset, there can be a rapid evolution of CT abnormalities, after which these findings recede gradually.

Laboratory testing also plays a role in the initial evaluation and diagnosis of COVID-19, especially in the workup of hospitalized patients. Multiple laboratory abnormalities are often seen in positive patients and can assist in assessing whether a patient is improving or declining. Among typical abnormal results are elevations in serum C-reactive protein, lactate dehydrogenase, ferritin, procalcitonin, creatine kinase, alanine aminotransferase, and aspartate aminotransferase. Many patients also present with a low albumin. Lymphocytopenia, which is associated with an increased risk of ICU care and acute kidney injury, is the most common hematologic abnormality seen, although leukopenia and leukocytosis are also common. A modest prolongation of prothrombin times, mild thrombocytopenia, and elevated D-dimer values often are seen and have also been associated with higher rates of ARDS and mortality. However, some of these laboratory findings are nonspecific, being common in pneumonia in general, and their clinical utility remains uncertain.

Differential Diagnosis
In its initial stages, COVID-19 appears clinically like many other viral and bacterial respiratory illnesses, presenting with a broad range of nonspecific and varied signs and symptoms. These other illnesses not only must be considered in the differential diagnosis but also may occur simultaneously with COVID-19 infection.

Viral infections in the differential diagnosis include influenza, parainfluenza, coronavirus, adenovirus, respiratory syncytial virus, infectious mononucleosis, acute human immunodeficiency virus, human rhinovirus/enterovirus, and human metapneumovirus. Bacterial pneumonias that should be considered in the differential diagnosis include *Streptococcus pneumoniae*, *Haemophilus influenza*, *Chlamydia pneumoniae*, and *Moraxella catarrhalis*. Atypical pneumonias in the differential include *Legionella pneumophila* and *Mycoplasma pneumoniae*. In immunocompromised

TABLE 1 High-Risk Clinical Conditions

- Cancer
- Cerebrovascular disease
- Chronic kidney disease
- Chronic lung diseases including:
  - Asthma
  - Interstitial lung disease
  - Pulmonary embolism
  - Pulmonary hypertension
  - Bronchiectasis
- Chronic obstructive pulmonary disease
- Chronic liver diseases including:
  - Cirrhosis
  - Nonalcoholic fatty liver disease
  - Alcoholic liver disease
  - Autoimmune hepatitis
  - Cystic fibrosis
  - Diabetes mellitus, type 1 and type 2
- Dementia and other neurologic conditions
  - Disabilities
  - Attention-deficit/hyperactivity disorder
  - Cerebral palsy
- Congenital malformations (birth defects)
- Down syndrome
- Limitations with self-care or activities of daily living
- Intellectual and developmental disabilities
- Learning disabilities
- Spinal cord injuries
- Heart conditions (such as heart failure, coronary artery disease, or cardiomyopathies)
- Human immunodeficiency virus
- Mental health disorders limited to:
- Mood disorders, including depression
- Schizophrenia spectrum disorders
- Neurologic conditions limited to dementia
- Obesity (body mass index $\geq 30 \text{ kg/m}^2$)
- Physical inactivity
- Primary immunodeficiencies
- Pregnancy and recent pregnancy
- Sickle cell disease or thalassemia
- Smoking, current and former
- Solid organ or hematopoietic cell transplantation
- Substance use disorder
- Tuberculosis
- Use of corticosteroids or other immunosuppressive medications

Modified from Centers for Disease Control and Prevention. Underlying Medical Conditions Associated with Higher Risk for Severe COVID-19: Information for Healthcare Professionals. Updated May 2023. Available at https://www.cdc.gov/coronavirus/2019-ncov/need-extra-precautions/people-with-medical-conditions.html

hosts, *Pneumocystis jirovecii* should be considered. If patients have returned from international travel, such illnesses as dengue and malaria should be considered.

In addition to these infectious illnesses, the differential diagnosis may include noninfectious disorders such as pulmonary embolism, COPD exacerbation, asthma, pulmonary edema, vasculitis, cor pulmonale, pneumonitis, ARDS, acute coronary syndrome, congestive heart failure, valvular disease, cancer, or acute chest syndrome in sickle cell disease.

Treatment
Outpatient Management
The majority of COVID-19 patients have a relatively mild illness and can be managed on an outpatient basis. It is essential to identify patients at highest risk of poor outcomes and evaluate them for treatment with monoclonal antibodies (mAbs) or oral SARS-CoV-2 antivirals. Those at highest risk include individuals with underlying immune suppression (regardless of vaccination status) and those 65 years of age and older. Numerous underlying medical conditions increase the risk of adverse outcomes. A summary of high-risk clinical conditions provided by the CDC is listed in Table 1. Clinically stable patients who are at increased risk for adverse

outcomes and do not require supplemental oxygen or increased oxygen should be evaluated for outpatient treatment. Current preferred therapies are oral nirmatrelvir/ritonavir (Paxlovid)[1] or intravenous (IV) remdesivir (Veklury). When these preferred treatments are not available, oral molnupiravir (Lagevrio)[1] is a recommended treatment option. Early diagnosis is key as most treatments must be provided early in the illness to be effective.

Nirmatrelvir/ritonavir is a viral protease inhibitor that has demonstrated activity against all known human coronaviruses. When used early in COVID-19 illness, this agent demonstrated an 88% decrease in death or hospitalization in the Evaluation of Protease Inhibition for COVID-19 in High Risk Patients trial. Nirmatrelvir/ritonavir is FDA approved for the treatment of COVID-19. This treatment consists of nirmatrelvir 300 mg and ritonavir 100 mg twice daily for 5 days (≥12 years and ≥40 kg) and must be started within 5 days of symptom onset. Doses must be adjusted for renal impairment, and this drug is not recommended for those with a creatinine clearance of less than 30 mL/min or those with advanced liver disease. Numerous potential drug-drug interactions with this treatment necessitate a thorough review of potential interactions with current medications. There also have been some case reports of a phenomenon called COVID-19 rebound, in which patients who completed a full course of nirmatrelvir/ritonavir and recovered with subsequent negative viral testing experienced a recurrent illness 2 to 8 days later with positive test results. This rebound usually resolved without additional COVID-19 treatment over 3 days. This rebound phenomenon also can be seen in the absence of treatment.

Remdesivir is a nucleotide analog that inhibits DNA-dependent RNA polymerase. This treatment is recommended for nonhospitalized patients with mild to moderate illness from COVID-19 at increased risk for adverse outcomes. This 3-day IV outpatient treatment is administered as a 200 mg dose on day 1 followed by 100 mg on days 2 and 3. Treatment with remdesivir has demonstrated similar efficacy to nirmatrelvir/ritonavir with an 87% reduction in hospitalization or deaths. Treatment must be provided within 7 days of onset of illness and is used for individuals who are 12 years of age and older and weigh at least 40 kg.

Molnupiravir (Lagevrio)[1] is recommended as a second-line outpatient treatment option for those unable to receive nirmatrelvir/ritonavir or remdesivir. Molnupiravir is a ribonucleoside that produces unstable mutagenesis in the replicating SARS-CoV-2 virus. It has demonstrated lesser efficacy than first-line recommended treatments, and it should not be used in pregnancy. Conception and pregnancy should be avoided for males and females during and immediately after treatment.

Corticosteroid treatment is not generally recommended for use in the outpatient setting, but it could be considered in circumstances when hospitalization is not available for patients with new oxygen requirements (i.e., overwhelmed hospital system capacity). Recommended treatment in this setting would be oral dexamethasone[1] 6 mg daily for the duration of oxygen requirement not to exceed 10 days.

Fluvoxamine (Luvox)[1], a selective serotonin reuptake inhibitor (SSRI), has demonstrated potential utility for treating COVID-19 but is currently only recommended for use in the context of clinical trials. Other treatment options, including hydroxychloroquine[1], azithromycin (Zithromax)[1], and ivermectin (Stromectol)[1] have been shown not to offer benefit for the treatment of COVID-19 in randomized controlled trials and are not recommended.

Inpatient Management
In addition to general supportive measures, specific therapeutic strategies are recommended to treat COVID-19 patients in the inpatient setting. For hospitalized patients not requiring supplemental oxygen, IV remdesivir for 5 days (200 mg on day 1 followed by 100 mg daily) is a recommended option and may be extended based on clinical circumstances. This treatment can be effective if started less than 10 days from symptom onset.

For patients with increasing oxygen requirements, the addition of oral dexamethasone[1], 6 mg daily until hospital discharge or up to a maximum of 10 days, is recommended and may be used in combination with remdesivir. For those with rapidly deteriorating hypoxemia or markedly elevated inflammatory markers, the addition of immune modulators (IL-6 inhibitors tocilizumab [Actemra][1] or sarilumab [Kevzara][1], or Janus kinase inhibitors baricitinib [Olumiant] or tofacitinib [Xeljanz][1]) should be considered as an intervention to modulate the inflammatory cascade.

In general, prophylactic doses of heparin for the prevention of venous thromboembolism should be initiated unless contraindicated. Therapeutic doses may be considered for those with elevated D-dimer levels and supplemental oxygen requirement if there is no elevated risk of bleeding.

Critical Illness
In general, the care of patients with critical illness from COVID-19 mirrors best practices of the management of critically ill patients with other inflammatory illness with additional approaches directed at treatment SARS-CoV-2 and the subsequent inflammatory response. High-flow nasal cannula oxygen is recommended over noninvasive ventilation for those with advanced oxygen requirements not requiring mechanical ventilation. Dexamethasone[1] should be administered to all patients requiring mechanical ventilation or extracorporeal membrane oxygenation. The addition of immune modulators (see the Inpatient Management section) is also recommended. Prophylactic doses of heparin for the prevention of venous thromboembolism should be initiated unless contraindicated.

Multisystem Inflammatory Syndrome in Children
MIS-C is defined as an inflammatory condition in individuals younger than 21 years of age with fever, laboratory evidence of inflammation, and clinically severe illness requiring hospitalization, with multisystem organ involvement within 4 weeks of COVID-19 infection. This is a severe illness that requires urgent intervention with management, preferably in a tertiary referral center. Treatment generally consists of IV immunoglobulin[1] and methylprednisolone[1]. Refractory cases may require additional immunomodulatory therapy. A similar syndrome in adults also occurs, but treatment recommendations are less well standardized.

Conclusions
Much remains unknown in our understanding of the transmission, infection, and management of this novel coronavirus (SARS-CoV-2). Several medical organizations, including the Infectious Diseases Society of America, the WHO, and the National Institutes of Health, have developed interim guidelines that are modified as more information becomes available during this rapidly evolving pandemic. Most of these guidelines emphasize that there are few proven treatments for COVID-19, that few randomized clinical trials have been published to guide effective management, and that further randomized trials are needed. The foundation of prevention of COVID-19 is vaccination, and the most effective current therapy centers on antiviral therapy and the early use of neutralizing mAbs. Because of the broad presence of some degree of immunity in the population and possibly fewer pathogenic COVID-19 variants, new cases have resulted in a lower proportion of deaths and hospitalizations. It remains to be seen how SARS-CoV-2 will settle into the landscape of other respiratory viruses and whether it will develop a clear seasonality as the pandemic shifts to more of an endemic phase. This unprecedented pandemic requires therapeutic flexibility and a continuous reshaping of treatment protocols and vaccine recommendations based on available scientific evidence for the most favorable patient outcomes.

---

[1] Not FDA approved for this indication.

[1] Not FDA approved for this indication.

References

Aiyegbusi OL, Hughes SE, Turner G, et al: Symptoms, complications, and management of long COVID: a review, *J R Soc Med*, 2021.

Altarawneh HN, Chemaitelly H, Ayoub HH, et al: Effects of previous infection and vaccination on symptomatic Omicron infections, *N Engl J Med*, 2022.

Al-Aly Z, Bowe B, Xie Y: Long COVID after breakthrough SARS-CoV-2 infection, *Nat Med*, 2022.

Azzolini E, Levi R, Sarti R, et al: Association between BNT162b2 vaccination and long COVID after infections not requiring hospitalization in health care workers, *JAMA*, 2022. *Published online*, July 01.

Bobrovitz N, Ware H, et al: Protective effectiveness of previous SARS-CoV-2 infection and hybrid immunity against the omicron variant and severe disease: a systematic review and meta-regression, *Lancet Infect Dis* 23(5):556–567, 2023.

Bruel T, Hadjadj J, Maes P, et al: Serum neutralization of SARS-CoV-2 Omicron sublineages BA.1 and BA.2 in patients receiving monoclonal antibodies, *Nat Med* 28:1297–1302, 2022.

Centers for Disease Control and Prevention. COVID Data Tracker. https://covid.cdc.gov/covid-data-tracker/#datatracker-home. Accessed August 1, 2023.

Coronavirus (COVID-19) at Centers for Disease Control and Prevention. Available at: https://www.cdc.gov/coronavirus/2019-nCoV/. Accessed on July 30, 2023.

Del Rio C, Malani PN: COVID-19 in 2022—the beginning of the end or the end of the beginning? *J Am Med Assoc* 327(24):2389–2390, 2022.

Drain PK: Rapid diagnostic testing for SARS-CoV-2, *N Engl J Med* 386:264–272, 2022.

Feldstein LR, Tenforde MW, Friedman KG, et al: Characteristics and outcomes of US children and adolescents with multisystem inflammatory syndrome in children (MIS-C) compared with severe acute COVID-19, *J Am Med Assoc* 325(11):1074–1087, 2021.

Gostin LO, Gronvall G: The origins of covid-19-- why it matters (and why it doesn't), *N Engl J Med* 388:2305–2308, 2023.

Hammond J, Leister-Tebbe H, Gardner A, et al: Oral nirmatrelvir for high-risk, nonhospitalized adults with covid-19, *N Engl J Med* 386(15):1397–1408, 2022.

Infectious Diseases Society of America. Infectious Diseases Society of America guidelines on the treatment and management of patients with COVID-19. Published May 27, 2021. Last updated, 6/26/23. https://www.idsociety.org/practice-guideline/covid-19-guideline-treatment-and-management/. Accessed July 30, 2023.

Johns Hopkins Coronavirus Resource Center. COVID-19 Dashboard by the Center for Systems Science and Engineering (CSSE) at Johns Hopkins University. https://coronavirus.jhu.edu/map.html. Accessed on July 29, 2023.

Labbé V, Contou D, Heming N, et al: Effects of standard-dose prophylactic, high-dose prophylactic, and therapeutic anticoagulation in patients with hypoxemic COVID-19 pneumonia: the ANTICOVID randomized clinical trial, *JAMA Intern Med* 183(6):520–531, 2023.

The COVID-19 pandemic in 2023: far from over." The Lancet. 401; January 14, 2023. https://www.thelancet.com/action/showPdf?pii=S0140-6736%2823%2900050-8.

Ma KC, Dorabawila V, León TM, et al: Trends in laboratory-confirmed SARS-CoV-2 reinfections and associated hospitalizations and deaths among adults aged ≥18 Years — 18 U.S. Jurisdictions, september 2021–december 2022, *MMWR Morb Mortal Wkly Rep* 72:683–689, 2023.

National Institutes of Health: Coronavirus disease 2019 (COVID-19) treatment guidelines, https://www.covid19treatmentguidelines.nih.gov/. Accessed July 4, 2023.

Plumb ID, Feldstein LR, Barkley E, et al: Effectiveness of COVID-19 mRNA vaccination in preventing COVID-19–associated hospitalization among adults with previous SARS-CoV-2 infection — United States, june 2021–february 2022, *MMWR Morb Mortal Wkly Rep* 71:549–555, 2022.

Shi DS, Whitaker M, Marks KH, et al: Hospitalizations of children aged 5–11 Years with laboratory-confirmed COVID-19 — COVID-NET, 14 States, march 2020–february 2022, *MMWR Morb Mortal Wkly Rep* 71:574–581, 2022.

World Health Organization: *Therapeutics and COVID-19: living guideline, January 13, 2023*, Geneva. 2022. WHO/2019-nCoV/therapeutics/2023.1).

World Health Organization. WHO Coronavirus (COVID-19) Dashboard. https://covid19.who.int. Accessed August 1, 2023.

Yu J, Collier AY, Rowe M, et al: Neutralization of the SARS-CoV-2 omicron BA.1 and BA.2 variants, *N Engl J Med* 386:1579–1580, 2022.

EBOLA VIRUS DISEASE

Method of
Uma Malhotra, MD

CURRENT DIAGNOSIS

- Detection of viral RNA in the blood by reverse transcriptase-polymerase chain reaction (RT-PCR) beginning 3 days after the onset of symptoms.
- Repeat testing may be necessary for patients with illness duration shorter than 3 days.
- Details on specimen collection and handling can be found on the Centers for Disease Control and Prevention (CDC), and World Health Organization (WHO) websites.

CURRENT THERAPY

- Intensive fluid management to correct volume losses and electrolyte abnormalities.
- Aggressive use of antiemetics, antidiarrheals, and rehydration solutions.
- Respiratory and hemodynamic support.
- Blood products for management of coagulopathy.
- Evaluate and treat any concomitant infections.
- Two monoclonal antibody therapies, REGN-EB3 (Inmazeb) and mAb114 (Ebanga), have been approved by the US Food and Drug Administration (FDA) for the treatment of adults and children with disease due to the *Zaire ebolavirus*.
- Strict infection control measures, with contact and droplet precautions, must be used.
- Personnel trained in the correct use of personal protective equipment (PPE) should care for the patients.
- The rVSV-ZEBOV Ebola vaccine (Ervebo), a replication-competent, live attenuated vaccine is now approved by the FDA for the prevention of disease caused by *Zaire ebolavirus* in adults aged ≥18 years at high risk for occupation exposure. A second two-component vaccine, Ad26.ZEBOV/MVA-BN-Filo (Zabdeno and Mvabea),[5] given in two doses 8 weeks apart, has been found to be safe and immunogenic when given to at-risk populations in regions where there is no active disease transmission and is expected to provide longer protection.

[5]Investigational drug in the United States.

Filoviridae, derived from the Latin word "filum," meaning thread-like, is a family of viruses with a filamentous structure that can cause severe hemorrhagic fever and fulminant septic shock. Filoviruses have been divided into three genera: Ebola-like viruses with six species—*Zaire, Sudan, Tai Forest, Bundibugyo, Reston*, and *Bombali*; Marburg-like viruses with a single species—*Marburg*, which has caused outbreaks in Central Africa; and Cuevavirus, detected only as viral RNA in bats in Spain. Using paleoviruses (genomic fossils) found in mammals, we can extrapolate that the viruses probably diverged several thousand years ago, and that the family itself is at least tens of millions of years old.

Epidemiology

Of the six Ebola virus species only four—*Zaire, Sudan, Tai Forest*, and *Bundibugyo*—cause disease in humans. Since its first recognition in 1976, *Zaire ebolavirus* has caused multiple outbreaks in Central Africa. It is the causative agent of the 2014 West African epidemic, with an initial estimated case fatality rate as high as 70%, although as the epidemic evolved, lower fatality rates in the range of 30% to 40% were observed. The 2014 epidemic began in Guinea, when a 2-year-old child became infected in late 2013, and *Zaire ebolavirus* subsequently spread to Liberia, Sierra Leone, Nigeria, Senegal, and Mali. The epidemic resulted in over 28,000 cases and 11,000 deaths, with more than 800 infections occurring in health care workers. Outbreaks due to the Zaire species continue to occur in the Democratic Republic of the Congo (DRC). *Sudan* virus has been associated with a case-fatality rate of approximately 50% in four epidemics, which occurred in Sudan and Uganda between 1970 and 2004. In 2022 there were two outbreaks of EVD. One caused by *Zaire ebolavirus* occurred in the DRC from April to July. Virus sequencing indicated that the outbreak was due to a new spillover event from an animal source. Another caused by *Sudan virus* occurred in Uganda from September 2022 to January 2023. In the latter outbreak, unrecognized transmission likely occurred over several weeks due to wide mobility of asymptomatic individuals and because the availability of vaccination was more limited than in recent outbreaks in the DRC. *Tai Forest* virus has been identified as the cause of illness in one person following exposure during a necropsy on a chimpanzee found dead in the Tai Forest. *Bundibugyo* virus, most closely related to the Ivory Coast species, emerged in Uganda in 2007, causing an outbreak with a case fatality rate of approximately 30%. *Reston* virus, discovered after an outbreak of lethal infection in macaques imported into the United States in 1989, is maintained in animal reservoirs in the Philippines. *Bombali* virus RNA has been found in African bats. Ebola virus outbreak updates can be found on the WHO website.

Risk Factors/Transmission

Outbreaks generally begin when an individual becomes infected through contact with the tissue or body fluids of an infected animal. The virus then spreads to others who come into contact with the infected individual's blood, skin, or other body fluids. Prior to the 2014 epidemic in West Africa, outbreaks occurred in remote regions with low population density and were controlled within short periods. However, this epidemic showed that movement of infected individuals facilitates the extensive and rapid spread of the virus.

Transmission occurs most commonly through direct contact of broken skin or mucous membranes with virus-containing body fluids from an infected person, the most infectious being blood, feces, and vomit. During the early phase of illness, the level of virus in the blood is typically quite low, but then increases rapidly to very high levels in advanced stages of the illness, when patients become highly infectious. In fact, corpses of persons who die from Ebola are highly infectious, and ritual washing of bodies at funerals has played a significant role in the spread of infection. The virus has also been detected in urine, semen, saliva, breast milk, tears, and sweat, and can persist in some of these fluids much longer than in blood. Ebola virus may also be transmitted through contact with contaminated surfaces where the virus can remain infectious from hours to days.

Transmission to health care workers may occur when appropriate PPE is not used, especially when caring for severely ill patients in advanced stages of illness. During the 2014 outbreak in West Africa, a large number of health care workers became infected. In Sierra Leone, the incidence of confirmed cases at the peak of the epidemic was about 100-fold higher in health care workers than in the general population. Several factors have contributed to the high rates of infections among health providers, including failure to recognize infection among patients and corpses, limited availability and training in the use of appropriate PPE, and inadequate management of contaminated waste and burial of corpses. Although there is no evidence of respiratory transmission, the virus is highly infectious when released in laboratory experiments as a small-particle aerosol, and therefore health care workers may be at risk if exposed to aerosols generated during procedures.

Human infection can occur through contact with infected wild animals during hunting, butchering, and preparing meat, with several episodes having occurred following contact with infected gorillas or chimpanzees. To prevent infection, food products should be properly cooked to inactivate the virus, and basic hygiene measures should be followed. Direct transmission of virus infection from bats to wild primates or humans has not been proven, although Ebola RNA sequences and antibodies have been detected in bats in Central Africa. Bats likely form a major reservoir.

Pathophysiology

Ebolavirus is a negative-sense, single-stranded RNA virus resembling rhabdoviruses and paramyxoviruses in its genome organization and replication mechanisms. The tubular virions contain the nucleocapsid surrounded by an outer envelope, which is derived from the host cell membrane and studded with viral glycoprotein spikes. The virions attach to host cell receptors through the spikes and are then endocytosed into vesicles. Initially, productive infection occurs primarily in dendritic cells, monocytes, and macrophages, resulting in impaired interferon production and release of proinflammatory cytokines, which have secondary effects on innate and adaptive immune responses, inflammation, and vascular integrity. Neutrophils are activated, with resultant degranulation, and lymphocytes

undergo apoptosis. The virus then spreads to regional lymph nodes, resulting in further rounds of replication, followed by dissemination to the liver, spleen, thymus, and other lymphoid tissues.

When the virus infects cells, it hijacks the cell and forces it to become a virus-producing factory, churning out new copies of the virus, which results in a loss of cellular function and eventual cell death by apoptosis. As the disease progresses, there is extensive tissue necrosis accompanied by a systemic inflammatory response induced by the release of various cytokines, chemokines, and proinflammatory mediators, as well as a severe coagulopathy triggered by the release of tissue factors. This systemic inflammatory response may contribute to gastrointestinal dysfunction, and ultimately there is a multisystem failure caused by the damage to vascular and coagulation systems.

Clinical Manifestations and Laboratory Findings

Patients with Ebola virus disease (EVD) typically have an abrupt onset of symptoms at an average of 8 to 10 days after exposure, with a range of 2 to 21 days. The first phase of the illness is characterized by high fever, chills, headaches, myalgia, and malaise. The second phase is marked by gastrointestinal symptoms, which develop by day 3 to 5, and includes watery diarrhea, nausea, vomiting, and abdominal pain. Patients may also develop chest pain, hiccups, shortness of breath, conjunctival injection, and rash. The rash is usually diffuse erythematous, maculopapular, involving the face, neck, trunk, and arms. Respiratory symptoms such as cough are rare. Common neurologic symptoms include delirium, manifested by confusion, slowed cognition, or agitation, and less frequently, seizures.

The final phase, beginning in the second week, is marked by either progression to shock and death or gradual recovery. Fatal disease is characterized by development of multisystem failure usually as a consequence of massive fluid losses that lead to shock, loss of consciousness, and renal failure. Major bleeding, typically hemorrhage from the gastrointestinal tract, is infrequent and seen in less than 5% during the terminal phase of illness. Patients who survive begin to improve during the second week of illness, with a prolonged convalescence marked by weakness, fatigue, myalgias, headache, and memory loss. About half of the survivors are plagued by chronic debilitating joint pain and a quarter experience eye problems. Other manifestations have included hearing loss, sloughing of skin, and hair loss, which may result from necrosis of dermal structures. The virus can persist in the eye for months, leading to uveitis, cataracts, and sometimes blindness. The prevalence of uveitis, unlike other causes, continues to increase until at least two years after symptom onset, with about 33% of the patients affected by that point.

During acute illness patients typically develop leukopenia, lymphopenia, thrombocytopenia, serum transaminase elevations, and proteinuria. They may develop renal insufficiency and electrolyte disturbances as a result of the gastrointestinal losses. Severe cases develop coagulation abnormalities with prolonged prothrombin and partial thromboplastin times, and elevated fibrin degradation products, consistent with disseminated intravascular coagulation.

Diagnosis

The approach to evaluating patients depends on whether or not appropriate signs and symptoms are evident, and if an exposure occurred within 21 days prior to the onset of symptoms. Infection control precautions must be used for all symptomatic patients with an identifiable risk for EVD. All symptomatic patients should be isolated in a single room with a private bathroom, and implementation of contact and droplet precautions. Only essential personnel who are well trained in the use of PPE should interact with the patient. Phlebotomy and laboratory testing should be limited to essential tests. Both the CDC and the WHO have provided detailed recommendations for approach to the evaluation of persons who may have been exposed to the virus.

Rapid diagnostic tests are the most commonly used tests for diagnosis. Viral RNA is generally detectable by RT-PCR in the blood 3 days after the onset of symptoms. Repeat testing may be necessary for patients with illness duration shorter than 3 days.

A negative RT-PCR test greater than or equal to 72 hours after the onset of symptoms rules out EVD. Details on specimen collection and handling can be found on the CDC website. For clinicians outside the United States, the WHO has issued guidance for the collection and shipment of specimens from patients with suspected disease.

Rapid immunoassays that detect virus antigen have also been developed. However, the tests are associated with both false positives and false negatives. Therefore they must be verified using RT-PCR test. The rapid immunoassays are mostly useful to make a provisional diagnosis in the appropriate clinical setting when RT-PCR is not readily available.

Differential Diagnosis

Acute onset of febrile illness in a person who lives or has recently been in West or Central Africa may be caused by a variety of local infectious diseases, which must be considered in the differential diagnosis. **Malaria** may have similar findings and might occur concurrently. Examination of blood smears and rapid antigen tests are typically used to diagnose malaria. **Typhoid** is characterized by fever and abdominal pain, and diagnosed by blood cultures.

Patients with **Lassa fever** may develop a severe clinical syndrome resembling EVD and progress to fatal shock. The illness is restricted to West Africa, where it is transmitted through exposure to the aerosolized excretions of rodents, and diagnosed by RT-PCR testing and/or serology. Clinical manifestations of **Marburg virus disease** are similar to EVD, and cases have been identified in Central Africa. The diagnosis is made by RT-PCR. Patients with **influenza** may have a similar initial presentation, but respiratory signs and symptoms are prominent.

Therapy

Good supportive care can significantly improve the chances of recovery from EVD. Mortality rates have been as low as 18% among those cared for in the US and Europe, receiving careful fluid and electrolyte management, nutritional support, and critical care. Large volumes of intravenous fluids and electrolytes are often needed to correct dehydration and electrolyte abnormalities resulting from gastrointestinal losses. Supportive care is required for complications such as shock, hypoxia, hemorrhage, and multiorgan failure. Patients may develop secondary bacterial infections, which may require concurrent management with antimicrobials. Infection prevention and control measures are critical; all bodily fluids and tissues must be considered potentially infectious. The illness is associated with high rates of pregnancy-associated hemorrhage and fetal death. The CDC and the American College of Obstetrics and Gynecology have issued recommendations for the care of pregnant women with EVD. However, there are no definitive data to recommend cesarean section versus vaginal delivery or the preferred timing for delivery. According to WHO guidelines from 2020, labor should not be induced. Additionally, procedures such as cesarean delivery, episiotomy, and vacuum extraction should only be performed for maternal indications, with the overall goal of reducing maternal morbidity and mortality.

Several monoclonal antibodies (mAbs) have been evaluated in animal studies and in clinical trials. Two products, mAb114 (ansuvimab-zykl, Ebanga) and REGN-EB3 (atoltivimab/maftivimab/odesivimab, Inmazeb) were approved for use by the FDA in 2020, and recommended for use by the WHO during the recent 2021 outbreak in the DRC. The first, mAb114, was isolated from a survivor of EVD and shown to protect 100 percent of macaques from lethal infection when administered up to five days after virus challenge. The second, REGN-EB3, contains three mAbs (atoltivimab, maftivimab, odesivimab) that target the virus surface glycoprotein, providing potent virus neutralization. In rhesus macaques, a single infusion prevented death, even when administered after the onset of illness. The antibodies showed modest reductions in overall mortality in the range 14.6%–17.8% when compared to ZMapp, a three mAb combo, that had previously shown a small reduction in mortality compared to placebo (22% versus 37%). Clinicians may contact the

CDC's Emergency Operations Center for additional information on use of experimental therapeutics for treatment of EVD.

Long-Term Follow-up

The WHO suggests close follow-up of patients after hospital discharge for the first year. A suggested schedule is first follow-up 2 weeks after discharge, then monthly for 6 months, and then every three 3 months to complete 1 year. Survivors with ocular findings require follow-up to assess for cataracts. Semen testing should be done at follow-up visits until negative for Ebola virus RNA. If semen testing is unavailable, then WHO recommends that men practice safe sex for 12 months from onset of illness.

If patients develop fever, then they should be assessed for relapse, while also being evaluated for other causes of infection. Development of uveitis and meningitis may suggest relapse. Spinal fluid analysis should be done when meningitis is suspected, even if the blood tests are negative for Ebola virus RNA.

Prevention

Two vaccines have shown promise in the prevention of EVD. The recombinant vesicular stomatitis virus-Zaire Ebola vaccine (rVSV-ZEBOV) has been found to have an efficacy of 97.5% when given as part of a ring vaccination strategy, where contacts of infected people are vaccinated, as are any subsequent contacts of those people. In November 2019, the WHO specified that the vaccine met standards for implementation in the prevention of EVD. The greatest role for the vaccine may be in disease prevention when given promptly post-exposure. The FDA approved rVSV-ZEBOV (Ervebo) in December, 2019. In the US, the vaccine is recommended for pre-exposure prophylaxis in adults at risk for occupation exposure to the *Zaire* virus species.

A second vaccine, Ad26.ZEBOV/MVA-BN-Filo (Zabdeno and Mvabea)[5], was introduced in the DRC in November 2019 in response to the ongoing Ebola epidemic. Given in two doses, Zabdeno and Mvabea 8 weeks apart, this prime-boost vaccine has been found to be safe and immunogenic. In contrast to the rVSV-ZEBOV vaccine, which is being employed in a ring vaccination strategy for health care workers in the outbreak area, the Ad26.ZEBOV/MVA-BN-Filo vaccine will be given to at-risk populations in regions where there is no active disease transmission and is expected to provide longer protection.

Recommendations for travelers to an area affected by an Ebola outbreak or those residing in such an area are as follows:
- Practice careful hand hygiene and avoid contact with an infected person's blood or body fluids, including personal items that may have come in contact with blood and body fluids.
- Avoid unprotected contact with the body of a deceased person who was infected with EVD.
- Avoid contact with bats and nonhuman primates, including blood, bodily fluids, and tissues from these animals.
- Monitor health for 21 days after return from an Ebola endemic region, and seek medical care immediately if any symptoms develop.

Health care workers at risk for exposure to Ebola must wear PPE and notify appropriate health officials at their institutions if they have unprotected contact with the blood or bodily fluids of a person infected with EVD. Finally institutions must have proper infection control and sterilization measures in place for handling of biohazardous materials. Clinicians may contact the CDC for additional information on use of experimental therapeutics and vaccines for prophylaxis following a high-risk occupational exposure to Ebola virus.

Monitoring

Local authorities may have specific regulations for management of asymptomatic individuals with Ebola virus exposure. This includes self-monitoring versus direct observation by a health official, and the need for quarantine. In general, asymptomatic

[5]Investigational drug in the United States.

persons who have had an exposure should be monitored for 21 days after the last known exposure, and should immediately report the development of fever or other clinical manifestations suggestive of EVD to the health authorities.

References

Bah EI, Lamah MC, Fletcher T, et al: Clinical presentation of patients with Ebola virus disease in Conakry, Guinea, *N Engl J Med* 372:40–47, 2015.

Chertow DS, Kleine C, Edwards JK, et al: Ebola virus disease in West Africa—clinical manifestations and management, *N Engl J Med* 371:2054–2057, 2014.

Lamontagne F, Fowler RA, Adhikari NK, et al: Evidence-based guidelines for supportive care of patients with Ebola virus disease, *Lancet* 391(10121):700, 2018.

Mulangu S, Dodd LE, Davey Jr RT, et al: A randomized, controlled trial of Ebola virus disease therapeutics, *N Engl J Med* 381:2293, 2019.

PREVAIL III Study Group, Sneller MC, Reilly C, Badio M, Bishop RJ, et al: A longitudinal study of Ebola sequelae in Liberia, *N Engl J Med* 380(10):924, 2019.

United States Centers for Disease Control and Prevention (CDC). Ebola (Ebola virus disease). Available at http://www.cdc.gov/vhf/ebola/.

WHO Ebola Response Team: Ebola virus disease in West Africa—the first 9 months of the epidemic and forward projections, *N Engl J Med* 371:1481–1495, 2014.

World Health Organization (WHO). Ebola. Available at https://www.who.int/health-topics/ebola/.

FOODBORNE ILLNESSES

Method of

Anita Devi K. Ravindran, MD; and Viswanathan K. Neelakantan, MD

CURRENT DIAGNOSIS

- Infective foodborne illnesses are innumerable and are caused by various microorganisms. Some microorganisms are established agents, several others are emerging pathogens, and the pathogenicity of the remainder is still under speculation.
- Classification of these illnesses is best done according to their incubation periods, the symptoms they produce, or both.
- Nausea and vomiting predominate in illnesses with short incubation periods caused by preformed toxins, whereas diarrhea predominates in those with long incubation periods caused by toxins produced in the intestine.
- Undercooked charcuterie, meat, poultry, and seafood account for a majority of foodborne illness, but dairy products, salads, pastries, fruits, and vegetables can also cause illness.
- Contaminated water acts as a vehicle in almost all instances.

CURRENT THERAPY

- The majority of infective foodborne illnesses with symptoms confined to the gastrointestinal tract, although apparently alarming, are self-limiting and need only supportive measures including replacement of water and electrolytes.
- Antimicrobial agents are indicated only in certain patients, including those with systemic illnesses, extremes of age, immunocompromised and malnourished states, and severe life-threatening illness.
- Antitoxin is useful in botulism poisoning.
- Vaccines are available against *Vibrio cholerae*, *Salmonella typhi*, hepatitis A virus, and rotavirus, but their effectiveness and cost-effectiveness are debatable.

The Centers for Disease Control and Prevention (CDC) estimates that each year roughly one in six Americans (about 48 million people) gets sick from foodborne illnesses; 128,000 are hospitalized, and 3000 die. These figures are higher in developing nations, and many cases are not brought to light because they occur in remote villages. The 2011 estimates provide the most accurate picture of infective foodborne illnesses, of which bacteria, viruses, and parasites account for the majority. Processing of ready-to-eat foods increases the risk of acquiring foodborne illness because of increased food handling, leading to introduction and growth of pathogens. Increased international travel and migration have also resulted in a greater risk because travelers are at high risk for developing foodborne gastroenteritis caused by pathogens to which they have not been exposed at home.

Classification of Foodborne Illnesses

Agents causing foodborne diseases may be classified in several ways. The most common scheme is a taxonomic combined with a classification based on mode of action (Tables 1 to 3).

Bacteria

Aeromonas Species

Species of *Aeromonas* are ubiquitous and autochthonous in aquatic environments, more so after the tsunami that followed the Indonesian earthquake in December 2004. These aeromonads share many biochemical characteristics with members of the Enterobacteriaceae. The mesophilic species *Aeromonas caviae*, *Aeromonas hydrophila*, and *Aeromonas veronii* are principally associated with gastroenteritis; *A. caviae* particularly infects children younger than 3 years.

Transmission is documented as occurring from a contaminated piped water source, as seen in community-based outbreaks, especially among children. The probability of occurrence of *Aeromonas* infection increased significantly when the mean seasonal temperature exceeded 14°C (57°F), and this was exacerbated where the mean free chlorine concentration fell below 0.1 mg/L.

Aeromonas species are potential food-poisoning agents. *A. hydrophila* is psychrotrophic and has been associated with spoilage of refrigerated animal products including chicken, beef, pork, lamb, fish, oysters, crab, and milk.

The incubation period for *Aeromonas*-associated traveler's diarrhea is 1 to 2 days. It usually causes a sporadic illness. Usually a mild to moderate but self-limiting diarrhea occurs, but it can be severe enough in children to require hospitalization. *Aeromonas* gastroenteritis can occur as a nondescript enteritis, as a more-severe form accompanied by bloody stools, as the etiologic agent of a subacute or chronic intestinal syndrome, as an extremely rare cause of cholera-like disease, or in association with episodic traveler's diarrhea. By far the most common presentation of *Aeromonas* gastroenteritis is watery enteritis. The most serious complication resulting from *Aeromonas* gastroenteritis is hemolytic uremic syndrome.

Pathogenesis

Mesophilic *Aeromonas* spp. can express a range of virulence factors, including attachment mechanisms and production of a number of toxins. Toxins include aerolysin (a pore-forming cytolysin that attaches to cell membrane, leading to leakage of cytoplasmic contents) and a cytotonic enterotoxin with activity similar to that of cholera toxin. Strains of *A. hydrophila* produce lectins and adhesins, which enable adherence to epithelial surfaces and gut mucosa.

Laboratory Diagnosis

Samples are best transported using Cary-Blair medium. *Aeromonas* forms a bull's-eye–like colony on the selective medium cefsulodin irgasan novobiocin (CIN) agar owing to fermentation of D-mannitol. Ampicillin blood agar has an advantage over CIN agar in that hemolytic colonies can readily be tested for oxidase. *Aeromonas* species produce hemolysis on sheep blood agar.

Treatment

In *Aeromonas* infections, ciprofloxacin (Cipro)[1] 500 mg PO or 400 mg IV twice daily is the antimicrobial treatment of choice. Piperacillin-tazobactam (Zosyn)[1] 4.5 g IV three times daily or

---

[1]Not FDA approved for this indication.

TABLE 1	Classification of Foodborne Illnesses	
SIGNS AND SYMPTOMS OR MECHANISM	**PATHOGENS**
Based on Symptoms and Duration of Onset	
Nausea and vomiting within 6 h	*Staphylococcus aureus, Bacillus cereus*
Abdominal cramps and diarrhea within 8–16 h	*Clostridium perfringens, Bacillus cereus*
Fever, abdominal cramps, and diarrhea within 16–48 h	*Salmonella, Shigella, Vibrio parahemolyticus,* enteroinvasive *Escherichia coli, Campylobacter jejuni*
Abdominal cramps and watery diarrhea within 16–72 h	Enterotoxigenic *E. coli, Vibrio cholerae* O1, O139 Bengal, *Vibrio parahemolyticus,* NAG (nonagglutinable) vibrios, *Norovirus*
Fever and abdominal cramps within 16–48 h	*Yersinia enterocolitica*
Bloody diarrhea without fever within 72–120 h	Enterohemorrhagic *E. coli* O157:H7
Nausea, vomiting, diarrhea, and paralysis within 18–36 h	*Clostridium botulinum*
Based on Pathogenesis	
Food intoxications resulting from the ingestion of preformed bacterial toxins	*Staphylococcus aureus, Bacillus cereus, Clostridium botulinum, Clostridium perfringens*
Food intoxications caused by noninvasive bacteria that secrete toxins while adhering to the intestinal wall	Enterotoxigenic *E. coli, Vibrio cholerae, Campylobacter jejuni*
Food intoxications that follow an intracellular invasion of intestinal epithelial cells	*Shigella, Salmonella*
Diseases caused by bacteria that enter the bloodstream via the intestinal tract	*Salmonella typhi, Listeria monocytogenes*
Based on Toxin Production	
The organisms responsible produce two major types of toxins, or they may be invasive, with no toxin production.	
Secretory toxins are enterotoxins produced by microbes that colonize the intestines in large numbers by attaching to the mucosal epithelial cells without invasion of mucosa, and, hence, there is no fever or other systemic symptoms as a result of lack of inflammatory response. Massive quantities of fluid and electrolytes are lost into the large bowel as its reabsorbing capacity is exceeded by the hypersecretion of isotonic fluid produced by the enterotoxins.	*Vibrio cholerae,* enterotoxigenic *E. coli, Shigella dysenteriae, Salmonella typhimurium*
Cytotoxins are those that destroy the epithelial cells of the mucosa.	*Shigella dysenteriae* elaborating Shiga toxin, causing destructive colitis, enterohemorrhagic *E. coli,* producing a similar toxin causing hemorrhagic colitis and hemolytic uremic syndrome (HUS), and *Vibrio parahemolyticus*) *Clostridium perfringens,* which produces a secretory enterotoxin, also has a cytotoxic action.
Secretory toxins, cytotoxins, and/or neurotoxins that are preformed are ingested directly in food.	*Bacillus cereus, Staphylococcus aureus, Clostridium botulinum*
Certain invasive microbes produce systemic symptoms such as fever, headache, and myalgia, in addition to gastrointestinal symptoms.	Salmonellosis typhoid fever, shigellosis, and brucellosis

ceftazidime (Fortaz)[1] 2 g IV daily may be added in severe infections. The organism is also susceptible to aminoglycosides and carbapenems. Resistance is now becoming a problem because *Aeromonas* can produce β-lactamases and carbapenemases. Therefore it is preferable to initiate therapy with a fluoroquinolone when the organism is isolated.

Bacillus cereus

Bacillus cereus is found abundantly in the environment and vegetation. It is known to produce two forms of food poisoning, emetic and diarrheal. The emetic (short-incubation) type of illness is associated with contaminated fried rice that is not refrigerated. The organism is present in uncooked rice, and the spores survive boiling. The illness is usually self-limiting, with recovery in a day. It is mediated by a heat-stable, preformed enterotoxin resembling that of *Staphylococcus aureus*. The first major outbreak of *Bacillus cereus* food poisoning was in 1971 in England. The diarrheal (long-incubation) type of illness is produced by a heat-labile diarrheal enterotoxin formed in the intestine, which activates adenylate cyclase, causing intestinal fluid secretion, similar to *Escherichia coli* LT toxin and the toxin of *Clostridium perfringens.*

Pathogenesis

During the slow cooling of cooked rice, spores germinate and vegetative bacteria multiply; then they sporulate again. Sporulation is also associated with toxin production. The toxin is heat stable and can easily withstand the temperatures used to cook fried rice.

Laboratory Diagnosis

The disease is diagnosed by the isolation of *B. cereus* from the incriminated food (emetic type) or from stool and food (diarrheal type). Isolation from stools alone is not sufficient because gastrointestinal colonization with *B. cereus* occurs in many persons.

Treatment

B. cereus food poisoning may be symptomatically managed with replacement of fluids and electrolytes. Antimicrobials have no

---

[1]Not FDA approved for this indication.

TABLE 2   Common Organisms Implicated in Infective Foodborne Illness

ETIOLOGIC AGENT	USUAL INCUBA-TION PERIOD	SYMPTOMS	DURATION OF SYMPTOMS	COMMON VEHICLES
Upper Gastrointestinal Tract Symptoms (Nausea, Vomiting) Occur First or Predominate				
Staphylococcus aureus (preformed toxin)	1–6 h	Sudden onset of severe nausea and vomiting Abdominal cramps, diarrhea, and fever may be present	24–48 h	Unrefrigerated or improperly refrigerated meat, potato and egg salads, cream pastries
Bacillus cereus (preformed toxin)	1–6 h	Sudden onset of severe nausea and vomiting Diarrhea may be present	24 h	Improperly refrigerated cooked or fried rice, meat
Lower Gastrointestinal Tract Symptoms (Abdominal Cramps, Diarrhea) Occur First or Predominate				
Bacillus cereus (diarrheal toxin)	10–16 h	Abdominal cramps, watery diarrhea, nausea	24–48 h	Meat, stew, gravy, vanilla sauce
Clostridium perfringens (toxin)	8–16 h	Watery diarrhea, nausea, abdominal cramps; fever is rare	24–48 h	Meat, poultry, gravy, dried or precooked foods, time- and/or temperature-abused food
Vibrio cholerae	2 h to 5 d	Rice-water purging diarrhea leading to dehydration, shock, acidosis, renal failure, abdominal pain Cholera sicca is a severe form; patient dies before diarrhea is manifest; ileus and abdominal bloating result	2–7 d	Sewage-contaminated water Seafood: fish, shellfish, crabs, oysters, clams Contaminated rice, millet gruel, vegetables
Vibrio parahaemolyticus	12–24 h	Watery diarrhea, abdominal cramps, nausea, vomiting Neurologic symptoms can occur, as with *Clostridium botulinum* and *Trichinella spiralis*	2–5 d	Raw or undercooked seafood
Shigella	1–4 d	Abdominal cramps, fever, diarrhea Stool might contain blood and mucus	4–7 d	Food or water contaminated with fecal matter Ready-to-eat food touched by infected food worker
Salmonella (not *typhi*)	1–3 d	Diarrhea, fever, abdominal cramps, vomiting	4–7 d	Contaminated eggs, unpasteurized milk or juice, cheese, contaminated raw fruits and vegetables
Enterotoxigenic *Escherichia coli*	1–3 d	Watery diarrhea, abdominal cramps, some vomiting	3–7 d (or longer)	Food or water contaminated with human feces
Shiga toxin–producing *E. coli*, including *E. coli* O157:H7	2–6 d	Severe diarrhea that is often bloody; abdominal pain and vomiting Usually little or no fever	5–10 d	Undercooked beef, especially hamburger, unpasteurized milk and juice, raw fruit and vegetables (e.g., sprouts), salami (rarely), contaminated water
Campylobacter jejuni	2–5 d	Diarrhea, cramps, fever, vomiting Diarrhea may be bloody	2–10 d	Raw and undercooked poultry, unpasteurized milk, contaminated milk
Vibrio vulnificus	1–7 d	Vomiting, diarrhea, abdominal pain Fever, bleeding within the skin, ulcers requiring surgical removal Can be fatal to people with liver disease or weakened immune systems	2–8 d	Undercooked or raw seafood, especially oysters
Yersinia enterocolitica	3–7 d	Appendicitis-like symptoms: diarrhea, vomiting, fever, abdominal pain	Can remit and relapse over weeks to 1 mo	Drinking water, food contaminated with human fecal matter
Cyclospora	7–10 d	Diarrhea (usually watery), loss of appetite, weight loss, stomach cramps, nausea, vomiting, fatigue	Can remit and relapse over weeks to 1 mo	Fresh herbs and produce (e.g., raspberries, basil, lettuce)
Giardia lamblia (beaver fever)	7–10 d	Diarrhea (acute or chronic), stomach cramps, flatulence, weight loss, malabsorption, developmental delay	Days to weeks	Drinking water, food contaminated with human fecal matter

TABLE 2 | Common Organisms Implicated in Infective Foodborne Illness—cont'd

ETIOLOGIC AGENT	USUAL INCUBA-TION PERIOD	SYMPTOMS	DURATION OF SYMPTOMS	COMMON VEHICLES
Entamoeba histolytica	1–4 wk	Intestinal: diarrhea, fever, abdominal pain, dysentery, colitis, bowel perforation, ameboma Extraintestinal amebiasis: liver abscess with anchovy-sauce pus, spread to viscera, lungs, and brain	Days to weeks	Drinking water Food contaminated with human fecal matter

Both Upper and Lower Gastrointestinal Tract Symptoms

Rotavirus	18–36 h	Acute onset of fever and vomiting followed 12–24 h later by frequent watery stools	3–7 d	Contaminated drinking water, food, fomites
Norovirus and other caliciviruses	12–48 h	Nausea, vomiting, cramping, diarrhea, fever, myalgia, some headache Diarrhea is more prevalent in adults; vomiting is more prevalent in children	12–60 h	Food (including shellfish) or water contaminated with human fecal matter Ready-to-eat food touched by an infected food worker

Generalized Symptoms

Listeria monocytogenes	9–48 h or GI symptoms; 2–6 wk for invasive disease	Fever, muscle aches, nausea or diarrhea Pregnant women can have mild flulike illness, and infection can lead to premature delivery or stillbirth Elderly and immunocompromised patients can have bacteremia or meningitis	Variable	Fresh soft cheese, unpasteurized milk, ready-to-eat deli meat, hot dogs
Balatidium coli	4–5 d	Mostly asymptomatic Chronic diarrhea, occasional dysentery, nausea, foul breath, colitis, abdominal pain, weight loss, deep intestinal ulcerations, possible perforation of the intestine, pneumonia-like illness	Variable	Water contaminated with pig feces
Salmonella typhi	8–14 d	Fever, anorexia, lethargy, malaise, headache, rose spots, constipation or diarrhea, hepatosplenomegaly	4–6 wk	Contaminated water; contaminated food, mainly via food handlers; shellfish from polluted water
Ascoris lumbricoides	4–16 d	Nausea, abdominal pain, intestinal obstruction, malnutrition, Loeffler's syndrome (cough, pneumonitis, eosinophilia), biliary colic, colangitis, pancreatitis, appendicitis	Variable (chronic)	Soil-contaminated raw food, food handlers, water
Trichinella spiralis	1–2 wk	Asymptomatic or chronic diarrhea, abdominal pain Allergy leading to rash, periorbital edema, vasculitis, intramural thrombi Weakness of jaw, biceps, diaphragm, intercostals Eosinophilia, subconjunctival, splinter hemorrhages Muscle penetration: myalgia, orbital pain, diplopia Chronic phase: neurologic symptoms	Variable Acute phase: 1–3 wk	Raw or undercooked meat of pig, horse, wild boar, bush pig, warthog, bear
Infective cysticerci of *Taenia solium* (pork tape worm)	2 months on average	Seizures, vasculitis, focal neurologic deficits, intracranial hypertension, hydrocephalus, mental changes, encephalitis and Brun's syndrome (intermittent obstruction of cerebral aqueduct), myosists, vasculitis	Highly variable	Undercooked charcuterie (pork), contaminated raw vegetables, salads, water
Hepatitis A	15–50 d	Diarrhea, dark urine, jaundice, flulike symptoms, fever, headache, nausea, aversion to food, vomiting, abdominal pain; distaste for cigarettes	Variable: 2 wk to 3 mo	Food (including shellfish) or water contaminated with human fecal matter Inadequately cooked clams, oysters, mussels, cockles Contaminated lettuce, slush beverages, frozen strawberries and salad items Ready-to-eat foods touched by an infected food worker

Continued

Foodborne Illnesses

601

TABLE 2 Common Organisms Implicated in Infective Foodborne Illness—cont'd

ETIOLOGIC AGENT	USUAL INCUBATION PERIOD	SYMPTOMS	DURATION OF SYMPTOMS	COMMON VEHICLES
Brucella species	1–8 wk	Flulike illness; undulating fever, malaise, arthralgia, anorexia, hepatosplenomegaly, pleurisy, nausea, vomiting, diarrhea, new onset of increased desire to sleep after lunch	Variable	Unpasteurized dairy products, undercooked meat, bone marrow Contact with laboratory cultures and tissue samples Accidental injection of live brucellosis vaccine
Hepatitis E	3–8 wk	Prodrome: anorexia, nausea, vomiting, arthralgia, myalgia, weight loss, dehydration, abdominal pain Icteric phase: jaundice, pruritus, light-colored stool Urticaria, diarrhea, malaise	Variable (several weeks)	Fecally contaminated drinking water and food Raw and undercooked shellfish incriminated in sporadic outbreaks Possibly zoonotic spread
Microsporidium: *Encephalitozoon,* *Pleistophora,* *Nosema,* *Vittaforma,* *Trachipleistophora,* *Brachiola,* *Microsporidium,* *Enterocytozoon*	Unknown	Watery or bloody or unspecified diarrhea, abdominal discomfort, cramps, flatulence, weight loss, loss of appetite, wasting syndrome, subfebrile temperatures Extraintestinal: pneumonitis, myositis, keratoconjunctivitis, seizures, nephritis, cholangiopathy	Variable; self-limiting (1–2 wk) in immunocompetent patients	Contaminated water, food, or inhalation

Abbreviation: GI=gastrointestinal.

TABLE 3 Rare and Emerging Infections

ETIOLOGIC AGENT	USUAL INCUBATION PERIOD	SYMPTOMS	DURATION OF SYMPTOMS	COMMON VEHICLES
Bacillus subtilis	10 min to 14 h (average, 2.5 h)	Vomiting, diarrhea, abdominal cramps, nausea, headache, flushing, sweating	1.5–8 h	Sausage rolls, meat pasties, turkey stuffing, chicken stuffing, pizza, whole-grain bread, steak pie, pork sandwiches
Cyanobacteria: *Microcystic aeuroginosa,* *Anabaena circinalis,* *Anabaena flosaquae,* *Aphanizomenon flosaquae,* *Cylindrospermopsis racibarskii*	3–6 h	Diarrhea, vomiting, allergic reactions, breathing difficulty, dizziness, tingling and numbness, liver and kidney toxicity	8–16 h	Drinking water from untreated surface sources, inhaling aerosols from jet-skis and boats, consuming dietary supplements contaminated by microcystin
Anisakis	Few hours to days	Gastric: abdominal pain, nausea, vomiting Allergic: urticaria, anaphylaxis Intestinal: ileus, perforation, peritonitis, stenosis	2 wk	Raw, lightly pickled, or salted marine fish: Mackerel, squid, horse mackerel, salmon, bonito Squid, cuttlefish Sushi, sashimi
Astrovirus	1–4 d	Watery diarrhea (especially in children), vomiting, fever, anorexia, abdominal pain	3–4 d	Sewage-polluted water and food
Pleisomonas shigelloides	5 d	Diarrhea with blood and mucus, abdominal pain, headache, nausea, chills, fever, vomiting	1–7 d	Contaminated water used for drinking or rinsing foods to be eaten raw Contaminated raw shellfish, salted fish, crabs, oysters
Cyclospora	7 d	Frequent watery diarrhea, weight loss, abdominal pain, bloating, flatulence, vomiting, nausea, low-grade fever, fatigue, malabsorption, cholecystitis	1–4 wk Relapse is common	Fecally contaminated fresh raspberries, snow peas, mesclun

TABLE 3 Rare and Emerging Infections—cont'd

ETIOLOGIC AGENT	USUAL INCUBATION PERIOD	SYMPTOMS	DURATION OF SYMPTOMS	COMMON VEHICLES
Iosospora belli	8–11 d	Diarrhea, steatorrhea, headache, fever, malaise, abdominal pain, vomiting, dehydration, weight loss Mesenteric lymph node, liver, spleen involvement	Variable; runs a chronic course in immunocompromised patients	Contaminated food and water
Edwardisella tarda	Not defined	Nausea, vomiting, diarrhea, dysentery, colitis, wound infections, septicemia	Variable: 1–2 wk or longer	Fecal contamination of food, water, raw fish
Citrobacter species	Not defined	Diarrhea, hemolytic uremic syndrome, thrombocytopenic purpura		Meat and milk Parsley (in green butter) from organic gardens using pig manure
Arizona	Not defined	Diarrhea		Cream pie, chocolate eclairs, custard, eggs, chicken, turkey
Achromobacter xylosoxidans	Not defined	Abdominal pain, diarrhea, headache, vomiting		Raw milk, spoiled canned food, contaminated well water

role in treatment. *B. cereus* is also known to produce a variety of ocular and systemic infections such as meningitis, osteomyelitis, pneumonia, and endocarditis. These are usually not foodborne, and it is in this situation that vancomycin (Vancocin)[1] becomes the drug of choice, with clindamycin (Cleocin)[1] and carbapenems being the alternative drugs, both being used along with aminoglycosides for synergistic action.

Campylobacter jejuni

Campylobacter jejuni are harbored in the reproductive and alimentary tracts of some animals. Other than gastrointestinal symptoms, the patient has malaise and headache. The organism may be shed in the patient's stool for up to 2 months. Bacteremia is observed in a small minority of cases. The disease is usually self-limiting. Guillain-Barré syndrome and Reiter's syndrome are recognized sequelae.

Pathogenesis
As few as 500 organisms can cause enteritis. The organism is invasive but generally less so than *Shigella*. *Campylobacter* produces adenylate cyclase–activating toxins resembling *E. coli* LT and cholera toxin.

Laboratory Diagnosis
The feces may be inoculated in enrichment medium or on selective media such as Campy-BAP or Skirrow's medium.

Treatment
Indications for antibiotic therapy in *C. jejuni* infections are prolonged fever, severe diarrhea, dysentery, and persistent symptoms for more than a week. Therapy of *Campylobacter* infection with ciprofloxacin (Cipro 500 mg orally twice daily for 7 days) early in the course of the illness shortens its duration. Unfortunately, this has led to the emergence of fluoroquinolone-resistant *Campylobacter* infections. Erythromycin eradicates carriage of susceptible *C. jejuni* and might shorten the duration of illness if given early in the disease. Erythromycin (Ery-Tab)[1] 250 mg PO four times daily is the drug of choice in *Campylobacter* enteritis. Azithromycin (Zithromax)[1] is also useful and has the advantage of shorter duration of therapy.

Gentamicin (Garamycin), carbapenems, amoxicillin-clavulanate (Augmentin),[1] and chloramphenicol[1] are useful in systemic infections. The usual duration of treatment is 2 weeks. The therapy is prolonged in immunocompromised persons and in patients with endovascular infections.

[1]Not FDA approved for this indication.

Clostridium botulinum

Clostridum botulinum is widely distributed in soil, in sediments of lakes and ponds, and in decaying vegetation. *C. botulinum* elaborates the most potent toxin known in humans. When the toxin is ingested, paralysis occurs, often requiring prolonged artificial ventilation. Common signs and symptoms include vomiting, thirst, dry mouth, constipation, ocular palsies, dysphagia, dysarthria, bulbar paralysis, and death due to respiratory paralysis. Coma or delirium occurs in some. Infants present with lethargy, poor feeding, loss of head control, and sometimes sudden infant death syndrome (SIDS).

The incriminated foods are corn syrup, home-canned or bottled meat, fruits, fish, vegetables, herb-infused oils, and cheese sauce. Infant botulism is associated with consumption of honey; honey should not be given to infants younger than 1 year.

Pathogenesis
Not all strains of *C. botulinum* produce botulinum toxin. Toxigenic types of the organism, designated A, B, C1, D, E, F, and G, produce immunologically distinct forms of botulinum toxin. Lysogenic phages encode toxin C and D serotypes.

Foodborne botulism is not an infection but an intoxication because it results from the ingestion of foods that contain the preformed clostridial toxin. If contaminated food has been insufficiently heated or canned improperly, the spores can germinate and produce botulinum toxin. The toxin is released only after cell lysis and death. The toxin resists digestion and is absorbed by the upper gastrointestinal tract and enters the blood. The toxin blocks release of acetylcholine by binding to receptors at synapses and neuromuscular junctions and causes flaccid paralysis.

Laboratory Diagnosis
Spoilage of food or swelling of cans or presence of bubbles inside the can indicate growth of *C. botulinum*. Food is homogenized in broth and inoculated in Robertson cooked meat medium and blood agar or egg-yolk agar, which is incubated anaerobically for 3 to 5 days at 37°C. The toxin can be demonstrated by injecting the extract of food or culture into mice or guinea pigs intraperitoneally.

Treatment
Hospitalization in an intensive care unit with immediate administration of botulinum antitoxin is vital in the management of botulism. The antitoxin neutralizes only toxin molecules unbound to nerve endings and does not reverse the paralysis. It should be given within 24 hours after the diagnosis is made. Penicillin is the

antimicrobial of choice. Intubation and mechanical ventilation are needed for respiratory failure. If swallowing difficulty persists, intravenous fluids or alimentation should be given through a nasogastric tube.

Clostridium perfringens

C. perfringens is heat resistant and elaborates two toxins that can induce specific pathology in the human intestinal tract. It is the third leading cause of foodborne illnesses in United States, after norovirus and *B. cereus*. It is present abundantly in the environment, vegetation, sewage, and animal feces.

Human diseases caused by this organism are the more common *C. perfringens* type A food poisoning and the less common, but more serious, *C. perfringens* type C food poisoning producing necrotic enteritis. Necrotic enteritis is characterized by vomiting, severe abdominal pain, and bloody diarrhea. The incubation period is 2 to 5 days. Progression to necrosis of the jejunum and death occur.

Pathogenesis

Spores in food can survive cooking and then germinate when the food is improperly stored. When these vegetative cells form endospores in the intestine, they release enterotoxins. Food poisoning is mainly caused by type A strains, which produce alpha and theta toxins. The toxins result in excessive fluid accumulation in the intestinal lumen.

Laboratory Diagnosis

Because the bacterium is present normally in intestines, isolation from feces might not be sufficient to implicate it as the cause of the illness. Similarly, isolation from food, except in large numbers ($>10^9$/g), might not be significant. The homogenized food is diluted and plated on selective medium, as well as Robertson cooked meat medium, and subjected to anaerobic incubation. The isolated bacteria must be shown to produce enterotoxin.

Treatment

Food poisoning due to *Clostridium perfringens* is managed conservatively with hydration and replacement of electrolytes. *C. perfringens* is susceptible to benzylpenicillin (penicillin G), which may be useful in managing severe infections (1 mU IV every 4 hours). Vancomycin,[1] clindamycin,[1] cefoxitin (Mefoxin), and metronidazole (Flagyl) are alternatives. *C. perfringens* type C toxoid vaccine[2] (two doses, 4 months apart) is preventive in pigbel.

Cronobacter sakazakii

Cronobacter sakazakii causes neonatal meningitis or necrotizing enterocolitis and bacteremia, which results in an alarming mortality rate. Surviving patients sometimes develop ventriculitis and cerebral abscess. *C. sakazakii* has been isolated from infant formulas.

Enterobacter species are generally resistant to the cephalosporins, except cefepime (Maxipime),[1] but are responsive to carbenicillin (Geocillin),[1] piperacillin (Pipracil),[1] ticarcillin (Ticar),[1] amikacin (Amikin),[1] and tigecycline (Tygacil).[1]

Enterohemorrhagic Escherichia coli

Many serogroups of *E. coli*, including O4, O26, O45, O91, O111, O145, and O157, are pathogenic, but the most common pathogenic serotype is O157:H7. Cattle are the main sources of infection; most cases are associated with the consumption of undercooked beef burgers and similar foods from restaurants and delicatessens. The latest outbreak of *E. coli* O157:H7 during the fall of 2019 and 2020 was linked to leafy greens (romaine salad greens). Several outbreaks of *E. coli* O157:H7 illnesses were identified as being caused by the REPEXH01 strain, which is classified as a "persistent" strain causing illness over many years.

Pathogenesis

Enterohemorrhagic *E. coli* (EHEC) strains can produce one or more types of cytotoxins, which are collectively referred to as Shiga-like toxins because they are antigenically and functionally similar to Shiga toxin produced by *Shigella dysenteriae*. (Shiga-like toxins were previously known as verotoxins.) The toxins provoke cell secretion and kill colonic epithelial cells, causing hemorrhagic colitis and hemolytic-uremic syndrome (HUS), leading occasionally to disseminated intravascular coagulation (DIC). A fibrin layer forms in the glomerular capillary bed, and acute renal failure occurs due to DIC. These are most likely to occur in children, elderly patients, and pregnant women. The young recover fully, but at times dialysis is warranted.

Laboratory Diagnosis

Laboratory diagnosis is performed by culturing the feces on McConkey's agar or sorbitol McConkey's agar. Strains can then be identified by serotyping using specific antisera. Shiga-like toxins can be detected by enzyme-linked immunosorbent assay (ELISA), and genes coding for them can be detected by DNA hybridization techniques.

Treatment

Hydration with electrolyte replacement is the mainstay of treatment in *E. coli* O157:H7 infection, and patients should be monitored closely and constantly for the development of HUS, which requires management in an intensive care setting with blood transfusion and dialysis. Although dysentery is self-limiting, the use of rifaximin (Xifaxan), a nonabsorbable agent, is recommended in those who are increasingly susceptible to infections. In the absence of dysentery, early institution of drugs like ciprofloxacin (Cipro) or azithromycin (Zithromax),[1] especially in traveler's diarrhea, decreases the duration of illness.

Enterotoxigenic Escherichia Coli

Enterotoxigenic *E. coli* (ETEC) is now ubiquitous in nature. Wild animals and cattle act as reservoirs of the organism. *E. coli* is carried normally in the intestine of humans and animals. Some specific serotypes harbor plasmids that code for toxin production. This bacterium is responsible for a majority of traveler's diarrhea. The disease is self-limiting and resolves in a few days.

Pathogenesis

The bacteria colonize the gastrointestinal tract by means of fimbriae, attaching to specific receptors on enterocytes of the proximal small intestine. Enterotoxins produced by ETEC include the LT (heat-labile) toxin and the ST (heat-stable) toxins. LTs are similar to cholera toxin in structure and mode of action, consisting of A and B subunits. The B (binding) subunit of LTs binds to specific ganglioside receptors (GM1) on the epithelial cells of the small intestine and facilitates the entry of the A (activating) subunit, which activates adenylate cyclase. Stimulation of adenylate cyclase causes an increased production of cyclic adenosine monophosphate (cAMP), which leads to hypersecretion of water and electrolytes into the lumen and inhibition of sodium reabsorption.

Laboratory Diagnosis

The sample of feces is cultured on McConkey's agar. The ETEC stains are indistinguishable from the resident *E. coli* by biochemical tests. These strains are differentiated from nontoxigenic *E. coli* present in the bowel by a variety of in vitro immunochemical, tissue culture, or DNA hybridization tests designed to detect either the toxins or the genes that encode for these toxins. With the availability of a gene probe method, foods can be analyzed directly for the presence of ETEC in about 3 days. LTs can be detected by ligated rabbit ileal loop test and by observing morphologic changes in Chinese hamster ovary cells and Y1 adrenal cells. ELISA, immunodiffusion, and coagglutination are also used in diagnosis.

---

[1]Not FDA approved for this indication.
[2]Not available in the United States.

---

[1]Not FDA approved for this indication.

Listeria monocytogenes

Listeria monocytogenes is quite hardy and resists the deleterious effects of freezing, drying, and heat remarkably well for a bacterium that does not form spores. It is capable of growing at 3°C and multiplies in refrigerated foods. The latest implicated food in a February 2021 outbreak is queso fresco cheese.

Pathogenesis

L. monocytogenes invades the gastrointestinal epithelium. Once the bacterium enters the host's monocytes, macrophages, or neutrophils, it is bloodborne and can grow. Its presence in phagocytes also permits access to the brain and transplacental migration to the fetus in pregnant women. Granulomatosis infantisepticum is a feature of listeriosis. The pathogenesis of *L. monocytogenes* centers on its ability to survive and multiply in phagocytic host cells.

Laboratory Diagnosis

The diagnosis of listeriosis is most commonly made by isolation of *L. monocytogenes* from a normally sterile site. β-Hemolytic colonies, which test negative for catalase, hydrolyze hippurate, and have a positive cAMP reaction, form on blood agar. Serologic testing is not useful in diagnosing acute invasive disease, but it can be useful in detecting asymptomatic disease and gastroenteritis in an outbreak or in other epidemiologic investigations. Stool testing is not commercially available.

Treatment

Ampicillin[1] (2 g IV every 4 hours) is the drug of choice in *Listeria monocytogenes* infections. Aminoglycosides are added for synergistic effect. Trimethoprim-sulfamethoxazole (TMP-SMX)[1] (Bactrim, 20 mg of trimethoprim/day IV every 6 hours) is an alternative for patients allergic to penicillin. Ampicillin and TMP-SMX may be used in combination. Vancomycin (Vancocin),[1] linezolid (Zyvox),[1] carbapenems, macrolides, and tetracyclines are also effective. Cephalosporins are ineffective in the treatment of listeriosis and should not be used. The duration of therapy is highly variable depending on the clinical situation and is 14 days for bacteremia, 21 days for meningitis, 42 days for endocarditis, and 56 days for neurologic infections. Patients whose disease is promptly diagnosed and treated recover fully, but permanent neurologic sequelae are common in patients with cerebral illnesses. Consuming only pasteurized dairy products and fully cooked meats, meticulously cleaning utensils, and thoroughly washing fresh vegetables before cooking will prevent foodborne listerial infections. Pregnant women and others at risk should avoid soft cheeses and thoroughly reheated ready-to-serve and charcuterie foods.

Nontyphoidal Salmonellosis

Nontyphoidal salmonellosis consists of several causative organisms classified under the family Enterobacteriaceae; one such organism is *Salmonella enteritidis*. It does not occur normally in humans, but several animals act as reservoirs.

The diarrhea may be watery, with greenish, foul-smelling stools. This may be preceded by headache and chills. Other findings include prostration, muscle weakness, and moderate fever. In August 2020, a multi-state outbreak of *Salmonella enteritidis* was linked to peaches packed or supplied by Prima Wawona packing company. An outbreak of *Salmonella stanley* infection was linked to wood ear mushrooms (dried mushrooms, also called kikurage/dried black fungus) imported to to the U.S. Yet another non-typhoidal Salmonella infection reported in July 2020 was caused by *Salmonella newport*. The likely source was identified as potentially contaminated red onions. A food-borne illness recently reported from Mexico was caused by *Salmonella poona* and linked to consumption of cucumbers. Newly reported include *Salmonella reading* and *Salmonella abony linked* to consumption of alfalfa sprouts.

---

[1]Not FDA approved for this indication.

Pathogenesis

The organism penetrates and passes through the epithelial cells lining the terminal ileum. Multiplication of bacteria in lamina propria produces inflammatory mediators, recruits neutrophils, and triggers inflammation. Release of lipopolysaccharides and prostaglandins causes fever and also loss of water and electrolytes into the lumen of the intestine, resulting in diarrhea.

Laboratory Diagnosis

Culture in selenite F broth and then subculture on deoxycholate citrate agar isolates the organisms. Plates are incubated at 37°C overnight, and growth is identified by biochemical and slide agglutination tests.

Treatment

The antibiotics recommended for gastroenteritis due to nontyphoidal salmonellosis are ciprofloxacin (Cipro)[1] 500 mg PO twice daily, and ceftriaxone (Rocephin) 2 g IV daily, for 3 to 7 days. Amoxicillin (Amoxil)[1] and TMP-SMX[1] are also effective. Therapy is prolonged in bacteremia, endocarditis, or meningitis.

Shigella Species

Shigella species belong to the family Enterobacteriaceae. Bacillary dysentery is caused by *Shigella flexneri*, *Shigella boydii*, *Shigella dysenteriae*, and *Shigella sonnei*. *S. flexneri* is most common in developing countries where hygiene is poor and clean drinking water is unavailable; *S. sonnei* is most common in developed countries. The watery diarrhea that is present initially becomes bloody after a day or two owing to spread of infection from the ileum to the colon. The illness is caused by exotoxin acting in the small bowel.

Extraintestinal manifestations are recognized, including HUS, Reiter's syndrome, meningitis, Ekiri syndrome (reported in Japanese children and consisting of a triad of encephalopathy due to cerebral edema, bizarre posturing, and fatty degeneration of liver), vaginitis, lung infections, and keratoconjunctivitis. Toxic megacolon, pneumatosis coli, perforation, and rectal prolapse are recognized complications.

Tossed salads, chicken, and shellfish are the commonly incriminated foods. Person-to-person spread by anal intercourse or oral sex also occurs. Prepared food acts as a vehicle of transmission. Spread of infection is also linked to flies.

Children are at high risk during the weaning period, and increasing age is associated with decreased prevalence and severity. Children in daycare centers, persons in custodial institutions, migrant workers, and travelers to developing countries are also at high risk.

Pathogenesis

The virulence factor is a smooth lipopolysaccharide cell wall antigen, which is responsible for the invasive features, and the Shiga toxin, which is both cytotoxic and neurotoxic. Shigellae survive the gastric acidity and invade and multiply within the colonic epithelial cells, causing cell death and mucosal ulcers, and spread laterally to involve adjacent cells but rarely invade the bloodstream.

Laboratory Diagnosis

Shigellosis can be correctly diagnosed in most patients on the basis of fresh blood in stool. Neutrophils in fecal smears strongly suggest infection. Any clinical diagnosis should be confirmed by cultivation of the etiologic agent from stools. Cary-Blair medium is the transport medium of choice, and MacConkey agar or deoxycholate citrate agar (DCA) as well as a highly selective medium such as xylose-lysin deoxycholate (XLD), Hektoen enteric (HE), or Salmonella-Shigella (SS) agar are also used.

Treatment

Ciprofloxacin (Cipro, 500 mg PO twice daily for 3 days) is the antibiotic of choice for shigellosis. Alternative agents are pivmecillinam (Selexid),[2] ceftriaxone (Rocephin),[1] and azithromycin (Zithromax).[1]

---

[1]Not FDA approved for this indication.
[2]Not available in the United States.

Staphylococcus aureus

A notable incident of staphylococcal food poisoning occurred in February 1975 when 196 of 344 passengers and one flight attendant aboard a jet from Tokyo to Copenhagen via Anchorage contacted a gastrointestinal illness characterized by nausea, vomiting, and abdominal cramps. The flight attendant and 142 passengers were hospitalized. Symptoms developed shortly after a ham and omelet breakfast had been served. *S. aureus* was incriminated as the offending agent and ham as the vehicle of the outbreak. The source was traced to a cook with pustules on his fingers.

S. aureus is ubiquitous in the environment. Only strains that produce enterotoxin cause food poisoning. Food is usually contaminated by infected food handlers.

Pathogenesis

If food is stored for some time at room temperature, the organism can multiply in the food and produce enterotoxin. Most food poisonings are caused by enterotoxin A, and the isolates commonly belong to phage type III. These are heat stable, and ingestion of as little as 23 μg of enterotoxin can induce symptoms. The toxin acts on the receptors in the gut, and sensory stimulus is carried to the vomiting center in the brain by vagus and sympathetic nerves.

Because the ingested food contains preformed toxin, the incubation period is very short. In severe illness, profound hypotension occurs. Death is known to occur at extremes of age and in the malnourished.

Laboratory Diagnosis

The presence of a large number of *S. aureus* in food can indicate poor handling or sanitation; however, it is not sufficient evidence to incriminate the food as the cause of food poisoning.

Staphylococcal food poisoning can be diagnosed if staphylococci are isolated in large numbers from the food and their toxins are demonstrated in the food or if the isolated *S. aureus* is shown to produce enterotoxins. Dilutions of food may be plated on Baird-Parker agar or mannitol salt agar. Enterotoxin may be detected and identified by gel diffusion.

Treatment

Therapy is mainly supportive. Antibiotics have no role in the treatment because they are not antitoxins. Intravenous fluids and electrolyte replacement are imperative in the severely dehydrated patient.

Yersinia Species

The *Yersinia* species that cause food poisoning are commonly *Yersinia enterocolitica* and rarely *Yersinia pseudotuberculosis*. Pigs and other wild or domestic animals are the hosts, and humans are usually infected by the oral route. Serogroups that predominate in human illness are O:3, O:5, O:8, and O:9.

Yersiniosis is common in children and occurs most often in winter. *Y. enterocolitica* is associated with terminal ileitis and *Y. pseudotuberculosis* with mesenteric adenitis, but both organisms can cause mesenteric adenitis and symptoms that cause a clinical picture resembling appendicitis, resulting in surgical removal of a normal appendix. Rarer strains of *Y. enterocolitica* are likely to cause systemic infections, especially in patients with diabetes or in iron overload states. In Japan, a form of vasculitis, called Izumi fever, occurs, and in Russia a scarlet fever–like illness has been reported.

Pathogenesis

Yersinia organisms can survive and grow during refrigerated storage. Strains that cause human yersiniosis carry a plasmid that is associated with a number of virulence traits. Ingested bacteria adhere and invade M cells or epithelial cells.

Laboratory Diagnosis

Suspect food is homogenized in phosphate-buffered saline and inoculated into selenite F broth and held at 4°C for 6 weeks. The broth is subcultured at weekly intervals on deoxycholate citrate (DCA) or *Yersinia*-selective agar plates. This is termed *cold-enrichment technique*.

Treatment

Antibiotics are not recommended for gastroenteritis caused by *Yersinia enterocolitica* and the less-common *Yersinia pseudotuberculosis*, but bacteremia and extraintestinal infections require treatment with ciprofloxacin[1] (500 mg PO or 400 mg IV twice daily for 2 weeks). Third-generation cephalosporins (cefotaxime[1] [Claforan]), amoxicillin[1] (Amoxil), TMP-SMX[1] (Bactrim), amoxicillin-clavulanate[1] (Augmentin), carbapenems, and gentamicin (Garamycin) are also effective agents in therapy.

Viruses

Noroviruses

Noroviruses (formerly called Norwalk or Norwalk-like viruses and small round structured viruses [SRSV]) and sapoviruses belong to the family Caliciviridae and are the most common cause of gastroenteritis. They account for about 90% of epidemic nonbacterial outbreaks of gastroenteritis around the world. Norovirus infection often affects people during the winter months and is therefore sometimes called winter vomiting disease; however, people may be affected at any time of the year. After a norovirus infection, immunity lasts only for 14 weeks and is incomplete. Persons with blood group O are more susceptible to infection, whereas those with groups B and AB are partially protected. Norovirus infection outbreaks more commonly occur in closed or semiclosed communities, such as prisons, dormitories, cruise ships, schools, long-term care facilities, and overnight camps—places where infection can spread rapidly from human to human or through tainted food and surfaces. Infection outbreaks can also result from food handled by an infected person.

Outbreaks have often been linked to consumption of cold foods, including salads, sandwiches, and bakery products. Salad dressing, cake icing, and oysters from contaminated waters have also been implicated in gastroenteritis outbreaks. Weight loss, lethargy, low-grade fever, headache, and (rarely) ageusia occur. Vomiting is more likely with infections caused by norovirus than sapovirus.

Pathogenesis

Norovirus strains that infect humans are found in genogroups I, II, and IV. GII.4 strains are more commonly associated with person-to-person transmission, and GI strains are identified more commonly in shellfish-associated outbreaks.

Noroviruses were shown to differentially bind to histo-blood group antigens, and the binding pattern correlates with susceptibility to infection and illness. A number of enzymes are important in the synthesis of histo-blood group antigens, including fucosyl transferase-2 (FUT-2, secretor enzyme), FUT-3 (Lewis enzyme), and the A and B enzymes. The glycan produced by FUT-2 H type 1, serves as a viral receptor for noroviruses.

Laboratory Diagnosis

The virus can be recovered from the infected person's stool and vomitus during illness for about 2 weeks. Electron microscopy and reverse-transcriptase polymerase chain reaction (RT-PCR) antigen-detection assays are performed on stool samples. Serologic assays are not available for clinical use. However, infection can be diagnosed by identifying a fourfold or greater increase in antibody titer between acute and convalescent sera using norovirus virus-like particles as antigen.

Treatment

There is no specific treatment for norovirus infection. Hydration is generally adequate for most patients. In developing countries, oral rehydration therapy is the treatment of choice. Effective hand washing, careful food processing, and education of food handlers along with chlorination of water are important preventive measures. A vaccine for norovirus is in clinical trials.

---

[1]Not FDA approved for this indication.

Rotavirus

Among the seven rotavirus species (A to G), rotavirus A, B, and C can cause disease in humans. Rotavirus A is the most common and is the major cause of waterborne outbreaks in humans. Infections are referred to as infantile diarrhea, winter diarrhea, or acute viral gastroenteritis. Children 6 months to 2 years of age, premature infants, the elderly, and the immunocompromised are particularly prone to more-severe symptoms caused by infection with group A rotavirus. Rotavirus can survive in water for days to weeks, depending on water quality and temperature. Waterborne outbreaks are most common, followed by spread by fomites. Rotaviruses infect intestinal enterocytes; diarrhea may be caused by malabsorption secondary to the destruction of enterocytes, villus ischemia and activation of the enteric nervous system, and intestinal secretion stimulated by the action of rotavirus nonstructural protein 4 (NSP4), a novel enterotoxin and secretory agonist with pleiotropic properties.

Outbreaks caused by group B rotavirus, also called adult diarrhea rotavirus, have also been reported in the elderly and adults. Such infections are rare and usually subclinical. Group C rotavirus has been associated with rare and sporadic cases of diarrhea in children in many countries. Subclinical infection to severe gastroenteritis leading to life-threatening dehydration can occur. The illness has an abrupt onset, with vomiting often preceding the onset of diarrhea. Up to one third of patients have fever of about 39°C. The stools are characteristically watery and only occasionally contain red or white cells. Symptoms generally resolve in a week.

Respiratory and neurologic features in children have been reported. Rotavirus infection has been associated with other clinical conditions including sudden infant death syndrome (SIDS), necrotizing enterocolitis, Kawasaki's disease, and type 1 diabetes.

Laboratory Diagnosis

Electron microscopy, direct antigen detection assays (ELISA, immunochromatography, latex agglutination), and nucleic acid detection (e.g., RT-PCR, polyacrylamide gel electrophoresis [PAGE]), are used mainly in epidemiologic studies during outbreaks.

Treatment

Dehydration due to group A rotavirus infection is treated with early institution of oral and intravenous fluids. The role of probiotics,[7] bismuth subsalicylate (Pepto Bismol),[1] inhibitors of enkephalinase, and nitazoxanide (Alinia)[1] are not clearly defined. Antimicrobials and antimotility agents should be avoided. A marked fall in deaths from childhood diarrhea following introduction of rotavirus vaccines (Rotarix, RotaTeq) has been reported from various parts of the world, and surveillance information has not revealed an association of any serious adverse reactions with the vaccine.

Other Pathogens

Cryptosporidium

Transmission of *Cryptosporidium* is usually by the fecal-oral route, often through food and water contaminated by livestock mammal feces. Persons most likely to be infected by *Cryptosporidium parvum* are infants and young children in daycare centers; those whose drinking water is unfiltered and untreated; those involved in farming practices such as lambing, calving, and muck-spreading; people engaging in anal sexual practices; patients in a hospital setting (from other infected patients or health care workers); veterinarians; and travelers.

Pathogenesis

Cryptosporidium spp. are believed to be noninvasive. Malabsorption resulting from the intestinal damage caused by prolonged protozoal infection can be fatal. Although host cells are damaged in cryptosporidiosis, the means by which the organism causes damage is not known. Mechanical destruction and the effects of toxins, enzymes, or immune-mediated mechanisms, working alone or together, may be instrumental. In the immunocompromised, the illness is much more debilitating, with cholera-like diarrhea.

Laboratory Diagnosis

Traditionally, cryptosporidiosis is diagnosed by microscopic observation of developmental stages of the organism in an intestinal biopsy specimen. Oocysts can be recovered from stool samples by formalin-concentration techniques, staining with a modified Ziehl-Neelsen acid-fast stain. Serologic tests (ELISA, immunofluorescence antibody, PCR) are of added value.

Treatment

Nitazoxanide (Alinia, 500 mg PO twice daily for 3 days) is recommended with antiretrovirals for HIV-positive patients. Fluid replacement and antidiarrheal agents are also given.

Trichinosis

Trichinosis is due to *Trichinella spiralis* infection, commonly as a result of consuming improperly cooked pork. Recent outbreaks in North America have been attributed to consumption of bear meat rather than pork. The parasite lodges in the extraocular muscles, deltoid, biceps, intercostals, diaphragm, tongue, or masseter and produces severe weakness with pain, fever, and cough along with splinter hemorrhages and eosinophilia.

Moderate *T. spiralis* infection is treated with mebendazole (Vermox 200–400 mg PO three times daily for 3 days) or albendazole[1] (Albenza 400 mg PO twice daily for 7–14 days). For severe infections, prednisone is added in a dose of 1 mg/kg/day for 5 days.

Neurocysticercosis

Neurocysticercosis is caused by *Taenia saginata* infection, commonly as a result of consuming improperly cooked pork or contaminated raw vegetables and water. The parasite lodges in the central nervous system and skeletal muscle and presents as intracranial calcifications and ring-enhancing lesions on radioimaging studies. Other than leukocytosis, eosinophilia, and raised erythrocyte sedimentation rate, antibodies to species-specific antigens of *T. solium* can be detected by immunosorbent assay and complement fixation-tests. Treatment is aimed at controlling seizures and relief of hydrocephalus. Albendazole (15 mg/kg/day for 8–28 days) or praziquantel (50–100 mg/kg/day in three divided doses for a month) are given for parenchymal cysticerci with glucocorticoids to suppress the inflammatory response around the dying parasites. Surgery may be required to reduce intracranial pressure.

Dinoflagellate toxins

Dinoflagellates, a very large and diverse group of eukaryotic algae in the marine ecosystem, are the major group producing toxins that impact humans. Dinoflagellate toxins are structurally and functionally diverse, and many present unique biological activities. Five major seafood poisoning syndromes caused by toxins have been identified from the dinoflagellates (Table 4): paralytic shellfish poisoning (PSP), neurotoxic shellfish poisoning (NSP), amnesic shellfish poisoning (ASP), diarrheic shellfish poisoning (DSP) and ciguatera fish poisoning (CFP). Symptoms include allergic manifestations, neurologic including paresthesia of the extremities, headache, ataxia, vertigo, cranial nerve palsies, and paralysis of respiratory muscles as well as gastrointestinal. Symptomatic treatment and antihistamines are the mainstay of treatment.

---

[1]Not FDA approved for this indication.
[7]Available as dietary supplement.

[1]Not FDA approved for this indication.

TABLE 4	Seafood Poisoning Caused by Neurotoxins Identified from Marine Dinoflagellate Species			
TYPE OF POISONING	**TOXINS**	**SOURCES OF TOXINS**	**PRIMARY VECTOR**	**ACTION TARGET**
PSP	Saxitoxins and gonyautoxins	*Alexandrium* spp., *Gymnodinium* spp., *Pyrodinium* spp.	Shellfish	Voltage-gated sodium channel 1
NSP	Brevetoxins	*Kerenia brevis, Chatonella marina, C. antiqua, Fibrocapsa japonica, Heterosigma akashiwo*	Shellfish	Voltage-gated sodium channel 5
	Yessotoxins	*Protoceratium reticulatum, Lingulodinium polyedrum Gonyaulax spinifera*	Shellfish	Voltage-gated calcium/sodium channel?
CFP	Ciguatoxins	*Gambierdiscus toxicus*	Coral reef fish	Voltage-gated sodium channel 5
CFP	Maitotoxins	*Gambierdiscus toxicus*	Coral reef fish	Voltage-gated calcium channel
AZP	Azaspiracids	*Protoperidinium crassipes*	Shellfish	Voltage-gated calcium channel
Palytoxin poisoning	Palytoxins	*Ostrepsis siamensis*	Shellfish	Na$_+$K$_+$ATPase

Tetrodotoxin poisoning

It is a neurotoxin concentrated in the skin and viscera of puffer fish, and other fishes of the order Tetraodontiformes and in some amphibian, octopus, and shellfish species. Human poisonings occur when the flesh or organs of the fish are improperly prepared and eaten. Tetrodotoxin acts by blocking the conduction of nerve impulses along nerve fibers and axons and interferes with the transmission of signals from nerves to muscles. Onset of symptoms usually is 30–40 minutes but may be as short as 10 minutes; it includes lethargy, paraesthesia, emesis, ataxia, weakness, and dysphagia; ascending paralysis occurs in severe cases with high mortality (1-2 mg is lethal). Management is symptomatic.

Group B Sreptococcus (GBS)

GBS bacteria is found in 15%–30% of adult human intestines and urinary tract. Rarely implicated in infections of skin, joints, heart and brain, a recent outbreak of food-borne illness caused by the Type III GBS ST283 strain was reported in Singapore during the period of January–July 2015. It is the largest of its kind and first association to food-borne transmission of GBS to people via consumption of "yusheng-style" raw fresh water fish. The primary case presented with giddiness and suffered bouts of vomiting and diarrhea. Further studies are ongoing to establish the link between increase in cases of Group B streptococcus (GBS) infection to consumption of raw fish. Treatment is symptomatic.

Newer Trends in Foodborne Illness

New or unusual pathogens and food hazards are identified in course of investigating outbreaks. In 2011, a novel outbreak of sprout-associated illness caused by a strain of *Escherichia coli* O104:H4 was reported from Germany and France. This enteroaggregative and Shiga toxin-producing strain caused severe illness leading to HUS and death. In 2008, an outbreak following consumption of chicken caused by *Arcobacter butzleri* (found in poultry) was reported from Wisconsin. The calcivirus Sapovirus is emerging as the likely cause of oyster-associated foodborne outbreaks in Japan. New and unsuspected food vehicles are also being identified that had not been previously recognized as problematic (Box 1).

Changing patterns of disease presentation have seen important foodborne challenges emerging. Chagas disease is emerging as a foodborne infection linked to fresh, unpasteurized acai and guava juice. Infected triatomid insects present in fruits are implicated. Outbreaks of Nipah virus encephalitis in Bangladesh and India

BOX 1	New Food Vehicles Identified in Outbreaks

Bagged spinach
Carrot juice
Peanut butter
Broccoli powder on a snack food
Dry dog food
Frozen potpies
Canned chilli sauce
Hot peppers
White and black pepper
Raw cookie dough (likely the flour)
Hazelnuts
Fenugreek sprouts
Papayas
Pine nuts
Raw scrapped tuna
Clover sprouts
Herbs
Avocado, guacamole

Reprinted from Braden C, Tauxe R: Emerging trends in foodborne diseases, *Inf Dis Clinics N Am* 27:517-533, 2013.

have been linked to drinking of palm sap, toddy, and well water contaminated with urine of feeding giant fruit bats, the vector of Nipah virus.

More syndromes and other systemic disease presentations are being linked to foodborne infection. The feco-oral transmission of pathogens leading to other systemic manifestation include Campylobacter sp. (Guillain-Barre syndrome, irritable bowel syndrome), Toxoplasma gondii (behavior changes and neuropsychiatric manifestations) and *Salmonella choleraesuis* (aortitis). Foodborne outbreak of Group G streptococci (GGS) pharyngitis in a school dormitory in Japan (2016) presented with sore throat and fever in a majority; implicated food was a broccoli salad.

Miscellaneous

Many other organisms are implicated in foodborne and waterborne illnesses (Box 2). Some are discussed elsewhere in this book. Amebiasis, brucellosis, cholera, hepatitis A and E,

BOX 2 Miscellaneous Organisms Implicated in Foodborne and Waterborne Illnesses

Adenovirus 40, 41
Bacillus anthracis
Bacillus mycoides
Burkholderia cepacia
Burkholderia pseudomallei
Clostridium bifermentans
Corynebacterium diphtheriae
Coxiella burnetii
Dientamoeba fragilis
Enterococcus faecalis, E. faecium
Erysipelothrix rhusiopathiae
Francicella tularensis
Henipa virus
Klebsiella spp.
Leptospira spp.
Mycobacterium bovis
Parvovirus B
Pediococcus
Pestivirus
Picobirnavirus
Proteus spp.
Pseudomonas aeruginosa
Pseudomonas cocovenanans
Reovirus
Streptobacillus moniliformis
Taenia solium, T. saginata
Torovirus
Toxoplasma gondii

giardiasis, typhoid fever, and other foodborne intestinal nematodes and cestodes are covered in the infectious diseases section of this text and are not covered in this section.

References

Baker AC, Goddard VJ, Davy J, et al: The identification of a diagnostic marker to detect freshwater cyanophages of filamentous cyanobacteria, *Appl Environ Microbiol* 72:5713–5719, 2003.

Braden CR, Tauxe RV: Emerging trends in foodborne diseases, *Infect Dis Clin North Am* 27(3):517–533, 2013.

Centers for Disease Control and Prevention: *A–Z index for foodborne illness*, 2012. http://www.cdc.gov/foodsafety/diseases/. 2012 [accessed August 11, 2016].

Centers for Disease Control and Prevention: *CDC Estimates of Foodborne Illness in the United States*, 2012. Available at: http://www.cdc.gov/foodborneburden/PDFs/FACTSHEET_A_FINDINGS.pdf. 2012 [accessed August 11, 2016].

Centers for Disease Control and Prevention. The National Institute for Occupational Safety and Health (NIOSH) Emergency Response Safety and Health Database; Category Index: Biotoxins, http://www.cdc.gov/niosh/ershdb/emergencyresponsecard_29750019.html. August 11, 2016.

Centers for Disease Control and Prevention: Tetrodotoxin Poisoning Associated with Eating Puffer Fish Transported from Japan — California, 1996, *Morb Mortal Wkly Rep* 45(19), 1996.

Gamarra RM. Food poisoning- Clinical presentation. Drugs and Diseases, Medscape. updated June 26, 2015, http://emedicine.medscape.com/article/175569-clinical#b5. [Accessed August 11, 2016].

Hajmeer MN, Fung DYC: Other bacteria. In Riemann H, Cliver DO, editors: *Foodborne Infections and Intoxications*, 3rd ed, New York, 2006, Academic Press, pp 341–363.

Hale TL, Keusch GT: Shigella, 1996: In Baron S, editor: *Medical Microbiology*, 4th ed, Galveston, 1996, TX: University of Texas Medical Branch at Galveston. PMID: 21413252 (PubMed). Available at: http://www.ncbi.nlm.nih.gov/books/NBK7627 (accessed August 11, 2016).

Hedberg CW, Osterholm MT: Outbreaks of food-borne and waterborne viral gastroenteritis, *Clin Microbio Rev* 6:199–210, 1993.

Janda JM, Abbott SL: The genus Aeromonas: Taxonomy, pathogenicity, and infection, *Clin Microbiol Rev* 23:35–73, 2010.

Juranek DD: Cryptosporidiosis: Sources of infection and guidelines for prevention, *Clin Infect Dis* 21:S57–61, 1995.

Ministry of Health, Singapore, National Environment Agency, Agri-food & Veterinary Authority of Singapore 24 July 2015. Update on Investigation into Group B Streptococcus Cases, https://www.moh.gov.sg/content/moh_web/home/pressRoom/pressRoomItemRelease/2015/update-on-investigation-into-group-b-streptococcus-cases.html. [Accessed August 11, 2016].

Nataro JP, Kaper JB: Diarrheagenic Escherichia coli, *Clin Microbiol Rev* 11:142–201, 1998.

Niyogi SK: Shigellosis, *J Microbiol* 43:133–143, 2005.

Ortega YR, Sanchez R: Update on Cyclospora cayetanensis, a food-borne and waterborne parasite, *Clin Microbiol Rev* 23:218–234, 2010.

Parashar UD, Bresee JS, Gentsch JR, Glass RI: Synopsis: Rotavirus, *Emerg Infect Dis* 4:561–570, 1998.

Sodha SV, Griffin PM, Hughes JM: Foodborne disease. In Mandell GL, Bennett JE, Dolin R, editors: *Principles and Practice of Infectious Diseases*, 7th ed, Philadelphia, 2009, Churchill Livingstone, pp 1413–1427.

University of Maryland: *Chemical Ecology: Tetrodotoxin- Mode of action*, 2001. http://www.life.umd.edu/grad/mlfsc/zctsim/ionchannel.html.

Wang D-Z: Neurotoxins from Marine Dinoflagellates: A Brief Review, *Marine Drugs* 6(2):349–371, 2008, https://doi.org/10.3390/md20080016.

Yamaguchi T, Kawahara R, et al: Foodborne outbreak of group G streptococcal pharyngitis in a school dormitory in Osaka, Japan, *J Clin Microbiol* 56(5):e01884–17, 2018. https://doi.org/10.1128/JCM.01884-17.

GIARDIASIS

Method of
Rodney D. Adam, MD

CURRENT DIAGNOSIS

- Giardiasis is the most common intestinal protozoan infection worldwide.
- Most cases result from exposure to contaminated drinking or recreational water.
- The clinical manifestations range from asymptomatic to chronic diarrhea with malabsorption and weight loss.
- The diagnosis can be established by stool microscopy or by immunoassays of fecal specimens.
- Occasionally, the trophozoites can be found in duodenal specimens when fecal assays are negative.
- Serologic testing plays no role in the diagnosis.
- Irritable bowel symptoms are very common after successful treatment of giardiasis.

CURRENT THERAPY

- The treatment of choice is metronidazole (Flagyl)[1] or tinidazole (Tindamax); tinidazole can be given as a single dose.
- Albendazole (Albenza)[1] and nitazoxanide (Alinia) are alternative agents.
- Paromomycin (Humatin),[1] a poorly absorbed aminoglycoside, is commonly recommended during early pregnancy when other agents are avoided.
- True drug resistance has not been documented, but refractory or recurrent cases can be treated by two drugs: a nitroimidazole combined with quinacrine (Atabrine)[2] or albendazole.[1]

[1]Not FDA approved for this indication.
[2]Not available in the United States.

Giardia lamblia is the most common parasitic cause of diarrhea. It is found globally with manifestations that range from asymptomatic to chronic diarrhea with weight loss and malnutrition. Infection occurs when cysts are ingested, most commonly from contaminated water or more direct fecal oral transmission. Less commonly, infections are acquired from food or from zoonotic sources. The cysts excyst in the small intestine and replicate as trophozoites, which cause the disease associated with the organism.

The diagnosis is made by the microscopic detection of cysts or trophozoites from fecal samples or by immunoassays of fecal samples. The treatment of choice for symptomatic patients is tinidazole (Tindamax) or metronidazole (Flagyl),[1] while treatment of asymptomatic people depends on the circumstances. Irritable bowel syndrome is common after symptomatic infection, so patients with persistent symptoms should only be treated when persistent infection is documented.

Background

Giardia lamblia (syn. *Giardia intestinalis, Giardia duodenalis*) was initially described by Leeuwenhoek in the 17th century while doing a microscopic examination of his own diarrheal feces. However, *G. lamblia* was not widely accepted as a human pathogen until the 1960s, when a number of outbreaks were reported in travelers to endemic areas. The presumed source of infection in these cases was contaminated drinking water. Subsequently, *Giardia* has become the most commonly identified parasitic cause of diarrhea, and, along with *Cryptosporidium* species, is among the most commonly identified parasitic causes of water-borne diarrheal disease.

Organism

Giardia species are members of the diplomonad (two bodies) group of flagellated protozoans. The life cycle consists of the environmentally resistant cyst, which infects its host on ingestion. It is oval in shape, is about 8 μm × 12 μm in size and contains four nuclei. It excysts into pear-shaped trophozoites in the proximal small intestine that are about 10 to 12 μm by 5 × 7 μm in size. Two symmetrically placed nuclei are in the body of the trophozoites and four pairs of flagella aid with motility. A ventral concave disk uses primarily mechanical means to attach to the intestinal wall of the host. While still in the small intestine, some of the trophozoites then encyst into the cyst form, which is passed in the feces to continue the cycle of infection. The *Giardia* species are all parasitic and were initially assigned to species on the basis of host of origin. However, in 1952, they were divided into three species (*Giardia agilis*, amphibians; *Giardia muris*, rodents; *G. duodenalis* [*G. lamblia*], mammals and birds) that could easily be distinguished on the basis of morphologic appearance of the trophozoites. Subsequently, the *G. lamblia* morphologic group has been divided into additional species based on differences that can be seen at the ultrastructural or molecular level. Of the organisms that remain assigned to *G. lamblia,* all are found in mammals but are divided into eight genotypes or assemblages (A through H) on the basis of molecular differences with varying host specificities. Only genotypes A and B have been found in humans. It is likely that at least some of these eight genotypes will eventually be assigned to separate species.

Epidemiology

Giardiasis is the most commonly diagnosed human protozoan infection and is one of the most commonly identified forms of gastroenteritis. Most cases occur from ingestion of contaminated water or by human-to-human transmission through the fecal–oral route. Thus the epidemiology of human infections can be understood by examining these mechanisms of transmission. In the United States most cases are sporadic and occur more often in the summer, probably reflecting infection from recreational water exposure. Infections were more commonly reported in children from ages 1 to 9 years, especially those younger than 4 years of age. In general, the incidence is higher in the northern states, perhaps because cysts survive longer in cool, moist environments.

Direct human-to-human transmission by the fecal oral route also occurs, leading to the higher prevalence found in children in daycare centers. The occasional reports of food-borne transmission most likely occurred because of food being contaminated by infected food handlers.

The greater incidence in children could reflect an increased use of recreational water facilities, daycare exposure, or increased susceptibility to symptomatic disease. The epidemiology of giardiasis in the United States is similar to that found in other developed countries located in temperate regions. However, in developing regions with inadequate availability of purified water, the epidemiology is very different. For example, in a shantytown near Lima, Peru, children were almost universally infected by the age of 2 years, and when treated, they were rapidly reinfected, but there were no symptoms that could clearly be correlated with their infections. Perhaps an outbreak at a ski resort town in the United States can explain these different epidemiologic patterns. In this water-borne outbreak, tourists were disproportionately affected despite drinking from the same water source as the local residents. The conclusion was that the local residents had repeatedly been exposed to water contaminated by *Giardia* cysts and were less susceptible to symptomatic disease.

The degree of zoonotic transmission of giardiasis remains controversial. Human acquisition of infection from dogs or cats has not been well documented, and usually the *Giardia* genotypes found in cats or dogs are distinct from those found in humans (A and B), even in regions where both are endemic. However, genotypes A and B have sometimes been identified in dogs or other animals, so the question is not totally resolved. On the other hand, beavers have been implicated as a source of contaminated water leading to human infections.

Risk Factors

People with hypogammaglobulinemia, and possibly those with IgA deficiency, are at increased risk for prolonged giardiasis. In animal models, deficiency in cell-mediated immunity (CMI) has been associated with increased risk, but in humans the increased risk has not been associated with defects in CMI.

Pathogenesis

Infection is initiated by the ingestion of as few as 10 cysts. After passage through the acidic environment of the stomach, each cyst excysts into two trophozoites in the proximal small intestine. However, gastric acidity is not required, and people with achlorhydria or who are treated with suppressors of gastric acid remain vulnerable to giardiasis. The trophozoites replicate in the proximal small intestine, where they attach to the intestinal mucosa by their ventral disks. The attachment appears to occur by mechanical means facilitated by the suction generated by the ventral disk and the four pairs of flagella as they provide motility. Although the trophozoites attach to the intestinal wall and leave imprints after separating from the wall, there is no well-documented evidence of invasion, either of the intestinal wall or at extraintestinal sites. Toxins have not been identified as causes of diarrhea. However, cysteine proteases, which are also involved in encystation, may be important contributors to the symptoms. The host parasite interaction leads to enterocyte apoptosis and epithelial barrier disruption. The host immune response is mediated through a TH17 response that includes IgA production. An inadequate immune response results in persistence of organisms and an excessive response may be responsibility for the prolonged diarrhea and malabsorption that is commonly found in symptomatic people. Irritable bowel syndrome as well as chronic fatigue are common after giardiasis with a rate over 30% in a large Norwegian outbreak in 2004. The trophozoites are coated with a cysteine-rich protein encoded by one of a family of related genes, and expression can be switched from one to another, perhaps contributing to the chronicity of the infection.

Prevention

The strategies for prevention should be determined by the most prevalent risk factors in specific situations. For travelers to endemic regions, the major risk is from the ingestion of contaminated water. Therefore drinking water should be purified by boiling for 1 minute or by filtration through a pore size of <1 μm.

---

[1]Not FDA approved for this indication.

Halogenization with iodine or chlorine requires a prolonged contact time (hours) to inactivate cysts and is not recommended. In daycare centers and for food handlers, the best preventive measure is effective hand washing. In addition, children or workers who are infected should be treated.

Clinical Features

Most people with giardiasis are symptom-free, but the percentages range from rates of diarrhea no higher than background among children in some highly endemic regions to attack rates of nearly 100% in visitors to endemic regions. Symptomatic patients typically present for evaluation only after several days or even weeks of illness because of the subacute onset. The symptoms of giardiasis typically develop after an incubation period of 1 to 2 weeks and consist of diarrhea that is characterized by loose, foul-smelling stools and abdominal discomfort described as cramping or bloating (Table 1). Fatigue is very common, but fever is unusual and, when present, is mild and occurs only within the first few days. Malabsorption and weight loss are often present. The majority of cases resolve within several weeks, but occasionally the symptoms will last for months in the absence of treatment. The prolonged symptoms are often due to postinfectious irritable bowel syndrome and/or chronic fatigue, especially if not accompanied by weight loss. Relapse is relatively uncommon after effective treatment.

Diagnosis

The gold standard of diagnosis has been the microscopic evaluation of three separate fecal samples, including concentrated specimens for cysts or, less commonly, trophozoites. The identification of trophozoites is typically associated with symptomatic infection, but cysts may be found in symptom-free persons. Because of the challenges in obtaining three fecal specimens and the interobserver variability in skill at identifying *Giardia* cysts, antigen detection tests have come into widespread use. The enzyme immunoassays are more commonly used and have high degrees of sensitivity and specificity. A direct fluorescent assay is slightly more sensitive than the enzyme immunoassays and can also detect *Cryptosporidium* species, but it requires the availability of fluorescent microscopy. Polymerase chain reaction (PCR) tests have also been described and are more sensitive but more expensive and not widely available. Some patients have negative workups of stool samples, but *Giardia* trophozoites can be detected in duodenal contents with the string test. The patient swallows a capsule on a string, which is left in situ for 4 hours to overnight. The string is then removed and examined microscopically for trophozoites. Alternatively, endoscopy with sampling of duodenal

contents and duodenal biopsy can be used. Endoscopy has the added advantage of being able to detect other possible diagnoses, such as celiac disease or tropical sprue.

Differential Diagnosis

The diagnosis of giardiasis should be suspected in patients presenting with prolonged (>5–7 days) diarrhea without blood in the stools and no fever. In patients presenting relatively early in the course of illness, the major considerations in the differential diagnosis are other infectious etiologies of diarrhea, particularly *Campylobacter jejuni*, *Salmonella*, *Cryptosporidium*, and *Cyclospora cayetanensis*. Thus patients presenting with compatible symptoms should have stool samples submitted for culture and for microscopic examination for ova and parasites (O and P). Watery diarrhea is uncommon, and bloody stools are not seen with giardiasis; thus these findings should prompt the search for other etiologies.

For patients presenting with more prolonged symptoms, a number of noninfectious illnesses should be added to the differential diagnosis. Irritable bowel syndrome and lactose intolerance are among the more common etiologies and should be considered in patients presenting with diarrhea but no weight loss. Gluten enteropathy, tropical sprue, and, rarely, Whipple's disease are among the noninfectious etiologies of diarrhea accompanied by weight loss.

Treatment

Patients with symptomatic giardiasis should be treated. The criteria for treatment of patients with asymptomatic giardiasis are not well defined, but in general, patients in regions with low prevalence or linked with outbreaks should be treated. On the other hand, in settings where the prevalence is high and recurrence rates are high, there is probably no value to treating asymptomatic infection.

The most commonly used agents for treatment of giardiasis are the nitroimidazoles. Metronidazole (Flagyl),[1] tinidazole (Tindamax), and secnidazole (Solosec)[1] are available in the United States, while orinidazole (Tiberal)[2] is available in other countries (Table 2). These agents are completely absorbed from the gastrointestinal tract and are inactivated primarily by hepatic metabolism. Metronidazole has been available in the United States for decades and has generally been considered the drug of choice for treatment of giardiasis in most situations. More recently, tinidazole has become available and is the only agent available in the United States with a high degree of efficacy when given as a single dose. A meta-analysis of 60 randomized clinical trials for treatment of giardiasis concluded that tinidazole was more effective than metronidazole or albendazole. Metronidazole is mutagenic in bacterial assays and showed some carcinogenic activity in an animal model. However, carcinogenicity in humans has not been documented. Serious adverse reactions to the nitroimidazoles are rare, but nausea and a metallic taste are common and may decrease the compliance of patients with metronidazole. The problem with noncompliance can be addressed by the use of tinidazole or the other agents that can be given as a single dose.

Albendazole (Albenza)[1] is a tubulin inhibitor that was introduced as a broad-spectrum antihelminthic, but it also has good activity against *Giardia* trophozoites. It is generally well tolerated and in areas with endemic helminth infections has the added advantage of antihelminthic activity.

The first trimester of pregnancy poses a special problem because none of the agents have been adequately studied or approved for use during this time. Paromomycin (Humatin)[1] is a nonabsorbed aminoglycoside and is expected to be safe during pregnancy. Therefore it is usually the preferred choice in that setting; however, it is somewhat less effective than other agents. Specialty consultation should be considered for treatment of patients in their first trimester. Metronidazole is used extensively during the second and third trimesters for other

TABLE 1	Symptoms of Giardiasis*
SYMPTOM	**AVERAGE (%)**
Diarrhea	95
Abdominal cramps	70
Weakness or malaise	70
Nausea	60
Weight loss	50
Anorexia (decreased appetite)	50
Abdominal distention (bloating/distension)	50
Flatulence	50
Vomiting	30
Fever	20

From Adam RD. Giardiasis. *Hunter's Tropical Medicine and Emerging Infectious Diseases*, Eds: Magill AJ, Ryan ET, Hill DR, Solomon T. Elsevier, 2019.

*The table includes the approximate frequency of the signs and symptoms reported in six studies of symptomatic giardiasis, but it is important to note that there is substantial variability of symptoms among studies.

[1]Not FDA approved for this indication.
[2]Not available in the United States.

	DOSE				
DRUG	**ADULT**	**PEDIATRIC***	**FREQUENCY**	**DURATION**	**EFFICACY (%)**
Metronidazole[1] (Flagyl)	250 mg	5 mg/kg	tid	5–7 days	90–100
Tinidazole (Tindamax)	2 g	50 mg/kg	Single dose	Single dose	90–100
Secnidazole[1] (Solosec)	1.5 g	30 mg/kg[†]	Single dose	Single dose	90–100
Quinacrine[2] (Atabrine)	100 mg	2 mg/kg	tid	5–7 days	80–100
Furazolidone[2] (Furoxone)	100 mg	1.5 mg/kg	qid	10 days	80–94
Paromomycin[1] (Humatin)	500 mg	8–10 mg/kg	tid	10 days	55–90
Albendazole[1] (Albenza)	400 mg qd	15 mg/kg	Daily	5 days	90–100
Nitazoxanide (Alinia)	500 mg bid	7.5 mg/kg	bid	3 days	70–80

TABLE 2 Treatment of Giardiasis

[†]Approved for adults and patients ≥12 years of age.
*The adult dose is the maximum pediatric dose.
[1]Not FDA approved for this indication.
[2]Not available in the United States.

indications; thus it can be considered the drug of choice for those patients.[1] Albendazole is known to be teratogenic and should be avoided during pregnancy.

Nitazoxanide (Alinia) has been approved in the United States for treatment of giardiasis (and cryptosporidiosis) and is very well tolerated. However, the somewhat lower efficacy compared with nitroimidazoles and albendazole, along with the requirement for twice daily dosing, limits its role.

Treatment failures are not uncommon but may or may not be due to true drug resistance because in vitro cultures are not routinely performed, and in vitro testing is not standardized. When treatment failure occurs, the patient may respond to the same or an alternative drug. Treatment-refractory cases have been treated successfully with a combination of metronidazole[1] plus quinacrine[2] or albendazole.[1] The most common reason for persistence of symptoms after treatment is due to postgiardiasis irritable bowel syndrome, which can occur in over 30% of patients. Thus it is important to reevaluate stool specimens from patients with symptoms that persist after therapy.

Diet

Lactose intolerance is quite common while patients have giardiasis and potentially for months thereafter, so lactose ingestion should be moderated or eliminated as needed.

[1]Not FDA approved for this indication.
[2]Not available in the United States.

References

Adam RD: Giardia duodenalis: biology and pathogenesis, *Clin Microbiol Rev* 34(4):e0002419, 2021.
Coffey CM, Collier SA, Gleason ME, Yoder JS, Kirk MD, Richardson AM, Fullerton KE, Benedict KM: Evolving epidemiology of reported giardiasis cases in the United States, 1995–2016, *Clinical Infectious Diseases* 72:764–770, 2020.
Cooper MA, Sterling CR, Gilman RH, Cama V, Ortega Y, Adam RD: Molecular analysis of household transmission of *Giardia lamblia* in a region of high endemicity in Peru, *J Inf Dis* 202:1713–1721, 2010.
Hanevik K, Dizdar V, Langeland N, Hausken T: Development of functional gastrointestinal disorders after giardia lamblia infection, *BMC Gastroenterology* 9:27, 2009.
Lengerich EJ, Addiss DG, Juranek DD: Severe giardiasis in the United States, *Clin Infect Dis* 18:760–763, 1994.
Morrison HG, McArthur AG, Gillin FD, Aley SB, Adam RD, Olsen GJ, Best AA, Cande WZ, Chen F, Cipriano MJ, et al: Genomic minimalism in the early diverging intestinal parasite, *Giardia lamblia Science* 317:1921–1926, 2007.
Ordonez-Mena JM, McCarthy ND, Fanshawe TR: Comparative efficacy of drugs for treating giardiasis: a systematic update of the literature and network meta-analysis of randomized clinical trials, *Journal of Antimicrobial Chemotherapy* 73:596–606, 2018.
Singer SM, Fink MY, Angelova VV: Recent insights into innate and adaptive immune responses to *Giardia*, *Advances in Parasitology* 106:171–208, 2019.

HUMAN IMMUNODEFICIENCY VIRUS: TREATMENT AND PREVENTION

Method of
Allison Cormier, MD; and Tyler K. Liebenstein, PharmD

CURRENT DIAGNOSIS

- National guidelines recommend universal screening for human immunodeficiency virus (HIV) infection for all adult and adolescent patients in all healthcare settings after notification that testing will be done, unless the patient specifically declines testing (opt-out testing). Patients with behavioral risk factors, sexually transmitted diseases, or tuberculosis should be screened annually.
- Revised HIV testing algorithms reflect the increased sensitivity of newer diagnostic assays during early infection, such as fourth-generation HIV-1/2 antigen/antibody combination immunoassays.
- Acute HIV infection is recognized as a variable syndrome including fever, pharyngitis, rash, and arthralgias. As many as one-half of patients may be asymptomatic during seroconversion and early infection.

CURRENT THERAPY

- Combination antiretroviral therapy (ART) should be offered to all patients with HIV infection, regardless of CD4 helper T-lymphocyte (CD4 T-cell) count.
- Initial ART regimens preferred for most patients include a combination of two nucleoside analogue reverse transcriptase inhibitors (NRTIs) and an integrase strand transfer inhibitor (INSTIs), which are often coformulated into single-tablet preparations that can be administered once daily.
- Although ART decisions are often made by providers with specialized training, all providers who care for people living with HIV should be aware of the risk of antiretroviral drug interactions, particularly interactions involving the pharmacokinetic-enhancing agents ritonavir (Norvir) and cobicistat (Tybost).
- All sexually active adult and adolescent patients should receive information about HIV preexposure prophylaxis (PrEP) to reduce the risk of HIV acquisition. Both oral and injectable medication options are available for PrEP.

Introduction

Remarkable advances in therapeutics, leading to the development of antiretroviral therapy (ART), have transformed human immunodeficiency virus (HIV) infection from an almost universally fatal illness to a chronic disease that can be managed over decades with an enlarging repertoire of treatment options. Further developments in ART have also provided opportunities for preventing HIV infection in high-risk individuals. This chapter provides an overview of the current understanding of HIV pathogenesis and epidemiology and discusses guidelines for the initial evaluation and long-term management of HIV infection in adult patients.

Pathophysiology

HIV is an enveloped, single-stranded RNA virus belonging to the family Retroviridae. It was recognized as the causative agent of AIDS within 3 years after the initial description of the syndrome in 1981, and ongoing characterization of its molecular biology has provided the identification of multiple targets for drug development. Two types of human immunodeficiency viruses exist: HIV-1 and HIV-2. HIV-1 has worldwide distribution, accounts for most infections outside western Africa, and is the focus of this chapter.

HIV-2 infection is endemic in West Africa and has limited spread outside this area. It should be considered in infections in patients of West African origin or those who have had sexual contact or shared needles with people of West African origin. HIV-2 generally has a longer asymptomatic stage, lower plasma HIV-2 viral loads, and overall lower mortality rate. Approximately 25% to 30% of patients with HIV-2 who do not receive ART will have HIV-2 RNA levels below the rate of detection, and some will also have clinical progression and a decreased CD4 helper T-lymphocyte (CD4 T-cell) count. HIV-2 can progress to AIDS over time. HIV-1 and HIV-2 coinfection may occur and should be a consideration in patients from high prevalence HIV-2 areas. Patients diagnosed with HIV-2 infection should be managed by an HIV specialist.

Genetic heterogeneity of HIV-1 is reflected in categorization of the virus into three groups (M, O, and N) and several subtypes (B, C, D, AE, and CRF01_AE), some of which have overlapping geographic distribution around the world. Subtype C is prevalent in southern and eastern Africa, China, India, South Asia, and Brazil and accounts for 50% of HIV subtypes, whereas subtype B, the most common subtype in the United States, accounts for 12%.

The HIV viral genome is encoded in single-stranded RNA, packaged in core protein structures, and surrounded by a lipid bilayer envelope that is derived from the cell membrane of the host cell as the virus buds from the cell surface after replication.

This outer viral membrane contains HIV-specific glycoproteins, including gp120 and gp41, which facilitate attachment and entry into host cells through interaction with the cell surface receptor, CD4, and coreceptors CCR5 and CXCR4. CD4 T cells are the predominant host cell affected by HIV; this molecular tropism explains the immune system destruction manifested in chronic HIV infection and provides the rationale for clinical staging of HIV infection using CD4 T-cell counts. After host cell entry, the key enzyme responsible for viral replication is reverse transcriptase, an RNA-dependent DNA polymerase that is packaged within the virion core. This enzyme facilitates conversion of the HIV genome into a double-stranded DNA intermediate molecule. The second key enzymatic step is integration of this intermediate nucleic acid product into the host genome, which is facilitated by the viral protein integrase. Protein synthesis with packaging of new viral particles ensues, utilizing an HIV-specific protease. The integrase inhibitor class of drugs acts by blocking this step of integration.

Natural History

Within 1 to 4 weeks after the initial HIV infection, seroconversion may be accompanied by a nonspecific, self-limiting illness, often referred to as *acute retroviral syndrome*. This illness has variable manifestations but may include fever, malaise, myalgias, arthralgias, generalized lymphadenopathy, pharyngitis, and rash. The associated rash may be maculopapular, urticarial, or roseola-like. An illness resembling acute infectious mononucleosis syndrome, similar to that caused by Epstein-Barr virus (EBV) or cytomegalovirus (CMV), and aseptic meningitis has been described. Diagnosis of acute HIV infection requires a high index of suspicion, which does not commonly occur unless the patient reports a recent history of high-risk exposure.

During the acute phase of infection, high levels of viremia are present (often exceeding 10 million copies/mL) as HIV becomes widely disseminated throughout the body and the host defenses begin to counteract circulating virus through cell-mediated and humoral (antibody-mediated) immune mechanisms. Antibodies against HIV usually become detectable 2 to 4 months after infection. The initial, high-level viremia plateaus and then begins to decrease as neutralizing antibodies are established. Ongoing replication is partially controlled by the immune response, resulting in a steady-state level of viremia. This virologic level differs from patient to patient and is one of the determinants of the rate of disease progression. A small number of HIV-infected persons are able to control viral replication to levels below the limit of detection, and they tend to have a more benign course of disease. In these patients, designated *elite suppressors* by researchers, HIV replication continues to occur, and HIV RNA can be isolated from latently infected cells by means of specialized laboratory techniques.

After the establishment of HIV infection and seroconversion, a period of asymptomatic infection ensues, during which patients are free from evidence of immune suppression and opportunistic infections (OIs) are uncommon. This phase of clinical latency lasts a median of 8 to 10 years, based on observational studies from the pre-ART era. Ongoing viral replication leads to a gradual decrease in CD4 T-cell counts.

The symptomatic stage of HIV infection can begin at any time after infection, but clinical manifestations become more likely as the CD4 count decreases farther below the normal range of 800 to 1200 cells/mm^3. For example, *Pneumocystis jirovecii* (formerly *Pneumocystis carinii*) pneumonia (PJP) usually occurs in patients with a CD4 count less than 200 cells/mm^3 or a percentage less than 10%. CMV retinitis occurs almost exclusively in patients with a CD4 count less than 50 cells/mm^3 or a percentage less than 5%. Mucocutaneous candidiasis (oral thrush), herpes zoster, HIV-associated nephropathy, peripheral neuropathy, tuberculosis, and community-acquired bacterial pneumonia occur with increased frequency at earlier stages of infection and are less reliably predicted by CD4+ T-cell measurement.

Diagnosis

The current recommended testing algorithm incorporates a fourth-generation antigen/antibody combination HIV-1/2 immunoassay with a confirmatory HIV-1/HIV-2 antibody differentiation immunoassay. The fourth-generation assay detects both HIV-1 and HIV-2 antibodies and HIV p24 antigen. It has increased sensitivity because of its ability to diagnose acute/early infection, because HIV p24 antigen is detected before seroconversion has occurred. If the fourth-generation combination assay is positive, the HIV-1 and HIV-2 antibody differentiation immunoassay both confirms the positive result and determines if the patient is infected with HIV-1 or HIV-2. If the fourth-generation assay is positive but the confirmatory antibody differentiation immunoassay is indeterminate or negative, a plasma HIV RNA level should be obtained.

In facilities where fourth-generation testing is not available, a two-step approach is utilized via enzyme-linked immunosorbent assay (ELISA) to detect HIV antibodies with subsequent confirmation using an HIV-1/HIV-2 differentiation assay. An ELISA can detect HIV IgM and IgG antibodies as early as 3 weeks after virus exposure. This modality has excellent sensitivity and specificity for diagnosing chronic HIV infection; however, diagnosis may be missed in patients with early HIV infection who have not yet had seroconversion. If concern exists for acute/early HIV infection, plasma HIV RNA can be assessed.

False-negative and false-positive tests occur rarely. False-negative screening tests can occur with ELISA-only testing during acute/early HIV infection. This occurs less often using the fourth-generation antigen/antibody assay, which is more sensitive in detecting early HIV infection by identifying the p24 antigen. False-positive screening test results can occur for several non-HIV reasons, including cross-reaction from alloantibodies in pregnant women, autoantibodies from autoimmune diseases or malignancy, and the influenza vaccine. False-positive results in both screening and confirmatory testing are particularly uncommon.

Indeterminate test results occur when the initial screening test is positive and subsequent confirmatory testing is indeterminate or negative. In the event of a positive fourth-generation antigen/antibody test and negative HIV differentiation assay, the detection of p24 antigen would yield a positive result, but the differentiation assay would be negative, as no antibody is present. In all patients with indeterminate test results, a plasma HIV RNA should be obtained, as viremia is present before antibody seroconversion. A detectable plasma HIV RNA level is diagnostic of HIV infection. If HIV RNA is negative, the patient should be reassured that HIV infection is unlikely. A repeat screening test can be repeated after 3 months for further reassurance. If the patient had a recent high-risk exposure, another plasma HIV RNA can be performed in 1 to 2 weeks. All patients with indeterminate testing should be counseled to avoid activities with potential to transmit HIV to others until evaluation is completed.

Consent

HIV screening should be voluntary and pursued only after discussion with the patient regarding testing. In the United States, written consent is no longer obligatory in any state, but individual states may have policies regarding documentation of the consent process and related counseling. Confidentiality, access to posttesting counseling, and services to support prompt linkage to HIV care for patients with positive results are important resources in HIV testing settings.

Screening

Early detection of HIV infection and subsequent initiation of ART can dramatically reduce morbidity and mortality of affected patients. A relatively normal life span is possible in patients in the United States who are diagnosed early in their infection and successfully treated. Such early treatment also can reduce the transmission of HIV. One-time testing is recommended for patients without high-risk factors for HIV exposure in patients 13 to 75 years of age. Pregnant women should be screened for HIV early in their pregnancy, even if they have been screened during prior pregnancies.

In patients with elevated risk of HIV exposure, more frequent testing is recommended. Men who have sex with men (MSM), along with patients who have sex with sexual partners who have HIV or with persons of unknown serostatus may benefit from HIV screening at least every 6 months. This is especially important in patients 13 to 24 years of age because this demographic group has experienced the highest rate of new infections in recent years. Other high-risk groups include patients who use injection drugs as well as sex workers.

Approach to the Patient with HIV Infection

HIV patient care is an ever-changing field, with routinely updated professional guidelines and new medications. The quality of care received by patients with HIV has been shown to correlate with the healthcare provider's experience and comfort in treating these patients. Referral to an HIV specialist is recommended for new HIV diagnoses, complications of HIV or antiretroviral drugs, and for treatment failure.

All patients with HIV should have a comprehensive history, physical examination, and laboratory evaluation when establishing care. This baseline evaluation can help establish and define the patient's goals and plan of care. In a patient who has already established treatment with ART and presents for initial evaluation with a new healthcare provider, it is important to document the complete antiretroviral history and drug resistance testing results, if available.

Patients with HIV are often faced with many medical, psychiatric, and social issues. These are best addressed through a patient-centered, multidisciplinary approach. In patients with a new diagnosis of HIV, it is important to counsel them regarding HIV infection and assess their understanding of the disease and its transmission. They should also be assessed for readiness to initiate ART, potential high-risk behaviors, mental illness, substance abuse, social support, medical comorbidities, and/or economic factors, because these are potential issues that may impair adherence to ART.

Antiretroviral Therapy

There are currently six major classes of antiretroviral medications used to treat patients with HIV. Although dozens of such medications are available, only a small selection of agents is currently preferred as initial treatment regimens (Table 1). For most patients, ART includes a combination of two NRTIs plus a third medication from a different class, although two-drug regimens are preferred for some patients.

When to Initiate Antiretroviral Therapy

Combination ART first became available in the mid-1990s and provided life-saving therapy for millions of patients suffering from HIV and AIDS. Although the early ART regimens were effective in helping patients with AIDS recover, they were also associated with many toxicities and side effects. In 2006, the U.S. Department of Health and Human Services, the International AIDS Society–USA, and the British HIV Society recommended CD4 counts of 200 cells/mm^3 as the threshold for initiating ART treatment in asymptomatic patients. More recently, the paradigm has shifted toward earlier initiation of ART based on accumulating evidence for the beneficial effects of treatment initiation earlier in the course of infection. Antiretroviral therapies have advanced significantly since their conception, consisting of multiple drug classes, fewer toxicities, less pill burden, and overall improved tolerance. Failure to suppress viral loads on these medications is more likely to result from therapy nonadherence than medication failure.

HIV patients are now achieving normal life spans, and non–AIDS-defining illnesses are becoming more prominent. Cardiovascular, renal, and hepatic disease complications are lower in patients who started ART at higher CD4 thresholds (>350 cells/mm^3). Earlier initiation of ART is also associated with reduced risk of transmission and improved immune restoration.

Current Recommendations for Antiretroviral Therapy

ART should be offered to all patients with HIV infection, regardless of CD4 T-cell count. The goal of ART is to prevent morbidity, mortality, and transmission associated with HIV. This is accomplished by maximally inhibiting HIV replication to achieve an undetectable HIV viral load. Based on guidelines from the U.S. Department of Health and Human Services, INSTI-based regimens are currently the first-line recommendation as initial therapy for most patients with HIV based on high rates of virologic suppression and tolerability demonstrated in large clinical trials. Nonnucleoside reverse transcriptase inhibitor (NNRTI) and protease inhibitor (PI) regimens are recommended in certain clinical situations (Table 2). Monotherapy with any antiretroviral drug is not recommended because of increased risk of drug resistance and therapy failure.

Selection of an Antiretroviral Regimen

ART regimens should be individualized based on a regimen's side-effect profile, pill burden, potential drug interactions, virologic efficacy, cost, and resistance testing results. Before starting ART in any patient with HIV, the following factors must be considered:

- Pretreatment HIV RNA level
- Pretreatment CD4 T-cell count
- HIV genotypic drug resistance testing results
- HLA-B*5701 status (if planning to use an abacavir-based ART regimen)

| TABLE 1 | Recommended Initial Regimens for Most People with HIV |

GENERIC NAME (TRADE NAME) AND RECOMMENDED ADULT DOSING	SINGLE TABLET REGIMEN?	IMPORTANT POINTS
INSTI + 2 NRTIs		
Bictegravir/emtricitabine/tenofovir alafenamide (Biktarvy)* 50/200/25 mg—1 tablet by mouth once daily	Yes	Bictegravir has been shown to increase serum creatinine from baseline by a median 0.1 mg/dL as a result of inhibition of creatinine secretion, not a true reduction in GFR
Dolutegravir/abacavir/lamivudine (Triumeq) 50/600/300 mg—1 tablet by mouth once daily	Yes	Dolutegravir has been shown to increase serum creatinine from baseline by a mean of 0.15 mg/dL as a result of inhibition of creatinine secretion, not a true reduction in GFR Dolutegravir has a drug interaction with metformin (maximum daily metformin dose is 1000 mg) Must be confirmed HLA-B*5701 negative before starting treatment to avoid abacavir hypersensitivity reaction
Dolutegravir (Tivicay)† 50 mg—1 tablet by mouth once daily *PLUS* Tenofovir alafenamide/emtricitabine (Descovy) 25/200 mg—1 tablet by mouth once daily *OR* Tenofovir disoproxil fumarate/emtricitabine (Truvada) 300/200 mg—1 tablet by mouth once daily	No	Dolutegravir has been shown to increase serum creatinine from baseline by a mean of 0.15 mg/dL because of inhibition of creatinine secretion, not a true reduction in GFR Dolutegravir has a drug interaction with metformin (maximum daily metformin dose is 1000 mg) Descovy generally preferred over Truvada because of fewer bone and kidney toxicities
INSTI + 1 NRTI		
Dolutegravir/lamivudine (Dovato) 50/300 mg—1 tablet by mouth once daily	Yes	This two-drug regimen should not be used in those with HIV RNA >500,000 copies/mL, HBV coinfection, or in whom ART is to be started before the results of HIV genotypic resistance testing for reverse transcriptase or HBV testing are available Dolutegravir has been shown to increase serum creatinine from baseline by a mean of 0.15 mg/dL as a result of inhibition of creatinine secretion, not a true reduction in GFR Dolutegravir has a drug interaction with metformin (maximum daily metformin dose is 1000 mg)

*Biktarvy [package insert]. Foster City, CA: Gilead Sciences, Inc.; 2021.
†Tivicay [package insert]. Research Triangle Park, NC: ViiV Healthcare; 2021.
ART, Antiretroviral therapy; *GFR,* glomerular filtration rate; *HBV,* hepatitis B virus; *HIV,* human immunodeficiency virus; *HLA,* human leukocyte antigen; *INSTI,* integrase strand transfer inhibitor; *NRTI,* nucleoside analogue reverse transcriptase inhibitor.
Modified from Panel on Antiretroviral Guidelines for Adults and Adolescents. Guidelines for the Use of Antiretroviral Agents in Adults and Adolescents with HIV. Department of Health and Human Services. Available at: https://clinicalinfo.hiv.gov/sites/default/files/guidelines/documents/adult-adolescent-arv/guidelines-adult-adolescent-arv.pdf (Table 6).

- Patient's individual preference
- Anticipated medication adherence

Other factors that are important to consider when choosing an initial regimen include the patient's medical comorbidities (cardiovascular, renal, psychiatric disease), pregnancy or the potential to become pregnant, and coinfections with tuberculosis, hepatitis C virus, and hepatitis B virus (HBV).

The currently recommended ART for most patients includes two NRTIs ("backbone"), abacavir/lamivudine (ABC/3TC [Epzicom]) or either tenofovir alafenamide/emtricitabine (TAF/FTC [Descovy]) or tenofovir disoproxil fumarate/emtricitabine (TDF/FTC [Truvada]), plus an INSTI (see Table 1). Single-tablet regimens coformulated with an INSTI and the NRTI backbone are available. INSTI-based regimens are well tolerated, have convenient dosing, and provide excellent virologic suppression. Regimens including NNRTI or PK-enhanced PIs remain effective but are now only recommended in certain clinical scenarios.

The NRTI combinations of ABC/3TC (Epzicom), TAF/FTC (Descovy), and TDF/FTC (Truvada) are available as fixed-dose combination tablets. The 3TC and FTC components have few adverse effects. The main differences among these combinations involve ABC, TAF, and TDF. The advantages of TAF and TDF include activity against HBV, and HLA-B*5701 testing is not required before use. TDF has some association with lower lipid levels compared with TAF, but also may cause decreased renal function and reduced bone mineral density. TAF is associated with less bone and kidney toxicity, and its use is preferred in patients with underlying bone and kidney disease or those at risk for these conditions. The advantage of ABC is that it has less bone mineral loss and less nephrotoxicity than TDF and does not require dose adjustment in patients with renal insufficiency. Potential drawbacks to ABC include an observed association with cardiovascular events in some studies and a hypersensitivity syndrome, necessitating screening for HLA-B*5701 before treatment initiation.

TABLE 2 Recommended Initial Regimens in Certain Clinical Situations

GENERIC NAME (TRADE NAME) AND RECOMMENDED ADULT DOSING	SINGLE TABLET REGIMEN?	IMPORTANT POINTS
INSTI + 2 NRTIs		
Elvitegravir/cobicistat/tenofovir alafenamide/emtricitabine (Genvoya) 150/150/10/200 mg—1 tablet by mouth once daily OR Elvitegravir/cobicistat/tenofovir disoproxil fumarate/emtricitabine (Stribild) 150/150/300/200 mg—1 tablet by mouth once daily	Yes	Genvoya generally preferred over Stribild because of fewer bone and kidney toxicities Drug interactions with other medications are prevalent with both products because of cobicistat, a CYP3A4 inhibitor
Raltegravir (Isentress HD) 600 mg—2 tablets by mouth once daily OR Raltegravir (Isentress) 400 mg—1 tablet by mouth twice daily PLUS Tenofovir alafenamide/emtricitabine (Descovy) 25/200 mg—1 tablet by mouth once daily OR Tenofovir disoproxil fumarate/emtricitabine (Truvada) 300/200 mg—1 tablet by mouth once daily	No	Isentress HD generally preferred over Isentress because of once-daily dosing Descovy generally preferred over Truvada (Isentress HD) because of fewer bone and kidney toxicities
NNRTI + 2 NRTIs		
Rilpivirine/tenofovir alafenamide/emtricitabine (Odefsey) 25/25/200 mg—1 tablet by mouth once daily OR Rilpivirine/tenofovir disoproxil fumarate/emtricitabine (Complera) 25/300/200 mg—1 tablet by mouth once daily	Yes	Rilpivirine should only be used if HIV RNA <100,000 copies/mL and CD4 >200 cells/mm^3 Odefsey generally preferred over Complera because of fewer bone and kidney toxicities PPIs contraindicated with rilpivirine H2 blockers may be used once daily but must be spaced 12 hours apart from rilpivirine Should be taken with food
Doravirine/tenofovir disoproxil fumarate/lamivudine (Delstrigo) 100/300/300 mg—1 tablet by mouth once daily OR Doravirine (Pifeltro) 100 mg—1 tablet by mouth once daily PLUS Tenofovir alafenamide/emtricitabine (Descovy) 25/200 mg—1 tablet by mouth once daily	Yes, for Delstrigo	May be taken with or without food Doravirine does not have any restrictions with acid-suppressive medications
Efavirenz/tenofovir disoproxil fumarate/emtricitabine (Atripla) 600/300/200 mg—1 tablet by mouth once daily	Yes	High rates of neuropsychiatric adverse effects (e.g., vivid dreams, depression, suicidal ideation)
PK-enhanced PI + 2 NRTIs		
Darunavir/cobicistat/emtricitabine/tenofovir alafenamide (Symtuza) 800/150/200/10 mg—1 tablet by mouth once daily OR Darunavir/cobicistat (Prezcobix) 800/150 mg—1 tablet by mouth once daily OR Darunavir (Prezista) 800 mg—1 tablet by mouth once daily + Ritonavir (Norvir) 100 mg—1 tablet by mouth once daily PLUS Tenofovir alafenamide/emtricitabine (Descovy) 25/200 mg—1 tablet by mouth once daily OR Tenofovir disoproxil fumarate/emtricitabine (Truvada) 300/200 mg—1 tablet by mouth once daily OR Abacavir/lamivudine (Epzicom) 600/300 mg—1 tablet by mouth once daily	Yes, for Symtuza	Prezcobix generally preferred over the combination of Prezista and Norvir because of single tablet and potentially fewer GI side effects and drug interactions Drug interactions with other medications are prevalent with both cobicistat and ritonavir because of CYP3A4 inhibition Ritonavir also inhibits and induces several other CYP enzymes Careful attention should be given to manage drug interactions Descovy generally preferred over Truvada because of fewer bone and kidney toxicities If using Epzicom, must be confirmed HLA-B*5701 negative before starting therapy to avoid abacavir hypersensitivity reaction
Atazanavir/cobicistat (Evotaz) 300/150 mg—1 tablet by mouth once daily OR Atazanavir (Reyataz) 300 mg—1 tablet by mouth once daily + Ritonavir (Norvir) 100 mg—1 tablet by mouth once daily PLUS Tenofovir alafenamide/emtricitabine (Descovy) 25/200 mg—1 tablet by mouth once daily OR Tenofovir disoproxil fumarate/emtricitabine (Truvada) 300/200 mg—1 tablet by mouth once daily	No	Darunavir-containing regimens generally preferred over atazanavir-containing regimens Atazanavir is known to increase serum bilirubin. This generally does not require further workup if the patient is asymptomatic Evotaz generally preferred over the combination of Reyataz and Norvir because of single tablet and potentially fewer GI side effects and drug interactions Drug interactions with other medications are prevalent with both cobicistat and ritonavir because of CYP3A4 inhibition. Ritonavir also inhibits and induces several other CYP enzymes. Careful attention should be given to manage drug interactions Descovy generally preferred over Truvada because of fewer bone and kidney toxicities

CYP3A4, Cytochrome P450 3A4; GI, gastrointestinal; H2, histamine H$_2$ receptor; HIV, human immunodeficiency virus; HLA, human leukocyte antigen; INSTI, integrase strand transfer inhibitor; NNRTI, non-nucleoside reverse transcriptase inhibitor; NRTI, nucleoside reverse transcriptase inhibitor; PI, protease inhibitor; PPI, proton pump inhibitor.
Modified from Panel on Antiretroviral Guidelines for Adults and Adolescents. Guidelines for the Use of Antiretroviral Agents in Adults and Adolescents with HIV. Department of Health and Human Services. Available at: https://clinicalinfo.hiv.gov/sites/default/files/guidelines/documents/adult-adolescent-arv/guidelines-adult-adolescent-arv.pdf (Table 6).

Once the combination NRTI backbone has been chosen, a third drug from another class must be added to the regimen. Current recommendations for most patients favor the INSTI class because of its high efficacy, fewer side effects, and no significant CYP3A4-associated drug interactions.

Darunavir (DRV [Prezista])–based regimens may still be preferred in certain patients with difficulty maintaining medication adherence, and a high genetic barrier to resistance is favored or in a situation when ART should be initiated before receiving resistance testing results. Darunavir boosted with ritonavir (Norvir) (DRV/r) or cobicistat (Tybost) (DRV/c [Prezcobix]) has a low rate of transmitted PI resistance, a high genetic barrier to resistance, and a low rate of treatment-emergent resistance. A dolutegravir (DTG [Tivicay])- or bictegravir (BIC)-containing regimen (BIC/TAF/FTC [Biktarvy]) is also a consideration for patients in whom it is necessary to initiate ART before receiving resistance testing results because of its high barrier of resistance.

NNRTI-based regimens include efavirenz (EFV [Sustiva]), rilpivirine (RPV [Edurant]), or doravirine (DOR [Pifeltro]) and may be appropriate choices in certain patients with good medication adherence. These medications have a low genetic barrier to resistance. EFV has minimal PK interactions with rifamycins, which makes it an excellent option in patients who require treatment for tuberculosis. EFV has a high rate of central nervous system–related side effects, which lowers its overall tolerability in some patients. RPV has fewer side effects than EFV, but its virologic efficacy is reduced in patients with high baseline HIV RNA and low CD4 T-cell counts. RPV also requires acid for absorption; it is contraindicated with proton pump inhibitors and must be spaced 12 hours apart from histamine 2 receptor antagonists.

More recently, two large, randomized controlled trials showed that a two-drug regimen of DTG plus lamivudine (DTG/3TC [Dovato]) was noninferior to DTG plus TDF/FTC. This two-drug regimen is another potential initial option for most people with HIV, except for patients with pretreatment HIV RNA greater than 500,000 copies/mL, who are known to have active HBV coinfection, or who will initiate ART before results of HIV genotype testing for reverse transcriptase or HBV testing are available.

Long-Acting Injectable Antiretroviral Therapy

In 2021, the first complete long-acting injectable ARV regimen, cabotegravir (CAB) and rilpivirine (RPV), Cabenuva, was approved as an option to replace the current ARV regimen in adults with HIV. Once-monthly or every-2-month CAB/RPV intramuscular (IM) injections can be used as an optimization strategy for people with HIV currently on oral ART with documented viral suppression (HIV-1 RNA less than 50 copies per mL) for at least 3 months. Candidates for CAB/RBV long-acting injections should have no baseline resistance to either medication, have no prior virologic failures, should not have HBV infection (unless also receiving an oral HBV active regimen), should not be pregnant or planning to become pregnant, and should not be receiving medications with significant drug interactions with CAB or RPV. Before initiation of the IM injection, patients should receive oral CAB (Vocabria) and oral RPV (Edurant) for approximately 1 month as an oral lead-in period to assess tolerance to these drugs. CAB/RPV (Cabenuva) injections should be administered by healthcare providers as gluteal IM injections. Administration variances of +/–7 days are allowed. The product is refrigerated and should be brought to room temperature before administration. Unopened vials may remain at room temperature for up to 6 hours. Medication drawn into a syringe may remain in the syringe for up to 2 hours.

Monitoring Response to Antiretroviral Therapy

HIV disease progression and response to ART can be monitored via CD4 T-cell count and HIV RNA (viral load). The CD4 T-cell count should be measured before initiation of ART and provides information regarding the patient's immune function and risk of OI. Recommendations for monitoring viral load and CD4 T-cell count are shown in Table 3.

CD4 T-cell counts can be highly variable, and significant change is only considered with 30% difference in absolute count or an increase or decrease in CD4 percentage by 3 percentage points. CD4 T-cell recovery is most rapid in the first 3 months after initiating ART, later followed by more gradual increases. For most patients on ART, adequate response is considered as an increase in CD4 count in the range of 50 to 150 cells/mm^3 during the first year of treatment. Subsequent increases may average 50 to 100 cells/mm^3 per year until a steady-state level is reached. Peripheral blood CD4 T-cell counts in most HIV patients will continue to increase over a decade as long as viral suppression is maintained. Most individuals will eventually recover CD4 counts within the normal range (>500 cells/mm^3). For approximately 15% to 20% of patients, especially those who initiate ART at very low CD4 counts (<200 cells/mm^3), low CD4 counts may persist, which is associated with increased morbidity and mortality. These patients should be evaluated for reversible causes of CD4-positive T-cell lymphopenia, including offending medications, untreated coinfections, and underlying malignancy. In patients with appropriate virologic suppression, the addition of more antiretroviral agents or transitioning to a different ART regimen has not been demonstrated to improve CD4 T-cell recovery.

CD4 T-cell counts should be repeated 3 months after ART initiation to monitor immune reconstitution and can be monitored in many patients at 3- to 6-month intervals for the first 2 years of ART. In virally suppressed patients with consistent CD4 counts between 300 and 500 cells/mm^3 for at least 2 years, CD4 counts can be checked annually. Although ART is recommended for all patients with HIV, patients who remain untreated should have CD4 counts monitored every 3 to 6 months to assess the need for OI prophylaxis.

Viral load functions as a marker for ART response and should be monitored at initiation of therapy and regularly thereafter. The pretreatment viral load can also provide useful information regarding selection of an initial ART. Commercially available HIV-1 RNA assays do not detect HIV-2 viral load. Decreases in viral load following ART initiation are associated with a reduction in risk of disease progression to AIDS or death. Optimal viral suppression is defined as a viral load persistently below the level of detection. Low-level viremia refers to a patient with confirmed detectable HIV RNA less than 200 copies/mL. This may be detected using real-time polymerase chain reaction (PCR) assays and may be predictive of developing viral rebound. Viral rebound, or virologic failure, is considered to occur when a patient with confirmed virologic suppression has HIV RNA greater than or equal to 1000 copies/mL. If virologic suppression occurs and the patient is found to have a single isolated detectable HIV RNA level with return to virologic suppression in subsequent tests, this is referred to as a *virologic blip*. This is not usually associated with virologic failure and does not require a change in ART. Acute illness, stress, and recent immunizations are a few potential causes of virologic blips. A repeat viral load can be rechecked in 3 months to confirm return to appropriate viral suppression.

If a patient has a very high HIV viral load at the time of ART initiation, it may take several weeks for a measurable virologic response to occur. Certain ART regimens may also have slower rates of virologic suppression than others. A patient who has received ART for at least 24 weeks and has not yet had documented virologic suppression should be evaluated for antiretroviral drug resistance.

The use of ART to prevent HIV transmission is called *treatment as prevention* (TasP), also known as *Undetectable = Untransmittable* (U = U). Maintaining HIV RNA levels less than 200 copies/mL with ART prevents HIV transmission to sexual partners. Patients who start ART should use another form of prevention with sexual partners for at least the first 6 months of treatment and until an HIV RNA level less than 200 copies/mL has been achieved. Patients who have HIV and who rely on ART for prevention require high ART adherence because transmission is possible during periods of poor compliance or treatment interruption.

TABLE 3	Recommendations on the Indications and Frequency of Viral Load and CD4 T-Cell Count Monitoring	
CLINICAL SCENARIO	**VIRAL LOAD MONITORING**	**CD4 T-CELL COUNT MONITORING**
Before initiating ART	At entry into care. If ART initiation is deferred, repeat before initiating ART. In patients not initiating ART, repeat testing is optional	At entry into care. If ART is deferred, every 3–6 months
After initiating ART	Preferably within 2–4 weeks (and no later than 8 weeks) after initiation of ART; thereafter, every 4–8 weeks until viral load is suppressed	3 months after initiation of ART
After modifying ART because of drug toxicities or for regimen simplification in a patient with viral suppression	4–8 weeks after modification of ART to confirm effectiveness of new regimen	Monitor according to prior CD4 count and duration on ART, as outlined below.
After modifying ART because of virologic failure	Preferably within 2–4 weeks (and no later than 8 weeks) after modification; thereafter, every 4–8 weeks until viral load is suppressed. If viral suppression is not possible, repeat viral load every 3 months or more frequently if indicated	Every 3–6 months
During the first 2 years of ART	Every 3–4 months	Every 3–6 months
After 2 years of ART (VL consistently suppressed, CD4 consistently 300–500 cells/mm^3) After 2 years of ART (VL consistently suppressed, CD4 consistently >500 cells/mm^3)	Can extend to every 6 months for patients with consistent viral suppression for greater than or equal to 2 years.	Every 12 months Optional
While on ART with detectable viremia (VL repeatedly >200 copies/mL)	Every 3 months or more frequently if clinically indicated	Every 3–6 months
Change in clinical status	Every 3 months	Perform CD4 count, and repeat as clinically indicated

ART, Antiretroviral therapy; *VL,* viral load.

Modified from Panel on Antiretroviral Guidelines for Adults and Adolescents. Guidelines for the Use of Antiretroviral Agents in Adults and Adolescents with HIV. Department of Health and Human Services. Available at: https://clinicalinfo.hiv.gov/sites/default/files/guidelines/documents/adult-adolescent-arv/guidelines-adult-adolescent-arv.pdf (Table 4).

Treatment Failure

Patients who are receiving ART and do not achieve HIV RNA levels below the lower limit of detection or are shown to have sustained virologic rebound are at risk for developing resistance mutations to their current ART regimen, especially at HIV RNA levels greater than 500 copies/mL. Virologic failure has a strong association with suboptimal medication adherence and drug intolerance/toxicity leading to self-discontinuation of ART.

Some factors that may increase the risk of ART nonadherence include active substance use, neurocognitive impairment, and mental illness. Unstable housing and other socioeconomic and psychosocial factors can make ART adherence particularly difficult. The patient's inability to afford the medication may lead to intermittent adherence or nonadherence. Some patients will stop taking ART as a result of adverse effects of their regimen. Others may not be able to adhere to a high pill burden or frequency of dosing.

Less common causes of treatment failure include existing or newly developed drug resistance. Patients with HIV-2 or HIV-1/HIV-2 coinfection can have innate resistance to certain ART regimens. Others may have adverse drug-drug interactions with other medications, suboptimal virologic potency, or error in their medication prescription.

If a patient is experiencing virologic failure, it is important to determine the cause because there is potential for choosing a subsequent therapy regimen that promotes better adherence. Management of a patient who is experiencing treatment failure is often complex; consultation with an HIV specialist can prove beneficial.

Drug Resistance and Resistance Testing

Two types of resistance assays exist to assess viral strains and direct treatment strategies: genotypic and phenotypic. These assays provide useful information in regard to resistance to NRTIs, NNRTIs, PIs, and INSTIs. In some settings, INSTI resistance tests must be ordered separately. In patients with newly diagnosed HIV infection, resistance testing can guide therapy selection to optimize virologic response. Genotypic assays detect drug resistance mutations by sequencing reverse transcriptase, protease, and integrase genes. Interpreting these test results requires knowledge of the mutations selected by different antivirals and the potential for cross-resistance to other drugs. Clinical trials have shown that consultation with HIV specialists regarding drug resistance interpretation improves virologic outcomes.

Adverse Drug Reactions and Drug-Drug Interactions

Adverse drug reactions to ART are common, especially when first initiating therapy. Generally, reactions such as nausea, fatigue, and headache often resolve within 1 to 2 weeks of starting ART. Severe or persistent adverse drug reactions should prompt consideration of change to a different agent. Each ART drug class has different characteristic adverse drug reactions. Additionally, each individual ART agent carries its own characteristic adverse drug reactions (Table 4). As drug therapies have evolved and new medications discovered, preferred agents have been updated to avoid those that have tended to cause more frequent and severe adverse effects. For example, older agents in the NRTI class (e.g., stavudine [Zerit] and didanosine [Videx]) were commonly

DRUG	TOXICITY	MONITORING
NRTIs		
Abacavir (Ziagen)	Liver Abacavir hypersensitivity syndrome	LFTs Screening for HLA-B*5701 (should be confirmed negative before abacavir initiation) Symptoms of abacavir hypersensitivity may include fever, rash, nausea, vomiting, diarrhea, abdominal pain, malaise, fatigue, or respiratory symptoms such as sore throat, cough, or shortness of breath
Emtricitabine (Emtriva)	Minimal toxicity Liver Hyperpigmentation/skin discoloration	Serum creatinine LFTs HBV (before initiation of therapy) Severe acute exacerbation of hepatitis may occur in patients with HBV/HIV coinfection who discontinue emtricitabine. For patients in whom discontinuation of tenofovir is necessary, ensure that an agent active against HBV is administered
Lamivudine (Epivir)	Minimal toxicity Liver	Serum creatinine LFTs HBV (before initiation of therapy) Severe acute exacerbation of hepatitis may occur in patients with HBV/HIV coinfection who discontinue lamivudine. For patients in whom discontinuation of tenofovir is necessary, ensure that an agent active against HBV is administered
Tenofovir (disoproxil fumarate [Viread], alafenamide [Vemlidy])	Renal toxicity (tubulopathy) Decreased bone mineral density Liver	Serum creatinine Urine glucose and protein (before initiation of therapy and as clinically indicated during therapy) Serum phosphorus (in patients with chronic kidney disease) Bone mineral density testing (if history of bone fracture or risk factors for bone loss) LFTs HBV (before initiation of therapy) Tenofovir alafenamide (Vemlidy) is associated with lower rates of bone and kidney toxicity compared with tenofovir disoproxil fumarate Severe acute exacerbation of hepatitis may occur in patients with HBV/HIV coinfection who discontinue tenofovir. For patients in whom discontinuation of tenofovir is necessary, ensure that an agent active against HBV is administered
NNRTIs		
Efavirenz (Sustiva)	Rash Neuropsychiatric symptoms Hyperlipidemia Hepatotoxicity Prolonged QT interval	LFTs Lipid panel (before initiation of therapy and as clinically indicated during therapy) Signs and symptoms of neuropsychiatric effects (e.g., vivid dreams, depression, suicidal ideation)
Rilpivirine (Edurant)	Rash Depression, insomnia, headache Hepatotoxicity Prolonged QT interval	LFTs Lipid panel
Doravirine (Pifeltro)	Nausea Dizziness Abnormal dreams	No specific tests
PIs		
All	GI intolerance, nausea, vomiting, diarrhea Hyperglycemia Insulin resistance Hepatotoxicity Fat maldistribution Hyperlipidemia	Serum glucose LFTs (before initiation of therapy and as clinically indicated during therapy)
Atazanavir (Reyataz)	Indirect hyperbilirubinemia	Bilirubin
Darunavir (Prezista)	Skin rash	Darunavir contains a sulfonamide moiety; Stevens-Johnson syndrome, toxic epidermal necrolysis, acute generalized exanthematous pustulosis, and erythema have been reported Risk of cross-reactivity between darunavir and sulfonamide medications is very low. However, use caution in patients with severe sulfonamide allergies

Continued

TABLE 4	Monitoring Recommendations for Antiretroviral Toxicity of Selected Drugs*—cont'd	
DRUG	**TOXICITY**	**MONITORING**
INSTIs		
All	INSTIs typically well tolerated for most patients GI intolerance Insomnia Headache Depression and suicidal ideation (rare, usually in patients with preexisting psychiatric conditions) CPK elevation, muscle weakness, and rhabdomyolysis (primarily reported with raltegravir [Isentress]) Possible association with weight gain	LFTs Serum creatinine (dolutegravir [Tivicay] and bictegravir) CPK (if signs of muscle toxicity)

CPK, Creatinine phosphokinase; *GI*, gastrointestinal; *HBV*, hepatitis B virus; *HIV*, human immunodeficiency virus; *HLA*, human leukocyte antigen; *INSTI*, integrase strand transfer inhibitor; *LFT*, liver function test; *NRTI*, nucleoside reverse transcriptase inhibitor; *NNRTI*, non-nucleoside reverse transcriptase inhibitor; *PI*, protease inhibitor. Table is not all inclusive.

https://clinicalinfo.hiv.gov/sites/default/files/guidelines/documents/AdultandAdolescentGL.pdf. Section accessed March 9, 2021 [Appendix B, table 20].

Modified from Panel on Antiretroviral Guidelines for Adults and Adolescents. Guidelines for the Use of Antiretroviral Agents in Adults and Adolescents with HIV. Department of Health and Human Services. Available at: https://clinicalinfo.hiv.gov/sites/default/files/guidelines/documents/adult-adolescent-arv/guidelines-adult-adolescent-arv.pdf.

associated with hepatic steatosis, lipodystrophy, and insulin resistance. Newer-generation NRTIs, which have much lower rates of these serious adverse effects, have largely supplanted the use of these older drugs.

All providers who care for patients who receive ART should be aware of the possibility of adverse drug-drug interactions of antiretroviral drugs with other medications. The use of the pharmacokinetic-enhancing agents ritonavir (Norvir) and cobicistat (Tybost) in many combination ART regimens can pose serious risks to patients who receive other drugs metabolized through the cytochrome P450 pathway, including numerous anticoagulant drugs and synthetic glucocorticoids. When prescribing or altering one or more drugs in an ART regimen, the potential for drug interactions must be explored. It is critical to carefully review the patient's other medications for potential interactions. If multiple drugs with similar or conflicting metabolic pathways are prescribed, healthcare providers should carefully monitor for appropriate therapeutic efficacy and concentration-related toxicities. Consultation with a pharmacist to evaluate drug interactions is recommended.

Viral Hepatitis Coinfection

Approximately 5% to 10% of patients with HIV in the United States have coinfection with chronic HBV. Disease progression to cirrhosis, end-stage liver disease, and hepatocellular carcinoma is more rapid in these patients. Some antiretroviral toxicities and complications may be attributed to flares of HBV after initiation or discontinuation of ART.

FTC, 3TC, TDF, and TAF[1] are approved for treatment of HIV and are also active against HBV. Discontinuation of these drugs can potentially cause significant hepatic damage resulting from reactivation of HBV. The anti-HBV drug entecavir (Baraclude) has activity against HIV.[1] When entecavir is used to treat HBV in patients with HBV/HIV coinfection who are not taking ART, the drug can select for the *M184V* mutation, resulting in HIV resistance to 3TC and FTC. When 3TC is the only active drug used to treat HBV in coinfected patients, 3TC resistance develops in approximately 40% to 90% of patients after 2 to 4 years on 3TC monotherapy.

Before ART is initiated, all patients who test positive for HBV surface antigen (HBsAg) should also be tested for HBV DNA using a quantitative assay. This test should be repeated every 3 to 6 months to ensure effective HBV suppression. In patients with HBV/HIV coinfection, immune reconstitution following initiation of treatment for HIV, HBV, or both can be associated with elevated transaminases.

Complications

Diagnosis and Management of Opportunistic Infections

The widespread availability and use of ART have significantly reduced OI-related mortality in persons with HIV infection. OIs continue to cause considerable morbidity and mortality, however, because of the increasing number of undiagnosed cases of HIV and patients who have known HIV infection but are not on ART or are unable to maintain adherence to ART.

PJP is an infection caused by a ubiquitous fungus, *P. jirovecii*. Most cases occur in patients with an advanced compromised immune system (CD4 count less than 100 cells/mm³). The most common manifestations are dyspnea, fever, nonproductive cough, and chest discomfort. Onset of symptoms is usually subacute and progressive over days to weeks. Patients with mild cases may present with normal pulmonary physical examination findings at rest but develop dyspnea, tachycardia, and rales with exertion. Hypoxemia is often present to varying severity. Laboratory findings are consistent with lactate dehydrogenase levels greater than 500 mg/dL and elevated serum 1,3 β-d-glucan. Chest radiography may show diffuse, bilateral, ground-glass interstitial infiltrates, but chest radiography can appear unremarkable in patients with early disease. In patients with normal chest plain films, computed tomography (CT) of the chest can show underlying abnormalities consistent with PJP. HIV-infected patients, including pregnant women and those on ART, should receive PJP chemoprophylaxis if they have CD4 counts less than 200 cells/mm³. Patients who receive pyrimethamine (Daraprim)-sulfadiazine for treatment or suppression of toxoplasmosis do not require additional prophylaxis for PJP. Trimethoprim-sulfamethoxazole (TMP-SMX [Bactrim]) is the first-line prophylactic agent at one double-strength tablet daily (which also confers prophylaxis against toxoplasmosis[1]) or three times weekly. In those who cannot tolerate TMP-SMX, alternative prophylactic options include atovaquone (Mepron), dapsone,[1] dapsone plus pyrimethamine (Daraprim)[1] plus leucovorin,[1] and aerosolized pentamidine (Nebupent).

Toxoplasma gondii is a protozoan infection and is associated with reactivation of latent tissue cysts. Patients at greatest risk have CD4 counts less than 50 cells/μL. Clinical disease is rare in patients with CD4 counts greater than 200 cells/μL. In patients with AIDS, the typical presentation of infection is focal encephalitis, including headache, confusion, focal motor weakness, and

[1] Not FDA approved for this indication.

[1] Not FDA approved for this indication.

fever. In the absence of treatment, disease progression may lead to seizures, coma, and death. CT and magnetic resonance imaging (MRI) of the brain may show multiple contrast-enhancing lesions within the gray matter of the cortex or basal ganglia, often with associated edema. HIV-infected patients with toxoplasma encephalitis are usually seropositive for toxoplasma IgG antibodies. Definitive diagnosis requires the combination of clinical presentation, identification of one or more mass lesions via CT or MRI, and detection of the organism in a sample, with brain biopsy being the most preferred method. The therapy of choice includes pyrimethamine plus sulfadiazine plus leucovorin.[1]

Disseminated *Mycobacterium avium* complex (MAC) disease typically occurs in patients with CD4 counts less than 50 cells/mm^3. Other factors associated with increased susceptibility to MAC disease include HIV RNA levels greater than 100,000 copies/mL, previous OIs, and previous colonization of the respiratory or gastrointestinal tract with MAC. In HIV-infected patients with AIDS who are not on ART, MAC disease usually presents as a disseminated, multiorgan infection. Symptoms may be minimal at first but may include fever, night sweats, weight loss, diarrhea, fatigue, and nonspecific abdominal pain. Laboratory abnormalities may include anemia out of proportion for that expected from HIV alone and an increase in liver alkaline phosphatase. Physical examination or imaging may note nonspecific hepatomegaly, lymphadenopathy, and/or splenomegaly. Diagnosis is based on a combination of clinical symptoms and the isolation of MAC from cultures obtained from blood, lymph nodes, bone marrow, or other sterile sites. Initial treatment should consist of at least two antimycobacterial medications in an effort to prevent the development of resistance. Infectious disease specialists should be consulted regarding treatment. MAC isolates should be tested for susceptibility to clarithromycin (Biaxin) and azithromycin (Zithromax).

Cryptococcus neoformans meningitis occurs more commonly in patients with CD4 counts less than 100 cells/μL. It can present as a subacute or acute meningoencephalitis associated with fever, headache, and malaise. Classic meningeal symptoms may be absent. Disseminated disease is usually present when diagnosed in a patient with HIV infection and can involve virtually any organ. Diagnosis of meningitis via cerebrospinal fluid (CSF) often demonstrates elevated opening pressure, elevated protein, low-to-normal glucose, and lymphocytic pleocytosis. Numerous yeast forms may be visualized on Gram stain or India ink preparations of CSF. The CSF cryptococcal antigen (CrAg) is often positive. Serum CrAg may be positive in both meningeal and nonmeningeal involving infections, and its presence can be detected weeks to months before the onset of symptoms. A positive serum CrAg should proceed to lumbar puncture to rule out meningeal disease. Treatment of cryptococcosis occurs in three stages: induction, consolidation, and maintenance therapy.

CMV disease can cause disseminated and localized end-organ damage in HIV-infected patients with suppressed immune states with CD4 counts less than 50 cells/mm^3. Clinical disease is usually the result of reactivation of latent infection. Risk factors include not receiving or failing to respond to ART, previous OIs, high level of CMV viremia, and high HIV viral load (>100,000 copies/mL). Retinitis is the most common clinical manifestation of CMV end-organ disease and is often unilateral, but it can progress to bilateral if therapy or immune recovery are not pursued. Retinitis may present with floaters, scotomata, or peripheral visual field defects. Colitis is another manifestation of CMV disease and may be associated with weight loss, abdominal pain, significant diarrhea, and malaise. Hemorrhage and bowel perforation can be life threatening. CMV viremia can be measured via PCR and is usually present in end-organ disease.

Mucocutaneous candidiasis of the oropharynx and esophagus occurs commonly in HIV-infected patients and is often an indication of underlying immune suppression (CD4 count <200 cells/mm^3). Oropharyngeal candidiasis is usually painless and affects the oropharyngeal mucosa and tongue surface. Esophageal candidiasis may be associated with retrosternal discomfort and odynophagia. Oropharyngeal candidiasis is usually diagnosed clinically. Diagnosis of esophageal candidiasis is made based on symptoms, response to therapy, or visualization of mucosal lesions on examination.

Many treatment guidelines recommend initiating ART within 2 weeks for most diagnosed OI. In patients with cryptococcal meningitis and possible tuberculous meningitis, ART should be deferred because of the risks of serious immune reconstitution syndrome outweighing the benefits of ART. In patients with AIDS-associated OI for which no effective therapy exists (e.g., progressive multifocal leukoencephalopathy [PML], cryptosporidiosis, and microsporidiosis), improvement in immune function with ART can potentially improve disease outcomes.

Neurologic Complications

Both central nervous system disease and peripheral nerve abnormalities are common in advanced AIDS. HIV infection can directly cause distal sensory neuropathy, which may manifest as dysesthesia or hypersensitivity, decreased reflexes, and chronic neuropathic pain. Inflammatory demyelinating polyneuropathy (e.g., Guillain-Barré syndrome) has known associations with some enteric pathogens and causes ascending motor weakness, typically without sensory involvement. CMV infection may cause polyradiculopathy, transverse myelitis, and encephalitis/ventriculitis in patients with CD4 counts lower than 50 cells/mm^3. CMV end-organ disease, including retinitis (a vision-threatening condition), requires prompt diagnosis and initiation of appropriate anti-CMV therapy.

Focal central nervous system lesions can arise from infectious and malignant conditions. Cerebral toxoplasmosis usually occurs in patients with prior exposure to *T. gondii* who develop reactivation disease when the CD4 count is less than 100 cells/mm^3. The main differential diagnosis for one or several enhancing brain lesions includes toxoplasmosis and primary central nervous system lymphoma (PCNSL). PCNSL is associated with EBV, and detection of nucleic acid for EBV in CSF carries a high specificity for this condition in the proper radiographic context. PML, a rare and potentially devastating demyelinating condition, is caused by reactivation of the JC virus and can manifest as focal neurologic deficit, seizures, or cognitive dysfunction. *C. neoformans* is a common cause of meningitis in AIDS patients and may manifest with central nervous system mass lesions, pulmonary disease, or gastrointestinal disease. Worldwide, tuberculosis accounts for a large proportion of HIV-associated meningitis cases; less commonly, it can manifest as single or multiple focal lesions (tuberculomas). Neurosyphilis should be considered in patients with unexplained neurologic disease and sexual risk factors.

Respiratory Complications

Respiratory illnesses are among the most common causes of morbidity in HIV-infected patients. Community-acquired bacterial pneumonia occurs at a significantly higher rate in HIV-infected patients compared with noninfected patients, regardless of CD4 T-cell count, and it is one of the most common reasons for hospitalization. *P. jirovecii* pneumonia (PJP) manifests with fever, cough, and dyspnea. Findings on physical examination and chest radiography can be variable, making the diagnosis difficult in the absence of high clinical suspicion. Elevated lactate dehydrogenase and oxygen desaturation with ambulation can be diagnostic clues. More than 90% of cases occur among patients with CD4 counts lower than 200 cells/mm^3. The diagnosis is established by visualization of organisms in induced sputum (sensitivity, 50% to 90%) or in bronchoalveolar lavage specimens (sensitivity, 90% to 99%), most commonly with the use of immunofluorescent staining.

The risk of reactivation of latent TB is increased 100-fold in patients with HIV infection. Patients with HIV infection who are latently infected have a 10% annual risk of developing symptomatic tuberculosis, compared with a 10% lifetime risk among the general population. The risk of reactivation increases with decreasing CD4 T-cell count, and patients with counts lower than

---

[1] Not FDA approved for this indication.

350 cells/mm^3 are more likely to have atypical radiographic presentations, including middle- and lower-lobe infiltrates without cavitation. Patients with low CD4 T-cell counts are more likely to have extrapulmonary tuberculosis. Diagnostic approaches to tuberculosis in patients with HIV infection are similar to those in patients without HIV infection. Tuberculin skin testing can be used to diagnose latent tuberculosis infection, although the recommended cutoff for a positive test is 5 mm of induration. Treatment of coinfection with *Mycobacterium tuberculosis* and HIV requires consultation with experienced clinicians and pharmacists because of extensive drug-drug interactions among antiretroviral drugs and rifamycins.

Gastrointestinal Complications

Oropharyngeal candidiasis (thrush) commonly manifests as white plaques on the tongue, palate, or buccal mucosa that are painless and are easily scraped off. Although thrush is typically uncomplicated and easily treatable with topical preparations such as nystatin (Mycostatin) and clotrimazole (Mycelex troche), in the proper clinical setting it can alert the clinician to the presence of esophageal candidiasis. Esophageal involvement should be suspected in patients with dysphagia and odynophagia; retrosternal chest pain may also be present. Thrush is usually present but is not required for the diagnosis, which is often made on clinical grounds rather than being confirmed with endoscopy. Patients with esophageal candidiasis typically respond after several days of treatment, and 7 to 14 days of antifungal therapy is usually sufficient. For cases not responsive to empiric treatment for candidiasis, referral for endoscopy should be considered. Esophagitis caused by CMV or herpes simplex virus requires a histopathologic diagnosis.

Acute diarrhea, defined as three or more loose or watery stools per day for 3 to 10 days, is common among patients with HIV infection, and more than 1000 different enteric pathogens have been described. Data from a large cohort indicate that the most common pathogens isolated are *Clostridium difficile*, *Shigella* spp., *Campylobacter jejuni*, *Salmonella* spp., *Staphylococcus aureus*, and MAC. Culture of the stool can yield a microbiologic diagnosis in many cases, particularly for acute diarrheal illnesses caused by *Campylobacter*, *Yersinia*, *Salmonella*, and *Shigella* species. Infection with C. *difficile*, the most common bacterial enteric pathogen in the United States for both HIV-infected and HIV-uninfected persons, is diagnosed in most settings by detection of cytotoxin in the stool by enzyme immunoassay (EIA) or PCR, although the more laborious tissue culture is considered the gold standard. Enteric viruses are present in 15% to 30% of HIV-infected persons with acute diarrhea. Definitive diagnosis is not feasible in most clinical laboratories; viral enteritis should be suspected in the setting of community outbreaks because of the high transmissibility of viral pathogens. Treatment is supportive with fluid resuscitation and antimotility agents.

Chronic diarrhea (duration 30 days) was a common manifestation of advanced-stage AIDS in the pre-ART era. Most pathogens that cause acute gastroenteritis can also cause chronic symptoms. Pathogens that should be suspected in cases of chronic watery diarrhea include protozoa such as *Cryptosporidium parvum*, *Isospora belli*, and *Microsporidia* spp. These entities are self-limiting in the absence of severe immunosuppression. In advanced HIV infection, pathogen-specific antimicrobial therapy is infrequently effective, and symptoms commonly do not improve without immune reconstitution in response to ART. *Giardia lamblia* causes watery diarrhea, abdominal bloating, and occasionally malabsorption syndrome, and it can occur at any CD4 T-cell count. CMV infection can affect any segment of the gastrointestinal tract and is a common cause of chronic diarrhea. Diagnosis of gastrointestinal CMV disease is difficult without biopsy. Detection of CMV viremia with PCR does not correlate well with presence of CMV disease in HIV-infected patients, and CMV can be undetectable in serum in patients with extensive gastrointestinal disease.

Other Conditions

ART has dramatically increased the survival of individuals living with HIV, and the older adult population with HIV is expanding. There are few clinical trials or studies systematically focused on this cohort. Older adults with HIV may develop comorbidities that can complicate their HIV management. ART-related CD4 T-cell recovery in older patients has been observed to be slower and to be of lower magnitude than in younger patients. Hepatic and renal functions decrease as the body ages and may lead to impaired drug elimination and increased drug exposure in older adult patients.

Immune Reconstitution Inflammatory Syndrome

Immune reconstitution inflammatory syndrome (IRIS) is a collection of inflammatory disorders often associated with paradoxical worsening of preexisting infectious diseases after initiation of ART. IRIS is usually accompanied by an increase in CD4 T-cell count and can occur at any CD4 count. It usually occurs in the first 4 to 8 weeks after initiation of ART. Clinical features are often associated with the type and location of the preexisting OI and can be localized or systemic. Patients should continue ART and should receive treatment for the underlying OI as quickly as possible. If the patient's presentation involves paradoxical worsening of a previously diagnosed OI that is already receiving treatment, OI therapy should also be continued. Disseminated MAC accounts for up to one-third of cases of IRIS in the United States. Other important causes of IRIS are tuberculosis, CMV infection, viral hepatitis, and candida infections.

Management of Human Immunodeficiency Virus in Pregnancy and Women of Childbearing Potential

Human Immunodeficiency Virus in Pregnant Women

Every pregnant woman with HIV should be given ART regardless of her immunologic or virologic status in order to improve her health and prevent transmission of HIV to the fetus. Increased perinatal transmission risk exists in pregnant women who experience early HIV infection and high-level viremia. Pregnant women with newly diagnosed HIV infection should start ART as soon as possible to prevent perinatal HIV transmission. The goal of ART is to achieve and sustain viral suppression throughout the pregnancy. Resistance testing should be performed before initiating ART, but therapy may be started before receiving resistance testing results. The ART regimen can be modified at a later date once resistance testing results are available.

Although there originally was a concern for increased risk of neural tube defects (NTDs) with DTG based on preliminary information from a study in Botswana in 2018, the most recent data from this study indicate that there is no longer a significant difference in NTDs with the use of DTG-based regimens compared with non–DTG-based regimens. Therefore, the U.S. Department of Health and Human Services guidelines on the use of antiretroviral drugs during pregnancy recommend DTG as a preferred agent in pregnant women with HIV.

In a patient already taking a regimen containing EFV [Sustiva] who presents for prenatal care during the first trimester and has virologic suppression, EFV can be continued. The risk of fetal NTDs is limited to the first 5 to 6 weeks of pregnancy, and pregnancy is often not recognized before weeks 4 to 6. Unnecessary changes to a patient's ART regimen during pregnancy may result in loss of viral suppression with increased risk of perinatal transmission.

In a pregnant patient with an HIV RNA viral load greater than or equal to 1000 copies/mL (or viral load is unknown) near delivery, IV infusion of zidovudine (Retrovir) during labor is recommended regardless of the patient's antepartum ART regimen or resistance profile. Maternal ART should be continued following delivery. Following delivery, patients should continue to follow up with their HIV healthcare provider as recommended for nonpregnant adults.

Maternal adherence to ART significantly reduces but does not completely eliminate the risk of transmission of HIV in breast milk. Postnatal HIV transmission can occur despite maternal ART adherence, and patients should be counseled to avoid breastfeeding. There have also been reports of mother-to-child transmission of HIV via mothers pre-masticating food and feeding it to their infants.

Preexposure Prophylaxis of Human Immunodeficiency Virus Infection

Globally, up to 2 million new HIV infections occur per year. It is estimated that up to 40,000 new HIV infections occur annually in the United States. The highest incidence of new HIV infections occur in MSM, especially among young African American males. For uninfected patients with a high risk of HIV acquisition, preexposure prophylaxis (PrEP) is an evidence-based method for preventing infections in those at risk. All sexually active adult and adolescent patients should receive information about PrEP and its role in preventing HIV acquisition. Clinicians should offer to prescribe PrEP to adults and adolescents whose sexual or injection behaviors and epidemiologic context place them at substantial risk of acquiring HIV infection. Available PrEP options include oral tenofovir disoproxil fumarate-emtricitabine (TDF/FTC [Truvada]), oral TAF/FTC (Descovy), and IM CAB (Apretude) (Tables 5 and 6). Efficacy is dependent on medication adherence; PrEP reduces the risk of acquiring HIV from sex by approximately 99% when taken as prescribed.

Before initiating PrEP, it is important to obtain a brief, targeted sexual and drug use history to identify patients likely to benefit from PrEP. The 2021 PrEP guidelines published by the U.S. Public Health Service recommend a dialogue around The "Five Ps": *partners, practices, protection* from sexually transmitted infections (STIs), *past* history of STIs, and *pregnancy* intention. It is important to determine sexual practices with a patient's main sexual partner, casual partners, or any anonymous partners. A drug history over the prior 6 months should be obtained and include injection drug use and sharing of needles. Clinicians should also briefly screen all patients for alcohol use disorder and the use of illicit non-injection drugs (e.g., amyl nitrite, stimulants) because use of these substances may affect sexual risk behavior. Clinicians should also consider the epidemiologic context of patient sexual practices as the risk of HIV acquisition is determined by both the frequency of specific sexual practices and the likelihood that a sex partner has HIV. Communities and populations that have higher HIV prevalence are more likely to lead to HIV exposure, indicating a greater need for risk-reduction methods (e.g., PrEP).

Patients screened for PrEP must be screened for common bacterial STIs, including serologic testing for syphilis and nucleic acid amplification tests for gonorrhea and chlamydia. This includes swabs of the oropharynx in patients who participate in oral sex and anal swabs for recipients of anal intercourse. Screening for trichomonas and bacterial vaginosis are not required before initiating PrEP because they lack strong correlation with HIV coinfection.

HIV testing with confirmed results within 1 week before initiating therapy is required to document that patients do not have HIV when they start taking PrEP medications. Plasma HIV testing with a fourth-generation antibody/antigen (Ab/Ag) test should be obtained to confirm that the patient does not have undiagnosed HIV infection. Additional HIV RNA testing should be performed in patients with signs or symptoms of acute HIV infection in the past 4 weeks, those with indeterminate antigen/antibody test results, and patients with high-risk HIV exposure in the preceding

TABLE 5	Guidance for Daily Oral Preexposure Prophylaxis Use	
	SEXUALLY ACTIVE ADULTS AND ADOLESCENTS	**PERSONS WHO INJECT DRUGS**
Identifying substantial risk of acquiring HIV infection	Anal or vaginal sex in the past 6 months *AND* any of the following: • HIV-positive sexual partner (especially if partner has an unknown or detectable viral load) • Bacterial STI in past 6 months • History of inconsistent or no condom use with sexual partner(s)	HIV-positive injection partner *OR* Sharing injection equipment
Clinically eligible	*All of the following conditions are met:* • Documented negative HIV test result within 1 week before initially prescribing PrEP • No signs/symptoms of acute HIV infection • Estimated creatinine clearance ≥30 mL/min • No contraindicated medications	
Dosage	• Daily, continuing, oral doses of FTC/TDF (Truvada), ≤90-day supply *OR* • For men and transgender women at risk for sexual acquisition of HIV; daily, continuing oral doses of FTC/TAF (Descovy), ≤90-day supply	
Follow-up care	*Follow-up visits at least every 3 months to provide the following:* • HIV Ag/Ab test and HIV-1 RNA assay, medication adherence and behavioral risk reduction support • Bacterial STI screening for MSM and transgender women who have sex with men • Access to clean needles/syringes and drug treatment services for PWID *Follow-up visits every 6 months to provide the following:* • Assess renal function for patients aged ≥50 years or who have an eCrCl <90 mL/min at PrEP initiation • Bacterial STI screening for all sexually active patients *Follow-up visits every 12 months to provide the following:* • Assess renal function for all patients • Chlamydia screening for heterosexually active women and men • For patients on FTC/TAF, assess weight, triglyceride and cholesterol levels	

eCrCl, Estimated creatinine clearance; *HIV,* human immunodeficiency virus; *MSM,* men who have sex with men; *PrEP,* preexposure prophylaxis; *PWID,* persons who inject drugs; *STI,* sexually transmitted infection.
Modified from Preexposure Prophylaxis for the Prevention of HIV Infection in the United States—2021 Update: A Clinical Practice Guideline. U.S. Public Health Service. Available at: https://www.cdc.gov/hiv/pdf/risk/prep/cdc-hiv-prep-guidelines-2021.pdf (Table 1a).

TABLE 6 Guidance for Cabotegravir Injection Preexposure Prophylaxis Use

	SEXUALLY ACTIVE ADULTS AND ADOLESCENTS	PERSONS WHO INJECT DRUGS
Identifying substantial risk of acquiring HIV infection	Anal or vaginal sex in the past 6 months AND any of the following: • HIV-positive sexual partner (especially if partner has an unknown or detectable viral load) • Bacterial STI in past 6 months • History of inconsistent or no condom use with sexual partner(s)	HIV-positive injection partner Sharing injection equipment
Clinically eligible	*All of the following conditions are met:* • Documented negative HIV test result within 1 week before initial CAB injection • No signs or symptoms of acute HIV infection • No contraindicated medications or conditions	
Dosage	• 600 mg CAB (one 3-mL injection in the gluteal muscle) • Initial dose • Second dose 4 weeks after first dose • Every 8 weeks thereafter	
Follow-up care	*At follow-up visit 1 month after first injection:* • HIV Ag/Ab test and HIV-1 RNA assay *At follow-up visits every 2 months (starting with third injection— month 3):* • HIV Ag/Ab test and HIV-1 RNA assay • Access to clean needles/syringes and drug treatment services for PWID *At follow-up visits every 4 months (starting with third injection— month 3):* • Bacterial STI screening for MSM and transgender women who have sex with men *At follow-up visits every 6 months (starting with fifth injection— month 7):* • Bacterial STI screening for all heterosexually active women and men *At follow-up visits every 12 months (after the first injection):* • Assess desire to continue injections for PrEP • Chlamydia screening for heterosexually active women and men *At follow-up visits when discontinuing CAB injections:* • Re-educate patients about the "tail" and the risks during declining CAB levels • Assess ongoing HIV risk and prevention plans • If PrEP is indicated, prescribe daily oral FTC/TDF or FTC/TAF beginning within 8 weeks after last injection • Continue follow-up visits with HIV testing quarterly for 12 months	

CAB, Cabotegravir; *HIV,* human immunodeficiency virus; *MSM,* men who have sex with men; *PrEP,* preexposure prophylaxis; *PWID,* persons who inject drugs; *STI,* sexually transmitted infection.
Modified from Preexposure Prophylaxis for the Prevention of HIV Infection in the United States—2021 Update: A Clinical Practice Guideline. U.S. Public Health Service. Available at: https://www.cdc.gov/hiv/pdf/risk/prep/cdc-hiv-prep-guidelines-2021.pdf. (Table 1b).

4 weeks. Testing for both HIV Ab/Ag and HIV-1 RNA should be obtained at least every 3 months after oral PrEP initiation or every 2 months when CAB injections are given.

TDF/FTC (Truvada) is generally tolerated well by most patients; however, screening for persons at increased risk of adverse effects should be performed before PrEP initiation. TDF is associated with renal and bone toxicity in some patients; serum creatinine should be measured as TDF/FTC is not recommended for PrEP in patients with creatinine clearance less than 60 mL/min. In patients without reduced kidney function but who have risk factors for developing renal disease, urinalysis to document baseline proteinuria can be obtained for monitoring purposes. A different formulation of tenofovir, TAF (tenofovir alafenamide fumarate), has less association with renal and bone toxicity compared with TDF. In the United States, once-daily TAF/FTC (Descovy) can be prescribed for PrEP in high-risk MSM and transgender women, particularly those who have bone or renal contraindications to TDF, including those with a creatinine clearance as low as 30 mL/min. CAB (Apretude), administered IM every 2 months, is another option for PrEP in those at risk for renal toxicity because it may be administered irrespective of renal function.

Screening for undiagnosed HBV infection should be performed via hepatitis B surface antigen, hepatitis B core antibody, and hepatitis B surface antibody. If the patient's serology shows nonimmunity, vaccination against HBV should be pursued, as individuals engaging in high-risk sexual and drug-use behaviors have an increased risk of HBV infection. If the patient's serology reveals chronic HBV, it must be determined whether the patient requires HBV treatment. TDF (Viread) and TAF (Vemlidy) are first-line treatment choices for chronic HBV and can be used for PrEP[1] and treatment of chronic HBV. In those with chronic HBV who do not require HBV treatment, there is a low risk of HBV flare if TDF or TAF is discontinued.

TDF is also associated with decreased bone density; therefore patients considering PrEP should be screened for osteoporosis risk factors. The greatest amount of bone loss has been associated with the first 6 months of treatment. In patients with known osteopenia or osteoporosis, the risk of acquiring HIV versus further bone loss should be considered. Because of a lack of clear benefit, neither baseline nor serial dual-energy x-ray absorptiometry (DEXA) scans are recommended before initiation of PrEP or for PrEP monitoring. Because of lower rates of bone and renal toxicity, TAF or CAB should be considered over TDF in patients with significant risk for bone-related complications.

Providers should offer PrEP with TDF/FTC (Truvada) to women seeking to conceive and to pregnant or breastfeeding women whose sexual partner has HIV, especially when the partner's viral load is detectable or unknown. In patients who are

[1] Not FDA approved for this indication.

pregnant, the risk of acquiring HIV must be considered against the risk of using antiretroviral medication during pregnancy. The 2021 PrEP guidelines published by the U.S. Public Health Service recommend that providers discuss the risks and benefits of all available alternatives for safer conception. Although each case should utilize shared decision making, generally the potential benefit of preventing HIV transmission to an infant during pregnancy outweighs theoretical risk to maternal or infant health.

Initiating Preexposure Prophylaxis

The combination tablet of TDF/FTC (Truvada) or TAF/FTC (Descovy) should be taken once daily for a duration of as long as the infection risk continues. It should be dispensed as a 90-day supply and renewed at each 3-month clinic follow-up. Condom use is encouraged while using PrEP. For patients who are not willing to use condoms consistently, the Centers for Disease Control and Prevention (CDC) recommends condom use to prevent acquisition of HIV (and other STIs) for the first 7 days after starting oral PrEP if engaging in receptive anal sex and 21 days if engaging in receptive vaginal sex. Common side effects of TDF/FTC and TAF/FTC include nausea and vomiting. These symptoms usually improve and resolve within the first 4 weeks of use.

CAB injections (Apretude) also be used for PrEP and may be especially appropriate for patients with significant renal disease, those who have difficulty with adherence to oral PrEP, and those who prefer injections every 2 months to an oral PrEP dosing schedule. CAB is administered as a 600 mg (3 mL) IM injection at baseline and at 1 month, followed by every 2 months thereafter. CAB injections should be administered in a healthcare setting; they should not be self-administered by patients. In studies, an oral CAB (Vocabria) lead-in phase was utilized before beginning IM injections, but this is not required before initiating CAB injections for PrEP unless patients are especially concerned about side effects with the first dose. Common side effects of CAB injections include injection site reactions, such as pain, tenderness, and induration. Over-the-counter pain medication and/or warm compresses or heating pads can be used if needed to manage injection site pain.

Preexposure Prophylaxis Monitoring and Follow-Up

Patients on oral PrEP should have routine follow-up with their prescribing medical provider approximately every 3 months, although some clinicians may wish to schedule contact more frequently at the beginning of PrEP, either by phone or clinic visit. More frequent follow-up should occur for patients with exposures or symptoms of STIs or medication side effects. Patients prescribed CAB for PrEP should return for follow-up visits 1 month after the initial injection and then every 2 months. Recommendations for follow-up screening tests are provided in Tables 5 and 6.

Postexposure Prophylaxis of Human Immunodeficiency Virus Infection

The most effective means to prevent HIV infection include preventing exposure to the virus. In the event that an isolated occupational, sexual, or injection drug–related exposure occurs, postexposure prophylaxis (PEP) can be a second line of defense against HIV acquisition.

Occupational Exposure

Healthcare personnel include all paid and unpaid persons working in a healthcare setting with potential for exposure to infectious materials such as bodily fluids, contaminated medical supplies, or environmental surfaces. In the occupational setting, prevention of exposures to blood and bodily fluids from infected sources is the key to preventing occupationally acquired HIV infection. The overall risk of becoming infected with HIV after inadvertent exposure to body fluids from an HIV-infected patient is low. It is estimated that the average risk for HIV transmission following percutaneous exposure to HIV-infected blood is 0.3% and after mucous membrane exposure is 0.09%. The average risk of HIV transmission following nonintact skin exposure has not

been defined; however, it is estimated to be lower than mucous membrane exposure. Healthcare personnel at the highest risk are those who received an accidental inoculation containing blood from a known HIV-infected source.

Initial Laboratory Evaluation

All patients initiating PEP after potential HIV exposure should be tested for HIV antigens and antibodies at baseline before PEP initiation. If baseline HIV testing indicates existing HIV infection, PEP should not be initiated. Repeat HIV testing should be performed at 4 to 6 weeks and 3 months following the exposure to determine if HIV infection has occurred. Administration of PEP should not be delayed while awaiting the results of HIV testing and can be discontinued if the source patient is found to not have HIV infection. PEP is most effective when taken as soon as possible following exposure.

Initiating Postexposure Prophylaxis/Choosing Appropriate Postexposure Prophylaxis Therapy

PEP is most effective when initiated as soon as possible following the exposure incident. If PEP is delayed, the effectiveness of therapy may be significantly reduced if initiated 72 hours or more following exposure. Initiating therapy after 72 hours might still be considered if the exposure is proven to be of an extremely high risk of transmission.

The current recommendation for PEP therapy is TDF/FTC (Truvada)[1] plus RAL (Isentress)[1] or DTG (Tivicay)[1] for 4 weeks. Overall, this regimen has acceptable tolerability, convenient dosing, and minimal drug interactions. In patients with significant underlying renal disease, an acceptable PEP alternative is zidovudine plus lamivudine (Combivir)[1] in addition to RAL or DTG.

PEP regimens include three (occasionally more) antiretroviral medications. Because of the potential for medication-related side effects, it is important to choose a PEP regimen with a lower toxicity profile to improve patient tolerance and encourage completion of PEP therapy.

HIV PEP should be offered to pregnant or breastfeeding healthcare providers based on the same criteria as any other provider with a similar exposure. Risk of HIV transmission from mother to child during acute HIV infection is increased during pregnancy and breastfeeding.

Additional resources regarding PEP are available (e.g., PEPline at https://nccc.ucsf.edu/clinician-consultation/pep-post-exposure-prophylaxis; 888-448-4911).

[1] Not FDA approved for this indication.

References

Baeten JM, Donnell D, Ndase P, et al: Antiretroviral prophylaxis for HIV prevention in heterosexual men and women, *N Engl J Med* 367(5):399–410, 2012.

Centers for Disease Control and Prevention: *HIV Surveillance Report*, vol.32. http://www.cdc.gov/hiv/library/reports/hiv-surveillance.html, 2019. Published May 2021.

Dominguez KL, Smith DK, Thomas V, et al: *Updated guidelines for antiretroviral postexposure prophylaxis after sexual, injection drug use, or other nonoccupational exposure to HIV-United States, centers for disease control and prevention*, U.S. Department of Health and Human Services, 2016.

Global UNAIDS: *AIDS Update*, 2021. https://www.unaids.org/sites/default/files/media_asset/2021-global-aids-update_en.pdf.

Grant RM, Lama JR, Anderson PL, et al: Preexposure chemoprophylaxis for HIV prevention in men who have sex with men, *N Engl J Med* 363(27):2587–2599, 2010.

Panel on Opportunistic Infections in Adults and Adolescents with HIV. Guidelines for the prevention and treatment of opportunistic infections in adults and adolescents with HIV: recommendations from the Centers for Disease Control and Prevention, the National Institutes of Health, and the HIV Medicine Association of the Infectious Diseases Society of America. Available at https://clinicalinfo.hiv.gov/sites/default/files/guidelines/documents/Adult_OI.pdf.

Kuhar DT, Henderson DK, Struble KA, et al: Updated US Public Health Service guidelines for the management of occupational exposures to human immuno- deficiency virus and recommendations for postexposure prophylaxis, *Infect Control Hosp Epidemiol* 34(9), 2013.

US Public Health Service: Preexposure prophylaxis for the prevention of HIV infection in the United States—2021. https://www.cdc.gov/hiv/pdf/risk/prep/cdc-hiv-prep-guidelines-2021.pdf.

INFECTIOUS MONONUCLEOSIS

Method of
Ben Z. Katz, MD

CURRENT DIAGNOSIS

- The classic triad of acute infectious mononucleosis consists of fever, lymphadenopathy, and pharyngitis.
- The diagnosis of infectious mononucleosis is usually based on the clinical picture, the presence of at least 10% atypical lymphocytes in the peripheral blood, and positive heterophil serology (monospot test).

CURRENT THERAPY

- In most patients, infectious mononucleosis is self-limited and requires only symptomatic treatment.
- Steroids and antiviral therapy have no place in the therapy of uncomplicated acute infectious mononucleosis in healthy persons.

Epidemiology and Risk Factors

One must distinguish between the epidemiology of Epstein-Barr virus (EBV) infection and that of infectious mononucleosis (IM), the most common symptomatic manifestation of primary EBV infection. Almost all adults have been infected with EBV. The symptomatology of primary EBV infection varies with the infected person's age at the time, with younger children usually having inapparent or mild infections. In developing countries and in lower socioeconomic groups in industrialized nations, up to 90% of children acquire primary EBV infection by 6 years of age, and IM frequently never develops. In contrast, in higher socioeconomic groups, only 40% to 50% of adolescents have previously experienced EBV infection. From 10% to 20% of susceptible adolescents and adults contract EBV every year thereafter, with IM developing in about half of these patients.

Pathophysiology

Saliva is the main vehicle for transmission of EBV, a double-stranded DNA herpesvirus. Transmission usually requires direct and prolonged contact with infected oropharyngeal secretions, with salivary exchange being the main mode of transmission. The infection begins with viral replication in oropharyngeal epithelial cells and then spreads to local B lymphocytes, which then disseminate throughout the reticuloendothelial system and induce vigorous T- and NK-cell responses and neutralizing antibodies. The atypical lymphocytes that are produced are mainly suppressor T cells directed against EBV-infected B cells.

It is thought that most of the clinical manifestations of IM are due to these T- and NK-cell responses, which might explain why young children, whose immune responses are incompletely developed, are often asymptomatic with primary EBV infection. It is also possible that viral load determines symptomatology, and, because young adults likely spread more virus via salivary exchange than toddlers, young adults are more likely to be symptomatic. All EBV-seropositive persons shed virus in saliva intermittently throughout their lives. EBV may rarely be spread via blood transfusion or transplantation.

Clinical Manifestations

IM is usually an acute, self-limited, benign lymphoproliferative disease. EBV is responsible for nearly all heterophil-positive and most heterophil-negative cases. Other causes of heterophil-negative mononucleosis include cytomegalovirus, toxoplasmosis, hepatitis A and B, adenovirus, HIV, rubella, and human herpesvirus 6.

The classic triad of IM consists of fever, lymphadenopathy, and pharyngitis. Other typical findings include lymphocytosis with atypical lymphocytes and the presence of heterophil antibodies. After a 4- to 6-week incubation period, the illness begins with a 3- to 5-day prodrome of malaise, headache, and fatigue, typically followed in about half of the cases by onset of the triad. Additional symptoms can include anorexia, nausea, vomiting, periorbital or facial edema, and generalized lymphadenopathy, which is usually symmetrical. Splenomegaly occurs by the second or third week of illness in about half of all cases; rarely, splenic rupture can occur, which very rarely may be fatal. Hepatomegaly occurs in 10% to 15%, with hepatitis occurring in about 5% of cases. Up to 20% of patients have a rash that may be erythematous, maculopapular, morbilliform, scarlatiniform, or urticarial, especially if ampicillin or one of its derivatives has been given. Other symptoms can include arthritis and jaundice.

IM is a self-limited disease in nearly all patients. Median illness duration is 16 days.

Diagnosis

The diagnosis is usually based on the clinical picture, atypical lymphocytosis, and positive heterophil serology. Most adolescents and young adults with IM have most or all of these features, as well as an elevated white blood cell count with a relative lymphocytosis. Atypical lymphocytes generally represent more than 9% to 10% of the white blood cell count. Many infected persons also have mild thrombocytopenia and elevated hepatocellular enzymes. Heterophil antibody positivity is usually measured as a positive monospot test. If IM is suspected and heterophil antibodies are negative, specific titers for EBV, including viral capsid antigen (VCA) IgM and IgG, early antigen (EA), and Epstein–Barr nuclear antigen (EBNA), should be obtained, as well as serologic testing for cytomegalovirus (CMV) and toxoplasmosis, the two most common causes of heterophil-negative infectious mononucleosis. Acute EBV infection is characterized by the presence of IgM and IgG VCA antibodies and EA antibodies and the absence of EBNA antibodies.

Differential Diagnosis

If liver chemistry values are markedly elevated and antibodies against EBV, CMV, and toxoplasmosis are unrevealing, serology for hepatitis A, B, and C should be measured. If risk factors are present, HIV antibodies should be checked. A throat culture is indicated in patients with pharyngitis or tonsillitis because the tonsillitis of acute IM can be indistinguishable from that of group A streptococcal pharyngitis.

Treatment

In most patients, IM is self-limited and requires only symptomatic treatment, including bed rest, acetaminophen (Tylenol, 10–15 mg/kg every 4–6 hours), aspirin (10–15 mg/kg every 4–6 hours), or nonsteroidal antiinflammatory agents such as ibuprofen (Advil, 5–10 mg/kg every 6–8 hours). Saline gargles can be useful in treating a sore throat. In severe cases, meperidine (Demerol, 1–1.5 mg/kg every 3–4 hours) may be required.

Although a short, tapering course of corticosteroid therapy (e.g., a Medrol Dosepak[1]) is often prescribed, there is little evidence for its clinical efficacy, and caution is warranted. Infection is ultimately self-limited in nearly all cases, and rare reports of neurologic or septicemic complications after steroid use have appeared. Long-term immune responses following steroid use appear to be normal. Corticosteroid therapy should, however, be considered for the treatment of severe cases of IM associated with hemolysis, respiratory embarrassment, or thrombocytopenic purpura. The use of corticosteroids in atypical or antibody-negative cases is inappropriate because the diagnosis of lymphoma can then be confounded.

Parenteral administration of acyclovir[1] (Zovirax, 10–20 mg/kg IV every 8 hours) to patients with acute IM secondary to EBV reduces the level of oropharyngeal viral replication; however, replication returns to the previously high levels after cessation of treatment, little or no reduction is seen in the number of EBV-infected B cells in the peripheral circulation, and the drug has little or no effect on the clinical course. Acyclovir administered in high doses orally (20 mg/kg, maximum dose of 800 mg qid for 5

---

[1]Not FDA approved for this indication.

days) is also ineffective. Antiviral therapy is therefore not recommended for acute IM in a normal host.

In immunosuppressed or severely ill patients, however, specific therapy has a role in many cases. For example, etoposide (VePesid)[1], a drug that reduces macrophage activation, is often used in cases of infection-associated hemophagocytic syndrome. In posttransplant lymphoproliferative disorders, first-line therapy is often a reduction in immunosuppression; other options include rituximab[1] (Rituxan, 375 mg/m[2] IV weekly for 4 weeks). Oral leukoplakia in patients with AIDS responds to oral acyclovir[1] (20 mg/kg, maximum dose of 800 mg qid for 20 days), whereas a tapering course of steroids (as recommended earlier) may be used for lymphocytic interstitial pneumonitis (see below).

Monitoring

Quarantine is not indicated. Ampicillin and related drugs should be avoided when treating secondary bacterial complications because of their association with rash in persons with IM. Contact sports should be avoided as long as splenomegaly is still evident because of the rare possibility of splenic rupture, which usually occurs within 3 weeks of onset of IM but has been reported as late as 7 to 10 weeks into the illness.

Complications

Complications of acute IM can be neurologic (seizures, cranial nerve palsies, aseptic meningitis, encephalitis, optic neuritis, transverse myelitis, infectious polyneuritis [Guillain-Barré syndrome], psychosis, Alice in Wonderland syndrome, or acute cerebellar ataxia), hematologic (hemolytic or aplastic anemia, thrombocytopenic purpura, agranulocytosis, or agammaglobulinemia), cardiac (pericarditis or myocarditis), pulmonary (cough or atypical pneumonia), renal (glomerulonephritis, acute kidney failure, or acute interstitial nephritis), or ophthalmologic (conjunctivitis) in nature. In about 10% of adolescents and young adults, fatigue can persist for 6 months or longer, and many of these patients meet the criteria for chronic fatigue syndrome. Young adults with more severe acute IM and certain predisposing symptoms and laboratory findings are more likely to meet criteria for chronic fatigue syndrome 6 months later.

Rare patients have very high titers of EBV antibodies, and a chronic active EBV infection associated with unusual clinical manifestations such as uveitis or lymphoma can occur. EBV is also associated with lymphoproliferative disorders in persons with underlying abnormal immune systems. These include X-linked lymphoproliferative syndrome, in which affected males usually die of acute EBV infection, and the related infection-associated hemophagocytic syndrome, which is most commonly (about 75% of the time) triggered by EBV and seems to be due to an overly exuberant macrophage response to EBV-infected lymphocytes. Transplant recipients can acquire EBV-associated lymphoproliferative disease that can range from an asymptomatic infection to fatal IM or lymphoma. Finally, although not seen much anymore due to combination antiretroviral therapy, patients with AIDS are susceptible to several serious complications of EBV infection, including lymphocytic interstitial pneumonitis, oral leukoplakia, leiomyosarcoma, and lymphoma.

References

Candy B, Hotopf M: Steroids for symptom control in infectious mononucleosis, *Cochrane Database Syst Rev*(3)CD004402, 2006.

Cohen JI, Jaffe ES, Dale JK, et al: Characterization and treatment of chronic active Epstein–Barr virus disease: A 28-year experience in the United States, *Blood* 117:5835–5849, 2011.

Jason LA, Cotler J, Islam MF, Sunnquist M, Katz BZ. Risks for developing ME/CFS in college students following infectious mononucleosis: a prospective cohort study. *Clin Infect Dis* 73:e3740-6, 2021.

Katz BZ: Commentary on "Steroids for symptom control in infectious mononucleosis (Review)" by B Candy and M Hotopf, *Evid Based Child Health* 7:447–449, 2012.

Katz BZ, Reuter C, Lupovitch Y, Gleason Y, McClellan D, Cotler J, Jason LA: A validated scale for assessing the severity of acute infectious mononucleosis, *J Pediatr* 209:130–133, 2019.

Odumade OA, Hogquist KA, Balfour Jr HH: Progress and problems in understanding and managing primary Epstein- Barr virus infections, *Clin Microbiol Rev* 24(1):193–209, 2011.

Rouphael N, Talati NJ, Vaughan C, et al: Infections associated with haemophagocytic syndrome, *Lancet Infect Dis* 7:814–822, 2007.

Soltys K, Green M: Posttransplant lymphoproliferative disease, *Pediatr Infect Dis J* 24:1107–1108, 2005.

INFLUENZA

Method of
Jeffrey A. Linder, MD, MPH

CURRENT DIAGNOSIS

- Influenza should be considered in any patient with respiratory symptoms between October and May in North America.
- The single most important piece of information when considering a diagnosis of influenza is the community prevalence of influenza.
- During influenza outbreaks, sudden onset of fever and cough has a positive predictive value of about 85%.
- Rapid testing should be done with molecular tests (e.g., reverse transcriptase polymerase chain reaction [RT-PCR]), which have a high sensitivity and specificity.

CURRENT THERAPY

- The influenza vaccine is the best means of preventing influenza. The inactivated influenza vaccine is recommended for all persons age 6 months and older.
- Influenza vaccination should be prioritized for essential workers and people at high-risk for influenza or COVID-19 complications.
- The antivirals zanamivir (Relenza) and oseltamivir (Tamiflu) can be used for prophylaxis of influenza in unimmunized patients, in close contacts of infected patients, and during institutional outbreaks of influenza.
- Early antiviral treatment should not be delayed and should be used for patients who are hospitalized; have severe, complicated, or progressive illness; or are at higher risk for complications.
- Antivirals may be prescribed within 48 hours of symptom onset for outpatients not at higher risk for influenza complications.

Influenza is a highly contagious viral infection that should be considered in any patient with respiratory symptoms between October and May in North America. Influenza infects 5% to 20% of the population of the United States in a typical year, sickens 3% to 11% of Americans, and is responsible for up to 810,000 hospitalizations and 61,000 deaths per year. Influenza can range in severity from mild illness to life-threatening disease. Those at highest risk of hospitalization, death, or complications from influenza are children younger than 2 years old, adults older than 65 years, people of any age who have underlying medical conditions or immune compromise, and pregnant women.

Information about influenza changes rapidly. Emergence of severe acute respiratory syndrome coronavirus 2 (SARS-CoV-2) and associated coronavirus disease 2019 (COVID-19) has complicated influenza diagnosis and management. To care optimally for patients with influenza-like illness during the influenza season, clinicians need to keep abreast of updated recommendations and the current prevalence of influenza and COVID-19 in their community. The influenza vaccine remains the best means of reducing the incidence, severity, and complications from influenza, but antiviral medications and symptomatic treatments have an important role in the prevention and treatment of influenza (Box 1).

Microbiology

There are two types of influenza viruses, A and B. Influenza A is separated into subtypes based on two surface antigens: hemagglutinin (H) and neuraminidase (N). The predominant circulating strains of influenza in recent decades have been influenza A (H1N1), influenza A (H3N2), and influenza B. Influenza

A (H3N2) subtypes generally cause more severe influenza and are associated with higher mortality than other types. Influenza viruses undergo slight genetic changes from year to year, termed *antigenic drift*. Major changes in surface glycoproteins are termed *antigenic shift* and can result in severe pandemic influenza in a nonimmune population, which happened with an antigenically novel influenza A (H1N1) virus in 2009. Because of antigenic drift, and because immunity to a given type or subtype of influenza provides limited cross-immunity to other types and subtypes, the influenza vaccine needs to be reformulated and administered most years.

Patients contract influenza by being exposed to small- and large-sized respiratory droplets and aerosols from an infected person or contact with surfaces harboring influenza virus. Influenza has a latency of 1 to 4 days before the onset of symptoms. Adults are infectious from the day before symptom onset through approximately day 7 of illness, but immunosuppressed adults and children shed the virus for longer periods. Symptoms generally last from 7 to 14 days.

Beyond the emergence of SARS-CoV-2 in 2019, several other novel, highly pathogenic respiratory viruses—avian influenza A (H5N1), avian influenza A (H7N9), and Middle East respiratory syndrome coronavirus (MERS-CoV)—have case-fatality rates ranging from 35% to 53%. Collectively there have been more than 5000 human cases. These pathogens, if they acquire the ability to be highly transmissible between humans, have the potential to cause pandemic respiratory disease.

Prevention

Influenza vaccination is between 20% and 90% effective in preventing influenza or complications of influenza. Influenza vaccination is highly cost-effective and can even be cost-saving in high-risk groups. Influenza vaccination is less effective in younger children, in adults older than 65 years, in adults with comorbid conditions, and when there is a poor match between the influenza vaccine and circulating influenza. The Centers for Disease Control and Prevention (CDC) Advisory Committee on Immunization Practices puts out annual recommendations and supplementary updates on the prevention and treatment of influenza (www.cdc.gov/flu). The Advisory Committee on Immunization Practices recommends vaccinating all persons 6 months of age and older.

At present in the United States, there are three commonly administered, recommended types of influenza vaccine: quadrivalent inactivated influenza vaccine (IIV4), quadrivalent recombinant influenza vaccine (RIV4), and quadrivalent live attenuated influenza vaccine (LAIV4). The IIV4 (Afluria Quadrivalent, Fluarix Quadrivalent, FluLaval Quadrivalent, Fluzone Quadrivalent, Flucelvax Quadrivalent, Fluzone High-Dose, Fluad Quadrivalent), adjuvant IV3 (Fluad), and RIV4 (Flublok Quadrivalent) vaccines are administered as an intramuscular injection.

Different products are approved for administration in different lower age limits. A high-dose IIV4 (Fluzone High-Dose Quadrivalent) and an adjuvanted IIV4 (Fluad Quadrivalent) are available for patients aged 65 years or older, who are less likely to respond immunologically to standard inactivated influenza vaccine (IIV). The RIV4 (Flublok Quadrivalent) is only licensed for persons age 18 years or older. The main adverse effect of the IIV is soreness at the injection site. Patients often report a mild immune response of fever, malaise, myalgia, and headache that can last for 1 to 2 days, but rates of most of these symptoms are no different from those in patients who receive placebo injection.

Allergic reactions to egg proteins or other vaccine components (e.g., antibiotics and inactivating compounds) include hives, angioedema, asthma, and anaphylaxis. For patients with egg allergy who have only hives, any otherwise appropriate IIV or RIV can be administered. For patients with more severe reactions to egg or who received treatment for an allergic reaction can also receive any recommended IIV or RIV in an inpatient or outpatient medical setting and observed for at least 15 minutes by a clinician able to recognize and manage severe allergic reactions. The

recombinant influenza vaccine (RIV4; FluBlok Quadrivalent) and cell culture derived quadrivalent (ccIIV4; Flucelvax, Quadrivalent) are considered egg free, but patients who had a severe allergic reaction to a previous dose of an egg-based vaccine should receive ccIIV4 or RIV4 in a supervised inpatient or outpatient setting. Patients who have had severe allergic reaction to influenza vaccine should not receive the vaccine.

Vaccination should be deferred in patients with confirmed or suspected COVID-19 or with any acute febrile illness, but patients with more moderate illness can be vaccinated. Guillain-Barré syndrome was associated with the 1976 swine flu vaccine, but there is no consistent evidence that modern influenza vaccines are associated with Guillain-Barré syndrome.

The LAIV4 (FluMist Quadrivalent) is administered as a nasal spray and is approved for patients ages 2 to 49 years. The LAIV4 is contraindicated in children aged 2 to 4 years with recurrent wheezing or asthma; children who are receiving aspirin or aspirin-containing products; patients with comorbid conditions or immunosuppression; pregnant women; family members or close contacts of severely immunosuppressed patients, who require a protected environment (e.g., hematopoietic stem cell transplant recipients); cerebrospinal leak or cochlear implants; and receipt of oseltamivir (Tamiflu) or zanamivir (Relenza) in the previous 48 hours, peramivir (Rapivab) in the previous 5 days, or baloxavir (Xofluza) in the previous 17 days. The LAIV4 should not be administered to those with severe nasal congestion. Adverse effects of the LAIV4 include runny nose, nasal congestion, headache, sore throat, chills, and tiredness, although these are only slightly more common than in patients receiving placebo. Those receiving the LAIV4 should avoid contact with severely immunosuppressed persons for 7 days.

Patients should be vaccinated in the fall when the seasonal vaccine becomes available, ideally before the end of October. In the event of vaccine shortages, higher-risk patients should receive priority (see Box 1). Patients should continue to be vaccinated until February and beyond because in the majority of recent influenza seasons the peak has been February or later.

BOX 1 | Influenza Vaccine Recommendations.

- All persons aged ≥6 months should be vaccinated annually
- Vaccination efforts should prioritize essential workers and people at higher risk of influenza and COVID-19 complications:
  - Age 6 months to 5 years
  - Age ≥50 years
  - Chronic pulmonary (including asthma), cardiovascular (except hypertension), renal, hepatic, neurologic, hematologic, or metabolic (including diabetes mellitus) disorders
  - Immunosuppressed
  - Pregnant during the influenza season
  - Age 6 months to 18 years old receiving long-term aspirin therapy and who therefore might be at risk for Reye syndrome
  - Residents of nursing homes and other long-term care facilities
  - American Indians/Alaska Natives
  - Morbidly obese (body mass index ≥40)
- Vaccination efforts should also prioritize those likely to transmit influenza to higher risk people:
  - Healthcare personnel
  - Household contacts and caregivers of children aged <5 years and adults aged ≥50 years, with particular emphasis on vaccinating contacts of children aged <6 months
  - Household contacts and caregivers of persons with medical conditions that put them at higher risk for severe complications from influenza

Children 6 months to 8 years of age who have not been previously immunized against influenza should be given two doses separated by at least 4 weeks.

Evaluation

Community Prevalence of Influenza

In caring for a patient with suspected influenza, the single most important piece of data is the community prevalence of influenza among patients with influenza-like illness. This ranges from near 0% during summer months to approximately 30% during a typical influenza seasonal peak. The prevalence may be higher during a particularly severe outbreak. In the United States clinicians can check the local prevalence of influenza and COVID-19 among patients with influenza-like illness through the CDC (www.cdc.gov/flu) and their state department of public health.

History and Physical Examination

Beyond the local prevalence of influenza, the diagnosis of influenza rests on the patient's history. All methods of diagnosing influenza—symptom complexes, clinician judgment, and testing—generally are highly specific but have poor sensitivity. Thus it is important to consider a diagnosis of influenza in any patient with respiratory symptoms during influenza season. Influenza is classically described as the very sudden onset of fever, headache, sore throat, myalgias, cough, and nasal symptoms. Children can also have otitis media, nausea, and vomiting. In differentiating influenza from nonspecific upper respiratory tract infections, it is most useful to consider the circulating prevalence of influenza, the abruptness of onset, and the severity of symptoms. Although COVID-19 and influenza symptoms overlap, COVID-19 may be more likely to include more profound shortness of breath, loss of taste or smell, nausea, vomiting, or diarrhea.

Certain symptom complexes have been shown in trials of antiviral treatment to strongly suggest influenza. For example, in an area with circulating influenza, prior to the emegence of SARS-CoV-2, the acute onset of cough and fever had a positive predictive value as high as 85%. Other studies have shown that clinician judgment performed as well as or better than hard-and-fast symptom complexes or rapid testing.

The physical examination in influenza primarily serves to identify the severity of influenza, complications, and worsening of underlying medical conditions. Clinicians should record vital signs and perform examinations of the ears, nose, sinuses, throat, neck, lungs, and heart for all patients suspected of having influenza.

Testing

Testing may not be required to make a diagnosis of influenza, but can help differentiate influenza from other respiratory viruses. Treatment for patients at high risk for influenza complications should not wait for test results. Testing may also help inform antiviral use, antibiotic prescribing, site-of-care decisions, and infection control measures. Specimens (nasopharyngeal swab, nasal swab, nasal wash, or nasal aspirate, depending on the particular test) should ideally be collected within 3 to 4 days of symptom onset.

Molecular assays such as reverse transcriptase polymerase chain reaction (RT-PCR) testing are highly sensitive (90% to 95%) and specific. Some can produce results in 15 to 45 minutes, and some can differentiate influenza types and subtypes. RT-PCR should be considered for hospitalized patients, institutional outbreaks, or other situations when clinicians are concerned about false-negative rapid test results. Other nucleic acid amplification tests, which can differentiate influenza from other respiratory pathogens, are becoming more available. The CDC recommends that all hospitalized patients with suspected influenza be tested with a high-sensitivity, high-specificity molecular assay.

Rapid influenza diagnostic tests (RIDTs) are much less sensitive (50% to 70%) and somewhat less specific (90%) than molecular tests. Negative results do not exclude the possibility of influenza, especially if the circulating prevalence of influenza is high (>30%). Some RIDTs can distinguish influenza A from influenza B and can provide a point-of-care result in less than 15 minutes.

In the event of a high prevalence of influenza or a high risk of complications from influenza, empiric antiviral treatment is indicated. Testing may be particularly helpful for hospitalized patients to rule out a need for antibiotics, but antiinfluenza treatment should not be withheld solely on the basis of a negative test result. Chest radiography, cultures, and blood tests are not routinely indicated, but they should be obtained for patients with suspected pneumonia or to identify other suspected complications.

Complications

Complications of influenza include primary complications, suppurative complications, and worsening of comorbid conditions. Primary complications of influenza include viral pneumonia, which is a feared complication and is likely a main cause of death in pandemic influenza. Other, less common primary complications of influenza include myositis and rhabdomyolysis, Reye syndrome, myocarditis, pericarditis, toxic shock syndrome, and central nervous system disease (e.g., encephalitis, transverse myelitis, and aseptic meningitis). Children can have a severe course with influenza, including signs and symptoms of sepsis along with febrile seizures. Suppurative complications of influenza include bacterial pneumonia, otitis media, and sinusitis. Influenza can cause worsening of comorbid conditions such as asthma, chronic obstructive pulmonary disease, congestive heart failure, and chronic kidney disease.

Chemoprophylaxis

Antiviral medications can be used to prevent influenza in patients who did not receive the influenza vaccine, cannot receive the influenza vaccine, received the vaccine in the prior 2 weeks (before reliable immunity develops), or in the event of poor matching between vaccine and circulating influenza strains (Table 1). Chemoprophylaxis should also be considered for close contacts of patients with confirmed influenza or for patients with immune deficiency who are unlikely to respond to the influenza vaccine but who are at high risk for having complications from influenza (see Box 1).

Amantadine (Symmetrel) and rimantadine (Flumadine) are not recommended for chemoprophylaxis or treatment because of a high prevalence of resistant influenza A strains. The neuraminidase inhibitors oseltamivir (Tamiflu), and zanamivir (Relenza) are approximately 80% effective in preventing influenza in household contacts of persons with influenza, and more than 90% effective in preventing influenza in institutional settings. Chemoprophylaxis should be taken for 7 days after last known exposure. For hospital or long-term care facility outbreaks, chemoprophylaxis should be taken and for a minimum of 2 weeks or until 1 week after the end of the outbreak. For patients allergic to or unable to respond to the vaccine, chemoprophylaxis should be used for the duration of circulating influenza. The IIV can be given to patients receiving chemoprophylaxis. The LAIV should not be given from 2 days before to 14 days after taking an antiviral medication. Patients who receive the LAIV in this window should be revaccinated at a later date.

Treatment

The influenza vaccine is the best means of reducing influenza-related morbidity and mortality, but its limitations include production problems, low vaccination rates, and variable effectiveness. Given these limitations, there is an important role in management for influenza-specific antiviral medications (see Table 1). Antiviral medications reduce the duration of influenza symptoms by approximately 1 day, reduce complications requiring antibiotics by 30% to 50%, might decrease hospitalizations, decrease mortality among hospitalized patients, and are cost-effective. Early antiviral treatment, which should not wait

ANTIVIRAL AGENT	TREATMENT*		PROPHYLAXIS†		COMMENTS
	CHILDREN	ADULTS	CHILDREN	ADULTS	
Oseltamivir (Tamiflu)	Any age‡ Dose for 5 days bid: <1 year: 3 mg/kg per dose; ≤15 kg: 30 mg; 16–23 kg: 45 mg; 24–40 kg: 60 mg; >40 kg: 75 mg	75 mg PO bid for 5 days	3 months to 1 year: 3 mg/kg/day‡ Dose qd: ≤15 kg: 30 mg; 16–23 kg: 45 mg; 24–40 kg: 60 mg; >40 kg: 75 mg	75 mg PO qd	For patients with creatinine clearance < 30 mL/min, oseltamivir adult dosing should be reduced to 30 mg qd for treatment and to 30 mg qod for prophylaxis
Zanamivir (Relenza)	Approved for children ≥7 years; 10 mg (2 inhalations) bid for 5 days	10 mg (2 inhalations) bid for 5 days	Approved for children ≥5 years; 10 mg (2 inhalations) qd	10 mg (2 inhalations) qd	Avoid in patients with chronic lung disease (e.g., asthma, chronic obstructive pulmonary disease)
Peramivir (Rapivab)	≥6 months: One 12-mg/kg dose, up to 600 mg maximum IV over minimum 15 min	≥13 years: One 600-mg IV dose over a minimum of 15 min	NA	NA	For patients with creatinine clearance 30–49 mL/min, the dose should be reduced to 200 mg; For patients with creatinine clearance 10–29 mL/min, the dose should be reduced to 100 mg
Baloxavir (Xofluza)	≥12 years: <80 kg: one 40-mg dose; ≥80 kg: one 80-mg dose	<80 kg: one 40-mg dose; ≥80 kg: one 80-mg dose	≥12 years: <80 kg: one 40 mg dose ≥80 kg: one 80 mg dose	<80 kg: one 40-mg dose; ≥80 kg: one 80-mg dose	For patients within 2 days of illness onset. Avoid in pregnant women or breastfeeding mothers

*Suspected or confirmed influenza among persons with severe influenza or for persons at higher risk for influenza complications up to 5 days after symptom onset. For outpatients not at higher risk for influenza complications, treatment should be started within 48 hours of symptom onset.
†Prophylaxis should be given for 7 days after last known exposure and for institutional outbreaks for at least 2 weeks or until 1 week after the end of the outbreak.
‡Oseltamivir is approved by the US Food and Drug Administration for treatment in children 14 days and older and prophylaxis in children 1 year and older. Treatment in children <14 days old and prophylaxis in children <1 year old is recommended by the Centers for Disease Control and Prevention and the American Academy of Pediatrics.
IV, Intravenous; *NA*, not approved; *PO*, per os (orally).
Adapted from Centers for Disease Control and Prevention. Influenza Antiviral Medications: Summary for Clinicians. Available at https://www.cdc.gov/flu/professionals/antivirals/index.htm (accessed July 7, 2022).

for test results, starting up to 5 days after symptom onset can reduce complications for patients who are hospitalized; have severe, complicated, or progressive illness; or are at higher risk for complications (see Box 1). For outpatients not at higher risk for complications, antiviral treatment must be started within 48 hours of symptom onset.

Oseltamivir (Tamiflu) is taken as a capsule or oral suspension. The dose of oseltamivir should be reduced in patients with renal disease. Adverse effects of oseltamivir include nausea, vomiting, and perhaps behavioral changes. Oseltamivir, oral or enterically administered, is the drug of choice for hospitalized patients and those with severe illness. Zanamivir (Relenza) is taken as an oral inhaled powder and is not recommended for patients with underlying lung or heart disease. Adverse effects of zanamivir include worsening of underlying lung disease and allergic reactions. Amantadine and rimantadine are not recommended because of a high prevalence of resistant influenza A strains.

Peramivir (Rapivab), an intravenous neuraminidase inhibitor, was approved in the United State in December 2014 for patients within 48 hours of symptom onset. Peramivir has been associated with diarrhea, rashes including Stevens-Johnson syndrome, and neuropsychiatric changes.

Baloxavir (Xofluza), a cap-dependent endonuclease inhibitor, is active against both influenza A and B. Baloxavir has been associated with diarrhea. It has the advantage of requiring only one dose.

Antibiotics are generally not necessary, but they should be prescribed to treat suppurative complications of influenza.

Antitussives such as guaifenesin with codeine (Robitussin AC) help coughing patients to sleep at night. β-Agonists, such as albuterol (Proventil)[1], can help patients with cough, especially if there is wheezing on examination. Analgesics and antipyretics such as acetaminophen (Tylenol) and ibuprofen (Motrin) reduce fever and generally help patients to feel better. Patients should be encouraged to rest and drink plenty of fluids.

Patients with suspected influenza should minimize contact with others to avoid spreading the infection. Use of face masks and hand hygiene can reduce the transmission of influenza.

---

[1]Not FDA approved for this indication.

References

Centers for Disease Control and Prevention: Influenza (Flu): information for health professionals, http://www.cdc.gov/flu/professionals/index.htm. Accessed 7 July 2022.

Ebell MH, Afonso AM, Gonzales R, et al: Development and validation of a clinical decision rule for the diagnosis of influenza, *J Am Board Fam Med* 25:55–62, 2012.

Falsey AR, Murata Y, Walsh EE: Impact of rapid diagnosis on management of adults hospitalized with influenza, *Arch Intern Med* 167:354–360, 2007.

Grohskopf LA, Alyanak E, Ferdinands JM, et al: Prevention and control of seasonal influenza with vaccines: Recommendations of the Advisory Committee on Immunization Practices — United States, 2021–22 Influenza Season, *MMWR Recomm Rep* 2021;70(No. RR-5):1–28. DOI: http://dx.doi.org/10.15585/mmwr.rr7005a1.

Tokars JI, Olsen SJ, Reed C: Seasonal incidence of symptomatic influenza in the United States, *Clin Infect Dis* 66:1511–1518, 2018.

LEISHMANIASIS

Method of
Luigi Gradoni, PhD

CURRENT DIAGNOSIS

- Infected tissues must be sampled for microscopy demonstration of *Leishmania* organisms in Giemsa-stained impression smears or cultures. Polymerase chain reaction (PCR) detection of *Leishmania* DNA increases diagnostic sensitivity.
- Different tissue samplings are performed depending on the clinical form of leishmaniasis: For visceral leishmaniasis, aspirate or biopsy specimens are obtained from spleen, bone marrow, the liver, or enlarged lymph nodes. For cutaneous and mucocutaneous leishmaniasis, the material is obtained by skin lesion scraping or biopsy.
- Serology is useful when the diagnosis of visceral leishmaniasis proves difficult with other methods.

CURRENT THERAPY

- The therapy of leishmaniasis relies on a limited number of drugs, most of which are old and relatively toxic. Systemic drug administration requires hospitalization and monitoring of the patient.
- The pentavalent antimony (Sb) drugs sodium stibogluconate (Pentostam)[10] and meglumine antimoniate (Glucantime)[2] are equivalent and used in all clinical forms of leishmaniasis. Dosage is Sb 20 mg/kg/day IM for 21 to 28 days. In cases of uncomplicated cutaneous leishmaniasis, use intralesional administration intermittently over 20 to 30 days.
- Liposomal amphotericin B (Ambisome) is the gold standard for treating visceral leishmaniasis. Dosage: Total dose of 18 to 21 mg/kg IV using one of the following schedules: 3 mg/kg/day on days 1 to 5 and 10; 3 mg/kg on days 1 to 5, day 14, and day 21; 10 mg/kg/day for 2 days.
- Amphotericin B desoxycholate (Fungizone) is used in visceral leishmaniasis[1] and mucocutaneous leishmaniasis. Dosage is 0.5 mg/kg IV every other day for 14 days.
- Other parenteral drugs: Pentamidine isethionate (Pentam 300)[1] is used to treat some forms of New World cutaneous leishmaniasis; dosage is 2 mg/kg IM every other day for 7 days. Paromomycin (aminosidine) sulfate[2] is used for Indian visceral leishmaniasis; dosage is 11 mg/kg/day IM for 21 days.
- Miltefosine (Impavido)[5] is recommended for visceral leishmaniasis therapy in India and Ethiopia and for cutaneous leishmaniasis therapy in Colombia and Bolivia. Dosage is 2.5 mg/kg/day (not exceeding 100 mg/day) PO for 28 days.

[1]Not FDA approved for this indication.
[2]Not available in the United States.
[5]Investigational drug in the United States.
[10]Available in the United States from the Centers for Disease Control and Prevention.

Epidemiology

Leishmaniases are diseases caused by members of the genus *Leishmania*, protozoan parasites infecting numerous mammal species, including humans. The flagellated forms (promastigotes) are transmitted by the bite of phlebotomine sand flies and multiply as aflagellated forms (amastigotes) within cells of the mononuclear phagocyte system. The diseases range over the intertropical zones of America and Africa and extend into temperate regions of Latin America, Southern Europe, and Asia. About 20 named *Leishmania* species and subspecies are pathogenic for humans, and 30

sand fly species are proven vectors. Each parasite species circulates in natural foci of infection where susceptible phlebotomines and mammals coexist. The epidemiology and clinical manifestations of the diseases are largely diverse, being usually grouped into two main entities: zoonotic leishmaniases, where domestic or wild animal reservoirs are involved in the transmission cycle and humans play a role of accidental host, and anthroponotic leishmaniases, where humans are the sole reservoir and source of the vector's infection.

Visceral leishmaniasis (VL) is caused by *Leishmania donovani* in the Indian subcontinent and East Africa (anthroponotic entity) and by *L. infantum (L. chagasi)* in the Mediterranan basin, parts of Central Asia, and Latin America (a zoonotic entity with domestic dogs acting as the main reservoir host). Several species of *Leishmania* cause cutaneous leishmaniasis (CL) or mucocutaneous (MCL) leishmaniasis. The most common are *L. major* (rural zoonotic entity) and *L. tropica* (urban anthroponotic entity) in the Old World and *L. mexicana, L. braziliensis, L. amazonensis, L. panamensis, L. guyanensis,* and *L. peruviana* (sylvatic zoonotic entities) in the New World.

Globally, 80 Old World and 21 New World countries are endemic for human leishmaniasis, with an estimated yearly incidence of 0.7 million to 1.2 million cases of CL forms and 0.2 million to 0.4 million cases of VL forms. Overall estimated prevalence is 12 million people with a disability-adjusted life years burden of 860,000 for men and 1.2 million for women. The disease affects the poorest people in the poorest countries: 72 are developing countries, of which 13 are among the least developed. The incidence is not uniformly distributed in endemic areas: 90% of CL cases are found in only seven countries (Afghanistan, Algeria, Brazil, Iran, Peru, Saudi Arabia, and Syria), whereas 90% of VL cases occur in rural and suburban areas of five countries (Bangladesh, India, Nepal, Sudan, and Brazil). These figures, however, must be regarded as underestimates; currently, it appears that the global incidence of human leishmaniases is higher than before, owing to environmental and human behavioral factors contributing to the changing landscape of these diseases.

Risk Factors

Risk factors for leishmaniasis are primarily associated with geographically and temporally defined human exposure to phlebotomine vectors. In the Old World, colonization and urbanization of desert areas have been identified as the major risk factor for outbreaks of zoonotic CL. Tourists and military personnel are often exposed to *L. major* or *L. tropica* infections in rural or urban endemic settings of North African and Middle Eastern countries. In the New World, the colonization of the primary forest associated with activities of deforestation, road building, mining, and tourism is responsible for the domestication of sylvatic cycles of CL and MCL agents. Increase in density and geographic range of phlebotomine vectors resulting from climate changes, together with the increased mobility of infected pet dogs, has been identified as a cause of northward spreading of zoonotic VL in Europe.

Individual risk factors play a major role in VL disease. Most of the *L. donovani* and *L. infantum* infections are asymptomatic or subclinical in well-nourished immunocompetent persons. Malnourished persons, infants younger than 2 years, and severely immunosuppressed adults are at high risk for acute VL when exposed to infection. Before the era of HAART (highly active antiretroviral therapy), the AIDS epidemics in southern Europe caused more than 2000 HIV and VL co-infection cases among men aged 39 years on average. Other conditions have been reported that influence the clinical outcome of VL, such as immunosuppressive therapies after organ transplantation, corticosteroid and anti–tumor necrosis factor α (TNF-α) treatments for immunologic disorders, hematologic neoplasia, and chronic conditions of hepatic cirrhosis. However, most acute VL episodes in adults remain unexplained. Other factors associated with impaired immune response to *Leishmania* (e.g., genetic factors) are probably involved.

Pathophysiology

Ingestion of metacyclic promastigotes inoculated by the vector in the skin is mediated by several types of receptors found in resident macrophages, monocytes, neutrophils, and dendritic cells. *Leishmania* lipophosphoglycan, the most abundant surface glycoconjugate, is the main factor of virulence. Once in the cell phagolysosome, amastigotes survive from hydrolase activity through pH acidification while selectively inhibiting production of reactive oxygen species. Multiplication of parasites, infection of new cells, and dissemination to tissues are contrasted by the host's inflammatory and specific immune responses. Even in most susceptible natural mammal hosts, most infections are efficiently controlled, giving rise to asymptomatic latent infections. Leishmaniases have typical immunologic polarity: Cure or control are associated with robust cellular immune responses driven by production of interleukin (IL) 12, whereas acute or chronic diseases are characterized by the absence of such responses and the presence of high levels of nonprotective serum antibodies, a condition often associated with high levels of IL-10 production. In spite of this polarity, analysis of cytokine patterns in tissues reveals a less-polar situation, as both T_H1 and T_H2 cytokines were found to be secreted in specimens from tissues infected with CL, MCL, and VL.

Prevention

There are no human vaccines available for the immune protection against leishmaniasis. Promising data on safety and immunogenicity have been provided for the only *Leishmania* candidate vaccine under development, consisting of the recombinant polyprotein antigen LEISH-F1 with MPL-SE as adjuvant. Preventive measures are thus limited to the individual protection from sand fly bites or to community protection through reservoir control. Individual protection is through the use of repellents or insecticide-impregnated nets. Reservoir control measures are largely diverse, depending on the epidemiologic entity of leishmaniasis. Examples related to zoonotic entities with synanthropic reservoir hosts are the destruction of rodent populations around human dwellings (e.g., to control zoonotic CL due to *L. major*) and the fight against canine infections through the mass use of topical insecticides or drug treatments (e.g., to control zoonotic VL due to *L. infantum*). Early diagnosis and treatment of human cases is the main control measure against anthroponotic entities of VL (*L. donovani*) and CL (*L. tropica*).

Clinical Manifestations

Visceral Disease

VL, also known as kala-azar, results from the multiplication of *Leishmania* in the phagocytes of the reticuloendothelial system. In endemic settings, the ratio of incident asymptomatic infections to incident clinical cases varies from 4:1 to 50:1 depending on the epidemiologic type (anthroponotic VL is normally more virulent) and the poverty of the affected country. Classic VL manifests as pallor, fever, and hard splenomegaly; hepatomegaly is less common. Laboratory findings document pancytopenia and hypergammaglobulinemia. The clinical incubation period ranges from 3 weeks (exceptional) to more than 2 years, but 4 to 6 months is average. Patients report a history of fever resistant to antibiotics; on physical examination, the spleen is typically appreciated 5 to 15 cm below the left costal margin. Symptomatic VL is 100% fatal when left untreated.

Cutaneous Disease

CL results from multiplication of *Leishmania* in the phagocytes of the skin. In the classic course of the disease, lesions appear first as papules, advance slowly to nodules or ulcers, and then spontaneously heal with scarring over months to years. The clinical incubation period ranges from 1 week (exceptional) to several months; lesions caused by *L. major* and *L. mexicana* tend to evolve and resolve quickly, whereas those caused by *L. braziliensis*, *L. tropica*, and dermotropic strains of *L. infantum* can have longer periods of incubation and spontaneous healing.

Mucosal Disease

MCL results from parasitic metastasis in the nasal mucosal that eventually extends to the oropharynx and larynx. It can develop from CL lesions caused by *L. braziliensis* and *L. panamensis*. Typically, MCL evolves slowly (3 years on average) and does not heal spontaneously.

Diagnosis

The standard diagnosis method for all forms of leishmaniasis is still the microscopy demonstration of *Leishmania* organisms in Giemsa-stained impression smears or cultures from samples of infected tissues. In general, sensitivity increases when both staining and culture are performed. Polymerase chain reaction (PCR) detection of *Leishmania* DNA on samples further increases the diagnostic sensitivity and also might allow species identification by target DNA sequencing or restriction fragment length polymorphism analysis.

Different tissue samplings must be performed depending on the clinical form of leishmaniasis. For VL, aspirate or biopsy specimens are obtained from the spleen, bone marrow, the liver, or enlarged lymph nodes. Higher diagnostic yields are obtained with spleen aspirates (more than 98%), although bone marrow aspirates (80% to 98% of yield) are usually preferred. For CL and MCL, material is obtained by scraping tissue juice from a nodular lesion or from the edge of an ulcer or by taking punch biopsies of inflamed tissue. Diagnostic yields of about 80% are obtained with impression smears and cultures during the first half of the natural course of the lesion. After that, standard parasitologic diagnosis becomes more difficult and PCR remains the only reliable method.

Serology is useful when the diagnosis of VL proves difficult with other methods. Commercially available dipstick tests using recombinant antigen K39 can be used in decisions for or against treatment. Negative serology results are common in CL and MCL, as well as in VL when patients are severely immunosuppressed.

Differential Diagnosis

Visceral Disease

The differential diagnosis depends on the local disease pattern associated with endemic areas. In many of them it includes chronic malaria, disseminated histoplasmosis, hepatosplenic schistosomiasis, typhoid fever, brucellosis, tuberculosis, endocarditis, relapsing fever, and African trypanosomiasis. Other cosmopolitan diseases include syphilis, lymphomas, chronic myeloid leukemia, sarcoidosis, malignant histiocytosis, and liver cirrhosis.

Cutaneous Disease

A typical history of CL—an inflammatory, slowly developing, and painless skin lesion associated with recent exposure to sand fly bites—can strongly support a clinical diagnosis of disease. However, there is an extensive differential diagnosis, which includes acute or chronic forms of CL. For the former, insect bites, furuncular myiasis, and bacterial tropical ulcers are the most common; for the latter, keloid, lupus vulgaris, discoid lupus erythematosus, and sarcoidosis.

Treatment

The therapy of leishmaniasis relies on a limited number of drugs, most of which are old and relatively toxic compounds. Systemic drug administration requires hospitalizing and monitoring the patient.

Pentavalent Antimonials

Organic salts of pentavalent antimony (Sb) are still the mainstay therapy for all clinical forms of leishmaniasis. Two preparations are available that are equal in efficacy and toxicity when used in equivalent Sb doses: sodium stibogluconate (Pentostam),[10] available in English-speaking countries, and meglumine antimoniate (Glucantime),[2] available in Southern Europe and Latin America.

[2]Not available in the United States.
[10]Available in the United States from the Centers for Disease Control and Prevention.

The recommended dosage of Sb is 20 mg/kg/day for 21 to 28 days, given intramuscularly or intravenously. Treatment should be prolonged for 40 to 60 days in areas with documented Sb-resistant VL (e.g., in Bihar State, India). The drugs can be administered intralesionally in cases of uncomplicated CL, intermittently over 20 to 30 days. Systemic toxicity caused by the antimonials relates to the total dose administered and includes anorexia, pancreatitis, and changes on electrocardiography (e.g., prolongation of the QT interval), which can precede dangerous arrhythmias.

Amphotericin B Drugs

Liposomal amphotericin B (Ambisome) is the current gold standard for VL treatment, being highly effective and nontoxic. However, the high cost of the drug precludes its use in developing countries where leishmaniasis is endemic. Liposomal amphotericin B is given intravenously at the total dose of 18 to 21 mg/kg, with various treatment schedules similarly effective: 3 mg/kg/day on days 1 to 5 and 10; 3 mg/kg on days 1 to 5, 14, and 21; or 10 mg/kg/day for 2 days.

Amphotericin B desoxycholate (Fungizone) is a relatively toxic compound used in Sb-resistant VL[1] and MCL, administered intravenously at the low dosage of 0.5 mg/kg every other day for 14 days. Doses in excess of 1 mg/kg/day commonly result in severe infusion-related side effects (fever, chills, and bone pain) and delayed side effects (toxic renal effects).

Other Parenteral Drugs

Other parenteral drugs include old second-line drugs whose use is limited. Pentamidine isethionate (Pentam 300)[1] is a toxic compound used to treat some forms of New World CL resistant to Sb therapy and is given intramuscularly at the low dose of 2 mg/kg every other day for 7 days. Treatment in excess of this dosage can result in common side effects such as myalgias, nausea, headache, and hypoglycemia. Paromomycin (aminosidine) sulfate injection[2] (manufactured by Gland Pharma, India, on behalf of Institute of One World Health) is an old aminoglycoside that is being reevaluated as a first-line drug for Indian VL. It is given intramuscularly at the dose of 11 mg base per kg per day for 21 days. Elevation of alanine aminotranferease (ALT) and aspartate aminotransferase (AST) liver enzymes is usually seen during therapy.

Miltefosine, the First Oral Drug for Leishmaniasis

Miltefosine (Impavido)[5] is a hexadecylphosphocholine originally developed as an anticancer agent. It is the first recognized oral treatment for leishmaniasis and is available in Germany and India. So far, it is recommended for VL therapy in India and Ethiopia and for CL therapy in Colombia and Bolivia. The drug is administered at 2.5 mg/kg/day (not exceeding 100 mg/day) for 28 days. Miltefosine administration does not require the patient to be hospitalized for monitoring. Mild gastrointestinal toxicity may be common. The drug is contraindicated in pregnancy.

Monitoring

In VL patients, fever recedes by day 3 to 5 of treatment, and well-being returns by the first week. Hematologic indices start to improve during the second week. Hemoglobin, serum albumin, and body weight are the most useful indicators of progress. The spleen tends to normalize 1 to 2 months after the end of therapy, although it can take up to 1 year to regress completely. Parasitologic assessment of cure is not normally necessary. Relapses can occur after apparent clinical cure from 2 to 8 months after treatment has been discontinued.

In CL patients, clinical response to drugs is rapid, but complete reepithelialization of lesions is observed in only one third of patients by the end of 3- to 4-week treatment courses.

---

[1]Not FDA approved for this indication.
[2]Not available in the United States.
[5]Investigational drug in the United States.

References

Alvar J, Aparicio P, Aseffa A, et al: The relationship between leishmaniasis and AIDS: The second 10 years, *Clin Microbiol Rev* 21:334–359, 2008.

Alvar J, Vélez ID, Bern C: Leishmaniasis worldwide and global estimates of its incidence, *PLoS One* 7:e35671, 2012.

Aronson N, Herwaldt BL, Libman L, et al: Diagnosis and treatment of leishmaniasis: clinical practice guidelines by the Infectious Diseases Society of America (IDSA) and the American Society of Tropical Medicine and Hygiene (ASTMH), *Clin Infect Dis* 63:e202–e264, 2016.

Berman JJ: Treatment of leishmaniasis with miltefosine: 2008 status, *Expert Opin Drug Metab Toxicol* 4:1209–1216, 2008.

Bern C, Adler-Moore J, Berenguer J, et al: Liposomal amphotericin B for the treatment of visceral leishmaniasis, *Clin Infect Dis* 43:917–924, 2006.

Bhattacharya SK, Sinha PK, Sundar S, et al: Phase 4 trial of miltefosine for the treatment of Indian visceral leishmaniasis, *J Infect Dis* 196:591–668, 2007.

Chappuis F, Sundar S, Hailu A, et al: Visceral leishmaniasis: what are the needs for diagnosis, treatment and control? *Nat Rev Microbiol* 5:873–882, 2007.

González U, Pinart M, Rengifo-Pardo M, et al: Interventions for cutaneous and mucocutaneous leishmaniasis, *Cochrane Database Syst Rev* (2), 2009, CD004834.

Gradoni L, Soteriadou K, Louzir H, et al: Drug regimens for visceral leishmaniasis in Mediterranean countries, *Trop Med Int Health* 13:1272, 2008.

Gramiccia M, Gradoni L: The current status of zoonotic leishmaniases and approaches to disease control, *Int J Parasitol* 35:1169–1180, 2005.

Sundar S, Agrawal N, Arora R, et al: Short-course paromomycin treatment of visceral leishmaniasis in India: 14-day vs 21-day treatment, *Clin Infect Dis* 49:914–918, 2009.

LEPROSY

Method of
Carolina Talhari, MD, PhD; Maria Lucia Penna, MD, PhD; and Gerson O. Penna, MD, PhD

CURRENT DIAGNOSIS

- Contact of susceptible person with untreated leprosy cases; travel to or residence in a leprosy-endemic country
- Skin lesion(s) with altered sensation
- Thickened or enlarged peripheral nerve, with sensory loss and/or weakness in the muscles supplied by the nerve
- Presence of acid-fast bacilli in a slit skin smear
- Skin biopsy with the presence of acid-fast bacilli or typical lesions, thereby aiding disease classification

CURRENT THERAPY*

Paucibacillary Leprosy (6 Months)
Adult (50–70 kg)
- Dapsone: 100 mg daily
- Rifampin (Rifadin)[1]: 600 mg once a month under supervision
- Clofazimine (Lamprene): 50 mg daily and 300 mg once a month under supervision

Child (younger than 10 years)
- Dapsone: 1 mg/kg daily
- Rifampin[1]: 10 mg/kg once a month under supervision
- Clofazimine: 1 mg/kg/day

Multibacillary Leprosy (12 Months)
Adult (50–70 kg)
- Dapsone: 100 mg daily
- Rifampin (Rifadin)[1]: 600 mg once a month under supervision
- Clofazimine (Lamprene): 50 mg daily and 300 mg once a month under supervision

Child (under younger than 10 years)
- Dapsone: 1 mg/kg daily
- Rifampin: 10 mg/kg once a month under supervision
- Clofazimine: 1 mg/kg/day

---

*As recommended by the World Health Organization (WHO).
[1]Not FDA approved for this indication.

Epidemiology

Leprosy is a chronic disease caused by *Mycobacterium leprae* that affects skin and nerves, often resulting in physical disabilities. The disease has been found around the world, showing that transmission occurs regardless of climate.

Disease transmission has ceased in nearly all developed nations, most likely because of better nutrition and socioeconomic development. Currently, new autochthonous cases are found in all tropical countries, with India, Brazil and Indonesia having the highest number of cases annually. Some insular countries located in the Pacific and Indian Oceans have the highest rates of new case detection, indicating a high risk of transmission. In 2020, there was a reduction of 27.7% in the global leprosy registered prevalence and 37.1% in the new cases detection rate compared with 2019. According to the World Health Organization (WHO), this decrease is probably caused by less detection and reporting during the coronavirus disease 2019 (COVID-19) pandemic.

In the Gulf region of the United States, mostly in the states of Louisiana and Texas, native cases are still diagnosed. There are armadillos *(Dasypus novemcinctus)* in the area that have been infected with strains of *M. leprae* found also in autochthonous human cases. This suggests that leprosy might be a regional zoonosis, even though *M. leprae* was introduced into the Americas by Europeans and Africans. There are also records of *M. leprae* infection in armadillos in Central and South America. Furthermore, cases in African chimpanzees raise the possibility that these animals could be helping maintain leprosy transmission in Africa.

The mechanisms of leprosy transmission are not well known because there is no easy way to diagnose infection. It is presumed that in endemic areas, infection is much more frequent than actual disease onset. The incubation period can vary from a few months to more than 10 years, with an average of 2 to 5 years for paucibacillary (PB) leprosy and 5 to 10 years for multibacillary (MB) leprosy.

It is known that MB cases excrete large numbers of viable bacilli through nasal mucus, suggesting that transmission may be by respiratory route; in fact, this is believed to be the main source of transmission. Because *M. leprae* can be eliminated from ulcerated skin lesions, breast milk, urine, and feces, and it remains viable in the environment for many days, especially in humid climates, it is possible to theorize the existence of many different forms of transmission. The role of insects as vectors of bacilli is arguable.

Leprosy cases are not uniformly distributed in a community but tend to form clusters within different geographic regions, villages, or groups of domiciles. In most countries, cases are more common among men, and the 15- to 29-year-old age group tends to present the highest risk of disease. In areas where transmission is decreasing, the incidence tends to be higher among older adults, affecting those who lived during a period with a higher risk of infection.

Until recently, *M. leprae* was the only agent responsible for leprosy. In 2008, a new species called *Mycobacterium lepromatosis* sp. was described in Mexico as responsible for a diffuse form of the disease associated with increased morbidity and mortality. However, the clinical significance of this new entity, both in magnitude and in distribution, as well as particularities of the immune response to this pathogen, are not well known.

Risk Factors

In endemic areas, the main risk factors are a history of household contact with leprosy cases and low socioeconomic status. It is estimated that home contacts of patients with MB leprosy show a 5 to 10 times increased risk of becoming ill; PB leprosy case contacts present a 2 to 3 times increased risk compared with a group with no history of home exposure. In general, the increased risk between contacts reflects the proximity of these individuals, inside the house, with the potential source of infection. Also important is the sharing of other factors by household members, such as genetic markers, behavior, diet, intercurrent infections, and contextual aspects related to socioeconomic and environmental conditions.

An important fact in leprosy is that, even when living for a long time and in the same house with an untreated MB leprosy patient, most people do not get sick. It is estimated that 90% of the population have natural defenses against *M. leprae*. Today, there is evidence that susceptibility and resistance to *M. leprae* are genetically determined. The low frequency of genetically determined susceptibility may be the cause of the wide difference between infection and disease that is believed to exist.

Recent studies confirmed the association between risk of incident leprosy and socioeconomic factors as demonstrated by the Norwegian study almost a century ago.

Prevention

Vaccination with bacille Calmette-Guerin (BCG)[1] reduces the risk of leprosy, with studies showing a variable efficacy of 20% to 80%. The revaccination of household contacts also provides protection, especially against the MB forms of the disease.

Chemoprophylaxis of contacts or high-risk groups with a single dose of rifampin (Rifadin)[1] has been shown to be effective for a period of 2 years. However, although the chemoprophylaxis trials reported a benefit, the relatively short duration of protection indicates functional limitations.

Combined strategies, including the active search for leprosy cases in the communities, integration of rapid diagnostic tests to facilitate the detection of early or asymptomatic cases, as well as both chemoprophylaxis and immunization, is suggested as an active control strategy with a great potential of reducing the incidence of leprosy.

Improving socioeconomic conditions in the general population in endemic areas is also a very effective strategy for disease control. This can be seen when comparing the current epidemiologic situation in the Hawaiian islands with Micronesia or the Marshall islands, where leprosy continues with a high incidence rate.

Pathophysiology

M. leprae is an intercellular microorganism with a specific tropism for skin and peripheral nerve cells. It cannot be cultivated in vitro, but can be inoculated in mouse footpads and armadillos, although growth is quite slow. Active *M. leprae* infection is characterized by a wide clinical range, varying from a disease in which few bacilli are present in the body to one in which a high bacterial load is found in skin lesions.

Upon entering the organism, *M. leprae*, through its pathogen-associated molecular patterns (PAMPs), is recognized by pattern recognition receptors (PRRs) expressed in antigen-presenting cells (APCs), mainly dendritic cells (DCs), macrophages, monocytes, fibroblasts, and Schwann cells. Thus, the innate immune response of the host is initiated, in which a local inflammatory response can eliminate the bacilli, avoiding the disease, or when this does not occur, the innate immunity can regulate the response of host adaptive immunity according to the pattern of cytokines produced by APCs.

In adaptive immunity, the bacilli multiply within macrophages, enter the lymph stream and bloodstream, reach the regional lymph nodes, and from there move on to the organs of the mononuclear phagocyte system. The mycobacterial antigens are then processed and presented by APCs that can be Langerhans cells, DCs, or others from the monocyte-macrophage system that induce the hapten-protein conjugates to link the HLA-DR class II molecules to the CD4 T lymphocytes. In patients in whom there is stimulation of the T-helper 1 cell response, these lymphocytes will produce interferon (IFN)-gamma cytokines, tumor necrosis factor (TNF-α), interleukin-2 (IL-2), IL-17, IL1-β, and IL-12, which will promote the differentiation of macrophages in epithelioid cells that will undergo a fusion process resulting in giant cells. This inflammatory response will be sufficient to reduce *M. leprae* in the tuberculoid form of leprosy. In the presence of massive tissue infiltration by CD4 T lymphocytes, large production of these cytokines occurs along with the chemokine CXCL-10, leading to edema and tissue inflammation of the leprosy type 1 reaction. The production of TNF-α and IFN-γ by Schwann cells will lead to neural damage, which is also more significant in the type 1 reaction.

---

[1] Not FDA approved for this indication.

On the other hand, in the presence of stimulation of the TH2 subpopulation of T lymphocytes, these will produce the cytokines IL-4, IL-5, IL-6, IL-13, TNF-α, IL-10, and TGF-β, the latter two produced by regulatory T lymphocytes (T-regs). TGF-β, IL-4, and IL-10 are suppressors of macrophage activation, leading to an insufficient immune cell response to combat the level of *M. leprae* proliferation within the macrophages. This characterizes the more infectious forms of the disease at the lepromatous end of the spectrum. The cytokines IL-4, IL-5, IL-6, and IL-13 activate plasma cells and B lymphocytes, which together with complement activation, will form the immunocomplexes that will trigger leprosy type 2 reactions.

Clinical Manifestations

Because of the complexity of the parasite-host relation and the variable efficacy of the host's cellular immune response, the clinical manifestations of the disease cross a wide spectrum. This can vary from an isolated nerve lesion or a single skin patch to a systemic disease with the presence of nodules or tubercles, generally on the face. The disease can affect several organs beyond skin and nerves, including eyes, testicles, and kidneys.

Ridley and Jopling, in 1966, proposed a case classification system that takes into consideration clinical, bacteriologic, histopathologic, and immunologic parameters: tuberculoid leprosy (TL), borderline-tuberculoid leprosy (BTL), borderline-borderline leprosy (BBL), borderline-lepromatous leprosy (BLL), and lepromatous leprosy (LL). Indeterminate leprosy (IL) can be considered the first clinical manifestation of the disease. Indeterminate leprosy can resolve spontaneously or evolve into one of the other clinical forms.

Indeterminate Leprosy

This is characterized by one or more hypochromic macules with imprecise borders and reduced thermal sensitivity, although pain and tactile sensation may be preserved (Figure 1). These may occur as areas of sensory disturbance with no alteration in skin color, sweat glands, or hair growth. Any alteration in nerve function is preliminary, therefore there are no physical disabilities described with this classification. Bacilloscopic readings are negative.

Tuberculoid Leprosy

This type is characterized by erythematous or hypochromic skin lesions with clear, raised borders (Figure 2). These are limited in number with an asymmetrical distribution and altered thermal sensation. Pain and tactile sensation may also be altered. Reduced perspiration and restricted partial or full alopecia may also be seen. Nerves can be affected intensively, but this usually only happens to a few. Slit skin smear results are negative.

Figure 1 Indeterminate leprosy.

Figure 2 Tuberculoid leprosy in a child.

Figure 3 Borderline-tuberculoid leprosy.

Among children, TL lesions may have the appearance of nodules or tubercles, generally only one on the face, named *nodular benign leprosy of childhood*. Although these lesions tend to regress spontaneously, treatment should continue as per standard ethical practice.

Borderline-Tuberculoid Leprosy

This form is characterized by lesions similar to those seen at the TL end of the spectrum, although they are more numerous. In general, there are more than five lesions with a diameter of 10 cm or more, less clearly defined borders, and containing possible satellite lesions (Figure 3). These lesions tend to be more symmetrical and several nerves may be affected. However, most patients with this disease type will still have a negative bacilloscopy.

Borderline-Borderline Leprosy

This is a relatively rare variation, given that it commonly evolves quickly toward the lepromatous pole, often spurred on by reaction episodes. There are usually many foveal lesions (infiltrated plaques with expanding outer borders and well-defined inner borders with apparently normal skin in the middle) (Figure 4). Generally, nerves are intensively affected, and skin smears are almost always positive.

Borderline-Lepromatous (Virchowian) Leprosy

A wide number of lesions are present with a range of possible clinical manifestations (infiltrations, papules, plaques, foveae, and nodules) that are common to the lepromatous form. However, with this type there is a tendency to see some delimitation

Figure 4 Borderline-borderline leprosy.

Figure 5 Lepromatous (Virchowian) leprosy.

between the lesions and areas of healthy skin. Bacilloscopy is positive with a high bacterial load.

Lepromatous (Virchowian) Leprosy
This form has the highest bacterial burden of human bacterial infections. Extensive lesions tend to be symmetrical, erythematous, infiltrated, and without clear delineation from normal skin areas. Simple lesions evolve to become papules, tubercles, and nodules that can eventually ulcerate and that are especially full of bacilli (Figure 5). There is diffuse infiltration of the face, with auricular appendages affected in the vast majority of cases and bilateral madarosis also common. Hands and feet may also be infiltrated or showing signs of xerodermia.

LL is a systemic disease that can affect, the liver, spleen, adrenal glands, lymph nodes, eyes, and nose when patients are not treated properly and opportunely. Nasal obstruction can be present with little or no response to vasoconstrictors. Often the nasal cavities will be affected, and the oropharynges will be full of nasal secretion highly abundant in bacilli. Subsequent nasal dryness can lead to secondary

ulceration and infection with possible perforation and destruction of the nasal septum, resulting in what is commonly referred to as *saddle nose*. With olfactory bulb dysfunction, anosmia will often be the outcome.

Lesions to the palate, lips, gum, and uvula can further compromise the pharynx, nasopharynx, and tonsils. The eyes may show erythema, dryness, dacryocystitis, lagophthalmos, and/or diminished sensation in the cornea. Likewise, iritis and iridocyclitis may be present, so proper intervention is necessary to ensure prevention of early onset of blindness.

The testes may also be directly affected by bacilli, as witnessed by atrophy of the testicular parenchyma and diffuse fibrosis with eventual sterility and alteration of sexual function. When secondary amyloidosis is present, renal insufficiency may result.

Variations of Lepromatous Leprosy
Histoid Lepromatous Leprosy (or Wade's Lepromatous)
This form of leprosy is rare. Nodular lesions are present, well defined, and of varying sizes. These may be round or oval with a reddish or pink color. These lesions contain a large number of bacilli and are normally associated with sulfone resistance. Histiocytes with a spongy appearance are present under histologic analysis.

Diffuse Lepromatous Leprosy
Described by Lucio, Alvarado, and Latapi, this is a diffuse form of LL, also called *beautiful leprosy* because this form confers a pinkish and healthy appearance to the skin. It is more frequently seen in Mexico and is characterized by the diffuse infiltration of the skin, altered sensation that starts in the hands and feet, loss of eyebrows, and telangiectasias in the face and torso. A mycobacterium was isolated in cases of diffuse lepromatous leprosy (DLL) with Lucio phenomenon, whose DNA cannot be amplified using usual *M. leprae* primers. As a result, a new species has been proposed under the name *M. lepromatosis*.

Pure Neural Leprosy
This type presents only nerve lesions without any cutaneous patches. The most common nerves affected are the ulnar, tibial, and fibular nerves. The radial, median, facial, trigeminal, and auricular nerves, among others, may also be damaged.

Neuropathic pain is often present spontaneously or when the nerve is palpated, either with or without thickening of the nerve. This can evolve to sensory loss, paresthesia, or muscular atrophy in the corresponding area, in addition to autonomic dysfunction and nerve abscess.

Leprosy Diagnosis
The patient is examined to locate any possible skin lesions with diminished sensation and/or areas of sensory alteration that may be caused by compromised peripheral nerves. Lighting must be adequate, and it is important to observe the entire body surface moving from head to toe. Where there are possible signs of disease, thermal, pain, and tactile sensation testing should be done, also looking for areas of alopecia and/or anhidrosis. It must be noted if there is any type of physical disability.

Bacilloscopy consists of collection and examination of skin smears taken from a suspected lesion, both earlobes, and both elbows, and helps classify a patient as PB with a negative examination result or MB when positive.

The bacilloscopic results will generally be negative in the IL, TL, and BTL, which are considered the PB group. Conversely, they tend to be positive in LL, BLL, and BBL, which are considered the MB group.

Ideally, the bacilloscopic reading should be expressed quantitatively as a bacteriologic index (BI) so it is possible to monitor the patient's progress during treatment. In patients with positive bacilloscopy at the time of diagnosis, it is recommended to repeat it at the end of therapy. Smear microscopy is important for differential diagnoses between reactions and relapse.

The histologic examination of a skin biopsy also helps provide a more precise disease classification and can help confirm the diagnosis in cases that are bacilloscopy negative. In

TABLE 1	Main Differential Diagnosis by Leprosy Forms	
INDETERMINATE LEPROSY	TUBERCULOID AND BORDERLINE-TUBERCULOID LEPROSY	BORDERLINE-BORDERLINE, BORDERLINE-LEPROMATOUS, AND LEPROMATOUS LEPROSY
Eczematidis (Pityriasis alba)	Seborrheic dermatitis	Erythema nodosum
Seborrheic dermatitis	Dermatofitosis	Diffuse (anergic) cutaneous leishmaniasis
Localized scleroderma (morphea)	Granuloma annulare	Cutaneous and mucosal leishmaniasis
Residual hypochromia and achromia	Cutaneous leishmaniasis	Systemic lupus erythematous and other rheumatologic diseases
Pityriasis versicolor	Discoid lupus erythematous	Neurofibromatosis (von Recklinghausen disease)
Vitiligo	Pityriasis rosea Gibert	Pityriasis rosea Gibert
Hypochromic nevus	Psoriasis	Congenital syphilis, secondary syphilis, tertiary syphilis
	Sarcoidosis	Cutaneous lymphoma (Mycosis fungoides)
	Secondary syphilis	
	Cutaneous tuberculosis	

IL, there is a nonspecific inflammatory infiltrate, consisting of lymphocytes and sometimes histiocytes, around superficial and deep vessels that affects the cutaneous appendages, especially the neural fillets. The TL and BTL forms are characterized histologically by the presence of granulomas-histiocytes, which differentiate into epithelioid cells, giant cells, and lymphocytes, located around vessels, cutaneous appendages, and nervous fillets. Bacillus research is almost always negative. In BLL and LL forms, the inflammatory infiltrate is characterized by the predominance of foamy or vacuolated histiocytes, with large numbers of bacilli that are isolated or grouped in structures called *globias*.

In regions with limited access to laboratory resources, clinical diagnosis is sufficient to warrant the beginning of the standard leprosy treatment regimen, keeping in mind that this is the only dermatologic disease with altered sensation in lesions. The WHO suggests the classification of cases as either PB or MB based on the number of skin lesions, with MB cases having five or more such patches.

Available serologic testing does not show sufficient accuracy for disease diagnosis or infection. A recent meta-analysis using a fixed model to estimate the association of phenolic glycolipid (PGL)-1 positivity and clinical leprosy demonstrated that PGL-1 does not appear to be a useful test to determine which contacts should receive chemoprophylaxis.

Real-time polymerase chain reaction is available for leprosy and can act as a means of confirmation for diagnosis of PB leprosy cases.

Differential Diagnosis

Differential diagnoses of leprosy include a variety of skin conditions, given the wide range of clinical manifestations in leprosy. The sensory loss symptomatic of leprosy can also be difficult to determine in children and in other diseases that produce changes in the normal skin characteristics (Table 1).

Treatment

Leprosy treatment, like tuberculosis treatment, must deal with the resistance of *M. leprae* and its persistence. Single-drug therapy selects drug-resistant bacilli and should be avoided. Therapy duration has, as a target, the reduction of the number of persistent bacilli that could lead to relapses.

Standard multidrug therapy (MDT) with dapsone, rifampin (Rifadin),[1] and clofazimine (Lamprene) for 12 months for MB cases and 6-month MDT with dapsone and rifampin for PB cases has dramatically changed the prognosis for leprosy patients. However, the evidence is rather weak on the efficacy of this drug regimen, especially regarding the necessary length of time for treatment, both in terms of the proportion of relapse cases and other outcomes, such as physical disability. The use of rifampin once a month was determined for financial reasons, and there is no study comparing this schedule with daily use. For this reason, research on new drugs and treatment regimens continues.

Shorter regimens were used but had shown high relapse rates: daily doses of rifampin[1] and ofloxacin (Floxin)[1] for 4 weeks; single-dose course of rifampin, ofloxacin, and minocycline (Minocin)[1] for single-lesion patients.

Fluoroquinolones (pefloxacin,[2] ofloxacin, and moxifloxacin [Avelox][1]), macrolides (clarithromycin [Biaxin][1]), and tetracycline (minocycline)[1] are effective against *M. leprae*. Only rifampin, its derivative rifapentine (Priftin),[1] and moxifloxacin are bactericidal drugs; all others are bacteriostatic.

In cases of intolerance or resistance to dapsone, this can be removed from the drug regimen, and for PB leprosy patients, clofazimine is used instead. For MB leprosy patients, in these cases, minocycline or ofloxacin can be used instead of dapsone, without alteration in treatment duration. When similar intolerance or resistance is related to rifampin, this should be substituted with a daily dose of 400 mg of ofloxacin. This alternate course lasts 6 months for PB leprosy cases and 24 months for MB leprosy cases.

For those who cannot take either dapsone or rifampin, PB leprosy patients can be treated with ofloxacin (400 mg/day) or minocycline (100 mg/day), and clofazimine (50 mg/day) in self-administered doses for 6 months. Similarly, MB patients can use ofloxacin plus minocycline plus clofazimine during the first 6 months of treatment (intensive phase), followed by 18 months with daily doses of ofloxacin or minocycline and clofazimine (maintenance phase).

Perspectives on the Use of a Uniform Treatment for All Forms, Regardless of Clinical or Laboratory Classification

Despite the success of MDT, the complexity of operationalization of the scheme throughout the healthcare system, the prolonged treatment time, and the difficulty of patient adherence reinforce the need for shorter regimens that can be easily implemented in primary care. Since 2002, the WHO recommended clinical studies to investigate the viability of uniform multidrug therapy (U-MDT) for all leprosy cases, regardless of classification, with 6 months' duration.

The first randomized and controlled study on U-MDT, "Estudo independente para determinar efetividade do esquema Uniforme de MDT de seis doses (U-MDT) em pacientes de hanseníase,

---

[1] Not FDA approved for this indication.

[2] Not available in the United States.

(U-MDT-CT-BR)," was performed in Brazil and evaluated the efficacy of daily intake of dapsone plus clofazimine and monthly rifampicin for 6 months for both PB and MB leprosy patients, regardless of classification criteria. Between 2012 and 2018, 14 scientific articles were published from U-MDT-CT-BR; these showed that reduction in the duration of treatment did not increase relapse rates, reaction frequency, or neural damage. The Brazilian study also demonstrated no statistical differences in BI decrease between regular MDT and U-MDT. Moreover, the same study showed that U-MDT reduced *M. leprae*–specific antibodies during and after treatment.

Together with the results from three previous studies performed in China, India, and Bangladesh, U-MDT-CT-BR support the premise that U-MDT is an acceptable option to be adopted in endemic countries to treat leprosy patients in the field worldwide. These studies led the WHO to recommend the addition of clofazimine to PB leprosy treatment in 2019.

A recent study showed the existence of a high susceptibility genetic profile among leprosy patients predisposing to disease recurrence. The authors showed that recurrence or reinfection is not related to time of treatment but rather to individual genetic susceptibility. Additionally, a population-based study for the search for *M. leprae* resistance reported the emergence and transmission of resistant strains in a former leprosy colony located in the Brazilian Amazon. Taken together, these studies demonstrated the need to save the unnecessary use of these drugs and strongly support the decision to adopt the shorter uniform treatment for leprosy.

Dapsone and rifampin resistance have been reported. Although reports of clofazimine-resistant isolates of *M. leprae* are rare, multidrug-resistant leprosy reports are increasing and should be regularly monitored.

Leprosy Reactions and Control

Over the course of this chronic disease, approximately 30% of the patients develop acute inflammatory episodes called *leprosy reactions*. These reactions can occur before diagnosis as well as during or after MDT treatment. They are commonly grouped into (1) type 1 (reversal) reactions (T1Rs) resulting from vigorous cell-mediated immune response and (2) type 2 reactions (T2Rs), the clinical manifestation of which is frequently erythematous nodosum leprosum (ENL) that comes about mainly from immunocomplex deposits. In patients with BBL and BLL, it is possible to have both reaction types simultaneously. There is also Lucio phenomenon, which is an immune system response with important clinical manifestations. Its physiopathology is not well understood, with abundant infection of *M. leprae* in endothelium, which can lead to thrombosis in the most superficial vases from immunocomplex deposits with hemorrhaging and cutaneous infarction.

In the literature, a robust association has been demonstrated between bacterial load and the frequency of leprosy reactions. A reaction can be set off by various factors, such as pregnancy, childbirth, vaccinations, puberty, intercurrent infections, stress (physical, psychological, or surgical), use of potassium iodate/iodide (SSKI), and immune reconstruction inflammatory syndrome (IRIS) linked to antiretroviral and/or immune-based therapies.

Those patients who experience leprosy reactions during MDT treatment should continue taking their regimen without modification while also beginning a specific and concurrent treatment for the appropriate reaction type.

Type 1 Reaction or Reversal Reaction

Clinically, lesions become more erythematous and infiltrated, and those with previously diminished sensation can become more sensitive to touch. Desquamation may occur, and some lesions may even ulcerate. New lesions can erupt along with edema in the hands, feet, and face, as well general systemic symptoms. These reactions can last for years in some patients. It is important to begin an immediate intervention given that neuritis is the most common, serious, and potentially disabling clinical manifestation of T1R.

The drug of choice for T1R treatment is prednisone (or prednisolone [Millipred]) with a dosage of 1 to 2 mg/kg/day for at least 12 weeks, at which point it can be tapered off until discontinuing the medication around the 24th week.

Alternative drugs for a type 1 reaction include the following:
- Azathioprine (Imuran)[1]: 1 to 2 mg/kg/day, until reaction control
- Cyclosporine (Neoral, Sandimmune)[1]: 5 to 8 mg/kg/day, until reaction control
- Clofazimine: 300 mg to 30 days/200 mg to 30 days/100 mg to 30 days

Type 2 Reaction

This occurs in MB leprosy patients, and ENL is the most frequent clinical manifestation of T2Rs. Other variations of T2R are polymorphic erythema and vasculitis.

Clinically, ENL is a systemic condition with the eruption of painful and often symmetrical erythematous nodules on the arms and legs. When deeper, these nodules are more easily palpated than the more visible ones but will often ulcerate. Neuritis is frequent, although it is less aggressive than seen in T1Rs. The systemic impact can produce edema, myalgia, fever, malaise, asthenia, weight loss, cephalalgia, iritis, episcleritis, iridocyclitis, glaucoma, epistaxis, arthralgia, and orchiepididymitis with testicular atrophy, glomerulonephritis, chronic renal insufficiency, hepatosplenomegaly, and amyloidosis.

The most common medication used for ENL is thalidomide (Thalomid) in variable dosage, from 100 to 400 mg/day, depending on the severity of the reaction. The distribution of thalidomide is restricted in some countries because of its teratogenic effects. For this reason, it should be given under strict supervision with proper medical, ethical, and legal measures in place.

For ENL associated with neuritis, iritis, orchitis, and/or hand-foot reactions or for women of childbearing age, a course of corticosteroids should be given (prednisone at 1 to 2 mg/kg/day).

In chronic cases and those that are nonresponsive to treatment, it is possible to administer clofazimine along with steroids at the initial dosage of 100 mg three times per day for a maximum of 12 weeks. This should be reduced to 100 mg twice daily for another 12 weeks and finally 100 mg/day for 12 to 24 weeks. Cyclosporine (Neoral, Sandimmune)[1] may also offer some benefit to the patient with serious ENL, as can the association of azathioprine (Imuran),[1] methotrexate,[1] and corticosteroids.

Alternative drugs for a type 2 reaction include the following:
- Azathioprine[1]: 1 to 2 mg/kg/day, until reaction control
- Cyclosporine[1]: 5 to 8 mg/kg/day, until reaction control
- Methotrexate[1]: 15 mg (IM/SC or PO)/week, until reaction control
- Pentoxifylline: (Trental)[1] 1200 mg/day, until reaction control
- Clofazimine: 300 mg to 30 days/200 mg to 30 days/100 mg to 30 days

Lucio Phenomenon

Lucio phenomenon can occur in LL patients. The skin lesions can be discrete and limited in number, pinkish or cyanotic, often very painful, and potentially necrotizing and ulcerative. This condition can lead to death. Treatment is based on a course of corticosteroid therapy appropriate for each patient.

Differential Diagnosis Between Relapse and Reaction

Relapse rates are very low, whereas reactions are quite frequent, even after completing treatment. Table 2 shows the main differences between reaction type 1 and type 2 relapse. Recently, an *M. leprae* whole-genome sequencing technique was used to discriminate between cases of relapse and reinfection.

---

[1] Not FDA approved for this indication.

TABLE 2 Differences Between Reaction Type 1 and Relapse	
REVERSAL REACTION	**RELAPSE**
Generally occurs during course of multidrug therapy or within 6 months of treatment completion	Occurs at least 2 years after treatment completion
Sudden and unexpected onset	Slow and insidious onset
Can be accompanied by fever and malaise	In general, no systemic symptoms present
Old lesions become erythematous, shiny, and infiltrated	Old lesions may present erythematous edges
In general, many new lesions	Few new lesions
There may be ulceration of the reaction lesions	Ulceration may occur on arms and legs in addition to the lesions
Regression with desquamation	No desquamation present
Can quickly affect several nerve trunks, with presence of pain, sensory alteration, and decreased motor function	May affect a single nerve, and functional alterations often take place very slowly
Excellent response to corticosteroid therapy	Does not respond well to corticosteroid therapy
Bacteriologic index stable or decreases	Bacteriologic index increases

Complications

Leprosy complications are the result of permanent nerve damage. Lesions to the large nerve trunks, such as the ulnar, median, and tibial, cause motor and sensory loss leading to disabilities such as claw hand and footdrop.

The absence of sensation in the hands, soles of the feet, and cornea leaves these areas predisposed to common wounds and pressure ulcers. This reality demands that patients take specific care to avoid ulcers and detect them as soon as possible to prevent secondary infection. In addition, corneal ulcers can result in blindness.

Acknowledgment

We thank Dr. Anna Maria Salles for the patient pictures.

References

Andrade KVF, Nery JS, Penna MLF, Penna GO, Pereira SM: Effect of Brazil's Conditional Cash Transfer Programme on the new case detection rate of leprosy in children under 15 years old, Lepr Rev 89:13–24, 2018, https://doi.org/10.1016/S1473-3099(19)30624-3.

Andrade KVF, Nery JS, Pescarini JM, et al: Geographic and socioeconomic factors associated with leprosy treatment default: an analysis from the 100 Million Brazilian Cohort, PLoS Negl Trop Dis 13(9):e0007714, 2019.

Becx-Bleumink M: Relapses among leprosy patients treated with multidrug therapy: experience in the leprosy control program of the All Africa Leprosy and Rehabilitation Training Center (ALERT) in Ethiopia; practical difficulties with diagnosing relapses; operational procedures and criteria for diagnosing relapses, Int J Lepr Other Mycobact Dis 60:421–435, 1992.

Butlin CR, Pahan D, Maug AKJ, et al: Outcome of 6 months MBMDT in MB patients in Bangladesh—preliminary results, Lepr Rev 87:171–182, 2016.

Cruz RCDS, Bührer-Sékula S, Penna GO, et al: Clinical trial for uniform multidrug therapy for leprosy patients in Brazil (U-MDT/CT-BR): adverse effects approach, An Bras Dermatol 93:377–384, 2018.

Cambau E, Perani E, Guillemin I, Jamet P, Ji B: Multidrug-resistance to dapsone, rifampicin, and ofloxacin in M leprae, Lancet 349:103–104, 1997.

Cruz RCDS, Bührer-Sékula S, Penna MLF, Penna GO, Talhari S: Leprosy: current situation, clinical and laboratory aspects, treatment history and perspective of the uniform multidrug therapy for all patients, An Bras Dermatol 92(6):761–773, 2017.

da Silva Rocha A, Cunha Dos Santos AA, Pignataro P, et al: Genotyping of Mycobacterium leprae from Brazilian leprosy patients suggests the occurrence of reinfection or of bacterial population shift during disease relapse, J Med Microbiol 60:1441–1446, 2011.

Ferreira IP, Bührer-Sékula S, De Oliveira MR, et al: Patient profile and treatment satisfaction of Brazilian leprosy patients in a clinical trial of uniform six-month multidrug therapy (U-MDT/CT-BR), Lepr Rev 85(4):267–274, 2014.

Fine PE: Leprosy: the epidemiology of a slow bacterium, Epidemiol Rev 4:161–188, 1982.

Gelber RH, Grosset J: The chemotherapy of leprosy: an interpretive history, Lepr Rev 83:221–240, 2012.

Gillis TP, Scollard DM, Lockwood DN: What is the evidence that the putative Mycobacterium lepromatosis species causes diffuse lepromatous leprosy? Lepr Rev 82:205–209, 2011.

Gonçalves H de S, Pontes MA, Bührer-Sékula S, et al: Brazilian clinical trial of uniform multidrug therapy for leprosy patients: the correlation between clinical disease types and adverse effect, Mem Inst Oswaldo Cruz 107(Suppl 1):74–78, 2012.

Guerra JG, Penna GO, Castro LCM: Eritema Nodoso Hansênico: atualização clínica e terapêutica, Erythema Nodosum Leprosum: clinical and therapeutic update, An Bras Dermatol 77:389–407, 2002.

Han XY, Sizer KC, Velarde-Félix JS, et al: The leprosy agents Mycobacterium lepromatosis and Mycobacterium leprae in Mexico, Int J Dermatol 51:952–959, 2012.

Hungria EM, Bührer-Sékula S, Oliveira RM, et al: Mycobacterium leprae-specific antibodies in multibacillary leprosy patients decrease during and after treatment with either the regular 12 doses multidrug therapy (MDT) or the uniform 6 doses MDT, Front Immunol 9:915, 2018.

Hungria EM, Bührer-Sékula S, de Oliveira RM, et al: Leprosy reactions: the predictive value of Mycobacterium leprae-specific serology evaluated in a Brazilian cohort of leprosy patients (U-MDT/CT-BR), PLoS Negl Trop Dis 11(2):e0005396, 2017.

Hungria EM, Oliveira RM, Penna GO, et al: Can baseline ML Flow test results predict leprosy reactions? An investigation in a cohort of patients enrolled in the uniform multidrug therapy clinical trial for leprosy patients in Brazil, Infect Dis Poverty 5(1):110–120, 2016.

International Federation of Anti-Leprosy Associations: Available at http://www.ilep.org.uk/about-ilep/. [Accessed July, 2022].

Kroger A, Pannikar V, Htoon MT, et al: International open trial of uniform multidrug therapy regimen for 6 months for all types of leprosy patients: rationale, design and preliminary results, Trop Med Int Health 13:594–602, 2008.

Lie H: Why is leprosy decreasing in Norway? Trans R Soc Trop Med Hyg 22(4):357–366, 1929.

Lockwood DN, Shetty V, Penna GO: Hazards of setting targets to eliminate disease: lessons from the leprosy elimination campaign, BMJ 348:1136, 2014.

Maeda S, Matsuoka M, Nakata N, Kai M, Maeda Y, et al: Multidrug resistant M leprae from patients with leprosy, Antimicrob Agents Chemother 45:3635–3639, 2001.

Matsuoka M, Kashiwabara Y, Namisato Y: A M leprae isolate resistant to dapsone, rifampicin, ofloxacin, and sparfloxacin, Int J Lepr 68:452–455, 2000.

Matsuoka M, Kahiwabara Y, Liangfen Z, Goto M, Kitajima S: A second case of multidrug-resistant Mycobacterium leprae isolated from a Japanese patient with relapsed lepromatous leprosy, Int J Lepr 71(3):240–243, 2003.

Moura RS, Penna GO, Cardoso LP, et al: Description of leprosy classification at baseline among patients enrolled at the uniform multidrug therapy clinical trial for leprosy patients in Brazil, Am J Trop Med Hyg 92(6):1280–1284, 2015.

Moura RS, Penna GO, Fujiwara T, et al: Evaluation of a rapid serological test for leprosy classification using human serum albumin as the antigen carrier, J Immunol Methods 412:35–41, 2014.

Nery JS, Ramond A, Pescarini JM, et al: Socioeconomic determinants of leprosy new case detection in the 100 Million Brazilian Cohort: a population-based linkage study, Lancet Glob Health 7(9):e1226–e1236, 2019.

Nery JS, Pereira SM, Rasella D, et al: Effect of the Brazilian conditional cash transfer and primary health care programs on the new case detection rate of leprosy, PLoS Negl Trop Dis 8:e3357, 2014. -e3360.

Norman G, Joseph G, Ebenezer G, et al: Secondary rifampin resistance following multi-drug therapy – a case report, Int J Lepr Other Mycobact Dis 71(1):18–21, 2003.

Opromolla DVA, Costa HC, Oliveira PRD: Resistência medicamentosa múltipla secundária na hanseníase, Hansen Int 18(1,2):11–16, 1993.

Pedrosa VL, Dias LC, Galban E, et al: Leprosy among schoolchildren in the Amazon region: a cross-sectional study of active search and possible source of infection by contact tracing, PLoS Negl Trop Dis 12:e0006261, 2018.

Penna GO, Bührer-Sékula S, Kerr LRS, et al: Uniform multidrug therapy for leprosy patients in Brazil (U-MDT/CT-BR): results of an open label, randomized and controlled clinical trial, among multibacillary patients, PLoS Negl Trop Dis 11:e0005725, 2017.

Penna GO, Pontes MA, Cruz R, et al: A clinical trial for uniform multidrug therapy for leprosy patients in Brazil: rationale and design, Mem Inst Oswaldo Cruz 107(Suppl 1):22–27, 2012.

Penna ML, Bührer-Sékula S, Pontes MA, et al: Primary results of clinical trial for uniform multidrug therapy for leprosy patients in Brazil (U-MDT/CT-BR): reactions frequency in multibacillary patients, Lepr Rev 83(3):308–319, 2012.

Penna ML, Bührer-Sékula S, Pontes MA, et al: Results from the clinical trial of uniform multidrug therapy for leprosy patients in Brazil (U-MDT/CT-BR): decrease in bacteriological index, Lepr Rev 83(4):262–266, 2014.

Penna ML, Penna GO: Leprosy frequency in the world, 1999–2010, Mem Inst Oswaldo Cruz 107(Suppl 1):3–12, 2012.

Penna ML, Penna GO, Iglesias PC, et al: Anti-PGL-1 positivity as a risk marker for the development of leprosy among contacts of leprosy cases: systematic review and metaanalysis, PLoS Negl Trop Dis 10:e0004703, 2016.

Pescarini JM, Strina A, Nery JS, et al: Socioeconomic risk markers of leprosy in high-burden countries: a systematic review and meta-analysis, *PLoS Negl Trop Dis* 12(7):e0006622, 2018.

Rosa PS, D'Espindula HRS, Melo ACL, et al: Emergence and transmission of drug/multidrug-resistant Mycobacterium leprae in a former leprosy colony in the Brazilian Amazon, *Clin Infect Dis ciz570*, 2019.

Santos SD, Penna GO, Costa MCN, et al: Leprosy in children and adolescents under 15 years old in an urban center in Brazil, *Mem Inst Oswaldo Cruz* 111:359–364, 2016.

Shen J, Yan L, Yu M, et al: Six years' follow-up of multibacillary leprosy patients treated with uniform multi-drug therapy in China, *Int J Dermatol* 54:315–318, 2015.

Shetty VP, et al: Primary resistance to single and multiple drugs in Leprosy—a mouse foot pad study, *Lepr Rev* 67, 1996.

Stefani MMA, Avanzi C, Bührer-Sékula S, et al: Whole genome sequencing distinguishes between relapse and reinfection in recurrent leprosy cases, *PLoS Negl Trop Dis* 11(6):e0005598, 2017.

Talhari C, Mira MT, Massone C, et al: Leprosy and HIV coinfection: a clinical, pathological, immunological, and therapeutic study of a cohort from a Brazilian referral center for infectious diseases, *J Infect Dis* 202:345–354, 2010.

Talhari C, Talhari S, Penna GO: Clinical aspects of leprosy, *Clin Dermatol* 33:26–37, 2015.

Talhari S, Gontijo B, Vale ECS, Marques SA: Editorial—new perspectives for the treatment of Hansen's disease, *An Bras Dermatol* 92(6):760, 2017.

Talhari S, Neves RG, Penna GO, Oliveira MLWR: *In Hanseníase, Manaus*, Gráfica Tropical, 2006.

Truman RW, Singh P, Sharma R, et al: Probable zoonotic leprosy in the southern United States, *N Engl J Med* 364:1626–1633, 2011.

Uaska Sartori PV, Penna GO, Bührer-Sékula S, et al: Human genetic susceptibility of leprosy recurrence, *Sci Rep* 10:1284, 2020.

Van Brakel W, Cross H, Declercq E, et al: Review of leprosy research evidence (2002–2009) and implications for current policy and practice, *Lepr Rev* 81:228–275, 2010.

Van Veen NH, Lockwood DN, Van Brakel WH, et al: *Interventions for erythema nodosum leprosum (Review)*, Cochrane Collaboration, John Wiley & Sons, 2012, p 53.

Vieira MCA, Nery JS, Paixão ES, Andrade KVF, Penna GO, Teixeira MG: Leprosy in children under 15 years of age in Brazil: a systematic review of the literature, *PLoS Negl Trop Dis* 12(10):e0006788, 2018.

WHO Expert Committee on Leprosy: *World Health Organ Tech Rep Ser* 968:1–61, 2012.

WHO: *In Global leprosy strategy 2016–2020: Accelerating towards a leprosy-Free world*, WHO, 2016.

WHO Global leprosy (Hansen disease) update: 2020: impact of COVID-19 on global leprosy control, *WER* 36:421–444, 2021.

LYME DISEASE AND POST-TREATMENT LYME DISEASE SYNDROME

Method of
Carlos R. Oliveira, MD, PhD; and Eugene D. Shapiro, MD

CURRENT DIAGNOSIS

- Lyme disease, caused by the spirochete *Borrelia burgdorferi*, is the most common vector-borne infection in both the United States and Europe.
- Early localized Lyme disease is a clinical diagnosis that is based on the presence of a single erythema migrans rash. The rash presents as an expanding circular macule that is often uniformly erythematous but occasionally can have central clearing that gives it the appearance of a target lesion. Erythema migrans usually appears 7 to 14 days after a tick bite (although the bite often is not recognized). If untreated, it persists for about 3 to 4 weeks.
- Early disseminated Lyme disease can present as multiple erythema migrans, cranial nerve palsy, lymphocytic meningitis, radiculomyelitis (Bannwarth syndrome), or carditis.
- Arthritis is the primary manifestation of late Lyme disease. Typically it is an oligoarthritis that most often involves a single knee.
- Patients with no objective signs but only nonspecific symptoms (e.g., arthralgia, myalgia, fatigue, or perceived cognitive difficulties) are highly unlikely to have active Lyme disease as the cause regardless of the result of antibody tests.

- Antibody test results for Lyme disease are usually negative in patients with erythema migrans (single or multiple); therefore testing for antibody generally is only indicated for patients with non-cutaneous manifestations of Lyme disease.
- The IgG antibody test has good sensitivity for patients with Lyme disease ≥4 weeks after initial infection.
- Tests for antibodies to *B burgdorferi* should use a two-tier procedure, first with a sensitive quantitative test, usually either a whole-cell or C-6 peptide enzyme-linked immunosorbent assay (ELISA); if that result is either positive or equivocal, a more specific test, the Western immunoblot, is done to confirm a positive test result. The presence of antibodies against at least either 2 (for IgM) or 5 (for IgG) proteins of *B burgdorferi* is required for the immunoblot result to be considered positive. Modified two-tier antibody tests, which use a second (different) ELISA assay as the second tier test, have been approved for use by the FDA and are available.
- In patients with symptoms present for 4-6 weeks or longer, Lyme disease should not be diagnosed based on a positive IgM antibody result alone.
- Sensitivity of PCR assays of both blood and CSF are poor because concentrations of *B burgdorferi* in these fluids are low.
- Once serum antibodies to *B burgdorferi* develop, both IgG and IgM antibodies may persist for decades despite adequate treatment; therefore elevated concentrations of antibodies in serum do not necessarily indicate active infection.

CURRENT THERAPY

- An oral course of doxycycline (Vibramycin)[1] for 10 days or of amoxicillin (Amoxil)[1] or cefuroxime axetil (Ceftin) for 14 days is highly effective for treating early localized Lyme disease.
- A 14-day course of the same antimicrobials also is highly effective in treating multiple erythema migrans and other manifestations of early disseminated Lyme disease, although patients with Lyme meningitis or complete atrioventricular block should be treated either parenterally with ceftriaxone (Rocephin)[1] or cefotaxime (Claforan)[1] or, in some instances, orally with doxycycline.[1]
- A 28-day course of an oral regimen is recommended for the treatment of Lyme arthritis.
- Doxycycline (Vibramycin) is contraindicated in women who are pregnant or are breastfeeding.
- The most effective preventive measure is avoidance of tick-infested areas. If exposure is unavoidable, visual inspection and prompt removal of embedded ticks, use of tick repellents with N, N-diethyl-3-methylbenzamide (DEET), and use of protective clothing have all been found to be modestly effective.
- An infected tick generally must be attached for 36 to 72 hours or longer for there to be a substantial risk of transmission of *B burgdorferi*. If a tick that has been embedded for at least 36 hours is removed, a single dose of doxycycline (Vibramycin) 8.8 mg/kg, maximum 200 mg,[1] given within 72 hours of removing the engorged tick, can be effective in preventing Lyme disease.
- Multiple or prolonged courses of antibiotics have not been shown to be effective and are not recommended for patients with only chronic, subjective symptoms after completing appropriate antibiotic treatment for Lyme disease.

[1]Not FDA approved for this indication.

Epidemiology and Ecology

Lyme arthritis was first described in 1977 when an unusual cluster of children with arthritis in Lyme, Connecticut, was reported. Soon after, Willy Burgdorfer identified the causative bacterial agent, a spirochete that was later named *Borrelia burgdorferi*, in *Ixodes scapularis*, the deer tick. Lyme disease, the most common vector-borne illness in both the United States and Europe, is transmitted by hard-bodied ticks of the *Ixodes* genus. In the United States, *Ixodes scapularis* (in the East and upper Midwest) and *Ixodes pacificus*, the Western black-legged tick (on the Pacific coast), can be vectors of Lyme disease. More than 90% of all cases in the United States occur in nine states: Connecticut, Maryland, Massachusetts, Minnesota, New Jersey, New York, Pennsylvania, Rhode Island, and Wisconsin. In Europe and in Asia, *Ixodes ricinus* (the sheep tick) and *Ixodes perscultatus* (the tiaga tick) can transmit *B burgdorferi*. *Ixodes* ticks feed once in each of the three stages of their 2-year life cycle: larva, nymph, and adult. There are a number of genomospecies of *Borrelia burgdorferi* sensu lato that cause Lyme disease. In the United States, Lyme disease is almost exclusively caused by *B burgdorferi* sensu stricto, whereas in Europe and in Asia, *Borrelia afzelii* and *Borrelia garinii*, in addition to *B burgdorferi* sensu stricto, are the major causes of Lyme disease.

Lyme disease is a zoonosis. The primary reservoir for *B burgdorferi* are small mammals, such as mice and chipmunks, although birds and other mammals, such as foxes and coyotes, can also serve as reservoirs of the organism. Deer are not a competent reservoir for *B burgdorferi*, but they are important for supporting the life cycle of the deer tick. Ticks are uninfected when they hatch. They can become infected after they feed on an infected animal. The bacteria live in the midgut of the tick, which must remain attached to a host for 36 to 48 hours or longer for the spirochete to travel to the salivary glands so it can be injected into the host. Although ticks may become infected at any stage of the life cycle, nymphs are more likely to transmit the organism. This is because their small size (<2 mm) makes them more difficult to detect than adult ticks. Consequently, nymphal ticks are less likely than are adult ticks to be removed before the organism can be transmitted. The most important risk factor for Lyme disease is exposure to ticks in an area in which the disease is endemic. Most cases of Lyme disease occur in the spring and summer, which correlates with peak activity of nymphal ticks and with frequent outdoor activity of humans.

Pathophysiology
The pathogenesis of Lyme disease is predominantly driven by the host immune response to the spirochete. During the first stage of infection, after transfer of the organism to the skin, inflammation ensues that leads to an erythematous lesion at the site of inoculation. The spirochete does not produce toxins; however, it can disseminate via the bloodstream or through the lymph vessels. After dissemination, the spirochete can adhere to distal tissues, and an immune-mediated inflammatory reaction at these sites leads to the characteristic clinical manifestations of Lyme disease.

Prevention
No vaccine is currently available to prevent Lyme disease in humans. The most effective preventive measure is avoidance of tick-infested areas. Tick repellents that contain N, N-diethyl-3-methylbenzamide (DEET) and the use of protective clothing (long sleeves and pants) have been found to be modestly effective at preventing Lyme disease. If exposure is unavoidable, frequent visual inspection with prompt removal of ticks is recommended. In endemic areas, if a nymphal or adult *Ixodes* tick is removed that is partially engorged (has been attached for at least 36 hours), a single dose of doxycycline (Vibramycin)[1] administered within 72 hours of removing the tick can be effective in preventing Lyme disease.

Clinical Manifestations
The clinical manifestations of Lyme disease can be divided into three stages: early localized disease, early disseminated disease, and late disease. About two-thirds of patients with Lyme disease in the

United States have early localized disease, which is characterized by a single erythema migrans (EM) rash at the site of the tick bite (although the tick bite is recognized in only a minority of cases). The rash starts as an erythematous macule or papule and then expands as an annular macule that is often uniformly erythematous (about two-thirds of cases of EM), although it can have central clearing that gives it the appearance of a classic target lesion. EM usually appears 7 to 14 days (range 3–30 days) after the tick bite and, if untreated, may expand to an average of 15 cm in diameter before resolving after 2 to 4 weeks or longer. The rash may be asymptomatic or it may be accompanied by systemic symptoms such as fever, malaise, headache, stiff neck, myalgia, or arthralgia.

The second most common manifestation of Lyme disease is multiple EM, which accounts for 15% to 23% of the reported cases in the United States. Multiple EM, a manifestation of early disseminated Lyme disease, occurs when the spirochete disseminates via the bloodstream and presents as multiple erythematous round or ovoid macules that are usually smaller than most single EM lesions and are often accompanied by fever and other systemic symptoms. Other manifestations of early disseminated Lyme disease include cranial nerve palsy (especially facial palsy), lymphocytic meningitis, radiculomyelitis, and carditis. Cranial nerve palsies, especially facial nerve palsy, occur more commonly in children and account for approximately 3% to 5% of all cases of Lyme disease. In most cases, facial nerve palsy resolves within 4 to 8 weeks usually leaving minor, if any, obvious residua. Lyme meningitis occurs less frequently (1% to 2% of cases) and typically has a subacute presentation similar to, though often of longer duration, than that of enteroviral meningitis. There is a mononuclear pleocytosis in cerebrospinal fluid. Increased intracranial pressure with papilledema is not uncommon. Neurologic involvement in Lyme disease is more common in Europe and in Asia, presumably because local strains of the bacteria are more neurotropic. Carditis, which is found in fewer than 1% of cases, typically causes various degrees of heart block, which usually is asymptomatic and may be detected only with an electrocardiogram, but may manifest as syncope, dyspnea, or dizziness due to complete heart block. Sudden death due to Lyme carditis has been reported but is very rare.

Arthritis is the main manifestation of late Lyme disease, and in North America accounts for approximately 6% to 8% of reported cases. Lyme arthritis typically is an oligoarthritis that involves a single knee about 90% of the time. Symptoms of arthritis develop 2 to 6 months after the tick bite and present with objective signs of inflammation of the joint. Arthritis typically resolves 2 to 6 weeks after appropriate treatment, although it may persist or recur in 10% to 20% of treated patients.

In Europe and in Asia, uncommon manifestations of Lyme disease include borrelial lymphocytoma, a painless nodule commonly located on the ear, breast, or scrotum; and acrodermatitis chronica atrophicans, a chronic fibrosing skin lesion typically found on the extensor surfaces of the extremities.

Diagnosis
Early localized Lyme disease is a clinical diagnosis based on a history of potential exposure to ticks in an endemic area and the presence of the characteristic EM rash. Antibodies to the organism typically appear 3 to 4 weeks after the initial infection. Consequently, serologic tests are not indicated in patients with EM because most will not have detectable antibodies. Although more patients with multiple erythema migrans may be seropositive at the time of presentation, a majority will still be seronegative early on. Moreover, detectable antibodies may never develop in patients who are treated early in their courses. In patients with extracutaneous manifestations of Lyme disease, serologic testing is useful in making a diagnosis. Tests for antibodies to *B burgdorferi* should use a two-tier procedure, in which a sensitive quantitative test, usually an enzyme-linked immunosorbent assay (ELISA) against either "whole cell" or C6 peptide antigens of the bacteria, is performed. If the result of the quantitative test is either positive or equivocal, a Western immunoblot is done to confirm the

---

[1] Not FDA approved for this indication.

specificity of the result. Modified two-tier antibody tests, which use a second (different) ELISA assay as the second tier test, have been approved for use by the FDA. As with most infections, once they develop, elevated concentrations of both IgM and IgG antibodies may persist for decades in symptom-free patients who have been cured of Lyme disease. A positive test result is evidence of prior exposure to the organism and is not evidence of active infection. In addition, false-positive antibody test results are common, especially in patients with a low prior probability of Lyme disease, such as those with chronic nonspecific symptoms such as arthralgia, myalgia, or fatigue, who do not have concomitant objective findings associated with Lyme disease. False-positive IgM test results are especially common. A diagnosis of Lyme disease should rarely be based on a positive IgM test result alone, especially in patients who have had symptoms for a month or longer.

Polymerase chain reaction (PCR) assays can detect the organism in skin biopsies, CSF, blood, or synovial fluid. However, because concentrations of the organism are low in both the blood and the CSF, sensitivity of PCR assays of these fluids is poor. Because the rash is so characteristic and because virtually all patients with Lyme arthritis will have a positive result for IgG antibodies to *B burgdorferi*, such assays rarely are needed to make a diagnosis. The organism can be cultured using special media, but sensitivity generally is poor, and it takes weeks for the organism to grow.

Differential Diagnosis

The differential diagnosis of Lyme disease depends on the clinical stage of the illness. Single EM may be confused with ringworm, cellulitis, nummular eczema, granuloma annulare or insect bites. Southern tick–associated rash illness (STARI) manifests in a rash identical to EM. However, it occurs at the site of a bite from the lone star tick (*Amblyomma americanum*) and is most common in the south-central United States. The cause of STARI is unknown, but, unlike with Lyme disease, it is not associated with significant extracutaneous manifestations. Multiple EM may look very similar to erythema multiforme. Lymphocytic meningitis occurs with numerous viral infections, most commonly enterovirus. There are many other causes of carditis, including a number of viruses, as well as rheumatologic diseases such as lupus and rheumatic fever. There is substantial variation in how Lyme arthritis presents. Most often it is a subacute arthritis that may mimic rheumatoid arthritis or other more chronic arthritides, with <50,000 white blood cells/mL in the synovial fluid. However, it can present acutely and may mimic acute bacterial arthritis (like that due to *Staphylococcus aureus*), with >100,000 white blood cells/mL in synovial fluid.

Relapse Versus Reinfection

Resistance of *B burgdorferi* to recommended antimicrobials has not been reported. First-line antimicrobial therapy for Lyme disease is highly efficacious, and bacteriologic treatment failures are very rare. In a study of patients with two or more episodes of EM that occurred years apart, it was shown that the episodes were caused by different strains of bacteria, indicating that reinfection, rather than persistence of the original organism, was the cause of repeated episodes of EM. Reinfection rarely occurs in patients with late Lyme disease, indicating that most such patients are immune. On the other hand, patients with early Lyme disease who are treated may become reinfected from a new tick bite, presumably because the organism was killed before a protective immune response could occur. Persistent or recurrent arthritis does occur in 10% to 20% of patients with Lyme arthritis. So-called antibiotic-refractory arthritis occurs when frank arthritis persists despite two or more courses of antimicrobial treatment. This may be due to either an autoimmune process or slow clearance of antigens of dead organisms. There is no evidence that the cause is failure of the antibiotic to kill the organisms.

Post-Treatment Lyme Disease Syndrome and "Chronic" Lyme Disease

A small minority of patients with Lyme disease who have completed appropriate treatment may continue to have nonspecific symptoms, such as fatigue, arthralgia, myalgia, or perceived cognitive difficulties, for weeks or months after completing treatment. These have been termed *post-treatment Lyme disease symptoms* and, if they persist for 6 months or longer and are disabling, they are referred to as *post-treatment Lyme disease syndrome* (PTLDS). It is not clear whether the frequency or the nature of these symptoms in patients with PTLDS is greater than that among the general population. In addition, several placebo-controlled, randomized clinical trials of prolonged courses (6 weeks or longer) of intensive antimicrobial treatment (e.g., with ceftriaxone) in patients with PTLDS have found there was virtually no benefit and substantial risk of adverse side effects of this treatment. Consequently, the Infectious Diseases Society of America, the American Academy of Pediatrics, the American Academy of Neurology, the American College of Rheumatology, and expert professional societies from many European countries do not recommend prolonged treatment with antimicrobials in patients with PTLDS. These patients are distinguished from patients with so-called "chronic" Lyme disease, who have complaints similar to those with PTLDS but who do not have evidence of ever having had Lyme disease. Of course, prolonged antimicrobial treatment is not indicated for these patients, who might better be described as having medically unexplained symptoms. Patients with either PTLDS or "chronic Lyme disease" are best managed by focusing on alleviating symptoms rather than with additional courses of antibiotic therapy. This is because long-term treatment with antibiotics has not been shown to provide benefit and is associated with substantial risks. Managing these patients can be challenging. Ideally, management decisions should be directed by a clinician who can both form a long-term therapeutic relationship with the patient, and who has substantial experience managing medically unexplained symptoms. Clinicians need to be aware that while there is no scientific evidence to support the existence of "chronic" Lyme disease, many of these patients are suffering, and thus, are vulnerable to those who would offer inappropriate and potentially harmful therapies.

Chemoprophylaxis

A single dose of doxycycline (Vibramycin; 8.8 mg/kg, maximum 200 mg)[1] taken within 72 hours of a deer tick bite was effective in preventing Lyme disease. However, because the risk of Lyme disease after a recognized tick bite is low, prophylaxis generally is not recommended routinely, but only for those at higher risk, such as someone in an endemic area who removes an engorged nymphal stage deer tick.

Treatment

Antimicrobial treatment of Lyme disease is highly effective and complications are rare (Table 1). The recommendations for treatment are summarized in the table. Antimicrobials that are highly effective and are considered first-line agents to treat Lyme disease orally include doxycycline (Vibramycin)[1], amoxicillin (Amoxil)[1] and cefuroxime axetil (Ceftin). Amoxicillin (Amoxil) is the preferred agent for women who are either pregnant or breastfeeding. Because the risk of staining of teeth is low, use of doxycycline for ≤21 days of treatment in children <8 years of age is now considered acceptable. Doxycycline (Vibramycin) is the preferred oral agent due to its good activity against other tick-borne illnesses such as human granulocytic anaplasmosis. Although macrolides such as azithromycin (Zithromax),[1] clarithromycin (Biaxin),[1] and erythromycin (EES)[1] are effective for treating early Lyme disease, they may not be as effective as the first-line agents. When parenteral treatment is indicated, ceftriaxone (Rocephin)[1] is the preferred agent because of once-a-day dosing. Alternative antimicrobials such as cefotaxime (Claforan)[1] and penicillin G (Pfizerpen-G)[1] also are highly effective, although penicillin G is rarely used because of frequent dosing due to its short half-life.

---

[1] Not FDA approved for this indication.

TABLE 1	Antimicrobials Recommended to Treat Lyme Disease		
MANIFESTATION	**FIRST-LINE AGENTS**	**ALTERNATIVE AGENTS**	**DURATION**
Single or multiple erythema migrans, cranial nerve palsy, carditis that is asymptomatic or for which the patient is not hospitalized	Doxycycline (Vibramycin)[1] 4.4 mg/kg/day in 2 divided doses (maximum 100 mg/dose)	Azithromycin (Zithromax)[1] 10 mg/kg/day in 1 dose (maximum 500 mg/dose)	14 days; for single EM, 10-days of doxycycline or 7–10 days of azithromycin is effective
	Amoxicillin (Amoxil)[1] 50 mg/kg per day in 3 divided doses (maximum 500 mg/dose)	Clarithromycin (Biaxin)[1] 7.5 mg/kg in 2 divided doses (maximum 500 mg/dose)	
	Cefuroxime axetil (Ceftin) 30 mg/kg PO in 2 divided doses (maximum 500 mg/dose)	Erythromyciin (E.E.S.)[1] 12.5 mg/kg in 4 divided doses (maximum 500 mg/dose)	
Severe carditis, meningitis,* radiculomyelitis	Ceftriaxone (Rocephin)[1] 50–75 mg/kg IV in 1 dose (maximum 2 g/dose)	Cefotaxime (Claforan)[1] 150–200 mg/kg/day IV in 3 divided doses (maximum 2 g/dose) Penicillin G (Pfizerpen)[1] 200,000-400,000 U/kg/day in 6 divided doses (maximum 4 million U/dose)	14 days; for severe carditis and for meningitis, an oral agent may be used to complete a course of treatment after substantial clinical improvement
Lyme arthritis†	Same oral agents used for EM	Same oral agents used EM	28 days

[1]Not FDA approved for this indication.
*Some experts treat Lyme meningitis with doxycycline (Vibramycin)[1], administered orally, 4.4 mg/kg/day in 2 divided doses (maximum 100 mg/dose), for 14 days.
†Patients with persistent or recurrent arthritis 4 weeks after completing treatment may receive either a second 4-week course of treatment orally or 2 weeks of treatment with a parenterally administered antimicrobial listed above.

For patients with single EM, a 10-day course of doxycycline or a 14-day course of either amoxicillin or cefuroxime is recommended. For multiple EM, cranial nerve palsy (without apparent meningitis) or carditis that is asymptomatic and for which the patient is not hospitalized, a 14-day course of an oral antimicrobial is recommended. For complicated carditis (complete heart block) and for meningitis, a 14-day course of a parental agent is recommended, althought there is evidence that 14 days of doxycycline orally may be adequate for treating meningitis. Some experts complete a course of initial parenteral treatment with oral therapy after the patient has improved clinically. Patients with Lyme meningitis should be carefully evaluated for increased intracranial pressure which, if present, should be managed appropriately. There is no evidence that steroids are beneficial for patients with facial palsy due to Lyme disease. For treatment of Lyme arthritis, a 28-day course of an oral antimicrobial is recommended. Nonsteroidal antiinflammatory drugs may be effective for treating the pain and inflammation associated with Lyme arthritis.

References

Centers for Disease Control. Lyme disease: *Data and statistics.* Available at https://www.cdc.gov/lyme/stats/index.html [Accessed April 10,2018].
Feder HM Jr, Johnson BJB, O'Connell S, et al: A critical appraisal of "chronic lyme disease." *N Engl J Med* 357:1422–1430, 2007.
Hatcher S, Arroll B: Assessment and management of medically unexplained symptoms, *BMJ* 336:1124–1128, 2008.
Klempner MS, Hu LT, Evans J, et al: Two controlled trials of antibiotic treatment in patients with persistent symptoms and a history of Lyme disease, *N Engl J Med* 345:85–92, 2001.
Lantos PM: Chronic Lyme disease: the controversies and the science, *Expert Rev Anti Infect Ther* 9:787–797, 2011.
Lantos PM, Rumbaugh J, Bockenstedt LK, Falck-Ytter YT, et al: Clinical practice guidelines by the Infectious Diseases Society of America (IDSA), American Academy of Neurology (AAN), and American College of Rheumatology (ACR): 2020 guidelines for the prevention, diagnosis and treatment of Lyme disease, *Clin Infect Dis* J.23;72(1):1–8, 2021.
Ljøstad U, Skogvoll E, Eikeland R, et al: Oral doxycycline versus intravenous ceftriaxone for European Lyme neuroborreliosis: a multicentre, non-inferiority, double-blind, randomised trial, *Lancet Neurol* 7:690–695, 2008.
Nadelman RB, Nowakowski J, Fish D, et al: Tick bite study group: prophylaxis with a single-dose doxycycline for the prevention of Lyme disease after an Ixodes scapularis tick bite, *N Engl J Med* 345:79–84, 2001.
Shapiro ED: Clinical practice: Lyme disease, *N Engl J Med* 370:1724–1731, 2014.
Steere AC, Strle F, Wormser GP, et al: Lyme borreliosis, *Nat Rev Dis Primers* 2:1–18, 2016.

MALARIA

Method of
José D. Suárez, MD; Nestor Sosa, MD, MS; and Laura Naranjo, MD

CURRENT DIAGNOSIS

- Malaria is endemic in tropical and subtropical areas of Africa, Asia, Oceania, and Central and South America.
- Suspect malaria in returning travelers and recently arrived immigrants from an endemic region with fever, accompanied by headaches, chills, malaise and body aches.
- The microscopic examination of Giemsa-stained thin and thick peripheral blood smears is the standard diagnostic method for malaria.
- Rapid antigen detection tests (RADTs) and polymerase chain reaction (PCR) testing can be used for initial diagnosis, but species confirmation and level of parasitemia require microscopy.

CURRENT THERAPY

- Treatment selection should be based on *Plasmodium* species involved, geographic area where the infection was acquired, presence of resistance to antimalarial drugs, and disease severity.
- Intravenous (IV) artesunate is the recommended therapy for severe malaria. Alternative treatments are artemether-lumefantrine (Coartem),[1] atovaquone-proguanil (Malarone),[1] or quinine (Qualaquin)[1] plus doxycycline[1] or clindamycin.[1]
- Uncomplicated malaria caused by chloroquine-sensitive *Plasmodium* species can be treated with chloroquine or hydroxychloroquine (Plaquenil). Radical cure of *Plasmodium vivax* and *Plasmodium ovale*[1] requires subsequent therapy with primaquine or tafenoquine (Krintafel).
- Artemisinin combination therapies (i.e., artemether-lumefantrine [Coartem]) are the primary regimens for uncomplicated malaria caused by chloroquine-resistant *P. falciparum* or *P. vivax*.[1]

[1]Not FDA approved for this indication.

Introduction

Malaria is an important parasitic disease caused by protozoa of the genus *Plasmodium* (phylum Apicomplexa) and transmitted primarily by the bite of female *Anopheles* mosquitoes.

Malaria remains a formidable health problem, especially in sub-Saharan Africa and in other tropical regions in Southeast Asia, Oceania, and Latin America. The World Health Organization (WHO) estimates that in 2020, there were 241 million cases of malaria and 627,000 malaria deaths worldwide. The WHO and partners had projected a doubling of malaria deaths if the worst-case scenario of service disruptions occurred during the early months of the coronavirus disease 19 (COVID-19) pandemic, but in April 2020, a good response to adapt and implement WHO guidance to maintain essential malaria services during the pandemic was put in place. Nevertheless, an increase of 69,000 deaths was estimated over the previous year, and about two-thirds of these deaths (47,000) were caused by moderated disruptions during the COVID-19 pandemic.

The WHO African Region carries a disproportionately high share of the global malaria burden. In 2020, the region had 95% of malaria cases and 96% of malaria deaths. Children younger than 5 years of age accounted for an estimated 80% of all malaria deaths in the region. The economic losses from the disease, only in Africa, are estimated to reach $12 billion per year.

In recent years, a significant investment has been made in malaria control and elimination efforts. According to the 2019 WHO World Malaria Report, governments of malaria-endemic countries and international partners invested an estimated $2.7 billion in 2018. The incidence rate of malaria decreased globally between 2010 and 2018 from 71 to 57 cases per 1000 population at risk; the number of countries with zero or less than 100 indigenous cases also increased in the same period. These advances in malaria control can be explained by the use of long-lasting insecticidal nets, indoor residual spraying programs, rapid diagnostic testing, and access to artemisinin combination therapy (ACT).

Epidemiology

Most cases of malaria occur in Africa, but cases are reported in other tropical and subtropical regions of Southeast Asia (the Greater Mekong region), Oceania, India, and Central and South America (Figure 1).

Five different species of *Plasmodia* have been associated with the disease: four human malaria parasites, *P. falciparum, P. vivax, P. ovale,* and *P. malariae,* and one simian plasmodia of macaque monkeys, *P. knowlesi,* which affects humans in Borneo and peninsular Malaysia.

P. falciparum is responsible for the great majority of cases overall, is the most prevalent in sub-Saharan Africa, and it is associated more frequently with the most severe and fatal forms of the disease. *P. vivax* is the most prevalent species in Southeast Asia and Central and South America; *P. ovale* circulates with a very low incidence in Africa, Asia, and Oceania; and *P. malariae* is rare but has been reported worldwide.

The infection is transmitted primarily from person to person via the bite of the female mosquito of the genus *Anopheles*. More than 30 different species of *Anopheles* have been associated with malaria transmission worldwide. Environmental factors, like relative humidity, elevation, and temperature, influence the transmission of malaria in the endemic areas. The highest transmission occurs during the wet or rainy season. Other less common modes of transmission include transmission from mother to child (congenital malaria), blood transfusions, needle sharing, and via solid organ transplants.

Most cases in nonendemic areas are reported in travelers and immigrants arriving from areas with local malaria transmission. Rarely, infected mosquitos can be accidentally transported in airplanes and cause cases in and around airport terminals in non-endemic regions, the so-called *airport malaria*. In the United States, the Centers for Disease Control and Prevention (CDC) reports about 2000 imported malaria cases every year, and it is a nationally reportable disease. Travelers to sub-Saharan Africa have the greatest risk of acquiring the disease. Sixty-nine percent of the cases reported in the United States in 2018 were caused by *P. falciparum,* 9.5% by *P. vivax,* 5.2% by *P. ovale,* and 2.6% by *P. malariae.* Of these cases for which the country of acquisition was known, 85% were acquired in Africa.

One of the greatest challenges for the prevention and treatment of malaria has been the development of drug resistance, especially among *P. falciparum,* but also reported with *P. vivax.* The patterns and geographical distribution of drug-resistant parasites is complex. Resistance to malaria medication continues to be an

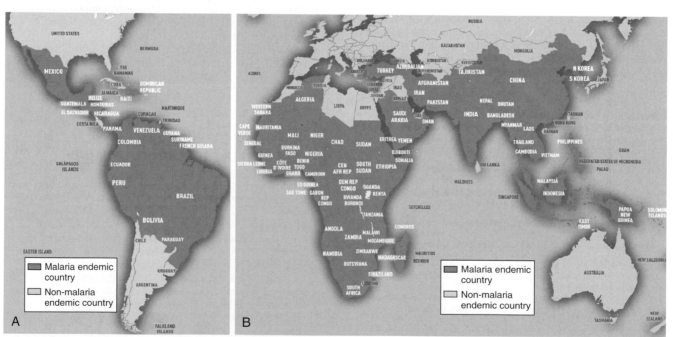

Figure 1 Malaria-endemic countries in the (**A**) western and (**B**) eastern hemispheres. Transmission occurs across most of Africa, Central and South America, Southern and Southeast Asia, as well as parts of the Caribbean, Eastern Europe, and the South Pacific. Countries are shaded completely, even if the area of endemicity is only in a small area of the country. (Modified from Centers for Disease Control and Prevention: *CDC Health Information for International Travel 2016,* New York, 2016, Oxford University Press. Public Domain.)

essential consideration when selecting drugs for treatment and chemoprophylaxis.

Since the 1970s, chloroquine resistance in *P. falciparum* has been confirmed in every continent where malaria is endemic, sparing only Mexico, Central America west of the Panama Canal, Haiti, the Dominican Republic, and a few Middle Eastern countries. High-grade chloroquine resistance in *P. vivax* has been reported in Papua New Guinea, the Solomon Islands, India, Myanmar, and Indonesia.

The emergence of resistance of *P. falciparum* to mefloquine (Lariam) has been documented in Myanmar (Burma), Lao People's Democratic Republic (Laos), Thailand, Cambodia, China, and Vietnam. Resistance to sulfadoxine/pyrimethamine (Fansidar)[2] and atovaquone/proguanil (Malarone) has also been reported. The resistance to these drugs has made ACT the treatment of choice for most cases of *P. falciparum* malaria. Unfortunately,

there have been recent reports of clinical failures and resistance to artemisinin derivatives from the five countries of Greater Mekong Subregions: Cambodia, Laos, Myanmar, Thailand, and Vietnam. There is now evidence of the clonal expansion of PfKelch13 mutations in Rwanda (R561H) and Uganda (C469Y and A675V). However, treatment failure rates in Rwanda and Uganda remain below 10%.

Parasite Life Cycle

The life cycle of the different species of *Plasmodia* are similar (Figure 2). The sexual cycle occurs in the mosquito, and repeated asexual cycles occur in the human host. The human infection starts when between 10 and 100 sporozoites—present in the salivary glands of the female Anopheles mosquito—enter the human host when the insect takes a blood meal. These sporozoites migrate from the dermis, invade the hepatocytes, and differentiate into hepatic schizonts that produce merozoites that later are liberated and invade circulating erythrocytes. *P. vivax* and *P.*

---

[2] Not available in the United States.

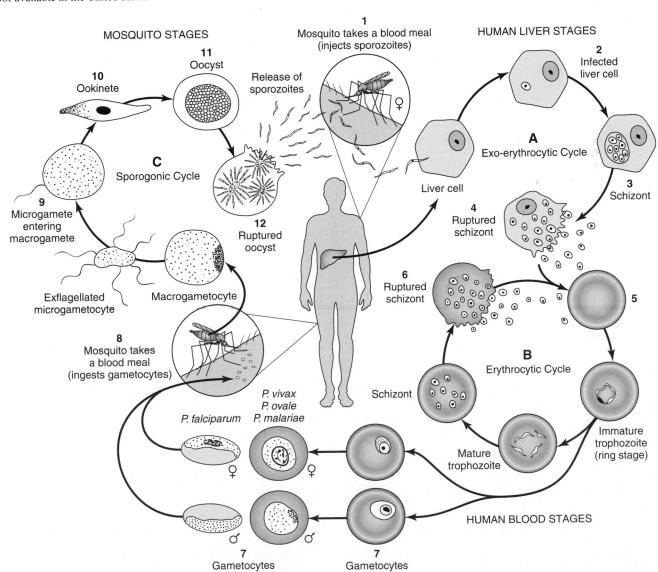

Figure 2 The malaria parasite life cycle involves two hosts. During a blood meal, a malaria-infected female *Anopheles* mosquito inoculates sporozoites into the human host (1). Sporozoites infect liver cells (2) and mature into schizonts (3), which rupture and release merozoites (4). (In *Plasmodium vivax* and *Plasmodium ovale*, a dormant stage [hypnozoites] can persist in the liver and cause relapses by invading the bloodstream weeks to years later.) After initial replication in the liver via exo-erythrocytic cycle or tissue schizogony (A), the parasites undergo asexual multiplication in erythrocytes via erythrocytic cycle or blood schizogony (B). Merozoites infect red blood cells (5). The ring stage trophozoites mature into schizonts, which rupture, releasing merozoites (6). Some parasites differentiate into sexual erythrocytic stages (gametocytes) (7). Blood-stage parasites are responsible for the clinical manifestations of the disease. The gametocytes—male (microgametocytes) and female (macrogametocytes)—are ingested by an *Anopheles* mosquito during a blood meal (8). The parasites' multiplication in the mosquito is known as the *sporogonic cycle* (C). While in the mosquito's stomach, the microgametes penetrate the macrogametes, generating zygotes (9). The zygotes in turn become motile and elongated (ookinetes) (10) and invade the midgut wall of the mosquito, where they develop into oocysts (11). The oocysts grow, rupture, and release sporozoites (12), which make their way to the mosquito's salivary glands. Inoculation of the sporozoites (1) into a new human host perpetuates the malaria life cycle.

ovale preferentially invade younger erythrocytes (reticulocytes); *P. falciparum* invades all types of erythrocytes.

Differences in the duration of these exo-erythrocytic cycles explain the variations in the incubation period of the different species of malaria. The incubation period is 9 to 12 days for *P. knowlesi*, 9 to 14 days for *P. falciparum*, 12 to 17 days for *P. vivax*, and 16 to 18 days for *P. ovale*. *P. malariae* is the most variable with ranges from 18 to 40 or more days.

The erythrocytic cycles of invasion and growth take approximately 24 hours in *P. knowlesi*; 48 hours in *P. falciparum*, *P. ovale*, and *P. vivax;* and 72 hours in *P. malariae*. These differences explain the periodicity of the fever paroxysm seen with the different parasites.

Once in the red blood cells, the merozoites develop into ring forms and mature into trophozoites, schizonts, and finally merozoites that rupture the cells and invade other erythrocytes, repeating and amplifying this erythrocytic asexual phase.

Some of the trophozoites in the red blood cells mature into gametocytes, the cell form that begins the sexual cycle when taken up by the mosquitoes. The sexual cycle takes approximately 1 to 2 weeks within the mosquito. The gametocytes cross-fertilize in the mosquito midgut and become diploid zygotes that form an ookinete, and finally close to 1000 sporozoites that migrate to the salivary glands and can infect another human host.

In *P. vivax* and *P. ovale* infection, parasites may remain latent in the liver as hypnozoites and reactivate after months, or even years, causing relapses of the disease.

Malaria Immunity

Acquired immunity to malaria is not sterilizing, but it protects against symptomatic and severe disease. It increases with age, number of episodes of the infection, and time spent living in the endemic area.

Several genetic polymorphisms seem to confer resistance to severe *P. falciparum* infection. Its relative increased prevalence in areas that are endemic for malaria demonstrates the natural selection forces of this disease over the human genome. Hemoglobin gene alterations like sickle cell disorders, thalassemia, hemoglobin C, hemoglobin E, and hemoglobin F; blood cell enzyme deficiencies like glucose-6-phosphate dehydrogenase; and certain blood group antigens (Duffy negative and ABO type O) have been associated with relative protection to infection or severe malaria.

Malaria is uncommon in neonates. The presence of fetal hemoglobin (hemoglobin F) and maternal antibodies may, in part, explain this observation.

Clinical Manifestations

The incubation period ranges from 9 to 40 days and it is influenced by the specific parasite species involved, the immune status of the host, the administration of chemoprophylaxis, and the infecting dose of sporozoites.

After a vague prodromal period of 2 to 3 days, malaria classically manifests as an acute febrile illness with episodes of paroxysms characterized by chills (classically described as "teeth-chattering, bed-shaking chills"), rigor, high temperature (≥40°C), and profuse sweating, usually followed by fatigue and sleep. Other common symptoms include headache, weakness, insomnia, arthralgia, myalgia, and, less frequently, diarrhea, abdominal pain, or respiratory symptoms.

Individuals with prior immunity and children may present only with fever and headache; infants and very young children may present with irritability and a decrease in food intake.

The malaria paroxysms may recur every 24 hours (*P. knowlesi*), 48 hours (tertian fever in *P. vivax* and *P. falciparum*), or 72 hours (quartan fever in *P. malariae*). In primary infections, this periodicity may take several days to become apparent. The patient may be relatively asymptomatic between these paroxysms.

On physical examination, the patient may exhibit pallor, hepatosplenomegaly and, in severe cases, jaundice, altered mental status, and convulsions. Rash, pulmonary manifestation, and lymphadenopathy are rare.

TABLE 1	Features of Complicated or Severe Malaria
FINDING	**DESCRIPTION**
Cerebral malaria	Diminished consciousness, Blantyre Coma Scale score of ≤2 in children, Glasgow Coma Scale score <9 in adults or seizures
Respiratory distress/ pulmonary edema	Radiographic evidence, hypoxemia
Hyperparasitemia	>2% or >100,000/μL in low-transmission settings; or >5% or >250,000 in high-transmission settings
Severe anemia	<5g Hgb or <15% Hct
Hypoglycemia	<2.2 mmol/L or 40 mg/dL
Jaundice/icterus	Clinically evident
Renal failure	Creatinine >265 mmol/L
Hemoglobinuria	
Metabolic acidosis or hyperlactatemia	HCO_3 <15 mmol/L or lactate >5 mmol/L
Shock	SBP <70 mm Hg in adults; SBP <50 mm Hg in children
Abnormal spontaneous bleeding	

HCO₃, Bicarbonate; *Hct*, hematocrit; *Hgb*, hemoglobin; *SBP*, systolic blood pressure.

Severe or Complicated Malaria

Nonimmune individuals such as children or travelers to endemic areas or pregnant females may develop more severe manifestations of malaria. Complicated malaria, more commonly associated with *P. falciparum* infection, has been recently reported with *P. knowlesi* and *P. vivax*. The most important clinical and laboratory findings of complicated malaria are listed in Table 1. In parasitemic patients, the presence of any of the clinical or laboratory features of severe malaria represents a medical emergency, and hospitalization, admission into critical care units, and rapid initiation of specific treatment are important. Even in patients with less severe disease, it is advisable to hospitalize all nonimmune individuals during their initial treatment period because of the ability of *P. falciparum* infection to progress in just a few hours to severe and life-threatening complications.

The clinical presentation of complicated malaria may be different in children and adults. Cerebral malaria (see later) is more common in children; multiorgan system involvement is more frequent in adults. Important clues in the physical examination are prostration, deep breathing, a decreased level of consciousness, slow capillary filling, signs of congestive heart failure, hepatosplenomegaly, pallor, and decreased urine output. Mortality rates of complicated or severe malaria range between 15% and 22% in adults and between 8.5% and 10.9% in children.

Cerebral Malaria

Parasite sequestration in the cerebral microvasculature is associated with a variable and potentially lethal constellation of symptoms that include a decreased level of consciousness, coma, generalized seizures, and/or focal neurologic deficits. Histopathologic findings frequently exhibit the presence of sequestered parasites, ring hemorrhages, perivascular leukocyte infiltrates, and immune-histochemical evidence of endothelial activation. In children with cerebral malaria, intracranial pressure is usually increased. Among those who survive, neurologic recovery can be rapid and complete, but sequelae have been reported in up to 15% of children with cerebral malaria. In patients with malaria who present with neurologic manifestations, it is important to exclude other conditions like meningitis, hypoglycemia, and other causes of encephalopathy. Fundoscopic examination may be useful, revealing retinal hemorrhages and white exudates suggestive of malarial retinopathy.

Respiratory Failure/Respiratory Distress Syndrome
Noncardiogenic pulmonary edema is a complication of severe *P. falciparum* malaria, seen more frequently in adults than in children. Sequestration of infected erythrocytes in the lungs is thought to be associated with the production of cytokines, increased vascular permeability, pulmonary edema, dyspnea, hypoxia and progression to acute lung injury, and respiratory distress syndrome. Patients may become hypoxemic and require mechanical ventilation.

Acute Kidney Injury
Although mild proteinuria and oliguria can be present in uncomplicated malaria, acute renal failure—secondary to decreased renal perfusion, intravascular hemolysis, hemoglobinuria, acute tubular necrosis, and anuria—is a complication of severe malaria. Renal replacement therapy and general support through the critical period is associated with complete recovery of renal function in the majority of patients.

Malaria During Pregnancy
Malaria during pregnancy, especially in nonimmune primigravidas, is associated with increased morbidity and mortality. Pregnant women are particularly vulnerable to *Plasmodium falciparum* infection because red blood cells infected with the parasite can sequester in the placenta and thereby cause adverse fetal effects. The relative immunosuppression of pregnancy and parasite accumulation in the placenta related to its affinity with abundant chondroitin sulfate A (CSA) seem to be contributing factors for this phenomenon. Complications such as premature delivery, intrauterine growth retardation, low neonatal birth weight, increased newborn mortality, and maternal hypoglycemia and pulmonary edema have been reported. Placental malaria during subsequent pregnancies tends to be less severe than in the first pregnancy because of the development of immunity to CSA-binding parasites. The increased risk for acquiring malaria and developing more severe disease persists for at least 60 to 70 days postpartum.

If anti-malarial drugs do not achieve therapeutic levels in the placenta, parasites sequestered there may be released intermittently into the peripheral blood and cause recurrent maternal infection.

Vertical Transmission
All species of malaria parasite can be transmitted in utero; congenital disease is most often associated with *P. falciparum* and *P. vivax*. Placental infection is a prerequisite for, but does not predict, congenital disease. Placental infection is more common than cord blood parasitemia, which is more common than detection of parasites in the infant's peripheral blood.

Non-*falciparum* Malaria
P. vivax and *P. ovale* are usually not associated with severe disease, but acute lung injury and splenic rupture may occur. Severe cases of *P. vivax* have been reported in Papua New Guinea and Indonesia, with complications like severe anemia, cerebral malaria, and respiratory distress. Relapses of *P. vivax* and *P. ovale* caused by reactivation of the hypnozoites months or years after the initial infection is another characteristic of these two *Plasmodium* species.

P. malariae, the etiology of quartan fever, is associated with very low parasitemia and chronic indolent infection; however, nephrotic syndrome has been reported in young children in endemic areas.

In *P. knowlesi*, the clinical presentation is similar to uncomplicated *P. falciparum* malaria, but approximately 10% of cases may present with daily fever spikes, hyperparasitemia, metabolic acidosis, hepatic and renal dysfunction, respiratory distress, severe anemia, and refractory hypotension.

Laboratory Diagnosis
The microscopic examination of Giemsa-stained thin and thick peripheral blood smears is the standard diagnostic method for malaria. Thick smears concentrate red cell layers by lysing the erythrocytes and are used to screen a relatively large amount of blood. Thin smears are used to determine the *Plasmodium* species based on the morphology and characteristics of the circulating forms.

P. falciparum infections are characterized by the presence of thin ring forms, frequently positioned at the red cell membrane; multiple infected cells; banana-shaped gametocytes; and the absence of trophozoites and schizonts that are sequestered in the microvasculature. The smears of *P. vivax* and *P. ovale* have thicker rings, ameboid trophozoites, schizonts, and round gametocytes. Erythrocyte enlargement and Schüffner dots are common in *P. vivax* and *P. ovale* but absent in other malaria species. *P. malariae* has characteristic band forms, and *P. knowlesi* rings are similar to *P. falciparum*, but its mature forms and gametocytes are indistinguishable from *P. malariae*.

In addition to direct microscopy, other diagnostic methods, such as rapid antigen detection tests (RADTs), PCR, and serology are used in different settings.

RADTs are increasingly useful, especially in situations in which microscopy is not immediately available. RADTs are immunochromatographic tests that detect *Plasmodium* antigens, like *P. falciparum* histidine-rich protein 2 (PfHRP2) or pan-malarial *Plasmodium aldolase* (PMA). Some of these tests are specific for *P. falciparum* or *P. vivax*, whereas others detect antigens common to several *Plasmodium* species.

The reported sensitivity and specificity of most RADTs are high, frequently around 95% and 99%, respectively. In patients with low parasitemia (less than 100 parasites/μL), the sensitivity decreases.

Even when RADTs are positive, direct microscopy is indicated to confirm the diagnosis to the species level (based on morphology) and to estimate the level of parasitemia. Most RADTs are not useful to evaluate treatment response because they may remain positive for several weeks after successful treatment.

Deletions in the parasite's *pfhrp2* and *pfhrp3* (*pfhrp2/3*) genes renders parasites undetectable by RADTs that are based on histidine-rich protein 2 (HRP2). The WHO recommends that countries with reports of *pfhrp2/3* deletions (Brazil, Democratic Republic of the Congo, Djibouti, Ethiopia, Ghana, Sudan, Uganda, United Republic of Tanzania) or neighboring countries conduct representative baseline surveys among suspected malaria cases to determine whether the prevalence of *pfhrp2/3* deletions causing false-negative RADT results has reached a threshold for a change in RADT (>5% *pfhrp2* deletions causing false negative RADT results).

PCR detects segments of the parasite DNA using amplification. It is very specific and may be useful in very low parasitemia, but it is not yet readily available in most clinical settings where malaria patients are diagnosed.

Serologic tests, like indirect fluorescent antibody (IFA) tests, are not useful for routine diagnosis of acute cases of malaria. Antibody positivity may take several days or weeks to develop. Serology is useful to screen blood donors in transfusion-related cases, to detect infection as part of an evaluation for tropical splenomegaly syndrome (TSS) when parasitemia is below the level of detection for microscopy or RADTs, and to test treated and cured malaria patients.

Other nonspecific clinical laboratory abnormalities frequently detected in patients with malaria are anemia, with decreased hemoglobin and hematocrit, increased lactic dehydrogenase (LDH) levels, and decreased haptoglobin levels. The anemia is normocytic normochromic, but microcytosis is not infrequent, especially in patients with iron deficiency or thalassemia. The white cell count may be increased, decreased, or normal. Platelet counts may be decreased or normal. Mild hyponatremia may be present secondary to inappropriate secretion of antidiuretic hormone, vomiting, or urinary losses.

In severe cases of malaria, hyperbilirubinemia, metabolic (lactic) acidosis, increased creatinine, albuminuria, and hemoglobinuria may be present. Hypoglycemia may occur in patients with malaria. Contributing factors to hypoglycemia are impaired hepatic neoglucogenesis, decreased oral intake, and increased glucose consumption caused by the hypermetabolic state and hyperinsulinemia secondary to drugs like quinine or quinidine.

In African children with malaria, secondary bacterial infection, including bacteremia, is not uncommon.

TABLE 2 Antimalarial Drugs: Activity and Side Effects

DRUG (TRADE NAME)	ACTIVITY	INDICATION	SIDE EFFECTS	COMMENTS
Chloroquine (Aralen), hydroxychloroquine (Plaquenil)	Blood schizonts (all *Plasmodia*) and gametocytes (*P. ovale, P. malariae, P. vivax, P. knowlesi*)	Treatment of choice for chloroquine-susceptible *Plasmodium*	GI symptoms, headache, dizziness, insomnia, visual changes, ototoxicity, retinopathy, and peripheral neuropathy	Safe in children and in pregnant patients
Atovaquone/Proguanil (Malarone)	Blood and tissue schizonts	Chemoprophylaxis and treatment of uncomplicated malaria outside endemic areas (in combination with artesunate[1] or primaquine[1])*	Headache, cough, GI upset, dizziness, mucosal ulcerations, increased enzymes in LFTs	Safe in children >5 kg of body weight Contraindicated in severe renal dysfunction
Artemisinin derivatives[†]: artemether, artesunate, dihydroartemisinin[2]	Blood schizonts and gametocytes	Treatment of choice for uncomplicated and severe *P. falciparum* malaria[1] in endemic areas	GI symptoms, dizziness, headache, neutropenia, increased enzymes in LFTs	Contraindicated in the first trimester of pregnancy
Quinine sulfate (Qualaquin) and Quinidine gluconate[‡]	Blood schizonts of all *Plasmodium* species, gametocytes of *P. vivax, P. ovale,* and *P. malariae*	Treatment of uncomplicated or severe malaria when ACTs are not available or cannot be used (early pregnancy)[1]	Tinnitus, hearing impairment or loss, nausea, headache, dizziness, dysphoria, visual changes, QT prolongation, angina, hypotension, vertigo, vomiting, diarrhea, hypoglycemia	Can be used in the first trimester of pregnancy
Tetracyclines: doxycycline (Vibramycin), tetracycline	Blood schizonts of all *Plasmodium* species	Chemoprophylaxis of *P. falciparum* Treatment of chloroquine-resistant *P. falciparum* and *P. vivax*[1] in combination with quinine	GI symptoms, dry mouth, stomatitis, photodermatitis, *Candida vaginitis,* anal pruritus	Contraindicated in children <8 years of age and in pregnant patients
Clindamycin (Cleocin)	Blood schizonts of all *Plasmodium* species	Severe[1] or uncomplicated malaria[1] in combination with artemisinin derivatives or quinine	GI symptoms (including *Clostridium difficile* colitis), rash	Not to be used as monotherapy
Mefloquine (Lariam)	Blood schizonts of all *Plasmodium* species	Chemoprophylaxis of all *Plasmodium* species[1] Treatment of *P. falciparum* malaria as part of ACT	GI symptoms, neuropsychiatric symptoms such as anxiety, irritability, paranoia, depression, hallucinations	Violent behavior reported with prolonged use Safe during pregnancy
Primaquine sulfate	Exo-erythrocytic forms (hypnozoites), gametocytes	Chemoprophylaxis of *P. vivax*–endemic areas[1] Treatment of *P. vivax* and *P. ovale* hypnozoites[1] (prevention of relapses or radical cure)	GI symptoms, severe hemolytic anemia in G6PD-deficient patients	Level of G6PD should be checked before primaquine use

*Not recommended in endemic areas because of resistance to atovaquone.

[†]Used in combination with other agents, ACT is considered the treatment of choice for *P. falciparum* malaria in endemic areas. Available ACT agents include artemether plus lumefantrine (Coartem), which is the only FDA-approved treatment; artesunate plus amodiaquine (Coarsucam)[2]; artesunate plus mefloquine (Artequin)[2]; artesunate plus sulfadoxine-pyrimethamine (Fansidar)[2]; and dihydroartemisinin plus piperaquine (Eurartesim).[2]

[‡]Quinidine gluconate intravenous formulation is the only FDA-approved treatment for severe malaria in the United States, but it is no longer available. Cardiac monitoring is recommended during treatment with this drug.

[1]Not FDA approved for this indication.

[2]Not available in the United States.

ACT, artemisinin combination therapy; *G6PD,* glucose-6-phosphate dehydrogenase; *GI,* gastrointestinal; *LFTs,* liver function tests.

Antimalarial Drugs

There are multiple drugs used in the treatment and prevention of malaria. Their indication depends on the species involved, availability of the medication, presence of drug resistance, and severity of the disease. Some of the drugs have activity against the erythrocytic phase or asexual forms and are referred to as *blood schizonticides.* Other antimalarial substances kill tissue or exoerythrocytic parasites in the liver and are called *tissue schizonticides.* Tissue schizonticides prevent disease relapses in patients with *P. vivax* and *P. malariae.* Finally, other drugs demonstrate activity against gametocytes and decrease disease transmission, preventing the sexual stage in the mosquito. See Table 2 for the name, activity, and side effects of the most commonly used antimalarial drugs.

Chloroquine (Aralen) and hydroxychloroquine (Plaquenil) are two of the oldest antimalarial drugs. They are considered blood schizonticides and also have gametocidal activity. They can be used in the prevention and treatment of all *Plasmodium* species in the absence of drug resistance, and they are considered the treatment of choice for *P. vivax*, *P. malariae*, *P. ovale*, and *P. knowlesi*. Unfortunately, chloroquine resistance in *P. falciparum* is widespread, and these drugs are no longer recommended for prevention or treatment, except in limited areas of Central America, the Caribbean, and the Middle East.

The combination of atovaquone/proguanil (Malarone) demonstrates activity against both tissue and blood schizonts and is frequently used in malaria prophylaxis or as part of multidrug regimens with primaquine[1] or artesunate[1] for the treatment of uncomplicated chloroquine-resistant malaria in returning travelers outside endemic areas. The emergence of resistance to the atovaquone component limits its use in endemic areas.

Artemisinin derivatives, like artemether, artesunate, and dihydroartemisinin,[2] have activity against blood schizonts and gametocytes. These substances are originally derived from the Chinese medicinal plant qinghaosu (*Artemisia annua*) and are frequently used in combination with other drugs. The available combinations are collectively referred to as *artemisinin combination therapy* (ACT) and include artemether plus lumefantrine (Coartem, approved by the U.S. Food and Drug Administration [FDA]); artesunate plus amodiaquine (Coarsucam, Arsuamoon),[2] artesunate plus mefloquine (Artequin),[2] dihydroartemisinin plus piperaquine (Eurartesim),[2] and sulfadoxina plus pyrimethamine (Fansidar).[2]

ACT is considered the first-line treatment of uncomplicated *P. falciparum* malaria in endemic areas. The recent emergence of *P. falciparum* resistant to ACT in Southeast Asia is compromising the efficacy of these two drug combinations. A recent study demonstrated improved efficacy of a three-drug regimen (dihydroartemisinin plus piperaquine plus mefloquine) in areas with artemisinin resistance. Artemisinin derivatives can be used in children and pregnant woman but are contraindicated during the first trimester of pregnancy. Oral monotherapy with artemisinin derivatives is strongly discouraged to prevent the development of resistance.

Quinine sulfate (Qualaquin) is one of the oldest antimalarial drugs and is derived from the bark of the Cinchona tree (*Cinchona calisaya*). Quinine sulfate demonstrates activity against blood schizonts and gametocytes of *P. vivax*, *P. ovale*, and *P. malariae*. It is used in combination with other drugs in severe malaria[1] and for uncomplicated chloroquine-resistant malaria species during pregnancy. Quinine has a narrow therapeutic index and can produce cardiac conduction disturbances (e.g., QT prolongation, angina) and lead to cardiac arrest. Hyperinsulinemic hypoglycemia has been observed in children, older adults and pregnant women. Intravenous (IV) preparations of quinine dihydrochloride and the antiarrhythmic quinidine gluconate were previously used as antimalarial drugs but are no longer available in the United States.

The antibiotics tetracycline and doxycycline (Vibramycin) display activity against blood schizonts; the latter is frequently used in travelers as prophylaxis for chloroquine- and mefloquine-resistant *P. falciparum* malaria. Tetracyclines can be employed in combination with quinine for the treatment of uncomplicated *P. falciparum* malaria and chloroquine-resistant *P. vivax* malaria.[1] These antibiotics should not be used as monotherapy against malaria, and they are contraindicated during pregnancy and for children younger than 8 years of age.

Clindamycin (Cleocin) is another antibiotic that acts as a blood schizonticide for all *Plasmodium* species. It is effective in combination with quinine for the treatment of uncomplicated *P. falciparum* malaria and for chloroquine resistant *P. vivax* when tetracyclines are contraindicated.[1]

Mefloquine (Lariam) is an antimalarial drug that is structurally related to quinine. It has a long half-life and has activity against blood schizonts of all *Plasmodium* species. It is used in prophylaxis of malaria but can be used as an alternative treatment of uncomplicated *P. falciparum* malaria and in combination with primaquine[1] (tissue schizonticide) in cases of chloroquine-resistant *P. vivax* infection. It is generally well tolerated, but central nervous system and psychiatric side effects, such as anxiety, depression, paranoia, hallucinations, and violent behavior, have been reported.

Primaquine is active against tissue or exoerythrocytic forms and gametocytes of malaria parasites. It is indicated in the radical cure of *P. vivax* and *P. ovale*[1] eliminating the hypnozoites and preventing relapses of the disease. Primaquine can be used for prophylaxis in travelers to areas when greater than 90% of the cases of malaria are caused by *P. vivax*.[1] In patients with glucose-6-phosphate dehydrogenase (G6PD) deficiency, primaquine administration may cause acute hemolytic anemia. The activity of the G6PD enzyme should be measured before its usage. Primaquine is also contraindicated during pregnancy and breast-feeding, unless the infant has been tested for G6PD deficiency.

Tafenoquine (Arakoda, Krintafel), an FDA-approved antimalarial drug related to primaquine. It is recommended for prophylaxis of all *Plasmodium* species (Arakoda) and as a radical cure of *P. vivax* infection combined with chloroquine only (Krintafel). Like primaquine, tafenoquine should not be used in individuals with G6PD deficiency, during pregnancy, or while breast-feeding.

Lumefantrine is an antimalarial drug used in combination with artemether (as Coartem) in the treatment of uncomplicated *P. falciparum* malaria. It is active against erythrocytic stages of all *Plasmodium* species. Possible serious adverse effects reported with this combination include QT prolongation, bullous eruption, urticaria, splenomegaly, hepatomegaly, hypersensitivity reaction, and angioedema. Artemether-lumefantrine (Coartem) is assigned a pregnancy category C by the FDA, and its use during pregnancy should only be considered when the benefits outweigh the risks.

For specific adult and pediatric dosing regimens, clinical indications, treatment duration, and primary and alternative antimalarial regimens, see Table 3.

Treatment of Uncomplicated Malaria

The CDC provides advice to healthcare providers on the diagnosis and treatment of malaria and can be reached Monday to Friday, 9 AM to 5 PM EST through the CDC Malaria Hotline (770) 488-7788, or toll free at (855) 856-4713. On off-hours, weekends, and federal holidays, call (770) 488-7100, and ask to have the on-call malaria clinician paged.

For *P. falciparum* or species not identified acquired in areas with chloroquine resistance, there are four regimens: Artemether-lumefantrine (Coartem) is the preferred regimen; alternatives are atovaquone-proguanil (Malarone); quinine plus either doxycycline,[1] tetracycline,[1] or clindamycin[1]; or mefloquine (Lariam). For cases of *P. falciparum* acquired in areas without chloroquine resistance, either chloroquine or hydroxychloroquine can be used. Alternatively, the same drugs used for chloroquine-resistant *P. falciparum* can be used.

---

[1] Not FDA approved for this indication.
[2] Not available in the United States.

[1] Not FDA approved for this indication.

TABLE 3	Antimalarial Regimens and Dosing by Clinical Diagnosis and Resistance

CLINICAL DIAGNOSIS/ PLASMODIUM SPECIES/ DRUG SUSCEPTIBILITY	DRUG/PRESENTATION	PEDIATRIC DOSE#	ADULT DOSE
Primary Regimens			
Uncomplicated malaria/*P. falciparum*/ chloroquine-sensitive or uncomplicated malaria/*P. malariae* or *P. knowlesi*	Chloroquine phosphate 1 tab = 500 mg (salt) (300 mg of base)	10-mg base/kg PO, then 5-mg base/kg PO at 6, 24, and 48 h. Total 25 mg base/kg	1 g salt (600-mg base) PO, then 500 mg in 6 h, and then 500 mg daily × 2 days. Total dose 2500 mg
	Hydroxychloroquine 1 tab = 200 mg (salt) (155 mg of base)		800 mg salt (620-mg base) PO, then 400 mg daily × 2 days. Total dose 2000 mg
Primary Regimens			
Uncomplicated malaria/*P. falciparum* or species not identified Chloroquine resistance or unknown resistance	Artemether/lumefantrine (Coartem)* 1 tab = 20 mg/120 mg	The patient should receive the initial dose, followed by the second dose 8 h later, and then 1 dose bid for the following 2 days: 5 to <15 kg: 1 tab per dose 15 to <25 kg: 2 tabs per dose 25 to <35 kg: 3 tabs per dose ≥35 kg: 4 tablets per dose	4 tabs PO in a single dose, then 4 tabs after 8 h, then 4 tabs every 12 h × 2 days
	Atovaquone/proguanil (Malarone)† Adult tab = 250 mg/100 mg Pediatric tab = 62.5 mg/25 mg	5 to <8 kg: 2 pediatric tabs PO qd × 3 days 8 to <10 kg: 3 pediatric tabs PO qd × 3 days 10 to <20 kg: 1 adult tab PO qd × 3 days 20 to <30 kg: 2 adult tabs PO qd × 3 days 30 to <40 kg: 3 adult tabs PO qd × 3 days ≥0 kg: 4 adult tabs PO qd × 3 days	4 adult tabs PO in a single dose daily × 3 days
	Quinine sulfate (Qualaquin) 1 tab = 324 mg either: Doxycycline[1] 100 mg‡ Tetracycline[1] 250 mg‡ Clindamycin[1] 450 mg	**Quinine sulfate:** 10 mg/kg PO tid × 3 days (7 days if Southeast Asia) plus one of the following: **Clindamycin:** 20 mg/kg/day divided tid × 7 days for children younger than 8 years *or* **Doxycycline:** 2.2 mg/kg/bid × 7 days *or* **Tetracycline:** 25 mg/kg/day PO divided qid × 7 days	**Quinine sulfate:** 648 mg PO tid × 3 days (7 days if Southeast Asia) plus **Doxycycline:** 100 mg PO bid × 7 days *or* Tetracycline: 250 mg PO qid × 7 days *or* **Clindamycin:** 20 mg/kg/day PO divided tid × 7 days
Alternative Regimens			
	Mefloquine§ 1 tab = 250 mg	15 mg salt/kg (13.7-mg base) PO as initial dose, and then 10 mg salt/kg (9.1-mg base/kg) PO given 6–12 h after initial dose. Total dose: 25 mg salt/kg	750 mg (684-mg base) PO as initial dose, and then 500 mg PO × 1 dose 6-12 h later.# Total 1250 mg
Primary Regimens			
Uncomplicated malaria/*P. vivax* or chloroquine-sensitive *P. ovale*	Chloroquine phosphate or hydroxychloroquine plus either primaquine[1] phosphate 1 tab = 15 mg (base) or tafenoquine[1] (Arakoda): 1 tab = 100 mg (Krintafel): 1 tab = 150 mg	**Chloroquine phosphate** or **hydroxychloroquine** see doses above Primaquine phosphate: 0.5 mg/kg base PO qd × 14 days *or* Tafenoquine succinate: 300 mg PO × 1 dose (children ≥16 years)	**Chloroquine phosphate:** see doses above Primaquine phosphate: 30 mg base = 2 tab PO qd × 14 days *or* Tafenoquine succinate:¶ 300 mg PO × 1 dose

CLINICAL DIAGNOSIS/ PLASMODIUM SPECIES/ DRUG SUSCEPTIBILITY	DRUG/PRESENTATION	PEDIATRIC DOSE#	ADULT DOSE
Primary Regimens			
Uncomplicated malaria/ *P. vivax* In case of suspected chloroquine-resistant *P. vivax*	1. Artemether- lumefantrine (Coartem)[1] plus either primaquine phosphate or tafenoquine	**Artemether-lumefantrine:** see doses above Primaquine phosphate: see doses above Tafenoquine: see doses above	**Artemether-lumefantrine:** see doses above **Primaquine phosphate:** see doses above Tafenoquine: see doses above
	2. Atovaquone-proguanil (Malarone)[1] plus either primaquine phosphate or tafenoquine	**Atovaquone-proguanil:** see doses above Primaquine phosphate or **Tafenoquine:** see doses above	**Atovaquone-proguanil:** see doses above Primaquine phosphate or **Tafenoquine:** see doses above
	3. Quinine sulfate[1] plus either doxycycline[1] or tetracycline[1] plus either primaquine phosphate or tafenoquine	**Quinine sulfate:** see doses above for 3 days Doxycycline or **Tetracycline:** see doses above Clindamycin: see doses above Primaquine phosphate: see doses above Tafenoquine can be used instead of primaquine in children ≥16 years: 300 mg PO × 1 dose	**Quinine sulfate:** see doses above for 3 days Doxycycline or **Tetracycline:** see doses above Clindamycin: see doses above Primaquine phosphate or **Tafenoquine:** see doses above
	4. Mefloquine plus either primaquine phosphate or tafenoquine	**Mefloquine:** see doses above Primaquine phosphate: see doses above Tafenoquine can be used instead of primaquine in children ≥16 years: 300 mg PO × 1 dose	**Mefloquine:** see doses above Primaquine phosphate or **Tafenoquine:** see doses above
Severe malaria	1. Artesunate IV 110-mg/ vial followed by a complete oral course of one of the following: Artemether/ lumefantrine[1] Atovaquone/proguanil[1] Quinine[1] plus doxycycline[1]	**Artesunate:** <20 kg 3.0 mg/kg IV at 0, 12, and 24 h. Continue q24h if unable to take oral medication **Atovaqoane/proguanil** × 3 days (see doses above) **Artemether/lumefantrine** × 3 days (see doses above) **Quinine sulfate:** × 3 days (7 days if Southeast Asia) plus **Doxycycline:** 2.2 mg/kg q12h × 7 days	**Artesunate:** 2.4 mg/kg IV at 0, 12, and 24 h. Continue q24h if unable to take oral medication **Atovaquane/proguanil** × 3 days (see doses above) **Artemether/lumefantrine** × 3 days (see doses above) **Quinine sulfate:** × 3 days (7 days if Southeast Asia) plus **Doxycycline:** 100 mg q12h × 7 days

#Pediatric dose should not be higher than adult dose.

*Artemether-lumefantrine: Take with food. Drug of choice in second/third trimester of pregnancy. Recommended by experts in the first trimester but not yet in the official guidelines.

†Atovaquone-proguanil: Take with food; repeat dose if patient vomits within 30 minutes; Not recommended in pregnancy.

‡Doxycycline and tetracycline: Not recommended during pregnancy or in children younger than 8 years of age. Avoid concomitant intake of divalent cations and antacids. The American Academy of Pediatrics now permits less than 21 days for any acute infection for children of all ages.

§Mefloquine: Not effective against strains of *P. falciparum* from Southeast Asia.

¶Tafenoquine succinate: Must have normal glucose-6-phosphate dehydrogenase activity.

#This is an off-label dose.

[1]Not FDA approved for this indication.

⁵Investigational drug in the United States.

Chloroquine or hydroxychloroquine can be used for most cases of malaria caused by *P. ovale* and *P. vivax*, *P. malariae*, and *P. knowlesi*. If these drugs are not available, artemether-lumefantrine (Coartem),[1] atovaquone-proguanil (Malarone),[1] mefloquine (Lariam),[1] or quinine[1] plus either doxycycline,[1] tetracycline,[1] or clindamycin[1] can be used. These regimens can be used for infections where chloroquine-resistant *P. vivax* has been reported (Papua New Guinea, Indonesia, Burma, and certain areas of Central and South America).

To eradicate *P. vivax* and *P. ovale* hypnozoites, patients should also be treated with either tafenoquine (Krintafel)[1] or primaquine phosphate.[1] Tafenoquine can be used in patients 16 years of age or older and is given as a single dose. If primaquine phosphate is used, the CDC recommends a dose of 30 mg (base) by mouth daily for 14 days. Because of reduced efficacy of primaquine in patients over 70 kg, the total dose of primaquine should be adjusted in these patients to 6 mg/kg. This total dose should be given in daily doses of 30 mg for the number of days needed to complete the total dose. As mentioned earlier, quantitative G6PD enzyme activity should be measured before the use of primaquine or tafenoquine.

[1]Not FDA approved for this indication.

Treatment of Severe Malaria

Patients with severe malaria should be treated promptly. IV artesunate is the treatment of choice regardless of the species involved. Clinicians caring for patients with suspected severe malaria should call the CDC to obtain IV artesunate as part of an expanded-use investigational new drug (IND) protocol (see the CDC contact information provided earlier in this chapter). Oral therapies should be started while waiting for IV artesunate to arrive. The preferred antimalarial drug for interim oral treatment is artemether-lumefantrine (Coartem)[1] because of its fast onset of action. Other oral options include atovaquone-proguanil (Malarone)[1], quinine[1] plus doxycycline (Vibramycin),[1] and mefloquine (Lariam).[1] Patients on treatment for severe malaria should have one set of blood smears (thick and thin) performed every 12 to 24 hours until a negative result (no *Plasmodium* parasites are detected) is reported.

After the course of IV artesunate is completed, if parasite density is ≤1% (assessed on a blood smear collected 4 hours after the last dose of IV artesunate), and the patient can tolerate oral treatment, a full treatment course with a follow-up regimen must be administered (see Table 3).

Antimalarial Drugs in Pregnancy

Monitoring the safety of antimalarial drugs and understanding their pharmacokinetics is particularly important in pregnancy because of altered maternal physiology and risks to the developing fetus. The scheme will depend on drug susceptibility, the region where infection was acquired, gestational age, severity of the disease, and drug category.

For infections with chloroquine-sensitive *P. falciparum, P. vivax, P. ovale,* and *P. knowlesi,* chloroquine or hydroxychloroquine can be used during pregnancy. If resistance to chloroquine is suspected, quinine sulfate[1] plus clindamycin[1] or mefloquine[1] can be used for treatment during the first trimester of pregnancy. Artemether-lumefantrine (Coartem)[1] is the treatment of choice during the second and third trimesters of pregnancy in chloroquine-resistant malaria infections.

Primaquine and tafenoquine should not be given during pregnancy. Pregnant patients with *P. vivax* and *P. ovale* infections should receive chloroquine prophylaxis[1] (300 mg [base] PO once a week) for the duration of the pregnancy to prevent relapses. After delivery, patients with normal G6PD activity should be treated with primaquine or tafenoquine or continue with chloroquine prophylaxis for a total of 1 year. For women who are breast-feeding, infants should be tested for G6PD deficiency and, if found to have normal activity, oral primaquine can be given to the mother. Tafenoquine is not recommended during breast-feeding.

Treatment of Pediatric Patients

The majority of cases and deaths, especially in sub-Saharan Africa, occur in young children. Prompt diagnosis and therapy initiation are key to prevent complications, like cerebral malaria in young children. Recommended treatment regimens are essentially the same as in adults, with few differences. Weight-based dose adjustments are necessary, and pediatric doses should not exceed those given to adults. Tetracycline and doxycycline should be avoided in children younger than 8 years of age. Tafenoquine is not indicated in those younger than 16 years of age. For complete details on dosing and treatment duration in pediatric patients, see Table 3.

Prevention of Malaria

Prevention of malaria includes both chemoprophylaxis and measures taken to reduce the number of mosquito bites and vaccines.

Travelers to endemic areas can reduce mosquito bites by using *N,N*-diethyl-meta-toluamide (DEET 10% to 50%) or 7% picaridin-containing insect repellents on exposed skin (applied after sunscreen), wearing permethrin-treated clothing, wearing clothes and footwear that cover as much skin as possible, sleeping under permethrin-treated bed nets, staying in housing with air-conditioning and well-screened areas cleared of mosquitoes, and refraining from outdoor activity during peak *Anopheles* biting hours (from dusk to dawn).

Recommendations for chemoprophylaxis based on the country being visited can be found on the CDC website (https://www.cdc.gov/malaria/travelers/country_table/a.html).

Several considerations must be taken into account for chemoprophylaxis in travelers to malarial areas. An individualized risk-benefit assessment should be conducted for every traveler, considering not only the region or country to be visited but also the itinerary and duration, specific cities or rural areas, types of accommodations, season (rainy or dry), and type of travel (adventure or business).

It is important to consider that no chemoprophylactic regimen is 100% effective, and other measures to decrease mosquito bites, as described previously, should be considered. If a person develops malaria while taking chemoprophylaxis, that particular drug should not be used as part of the treatment regimen.

The main drugs used for prophylaxis are atovaquone/proguanil, doxycycline, mefloquine, and tafenoquine. Recommended regimens according to the *Plasmodium* species and its pattern of resistance are detailed in Table 4.

Malaria vaccines have been studied primarily in children in endemic areas. In January 2016, the WHO recommended the RTS,S malaria vaccine for pilot introduction in selected areas of three African countries: Ghana, Kenya, and Malawi. The data showed that the vaccine has a favorable safety profile and significantly reduces severe, life-threatening malaria. Therefore on October 6, 2021, the WHO recommended that the RTS,S malaria vaccine be used for the prevention of *P. falciparum* malaria in children living in regions with moderate to high transmission. RTS,S/AS01 (Mosquirix) is a pre-erythrocytic recombinant protein vaccine based on the RTS,S recombinant antigen. It comprises the hybrid polypeptide RTS in which regions of the *P. falciparum* circumsporozoite protein, known to induce humoral (R region) and cellular (T region) immune responses, are covalently bound to the hepatitis B virus surface antigen (S). This recombinant fusion protein (RTS) is expressed in *Saccharomyces cerevisiae* together with free hepatitis B surface antigen (S) to form RTS,S virus-like particles. The formulation contains 25 μg of RTS,S with the AS01 adjuvant system. The first dose of the vaccine is given to children from 6 weeks to 17 months of age. The first dose is given at 5 months of age. The first three doses are administered monthly, and the third should be completed by 9 months of age. The fourth dose should be administered at 15 to 18 months.

Two vaccine candidates are approaching late-stage clinical evaluation: the R21/Matrix-M vaccine targeting the *Plasmodium falciparum* circumsporozoite protein (PfCSP) and the attenuated whole-sporozoite *Plasmodium falciparum* sporozoites (PfSPZ) vaccine.

---

[1] Not FDA approved for this indication.

TABLE 4 Chemoprophylaxis of Malaria

LOCAL RESISTANCE PATTERN	DRUG	PEDIATRIC DOSE	ADULT DOSE
Primary Regimens			
Chloroquine-sensitive *Plasmodium falciparum*	1. Chloroquine phosphate 1 tab = 500 mg (salt) (300 mg of base)	8.3 mg/kg (5 mg/kg of base) PO 1×/week up to 300 mg (base) max dose. 1–2 weeks before travel, during travel, and for 4 weeks post-travel	500 mg (300-mg base) PO per week. 1–2 weeks before travel, during travel, and 4 weeks post-travel
	2. Atovaquone/proguanil (Malarone)* 1 adult tab = 250/100 mg 1 pediatric tab = 62.5/25 mg	5–8 kg: ½ pediatric tab 9–10 kg: ¾ pediatric tab 11–20 kg: 1 pediatric tab 21–30 kg: 2 pediatric tabs 31–40 kg: 3 pediatric tabs >40 kg: 1 adult tab per day with food 1 day before travel, during travel, and for 7 days post-travel	1 adult tab (250/100 mg) per day with food 1 day before travel, during travel, and 7 days post-travel
	Alternative Regimens		
	1. Tafenoquine[†] (Arakoda) ≥16 years only 1 tab = 100 mg		Before travel to malaria-endemic area (loading regimen): 200 mg once daily × 3 days (starting 3 days before travel) In endemic area (maintenance regimen): 200 mg once weekly (starting 7 days after last loading regimen dose) Post-travel: 200-mg one-time dose (7 days after last maintenance dose)
	2. Doxycycline 1 tab = 100 mg[‡]	8–12 years: 2.2 mg/kg once/day up to 100 mg/day 1–2 days before travel, during travel, and for 4 weeks post-travel	100 mg PO qd 1–2 days before travel, during travel, and for 4 weeks post-travel
	3. Mefloquine 1 tab = 250 mg[§]	Weekly dose by weight in kg 5 to <10 kg: 31.25 mg (⅛ tab) 10 to <20 kg: 62.5 mg (¼ tab) 20 to <30 kg: 125 mg (½ tab) 30–45 kg: 187.5 mg (¾ tab) >45 kg: 250 mg (1 tab) 1–2 weeks before travel, during travel, and 4 weeks post-travel	250 mg (228-mg base) 1 tab PO once per week 1–2 weeks before travel, during travel, and 4 weeks after travel
Nonchloroquine-resistant *Plasmodium vivax*	Primaquine phosphate[1] 1 tab = 15 mg (base)	0.5 mg/kg base (0.8 mg/kg salt) up to adult dose 30-mg base (52.6 mg salt) daily 1–2 days before travel, during travel, and 7 days post-travel	30 mg base PO daily in nonpregnant, G6PD-normal travelers 1–2 days before travel, during travel, and for 7 days post-travel
Primary Regimens			
Chloroquine-resistant *P. falciparum*	1. Atovaquone/proguanil* 1 adult tab = 250/100 mg 1 pediatric tab = 62.5/25 mg	5–8 kg: ½ pediatric tab 9–10 kg: ¾ pediatric tab 11–20 kg: 1 pediatric tab 21–30 kg: 2 pediatric tab 31–40 kg: 3 pediatric tab >40 kg: 1 adult tab Daily with food 1–2 days before travel, during travel, and for 7 days post-travel	1 adult tab/day with food 1–2 days before travel, during travel, and for 7 days after travel
	Alternative Regimens		
	1. Tafenoquine (Arakoda) 1 tab = 100 mg[†]	Not approved for malaria prophylaxis in patients <18 years of age	Before travel to malaria-endemic area (loading regimen): 200 mg once daily × 3 days (starting 3 days before travel) In endemic area (maintenance regimen) 200 mg once weekly (starting 7 days after last loading regimen dose) Post-travel: 200 mg one-time dose (7 days after last maintenance dose)
	2. Doxycycline 1 tab = 100 mg[‡]	8–12 years: 2.2 mg/kg once/day up to 100 mg/day 1–2 days before travel, during travel, and for 4 weeks post-travel	100 mg PO qd Start 1–2 days before travel, during travel, and 4 weeks post-travel
	3. Mefloquine 1 tab = 250 mg[§]	Weekly dose by weight in kg <9 kg: 5 mg/kg 15–19 kg: ¼ adult dose 20–30 kg: ½ adult dose 31–45 kg: ¾ adult dose >45 kg: adult dose	250 mg (228 mg base) 1 tab PO once per week, 2–3 weeks before travel, during travel, and for 4 weeks post-travel

*Atovaquone-proguanil: preferred for short trips because of increase adherence.

[†]Tafenoquine: must have glucose-6-phosphate activity greater than 70% normal on a quantitative test. Preferred for longer trips because of few adverse effects.

[‡]Doxycycline: the American Academy of Pediatrics now recommends that doxycycline can safely be administered for short durations (≤21 days) regardless of patient age; this does not apply to malaria prophylaxis because of required duration of dosing.

[§]Mefloquine: start 3 weeks ahead, if feasible, to assess for intolerance. This is the current best option for pregnancy.

[1]Not FDA approved for this indication.

References

Ansong D, Seydel K, Taylor T: Malaria. In Ryan E, Hill D, Solomon T, editors: *Hunter's Tropical Medicine and Emerging Infectious Diseases, 2020,* ed 10, Syracuse, 2020, Elsevier, pp 734–754.

Centers for Disease Control and Prevention: Malaria and travelers for U.S. residents. Available at: https://www.cdc.gov/malaria/travelers/index.html.

Centers for Disease Control and Prevention: Malaria treatment (United States). Available at: https://www.cdc.gov/malaria/diagnosis_treatment/treatment.html.

Diagne N, Rogier C, Sokhna CS, et al: Increased susceptibility to malaria during the early postpartum period, *N Engl J Med* 343(9):598, 2000.

Fairhurst R, Wellems T: Malaria (Plasmodium species). In Bennett J, Dolin R, Blaser M, editors: *Mandell, Douglas and Bennett's Principles and Practice of Infectious Diseases, 2019,* ed 9, Philadelphia, 2019, Elsevier, pp 3299–3320.

Mace KE, Lucchi NW, Tan KR: Malaria Surveillance — United States, 2018, *MMWR Surveill Summ* 71(No. SS-8):1–29, 2022.

Ramharter M, Grobusch MP, Kiessling G, et al: Clinical and parasitological characteristics of puerperal malaria, *J Infect Dis* 191(6):1005, 2005.

Tan KR. Arguin PM. Malaria. In *CDC Yellow Book,* Chapter 4. Travel-Related Infectious Diseases https://wwwnc.cdc.gov/travel/yellowbook/2020/travel-related-infectious-diseases/malaria

Van Der Pluijm R, Tripura R, Hoglund R, et al: Triple artemisinin-based combination therapies versus artemisinin-based combination therapies for uncomplicated Plasmodium falciparum malaria: a multicenter, open label, randomized clinical trial, *www.thelancet.com Lancet* 395:1345–1360, 2020, Available at: https://doi.org/10.1016/S0140-6736(20)30552-3.

World Health Organization: Malaria vaccine: WHO position paper-March 2022, Weekly Epidemiological Record No 9, 97:61–80, 2022.

World Health Organization: Malaria. Available at: https://www.who.int/news-room/fact-sheets/detail/malaria

World Health Organization: World malaria report 2021. Available at: https://www.who.int/teams/global-malaria-programme/reports/world-malaria-report-2021

WHO Guidelines for malaria, 18 February 2022. Geneva: World Health Organization; 2022 (WHO/UCN/GMP/2022.01)

MEASLES (RUBEOLA)

Method of
Jane A. Weida, MD

CURRENT DIAGNOSIS

- Measles is a highly contagious viral illness with a prodrome of high fever, cough, conjunctivitis, and coryza.
- A pathognomonic enanthem (Koplik spots—small clustered white lesions) may appear on buccal mucosa during the prodromal period.
- The incubation period is about 10 days to the onset of fever; the typical rash appears after about 14 days.
- Measles produces a red maculopapular rash beginning on the face and then becoming generalized.
- Patients usually have a history of exposure, particularly of travel to an endemic area or of contact with carriers or non-immunized individuals.

CURRENT THERAPY

- No specific antiviral therapy is available
- Adequate hydration
- Bed rest
- Antipyretics
- Antibiotics if needed for bacterial complications

Epidemiology

Before measles vaccines were introduced, measles caused millions of deaths worldwide each year. In the decade before the first measles vaccine was licensed in 1963, there were about 549,000 reported measles cases and 495 deaths annually in the United States. It is estimated that the actual incidence was much higher, possibly 3 to 4 million.

Measles was declared to have been eliminated from the United States in 2000, but outbreaks have occurred since then. As of February 28, 2023, there were 3 measles cases reported in the United States in 2023. There were 121 cases reported in 2022, 49 in 2021, and 13 in 2020. Conversely, in 2019 there were 1282 cases of measles in 31 states, the largest outbreak since 1992. The majority of these cases involved people who had not been vaccinated. The risk of measles for the majority of the U.S. population remains low.

Most measles cases are caused by either travel to endemic areas or exposure to carriers or persons who have not been immunized. Travelers with measles continue to bring the disease to the United States. Measles can spread when it reaches an area where groups of people are unvaccinated, including areas where immunity dips below 95%.

Measles continues to be a major problem in many regions of the world. Worldwide, from 2000 to 2021, measles vaccination prevented an estimated 56 million deaths, a reduction in measles mortality of 83%. By the end of 2019, 83 countries had achieved or maintained measles elimination. However, in 2021, only 81% of children worldwide received their first dose of measles-containing vaccine, the lowest coverage reported since 2008. This leaves 25 million children worldwide at risk for measles. Large outbreaks continue in 22 countries.

Risk Factors

Being unvaccinated is the largest risk factor for measles in the United States. Infants who have lost maternal immunity but are too young to be immunized are at higher risk, as are individuals with vitamin A deficiency. Travel to international areas where measles is more common or where there is an outbreak also increases the risk of contracting the disease. If measles is suspected in a patient, a careful travel history should be obtained.

Pathophysiology

Measles is caused by an RNA respiratory virus of the family *Paramyxoviridae* and genus *Morbillivirus*. It is one of the most highly contagious of the communicable diseases. The virus spreads from person to person via respiratory droplets from coughing or sneezing or via direct contact. Patients are usually contagious from about 4 days before to about 4 days after the rash appears. The fact that the disease is contagious before the onset of symptoms makes quarantining particularly difficult. The incubation period is generally 10 days before the prodrome and 14 days before the onset of the rash, but it may vary from 6 to 21 days.

The virus triggers an aggressive immune response. This leads to a suppression of the immune response to other pathogens, which can make the individual susceptible to secondary infections. This immune suppression can last for a few weeks to a few months, but, in some cases, it may last for 2 to 3 years. These individuals may have increased mortality rates, another reason why immunization is so important.

Once a measles infection has cleared, the affected person gains lifelong immunity provided that they remain immunocompetent. Infants are protected by maternal antibodies for about 1 month in the case of an immunized mother and for about 4 months in the case of a mother who had a prior measles infection.

Prevention

The best way to prevent measles is with measles vaccination. The Centers for Disease Control and Prevention (CDC) recommends measles-mumps-rubella (MMR) vaccination at 12 to 15 months of age, with the second dose at 4 to 6 years of age. Two doses are more than 99% effective. Students at post–high school institutions who are not immune to measles should have two doses of MMR vaccine at least 28 days apart. Adults born during or after 1957 who do not have evidence of immunity should receive at least one dose of MMR vaccine. Adults born before 1957 are assumed to have herd immunity. The vaccine should not be given to pregnant women or immunocompromised individuals.

International travelers should be protected against measles. Infants 6 to 11 months of age who are traveling internationally should receive one dose of MMR vaccine. Children 12 months of age and older should have documentation of two doses of MMR vaccine at least 28 days apart. Adults born during or after 1957 and teenagers without evidence of immunity should have two documented doses of MMR vaccine.

Despite the importance of measles prevention, some parents refuse to vaccinate their children. A study published in the United Kingdom in 1998 claimed to find a link between autism and MMR vaccine. The study was later proven to be erroneous and fraudulent. Subsequent repeated studies have consistently shown that there is no link between vaccines and autism. It is vital for clinicians to educate parents about the importance—which cannot be overstated—of MMR vaccination.

Clinical Signs and Symptoms

Measles generally presents with a prodrome that includes high fever, malaise, anorexia, conjunctivitis, coryza, and nonproductive cough. Fever may reach over 40°C. Conjunctivitis may include redness, swelling, photophobia, and discharge. Koplik spots, which are small, clustered white spots surrounded by a red ring that appear on the buccal mucosa, are pathognomonic but are not always present.

The measles rash is erythematous and maculopapular. It usually appears first on the face and behind the ears and then spreads to the trunk and extremities. The rash lasts 3 to 7 days. Recovery begins soon after the rash appears.

Diagnosis

Measles is usually diagnosed clinically, based on the presenting signs, vaccination history, and travel exposure history. Clinical diagnosis can be difficult when the incidence of measles is low. The World Health Organization (WHO) clinical case definition for measles is a person with fever and maculopapular rash and at least one of the symptoms of cough, coryza, or conjunctivitis.

Laboratory findings include leukopenia unless there is a secondary bacterial infection, as well as thrombocytopenia and proteinuria. The most commonly used serologic test is virus-specific immunoglobulin M (IgM) in serum or oral fluid. IgM antibodies generally appear at the time of the rash, but they may not be detectable until 4 or more days after the rash appears. IgG antibodies appear a few days later. Throat or nasopharyngeal viral cultures may be obtained, although measles is technically difficult to culture. Throat or nasopharyngeal swabs may also be obtained for detection of virus by polymerase chain reaction (PCR).

Measles is a reportable illness in the United States; therefore suspected cases must be reported to the local health department without delay. The CDC recommends that serologic and viral specimens be collected in suspected cases of measles; clinicians can contact their local health department laboratories to find out which specimens to collect.

Differential Diagnosis

During the prodromal stage, measles can easily be mistaken for other viral upper respiratory illnesses. Although Koplik spots are pathognomonic, they are easy to overlook. Once the rash has appeared, measles can still be mistaken for other illnesses, including erythema infectiosum, infectious mononucleosis, enterovirus, Kawasaki disease, chikungunya, Rocky Mountain spotted fever, rubella, and scarlet fever.

Treatment

No specific antiviral treatment is available for measles. Treatment is supportive, including rest, adequate fluids, and antipyretics. Patients should be kept on bed rest until they are afebrile.

Prompt recognition and treatment of secondary bacterial infections is essential. The WHO recommends the administration of vitamin A[1] to individuals with measles who are under the age of 5. In the United States vitamin A is not routinely given for milder cases of measles. The CDC recommends treatment with vitamin A for children with severe cases of measles, such as those who are hospitalized. The dosage is 200,000 IU for children 12 months of age and older, 100,000 IU for infants 6 through 12 months, and 50,000 IU for infants younger than 6 months. It is given immediately when the disease is diagnosed and then repeated the following day.

Monitoring

Most patients with measles do not need hospitalization. For those who do, both standard and respiratory precautions should be initiated. Respiratory precautions should continue for 4 days after onset of rash for healthy children and for the duration of the illness for patients who are immunocompromised.

For those who have been exposed to measles and are not immune, MMR should be administered within 72 hours of exposure or immune globulin (Ig, GamaSTAN) administered within 6 days of exposure.

Complications

Complications of measles can occur in up to 40% of patients; complications are highest in the very young, the very old, and those who are malnourished. Often the complications affect the respiratory tract, with pneumonia being the leading cause of death associated with measles. Pneumonia may be caused by a secondary bacterial or viral infection or by the measles virus itself. Otitis media is another common complication. Gastrointestinal complications include diarrhea and stomatitis. Measles keratoconjunctivitis is a common complication, especially in children with vitamin A deficiency.

Rarely, measles can cause severe central nervous system (CNS) complications. About 1 in 1000 cases of measles results in measles inclusion body encephalitis (MIBE), leading to fever, seizures, and progressive neurologic abnormalities seen over weeks to months. Measles causes about 1 to 2 deaths per 1000 as a result of respiratory or neurologic complications. Subacute sclerosing panencephalitis is a rare delayed neurologic complication of measles, occurring in about 1 in 10,000 to 100,000 patients. This fatal complication causes seizures and progressive intellectual and behavioral deterioration about 7 to 10 years following a measles infection.

The complications of measles as well as the disease itself are best managed by prevention with immunization. Clinicians must continue to work with patients to stress the importance of measles immunization.

---

[1] Not FDA approved for this indication.

References

Akamine C, Clark E, Shandra WX: Vital & Rickettsial infections: measles. In Papadakis MA, McPhee SJ, Rabow MW, editors: *Current medical diagnosis and treatment 2023*, 62 ed, McGraw Hill, 2023, pp 1368–1371.

Bester J: Measles and measles vaccination a review, *JAMA Pediatr* 170(12):1209–1215, 2016.

Centers for Disease Control and Prevention. Measles Cases and Outbreaks. Available at: https://www.cdc.gov/measles/cases-outbreaks.html.

Centers for Disease Control and Prevention: Measles Elimination. Available at: https://www.cdc.gov/measles/elimination.html.

Centers for Disease Control and Prevention: Measles for Healthcare Providers. Available at: https://www.cdc.gov/measles/hcp/index.html.

Centers for Disease Control and Prevention: Progress toward regional measles elimination – worldwide, 2000 - 2021. Available at: https://www.cdc.gov/mmwr/volumes/71/wr/mm7147a1.htm.

Hubschen JM, Vasilache IG, Dina J: Measles, *The Lancet* 399(10325):678-690, 2022

Moss W: *Measles, Lancet* 390:2490–2502, 2017.

METHICILLIN-RESISTANT *STAPHYLOCOCCUS AUREUS*

Method of
Elissa Rennert-May, MD, MSc; and John M. Conly, MD

CURRENT DIAGNOSIS

- Healthcare-associated methicillin-resistant *Staphylococcus aureus* (HA-MRSA) is endemic in many hospital settings. The strains are polyclonal, resistant to many non–β-lactam antimicrobials, and typically cause pneumonia, line-related infection, surgical site infection, bacteremia, and infrequently skin and soft tissue infections.
- Strains of community-associated MRSA (CA-MRSA) have risen exponentially. The strains are clonal, sensitive to many non–β-lactam antimicrobials, harbour multiple virulence factors, and typically cause pyogenic skin and soft tissue infections and occasionally severe necrotizing pneumonia, fasciitis, and multifocal osteomyelitis.
- HA-MRSA infections typically affect patients with multiple co-morbidities in the healthcare setting, but CA-MRSA typically affects previously healthy persons.
- It can be difficult to differentiate infectious syndromes due to β-hemolytic streptococci versus CA-MRSA.

CURRENT THERAPY

- Methicillin-resistant *Staphylococcus aureus* (MRSA) strains harbor resistance to the β-lactam antimicrobials, including oxacillin, dicloxacillin, cloxacillin[2], nafcillin, methicillin[2], and first-, second-, and third-generation cephalosporins.
- Healthcare-associated MRSA (HA-MRSA) strains are typically resistant to macrolides, clindamycin (Cleocin), aminoglycosides, and quinolones (with the exception of delafloxacin [Baxdela]) and are variably resistant to tetracycline and trimethoprim-sulfamethoxazole (Bactrim). They are sensitive to vancomycin (Vancocin) and the lipoglycopeptides, fusidic acid[2], rifampin (Rifadin)[1], the oxazolidinones linezolid (Zyvox) and tedizolid (Sivextro), daptomycin (Cubicin), ceftaroline (Teflaro), and ceftobiprole (Zevtera)[2].
- Community-associated MRSA (CA-MRSA) strains are resistant to macrolides and quinolones (with the exception of delafloxacin [Baxdela]) but usually are sensitive to aminoglycosides such as gentamicin (Garamycin), clindamycin, (Cleocin) and trimethoprim-sulfamethoxazole (Bactrim)[1], in addition to vancomycin (Vancocin), the lipoglycopeptides, fusidic acid[2], rifampin (Rifadin)[1], the oxazolidinones linezolid (Zyvox) and tedizolid (Sivextro), daptomycin (Cubicin), ceftaroline (Teflaro), and ceftobiprole (Zevtera)[2].
- Empiric antimicrobial therapy should be guided by the clinical presentation, and when full sensitivities are available, the antimicrobials may be tailored accordingly.

[1]Not FDA approved for this indication.
[2]Not available in the United States.

Epidemiology

Staphylococcus aureus is one of the most frequently encountered bacteria causing human infections and may be considered as either methicillin-sensitive *S. aureus* (MSSA) or methicillin-resistant *S. aureus* (MRSA). MRSA was first described in 1961 and is resistant not only to the traditional antistaphylococcal β-lactam antibiotics (methicillin[2], nafcillin, oxacillin, cloxacillin[2],

[2]Not available in the United States.

and dicloxacillin) but also other important β-lactam antibiotics, including the first- to fourth-generation cephalosporins and the carbapenem family, thus eliminating an important class of antibiotics from the clinician's armamentarium. The only β-lactams that have activity against MRSA are the advanced-generation cephalosporin agents ceftaroline (Teflaro) and ceftobiprole (Zevtera)[2].

MRSA strains acquired in the hospital or other healthcare settings have traditionally been referred to as healthcare-associated MRSA (HA-MRSA), whereas community-associated MRSA (CA-MRSA) has referred to isolates acquired in the community setting and in the absence of traditional hospital or healthcare exposures for at least 1 year (overnight stays in an acute care or long-term care facility, surgery, dialysis, or presence of a central venous catheter). The term *community-onset HA-MRSA* has been used to describe the occurrence of MRSA infection in the setting of the presence of a healthcare exposure within the past year. MRSA has been recognized as a healthcare-associated pathogen since the 1970s and became endemic in hospitals in many countries, including the United States, United Kingdom, and many European countries, with exceptions being Denmark, the Netherlands, Scandinavia, and Canada. For several decades, MRSA was typically considered a hospital pathogen. Novel and virulent MRSA strains arising in the community and not associated with any traditional healthcare exposure risks were first encountered in the late 1990s in the United States, Australia, and some European countries and have since risen explosively on a global basis to become the predominant clone of *S. aureus* associated with community infections. Methicillin resistance among community isolates of *S. aureus* has been reported to be as high as 75% in some US communities. More recently livestock-associated MRSA (LA-MRSA) has been reported on a global basis, and transmission of these strains from swine, cattle, and horses has been implicated as a source of human infections, particularly in farmers, abattoir workers, and veterinarians.

Specific genetic and molecular distinctions initially distinguished the HA- and CA-MRSA strains (Table 1) and have been used to characterize MRSA strains as likely of community versus healthcare origin. The HA-MRSA strains were found to harbor large staphylococcal cassette chromosome (SCC*mec*) types known as SCC*mec* types I, II, or III; to have multidrug resistance to non–β-lactam antimicrobials; to have the absence of specific virulence characteristics such as carriage of the Panton-Valentine Leukocidin *(PVL)* gene; and to have varying multilocus sequence types (ST5, ST239, ST 247, ST250). On the other hand, the CA-MRSA strains have been found to harbor SCC*mec* types IV, V, and more recently VI to XV have been described; to have paucidrug resistance to non–β-lactam antimicrobials; to have the presence of specific virulence characteristics such as carriage of the *PVL* gene, and to have multilocus sequence types ST1, ST8, and ST80. LA-MRSA strains often are nontypeable or harbor SCC*mec* V, have high rates of tetracycline resistance, carry multiple virulence factors, and are most often multilocus sequence types ST398 or ST9. However, over the past few years, healthcare-associated strains have moved into the community and likewise community strains have spread rapidly within hospitals, and the original distinctions between CA-MRSA and HA-MRSA from an epidemiologic perspective have become increasingly blurred. The point of transmission of MRSA is not always possible to identify with certainty, making the classification of CA and HA strains increasingly imprecise.

Risk Factors

The risk factors for HA-MRSA may be viewed from the perspective of the healthcare environment and patient-specific risk factors. A major risk factor for acquiring HA-MRSA is exposure to a healthcare setting and particularly in hospital or other institutional settings where the prevalence of carriage of MRSA among patients is high. Additional risk factors in the healthcare environment include poor hand hygiene practices among hospital employees, contaminated bedside equipment and surfaces, overcrowding, and reduced healthcare worker-to-patient ratios. Patient risk factors (see Table 1) include aging, multiple comorbidities, receipt of antibiotics within the preceding 3 months, prolonged duration of hospital stay, admission

VIII Infectious Diseases

TABLE 1 General Features Differentiating HA- and CA-MRSA*

CHARACTERISTIC	HA-MRSA	CA-MRSA
Drug resistance to non–β-lactams	Multiresistance	Pauciresistance
Pathogenicity islands	Few	Multiple
Age predilection	Older	Younger
Comorbidities	Multiple	None
Traditional risk factors	Healthcare contact, prolonged hospital stay, poor hand hygiene, contaminated equipment, invasive procedures, medical devices, recent antibiotic use	Crowded community environment, lack of cleanliness, loss of skin integrity, intravenous drug user, homelessness, incarceration, aboriginal, HIV+, contact sports, athletes, military, chronic skin disorder, veterinary worker

*Features are generalizations only given the appearance of community strains replacing traditional hospital strains in the health care setting and the appearance of typical HA strains in the community setting.
CA, Community-associated; HA, healthcare-associated; HIV, human immunodeficiency virus; MRSA, methicillin-resistant *Staphylococcus aureus*.

The "5 Cs" for Transmission of CA-MRSA

- **C**rowding
- **C**ontact with skin
- **C**ompromised skin
- **C**ontaminated personal care items
- **C**leanliness lack

Figure 1 The five Cs implicated in transmission of community-associated methicillin-resistant *S. aureus*. Adapted from the US Centers for Disease Control and Prevention.

to a long-term care facility or hospital in the previous year, invasive procedures, and the presence of indwelling catheters or other devices. In addition, the recent COVID-19 pandemic has led to some settings experiencing increased nosocomial rates of MRSA and with strains with increased numbers of virulence genes and may be considered an additional risk factor. Initial risk groups for CA-MRSA were injection drug users, homeless populations, incarcerated persons, and indigenous peoples. The Centers for Disease Control and Prevention have suggested the five Cs (Figure 1 and Table 2) as contributing factors implicated in the transmission among these groups. The initial risk groups have expanded (Table 3) to include men who have sex with men (MSM), athletes (especially those involved in team and contact sports), military personnel, those with a prior history of abscesses, individuals with chronic skin disorders, individuals with recent antibiotic receipt, underserved urban populations, individuals who have contact with colonized pets or livestock, and veterinary workers. In the drug-using and underserved urban populations, prevalence and social networking studies have identified hospices, shooting galleries, and crack houses as key sites in which CA-MRSA transmission may occur. Recent outbreaks have been reported in hospital nurseries, daycare settings, nursing home workers, schools, and college dormitories. Sexual transmission has been reported, but it may reflect close skin-to-skin genital contact rather than a true sexually transmitted pathogen. CA-MRSA has now become endemic in the general population in many communities, and the elderly and the very young seem to have a predilection for infection, especially if other risk factors are present. Risk groups for LA-MRSA include farmers, their family members and farm hands who are engaged in livestock production (especially swine and cattle), abattoir workers, veterinarians, and veterinary assistants. There is concern about increasing threats to food safety and public health with the rise in strains of both LA-MRSA and LA-MSSA in livestock farms, especially in swine populations. Recent transmission of strains of LA-MRSA has been reported in the hospital setting as well.

Pathophysiology

The resistance to the antistaphylococcal β-lactam antibiotics in MRSA strains is imparted by the presence of an altered configuration for a specific penicillin-binding protein (PBP) known as PBP2a in the cell wall of staphylococci. Normally the PBPs would act as a site for the attachment of the active moieties of the β-lactam agent, which then would inhibit further cell wall assembly. The alteration in the configuration of PBP2a occurs as the result of the presence of the SCC*mec* gene in *S. aureus*, which confers resistance to the β-lactam antibiotics. The origins of the *mec* gene and its insertion into the SCC*mec* element are not known with certainty. Once the MRSA strains acquired resistance to the antistaphylococcal β-lactam antibiotics in the healthcare setting, it is not difficult to appreciate how it emerged as a predominant pathogen in the hospital setting over the years, with increasing acuity of illness in the patient populations and increased use of broad-spectrum antimicrobials.

The appearance and rapid spread of CA-MRSA with the clinical impression of more virulent and lethal infections than what had been seen with traditional HA-MRSA strains may be explained by several factors. The SCC*mec* IV genetic element is very widely distributed among *S. aureus* isolates, which may explain its appearance in multiple settings globally, and these strains appear to have more rapid growth rates than typical HA-MRSA strains, larger numbers of virulence factors, pathogenicity islands, and higher levels of expression of the virulence factors produced. Recently α-type phenol-soluble modulins were described in strains of CA-MRSA, which are produced at very high levels and are potent lysins of neutrophils. High levels of α-toxin production by these strains, which act as pore-forming toxins for multiple cell types, may also contribute to their virulence. The vast majority of CA-MRSA strains also produce the genes for PVL and it functions as a dermonecrotic factor in skin lesions, a potent cell lysin in high concentrations, and a potent inflammatory mediator in lower concentrations. However, there is controversy about the role of PVL as a single predominant virulence factor, because strains of CA-MRSA that have this gene knocked out have demonstrated no difference in pathogenicity in both vertebrate and invertebrate animal models and in human settings when the PVL is not present.

Prevention

Controlling the spread of HA-, CA-, or LA-MRSA from an infected or colonized person to others in the hospital, family, or community is a key goal of prevention. In the hospital setting, strict adherence to hand hygiene, application of barrier precautions (gloves, gowns, and private rooms) for patients colonized or infected with MRSA, environmental and equipment cleaning, and antimicrobial stewardship are the key preventive strategies. Active surveillance cultures to identify colonized patients and decolonization may be effective in selected settings, but its general application is controversial. In the community setting, practicing hygienic measures including good personal hygiene,

TABLE 2 Risk Factor Associations Reported for CA-MRSA Infections

RISK CATEGORIES	FACTOR	DETAILS FROM REPORTS
High-risk populations	Younger and older age	Age distribution in CA-MRSA younger than HA-MRSA High rate of CA-MRSA in children under 2 years CA-MRSA more common in children compared to adults Outbreaks in hospital nurseries Outbreaks in nursing homes with elderly residents
	Indigenous populations: Native or Aboriginal or African American	Aboriginal communities in midwestern United States, Canada, and Australia Alaskan natives More common in African Americans
	Athletes (predominantly contact sports)	Outbreaks on football teams Outbreaks on wrestling team Other competitive sports
	Injection (intravenous) drug users (IVDUs)	San Francisco IVDUs Canadian report of USA300 strain outbreak
	Men who have sex with men (MSM)	CA-MRSA described in HIV+ population of MSM
	HIV+ individuals	Risk associated with overlapping social networks, intravenous drug use, hemodialysis, and CD4 counts <200 reported as independent risks
	Military personnel	3% of US Army soldiers colonized
	Inmates of correctional facilities	Reports of outbreaks in US prisons Two outbreaks (total 10 inmates) in Canada
	Students in elementary schools and college dormitories	Reports of outbreaks in schools and college dormitories
Previous positive MRSA cultures	MRSA carriage Past MRSA infection	Colonized soldiers more likely to get CA-MRSA disease Prior abscess risk factor for CA-MRSA
Medical history	Chronic skin disorder	Dermatologic condition most common underlying medical disorder for CA-MRSA infection Classroom contact of index CA-MRSA case had chronic dermatitis
	Recurrent or recent antibiotic use	Antibiotic use associated with CA-MRSA infection in rural Alaska
Environmental	Homelessness and living in shelters Overcrowding Contact with colonized pet Veterinary workers and family members	Medically underserved populations at higher risk of CA-MRSA Reports of USA300 strain outbreak involving individuals living in shelters or homeless Close contact implicated in jail outbreaks Neonatal intensive care unit transmission Family dog source of recurrent infection Veterinarians working with horses and livestock Family members of animal care workers Small animal veterinarians Swine farmers

CA, Community-associated; *HA,* healthcare-associated; *HIV,* human immunodeficiency virus; *MRSA,* methicillin-resistant *Staphylococcus aureus.*
Adapted from Barton-Forbes M, Hawkes M, Moore D, et al. Guidelines for the prevention and management of community associated methicillin resistant *Staphylococcus aureus* (CA-MRSA): a perspective for Canadian Health Care Practitioners. *Can J Infect Dis Med Microbiol.* 2006;17(suppl C):1B–24B.

TABLE 3 Principles of Empiric Treatment of Minor Skin and Soft Tissue Infections (Folliculitis, Furuncles, Small Abscesses Without Cellulitis, Impetigo, Secondarily Infected Lesions Such as Eczema, Ulcers, or Wounds) Where the Etiology Is Unknown But May Include MRSA as a Possibility

Recommendations

One or more of the following measures may be employed:
- Local therapy using hot soaks, elevation, and dressings as appropriate
- Incision and drainage of furuncles or small abscesses without antimicrobial therapy
- Topical 2% mupirocin ointment (Bactroban) or fusidic acid[2] for impetigo and secondarily infected lesions if local strains are likely sensitive
- Topical antiseptics may be considered
- Antimicrobial therapy is recommended in addition to local measures if one or more of the following is present: multiple sites of infection, evidence of progression, clinical evidence of systemic symptoms and signs, presence of comorbidities, extremes of age, immunosuppression, septic phlebitis, or difficult site for incision and drainage.
- In follow-up, routine screening for colonization of the nares or other body sites is not recommended.

[2]Not available in the United States.
MRSA, Methicillin-resistant *Staphylococcus aureus.*

consistent hand hygiene, ensuring all draining skin and soft tissue lesions have adequate dressings, not sharing potentially contaminated personal articles, and keeping the household environment hygienic are important. Public health organizations may also contribute to the prevention of CA-MRSA by instituting education programs targeting healthcare providers and individuals in high-risk groups in the community, and by promoting appropriate antimicrobial use. In sports settings, in addition to the basic hygienic measures mentioned previously, avoidance of sharing of towels and other personal items, showering after every practice or tournament, cleaning of communal showering and bathing areas, and cleaning or laundering of equipment after each use are also important.

Clinical Manifestations

The specific clinical infections associated with MRSA parallel those associated with MSSA. Almost any body site, organ, or appendage may be affected by infections due to *S. aureus*, but there are specific predilections associated with HA- and CA-MRSA. In the hospital or other healthcare setting, the most commonly encountered infections include pneumonia, line-related infection, surgical site infection, bacteremia, and less often skin and soft tissue infections. In the community setting, the most common sites (>80%) are skin and soft tissue infections (furuncles, cellulitis, and soft tissue abscesses) and less commonly severely invasive infections such as necrotizing pneumonia, necrotizing fasciitis, multifocal osteomyelitis/septic arthritis, epidural abscess, pelvic septic thrombophlebitis, and bacteremia with toxic shock syndrome. The skin and soft tissue infections often affect young previously healthy patients and are characteristically very painful and pyogenic with an initial black eschar that patients presume was a "spider bite" as the initiating process.

Diagnosis

The diagnosis of MRSA infections is based on the clinical presentation and the isolation of the causative organism from purulent discharge, sputum, or urine, or from specimens obtained from normally sterile body fluids (joint fluid, abscess or tissue aspirates, and blood). The organism appears on Gram stain as a gram-positive organism in clusters and is usually seen in association with neutrophils and may be either intracellular or extracellular. The organism is very hardy and grows readily on typical media in the microbiology laboratory within 24 to 48 hours. Some laboratories are using rapid agglutination tests to detect the PBP2a protein or polymerase chain reaction (PCR)-based techniques to provide same-day or next-day identification. In settings where no cultures have been obtained or in the setting of toxic shock syndrome where cultures are often negative, the diagnosis may be difficult and only suspected based on a typical clinical presentation.

Treatment

MRSA strains harbor resistance to the β-lactam antimicrobials, including oxacillin, dicloxacillin, cloxacillin[2], nafcillin, methicillin[2], and first-, second-, and third-generation cephalosporins.

The newer advanced-generation cephalosporin antimicrobials ceftaroline (Teflaro) and ceftobiprole (Zevtera)[2] have activity against MRSA strains. The majority of HA-MRSA strains are resistant to macrolides, clindamycin (Cleocin), aminoglycosides, and quinolones (with the exception of delafloxacin [Baxdela]) and are variably resistant to tetracycline and trimethoprim-sulfamethoxazole (Bactrim)[1], depending on local epidemiologic patterns. They are sensitive to vancomycin (Vancocin) and the lipoglycopeptides such as dalbavancin (Dalvance), telavancin (Vibativ), and oritavancin (Orbactiv) and usually sensitive to fusidic acid[2], rifampin (Rifadin)[1], the oxazolidinones linezolid (Zyvox) and tedizolid (Sivextro), and daptomycin (Cubicin). For hospitalized patients where *S. aureus* is considered a possible etiology of any major infectious syndrome, it should be considered as methicillin-resistant until proven otherwise. Empiric choices of vancomycin or lipoglycopeptides such as dalbavancin (Dalvance), telavancin (Vibativ) or oritavancin (Orbitactiv), linezolid (Zyvox) or tedizolid (Sivextro), daptomycin (Cubicin) or advanced-generation cephalosproins such as ceftaroline (Teflaro) or ceftobiprole (Zevtera)[2] should be considered as appropriate to the presenting syndrome. CA-MRSA strains are resistant to macrolides and often quinolones (with the exception of delafloxacin [Baxdela]) but usually are sensitive to aminoglycosides such as gentamicin (Garamycin), clindamycin, and trimethoprim-sulfamethoxazole (Bactrim)[1], but the resistance patterns vary depending on local resistance patterns. In addition, these strains are sensitive to vancomycin (Vancocin) and the lipoglycopeptides, fusidic acid[2], rifampin (Rifadin)[1], linezolid (Zyvox), daptomycin (Cubicin), ceftaroline (Teflaro), and ceftobiprole (Zevtera)[2]. LA-MRSA strains are almost always resistant to tetracyclines; often resistant to quinolones, macrolides, and clindamycin, and variably resistant to aminoglycosides and trimethoprim-sulfamethoxazole. In addition, these strains are sensitive to vancomycin (Vancocin) and the lipoglycopeptides, fusidic acid[2], rifampin (Rifadin)[1], the oxazolidinones linezolid (Zyvox) and tedizolid (Sivextro), daptomycin (Cubicin), ceftaroline (Teflaro) and ceftobiprole (Zevtera)[2]. Treatment guidelines for MRSA with a focus on the ambulatory setting have been published in Canada, the United Kingdom, and the United States, and provide both empiric choices for common infectious presentations of unknown etiology and definitive treatment once an etiology of MRSA is known. New guidelines for *S. aureus* bacteremia are currently under development by the Infectious Diseases Society of America. The treatment options for both empiric and definitive use where MRSA is considered or proven are presented in Tables 3 through 6 and represent a constellation of the various guidelines that have been published. A recent

[2]Not available in the United States

[2]Not available in the United States

TABLE 4 Principles of Empiric Treatment of Non–Life-Threatening Skin and Soft Tissue Infections Other Than Minor Skin Infections Where the Etiology Is Unknown But May Include MRSA as a Possibility

Recommendations
- Antibiotic choice should be based on the severity of illness at presentation, clinical judgment, and regional susceptibility patterns of strains
- Empiric therapy for CA-MRSA and β-hemolytic streptococci is recommended*

*The IDSA guideline suggests to differentiate purulent and nonpurulent cellulitis and reserve empiric therapy for β-hemolytic streptococci only in nonpurulent cellulitis but acknowledges it is an area of controversy. The previous UK and Canadian guidelines explicitly recommend coverage for β-hemolytic streptococci and do not differentiate cellulitis into different types. The guidelines that exist have not been updated and hence knowledge of local susceptibility patterns is important.
CA, Community-associated; *IDSA*, Infectious Diseases Society of America; *MRSA*, methicillin-resistant *Staphylococcus aureus.*

TABLE 5 Principles of Empiric Treatment of Life-Threatening Infections Where the Etiology Is Unknown But May Include MRSA as a Possibility

Recommendations
- Include MRSA coverage, regardless of prevalence rates of CA-MRSA in the community
- Include an agent effective against MSSA until susceptibility results become available

CA, Community-associated; *MRSA*, methicillin-resistant *Staphylococcus aureus*; *MSSA*, methicillin-sensitive *Staphylococcus aureus.*

TABLE 6 Guidelines for the Management of MRSA Infections

CLINICAL DISEASE	KEY FEATURES	MANAGEMENT PRINCIPLES	ANTIMICROBIAL CHOICES AND COMMENTS*
Skin and Soft Tissue Infection (SSTI)			
Localized lesion	Infected scratches and minor wounds Insect bites Furuncles Small abscesses Absence of systemic illness	Culture selectively† No antibiotic therapy recommended *Exceptions: multiple sites of infection, evidence of progression, systemic symptoms and signs, presence of comorbidities, extremes of age, immunosuppression, septic phlebitis, or difficult site for incision and drainage: antimicrobial therapy is recommended in addition to local measures* Cover draining lesions Emphasize personal hygiene Close follow-up Return if worsening	Generally not indicated, although some evidence exists for treatment with clindamycin PO or trimethoprim-sulfamethoxazole (Bactrim)[1] PO, in conjunction with incision and drainage for small simple abscesses Topical antibacterial (e.g., mupirocin [Bactroban] or fusidic ointment[2]) therapy may be considered Systemic antimicrobial therapy indicated if one or more of the following: multiple sites of infection, evidence of progression, systemic symptoms and signs, presence of comorbidities, extremes of age, immunosuppression, septic phlebitis, or difficult site for incision and drainage
Cellulitis (not extensive) or multiple abscesses with minimal or no associated systemic features for oral treatment consideration	Classic features of rubor, dolor, calor, and swelling suggesting cellulitis with or without associated drainage or exudate	Culture site (if purulent or drainage) Drainage of abscess or needle aspiration Oral therapy in older child and adult Appropriate infection control measures Imaging for extent and complications as appropriate Close follow-up Return if worsening	*Empiric:* Include coverage for β-hemolytic streptococci¶ Clindamycin (Cleocin) 300–450 mg tid-qid PO for adults and 30–40 mg/kg/day[3] ÷ q6–8h PO for children TMP-SMX (Bactrim)[1] 1–2 DS tab bid PO for adults and 8–12 mg/kg/day (of TMP) ÷ q12h PO for children PLUS coverage for β-hemolytic streptococci (e.g., amoxicillin, cephalexin [Keflex]) Doxycycline (Vibramycin) 100 mg bid PO for adults and 4.4 mg/kg/day mg/kg/day ÷ q12h PO for children** PLUS coverage for β-hemolytic streptococci (e.g., amoxicillin, cephalexin) Delafloxacin (Baxdela) 450 mg bid PO for adults *Comment:* Recently became the first fluoroquinolone approved by the FDA for MRSA SSTI Linezolid (Zyvox) 600 mg bid PO for adults and 30 mg/kg/day ÷ q8h PO for children, not to exceed 600 mg/dose; for children older than 12 years of age 600 mg bid PO *Comment:* Linezolid is more expensive than the other options and may not always be readily available depending on the setting *Comment:* If parenteral therapy considered, see choices for severe SSTI Tedizolid (Sivextro) 200 mg PO/IV once daily for 6 days; safety and efficacy have not been established for children *Proven MRSA:* As above, based on sensitivity testing If parenteral therapy necessary, see choices for SSTI with systemic features Lefamulin (Xenleta) was recently approved for community acquired neumonia related to *S. aureus* and ABSSSI[1] in the United States.
Cellulitis (severe or rapidly spreading or extensive) or complicated SSTI (deep soft tissue infection, surgical or traumatic wound infection, large or multiple abscesses, or infected ulcers and burns) and/or associated systemic features for parenteral treatment consideration	Classic features of rubor, dolor, calor, and swelling suggesting cellulitis with or without associated drainage or exudate with systemic features of fever, chills, malaise, prostration	Culture (blood if febrile, site if purulent) Hospitalize as appropriate Drainage of abscess or needle aspiration Parenteral therapy Imaging for extent and complications as appropriate Appropriate infection control measures Consultation as indicated	*Empiric:* Include coverage for β-hemolytic streptococci¶ Vancomycin (Vancocin) 15–20 mg/kg/dose q8–12h IV for adults and 40–60[3] mg/kg/day ÷ q6h IV for children *Proven MRSA:* Based on sensitivity testing Vancomycin 15–20 mg/kg/dose q8–12h IV for adults and 40–60[3] mg/kg/day ÷ q6h IV for children Clindamycin 600–900 mg q8h IV/IM for adults and 30–40 mg/kg/day[3] ÷ q6–8h IV for children Linezolid 600 mg q12h PO/IV for adults and 30 mg/kg/day ÷ q8h PO/IV for children, not to exceed 600 mg/dose; for children older than 12 years of age 600 mg bid PO/IV Tedizolid (Sivextro) 200 mg PO/IV once daily for 6 days; safety and efficacy have not been established for children Ceftaroline (Teflaro) 600 mg IV q12h for adults; safety and efficacy have not been established for children Daptomycin (Cubicin) 4 mg/kg/dose once daily IV for adults and under investigation in children Dalbavancin (Dalvance) 1000 mg IV followed by 500 mg IV 1 week later for adults; safety and efficacy not established in children Telavancin (Vibativ) 10 mg/kg/dose IV once daily Oritavancin (Orbactiv), given as a single 1200 mg 3-hour infusion; not approved for children Delafloxacin (Baxdela) 300 mg bid IV *Comment:* Linezolid, tedizolid, daptomycin, ceftaroline, ceftobiprole,[2] dalbavancin, oritavancin and telavancin are more expensive than the other options and may not always be readily available depending on the setting

TABLE 6 Guidelines for the Management of MRSA Infections—cont'd

CLINICAL DISEASE	KEY FEATURES	MANAGEMENT PRINCIPLES	ANTIMICROBIAL CHOICES AND COMMENTS*
Necrotizing fasciitis (NF)	Clinically indistinguishable from group A streptococcus NF disease Extreme toxicity High complication rate	Cultures (blood, tissue) Imaging for extent and complications Surgical débridement Consultation as indicated Parenteral therapy Infection control measures	*Empiric:* Include coverage for β-hemolytic streptococci Vancomycin 15–20 mg/kg/dose q8–12h IV for adults and 40–60[3] mg/kg/day ÷ q6h IV for children Clindamycin 600–900 mg q8h IV/IM for adults and 30–40 mg/kg/day[3] ÷ q6–8h IV for children *Proven MRSA:* Based on sensitivity testing Vancomycin 15–20 mg/kg/dose q8–12h IV for adults and 40–60[3] mg/kg/day ÷ q6h IV for children Clindamycin 600–900 mg q8h IV/IM for adults and 30–40 mg/kg/day[3] ÷ q6–8h IV for children Linezolid 600 mg q12h PO/IV for adults and 30 mg/kg/day ÷ q8h PO/IV for children, not to exceed 600 mg/dose; for children older than 12 years of age 600 mg bid PO/IV TMP/SMX[1] 8–12 mg/kg/day (of TMP) ÷ q8–12h IV for adults and 8–12 mg/kg/day (of TMP) ÷ q6h IV for children *Comments:* Adjuncts such as IVIG (Gamunex)[1] may be considered in severe cases with septic shock Few data available for the use of TMP-SMX in this indication

Musculoskeletal Infection (MSI)

CLINICAL DISEASE	KEY FEATURES	MANAGEMENT PRINCIPLES	ANTIMICROBIAL CHOICES AND COMMENTS*
Osteomyelitis/septic arthritis	Preceding trauma Tendency for multifocal involvement Disease in adjacent muscle not uncommon Progression to chronic osteomyelitis possible May be complicated by deep venous thrombosis	Cultures (blood, bone, and tissue) Imaging for extent and complications Involve surgical team (early débridement and drainage) Consultation as indicated Parenteral therapy Consider combination therapy for severe cases or if slow to respond Infection control measures Look for other infected sites (imaging)	*Empiric:* Vancomycin 15–20 mg/kg/dose q8–12h IV for adults and 40–60[3] mg/kg/day ÷ q6h IV for children Clindamycin 600–900 mg q8h IV/IM for adults and 30–40 mg/kg/day[3] ÷ q6–8h IV for children Linezolid[1] 600 mg q12h PO/IV for adults and 30 mg/kg/day ÷ q8h PO/IV for children, not to exceed 600 mg/dose; for children older than 12 years of age 600 mg bid PO/IV Daptomycin[1] 6 mg/kg/dose once daily IV for adults and 6–10 mg/kg once daily for children TMP/SMX[1] 8–12 mg/kg/day (of TMP) ÷ q8–12h IV for adults and 8–12 mg/kg/day (of TMP) ÷ q6h IV for children *Comments:* Linezolid and daptomycin are more expensive than the other options and may not always be readily available depending on the setting Few data available for the use of TMP-SMX in these indications for children *Proven MRSA:* As above, based on sensitivity testing Addition of rifampin (Rifadin)[1] may be considered for osteomyelitis
Pyomyositis	May be extensive Tendency for multifocal involvement	Cultures (blood, tissue) Imaging for extent and complications Surgical drainage Consultation as indicated Parenteral therapy Infection control measures	

Respiratory Tract Infection (RTI)

CLINICAL DISEASE	KEY FEATURES	MANAGEMENT PRINCIPLES	ANTIMICROBIAL CHOICES AND COMMENTS*
Pneumonia	Influenza-like prodrome, hemoptysis, fever, shock, leukopenia, pneumatoceles, multifocal abscesses, consolidation, frequent empyema, respiratory failure, and high mortality	Cultures (blood, pleural fluid, sputum) Imaging for extent and complications Consultation as indicated Intensive care unit as appropriate Infection control measures Combination parenteral therapy Chest tube drainage for empyema	*Empiric:* Vancomycin 15–20 mg/kg/dose q8–12h IV for adults and 40–60[3] mg/kg/day ÷ q6h IV for children Linezolid 600 mg q12h PO/IV for adults and 30 mg/kg/day ÷ q8h PO/IV for children, not to exceed 600 mg/dose; for children older than 12 years of age 600 mg bid PO/IV Clindamycin 600–900 mg q8h IV/IM for adults and 30–40 mg/kg/day[3] ÷ q6–8h IV for children TMP/SMX[1] 8–12 mg/kg/day (of TMP) ÷ q8–12h IV for adults and 8–12 mg/kg/day (of TMP) ÷ q6h IV for children Telavancin (Vibativ) 10 mg/kg/dose IV once daily for adults for hospital or ventilator acquired pneumonia Ceftaroline (Teflaro) 600 mg IV q12h for adults with community-acquired pneumonia; safety and efficacy have not been established for children Ceftobiprole (Zevtera)[2] 500 mg IV q8h for adults with community-acquired and hospital-acquired pneumonia; safety and efficacy have not been established for children *Comment:* Daptomycin not indicated because it is inactivated by lung surfactant *Proven MRSA:* As above, based on sensitivity testing

Continued

TABLE 6 Guidelines for the Management of MRSA Infections—cont'd

CLINICAL DISEASE	KEY FEATURES	MANAGEMENT PRINCIPLES	ANTIMICROBIAL CHOICES AND COMMENTS*
Other			
Sepsis syndrome Bacteremia Native valve endocarditis	Shock Multiple-organ failure May have purpura fulminans Associated SSTI, MSI, and RTI May be complicated by Waterhouse-Friedrichsen syndrome High mortality	Blood cultures Culture any pus or fluid collection Look for primary or secondary focus Imaging for identification of source including echocardiography Consultation as indicated ICU care Imaging: look for occult abscesses, bone infection, or endocarditis Involve surgery and other specialists as needed Infection control measures Parenteral, multidrug therapy Prolonged therapy for endovascular source infections	*Empiric:* Vancomycin 15–20 mg/kg/dose q8–12h IV for adults and 40–60[3] mg/kg/day ÷ q6h IV for children Daptomycin 6 mg/kg/dose once daily IV for adults and 4–10[3] mg/kg/dose once daily for children[1] *Comments:* Doses of daptomycin of up to 10 mg/kg/dose[3] once daily have been used in adults in this indication Some recommendations have included linezolid in this setting at the doses described above *Proven MRSA:* As above, based on sensitivity testing. *Comment:* New IDSA guidelines for the treatment of *S. aureus* bacteremia are in progress

*Choice of antimicrobial therapy depends on local susceptibility patterns.

†Patients with risk factors, as a part of an outbreak investigation, patients with slowly responding or recurrent lesions.

¶The IDSA guideline suggests to differentiate purulent and nonpurulent cellulitis and reserve empiric therapy for β-hemolytic streptococci only in nonpurulent cellulitis but acknowledges it is an area of controversy. The UK and Canadian guidelines explicitly recommend empiric coverage for β-hemolytic streptococci and do not differentiate cellulitis into different types. A recent randomized controlled trial in the United States found no significant difference in efficacy between clindamycin and trimethoprim-sulfamethoxazole when used for treatment of uncomplicated skin and soft tissue infections, which were thought to be secondary to either β-hemolytic streptococci or *S. aureus*. Another recent placebo-controlled trial in the United States found that clindamycin or trimethoprim-sulfamethoxazole in conjunction with incision and drainage improved outcomes in patients with simple small abscesses (<5 cm) compared with incision and drainage alone.

[1]Not FDA approved for this indication. Dosing has varied in published reports and specific dosing guidelines are not available.

[2]Not available in the United States.

[3]Exceeds dosage recommended by the manufacturer.

**Not recommended for pediatric patients younger than 8 years of age or in pregnancy.

ICU, Intensive care unit; *IDSA,* Infectious Diseases Society of America; *IVIG,* intravenous immunoglobulin; *MRSA,* methicillin-resistant *Staphylococcus aureus; TMP-SMX,* trimethoprim-sulfamethoxazole.

randomized controlled trial assessed the efficacy of combination therapy in patients with MRSA bacteremia (vancomycin or daptomycin with flucloxacillin[2]). They found that the number of patients with persistent bacteremia after 5 days was lower in the combination arm. However, due to increased nephrotoxicity in the combination arm the trial was stopped early. Further studies are required to determine the role and benefit of combination therapy for MRSA infections.

---

[2]Not available in the United States.

References

Barton-Forbes M, Hawkes M, Moore D, et al: Guidelines for the prevention and management of community associated methicillin resistant *Staphylococcus aureus* (CA-MRSA): a perspective for Canadian Health Care Practitioners, *Can J Infect Dis Med Microbiol* 17(Suppl. C):1B–24B, 2006.

Brown NM, Brown EM: Guideline Development Group: Treatment of methicillin-resistant Staphylococcus aureus (MRSA): updated guidelines from the UK, *J Antimicrob Chemother* 76(6):1377–1378, 2021.

Chambers HF, Deleo FR: Waves of resistance: *Staphylococcus aureus* in the antibiotic era, *Nat Rev Microbiol* 7:629–641, 2009. https://doi.org/10.1038/nrmicro2200.

Daum RS, Miller LG, Immergluck L: A placebo-controlled trial of antibiotics for smaller skin abscesses, *N Engl J Med* 376(26):2545–2555, 2017.

David MZ, Daum RS: Community-associated methicillin resistant *Staphylococcus aureus*: epidemiology and clinical consequences of an emerging epidemic, *Clin Microbiol Rev* 23:616–687, 2010. https://doi.org/10.1128/CMR.00081-09.

File TM, Goldberg L, Das A, et al: Efficacy and safety of intravenous-to-oral lefamulin, a pleuromutilin antibiotic, for the treatment of community-acquired bacterial pneumonia: the phase III Lefamulin Evaluation Against Pneumonia (LEAP 1) trial, *Clin Infect Dis* 69:1856–1867, 2019.

Fluit AC: Livestock-associated *Staphylococcus aureus*, *Clin Microbiol Infect* 18:735–744, 2012. https://doi.org/10.1111/j.1469-0691.2012.03846.x.

Geriak M, Haddad F, Khulood R, et al: Clinical data on daptomycin plus ceftaroline versus standard of care monotherapy in the treatment of methicillin-resistant *Staphylococcus aureus* bacteremia, *Antimicrob Agents Chemother*, 2019. https://doi.org/10.1128/AAC.02483-18.

Gorwitz RJ, Jernigan DB, Powers JH, et al: *Strategies for clinical management of MRSA in the community: summary of an experts' meeting convened by the Centers for Disease Control and Prevention, 2006:* 2006. Available at www.cdc.gov/%20ncidod/dhqp/pdf/ar/CAMRSA_ExpMtgStrategies.pdf (accessed 02.01.2013).

Gould FK, Brindle R, Chadwick PR, et al: Guidelines (2008) for the prophylaxis and treatment of methicillin resistant *Staphylococcus aureus* (MRSA) infections in the United Kingdom, *J Antimicrob Chemother* 63:849–861, 2009. https://doi.org/10.1093/jac/dkp065.

Gu J, Shen S, Xiong M, et al: ST7 Becomes One of the Most Common Staphylococcus aureus Clones After the COVID-19 Epidemic in the City of Wuhan, China, *Infect Drug Resist* 16:843–852, 2023.

Kaplan SL, Hulten KG, Gonzalez BE, et al: Three-year surveillance of community-acquired *Staphylococcus aureus* infections in children, *Clin Infect Dis* 40:1785–1791, 2005.

Klevens RM, Morrison MA, Nadle J, et al: Invasive methicillin resistant *Staphylococcus aureus* infections in the United States, *JAMA* 298:1763–1771, 2007.

Kock R, Becker K, Cookson B, et al: Methicillin resistant *Staphylococcus aureus* (MRSA): burden of disease and control challenges in Europe, *Euro Surveill* 15:19688, 2010.

Lakhundi S, Zhang K: Methicillin-resistant *Staphylococcus aureus*: molecular characterization, evolution, and epidemiology, *Clin Microbiol Rev* 31, 2018. e00020-18. https://doi.org/10.1128/CMR.00020-18.

Lastinger LM, Alvarez CR, Kofman A, et al: Continued increases in the incidence of healthcare-associated infection (HAI) during the second year of the coronavirus disease 2019 (COVID-19) pandemic, *Infect Control Hosp Epidemiol* 20:1–5, 2022.

Lee SI, Lee GY, Park JH, Yang SJ: High prevalence of clonal complex 398 methicillin-susceptible and -resistant Staphylococcus aureus in pig farms: clonal lineages, multiple drug resistance, and occurrence of the staphylococcal cassette chromosome mec IX, *Foodborne Pathog Dis* 20(3):100–109, 2023.

Liu C, Bayer A, Cosgrove SE, et al: Clinical practice guidelines by the Infectious Diseases Society of America for the treatment of methicillin resistant *Staphylococcus aureus* infections in adults and children: executive summary, *Clin Infect Dis* 52:285–292, 2011. https://doi.org/10.1093/cid/cir034.

Miller LG, Daum RS, Creech CB, et al: Clindamycin versus trimethoprim-sulfamethoxazole for uncomplicated skin infections, *N Engl J Med* 372(12):1093–1103, 2015.

Muto CA, Jernigan JA, Ostrowsky BE, et al: SHEA guideline for preventing nosocomial transmission of multidrug-resistant strains of *Staphylococcus aureus* and enterococcus, *Infect Control Hosp Epidemiol* 24:362–386, 2003.

Nathwani D, Morgan M, Masterton RG, et al: Guidelines for UK practice for the diagnosis and management of methicillin resistant *Staphylococcus aureus* (MRSA) infections presenting in the community, *J Antimicrob Chemother* 61:976–994, 2008. https://doi.org/10.1093/jac/dkn096.

Prince WT, Ivezic-Schoenfeld Z, Lell C, et al: Phase II clinical study of BC-3781, a pleuromutilin antibiotic, in treatment of patients with acute bacterial skin and skin structure infections, *Antimicrob Agents Chemother* 57:2087–2094, 2013.

Tong SYC, Lye DC, Yahav D, et al: Effect of vancomycin or daptomycin with vs without an antistaphylococcal β-lactam on mortality, bacteremia, relapse, or treatment failure in patients with MRSA bacteremia: a randomized clinical trial, *JAMA* 323(6):527–537, 2020.

Urushibara N, Aung MS, Kawaguchiya M, Kobayashi N. Novel staphylococcal cassette chromosome mec (SCCmec) type XIV (5A) and a truncated SCCmec element in SCC composite islands carrying speG in ST5 MRSA in Japan, *J Antimicrob Chemother* 75(1):46–50, 2020.

Weidmann MD, Berry GJ, Zucker JE, et al: Bacterial pneumonia and respiratory culture utilization among hospitalized patients with and without COVID-19 in a New York City hospital, *J Clin Microbiol* 60(7):e0017422, 2022.

MPOX

Method of
Scott Kellermann, MD, MPH; and Rick D. Kellerman, MD

CURRENT DIAGNOSIS

- Clinical suspicion is based on history and symptoms, including suggestive skin lesions and high-risk epidemiologic characteristics.
- Clinical manifestations are usually mild but may be life-threatening.
- Prodromal symptoms may include fatigue, headache, fever, chills, myalgias, and backache. A rash may develop at the site of inoculation, including the anogenital and perioral areas, and may or may not spread to the trunk and acral areas. The total number of lesions may be a few or thousands and evolve from macular to papular, vesicular, pustular, and pseudopustular phases. The lesions are firm and deep-seated and 2 to 10 mm. in size. Pseudopustules are filled with solid material, not pus, and are actually papules.
- Confirmed by polymerase chain reaction testing of fluid from open lesions or other testing, including electron microscopy, immunohistochemical analysis, culture, or genomic sequencing.
- Histopathologic diagnosis is nonspecific.

CURRENT THERAPY

- JYNNEOS vaccine is Food and Drug Administration (FDA) approved and preferred for prevention.
- Vaccination prior to exposure and postexposure prophylaxis protocols exist.
- Certain high-risk individuals should be considered for treatment with tecovirimat.

In November 2022, following the current best practice of not naming diseases after animals or geographic locations, the World Health Organization changed the name of the disease previously referred to as "monkeypox" to "mpox." Until the International Committee on the Taxonomy of Viruses decides on a different name, the virus will continue to be called monkeypox virus. The monkeypox virus is an *Orthopoxvirus*, the same genus as smallpox (variola) and cowpox (vaccinia). Mpox is a contagious zoonotic disease and is endemic in certain parts of Africa. It was first isolated in 1958 in Copenhagen from a colony of laboratory monkeys sent from Singapore for polio virus research. In 1970 the first proven case of human mpox was diagnosed in the Democratic Republic of the Congo (formerly the Republic of Zaire). Despite initially being named *monkeypox*, African rodents such as Gambian pouched rats, dormice, and African squirrels, rather than monkeys, are considered to be the most likely reservoir of the virus.

There have been isolated cases and a few outbreaks of mpox in various countries, including the United Kingdom and the United States. In 2003 the United States reported an outbreak of 71 probable cases (35 laboratory-confirmed) that resulted from direct contact with prairie dogs sold as pets. The prairie dogs were found to have been infected when they were housed with Gambian pouched rats imported from Ghana. There were no reported deaths in the 2003 outbreak. Cases in a 2018 outbreak in the United Kingdom were eventually traced back to travelers who had visited Nigeria. From January to May 2022, most suspected cases of mpox occurred in the Democratic Republic of the Congo, with 1284 cases and 58 deaths reported.

In May 2022, cases of mpox were confirmed in the United Kingdom and traced to an individual who had traveled from Nigeria. Since then, tens of thousands of cases have been confirmed in North America, South America, Europe, Asia, Africa, and Australia. The majority of these cases had no history of travel to an endemic African country. The 2022 outbreak is considered the first example of widespread community transmission outside of Africa. On July 23, 2022, the World Health Organization declared this outbreak of mpox a public health emergency of international concern. As of August 30, 2023, there have been 89,581 confirmed cases worldwide, with 160 total confirmed deaths. The U.S. disease burden is 30,794 cases, with 53 deaths.

Epidemiology

The eradication of smallpox in 1977 and the discontinuation of routine smallpox immunization paved the way for mpox to gain worldwide clinical relevance. This hypothesis was supported by a 2005 to 2007 study in the Democratic Republic of the Congo that reported a 20-fold increase in mpox compared with the incidence seen in the 1980s. Those who were not immunized for smallpox had a fivefold higher risk of mpox infection compared with those who were vaccinated.

Two distinct clades of mpox exist in different geographic regions of Africa. The mortality risk associated with mpox varies with respect to the clade. Clade I is prevalent in Central Africa, demonstrates little human-to-human spread, but has a fatality rate of approximately 11%, with deaths generally occurring during the second week of illness. Clade II, which has been isolated in West Africa, lacks several genes present in the strain from Central Africa and is a milder disease with a fatality rate of around 1%. Clade II consists of two subclades, clades IIa and IIb. Clade IIa exists in West Africa. Clade IIb is spreading globally by human-to-human transmission. Sequencing analyses of viruses from the 2022 worldwide outbreak reveal similarities to strains circulating in Nigeria during the 2018 to 2019 outbreak.

Outcomes in the United States are favorable. Of the initial 10,000 cases reported, there were no deaths. This may be a result of milder clade II, subclade IIb, infections and also could be related to a healthier patient population and greater availability of supportive medical care and because most of the older adult population in the United States are vaccinated against smallpox.

As a zoonotic infection, animal-to-human transmission of mpox has been confirmed. Animal-to-human transmission can result from contact with infected papules, vesicles, pustules, or body fluids; ingesting infected meat; or bites and scratches.

A variety of animals, including nonhuman primates, and especially rodents, may contract mpox. Symptoms and severity of symptoms may differ among animals. Some may have symptoms that are mild, and others may have fever, upper respiratory illness, cough, and a papular-pustular rash. Animal-to-animal transmission may occur through the fecal-oral route, respiratory droplets, contact with wounds, and eating infected meat.

Human-to-human transmission of monkeypox virus occurs primarily from transfer of infectious material through microabrasions in the skin and/or mucous membranes during physical contact. This mainly occurs during sexual and/or close intimate contact. Sexual activity, largely among gay or bisexual men, is the main mode of transmission.

There is also the potential for spread through large respiratory droplets during prolonged face-to-face contact (e.g., within a 6-foot radius for ≥3 hours in the absence of personal protective equipment).

Fomites may present a transmission risk through resuspension of dried material from infected lesions (e.g., shaking contaminated linens).

Transmission may occur through an inadvertent needle-stick injury while collecting samples from a cutaneous lesion.

Vertical transmission of monkeypox virus from mother to child has been proven.

Though the virus has been found in semen and vaginal secretions, it is uncertain whether the disease can be transmitted through these fluids.

It has not been determined whether infected asymptomatic patients can spread the virus.

In a review of 528 mpox cases from multiple countries, only 0.8% were likely owing to nonsexual close contact, and 0.6% were due to household contact. One study noted that the reproductive number of the virus ranged from 1.40 to 1.80, implying a potential for sustainable local transmission.

Risk Factors

In a U.S. study of 7500 cases of mpox from May 17 to July 22, 2022, 99% of the cases were male, and 94% reported recent male-to-male sexual or intimate conduct. Similar to data from other countries, 41% of these patients were HIV-positive. It is unknown whether HIV infection increases a person's risk of acquiring mpox disease after exposure; however, the risk of progressing to severe mpox disease has been reported to be higher in those who are virologically suppressed. During the outbreak that began in 2022, persons who experienced severe manifestations of mpox and who had HIV with CD4 counts <200 cells/mL presented significant treatment challenges.

Coinfections with sexually transmitted infections ranged from 16% to 29%, with gonorrhea, chlamydia, and syphilis the most commonly reported.

Mpox is disproportionately spread among men who have sex with men, suggesting amplification of transmission through sexual networks.

Pathophysiology

Monkeypox virus is a large, linear, double-stranded DNA virus with a genome size of around 190 kb. The virus replicates in the cytoplasm of vertebrate and invertebrate cells, although DNA viruses typically replicate and express their genomes in the nucleus. The virus invades the cell, replicates in the cytoplasm, and causes cell death.

Following viral entry through skin or mucous membranes, the monkeypox virus replicates at the inoculation site and then spreads to local lymph nodes. This is followed by a viremia that leads to viral spread and seeding at other sites.

The large size of the monkeypox virus readily generates an immune response. Monkeypox virus infection stimulates an adaptive immune response comprising activated effector CD4+ and CD8+ T cells, neutralizing IgM and IgG antibodies and the production of Th1-inflammatory cytokines. Genomic analysis reveals that the virus may be actively mutating and adapting to human host immune responses.

Prevention

General safety measures such as use of personal protective equipment should be employed by healthcare workers and laboratory researchers who may come in contact with the monkeypox virus. Hospitalized patients with confirmed or suspected mpox should be isolated. Lesions should be covered by gloves, a gown, or a sheet. Routine cleaning and disinfection procedures should be followed, and special attention should be paid to soiled laundry. Intubation, extubation, and any procedures likely to spread oral secretions should be performed in an airborne infection isolation room. To date, there have been no cases of mpox transmitted by blood transfusion, organ transplantation or implantation, infusion, or transfer of human cells, tissues, or cellular or tissue-based products.

Patients and household members who are isolated at home should use face masks and gloves. Lesions should be covered and good hand hygiene should be routine. Laundering linens and towels with detergent and water should be sufficient.

Activities that could aerosolize dried material from lesions (e.g., use of portable fans, dry dusting, sweeping, vacuuming) should be avoided. If possible, use a separate bathroom if there are others living in the same household. Those infected with mpox should avoid contact with animals (specifically mammals), including pets.

Though it is uncertain whether the disease can be transmitted through intercourse, it is recommended that condoms be used for 12 weeks after contracting the illness.

Vaccinations

Immunization against smallpox will confer cross-reactive protection against mpox.

There are two available vaccines that can reduce the risk of developing mpox: the modified vaccinia Ankara (MVA) vaccine (JYNNEOS in the United States, IMVANEX in the European Union, and IMVAMUNE in Canada) and the ACAM2000 vaccine.[1] Supplies of both vaccines are limited.

JYNNEOS

The JYNNEOS vaccine is recommended as the primary vaccine to prevent mpox because it is associated with fewer side effects than the ACAM2000 vaccine. JYNNEOS is a live, nonreplicating MVA virus that was approved in 2019 by the U.S. Food and Drug Administration (FDA) for the prevention of mpox. JYNNEOS is administered subcutaneously as a two-dose series delivered 28 days apart. The standard FDA-approved regimen involves a *subcutaneous route* of administration with an injection volume of 0.5 mL per dose. In the context of the current national public health emergency, an alternative regimen may be used for people age 18 years or older under an emergency use authorization. This alternative regimen involves an *intradermal route* of administration with an injection volume of 0.1 mL per dose. Experience with JYNNEOS is limited, but serious side effects are minor and rare. Booster doses[1] are recommended. Peak immunity is expected to be reached 14 days after the second dose of JYNNEOS vaccine. Because JYNNEOS is based on a live, attenuated, nonreplicating orthopoxvirus, JYNNEOS may be administered without regard to timing of other vaccines.

Across 32 U.S. jurisdictions, among males aged 18 to 49 years eligible for JYNNEOS vaccination, mpox incidence was 14 times higher among unvaccinated males compared with those who had received a first vaccine dose ≥14 days earlier.

Vaccine considerations for specific populations can be found at: (https://www.cdc.gov/poxvirus/mpox/interim-considerations/special-populations.html).

ACAM2000

ACAM2000 is a single-dose vaccine administered through the scarification (multiple puncture) technique. It requires 15 percutaneous jabs with a stainless steel bifurcated needle that is dipped into the reconstituted vaccine. The technique produces a severe cutaneous reaction (development of a pustule or ulcer that will eventually scab over) known as a *take*, eventually leaving a dime-sized scar. This vaccination is a derivative of the Dryvax method that was used to eradicate smallpox worldwide.

Because the ACAM2000 vaccine is a replicating live virus, it has a number of contraindications: immunocompromise, age younger than 1 year, pregnancy, breastfeeding, atopic dermatitis and exfoliative skin conditions, known underlying cardiac disease or significant cardiac risk factors, and serious allergy to a vaccine component. Individuals should isolate after immunization with the ACAM2000 vaccine if potential close contacts have any of the aforementioned conditions. If possible, because of the reactogenicity profile of ACAM2000, consider delaying other vaccines when administering ACAM2000. Live vaccines and ACAM2000 should be separated by at least 28 days. Healthcare workers scheduled to receive an annual purified protein derivative (PPD) skin test for tuberculosis screening should not receive the skin test until more than 1 month after ACAM2000 vaccination.

Myopericarditis has been associated with the ACAM2000 vaccine. The risk of myopericarditis resulting from the JYNNEOS

---

[1]Not FDA approved for this indication.

vaccine is uncertain. As a precaution, it is recommended that the mRNA SARS-CoV-2 vaccine be administered no sooner than 4 weeks after the ACAM2000 or JYNNEOS vaccine.

Adverse reactions to either vaccine should be reported to the Vaccine Adverse Event Reporting System.

Vaccination Prior to Exposure
The JYNNEOS vaccine has been recommended as vaccination prior to exposure to select persons at risk for orthopoxvirus infection in the occupational setting, such as research laboratory personnel working with poxviruses, specialized clinical laboratory personnel performing diagnostic testing for orthopoxviruses, and designated response team members.

Postexposure Prophylaxis
JYNNEOS and ACAM2000 may be used for postexposure prophylaxis (PEP). Exposures in both community and healthcare settings should be assessed to determine the risk of monkeypox virus transmission.

Mpox vaccination should be offered to the following:
- People who had known or suspected exposure to someone with mpox
- People who had a sex partner in the past 2 weeks who was diagnosed with mpox
- Gay, bisexual, and other men who have sex with men, and transgender or nonbinary people (including adolescents who fall into any of the these categories) who, in the past 6 months, have had:
  - A new diagnosis of one or more sexually transmitted diseases (e.g., chlamydia, gonorrhea, syphilis) or
  - More than one sex partner
- People who have had any of the following in the past 6 months:
  - Sex at a commercial sex venue
  - Sex in association with a large public event in a geographic area where mpox transmission is occurring
  - Sex in exchange for money or other items
- People who are sexual partners of people with the above risks
- People who anticipate experiencing any of the above scenarios
- People with HIV infection or other causes of immunosuppression who have had recent or anticipate potential mpox exposure
- People who work in settings where they may be exposed to mpox, such as those who work with orthopoxviruses in a laboratory

To be most effective, mpox vaccination should be included as part of broader prevention activities and sexual health care.

If administered within 4 days of exposure, PEP with JYNNEOS may prevent disease. If given between days 4 and 14 of exposure, vaccination is thought to reduce the symptoms of mpox but not prevent the disease.

The CDC Components of the U.S. National Mpox Vaccination Strategy can be accessed at: (https://www.cdc.gov/poxvirus/mpox/clinicians/vaccines/vaccine-basics-healthcare.html).

Pregnancy/Breastfeeding
Mpox can pose considerable risks to the fetus. Miscarriages, stillbirth, preterm birth, and neonatal mpox have been reported when pregnant women contract mpox. Fetal ultrasound monitoring is recommended in cases of maternal monkeypox virus infection, and subsequent management should be based on the presence of ultrasound anomalies such as fetal hepatomegaly or hydrops. The sensitivity of molecular detection of monkeypox virus in the amniotic fluid is unknown though, by analogy with cytomegalovirus, toxoplasmosis, and Zika virus infections, it is likely that monkeypox virus is shed in the amniotic fluid when the fetal kidneys produce sufficient urine (i.e., after 18 to 21 weeks gestation).

Though most nonpregnant adults with mpox experience mild illness, those with the infection who are pregnant, recently pregnant, or breastfeeding should be prioritized for treatment. These individuals may be at increased risk of severe disease and

TABLE 1	High-Risk Children and Adolescents With Monkeypox to Be Considered for Treatment*

While most cases of mpox resolve without treatment, treatment should be considered, based on interim guidance for clinical treatment, for children and adolescents who have the following clinical manifestations:
- Severe disease, including disseminated rash, a large number of lesions that are confluent, hemorrhagic or necrotic lesions, severe lymphadenopathy that can cause airway obstruction, involvement of multiple organ systems and associated comorbidities (e.g., pulmonary involvement with nodular lesions, encephalitis, ocular disease, myocarditis, neurologic involvement), sepsis, or if the disease requires hospitalization.

Treatment should also be considered for children and adolescents who may be at high risk for severe disease:
- Children under 1 year of age
- Children and adolescents experiencing severe immunodeficiency or immunocompromise
- Adolescents who are pregnant or breastfeeding
- Children and adolescents with a condition affecting skin integrity

*Modified from Centers for Disease Control and Prevention. *Clinical Considerations for Monkeypox in Children and Adolescents.* Available at: https://www.cdc.gov/poxvirus/mpox/clinicians/pediatric.html#print. Updated September 1, 2023.

transmitting infection to the fetus or newborn. Following consultation with the CDC, tecovirimat (Tpoxx)[1] should be considered for first-line treatment. Animal studies have suggested the risk of teratogenicity from brincidofovir (Tembexa)[1] and cidofovir.[1]

JYNNEOS can be offered to people who are pregnant or breastfeeding who are otherwise eligible. The risks and benefits of JYNNEOS should be discussed with the patient using shared decision making.

ACAM2000 is a replicating live viral vaccine; therefore ACAM2000 is contraindicated in people who are pregnant or breastfeeding.

Given the risk of neonatal transmission of monkeypox virus from close contact and the potential for severe disease in newborns, direct contact between a mother with mpox and her newborn is not advised.

Children
Though most cases will resolve without a problem, treatment should be considered for the following children: those under 1 year of age, children and adolescents with severe immunodeficiency or immunocompromise, adolescents who are pregnant or breastfeeding, and children and adolescents with a condition affecting skin integrity (Table 1).

Covering lesions and attempting to prevent scratching are especially important in children because of the risk of autoinoculation and the risk of spreading the pox to the eyes. Maintenance of hydration is important. Fluid intake may be limited because of mouth lesions and general malaise, and fluid loss may be significant as a result of multiple and open lesions. Children should be closely monitored for complications and severe illness.

Clinical Manifestations
In patients with classic mpox, the incubation period from time of exposure to clinical illness is usually 5 to 13 days, but it may be up to 21 days.

The clinical manifestations of mpox are usually mild, and patients may have subclinical infection or be asymptomatic. In rare situations, patients may develop life-threatening illness. The duration of symptoms is usually 2 to 4 weeks. Most patients recover without specific treatment. Systemic symptoms are common and may occur before the rash appears, during a prodromal

[1] Not FDA approved for this indication.

stage, or shortly thereafter. Common prodromal symptoms include headache, fatigue, fever, chills, myalgias, backache, and sore throat. During the 2022 outbreak, it was noted that patients frequently presented with lesions located on the anogenital and perioral areas alone, presumably at the site of inoculation, with some developing a small number of lesions on the trunk or acral areas of the body. The rash may or may not spread to the rest of the body, and the total number of lesions may vary from a few to thousands. Over the following 2 to 4 weeks, the lesions evolve in 1- to 2-day increments through macular, papular, vesicular, and pustular phases. The lesions are characterized as firm, deep-seated, and 2 to 10 mm in size. Peudopustules have also been described. These pseudopapules are solid, white, raised, and non-pustular. Lesions are often described as painful until the healing phase when they become itchy. The evolution of the lesions may vary. They may evolve in the same stage on the same area of the body, or different areas of the body may have lesions at different stages of development. Lesions remain in the pustular phase for 5 to 7 days before crusts begin to form. Healing lesions may itch. Crusts form and desquamate over the subsequent 7 to 14 days, and the condition resolves around 3 to 4 weeks after symptom onset in most cases. Patients are no longer considered infectious after all crusts have sloughed off and the lesions have reepithelialized. An excellent monograph can be found at: https://www.cdc.gov/poxvirus/mpox/clinicians/clinical-recognition.html.

Other symptoms may include conjunctivitis, cough, dyspnea, nausea, vomiting, dysphagia, and photophobia. During the 2003 U.S. outbreak, a detailed review of 34 patients reported that the predominant signs and symptoms were rash (97%), fever (85%), chills (71%), lymphadenopathy (71%), headache (65%), and myalgias (56%). During the prodromal or early clinical stages in the 2022 outbreak, generalized swelling of the lymph nodes was uncommon, although regional lymphadenopathy is often associated with the skin rash.

Rectal symptoms (e.g., purulent or bloody stools, rectal pain, or rectal bleeding) have been reported.

Diagnosis

The diagnosis can be most easily confirmed by polymerase chain reaction testing of fluid from open lesions. Unlike the lesions seen in herpes simplex virus, which are usually filled with fluid and easily unroofed, mpox lesions may contain solid material, making them difficult to unroof with a swab. Two swabs from each of two to three lesions should be collected for testing. Using two sterile synthetic swabs (including, but not limited to, polyester, nylon, or Dacron with a plastic, wood, or thin aluminum shaft), swab the lesion vigorously to collect adequate DNA. Do not use cotton swabs. Unroofing or aspiration of lesions before swabbing is not necessary, nor is it recommended owing to the risk for sharps injury. All recommended personal protective equipment (PPE) should be worn when collecting a specimen from a person with suspected or confirmed mpox.

Diagnosis may also be confirmed through the use of electron microscopy, culture, and immunohistochemical analysis. Genomic sequencing may be used in some situations. The use of serum IgM and IgG antibody testing may provide supportive information. Histopathologic diagnosis is nonspecific.

The CDC uses case definitions for mpox as follows (https://ndc.services.cdc.gov/case-definitions/monkeypox-virus-infection/):

- Suspect case: a new characteristic rash OR history and symptoms suggesting a high clinical suspicion of mpox PLUS one of the following epidemiologic criteria:
  - contact with a person or people with a similar rash who have received a diagnosis of confirmed or probable mpox
  - close or intimate in-person contact with individuals in a social network experiencing mpox activity
  - travel outside the United States to a confirmed country with confirmed cases of mpox or where mpox is endemic
  - contact with a dead or wild animal or exotic pet that is an African endemic species or use of a product derived from such an animal such as game meat, cream or lotion, etc.

- Probable case: no suspicion of other recent *Orthopoxvirus* exposure (e.g., *Vaccinia* virus in ACAM2000 vaccination) AND demonstration of the presence of *Orthopoxvirus* DNA by polymerase chain reaction of a clinical specimen or *Orthopoxvirus* using immunohistochemical or electron microscopy testing methods or demonstration of detectable levels of anti-orthopoxvirus IgM antibody during the period of 4 to 56 days after rash onset
- Confirmed case: demonstration of the presence of monkeypox virus DNA by polymerase chain reaction testing or next-generation sequencing of a clinical specimen OR isolation of monkeypox virus in culture from a clinical specimen

Differential Diagnosis

The differential diagnosis of mpox includes other poxviruses, particularly smallpox and chickenpox. Other conditions to be considered in the differential diagnosis include hand, foot, and mouth disease; herpes zoster; herpes simplex; measles; impetigo; scabies; candidiasis; dermatitis herpetiformis; orf; bullous disease; insect bites; contact dermatitis; molluscum contagiosum; and drug eruptions. Pharyngeal features of mpox may be mistaken for bacterial tonsillitis or primary syphilis. The symptoms during the prodromal period may be similar to those of influenza, COVID-19, and other viral respiratory illnesses. Symptoms may be particularly variable in patients with HIV or other types of immunocompromise. Papules, vesicles, and pustules may be present in the genital and perianal areas and can be confused with sexually transmitted illnesses such as herpes, syphilis, chancroid, or lymphogranuloma venereum. Distinguishing between varicella and mpox might be challenging; however, lymphadenopathy is a distinctive feature of mpox compared with varicella. Also, unlike varicella lesions, which are vesicular fluid filled lesions, mpox lesions may be pseudopustules that simulate the appearance of pustules but do not contain fluid or pus.

Treatment

Treatment of mpox is usually aimed at reducing symptoms. In rare situations, supportive treatment is required for those who experience severe disease. Currently, there is no treatment approved specifically for mpox virus infections. Certain high-risk individuals should be considered for antiviral treatment with tecovirimat (TPOXX, ST-246)[1] or brincidofovir,[1] which are approved for the treatment of smallpox. Treatment should be considered for use in people who have the following clinical manifestations:

- Severe disease—consider severe disease when a patient has conditions such as hemorrhagic disease; a large number of lesions such that they are confluent; necrotic lesions; severe lymphadenopathy that can be necrotizing or obstructing (such as in airways); involvement of multiple organ systems and associated comorbidities (e.g., pulmonary involvement with nodular lesions, sepsis, encephalitis, myocarditis, ocular or periorbital infections); or other conditions requiring hospitalization
- Involvement of anatomic areas that might result in serious sequelae that include scarring or strictures—these include lesions directly involving the pharynx causing dysphagia, inability to control secretions, or need for parenteral feeding; penile foreskin, vulva, vagina, urethra, or anorectum with the potential for causing strictures or requiring catheterization; anorectal lesions interfering with bowel movements (e.g., severe pain); and severe infections (including secondary bacterial skin infections), especially those that require surgical intervention such as debridement.

Treatment should also be considered for use in people who are at high risk for severe disease:

- People currently experiencing severe immunocompromise due to conditions such as advanced or poorly controlled HIV, leukemia, lymphoma, generalized malignancy, solid organ transplantation, therapy with alkylating agents, antimetabolites,

---

[1] Not FDA approved for this indication.

radiation, tumor necrosis factor inhibitors, high-dose corticosteroids, being a recipient of a hematopoietic stem cell transplant <24 months post-transplant or ≥24 months but with graft-versus-host disease or disease relapse, or having autoimmune disease with immunodeficiency as a clinical component[1]

- Pediatric populations, particularly patients younger than 1 year of age
- Pregnant or breastfeeding people[2]
- People with a condition affecting skin integrity—conditions such as atopic dermatitis, eczema, burns, impetigo, varicella zoster virus infection, herpes simplex virus infection, severe acne, severe diaper dermatitis with extensive areas of denuded skin, psoriasis, or Darier disease (keratosis follicularis)

For patients at high risk for progression to severe disease, treatment should be administered early in the course of illness along with supportive care and pain control (https://www.cdc.gov/poxvirus/mpox/clinicians/treatment.html; updated July 10, 2023). Animal studies have suggested a risk of teratogenicity from brincidofovir (Tembexa),[1] and it is recommended that it not be used for the treatment of pregnant women and used with caution in women of childbearing age.

Tecovirimat (TPOXX, ST-246) is a potent inhibitor of an orthopoxvirus protein required for the formation of infectious virus particles that are essential for dissemination within an infected host. Tecovirimat was approved for the treatment of smallpox under a regulation known as the Animal Rule. Under the Animal Rule, efficacy is established on the basis of adequate and well-controlled studies in animal models of the human disease or condition of interest. The CDC, in partnership with the FDA, has made it easier for healthcare providers to access tecovirimat treatment under the Expanded Access Investigational New Drug protocol. Tecovirimat can be administered as an oral drug or an intravenous injection based on weight of the patient. The duration of treatment is 14 days. Tecovirimat is well tolerated; the most common side effects are headache and nausea.

Brincidofovir (Tembexa, CMS001) is an oral drug approved by the FDA for treatment of smallpox in adults, children, and neonates. Its effectiveness against mpox in humans is not proven, though in vitro and animal studies have demonstrated its effectiveness against orthopoxviruses. Brincidofovir is a prodrug of cidofovir (Vistide), an antiviral medication used to treat cytomegalovirus retinitis in patients with AIDS. However, the use of cidofovir can result in renal toxicity and other adverse events. Animal studies have suggested that brincidofovir and cidofovir may have teratogenic effects.

The vaccinia immune globulin intravenous (VIGIV [CNJ-016]) may be considered for use in patients with severe disease. The use of VIGIV has no proven benefit in the treatment of mpox, and it is unknown whether a person with severe mpox infection will benefit from treatment with VIGIV. However, healthcare providers may consider its use in severe cases where the development of a robust antibody response may be impaired.[1]

Because of the developing evidence base to support these therapies and because treatment of mpox will evolve with time, consultation with state health department authorities and the CDC Emergency Operations Center (1-800-488-7100) is recommended before initiation of treatment. Updated information regarding indications for treatment of mpox can be found on the CDC website (https://www.cdc.gov/poxvirus/mpox/clinicians/treatment.html; updated July 10, 2023).

Complications
Serious complications are uncommon, and death is rare. Complications may include pneumonia, sepsis, or encephalitis. Mpox may be life threatening in the severely immunocompromised and in young children. Secondary infections of the mpox lesions may occur. Corneal infection with loss of vision has been reported. Mpox can be transmitted to the fetus during pregnancy, and newborns may contract it through close contact during and after birth. Miscarriages and stillbirth have been associated with mpox contracted during pregnancy.

References
Centers for Disease Control and Prevention. Monkeypox: Information for Health Care Professionals. Available at: https://www.cdc.gov/poxvirus/monkeypox/clinicians/index.html. Updated August 19, 2022.

Dashraath P, Nielsone-Saines K, Mattar C, et al: Guidelines for pregnant individuals with monkeypox exposure (correspondence), *Lancet*, 2022. https://doi.org/10.1016/S01406736(22)01063-7. Published online June 21.

Huhn GD, Bauer AM, Yorita K, et al: Clinical characteristics of human monkeypox, and risk factors for severe disease, *Clin Infect Dis* 41:1742, 2005.

Kaler J, Hussain A, Flores G, et al: Monkeypox: a comprehensive review of transmission, pathogenesis, and manifestation, *Cureus* 14(7):e26531, 2022, https://doi.org/10.7759/cureus.26531.

Kwok KO, Wei WI, Tang A, et al: Estimation of local transmissibility in the early phase of monkeypox epidemic in 2022, *Clin Microbiol Infect* 28:1653.e1, 2022.

Miller MJ, Cash-Goldwasser S, Marx GE, et al. Severe monkeypox in hospitalized patients — United States, august 10–October 10, 2022. *MMWR Morb Mortal Wkly Rep*. ePub: October 26, 2022

Minhaj FS, Ogale YP, Whitehill F, et al: Monkeypox outbreak — nine states, May 2022, *MMWR Morb Mortal Wkly Rep* 71:764–769, 2022, https://doi.org/10.15585/mmwr.mm7123e1.

Moore MJ, Rathish B, Zahra F: Monkeypox. [Updated 2022 Jul 16]. In *StatPearls [internet]*, Treasure Island (FL), 2022, StatPearls Publishing. Available from: https://www.ncbi.nlm.nih.gov/books/NBK574519/.

Philpott D, Hughes CM, Alroy KA, et al: Epidemiologic and clinical characteristics of monkeypox cases — United States, May 17–July 22, 2022, *MMWR Morb Mortal Wkly Rep* 71:1018–1022, 2022, https://doi.org/10.15585/mmwr.mm7132e3.

Rao AK, Petersen BW, Whitehill F, et al: Use of JYNNEOS (smallpox and monkeypox vaccine, live, nonreplicating) for preexposure vaccination of persons at risk for occupational exposure to orthopoxviruses: recommendations of the Advisory Committee on Immunization Practices — United States, 2022, *MMWR Morb Mortal Wkly Rep* 71:734–742, 2022, https://doi.org/10.15585/mmwr.mm7122e1.

Sherwat A, Brooks JT, Birnkrant D, Kim P: Tecovirimat and the treatment of monkeypox— past, present, and future considerations, *N Engl J Med* 387:579–581, 2022, https://doi.org/10.1056/NEJMp2210125.

Thornhill JP, Barkati S, Walmsley S, et al: For the SHARE-net Clinical Group. Monkeypox virus infection in humans across 16 countries — april–June 2022, *N Engl J Med* 387:1–14, 2022, https://doi.org/10.1056/NEJMoa2207323.

Weaver JR, Isaacs SN: Monkeypox virus and insights into its immunomodulatory proteins, *Immunol Rev* 225:96–113, 2008, https://doi.org/10.1111/j.1600-065X.2008.00691.x. PMID: 18837778; PMCID: PMC2567051.

MUMPS

Method of
Kristen Rundell, MS, MD

CURRENT DIAGNOSIS

- Parotitis (swelling of the parotid salivary glands): unilateral or bilateral
- Fever
- Headache
- Malaise
- Myalgias
- Anorexia
- Increased serum amylase

CURRENT THERAPY

- Supportive care
- Warm or cold packs on the parotid
- Analgesics and/or antipyretics (such as acetaminophen [Tylenol] or ibuprofen [Motrin])
- IV fluids or hospitalization for cases of pancreatitis, meningitis, or severe orchitis

---

[1] Not FDA approved for this indication.

Epidemiology

Mumps is an extremely contagious, self-limiting virus that had disease rates of 99% until the vaccine was introduced in 1967. Since 2006, there have been several outbreaks, in the United States, these usually present in young people and those who are not vaccinated, and have increased transmissibility on college campuses, in close knit communities and large social gatherings. For the United States and Finland, mumps is almost eradicated. For the rest of the world, mumps is still endemic as a result of a vaccination rate of only 61%.

Pathophysiology

Mumps is a single-stranded RNA virus and a member of the *Paramyxovirus* genus. It is transmitted through respiratory secretions, saliva, and contact with contaminated fomites.

Prevention

With the high rate of transmission and no antiviral therapy, prevention for mumps relies on community immunity as a result of high vaccine rates. There are two formulations of the mumps vaccine currently available in the United States: the measles-mumps-rubella vaccine (MMR) and the measles-mumps-rubella-varicella vaccine (MMRV, ProQuad). The dosing schedule for children calls for the first dose at age greater than 12 months to 15 months, and the second dose for children greater than 4 years to 6 years of age. For infants aged 6 through 11 months who are traveling internationally, a single MMR vaccine is recommended. These children should be revaccinated with 2 doses of MMR vaccine with the first dose at ages 12 months to 15 months and the second dose at ages 4 years to 6 years. During an epidemic, a single dose for adults born before 1957 is recommended and may be required by some health care professionals. The first dose gives approximately 80% immunity. Persons receiving both doses may still get the mumps virus if there is outbreak or if they travel to an endemic area. To avoid exposure or contraction of the disease during travel, it is suggested that travelers wash hands frequently and use alcohol-based sanitizers to decrease the contraction or spread of disease.

The vaccine is contraindicated for patients who are pregnant or planning to conceive in the 28 days after vaccination. Vaccine administration is also contraindicated for those who have a severe anaphylactic reaction to the vaccine or one of the components, and those individuals who are severely immunocompromised.

Clinical Manifestations

The incubation period for the mumps virus is 16 to 18 days. At the onset of the illness, patients may develop acute viral infection symptoms of fever, headache, and malaise. The parotitis, swelling of the parotid gland, is the diagnostic hallmark of the mumps virus. This is caused by the infection and inflammation of the parotid ductal epithelium. The swelling may last up to 10 days. Close to 30% of persons may not have this symptom and may be only mildly symptomatic.

Diagnosis

Diagnosis is made by the history and the constellation of symptoms and physical findings. It is difficult to use IgM to determine active infection, because the response may be short in duration, delayed, or even absent. PCR testing is available and requires early sampling.

Differential Diagnosis

Viral infections such as parainfluenza (also in the paramyxovirus genus) coxsackievirus, influenza A, Epstein-Barr, adenovirus, HIV, and cytomegalovirus may present with similar symptoms as mumps. There are also noninfectious etiologies of parotitis, which include salivary stones or tumors, sarcoid, Sjögren's syndrome, and thiazide diuretics.

Therapy (or Treatment)

Treatment for mumps virus is largely supportive. For complicated cases of pancreatitis, meningitis, encephalitis, and orchitis, patient may need to be hospitalized for additional care. The additional care usually includes fever reduction, analgesia, fluid resuscitation, and treatment of secondary bacterial infections.

Monitoring

For persons with active mumps, it is suggested that they be isolated from school or work for 5 days after the onset of symptoms. Shedding of virus usually occurs 4 days prior to the onset of symptoms. For this reason, it is difficult to slow down outbreaks of the disease. The last outbreak in the United States was in 2010.

Complications

Complications from mumps are rare. In children, pancreatitis and hearing loss are the sensorineural complications most often diagnosed. For adolescents and adults the complications are more common and usually more severe. These include aseptic meningitis; orchitis in males, which rarely leads to sterility; oophoritis in females; pancreatitis; and arthritis. Even more uncommon are Guillain–Barré/ascending polyradiculitis, transverse myelitis, facial palsy, interstitial nephritis, and myocardial involvement.

Mumps in pregnancy has been associated with increased fetal loss. There are no known teratogenic effects.

References

American Academy of Pediatrics: Mumps. In Pickering LK, Baker CJ, Kimberlin DW, Long SS, editors: *Red Book: 2009 Report of the committee on Infectious Diseases*, ed 28, Elk Gove Village IL, 2009, American Academy of Pediatrics, pp 468–472.

Centers for Disease Control and Prevention (CDC): Exposure to mumps during air travel—United States, April 2006, *MMWR Morb Mortal Wkly Rep* 55(401), 2006.

Centers for Disease Prevention and Control Website 5/1/2021.

Dayan GH, Rubin S: Mumps outbreaks in vaccinated population: are available mumps vaccines effective enough to prevent an outbreak? *Clin Infect Dis* 47:1458, 2008.

Kleiman MB: Mumps virus. In Lenette EH, editor: *Laboratory Diagnosis of Viral Infections*, ed 2, New York, 1992, Marcel Dekker. p. 549.

Kutty PK, Barskey AE, Gallagher KM: *Mumps. Infectious diseases related to travel*, CDC Yellowbook, 2012(chapter 3).

Wharton M, Cochi SLK, William S: Measles, mumps and rubella vaccines, *Infect Dis Clin North Am* 4:47, 1990. www.cdc.gov/travel/yellowbook.

MYALGIC ENCEPHALOMYELITIS/CHRONIC FATIGUE SYNDROME

Method of
Stephen J. Gluckman, MD

CURRENT DIAGNOSIS

- Myalgic encephalomyelitis/chronic fatigue syndrome is defined as
  - a substantial new-onset reduction in the ability to engage in preillness levels of occupational, educational, social, or personal activities
  - accompanied by (often profound) fatigue that is not alleviated by rest
  - associated with unrefreshing sleep
  - worsened with physical or mental exertion
  - persisting for more than 6 months
  - frequently associated with cognitive impairment, orthostatic intolerance, joint and muscle pain, and depression.
- A typical story is a previously highly functioning individual who develops characteristic symptoms after an acute illness or significant stress.
- Should be differentiated from an isolated symptom of fatigue.
- The diagnosis is clinical, and individual patients may not completely fit the definition which was established for research purposes.
- There is no proven etiology and no specific diagnostic test or physical finding.

Myalgic encephalomyelitis/chronic fatigue syndrome (ME/CFS) is an often-misunderstood syndrome that should not be confused with malingering, hypochondriasis, or just fatigue. Patients with ME/CFS are truly suffering from their often-disabling symptoms. The absence of an objective finding does not alter the validity of the patient's symptoms. It is impossible to successfully treat a patient with ME/CFS unless the clinician believes the patient is genuinely symptomatic. ME/CFS also should not be confused with the isolated symptoms of fatigue. Fatigue is a common patient complaint, whereas ME/CFS has a much lower prevalence.

Definition

ME/CFS is not a new disease; the syndrome has been described since at least the mid-1700s. However, since that time, it has been mistakenly ascribed to a number of incorrect pathologic and infectious causes. In the past, it has been called *febricula, neurasthenia, effort syndrome, Da Costa syndrome, chronic brucellosis, chronic Lyme disease, chronic Epstein-Barr syndrome, total allergy syndrome, chronic candidiasis,* and *multiple chemical sensitivity syndrome.* More recently, it has been falsely attributed to infection with xenotropic murine leukemia virus–related virus (XMRV) and related retroviruses, such as murine leukemia virus (MLV). None of these possible causes has proved to be correct.

In 1988, in an attempt to be descriptive rather than to attribute an incorrect etiology to the disease, the term *chronic fatigue syndrome* was coined. Therefore the name is relatively new, but the syndrome is not. The disease is chronic, and fatigue is a cardinal feature, but it is more than being chronically tired. This working case definition was published by the Centers for Disease Control and Prevention and then modified in 1992 by the National Institute of Allergy and Infectious Diseases. In March 2015 the Institute of Medicine (IOM; now the National Academy of Medicine [NAM]) issued an extensive and thorough review of the topic. As a result of this review, they proposed a name change to *systemic exertion intolerance disease* (SEID). This comprehensive report has three major themes: (1) ME/CFS has acquired a great deal of negative connotation with associated misunderstanding and prejudice. The name change to SEID is an attempt to disconnect this disease from past misunderstandings. However, this name change has not caught on. (2) The criteria for diagnosis were greatly simplified, with emphasis on the major features (Box 1). (3) By using the term *disease* and by supplying ample reference support in the document, the IOM unequivocally underscores the very real nature of this malady. The IOM report is by far the most thorough examination of the topic, and it unequivocally supports the validity of this disease.

One note of caution: This case definition is an epidemiologic and research tool and not a strict clinical tool. It is useful for studying the disease. However, some patients do not completely fit this definition. ME/CFS can nonetheless be diagnosed by a knowledgeable clinician who is willing to consider this diagnosis.

Because some immune abnormalities are often seen in these patients, some people have called this *chronic fatigue and immune dysregulation syndrome.* The immune abnormalities seen in

patients with ME/CFS are mild and differ from patient to patient. Most significant, these patients are not immunosuppressed or at risk for opportunistic infections.

It has been noted that many of the symptoms of fibromyalgia overlap with ME/CFS, and some clinicians consider fibromyalgia and ME/CFS to be different aspects of the same disease because both often include pain and fatigue. These different names for the same syndrome can be confusing to patients and clinicians, and it is important to explain this when managing patients with ME/CFS.

A mention should be made in regard to long-haul COVID-19. In this entity, patients have persistent symptoms after recovering from acute COVID-19. There are a number of reasons for persistent symptoms, including lingering or permanent organ damage as the result of a severe episode of COVID and/or posttraumatic stress disorder (PTSD) related to the trauma of being intubated in an intensive care setting. In addition, COVID-19 triggers typical ME/CFS in some persons.

Epidemiology

Although chronic fatigue is an extremely common symptom, ME/CFS is not. The former has been noted to have a prevalence of 10% to 25% in a number of studies. However, the point prevalence of ME/CFS has been estimated to be in the range of 0.1%. ME/CFS is overrepresented in young and middle-age women, but it has been described in both men and women and in all age groups.

Pathophysiology

The cause of ME/CFS is unknown. Much effort has gone into trying to discern an infectious, endocrine, immune, or psychiatric cause, but to date none has been proven. Studies have shown a link between ME/CFS and the presence of certain genes that mediate immune and stress responses. The findings suggest that difficulty managing stress may be linked to the development of ME/CFS. They also suggest that there may not be a single cause of ME/CFS but that there may be a number of stress-related triggers (physical or emotional) in those with a genetic predisposition. This is consistent with the typical course, in which a previously healthy person develops an acute illness that resolves but initiates ME/CFS.

Clinical Features and Diagnosis

Although there is, as yet, no diagnostic test, the history, physical examination, and laboratory testing are generally very characteristic and allow a clinician to confidently make the diagnosis in most cases. The typical story is one of a previously highly functioning person who develops an acute illness or other stressor. The acute problem resolves; however, from that time on, symptoms of

ME/CFS are triggered. Despite often-profound symptoms, physical examination is persistently normal, as is laboratory testing. *In fact, if there are significant abnormalities on physical examination or testing, those abnormalities are not consistent with ME/CFS and should be further evaluated.* Symptoms are exacerbated by physical activity. The pre-ME/CFS medical history of the patient is not one of multiple medical problems. Affected patients are typically high-functioning persons who are "struck down" with this disease. Features to emphasize in addition to the case definition noted in Box 1 are included in Box 2.

In a patient with a typical history and examination, laboratory testing should be limited (Box 3). Testing for diseases with a low pretest likelihood runs the serious risk of false positive results. This can result in further testing, diagnostic confusion, and unnecessary treatments. Specifically, the signs and symptoms of ME/CFS are not those of systemic lupus, Lyme disease, cytomegalovirus, bartonellosis, ehrlichiosis, or babesiosis, among others. Serologic testing for these diagnoses is not helpful and can be harmful if the presence of antibodies results in the initiation of unwarranted medications. The presence of antibodies does not mean active disease. The analogy that patients can relate to is to remind them that they likely have antibodies to chickenpox but that they clearly do not have active chickenpox. For similar reasons, neuroimaging without objective clinical findings is not indicated. Although abnormalities can be found, they are nonspecific and of no clinical utility. Tilt-table testing is abnormal in many patients with ME/CFS; however, testing is expensive and uncomfortable, and abnormal results do not alter management. Of course, if history, physical examination, and initial laboratory testing do reveal abnormalities, as noted earlier, further laboratory evaluation should be undertaken to elucidate the cause of the aberration(s).

Treatment

There is no established cure for ME/CFS, but patients should be counseled that a number of things can be done to manage this often-disabling illness (Box 4). These can be divided into things the clinician should do and things the patient should do.

Things the Clinician Should Do

To successfully manage ME/CFS, a clinician must believe that the patient is truly symptomatic. Patients with ME/CFS are not malingering. Because they often appear well and have consistently normal objective testing, they often become very defensive about their limitations. They are sensitive to the validity of their symptoms. Not only are they suffering but they are also blamed for it. Many patients with ME/CFS are partially or totally disabled. Their outward healthy appearance belies the internal sense of ill health. It is common for relatives and colleagues to believe they are malingering. A vicious cycle of frustration, anger, and depression commonly ensues.

As part of establishing the validity of the diagnosis, a clinician should review the history of ME/CFS, emphasizing that this is not a new disease but was originally described centuries ago.

For successful management, the clinician should give the patient enough time, specifically inquire about other diagnoses the patient is concerned about, and explain why they are not correct. The clinician should see the patient at regular intervals.

The clinician should also ensure that the patient has reasonable expectations. Most patients with ME/CFS have not had previous chronic illnesses or significant prolonged limitations. It is often necessary to review the information about ME/CFS with the patient's family and to emphasize that this disabling illness is not volitional.

Although it is generally wise to avoid a discussion about whether the origin of ME/CFS is psychiatric or organic, depression is an expected consequence of any chronic illness. Depression has specific treatments, and it should be aggressively diagnosed

---

| BOX 2 | Frequent Features of Chronic Fatigue Syndrome |

- Sudden onset of fatigue after a relatively common illness or other stressor
- Previously active and healthy person
- Symptoms very sensitive to exacerbation by physical activity
- Normal physical examination and laboratory testing
- Altered sleep
- "Foggy" thought processes
- Lack of progression to organ failure or any significant objective organ abnormality
- Joint and muscle aching without physical evidence of inflammation
- Feverish feeling (sustained elevated temperatures [>37.4°C] should prompt a search for an alternative diagnosis because the patient with chronic fatigue syndrome is not truly febrile)
- Diffuse aching that is not well localized to joints or muscles but without erythema, effusion, or limitation of motion
- Muscles that are easily fatigued (however, strength is normal, as are biopsies and electromyograms)
- Occasional mild cervical and/or axillary lymphadenitis (painful lymph nodes [lymphadenia] are a common complaint, but this is not a true lymphadenopathy)

| BOX 3 | Diagnostic Testing |

Tests to Perform
- Complete blood count
- Comprehensive chemistry screen
- Thyroid-stimulating hormone
- Perhaps: Cosyntropin (Cortrosyn) stimulation test, sleep study
- Additional testing *only* with specific clinical indications

Do Not Routinely Perform
- ANA testing
- Serology for cytomegalovirus, Epstein-Barr virus, *Bartonella, Babesia, Ehrlichia,* and *Anaplasma*
- MRI, SPECT, or PET scans
- Tilt-table testing

ANA, Antinuclear antibody; *MRI,* magnetic resonance imaging; *PET,* positron emission tomography; *SPECT,* single-photon emission computed tomography.

| BOX 4 | Therapy for Chronic Fatigue Syndrome |

- Educate the patient and his or her support system about the diagnosis of chronic fatigue syndrome. Emphasize the validity of the diagnosis and of the patient's symptoms. Make sure there is an understanding about expectations.
- Aggressively manage specific symptoms of sleep disturbance, pain, and depression.
- Consider cognitive behavioral therapy.
- Emphasize the need for gradual, graded exercise. Give the patient a specific "prescription" for this.
- Avoid the temptation to prescribe antimicrobials, corticosteroids, or other medications with no proven benefit and the potential to do harm.
- Discuss the pros and cons of using unstudied, expensive, or potentially dangerous "alternative therapies."

and treated. The patient should be told that successful management of depression will help him or her cope with ME/CFS.

If a sleep disturbance exists, it also should be aggressively managed, if necessary, by a sleep specialist. Sleep deprivation makes other symptoms more difficult to deal with.

Chronic pain is very enervating. If pain is prominent, that also should be aggressively managed, often by a pain specialist.

It is important for the clinician to be cautious about ascribing all of a patient's symptoms to ME/CFS. Such patients are, of course, not protected from getting additional, unrelated illnesses. Each symptom should be considered on its own before defaulting it to ME/CFS.

Complementary therapies must be discussed, or the patient might get the impression that the clinician is not comfortable in considering them; this can partially undermine the clinician-patient relationship. Although all are of unproved benefit and often undetermined risk, "complementary" therapies that are not dangerous (e.g., acupuncture) or expensive are reasonable to consider.

Things the Patient Should Do
Of the 350 studies that have looked at treatment options for ME/CFS, only cognitive behavioral therapy and graded exercise therapy have been shown to be of possible benefit. In cognitive behavioral therapy, the patient undergoes a series of 1-hour sessions designed to alter beliefs and behaviors that might delay recovery. Although exercise can exacerbate symptoms, deconditioning will also do so. Limiting activity can worsen weakness and depression. The risk of exacerbating symptoms can be reduced by cautiously setting less-ambitious activity/exercise goals. Because many patients with ME/CFS were particularly active before the onset of their illness and are impatient to get their former lives back, they often need strict guidelines to try to prevent overdoing exercise while at the same time getting a clear prescription to exercise. The exercise prescription should be individualized based on the degree of impairment, but it is wise to initially set goals on the low side to avoid exacerbating symptoms. It is important to acknowledge that both cognitive behavioral therapy and graded exercise are controversial, with several interest groups opposed to these modalities. As for cognitive behavioral therapy, it is safe and there is nothing to lose. As for exercise, the emphasis should be on very gradual to minimize the risk for exacerbation.

As part of the management of ME/CFS, patients, their families, and, when appropriate, their employers must reframe their expectations. Patients with ME/CFS have a chronic, disabling illness. Families and others must understand that patients cannot do all that they were able to do before the onset of ME/CFS and that patients cannot "will" the disease away any more than they could will away a more visible disability.

Things That Should Not Be Done
There are many suggested remedies for ME/CFS. Most are either unstudied or disproved. In particular, treatments that are expensive or potentially harmful should be avoided. There is no role for antimicrobial therapy. There is no role for antiviral therapy, including treatment for retroviruses. There is no role for intravenous immunoglobulin, corticosteroids, special diets, or vitamin treatments.

Prognosis
The likelihood of complete recovery from ME/CFS is only fair. The disease tends to wax and wane over time, but in only a minority of patients does it completely resolve. If sustained improvement occurs, it is generally over several years. Several features have been associated with a poorer prognosis, including age older than 38 years, more than eight symptoms, duration longer than 1.5 years, less than 16 years of formal education, a history of a dysthymic disorder, and a sustained belief that the disease results from a physical cause.

Monitoring
Despite the lack of very effective treatment, many patients benefit from regular monitoring of their condition. Knowing they have scheduled visits minimizes the number of crises and emergency visits and allows the patient to reconnect with a validating physician. Follow-up on a quarterly basis is a reasonable interval.

References
Bouquet J, Gardy JL, Brown S, et al: RNA-seq analysis of gene expression, viral pathogen, and B-cell/T-cell receptor signatures in complex chronic disease, *Clin Infect Dis* 64:476, 2017.

Clark MR, Katon W, Russo J, et al: Chronic fatigue: risk factors for symptom persistence in a 212-year follow-up study, *Am J Med* 98:187–195, 1995.

Fulcher KY: White PD: Randomised controlled trial of graded exercise in patients with the chronic fatigue syndrome, *BMJ* 314:1647–1652, 1997.

Goertzel BN, Pennachin C, de Souza Coelho L, et al: Combinations of single nucleotide polymorphisms in neuroendocrine effector and receptor genes predict chronic fatigue syndrome, *Pharmacogenomics* 7:475–483, 2006.

Goldenberg DL, Simms RW, Geiger A, et al: High frequency of fibromyalgia in patients with chronic fatigue seen in a primary care practice, *Arthritis Rheum* 33:381–387, 1990.

Green CR, Cowan P, Elk R, et al: National Institutes of Health pathways to prevention workshop: advancing the research on myalgic encephalomyelitis/chronic fatigue syndrome, *Ann Intern Med* 162:860, 2015.

Haney E, Smith ME, McDonagh M, et al: Diagnostic methods for myalgic encephalomyelitis/chronic fatigue syndrome: a systematic review for a National Institutes of Health Pathways to Prevention Workshop, *Ann Intern Med* 162:834, 2015.

IOM (Institute of Medicine): *Beyond Myalgic encephalomyelitis/chronic fatigue syndrome: redefining an illness*, Washington, DC, 2015, The National Academies Press. https://www.ncbi.nlm.nih.gov/25695122.

Lightfoot Jr RW, Luft BJ, Rahn DW, et al: Empiric parenteral antibiotic treatment of patients with fibromyalgia and fatigue and a positive serologic result for Lyme disease. A cost-effectiveness analysis, *Ann Intern Med* 119:503–509, 1993.

Schwartz RB, Garada BM, Komaroff AL, et al: Detection of intracranial abnormalities in patients with chronic fatigue syndrome: comparison of MR imaging and SPECT, *Am J Roentgenol* 162:935–941, 1994.

Wessely S, Chalder T, Hirsch S, et al: The prevalence and morbidity of chronic fatigue and chronic fatigue syndrome: a prospective primary care study, *Am J Public Health* 87:1449–1455, 1997.

White PD, Goldsmith KA, Johnson AL, et al: Comparison of adaptive pacing therapy, cognitive behaviour therapy, graded exercise therapy, and specialist medical care for chronic fatigue syndrome (PACE): a randomised trial, *Lancet* 377:823–836, 2011.

NECROTIZING SKIN AND SOFT-TISSUE INFECTIONS

Method of
Kalyanakrishnan Ramakrishnan, MD

CURRENT DIAGNOSIS

- Physical examination of the affected area may detect:
  - Exquisite pain and tenderness out of proportion to local signs of infection.
  - Cutaneous anesthesia, firm woody subcutaneous tissue, edema, and tenderness extending outside involved skin margins, hemorrhage or bullae of the overlying skin, and soft tissue crepitus.
  - Laboratory Risk Indicator for Necrotizing Fasciitis (LRINEC) score is useful in diagnosing necrotizing fasciitis. Imaging (computed tomography [CT] or magnetic resonance imaging [MRI] in adults; ultrasonography [US] in children) is usually confirmatory. Imaging should not delay surgery if indicated based on suspicion.

CURRENT TREATMENT

- Empiric high-dose intravenous polymicrobial antibiotics and surgical debridement remain the cornerstones of initial management of necrotizing skin and soft-tissue infections. Organism-specific antibiotics are continued until resolution of infection and debridement complete (usually 7–14 days).

Epidemiology

Necrotizing skin and soft tissue infections are rare with an estimated annual incidence of 1000 cases in the United States. These infections may be polymicrobial or monomicrobial. Polymicrobial infections are more common (70%–80%) and generally caused by synergistic activity of aerobes and anaerobes originating from the bowel or genitourinary tracts. They are more prevalent among older and immunocompromised patients, individuals with significant comorbidities, and those with underlying abdominal pathology. These infections typically involve the trunk and perineal regions, and follow penetrating abdominal injuries or surgery, genital or perianal sepsis, or decubitus ulcers. They have a more indolent course and thus are easier to diagnose. Monomicrobial infections (20%–30%) frequently follow minor trauma and are usually caused by group A streptococcus (GAS), occasionally by methicillin-resistant *Staphylococcus aureus* (MRSA), or by clostridia. They are more aggressive, involve the extremities and occur more often in younger healthy individuals. Type 3 infections follow exposure to contaminated fresh or warm seawater or ingestion of raw seafood; organisms responsible include *Aeromonas hydrophila*, *Vibrio vulnificus*, *Mycobacterium marinum*, *Pasteurella multocida*, *Haemophilus* and *Klebsiella* species. Type 4 (fungal) infections generally follow burns or major trauma. Both types 3 and 4 infections are rare, progress rapidly, and have a high mortality rate, especially in immune-suppressed patients.

Risk Factors

Cardiopulmonary disease, debility, diabetes mellitus, hepatorenal disease, immunocompromised states, obesity, arteriovenous/lymphatic insufficiency, and senescence all increase risk of skin and soft tissue infections by reducing tissue vascularity and oxygenation, increasing fluid stasis and risk of trauma, and decreasing ability to counter infections. Diabetes mellitus and hepatic cirrhosis favor polymicrobial infections due to staphylococcus and streptococcus species, anaerobes, and gram-negative bacilli. Neutropenia, intravenous drug use, and hot tub exposure promote pseudomonas infection. Human and animal bites cause infections with oral flora, staphylococci, *Pasteurella multocida*, and anaerobes. Poor sanitation and soil contamination propagate clostridial infections. Postoperative infections typically follow wound contamination with microorganisms from the patient during surgery.

Pathophysiology

Necrotizing skin and soft tissue infections advance rapidly, breaking down and traversing anatomic barriers, initiating extensive destruction of the subcutaneous tissue, fascia, and muscle and damaging the neurovascular bundle, thrombosing the subcutaneous vessels, and causing overlying skin necrosis. Most infections follow a rift in the protective cutaneous barrier due to trauma or increased tissue tension. Necrotizing fasciitis may also result from blunt injuries (bruise, muscle strain) and, occasionally vascular or lymphatic spread from a distant focus of infection. Various toxins expressed by the organisms (GAS and clostridia) display local and systemic effects (platelet aggregation and thrombosis, decreasing phagocytosis, neutrophil function and vascular tone, myocardial inhibition) triggering the systemic inflammatory response syndrome (SIRS) and multiple organ failure.

Prevention

Preserving cutaneous integrity prevents infection. Abrasions and lacerations should be washed with antibacterial solutions, foreign bodies should be removed, and dead/devitalized tissue excised to minimize infection risk. Preoperative skin cleansing with chlorhexidine/alcohol (Hibiclens) or povidone iodine diminishes rates of superficial and deep incisional infections. Intranasal 2% mupirocin ointment (Bactroban) twice daily with chlorhexidine total body wash daily for 5 days in nasal carriers of MRSA reduces hospital-acquired deep surgical–site infections, as does administering antibiotics (aminopenicillins, a second- or third-generation cephalosporin) 60 minutes before incision, sterile surgical technique, minimal tissue handling, and minimally invasive surgery.

Clinical Manifestations

Features of inflammation (redness, warmth, swelling, pain) and loss of function characterize necrotizing skin and soft tissue infections. Altered mental status, anorexia, diaphoresis, fatigue, fever, hypotension, nausea, and tachycardia suggest systemic spread of infection. The extremities, trunk, or anogenital regions are usually involved. Induration denotes cutaneous involvement. Patients with necrotizing fasciitis have severe pain disproportionate to the physical findings and rapid progression of infection. Examination reveals cutaneous anesthesia, firm and woody subcutaneous tissue, edema and tenderness extending beyond involved skin, hemorrhage or bullae of the overlying skin, and crepitus (indicates soft tissue gas; seen especially with gas-forming organisms such as clostridia). Tense edema and bullae have high specificity and positive predictive value for necrotizing fasciitis. Fournier gangrene is a form of polymicrobial necrotizing soft-tissue infection involving the loose groin and genital skin, where subcutaneous vessel thrombosis causes extensive tissue loss.

Diagnosis

Diagnosis is based on a strong clinical suspicion followed by confirmatory laboratory and imaging studies (if time permits), and surgery. Leukocytosis with a marked left shift, elevated C-reactive protein, elevated serum creatinine and creatine phosphokinase (denotes muscle injury), and low serum bicarbonate (suggests acidosis) signify severe infection. The LRINEC score (https://www.mdcalc.com/lrinec-score-necrotizing-soft-tissue-infection) uses six different laboratory parameters (hemoglobin, white blood cell count, C-reactive protein, glucose, creatinine, sodium) to predict risk of necrotizing fasciitis (score ≥ 6 suggestive, ≥ 8 strongly predictive). White blood cell count (< 15,000 mm^3) and serum sodium (> 135 mmol/L) levels alone are useful in ruling out necrotizing fasciitis (99% negative predictive value). Gram stains and cultures of aspirates or tissue biopsies, and blood cultures are valuable for detecting the infecting organisms and systemic spread; contamination may yield false-positive results. Biopsy or debridement typically demonstrates swollen gray soft tissue with undermining of the overlying skin, a brownish and odorous exudate and non-contractile muscle. Imaging (plain x-rays, ultrasonography [US], computed tomography [CT], magnetic resonance imaging [MRI]) may show edema or thickening, fluid collections or free air in the soft tissues. US, CT and MRI are highly sensitive (MRI highest) in detecting deep soft tissue involvement characteristic of necrotizing fasciitis; specificity is lower. US is sufficient in children, whose tissues are thin enough to allow adequate evaluation on imaging. Imaging should not delay debridement, if considered necessary.

Therapy

Patients with necrotizing skin and soft-tissue infections typically require in-hospital management, because many have underlying unstable comorbid illnesses, systemic sepsis, severe dehydration and acidosis, muscle breakdown, and organ dysfunction. Initial resuscitation may require airway and oxygen support, large-volume rehydration, and invasive monitoring. High-dose intravenous (IV) broad-spectrum antibiotics effective against the usually infecting polymicrobial spectrum of pathogens are commenced, followed by early and aggressive debridement of all necrotic tissue. IV antibiotics are maintained until the patient is afebrile for 48 to 72 hours and tolerates oral intake, debridement is completed and culture results are available. For polymicrobial necrotizing fasciitis acceptable antimicrobial choices include vancomycin plus piperacillin/tazobactam (Zosyn), a carbapenem (meropenem [Merrem], ertapenem [Invanz] or imipenem-cilastatin [Primaxin]), or cefotaxime (Claforan) with metronidazole (Flagyl) or clindamycin (Cleocin). Streptococcal and clostridial infections are treated with penicillin G and clindamycin. Antibiotic options in methicillin-susceptible *S. aureus* infections include nafcillin oxacillin or cefazolin. Options for methicillin-resistant *S. aureus* (MRSA) infections and in penicillin-allergic patients include vancomycin, daptomycin (Cubicin), or linezolid (Zyvox). Antibiotic doses are modified in children. Recommended duration is 7 to 14 days; longer as needed. Doxycycline combined with ciprofloxacin (Cipro) treats *Vibrio vulnificus* infection. Ceftriaxone (Rocephin) or cefotaxime combined with doxycycline is useful in aeromonos infections. Doxycycline is contraindicated in children (< 8 years), as is ciprofloxacin (< 17 years), unless the infection is considered life-threatening. Fungal infections respond well to fluconazole (Diflucan), voriconazole (Vfend) or amphotericin B; the antifungals usually continued for 2 weeks after resolution of symptoms. Debridement/drainage is repeated until all diseased tissue or collections are eliminated and healing begins. Wound vacuum dressings help remove drainage and encourage formation of healing granulation tissue. The tissue defect heals by secondary intention or may require skin grafting or flap closure. Hyperbaric oxygen (3–4 daily treatments at 2–3 atmosphere pressure for 30–90 minutes each) is useful, especially in clostridium-related synergistic infections. Adding intravenous immunoglobulin[1] 0.5–2 g/kg daily for 3 days has shown some success, and is an option in critically ill hemodynamically unstable patients not responding to conventional measures, especially in those with streptococcal toxic shock syndrome. Fournier gangrene is managed along the same principles as above.

Monitoring

Patients in shock or with acute respiratory distress syndrome, SIRS, or multi-organ failure are best managed in an intensive care unit and often require invasive monitoring, cardiorespiratory and renal support, and occasionally, endotracheal intubation.

Complications

Significant disfigurement, limb loss, respiratory and renal failure, and mortality (14%–50%) may eventuate despite timely and appropriate treatment; the mortality influenced by age, extent of infection, degree of biochemical/acid-base imbalance, presence of comorbidities, and treatment delay.

---

[1]Not FDA approved for this indication.

References

Kaafarani HMA, King DR: Necrotizing skin and soft tissue infections, *Surg Clin North Am* 94:155–163, 2014.

Hakkarainen TW, Kopari NM, Pham TN, Evans HL: Necrotizing soft tissue infections: review and current concepts in treatment, systems of care and outcomes, *Curr Probl Surg* 51:344–362, 2014.

Morgan MS: Diagnosis and management of necrotizing fasciitis: a multiparametric approach, *J Hosp Infect* 75:249–257, 2010.

Stevens DL, Bisno AL, Chambers HF, et al: Practice guidelines for the diagnosis and management of skin and soft tissue infections: 2014 update by the Infectious Diseases Society of America, *Clin Infect Dis* 59:e10–e52, 2014.

Ramakrishnan K, Salinas RC, Agudelo Higuita NI: Skin and soft tissue infections, *Am Fam Physician* 92:474–483, 2015.

OSTEOMYELITIS

Method of
Wissam El Atrouni, MD, MSc; John Sojka, MD; Mitchell Birt, MD; and Kim Templeton, MD

CURRENT DIAGNOSIS

- Osteomyelitis in adults typically occurs as a result of spread from adjacent soft tissues or direct inoculation of bone, such as after trauma or surgery. Hematogenous bacterial seeding leading to osteomyelitis is more common in children than in adults. When it occurs in adults, it is almost exclusively in the spine.
- Open fractures can lead to osteomyelitis due to contamination of bone at the time of injury; even small soft tissue wounds can indicate the presence of an open fracture. Due to the risk of infection, open fractures should be treated emergently.
- Infections around implanted hardware, especially joint arthroplasties or hardware in the spine, require urgent referral. These infections can occur at the time of hardware placement or later due to hematogenous seeding from distant infections. Patients with late arthroplasty infections usually demonstrate new pain in the area of a previously well-functioning joint.
- Diabetes mellitus is one of the more common chronic health conditions that increases the risk of developing osteomyelitis. Osteomyelitis in this population of patients usually occurs in the foot as a result of progressively deepening soft tissue ulcers and secondary infection. These infections are frequently polymicrobial.
- Initial evaluation of patient suspected of having osteomyelitis includes obtaining plain films. However, plain film findings are usually not specific for infection. Additional radiographic modalities, such as magnetic resonance imaging (MRI) scan and/or a variety of nuclear medicine studies, can provide additional information regarding diagnosis and extent of involvement.

CURRENT THERAPY

- In the absence of sepsis, antibiotics for patients with suspected osteomyelitis are not started until adequate cultures can be obtained, through aspiration or biopsy of the bone or during surgical debridement of the affected area.
- Antimicrobial therapy for osteomyelitis in adults typically lasts 4–6 weeks, while in children it may only be needed for 2–3 weeks, depending on the clinical picture.
- Surgical intervention for osteomyelitis of long bones is indicated for patients with chronic infections, infections adjacent to joint replacements, or to address bone abscesses. Surgery in these instances requires extensive debridement of infected and necrotic bone to remove all microabscesses and then irrigation to dilute any remaining bacterial load.
- Treatment of patients with diabetes-related foot infections and underlying osteomyelitis may require revascularization of the affected limb to decrease the need for amputation.

Introduction

Normal bone is typically highly resistant to infection. Infections in bone can arise when the host immune system is compromised or there is injury to the bone. Osteomyelitis occurs either due to hematogenous spread, extension from infections in adjacent soft tissues or joints, or as a result of direct inoculation of the bone due to trauma or surgery. Osteomyelitis can lead to devastating outcomes, including amputation or sepsis, if not addressed early, especially in patients with other health conditions.

Various classification systems have been developed to describe osteomyelitis. The Lew and Waldvogel classification described the etiology of the infection (in order of decreasing frequency: contiguous focus, vascular insufficiency, or hematogenous); however, this classification system does not guide or indicate the results from treatment. The Cierny-Mader system is based on the location (intramedullary) and extent (localized vs. diffuse) of the infection, as well as the degree of compromise of the patient. Unlike the Lew and Waldvogel classification, the Cierny-Mader (C-M) staging systems correlates with outcomes and can help guide treatment. Mandell et al. recommend considering C-M type 1 as early (intramedullary) hematogenous osteomyelitis, type 2 as early contiguous spread, and types 3 (localized) and 4 (diffuse) as more advanced disease.

Osteomyelitis can be described as acute, usually being present for 2 weeks or less, subacute, and chronic. Chronic osteomyelitis can be more challenging to eradicate due to the development of avascular areas of bone (sequestra) and surrounding bone sclerosis (involucra) that help to wall off the sequestra, making it difficult to adequately address these areas with systemic antibiotics.

Epidemiology

The incidence of osteomyelitis appears to be increasing, especially among adults. This may reflect better evaluation and diagnostic measures or the increased prevalence of comorbidities, such as diabetes mellitus, or the aging of the population, as the risk increases with age. The reported age- and sex-adjusted annual incidence has been reported to be approximately 24 cases per 100,000 person-years and is higher among men than women.

No similar increased prevalence of osteomyelitis has been identified among children or young adults. However, other demographic differences have been noted. African American children have the highest rates of hospitalization related to osteomyelitis, while the lowest rates are among children of Asian or Hispanic descent. In addition, children who live in households with low median incomes or whose care is covered by private funds or Medicaid are more likely than children from other socioeconomic backgrounds to be hospitalized with acute osteomyelitis.

Pathogenesis

Osteomyelitis can occur via hematogenous seeding, direct extension from an adjacent area of infection, or due to inoculation of the bone as a result of trauma or surgery (Figure 1). *Staphylococcus aureus*, in particular, has receptors for fibronectin, laminin, collagen, and sialoglycoproteins that are present in the bone matrix, leading to seeding of the bone and consequent inflammatory reaction. Hematogenous osteomyelitis is more common among children than among adults. In adults, hematogenous osteomyelitis is almost exclusively seen in the spine, resulting from seeding of the disc space from a distant infected site (Figure 2). This can then involve the adjacent vertebral bodies and, with time, result in epidural extension. When hematogenous osteomyelitis occurs in the long bones of children and adolescents, it is almost always in the metaphysis. It is thought that this reflects the

Figure 1 A diagram showing three categories of osteomyelitis. **A** and **B,** Primary hematogenous (bloodborne) spread of bacteria mainly afflicts the vertebral bodies at all ages or the metaphysis of skeletally immature patients. **C** and **D,** Contiguous bone infection is most commonly seen with direct contamination of bacteria in open fractures or joint replacement surgery with prosthetic implants. **E,** Vascular or neurologic disease associated osteomyelitis most commonly affects the lower extremity. (From Birt MC, Anderson DW, Toby WB, et al: Osteomyelitis: recent advances in pathophysiology and therapeutic strategies, *J Orthop* 14:45–52, 2017.)

Figure 2 **A,** Sagittal computed tomography scan demonstrating C6-8 spondylodiskitis. Note the cortical irregularity of the vertebral end plates. There is disc space narrowing and loss of the normal cervical spine curvature. Severe cortical destruction is present due to bacterial infection of the bone and intervertebral disc. **B,** Sagittal T2 magnetic resonance imaging reveals diffuse T2 signal throughout the vertebral body and disc. Evident is loss of the normal cortical line of the endplates compared to adjacent levels and hyperintensity that extends posteriorly to the soft tissues.

circulation in that area, with slowing of bone flow in the terminal capillaries along the area of the physis. In young children, there is connection between the metaphyseal and epiphyseal vessels that can allow infection of the epiphysis and eventually the adjacent joint. This is much less likely to occur in adults.

Bone infections due to trauma are typically related to presence of open fractures. Open fractures usually reflect significant levels of trauma to the bone and secondary soft tissue involvement. Infections can arise in these situations due to direct contamination of the soft tissues and bone with materials from the environment, including clothing, grass, and dirt, with contained bacteria. Open fractures are graded with the system described by Gustilo and Anderson and range from small puncture wounds over the fracture site to soft tissue stripping from the bone to open fractures with associated vascular injury. This classification system can help in determining the prognosis: patients with higher grade injuries typically have a greater incidence of subsequent infection—up to 50% among patients with concomitant vascular injury. While a small puncture wound over a fracture may seem inconsequential, these wounds usually indicate that bone was exposed at some point and was at risk for bacterial contamination. Open fractures are surgical emergencies and need immediate referral.

Bone infections can develop at sites of prior surgery, especially past surgical sites that include implantation of hardware. Many of these infections are thought to occur during the time of hardware placement. While such infections can occur at the site of any hardware, it is most common among patients who have undergone joint arthroplasty and is one of the most devastating complications of these procedures. The rate of infection after primary joint arthroplasty ranges from 0.3% to 2.4% for total hip arthroplasties (THAs) and 1.0% to 3.0% for total knee arthroplasties. Infection rates are higher among patients who undergo revision surgeries. Patients with infected arthroplasties may present in the first few weeks after surgery or may note onset of new pain in a previously well-functioning joint. The bacteria in these cases not only exist on the surface of the implant but also extend into adjacent bone and soft tissues (Figure 3). Patients with prior surgery of the spine, with or without the placement of hardware, are also at risk of developing late infections in the range of 0.2% to 9%. Suspected infections in areas of prior surgery, especially if implants are in place, require urgent referral.

Osteomyelitis is more likely to occur in patients with serious and/or chronic health conditions, including obesity, malignancy, immune compromise, substance abuse, and malnutrition. One of the most common of conditions increasing the risk for development of osteomyelitis is diabetes mellitus. An estimated 25% of diabetic patients will develop a foot ulcer at some point in their lifetime, with increased morbidity and mortality, compared to patients with diabetes without foot ulcers. Of these foot ulcers, 20% to almost 60% will harbor underlying osteomyelitis (Figure 4). Infected foot ulcers are the most common risk factor for lower extremity amputations in this population. Diabetic foot ulcers usually start as superficial breaks in the skin or ulcers, which, if they become chronic, are at risk of infection. Infections of foot ulcer in the setting of diabetes are greater among patients with peripheral neuropathy or peripheral vascular disease; these comorbidities can also lead to masking of the signs and symptoms of inflammation, making a diagnosis of infection more challenging. Superficial infections in diabetic foot ulcers can eventually affect deeper tissues, in some patients progressing to osteomyelitis. Depth of the ulcer, especially in the presence of elevated inflammatory markers, can aid in the diagnosis of osteomyelitis. Involvement of bone can be confirmed with plain films; other imaging modalities, such as magnetic resonance imaging (MRI), white blood cell (WBC) scintigraphy, and 18F-fluorodeoxyglucose (18F) positron emission tomography (FDG-PET)/computed tomography (CT) may be useful in confirming the diagnosis but have variable reported sensitivities and specificities. Treatment of these ulcers and associated infections is multidisciplinary: in addition to administration of antibiotics for culture-confirmed infections and potential surgical debridement of involved tissue, treatment includes local wound care (although evidence of type of wound care is mixed), evaluating and addressing, if needed or possible, peripheral vascular disease; off-loading of the involved portion of the extremity; and appropriate glycemic control.

Etiology

In children, most cases of acute hematogenous osteomyelitis are caused by a single organism, most commonly *S. aureus*. These cases typically involve the vascular metaphysis of long bones. Coagulase-negative staphylococci can also be an etiology in infants in intensive care with vascular catheters. Other

Figure 3 A, Anteroposterior radiograph of an infected total knee arthroplasty. The radiograph shows resorption of the bone, especially the femur, adjacent to the implant. B, Lateral radiograph of the knee demonstrating lucencies extending posterior along the femur and interface between the femur and implant.

Figure 4 Osteomyelitis associated with diabetes/vascular insufficiency. A, Anteroposterior radiograph revealing diffuse osteopenia within the fifth toe and subtle cortical disruption along lateral aspect of the proximal phalanx. Note previous amputation of third toe. Patients with loss of protective sensation and poor vascular supply have recurrent or multiple episodes of wound infections that can extend to involve adjacent bone. B and C, Coronal and axial short tau inversion recovery (STIR) magnetic resonance images. Hyperintense STIR signal along the proximal phalanx and adjacent soft tissues of the fifth toe, consistent with infection and inflammation.

gram-positive cocci include Streptococci: *Streptococcus pneumoniae* in incompletely immunized children, or young children with underlying conditions and *Streptococcus pyogenes* (group A), especially following primary varicella-zoster and *Streptococcus agalactiae* (group B) in neonates. Culture-negative cases occur frequently, and these are usually presumed to be due to *S. aureus* and treated as such. In children 6 to 36 months old, *Kingella kingae*, a gram-negative component of the oral flora, is a major pathogen that causes non-long bone osteomyelitis. *Haemophilus influenzae* type b (Hib) is a rare cause of hematogenous osteomyelitis in young children after the wide implementation of Hib vaccination. Enteric gram-negative bacilli can cause osteomyelitis in infants and children with sickle cell disease. Those with hemoglobinopathies and HIV infection are also at risk for Salmonella osteomyelitis.

In adults, hematogenous osteomyelitis primarily presents as vertebral osteomyelitis and is caused by *S. aureus* in more than half of cases in case series in developed countries. The proportion of the cases of hematogenous osteomyelitis due to methicillin-resistant *S. aureus* (MRSA) depends on local epidemiology. Other etiologic organisms include aerobic gram-negative bacilli after genitourinary instrumentation, pyogenic streptococci including group B and C/G in diabetics, viridans and anginosus-group streptococci, enterococci, *Pseudomonas aeruginosa*, coagulase-negative staphylococci in patients with indwelling venous catheters, and injection drug users. In endemic areas, *Brucella* species and *Mycobacterium tuberculosis* should be considered. Disseminated *Mycobacterium avium complex* (MAC) can involve the spine in patients with AIDS. Fungal vertebral osteomyelitis is rare but can occur in people at risk such as individuals who live in endemic areas for dimorphic fungi like *Histoplasma, Blastomyces,* and *Coccidioides*; intravenous drug users who can get *Candida* osteomyelitis; and immunocompromised hosts who can develop infections with Aspergillus.

Among adults with trauma or open fractures, diabetic and vascular insufficiency foot infections are more likely to develop

TABLE 1	Microbiology of Osteomyelitis

Common >50%	Rare <5%
• *Staphylococcus aureus* (MSSA, CA-MRSA) • Coagulase-negative staphylococci	• *Salmonella* • *Mycobacterium tuberculosis* • *Brucella* • *Coxiella* • Dimorphic fungi • *Mycobacterium avium* complex • Atypical mycobacteria • *Aspergillus* • *Mycoplasma* • *Tropheryma* • *Actinomyces* • *Bartonella* • *Pasteurella* • *Eikenella*
Occasional 25%–50%	
• *Streptococci* • *Enterococci* • *Pseudomonas* • *Enterobacter* • *Proteus* • *Escherichia coli* • *Serratia* • Anaerobes (*Finegoldia*, *Clostridium*, *Bacteroides*)	

CA, Community-associated; MRSA, Methicillin-resistant *Staphylococcus aureus*; MSSA, Methicillin-susceptible *Staphylococcus aureus*.
Adapted from *Mandell, Douglas, and Bennett Principles and Practice of Infectious Diseases*, 9th edition, chapter 104, pages 1418–1429.

polymicrobial osteomyelitis with staphylococci, streptococci, enterococci, gram-negative bacilli, and anaerobes (Table 1). After animal or human bites, *Pasteurella multocida*, *Eikenella corrodens*, and oral anaerobic gram-positive cocci are usually identified.

Clinical Manifestations

Patients with osteomyelitis typically present with pain and tenderness in areas with or without prior injury. They may experience pain with activity but also note pain at rest and that awakens them at night. Symptoms may be acute and localized or gradual onset and nonspecific; the latter may be subtle, making clinical suspicion crucial. There may be noted warmth and erythema, especially in more superficial bones. Patients may also present with fever and other systemic signs of infection. Symptoms of pain at rest and constitutional signs may be interpreted as representing an underlying neoplasm, especially in children, in whom osteomyelitis and Ewing sarcoma often have nearly identical presentations. Patients whose bone infection has involved an adjacent native joint are reluctant to use that joint and have significant pain, even with limited attempts at range of motion. Patients with long bone infections, especially children, are reluctant to utilize that extremity, including bearing weight, if the infection involves a lower extremity. Patients with new onset pain in the setting of implanted hardware, especially joint arthroplasties, should be assumed to have an infection until proven otherwise. Patients with vertebral osteomyelitis usually present with unremitting back pain. The diagnosis can be difficult to make, because the symptoms may seem consistent with degenerative changes in the spine and initial plain radiographs prove nondiagnostic. However, continued infections in this area can lead to epidural extension, with neurologic changes that require rapid referral.

Diagnosis/Confirmation

The clinical diagnosis of osteomyelitis is confirmed by a combination of serum studies, radiographic findings, microbiology or culture results, and pathology, if the patient undergoes surgery. Plain radiographs are an inexpensive initial study; however, their sensitivity in diagnosing osteomyelitis is limited, as the findings of bone loss and periosteal reaction can be attributed to a number of aggressive bone conditions, including neoplasms. In addition, bone loss of approximately 30% to 40% is required before being noted on plain radiographs. MRI provides additional sensitivity and specificity in diagnosis, even in early osteomyelitis, especially if obtained with and without contrast. MRI findings include reduced T1- and heightened T2-weighted bone marrow signals, representing fatty marrow replaced by inflammation. Contrast enhancement patterns can also help to differentiate infection from neoplasia. CT is an alternative to MRI if the latter is not available or the patient is unable to tolerate the examination. CT findings can include gas along fascial plains, decreased density of infected bone, soft tissue masses, and abscesses, as well identifying the course of overlying sinus tracts. Nuclear medicine imaging modalities are more expensive than other imaging options. While in some reports nuclear medicine imaging modalities have been noted to be more sensitive in identifying osteomyelitis, they are less specific, with high false-positive rates. However, they can be useful in imaging areas in which hardware is present, because such metal can significantly limit the details seen on MRI or CT. Nuclear medicine imaging modalities include three-phase Tc99m MDP scan—ideal for bones not affected by underlying conditions, gallium 67 scan (usually performed as sequential bone then gallium scan for comparison), 111-indium radiolabeled WBC scans, or Tc99m sulfur colloid bone marrow scans performed in sequence with WBC scans. These additional imaging modalities are usually used in complicated cases or cases in which the diagnosis is unclear based on other, less expensive tests.

The identification of the infecting organism is crucial to optimal medical management. In cases of presumed osteomyelitis, antibiotics should be withheld until material for culture is obtained, usually via needle aspiration of the area. If the patient requires surgical debridement, tissue can be sent for culture and for pathologic evaluation. Pathology in these instances can help to rule out neoplasia and will demonstrate acute, chronic, or acute on chronic inflammatory cells. Swab cultures of draining sinuses demonstrate poor correlation with adjacent bone cultures, except for S. aureus. Material obtained for culture should be sent for both aerobic and anaerobic assessment.

Treatment

Medical Treatment

Vertebral osteomyelitis without associated neurologic deficit or nerve compression, and acute hematogenous osteomyelitis in children, are usually treated with systemic antimicrobials without the need for surgical debridement. Most other osteomyelitis syndromes in adults require a combination of medical and surgical treatments to eradicate infection and restore function. A cornerstone of medical therapy for osteomyelitis is identification of the causative organisms in culture. In the absence of associated active soft tissue infection or sepsis, antimicrobials are usually held until adequate cultures are obtained either by aspiration/biopsy or during surgical debridement of the affected bone. Vancomycin (Vancocin) and beta-lactams including cephalosporins have been used extensively for the treatment of osteomyelitis (Table 2). Although most experience is with intravenous antimicrobials, some data support the use of highly orally bioavailable antibiotics like trimethoprim-sulfamethoxazole (Bactrim)[1], rifampin[1], clindamycin, and quinolones. Duration of antimicrobial treatment is generally 4 to 6 weeks based on experimental models and limited prospective studies. Parenteral antimicrobials can be continued outside the hospital using peripherally inserted central catheters (PICCs). In children with hematogenous osteomyelitis, parenteral therapy can be changed to oral when the child is afebrile and able to tolerate oral medications, and duration of therapy as short as 2 to 3 weeks has been reported to be effective.

Fracture site infections following open fractures are treated with debridement, cultures, and organism-directed antimicrobial therapy. Considering that it is common to use or retain fracture fixation devices, long-term oral antimicrobial suppression following induction treatment for 6 weeks is used until fracture healing is documented on imaging. At that point, antimicrobial suppression can be stopped.

Vertebral osteomyelitis treatment might require drainage of associated paravertebral or psoas abscesses by radiology. Duration of antimicrobial therapy might be longer than 6 weeks in patients with undrained abscesses, MRSA infections, or end-stage renal disease. Follow-up at the end of treatment includes

[1]Not FDA approved for this indication.

TABLE 2 Medical Treatment of Osteomyelitis

ORGANISM	FIRST CHOICE	ALTERNATIVE
MSSA	Nafcillin, oxacillin or cefazolin	Vancomycin, some add rifampin to nafcillin/oxacillin
MRSA	Vancomycin or daptomycin	Linezolid or levofloxacin + rifampin
Penicillin susceptible Streptococci	Penicillin G, ceftriaxone, or cefazolin	Vancomycin
Enterococci and Streptococci with Penicillin MIC >0.5	Penicillin G, ampicillin with optional gentamicin	Vancomycin with addition of gentamicin
Enterobacteriaceae	Ceftriaxone or ertapenem	Ciprofloxacin or levofloxacin
Pseudomonas aeruginosa	Cefepime, meropenem, or imipenem	Ciprofloxacin or ceftazidime

MIC, Minimum inhibitory concentration; MRSA, Methicillin-resistant *Staphylococcus aureus*; MSSA, Methicillin-susceptible *Staphylococcus aureus*.
Adapted from *Mandell, Douglas, and Bennett Principles and Practice of Infectious Diseases*, 9th edition, chapter 104, page 1418–1429.

assessment of resolution or improvement in pain and in level of inflammation markers in the erythrocyte sedimentation rate C-reactive protein (ESR, CRP) test. A 25% or more reduction in these inflammation markers at the end of therapy is associated with treatment success. Repeat MRI is not routinely recommended and is reserved for patients with failure to improve or worsening symptoms. In 1 to 2 years after successful therapy, spontaneous fusion of the affected vertebral levels usually occurs.

Diabetic foot osteomyelitis management requires evaluation of the vascular supply to the affected area and revascularization is needed in patients with peripheral arterial disease to optimize surgical outcome and minimize need for amputation. Because most of these infections are polymicrobial, use of antimicrobials with anaerobic spectrum of activity is recommended (piperacillin-tazobactam [Zosyn][1], ampicillin-sulbactam [Unasyn][1], ertapenem [Invanz][1], cephalosporins with metronidazole [Flagyl], quinolones with metronidazole or clindamycin).

Surgical Treatment

Surgery is often performed in conjunction with antibiotic treatment in cases of osteomyelitis of long bones, especially in cases of chronic osteomyelitis or in the presence of bone abscesses, typically in cases of chronic osteomyelitis or in the presence of bone abscesses, especially in the presence of implanted hardware. Surgery for osteomyelitis of the spine is usually reserved for patients whose infection does not completely respond to antibiotic treatment or who develop neurologic deficits. Surgical treatment of osteomyelitis of long bones is primarily performed with wide excisional debridement and copious irrigation. The order in which the operations are performed is very important because a large bacterial load can be pushed further into surrounding bone and soft tissues by irrigating before debridement. The adage "the solution to pollution is dilution" accurately describes the intent of copious irrigation at a site of bone infection.

Bacteria identified within bone, either causing a biologic breakdown of the structure of the bone (infection) versus bacteria on or near bone (colonization), are two distinct clinical pictures. The structure of bone is similar to that of sponge; bacteria resulting in osteomyelitis can "hide" in the caverns and nooks of cancellous bone quite readily, leading to small local abscess communities in the bone, bone marrow, and surrounding soft tissues, making it difficult to eradicate them through the host inflammatory response or with systemic antibiotics. In addition, bacteria in these areas may not be exposed to antibiotic agents, WBCs, or irrigation solutions. Therefore, they can exist and multiply until the bone reacts and begins to break down at the site of the infection. Given this analogy, it is understandable that there is the need to irrigate a site of osteomyelitis thoroughly to dilute the bacterial load and then allow antibiotics the opportunity to work to eliminate the remaining pathogens from the infected bone.

To rid the bone of infection, surgeons typically debride bone that is obviously infected and/or necrotic, while healthy bone can and will be removed up to the margin of infected bone to improve the likelihood of healing in the absence of infection. This is critical to the success of the procedure but can lead to large defects. In addition, adjacent soft tissues should be sharply debrided back to healthy, bleeding tissue. As a result, WBCs can come into the area along with antibiotic agents delivered via the healthy, small blood vessels to complete the task of eliminating the bacteria. It is important that tissue removed during these procedures is sent for culture, as well as for pathologic examination.

Debridement involving infected bone with orthopedic implants adjacent to the site can be challenging. These implants and any surrounding necrotic tissue can be colonized by bacteria, often in the form of a surrounding glycocalyx or exopolysaccharide coating that envelops the bacteria. In some patients, this can necessitate the removal of rods, plates, screws, or the components of a joint replacement, as systemic antibiotics are unable to access bacteria housed in this biofilm. Removing the implant results in removal of the glycocalyx and reduces the bacterial load but frequently necessitates subsequent reconstructive surgeries.

Often, with obvious purulent infections, several surgical procedures are required to accomplish the task of bacterial elimination. The initial bacterial load can be so great that even after significant tissue (both bone and soft tissue) has been excised and irrigated, the surgeon cannot confidently close the wound for the completion of the case. Surgical decision making may include a second or third procedure to assess the site and determine the need for further tissue removal and irrigation versus wound closure. When multiple (staged) procedures are performed, wound coverage techniques can help to continue to minimize or eliminate bacteria during the patient's hospitalization.

A vacuum-assisted closure (VAC) device is one such coverage technique. These devices apply a vacuum or negative pressure environment to the wound with an evenly applied suction level to allow for continued bacterial debridement while keeping the wound covered during the time that the patient is out of the operating room. The VAC can be applied after the excisional debridement and irrigation procedure has been completed. VACs are typically used in anticipation of a return to the operating room for a second or third procedure.

A wound VAC device is applied to the bed of the wound utilizing three key elements: (1) a sponge substrate (for even application of the suction), (2) a plastic tape to seal the wound edges, and (3) a suctioning device or pump to apply the negative pressure to the wound. Once applied, these devices can continue to promote healthy tissue growth and create a hostile environment for bacteria, thereby limiting bacterial proliferation.

Conclusion

Patient outcomes after treatment of osteomyelitis have improved over the years with development of new imaging technologies to improve diagnostic accuracy, development of new antibiotics and antibiotic delivery methods, and expanded surgical techniques. Most importantly, treatments, both medical and surgical, are based on a better understanding of the pathogenesis of this

[1] Not FDA approved for this indication.

infection. However, given the continued increase in prevalence of this condition, we need additional research to better understand the contribution of various risk factors and comorbidities so that we can improve prevention efforts and continue to tailor multidisciplinary interventions.

References

Birt MC, Anderson DW, Toby EB, Wang J, Osteomyelitis: Recent advances in pathophysiology and therapeutic strategies, *J of Orthopaedics* 14:45–52, 2017.

Bouchoucha S, Gafsi K, Trifa M, et al: Intravenous antibiotic therapy for acute hematogenous osteomyelitis in children: a short versus long course, *Arch Pediatr* 20:464–469, 2013.

Chong BSW, Brereton CJ, Gordon A, Davis JS: Epidemiology, microbiological diagnosis, and clinical outcomes in pyogenic vertebral osteomyelitis: a 10-year retrospective cohort study, *Open Forum Infect Dis* 5(3), ofy037, 2018 Epub.

Cierny G, Mader JT, Penninck JJ: The Classic: A clinical staging system for adult osteomyelitis, *CORR* 414:7–24, 2003.

Crenshaw AH, ed: *Campbell's Operative Orthopedics*, 8th ed. edition

Dartnell J, Ramachadran M, Katchburian M: Haematogenous acute and subacute paediatric osteomyelitis: a systemic review of the literature, *J Bone Joint Surg Br* 94(5):584, 2012.

Euba G, Murillo O, Fernandez-Sabe N, et al: Long-term follow up trial of oral rifampin-cotrimoxazole combination versus intravenous cloxacillin in treatment of chronic staphylococcal osteomyelitis, *Antimicrob Agents Chemother* 53:2672–2676, 2009.

Gehrke Alijanipour P, Parvizi J: The management of an infected total knee arthroplasty, *Bone Joint J* 97-B(10 Suppl A):20–29, 2015.

Gustilo RB, Mendoza RM, Williams DN: Problems in management of type III (severe) open fractures: a new classification of type III open fractures, *J Trauma* 24:742–746, 1984.

Kim UJ, Bae JY, Kim S-E, et al: Comparison of pyogenic postoperative and native vertebral osteomyelitis, *Spine J* 19:880–887, 2019.

Kremers HM, Nwojo ME, Ransom JE, et al: Trends in the epidemiology of osteomyelitis: a population-based study, 1969 to 2009, *JBJS(A)* 97:837–845, 2015.

Lew DP, Waldvogel FA: Osteomyelitis. *Lancet* 364(9431):369–379, 2004.

Lew DP: Waldvogel FA: Current concepts: osteomyelitis, *NEJM* 336:999–1007, 1997.

Lindbloom BJ, James ER, McGarvey WC: Osteomyelitis of the foot and ankle: diagnosis, epidemiology, and treatment, *Foot Ankle Clin N Am* 19:569–588, 2014.

Lipsky BA, Senneville E, Abbas ZG, et al: Guidelines on the diagnosis and treatment of foot infection in persons with diabetes (IWGDF 2019 update), *Diabetes Metab Res Rev* 36(S1):e3280, 2020.

Mandell JC, Khurana B, Smith JT, et al: Osteomyelitis of the lower extremity: pathophysiology, imaging, and classification, with an emphasis on diabetic foot infection, *Emerg Radiol* 25:175–188, 2018.

Masters EA, Trombetta RP, de Mesy Bentley KL, et al: Evolving concepts in bone infection: redefining "biofilm", "acute vs. chronic osteomyelitis", "the immune proteome" and "local antibiotic therapy", *Bone Res* 7:20, 2019.

Okubo Y, Nochioka K, Testa M: Nationwide survey of pediatric acute osteomyelitis in the USA, *J Pediatric Ortho* 26:501–506, 2017.

Park KH, Cho OH, Lee JH, et al: Optimal duration of antibiotic therapy in patients with hematogenous vertebral osteomyelitis at low risk and high risk of recurrence, *Clin Infect Dis* 262:1262–1269, 2016.

Miller M, ed: *Review of Orthopaedics*, 3rd ed.

Samara E, Spyropoulou V, Tabard-Fougère A, et al: Kingella kingae and osteoarticular infections, *Pediatrics* 144(6), 2019, Epub.

Senneville E, Lipsky BA, Abbas ZG, et al: Diagnosis of infection in the foot in diabetes: a systematic review, *Diabetes Metab Res Rev* 36(S1):e3281, 2020.

Zalavras CG, Marcus RE, Levin LS, Patzakis MJ: Management of open fractures and subsequent complications, *JBJS (A)* 4:884–895, 2007.

PLAGUE

Method of

Nelson Iván Agudelo Higuita, MD; Douglas A. Drevets, MD; and Deidra Bowman, MD

CURRENT DIAGNOSIS

- Plague should be suspected when a person develops abrupt onset of fever, lymphadenopathy, or sepsis and there is history of a flea bite or possible exposure to an infected animal or person.
- *Yersinia pestis* is an aerobic gram-negative coccobacilli that exhibits bipolar staining with Giemsa, Wright's, and Wayson stains.
- Automated diagnostic systems may misidentify *Y. pestis* as another organism.

CURRENT THERAPY

- Timely and appropriate management is imperative for a good outcome.
- Despite their toxicities, aminoglycosides are the treatment agents of choice.
- Respiratory droplet precautions should be instituted when pneumonic plague is suspected.
- Postexposure prophylaxis is indicated for close contacts.

Historical descriptions indicate that *Yersinia pestis* probably caused Justinian's Plague (AD 541), which led into the first plague pandemic. The second plague pandemic, also known as the Black Death, began in Central Asia in 1347 and then spread to Europe, Asia, and Africa. It killed an estimated 50 million people. The current (third) plague pandemic began in China and then spread worldwide along shipping routes in 1899–1900. *Y. pestis* is a gram-negative, nonmotile, facultatively anaerobic, non-spore-forming coccobacillus that is approximately 0.5 to 0.8 μm in diameter and 1 to 3 μm in length. Genomic sequencing shows that *Y. pestis* is a recently emerged clone of *Y. pseudotuberculosis*.

Epidemiology

Plague is a zoonosis for which urban and sylvatic rodents (e.g., rats, prairie dogs, and marmots) are the most important enzootic reservoirs. Additionally, domestic cats and dogs have been linked to human disease. Human plague occurs in North and South America, Asia, and Africa. Recent outbreaks reported to the World Health Organization (WHO) have occurred in the Democratic Republic of Congo (2005, 2006), China (2009), and Peru (2010). Plague is endemic in Madagascar, and between 2004 and 2009, 30% of all human cases worldwide were reported from this country. The largest epidemic in a quarter of a century was identified August 1, 2017, and was contained November 27, 2017. A total of 2417 cases (77% pneumonic) with a 9% case fatality ratio were reported. From 2000 to 2009, a total of 21,725 cases of plague with a 7.4% fatality rate were reported worldwide. The incidence of plague in most of the world is otherwise declining. In 2018, only 5 countries reported cases of plague. In North America, most human cases occur in New Mexico, Arizona, California, Colorado, and Texas. Between 1900 and 2012, 1006 confirmed or probable cases have occurred in the U.S. with over 80% of these attributable to bubonic plague. In the United States, an average of seven human cases have been reported annually. More information can be found on the WHO and Centers for Disease Control and Prevention websites.

Modes of Transmission

Most human infections are transmitted from rodent to humans via the bite of an infected flea. Infection also can be acquired by contact with body fluids from infected animals, such as during field dressing of game or by inhalation of respiratory droplets from animals, particularly cats, or humans with pneumonic plague.

Bioterrorism Threat

Plague was used as an agent of biowarfare by the Japanese in World War II and was a focus of intensive research and development in the former Soviet Union during the Cold War. Primary pneumonic plague is the most likely form of exposure because of biowarfare or bioterrorism. Recent increases in terrorism worldwide have increased the focus of public health management groups to develop comprehensive statements regarding plague as a biological weapon.

Pathogenesis and Clinical Syndromes

Transdermal inoculation of bacilli from the bite of an infected flea ultimately leads to infection of the regional lymph nodes in which massive replication of bacteria creates the bubo (derived from the Greek *bubon* or "groin"), a swollen, erythematous, and painful lymph node in the groin, axilla, or cervical region. Bacteremia and septicemia frequently develop and lead to secondary infection of other organs including the lungs, spleen, and central nervous system. Primary pneumonic plague is a rare natural occurrence and results from the inhalation of respiratory droplets containing *Y. pestis* bacilli from another case of pneumonic plague, usually in humans or in cats. Although plague in dogs is rare, human outbreaks have been traced to sick dogs with wildlife exposure. Secondary pneumonic plague results from seeding of the lungs by blood-borne bacteria in the setting of either bubonic or septicemic plague. Septicemic plague also begins with transdermal exposure but manifests as primary bacteremia/septicemia without the bubo. Less common manifestations include meningitis, pharyngitis, and gastroenteritis. In addition, inhalation of respiratory droplets produced by intense manipulation of human corpses or animal carcasses are another potential form of infection. Direct skin contact with infected blood from a corpse or carcass could also result in bubonic plague. Finally, transmission of antimicrobial resistant *Y. pestis* has been documented during outbreaks of pneumonic plague.

Bubonic plague is an acute febrile lymphadenitis that develops 2 to 8 days after inoculation. Inflamed lymph nodes are usually 1 to 6 cm in diameter and painful. Abrupt onset of fever is an almost universal finding and occurs simultaneously with, or up to 24 hours before, the appearance of the bubo. Headache, malaise, and chills are frequent, along with nausea, vomiting, and diarrhea. Most patients are tachycardic, hypotensive, and appear prostrate and lethargic with episodic restlessness. Leukocytosis with a left shift is typical. Complications include pneumonia, shock, disseminated intravascular coagulation, purpuric skin lesions, acral cyanosis, and gangrene. The differential diagnosis of bubonic plague includes tularemia and Group A β-hemolytic streptococcal adenitis with bacteremia.

Symptoms of septicemic plague are similar to those caused by other gram-negative bacteria, and are very similar to those of bubonic plague except that abdominal pain is more common in septicemic plague. Septicemic plague must be differentiated from fulminating septicemia caused by other gram-negative bacteria. Primary pneumonic plague has an abrupt onset of fever and influenza-like symptoms 1 to 5 days after inhalation exposure. Symptoms include shortness of breath, cough, chest pain, and bloody sputum with rapid progression to fulminating pneumonia and respiratory failure. Patients with secondary pneumonic infection show respiratory symptoms in addition to those attributed to the bubo or sepsis. Radiographic findings include patchy bronchopneumonia, multilobar consolidations, cavitations, and alveolar hemorrhage and are not pathognomonic of *Y. pestis*. Plague pneumonia must be differentiated from severe influenza, inhalation anthrax, and overwhelming community-acquired pneumonia.

Plague meningitis is rare but almost always universally fatal if untreated. This entity is most commonly seen as a complication of primary axillary bubonic plague. Plague meningitis can develop during appropriate treatment administration, particularly if treatment initiation was delayed or if the clinical course has been protracted.

Diagnosis

Plague is diagnosed by demonstrating *Y. pestis* in blood or body fluids such as a lymph node aspirate, sputum, or cerebrospinal fluid. A tentative diagnosis of bubonic plague can be made rapidly with fluid aspirated from a bubo showing gram-negative coccobacilli with bipolar staining. It is important to remember that automated diagnostic systems might misidentify *Y. pestis*. In an outbreak in Colorado, the misidentification of *Y. pestis* as *Pseudomonas luteola* delayed the recognition of the outbreak. *Y. pestis* has also been misidentified as *Y. pseudotuberculosis* with matrix-assisted laser desorption/ionization time-of-flight mass spectrometry (MALDI-TOF). Serology showing a fourfold rise in antibody titers to F1 antigen or a single titer of more than 1:128 is also diagnostic. Rapid tests using monoclonal antibodies to detect *Y. pestis* F1 antigen in bubo aspirates and sputum have been developed and field tested. The use of mass spectrometry as a more rapid and cost-effective diagnostic tool has also been studied.

Treatment

The aminoglycosides (gentamicin[1] and streptomycin), the fluoroquinolones (ciprofloxacin [Cipro] moxifloxacin [Avelox] and levofloxacin [Levaquin]) and doxycycline (Vibramycin) are considered first

---

[1]Not FDA approved for this indication.

line therapy for all forms of plague with the exception of pneumonic and septicemic plague, in which doxycycline is considered an alternative agent. For plague meningitis, the first line therapy consists of levofloxacin or moxifloxacin with chloramphenicol. Typical minimal inhibitory concentrations for 90% (MIC_{90}) of tested strains for the fluoroquinolones are less than 0.03 to 0.25 μg/mL compared with less than 1.0 μg/mL and less than 1.0 μg/mL to 4.0 μg/mL for gentamicin and streptomycin, respectively, and less than 1.0 μg/mL for doxycycline. Streptomycin (15 mg/kg up to 1 g intramuscularly [IM] every 12 hours) and gentamicin (5 to 7 mg/kg/day intravenously [IV]/IM in one or two doses daily) are the drugs of choice for severe infection. For adults, standard fluoroquinolone dosing includes ciprofloxacin 400 mg IV every 8 hours or 750 mg orally every 12 hours; levofloxacin 750 mg IV/orally daily; and moxifloxacin 400 mg IV/orally daily. Doxycycline is administered starting with a 200 mg loading dose followed by 100 mg IV/orally every 12 hours. Chloramphenicol (25 mg/kg IV/orally every 6 hours) can be used in select circumstances. Antibiotic therapy should be continued for a total of 10 days; some experts will extend the duration of therapy to 14 days when a bacteriostatic agent like a tetracycline is used.

Prevention and Control

Standard infection control procedures should include a disposable surgical mask, latex gloves, devices to protect mucous membranes, and good hand washing. Hospitalized patients with known or suspected pneumonic plague should be isolated under respiratory droplet precautions for at least 48 hours after appropriate antibiotics are initiated. Patients without respiratory plague can be managed under standard precautions. Pre-exposure prophylaxis is not routinely recommended but can be considered under certain circumstances and for up to 48 hours after the last potential exposure. Postexposure prophylaxis should be given to individuals with close contact (less than 2 meters) with an infectious case or who have had a potential respiratory exposure. The recommended adult antibiotics for prophylaxis are doxycycline or ciprofloxacin in the same doses used for treatment. Postexposure prophylaxis can be given orally and should be continued for 7 days following exposure. Currently, there is no licensed plague vaccine. An encapsulated *Y. pseudotuberculosis*, strain V674pF1, is an efficient live oral vaccine against pneumonic plague in mice. Recently, flea resistance to insecticides such as DDT and Deltamethrin in Madagascar has prompted an immediate need for alternative insecticides to prevent future plague outbreaks.

References

Andrianaivoarimanana V, et al: Understanding the persistence of plague foci in Madagascar, *PLoS Negl Trop Dis.* 7(11):e2382, 2013.

Boyer S, et al: Xenopsylla cheopis (Siphonaptera: Pulicidae) susceptibility to deltamethrin in Madagascar, *PLoS One* 9(11), 2014, e111998.

Butler T: A clinical study of bubonic plague. Observations of the 1970 Vietnam epidemic with emphasis on coagulation studies, skin histology and electrocardiograms, *Am J Med* 53:268–276, 1972.

CDC. Maps and Statistics. http://www.cdc.gov/plague/maps/index.html.

Cooley KM, Fleck-Derderian S, McCormick DW, Nelson CA: Plague meningitis: a systematic review of clinical course, antimicrobial treatment, and outcomes, *Health Security* 21(1):22–33, 2023.

Dale AP, Kretschmer M, Ruberto I, et al: Notes from the field: delays in identification and treatment of a case of septicemic plague--Navajo County, Arizona, 2020, *MMWR Morb Mortal Wkly Rep* 70(31):1063–1064, 2021.

Derbise A, Cerdà Marín A, et al: An encapsulated *Yersinia* pseudotuberculosis is a highly efficient vaccine against pneumonic plague, e1528 *PLoS Negl Trop Dis* 6(2), 2012. Feb.

Gage KL, Dennis DT, Orloski KA, et al: Cases of cat-associated human plague in the Western US, 1977–1998, *Clin Infect Dis* 30:893–900, 2000.

Inglesby TV, Dennis DT, Henderson DA, et al: Plague as a biological weapon: Medical and public health management. Working Group on Civilian Biodefense, *JAMA* 283:2281–2290, 2000.

Jullien S, de Silva NL, Garner P: Plague transmission from corpses and carcasses, *Emerg Infect Dis* 27(8):2033–2041, 2021.

Nelson CA, Meaney-Delman D, Fleck-Derderian, et al: Antimicrobial treatment and prophylaxis of plague: recommendations for naturally acquired infections and bioterrorism response, *MMWR Recomm Rep* 70(3):1–27, 2021.

Prentice MB, Rahalison L: Plague, *Lancet* 369:1196–1207, 2007.

Runfola JK, et al: Outbreak of human pneumonic plague with dog-to-human and possible human-to-human transmission, *MMWR Morb Mortal Wkly Rep* 64(16):429–434, 2015.

Wang H, et al: A dog-associated primary pneumonic plague in Qinghai Province, China, *Clin Infect Dis* 52(2):185–190, 2011.

Wong JD, Barash JR, Sandfort RF, Janda JM: Susceptibilities of *Yersinia pestis* strains to 12 antimicrobial agents, *Antimicrob Agents Chemother* 44:1995–1996, 2000.

World Health Organization: Plague around the world in 2019, *Weekly Epidemiological Record* 94(25):289–292, 2019.

POST-ACUTE COVID SYNDROME

Method of
Victor S. Sierpina, MD; Justin Seashore, MD; Sagar Kamprath, MD; and Cathy Xie, DO

CURRENT DIAGNOSIS

- *Post-acute COVID syndrome* is defined as symptoms extending 3 weeks to 3 months after the acute disease occurs, and *long-haul COVID* is defined as symptoms persisting beyond 3 months after the infection has resolved.
- Predominant symptoms are new-onset shortness of breath, cough, palpitations, fatigue, and brain fog. Other common symptoms include gastrointestinal disturbances, headache, hair loss, new-onset nondescript pain, depression, anxiety, and posttraumatic stress disorder.
- Results of testing are not part of the current definition as many patients were not tested and are or were asymptomatic carriers.
- The broad spectrum of clinical manifestations of post-acute COVID syndrome should encourage clinicians and medical educators to include it in the differential diagnosis of any of a number of new or worsening complaints.

CURRENT TREATMENT

- Evidence for optimal management of long-haul COVID may be lacking at this time but is evolving, with best practices being described by multiple professional bodies.
- Multidisciplinary management and rehabilitation are essential to whole-person care.
- Organ- and system-specific care is appropriate and must be prioritized as to serious versus milder long-term problems.
- Self-management and peer support can plan important roles and must include shared decision making.
- Appropriate consultation and use of currently established disease-specific and organ-specific practice guidelines are foundational to optimal treatment planning.
- Quality-of-care principles for long-haul COVID include providing access to care, reducing the burden of illness, taking clinical responsibility, offering continuity of care, providing multidisciplinary rehabilitation, conducting evidence-based investigation and management, and continuing further research and development on appropriate and evidence-based clinical services.

Over the past 3 years, we have endured an ever-changing multimodal disease process, devastating millions of people not only with severe infection but also with mild or asymptomatic forms of the disease. Our understanding and definitions of the spectrum of conditions that encompasses post-acute COVID syndrome and long-haul COVID is an ongoing discovery. It is estimated that 10% to 30% of COVID-infected patients may be left with residual symptoms. With over 500,000 million worldwide known cases and many not reported, untested, or asymptomatic, post-acute COVID syndrome can be expected to affect a huge number of people.

Equally concerning is the puzzling discovery that those with even mild or asymptomatic COVID infections may develop post-acute COVID syndrome. Vaccination is largely protective of severe disease, though the syndrome may still occur in a small number of these patients. Children generally do not experience severe post-acute COVID syndrome, although psychological, mental health, and gastrointestinal symptoms are of increasing concern in this group and are often difficult to dissect from pre-existing conditions.

Some key ongoing questions include the following:
- What is the underlying biology of long-haul COVID?
- How many people become infected with long-haul COVID and who is most at risk?
- What is the relationship between long-haul COVID and other post-infection syndromes?

We endeavor to address these questions, though much further research is needed. We present here a holistic and methodical foundational program that uses minimally invasive procedures and management strategies. This approach will offer patients with post-acute COVID syndrome an improved quality of life with low-risk, cost-effective, common-sense healthcare approaches. The evidence base for this approach is grounded in current best practices but continues to evolve with new knowledge about the course of post-acute COVID syndrome. In parallel, we must guide patients away from high-risk, high-cost invasive therapies that have no proven benefit.

Healthcare professionals must be cognizant of the range of real physical long-term effects of COVID-19 and should address them with clinical discernment, understanding, and empathy. They should be careful not to label all such presentations as related to stress, anxiety, depression, or other psychological epiphenomena. The role of peer support is clearly important to those with post-acute COVID syndrome who may otherwise feel isolated and misunderstood.

Pathophysiology

COVID-19 is caused by the severe acute respiratory syndrome coronavirus 2 (SARS-CoV-2) and is genetically similar to the severe acute respiratory syndrome (SARS) and Middle East respiratory syndrome (MERS) coronaviruses that were responsible for the SARS outbreaks earlier in the century. SARS and MERS infections have been found to result in long-term postviral syndromes, some extending a decade a more after the initial disease. Coronaviruses that circulate among humans are usually benign and are responsible for about one-fourth of all common cold illnesses, with a total of seven human coronaviruses in known existence. However, it is likely that bats, a natural animal reservoir, facilitated mutation of the virus in China in late 2019. Another spillover possibility, escape of modified virus from a research laboratory in Wuhan, is still being debated. This novel coronavirus is composed of single-stranded RNA with its envelope surrounded by spike proteins resembling a crown, typically transmitted through respiratory droplets as well as fecal-oral transmission. The incubation period is about 5 days, though some variants such as the Delta variant have a shorter cycle and are potentially followed by 1 week of worsening symptoms that may lead to hospitalization in severe cases. Interferon is a key component that affects the mechanism of viral infection. Higher viral loads and delayed interferon responses are seen in severe infection, and it may be likely that patients most susceptible to severe disease cannot adequately mount an effective early antiviral response.

The virus attaches to cells via the ACE2 receptor, found in our tongue, nose, throat, stomach, small intestine, liver, brain, kidneys, and lungs. In the lungs, it binds to type 2 alveolar cells, where it replicates. The cells subsequently send a distress signal of cytokines and downregulate the ACE2 receptor, decreasing angiotensin 1 to 9 and angiotensin 1 to 7 (pro-vasodilation and antifibrotic). Angiotensin 1 receptors become more stimulated, which leads to a proinflammatory and profibrotic stage. COVID-19 also favors disordered endothelial function, which contributes to protein accumulation in the alveolar space seen in the "cytokine storm" directly related to capillary leak and the cases of ARDS seen in advanced states of the disease. Unfortunately, this is not only limited to the lungs, but predisposes the entire body system to a prothrombotic state, as seen in cases of stroke and other types of ischemic dysfunction. In this inflammatory state, vascular endothelial and smooth muscle cells produce large amounts of IL-6. This stimulates the acute-phase response, increasing fibrinogen production and favoring clot formation.

COVID-19 remains a complex disease process of the endothelium, and future treatments may focus on antiinflammatory therapies and promoting endothelial homeostasis. Obesity is one of the major risk factors for the cytokine storm as it induces a constant state of low-grade inflammation characterized by acute-phase reactants, reactive oxygen species, and proinflammatory cytokines. However, moderate exercise over time enhances the immune system, mobilizing NK and CD8+ T cells, and overall improves immunosurveillance and lowers inflammation.

Prevention

Conventional prevention includes the well-known guidelines from the Centers for Disease Control and Prevention (CDC) regarding masking, social distancing, hand washing/avoidance of touching the face, various isolation and quarantine measures, and vaccination. Large droplets are the primary mode of spread, which can be greatly mitigated with widespread mask wearing in addition to adequate ventilation.

Monoclonal antibodies may also be used in acute infection as they bind to the spike proteins of the coronavirus and can reduce the viral load, theoretically reducing the severity of the illness. Immunotherapy continues to evolve as certain formulations are more or less effective against emerging variants.

Given that over 99% of the recent cases in 2022 within the United States were caused by the omicron variant, bamlanivimab[5] and etesevimab[5] (administered together)[5] and REGEN-COV (casirivimab and imdevimab)[5] are not recommended because they have reduced activity against this variant. Paxlovid[5] (nirmatrelvir and ritonavir, approved for Emergency Use Authorization [EUA] by the U.S. Food and Drug Administration [FDA]), sotrovimab[5] (no longer has EUA), remdesivir (Veklury), molnupiravir[5] (Lagevrio, approved for EUA), and most recently bebtelovimab[5] (approved for EUA) are recommended for those with mild-to-moderate COVID-19 who are at risk for progression to severe disease. The monoclonal antibodies leronlimab[5] and tocilizumab (Actemra),[1] which have been efficacious in treating HIV, have been shown to reduce IL-6 levels in COVID-19 and are being further studied. Healthcare providers can consult with the National Institutes of Health's COVID-19 guidelines to decide whether these therapies are beneficial for individual patients as they are expected to evolve with new variants.

These measures may be used for patients with COVID-19 who are not sick enough to be hospitalized but are at risk for hospitalization because of medical comorbidities such as diabetes, immunosuppression, or obesity. Vaccination along with booster are still recommended for these patients. Access, cost, and administration hurdles impede the availability of immunotherapies worldwide.

The recent mRNA vaccines offer hope for prevention of infection and transmission, with current projections of 94.5% efficacy in reducing severe disease. Additionally, as new variants occur, these newly developed vaccines continue to protect up to 100% against severe COVID-19 infections. However, it is recommended to continue masking and engaging in social distancing even after vaccination. Some recent reports have indicated that patients suffering with post-acute COVID symptoms found that getting the COVID vaccine relieved these symptoms. The exact mechanism of this is unknown and bears further study but may have to do with clearing residual virus or reducing autoimmune and inflammatory processes.

Rates of anxiety and depression have increased during the pandemic, and this subsequently attenuates the immune system. Managing these appropriately and promptly can improve immunity as well as quality of life. Spending time outside and engaging in physical activity can also help strengthen the immune system and mitigate the cabin fever of COVID-19. Breathing techniques such as resonant breathing, singing, or 4-7-8 breathing can also help increase parasympathetic tone, increase heart rate variability, and decrease stress. At least 7 hours of sleep before vaccination provides a more robust antibody response from the immune system.

Other less proven but widely used methods include use of various supplements such as vitamin C,[1] vitamin D,[1] quercetin,[7] zinc,[1] probiotics,[7] luteolin,[7] melatonin,[7] and other supplements. None of these methods have been proven in prospective trials, but they are widely used, and there is some historical evidence for their utility and mechanisms of action in other coronavirus-like infections such as the common cold. An open discussion with patients regarding the limited evidence for them may be helpful while respecting patient autonomy and desire for agency in selecting self-care strategies in the presence of fear and uncertainty.

Vitamin C remains a potent antioxidant and anecdotally beneficial in several studies. The ongoing Lessening Organ Dysfunction With VITamin C—COVID-19 (LOVIT-COVID) clinical trial (NCT04401150) is assessing high-dose intravenous vitamin C for inpatients with COVID-19. For prevention, one may focus on increasing consumption of foods high in vitamin C such as citrus.

Vitamin D is an important regulator of human immune function and may stimulate the innate immune response to provide front-line protection against infectious agents. On the whole, people are spending less time outside in the sunlight, which hampers the production of the active form of vitamin D. Recently it was noted that higher vitamin D levels correlated with fewer COVID-19 cases and mortality. This could be a result of low vitamin D being a marker of a sedentary lifestyle and thus likely overall health risk. Whether or not one is COVID positive, taking vitamin D may be beneficial in a dose of around 4000 IU daily. There is also evidence that vitamin K_2[1] may be helpful in the absorption of vitamin D, but it should be avoided in patients on blood thinners.

Quercetin is a naturally occurring dietary flavonoid with antiviral properties and may disrupt the infectious mechanism of the coronavirus. It is an antioxidant found in many plant foods including capers, red onions, apples, leafy greens, dill, cilantro, fennel, berries, sweet potato, tomatoes, broccoli, and tea. Quercetin can also be purchased as a supplement. It is often combined with vitamin C to increase absorption and taken up to 500 mg twice a day.

Zinc impairs replication in RNA viruses and may enhance cytotoxicity when used with a zinc ionophore such as quercetin. Long-term zinc supplementation may result in copper deficiency, thus replacing copper is recommended.

N-acetylcysteine,[1] a glutathione precursor, at 600 mg orally twice per day, may help improve oxidative stress and inflammatory response in patients with upper respiratory tract infections. N-acetylcysteine assists the liver in reducing glutathione, which in turn helps the liver in removing toxins. A case report has noted that glutathione supplementation has improved dyspnea in COVID-19 patients. These may represent a novel treatment approach in blocking nuclear factor kappa B (NF-κB) and attenuating the cytokine storm seen in COVID-19.

Several trials to assess various adaptogens, probiotics, and dietary supplements such as nicotinamide riboside[7] are currently underway as additional therapies for long-haul COVID. Hyperbaric oxygen therapy, montelukast (Singulair),[1] and deupirfenidone[5] are being evaluated to help with COVID-related respiratory complaints. Histamine-1 and histamine-2 antagonists show promise by inhibiting the virus from entering ACE-2–expressing cells. In addition, use of selective serotonin reuptake inhibitors (SSRIs) and serotonin-norepinephrine reuptake inhibitors (SNRIs) has been associated with reduced risk of intubation or death in COVID-19. As future trials ensue, we may have clearer direction in treating the long-term effects of COVID-19.

---

[1] Not FDA approved for this indication.
[5] Investigational drug in the United States.

[1] Not FDA approved for this indication.
[5] Investigational drug in the United States.
[7] Available as dietary supplement.

Clinical Manifestations

The multifaceted aspects of long-haul COVID are shown in Figure 1. According to the CDC, the most commonly reported long-term post-acute COVID symptoms are outlined in Box 1.

Diagnosis

The predominant symptoms leading patients to seek help are focused on new-onset shortness of breath, cough, palpitations, fatigue, and brain fog. Other common symptoms include gastrointestinal disturbances, headache, hair loss, new-onset nondescript pain, depression, anxiety, and posttraumatic stress disorder (PTSD).

Post-acute COVID syndrome is defined as symptoms extending 3 weeks to 3 months after the acute disease occurs, and *long-haul COVID* is defined as symptoms persisting beyond 3 months after the infection has resolved. Results of testing are not part of the current definition as many patients were not tested and are or were asymptomatic carriers. Even antibody testing is not entirely reliable as we are unsure of the durability of post-infection IgG results.

Persons with the following risks were two to three times more likely to develop long-haul COVID: persistent cough, hoarseness, headache, diarrhea, loss of appetite, and shortness of breath in the first week.

Persons with more than five symptoms in the first week of illness were four times more likely to develop long-haul COVID than those with fewer symptoms. The five most predictive symptoms of long-haul COVID in the first week of illness were fatigue, headache, shortness of breath, hoarse voice, and myalgia. Long-haul COVID was also more likely to occur in women, older adults, and those with obesity. An autoimmune component may explain the higher rate of post-acute COVID syndrome in women.

Indeed, post-acute COVID syndrome may comprise four or more syndromes rather than one distinct postviral entity, and it may include post–intensive care syndrome, post–viral fatigue syndrome, and long-haul COVID. Symptoms may fluctuate and present in nonlinear and nonsequentially unpredictable ways.

Such conditions have been seen in other post-infectious conditions, largely as a result of the persistence of the immune response, ongoing inflammation, and effects on blood coagulation.

After the Spanish flu of 1918, which killed an estimated 50 million people, late-occurring neurologic sequela included long-lasting brain damage in up to 1 million people. SARS and MERS as well as myalgic encephalomyelitis or chronic fatigue syndrome are other syndromes that share overlapping symptoms with post-acute COVID syndrome.

Long-haul COVID is an evolving clinical problem that has important public health and long-term considerations as the pandemic continues and it becomes endemic.

Therapy

Once post-acute COVID syndrome or long-haul COVID is suspected or diagnosed, determining the patient's baseline status helps organize and systematize clinical interventions. Addressing evolving exacerbations and life-threatening manifestations must take priority. It is important to avoid unproven, high-cost,

Figure 1 An overview of the symptoms, putative pathophysiology, associated risk factors, and potential treatments involved in long-haul COVID. *Dashed lines* represent areas where evidence is relatively lacking compared with the *solid lines*. (Modified from Yong SJ: Long COVID or post-COVID-19 syndrome: putative pathophysiology, risk factors, and treatments, *Infect Dis (Lond)* 53(10):737–754, 2021.)

BOX 1 — Symptoms Commonly Reported Among Patients with Post-Acute COVID Conditions

- Dyspnea or increased respiratory effort
- Fatigue
- Post-exertional malaise* and/or poor endurance
- "Brain fog," or cognitive impairment
- Cough
- Chest pain
- Headache
- Palpitations and/or tachycardia
- Arthralgia
- Myalgia
- Paresthesia
- Abdominal pain
- Diarrhea
- Insomnia and other sleep difficulties
- Fever
- Lightheadedness
- Impaired daily function and mobility
- Pain
- Rash (e.g., urticaria)
- Mood changes
- Anosmia or dysgeusia
- Menstrual cycle irregularities

*Post-exertional malaise (PEM) is the worsening of symptoms following even minor physical or mental exertion, with symptoms typically worsening 12 to 48 hours after activity and lasting for days or even weeks.

From Centers for Disease Control and Prevention: Clinical Care Information for COVID-19. Post-COVID Conditions: Overview for Healthcare Providers. Available at: https://www.cdc.gov/coronavirus/2019-ncov/hcp/clinical-care.html.

invasive experimental therapies outside of clinical trials. The general principles of management are described in a monograph by the National Institute for Health and Care Excellence (NICE) (Box 2).

For clinicians, a standardized approach to patients in the initial setting is important. Functional and behavioral assessments are of central importance as the rehabilitation of patients requires management of both. Multidisciplinary teams to direct care and address newly developing symptoms should be utilized when available.

To begin evaluation of the patient with post-acute COVID syndrome, the clinician should perform initial screening with standardized questionnaires including shortness-of-breath scales, such as the University of California, San Diego Shortness of Breath Questionnaire (SOBQ), and activity scales that assess activities of daily living (ADLs) and instrumental activities of daily living (iADLS). Nutritional evaluation (e.g., the subjective global assessment [SGA]), the Generalized Anxiety Disorder 7-Item Questionnaire (GAD-7), the Patient Health Questionnaire-9 (PHQ-9), the International Education Standard-6 (IES-6), and the Impact of Event Scale-Revised (IES-R) are examples of behavioral assessments that can be used to evaluate anxiety, depression, and PTSD along with an ongoing symptoms evaluation. Use of these scales with each visit allow for individualized evaluations of improvement (Box 3).

Utilizing a multidisciplinary rehabilitation team including physicians, rehabilitation therapists, psychologists, nutritionists, and social workers to review these screenings allows the healthcare provider to develop a personalized, patient-centered approach to care.

Shared decision making with patients is key, given the vast number of symptoms patients may be experiencing. Discussing which are most troubling and limiting to the patient is of importance

BOX 2 — Management of Post-Acute COVID Syndrome

These recommendations are for healthcare professionals who provide care for patients with ongoing symptomatic COVID-19 or post-acute COVID syndrome in primary care and community settings or in multidisciplinary assessment and rehabilitation services.

Self-Management and Supported Self-Management

- Give advice and information on self-management to people with ongoing symptomatic COVID-19 or post-acute COVID syndrome, starting from their initial assessment. This should include the following:
  - Ways to self-manage their symptoms, such as setting realistic goals
  - Who to contact if they are worried about their symptoms or if they need support with self-management
  - Sources of advice and support, including support groups, social prescribing, online forums, and apps
  - How to obtain support from other services, including social care, housing, and employment, and advice about financial support
  - Information about new or continuing symptoms of COVID-19 that patients can share with their family, careers, and friends (see the section on common symptoms of ongoing symptomatic COVID-19 and post-acute COVID syndrome [https://www.nice.org.uk/guidance/NG188]).
- Explain that it is not known if over-the-counter vitamins and supplements are helpful, harmful, or have no effect in the treatment of new or ongoing symptoms of COVID-19.
- Support patients in discussions with their employer, school, or college about returning to work or education, for example by having a phased return. For advice on returning to work, follow national guidelines such as the NICE guideline on workplace health: long-term sickness absence and capability to work.

Multidisciplinary Rehabilitation

- Assess patients who have been referred to integrated multidisciplinary rehabilitation services to guide management. Include the physical, psychological, and psychiatric aspects of rehabilitation. Ensure that any symptoms that could affect the patient's ability to safely start rehabilitation have been investigated first (see recommendations for multidisciplinary rehabilitation teams [https://www.nice.org.uk/guidance/NG188]).
- Work with the patient to develop a personalized rehabilitation and management plan that is recorded in a rehabilitation prescription and includes the following:
  - Areas of rehabilitation and interventions based on their assessment
  - Helping the patient decide and work toward goals
  - Symptom management for all presenting symptoms, for example advice and education on managing breathlessness, fatigue and "brain fog."
- Encourage patients to keep a record or use a tracking app to monitor their goals, recovery, and any changes in their symptoms (see recommendations for follow-up and monitoring [https://www.nice.org.uk/guidance/NG188]).

Support for Older Adults and Children

- Consider additional support for older adults with ongoing symptomatic COVID-19 or post-acute COVID syndrome, for example short-term care packages, advance care planning and support with social isolation, loneliness, and bereavement, if relevant.
- Consider referral from 4 weeks for specialist advice for children with ongoing symptomatic COVID-19 or post-COVID-19 syndrome.

Modified from National Institute for Health and Care Excellence: COVID-19 rapid guideline: managing the long-term effects of COVID-19. Nice Guideline [NG188] Published: 18 December 2020. Last updated: 11 November 2021. Available at: https://www.nice.org.uk/guidance/NG188.

University of Texas Medical Branch Health (UTMB) Post COVID Recovery Clinic intake questionnaire
https://www.utmbhealth.com/post-covid-19-clinic
University of California, San Diego Shortness of Breath Questionnaire (SOBQ)
https://doi.org/10.1378/chest.113.3.619
Activities of Daily Living/Instrumental Activities of Daily Living
https://www.alz.org/careplanning/downloads/lawton-iadl.pdf
Subjective Global Assessment (SGA)
https://nutritioncareincanada.ca/sites/default/uploads/files/SGA%20Tool%20EN%20BKWT_2017.pdf
Generalized Anxiety Disorder 7-Item Questionnaire (GAD-7)
https://adaa.org/sites/default/files/GAD-7_Anxiety-updated_0.pdf
Patient Health Questionnaire-9 (PHQ-9)
https://www.apa.org/depression-guideline/patient-health-questionnaire.pdf
Impact of Event Scale-Revised (IES-R)
https://emdrfoundation.org/toolkit/ies-scoring.pdf

| BOX 4 | Breathing Techniques for Post-COVID Syndrome |

About 80% of the work of breathing is done by the diaphragm. After illness or general deconditioning, the breathing pattern may be altered, with reduced diaphragmatic movement and greater use of neck and shoulder accessory muscles. This results in shallow breathing, increasing fatigue and breathlessness, and higher energy expenditure. The "breathing control" technique is aimed at normalizing breathing patterns and increasing the efficiency of the respiratory muscles (including the diaphragm), resulting in less energy expenditure, less airway irritation, reduced fatigue, and improvement in breathlessness. The patient should sit in a supported position and breathe in and out slowly, preferably in through the nose and out through the mouth, while relaxing the chest and shoulders and allowing the tummy to rise. They should aim for an inspiration to expiration ratio of 1:2. This technique can be used frequently throughout the day, in 5–10 minute bursts (or longer if helpful).

Other breathing techniques—such as diaphragmatic breathing, slow deep breathing, pursed lip breathing, yoga techniques, Buteyko—are used in strategies to manage patients' breathing patterns and breathlessness but require specialist advice to identify which technique best suits each patient.

From Greenhalgh T, Knight M, A'Court C, Buxton M, Husain L. Management of post-acute covid-19 in primary care. BMJ. 2020;370:m3026.

in goal setting. From this baseline, the healthcare provider can establish plans to address the most severe symptoms initially and determine those that can be readdressed in the future.

Acute COVID-19 presents with a broad range of symptoms, therefore patients recovering from this illness show heterogeneity that may be phenotypic. Some have few or no residual symptoms after the acute infection, while others show sustained symptoms at higher or lesser clinical penetrance.

Pulmonary

For many, respiratory symptoms may be the predominating indication, therefore a proper pulmonary examination is important. Pulse oximetry, pulmonary function testing, a 6-minute walk test, and chest x-ray are good starting points. Utilization of pulmonary rehabilitation will guide patients through this new sensation of shortness of breath and reduce symptom burden. This aspect of rehabilitation should not be limited to patients with only abnormal pulmonary function testing. Home monitoring with pulse oximetry is recommended. It is also important to eliminate other factors for dyspnea such as smoking, air pollutants, extremes in temperature, or excess exercise.

Several breathing techniques have been offered to help patients deal with breathlessness, improve diaphragmatic breathing, and help normalize lung function (Box 4).

The question of whether to use inhaled bronchodilators remains. A potential practice is to begin a trial with a short-acting agent to be used when symptomatic, and if the patient notes temporary benefit and the need to use it frequently, a long-acting beta agonist plus an inhaled corticosteroid can be considered. COVID-19 is known to induce an inflammatory response, and this may abate symptoms. Step-down therapy should be planned as one would do for asthma.

As pulmonary symptoms such as cough and shortness of breath have predominated presenting concerns in patients with post-acute COVID syndrome, a program at Yale called RECOVERY has been developed that could be a model for approaching pulmonary and other systems (Figure 2).

Cardiac

Another key organ affected by COVID-19 infection is the heart. Cardiotoxicity from the infection can cause inflammation of the heart (myocarditis), rhythm disturbances, and damage to the heart muscle (cardiomyopathy). Sudden cardiac death, heart attacks, and heart failure have all been observed, including Takotsubo heart syndrome. Beta blockers and immunotherapy may be indicated.

Cardiac symptoms such as palpitations or increased resting heart rate can be further evaluated with long-term ambulatory cardiac monitoring. A cardiopulmonary exercise test or echocardiogram can assist in delineating cardiac from pulmonary symptoms.

The appropriate type of testing and therapy for post-COVID cardiac syndrome will need to be determined. Electrocardiogram and rhythm monitoring, echocardiography, cardiac biomarkers, and close clinical observation with directed questions about cardiac function will be required for months and perhaps years. Cardiac biopsy may be needed in select cases as well as special imaging such as cardiac magnetic resonance imaging.

Long-term physiotherapy and ongoing cardiology consultation may be needed. Special consideration to cardiac rehabilitation must be given to patients with post-acute COVID syndrome, and modifying or suspending rehabilitation exercises is indicated for the following:

- Saturation <88% to 93%
- Heart rate <40 beats per minute or >120 beats per minute
- Systolic blood pressure <90 mm Hg or >180 mm Hg
- Body temperature fluctuations >37.2°C
- Respiratory symptoms and fatigue that worsen during exercise and do not alleviate after rest
- Symptoms such as chest tightness or pain, difficulty breathing, severe cough, dizziness, headache, unclear vision, palpitations, sweating, and instability

Fatigue

Prevention of deconditioning while considering the risks associated with overexertion can be a balancing act in the patient with post-acute COVID syndrome.

Exercise rehabilitation for athletes and others requires careful titration and personalization as excessive exercise can set back progress. This is also seen in treatment of fibromyalgia and chronic fatigue syndrome in which even slowly graded increases in exercise can cause worsening. It is likely that what we have learned from other conditions such as fibromyalgia and chronic fatigue syndrome, now called *myalgic encephalomyelitis/chronic fatigue syndrome* (ME/CFS), may be transferrable and helpful.

NICE guidelines for these conditions were revised in 2021 and may inform care for patients with post-acute COVID syndrome,

Figure 2 The RECOVERY Clinic Model. (From Lutchmansingh DD, Knauert MP, Antin-Ozerkis DE, et al.: A clinic blueprint for post-coronavirus disease 2019 RECOVERY: Learning from the past, looking to the future, *Chest* 159(3):949–958, 2021.

but they are still controversial. It is important to consider safe approaches from complementary and integrative medicine, including mind-body therapies, yoga, tai chi, acupuncture, personalized nutritional and fitness prescriptions, and carefully selected supplements, minerals, and vitamins.

A general rule of thumb for rehabilitation of patients with post-acute COVID syndrome is that if a patient feels excessively fatigued the day following exercise, so-called *postexercise malaise,* the program must be backed down to prevent overdoing. Controlled breathing exercises, careful pacing, goal setting, low intensity of exercise, and stress reduction are all critical.

Detailed guidelines on returning to sports activities are provided in the Stanford Hall consensus statement (see references). These guidelines can help address appropriate measures, timing, and rehabilitation of multiple systems (i.e., pulmonary, cardiac, neurologic, psychological, musculoskeletal) and overall exercise rehabilitation for returning to vigorous activities. The risk associated with post-acute COVID syndrome deconditioning is significant and must be considered on returning athletes to activity.

Dysautonomia

Providers should be familiar with syndromes such as chronic fatigue syndrome, postural orthostatic tachycardia syndrome, and mast cell activation syndrome. These syndromes are commonly brought up within the post-acute COVID syndrome community.

Dysautonomia may be particularly challenging as it presents with rapid heartbeat, anxiety, numbness, dizziness, low blood pressure, and extreme fatigue. Orthostatic intolerance, a postural orthostatic tachycardia (POT)-like syndrome, may be caused by viral or autoimmune damage to the autonomic nervous system. This condition is best managed with established measures such as patient education, maintaining volume and vascular tone, gradually adjusting positional changes, performing structured exercises including isometrics, wearing compression garments, and in some cases using pharmacologic agents to manage palpitations and to retain sodium and fluid. These pharmacologic agents include fludrocortisone (Florinef),[1] midodrine

(Proamatine), and others affecting adrenergic surge such as beta blockers, methyldopa,[1] and clonidine (Catapres).[1]

Neurologic

Patients with COVID-19 may suffer severe central nervous system insults resulting in strokes, severe brain inflammation (encephalomyelitis, a multiple sclerosis–like or Guillain-Barré type of demyelination), weakness, numbness, confusion, delirium, memory loss, headache, and psychosis. A complaint of enduring "brain fog" is common. Some of these problems occur early, and others occur late. They may be difficult to detect in patients in the intensive care unit who are very sick, hypoxemic, or sedated and when magnetic resonance imaging is difficult to obtain. The Mayo Clinic recommends that brain fog be managed like chemobrain including coping strategies and stress relief. Methylphenidate (Ritalin),[1] donepezil (Aricept),[1] modafinil (Provigil),[1] and memantine (Namenda)[1] have been suggested as options. Luteolin,[7] a flavonoid, has some promise of benefit.

Full neuropsychological testing and/or neurologic consultation should be considered in cases in which post-COVID cognitive changes persist. Occupational, physical, and speech/language therapy may play an important role.

Anosmia is another neurologic symptom of COVID and can be quite debilitating, though patients often recover with time. It can lead to loss of appetite, weight loss, and depression. Therapy for persistent anosmia can include olfactory training, which includes repeated sniffing of a set of odorants to speed recovery.

Mental Health

Mental health support for many will be of importance as patients cope with so many unknowns in their post-COVID world. Sorting out somatic from psychosomatic problems requires clinical acumen, patience, perseverance, and continuity of care. Psychiatric consequences may be severe and related to the immune response and/or from psychological stressors such as social isolation, worries about a potentially fatal illness, concerns about infecting others, stigma of disease, impact on employment, finances, and relationships in general.

---

[1] Not FDA approved for this indication.

[1] Not FDA approved for this indication.
[7] Available as dietary supplement.

The immune response to coronaviruses induces local and systemic production of cytokines, chemokines, and other inflammatory mediators, all of which combine to worsen the burden of preexisting depression, anxiety, PTSD, and other mental health disorders, particularly in female patients.

Mental health issues may end up being one of the most serious, enduring, yet largely hidden impacts seen in the post-COVID patient; thus management and monitoring must address this domain to maintain a holistic approach. Children and adolescents may be most affected.

Therapeutic trials of holistic, integrative, and functional medicine are appropriate given low harm and potential benefit. These may include antiinflammatory diets, acupuncture, meditation, and selected supplements such as fish oil,[1] magnesium,[1] SAMe,[7] valerian,[7] B vitamins,[1] and others.

Hematologic

Thrombotic sequelae and hypercoagulable states require monitoring and management, and prolonged anticoagulation may be required, especially in those with significant deep venous thromboses or pulmonary or cardiac emboli. Many patients will need transient anticoagulation, though some may require ongoing therapy if clotting abnormalities persist. Endothelial damage is now recognized as a perpetuating factor in post-acute COVID syndrome.

Gastrointestinal

If diarrhea and other gastrointestinal complaints continue, this likely reflects viral impact on the microbiota. Gastrointestinal symptoms are prominent in affected children. An antiinflammatory diet, Mediterranean-type diet, hypoallergenic elimination diet, or other personalized nutritional strategies should be considered. Optimizing nutritional support for vulnerable older adults and those with continued anosmia and dysgeusia is likewise vital. Though not yet well defined in terms of dosing and speciation, replacing microbiota with food-sourced or encapsulated prebiotics[7] and probiotics is worth considering as a safe and potentially useful strategy in this population. Microbiome changes also affect cognitive and mood function in the central nervous system via the gut-brain axis.

Renal

Acute kidney injury during the infectious stage may result in longer-term decreases in glomerular filtration rate and other renal parameters. This is likely to be worse in those already at risk with existing chronic kidney disease, diabetes, or hypertension. Nephrology consultation should be sought in appropriate cases.

Endocrine

Loss of control of diabetes and even diabetic ketoacidosis has been observed after resolution of acute COVID-19 symptoms, sometimes weeks or months later. New cases of prediabetes and diabetes types 1 and 2 have been reported. COVID-19 may also activate latent autoimmune thyroid disease, resulting in thyroiditis or thyrotoxicosis in the aftermath and resolution of respiratory disease. Risks for osteoporosis may also increase as a result of a multiplicity of factors such as immobilization, inflammation, steroid use, and other lifestyle or dietary factors. Weight gain and inactivity during lockdowns contributed to these conditions as well.

Being alert to the potential for the development or exacerbation of endocrinologic issues will enhance the healthcare provider's ability to respond quickly and appropriately when managing these patients.

Dermatologic

There is broad range of dermatologic presentations that include rash, chilblains, urticaria, and "COVID-toe," but they are usually self-limiting and not prolonged. They are treated with topical steroids, antihistamines, or oral steroids. Hair loss (telogen effluvium) is a particularly distressing problem from COVID and must be addressed for its emotional and cosmetic impact. It may be short-lived, but if prolonged it must be part of a holistic program of care including dermatologic consultation, particularly if there is an ongoing autoimmune or inflammatory etiology.

Monitoring

Supportive and rehabilitative care are still the mainstay of treatment for post-acute COVID syndrome. This includes adequate rest, nutrition, immune support, activity modification, mental and cognitive stimulation, stress management, and heart and lung rehabilitation, including supplemental oxygen for some patients. Utilizing standard and evidenced treatments for lung, heart, neurologic, and renal problems is a logical start. Given protracted and relapsing symptoms, it is important to reassure patients that most cases will recover with time and supportive symptomatic care. Registries and post-COVID clinics are needed to track and manage these serious sequelae of COVID-19. Our awareness is the first line of defense. The diffuse and protean manifestations of PCS should motivate our clinicians and medical educators to include it in the differential diagnosis of many other presenting complaints.

Multidisciplinary teams are key to long-term management but are not always easily accessible. Self-care, online, and other forms of support groups have sprung up widely for emotional, social support and peer-led practical advice in managing post-acute COVID syndrome. Much of the knowledge about this syndrome has been brought to public and professional awareness by such peer groups. Further research support in this area will be helpful.

Quality-of-care principles for long-haul COVID include providing access to care, reducing the burden of illness, taking clinical responsibility, offering continuity of care, providing multidisciplinary rehabilitation, conducting evidence-based investigation and management, and continuing further research and development on appropriate and evidence-based clinical services. Given the disproportionate impact of COVID on communities of color, additional attention must be given to social determinants of health, healthcare access, and enhanced research efforts regarding the genetic and racial differences in disease impact, both acute and long-term. Determining phenotypic differences in susceptibility to post-acute COVID syndrome and personalized rehabilitation are key future directions.

Complications

Understanding of COVID-19 and its potential long-term complications is evolving and offers many opportunities for clinicians and researchers to examine. As with COVID-19 infection itself, long-term complications may broadly affect multiple body systems. Addressing these symptoms starts with recognition.

One persistent neurologic complication that remains of concern is cognitive decline, which many describe as "brain fog." Additional symptoms of neuropathic pain and headaches may require further evaluation by a neurologist.

Myocardial inflammation seen in some COVID-19 infections may lead to future reduced cardiac function, arrhythmias, scarring, or cardiomyopathy. The prevalence currently remains unknown but is a major concern in our younger population and athletes.

Pulmonary complications are common in hospitalized patients who require ventilatory assistance. Our experience in the post-COVID population shows that fibrotic conversion, if it occurs, is rare, but reduction in diffusion capacity may persist. This reduction is a sign of parenchymal disease and should be monitored if patients develop future reductions in lung volumes compared with the standard population.

Hematologic complications such as thrombosis and long-term risk remain unknown, and further study is necessary. For example, it is unknown whether COVID-19 and a thrombosis can be safely considered a short-term event and managed as a provoked clot or if there is a prolonged inflammatory cascade that leaves a sustained risk.

The behavioral health component also remains of utmost importance because so much is not known, and the duration of symptoms is not clear. Management of PTSD, anxiety, and depression for patients with long-term complications should be included in strategies addressing the care of this new and ever-growing at-risk population.

---

[1] Not FDA approved for this indication.
[7] Available as dietary supplement.

Acknowledgment

We wish to thank Ms. Julie Trumble of the University of Texas Medical Branch Moody Medical Library for her incredibly diligent work on helping us assemble and keep updated on the literature on this evolving topic with weekly literature reviews in the past year.

References

Alwan NA: Surveillance is underestimating the burden of the COVID-19 pandemic, *Lancet* 396(10252):e24, 2020.

Barker-Davies RM, O'Sullivan O, Senaratne KPP, et al: The Stanford Hall consensus statement for post-COVID-19 rehabilitation, *Br J Sports Med* 54(16):949–959, 2020.

Calabrese M, Garofano M, Palumbo R, et al: Exercise training and cardiac rehabilitation in COVID-19 patients with cardiovascular complications: state of art, *Life (Basel)* 11(3):259, 2021.

Centers for Disease Control and Prevention. Post COVID Conditions. https://www.cdc.gov/coronavirus/2019-ncov/hcp/clinical-care/post-covid-conditions.html. Accessed 3/12/22.

COVID-19 rapid guideline: managing the long-term effects of COVID-19, London, 2020, National Institute for Health and Care Excellence (UK).

Crook H, Raza S, Nowell J, Young M, Edison P: Long covid—mechanisms, risk factors, and management—state of the art review, *BMJ* 374:n1648, 2021, https://doi.org/10.1136/bmj.n1648.

Dani M, Dirksen A, Taraborrelli P, et al: Autonomic dysfunction in 'long COVID': rationale, physiology and management strategies, *Clin Med (Lond)* 21(1):e63–e67.d, 2021.

Flottorp A, Brurber K, Fink P, Knoops H, Wyller V: New NICE guideline on chronic fatigue syndrome: more ideology than science? *Lancet* 399(Feb 12):611–613, 2022. https://www.thelancet.com/journals/lancet/article/PIIS0140-6736(22)00183-0/fulltext.

Greenhalgh T, Knight M, A'Court C, Buxton M, Husain L: Management of post-acute covid-19 in primary care, *BMJ* 370:m3026, 2020.

Logue JK, Franko NM, McCulloch DJ, et al: Sequelae in Adults at 6 Months after COVID-19 infection, *JAMA Netw Open* 4(2):e210830, 2021.

Mahase E: Long covid could be four different syndromes, review suggests, *BMJ* 371:m3981, 2020.

Mendelson M, Nel J, Blumberg L, et al: Long-COVID: an evolving problem with an extensive impact, *S Afr Med J* 111(1):10–12, 2020.

Nabavi N: Long covid: How to define it and how to manage it, *BMJ* 370:m3489, 2020.

Nalbandian A, Sehgal K, Gupta A, et al. Post-acute COVID-19 syndrome. *Nature Medicine*. Available at https://doi.org/10.1038/s41591-021-1283-z

NIHR Themed Review, Living with Covid19. 2020:1-29.

PSITTACOSIS

Method of
Christopher C. McGuigan, MBChB, MPH

CURRENT DIAGNOSIS

- The key to successful management of psittacosis is to consider this diagnosis, particularly in cases of community-acquired pneumonia (CAP), especially given a history of bird contact.
- The typical clinical pictures are of CAP, influenza-like illness, or fever of unknown origin. Psittacosis causes 1% of incident CAP cases. Onset is usually sudden with fever, chills and a prominent headache. Consider this diagnosis in a patient with CAP unresponsive to β-lactam antibiotics.
- Investigation will typically reveal a normal or slightly elevated white blood cell count with a left shift or toxic changes, increase in C-reactive protein (CRP) or erythrocyte sedimentation rate (ESR), mildly abnormal liver function tests, hyponatremia, and mild renal impairment. Chest x-ray may be more abnormal than examination alone would predict.
- Diagnosis can be confirmed with (ideally) paired serum samples: using either the complement fixation test (widely used but unable to differentiate between *Chamydophila* species), or the microimmunofluorescence test, which is specific for individual *Chamydophila* species. Either a single high titer or a fourfold rise in titer using samples collected at least 14 days apart are interpreted as positive. More recently, real-time polymerase chain reaction (rt-PCR) tests are used to detect specific DNA. These can provide a more rapid diagnosis, as well as subspecific genotype.

CURRENT THERAPY

- Therapy should commence when the diagnosis is suspected on clinical presentation and initial investigation.
- Tetracyclines are the drugs of choice; for example, doxycycline (Vibramycin) 100 mg bid for 10 to 14 days.
- Macrolides are suitable (but probably less effective) alternatives in those intolerant of tetracyclines (e.g., children and pregnant women).
- Notification to health authorities facilitates public health investigation and interventions to reduce transmission and control outbreaks.

Psittacosis is caused by infection with the bacterium *Chlamydophila psittaci* (formerly *Chlamydia psittaci*). It is twice as common in men than in women, and mainly affects adults typically aged 40 to 50 years. The main reservoir for psittacosis is birds, particularly psittacine birds (parrots, parakeets, budgerigars and cockatoos), but other bird species and mammals can be infected.

Risk Factors

The most common etiological factor is exposure to infected birds—especially a new, sick, or dead one—typically a pet or via occupational exposure (e.g., work as a veterinarian, zoo keeper, or poultry-worker). Most cases are sporadic, but outbreaks have occurred associated with pet shops, aviaries, and poultry-processing plants and with mowing lawns in areas with large numbers of psittacine birds. Person-to-person transmission is rare. Ingestion of poultry products is *not* a risk factor.

Pathophysiology

C psittaci infection is via the respiratory tract and is typically thought to be by inhalation of an aerosol of dried feces or other avian secretion. It then either travels via the blood to the liver and spleen (where it replicates, causing a secondary bacteremia) or directly infects respiratory epithelial cells.

Prevention

Prevention is aimed at controlling disease or colonization in susceptible host species: usually birds. This is facilitated by import restrictions including quarantine and treatment of suspected infections with tetracycline-impregnated feeds. Notification of health authorities is important for initiating public health investigations and interventions to reduce transmission and control of outbreaks.

Clinical Manifestations

The incubation period varies from 4 to 14 or more days. The typical presentation of psittacosis is of an influenza-like illness with sudden onset of fever, chills, and prominent headache, with or without rigors. A more gradual onset is also seen. A typically mild, dry cough usually starts later. There may also be diarrhea, pharyngitis, altered mental state, or shortness of breath. Chest examination is usually abnormal, but the findings are often minimal and less prominent than symptoms or x-ray findings would suggest. Pleural effusion is rare.

Patients might present with a fever of unknown origin without obvious respiratory involvement, or the disease can be misdiagnosed as meningitis because of prominent headache, sometimes with photophobia.

The white blood cell count is usually normal or slightly raised, but there is often a left shift or toxic changes. Increases in the C-reactive protein (CRP) and erythrocyte sedimentation rate (ESR) are common. Mildly abnormal liver function tests, hyponatraemia, and mild renal impairment are also common. The cerebrospinal fluid sometimes contains a few mononuclear cells but is otherwise normal. The chest x-ray usually shows more (nonspecific) abnormality than examination findings might predict. The most common finding is lobar consolidation, but bilateral consolidation and interstitial opacities are also common.

Confirmation of diagnosis is more commonly performed using serology. The complement fixation (CF) test is widely used, but cannot differentiate between *Chlamydophila* species. A fourfold rise in titer, using samples collected at least 14 days apart, or a single titer of 1:128 or higher, is interpreted as positive, but this test is not widely available. Culture of C *psittaci* is difficult and hazardous. Polymerase chain reaction (PCR) assays have been developed, but are not yet widely available for routine clinical use.

Diagnosis

Diagnosis is facilitated by eliciting a history of recent bird contact from a patient with a compatible clinical syndrome, most commonly an influenza-like presentation, community acquired pneumonia (CAP), or a fever of unknown origin. The diagnosis should be considered in a patient with CAP and prominent headache, splenomegaly, or failure to respond to β-lactam antibiotics.

Differential Diagnosis

Differential diagnosis of an atypical CAP, includes infection with *Legionella* species, *Mycoplasma pneumoniae,* or *Chlamydophila pneumoniae.*

Treatment

When the diagnosis is suspected on clinical presentation and initial investigations, empiric therapy should be commenced. Tetracyclines are the drugs of choice, for example doxycycline (Vibramycin) 100 mg bid for 10 to 14 days. Tetracycline treatment usually leads to improvement in symptoms (including fever) within 24 to 48 hours. Macrolides are usually recommended for pregnant women, children, and other patients intolerant of tetracyclines. However, erythromycin (Erythrocin)[1] has been shown to fail in situations where a tetracycline was effective, and there are few clinical data on the efficacy of the other agents in this class. Some data suggest that quinolones may be effective. Tetracycline hydrochloride or doxycycline (4.4 mg/kg/d divided into two infusions) may be given intravenously for critically ill patients.

Monitoring

Symptomatic improvement usually occurs within 24 to 48 hours of starting a tetracycline; typically including reduction of fever.

Complications

The degree of illness varies from asymptomatic to life threatening. Given appropriate antimicrobial therapy, subsequent case-fatality is less than 1%. Elderly persons and pregnant women are susceptible to more severe illness. Neurologic consequences (e.g., meningo-encephalitis) are recognized but rare. Other less-common sequellae include hemoptysis, proteinuria, hepato-splenomegaly, and encephalitis. Cardiac manifestations include relative bradycardia and, rarely, myocarditis, culture-negative endocarditis, and pericarditis. Erythema nodosum and other skin manifestations have also been described. C *psittaci* has been demonstrated by PCR to be present in ocular adnexal lymphoma (OAL) in parts of Eurasia. Up to one half of such cases respond to antibiotic treatment. However, studies elsewhere suggest that this organism might not commonly play a role in OAL. Recovery with minimal residual deficit is normal.

---

[1]Not FDA approved for this indication.

References

Contini C, Seraceni S, Carradori S, et al: Identification of *Chlamydia trachomatis* in a patient with ocular lymphoma, *Am J Hematol* 84:597–599, 2009.

Grayston JT, Thom DH: The chlamydial pneumonias, *Curr Clin Top Infect Dis* 11:1–18, 1991.

Heddema ER, Beld MG, De Wever B, et al: Development of an internally controlled real-time PCR assay for detection of *Chlamydophila psittaci* in the LightCycler 2.0 system, *Clin Microbiol Infect* 12:571–575, 2006.

Hogerwerf L, DE Gier B, Baan B, Van Der Hoek W: Chlamydia psittaci (psittacosis) as a cause of community-acquired pneumonia: a systematic review and meta-analysis. [Review], *Epidemiol Infect* 145(15):3096–3105, 2017.

Hughes P, Chidley K, Cowie J: Neurological complications in psittacosis: a case report and literature review, *Respir Med* 89:637–638, 1995.

National Association of State Public Health Veterinarians. Compendium of measures to control *Chlamydophila psittaci* infection among humans (psittacosis) and pet birds (avian chlamydiosis), 2010. Available at: http://www.nasphv.org/Documents/Psittacosis.pdf [accessed July 9, 2015].

Richards M. Psittacosis, Up to date 2006; Available at http://www.uptodate.com/physicians/pulmonology_toclist.asp [accessed 31.12.12; subscription required].

Wallensten A, Fredlund H, Runehagen A: Multiple human–to–human transmission from a severe case of psittacosis, Sweden, January–February 2013, *Euro Surveill* 19(42):20937, 2014.

Williams J, Tallis G, Dalton C, et al: Community outbreak of psittacosis in a rural Australian town, *Lancet* 351:1697–1699, 1998.

Yung AP, Grayson ML: Psittacosis: a review of 135 cases, *Med J Aust* 148:228–233, 1988.

Q FEVER

Method of
Didier Raoult, MD, PhD

Q fever is a widespread zoonosis caused by *Coxiella burnetii*, a small, coccoid, strict intracellular gram-negative bacterium. It lives within the phagolysosome of its eukaryotic host cell at very low pH (4.5–4.8). It had previously been classified in the rickettsial family; however, recent phylogenic data based on study of the 16S rRNA gene sequence have shown that it belongs to *Legionellales* with the *Legionella* species and *Francisella tularensis*.

The bacterium has a sporelike life cycle, which explains its marked resistance to physicochemical agents. In cultures, *C. burnetii* exhibits a phase variation (from virulent phase I to avirulent phase II) caused by a spontaneous chromosome deletion. The avirulent form paradoxically generates high antibody levels in patients, but only patients with chronic infection have high antiphase I immunoglobulin G (IgG) and IgA antibody titers.

The reservoir of *C. burnetii* is wide, and nearly all tested mammals, birds, and ticks can be infected. Outbreaks have also been reported in association with the birth products of mammals (including ungulates and pets), raw milk, slaughterhouses, and farm work. Laboratory outbreaks have been reported. The disease is prevalent everywhere in the world but in New Zealand and South Pacific Islands, but because its clinical spectrum is wide and nonspecific, the observed incidence is directly related to physician interest in Q fever. A recent outbreak has been observed in the Netherlands.

Clinical Features

Q fever is a reportable disease in the United States. In humans, infection is symptomatic in only 50% of patients. Most symptomatic patients experience a flulike syndrome lasting 2 to 7 days and consisting of severe headaches and cough; 5% to 10% of infected patients may be sick enough to be investigated. They initially have high fever and one or several of pneumonia, hepatitis, meningoencephalitis, rash, myocarditis, and pericarditis. Routine laboratory investigation commonly shows mildly elevated transaminase levels and mild thrombocytopenia. The local strain may influence the clinical manifestations. In French Guyana, the disease is more commonly symptomatic and severe.

In special hosts such as immunocompromised patients (specifically those with splenectomy), *C. burnetii* can cause endocarditis. In pregnant women it can lead to recurrent miscarriage, low-birth-weight offspring, and prematurity. *C. burnetii* could contribute to the evolution of lymphoma.

In patients with valvular heart disease and those with arterial aneurysms or a vascular prosthesis, it can cause chronic endocarditis or vascular infection in patients in the 2 years following primary infection. The clinical picture is that of a chronic blood culture–negative endocarditis; the modified Duke criteria are of diagnostic value in such cases. It is spontaneously fatal in most cases. Recently, acute endocarditis associated with anticardiolipin antibodies was described. Criteria specifically adapted to Q fever may be used to diagnosed focalized infections. This denomination appears to be more appropriate than "chronic Q fever."

Diagnosis

Because Q fever is pleomorphic, the diagnosis is based mainly on comprehensive serum testing in patients with an unexplained infectious syndrome. Liver biopsy may be of diagnostic value, because the typical doughnut granuloma is quasispecific to acute Q fever. Valves obtained at surgery or autopsy can be used for culture, direct immunostaining, and polymerase chain reaction (PCR).

Three serologic techniques are used. Complement fixation lacks sensitivity, and one-third of patients with acute Q fever do not exhibit complement-fixing antibodies within 1 month after onset of the disease. However, a fourfold increase in antibodies to phase II antigen indicates acute Q fever, and antibody levels against phase I that are higher than 1:200 indicate persistent focalized Q fever. Indirect immunofluorescence assay is the reference method. A single titer of 1:200 for IgG antiphase II associated with a titer of 1:50 for IgM is diagnostic of acute infection. IgG antibody levels against phase I that are greater than 1:800 and IgA antibody levels greater than 1:50 are highly predictive of endocarditis or vascular infection. Enzyme-linked immunosorbent assay (ELISA) is useful for diagnosing acute infection in detecting IgM antiphase II.

PCR has recently been developed to detect *C. burnetii* DNA in the sera of patients with Q fever. Real-time PCR using multicopy gene *IS1111* is the more-sensitive technique. It is positive in the sera of patients with acute Q fever before IgG antibodies to *C. burnetii* become apparent. It is also positive in patients with untreated endocarditis. Contamination of PCR can occur, and many unconfirmed results are reported in the literature. Detection of patients at risk for endocarditis may be provided by systematic echocardiography in patients with acute Q fever specifically seeking for aortic bicuspidy and serologic follow-up at 3 and 6 months after acute infection. Antiphospholipid antibodies are relatively common during acute Q fever and predictive of endocarditis and deep vein thrombosis.

Use of a positron emission tomography (PET) scanner may help in the diagnosis of endocarditis (and may reveal mycotic aneurisms), vascular infection, and joint infection.

Treatment

To be active against Q fever, an antibiotic compound has to enter the cell, be effective at an acidic pH (where *C. burnetii* multiplies), and have activity against *C. burnetii*. No antibiotic is bactericidal, but bactericidal activity can be achieved by the addition of hydroxychloroquine (Plaquenil)[1] to doxycycline (Vibramycin).

For acute Q fever, the reference treatment is doxycycline 100 mg orally twice daily for 2 to 3 weeks. Other compounds have been reported to be effective, such as trimethoprim-sulfamethoxazole (TMP-SMX) (Bactrim)[1], Rifampin (Rifadin)[1] 300 mg twice daily, and ofloxacin (Floxin)[1] 200 mg twice daily. In the case of Q fever in pregnant women, one double-strength TMP-SMX tablet (trimethoprim 160 mg, sulfamethoxazole 800 mg)[1] twice daily until delivery prevents fetal death (Table 1). Patients with acute Q fever and high antiphospholipid antibodies may be treated with hydroxychloroquine[1] until normalization.

---

[1] Not FDA approved for this indication.

TABLE 1	Treatment	
Q FEVER	**RECOMMENDED TREATMENT**	**ALTERNATIVE TREATMENT**
Acute	Doxycycline (Vibramicyn) 100 mg PO q12h × 14 d	Ofloxacin (Floxin)[1] 200 mg PO q8h[3] × 14 d Cotrimoxazole (Bactrim)[1] 160/800 mg/PO q12h × 14 d
Acute Q fever with high antiphospholipid antibodies	Hydroxychloroquine (Plaquenil)[1] 200 mg PO q8h as long as high antiphospholipid antibodies persist	
Endocarditis	Doxycycline 100 mg PO q12h *plus* hydroxychloroquine (Plaquenil)[1] 200 mg PO q8h[3] × 18–24 mo	Doxycycline 100 mg PO q12h *plus* ofloxacin[1] 200 mg PO q8h[3] for 3 y to lifetime
Acute in a patient with a valvular lesion	Same as chronic Q fever for 12 mo	
In pregnancy	Trimethoprim/ Sulfamethoxazole (Bactrim)[1] 160/800 mg PO q12h until term	

[1] Not FDA approved for this indication.
[3] Exceeds dosage recommended by the manufacturer.

Persistent focalized and acute endocarditis should be treated for 18 months to 2 years, and antibody levels should be monitored. Patients with prosthetic valves may be treated for 2 years. Two protocols have been evaluated: doxycycline 200 mg daily combined with ofloxacin[1] 400 mg daily for 4 years to lifetime, and doxycycline combined with hydroxychloroquine[1] for 1.5 to 2 years in an amount to achieve a 1 ± 0.20 µg/mL plasma concentration. Doxycycline serum levels greater than 4.5 µg/mL are associated with a more rapidly favorable outcome. This last regimen is apparently more efficacious in terms of relapse. However, regular ophthalmologic surveillance is critical to detect the accumulation of chloroquine in the retina. Both regimens expose the patient to a major risk of photosensitization.

The combination of doxycycline and hydroxychloroquine for 1 year has demonstrated efficacy in preventing endocarditis. Patients with high-level antiphospholipid antibodies may be treated by the same treatment until normalization of the antibody level.

Prevention

Prevention depends on avoiding exposure, particularly by pregnant women and patients with valvulopathy. No vaccine is currently available outside Australia.

---

[1] Not FDA approved for this indication.

References

Eldin C, Melenotte C, Mediannikov O, et al: From Q fever to *Coxiella burnetii* infection: a paradigm shange, *Clin Microbiol Rev* 30:115–190, 2017.

Klee SR, et al: Highly sensitive real-time PCR for specific detection and quantification of Coxiella burnetii, *BMC Microbiol* 19:2, 2006.

Maurin M, Raoult D: Q fever, *Clin Microbiol Rev* 12:518–553, 1999.

Merhej V, Cammilleri S, Piquet P, et al: Relevance of the positron emission tomography in the diagnosis of vascular graft infection with *Coxiella burnetii*, *Comp Immunol Microbiol Infect Dis* 35(1):45–49, 2012.

Melenotte C, Epelboin L, Million M, et al: Acute Q fever endocarditis: a paradigm shift following the systematic use of transthoracic echocardiography during acute Q fever, *Clin Infect Dis* 13;69(11):1987-1995, 2019.

Million M, Bardin N, Bessis S, et al: Thrombosis and antiphospholipid antibody syndrome during acute Q fever: a cross-sectional study, *Medicine (Baltimore).* 96(29):e7578, 2017 Jul.

Million M, Roblot F, Carles D, et al: Reevaluation of the risk of fetal death and malformation after Q fever, *Clin Infect Dis* 59(2):256–260, 2014.

Million M, Thuny F, Richet H, Raoult D: Long-term outcome of Q fever endocarditis: a 26-year personal survey, *Lancet Infect Dis* 10:527–535, 2010.

Million M, Walter G, Thuny F, et al: Evolution from acute Q fever to endocarditis is associated with underlying valvulopathy and age and can be prevented by prolonged antibiotic treatment, *Clin Infect Dis* 57(6):836–844, 2013.

Raoult D: Chronic Q fever: expert opinion versus literature analysis and consensus, *J Infect* 65:102–108, 2012.

Rolain JM, Maurin M, Raoult D: Bacteriostatic and bactericidal activities of moxifloxacin against Coxiella burnetii, *Antimicrob Agents Chemother* 45:301–302, 2001.

RABIES

Method of
Alan C. Jackson, MD

CURRENT DIAGNOSIS

- A history of animal bite or exposure is often absent in rabies acquired in North America.
- Pain, paresthesias, and pruritus are early neurologic symptoms of rabies, probably reflecting infection in local sensory ganglia.
- Autonomic features are common including hypersalivation, gooseflesh, cardiac arrhythmias, and priapism.
- Hydrophobia is a highly specific feature of rabies.
- Paralytic features may be prominent, and the clinical presentation can resemble that of Guillain-Barré syndrome.
- Saliva samples for reverse transcription polymerase chain reaction (RT-PCR) and a skin biopsy should be obtained to detect rabies virus antigen or RNA to make a laboratory diagnosis of rabies.

CURRENT THERAPY

Rabies Prophylaxis

Details of an exposure determine whether postexposure rabies prophylaxis should be initiated.

- Wound cleansing is important after potential rabies exposure.
- Active immunization with a schedule of four doses of rabies vaccine (RabAvert or Imovax Rabies) at intervals is recommended. The four-dose series is a new Centers for Disease Control and Prevention (CDC) recommendation and is not yet reflected in the package insert, which calls for five doses.
- Passive immunization (if previously the patient was not immunized) consists of infiltrating human rabies immune globulin (HyperRAB, Imogam Rabies, or KamRAB) into the wound, with the remainder of the 20 IU/kg dosage given intramuscularly.

Rabies Cases

- There is no established effective therapy for rabies, but there is an increasing number of survivors who received supportive care in critical care units, particularly in India.
- Palliation is important for many fatal cases of rabies.

Rabies is an acute infection of the nervous system caused by rabies virus, which is a member of the family Rhabdoviridae in the genus *Lyssavirus*. Other lyssaviruses have only very rarely caused rabies in locations outside of the Americas.

Pathogenesis

Rabies virus is usually transmitted by bites from rabid animals. Transmission has rarely occurred through an aerosol route (in a laboratory accident or in a cave containing millions of bats) or by transplantation of infected organs or tissues (e.g., corneas). The virus is in the saliva of the rabid animal and is inoculated into subcutaneous tissues or muscles via a bite.

During most of the long incubation period (lasting 20–90 days or longer), the virus is close to the site of inoculation. The virus binds to the nicotinic acetylcholine receptor at the postsynaptic neuromuscular junction and travels toward the central nervous system (CNS) in peripheral nerves by retrograde fast axonal transport. There is rapid dissemination throughout the CNS by fast axonal transport. Under natural conditions, degenerative neuronal changes are not prominent, and it is thought that the rabies virus induces neuronal dysfunction by mechanisms that are not well understood. Oxidative stress due to mitochondrial dysfunction is thought to play an important role. In rabies vectors, the encephalitis is associated with behavioral changes that lead to transmission by biting. After the CNS infection is established, the virus spreads by autonomic and sensory nerves to multiple organs, including the salivary glands of rabies vectors in which the virus is secreted in saliva.

Clinical Features

In North America, where the bat is the most common rabies vector for human disease, a history of an animal bite is often absent, and there may be no known contact with animals. The incubation period is usually between 20 and 90 days, but it rarely lasts 1 year or longer. Prodromal features are nonspecific and include malaise, headache, and fever, and patients can also have anxiety or agitation. Approximately half of patients experience pain, paresthesias, or pruritus at the site of the wound, which has often healed, and these symptoms likely reflect infection and inflammation involving local sensory ganglia. Approximately 80% of patients with rabies have encephalitic rabies; approximately 20% have paralytic rabies.

In encephalitic rabies, there are characteristic periods of generalized arousal or hyperexcitability separated by lucid periods. Autonomic dysfunction is common and includes hypersalivation, gooseflesh, cardiac arrhythmias, and priapism. Hydrophobia is the most characteristic feature of rabies and occurs in 50% to 80% of patients; contractions of the diaphragm and other inspiratory muscles occur on swallowing. This can become a conditioned reflex, and even the sight or thought of water can precipitate the muscle contractions. Hydrophobia is thought to be caused by inhibition of inspiratory neurons near the nucleus ambiguus.

In paralytic rabies, prominent muscle weakness usually begins in the bitten extremity and progresses to quadriparesis; typically there is sphincter involvement. Patients have a longer clinical course than in encephalitic rabies. Paralytic rabies is often misdiagnosed as Guillain-Barré syndrome.

Coma subsequently develops in both clinical forms. With aggressive medical therapy, a variety of medical complications develop, and multiple organ failure is common. Survival is very rare and has usually occurred in the context of incomplete postexposure rabies prophylaxis that included administration of one or more doses of rabies vaccine.

Epidemiology

Worldwide about 60,000 human deaths per year are attributed to rabies. The impact is particularly significant in terms of years of life lost because children are commonly the victims. Most human rabies cases occur through transmission from dogs in developing countries with endemic dog rabies, particularly in Asia and Africa. Travelers to endemic regions may develop rabies after they return home if they have not received effective postexposure rabies prophylaxis after an exposure. In the United States and Canada, transmission of rabies virus occurs most commonly in human cases from insect-eating bats, and often there is no known history of a bat bite or exposure to bats.

cannot be grown using synthetic media, and thus microbiologic diagnosis rests on visualization of these organisms in infected tissues.

Diagnosis

Diagnosis is difficult and requires a high clinical index of suspicion. The initial symptoms of rat-bite fever are nonspecific, triggering a broad differential diagnosis. Additionally, the fastidious nature of this organism makes isolation from blood cultures difficult. Clinicians should ask about rodent exposure when compatible symptoms are seen in patients. Rat-bite fever should not be ruled out in the absence of bite history, because transmission can occur without a bite, and pet owners or laboratory workers can minimize the significance of the bite, especially in the absence of a local reaction.

No reliable serologic test is available, and the definitive diagnosis requires isolation of *S moniliformis* from the wound, blood, or synovial fluid in patients with septic arthritis. The microbiology laboratory should be specifically notified of any clinical suspicion to enhance the chances of recovering the pathogen.

S moniliformis is a highly pleomorphic, nonencapsulated, nonmotile, gram-negative rod, which can stain positively on Gram stain (Figure 1). It is often dismissed as proteinaceous debris because of its numerous bulbous swellings with occasional clumping (*moniliformis*="necklace-like"). It grows slowly and requires a microaerophilic environment with 5% to 10% CO_2 or anaerobic conditions and media supplementation with 20% normal rabbit serum. Cultures can take up to 7 days to turn positive. Some experts recommend holding blood cultures for 21 days to permit sufficient time to grow this organism. *S moniliformis* is also inhibited by sodium polyanethol sulfonate, a common adjunct in most commercial blood culture media at a concentration as low as 0.0125%. *S moniliformis* has been identified using polymerase chain reaction amplification and 16S ribosomal ribonucleic acid (rRNA) sequencing, which shows great promise though it is available at reference laboratories. Fatty acid profiles obtained by gas-liquid chromatography can also be used for identification.

S minus, the other etiologic agent of rat-bite fever, is a short, thick, gram-negative, tightly coiled spiral rod that measures 0.2 to 0.5 μm and has two to six helical turns.

Differential Diagnosis

Differential diagnosis for fever, rash, and polyarthritis is broad. Malaria, typhoid fever, and neoplastic disease can cause relapsing fevers, and the presence of a rash and polyarthritis might suggest viral and rickettsial diseases including Rocky Mountain spotted fever. An asymmetric oligoarthritis suggests disseminated gonococcal and meningococcal diseases in the context of cutaneous lesions on the palms and soles. Lyme disease, leptospirosis, or secondary syphilis can have a similar clinical presentation. Finally, when classic infectious symptoms such as fever or rash are missing, any causes of polyarthritis, from crystal-induced arthropathies to rheumatoid arthritis, should be considered.

Treatment

All established cases of rat-bite fever should be treated with antibiotics because of the associated mortality and potential for complications. Intravenous penicillin G at a dose of 1.2 million units per day should be initiated as soon as the clinical diagnosis is made. Empiric therapy is necessary and should not be delayed for laboratory confirmation of this bacterial infection. The intravenous treatment should continue for 5 to 7 days. After treatment with IV penicillin and suitable clinical response, therapy should be continued with oral penicillin (PenVK)[1] or ampicillin (Omnipen)[1] at a dose of 500 mg qid for an additional 7 days. For patients allergic to penicillin, intravenous doxycycline (Vibramycin)[1] at a dose of 100 mg every 12 hours or oral tetracycline (Achromycin)[1] at a dose of 500 mg four times a day can be used.

Streptomycin[1] and cephalosporins including cefotamxine (Claforan)[1] have been reported to be potentially useful. Other antibiotics including azithromycin (Zithromax),[1] erythromycin,[1] carbapenems,[1] aztreonam (Azactam),[1] clindamycin (Cleocin),[1] vancomycin (Vancocin),[1] and nitrofurantoin (Macrodantin)[1] have shown efficacy in vitro, but they lack good clinical correlation to recommend them for routine use. Erythromycin has been associated with treatment failures. Trimethoprim-sulfamethoxazole (Bactrim),[1] polymyxin B,[1] gentamicin (Garamycin),[1] tobramycin (Nebcin),[1] ciprofloxacin (Cipro),[1] and levofloxacin (Levaquin)[1] should not be used because in vitro resistance has been demonstrated.

Typically, the bite site heals promptly. It should be cleaned and disinfected, as is typical for management of other wounds. Tetanus prophylaxis (tetanus-diphtheria toxoids, Td) administration is indicated as required by the patient's immunization record. Rabies prophylaxis (Imovax Rabies) is usually not required for rodent bite, but consultation with local public health authorities is encouraged. There are no reports of transmission of the rabies virus from rats to humans.

[1]Not FDA approved for this indication.

Figure 1 Gram stain of *Streptobacillus moniliformis*. Gram stain of growth from anaerobic bottle, ×100 magnification [microphotography]. Reprinted with permission from Partners' Infectious Disease Images; accessed on August 11, 2016, from http://www.idimages.org/images/detail/?imageid=373.

References

Abusalameh M, Mahankali-Rao P, Earl S, et al: Discitis caused by rat bite fever in a rheumatoid arthritis patient on tocilizumab-first ever case, *Rheumatology (Oxford)* 57:1118–1120, 2018.

Adam JK, et al: Notes from the field: fatal rat-bite Fever in a child - San Diego County, California, 2013, *MMWR Morb Mortal Wkly Rep* 63(50):1210–1211, 2014.

Chen PL, Lee NY, Yan JJ, et al: Prosthetic valve endocarditis caused by *Streptobacillus moniliformis*: A case of rat bite fever, *J Clin Microbiol* 45:3125–3126, 2007.

Crews JD, Palazzi DL, Starke JR: A teenager with fever, rash, and arthralgia. *Streptobacillus moniliformis* infection, *JAMA Pediatr* 168(12):1165–1166, 2014.

Elliott SP: Rat bite fever and *Streptobacillus moniliformis*, *Clin Microbiol Rev* 20:13–22, 2007.

Fenn DW, et al: An unusual tale of rat-bite fever endocarditis, *BMJ Case Rep.* 2014, 2014.

Gaastra W, Boot R, Ho HT, Lipman LJ: Rat bite fever, *Vet Microbiol* 133:211–228, 2009.

Giorgiutti S, Lefebvre N: Rat bite fever, *N Engl J Med* 381(18):1762, 2019.

Graves MH, Janda JM: Rat-bite fever (*Streptobacillus moniliformis*): A potential emerging disease, *Int J Infect Dis* 5:151–155, 2001.

Holroyd KJ, Reiner AP, Dick JD: *Streptobacillus moniliformis* polyarthritis mimicking rheumatoid arthritis: An urban case of rat bite fever, *Am J Med* 85:711–714, 1988.

King HY. Rat Bite Fever. UpToDate. http://www.uptodate.com/contents/rat-bitefever; [accessed April 21, 2018].

Lambe DW Jr, McPhedran AM, Mertz JA, Stewart P: *Streptobacillus moniliformis* isolated from a case of Haverhill fever: Biochemical characterization and inhibitory effect of sodium polyanethol sulfonate, *Am J Clin Pathol* 60:854–860, 1973.

Miura Y, Nei T, Saito R, Sato A, Sonobe K, Takahashi K: Streptobacillus moniliformis bacteremia in a rheumatoid arthritis patient without a rat bite: a case report, *BMC Res Notes* 8(1):694, 2005 Nov 19, https://doi.org/10.1186/s13104-015-1642-6.

Schachter ME, Wilcox L, Rau N, et al: Rat-bite fever, Canada, *Emerg Infect Dis* 12:1301–1302, 2006.

Stehle P, Dubuis O, So A, Dudler J: Rat bite fever without fever, *Ann Rheum Dis* 62:894–896, 2003.

Torres-Miranda D, Moshgriz M, Siegel M: Streptobacillus moniliformis mitral valve endocarditis and septic arthritis: the challenges of diagnosing rat-bite fever endocarditis, *Infect Dis Rep* 10(2):7731, 2018.

Washburn RG: Streptobacillus moniliformis (rat–bite fever). In Mandell GL, Bennett JE, Dolin R, editors: *Principles and Practice of Infectious Diseases*, vol 2, 6th ed, Philadelphia, 2005, Elsevier, pp 2708–2710.

RELAPSING FEVER

Method of
Diego Cadavid, MD

CURRENT DIAGNOSIS

- There are two forms of relapsing fever: epidemic and endemic.
- Epidemic relapsing fever is transmitted from person to person by the body louse *Pediculus humanus*.
- Endemic relapsing fever is transmitted from rodent reservoirs to humans exposed to endemic areas by soft-bodied ticks of the genus *Ornithodoros*.
- The hallmark of relapsing fever is two or more febrile episodes separated by periods of relative well-being.
- The diagnosis is confirmed by visualization of the etiologic spirochetes in thin peripheral blood smears prepared at times of febrile peaks by phase-contrast or darkfield microscopy or light microscopy after Wright or Giemsa staining.

CURRENT THERAPY

- The antibiotic of choice for treatment of relapsing fever is doxycycline except in children or pregnant women. In children <8 years of age, erythromycin[1] or oral penicillin is used instead of tetracycline (Table 3).
- Relapsing fever, if severe or complicated with neuroborreliosis, requires treatment with the intravenous antibiotics ceftriaxone or penicillin G (Table 3).
- The louse-borne epidemic form is treated with a single dose, whereas the endemic tick-borne form is treated with multiple doses for at least 1 week (Table 3).
- Antibiotic treatment of relapsing fever results in the Jarisch-Herxheimer reaction (JHR) in as many as 60% of cases, more often in the epidemic than in the endemic forms. It is characterized by the sudden onset of tachycardia, hypotension, chills, rigors, diaphoresis, and high fever. To reduce the risk of JHR, antibiotics should be started between but not at times of febrile peaks.

[1]Not FDA approved for this indication.

Relapsing fever is one of several diseases caused by spirochetes. Other human spirochetal diseases are syphilis, Lyme disease, and leptospirosis. Notable features of spirochetes are wavy and helical shapes, length-to-diameter ratios of as much as 100 to 1, and flagella that lie between the inner and outer cell membranes. The spirochetes that cause relapsing fever are in the genus *Borrelia*. Other *Borrelia* species cause Lyme disease, avian spirochetosis, and epidemic bovine abortion. Table 1 shows the main *Borrelia*

species of relapsing fever, their vectors, and an estimate of their geographic ranges. In the United States, relapsing fever was considered a disease endemic only in the West. However, the recent finding of relapsing fever–like *Borrelia* in ticks and dogs in the eastern United States suggests that the risk of relapsing fever may extend into the East.

Epidemiology

There are two forms of relapsing fever: epidemic transmitted to humans by the body louse *Pediculus humanus* (louse-borne relapsing fever [LBRF]) and endemic transmitted to humans by soft-bodied ticks of the genus *Ornithodoros* (tick-borne relapsing fever [TBRF]). In LBRF, itching caused by skin infestation with lice leads to scratching, which may result in crushing of lice and release of infected hemolymph into areas of skin abrasion. Louse infestation is associated with cold weather and a lack of hygiene. Migrant workers and soldiers at war are particularly susceptible to this infection. Historically, massive outbreaks of LBRF occurred in Eurasia, Africa, and Latin America, but currently the disease is found only in Ethiopia and neighboring countries. However, immigrants can spread LBRF to other parts of the world.

The main risk factor for TBRF is exposure to endemic areas (Table 1). The risk of infection increases with outdoor activities in areas where rodents nest, like entering caves or sleeping in rustic cabins. *Ornithodoros* ticks are soft-bodied and feed for short periods of time (minutes), usually at night. They can live many years between blood meals and may transmit spirochetes to their offspring transovarially. Infection is produced by regurgitation of infected tick saliva into the skin wound during tick feeding. There are several natural vertebrate reservoirs for TBRF, but most common are rodents (deer mice, chipmunks, squirrels, and rats). In contrast, the body louse *Pediculus humanus* is a strict human parasite, living and multiplying in clothing. Hard-tick-borne relapsing fever (HTBRF) is an emerging infectious disease throughout the temperate zone caused by *Borrelia miyamotoi*. *Borrelia miyamotoi* is a spirochete closely related to the bacteria that cause TBRF. It is more distantly related to the bacteria that cause Lyme disease. First identified in 1995 in ticks from Japan, *B miyamotoi* has since been detected in two species of North American ticks, the black-legged or "deer" tick (Ixodes scapularis) and the western black-legged tick (Ixodes pacificus). These ticks are already known to transmit Lyme disease, anaplasmosis, and babesiosis.

Clinical Diagnosis

Relapsing fever should be suspected in any patient presenting with two or more episodes of high fever and constitutional symptoms spaced by periods of relative well-being. The index of suspicion increases if the patient has been exposed to endemic areas for TBRF or to countries where LBRF still occurs (Table 1). Whereas LBRF is usually associated with a single febrile relapse, TBRF usually has multiple relapses (up to 13). Only about 10% of cases of HTBRF have febrile relapses. In LBRF the second episode of fever is typically milder than the first; in TBRF the multiple febrile periods are usually of equal severity. The febrile periods last from 1 to 3 days, and the intervals between fevers last from 3 to 10 days. During the febrile periods, numerous spirochetes are circulating in the blood. This is called *spirochetemia* and is sometimes unexpectedly detected during routine blood smear examinations. Between fevers, spirochetemia is not observed because the numbers are low. The fever pattern and recurrent spirochetemia are the consequences of antigenic variation of abundant outer membrane lipoproteins of relapsing fever *Borrelia* species that are the target for serotype-specific antibodies.

The mean latency between exposure to ticks in the endemic form or to lice in the epidemic form and onset of symptoms is 6 days (range, 3–18 days). Because *Ornithodoros* ticks feed briefly and painlessly at night, patients with TBRF may not be able to recall having been bitten by a tick. The clinical manifestations of TBRF and LBRF are similar, although some differences do exist. Table 2

TABLE 1 — Relapsing Fever *Borrelia* Species Pathogenic to Humans

RELAPSING FEVER	*BORRELIA* SPECIES	ARTHROPOD VECTOR	DISTRIBUTION OF DISEASE
Endemic	*Borrelia hermsii*	*Ornithodoros hermsi*	Western North America
	Borrelia turicatae	*Ornithodoros turicata*	Southwestern North America and northern Mexico
	Borrelia venezuelensis	*Ornithodoros rudis*	Central America and northern South America
	Borrelia hispanica	*Ornithodoros marocanus*	Iberian peninsula and northwestern Africa
	Borrelia crocidurae	*Ornithodoros erraticus*	North and East Africa, Middle East, southern Europe
	Borrelia duttoni	*Ornithodoros moubata*	Sub-Saharan Africa
	Borrelia persica	*Ornithodoros tholozani*	Middle East, Greece, Central Asia
	Borrelia uzbekistan	*Ornithodoros pappilipes*	Tajikistan, Uzbekistan
	Borrelia miyamotoi	*Ixodes* spp.	Asia, Europe, North America
Epidemic	*Borrelia recurrentis*	*Pediculus humanus*	Worldwide (recently only in East Africa including immigrants to Europe)

TABLE 2 — Frequent Clinical Manifestations of Tick-Borne Relapsing Fever

SIGN OR SYMPTOM	FREQUENCY (%)
Headache	94
Myalgia	92
Chills	88
Nausea	76
Arthralgia	73
Vomiting	71
Abdominal pain	44
Confusion	38
Dry cough	27
Ocular pain	26
Diarrhea	25
Dizziness	25
Photophobia	25
Neck pain	24
Rash	18
Dysuria	13
Jaundice	10
Hepatomegaly	10
Splenomegaly	6

disease progresses, fever, jaundice, hepatosplenomegaly, cardiac arrhythmias, and cardiac failure may occur, especially with LBRF. Jaundice is more common at times of relapses. Patients with LBRF are more likely to develop petechiae on the trunk, extremities, and mucous membranes; epistaxis; and blood-tinged sputum. Rupture of the spleen may rarely occur. Multiple neurologic complications can occur as a result of disseminated intravascular coagulation in LBRF and as a result of infection of the meninges and cranial and spinal nerve roots by spirochetes in TBRF. The most common neurologic complications of TBRF are aseptic meningitis and facial palsy. Relapsing fever in pregnant women can cause abortion, premature birth, and neonatal death. Sometimes patients can have nonfebrile relapses, consisting of periods of severe headache, backache, weakness, and other constitutional symptoms without fever that occur at the time of expected relapses. Delirium may persist for weeks after the fever resolves, and, rarely, symptoms may be protracted.

Relapsing fever may be confused with many diseases that are relapsing or cause high fevers. These include typhoid fever, yellow fever, dengue, African hemorrhagic fevers, African trypanosomiasis, brucellosis, malaria, leptospirosis, rat-bite fever, intermittent cholangitis, cat-scratch disease, and echovirus 9 infection, among others. Relapsing fever *Borrelia* spp. have antigens that are cross reactive with Lyme disease *Borrelia* spp. and inasmuch as the endemic areas of relapsing fever and Lyme disease overlap to some extent, confusion between the two infections can be expected. In fact, the same species of ticks can transmit HTBRF and Lyme disease, although erythema migrans rash is rare in the former and common in the latter.

Laboratory Diagnosis

Although the pattern of recurring fever is the clue to diagnosing relapsing fever, confirmation of the diagnosis requires demonstration of spirochetes in peripheral blood taken during an episode of fever. The comparatively large number of spirochetes in the blood during relapsing fever provides the opportunity for the simplest method for laboratory diagnosis of the infection, light microscopy of Wright- or Giemsa-stained thin blood smears or darkfield or phase-contrast microscopy of a wet mount of plasma. The blood should be obtained during or just before peaks of body temperature. Between fever peaks, spirochetes often can be demonstrated by inoculation of blood or cerebrospinal fluid (CSF) into special culture medium (BSK-H with 6% rabbit serum available from Sigma) or experimental animals. Enrichment for spirochetes is achieved by using the platelet-rich fraction of plasma or the buffy coat of sedimented blood. In the United States the most common causes of relapsing fever are *Borrelia*

lists the frequency of the most common manifestations of TBRF. The usual initial presentation is sudden onset of chills followed by high fever, tachycardia, severe headache, vomiting, myalgia and arthralgia, and often delirium. In the early stages, a reddish rash may be seen over the trunk, arms, or legs. The fever remains high for 3 to 5 days, and then it clears abruptly. After an asymptomatic period of 7 to 10 days, the fever and other constitutional symptoms can reappear suddenly. The febrile episodes gradually become less severe, and the person eventually recovers completely. As the *hermsii* and *Borrelia turicatae*; both grow in BSK-H medium and in young mice or rats. Whereas direct visual detection of organisms in the blood is the most common method for laboratory confirmation of relapsing fever, immunoassays for antibodies are the most common means of laboratory confirmation for Lyme disease. Although serologic assays have been developed for the agents of relapsing fever, these are not widely available and of dubious utility. The antigenic variation displayed by the relapsing fever species means there are hundreds of different "serotypes." If a different serotype or species is used for preparing the antigen, only antibodies to conserved antigens may be detected. For this reason, a standardized enzyme-linked immunosorbent assay (ELISA) with Lyme disease *Borrelia* as antigen may be the best available serologic assay for relapsing fever. ELISA for *Borrelia burgdorferi* antibodies is routinely done across the United States and Europe. If a positive result for IgM or IgG antibodies is obtained, the Western blot for antibodies to *B burgdorferi* antigens would be expected to discriminate current or past Lyme disease from relapsing fever, as well as from syphilis, another cause of false-positive Lyme disease ELISA results. Other frequent laboratory abnormalities can occur in relapsing fever but are not diagnostic. These include elevated white blood cell count with increased neutrophils, thrombocytopenia, increased serum bilirubin, proteinuria, microhematuria, prolongation of the prothrombin time (PT) and partial thromboplastin time (PTT), and elevation of fibrin degradation products.

It may also be possible to confirm infection with relapsing fever borrelias, including *Borrelia miyamotoi*, by directly probing blood and/or CSF samples for fragments of the bacterium's genetic sequence, which few laboratories may be able to do.

Treatment

Relapsing fever *Borrelias* are very sensitive to several antibiotics, and antimicrobial resistance is rare. Table 3 summarizes the treatment options for adults and children younger than 8 years. Children older than 8 years can be treated with the same antibiotics as adults, but the doses should be adjusted by weight. Before antibiotics are given, the possibility of causing the Jarisch-Herxheimer reaction (JHR) should be considered (see later). The tetracycline antibiotics are most commonly used for treatment of LBRF and TBRF. The first antibiotic of choice in adults and children older than 8 years is doxycycline (Doryx). In general, shorter treatments are needed for LBRF than for TBRF. Single-dose therapy is usually recommended for LBRF. In contrast, in TBRF even multiple doses of tetracyclines for up to 10 days may fail to prevent relapses, and retreatment can be required. *B. miyamotoi* is susceptible in vitro to doxycycline, azithromycin, and ceftriaxone. Physicians have successfully treated patients infected with *B miyamotoi* with a 2 to 4-week course of doxycycline.

Alternative oral antibiotics to the tetracyclines are erythromycin (E-Mycin)[1], azithromycin (Zithromax)[1], amoxicillin (Amoxil)[1], penicillin[1], and chloramphenicol (Chloromycetin)[1]. However, oral chloramphenicol is not available in the United States. Erythromycin, azithromycin, and penicillin do not appear as effective as the tetracyclines; however, they are recommended for children younger than 8 years and for pregnant women. Amoxicillin is another alternative for young children with early Lyme disease; however, it is ineffective for human granulocytic ehrlichiosis, which sometimes occurs as a co-infection with Lyme disease. *Borrelia miyamotoi* may be resistant to amoxicillin.

Although treatment with antibiotics is usually given orally, they may need to be given intravenously if severe vomiting makes swallowing impractical. If there are symptoms and signs of meningitis or encephalitis without clinical or radiologic signs of increased intracranial pressure, the CSF should be examined to rule out central nervous system (CNS) infection. The finding of elevation of CSF cells and protein demands the use of parenteral antibiotics, such as penicillin G[1] or ceftriaxone (Rocephin).[1]

[1]Not FDA approved for this indication.

TABLE 3 Treatment Options for Tick-Borne Relapsing Fever*

Adults

Nonsevere forms

1. Doxycycline (Doryx oral), 100 mg PO bid for 1–2 wk[†]
2. Tetracycline (Sumycin), 500 mg PO qid for 1–2 wk
3. Erythromycin (Erythrocin),[1] 500 mg PO tid for 1–2 wk

Severe forms

1. Ceftriaxone (Rocephin),[1] 2 g IV qd for 1–2 wk
2. Penicillin G parenteral aqueous (Pfizerpen),[1] 4 million U IV q4h for 1–2 wk

Children (≤8 y)

Nonsevere forms

1. Erythromycin suspension oral (EryPed),[1] 30–50 mg/kg/d divided tid for 1–2 wk
2. Azithromycin oral suspension (Zithromax),[1] 20 mg/kg on the first day followed by 10 mg/kg/d for 4 more days
3. Penicillin V (Pen-Vee K),[1] 25–50 mg/kg/d divided qid for 1–2 wk
4. Amoxicillin (Amoxil),[1] 50 mg/kg/d divided tid for 1–2 wk

Severe forms

1. Ceftriaxone (Rocephin),[1] 75–100 mg/kg/d IV for 1–2 wk
2. Penicillin G parenteral aqueous (Pfizerpen),[1] 300,000 U/kg/d given IV in divided doses q4h for 1–2 wk

Abbreviations: IV = intravenous; PO = orally.
[1]Not FDA approved for this indication.
*The same oral agents are used for treatment of louse-borne (epidemic) relapsing fever but given as a single dose.
[†]In general, treatment for 1 wk is recommended in early/milder cases and for up to 2 wk for more severe cases.

Optimally, antibiotic treatment should be started during afebrile periods when the spirochetemia is low. Starting therapy near the peak of a febrile period may induce JHR, in which high fever and a rise and subsequent fall in blood pressure, sometimes to dangerously low levels, may occur. Dehydration should be treated with fluids given intravenously. Severe headache can be treated with pain relievers such as codeine, and nausea or vomiting can be treated with prochlorperazine (Compazine).

Jarisch-Herxheimer Reaction

Antibiotic treatment of relapsing fever causes JHR in as many as 60% of cases. JHR is more common in LBRF than in TBRF. It can also occur in HTBRF. It is characterized by the sudden onset of tachycardia, hypotension, chills, rigors, diaphoresis, and high fever. Patients with JHR have said that they felt as if they were going to die. JHR is caused by the rapid killing of circulating spirochetes 1 to 4 hours after the first dose of antibiotic, which results in the release of large amounts of *Borrelia* lipoproteins in the circulation followed by massive release of tumor necrosis factor and other cytokines. If possible, patients with JHR should be transferred to an intensive care unit for close monitoring and treatment. Over several hours, the temperature declines and the patient feels better. Large amounts of intravenous fluids (0.9% sodium chloride solution) may be required to treat hypotension. Steroids and nonsteroidal antiinflammatory agents have no effect on the frequency or severity of the JHR. One study found that pretreatment with anti-TNF-alpha monoclonal antibody (Humira)[1] suppressed JHR after penicillin treatment for LBRF and reduced the associated increases in plasma cytokines.

Death can occur as a result of JHR secondary to cardiovascular collapse in up to 5% of patients with treated LBRF and much less frequently in TBRF.

Outcome

Complete recovery occurs in 95% or more of adequately treated patients. The prognosis for untreated cases or if treatment is delayed varies. A mortality rate as high as 40% is reported in untreated epidemics of LBRF. Relapsing fever also has a high mortality rate in neonates. Some neurologic sequelae can occur in patients with TBRF complicated with neuroborreliosis.

Prevention

Prevention of TBRF involves avoidance of rodent- and tick-infested dwellings such as animal burrows, caves, and abandoned cabins. Wearing clothing that protects skin from tick access (e.g., long pants and long-sleeved shirts) is also helpful. Repellents and acaricides provide additional protection. Diethyltoluamide (DEET) repels ticks when applied to clothing or skin, but it must be used with caution. It loses its effectiveness within 1 to several hours when applied to skin and must be reapplied; it is absorbed through the skin and may cause CNS toxicity if used excessively. Picaridin (KBR 3023), which has been used as an insect repellent for years in Europe and Australia, is now available in the United States in 7% solution as Cutter Advanced Repellent (Spectrum Brands). The US Centers for Disease Control and Prevention (CDC) is recommending it as an alternative to DEET. Permethrin Insect Repellent, an acaricide, is more effective than DEET but should not be applied directly to skin. When applied to clothing, it provides good protection for 1 day or more. In LBRF, prevention can be achieved by promoting personal hygiene and by dusting undergarments and the inside of clothing with malathion[1] powder[2] or lindane[1] powder[2] when available. Widespread antibiotic use may be necessary to control epidemics of LBRF, using one or two doses of 100 mg doxycycline[1] given within 1 week of exposure.

---

[1]Not FDA approved for this indication.

[2]Not available in the United States

References

Barbour AG, Hayes SF: Biology of *Borrelia* species, *Microbiol Rev* 50:381–400, 1986.
Bryceson AD, Parry EH, Perine PL, et al: Louse-borne relapsing fever, *Q J Med* 39:129–170, 1970.
Cadavid D, Barbour AG: Neuroborreliosis during relapsing fever: Review of the clinical manifestations, pathology, and treatment of infections in humans and experimental animals, *Clin Infect Dis* 26:151–164, 1998.
Fekade D, Knox K, Hussein K, et al: Prevention of Jarisch-Herxheimer reactions by treatment with antibodies against tumor necrosis factor alpha, *N Engl J Med* 335:311–315, 1996.
Kazragis RJ, Dever LL, Jorgensen JH, Barbour AG: In vivo activities of ceftriaxone and vancomycin against *Borrelia* spp. in the mouse brain and other sites, *Antimicrob Agents Chemother* 40:2632–2636, 1996.
Melkert PW: Fatal Jarisch-Herxheimer reaction in a case of relapsing fever misdiagnosed as lobar pneumonia, *Trop Geogr Med* 39:92–93, 1987.
Southern P, Sanford J: Relapsing fever, *Medicine* 48:129–149, 1969.
Taft W, Pike J: Relapsing fever. Report of a sporadic outbreak including treatment with penicillin, *JAMA* 129:1002–1005, 1945.

RUBELLA AND CONGENITAL RUBELLA

Method of
Dee Ann Bragg, MD

CURRENT DIAGNOSIS

- Given its clinical overlap with other viral syndromes, suspected rubella infection must be confirmed with laboratory testing.
- Rubella serology or viral polymerase chain reaction (PCR) testing are available options for confirming a suspected diagnosis.

CURRENT THERAPY

- Rubella infection is largely self-limited with no specific treatment indicated.
- Infection during pregnancy should prompt further evaluation and counseling regarding risks and potential outcomes.
- Treatment of children with congenital rubella syndrome requires a multidisciplinary effort based on individual manifestations.
- Vaccination is essential in reducing the risk of rubella and congenital rubella syndrome.

Rubella typically presents in children and adults as a mild viral illness, but is one of the TORCH infections (toxoplasmosis, other, rubella, cytomegalovirus, herpes) known to cause congenital anomalies. Although vaccination efforts have led to the successful eradication of rubella in the United States, it remains a significant cause of morbidity and death worldwide. Its name is derived from Latin and means "little red." Initially considered a variant of measles or scarlet fever, rubella was first described as its own entity in the German medical literature in 1814. Thus it is still often referred to as "German measles" in common nomenclature.

Pathophysiology and Virology

Rubella virus, a single-stranded RNA virus and the only member of the Rubivirus genus, is part of the Togaviridae family and is the causative agent of rubella infection. There are 13 recognized genotypes of rubella, each with minor differences in nucleotide sequencing and gene expression. Rubella typically presents as a mild and self-limited illness. During pregnancy, however, it can infect the placenta and disrupt organogenesis by creating systemic inflammation and inhibiting actin assembly. Outcomes of antenatal infection are variable but can include miscarriage, fetal death, and congenital rubella syndrome (CRS).

Multiple factors are involved in the pathogenesis of CRS. Rubella infection can cause necrosis of the chorionic epithelial and endothelial cells. These cells then enter fetal circulation and can incite thrombotic or ischemic lesions in the eyes, ears, brain, and heart. The virus also appears to trigger an immune-modulated upregulation of interferon and cytokines, which can alter the normal development and differentiation of fetal cells.

Epidemiology

Although rubella is less contagious than other viruses such as influenza or measles, large epidemics are associated with significant morbidity from complications including encephalitis, fetal loss, deafness, and blindness. Norman Gregg, an Australian ophthalmologist, was the first to recognize the teratogenic potential of rubella when in 1941 he noted an unusually high incidence of congenital cataracts after an area outbreak.

Rubella was successfully eradicated from the United States in 2004 due to widespread vaccination efforts, and most sporadic cases since that time have been documented in foreign-born young adults. In endemic areas, annual springtime outbreaks are common. However, sporadic cases can occur year-round in temperate climates. Outbreaks typically affect early school–aged children, and the mean age for an infected host is 5 to 9 years. Because lifelong immunity develops after natural infection, large cyclical epidemics tend to occur every 3 to 8 years as population immunity wanes.

Humans are the only known host of rubella infection, and the virus is transmitted from person to person through respiratory droplets. After transmission, rubella virus replicates in the respiratory mucosa and cervical lymph nodes before entering systemic circulation and spreading to target organs.

Clinical Manifestations
Acquired Rubella

After an incubation period of about 14 days (range, 12–23), a variety of clinical symptoms can appear. These are generally mild, and about 50% of cases are asymptomatic. In children, a skin rash is typically the initial manifestation of rubella. The rash usually appears on the face and then progresses downward from the head to the feet. It lasts about 3 days and is characteristically maculopapular, presenting with small pink non-coalescing papules that are occasionally pruritic. Bathing or showering in hot water tends to make the rash more evident.

Adults more often have a prodromal period of low-grade fever, malaise, and adenopathy lasting 1 to 5 days before the onset of skin findings. Lymphadenopathy may begin up to a week before the rash and can last for several weeks. The postauricular nodes are particularly commonly involved, and posterior cervical or suboccipital nodes may also be affected.

Sequelae
Polyarthritis and polyarthralgia are the most common complications of rubella, particularly in adult women, in whom they are seen up to 70% of the time. They appear with such frequency that they are often considered intrinsic to the virus itself rather than complications. Joint symptoms typically present around the same time or just after the onset of the rash. They usually last 3 to 4 days but can remain for up to 1 month. The most commonly affected joints are fingers, wrists, and knees. Chronic arthritis is rarely observed.

Other complications are uncommon but can carry a high degree of morbidity and death. Hemorrhagic events are more likely in children than adults and occur in about 1 in 3000 cases. They manifest as a result of vascular damage or thrombocytopenia. Skin purpura is the most common presentation, but gastrointestinal, cerebral, or intrarenal hemorrhage can occur. Encephalitis occurs in about 1 in 6000 cases, more commonly in adults than children. Rare complications include orchitis, neuritis, progressive panencephalitis, and Guillain-Barré syndrome.

Congenital Rubella Syndrome (CRS)
CRS can present transiently with low birth weight, thrombocytopenic purpura, or hemolytic anemia. However, permanent defects are the hallmark of CRS because it classically involves a triad of cataracts, cardiac anomalies, and sensorineural deafness. Of these, hearing loss is the most common and sometimes the only complication observed. Cardiac abnormalities can include patent ductus arteriosus, ventricular septal defect, pulmonary artery hypoplasia, and coarctation of the aorta. Other ocular defects such as glaucoma, retinopathy, and microphthalmia can also occur. Additional manifestations can include microcephaly, intellectual disability, psychomotor retardation, and delayed speech.

Notably, it can take 2 to 4 years for certain neurologic, endocrine, or cardiac abnormalities associated with CRS to manifest. Diabetes mellitus, thyroid disease, autism, and progressive panencephalopathy can all occur as late effects of CRS.

The risk of CRS and its associated congenital defects is greatest when infection occurs in the first trimester. Up to 85% of infants born under these conditions are found to be affected, whereas defects are rare when infection occurs after 20 weeks' gestation.

Diagnosis
Given its nonspecific nature and similarity to other viral infections, clinical diagnosis of rubella is challenging and largely unreliable. Suspected infection should be confirmed by 1 of 3 diagnostic methods: (1) rubella immunoglobulin M (IgM) serology, (2) a demonstrated rise in rubella virus immunoglobulin G (IgG) between acute and convalescent phases, or (3) detection of rubella virus by PCR.

Among the existing options for laboratory diagnosis, rubella IgM is the most accessible and widely used. However, collection timing is important to consider. Rubella IgM will only be detectable in about 50% of cases on the day of rash appearance but will be present in nearly all cases by 7 to 10 days after the rash. It will then remain positive for 4 to 12 weeks. Importantly, serum IgM testing is most sensitive and specific in the setting of local

outbreaks. False-positive results occur more frequently in sporadic cases, and in those instances, additional means of analysis should be performed to confirm diagnosis.

Rubella IgG testing can be used to diagnose acute rubella infection under two circumstances: either (1) a negative rubella IgG during acute infection followed by a positive IgG in the convalescent phase, or (2) a fourfold increase in IgG titer over 10 to 14 days. IgG avidity testing may also be useful. This measures the strength of antigen-antibody binding, which is typically weaker in acute infection and increases over time. Therefore a low avidity index would indicate a more recent infection.

Viral isolation of rubella by PCR is quite valuable for diagnostic confirmation and can be performed on samples obtained from throat or nasopharyngeal swabs. These tests are not as widely available in postvaccination settings and may need to be performed in conjunction with local health departments or national epidemiology centers.

Diagnosis of CRS in infants can similarly be confirmed by one of three methods: (1) rubella IgM detection in serum or cord blood, (2) persistence of rubella IgG >6 months of age (past the time frame of passive maternal immunity), or (3) PCR isolation of rubella virus from respiratory or urinary samples. Because both rubella virus and IgM remain positive for several months in patients with CRS, the time frame for testing is less crucial than in cases of postnatal infection.

Treatment
There is no specific treatment for rubella and, because acquired cases are generally mild and self-limiting, basic supportive care is recommended. Detection of rubella infection in pregnancies before 18 weeks' gestation should prompt further investigation including maternal-fetal medicine referral, detailed ultrasound examination, support for adverse outcomes including neonatal hospice services, and follow-up examination and screening of the newborn. Maternal infections after 18 weeks can be followed with routine ultrasound monitoring along with newborn evaluation and testing.

Prevention
Rubella Vaccine
The first rubella vaccines became available in 1969, and a number of strains have been developed since that time. Of these, the RA 27/3 vaccine has been the most enduring, and all other strains were discontinued at the time of its introduction in 1979. The RA 27/3 rubella vaccine is a live attenuated virus that is administered in conjunction with measles and mumps as MMR, or with measles, mumps, and varicella as MMRV (ProQuad). Single-antigen rubella vaccine is not available in the United States.

Vaccination against rubella is safe and effective. Adverse events such as fever and rash are mild and are generally attributable to the measles and mumps portions of the vaccines. After a single dose, more than 95% of those vaccinated have serologic confirmation of rubella immunity, with evidence of lifelong immunity in the vast majority of responders. MMR or MMRV is recommended for all children at 12 months of age, followed by a second dose between 4 and 6 years of age. The second dose is generally indicated to stimulate measles and mumps immunity in those who did not respond to the first vaccine. MMR and MMRV are contraindicated in immunosuppression, pregnancy, and in patients with a history of anaphylaxis to neomycin or other vaccine components.

Preconception Counseling and Prenatal Care
Rubella immunity, defined as serum rubella IgG of 10 IU/mL or greater, should be documented in all women attempting to conceive. MMR vaccine should be given in cases of nonimmunity, and although it is recommended at least 4 weeks before conception, inadvertent vaccination after that time is unlikely to be associated with adverse events. Rubella IgG should likewise be checked in all pregnant females as part of routine obstetric care, and MMR should be administered postpartum to nonimmune women.

Eradication and Future Goals

Despite widely available effective vaccines and evidence of sustained eradication in the Western Hemisphere, there are still approximately 100,000 cases of CRS annually worldwide. Although some African and Asian nations have introduced routine rubella vaccination, public health efforts have been inconsistent in many developing countries. Dedicated personnel and funding will likely be necessary to decrease rubella incidence and its complications on a global scale.

References

Baltimore RS, Nimkin K, Sparger K, et al: Case 4-2018: a newborn with thrombocytopenia, cataracts, and hepatosplenomegaly, *N Engl J Med* 378:564–572, 2018.

Bouthry E, Picone O, Hamdi G, et al: Rubella and pregnancy: diagnosis, management and outcomes, *Prenat Diagn* 34:1246–1253, 2014.

Centers for Disease Control and Prevention: *Epidemiology and Prevention of Vaccine-Preventable Diseases, 13th Edition*. Hamborsky J, Kroger A, Wolfe S, eds. Washington, DC: Public Health Foundation, pp 325–340, 2015.

Lambert N, Strebel P, Orenstein W, et al: *Rubella, Lancet* 385(9984):2297–2307, 2015.

Papania M, Wallace G, Rota P, et al: Elimination of endemic measles, rubella, and congenital rubella syndrome from the western hemisphere: the US experience, *JAMA Pediatr* 168:148–155, 2014.

Tipples G: Rubella diagnostic issues in Canada, *J Infect Dis* 204(Suppl 2):S659–S663, 2011.

SALMONELLOSIS

Method of
Arelis Santana, MD, MPH

CURRENT DIAGNOSIS

- Nontyphoidal Salmonellae (NTS) represent a significant cause of infectious diarrhea globally.
- Underlying comorbidities, the virulence of the pathogen, and the size of inoculum can affect the severity of the infection.
- The most common clinical manifestation of NTS is self-limited acute gastroenteritis.
- Bacteremia and invasive infections (mycotic aneurysms, aortitis, among others) should be suspected in patients with high-grade fevers and predisposing risk factors (e.g., aneurysms and atherosclerotic disease).
- Diagnosis of NTS infection is confirmed by laboratory isolation of Salmonellae from the stool, blood, or sterile body fluid.

CURRENT THERAPY

- Treatment for uncomplicated Salmonella gastroenteritis is based on supportive care with fluid and electrolyte replenishment.
- Antimicrobial therapy may be warranted for those with severe infection (severe diarrhea, high fever, need for hospitalization) or risk factors for invasive disease.
- Chronic carriage of NTS can occur in less than 1% of patients. Antimicrobial therapy may be of some utility in patients with chronic carriage; however, there is no strong evidence yet supporting its routine use.
- Adequate hand hygiene practices, appropriate food handling, and standard precautions are still the best way to avoid NTS spread.

Salmonellae was named after Dr. Daniel Elmer Salmon, a veterinary pathologist chief of the Bureau of Animal Industry, who helped with the eradication of contagious bovine pleuropneumonia in the United States. His colleague and professor, Dr. Theobald Smith, was the first to isolate *Salmonella choleraesuis* from porcine intestines in 1885. This microorganism can grow in both humans and animals, causing a broad range of clinical manifestations. Clinical presentations comprise gastroenteritis, bacteremia, endovascular infections, localized infections, and chronic carrier state. However, the most common presentation of salmonellosis is uncomplicated gastroenteritis.

Microbiology

Salmonella is a genus of gram-negative bacilli belonging to the family of Enterobacteriaceae. The genus of Salmonellae is divided into two species: *enterica and bongori. Salmonella enterica* is further divided into six different subspecies based on DNA resemblances. Subspecies are also differentiated into serotypes. Salmonellae serotypes are designated based on the immunoreactivity of cell surface structures, the O and H antigens. These serotypes are classified using the Kauffmann–White classification scheme. Salmonella has more than 2500 serotypes. However, less than 100 have been found to be pathogenic in humans.

Salmonellae species are nonspore forming, motile, facultative anaerobes that can measure 2 to 3 µm by 0.4 to 0.6 µm in size. All Salmonellae are motile utilizing a flagellum, except for *S. Gallinarum-and S. Pullorum*. Similar to other Enterobacteriaceae, they can produce acid on glucose fermentation. Most of the species do not ferment lactose and appear white on MacConkey agar plates, except for approximately 1% of them, which can make their identification challenging. Another important feature of identification is that most of the species, except for *S. Typhi*, produce hydrogen sulfide on sugar fermentation, which can be detected on the selective indicator plates.

Epidemiology

Nontyphoidal Salmonellae (NTS) represent a significant cause of infectious diarrhea globally. Approximately, there are 93.8 million cases of gastroenteritis Salmonella species and 155,000 deaths per year. According to the Centers for Disease Control and Prevention (CDC), there are approximately 1.35 million illnesses and 420 deaths due to NTS yearly in the United States, with an estimate of 39 cases of salmonellosis for each culture-confirmed case. The Salmonella serotypes most frequently isolated are *S. enteritidis, S. typhimurium,* and *S. newport.*

Salmonellae can inhabit the intestinal tract and can be found in the feces of humans and animals. These include but are not limited to birds (including poultry), reptiles, and amphibians. Infection can occur from the ingestion of animal food products such as undercooked meat, poultry, eggs, and dairy products, or from cross-contamination due to improperly handled food or water. Other possible sources include animal bodies contaminated with Salmonella. For example, reptiles can commonly harbor this organism. Also, areas where animals live, such as water tanks and cages, may be contaminated with these organisms and can be potential sources of infection. NTS outbreaks have also been associated with fresh produce, milk, nuts, fruits, and raw vegetables. These products can become contaminated by manure or water and then are distributed.

The emergence of antibiotic resistance in NTS has been on the rise and is currently a global concern as antibiotic treatment options are becoming limited and ineffective. Antibiotic resistance has been associated with the use of antimicrobials in animal feeds. The mechanisms of resistance described in NTS include active efflux pumps to remove antibiotics from inside the cell, hydrolytic enzyme production, mutations in target genes to evade the action of antibiotics, and decreased permeability of the outer membrane, among others.

In the United States, the National Antimicrobial Resistance Monitoring System (NARMS) monitors antibiotic resistance, including Salmonella. According to their last report in 2015, approximately 4% of NTS isolates were resistant to five or more antimicrobials, 4.7% of NTS strains were nalidixic acid resistant, 0.4% were resistant to ciprofloxacin, and 2.7% were resistant to ceftriaxone. Resistance to nalidixic acid is a good indicator of a decreased susceptibility to fluoroquinolones. In summary, resistance rates to fluoroquinolones or third-generation cephalosporins in the United States are not high but warrant careful monitoring.

Pathogenesis

A combination of factors related to both the pathogen and the host affects the pathogenesis of Salmonella infection and clinical presentation. Underlying conditions and the size of inoculum can affect the severity of the infection. NTS infection commences with the ingestion of organisms in contaminated food or water and usually requires approximately 10^6 organisms to produce the disease. However, infants or persons with certain underlying predisposing factors could develop the disease with smaller inoculums. Some of these predisposing risk factors include impaired cellular immunity, achlorhydria, alteration in the intestinal flora and integrity, and the extreme of ages (Table 1). These risk factors can lead to a more severe initial infection and complications such as bacteremia and/or

TABLE 1	Predisposing Factors for Salmonellosis
Gastrointestinal	
Achlorhydria	
Gastric surgery	
Inflammatory bowel disease	
Infections	
HIV/AIDS (decreased T-cells)	
Bartonellosis	
Malaria	
Schistosomiasis	
Immune or structural compromise	
Age (<6 months, >60 years)	
Lymphoma	
Splenectomy	
Cirrhosis with portal hypertension	
Diabetes mellitus	
Chronic uremia	
Hemolytic anemia (iron overload)	
Sickle cell (bone infarct, autosplenectomy)	
Systemic lupus	
Atheromata, aortic aneurysm	
Drugs	
H2-blockers, proton pump inhibitors	
Antibiotic administration	
Antimotility agents	
Chemotherapy	
Corticosteroids	
Transplant antirejection agents	

metastatic infection. Gastric acidity is the initial barrier to Salmonellae; therefore, underlying conditions or medications that increase the pH of the stomach can predispose a person to infection. Salmonellae invade by binding to the gastrointestinal mucosa and submucosal lymphoid systems. After the invasion of Salmonella and the translocation of bacterial proteins into the host cell cytoplasm, the intestinal mucosa secretes interleukin-8 (IL-8), a strong neutrophil chemotactic factor. This causes an extensive polymorphonuclear leukocyte infiltration in both small and large intestinal mucosa. Degranulation and release of toxic neutrophils result in damage to the intestinal mucosa, producing diarrhea.

Clinical Presentation

Gastroenteritis

The most common clinical manifestation of NTS is self-limited acute gastroenteritis. The incubation period is usually 6 to 48 hours following the exposure, but more extended incubation periods of up to 7 days have been reported. Symptoms include sudden onset of nausea and vomiting, followed by fever, constitutional symptoms, abdominal pain, and watery diarrhea. On rare occasions, bloody diarrhea can also be present. Symptoms subside within 3 to 7 days in uncomplicated gastroenteritis. In patients with predisposing factors (see Table 1), the clinical illness may be more complex, including bacteremia. Patients with inflammatory bowel disease can have serious complications like toxic megacolon that can potentially be life-threatening.

Higher inoculum of bacteria and virulence of different strains may correlate with the severity of diarrhea and the length of the disease course. The stool can contain polymorphonuclear leukocytes, or occult blood and leukocytosis can also be seen in the complete blood cell count.

Invasive Infections

Bacteremia can result as a complication from Salmonella gastroenteritis in up to 5% of the patients, and it should be suspected in patients with high-grade fevers or with predisposing risk factors. Bacteremia can lead to a variety of extraintestinal manifestations such as endocarditis, mycotic aneurysm, hepatic abscesses, or osteomyelitis. *S. choleraesuis and S. Dublin* are commonly associated with more invasive infections.

Although these are uncommon, NTS endovascular infection, including aortitis and mycotic aneurysms, should be suspected in patients with high-grade bacteremia or persistent bacteremia, or with pre-existing valvular heart disease, prosthetic vascular graft, or aortic aneurysm.

Intraabdominal infections due to NTS are also rare but can occur as hepatic and/or splenic abscesses, or cholecystitis, more commonly in patients with underlying hepatobiliary abnormalities. Other rare manifestations of invasive disease are meningitis (more common in infants 1 to 4 months old), pneumonia, and urinary tract infections. Salmonella osteomyelitis is most commonly seen with sickle cell disease, or underlying bone disease.

Diagnosis

Diagnosis of NTS infection is confirmed by laboratory isolation of Salmonellae from the stool, blood, or sterile body fluid. The definitive diagnosis of NTS gastroenteritis requires the identification in stool culture. Blood cultures should be performed whenever a patient has a prolonged or recurrent fever with NTS gastroenteritis. Endovascular infection should be suspected if there is high-grade bacteremia or persistent bacteremia. If an aortic or vascular infection is suspected, further imaging with computed tomography or magnetic resonance imaging (preferably with contrast angiographic analysis) should be performed.

Additionally, if a localized infection is diagnosed, such as an intraabdominal abscess or osteomyelitis, a body fluid drainage and culture is recommended. Salmonellosis is a nationally

TABLE 2	Recommended Antibiotic Therapy for Nontyphoidal Salmonella Infection in Adults		
	ANTIBIOTIC	**DOSE**	**DURATION**
Severe gastroenteritis	Ceftriaxone (Rocephin)[1]	1–2 g IV daily	3–7 days (Immunosuppressed patients may require longer treatment of 2–6 weeks)
	Cefotaxime (Claforan)[1]	2 g IV Q8h	
	Amoxicillin[1]	1 g PO TID	
	Trimethoprim-sulfamethoxazole Bactrim DS[1]	160/800 mg PO BID	
	Azithromycin (Zithromax)[1]	1000 mg PO on day 1, then 500 mg PO daily	
	Ciprofloxacin (Cipro)[1]	500 mg PO BID or 400 mg IV Q12h	
Bacteremia	Ceftriaxone[1]	2 g IV daily	7–14 days (Immunosuppressed patients may require longer treatment of 2–6 weeks)
	Cefotaxime[1]	2 g IV Q8h	
	Ciprofloxacin[1]	400 mg IV Q12h	
	Trimethoprim-sulfamethoxazole[1]	8–10 mg/kg/day of TMP component IV TID	
	Ampicillin	2 g IV Q4h	
Endovascular infection*	Ceftriaxone[1]	2 g IV daily	6–8 weeks
	Cefotaxime[1]	2 g IV Q8h	
	Ciprofloxacin[1]	400 mg IV Q12h	
	Ampicillin	2 g IV Q4h	
Extraintestinal focal infection**	Ceftriaxone[1]	2 g IV daily	4–6 weeks
	Ampicillin	2 g IV Q4h	
	Ciprofloxacin[1]	400 mg IV Q12h or 750 mg PO BID	

*Treatment includes antibiotic regimen with surgical intervention.
**Bone and joint infection should be treated for 4–6 weeks along with surgical intervention if clinically indicated.
[1]Not FDA approved for this indication.

Treatment

notifiable disease for which most states require that isolates of Salmonella be sent for serotyping to the local public health laboratory.

Treatment

NTS gastroenteritis is usually self-limited; therefore, antibiotics are routinely not recommended for an uncomplicated infection. Antibiotic therapy has been associated with prolonged bacterial shedding and potentially extending carriage.

Supportive care with fluid and electrolyte replenishment, preferably via the oral route, is the mainstay of treatment for Salmonella gastroenteritis. Patients that present with severe dehydration or profuse vomiting should initially receive intravenous fluid repletion and may require hospitalization. Antiemetics such as, but not limited to, prochlorperazine (Compazine) or promethazine (Phenergan) may be helpful for symptom control. Antimotility agents are not recommended as they can increase the risk of complications.

There are specific clinical settings where antimicrobial therapy may be warranted for those with severe disease (severe diarrhea, high fever, need for hospitalization) or risk factors for invasive disease. When antimicrobial therapy is indicated, empiric treatment is started, and it must be tailored to susceptibility data once results are available.

Fluoroquinolones are usually the agents commonly used for adults and adolescents without contraindications to such antibiotics (Table 2). Fluoroquinolones are often avoided in children due to association with the development of cartilage defects. Additionally, note that serious adverse reactions have been associated with fluoroquinolones, including tendonitis, tendon rupture, peripheral neuropathy, and QT prolongation, among others. Other antibiotic options (see Table 2) include trimethoprim-sulfamethoxazole (Bactrim)[1], amoxicillin[1], ceftriaxone (Rocephin)[1], or azithromycin (Zithromax)[1]. For patients with severe infection who cannot tolerate oral intake, intravenous fluoroquinolone or a third-generation cephalosporin such as ceftriaxone[1] is a good option. The duration of antibiotic therapy for NTS gastroenteritis in the absence of bacteremia is 3 to 7 days, depending on clinical response.

In the case of NTS bacteremia without other focal infection or immunocompromised state, 14 days of antibiotics are appropriate. Longer duration of antibiotics of 2 to 6 weeks of antibiotic therapy is recommended in patients with an immunocompromised state, including patients with advanced HIV with CD4 cell counts less than 200 cells/µL and organ transplant recipients in order to prevent a relapse of the infection.

Prolonged antibiotic therapy may be needed in patients with extraintestinal and endovascular infections, and eradication of the infection may require surgical intervention. Focal infections may require removal of the fluid collection like joint lavage in septic arthritis or abscess drainage if clinically indicated. In addition, graft or prosthetic material removal may be necessary for the eradication of the infection. The duration of the antibiotic course will depend on the infection site (see Table 2).

---

[1]Not FDA approved for this indication.

Chronic Carriage

Asymptomatic excretion or carriage of Salmonella can occur after NTS infection. This can last up to 5 weeks; however, more extended periods have been reported. Chronic carriage of NTS is defined as excretion of the organism for more than 12 months, identified in stool culture 1 month after illness, followed by repeat positive cultures. Less than 1% of patients develop NTS chronic carriage. Routine follow-up cultures are not recommended after an uncomplicated Salmonella gastroenteritis in immunocompetent patients after the resolution of symptoms. However, in the United States, public health departments may require one or more negative stool cultures for individuals who work in specific settings such as childcare, food preparation, or health care in order to return to work.

An antibiotic course for asymptomatic carriage has not been proved to be effective and may promote resistance; hence, it is not recommended. Antimicrobial therapy may be of some utility in patients with chronic carriage; however, there is no strong evidence yet supporting its routine use.

Prevention

Prevention of NTS infections involves personal and institutional efforts. Currently, there are no vaccines to prevent NTS infection. Adequate hand hygiene practices and standard precautions are still the best way to avoid NTS spread. Individuals with the condition should remain out of work until the symptoms of gastroenteritis and diarrhea resolve, especially individuals that work in food handling, childcare, health care, or direct contact with immunosuppressed patients. This approach will decrease the possibility of outbreaks. Cross-contamination can occur when uncooked meat or poultry is being prepared. Therefore, utensils and the cutting board used in the preparation of these should be washed to prevent other foods from contamination.

Additionally, the CDC advises that children less than 5 years old, adults older than 65 years of age, and immunosuppressed individuals should not handle or touch amphibians or reptiles. They also recommend keeping the equipment used to handle reptiles out of the kitchen. The CDC also recommends that live poultry should not be kept inside the house, particularly in areas of food preparation. Also, strict hand hygiene precautions are recommended after touching live fowl. Children under 5 years of age or immunocompromised patients should not handle live poultry.

References

Benenson S, Raveh D, Schlesinger Y, et al: The risk of vascular infection in adult patients with nontyphi Salmonella bacteremia, *Am J Med* 110:60–63, 2001.

Center for Disease Control and Prevention (CDC): *National Antimicrobial Resistance Monitoring System for Enteric Bacteria (NARMS): Human Isolates Surveillance Report for 2015 (Final Report)*, Atlanta, GA, 2018, US Department of Health and Human Services. https://www.cdc.gov/narms/pdf/2015-NARMS-Annual-Report-cleared_508.pdf. Accessed 29 April 2020.

Eaves DJ, Randall L, Gray DT, et al: Prevalence of mutations within the quinolone resistance-determining region of gyrA, gyrB, parC, and parE and association with antibiotic resistance in quinolone-resistant Salmonella enterica, *Antimicrob Agents Chemother* 48:4012–4015, 2004.

Hohmann EL: Nontyphoidal salmonellosis, *Clin Infect Dis* 32:263, 2001.

Majowicz SE, Musto J, Scallan E, et al: The global burden of nontyphoidal Salmonella gastroenteritis, *Clin Infect Dis* 50:882, 2010.

Panel on Opportunistic Infections in HIV-Infected Adults and Adolescents. Guidelines for the prevention and treatment of opportunistic infections in HIV-infected adults and adolescents: Recommendations from the Centers for Disease Control and Prevention, the National Institutes of Health, and the HIV Medicine Association of the Infectious Diseases Society of America. http://aidsinfo.nih.gov/contentfiles/lvguidelines/adult_oi.pdf. Accessed on April 28, 2020.

Pegues D, Miller S: Salmonella species. In Bennett J, Dolin R, Blaser M, Mandell, Douglas, editors: *Bennett's Principles and Practice of Infectious Diseases*, ed 8, Philadelphia, PA, 2015, Elsevier/Saunders, pp 2559–2568.

Riddle MS, DuPont HL, Connor BA: ACG clinical guideline: diagnosis, treatment, and prevention of acute diarrheal infections in adults, *Am J Gastroenterol* 111:602, 2016.

Schultz M: Theobald Smith, *Emerg Infect Dis* 14(12):1940–1942, 2008. https://doi.org/10.3201/eid1412.081188.

Tindall BJ, Grimont PA, Garrity GM, Euzéby JP: Nomenclature and taxonomy of the genus Salmonella, *Int J Syst Evol Microbiol* 55:521, 2005.

SEPSIS

Method of
Rabab Nasim, MD; Jeannina Smith, MD; and Hilary Faust, MD, MS

CURRENT DIAGNOSIS

Sepsis
- Evidence of end organ dysfunction caused by dysregulated inflammatory response from an infection

Septic Shock
- Persistent hypotension caused by sepsis despite adequate fluid resuscitation (defined as 30 mL/kg)

Sequential Organ Failure Assessment Score
- Mortality prediction score (https://www.mdcalc.com/calc/691/sequential-organ-failure-assessment-sofa-score)
- Includes respiratory, cardiovascular, central nervous system, renal, coagulation, and liver dysfunction
- Assessment of severity of sepsis and not diagnosis
- Validated as a predictor of mortality and prolonged intensive care unit (ICU) stay
- May apply less favorably in certain populations, including African American patients

Quick Sequential Organ Failure Assessment Score
- Screening tool for organ dysfunction (https://www.mdcalc.com/calc/2654/qsofa-quick-sofa-score-sepsis)
- May apply less favorably to patients in the emergency department and ICU
- A score >2 prompts for evaluation for sepsis and is used for screening and not diagnosis
  - Altered mental status (Glasgow Coma Scale score <15)
  - Respiratory rate >22/min
  - Systolic blood pressure <100 mm Hg

Laboratory Findings
- Lactic acidosis (≤2 mmol/L)
- Hypoxia (Pao_2:Fio_2 <400)
- Hyperbilirubinemia (≥1.2 mg/dL)
- Acute kidney injury (creatinine ≥1.2)
- Thrombocytopenia (<150,000/µL)
- Leukocytosis or leukopenia (white blood cell count <4000 or >12,000/µL)
- Elevated erythrocyte sedimentation rate or C-reactive protein

Physical Findings
- Altered mental status (Glasgow Coma Scale score <15)
- Increased capillary refill (>2 seconds)
- Anuria and oliguria (urine output <500 mL/day)
- Tachypnea (respiratory rate >22 breaths/minute)
- Tachycardia (heart rate >90 beats/minute)
- Hypothermia or hyperthermia (temperature <36°C or >38°C)

CURRENT THERAPY

Initial 3 Hours of Triage (or Within 1 Hour of Presumptive Diagnosis)
- All interventions should be undertaken simultaneously and initiated within 1 hour after making a presumptive diagnosis of sepsis.
- Initiate adequate fluid resuscitation with crystalloid solution (lactated Ringer's preferred to normal saline solution) at 30 mL/kg.
- Obtain blood, urine, and other appropriate cultures (cerebrospinal fluid, abscess drainage, catheter tip, tissue, sputum).

- Administer empiric antimicrobial therapy.
- Perform appropriate imaging studies with urgent source control as indicated and allowed by clinical status; remove potentially infected foreign bodies.

Subsequent Interventions
- Add norepinephrine (Levophed) as a first-line pressor for persistent hypotension (mean arterial pressure <65 mm Hg) despite adequate fluid resuscitation.
- Initiate therapy with dobutamine (Dobutrex) for ionotropic support if there is suspicion of contributory cardiogenic shock.
- Consider therapy with hydrocortisone (Solu-Cortef) for patients with continued hypotension despite adequate fluid resuscitation and vasopressors.
- Maintain glycemic control with a target blood glucose level <180 mg/dL.
- Use unfractionated or low-molecular-weight heparin for prophylaxis against deep venous thrombosis.
- Use a proton pump inhibitor for gastric ulcer prophylaxis.

Epidemiology

Sepsis and septic shock are leading causes of mortality both globally and domestically. The mortality exists on a continuum, with more modest mortality rates in patients with early sepsis and much higher rates in those with septic shock, in whom >40% to 50% may not survive. Although community-acquired sepsis is more common, hospital-acquired sepsis is associated with higher morbidity and mortality rates. The incidence of sepsis has increased over time, although the overall mortality rate among patients with sepsis has decreased. Studies have shown that sepsis affects all age groups, with older adults and patients who are immunocompromised being at the highest risk. Indeed, the majority of episodes of sepsis and mortality occur in individuals older than 65 years of age. Rates of sepsis and associated mortality demonstrate differences by demographic group. For example, in the United States, rates are greatest among African American men.

Etiology

Pneumonia is the leading cause of sepsis, followed by abdominal infections, bloodstream infections, and sepsis from a urinary source. The incidence of sepsis is highest during the winter, most likely reflecting increased respiratory viral infections that precede the development of bacterial pneumonia.

Microbiology

Sepsis can be caused by infection with viruses, bacteria, or fungi. The role of viruses in sepsis has been underappreciated, perhaps because of diagnostic challenges. The coronavirus disease 19 pandemic made it clear that viral sepsis can be highly morbid, but a number of common viruses can cause sepsis, including influenza and noninfluenza respiratory viruses such as parainfluenza viruses, coronaviruses, and adenoviruses.

Common bacterial causes of sepsis include gram-positive pathogens such as *Staphylococcus aureus* and *Streptococcus pneumoniae*. Among gram-negative pathogens, *Escherichia coli, Klebsiella* spp., and *Pseudomonas aeruginosa* are most commonly reported. The emergence of resistant organisms, particularly methicillin-resistant *S. aureus* and gram-negative bacteria harboring extended-spectrum β-lactamases, increases the risk of antibiotic failure and attendant mortality. Fungal pathogens may cause sepsis as well. In recent years, non-*Candida albicans* species continue to increase in incidence, particularly among patients who are immunocompromised.

It is important to note that cultures are often negative in the setting of sepsis. Indeed, nearly 50% of the time, a specific pathogen is not identified. Culture negativity is an independent predictor

of death in patients with sepsis. The relative paucity of definitive etiologic pathogens has implications for empiric antimicrobial therapy.

Definitions

The term *sepsis* is defined as a dysregulated inflammatory response of the body caused by an infection and resulting in end organ damage. Sepsis was usually fatal in the preantibiotic era, and its morbidity and mortality remain substantial. The cardinal finding is organ dysfunction that is unrelated to the primary site of infection. Organ systems affected by sepsis most commonly include the heart, kidney, lung, and central nervous system. Other systems that may be affected include endocrine, hematologic, and gastrointestinal systems.

Uncontrolled sepsis progresses to septic shock, implying a progressively graver degree of illness with associated increasing mortality. Septic shock is persistent hypotension caused by sepsis with either a systolic blood pressure less than 90 mm Hg or a mean arterial pressure (MAP) less than 65 mm Hg and a serum lactate greater than 2 mmol/L despite adequate fluid resuscitation. No single symptom, physical finding, organ dysfunction, or laboratory abnormality serves to make or exclude the diagnosis, although isolation of a microorganism in the setting of such findings is highly suggestive. Increasing numbers of physical findings and other abnormalities correlate with an increasing likelihood of the diagnosis of sepsis.

Typical clinical findings include hypoxia and/or hypercarbia, oliguria, acute kidney injury, poor perfusion, sepsis-induced cardiomyopathy, hyperglycemia or hypoglycemia, thrombocytopenia, anemia, coagulopathy, ileus, acute liver injury, hyperbilirubinemia, acidosis, elevated lactate, edema, hyperthermia or hypothermia, and hypotension.

Pathophysiology

Infection of the host by a microorganism leads to innate and then adaptive immune activation. This process serves to isolate the site and source of infection. As a consequence, local tissue is often damaged, but eventually the infection is cleared, allowing for repair and regeneration. This process is highly regulated, with a number of different cell types and mediators involved, all in delicate balance between proinflammatory and antiinflammatory effects. The patient may have few or no symptoms, or there may be systemic evidence of infection.

Sepsis is the failure of localization such that the process becomes generalized and leads to tissue destruction remote from the site of infection. Why the immune system enters this state of dysregulation currently remains poorly understood. Some microbes contribute to this process through the elaboration of pathogen-associated molecular patterns by the innate immune system or the elaboration of toxins (typically by gram-positive organisms) and endotoxins (gram-negative–derived lipopolysaccharide). Immune recognition of these mediators leads to tissue destruction as a result of ischemic insult, direct cytotoxicity, and accelerated programmed cell death including apoptosis, necroptosis, pyroptosis, and ferroptosis. Generation of damage-associated molecular patterns from lytic cell death may further amplify the inflammatory response, leading to increased tissue injury and organ dysfunction and higher mortality. Genetic predisposition to sepsis and sepsis mortality has long been recognized, with specific genetic loci increasingly identified as risk factors.

The host response is highly heterogenous, making it difficult to predict who will be at a higher risk of developing sepsis or having poor outcomes. An enormous amount of research over the past four decades has elucidated many of the pathways and mediators involved. Tumor necrosis factor-alpha; platelet-activating factor; interleukin (IL)-1, IL-6, and IL-8; eicosanoids; complement pathway proteins; interferons; and nitric oxide are among the biologically active molecules characterized to date. Recent studies using integrated genomics have identified genetic variants more likely to have a pathogenic response to infections. Certain endotypes within sepsis reflecting differential gene expression such as sepsis response syndromes 1 and 2 and the Dutch molecular diagnosis and risk stratification of sepsis (MARS) 1 to 4 endotypes are noted to have differential mortality rates and treatment response. These studies provide a platform for future exploration of a "precision medicine approach" to targeted therapeutic intervention in this population to improve sepsis outcomes, but they are not yet clinically relevant.

Diagnosis

The diagnosis of sepsis ultimately relies on the clinical suspicion of infection in the setting of end organ dysfunction. The quick Sequential Organ Failure Assessment screening tool (https://www.mdcalc.com/calc/2654/qsofa-quick-sofa-score-sepsis) identifies organ dysfunction, which distinguishes uncomplicated infection from sepsis. A constellation of other supportive evidence establishes a greater or lesser likelihood of the presence of sepsis (see the Current Diagnosis box). If clinical suspicion of an underlying infection warrants drawing of culture of body fluids, the diagnosis of sepsis is presumed and justifies the initiation of empiric antibiotics and fluid resuscitation in the setting of hypotension. It is rare that specific microbiologic identification and antibiotic susceptibilities are available to guide initial therapy; therefore sepsis diagnosis relies on careful history taking, a high index of suspicion, and appropriate evaluation for end organ dysfunction.

Treatment

Screening and Early Treatment

The 2021 guidelines from the Surviving Sepsis Campaign, an international initiative to improve sepsis outcomes, emphasize the importance of early screening and initiation of treatment. Protocolized sepsis resuscitation became common after the success of early goal-directed therapy (EGDT). However, the Australasian Resuscitation in Sepsis Evaluation, Protocolised Management In Sepsis, and Protocolized Care for Early Septic Shock randomized clinical trials did not demonstrate a benefit to EGDT or protocolized sepsis management over "usual standard care," which may reflect the extent to which EGDT and protocolized resuscitation influenced usual practices. Nevertheless, the mandated introduction of a sepsis bundle including early sepsis identification, initial lactate measurement, cultures, and timely and empiric antimicrobial therapy in the state of New York was associated with reductions in sepsis morbidity and mortality. Based on this, recent recommendations have advocated for performance improvement programs for sepsis, including screening of high-risk acutely ill patients for sepsis and implementation of standard operating procedures for evaluation and treatment, commonly referred to as *sepsis bundles* or *sepsis resuscitation bundles*. The sepsis resuscitation bundle is a combination of evidence-based objectives that must be completed within 1 to 6 hours for patients presenting with severe sepsis, septic shock, and/or elevated lactate, defined as >4 mmol/L (36 mg/dL). Sepsis bundles aim to deliver efficient and effective sepsis care in a timely manner, and studies have shown improved mortality with higher compliance with sepsis bundles.

Initial Resuscitation

Sepsis and septic shock are medical emergencies, and it is recommended to begin treatment and resuscitation immediately (within the first 3 hours of triage or within 1 hour of presumed diagnosis). Clinicians should not wait for microbiological confirmation or evidence of an increasing Sequential Organ Failure Assessment score to initiate therapy. For all patients with sepsis and septic shock, recommended treatment includes measuring lactate, obtaining blood cultures, and administering broad-spectrum antibiotics. If the lactate exceeds 2 mg/dL, it should be repeated within 6 hours of presentation. For patients with evidence of septic shock, including hypotension or hypoperfusion as defined by a lactate level >4 mg/dL, it is additionally recommended to give at least 30 mL/kg of intravenous crystalloid solution.

After initial fluid resuscitation of 30 mL/kg in the first 3 hours, fluid status should be reassessed with a goal of resuscitation directed toward a MAP >65 mm Hg, urine output >0.5 mL/kg, or decreasing lactate by 20%.

If hypotension does not respond to the initial 30 mL/kg fluid resuscitation within 6 hours of diagnosis, administration of vasopressors is recommended with a goal of resuscitation directed toward a MAP goal >65 mm Hg. If the initial lactate was elevated, it should be remeasured within 6 hours.

Choice of Fluid Administered

In patients with septic shock, normal saline solution was previously one of the most common intravenous fluids used for resuscitation. However, recent data suggest that the use of normal saline is associated with increased rates of acute kidney injury, hyperchloremic acidosis, and requirement for renal replacement therapy. Balanced crystalloid solutions like lactate Ringer's solution or Plasma-Lyte A, which have electrolyte compositions more similar to that of plasma, have improved performance over normal saline solution and represent an increasingly used alternative.

Colloids are more effective at volume resuscitation compared with crystalloids in septic shock, although the translation of this finding to improved outcomes remains uncertain. The Saline versus Albumin Fluid Evaluation trial of 4% albumin and the Albumin Italian Outcome Sepsis trial of 20% albumin did not show a mortality benefit of using albumin solution for fluid resuscitation compared with crystalloid solution, although decreased mortality was observed in patients with sepsis in the Saline versus Albumin Fluid Evaluation trial and in septic shock in the Albumin Italian Outcome Sepsis trial in post hoc analyses. The Surviving Sepsis Campaign suggested the use of albumin in patients requiring large volumes of fluid resuscitation based on these data, and other populations such as patients with cirrhosis may also benefit from albumin resuscitation. Data have shown serious adverse events including increased risk of acute kidney injury and mortality with the use of pentastarch or hydroxyethyl starch, both of which should be definitively avoided in sepsis patients.

Monitoring Treatment Response

Static parameter targets include a central venous pressure of 8 to 12 mm Hg and a central venous oxygenation ($ScvO_2$) greater than 70%. Since the publication of the Protocolized Care for Early Septic Shock, Australasian Resuscitation in Sepsis Evaluation, and Protocolised Management In Sepsis trials, which reported no mortality benefit in association with use of these static measures, dynamic parameters have been emphasized in guidelines such as the Surviving Sepsis Campaign.

Dynamic parameters such as pulse pressure variation, stroke volume variation, respirophasic variation of the inferior vena cava (IVC), and the passive leg raise test may be used to guide fluid resuscitation to predict fluid responsiveness and avoid complications such as volume overload and pulmonary edema, particularly in patients who have concomitant heart failure and chronic kidney disease.

Pulse pressure variation is calculated as a difference in systolic and diastolic arterial blood pressure and for mechanically ventilated patients is a good indicator of volume responsiveness. A systematic review of 29 studies reported a higher area under the receiver operating characteristic curve for pulse pressure variation compared with central venous pressure (0.94 vs. 0.55) as an indicator of fluid responsiveness. Stroke volume variation greater than 10% measured by echocardiography is also associated with fluid responsiveness. According to one study, stroke volume variation showed a sensitivity and specificity of 94% each, and another meta-analysis reported that it resulted in shorter length of hospital stay. Point-of-care ultrasonography can be used to assess respirophasic variation in the IVC. Change in IVC diameter with respiration of 12% to 18% has been associated with fluid responsiveness. Other maneuvers include the passive leg raising test, which demonstrates similar performance. Although these methods are promising for prediction of fluid responsiveness, none have demonstrated clear superiority or mortality benefit; thus optimal assessment of fluid resuscitation remains an area of active research.

Serial measurement of lactate to determine whether clearance is achieved along with serial assessment of capillary refill time as a marker of perfusion may be useful to guide resuscitation and fluid or vasopressor administration. Some studies have shown the use of serial measurement of lactate and capillary refill time as markers of resuscitation to be associated with less intravenous fluid administration and possible 28-day mortality benefit.

Vasopressor Support

If there is persistent hypotension despite adequate fluid resuscitation, it is recommended to initiate vasopressor support. Norepinephrine is the first-line agent recommended for septic shock, and addition of vasopressin and epinephrine are recommended as second-line agents. Norepinephrine is superior to dopamine, resulting in a lower risk of mortality and arrhythmias in a large meta-analysis, an effect that is particularly pronounced in patients with cardiogenic shock. Use of low-dose dopamine for renal protection is no longer recommended. Dobutamine is recommended if evidence of hypoperfusion persists after adequate fluid resuscitation and vasopressor administration.

Randomized controlled trials of early vasopressor initiation in early sepsis and patients in the intensive care unit (ICU) have not demonstrated a benefit over protocolized fluid resuscitation in the CLOVERS and CLASSIC trials. Choice of fluid resuscitation or early vasopressor initiation should therefore be tailored based on individual patient characteristics, such as history of clinical evidence of volume depletion, history of end stage renal disease or congestive heart failure, or evidence of volume overload. A MAP goal of >65 mm Hg is appropriate for most patients; patients with chronic hypertension treated with a MAP goal of 80 to 85 mm Hg had lower rates of acute kidney injury requiring renal replacement therapy but higher rates of arrhythmias compared with those treated with a MAP goal of 60 to 65 mm Hg. A subsequent pooled analysis demonstrated increased mortality in patients treated with a higher MAP goal for greater than 6 hours, necessitating an individualized approach.

Antimicrobial Therapy

National and international quality measures and guidelines recommend immediate empiric broad-spectrum antibiotics for all patients with suspected sepsis. Timely initiation of appropriate antimicrobials is critical because the risk of mortality increases with every hour delay. Inadequate therapy is much more likely in patients with resistant pathogens including methicillin-resistant *S. aureus*, vancomycin-resistant enterococci, and resistant gram-negative bacteria, as well as in nosocomial versus community-acquired sepsis. It is less well appreciated that "overly broad" antimicrobial treatment for sepsis is also associated with an increased risk of poor outcome. A careful review of the history and physical examination and the prior culture results may help with the selection of empiric antimicrobials. The increasing availability of molecular detection methods is hoped to assist in selecting appropriate antimicrobial therapy in the future. This in turn can decrease the time to correct treatment for patients with sepsis and the incidence of multidrug-resistant organisms, *Clostridium difficile* infection, organ failure resulting from ineffective treatment, and deleterious effect on the gut microbiota.

Source Control

A survey for potential sources of infection should be performed, and early resuscitation efforts should occur concomitantly. Elimination of the source of infection is critical to reversing septic shock. Conditions that require emergent intervention, such as necrotizing fasciitis, cholangitis, and intestinal infarction, should be ruled out within the first 6 hours after presentation. Potentially infected indwelling devices should be removed as soon as possible. Necrotic tissue should be debrided and abscesses drained if either condition is detected. Practitioners must consider the risks and benefits of the specific invasive procedures and the timing of such interventions for each patient individually. Imaging studies such as computed tomography of the head, chest, abdomen, and pelvis are commonly necessary to assess for potential sources or sequelae of infection. An exception to the mandate to drain or debride infected collections is the presence of infected pancreatic necrosis, in which case a step-up approach including endoscopic and/or percutaneous drainage, preferably delayed by at least 2 weeks, is preferred.

Biomarkers in Sepsis

The need for a prompt diagnosis and treatment of sepsis has led to intense research into biomarkers for diagnosis and prognostication in sepsis. Over 250 biomarkers have been identified in sepsis, although procalcitonin and C-reactive protein remain the principal biomarkers in clinical use. Procalcitonin is a precursor to calcitonin that is often upregulated in sepsis. Data show that the use of procalcitonin is beneficial as a tool to deescalate antibiotics in patients with sepsis, particularly those with community-acquired pneumonia, rather than as a diagnostic tool. A randomized trial has shown use of procalcitonin to guide discontinuation of antibiotic therapy to be associated with a reduction in 28-day mortality in patients with pneumonia, pyelonephritis, or primary bloodstream infections, suggesting that this may be a useful approach to antimicrobial deescalation for patients with septic shock. Identifying sepsis biomarkers with superior diagnostic performance to procalcitonin and C-reactive protein is an area of active study. Some promising examples include decoy receptor 3, group II phospholipase A2, sCD163, CD64, and heparin-binding protein, but they will require further research and validation before they become available for widespread clinical use.

Steroid Use

Patients with critical illness can develop absolute or relative adrenal insufficiency. Although absolute adrenal insufficiency is rare, relative adrenal insufficiency caused by hypothalamic-pituitary-adrenal dysfunction may occur in critically ill patients. Administration of low-dose glucocorticoids, typically hydrocortisone 200 to 300 mg in divided doses, has consistently been associated with faster reversal of septic shock. However, the data conflict as to whether there is a mortality benefit associated with steroid use. A large meta-analysis found that there was no overall association of glucocorticoid use with improved mortality but did find improved 28-day, ICU, and hospital mortality with combined administration of hydrocortisone and fludrocortisone. Subsequent studies have found that response to steroids interacts with underlying endotype, with associated harm in the SRS2 endotype. Thus steroid administration should be considered on a personalized basis. Steroids should be tapered as soon as vasopressor support is no longer required.

Conservative Transfusion Threshold

Blood transfusions are immunomodulatory and associated with volume overload. Guidelines recommend limiting red blood cell transfusion to patients with septic shock with a hemoglobin level less than 7 g/dL, which is based on data derived from randomized controlled trials. A large randomized trial of nearly 1000 patients demonstrated no increased mortality with a restrictive strategy using transfusion triggers of hemoglobin <7 g/dL (conservative strategy) versus hemoglobin <9 g/dL (liberal strategy). The restrictive group additionally did not have higher ischemic adverse effects. However, evidence extrapolated from studies of transfusion thresholds in patients with stable cardiovascular disease and patients post cardiac surgery suggests the use of a transfusion threshold of hemoglobin <8 g/dL in patients with sepsis with known coronary artery disease.

Nutrition in the Critically Ill Patient

Critically ill patients are in a state of catabolism, and studies have shown that early enteral nutrition, which is defined as within 48 hours of admission to the critical care unit, may decrease the risk of infection, specifically pneumonia, and mortality. However, if there is ongoing shock with MAPs <50 mm Hg and escalating vasopressor support, initiating enteral feeding may theoretically precipitate mesenteric ischemia and nonocclusive bowel necrosis. Enteral nutrition should be initiated only in patients who have been well resuscitated and are on stable levels of vasopressor support.

Glycemic Control

It is recommended for critically ill patients to have blood glucose target between 140 and 180 mg/dL rather than tighter control with intensive insulin therapy because studies have shown that tighter blood glucose control has no benefit and is associated with increased incidences of hypoglycemia and a higher risk of mortality. More recent data demonstrated that the use of individualized glucose targets based on pre-ICU glycated hemoglobin levels resulted in higher rates of severe hypoglycemia and increased mortality in nondiabetic patients; thus a goal of <180 mg/dL is appropriate for this population.

Summary

Sepsis remains a life-threatening medical emergency and a leading cause of death in the United States and worldwide. Early recognition and aggressive management are vital to improving outcomes, yet the diagnosis continues to require a high index of suspicion, timely evaluation, and robust clinical judgment. Major challenges include diagnostic uncertainty, low yield of current culture techniques, and antimicrobial overuse and resistance. Improvements in diagnostic and prognostic biomarkers, technologies to identify responsible microbes, identification of biologically based endotypes, and precision therapies are promising areas for future inquiry and improvement in sepsis care.

References

Antcliffe DB, Burnham KL, Al-Beidh F, et al: Transcriptomic signatures in sepsis and a differential response to steroids. From the VANISH randomized trial, *Am J Respir Crit Care Med* 199(8):980–986, 2019.

Davenport EE, Burnham KL, Radhakrishnan J, et al: Genomic landscape of the individual host response and outcomes in sepsis: a prospective cohort study, *Lancet Respir Med* 4(4):259–271, 2016.

Evans L, Rhodes A, Alhazzani W, et al: Surviving sepsis Campaign: international guidelines for management of sepsis and septic shock 2021, *Crit Care Med* 49(11):e1063–e1143, 2021.

Kyriazopoulou E, Liaskou-Antoniou L, Adamis G, et al: Procalcitonin to reduce long-term infection-associated adverse events in sepsis. A randomized trial, *Am J Respir Crit Care Med* 203(2):202–210, 2021.

Liu VX, Fielding-Singh V, Greene JD, et al: The timing of early antibiotics and hospital mortality in sepsis, *Am J Respir Crit Care Med* 196(7):856–863, 2017.

Lyu QQ, Chen QH, Zheng RQ, Yu JQ, Gu XH: Effect of low-dose hydrocortisone therapy in adult patients with septic shock: a meta-analysis with trial sequential analysis of randomized controlled trials, *J Intensive Care Med* 35(10):971–983, 2020.

Meyhoff TS, Hjortrup PB, Wetterslev J, CLASSIC Trial Group, et al: Restriction of intravenous fluid in ICU patients with septic shock, *N Engl J Med* 386(26):2459–2470, 2022.

Mouncey PR, Osborn TM, Power GS, et al: Protocolised Management in Sepsis (ProMISe): a multicentre randomised controlled trial of the clinical effectiveness and cost-effectiveness of early, goal-directed, protocolised resuscitation for emerging septic shock, *Health Technol Assess* 19(97):i–xxv, 1–150, 2015.

National Heart, Lung, and Blood Institute Prevention and Early Treatment of Acute Lung Injury Clinical Trials Network, Shapiro NI, Douglas IS, Brower RG, et al: Early restrictive or liberal fluid management for sepsis-induced hypotension, *N Engl J Med* 388(6):499–510, 2023.

Peake SL, Delaney A, Bailey M, et al: Goal-directed resuscitation for patients with early septic shock, *N Engl J Med* 371(16):1496–1506, 2014.

Rudd KE, Johnson SC, Agesa KM, et al: Global, regional, and national sepsis incidence and mortality, 1990-2017: analysis for the Global Burden of Disease Study, *Lancet* 395(10219):200–211, 2020.

Yealy DM, Kellum JA, Huang DT, et al: A randomized trial of protocol-based care for early septic shock, *N Engl J Med* 370(18):1683–1693, 2014.

SMALLPOX

Method of
Raul Davaro, MD

CURRENT DIAGNOSIS

- Human-to-human transmission of variola virus occurs by inhalation of large, virus-containing airborne droplets of saliva from an infected person.
- Before smallpox was eradicated, the disease had a secondary household or close contact attack rate of approximately 60% among unvaccinated individuals.
- There are four main clinical forms of smallpox, each with different characteristics.
- During the smallpox era, the case-fatality rate differed for the different clinical forms, but it was approximately 30% overall in unvaccinated individuals.

CURRENT THERAPY

- There is no proven treatment for smallpox disease in people sick with smallpox.
- Isolating patients in a negative-pressure room and insuring vaccination is the main course of therapy.

Smallpox is caused by the variola virus (VARV) and is highly infectious by the respiratory route. Susceptible persons have up to a 90% chance of contracting the disease if they are exposed to someone who is infected, and the overall fatality rate is estimated at 30% among those who have not been vaccinated. The VARV is unique among the orthopoxviruses in that it is known to be a sole human pathogen.

The World Health Organization (WHO) declared smallpox eradicated in 1980 and today is the only human disease to be eliminated by the WHO. The eradication of smallpox through vaccination has not eliminated the risk of reintroduction of the infection by the accidental or intentional release of the VARV.

This viral infection, spread by respiratory droplets, continued to have worldwide distribution at the beginning of the 20th century. Because smallpox confers immunity in the survivors of an attack, its persistence depends on the contact of nonimmune persons with infected persons in the initial 2 weeks of acquiring the infection.

The WHO designed an Intensified Eradication Program based on a ring vaccination strategy that began in 1966 and eradicated smallpox from humans in an unprecedented effort in less than 10 years. The last natural case was documented in Somalia in 1977. Routine immunization against smallpox ceased in the United States in 1972 and worldwide in 1980. It was thought that without a human reservoir, the reemergence of this infection would not occur.

Smallpox virus stocks are still available in the United States at the Centers for Disease Control and Prevention (CDC) in Atlanta, Georgia, and in Russia at the State Center for Virology and Biotechnology in Novosibirsk, Siberia. These stocks are maintained under strict biocontainment measures. In the aftermath of the terrorist attacks on September 11, 2001, and the deliberate distribution of *Bacillus anthracis* afterward, President Bush announced plans to immunize health care workers and first responders against smallpox by 2003. Although the plan fell short of its goals, 40,000 first responders and health care workers were vaccinated by the end of 2003.

The Agent

Smallpox is a single, linear, double-stranded DNA virus that belongs to the *Orthopoxvirus* genus, family Poxviridae. The poxviruses replicate in the cell cytoplasm. They are brick shaped and measure about 300 by 250 by 200 nm.

Epidemiology

The natural reservoir of smallpox is the patient suffering from the disease. Smallpox spreads from person to person through droplet nuclei or fine-particle aerosols released from the pharynx of infected persons. Smallpox can also be transmitted by fomites such as clothing and bedding. Smallpox patients are not infectious until the third day of the clinical disease, typically 1 day before the skin eruption. The secondary attack rate of smallpox is 37% to 88% among unvaccinated contacts, depending on many variables.

Clinical Presentation

Smallpox occurs as either variola major or variola minor (alastrim). Variola major had a mortality rate of 30% compared with 1% for variola minor.

After an incubation period of 10 to 14 days, the illness begins with intense prostration and high fever lasting 4 to 6 days (Figure 1). Headache, photophobia, and vomiting are noted. During the prodrome phase, most patients are bedridden. Around the fourth day, the fever breaks and the patient feels better.

The eruptive phase is signaled by an enanthem involving the buccal mucosa and pharynx and a centrifugal exanthem that begins on the face and forearms. The initial rash is macular and turns pustular in 1 to 2 days. Within 2 days, the papules evolve into vesicles that become cloudy and pustular. Most patients exhibit lesions on their soles and palms. A typical feature of variola is that the exanthem everywhere is in the same state of evolution, unlike the exanthem of chickenpox, in which lesions exhibit all stages of evolution. At the end of days 8 to 10, the skin rash crusts and dries; it takes 3 to 4 weeks from the onset of the disease for all the scabs to fall off. The period of contagiousness ends when the last scab falls off. Scarring and pitting of the skin are common sequelae.

Patients with the hemorrhagic disease develop severe prostration, high fever, abdominal pain, petechiae, and extensive cutaneous ecchymoses. In the malignant or flat form, the lesions fail to progress to the pustular stage. In the hemorrhagic and the malignant forms, death invariably occurs within 1 week.

Complications

Bacterial infections of the skin and other organs are common. Ocular involvement may result in blindness. Encephalitis (1 in 500 cases of variola major) is a devastating complication.

Differential Diagnosis (Figure 2)

Many rashes can be confused with smallpox, especially at the outset of the eruption, when the rash is maculopapular. Herpes zoster, chickenpox, herpes simplex, impetigo, scabies, erythema multiforme, and syphilis are some of the conditions that can be confused with smallpox (Box 1). When smallpox was endemic, chickenpox was the most common condition confused with smallpox. The most useful clinical points of smallpox are the following:

- Centrifugal distribution of the lesions
- All the lesions in the same stage of development
- Progression of the rash from the face to the arms, trunk, and legs
- A severe prodrome phase that lasts 4 days
- In an epidemic, known contact with an active case

Diagnosis

The identification of a suspected case of smallpox should be treated as an international health emergency. Clinical samples may be collected from vesicular or pustular fluid, blood, tonsillar swabs, and skin biopsy and must be transported to a biosafety level 4 facility for processing and testing with real-time polymerase chain reaction (PCR) assays to detect virus DNA.

Lesions of varicella zoster virus (chickenpox, herpes zoster) demonstrate multinucleated giant cells on Tzanck smears; lesions of smallpox do not. Serology or electronic microscopy is not recommended for the diagnosis of smallpox

Figure 1 Clinical manifestations and pathogenesis of smallpox and the immune response. **A,** The initial phases of infection and the clinical manifestations include temperature spikes and progressive skin lesions (photographs of lesions courtesy of Dr. David Heymann, World Health Organization). **B,** The pathogenesis of the infection. The photographs on the *right* show the characteristic features of the vesicles caused by smallpox (H&E, × 90). **C,** The immune response to smallpox and the period of infectiousness. *CF,* Complement fixation; *HI,* hemagglutination inhibition. (Reprinted with permission from Breman JG, Henderson DA: Diagnosis and management of smallpox, *N Eng J Med* 346:1300–1308, 2002.)

Figure 2 Algorithm for assessing patients for smallpox. (Reprinted with permission from Moore ZS, Seward JF, Lane JM: Smallpox, *Lancet* 367:425–435, 2006.)

BOX 1   Conditions That Might Be Confused with Smallpox

Maculopapular stage
Measles
Rubella
Drug eruptions
Secondary syphilis
Erythema multiforme
Scabies, insect bites
Acne
Scarlet fever

Vesicular/Pustular stage
Chickenpox
Disseminated herpes zoster
Disseminated herpes simplex virus
Drug eruptions
Contact dermatitis
Erythema multiforme (including Stevens-Johnson syndrome)
Enteroviral infections
Secondary syphilis
Acne
Generalized vaccinia
Monkeypox
Impetigo
Scabies, insect bites
Disseminated molluscum contagiosum

---

because these modalities cannot distinguish among different orthopoxviruses.

Treatment

A suspected case of smallpox should be placed in a negative-pressure room with strict respiratory and contact isolation precautions. Ideally, to minimize the risk of contagion in health care personnel, patients with smallpox should be assisted by providers documented to have been immunized against this condition. Patients with smallpox require careful care of their eyes to avoid complications, and this is accomplished with daily eye rinsing. Patients must receive adequate nutrition and hydration. Skin and soft tissue infections must be treated with an antistaphylococcal β-lactam and, initially pending results of cultures, an antimicrobial with activity against methicillin-resistant *Staphylococcus aureus*. Tecovirimat (TPOXX) is an inhibitor of the orthopoxvirus VP37 envelope wrapping protein and is indicated for the treatment of human smallpox disease in adults and pediatric patients weighing at least 13 kg. The effectiveness of TPOXX for treatment of smallpox disease has not been determined in humans because adequate and well-controlled field trials have not been feasible, and inducing smallpox disease in humans to study the drug's efficacy is not ethical. TPOXX efficacy may be reduced in immunocompromised patients based on studies demonstrating reduced efficacy in immunocompromised animal models. The recommended dosage of tecovirimat in adults weighing at least 40 kg is 600 mg (three 200-mg capsules) taken twice daily orally for 14 days. No adequate and well-controlled studies in pregnant women were conducted; therefore, there are no human data to establish the presence or absence of tecovirimat-associated risk. Common adverse reactions in healthy adult subjects (≥2%) were headache, nausea, abdominal pain, and vomiting.

Vaccines and Vaccination

The current smallpox live vaccine, ACAM2000 (Sanofi Pasteur Biologics), is based on the traditional Jenner vaccine (using the related virus, vaccinia) and is administered in a single percutaneous dose. Vaccination after exposure—but before the rash is present—can abort or attenuate the clinical manifestations of the disease. This live vaccine is contraindicated for persons with severe immunosuppression, and newer-generation vaccinations have been developed for these populations. The virus begins growing at the injection site causing a localized infection or "pock" to form. A red, itchy sore spot at the site of the vaccination within 3 to 4 days is an indicator that the vaccination was successful; that is, there is "a take." A blister develops at the vaccination site and then dries up, forming a scab that falls off in the third week, leaving a small scar. If no evidence of vaccine take is apparent after 7 days, the person can be vaccinated again.

The vaccine causes local and systemic symptoms. There is an eruption at the injection site with redness and pain, systemic symptoms such as fever, and headaches. Swelling and tenderness of regional lymph nodes begin 3 to 10 days after vaccination and can last up to a month.

The Modified Vaccinia Ankara (MVA [JYNNEOS]) was compared with ACAM2000. The immune responses and attenuation of the major cutaneous reaction suggest that this MVA vaccine protected against variola infection.

Complications

The vaccine (ACAM2000) is not without risk: it is estimated that pericarditis or myocarditis may develop in 5.7 per 1000 vaccinees. In addition, eczema vaccinatum, generalized vaccinia, progressive vaccinia, and vaccinia encephalitis can also occur (Table 1). The most common complication is inadvertent autoinoculation causing self-limited satellite lesions. Generalized vaccinia results from viremia and may be life threatening in immunocompromised patients. Progressive vaccinia is characterized by necrosis at the inoculation site and distal sites such as bones and internal organs. Progressive vaccinia is often a fatal complication. Myopericarditis was observed with the use of adult vaccines in the United States in 2002 (see Table 1).

Contraindications to Vaccination

Persons who are immune compromised or who have severe eczema or who are pregnant should not receive postexposure vaccination against smallpox. However, in the event of exposure to a patient with smallpox, no absolute contraindication is applicable.

Use in Warfare

Because natural smallpox has been eradicated, the only possibility of a smallpox outbreak is the deliberate release of smallpox in a population by a nation or a terrorist group to inflict casualties in a civilian population. Preemptive vaccination of first responders and ring immunization of those exposed are the means available to avoid the massive propagation of smallpox. Smallpox stocks have been earmarked for destruction since the eradication of the disease in 1980. Yet, successive meetings of the World Health Assembly have postponed making a final recommendation while the threat of reemergence from elsewhere remains. At its last meeting in September 2018, the Advisory Committee on Variola Virus Research told WHO that live virus is still needed for the development of new antivirals, with split opinions on whether it is needed for diagnostics.

References

Adalja AA, Toner E, Inglesby TV: Clinical management of potential bioterrosism related conditions, *N Engl J Med* 372:954–962, 2015.

Behbehani A: The smallpox story: Life and death of an old disease, *Microbiol Rev* 47:455–509, 1983.

Breman JG, Henderson DA: Diagnosis and management of smallpox, *N Engl J Med* 346:1300–1308, 2002.

Bronze MS, Huycke MM, Machado LJ, et al: Viral agents as biological weapons and agents of bioterrorism, *Am J Med Sci* 323:316–325, 2002.

Centers for Disease Control and Prevention: Smallpox vaccination. Information for Health Care professionals. Available at http://www.bt.cdc.gov/agent/smallpox/vaccination/ [accessed 05.05.15].

Cleri DJ, Porwancher RB, Ricketti AJ, et al: Smallpox as a bioterrorist weapon: Myth or menace? *Infectious Dis Clin North Am* 20:329–358, 2006.

Grosenbach DW, Honeychurch K, Rose EA, et al: Oral tecovirimat for the treatment of smallpox, *N Engl J Med* 379:44–53, 2018.

Kempe HC: Variola. In Beeson PB, McDermott W, editors: *Textbook of Medicine*, ed 12, Philadelphia, 1967, WB Saunders, pp 44–46.

Lofquist J, Weimert NA, Hayney MS: Smallpox: a review of clinical disease and vaccination, *Am J Health Syst Pharm* 60:749–758, 2003.

Moore ZS, Seward JF, Lane JM: Smallpox, *Lancet* 367:425–435, 2006.

Pittman PR, Hahn M, HeeChoon S Lee, et al: Phase 3 efficacy trial of modified vaccinia ankara as a vaccine against smallpox, *N Engl J Med* 381:1897–1908, 2019.

Weiss MM, Weiss PD, Mathisen G, et al: Rethinking smallpox, *Clin Infect Dis* 29:1668–1673, 2004.

Whitley RJ: Smallpox: a potential agent of bioterrorism, *Antiviral Res* 57(7–12), 2003.

TABLE 1 | Rates of Complications from Vaccinia, According to Vaccination Status and Age[a]

Complications	PRIMARY VACCINATION (*N* = 650,000)				REVACCINATION (*N* = 996,000)			
	0–4 Years	5–19 Years	> 20 Years	All Ages	1–4 Years[b]	5–19 Years	> 20 Years	All Ages
Accidental infection	564	371	606	529	198	48	25	42
Generalized vaccinia	263	140	212	242	0	10	9	9
Erythema multiforme	299	87	30	165	73	2	9	10
Eczema vaccinatum	39	35	30	39	0	2	5	3
Postvaccinal encephalitis	15	9	0	12	0	0	5	2
Progressive vaccinia	3	0	0	2	0	0	7	3
Other	222	214	6636	266	18	24	55	39

[a]Data are from a 1968 survey of 10 states. No deaths occurred.
[b]No children younger than 1 year were revaccinated.
Reprinted with permission from Breman JG, Henderson DA: Diagnosis and management of smallpox, *N Engl J Med* 346:1300–1308, 2002.

TETANUS

Method of
Dilip R. Karnad, MD

Tetanus is a potentially fatal illness caused by the neurotoxin produced by the spore-bearing anaerobic bacterium *Clostridium tetani*. As the causative organism and its spores are ubiquitous, nonimmune individuals in any part of the world may get tetanus unless they are protected by the highly effective vaccine.

Epidemiology

As a result of effective universal immunization, tetanus is rare in the developed world. Twenty to 40 cases of tetanus occur annually in the United States and 12 to 15 cases per year have been reported from the United Kingdom in the last 10 years. Although progressively declining in the developing world due to improved immunization coverage, according to WHO figures, more than 500 cases were reported in 2012 from each of these nations: Angola, Bangladesh, Congo, India, and Uganda. While tetanus may affect individuals of all ages, a significant number of cases in developed countries are elderly people who did not receive a primary immunization or lacked the booster dosage needed to maintain protective immunity. In developing countries, most cases are neonates (*tetanus neonatorum*), children who are born to nonimmunized mothers and thus lack transplacentally acquired passive immunity. Infection of the umbilical stump due to poor hygiene results in severe tetanus that has mortality in excess of 60%.

The infection is caused by the gram-positive, spore-bearing bacterium *C. tetani*, the spores of which exist in the soil, in animal feces, and even in the human gastrointestinal tract. Spores remain dormant and viable for several months and are destroyed by autoclaving at 1 atmosphere pressure at 120°C for 15 minutes. When inoculated into human or animal tissues, they transform into motile bacilli in an anerobic environment that produce a potent exotoxin, tetanospasmin, which produces the manifestations of tetanus. It must be emphasized that tetanus is not transmitted from human to human, and patients do not require isolation.

Risk Factors

Elderly individuals are at increased risk, as they may not have received adequate immunization or may have waning immunity. Other predisposed groups include immigrants from countries with an unreliable immunization program, immunosuppressed individuals (with HIV infection or receiving immunosuppressive drugs), and intravenous drug addicts. Local factors include wounds with crushed, devitalized tissue or contaminated by dirt or rust, such as open fractures, punctures, and abscesses. However, even scratches, chronic ulcers, or tattooing may cause tetanus. In developing countries, unsafe practices related to termination of pregnancy may cause maternal tetanus; newborn babies born outside of medical facilities are at risk of neonatal tetanus.

Pathophysiology

Tetanospasmin is a highly toxic protein released by *C. tetani*. It is absorbed into the circulation and reaches the ends of motor axons all over the body, from where it is transported proximally along the axonal cytoplasm to motor nuclei in the brainstem and spinal cord at a rate of 3 to 13 mm/hour. A fragment of the toxin then binds inhibitory interneurons that produce gamma-amino butyric acid (GABA) and glycine and inactivates synaptobrevin, a protein that is essential for the release of these neurotransmitters from presynaptic vesicles.

The loss of normal inhibition at motor and autonomic neurons results in spontaneous discharge of nerve impulses as well as exaggerated responses to stimuli manifesting as tonic muscle contraction with superadded intermittent muscle spasms. As tetanospasmin reaches the motor nuclei of the shortest motor axons first, muscles innervated by motor cranial nerves are affected first, followed by trunk muscles, and finally the extremities. Autonomic overactivity results in severe tachycardia, swings in blood pressure, profuse sweating, and (rarely) ileus. An exaggerated startle-like response to stimuli with motor and autonomic components is also typical. Generalized spasms may mimic tonic seizures.

Clinical Manifestations

An attempt should be made to locate the predisposing wound, such as cuts, abrasions, burns, puncture wounds, and other skin lesions. Uncommon causes include needle-sticks in intravenous drug abusers, ulcerated malignant tumors, and chronic middle-ear infection in children (otogenic tetanus). In up to 30% of patients, no site of infection is discovered. The incubation period is the interval between the injury and the onset of symptoms and can range from a few days to a few months (usually 3–21 days). A short incubation period (<7 days) suggests the likelihood of developing severe tetanus; however, a long incubation period does not necessarily indicate a milder disease. The period of onset (the interval between the first symptom and first paroxysmal muscle spasm) is a better predictor of severity: early elective tracheal intubation and mechanical ventilation are usually required if the interval is <48 hours.

Generalized Tetanus

Initial symptoms include an inability to open the mouth (lockjaw or trismus), difficulty in chewing and swallowing, and stiffness of neck muscles. The contraction of facial muscles produces the characteristic sneering smile (*risus sardonicus*) (Figure 1). In severe cases, intermittent spasms are provoked by attempts to speak or swallow. Pooled saliva from hypersalivation and dysphagia may trigger cough and laryngeal spasms; if prolonged, these may prove fatal. Rigidity of paraspinal muscles follows, and hyperextension of the spine results in opisthotonus (Figure 2). Finally, proximal muscles of the extremity are also affected. Deep tendon reflexes are always exaggerated and ankle clonus is common. Tonic muscle spasms may affect head and neck muscles and laryngeal muscles, or may be generalized. Paroxysmal spasms occur spontaneously or in response to loud noise, bright lights, or attempts to speak or swallow. Prolonged spasms may compromise breathing.

The Ablett classification is commonly used to grade the severity of tetanus. Grade I (mild) tetanus is characterized by moderate trismus and general spasticity without spasms, dysphagia, or respiratory distress. Grade II (moderate) tetanus has severe trismus, intermittent short spasms, mild tachypnea, and dysphagia. Grade III (severe) tetanus is associated with severe rigidity, prolonged spasms, severe dysphagia, tachypnea, apneic spells, and tachycardia. The presence of additional violent autonomic disturbances with persistent or intermittent episodes of severe hypertension and tachycardia alternating with hypotension and bradycardia is classified as Grade IV (very severe) tetanus. Cardiac arrhythmias, peripheral vasoconstriction, and sudden asystole may also occur in very severe tetanus.

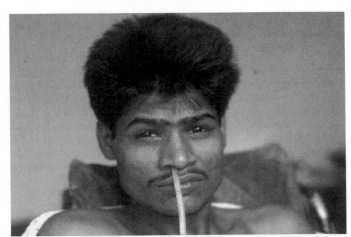

Figure 1 Typical facial expression with the sneering smile (*risus sardonicus*), wrinkled forehead, narrow palpebral fissures, and "crow's feet" at the lateral palpebral margins from the tonic contraction of muscles of facial expression in moderate tetanus.

Figure 2 Spasm of paraspinal muscles, producing the hyperextended opisthotonic posture in severe tetanus.

Figure 3 Cephalic tetanus: This 6-year-old child developed mild tetanus 3 weeks after a wound on his right cheek was sutured. He had cephalic tetanus characterized by partial paralysis of the right facial nerve along with overactivity of the unaffected nerve fibers. **A,** Note the overactivity of the facial muscles with a narrow palpebral and prominent nasolabial fold on the same side as the injury. On asking him to shut his eyes tight (**B**), weakness of the orbicularis oculi and other facial muscles on the right side become manifest.

Despite the use of antitetanus immune globulin (HyperTET) to neutralize circulating tetanus toxin, the disease may progress for up to 2 weeks as more intraaxonal toxin continues to reach the central nervous system. Manifestations persist for another 2 to 3 weeks before gradually subsiding. During this period, an apparently stable patient is at risk of developing sudden asphyxia due to severe generalized or laryngeal spasms. Patients may develop fever, rhabodomyolysis, and hyperthermia due to excessive muscular activity.

Cephalic Tetanus
Following injuries to the head or face, in some patients, the toxin reaches the local motor nuclei earlier and produces a combination of partial paralysis and overactivity—more severely affected motor neurons stop functioning while the remaining fibers are overactive and cause muscle spasm (Figure 3).

TABLE 1	Conditions that Mimic Clinical Manifestations of Tetanus
CLINICAL FEATURE	**DIFFERENTIAL DIAGNOSIS**
Trismus	Acute tonsillar abscess, temporomandibular joint disease, extraptramidal reaction to drugs, dental pathology
Neck stiffness	Cervical spine disease; extrapyramidal reaction to drugs such as antipsychotics, antiemetics, or metoclopramide; meningitis; subarachnoid hemorrhage
Abdominal rigidity	Acute abdomen
Dysphagia	Myasthenia gravis, acute bulbar paralysis, rabies
Muscle spasms	Seizures, spasticity due to spinal cord disease, stiff man syndrome

Localized Tetanus
In this rare form of tetanus, manifestations are restricted to muscles in the region of the wound. These patients have a good prognosis.

Diagnosis
C. tetani can be isolated from the wound in <30% of cases, and microbiological and other laboratory tests do not help in confirming the diagnosis. The diagnosis is entirely clinical. In an individual with a predisposing injury, the presence of trismus, rigidity of neck, abdominal and paraspinal muscles, and severe hyperreflexia are suggestive. The spatula test is a useful bedside test: A spatula (tongue depressor) is inserted into the mouth to touch the posterior pharyngeal wall. Normally, a gag reflex is activated in an attempt to expel the spatula. In tetanus, severe spasms of the masseters results in the patient biting on the spatula, making it difficult to withdraw—a positive test. In one study, the spatula test was positive in 94% of patients with tetanus and in none without tetanus. The electromyogram shows the continuous discharge of motor units in moderate tetanus and the absence of the normal silent period.

Differential Diagnosis
While the diagnosis of tetanus is easy in severe tetanus, it may be mistaken for other conditions in its initial stages (Table 1). The spatula test is negative in other conditions causing trismus. Abdominal muscles usually relax after adequate sedation. As in spasticity due to cord compression, deep reflexes are exaggerated; however, the plantar response, which is extensor in spinal cord disorders, is always flexor with tetanus. Unlike seizures or other intracranial diseases, the patient with tetanus is always fully alert and awake.

Treatment
In patients with life-threatening spasms, prompt, adequate sedation is the first step in management. Patients must be observed in an intensive care unit because the disease may rapidly worsen. They should be nursed in a quiet, dimly lit room in order to keep external stimuli to a minimum—this is difficult in modern intensive care units.

Neutralization of Toxin
Although unsupported by randomized studies, human tetanus immune globulin (HyperTET) (3000–6000 units) is administered intramuscularly to neutralize the circulating toxin. This does not bind to the toxin that has already entered neurons. There is insufficient evidence favoring intrathecal administration[1] of tetanus immune globulin over the usual intramuscular route, although one randomized study showed a shortening of the course of tetanus. Equine antiserum[2] (10,000–20,000 units) may be administered after skin testing for hypersensitivity. Though rarely used

[1]Not FDA approved for this indication.
[2]Not available in the United States.

today due to the risk of anaphylaxis or serum sickness, it has the advantage of being administered intravenously.

Control of Clostridial Infection
Benzylpenicillin (Penicillin G) in a dose of 10 to 12 million units per day is given intravenously for 10 days. In one study, metronidazole (Flagyl) (500 mg every 6 hour for 10 days) was superior to procaine penicillin (Wycillin),[1] presumably because procaine and penicillin are GABA antagonists and may worsen manifestations of tetanus. However, a more recent study showed that a single intramuscular injection of 1.2 million units of benzathine penicillin (Bicillin LA)[1] was as effective as benzylpenicillin or metronidazole. Fortunately, resistance to these antibiotics has not been reported. Debridement of the infected wound and abscess drainage should be performed after spasms have been adequately controlled.

Control of Muscle Spasms
Benzodiazepines (diazepam [Valium] or lorazepam [Ativan][1]) are the preferred drugs and act by enhancing the effect of GABA on its receptor on the postsynaptic membrane, thus potentially antagonizing the effect of tetanospasmin. However, as very little GABA is released in tetanus, large doses (up to 1000 mg/day[3]) of diazepam may be required to achieve adequate sedation and muscle relaxation. Diazepam may be administered intravenously (10–30 mg in 5 mg boluses every 5 minutes)[3] or through a nasogastric tube (10–40 mg every 1 to 2 hours).[3] Barbiturates and chlorpromazine (Thorazine)[1] are alternative agents. Other sedative hypnotic agents such as midazolam (Versed)[1] and propofol (Diprivan)[1] have also been used with good effect. In mild to moderate tetanus, drug doses can be titrated to achieve moderate sedation and control rigidity and spasms without causing respiratory depression. In severe cases, however, spasms may not be controlled despite large doses, increasing the risk of severe central nervous system (CNS) depression. In these patients, heavy sedation combined with neuromuscular blockade and mechanical ventilation is required. In about 10% of cases, benzodiazepines may produce paradoxical excitation instead of sedation; increasing doses make the patient more wakeful, agitated, and delirious, with increased spasms. Discontinuation of diazepam and the use of barbiturates and chlorpromazine may prevent the need for paralysis and mechanical ventilation. Pancuronium (Pavulon),[1] vecuronium (Norcuron),[1] and rocuronium (Zemuron)[1] are often used for neuromuscular blockade. Atracurium (Tracrium)[1] could also be used but may have unfavorable cardiovascular effects. Intravenous and intrathecal baclofen (Lioresal Intrathecal)[1] have been used in some case.

Airway Management
Tracheostomy or endotracheal intubation is required in moderate and severe tetanus to prevent respiratory failure due to laryngeal spasm and aspiration of oropharyngeal secretions. In most developing countries, elective tracheostomy is performed early in severe tetanus. In countries with superior intensive care facilities, heavy sedation, neuromuscular blockade, endotracheal intubation, and mechanical ventilation are preferred, with tracheostomy being reserved for those who need prolonged ventilation.

Control of Autonomic Disturbances
With good intensive care, mortality due to respiratory failure has been drastically reduced. Autonomic dysfunction is now the major challenge in patients with severe tetanus; it is common even in sedated and paralyzed patients. Various measures to control autonomic fluctuations include intravenous fluid loading, oral and parenteral beta-blockers, alpha-blockers, centrally acting sympatholytics such as clonidine (Catapres)[1] or dexmedetomidine (Precedex),[1] and epidural or spinal bupivacaine (Marcaine).[1] More recently, infusion of dexmedetomidine has been used by some authors. Many patients may develop sudden asystole, possibly due to sudden parasympathetic discharge, catecholamine-induced myocardial damage, or sudden loss of sympathetic drive. Consequently, the use of long-acting

antiadrenergic drugs should be avoided. Increasing the level of sedation itself is also effective, to a significant extent.

The agent most frequently used for autonomic dysfunction is intravenous magnesium sulfate.[1] A randomized controlled trial in Vietnamese patients showed that magnesium sulfate did not decrease mortality, ICU stay, or the need for mechanical ventilation but did reduce the dose of sedatives and neuromuscular blocking drugs required. This study used a loading dose of 40 mg/kg over 30 minutes, followed by intravenous infusion of 2 g/hour in patients >45 kg and 1 to 5 g/hour in patients ≤45 kg. Infusion was titrated to maintain serum magnesium levels between 2 and 4 mmol/L.

Other Measures
Continuous muscle hyperactivity and spasms greatly increase caloric requirements. Most patients require nasogastric tube feeding because of trismus and dysphagia. A catabolic state similar to sepsis may develop in very severe tetanus. Consequently, patients lose up to 15% of their body weight during the illness. Good nursing care is essential to prevent pressure sores, deep vein thrombosis, stress ulcers, and aspiration pneumonia. Urinary catheterization is required in most patients as urinary retention is common and distension of the urinary bladder may provoke spasms and autonomic overactivity. All patients should be started on a primary immunization schedule against tetanus.

Complications
Respiratory failure may occur due to laryngeal obstruction, prolonged spasm of respiratory muscles, aspiration pneumonia, or sedative drugs. Severe spasms may result in tongue-bite, compression fractures of midthoracic vertebrae, rhabdomyolysis, myoglobinuria, and renal failure. Rarely, patients may develop acute respiratory distress syndrome (ARDS) either due to tetanus itself or as a result of secondary bacterial sepsis. Cardiac arrhythmias and sudden asystole are common in patients with autonomic dysfunction. Acute myocardial infarction may occur in elderly patients with underlying coronary artery disease due to sympathetic overactivity. Deep vein thrombosis and pressure sores are preventable complications. The overall mortality ranges from 40% to 60% in countries with inadequate health care facilities. With good intensive care, mortality as low as 10% is reported in some series. Mortality is higher in neonates, the elderly, and patients with a short incubation period and period of onset.

Prevention
Adsorbed tetanus toxoid (Tt), derived from formaldehyde-treated tetanus toxin, is extremely effective in inducing active immunity. It is available as a single-antigen preparation or in combination with diphtheria toxoid as pediatric diphtheria-tetanus toxoid (DT) or adult tetanus-diphtheria (Td), and with both diphtheria toxoid and acellular pertussis vaccine as DTaP (Infanrix, Tripedia) or Tdap (Adacel, Boostrix) (lower-case alphabets indicate lower doses of antigens). Pediatric vaccines (DT and DTaP) contain identical amounts of tetanus toxoid as adult vaccines, but three to four times as much diphtheria toxoid. The usual schedule for primary immunization in children <7 years consists of four doses of DTaP or DT at age 2, 4, 6, and 15 to 18 months. A booster dose is recommended at 4 to 6 years of age. In individuals aged 7 years or older, three doses of the adult formulation are administered; the second dose is given 4 to 8 weeks after the first, and the third dose after another 4 to 6 months. Further booster doses are needed every 10 years to maintain antibody titers above the protective level of 0.1 IU/mL.

After administration of Tt to individuals with wounds, protective titers of antibody are achieved after at least 2 weeks. Consequently, passive immunization with 250 units of human tetanus immune globulin (HyperTET) or 1500 units of equine antitetanus serum[2]

---

[1]Not FDA approved for this indication.
[3]Exceeds dosage recommended by the manufacturer.

[1]Not FDA approved for this indication.
[2]Not available in the United States.

administered intramuscularly is needed to confer protection during these initial few weeks. This is especially required in individuals with tetanus-prone wounds who have not received at least three doses of tetanus toxoid in the past. Previously unimmunized individuals with clean, minor, nontetanus prone wounds do not need any passive immunization, but should receive active immunization. Passive immunization is not necessary in those who have received three or more doses of the toxoid. These individuals should receive a dose of Tt (or Td) if more than 10 years have elapsed since the last booster dose and they have nontetanus prone wounds or if >5 years have elapsed after the booster dose and they have a tetanus-prone wound. In countries where neonatal tetanus is common, primary immunization of women during pregnancy has been advocated as a public health program to prevent neonatal tetanus.

References

Apte NM, Karnad DR: The spatula test: A simple bedside test to diagnose tetanus, *Am J Trop Med Hyg* 53:386–387, 1995.

Centers for Disease Control and Prevention: In Atkinson W, Wolfe S, Hamborsky J, editors: *Epidemiology and Prevention of Vaccine-Preventable Diseases*, ed 12, Washington, DC, 2011, Department of Health and Human Services, Centers for Disease Control and Prevention, pp 291–299.

Farrar JJ, Yen LM, Cook T, et al: Tetanus, *J Neurol Neurosurg Psychiatry* 69:292–301, 2000.

Gibson K, Uwineza JB, Kiviri W, Parlow J: Tetanus in developing countries: A case series and review, *Can J Anaesth* 56:307–315, 2009.

Lisboa T, Ho YL, Filho GTH, et al: Guidelines for the management of accidental tetanus in adult patients, *Rev Bras Ter Intensiva* 23:394–409, 2011.

Rodrigo C, Samarakoon L, Fernando SD, Rajapakse S: A meta-analysis of magnesium for tetanus, *Anaesthesia* 67:1370–1374, 2012.

Roper MH, Vandelaer JH, Gasse FL: Maternal and neonatal tetanus, *Lancet* 370:1947–1959, 2007.

Thwaites CL, Yen LM, Loan HT, et al: Magnesium sulphate for treatment of severe tetanus: A randomized controlled trial, *Lancet* 368:1436–1443, 2006.

Trujillo MH, Castillo A, Espana J, et al: Impact of intensive care management on the prognosis of tetanus. Analysis of 641 cases, *Chest* 92:63–65, 1987.

TICKBORNE RICKETTSIAL DISEASES (ROCKY MOUNTAIN SPOTTED FEVER AND OTHER SPOTTED FEVER GROUP RICKETTSIOSES, EHRLICHIOSES, AND ANAPLASMOSIS)

Method of
Robert Wittler, MD

CURRENT DIAGNOSIS

- Early diagnosis of Rocky Mountain spotted fever (RMSF) and other tickborne rickettsial diseases is made clinically. RMSF should be considered in the setting of fever, headache, rash, and a history of possible tick exposure. The rash is not always present and typically occurs 2 to 4 days after the onset of fever.
- Diagnostic laboratory tests for rickettsial diseases, particularly RMSF, are usually not helpful in making a timely diagnosis during the initial states of illness.
- Tickborne rickettsial diseases can be confirmed by polymerase chain reaction (PCR) during the acute stage if readily available (whole blood for ehrlichiosis and anaplasmosis and skin biopsy or whole blood for RMSF) or at later stages by subsequently demonstrating a fourfold increase between acute and convalescent (ideally 2 to 4 weeks apart) serum immunoglobulin G (IgG) indirect immunofluorescence antibody titers. PCR of whole blood for RMSF has low sensitivity, although sensitivity increases in patients with severe disease.
- Typical findings of ehrlichiosis and anaplasmosis include fever, headache, malaise, leukopenia, thrombocytopenia, and elevated serum transaminases. Rash is often not present.

CURRENT THERAPY

- Treatment of choice for all tickborne rickettsial diseases in patients of all ages (including children less than 8 years of age) is doxycycline (Vibramycin).
- The dose for doxycycline is 100 mg twice daily (intravenously [IV] or orally depending on severity of illness) for adults. For children weighing <45 kg,[1] the recommended dose is 2.2 mg/kg/dose IV or orally twice daily.
- Delay in recognition and appropriate treatment is the most important factor associated with death from RMSF. Empiric treatment within 5 days of the onset of symptoms with doxycycline is the best way to prevent morbidity and death. Treatment decisions should never be delayed while awaiting laboratory confirmation, nor should treatment be discontinued solely on the basis of a negative test result with an acute-phase specimen.
- Although optimal duration of therapy has not been well studied, a common treatment course for RMSF and ehrlichiosis is at least 3 days after the patient defervesces (typically the minimum total course is 5–7 days) or longer for severe illness. Anaplasmosis should be treated for 10 days to provide appropriate therapy for possible coinfection with *Borrelia burgdorferi*.
- Historically chloramphenicol has been recommended for the treatment of RMSF during pregnancy based on adverse effects of older tetracycline drugs (but not specifically doxycycline). Although there is limited evidence, doxycycline has not been associated with teratogenicity or maternal hepatic toxicity during pregnancy, and doxycycline has been used successfully to treat tickborne rickettsial disease in several pregnant women without adverse effects.
- Chloramphenicol is not an alternative treatment for human monocytic ehrlichiosis (HME) or HGA. Chloramphenicol treatment of RMSF has been associated with a greater risk of death compared with doxycycline treatment.
- Limited case report data suggest that rifampin[1] can be used as an alternative to doxycycline for the treatment of confirmed (RMSF ruled out) mild anaplasmosis during pregnancy or with documented tetracycline allergy.

[1]Not FDA approved for this indication.

Tickborne rickettsial diseases in humans often share clinical features but are epidemiologically and etiologically distinct. In the United States included diseases are (1) Rocky Mountain spotted fever (RMSF) caused by *Rickettsia rickettsii*; (2) other spotted fever group (SFG) rickettsioses, caused by *Rickettsia parkeri* and *Rickettsia* species 364D; (3) *Ehrlichia chaffeensis* ehrlichiosis, also called human monocytic ehrlichiosis (HME); (4) other ehrlichioses, caused by *Ehrlichia ewingii* and *Ehrlichia muris*-like agent; and (5) anaplasmosis, caused by *Anaplasma phagocytophilum*, also called human granulocytic anaplasmosis (HGA). The reported incidence of tickborne rickettsial diseases has increased in the United States. Tickborne rickettsial diseases, especially RMSF, continue to cause severe illness and death in otherwise healthy adults and children, despite the availability of effective antibiotic therapy. SFG rickettsioses (including RMSF), ehrlichioses, and anaplasmosis are nationally notifiable diseases in the United States. Providers report potential cases to state or local health departments. In 2010, the reporting category of RMSF was changed to spotted fever rickettsiosis, as serology does not readily distinguish RMSF from other SFG rickettsioses.

Epidemiology

Tickborne rickettsial pathogens are maintained in natural cycles involving domestic or wild vertebrates and ticks. The epidemiology of each disease reflects the geographic distribution and seasonal activities of the tick vectors and the natural vertebrate hosts, as well as the human activities resulting in tick exposure. Although cases have been reported in every month, most cases occur during April to September, coincident with peak levels of tick host-seeking activity.

RMSF is the rickettsiosis in the United States that is associated with the highest rates of severe and fatal outcomes. The case-fatality rate in the preantibiotic era was ~25%. Current case-fatality rates are estimated at 5% to 10%. From 2008–2012, the estimated average annual incidence from passive surveillance of SFG rickettsioses was 8.9 cases per million persons. Reported annual incidence has increased during the past two decades. The highest incidence occurs in persons aged 60 to 69 years, and the highest case-fatality rate is among children aged <10 years. Additional epidemiologic risk factors for fatal RMSF include age ≥40 years, alcohol abuse, and glucose-6-phosphate dehydrogenase deficiency. From 2008 to 2012, 63% of reported SFG rickettsiosis cases came from Arkansas, Missouri, North Carolina, Oklahoma, and Tennessee. SFG rickettsiosis has been reported from all the contiguous 48 states and the District of Columbia.

In the United States, the tick species most frequently associated with transmission of *R rickettsii* is the American dog tick, *Dermacentor variabilis*, which is found primarily in the eastern, central, and Pacific Coast regions. The Rocky Mountain wood tick, *Dermacentor andersoni*, is associated with transmission in the western United States. Larval and nymphal stages of most *Dermacentor* spp ticks usually do not bite humans. Adult *D variabilis* and *D andersoni* ticks bite humans, but the principal hosts are deer, dogs, and livestock.

The brown dog tick, *Rhipicephalus sanguineus*, which is located throughout the United States, is an important vector in parts of Arizona and along the United States–Mexico border. All stages (larvae, nymphs, and adults) of *Rh sanguineus* bite humans and can transmit *R rickettsia*. Domestic dogs are the preferred host. On Arizona tribal lands, the warm climate and proximity of ticks to domiciles (tick-infested dogs) provide a suitable environment for *Rh sanguineus* to remain active year-round, resulting in cases of RMSF in Arizona every month of the year.

Rickettsia parkeri is transmitted by the Gulf Coast tick, *Amblyomma maculatum*. *R parkeri* rickettsiosis cases have not been documented in children, and no fatal cases have been reported. The first confirmed case of Rickettsia species 364D was in 2010 and likely transmitted by the Pacific Coast tick, *Dermacentor occidentalis*. All reported cases have been from California.

The average annual incidence of ehrlichiosis from 2008 to 2012 was 3.2 cases per million persons, with the most common cause being *E chaffeensis*. The highest incidence is in persons aged 60 to 69 years. The case fatality rate is ~3% and is highest among children aged <10 years, adults aged ≥70 years, and immunosuppressed persons. *E chaffeensis* is transmitted to humans by the lone star tick, *Amblyomma americanum*, which is the most commonly encountered tick in the southeastern United States, with a range that extends into areas of the Midwest and New England. Arkansas, Delaware, Missouri, Oklahoma, Tennessee, and Virginia have the highest reported incidence. The white-tailed deer is an important natural reservoir for *E chaffeensis*, and most cases occur during May to August.

The principal vector for *E ewingii* ehrlichiosis is also *A americanum*. Cases have primarily been reported from Missouri. No fatal cases of *E ewingii* ehrlichiosis have been reported. *Ehrlichia muris*–like agent (EML) has recently been recognized as a human pathogen. Reported cases have been from Minnesota and Wisconsin. The blacklegged tick, *Ixodes scapularis*, is an efficient vector for EML in experimental studies. EML agent DNA has been detected in *I scapularis* collected in Minnesota and Wisconsin but has not been detected in *I scapularis* from other states.

The incidence of human anaplasmosis during 2008–2012 was 6.3 cases per million persons. Incidence is highest in the northeastern and upper midwestern states, and the geographic range seems to be expanding. The case fatality rate is <1%. *I scapularis* is the vector for *Anaplasma phagocytophilum* in the northeastern and midwestern United States, whereas the western blacklegged tick, *Ixodes pacificus*, is the principal vector along the West Coast. The seasonality is bimodal, with the first peak June–July and a smaller peak in October, corresponding to the emergence of the adult stage of *I scapularis*. *I scapularis* also transits *Borrelia burgdorferi* (Lyme disease), *Babesia microti* (babesiosis), *Borrelia miyamotoi* (tickborne relapsing fever), and deer tick virus (a cause of tickborne encephalitis). Simultaneous infections with *A phagocytophilum* and *B burgdorferi* or *B microti* have occurred.

Pathophysiology

The agents causing RMSF, ehrlichiosis, and anaplasmosis are all obligate intracellular pathogens, but the target host cells they infect and subsequent pathology vary by organism.

R rickettsii is transmitted from the tick to humans via a painless bite, which often goes unrecognized. The organism resides in the salivary gland of the tick and is passed during acquisition of a blood meal. *R rickettsii* can be transmitted as early as 10 to 24 hours after tick attachment. When transmitted to a human host, *R rickettsia* localize and multiply in vascular endothelial cells, and, less commonly, underlying smooth muscle cells of small and medium vessels, resulting in vasculitis. The vasculitis is the underlying mechanism for most of the clinical features and laboratory abnormalities of RMSF. Injury to the vascular endothelium results in increased capillary permeability, microhemorrhage, and platelet consumption. Late-stage complications of pulmonary edema (acute respiratory distress syndrome) and cerebral edema are consequences of the microvascular leakage.

E chaffeensis predominantly infects monocytes and tissue macrophages and replicates in cytoplasmic vacuoles called morulae. Unlike RMSF, direct vasculitis and endothelial injury are rare in human monocytic ehrlichiosis. Frequent pathologic findings include granuloma formation, myeloid hyperplasia, and megakaryocytosis in the bone marrow. The severe pathology and multiorgan involvement in severe and fatal HME in immunocompetent patients is believed to be due to dysregulation of the host immune response that leads to tissue damage and eventually multiorgan failure. *E ewingii* has a predilection for neutrophils, and morulae can be observed in granulocytes of the blood, cerebrospinal fluid (CSF), and bone marrow.

A phagocytophilum is found predominantly in neutrophils in the peripheral blood and tissues from infected individuals. *A phagocytophilum* has the unique ability to selectively survive and multiply within cytoplasmic vacuoles (morulae) of polymorphonuclear cells by delaying their apoptosis. Infection with *A phagocytophilum* induces a systemic inflammatory response, which is believed to be the mechanism for tissue damage. Pathologic findings with human granulocytic anaplasmosis include normocellular or hypercellular bone marrow, erythrophagocytosis, hepatic apoptosis, focal splenic necrosis, and mild interstitial pneumonitis and pulmonary hemorrhage.

Clinical Manifestations

A detailed history should include information about known tick bites or activities that might be associated with tick exposure. Unrecognized tick bites are common. A history of a tick bite within 14 days of illness onset is reported in only 50% to 60% of RMSF cases and 68% of ehrlichiosis cases. Absence of a tick bite should never dissuade providers from considering tickborne rickettsial disease in the appropriate clinical context. Contact with pets, especially dogs, and a history of tick attachment or recent tick removal from pets can be useful in assessing human tick exposure.

Tickborne rickettsial diseases commonly have nonspecific clinical signs and symptoms early in the course of disease. Although there is overlap in the clinical presentations of tickborne rickettsial diseases, the frequency of certain associated signs and symptoms (e.g., rash and other cutaneous findings) and typical laboratory findings differ by pathogen and assist providers in developing a differential diagnosis, beginning appropriate antibacterial treatment, and ordering confirmatory diagnostic tests.

Symptoms of RMSF typically begin 3 to 12 days after the bite of an infected tick or 4 to 8 days after discovery of an attached tick. The incubation period is generally shorter (≤5 days) in patients who develop severe disease. Initial symptoms are often nonspecific and include the sudden onset of fever, chills, malaise, and myalgia. Clinical suspicion for RMSF should be maintained in cases of nonspecific febrile illness and sepsis of unclear cause, particularly during the spring and summer months.

The classic triad of fever, rash, and reported tick bite is present in only a minority of RMSF patients during the initial presentation to health care; therefore it is crucial not to wait for development of this triad before considering a diagnosis of RMSF and beginning treatment. A rash typically occurs 2 to 4 days after the onset of fever; however, many patients initially seek medical care before the rash. In one large series of patients with RMSF, 88% of patients had a rash, but only 49% had a rash in the first 3 days. Children more frequently have rash (97%) and develop the rash earlier. The rash typically begins as small, blanching macules on the ankles, wrists, or forearms that then spreads to the palms, soles, arms, legs, and trunk, usually sparing the face. The generalized petechial rash appears later (day 5 or 6) and is indicative of advanced disease. An inoculation eschar is rarely present with RMSF. In addition to rash, the most frequent clinical findings at any point in the illness are fever (99%), headache (91%), and myalgia (82%).

The total white blood cell count is typically normal or mildly increased with RMSF, and increased numbers of immature neutrophils are often present. Thrombocytopenia, slight elevations of AST or ALT, and hyponatremia might be present, particularly as the disease advances. Laboratory values cannot be relied on to guide early treatment decisions because they are often within or slightly deviated from normal reference values early in the course. When CSF is obtained, a lymphocytic (less commonly neutrophilic) pleocytosis can be present, along with a moderately elevated CSF protein. CSF glucose is generally normal.

R parkeri rickettsiosis is a milder illness compared with RMSF; no severe manifestations or death has been reported. Symptoms develop a median of 5 days (range, 2–10 days) after the bite of an infected tick. The first manifestation in nearly all patients is an inoculation eschar, which generally is nonpruritic, nontender or mildly tender, and surrounded by an indurated, erythematous halo and occasionally a few petechiae. Shortly after the onset of fever (0.5–4 days later), a nonpruritic maculopapular or vesicopustular rash develops in 90% of patients. The rash primarily involves the extremities and trunk and in ~half of patients involves the palms and soles. Headache (86%) and myalgia (76%) are common. Laboratory findings include modest elevation of hepatic transaminases (78%), mild leukopenia (50%), and thrombocytopenia (40%).

Few patients with *Rickettsia* species 364D have been reported, so the full clinical spectrum has yet to be described. It does appear to be relatively mild and characterized by an eschar or ulcerative skin lesion with regional lymphadenopathy. Fever, headache, and myalgia occur, but rash has not been a notable feature.

Symptoms of *E chaffeensis* ehrlichiosis typically occur a median of 9 days (range, 5–15 days) after an infected tick bite. Fever (96%), headache (72%), malaise (77%), and myalgia (58%) are common. Abdominal pain, vomiting, and diarrhea can occur, particularly in children. Rash (maculopapular, petechial, or diffuse erythema) occurs in approximately one-third of patients and is more frequent in children. The rash occurs a median of 5 days after illness onset and can involve the palms and soles. Neurologic manifestations are present in ~20% of patients. Characteristic laboratory findings in the first week include leukopenia, thrombocytopenia, and elevated levels of hepatic transaminases. *Ehrlichia ewingii* and *Ehrlichia muris*-like agent ehrlichiosis have similar clinical and laboratory features as *E chaffeensis* ehrlichiosis, although rash and gastrointestinal symptoms are less common.

Symptoms of human granulocytic anaplasmosis typically occur 5 to 14 days after an infected tick bite. Fever (92%–100%), headache (82%), malaise (97%), and myalgia (77%) are common.

Rash is present in <10% of patients, and central nervous system involvement is rare. Laboratory findings are similar to ehrlichiosis.

Diagnosis

Early diagnosis and initiation of treatment of tickborne rickettsial diseases is based on clinical and epidemiologic findings, as rapid confirmatory assays are often not available or reliable to guide treatment decisions early in the clinical course. Confirmatory diagnostic tests are serologic assays, nucleic acid detection, immunostaining of biopsy tissue, blood-smear microscopy, and culture.

Assays using paired acute and convalescent sera (ideally collected 2–4 weeks apart) are the standard for serologic confirmation. Assays are insensitive during the first week of rickettsial infection. After 7 days of illness, the sensitivity increases. Assays are highly sensitive 2 to 3 weeks after illness onset. Early therapy with doxycycline may diminish or delay the development of antibodies in RMSF.

A diagnosis of tickborne rickettsial diseases is confirmed with a ≥fourfold increase in antibody titer in patients with a clinically compatible acute illness. A single IgG antibody reciprocal titer ≥64 is supportive of, but not confirmatory for, the diagnosis. In the United States, R rickettsia–reactive IgG antibody reciprocal titers ≥64 can be found in 5% to 10% of the population who do not acutely have RMSF. Some laboratories also perform assays for IgM antibodies. However, because of the lower specificity of IgM compared with IgG assays, IgM titers should not be used as a stand-alone method for diagnosis.

PCR amplification of DNA from whole blood specimens collected during the acute stage of illness is particularly useful for confirming E chaffeensis, A phagocytophilum, E ewingii, and EML agent infections due to the tropism of those organisms for circulating cells. PCR detection of R rickettsia in whole blood is less sensitive, as low numbers of rickettsiae typically circulate in the blood in the absence of advanced disease. Tissue specimens such as a skin biopsy are a more useful source of SFG rickettsial DNA compared with blood samples. Doxycyline treatment decreases the sensitivity of PCR. Obtaining blood before treatment is recommended to decrease false-negative results.

Immunostaining of a skin punch biopsy is useful for diagnosing RMSF with 100% specificity and 70% sensitivity. Microscopic examination of blood smears or buffy-coat preparations during the first week of illness may reveal leukocyte morulae in patients infected with E chaffeensis or anaplasmosis, although it is relatively insensitive, and accuracy is dependent on having experienced microscopists. Culture is the reference standard for microbiologic diagnosis, but the agents that cause tickborne rickettsial diseases require cell culture techniques that are not widely available.

Differential Diagnosis

The differential diagnosis of fever and rash is broad, and during the early stages of illness tickborne rickettsial diseases can be indistinguishable from many viral exanthams, particularly in children. In addition to viral infections, conditions that should be considered include meningococcemia, Kawasaki disease, secondary syphilis, disseminated gonococcal infection, bacterial endocarditis, scarlet fever, leptospirosis, typhoid, drug eruptions, Stevens-Johnson syndrome, toxic shock syndrome, and thrombotic thrombocytopenic purpura.

Treatment

Doxycycline is the drug of choice for treatment of all tickborne rickettsial diseases in patients of all ages and should be initiated immediately in persons with signs and symptoms suggestive of rickettsial disease. Treatment decisions should never be delayed awaiting laboratory confirmation. Multiple studies have noted a delay in appropriate treatment of tickborne rickettsial diseases, particularly after the fifth day of illness for RMSF, to be a significant potentially preventable risk factor for severe disease, increased mortality rates, and long-term sequelae. Because of the nonspecific signs and symptoms of tickborne rickettsial diseases, concomitant empiric treatment for other conditions in the differential diagnosis should be administered (e.g., treatment with ceftriaxone for meningococcemia).

The recommended dose of doxycycline is 100 mg twice daily (IV or oral) for adults and 2.2 mg/kg twice daily (IV or oral) for children weighing <45 kg.[1] Oral therapy is appropriate for patients with early-stage disease who can be treated as outpatients. The recommended duration of therapy for RMSF and ehrlichiosis is at least 3 days after fever resolves and until evidence of clinical improvement is noted; typically, the minimum total course is 5 to 7 days. Severe or complicated disease could require a longer course. HGA should be treated for 10 days to provide appropriate therapy for possible coinfection with Lyme disease.

The use of doxycycline to treat children with suspected tickborne rickettsial disease should no longer be a subject of controversy. The American Academy of Pediatrics and CDC recommend doxycycline as the treatment of choice for children of all ages with suspected tickborne rickettsial disease. Doxycycline used at the recommended dose and duration for RMSF in children aged <8 years, even after multiple courses, has not resulted in tooth staining or enamel hypoplasia.

Chloramphenicol in the past was used as an alternative drug for treating RMSF. However, chloramphenicol has been associated with a higher risk of death compared to patients treated with a tetracycline; in vitro evidence indicates that chloramphenicol is not effective treatment for ehrlichiosis or anaplasmosis. Chloramphenicol is no longer available in the oral form in the United States, and the IV form is not readily available at all institutions.

Chloramphenicol has been recommended for the treatment of RMSF during pregnancy based on adverse effects of older tetracycline drugs (but not specifically doxycycline). Although there is limited evidence, doxycycline has not been associated with teratogenicity or maternal hepatic toxicity during pregnancy, and doxycycline has been used successfully to treat tickborne rickettsial diseases in several pregnant women without adverse effects.

Rifamycins demonstrate in vitro activity against *E chaffeensis* and *A phagocytophilum*. Case reports document favorable outcomes in small numbers of pregnant women treated with rifampin for anaplasmosis. Rifampin[1] could be an alternative for treatment of confirmed mild anaplasmosis (RMSF ruled out) during pregnancy or documented allergy to tetracycline-class drugs. Rifampin is not acceptable treatment for RMSF or potential coinfection with *B burgdorferi*.

Treatment of symptom-free persons seropositive for tickborne rickettsial disease is not recommended, regardless of past treatment, because antibodies can persist for months to years after infection.

Monitoring and Complications
Fever with tickborne rickettsial diseases typically subsides within 24 to 48 hours when treated with doxycycline in the first 4 to 5 days of illness. Lack of a clinical response within 48 hours of early treatment with doxycycline could indicate the illness is not a tickborne rickettsial disease, and alternative diagnoses or coinfection should be considered. Severely ill patients may require >48 hours of treatment before clinical improvement is noted. Patients

with mild disease treated on an outpatient basis need close follow-up to ensure they are responding appropriately.

Patients with evidence of organ dysfunction, severe thrombocytopenia, mental status changes, or the need for supportive therapy should be hospitalized. Other considerations for hospitalization include the likelihood and ability to take oral medication and existing comorbid conditions, including the patient's immune status. Infection with RMSF and to a somewhat lesser extent HME are most likely to have a severe disease or death. Severe, late-stage manifestations of RMSF include meningoencephalitis, acute respiratory distress syndrome (ARDS), acute renal failure, arrhythmia, and seizures. Severe manifestations of HME include ARDS, shock-like syndromes, renal failure, hepatic failure, coagulopathies, and hemorrhagic complications.

Severe or life-threatening manifestations are less frequent with anaplasmosis than with RMSF or HME. Predictors of a more severe course of anaplasmosis include advanced age, immunosuppression, comorbid medical conditions, and delay in diagnosis and treatment. Confirmed *A phagocytophilum* coinfection has been reported in <10% of patients with Lyme disease. Response to treatment can provide clues to possible coinfection with Lyme disease or babesiosis. If the clinical response to treatment with doxycycline is delayed, coinfection or an alternate infection should be considered. Conversely, if Lyme disease is treated with a beta-lactam antibiotic in a patient with unrecognized *A phagocytophilum* infection symptoms could persist.

Prevention
The best prevention for all the tickborne rickettsial diseases is to avoid tick bites, perform regular tick checks on humans and pets, and promptly remove attached ticks. Longer periods of tick attachment increase the probability of transmission of tickborne diseases. Repellents and protective clothing can reduce the risk for tick bites. Products containing 20% to 30% N,N-Diethyl-meta-toluamide (DEET) effectively repel ticks and can be applied directly to the skin. DEET is not recommended for use on infants younger than 2 months. Permethrin-treated or -impregnated clothing can significantly reduce tick bites. Prophylactic treatment is not recommended in persons who have had recent tick bites and are well.

References
Biggs HM, Behravesh CB, Bradley KK, et al: Diagnosis and management of tickborne rickettsial diseases: Rocky Mountain spotted fever and other spotted fever group rickettsioses, ehrlichioses, and anaplasmosis—United States, *MMWR Recomm Rep* 65:1–44, 2016.

Buckingham SC, Marshall GS, Schutze GE, et al: Clinical and laboratory features, hospital course, and outcome of Rocky Mountain spotted fever in children, *J Pediatr* 150:180–184, 2007.

Cross R, Ling C, Day NPJ, McGready R, Paris DH: Revisiting doxycycline in pregnancy and early childhood—time to rebuild its reputation? *Expert Opin Drug Saf* 15:367–382, 2016.

Dahlgren FS, Holman RC, Paddock CD, Callinan LS, McQuiston JH: Fatal Rocky Mountain spotted fever in the United States, 1999–2007, *Am J Trop Med Hyg* 86:713–719, 2012.

Hamburg BJ, Storch GA, Micek ST, Kollef MH: The importance of early treatment with doxycycline in human ehrlichiosis, *Medicine (Baltimore)* 87:53–60, 2008.

Helmick CG, Bernard KW, D'Angelo LJ: Rocky Mountain spotted fever: clinical, laboratory, and epidemiological features of 262 cases, *J Infect Dis* 150:480–488, 1984.

Ismail N, McBride JW: Tick-borne emerging infections: ehrlichiosis and anaplasmosis, *Clin Lab Med* 37:317–340, 2017.

Kirkland KB, Wilkinson WE, Sexton DJ: Therapeutic delay and mortality in cases of Rocky Mountain spotted fever, *Clin Infect Dis* 20:1118–1121, 1995.

Kjemtrup AM, Padgett K, Paddock CD, et al: A forty-year review of Rocky Mountain spotted fever cases in California shows clinical and epidemiologic changes, *PLoS Negl Trop Dis* 16:1–18, 2022.

Marshall GS, Stout GG, Jacobs RF, et al: Antibodies reactive to Rickettsia rickettsii among children living in the southeast and south central regions of the United States, *Arch Pediatr Adoles Med* 157:443–448, 2003.

---

[1] Not FDA approved for this indication.

TOXIC SHOCK SYNDROME

Method of
Alwyn Rapose, MD

CURRENT DIAGNOSIS

- Clinical diagnosis: High index of suspicion when there is a combination of fever, rash—initially erythematous followed by desquamation, hypotension, and multiorgan injury.
- There needs to be a thorough search for a focus of infection like retained foreign body or tampon, deep-seated abscess or peritonitis, necrotizing fasciitis, or postoperative wound infection.
- Blood cultures and deep tissue cultures (from the site of the suspected infection) are recommended in all cases.

CURRENT THERAPY

- Aggressive fluid resuscitation.
- Broad antibiotic coverage initially, followed by deescalation to target the organism identified in cultures.
- Intravenous immunoglobulin may help in patients who fail to respond to standard care.

Introduction

Toxic shock syndrome (TSS) is an acute illness, which as the name suggests is caused by a toxin, and the patient presents with hypotension (shock) and multiorgan involvement (syndrome). It was initially described in children with *Staphylococcus aureus* infection, but a similar syndrome is associated with *Streptococcus* infections as well as clostridial infections in children and adults. Different toxins—acting either directly or via different cytokine pathways—have been implicated in the pathogenesis of the disease. TSS carried a high mortality risk (40% to 60% in streptococcal TSS). However, early recognition and aggressive interventions have resulted in much improved outcomes in the era of modern medicine.

Historical Aspects

A review of the medical literature indicates this was first described in 1978 when J. Todd and colleagues reported a collection of seven cases in children. In the early years following its description, a majority of cases were seen in young menstruating women who used tampons, with the onset of illness within a few days of onset of their menstrual period. A large number of investigators evaluated tampons, contraceptive sponges, sanitary pads, and other medical and surgical materials and as the medical community became more familiar with this syndrome, there was a decrease in tampon-associated TSS and an increased incidence of nonmenstrual TSS associated with respiratory infections, necrotizing skin infections, deep-seated abscesses, and postoperative infections including gynecologic surgeries.

TSS is classically associated with *S. aureus* infection. The clinical features included fever, skin rash, hypotension, and multiorgan involvement with various combinations of respiratory, renal, and hepatic injury. Similar features following infection with *Streptococcus pyogenes* (group A *Streptococcus* [GAS] as well as other streptococci) resulted in a description of streptococcal toxic shock–like syndrome (TSLS). In patients with complications of medical or spontaneous abortions and infection with *Clostridium species* similar clinical features were seen along with very high mortality, and this condition was also included when describing TSS.

Pathogenesis

The *S. aureus* isolates from patients with menstruation-related TSS revealed a toxin that was first called toxic shock syndrome toxin 1 (TSST-1). Since then, however, multiple other toxins associated with *S. aureus* (enterotoxins B-F) have been described to be associated with TSS. Similarly, streptococcal exotoxins (A, B, and C)—superantigens—are potent activators of T lymphocytes and can also directly cause high fever (pyrotoxins) and shock, as well as tissue damage.

These bacterial toxins induce production of tumor necrosis factor (TNFα), interferons (IFNγ), interleukins (IL-1, IL-2), and other cytotoxins by human monocytes and lymphocytes that result in a cascade of proinflammatory cytokines (cytokine storm). These cytokines are responsible for fever, damage to vascular endothelium resulting in tissue injury, as well as the loss of intravascular volume and hypotension.

In contrast, clostridial infection is associated with direct tissue damage by secreted clostridial toxins.

Clinical Features

The surveillance case definition developed by the Centers for Disease Control and Prevention (CDC) included five clinical criteria: Fever, rash, hypotension, and involvement of three or more organ systems. The rash usually subsided with desquamation, which is the fifth clinical criterion. The patient may have prodromal symptoms like myalgia, arthralgia, and headache. Fever associated with a diffuse erythematous skin rash (sheets of erythema) involving the face trunk and extremities is rapidly followed by hypotension, decreased urine output, and features of septic shock (Figures 1 through 3). Detailed history taking and a thorough clinical examination is essential to determine the focus of infection—either menstrual tampon, retained foreign body, necrotizing infection in a closed space (fasciitis), postoperative wound infection, or, more recently described, peritonitis-associated TSS. Subtle differences between TSS and TSLS have been described. Clostridial infection following septic abortion or other gynecologic surgery is associated with severe abdominal and pelvic pain, uterine tenderness (endometritis), and a foul-smelling vaginal discharge. A delay in diagnosis and intervention results in a rapid progression of systemic involvement. A cytokine storm in the lungs can result in respiratory complications like acute respiratory distress syndrome (ARDS), and there can be acute renal injury secondary to hypotension or toxin-induced acute interstitial nephritis, shock liver, and in severe situations, altered mental status. In the recovery phase, the erythematous rash subsides with desquamation.

Management

Early diagnosis, rapid intervention with intravenous (IV) fluids, IV antibiotics as well as IV immunoglobulin (IVIG)[1] in some circumstances, along with supportive therapy like mechanical ventilation in patients with respiratory failure and dialysis for patients with severe renal injury, are key to survival in patients with TSS. Patients in circulatory shock are treated in an intensive care unit with ionotropic agents such as norepinephrine (Levophed) and vasopressin (Pitressin) to provide pressor support. A multidisciplinary team, including intensivists, infectious disease specialists, pulmonologists, and nephrologists, is required for the management of these patients because they often develop respiratory failure and acute renal injury.

Removal of the focus of infection—be it an infected tampon, retained products of conception, surgical drainage of deep-seated abscess, aggressive debridement in patients with necrotizing fasciitis, or postoperative wound infection—is an essential component in the management of TSS.

Blood cultures should be obtained at presentation, and tissue cultures should be obtained at the time of surgery. Ascitic fluid cultures are essential in cases with suspected peritonitis.

---

[1]Not FDA approved for this indication.

Figure 1 Diffuse erythematous rash on the trunk.

Figure 2 Diffuse erythematous rash on the lower extremity.

Figure 3 Diffuse erythematous rash on the upper extremity.

Patients should be initially treated with aggressive IV fluid resuscitation along with antibiotic combinations that will provide broad coverage against *Staphylococcus*, *Streptococcus*, and anaerobic organisms. Vancomycin (15 to 20 mg/kg every 12 hours) along with a carbapenem (meropenem [Merrem] 1 g every 8 hours, imipenem [Primaxin] 500 mg every 6 hours, or ertapenem [Invanz] 1 g every 24 hours), or vancomycin along with

piperacillin-tazobactam (Zosyn 4.5 g every 6 to 8 hours) (though there has been reported a higher risk of nephrotoxicity with this compared to the combination of vancomycin with carbapenem) is often the first choice for broad coverage. These antibiotics need dose adjustments based on a patient's renal function. In addition, antibiotics like clindamycin (600 to 900 mg every 8 hours) and linezolid (Zyvox 600 mg every 12 hours) are included because of their direct antitoxin effect (suppress toxin production and accelerate phagocytosis). These antibiotics do not need renal dose adjustments. When the patient is on vancomycin, there should be close monitoring of vancomycin troughs or vancomycin area under the curve, as well as creatinine, to optimize vancomycin dosage and reduce the risk of nephrotoxicity. If linezolid is used, vancomycin will not be required. Newer agents like ceftaroline (Teflaro 600 mg every 12 hours) also provide coverage against methicillin-resistant *S. aureus* (MRSA). The results of microbiology cultures help guide the final antibiotic choice (deescalation of antibiotics). If an infection is caused by a *Streptococcus* species, and no *S. aureus* is identified, vancomycin/ceftaroline can be discontinued and IV penicillin (12 to 24 million units per day as a continuous infusion or in six divided doses) combined with clindamycin is recommended. The duration of antibiotic therapy depends on the patient's clinical response. IVIG[1] has been used in patients who are failing standard therapy. It probably acts by providing antiinflammatory mediators and antibodies against some of the toxins and superantigens and has been shown to improve survival especially in TSLS.

New Research and Developments

Newer antibiotics recently approved for use in skin and skin structure infections, including dalbavancin (Dalvance), oritavancin (Orbactiv), delafloxacin (Baxdela), and omadacycline (Nuzyra), have great coverage against *S. aureus*, including MRSA and *Streptococcus*. However, these have not been approved for use in TSS.

There is ongoing research into the development of immunological agents (monoclonal antibodies and vaccines) that can target toxins and other superantigen-induced cytokine pathways. These nonantibiotic therapies have the potential to block the toxin-induced shock without the side effects commonly associated with antibiotic use.

---

[1]Not FDA approved for this indication.

References

Burnham JP, Kollef MH: Understanding toxic shock syndrome, *Intensive Care Med* 41(9):1707–1710, 2015.

Emgard J, Bergsten H, McCormick JK, et al: MAIT cells are major contributors to the cytokine response and group A streptococcal toxic shock syndrome, *Proc Natl Acad Sci USA* 116(51):25923–25931, 2019.

Jayouhey E, Bolze PA, Jamen C, et al: Similarities and differences between staphylococcal and streptococcal toxic shock syndromes in children: results from a 30-case cohort, *Front Pediatr* 6:360, 2018.

Krakauer T: FDA-approved immunosuppressants targeting staphylococcal super antigens: mechanisms and insights, *Immunotargets Ther* 6:17–29, 2017.

Krakauer T: Staphylococcal superantigens: pyrogenic toxins induced toxic shock, *Toxins (Basel)*. 11(3), 2019.

Linner A, Darenberg J, Sjolin J, et al: Clinical efficacy of poly-specific intravenous immunoglobulin therapy in patients with streptococcal toxic shock syndrome: a comparative observational study, *Clin Infect Dis* 59(6):851–857, 2014.

Reingold AL, Hargrett NT, Shands KN, et al: Toxic shock syndrome surveillance in the United States. 1980 to 1981, *Ann Intern Med* 96(6 Pt 2):875–880, 1982.

Shibl AM: Effect of antibiotics on production of enzymes and toxins by microorganisms, *Rev Infect Dis* 5(5):865–875, 1983.

Tierno Jr PM, Hanna BA: Ecology of toxic shock syndrome: amplification of toxic shock syndrome toxin 1 by materials of medical interest, *Rev Infect Dis* 11(Suppl 1):S182–S186, 1989.

Todd J, Fishaut M: Toxic-shock syndrome associated with phage-group-1 staphylococci, *Lancet* 2:1116–1118, 1978.

Wannamaker LW: Streptococcal toxins, *Rev Infect Dis* (5 Suppl 4)S723–S732, 1983.

Zumla A: Super antigens, T cells and microbes, *Clin infec Dis* 15(2):313–320, 1992.

TOXOPLASMOSIS

Method of
Jihoon Baang

Introduction

Toxoplasma gondii, a widespread protozoan parasite, infects a significant portion of the global population. Its interaction with humans can result in a wide array of presentations, ranging from asymptomatic dormant forms and illnesses resembling acute mononucleosis to reactivation of the dormant organism, causing disease in various body parts, particularly the brain. In pregnant women, the parasite can infect the fetus, leading to substantial morbidity worldwide. Although most infections fortunately remain dormant, toxoplasmosis continues to be a major cause of morbidity, particularly in pregnant patients in resource-limited settings and among immunocompromised individuals.

Epidemiology and Risk Factors

Toxoplasmosis is a cosmopolitan zoonotic disease that has important implications for public health because it affects one-third of the world's population. The prevalence of *Toxoplasma gondii* varies widely depending on geographic area. For example, the United States has a prevalence of roughly 10% compared with other places such as Brazil and France, which has a prevalence of greater than 50%.

Toxoplasma gondii, a parasitic protozoan, relies on cats and their relatives as its sole definitive hosts, making them instrumental in the parasite's propagation. Three primary transmission routes contribute to the spread of toxoplasmosis. Firstly, foodborne transmission occurs when undercooked meat (particularly pork, lamb, and venison) from an infected animal is consumed. This mode of transmission is more prevalent in countries and cultures with a preference for undercooked meat. Secondly, cats, particularly kittens, can directly spread the parasite. An infected kitten may shed millions of oocysts for up to 3 weeks, contaminating soil, water, and its litter box. The third route involves congenital transmission from an infected mother to her unborn child, particularly when the infection is newly acquired. This can result in significant morbidity for the fetus. Though rare, additional transmission methods include organ transplantation from an infected donor, blood transfusions, and improper handling of infected tissue or blood within a laboratory setting.

Pathophysiology

T. gondii exists in three forms: the oocysts, tachyzoites and bradyzoites, and they all play a different role in the life cycle of this disease. The major route of infection for *T. gondii* is the gastrointestinal tract. The parasite gains access through the gastrointestinal tract, most commonly through oocysts (i.e., the egg stage) that can exist in contaminated soil, food, and water or through bradyzoites, which exist in tissue and can be transmitted through the ingestion of meat harboring *T. gondii*. Once the parasite enters the gastrointestinal tract, it transforms into tachyzoites which can rapidly multiply within the intestinal epithelium and spread throughout the body. Patients are often asymptomatic but can also develop a mononucleosis-like syndrome of fever, myalgias, and night sweats during this phase.

T. gondii tachyzoites can infect mammalian cells, but, in a normal host, the immune system can effectively reduce the burden of tachyzoites, leading to the elimination of the majority of tachyzoites in human tissue. Murine models suggest T cells, macrophages, and type 1 cytokines such as IFN-gamma and IL-12 play an important role in controlling *T. gondii*. Tachyzoites can change into bradyzoites and remain dormant in various tissues of the body, primarily the brain, skeleton, heart muscle and eye, without causing any symptoms for the remainder of a person's life. Bradyzoites can reactivate when a person who is harboring *T. gondii* becomes immunosuppressed and can lead to diseases in various parts of the body, mainly the brain, skeletal muscle, myocardium, and eye. The tissue cyst form will differentiate into tachyzoites, leading to uncontrolled proliferation that results in tissue destruction, most commonly in the brain and eye.

Clinical Presentation

When thinking about the diagnosis of *T. gondii* infection, there are a few clinical points that should be considered in the clinical reasoning process. The first is that the clinical presentation is influenced by the immune status of the host that it infects. The second is appreciation of the protean clinical manifestation of this cosmopolitan protozoan. The third is understanding the life cycle of this protozoan. And last, but not least, is understanding the limitations of various available diagnostic tests and how to interpret them in a certain clinical setting.

Clinical presentation will be categorized as presentation in a normal host, an immunocompromised host, and a pregnant patient for the convenience of this chapter. The genotype of *T. gondii* also influences the clinical presentation but it is seldom checked in clinical practice.

Clinical Presentation in the Normal Host

When a normal host encounters this protozoan, usually through soil and water contaminated with oocysts excreted from cats or the ingestion of undercooked meat harboring cyst bradyzoites, most of the time, they will have little to no symptoms. When they do have symptoms, they can develop flulike symptoms characterized by fevers, myalgias, and painless enlargement of cervical lymph nodes although rarely larger than 3 cm. Diffuse lymphadenopathy can also be observed but is less common. It can mimic other "mononucleosis-like syndromes," such as acute HIV; viral hepatitis, such as hepatitis A virus; acute Epstein Barr virus (EBV); or acute cytomegalovirus (CMV) infection, and these should be considered in the differential diagnosis when considering acute toxoplasmosis. Symptoms can last for weeks and months but are almost always self-limiting. More severe presentations, such as hepatitis, pneumonitis, and myocarditis, have been reported but these are relatively rare manifestations in a normal host and other more common causes should be considered before considering acute toxoplasmosis. Not uncommonly, chorioretinitis can be the sole presentation of acute toxoplasmosis in a normal host and can manifest itself as visual disturbances or floaters. There have been epidemiologic and animal studies suggesting a link between psychiatric illnesses such as schizophrenia with toxoplasmosis, but a definitive link has not been established.

Clinical Presentation in the Immunocompromised Host

In marked contrast, toxoplasmosis has a much more morbid clinical course in the immunocompromised host, with a wider range of clinical presentations. The compromised immune system either cannot contain the infection when it happens, or the mechanism involved in keeping the infection dormant breaks down, leading to reactivation of the infection. Acute toxoplasmosis can lead to more severe disease in the immunocompromised host, sometimes leading to disseminated disease and ultimately death if left untreated. Dormant bradyzoites can reactivate and change to tachyzoites, the invasive form of *T. gondii*. This can lead to a wide range of clinical syndromes depending on the anatomic site it reactivates in. The protean clinical manifestation of toxoplasmosis is impressive and can involve any organ but most commonly involves the eye or the brain. Diagnosis can be challenging because it can often mimic other infections, routine culture data are unrevealing, and the diagnostic studies are often not as reliable in the immunocompromised host. A thorough exposure (e.g., adopted new kittens recently) history based on the life cycle of this protozoan can sometimes be helpful in the diagnostic reasoning process. A high index of clinical suspicion is needed in the early diagnosis of this disease.

The most common site of reactivation is the brain, in which reactivation leads to toxoplasma encephalitis (TE). It is the most common central nervous system (CNS) infection in patients with HIV with a CD4 count less than 100 cells/mm^3 who are not taking any prophylactic regimen. TE can present with a wide range of signs and symptoms depending on the anatomic lesion that it reactivates in the brain. It can present with mild headaches to various degrees of confusion and focal neurologic deficits including cranial nerve abnormalities. Symptoms often will progress over weeks and sometimes months. Patients can present acutely with seizures and cerebral hemorrhage. Sometimes they can present with neuropsychiatric symptoms with paranoid psychosis. In short, there are no pathognomonic clinical findings in TE, emphasizing the importance of maintaining an index of suspicion. It leads to a variety brain pathology, including ventriculitis and meningo-encephalomyelitis, rarely hydrocephalus, and, most commonly, focal areas of enhancing lesions in the brain. It often will present as ring enhancing lesions on brain imaging studies but can be difficult to differentiate between other diseases, such as CNS lymphoma, and other more indolent infections, such as tuberculosis and fungal infections.

T. gondii can involve the lungs and lead to pneumonia. The symptoms are nonspecific, and patients will often present with a worsening cough and shortness of breath that progresses over days to weeks. It is not uncommon to present without fevers. The clinical presentation and imaging findings can look nearly identical to *Pneumocystis jirovecii* pneumonia. The imaging findings can also resemble viral pneumonitis, pulmonary tuberculosis, and fungal pneumonias from histoplasmosis, coccidioidomycosis, and mycoplasma pneumonia.

The impressive range of manifestation is owing to the protozoan's ability to infect and remain dormant in any organ tissue in the form of bradyzoites. Because of this, although much less common, toxoplasmosis can present as myocarditis, pancreatitis, myositis, hepatitis and various ocular findings, most commonly chorioretinitis. We will discuss ocular toxoplasmosis separately because of the unique challenges it poses.

Toxoplasmosis of the Eye

Toxoplasmosis, a protozoal infection caused by *Toxoplasma gondii*, is a leading cause of posterior uveitis worldwide. The infection can occur following an episode of acute infection or reactivation of a dormant bradyzoite, and congenital transmission is also possible. Though some patients with ocular toxoplasmosis may be asymptomatic, others may experience eye pain, photophobia, blurry vision, and floaters. Early diagnosis and treatment of subclinical congenital toxoplasmosis is crucial because untreated chorioretinitis, the most common late manifestation of congenital toxoplasmosis, can result in blindness. In patients who are immunocompromised, larger retinal lesions with diffuse retinal necrosis may be present and may indicate a prodrome to the development of toxoplasma encephalitis.

Toxoplasmosis in Pregnancy

Congenital toxoplasmosis occurs when a pregnant mother with an acute infection transmits the disease to her fetus through the placenta. The incidence and severity of the disease depend on the gestational age at the time of maternal infection. The transmission risk is inconsistent throughout pregnancy. Congenital infection during early pregnancy is rare. However, when the primary maternal infection occurs in the latter half of pregnancy, congenital infection is more frequently observed. Most infected infants are born healthy, but around 22% may develop clinical disease by 3 years of age. Fetal outcomes associated with congenital toxoplasmosis can be severe, including miscarriage, stillbirth, or severe CNS sequelae. It is crucial to monitor and manage maternal infections during pregnancy to minimize the risk of congenital transmission and its associated complications.

Diagnosis

The diagnosis of toxoplasmosis is typically made through a combination of a clinical syndrome compatible with toxoplasmosis and positive serologic studies. In certain clinical scenarios, especially in congenital infections in utero, the detection of *T. gondii* DNA in various body fluids and tissue can provide a definitive diagnosis. Histopathologic diagnosis through a biopsy of affected tissue is also possible but often pursued in a clinical scenario where other diagnoses need to be excluded. It is essential to consider a patient's immune status because the presentation of toxoplasmosis can vary depending on the host's immune response.

The detection of antibodies against *T. gondii* is the most common laboratory test used in the diagnosis of toxoplasmosis. Both immunoglobulin (Ig)M and IgG antibody tests should be performed initially, and the results should be combined with the patient's clinical presentation to establish a diagnosis. It is important to note that a single serologic test is rarely sufficient to confirm acute or chronic toxoplasmosis. Often, multiple tests at different time points are required. Accurately differentiating between acute and chronic infections is particularly crucial for pregnant patients because chronic infections pose minimal risk to the fetus and acute infections are more likely to result in congenital toxoplasmosis.

IgG and IgM antibodies against *T. gondii* can be easily detected in most laboratories using commercially available kits. If toxoplasmosis is suspected, *Toxoplasma*-specific IgG testing serves as a convenient initial step to determine the host's immune response to the organism. A positive IgG test signifies past exposure to *T. gondii* and the presence of the parasite in the host's body. A negative IgG test often implies no exposure to *T. gondii*, but it can also represent an early infection or, rarely, a false-negative test result, typically in individuals with compromised immune systems.

The IgM plays a role in differentiating between acute and chronic infections. A negative test result generally indicates a chronic infection, though a positive IgM test is less informative due to its lack of specificity. Because the IgM antibody can persist for over 18 months, it is less useful for determining the infection's timing. In pregnant patients, the timing of infection is crucial. One test that can be used is the IgG avidity test. This is based on the observation that the functional affinity of *T. gondii*–specific IgG antibodies is initially low after infection and increases over time, which can help ascertain the infection's age. A high avidity pattern reliably predicts an infection older than 4 months, whereas a low avidity pattern suggests an acute infection but is not as reliable. IgE antibodies can also be checked. These antibodies have shorter half-lives, which makes it more useful than IgM in determining whether someone has an acute infection. The IgA antibodies do not bring value in adults compared with the IgM as it can persist in recently infected patients for more than a year. However, IgA antibodies are more sensitive in detecting congenital toxoplasmosis and should be checked in fetuses and newborns with a high clinical suspicion for the condition. The avidity test, along with IgA and IgE antibodies, is not widely available in most labs; however, it can be performed at the Palo Alto Medical Foundation in the United States. None of the current commercial assays in the United States have been approved by the U.S. Food and Drug Administration for the use in infants, and all specimens from neonates should be sent to the Palo Alto Medical Foundation for testing. Table 1 summarizes the basic interpretation of serologic studies in individuals greater than a year old.

Polymerase chain reaction (PCR) amplification serves as an important tool for detecting *T. gondii* DNA in a variety of body fluids and tissues. This method has proven to be effective in diagnosing diverse forms of toxoplasmosis, including congenital, ocular, cerebral, and disseminated cases. The use of PCR on amniotic fluid has significantly transformed the diagnosis of fetal *T. gondii* infection by enabling early detection, thereby circumventing the need for more invasive procedures on the fetus. PCR allows for the precise identification of *T. gondii* DNA in numerous sample types, such as brain tissue, cerebrospinal fluid (CSF), vitreous and aqueous fluid, bronchoalveolar lavage (BAL) fluid, urine, amniotic fluid, and peripheral blood.

Histopathologic diagnosis of toxoplasmosis has become less common owing to the invasive techniques required for tissue collection and the growing prevalence of PCR usage. Detecting tachyzoites in body fluids and tissue samples can confirm the presence of an acute infection, although this can be challenging to demonstrate. Meanwhile, the identification of bradyzoites may

TABLE 1	Toxoplasmosis Laboratory Diagnosis	
IGG RESULT	**IGM RESULT**	**REPORT/INTERPRETATION FOR HUMANS***
Negative	Negative	There is no serologic evidence of infection with *Toxoplasma*.
Negative	Equivocal	This is a possible early acute infection or a false-positive IgM reaction. Obtain a new specimen for IgG and IgM testing. If results for the second specimen remain the same, the patient is probably not infected with *Toxoplasma*.
Negative	Positive	This is a possible acute infection or a false-positive IgM result. Obtain a new specimen for IgG and IgM testing. If results for the second specimen remain the same, the IgM reaction is probably a false-positive.
Equivocal	Negative	This is indeterminate. Obtain a new specimen for testing, or retest this specimen for IgG in a different assay.
Equivocal	Equivocal	This is indeterminate. Obtain a new specimen for both IgG and IgM testing.
Equivocal	Positive	This is a possible acute infection with *Toxoplasma*. Obtain a new specimen for IgG and IgM testing. If results for the second specimen remain the same or if the IgG becomes positive, both specimens should be sent to a reference laboratory with experience in diagnosis of toxoplasmosis for further testing.
Positive	Negative	This individual is infected with *Toxoplasma* for 6 months or more.
Positive	Equivocal	This individual is infected with *Toxoplasma* for probably more than 1 year, or this is a false-positive IgM reaction. Obtain a new specimen for IgM testing. If results with the second specimen remain the same, both specimens should be sent to a reference laboratory with experience in the diagnosis of toxoplasmosis for further testing.
Positive	Positive	This is a possible recent infection within the last 12 months or a false-positive IgM reaction. Send the specimen to a reference laboratory with experience in the diagnosis of toxoplasmosis for further testing.

*Except infants.
Source: NCCLS. Clinical Use and Interpretation of Serologic Tests for *Toxoplasma gondii*; Approved Guideline. NCCLS document M36-A [ISBN 1-56238-523-2]. NCCLS, 940 West Valley Road, Suite 1400, Wayne, PA 19087-1898 USA, 2004.

indicate either chronic infection or reactivation disease, depending on the host's condition.

Therapeutic response can serve as a diagnostic tool in certain cases. For patients presenting with ring-enhancing lesions in the brain who cannot undergo a brain biopsy and have inconclusive cerebrospinal fluid (CSF) results, a course of treatment for toxoplasma encephalitis should typically yield clinical and radiologic improvements within 14 days. If a clinical response is observed, it is generally considered sufficient for confirming the diagnosis of toxoplasma encephalitis.

Treatment

Treatment for *T. gondii* primarily targets the tachyzoite stage of the parasite but is unable to eliminate bradyzoites embedded within tissue, which can result in relapse in certain scenarios. In immunocompetent individuals, acute toxoplasmosis usually does not warrant treatment. However, if visceral involvement or severe symptoms are present, a 2- to 4-week course of therapy might be advantageous. On the other hand, treatment is typically necessary for acute toxoplasmosis and reactivation disease in immunocompromised hosts, ocular toxoplasmosis with visual disturbances, acute toxoplasmosis in pregnant patients, and cases of congenital toxoplasmosis.

The treatment regimen remains consistent across various clinical scenarios except for pregnant patients in their first trimester owing to the teratogenicity of pyrimethamine. Nevertheless, the dose and duration of treatment can vary depending on the specific situation and immune status of the host. The dose is typically higher and duration of treatment longer in patients who are immunocompromised.

Pyrimethamine (Daraprim) serves as the cornerstone of toxoplasmosis treatment and should be incorporated when possible. As a folic acid antagonist, it is associated with dose-dependent bone marrow suppression. This side effect can be mitigated through the coadministration of folinic acid (leucovorin).[1] Pyrimethamine

monotherapy is not recommended owing to the high doses required for effective treatment. The addition of a second drug, such as sulfadiazine, adds synergy, allowing pyrimethamine to be used at substantially lower, nontoxic levels compared with when administered alone. Clindamycin,[1] atovaquone (Mepron),[1] and azithromycin (Zithromax)[1] can be used to replace sulfadiazine, if the patient is unable to tolerate sulfadiazine. Trimethoprim-sulfamethoxazole (Bactrim)[1] monotherapy has been shown in a small trial to be as effective as pyrimethamine combined with sulfamethoxazole and can be used if the patient is unable to tolerate pyrimethamine. For ocular toxoplasmosis, intravitreous injection of clindamycin[1] and dexamethasone[1] can be used, although a small, randomized trial did not show any difference in outcome compared with an oral regimen.

In pregnant patients, chronic *T. gondii* infection poses little risk to the fetus and does not need treatment. In acute or recent infection, treatment should be initiated. If a patient is in their first trimester (<14 weeks), spiramycin (Rovamycine)[2] should be started. In their second and third trimesters (>14 weeks), a pyrimethamine-sulfadiazine regimen can be used.

Because of the inability to eradicate bradyzoites embedded in tissue, secondary prophylaxis is recommended for immunocompromised patients to prevent relapse until immune reconstitution is achieved. For patients with HIV, this typically involves maintaining a CD4 count greater than 200/mm^3 for over 6 months. Transplant recipients, on the other hand, may require lifelong secondary prophylaxis to prevent the recurrence of infection.

Effective management of toxoplasmosis necessitates not only addressing the various side effects associated with treatment but also possessing the flexibility to switch to alternative regimens when a patient's tolerance to the initial therapy proves inadequate. This adaptability is crucial in optimizing patient outcomes and ensuring successful treatment. A summary of treatment for toxoplasmosis is provided in Table 2.

---

[1] Not FDA approved for this indication.

---

[1] Not FDA approved for this indication.
[2] Not available in the United States.

TABLE 2 Summary of Treatment Regimens for Toxoplasmosis

HOST	REGIMEN AND DURATION
Primary infection in immunocompetent host	No treatment in general but can treat with same regimen as below for 2–4 weeks in severe disease
Treatment of immunocompromised host/reactivation disease/ocular toxoplasmosis	Preferred: Pyrimethamine[1] (PO) 200 mg loading dose followed by 50 mg (<60 kg); 75 mg (≥60 kg) daily + sulfadiazine 1 g (<60 kg); 1.5 g (≥60 kg) + folinic acid (leucovorin)[1] 10–25 mg PO daily for 6 weeks or longer depending on clinical response and then secondary prophylaxis If unable to tolerate pyrimethamine: Trimethoprim/sulfamethoxazole[1] 10 mg/kg/day (trimethoprim component) divided in two to three doses for monotherapy for 6 weeks If unable to tolerate sulfadiazine: Can change to clindamycin[1] 600 mg IV/PO q8–q6h or atovaquone (Mepron)[1] 1500 mg PO q12h or azithromycin[1] 900–1200 mg PO daily with pyrimethamine 25–50 mg and leucovorin for 6 weeks or longer
Secondary prophylaxis	Sulfadiazine 500–1000 mg PO qid + primethamine[1] 25–50 mg PO daily + folinic acid[1] 10–25 mg PO daily until immune reconstitution Clindamycin[1] 300–450 mg PO q6-q8h + primethamine[1] 25–50 mg PO daily + folinic acid[1] 10–25 mg PO daily Atovaquone[1] 1500 mg PO daily with food
Pregnancy	First trimester: Spiramycin (Rovamycine)[2] 1 g q8h Second and 3rd trimester: Pyrimethamine (PO) 50 mg twice daily loading dose for 2 days then 50 mg daily + sulfadiazine 75 mg/kg/d in two divided doses for 2 days then 50 mg/kg twice daily + folinic acid[1] 10–20 mg PO daily until delivery
Fetal/congenital toxoplasmosis	Pyrimethamine + sulfadiazine + leucovorin[1]: expert consultation is recommended

[1]Not FDA approved for this indication.
[2]Not available in the United States.

Prevention

Currently, no vaccines are available for the prevention of toxoplasmosis or for reducing the risk of reactivation. Preventative measures are crucial, particularly for seronegative pregnant women and individuals who are immunocompromised. Toxoplasmosis can occasionally be transmitted through donor organs, and routine screening is a standard practice in many transplant programs. Familiarity with the modes of transmission is the first step in mitigating the risk of acquiring toxoplasmosis. This includes avoiding areas potentially contaminated with cat feces or wearing gloves when exposure is unavoidable, such as when cleaning a kitten's litter box. Freezing meat to –20°C (–4°F) for at least 48 hours or cooking meat thoroughly is sufficient to eliminate bradyzoites that may be present within the meat. Washing fruits and vegetables under running water and consistently washing hands after outdoor activities are simple interventions that can minimize the risk of acquiring oocysts.

References

Bennett JE, Dolin R, Blaser MJ: Preface to the eighth edition. In Bennett JE, Dolin R, Blaser MJ, editors: *Mandell, douglas, and bennett's principles and practice of infectious diseases*, Eighth Edition, xxvii. Philadelphia, 2015, W.B. Saunders, pp 3355–3387.
CDC - DPDx Homepage, February 21, 2023. https://www.cdc.gov/dpdx/index.html, 2023. Accessed 03/01/2023.
Montoya JG, Liesenfeld O: Toxoplasmosis, *Lancet.* 363(9425):1965–1976, 2004.
NCCLS: *Clinical Use and interpretation of serologic tests for toxoplasma gondii; approved guideline.* NCCLS document M36-A [ISBN 1-56238-523-2], 2004. NCCLS, 940 West Valley Road, Suite 1400, Wayne, PA 19087-1898 USA.
Panel on Guidelines for the Prevention and Treatment of Opportunistic Infections in Adults and Adolescents with HIV. Guidelines for the Prevention and Treatment of Opportunistic Infections in Adults and Adolescents with HIV. National Institutes of Health, Centers for Disease Control and Prevention, HIV Medicine Association, and Infectious Diseases Society of America. Year. Available at https://clinicalinfo.hiv.gov/en/guidelines/adult-and-adolescent-opportunistic-infection. Accessed 03/01/2023 [pp CC-1 – CC-15].

TYPHOID FEVER

Method of
Tamilarasu Kadhiravan, MD

CURRENT DIAGNOSIS

- Typhoid fever typically manifests as an undifferentiated acute febrile illness.
- Soft splenomegaly, normal or low white blood cell count, and elevated liver enzymes are subtle diagnostic pointers.
- Blood culture, drawn before antibiotic administration, is the most useful investigation.
- Consider presumptive treatment in appropriate epidemiologic settings.

CURRENT THERAPY

- Intermediate susceptibility and resistance to fluoroquinolones are widespread among *Salmonella enterica* Typhi.
- High-dose fluoroquinolones are suboptimal for treating such infections.
- Azithromycin (Zithromax)[1] is the preferred drug for uncomplicated typhoid fever.
- Ceftriaxone (Rocephin)[1] is preferred for treating hospitalized and seriously ill patients.
- Extensively drug-resistant (XDR) typhoid fever, which is resistant to ceftriaxone and fluoroquinolones, is an emerging threat.

[1]Not FDA approved for this indication.

Typhoid fever is a bacteremic infection caused by the gram-negative bacillus *Salmonella enterica* serovar Typhi. *S enterica* Paratyphi also causes an illness clinically indistinguishable from typhoid fever. Humans are the only known host of *S enterica* Typhi, and it is transmitted by ingestion of contaminated food or water. Improvement in sanitation and hygiene led to the elimination of typhoid fever from the developed world long before the advent of antibiotics. On the other hand, in parts of the world lacking sanitation, it continues to be an important cause of febrile illness despite the availability of effective antibiotics.

Epidemiology

Typhoid fever is endemic in the developing world, especially the South and South East Asian countries of India, Nepal, Pakistan, Bangladesh, Vietnam, and Indonesia. Annual incidence in endemic settings is typically more than 100 cases per 100,000 population, and it predominantly affects children and young adults. Apart from sick persons with typhoid fever, convalescent carriers and asymptomatically infected food handlers (long-term carriers) are the sources of infection. Potential vehicles of infection include food or water consumed from roadside eateries, ice cubes and ice cream made from contaminated water, and raw vegetables and fruits. In contrast, most cases of typhoid fever in developed countries are imported by travel, especially to the Indian subcontinent.

Pathogenesis and Clinical Features

Following ingestion, the bacilli invade and multiply in the small-intestinal lymphoid tissue before entering the bloodstream. This primary bacteremia leads to widespread seeding of the reticuloendothelial system and intestinal lymphoid tissue, where the infection is amplified and spills over into the circulation. Onset of symptoms usually coincides with this secondary bacteremia. Interestingly, unlike other gram-negative bacteremic infections, septic shock develops relatively late in the course of illness, and the infection can be eminently cured by oral antibiotic therapy. Nonetheless, it should be emphasized that any delay in initiating antibiotic therapy increases the risk of complications (Box 1).

During the first week, temperature gradually increases in a stepladder fashion. Localizing symptoms are usually minimal. Anorexia, lassitude, and malaise are often marked. Headache and vomiting are common; however, a supple neck helps rule out meningitis. Abdominal symptoms such as constipation, loose stools, and abdominal pain are not infrequent, but they are nonspecific and often overlooked. Soft, tender enlargement of liver or spleen is seen in about half the patients. Rose spots and relative bradycardia, though classic, are rare. When the infection goes untreated, the hypertrophied lymphoid tissue of the Peyer's patches can ulcerate toward the end of the second week, resulting in torrential gastrointestinal bleeding, small intestinal perforation, and secondary bacterial peritonitis. Patients with severe illness can present with a muttering delirium described as *coma vigil*. Untreated typhoid fever often resolves spontaneously in about 4 to 6 weeks. However, the risk of death is high (>10%), and relapses are frequent. Many patients excrete *S enterica* Typhi in feces and urine during convalescence (convalescent carriers), and some of them continue to excrete beyond 1 year (long-term carriers).

Current Pattern of Antimicrobial Susceptibility

Since 1990, a sea change has occurred in the antimicrobial susceptibility of *S enterica* Typhi in endemic countries and elsewhere. Unregulated use of fluoroquinolones initially led to the emergence of *S enterica* Typhi strains with decreased susceptibility. These strains had a subthreshold increase in minimal inhibitory concentration (MIC) that was not detected by conventional disk-diffusion testing. Hence, resistance to nalidixic acid (NegGram)[2] (a quinolone) was often used as a surrogate marker for such strains. Currently, determination of MIC is recommended to identify fluoroquinolone susceptibility. Most infections in endemic countries are now caused by *S. enterica* Typhi with intermediate susceptibility or resistance to fluoroquinolones. Not surprisingly, this change is reflected in far-away geographic locales such as the United States and the United Kingdom. Of late, sporadic instances of resistance to azithromycin and third-generation cephalosporins have been reported. Notably, an ongoing outbreak of extensively drug-resistant (XDR) *S. enterica* Typhi with extended-spectrum β-lactamase–mediated resistance to third-generation cephalosporins has been reported in the Sindh province of Pakistan. In 2019, two-thirds of *S. enterica* Typhi isolates from Karachi, Pakistan, were resistant to third-generation cephalosporins. Travel-associated XDR-typhoid cases have been reported from several countries in the Europe and North America.

Diagnosis

Clinical features are nonspecific, and laboratory testing is essential to confirm a diagnosis of typhoid fever. A soft splenomegaly, absence of leukocytosis, mild leukopenia, and modest elevation of transaminases are subtle pointers to a diagnosis of typhoid fever. Blood culture drawn early in the illness before initiation of antibiotics is often fruitful and is the gold standard for the diagnosis of typhoid fever. The time-honored Widal test, which detects agglutinating antibodies to somatic and flagellar antigens of *S enterica* Typhi, adds little to decision making. Initial enthusiasm about rapid serologic tests such as Typhidot and Tubex TF has not been confirmed in community-based studies. None of these tests are sensitive enough to rule out typhoid. In a patient who has non-localizing acute febrile illness lasting more than 5 to 7 days in a suggestive epidemiologic setting (residence in or travel to endemic area; outbreaks), it is prudent to treat presumptively for typhoid fever, after reasonably ruling out competing diagnoses such as malaria, dengue, leptospirosis, and rickettsial infection.

Treatment

Fluoroquinolones (ciprofloxacin [Cipro] or ofloxacin [Floxin][1] 7.5 mg/kg twice a day for 5–7 days) were unparalleled in efficacy for treating fully susceptible *S enterica* Typhi strains. However, their use was associated with frequent treatment failures, prolonged defervescence, and higher rates of complications in nalidixic acid-resistant *S. enterica* Typhi (NARST) infections. Given the widespread emergence of reduced susceptibility, fluoroquinolones are no longer considered the drug of choice. Several alternatives have been evaluated in randomized, controlled trials for treating uncomplicated typhoid fever caused by NARST (Table 1). Ease of oral administration, proven efficacy, and safety (under FDA review) make azithromycin (Zithromax)[1] a good first choice for

---

BOX 1 Complications of Typhoid Fever

Abdominal
Paralytic ileus
Intestinal hemorrhage
Intestinal perforation
Secondary peritonitis
Symptomatic liver dysfunction
Acalculous cholecystitis

Extra abdominal
Encephalopathy
Cerebellar dysfunction
Myocarditis
Osteomyelitis and soft tissue abscesses
Multiorgan dysfunction syndrome
Hemophagocytic syndrome
Hemolysis
Glomerulonephritis

Long-term
Gallbladder cancer

---

[1] Not FDA approved for this indication.
[2] Not available in the United States.

TABLE 1	Outcomes of Alternative Treatments for Nalidixic Acid–Resistant *S enterica* Typhi (NARST) Infection Evaluated in Randomized, Controlled Trials				
DRUG	**DOSAGE**	**FEVER CLEARANCE TIME (MEDIAN OR MEAN)**	**RATE OF TREATMENT FAILURE**	**RELAPSE RATE**	**COMMENTS**
High-dose ofloxacin (Floxin)[1]	10 mg/kg[3] bid × 7 d	8.2 d	36%	<1%; insufficient data	Not recommended
Gatifloxacin (Tequin)[2]	10 mg/kg qd × 7 d	4.4 d	9%	3%	Serious concerns about dysglycemia; resistance emerging in Nepal
Azithromycin (Zithromax)[1]	10–20[3] mg/kg qd × 7 d	4.4 d	9%	<1%; insufficient data	Effective in XDR-typhoid. Unproven in complicated typhoid fever
Cefixime (Suprax)[1]	10 mg/kg[3] bid × 7 d	5.8 d	27%	9%	High cost; not recommended
Ceftriaxone (Rocephin)[1]	60 mg/kg qd × 7 d	2.8 d	7%	7%	Experts suggest treatment for 10–14 d

Data from Arjyal A, Basnyat B, Nhan HT, et al: Gatifloxacin versus ceftriaxone for uncomplicated enteric fever in Nepal: an open-label, two-centre, randomised controlled trial. Lancet Infect Dis 2016;16:535. Dolecek C, Tran TP, Nguyen NR, et al: A multi-center randomised controlled trial of gatifloxacin versus azithromycin for the treatment of uncomplicated typhoid fever in children and adults in Vietnam. PLoS One 2008;3:e2188; Pandit A, Arjyal A, Day JN, et al: An open randomized comparison of gatifloxacin versus cefixime for the treatment of uncomplicated enteric fever. PLoS One 2007;2:e542; and Parry CM, Ho VA, Phuong le T, et al: Randomized controlled comparison of ofloxacin, azithromycin, and an ofloxacin-azithromycin combination for treatment of multidrug-resistant and nalidixic acid-resistant typhoid fever. Antimicrob Agents Chemother 2007;51:819.

[1]Not FDA approved for this indication.
[2]Not available in the United States.
[3]Exceeds dosage recommended by the manufacturer.

uncomplicated typhoid fever. In hospitalized seriously ill patients and treatment failures, parenteral ceftriaxone (Rocephin)[1] is preferred. Usually, it takes about 4 to 7 days for defervescence after the initiation of antibiotics.

Recently, combining oral azithromycin (500 mg qd) with ceftriaxone (2 g qd) for inpatient or cefixime (Suprax)[1] (400 mg qd) for outpatient treatment was found to shorten the fever clearance time by about 7 hours, and fewer patients had persistent bacteremia on Day 3 (17% vs 4%). This clinical trial had certain limitations, and I do not recommend using a combination of antibiotics to treat typhoid fever. Despite in vitro susceptibility, aminoglycosides and first- and second-generation cephalosporins are not effective clinically for treating typhoid fever. Azithromycin (20 mg/kg qd for 7 days)[3] and meropenem (Merrem[1]; 20 mg/kg tid for 14 days) are the only options currently available for the treatment of XDR-typhoid. Antipyretics should be used for symptom relief; ibuprofen (Motrin; 10 mg/kg every 6 hours) is superior to acetaminophen (Tylenol; 12 mg/kg every 6 hours). However, ibuprofen should be avoided when dengue fever is a possibility. A soft, low-residue diet is traditionally advised to prevent intestinal perforation. Such a practice, however, is not founded on scientific evidence. Treatment of *S enterica* Paratyphi infection is identical to that of *S enterica* Typhi infection.

Prevention
Sustained improvement in sanitation and access to safe drinking water are essential to control typhoid fever in endemic areas. Avoiding potentially contaminated food and beverages and being vaccinated before travel decrease the risk of typhoid fever among travelers (see the article on travel medicine). Mass administration of the Vi polysaccharide vaccine (Typhim Vi, Typherix [outside United States]) has been found to confer herd immunity and is a potential tool for the control of typhoid fever in endemic settings.

---

[1]Not FDA approved for this indication.
[3]Exceeds dosage recommended by the manufacturer.

References
Azmatullah A, Qamar FN, Thaver D, et al: Systematic review of the global epidemiology, clinical and laboratory profile of enteric fever, *J Glob Health* 5:020407, 2015.
Basnyat B, Qamar FN, Rupali P, et al: Enteric fever, *BMJ* 372:n437, 2021.
Britto CD, Wong VK, Dougan G, et al: A systematic review of antimicrobial resistance in *Salmonella enterica* serovar typhi, the etiological agent of typhoid, *PLoS Negl Trop Dis* 12:e0006779, 2018.
Chatham-Stephens K, Medalla F, et al: Emergence of extensively drug-resistant *Salmonella* Typhi infections among travelers to or from Pakistan - United States, 2016-2018, *MMWR Morb Mortal Wkly Rep* 68:11, 2019.
Jin C, Gibani MM, Pennington SH, et al: Treatment responses to azithromycin and ciprofloxacin in uncomplicated *Salmonella* typhi infection: a comparison of clinical and microbiological data from a controlled human infection model, *PLoS Negl Trop Dis* 13:e0007955, 2019.
Qamar FN, Yousafzai MT, Dehraj IF, et al: Antimicrobial resistance in typhoidal *Salmonella*: surveillance for enteric fever in asia project, 2016-2019, *Clin Infect Dis* 71(Supplement_3):S276, 2020.
Qureshi S, Naveed AB, Yousafzai MT, et al: Response of extensively drug resistant *Salmonella* Typhi to treatment with meropenem and azithromycin, in Pakistan, *PLoS Negl Trop Dis* 14:e0008682, 2020.
Vinh H, Parry CM, Hanh VT, et al: Double blind comparison of ibuprofen and paracetamol for adjunctive treatment of uncomplicated typhoid fever, *Pediatr Infect Dis J* 23:226, 2004.
Wijedoru L, Mallett S, Parry CM: Rapid diagnostic tests for typhoid and paratyphoid (enteric) fever, *Cochrane Database Syst Rev*(5), 2017:CD008892.
Zmora N, Shrestha S, Neuberger A, et al: Open label comparative trial of mono versus dual antibiotic therapy for typhoid fever in adults, *PLoS Negl Trop Dis* 12:e0006380, 2018.

VARICELLA (CHICKENPOX)

Method of
Martha Riese, MD

CURRENT DIAGNOSIS

- Historically, varicella has been diagnosed clinically. Symptoms include a pruritic vesicular rash, fever, malaise, abdominal pain, and anorexia.
- Polymerase chain reaction (PCR) testing is available for confirmation of the diagnosis. An open vesicular lesion is swabbed for specimen collection.

TABLE 1	Pertussis Treatment	
ANTIBIOTIC	**DOSING**	**COMMENTS**
Azithromycin (Zithromax)	Children: 10 mg/kg/day for 3 days, or 10 mg/kg on day 1, then 5 mg/kg/day on days 2 through 5 Adults: 500 mg/day for 3 days, or 500 mg on day 1, then 250 mg/day on days 2 through 5	Preferred therapy due to ease of use and tolerability. Preferred agent for infants younger than 1 month Prolongation of the QT interval
Clarithromycin (Biaxin)	Children: 7.5 mg/kg twice daily for 7 days Adults: 500 mg twice daily for 7 days	Fewer adverse effects than erythromycin, but typically more than azithromycin Prolongation of the QT interval CYP3A4 inhibitor; use with caution with other CYP3A4 medications
Erythromycin, delayed release (Ery-Tab)	Children: 40 to 60 mg/kg/day in three or four divided doses for 7 to 14 days Adults: 666 mg three times per day for 7 to 14 days	Gastrointestinal adverse effects limit use Risk of hypertrophic pyloric stenosis in infants CYP3A4 inhibitor; use with caution with other CYP3A4 medications
Trimethoprim/ sulfamethoxazole	Children: 8/40 mg/kg/day divided into two doses for 14 days Adults: one double-strength tablet (160/800 mg) twice daily for 14 days	May be effective for those with intolerance to macrolide antibiotics Caution in pregnancy; contraindicated in infants younger than 2 months, or in mothers breastfeeding infants younger than 2 months

CYP, Cytochrome P450.

From Kline JM, Lewis WD, Smith EA, Tracy LR: Pertussis: A reemerging infection, *Am Fam Physician* 88:507–514, 2013.

and first- and second-generation cephalosporins are not effective against *B. pertussis*.

Trimethoprim-sulfamethoxazole (Bactrim)[1] is an alternative for patients older than 2 months who cannot tolerate macrolides or who are infected with a macrolide-resistant strain, but studies evaluating trimethoprim-sulfamethoxazole as treatment for pertussis are limited (Table 1).

Hospitalized young infants with pertussis should be managed in a setting/facility where these complications can be recognized and managed urgently. Exchange transfusions or leukapheresis have been reported to be life-saving in infants with progressive pulmonary hypertension and markedly elevated lymphocyte counts.

Prevention

In the United States, all vaccines available for preventing pertussis are acellular pertussis formulations combined with tetanus and diphtheria toxoids. Five doses of pertussis-containing vaccine (DTaP [Daptacel, Infanrix]) are recommended prior to entering school: four doses of DTaP before 2 years of age and one dose of DTaP before school entry. Adolescent and adult formulations, known as Tdap vaccines (Adacel, Boostrix), contain reduced quantities of diphtheria toxoid and some pertussis antigens compared with DTaP. A single dose is recommended universally for people 11 years and older, including adults of any age, in place of a decennial tetanus and diphtheria vaccine (Td). Booster doses of Tdap are not recommended for any group of people except pregnant women. The Centers for Disease Control and Prevention (CDC) recommends the use of PEP with antimicrobials in persons at high risk of developing severe pertussis and those who will have close contact with those at high risk of developing severe pertussis.

---

[1]Not FDA approved for this indication.

References

American Academy of Pediatrics. Pertussis. In: Kimberly DW, Brady MT, Jackson MA, Long SS, eds. *Red Book: 2018 Report of the Committee on Infectious Diseases.* 31st ed. Itasca, IL: AAP.

Ebell MH, Marchello C, Callahan M: Clinical diagnosis of bordetella pertussis infection: A systematic review, *J Am Board Fam Med* 2017; 30:308–319.
Hewlett EL, Edwards KM: Pertussis—not just for kids, *N Engl J Med* 2005; 32:1215–1222.
Kilgore PE, Salim AM, Zervos MJ, Schmitt HJ: Pertussis: microbiology, disease, treatment and prevention, *Clin Microbiol Rev* 2016; 29:449–486.
Kline JM, Lewis WD, Smith EA, Tracy LR: Pertussis: A reemerging infection, *Am Fam Physician* 2013; 88:507–514.
Liang JL, Tiwari T, Moro P, et al: Prevention of pertussis, tetanus, and diphtheria with vaccines in the united states: recommendations of the Advisory Committee on Immunization Practices (ACIP), *MMWR Recomm Rep* 2018; 67(No. RR-2):1–44.
Skoff TH, Hadler S, Hariri S: The epidemiology of nationally reported pertussis in the United States, 2000-2016, *Clin InfecDis* 2019; 68:1634–1640.

YELLOW FEVER

Method of
Lucius M. Lampton, MD

CURRENT DIAGNOSIS

- Yellow fever is a historically important mosquito-borne Flavivirus with high morbidity and mortality.
- Travel to yellow fever–endemic areas in Sub-Saharan Africa and tropical Central and South America is the essential risk factor.
- Symptoms may include abrupt onset of fever, relative bradycardia, headache, and, if severe, jaundice, hemorrhage, and multiorgan failure.
- Diagnosis is with viral culture and serologic tests.
- Although infectious disease experts consider it improbable that yellow fever outbreaks will return to the continental United States, this reemerging disease is threatening to become more prevalent and deadly in tropical South America and Africa. Travel-related cases should be anticipated in the United States and its territories, as well as the possibility of brief episodes of local dissemination in areas bordering the Gulf of Mexico, where the vector, the *Aedes aegypti* mosquito, can be found.

CURRENT THERAPY

- Prevention is key and accomplished by vaccination and mosquito avoidance and control.
- Supportive care is the only treatment.

Epidemiology

Yellow fever is one of the great epidemic diseases of tropical Africa and the Americas. It receives its appellation "yellow" from the symptom of jaundice, which appears in severe disease, and it is caused by an RNA virus, specifically a Flavivirus (a family name derived from yellow fever, with *flavus* Latin for yellow), that is held in natural reservoirs by forest monkeys and spread to people via mosquitoes. The disease, termed an acute hemorrhagic fever, infects humans, all species of monkeys, and certain other small mammals and is transmitted among its hosts by several species of mosquitoes.

There are three types of yellow fever infection: urban, jungle, and intermediate. In urban or classical yellow fever, human-to-human spread occurs by the bite of the *A. aegypti* mosquito, which breeds in urban unpolluted water and bites principally in the daytime. Reinvasion of this mosquito in Central and South America has occurred beginning in the 1970s owing to increases in breeding sites resulting from urbanization and the collapse of vector control efforts. In jungle or sylvatic yellow fever, which was first recognized in 1933, the disease is perpetuated by enzootic infection of mammalians, usually monkeys, disseminated by several different mosquitoes: in South America via the *Haemagogus* and *Sabethes* spp.; in East Africa via *Ae. africanus*; and in West Africa via a variety of species of *Aedes*. Human infection arises by jungle exposure to these mosquitoes. In intermediate or savannah yellow fever, which commonly occurs in Africa, the virus disseminates from mosquitoes to humans residing or working in areas bordering jungles. This cycle also involves spread of the virus from monkey to human or from human to human via the bite of a mosquito.

Yellow fever, also termed Yellow Jack, the Saffron Scourge, fièvre jaune, Bronze John, and Black Vomit (the Spanish name is vómito negro), is the deadliest arthropod virus ever to emerge in the Americas. Both the molecular taxonomic research of viral strains and the annals of history reveal an African origin. Most authorities assert it was introduced to the new world by *A. aegypti*–infested slave ships voyaging from West Africa, with its first recognition in the Americas occurring in Yucatan, Mexico, in 1648 (although research suggests the disease was present in the Americas as early as 1498). Over the next two and a half centuries, yellow fever erupted with regularity in American and European port cities, with hundreds of thousands of deaths, earning the virus deserved recognition as one of the worst plagues the world had ever seen. Two of the most significant North American epidemics occurred in Philadelphia in 1793 and in the Mississippi Valley in 1878. American epidemics were the result of the introduction of the mosquito vector and infected humans along routes of trade, especially sea and river ports and rail lines, with particular virulence associated with the Gulf region where *A. aegypti* resided. Early attempts at control focused on quarantine and sanitary measures. The devastation associated with American epidemics was an important impetus in the nation's early public health and sanitation movements for the creation of city, state, and national boards of health.

Although two 19th-century physicians, Josiah Nott and Carlos Juan Finlay, suggested the mosquito was the infectious agent for yellow fever, it was not until 1900 that the work of the US Army Commission in Cuba under Major Walter Reed established that the vector of the urban form of this disease was the *A. aegypti* mosquito, with its viral cause not established until after 1928. Max Theiler developed an attenuated vaccine strain in 1937, which was recognized with a Nobel Prize. In what is acknowledged as one of the most successful campaigns in history against infectious disease, mosquito eradication efforts and this vaccine effectively controlled and eliminated urban yellow fever in the Americas and the West Indies, with the last large outbreak occurring in the continental United States in New Orleans in 1905. However, the disease persisted in its jungle form in forest areas in Africa and South America. Vaccine administration remains incomplete in endemic areas, and outbreaks periodically recur. As well, mosquito eradication efforts in both the Americas and Africa have recently slackened, with the resulting resurgence of *A. aegypti* into nearly all of the tropical American countries, placing this region at extraordinary risk for urban outbreaks. While only travel-related cases have been documented in Asia, theoretic anthroponotic dissemination could also take place there in the many areas where the urban vector resides.

Official statistics suggest the incidence of yellow fever fluctuates, with 90% of the 200,000 annual cases reported in Africa. However, authorities warn that these statistics considerably underestimate (owing to underreporting) the true magnitude of epidemics, which field studies estimate as 50 times greater. A frightening prospect associated with failing mosquito control in urban habitats is the potential reemergence of yellow fever similar to the recent rapid resurgence of dengue, which is also transmitted by the vector *A. aegypti*. Experts contend that one of the most profound mysteries of tropical medicine is that this dangerous virus has not emerged more frequently where a susceptible, unimmunized human population and the vector density coexist. However, since the 1980s, a resurgence of yellow fever has been seen across South America and Africa, which augurs potential risk for the United States. While yellow fever outbreaks remain unlikely in the Unites States, travel-related cases should be expected, as well as the possibility of brief urban cycle transmission in the American Southeast.

The 2015–2023 outbreaks in Brazil and Africa portend ominously that yellow fever appears to be moving from its typical rural setting toward urban areas. A large urban outbreak in Angola, which began in December 2015 and subsequently spread to the Democratic Republic of the Congo, resulted in 962 confirmed cases and 393 deaths and included multiple travel-related cases appearing in nonendemic areas internationally such as China. The outbreak in Brazil was first recognized in December 2016, with more than 2251 confirmed cases and 772 deaths noted as of June 1, 2019, including two dozen travel-related cases. This upsurge of human cases, which is the highest observed in the Americas for decades, reflects the spread into densely populated metropolitan areas, such as Rio de Janeiro and Sao Paulo, which in the past were not considered at risk for transmission. In the current outbreak, all human cases have been linked only to *Haemagogus* and *Sabethes* mosquitoes. As of 2023, according to World Health Organization (WHO) data, 13 countries in South and Central America and 34 countries in Africa are endemic for, or have large areas that are endemic for, yellow fever.

In response to yellow fever's reemergence in Africa, the WHO launched the Yellow Fever Initiative. This campaign, which has primarily utilized fractional dosing, appears to be currently successful in holding the virus to lower numbers of cases. in 2006, vaccinating in mass campaigns more than 105 million people in West Africa and attempting to secure a global vaccine supply. In 2017, the Eliminate Yellow Fever Epidemics (EYE) strategy was initiated with more than 50 partners supporting 40 at-risk countries in the Americas and Africa to prevent, detect, and contain global outbreaks. By 2026, it is projected that 1.38 billion people will be vaccinated against the disease. In March 2018, Brazil's health minister announced that all of the country's 78 million people will be targeted in a large-scale vaccination campaign.

Yellow fever remains the most dangerous arbovirus ever to inhabit the Western Hemisphere. Despite ongoing vaccination and mosquito control efforts in endemic areas, sylvatic and intermediate transmission cycles persist and appear to be expanding toward urban spread. Public health leaders encourage clinicians to utilize heightened suspicion and awareness for the virus, especially among travelers to tropical areas. Recent yellow fever

TABLE 4   FDA-Approved Medications for Treating Cognitive Symptoms of Alzheimer's Disease*

	DONEPEZIL (ARICEPT)		RIVASTIGMINE (EXELON)		GALANTAMINE (RAZADYNE)	MEMANTINE (NAMENDA)	COMBINED MEMANTINE-DONEPEZIL (NAMZARIC)
Stage of AD	Mild to moderate	Moderate to severe	Mild to moderate	Mild to moderate	Mild to moderate	Moderate to severe	Moderate to severe
Mechanism	Acetylcholinesterase inhibitor (AChEI)					NMDA receptor antagonist	Shared characteristics of component medications
Route of administration	Tablet ODT (orally disintegrating tablets)		Oral capsules Oral solution	Patch	Tablet XR tablet Oral solution	Tablet Oral solution	XR tablet
Doses	5 mg, 10 mg ODT: 5 mg, 10 mg Transdermal weekly patch (Adlarity): 5 mg/day, 10 mg/day	10 mg, 23 mg	1.5 mg, 3 mg, 4.5 mg, or 6 mg Oral sol: 2 mg/mL	Patch 4.6 mg/24hr (9 mg rivastigmine) Patch 9.5 mg/24hr (18 mg rivastigmine)	4 mg, 8 mg, 12 mg Oral sol: 4 mg/mL XR: 8 mg, 16 mg, 24 mg	5 mg, 10 mg Oral sol: 2 mg/mL XR: 7 mg, 14 mg, 21 mg, 28 mg	XR: 7 mg–10mg, 14 mg–10 mg, 21 mg–10 mg, 28 mg–10 mg
Target daily dose	10 mg	23 mg	6 mg BID	9.5 mg/24 hours once daily	Tabs: 12 mg BID XR: 24 mg QD	10 mg XR: 28 mg	28 mg–10 mg
Renal impairment	No dose adjustment	No dose adjustment	May be able to tolerate lower doses	No dose adjustment	Do not exceed 16 mg/day; none if CrCl < 9 mL/min	5 mg BID XR: 14 mg	14 mg–10 mg
Hepatic impairment	Use with caution	Use with caution	May be able to tolerate lower doses	No dose adjustment	Do not exceed 16 mg/day	Use with caution	Use with caution
Frequency	Once daily	Once daily	BID	Daily	Varies	Once daily in evening	Once daily in evening
Minimum interval between dose increases	4–6 weeks between 5 mg and 10 mg	at least 3 months at 10 mg before increasing to 23 mg	2 weeks	4 weeks	4 weeks	1 week	1 week
Administration cautions		23 mg tablet should not be split, crushed, or chewed because this may increase its rate of absorption	Should be taken with meals	The patch should be replaced with a new one every 24 hours. The same site should not be used within 14 days.	Should be taken with meals	XR: do not divide, crush, or chew	Do not divide, crush or chew
Most common adverse effects	Nausea, diarrhea, insomnia, vomiting, muscle cramps, fatigue, and anorexia. May cause bladder outflow obstructions		Nausea, vomiting, anorexia, dyspepsia, and asthenia	Nausea, vomiting and diarrhea	Nausea, vomiting, diarrhea, dizziness, headache, decreased appetite, and weight decreased. May cause bladder outflow obstructions.	Dizziness, headache, confusion, and constipation	Headache, diarrhea, dizziness. May cause bladder outflow obstructions

*See chapter text for aducanumab commentary.

symptoms, not alter the progression of the disease. There are two classes of these medications: acetylcholinesterase inhibitors (AChEIs) and NMDA-receptor antagonists (Table 4).

AChEIs increase the available acetylcholine between neuronal synapses, enhancing neurotransmission. These medications are most effective in mild to moderate AD. Donepezil (Aricept), rivastigmine (Exelon), and galantamine (Razadyne) are AChEIs currently approved by the FDA. Historically, the first FDA-approved medication for treating AD was tacrine, but this was withdrawn later due to hepatotoxicity.

NMDA-receptor antagonists function by inhibiting the excitation of NMDA receptors by the neurotransmitter glutamate, preventing influx of Ca^{2+}. This inhibition has the effect of both decreasing excitotoxicity of the neurons involved (reducing symptoms) and restoring the amyloid-β induced Ca^{2+} imbalance (potential neuroprotective role).

A new class of medications became available to select patients in 2021: monoclonal antibodies directed against amyloid. The first of this class was aducanumab (Aduhelm), a recombinant human immunoglobulin gamma 1 (IgG1) monoclonal antibody directed against aggregated soluble and insoluble forms of amyloid beta. As the accumulation of amyloid beta plaques in the brain is part of the AD disease process, there is hope that this new class of drug could provide clinical benefit. A second drug in this class, lecanemab (Leqembi), received accelerated approval by the FDA and was traditionally FDA approved in July of 2023 for the treatment of AD initiated in early AD (mild cognitive impairment due to AD or mild AD). Approval of these medications was controversial since the amyloid hypothesis of Alzheimer's disease is only part of the complex physiology of this condition.

Although numerous vitamins and supplements have been studied in prevention and treatment of cognitive behaviors in Alzheimer's disease, the evidence of benefit is inconclusive and not subject to FDA scrutiny.

Multiple studies have shown aerobic exercise has a positive overall effect on cognitive function and may even slow the progression of Alzheimer's disease. Cognitive stimulation (engagement in a range of activities aimed at general enhancement of cognitive and social functioning) has also been shown to have beneficial effects on cognitive function, while music-based therapies and psychological treatment can improve symptoms of anxiety, depression, and quality of life in those suffering from AD. Cognitive training (guided practice of standard tasks designed to engage particular cognitive functions with a range of difficulty levels to suit the individual's level of ability) has been shown to provide a few months of benefit to cognitive function.

Management of Behavioral Symptoms

Behavioral symptoms in AD are the most common reason for acute care appointments, emergency room visits, or psychiatric admissions in persons with major neurocognitive disorders. Although admittedly more difficult to implement, the most effective treatment is nonpharmacologic.

Some behavior disturbances are induced by brain changes due to AD. In early stages of the disease, these are repetition, wandering, and refusing assistance. In moderate AD, pacing, agitation, antisocial or oversexualized behavior, resistance to care, and aggression can be common. Lastly, in late AD, resistance to care and repetitive vocalizations such as moaning or screaming may appear. The disease process notwithstanding, the most common cause of new behavioral symptoms is an environmental trigger, either internal (e.g., infection, pain) or external (e.g., new housing, change in caregivers or daily routine). To manage the behavior, the trigger must be identified.

Patient-centered and adaptive dementia communications skills are key to solving most behavioral symptoms of AD: making eye contact before speaking, using simple language, speaking slowly and clearly, communicating empathy through actions (smiling), asking only one question at a time, and allowing adequate time for the patient to respond (Table 5).

Although it is appropriate to consider anxiolytics and antidepressants in the treatment of anxiety and depression

TABLE 5	Initial Treatment of Common Behavioral Symptoms in Alzheimer's Disease			
BEHAVIORAL SYMPTOM	**CONSIDERATIONS**	**TREATMENT**	**FOLLOW-UP**	**CAUTION**
Agitation	Change in patient's environment (most common cause)	If possible, remove the new trigger. If not, caution 3–4 week adjustment period.	1–2 weeks	Reassure caregiver and allow for more frequent contact.
	Lack of caregiver training/knowledge	Provide in office training on redirection, reassurance, de-escalation. Alzheimer's Association offers free online classes on Living with Alzheimer's for Caregivers.	1–2 weeks	Evaluate for caregiver strain as this will have lasting impact on both caregiver and patient health and may lead to early institutionalization of patient.
	Unreported pain	Acetaminophen 500 mg daily. Can slowly scale up to 1000 mg BID. Use the lowest effective dose.	3–4 weeks	Medication review of other APAP containing medications; contraindicated in concurrent hepatic illness
	Infection	Determine source and treat appropriately	After treatment	Many common antibiotics can trigger behavioral issues; review Beers criteria and use with caution
	Drug reaction	Review medications with Beers criteria	1–2 weeks	Due to lower renal and hepatic clearances, drug effect may last longer than expected
Anxiety	Start at half of recommended adult dose, and taper slowly.	Cognitive behavioral therapy, anxiolytics	3–4 weeks	Avoid benzodiazepines or sedative-hypnotics
Depression	Start at half of recommended adult dose, and taper slowly	Cognitive behavioral therapy, antidepressants	3–4 weeks	

Continued

TABLE 4 Pituitary Adenomas, Frequency, Secretion Profile, and Clinical Manifestations

ADENOMA SUBTYPE	FREQUENCY	SECRETION PROFILE	CLINICAL SYMPTOMS
Prolactinoma	27%	Prolactin	Amenorrhea-galactorrhea
Somatotroph adenoma	15%–18%	Growth hormone	Acromegaly
Corticotroph adenoma	10%	ACTH	Cushing disease
Gonadotroph adenoma	10%	FSH, LH	Nonfunctional
Thyrotroph adenoma	1%	TSH	Hyperthyroidism, hypothyroidism, or silent
Other	30%–40%	–	Nonfunctional

ACTH, Adrenocorticotropic hormone; *FSH,* follicle-stimulating hormone; *LH,* luteinizing hormone; *TSH,* thyroid-stimulating hormone.
Mete O, Lopes MB. Overview of the 2017 WHO Classification of Pituitary Tumors. *Endocr Pathol.* 2017;28:228-243.

early experience with traditional therapy regimens for diffuse large B-cell lymphoma was ineffective in PCNSL. However, in high doses methotrexate effectively traverses the BBB and continues to be the backbone of current chemotherapy regimens. Although radiotherapy (specifically WBRT) has fallen out of favor because of cognitive impairment, this remains an active area of study with several ongoing trials. Despite maximal therapy, disease recurrence is common with 5-year survival between 30% and 40%.

Pituitary Adenomas

Tumors of the pituitary are a diverse group of tumors and account for a growing number (17.2%) of newly discovered CNS tumors. Patients often present with endocrinopathies and/or vision changes, which occurs because of the proximity of the dorsum sellae and the nearby optic chiasm. Tumors less than 1 cm are considered microadenomas, whereas growth greater than 1 cm defines a macroadenoma. When tumors grow large enough to displace the optic chiasm, patients classically present with bitemporal peripheral vision loss. Initial workup includes a full endocrine workup. Tumors are classified by their secretory activity (functional tumors), or lack thereof (nonfunctional tumors). Table 4 shows the typical laboratory findings among the most common subtypes. Small asymptomatic (nonfunctional) microadenomas may be managed conservatively with routine surveillance. However, treatment for most symptomatic pituitary adenomas is surgical. Prolactinomas are an exception, due to highly efficacious medical therapy with dopaminergic agonists (cabergoline [Dostinex] and bromocriptine [Parlodel]). Yet, all large pituitary adenomas causing significant mass effect should be urgently referred for surgery to preserve vision. Surgery is often performed transnasally using endoscopes with high success. However, very large tumors may require craniotomy for successful resection. Similar to other CNS tumors, patients with pituitary adenomas require close follow-up with a multidisciplinary team involving both neurosurgery and endocrine.

References

Bang A, Schoenfeld JD: Immunotherapy and radiotherapy for metastatic cancers, *Ann Palliat Med* 8:312–325, 2019.
Brown PD, et al: Postoperative stereotactic radiosurgery compared with whole brain radiotherapy for resected metastatic brain disease (NCCTG N107C/CEC.3): a multicentre, randomised, controlled, phase 3 trial, *Lancet Oncol* 18:1049–1060, 2017.
Baumert BG, et al: Temozolomide chemotherapy versus radiotherapy in high-risk low-grade glioma (EORTC 22033-26033): a randomised, open-label, phase 3 intergroup study, *Lancet Oncol* 17:1521–1532, 2016.
Buckner JC, et al: Radiation plus procarbazine, CCNU, and vincristine in low-grade glioma, *N Engl J Med* 374:1344–1355, 2016.
Fabian D, et al: Treatment of glioblastoma (GBM) with the addition of tumor-treating fields (TTF): a review, *Cancers* 11, 2019.
Garzon-Muvdi T, Bailey DD, Pernik MN, Pan E: Basis for immunotherapy for treatment of meningiomas, *Front Neurol* 11:945, 2020.
Grabowski MM, et al: Combination laser interstitial thermal therapy plus stereotactic radiotherapy increases time to progression for biopsy-proven recurrent brain metastases, *Neurooncol Adv* 4:vdac086, 2022.
Mete O, Lopes MB: Overview of the 2017 WHO classification of pituitary tumors, *Endocr Pathol* 28:228–243, 2017.
Mitchell DK, et al: Brain metastases: an update on the multi-disciplinary approach of clinical management, *Neurochirurgie* 68:69–85, 2022.
Mittal S, et al: Alternating electric tumor treating fields for treatment of glioblastoma: rationale, preclinical, and clinical studies, *J Neurosurg* 128:414–421, 2018.
Nieder C, Grosu AL, Gaspar LE: Stereotactic radiosurgery (SRS) for brain metastases: a systematic review, *Radiat Oncol* 9:155, 2014.
Ostrom QT, et al: CBTRUS statistical report: primary brain and other central nervous system tumors diagnosed in the United States in 2015-2019, *Neuro Oncol* 24:v1–v95, 2022.
Patchell RA, et al: A randomized trial of surgery in the treatment of single metastases to the brain, *N Engl J Med* 322:494–500, 1990.
Putora PM, et al: Treatment of brain metastases in small cell lung cancer: decision-making amongst a multidisciplinary panel of European experts, *Radiother Oncol* 149:84–88, 2020.
Schaff LR, Grommes C: Primary central nervous system lymphoma, *Blood* 140:971–979, 2022.
Stupp R, et al: Radiotherapy plus concomitant and adjuvant temozolomide for glioblastoma, *N Engl J Med* 352:987–996, 2005.
Stupp R, et al: Effect of tumor-treating fields plus maintenance temozolomide vs maintenance temozolomide alone on survival in patients with glioblastoma: a randomized clinical trial, *JAMA* 318:2306–2316, 2017.
Wick W, et al: Lomustine and bevacizumab in progressive glioblastoma, *N Engl J Med* 377:1954–1963, 2017.

GILLES DE LA TOURETTE SYNDROME

Method of
Alonso G. Zea Vera, MD; Steve W. Wu, MD; and Donald L. Gilbert, MD

CURRENT DIAGNOSIS

- Multiple motor tics and one or more phonic tics have been present for some time during the illness, although not necessarily concurrently.
- The tics may wax and wane in frequency but have persisted for more than 1 year since the first tic onset.
- Onset occurs before 18 years of age.
- The disturbance is not caused by the direct physiologic effects of a substance or a general medical condition.

CURRENT THERAPY

- Educate the patient and family about tics, their waxing and waning course, and its natural history. Long-term reductions in tics may occur in the late teens, irrespective of pharmacologic therapy.
- If necessary, provide information to educate teachers and classmates to reduce social impairment.

IX Neurological System

- Assess for the presence of comorbidities including attention-deficit/hyperactivity disorder (ADHD), obsessive-compulsive disorder (OCD), anxiety, mood problems, learning problems, and behavior problems.
- Consider nonpharmacologic and pharmacologic treatment for the most impairing symptoms first. Tics do not always need to be treated, and other comorbidities may be more impairing.
- Treatment of ADHD, OCD, anxiety, mood problems, learning problems, and behavior problems should follow evidence-based guidelines and may require specialty evaluation (neurology, psychiatry, and psychology). Stimulants are not contraindicated in patients with Tourette syndrome.
- Comprehensive Behavioral Intervention for Tics could be considered in motivated families and can be offered even if tics are not impairing. Families should be counseled about the time and effort required and the scarcity of trained providers in some areas. Patients who are very young or have severe untreated comorbidities may not be able to participate in this therapy.
- Alpha-agonists are the most common first-line medications used in the treatment of tics and are particularly beneficial for patients with comorbid ADHD. Commonly used second-line medications include topiramate (Topamax)[1] or baclofen (Lioresal).[1] Dopamine receptor antagonists are usually restricted to severe and refractory cases.
- Monitor the benefits and side effects at regular intervals. Counsel parents that tics fluctuate and that brief worsening of symptoms is common. Brief exacerbations do not necessarily require a change in therapy.
- Do not begin treatment with more than one central nervous system drug simultaneously, and avoid changing medication regimens too fast. Start one medication, wait 2 to 4 weeks, and then reassess all symptoms before starting the next medication.
- Maintain stable dosing during the school year; consider tapering medications in the summer.
- Consider weaning tic-suppressing medications in the middle to late teen years if tics are well controlled.

---

[1]Not FDA approved for this indication. Tourette syndrome (TS) is a neuropsychiatric illness characterized by multiple motor and phonic tics that persist for longer than 1 year (see the Current Diagnosis box). Transient tics have been reported in up to ~25% of children from kindergarten to sixth grade. However, the prevalence of TS is closer to 0.3% to 1.5% of the population, and boys are three to four times more likely to be affected than girls. The prevalence of tic disorders is even higher in children with intellectual disabilities.

Clinical Manifestations

Tics are sudden, recurrent, nonrhythmic, patterned movements (i.e., motor tics) or vocalizations (i.e., phonic tics; also called *vocal tics*). Tics are fragments of normal behavior that present out of context and are not goal-directed. What separates tics from normal actions is their exaggerated character in intensity, frequency, and repetition. Tics usually follow a somatotopic distribution, with tics being more frequent in the eyes, face, neck, phonic muscles (i.e., phonic tics), and shoulders compared with the trunk and extremities.

Tics can be divided into simple or complex tics. Simple tics are brief and involve a single muscle or small group of muscles. Common simple motor tics include eye blinking, facial grimace, head jerk, and shoulder shrug. Common simple phonic tics include throat clearing, sniffing, and coughing. Complex tics can be a series of simple tics or a seemingly purposeful coordinated sequence of actions or sounds. Examples of complex motor tics include jumping, touching, or copropraxia (i.e., performing obscene gestures). Examples of complex phonic tics include echolalia (i.e., repeating others' words), palilalia (i.e., repeating their own words), or coprolalia (i.e., utterance of foul language). Simple tics are more frequent than complex tics.

The possibility of developing coprolalia or copropraxia often causes significant distress in patients and families. These phenomena are commonly considered a core symptom of TS by the general population leading to names like *the cursing disease*. This perception has been fueled by inaccurate and exaggerated portrayals of people with TS in the media. Coprophenomena is only present in 10% to 20% of patients.

Tics have a characteristic waxing and waning pattern. Patients frequently report the resolution of old tics (although they may recur later) and the appearance of new tics. Tics tend to be exacerbated by stress, anxiety, excitement, anger, fatigue, and acute illnesses. Parents often notice more tics when the child is bored or unoccupied with an activity. On the contrary, tics are often diminished during focused mental or physical activities, and they usually do not affect activities of daily living, occupational activities, or recreational activities. Although tics are commonly reported to be absent during sleep, studies using polysomnography have shown that they may persist during it.

Patients with tics often describe an uncomfortable sensation preceding the tics, known as a premonitory urge, that remits once the tic is performed. This urge can be described as a physical sensation (i.e., itch or pressure) in a specific body area or a general ill-defined feeling. The majority of older children and adults report premonitory urges associated with at least one of their tics. However, younger children are less likely to report it. It is unclear if this is caused by the absence of an urge or the lack of awareness of the urge. Some young children that deny urges may report that their tics are "painful," even with mild tics. Further questioning may reveal that the pain appears shortly before the tic and disappears after the tic, suggesting a premonitory urge.

Tics can often be suppressed, although only momentarily, leading to the misinterpretation that tics are voluntary actions. The ability to suppress tics improves with age. Patients frequently report that the premonitory urge worsens when suppressing their tics and that the release of the tic brings relief. Some patients report a "rebound effect" with many tics occurring after a prolonged period of tic suppression. For example, some children who suppress their tics in school report an increased frequency of tics when they get home.

A natural course has been described in TS. The onset of tics is usually between 4 and 8 years of age. Children often present with motor tics first, followed by the development of phonic tics. Tic severity usually increases in the later elementary school years and early adolescence and decreases by late adolescence and early adulthood. Most TS patients have minimal tics or may "outgrow" their tics when they become adults. However, a minority of patients may continue to have bothersome tics throughout life.

Comorbidities

About 85% of patients with Tourette syndrome have at least one psychiatric comorbidity and ~60% have 2 or more. The most common comorbidities are obsessive-compulsive disorder (~65%; OCD) and attention deficit and hyperactivity disorder (~55%; ADHD). Anxiety, mood disorders, and sleep problems are also common. ADHD symptoms frequently are present before tic onset, but OCD symptoms are more likely to appear after the onset of tics. TS patients should be screened for these conditions regularly.

Diagnosis

TS is a primary tic disorder diagnosed based on clinical criteria (see Current Diagnosis box) listed in the *Diagnostic and Statistical Manual of Mental Disorders*, fifth edition (DSM-5). Other primary tic disorders include *provisional tic disorder, persistent (chronic) motor* or *vocal tic disorder, other specified tic disorder,* and *unspecified tic disorder.* The diagnosis depends on correctly recognizing that the abnormal movements are tics through a careful history and physical examination. Laboratory and imaging studies can be used to rule out other conditions but are rarely needed. Sometimes tics are interpreted as a symptom of a different condition. Coughing or sniffing tics may be attributed to

INTRACEREBRAL HEMORRHAGE

Method of
Ronda Lun, MD; and Dar Dowlatshahi, MD, PhD

CURRENT DIAGNOSIS

- Intracerebral hemorrhage is a medical emergency; immediate imaging must be obtained in anyone with acute onset focal neurologic deficits.
- Noncontrast computed tomography (CT) is the gold standard; CT angiography can be helpful for prognostic factors and to rule out underlying vascular malformations.
- Obtain magnetic resonance imaging (MRI) +/− MR venogram (MRV) if etiology of bleed is unclear.

CURRENT THERAPY

- Ensure the airway is protected because level of consciousness could deteriorate rapidly.
- Medical treatment:
  - Hemostasis by correcting coagulopathies
  - Blood pressure (BP) lowering
- Surgical treatment:
  - Posterior fossa decompression for cerebellar hemorrhages
  - Extraventricular drainage for hydrocephalus
  - Evacuation of hematoma may be necessary as a life-saving measure

Figure 1 Types of intracranial hemorrhage. From Zebian B, Critchley G: Spontaneous intracranial haemorrhage. Surgery (Oxford) 2015; 33(8):363–368.

TABLE 1 Spontaneous vs Secondary Causes of ICH

SPONTANEOUS ICH	SECONDARY ICH
Hypertensive vasculopathy	Vascular malformations (dural arteriovenous fistula, arteriovenous malformation, cavernous malformation, capillary telangiectasias)
Cerebral small vessel disease	Cerebral venous thrombosis
Cerebral amyloid angiopathy	Hemorrhagic conversion of ischemic infarct
	Moyamoya disease
	Septic emboli/mycotic aneurysm
	Brain tumors
	Vasculitis (infectious, systemic autoimmune disease, primary CNS)
	Reversible cerebral vasoconstriction syndrome
	Drugs/toxins (cocaine, amphetamines)

Introduction

Intracranial hemorrhage (ICH) refers to bleeding within the skull in any intracranial compartment (i.e., subdural, subarachnoid, epidural, or intraparenchymal) (Figure 1). However, the term is commonly used for intraparenchymal hemorrhages specifically, which will be the focus of this chapter. ICH can be further categorized as "spontaneous" or "secondary," with the latter inferring that there is an underlying lesion (i.e., vascular malformation, tumor) or alternative explanation (i.e., trauma) for the bleed (Table 1). Spontaneous ICH is synonymous with hemorrhagic stroke, referring to spontaneous intraparenchymal bleeding in the absence of identifiable secondary causes. It represents 10% to 15% of all strokes and is the second most common subtype after ischemic strokes. Although its incidence has been increasing in recent years, likely as a result of the aging population and increased use of antithrombotic medications, long-term outcomes from ICH have remained largely unchanged, with mortality rates of 50% at 1 year, and loss of functional independence in almost 75% of patients.

Pathophysiology

ICH occurs when an arterial intracranial blood vessel bursts and a hematoma is formed as a result of accumulation of extravasated blood. The hematoma then causes mass effect with compression of adjacent healthy brain tissue, causing neuronal dysfunction and cell death from cytotoxic edema. Hematoma expansion (HE) occurs in up to 1/3 of patients with ICH in the first 6 hours and is a potentially targetable surrogate outcome for improving survival and preventing disability. The risk for hematoma expansion is greatest at within 3 hours after symptom onset, and the predicted probability of HE is inversely associated with time, although delayed expansion after 24 hours can rarely be encountered. Concurrent with the cessation of active bleeding, vasogenic edema will develop and peak over the next 2 to 7 days. Extension of the blood into the ventricular system may cause acute hydrocephalus because of obstruction of venous outflow. Even small volumes of HE are associated with an increased risk for adverse outcomes; the development of a teaspoon of new parenchymal hemorrhage is associated with quadruple the odds of mortality, and the development of even 1 mL of new ventricular hemorrhage has been shown to be associated with increased risk of disability and death. Ultimately, increased intracranial pressure from the mass effect may cause supratentorial herniation, midline shift, and secondary brain injury.

Location of ICH is a helpful predictor in determining the underlying pathogenesis of the ICH. Chronic hypertension is the most common risk factor responsible for subcortical and infratentorial hemorrhages, such as those in the basal ganglia, thalamus, brainstem, and cerebellum. The pathogenesis of hypertensive hemorrhages is attributed to chronic exposure to high pressures in the branching arterioles from major intracranial vessels, resulting in lipohyalinosis of the small arterioles. These relatively fragile vessel walls may then rupture and result in ICH. On the contrary, lobar hemorrhages and convexity subarachnoid hemorrhages in adult patients over the age of 55 are often attributed to cerebral amyloid angiopathy. This disease process is characterized by the deposition of abnormal amyloid beta proteins in the small to medium-sized vessels of the brain, resulting in weakened vascular integrity over time, which increases the risk for arterial rupture. Amyloid-related hemorrhages typically spare the deep gray matter and brainstem, reflecting the distribution of amyloid deposits, most of which are detected only on MRI sequences sensitive for blood byproducts (see Diagnosis section). They are thought to represent clinically silent cerebral microbleeds and are an important risk factor to recognize for increased risk for recurrent ICH.

Although this chapter focuses on arterial ICH, it is important to recognize that bleeding from a ruptured venous blood vessel may occur rarely and that venous hemorrhages are not considered a subtype of ICH. However, it needs to be ruled out as a potential secondary etiology for parenchymal hemorrhage because the treatment and prognosis are drastically different. Counterintuitively, the mechanism by which venous hemorrhages occur is caused by formation of thrombus in the venous drainage of the brain, leading to buildup of intracranial pressure and blockage of cerebral spinal fluid (CSF)/blood outflow from the brain. The backlog of pressure leads to venous infarction, petechial hemorrhage, and ICH. In any patient with a lobar ICH of unknown origin or ICH that crosses typical arterial territories, immediate neuroimaging with CTV or MRV should be pursued to rule out underlying cerebral venous sinus thrombosis as the ultimate culprit.

Clinical Manifestations

Neurologic deficits caused by ICH are sudden in onset, but unlike its ischemic stroke counterpart—where stroke deficits are maximal at onset—neurologic signs and symptoms attributed to ICH tend to worsen with time. As the hematoma expands, patients can rapidly deteriorate, resulting in decreased level of consciousness and requiring intubation. Initial clinical manifestations vary depending on hemorrhage location. The most frequent location for ICH related to chronic hypertension is within the basal ganglia, more specifically the internal capsule/thalamus/putamen/pons. Thus the most common symptomatology includes hemiplegia, hemi-body sensory loss, dysarthria, ataxia, and visual field loss. Cortical bleeds are most frequently associated with cerebral amyloid angiopathy and may clinically manifest with aphasia, apraxia, and hemianopia, in addition to the symptomatology mentioned previously. Epileptic seizures may be seen either at the onset of disease or later, as a manifestation of cortical irritation from blood/scar tissue. Headaches, nausea, vomiting, and decreased level of consciousness are common in the context of increased intracranial pressure (ICP) but may result from other mechanisms such as brainstem compression, development of hydrocephalus, or herniation.

Diagnosis

ICH is a medical emergency. The development of acute neurologic deficits should immediately raise concern for stroke, thus rapid assessment and management are crucial. Initial assessment should prioritize the ABCs of resuscitation—airway, breathing, and circulation—before proceeding with assessment for neurologic deficits. The most commonly used rapid stroke assessment scale is the National Institute of Health Stroke Severity (NIHSS) scale, which can be found in Table 2. However, another frequently used clinical assessment tool is the Glasgow Coma Scale (GCS), which is often used to assess indications for intubation in the context of decreased level of consciousness. A threshold of GCS 8 or less is used as an indication for intubation. Immediate neuroimaging should be obtained to confirm the diagnosis and rule out other diseases that may present in a similar manner, including ischemic stroke and subarachnoid hemorrhage. The noncontrast CT scan is the gold standard for emergent assessment of ICH. Administration of CT iodinated contrast to facilitate CT angiography may be pursued to look for active contrast extravasation (known as the *spot sign*) and to investigate for underlying lesions such as tumor or vascular malformations. Emergent MRI may be used as the initial imaging modality in select centers, although more commonly MRI is obtained in a

TABLE 2	NIHSS Stroke Scale
CATEGORY	**SCORE/ DESCRIPTION**
1a. Level of consciousness (awake, drowsy, comatose, etc.)	0 = alert 1 = drowsy 2 = stuporous 3 = coma
1b. LOC questions (month, age)	0 = answers both correctly 1 = answers one correctly 2 = incorrect
1c. LOC commands (open/close eyes, make fist/let go)	0 = obeys both correctly 1 = obeys one correctly 2 = incorrect
2. Best gaze (eyes open and tracks)	0 = normal 1 = partial hemianopia 2 = complete hemianopia 3 = bilateral hemianopia (blind)
3. Visual fields (introduce visual stimulus to all 4 visual field quadrants)	0 = normal 1 = minor 2 = partial 3 = complete
4. Facial paresis (show teeth, raise eyebrows and squeeze eyes shut)	0 = normal 1 = minor 2 = partial 3 = complete
5a. Motor arm (left) 5b. Motor arm (right) (elevate arm to 90°)	0 = no drift 1 = drift 2 = can't resist gravity 3 = no effort against gravity 4 = no movement X = untestable (joint fusion or limb amputation)
6a. Motor leg (left) 6b. Motor leg (right) (elevate leg 30°)	0 = no drift 1 = drift 2 = Some effort against gravity 3 = no effort against gravity 4 = no movement X = untestable (joint fusion or limb amputation)
7. Limb ataxia (finger-nose, heel-shin)	0 = no ataxia 1 = present in one limb 2 = present in two limbs
8. Sensory (pinprick to face/arm/trunk/leg)	0 = normal 1 = partial loss 2 = severe loss
9. Best language (naming, fluency, reading)	0 = no aphasia 1 = mild to moderate aphasia 2 = severe aphasia 3 = mute
10. Dysarthria (evaluate speech clarity by repeating listed words)	0 = normal articulation 1 = mild or moderate slurring of speech 2 = near unintelligible or worse X = intubated or other physical barrier
11. Extinction and inattention	0 = no neglect 1 = partial neglect (visual, tactile, auditory, spatial, or personal inattention or extinction to bilateral stimulus in one sensory modality) 2 = profound hemi-attention or extinction to more than one modality

delayed fashion to investigate the etiology of the bleed. Useful MRI sequences include T2* susceptibility-weighted images (SWI) or gradient-echo (GRE) sequences, which are sensitive for the detection of deoxyhemoglobin, a byproduct of blood. Additional pursuit of imaging such as CTV or MRV should be considered when there is clinical or radiologic suspicion for

CVST. Catheter angiography may be pursued when diagnostic suspicion for underlying vascular malformation is high and no etiology for the ICH can be found.

Therapy

Treatment of ICH is composed of a combination of medical and surgical approaches and generally follows two important principles. During the acute period, stabilizing the hematoma and decreasing the risk for hematoma expansion is crucial and may be achieved through hemostasis and blood pressure (BP) control. Secondly, addressing mass effect and its downstream complications may be done through surgery and osmolar therapies.

Emergency Medical Treatment

The two mainstays of medical treatment in ICH are hemostasis and BP control. Hemostatic abnormalities may not only cause ICH but potentially worsen outcomes if not corrected. Patients with known coagulation factor deficiency or platelet disorders should have replacement of the appropriate factor(s). Patients with significant thrombocytopenia should be considered for platelet transfusion. Those taking vitamin K antagonists (i.e., warfarin) with elevated international normalized ratio (INR) should have their INR corrected rapidly. Either fresh frozen plasma (FFP) or prothrombin complex concentrates (PCC) may be used, although PCC may be superior in achieving a faster INR normalization rate than FFP and is the preferred agent. Vitamin K (phytonadione) needs to be given concurrently because of the short half-life of PCC; the onset of action of vitamin K starts approximately 2 hours after administration and will continue to peak over the next 12 to 14 hours. Other hemostatic factors such as rFVIIa are not currently recommended, although there are ongoing clinical trials evaluating its efficacy in patients presenting in an early time window from symptom onset. Patients taking direct-oral anticoagulants (DOACs) may be eligible for specific reversal agents, such as idarucizumab (Praxbind) for dabigatran (Pradaxa) and andexanet alfa (Andexxa) for factor Xa inhibitors (such as rivaroxaban [Xarelto], edoxaban [Savaysa, Lixiana],[1] or apixaban [Eliquis]). If andexanet alfa is not available, some clinicians may choose to use PCC to reverse factor Xa inhibitors if there is biochemical evidence of activity at time of presentation or confirmed recent ingestion. Patients taking antiplatelet agents prior to development of their ICH should not routinely receive platelet transfusion if their platelet count is normal because it has been found to be harmful rather than beneficial.

Elevated BP is frequently encountered in acute ICH as a result of a variety of physiologic responses. However, high BP is a major risk factor for developing hematoma expansion and thereby worse outcomes after ICH. For patients presenting with systolic blood pressure (SBP) between 150 and 220, lowering the SBP to <140 mm Hg is safe and may be effective for improving functional outcomes at 3 months. However, more aggressive BP lowering may be associated with increased risk for renal insufficiency, and therefore the potential benefit achieved from BP reduction should be balanced with feasibility and maintenance of systemic perfusion pressure to all organs. For those presenting with severely elevated SBP (>220 mm Hg), lowering to 140 mm Hg is practically challenging and may be harmful, thus many clinicians may choose to target a BP that is 25% lower than the patient's initial SBP instead.

Inpatient Medical Treatment

Medical treatment of ICH should be continued beyond the emergency setting to prevent further complications during hospitalization. Maintenance of normoglycemia and normothermia should be standard of care because hyperglycemia and hypothermia have both been associated with poorer long-term outcomes. Universal dysphagia screening before initiation of an oral diet should be implemented to reduce the risk of aspiration pneumonia, a common complication during the first weeks of hospitalization. To mitigate the risk for urinary tract infections, indwelling foleys should not be inserted without appropriate clinical indication. All patients should have intermittent pneumatic compression devices for prevention of venous thromboembolism (VTE) beginning the day of hospital admission. Once the patient has been deemed clinically and radiologically stable, the patient may be transitioned to a pharmacologic agent for VTE prophylaxis. Osmolar therapies such as hypertonic saline[1] and mannitol (Osmitrol) should be considered in patients with concern for increased intracranial pressure, but these are considered temporizing measures until definitive surgical intervention.

Surgical Management

Although the evidence for indications and timing of surgical treatment of ICH remains somewhat controversial, surgery is often indicated for cerebellar hemorrhages, intraventricular extension, and hydrocephalus. Because of the limitations in room for expansion in the posterior fossa, it is generally accepted that any cerebellar hemorrhage with brainstem compression and/or hydrocephalus and/or neurologic deterioration should have immediate surgical decompression. A threshold of 3 cm in the diameter of the hematoma is commonly used for consideration of surgery. On the contrary, the evidence for supratentorial and deep hemorrhages is much less robust. Hematoma evacuation with decompressive craniotomy/craniectomy may be considered a life-saving measure in deteriorating patients; however, its efficacy for prevention of functional disability has not been well established. In patients with intraventricular hemorrhage causing hydrocephalus and deteriorating level of consciousness, extraventricular drainage (EVD) should be considered. There is limited evidence for irrigation of extraventricular drains with alteplase (Activase)[1] and its use is not routinely recommended based on the current level of evidence. Other surgical interventions such as minimally invasive clot evacuation have demonstrated promising results, and research in this field is active and ongoing. A summary of therapeutic options for ICH are outlined in Table 4.

Monitoring

ICH patients should be cared for in a dedicated stroke or intensive care unit wherever possible, as this has been shown to be associated with better outcomes. Frequent vital sign checks, neurologic assessments with validated scales such as GCS and NIHSS, and continuous cardiopulmonary monitoring should be part of the standard treatment plan. BP monitoring is especially crucial because it is the only therapy that has the potential to improve functional outcomes; thus hypertensive patients should have repeat BP checks every 15 minutes until the desired BP target is achieved and maintained for 24 hours. Electroencephalogram (EEG) monitoring should be considered in any patient who has persistent unexplained decreased loss of consciousness (LOC) caused by frequent subclinical seizures in ICH patients. Continuous monitoring of ICP is not universally indicated but may be considered in patients with evidence of transtentorial herniation, significant intraventricular hemorrhage (IVH), hydrocephalus, or decreased level of consciousness (i.e., Glasgow Coma Scale [GCS] of ≤8).

Complications

Prognostication

ICH patients typically present very severely (i.e., decreased LOC, debilitating deficits), and recovery in ICH tends to be much slower than its ischemic stroke counterpart. It is a devastating disease with limited treatment options, and a vital role for the clinician is providing accurate prognostication to family members/patients. The most widely used prognostication tool is the ICH score, which was initially developed to predict 30-day mortality

---

[1]Not FDA approved for this indication.

[1]Not FDA approved for this indication.

TABLE 3   Glasgow Coma Scale

RESPONSE	SCALE	SCORE
Eye opening response	Eyes open spontaneously	4 points
	Eyes open to verbal command	3 points
	Eyes open to pain	2 points
	No eye opening	1 point
Verbal response	Oriented	5 points
	Confused conversation, but able to answer questions	4 points
	Inappropriate responses, words discernible	3 points
	Incomprehensible sounds or speech	2 points
	No verbal response	1 point
Motor response	Obeys verbal command for movement	6 points
	Purposeful movement to painful stimulus	5 points
	Withdraws from pain	4 points
	Flexion response, decorticate posture	3 points
	Extensor response, decerebrate posture	2 points
	No motor response	1 point
Total possible points		15 points

TABLE 4   Components of ICH Score and FUNC Score and Their Associations With Outcomes*

	ICH SCORE	FUNC SCORE
Scoring	Glasgow coma scale: 3–4: 2 points 5–12: 1 point 13–15 0 points	Glasgow coma scale: ≥ 9: 2 points ≤ 8: 0 points
	ICH Volume (cm³): ≥30: 1 point <30: 0 points	ICH Volume (cm³): <30: 4 points 30–60: 2 points >60: 0 points
	Intraventricular hemorrhage: Yes: 1 point No: 0 points	Pre-ICH cognitive Impairment: No: 1 point Yes: 0 points
	ICH location: Infratentorial: 1 point Not infratentorial: 0 points	ICH location: Lobar: 2 points Deep: 1 point Infratentorial: 0 points
	Age (years): ≥80: 1 point <80: 0 points	Age (years): <70: 2 points 70–79: 1 point ≥80: 0 points
	Total: 0–6 (higher score suggests worse prognosis)	Total: 0–11 (lower score suggests worse prognosis)
Association with outcomes in original publication	Association with 30-day mortality: 0: 0% mortality 1: 13% mortality 2: 26% mortality 3: 72% mortality 4: 97% mortality >5: 100% mortality	Association with 90-day functional independence: 0–4: 0% independent 5–7: 13% independent 8: 42% independent 9–10: 66% independent 11: 75% independent

*Prognostication and decisions around withdrawal of care should not be made for at least 48 hours.

but has since then been validated to predict long-term mortality up to 1 year (Table 3). Other prediction scores include the FUNC score, originally developed to predict the chances of meaningful functional recovery (see Table 3), although its use is less widely implemented. It is generally recommended that prognostication should be deferred to at least 48 to 72 hours after time of presentation to optimally assess the patient's clinical trajectory and to allow time for radiographic stability to ensue.

Acute Neurologic Deterioration
Acute neurologic deterioration is associated with increased risk for long-term disability and mortality and may result from hematoma expansion, seizures, increasing mass effect, development of ventricular hemorrhage, and cerebral herniation. Approximately 1/5 patients will experience early neurologic deterioration. Antiepileptic medications should not be initiated unless a clinical seizure is witnessed or suspected and confirmed with EEG. Important inpatient complications were discussed under "Therapy: Inpatient Medical Treatments."

Long-Term Complications
The long-term sequelae of ICH include physical disability, cognitive impairment, mood disorders, localization-related epilepsy, and increased risk for recurrent ICH. There may be an increased risk for ischemic stroke in patients with a history of ICH caused by avoidance of antithrombotic medications. Important predictors for recurrent ICH include microhemorrhages detected on MRI, uncontrolled hypertension, prior lacunar stroke, older age, and ongoing anticoagulation therapy, although it is still an ongoing, active area of research. Patients with ICH who require long-term anticoagulation (i.e., atrial fibrillation, mechanical heart valves, hypercoagulable disorders) should be assessed by a neurologist or thrombosis specialist to optimize risk factor control and the risk for future ICH should be weighed against the need for antithrombotic therapy.

Prevention
Primary Prevention
Hypertension is the major modifiable risk factor for hemorrhagic strokes. Uncontrolled hypertension accounts for approximately 74% of ICH worldwide, and treatment of hypertension is effective as both primary and secondary prevention. Use of antithrombotic medication is another modifiable risk factor for ICH. For patients who require long-term anticoagulation for atrial fibrillation or venous thromboembolism, direct oral anticoagulants (DOACs) carry a much lower risk for ICH than warfarin and should be first line therapy unless patients have a specific indication otherwise (i.e., valvular atrial fibrillation, mechanical valve). Patients should not be on antiplatelet agents without appropriate clinical indication because chronic antiplatelet therapy is a known risk factor for ICH.

Secondary Prevention
Hypertension is not only an important risk factor for ICH but is also implicated in other cardiovascular diseases. Treatment of hypertension is effective for attenuating the risk for recurrent hemorrhagic strokes and prevention of ischemic strokes. For patients at a high risk for cardiovascular events who previously experienced an ICH, recent research has shown that antiplatelet therapy may be resumed without an increased risk of recurrent ICH. The decision to start anticoagulants after an ICH, however, is not as clear cut and will depend on the balance of risk for ICH occurrence and clinical indications for requiring anticoagulation. Important factors to consider include the suspected etiology of ICH, control of risk factors prior to the last ICH, age/comorbidities, and patient preference. Lastly, statin therapy is not currently indicated for primary or secondary prevention of intracerebral hemorrhage. Traditionally lower levels of low-density lipoprotein (LDL) have been associated with increased risk for ICH, but research is ongoing to better understand this relationship.

TABLE 5 Summary of Therapies in the Treatment of ICH

MEDICAL TREATMENT OPTIONS

Hemostasis	Known coagulation factor deficiency: replacement of appropriate factors
	Vitamin-K antagonist related ICH: Fresh frozen plasma (FFP) or prothrombin complex concentrates Vitamin K
	DOAC related ICH: Idarucizumab (Praxbind) for dabigatran (Pradaxa) Andexanet alfa (Andexxa) for rivaroxaban (Xarelto), edoxaban (Savaysa, Lixiana),[1] or apixaban (Eliquis) Consider using FFP if andexanet alfa is not available
	Antiplatelet related ICH: Do not give platelet transfusion
	Ongoing trials for rFVIIa: not currently recommended
Blood pressure control	SBP between 150–220 mm Hg: Lowering SBP to 140 mm Hg is safe and may improve functional outcomes Be aware of maintenance of systemic perfusion pressures to other organs (i.e., kidneys) SBP >220 mm Hg: Lowering SBP is still indicated, although practically challenging to 140 mm Hg. Consider lowering SBP by 25% reduction

SURGICAL TREATMENT OPTIONS

Decompressive surgery	Posterior fossa/cerebellar hemorrhages: Surgery is indicated for any cerebellar hemorrhage with brainstem compression and/ or hydrocephalus and/ or neurologic deterioration Threshold of 3 cm in hematoma diameter for surgical intervention Supratentorial/deep hemorrhages: Surgery may be considered a life-saving measure in deteriorating patients but does not improve functional outcomes
Extraventricular drainage	Indicated for patients with hydrocephalus and decreased level of consciousness Irrigation with alteplase (Activase)[1] is not currently indicated
Minimally invasive surgery	Not currently indicated

PREVENTION OF SECONDARY INJURY AND COMPLICATIONS

Monitoring	Dedicated stroke unit or intensive care unit with neuroscience expertise Frequent vital sign checks (including blood pressure), neurologic assessments, and continuous cardiopulmonary monitoring if on continuous IV antihypertensives EEG should be considered for decreased level of consciousness Continuous intracranial pressure monitoring may be considered for transtentorial herniation, significant intraventricular hemorrhage (IVH), hydrocephalus, or decreased level of consciousness
Glucose	Maintenance of normoglycemia is recommended
Temperature	Maintenance of euthermia is recommended
Seizure control	Antiepileptics should be considered in those with clinical seizures. It is not routinely recommended as prophylaxis
Dysphagia	Dysphagia assessment needs to be performed before initiation of oral diet to prevent aspiration pneumonia
Urinary tract infection	Foley catheters should not be routinely used
Venous thromboembolism	Intermittent pneumatic compression devices are indicated on first day of hospitalization

[1]Not FDA approved for this indication.

References

Greenberg SM, Ziai WC, Cordonnier C, et al: 2022 Guideline for the management of patients with spontaneous intracerebral hemorrhage: a guideline from the American Heart Association/American Stroke Association. *Stroke.* 2022; 53(7):e282–e361. https://doi.org/10.1161/STR.0000000000000407.

Hemphill JC, Bonovich DC, Besmertis L, Manley GT, Johnston SC: The ICH score: a simple, reliable grading scale for intracerebral hemorrhage, *Stroke* 32(4):891–897, 2001, https://doi.org/10.1161/01.str.32.4.891.

O'Donnell MJ, Xavier D, Liu L, et al: Risk factors for ischaemic and intracerebral haemorrhagic stroke in 22 countries (the INTERSTROKE study): a case-control study, *Lancet Lond Engl* 376(9735):112–123, 2010, https://doi.org/10.1016/S0140-6736(10)60834-3.

Primary and secondary prevention of ischemic stroke and cerebral hemorrhage: JACC focus seminar, *J Am Coll Cardiol* 75(15):1804–1818, 2020, https://doi.org/10.1016/j.jacc.2019.12.072.

Rordorf G, McDonald C: Spontaneous intracerebral hemorrhage, *Pathogenesis, clinical features, and diagnosis*, 2020. UpToDate. Available at: https://www.uptodate.com/contents/spontaneous-intracerebral-hemorrhage-pathogenesis-clinical-features-and-diagnosis. [Accessed Dec 31, 2020].

Rost NS, Smith EE, Chang Y, et al: Prediction of functional outcome in patients with primary intracerebral hemorrhage: the FUNC score, *Stroke* 39(8):2304–2309, 2008, https://doi.org/10.1161/STROKEAHA.107.512202.

Salman RA-S, Frantzias J, Lee RJ, et al: Absolute risk and predictors of the growth of acute spontaneous intracerebral haemorrhage: a systematic review and meta-analysis of individual patient data, *Lancet Neurol* 17(10):885–894, 2018, https://doi.org/10.1016/S1474-4422(18)30253-9.

Shoamanesh (Co-chair) A, Patrice Lindsay M, Castellucci LA, et al. Canadian stroke best practice recommendations: management of spontaneous intracerebral hemorrhage, 7th Edition Update 2020. *Int J Stroke*. Published online November 11, 2020:1747493020968424, https://doi.org/10.1177/1747493020968424.

Yogendrakumar V, Ramsay T, Fergusson DA, et al: Redefining hematoma expansion with the inclusion of intraventricular hemorrhage growth, *Stroke* 51(4):1120–1127, 2020, https://doi.org/10.1161/STROKEAHA.119.027451.

Ziai WC, Carhuapoma JR: Intracerebral hemorrhage, *Contin Minneap Minn* 24(6):1603–1622, 2018, https://doi.org/10.1212/CON.0000000000000672.

ISCHEMIC CEREBROVASCULAR DISEASE

Method of
Alvaro Cervera, MD, PhD; and Geoffrey A. Donnan, MD

CURRENT DIAGNOSIS

- Early recognition of stroke is crucial to transport patients to hospitals with dedicated stroke units.
- Advanced neuroimaging allows the use of reperfusion therapies with a prolonged time window.

CURRENT THERAPY

- Admission to a stroke unit is the most effective and widely available resource for the majority of patients.
- Thrombolysis and thrombectomy have revolutionized the management of acute stroke, greatly improving the outcome.

Treatment of ischemic stroke has improved significantly in the past few years, and mortality and disability rates owing to this condition have decreased. The management of patients in stroke units and the demonstration of the efficacy of thrombolysis and thrombectomy have been crucial in this achievement. Control of vascular risk factors has decreased the number and severity of events. However, recent studies have found an increased incidence of ischemic stroke in the young. Improved management has included high-quality rehabilitation, which has to start early to improve the recovery (i.e., functional independence) of stroke survivors. The multidisciplinary management of stroke can be improved with specific educational programs aimed at increasing awareness of stroke in the general population and among professionals. The concept of "Time is Brain" has great value in emphasizing that stroke is an emergency. Because the window for the available time-dependent treatments is very narrow, avoiding delay is the major goal in the prehospital phase of acute stroke care. Therefore it is important to transport all stroke patients as soon as possible to the closest hospital with a stroke unit. In rural or remote areas with no stroke unit facilities, telemedicine has proven to be a valid alternative.

Prevention

Lifestyle modification can be a major contributor to reducing the risk of ischemic stroke. Strategies to achieve this protection include avoiding smoking and excessive alcohol consumption, keeping a low/normal body mass index, practicing regular exercise, and having a diet low in salt and saturated fat, high in fruits and vegetables, and rich in fiber. In addition, a Mediterranean diet supplemented with nuts is associated with a decreased risk of vascular events. There is no need to add vitamin supplements to the diet because they do not affect stroke prevention.

Regular assessment of vascular risk factors (e.g., hypertension, diabetes, hypercholesterolemia) is important because their control can significantly reduce the incidence of vascular events. In the case of blood pressure, this can be done with diet and pharmacologic therapy, aiming at normal levels of 120/80 mm Hg. After an ischemic stroke, blood pressure should be lowered even in patients with normal blood pressure. Diabetes should be managed with lifestyle modification and pharmacologic therapy as required, and blood pressure needs to be more tightly controlled in these patients (<130/80 mm Hg). The best antihypertensive treatments for diabetics are angiotensin-converting enzyme inhibitors or angiotensin receptor antagonists. Hypercholesterolemia should be managed with lifestyle modification and a statin. After a noncardioembolic ischemic stroke, high-dose statins are beneficial in all patients for secondary prevention.

TABLE 1	Prevention of Stroke in Patients With Atrial Fibrillation
CHA2DS2-VASc SCALE	
RISK FACTOR	**SCORE**
Congestive heart failure	1
Hypertension	1
Age ≥75	2
Age 65–74	1
Diabetes mellitus	1
Stroke or transient ischemic attack	2
Vascular disease	1
Female sex	1

Postmenopausal hormone replacement therapy should be avoided for the primary or secondary prevention of stroke because it can increase the risk of new vascular events. Other strategies to prevent stroke include the treatment of obstructive sleep apnea with continuous positive airway pressure breathing.

Antithrombotic Therapy

Low-dose aspirin[1] can be used for the primary prevention of stroke in women or of myocardial infarction in men. Nevertheless, its effect is very small, and it cannot be recommended on a population-wide basis. Aspirin is beneficial for the prevention of stroke in patients with asymptomatic carotid stenosis.

In patients with atrial fibrillation, the CHA2DS2-VASc scale (Table 1) is used to decide whether to use anticoagulation. If the score (https://www.mdcalc.com/chads2-score-atrial-fibrillation-stroke-ris) is 2 or more, treatment with oral anticoagulants is indicated. With a score of 1, the decision should be made according to the presence of risk factors, risk of bleeding, and patient choice. If the score is 0, there is no need to start antithrombotic treatment, neither antiplatelets nor anticoagulants. All patients with stroke or transient ischemic attack (TIA) should be anticoagulated, unless strictly contraindicated. Patients with valvular atrial fibrillation require anticoagulation with warfarin, aiming at an international normalized ratio (INR) of 2.0 to 3.0. Patients with prosthetic heart valves should also receive warfarin, and the target INR depends on the prosthesis type. In nonvalvular atrial fibrillation, the treatment options include warfarin (INR 2.0 to 3.0) or a direct oral anticoagulant (dabigatran [Pradaxa], apixaban [Eliquis], rivaroxaban [Xarelto], and edoxaban [Savaysa]). The direct oral anticoagulants are associated with a decreased risk of intracranial hemorrhage compared with warfarin. Dabigatran (150 mg, twice daily) and apixaban (5 mg, twice daily) have shown to be superior to warfarin in stroke prevention. The dose of the direct oral anticoagulants needs to be adjusted depending on age, renal function, and/or weight.

After an ischemic stroke, all patients should receive antithrombotic therapy. Antiplatelet agents are the first choice unless anticoagulation is required. The most effective regimen is clopidogrel (Plavix) or aspirin plus dipyridamole (Aggrenox). However, low-dose aspirin is a reasonable alternative. During the first 3 weeks after a minor stroke or TIA, the combination of aspirin plus clopidogrel can be more effective in reducing ischemic events than clopidogrel alone, although the evidence is scarce. However, dual antiplatelet treatment is not recommended in the long term, except if there is an association with unstable angina or non–Q wave myocardial infarction, or if there has been a recent stenting. Anticoagulation is usually indicated for secondary prevention if the stroke cause is cardioembolic and in specific situations,

---

[1] Not FDA approved for this indication.

Ischemic Cerebrovascular Disease

such as aortic arch atheroma or fusiform aneurysms of the basilar artery. However, level 1 evidence is lacking for these approaches.

Management of Carotid Stenosis

In patients with asymptomatic carotid stenosis (≥60%), surgery is indicated only if the risk of stroke is high. Endarterectomy is the treatment of choice if the stenosis is symptomatic (i.e., has been associated with an ipsilateral stroke or TIA), and severe (70% to 99%). Surgery should be performed in centers with a perioperative complication rate of less than 6% and as soon as possible after the last ischemic event.

Endarterectomy may be indicated for certain patients with moderate stenosis (50%–69%), although it should be performed only in centers with a perioperative complication rate of less than 3% to be effective. In cases of symptomatic carotid lesions, angioplasty plus stenting is a reasonable alternative, mainly in patients younger than 70 years. If stenting is performed, a combination of clopidogrel and aspirin is required immediately before the procedure and for at least 1 month after to prevent stent thrombosis.

In patients with intracranial atheromatosis and stroke recurrences, intensive medical treatment is the preferred option. Angioplasty and stenting are not recommended.

Management of Patent Foramen Ovale

The presence of a patent foramen ovale (PFO) is associated with cryptogenic stroke in the young. There is evidence that in selected patients with stroke or TIA (<60 years of age, nonlacunar stroke, and exclusion of other causes of stroke) the percutaneous transcatheter closure of the PFO is associated with a significant reduction of new vascular events, although with more frequent atrial fibrillation postprocedure, usually transient. Otherwise, there is no evidence indicating that anticoagulation is more effective than antiplatelets for stroke prevention in patients with PFO.

Management of Acute Ischemic Stroke

All stroke patients should be treated in a stroke unit, because this is associated with a reduction of death, dependency, and the need for institutional care. This effect is present in all stroke patients, irrespective of gender, age, stroke subtype, and stroke severity. Patients with stroke should have a careful clinical assessment, including a neurologic examination. The use of a stroke rating scale, such as the National Institutes of Health Stroke Scale, provides important information about the severity of stroke.

Urgent cranial computed tomography (CT) is mandatory after an ischemic stroke before starting any therapy. Alternatively, magnetic resonance imaging (MRI) or CT perfusion (CTP) can be performed, providing additional information about the selection of patients for mechanical thrombectomy within 6 to 24 hours from symptom onset. However, there is not enough evidence to recommend its routine use in the acute stroke setting.

For the detection and early management of the medical complications of stroke, neurologic status, pulse, blood pressure, temperature, and oxygen saturation should be monitored. Similarly, serum glucose levels need to be monitored and hyperglycemia needs to be treated with insulin accordingly. Normal saline is recommended for fluid replacement during the first 24 hours after stroke. If the patient has a fever, treatment with acetaminophen (paracetamol) may be used while sources of infection are being sought. Reducing blood pressure is recommended only in patients with extremely high blood pressure or when indicated by other medical conditions. Blood pressure should be lowered gradually, avoiding abrupt changes.

Thrombolysis

All patients suffering an ischemic stroke within 4.5 hours of onset should receive thrombolytic treatment, with intravenous tissue plasminogen activator (tPA [Activase]) unless contraindicated, because it is effective in improving stroke outcome (Box 1). It is very important to start treatment as soon as possible, because pooled analysis has demonstrated that earlier treatment results in a better outcome. Thrombolysis with tPA is effective in all

---

> ### BOX 1 Treatment of Acute Ischemic Stroke: Intravenous Administration of Tissue Plasminogen Activator
>
> - Infuse 0.9 mg/kg (maximum dose 90 mg) of tPA (Activase) over 60 minutes, with 10% of the dose given as a bolus over 1 minute.
> - Admit the patient to a stroke unit for monitoring. Perform neurologic assessment and blood pressure measurement every 15 minutes during the infusion, every 30 minutes thereafter for the next 6 hours, and then hourly until 24 hours after treatment. Administer antihypertensive medications to maintain systolic blood pressure ≤180 mm Hg and diastolic ≤105 mm Hg.
> - If intracranial hemorrhage is suspected, discontinue the infusion and obtain an emergency CT scan.
> - Obtain a follow-up CT scan at 24 hours before starting anticoagulants or antiplatelet agents.
>
> *CT,* Computed tomography; *tPA,* tissue plasminogen activator.

different population subgroups, including the very elderly, even with significant comorbidities. The therapeutic window can be extended up to 9 hours from onset when using advance imaging, such as perfusion-diffusion MRI or CTP. This approach has also been shown to be effective in wake-up strokes. Tenecteplase (TNKase)[1] is an alternative treatment to tPA, with the advantage of being administered in a single bolus (0.25 mg/kg).

Endovascular Thrombectomy

Mechanical thrombectomy using stent retrievers, in addition to thrombolysis, is more effective in improving outcomes than thrombolysis alone in anterior circulation strokes and a large artery occlusion, with a time window of up to 6 hours. This treatment is also effective when there are contraindications for intravenous thrombolysis. In a recent metaanalysis of five major trials (MR CLEAN, ESCAPE, REVASCAT, SWIFT PRIME, and EXTEND IA), endovascular thrombectomy led to significantly reduced disability at 90 days compared with control (odds ratio 2.49), with a number needed to treat of 2.6. All subgroups of patients benefit from this effect. Therefore health authorities have to implement access to thrombectomy within a reasonable time frame in a network, including stroke centers. Recent evidence shows that similar results are obtained when treating basilar artery occlusion.

There is recently published evidence indicating that the therapeutic window could be extended significantly when using multimodal imaging to select patients who have marked penumbra. Thus the DAWN trial showed that patients with ischemic penumbra could benefit from thrombectomy up to 24 hours since symptom onset, in comparison with standard care. This result was replicated by the DEFUSE 3 trial, although it included patients up to 16 hours from onset. Also, recent studies showed that thrombectomy can be beneficial in patients with a large ischemic core, although there is a higher risk of vascular complications. In Box 2, there is a simplified algorithm for the use of reperfusion therapies in acute ischemic stroke.

In large urban areas, mobile stroke units can significantly improve the management of acute stroke patients. These specialized units are ambulances equipped with CT scans and staff expert in acute stroke care. The use of mobile stroke units is associated with a faster thrombolytic treatment and a better functional outcome in comparison with the standard of care (transferring patients to emergency services). Also, these mobile units could facilitate a faster access to endovascular thrombectomy.

---

[1] Not FDA approved for this indication.

BOX 2   Reperfusion Therapies in Acute Ischemic Stroke

Symptom onset between 0 and 4.5 hours:
- No contraindications for thrombolysis.
  - Perform CT scan.
  - Administer IV tPA (Activase).
  - Perform multimodal imaging (this could be done beforehand if it does not delay treatment with IV tPA).
  - MT: if occlusion of intracranial internal carotid artery or middle cerebral artery (segment 1, M1), NIHSS score ≥ 6, no premorbid disability (mRS 0–1), and ASPECTS ≥ 6. Groin puncture within 6 hours of symptom onset.

Contraindications for thrombolysis:
- Perform multimodal imaging.
  - Proceed to MT: if occlusion of intracranial internal carotid artery or middle cerebral artery (M1), NIHSS score ≥ 6, no premorbid disability (mRS 0–1), and ASPECTS ≥ 6. Groin puncture within 6 hours of symptom onset.

Symptom onset between 4.5 and 9 hours or wake-up stroke:
- Perform multimodal imaging.
  - If no contraindications for thrombolysis, administer IV tPA (Activase) if significant penumbra according to EXTEND or WAKE-UP trials.
  - Proceed to MT if significant penumbra according to DAWN or DEFUSE 3 trials (this varies depending on age, NIHSS, and size of infarct core).
  - Standard medical management if no criteria for thrombolysis or MT.

Symptom onset between 9 and 24 hours:
- Perform multimodal imaging.
  - If occlusion of the intracranial internal carotid artery, middle cerebral artery (M1), or both.
  - Proceed to MT if significant penumbra according to DAWN or DEFUSE 3 trials (this varies depending on age, NIHSS, and size of infarct core).
  - Otherwise, standard medical management.

Other circumstances:
1. MT could be a reasonable option in selected cases with distal occlusion of the middle cerebral artery (M2 or M3).
   - MT is a reasonable therapeutic option for selected patients with occlusion of the anterior cerebral arteries, vertebral arteries, basilar artery, or posterior cerebral arteries.
   - Selected patients could benefit from MT even with premorbid conditions (mRS > 1), ASPECTS < 6, or NIHSS score < 6.
2. Patients with large ischemic cores can also benefit from MT, although there is a higher risk of vascular complications.

ASPECTS, Alberta stroke program early CT score; *CT,* computed tomography; *IV,* intravenous; *mRS,* modified Rankin Scale; *MT,* mechanical thrombectomy; *NIHSS,* National Institutes of Health Stroke Scale; *tPA,* tissue plasminogen activator.

Antithrombotic Drugs

All ischemic stroke patients should receive a low dose of aspirin daily. This can be started as soon as possible in patients who have not received reperfusion therapies, but always within 48 hours after onset. However, in patients who received thrombolysis, aspirin should be delayed for 24 hours. The use of other antiplatelet agents during the acute phase of stroke cannot be recommended based on available evidence. Similarly, early administration of unfractionated heparin, low-molecular-weight heparin, or heparinoids is not indicated in patients with acute ischemic stroke.

Treatment of Stroke Complications

Brain edema develops between the second and fifth day after stroke onset and is the cause of early deterioration and death. In the case of a malignant infarction of the middle cerebral artery, the mortality rate is 80%. In patients younger than 60 years, with this pattern of cerebral infarction, hemicraniectomy has been effective in reducing mortality and severe disability, as shown in the pooled analysis of the DECIMAL, DESTINY, and HAMLET trials. Decompressive hemicraniectomy is also effective in reducing mortality in patients older than 60 years, although the rates of severe disability are very high. Surgery needs to be performed within 48 hours after symptom onset. Surgical decompression is also indicated in the case of large cerebellar infarctions that compress the brainstem.

Stroke-associated infections require appropriate antibiotics, but prophylactic administration is discouraged. Venous thromboembolism is a frequent complication after stroke, but its incidence can be reduced with appropriate hydration and graded compression stockings. If the risk of deep venous thrombosis or pulmonary embolism is high, the use of subcutaneous heparin or low-molecular-weight heparin is beneficial. Early mobilization is an effective way of preventing complications, such as aspiration pneumonia or pressure ulcers. Anticonvulsants are administered only to prevent recurrent seizures but are not used prophylactically.

In the case of urinary incontinence, specialist assessment and management are recommended. Dysphagia is common after stroke and is associated with a higher incidence of medical complications and increased mortality. Malnutrition also predicts a poor functional outcome and increased mortality, and it is important to assess the swallowing capacity and the nutritional status of the patient.

Rehabilitation should be started after admission to the stroke unit. The optimal timing of first mobilization is unclear, but mobilization within the first few days appears to be well tolerated. However, very early mobilization can be associated with a worse outcome, as shown in the AVERT trial. An early, lower-dose, out-of-bed activity regimen is preferable to very early, frequent, higher-dose intervention. It is important to assess cognitive deficits and depression during the patient's hospital stay, because this may require specific intervention, although evidence about the type is lacking.

References

Albers GW, Marks MP, Kemp S, et al: DEFUSE 3 Investigators. Thrombectomy for stroke at 6 to 16 hours with selection by perfusion imaging, *N Engl J Med* 378(8):708–718, 2018.

AVERT Trial Collaboration Group, Bernhardt J, Langhorne P, et al: Efficacy and safety of very early mobilisation within 24h of stroke onset (AVERT): a randomised controlled trial, *Lancet* 386(9988):46–55, 2015.

Campbell BCV, Ma H, Ringleb PA, et al: EXTEND, ECASS-4, and EPITHET Investigators. Extending thrombolysis to 4·5-9 h and wake-up stroke using perfusion imaging: a systematic review and meta-analysis of individual patient data, *Lancet* 394(10193):139–147, 2019.

Campbell BCV, Mitchell PJ, Churilov L, et al: Tenecteplase versus alteplase before thrombectomy for ischemic stroke, *N Engl J Med* 378(17):1573–1582, 2018.

Goyal M, Menon BK, van Zwam WH, et al: Endovascular thrombectomy after large-vessel ischaemic stroke: a meta-analysis of individual patient data from five randomised trials, *Lancet* 387(10029):1723–1731, 2016.

Jovin TG, Li C, Wu L, et al: Trial of thrombectomy 6 to 24 hours after stroke due to basilar-artery occlusion, *N Engl J Med* 387(15):1373–1384, 2022.

Nogueira RG, Jadhav AP, Haussen DC, et al: DAWN Trial Investigators. Thrombectomy 6 to 24 hours after stroke with a mismatch between deficit and infarct, *N Engl J Med* 378(1):11–21, 2018.

Powers WJ, Rabinstein AA, Ackerson T, et al: American Heart Association stroke council. 2018 guidelines for the early management of patients with acute ischemic stroke: a guideline for healthcare professionals from the American Heart Association/American Stroke Association, *Stroke* 49(3):e46–e110, 2018.

Sarraj A, Hassan AE, Abraham MG, et al: SELECT2 investigators. Trial of endovascular thrombectomy for large ischemic strokes, *N Engl J Med* 388(14):1259–1271, 2023, https://doi.org/10.1056/NEJMoa2214403. Epub 2023 Feb 10. PMID: 36762865.

Stroke Foundation: *Clinical guidelines for stroke management,* 2022. Melbourne Australia.

Turc G, Hadziahmetovic M, Walter S, et al: Comparison of mobile stroke unit with usual care for acute ischemic stroke management: a systematic review and meta-analysis, *JAMA Neurol* 79(3):281–290, 2022.

Vahedi K, Hofmeijer J, Juettler E, et al: Early decompressive surgery in malignant infarction of the middle cerebral artery: a pooled analysis of three randomised controlled trials, *Lancet Neurol* 6:215–222, 2007.

MIGRAINE

Method of
Natalia Murinova, MD

CURRENT DIAGNOSIS

- Migraine is a primary headache disorder, with severe one-sided headache associated with nausea, vomiting, and/or light and sound sensitivity.
- Migraine is highly prevalent: it affects more than a billion people worldwide. It is highly disabling and constitutes the second leading cause of years lost to disability.
- The aftermath of the COVID-19 pandemic continues to be challenging for migraineurs.

CURRENT THERAPY

- Acute treatment of migraine
  - Nonspecific
    - Acetaminophen; nonsteroidal antiinflammatory drugs (NSAIDs); antiemetics
  - Specific migraine medication classes
    - U.S. Food and Drug Administration–approved for acute treatment of migraine with or without aura in adults
      - Triptans, serotonin (5-HT1B, 5-HT1D, 5-HT1F) receptor agonists
      - Ditans, oral serotonin (5-HT1F) receptor agonists
      - Gepants, oral calcitonin gene-related peptide (CGRP) receptor antagonists
- Preventive treatment of migraine
  - Nonspecific therapies
    - Beta-blockers; tricyclics; antiepileptics; *N*-methyl-D-aspartate (NMDA)
  - Specific therapies
    - Anti-CGRP medications
    - OnabotulinumtoxinA (Botox) injections

Definition

Migraine is a primary headache disorder, not caused by any known structural cause. International Headache Society (IHS) criteria define migraine and explain clinical variability seen in patients.

The headache episode in migraine as defined by the IHS has at least two of four defining features (one-sided, pulsating, moderate to severe, and aggravated by movement) and at least one of two associated features (nausea and/or vomiting, light and sound sensitivity). In its most common form, migraine is an episodic, recurrent headache lasting 4 hours or longer per episode if left untreated. The frequency varies from rare episodes to everyday headache.

In its more malignant forms, migraine is chronic, daily, non-stop pain with rare or no pain-free time. There is significant clinical variability: unilateral location and pulsating pain is present in around 50% of migraine sufferers. Most patients are disabled from pain; environmental oversensitivity to light, sound, and smell; inability to function; and often transient cognitive dysfunction such as difficulty with concentration. There is a subset of migraine with aura, most commonly the visual symptoms associated with fully reversible visual changes that can mimic transient ischemic attack or stroke.

Many medical providers fail to recognize migraine because they default to the most classic migraine presentation with visual aura with unilateral, pulsating pain with nausea and vomiting. Because migraine can manifest in different ways, this makes diagnosis more challenging. If a patient presents to a medical provider with recurrent moderate-to-severe headaches, migraine diagnosis should be considered. In general, most migraine experts consider a headache migraine unless there is a warning sign or some atypical feature. However, there are a number of neurologic disorders that mimic migraine. For example, stroke can present with migraine-like headache. The majority of people with "sinus headache" can also suffer from migraine. For patients' safety, other causes of headache and other neurologic disorders need to be ruled out. The clinical presentation differs from person to person, and we should consider migraine diagnosis as a possibility in anyone with recurring, disabling headaches and impaired function.

Epidemiology

Migraine affects more than 1 billion people worldwide. In the United States, migraine affects more than 45 million adults, encompassing 18% to 23% of women and 6% to 9% of men. Onset can occur as early as age 5 years and prevalence peaks in young people, but it can occur at any age. Though migraine can be transient, migraine affects people during their most productive years of life. The Global Burden of Disease Study 2016 measured how disabling various disorders are across the world and assessed how disorders affect disability-adjusted life years. In Global Burden of Disease 2016, migraine was the second-most disabling disorder, after low back pain. In one study, 88% of patients diagnosed with sinus headache had migraine.

Risk Factors

Migraine is most commonly seen in young White women with family history of migraine. There are many risk factors that can be cumulative for a given individual who presents with migraine. Lifestyle factors that lead to migraine include high-stress work, nutrition (high carbohydrate diet), physical inactivity, and chronic stress. Therefore a young person with genetic susceptibility to migraine with stress at work, physical inactivity, poor nutrition, and sleep deprivation has increased risk for developing migraine. It is estimated that in 1 year, up to 3% of episodic migraine cases become chronic. Risk factors for migraine chronification are obesity, acute medication overuse, caffeine overuse, stressful life events, depression, and sleep disorders. Comorbid conditions often seen in migraine include anxiety, depression, and insomnia, and these conditions have bidirectional effect.

Pathophysiology

Although migraine was once considered exclusively a disorder of the blood vessels, compelling evidence has led to the realization that a migraine represents a highly choreographed interaction between major inputs from both peripheral and central nervous systems, with the trigeminovascular system and the cerebral cortex among the main players. Migraine was initially thought to be a purely vascular disorder, but it is understood that migraine involves the neurotransmitter calcitonin gene-related peptide (CGRP). The pain of a migraine attack seems to be caused by the release of CGRP in the dura mater, which results in vasodilation and inflammation. Studies have shown that if CGRP is given intravenously to people with migraine, most will have a migraine episode in the next few hours.

Diagnosis and Workup

The main questions are whether the patient presents with headache that meets migraine criteria and whether he or she needs neuroimaging (Table 1). We diagnose migraine using IHS criteria (https://ichd-3.org/1-migraine/). Migraine is divided into two major subtypes. Migraine without aura is the most common, characterized by a headache with severe unilateral pain, photophobia, phonophobia, and functional impairment. Migraine with aura is most commonly characterized by reversible visual changes that precede and sometimes accompany the migraine pain. The success of migraine treatment depends on making the correct diagnosis. This requires careful headache history, because many

TABLE 1	Precision Questions Helpful in Migraine Diagnosis
1. Is this a new kind of headache?	New headache needs further history; make sure this is not a migraine mimic.
2. Use "red flag" questions, such as do you have any other condition such as cancer?	"Red flag" questions are used to exclude secondary headache.
3. How many total headache days do you have per month? Lump all headache days.	Total headache days >15 days per month are suggestive of chronic migraine.
4. How long do your headaches last with no treatment?	Duration of headache without therapy should be more than 4 h for migraine diagnosis. With shorter duration, consider other diagnosis, such as trigeminal autonomic cephalgia.
5. What associated symptoms do you have?	For migraine, look for associated nausea and light and sound sensitivity.
6. How many days per month do you use an acute therapy for any pain?	Medication overuse headache is commonly seen with chronic migraine, and any medication used for any pain can cause this.

patients diagnose themselves with sinus headache or tension-type headache or other type of headache. Identifying classic symptoms has a high probability of accurate diagnosis. The headache pattern should distinguish migraine from other primary headaches (tension or cluster headache). The clinical history and neurologic examination target need to exclude secondary headache that can present as migraine. In most patients the diagnosis is made using their history and IHS criteria. Diagnostic imaging is not indicated in otherwise healthy patients with migraine with normal neurologic examination. Patients with "red flags" such as abnormalities during the neurologic examination, fever, unintentional weight loss, history of cancer, transplant, or immunodeficiency need further workup with neuroimaging. Which kind of neuroimaging should be performed is a common question: Magnetic resonance imaging of the brain with and without contrast is the preferred imaging modality.

Treatment

The pharmacologic treatment addresses acute treatment, used for management of acute exacerbations, and preventive treatments that have shown efficacy in decreasing migraine attacks in the long term. Preventive medications are taken daily for at least several months, sometimes years, to reduce the severity and frequency of migraines before they start.

The treatment strategy for migraines has shifted from using mostly nonspecific pain medications such as aspirin and acetaminophen to migraine-specific therapies such as triptans, ditans, and gepants and other treatments such as neuromodulation (Table 2; Boxes 1–3).

Acute Treatment

Mechanism of Acute Migraine Medications

Migraine pain is considered to be caused by dura mater release of CGRP, with subsequent vasodilation and neurogenic inflammation. Triptans and ergots are agonists of serotonin 5-HT1D receptors, and their activation prevents CGRP release. Agonism at 5-HT1B receptors results in vasoconstriction, which opposes the action of CGRP. Ditans are selective nontriptan oral serotonin (5-HT1F) receptor agonists, which is thought to stop plasma protein release by action of the trigeminal ganglion. 5-HT1F receptors are not present in vessels. Ditans also inhibit trigeminal nucleus caudalis. Gepants such as ubrogepant (Ubrelvy), rimegepant

(Nurtec ODT), and atogepant (Qulipta) are oral CGRP receptor antagonists.

The American Headache Society guideline for acute treatment in 2015 summarized evidence-based assessment of acute treatments for migraine: "The specific medications—triptans and dihydroergotamine (nasal spray [Migranal, Trudhesa], inhaler[5]) are effective (level A)," whereas "effective nonspecific medications include acetaminophen, NSAIDs (nonsteroidal antiinflammatory drugs), opioids (butorphanol nasal spray)[1] (not recommended), sumatriptan/naproxen (Treximet), and the combination of acetaminophen/aspirin/caffeine (e.g., Excedrin Migraine)" also have level A evidence. "Ergotamine tartrate (Ergomar) and other forms of dihydroergotamine, ketoprofen (Orudis),[1] intravenous and intramuscular ketorolac (Toradol),[1] flurbiprofen (Ansaid),[1] intravenous magnesium (in migraine with aura),[1] and the combination of isometheptene compounds, codeine/acetaminophen,[1] tramadol/acetaminophen (Ultracet),[1] prochlorperazine (Compazine),[1] droperidol (Inapsine),[1] chlorpromazine (Thorazine),[1] and metoclopramide (Reglan)[1] are probably effective (level B)."

It is important to educate patients on appropriate use of acute therapy, because medication overuse headache (MOH) can develop. This is defined as the presence of headache while taking any acute medications for any pain, even if not headache related, more than 15 days per month. MOH is often difficult to treat and is medication and procedure refractory. We strongly recommend monitoring days per month of acute medication use and setting a limit on maximum monthly use. An electronic headache diary app, such as https://migrainebuddy.com/, can be helpful in documenting headache days and medication use.

An oral nonopioid analgesic, such as naproxen (Aleve),[1] is often adequate for acute treatment of mild to moderate migraine without nausea or vomiting. Migraine-specific agents should be considered when migraine episodes are moderate to severe. The acute migraine-specific pharmacotherapies include triptans, ergotamines, ditans, and gepants.

Many acute therapies are effective only for some patients and can cause significant side effects. Patients who do not respond to one triptan may respond to another triptan or a different mode of administration of the same triptan. Note that triptans are contraindicated in patients with vascular risk factors.

- Sumatriptan (Imitrex) (6 mg SQ injections; 20 mg nasal solution; 25, 50, and 100 mg oral tablet)
- Zolmitriptan (Zomig) (2.5, 5 mg nasal solution; oral tablet or oral disintegrating tablet)
- Rizatriptan (Maxalt) (5, 10 mg oral tablet; oral disintegrating tablet)
- Naratriptan (Amerge) (1, 2.5 mg oral tablet)
- Eletriptan (Relpax) 20, 40 mg oral tablet
- Almotriptan (Axert) (6.25, 12.5 mg oral tablet)
- Frovatriptan (Frova) (2.5 mg oral tablet)

Dihydroergotamine (D.H.E. 45, Migranal, Trudhesa) should be considered in patients who are refractory to triptans, although they have the same vascular disease contraindication.

- Dihydroergotamine (D.H.E. 45, 1 mg SQ or IV; Migranal 0.5 mg/spray into each nostril; Trudhesa 0.725 mg/spray into each nostril) A number of new agents became available in 2020.
- New acute migraine treatment: ditans and gepants

The one approved ditan is lasmiditan (Reyvow), which is an oral serotonin (5HT1F) receptor agonist. The gepants approved for acute migraine treatment are ubrogepant (Ubrelvy) and rimegepant (Nurtec ODT), which are oral CGRP receptor agonists. These drugs were approved by the U.S. Food and Drug Administration (FDA) in 2020 for acute migraine treatment with and without aura in adults.

Ditans for Acute Migraine Treatment

Ditans are the only group of medications known to selectively bind serotonin 1F receptor (5-HT1F) on the trigeminal neurons.

---

[5] Investigational drug in the United States.
[1] Not FDA-approved for this indication.

TABLE 2	Migraine Treatment by Severity and Phenotype		
	CLINICAL MIGRAINE PHENOTYPE	**STRATEGY**	**MEDICATION**
Increasing migraine severity	Mild to moderate	Acetaminophen	Acetaminophen (Tylenol)[1] 1000 mg
		NSAID	Naproxen sodium (Aleve)[1] 220–660 mg Ibuprofen (Motrin) 800 mg
	Moderate to severe	NSAID + triptan + antinausea	Naproxen (Aleve) 440 mg + ondansetron (Zofran)[1] 8 mg ODT + triptan later for rescue if necessary
		Triptan (5HT1B agonist 5HT1D agonist)	Sumatriptan (Imitrex) (6 mg SQ injection; 20 mg nasal solution; 25, 50, and 100 mg oral tablet) Zolmitriptan (Zomig) (2.5, 5 mg nasal solution; oral tablet; ODT) Rizatriptan (Maxalt) (5 mg, 10 mg oral tablet; ODT) Naratriptan (Amerge) (1, 2.5 mg PO tablet) Eletriptan (Relpax) (20, 40 mg PO tablet) Almotriptan (Axert) (6.25, 12.5 mg PO tablet) Frovatriptan (Frova) (2.5 mg PO tablet)
		Ditan (5HT1F agonist) Gepant (CGRP antagonist)	Lasmiditan (Reyvow) 50, 100, 200 mg PO tablet Ubrogepant (Ubrelvy) 50, 100 mg PO tablet Rimegepant (Nurtec ODT) 75 mg ODT
	Severe attack difficult to treat and refractory migraine		Triptan + NSAID + antinausea drug Gepant + NSAID + antinausea drug Ditan + NSAID + antinausea drug Ketorolac (TORADOL)[1] IM 60 mg Indomethacin[1] oral or rectal Prochlorperazine (COMPAZINE)[1] 5, 10 mg Dexamethasone[1] or prednisone[1]

[1]Not FDA approved for this indication.
ODT, Oral disintegrating tablet.
From Pringsheim T, Davenport W, Mackie G, et al. Canadian Headache Society guideline for migraine prophylaxis. *Can J Neurol Sci.* 2012;1;39(Suppl 2):S1–59.

BOX 1	First-Line Acute Therapy of Migraine

Naproxen (Aleve)[1] 440 mg + ondansetron (Zofran)[1] 8 mg ODT + triptan later for rescue if necessary

Triptans:
- Sumatriptan (Imitrex) 6 mg SQ injection; 20 mg nasal solution; 25, 50, and 100 mg oral tablet
- Zolmitriptan (Zomig) 2.5, 5 mg oral tablet; ODT; nasal spray
- Rizatriptan (Maxalt) 5, 10 mg oral tablet; ODT
- Naratriptan (Amerge) 1, 2.5 mg oral tablet
- Eletriptan (Relpax) 20, 40 mg oral tablet
- Almotriptan (Axert) 6.25, 12.5 mg oral tablet
- Frovatriptan (Frova) 2.5 mg oral tablet

Ditans:
- Lasmiditan (Reyvow) 50, 100, 200 mg oral tablet

Gepants:
- Ubrogepant (Ubrelvy) 50, 100 mg oral tablet
- Rimegepant (Nurtec ODT) 75 mg oral disintegrating tablet

[1]Not FDA approved for this indication.
ODT, Oral disintegrating tablet.

Ditans do not cause vasoconstriction via the serotonin 1B receptor on blood vessels as triptans do and therefore are not contraindicated in patients with known vascular risk factors. A majority of patients in clinical studies had at least one cardiovascular risk factor, only a few of the subjects had ischemic heart disease, and none had ischemic events attributed to lasmiditan during the trial within 48 hours. To date, no clinical trials are available that have compared lasmiditan to other acute headache treatments. The most common side effects in clinical trials were dizziness, paresthesias, and sedation. Cognitive changes and confusion were also reported. Lasmiditan can cause impaired driving ability, and there is a drug warning against driving and operating machinery for at least 8 hours after taking this drug. It is important to mention this to the patient. Because of the central nervous system (CNS) action, other concomitant CNS depressants should be avoided. Caution is also advised with heart rate–lowering medications. It is not known whether ditans can cause serotonin syndrome.

There is no available evidence that supports limiting the use of ditans with selective serotonin reuptake inhibitors or serotonin-norepinephrine reuptake inhibitors because of concerns for serotonin syndrome. However, given the seriousness of serotonin syndrome, caution is warranted, especially in a patient taking other medications and supplements. No data for pregnancy and breastfeeding are available at this time.
- Lasmiditan (Reyvow 50, 100, or 200 mg PO as a single dose; maximum: one dose in 24 hours)

Gepants for Acute Migraine Treatment

Gepants are the only group of oral medications known to selectively bind and antagonize CGRP receptor. Gepants do not cause vasoconstriction, because they do not bind to serotonin 1B receptor on blood vessels as triptans do and therefore are not contraindicated in patients with known vascular risk factors. CGRP levels tend to increase with migraine, and patients with migraine injected with CGRP develop migraine within 4 hours. No clinical trials are available that have compared gepants to other acute headache treatments. Gepants are well tolerated, and the most commonly reported side effect compared with placebo is nausea in ubrogepant trials. Because gepants are metabolized via CYP3A4 via liver, coadministration with strong inhibitors of CYP3A4 such as ketoconazole and CYP3A4 inducers such as rifampin should be avoided. No data for pregnancy and breastfeeding are available at this time.
- Ubrogepant (Ubrelvy 50 to 100 mg PO as a single dose; may repeat once based on response and tolerability after ≥2 hours)

BOX 2 — Steps for Acute Treatment for Migraine Headache

Step 1: Choose options that are not known to lead to MOH.
- Antiemetics: Ondansetron (Zofram)[1] (tablet, dispersible tablet), prochlorperazine (Compazine)[1] (tablet, suppository), promethazine (Phenergan)[1] (tablet, suppository), metoclopramide (Reglan)[1]
- Natural supplements/herbs: Feverfew tea,[1] Boswellia,[7] magnesium[7]
- Anesthetic: Lidocaine nasal spray[1]
- Neuromodulation: Cefaly (supraorbital stimulation), Gammacore (vagal nerve stimulation), SpringTMS (transcranial magnetic stimulation), Relivion (external combined occipital and trigeminal neurostimulation), Nerivio (remote electrical neuromodulation)
- Nonmedication options: Rest, ice, meditation, biofeedback, distraction, essential oils[7]

Step 2: NSAIDs, longer acting are generally considered less likely to lead to MOH.
- Diclofenac (tablet,[1] capsule,[1] powder), ketorolac,[1] naproxen,[1] ibuprofen

Step 3: Limit any acute medications such as triptans to 1–2 days per week to avoid MOH.
- Triptans: Sumatriptan (Imitrex) (tablet, nasal spray, injection), rizatriptan (Maxalt) (tablet, dispersible tablet), eletriptan (Relpax), zolmitriptan (Zomig) (tablet, dispersible tablet, nasal spray), almotriptan (Axert), frovatriptan (Frova), naratriptan (Amerge)
- Ergotamines: dihydroergotamine DHE 45 injection, Migranal nasal spray

---

[1] Not FDA approved for this indication.
[7] Available as dietary supplement.
MOH, Medication overuse headache.

BOX 3 — Preventive Medications for Episodic Migraine

Level A Therapies, Established as Effective and FDA Approved for EM
- AEDs: Topiramate (Topamax) (caution if low weight or history of kidney stones), divalproex sodium (Depakote) (caution of weight gain), sodium valproate (Depakene)
- Beta-blockers: Propranolol (Inderal), timolol (Blocadren), metoprolol (Lopressor) (the only Level A medication that is not FDA approved)

Specific Preventive Migraine Therapies FDA Approved for EM and CM
- Anti-CGRP monoclonal antibodies: erenumab-aooe (Aimovig), fremanezumab-vfrm (Ajovy), galcanezumab-gnlm (Emgality)
- Gepants: Rimegepant (Nurtec ODT)
- Neuromodulation devices: Cefaly (supraorbital stimulation), Gammacore (vagal nerve stimulation)

Level B Therapies, Probably Effective for EM, not FDA Approved for EM
- Antidepressants: Amitriptyline, venlafaxine (Effexor XR)
- Beta-blockers: Atenolol (Tenormin), nadolol (Corgard)

Level C Therapies, Possibly Effective for EM, not FDA Approved
- Calcium channel blockers and angiotensin-converting-enzyme inhibitors: Verapamil (Calan), lisinopril (Prinivil)
- AEDs: Carbamazepine (Tegretol)
- Beta-blockers: Pindolol (Visken)
- Antihistamines: Cyproheptadine (Periactin)
- Angiotensin-receptor blockers: candesartan (Atacand), clonidine (Catapres)

AED, Antiepileptic drug; CM, chronic migraine; EM, episodic migraine.

- Rimegepant (Nurtec 75 mg PO as a single dose; maximum: 75 mg/24 hours)
- Zavegepant (Zavzpret 10 mg intranasally one spray/dose/24 hours) is the first intranasal gepant.

Neuromodulation Therapies for Migraine

There are currently several FDA-approved neuromodulation devices for use in migraine, all of which use noninvasive stimulation to modulate brain function. All are considered to have nonsignificant risks and are generally well tolerated by patients. Neuromodulation can be used for acute treatment of migraine. These devices generally require patient payment, although they are generally free of charge for veterans or military active duty personnel.
- Remote electrical neuromodulation device (Nerivio)
- External trigeminal neurostimulation device (Cefaly)
- Single-pulse transcranial magnetic stimulation device (Savi Dual)
- External vagal nerve stimulation device (GammaCore)
- External combined occipital and trigeminal neurostimulation device (Relivion)

Preventive Treatment

There is emphasis on prevention of migraine attacks for many patients, because acute therapy is often less effective in more severe cases. Consider preventive treatments for patients who are disabled by migraine, who are missing work, who are using the emergency room for headache treatment, who have five or more migraine days per month, or who are prone to overusing acute medications. Preventive treatments should also be considered for patients with serious medical problems, such as heart disease or stroke.

Medical providers should consult the American Academy of Neurology/American Headache Society guidelines. All guidelines were consistent in their recommendations of treatments for first-line use. All rated topiramate, divalproex/sodium valproate, propranolol, and metoprolol as having the highest level of evidence.

Level A: Effective
- Divalproex (Depakote ER)/sodium valproate (Stavzor) 500 to 1000 mg/day
- Metoprolol (Lopressor)[1] 25 to 200 mg/day
- Petasites (butterbur)[7] 50 to 75 mg bid
- Propranolol (Inderal) 40 to 240 mg/day
- Timolol (Blocadren) 10 to 15 mg bid
- Topiramate (Topamax) 25 to 200 mg/day

Level B: Probably Effective

Should be considered for patients requiring migraine prophylaxis
- Amitriptyline (Elavil)[1] 10 to 150 mg/day
- Fenoprofen (Nalfon)[1] 200 to 600 mg three times per day[a]
- Feverfew[7] 50 to 150 mg bid; 2.08 to 18.75 mg three times per day for MIG-99 preparation
- Ibuprofen (Advil, Motrin)[1] 200 mg twice a day[a]
- Ketoprofen (Orudis)[1] 50 mg three times per day[a]
- Magnesium[1] 600 mg per day
- Naproxen (Naprosyn)[1]/naproxen sodium (Anaprox DS)[1] 500 to 1100 mg/day or naproxen sodium 550 mg twice a day[a]
- Riboflavin (Vitamin B_2)[7] 400 mg/day
- Venlafaxine (Effexor ER)[1] 150 mg extended release/day
- Atenolol (Tenormin)[1] 25 to 100 mg/day

Anti-Calcitonin Gene-Related Peptide Monoclonal Antibodies for Preventive Treatment

Since 2018, CGRP receptor antagonist monoclonal antibodies have been FDA approved for preventive treatment of both

---

[1] Not FDA approved for this indication.
[7] Available as dietary supplement.
[a] Used for 1 month or less.

episodic and chronic migraine: erenumab-aooe (Aimovig), galcanezumab-gnlm (Emgality), fremanezumab-vfrm (Ajovy), and eptinezumab-jjmr (Vyepti). The first three are intended for self-injection at home. Before covering, most medical insurances require trial of at least three classes of preventive therapies with highest level of evidence including beta-blockers (propranolol or timolol), antiseizure medications (divalproex sodium or topiramate), and tricyclics or SNRIs. They are effective in about one-third of patients with migraine with super-responders, have low side effect profile, and do not interact with any medications. They are not indicated during pregnancy or breastfeeding owing to lack of evidence.

- Erenumab-aooe (Aimovig) 70, 140 mg SQ once a month self-administered by patient
- Fremanezumab-vfrm (Ajovy) 225 mg SQ monthly or 675 mg every 3 months (quarterly), which is administered as three consecutive subcutaneous injections of 225 mg each
- Galcanezumab-gnlm (Emgality) 240 mg (two consecutive subcutaneous injections of 120 mg each) once as a loading dose, followed by monthly doses of 120 mg injected subcutaneously

Gepant Anti-CGRP Receptor Antagonists for Migraine Prevention

Atogepant (Qulipta) was approved in 2021 for prevention of migraine at doses from 10 mg to 60 mg a day. Rimegepant (Nurtec ODT) received additional FDA approval for migraine prevention in 2021 at the dose of 75 mg every other day.

Chronic Migraine Treatment

Patients with chronic forms of migraine are especially difficult to treat. They are prone to chronic MOH. Overuse is defined as taking acute medication 15 or more days per month for nonopioid analgesics (including aspirin, NSAIDs, and acetaminophen) and 10 or more days per month for triptans, ergotamines, opioids, and combination analgesics. People can develop MOH at much lower levels of regular medication use. Medical providers should ensure that patients are aware of the risk of MOH and limit medication use well below these levels. We recommend not using acute medication more than 1 to 2 days per week on average, and this includes all acute medications. Neuromodulation is a great option for management of acute exacerbation in patients with chronic migraine because daily use does not lead to rebound and worsening headaches. Always consider preventive medications and lifestyle changes in patients with chronic migraines, because acute medications cause MOH when used 15 or more days per month.

MOH often leads to clinically refractory migraine. Taking acute medications to abort migraine attacks more than 10 days per month can lead to increased neuronal excitability, depletion of central serotonin production, and increased release of CGRP. Clinical observation suggests that both preventive and acute treatment for the primary headache usually fail unless the offending medication or medications that caused MOH are stopped.

Treatments for chronic migraine include:

- Topiramate (Topamax)[1] 25 to 200 mg/day
- OnabotulinumtoxinA (Botox)[1] 155 units injections by medical providers every 3 months
- Erenumab-aooe (Aimovig)[1] 70, 140 mg SQ once a month self-administered by patient
- Fremanezumab-vfrm (Ajovy)[1] 225 mg SQ monthly, or 675 mg every 3 months (quarterly), which is administered as three consecutive subcutaneous injections of 225 mg each.
- Galcanezumab-gnlm (Emgality)[1] 240 mg (two consecutive subcutaneous injections of 120 mg each) once as a loading dose, followed by monthly doses of 120 mg injected subcutaneously
- Atogepant (Qulipta)[1] 10 to 60 mg daily orally

---

[1] Not FDA approved for this indication.

Monitoring

Primary care providers should consider regular follow-up of their patients every few months or more frequently until patients are stable and have gained therapeutic success. We recommend adding multimodal therapy at each visit, and this can include exercise, sleep therapy, nutrition therapy, stress reductions, and supplements in addition to pharmacotherapy reevaluation. We use the visits to address migraine comorbidities, especially anxiety and sleep. With regular monitoring, medication dose can be optimized for maximum efficacy and the least possible side effects. Acute pharmacotherapy escalation in patients who are not optimally controlled can backfire and lead to development of MOH. When a patient experiences significantly worsening headache on 15 or more days per month and has history of migraine, acute medication frequency of use needs to be assessed. MOH may resolve after the acute medication is stopped; however, in many patients with comorbid anxiety and insomnia, more treatment should be considered. In patients with MOH we should consider preventive therapy and neuromodulation therapy. Compliance with medication therapy can be improved by education offered by caring providers and establishing therapeutic alliance with patients by using motivational interviewing skills.

References

Chou DE, Shnayderman Yugrakh M, Winegarner D: Acute migraine therapy with external trigeminal neurostimulation (ACME): a randomized controlled trial, *Cephalalgia* 39:3–14, 2019.

Dodick DW, Lipton RB, Ailani J, et al: Ubrogepant for the treatment of migraine, *N Engl J Med* 381:2230–2241, 2019.

Goadsby PJ, Wietecha LA, Dennehy EB, et al: Phase 3 randomized, placebo-controlled, double-blind study of lasmiditan for acute treatment of migraine, *Brain* 142:1894–1904, 2019.

Halker Singh RB, Ailani J, Robbins MS: Neuromodulation for the acute and preventive therapy of migraine and cluster headache, *Headache* 59(Suppl 2):33–49, 2019.

Headache Classification Committee of the International Headache Society: The international classification of headache disorders, 3rd edition (beta version), *Cephalalgia* 33(9):629–808, 2013.

Kuca B, Silberstein SD, Wietecha L, Berg PH, Dozier G, Lipton RB: Lasmiditan is an effective acute treatment for migraine: a phase 3 randomized study, *Neurology* 91:e2222–e2232, 2018.

Lipton RB, Croop R, Stock EG, et al: Rimegepant, an oral calcitonin gene-related peptide receptor antagonist, for migraine, *N Engl J Med* 381:142–149, 2019.

Lipton RB, Dodick DW, Silberstein SD, et al: Single pulse transcranial magnetic stimulation for acute treatment of migraine with aura: a randomised, double-blind, parallel-group, sham-controlled trial, *Lancet Neurol* 9:373–380, 2010.

Loder E, Burch R, Rizzoli P: The 2012 AHS/AAN guidelines for prevention of episodic migraine: a summary and comparison with other recent clinical practice guidelines, *Headache J Head Face Pain* 52(6):930–945, 2012.

Marmura MJ, Silberstein SD, Schwedt TJ: The acute treatment of migraine in adults: the American headache society evidence assessment of migraine pharmacotherapies, *Headache* 55:3–20, 2015.

Misra UK, Kalita J, Bhoi SK: High-rate repetitive transcranial magnetic stimulation in migraine prophylaxis: a randomized, placebo-controlled study, *J Neurol* 1–9, 2013.

Pierelli F, Iacovelli E, Bracaglia M: Abnormal sensorimotor plasticity in migraine without aura patients, *Pain*, 2013.

Pietrobon D, Moskowitz MA: Pathophysiology of migraine, *Ann Rev Physiol* 75:365–391, 2013.

Stovner LJ, Nichols E, Steiner TJ, et al: Global, regional, and national burden of migraine and tension-type headache, 1990–2016: a systematic analysis for the Global Burden of Disease Study 2016, *Lancet Neurol* 17(11):954–976, 2018.

Stovner LJ, Nichols E, Steiner TJ, Vos T: Headache in the Global Burden of Disease (GBD) studies. In *Societal impact of headache*, New York, NY, 2019, Springer, Cham, pp 105–125.

Sussman M, Benner J, Neumann P, Menzin J: Cost effectiveness analysis of erenumab for the preventive treatment of episodic and chronic migraine: results from the US societal and payer perspectives, *Cephalalgia* 38:1644–1657, 2018.

Szperka CL, et al: Migraine care in the era of COVID-19: clinical pearls and plea to insurers, *Headache*, 2020.

Tassorelli C, Grazzi L, de Tommaso M, et al: Noninvasive vagus nerve stimulation as acute therapy for migraine: the randomized PRESTO study, *Neurology* 91:e364–e373, 2018.

Tepper SJ: Debate: analgesic overuse is a cause, not consequence, of chronic daily headache. Analgesic overuse is a cause of chronic daily headache, *Headache* 42:543–547, 2002.

Vollbracht S, Rapoport AM: The pipeline in headache therapy, *CNS Drugs* 1–13, 2013.

Yarnitsky D, Dodick DW, Grosberg BM, et al: Remote electrical neuromodulation (REN) relieves acute migraine: a randomized, double-blind, placebo-controlled, multicenter trial, *Headache* 59:1240–1252, 2019.

MULTIPLE SCLEROSIS

Method of
Caitlin Jackson-Tarlton, MD

CURRENT DIAGNOSIS

- Multiple sclerosis (MS) is an immune-mediated demyelinating disease of the central nervous system (CNS).
- The McDonald criteria, the most widely used diagnostic criteria, incorporate a patient's symptoms, physical examination, magnetic resonance imaging (MRI) findings, and, when applicable, cerebrospinal fluid (CSF) analysis and other ancillary tests.
- The core MS phenotypes are relapsing and progressive MS. Diagnosis of relapsing-remitting multiple sclerosis (RRMS) requires recurrent episodes of acute CNS demyelinating attacks (also referred to as *relapses* or *flares*). Clinically isolated syndrome (CIS), a single demyelinating episode and often first attack of MS, may meet McDonald criteria for RRMS based on MRI and CSF results.
- Primary progressive multiple sclerosis (PPMS) is heralded by progressive neurologic impairment from disease onset in the absence of any preceding attacks. Secondary progressive multiple sclerosis (SPMS) is progressive neurologic disease following a history of relapsing MS.
- Radiologically isolated syndrome (RIS) is the presence of CNS demyelinating lesions on MRI in a patient lacking symptoms and physical examination findings typical of demyelination. RIS and CIS not meeting McDonald criteria may later develop into clinically definite MS requiring clinical and radiologic monitoring.

CURRENT THERAPY

- Acute attacks of MS are treated with high-dose corticosteroids and, in severe cases, plasma exchange. These therapies facilitate time to recovery but do not prevent future relapses.
- Disease-modifying therapies (DMTs) reduce the number of new attacks and new MRI lesions. To date, there are no curative treatments.
- There are many distinct and effective DMT choices approved for CIS, RRMS, and SPMS with activity (ongoing clinical attacks and/or new MRI lesions).
- The single approved therapy for PPMS is ocrelizumab (Ocrevus). Treatment for RIS remains uncertain with trials ongoing.
- Medications vary in their mechanism of action, efficacy, side effect profile, and mode of delivery. DMT choice should be individualized considering the patient's age, severity of MS, presence of comorbidities, family planning, and patient preference. Insurance coverage often plays a role given the substantial cost of these medications.
- Novel MS medications, including further oral medications, and infusion-based monoclonal antibodies are currently under scientific evaluation.

Multiple sclerosis (MS) is an immune-mediated inflammatory demyelinating disease of the central nervous system (CNS) that affects approximately 1 million people in the United States alone.

Risk Factors

Women are at least twice as likely as men to develop of MS. Other known risk factors for development of MS include ethnicity, genetic background, and socioeconomic and environmental exposures. Persons of European ethnicity, particularly those born and reared in extreme northern or southern latitudes, are particularly susceptible to MS, although recent data suggest that African Americans may have a more severe clinical course. Genetic susceptibility is associated with the *HLA-DRB1* major histocompatibility allele as well as interleukin-2 and interleukin-7 receptors. Obesity, particularly during adolescence, and low serum vitamin D levels are both associated with an increased risk of development of MS and may influence the severity of its clinical course. The association between MS and infection with Epstein-Barr virus (infectious mononucleosis) has been studied extensively. A recent large longitudinal study of U.S. military recruits strengthened this association by demonstrating that Epstein-Barr infection preceded the development of MS in those who were subsequently diagnosed with MS. Further, the risk of developing MS was increased 32-fold after Epstein-Barr infection but was not increased by other viruses such as cytomegalovirus. Given that Epstein-Barr infection is very common and MS quite uncommon, this suggests that exposure to the virus may be necessary but insufficient for developing MS. Comorbid chronic vascular diseases and mood disorders complicate and worsen the MS disease course. Cigarette smoking is associated with an increased risk for development of MS and likely is associated with an increased severity and clinical course.

Pathophysiology

The etiology and pathophysiology of MS as a whole remains uncertain. However, most evidence supports an inflammatory autoimmune demyelinating disease induced by environmental factors in a genetically susceptible host. Animal models including experimental allergic encephalomyelitis and Theiler murine encephalomyelitis virus also point to an autoimmune inflammatory demyelinating etiology, most likely associated with viral infection. Studies that suggested chronic cerebrospinal vascular insufficiency has an important association with MS have been refuted.

Pathophysiology likely varies among individual patients with MS. Four distinct pathologies in active demyelinating MS lesions have been described. Pattern 1 displays marked macrophage infiltration without humoral abnormalities. Pattern 2 shows distinct humoral abnormalities with complement activation and immunoglobulin (Ig) deposition. Pattern 3 involves primary oligodendrocyte degeneration and early loss of myelin-associated glycoprotein. Pattern 4 reveals oligodendrocyte dystrophy in periplaque white matter. Early studies suggest that there could be a therapeutic advantage with different therapies for different types of demyelinating disease.

Prevention

Currently, there is no known way to definitively prevent the development of MS. Patients with a single clinical attack of demyelination and abnormal magnetic resonance imaging (MRI) ("high-risk" clinically isolated syndrome) have a delayed onset to MS diagnosis with immunomodulatory therapy. A recent small randomized, double-blinded, placebo-controlled trial of individuals with radiologically isolated syndrome (RIS) showed treatment with dimethyl fumarate (Tecfidera)[1] substantially reduced the risk of clinical demyelinating attacks. Additional studies on the treatment of RIS are ongoing but currently no agent has a U.S. Food and Drug Administration (FDA)-approved indication for RIS.

Clinical Manifestations

The clinical course of MS is varied. Approximately 85% of patients present with a relapsing-remitting course. This entails an acute impairment within the CNS, with symptoms depending on the area of inflammation. An acute demyelinating cause of a focal neurologic symptom is suggested by an onset over hours to days, with a plateau of impairment over a few weeks. Symptoms then improve either spontaneously or with the use

---

[1]Not FDA approved for this indication.

of corticosteroids over a number of days to weeks or longer. However, symptoms might not completely resolve, leaving an individual with permanent neurologic disability. Inflammation within the optic nerve (optic neuritis) is heralded by painful, unilateral, central monocular visual deficit (central scotoma). Symptoms of brainstem dysfunction include binocular diplopia, sensory deficits unilaterally on the face and contralaterally on the arm and leg, significant dysarthria, and vertigo. Cerebellar dysfunction is seen with pure ataxia that is typically unilateral. Spinal cord inflammation is indicated by a distinctive, usually gradually rising sensory level of deficit that commonly is accompanied by bowel and bladder impairment and paraparesis or quadriparesis, depending on a thoracic versus cervical level of the lesion.

Progressive forms of MS include secondary progressive multiple sclerosis (SPMS) and primary progressive multiple sclerosis (PPMS). These are heralded by a slow (months to years) but steady and insidious, progressive neurologic deficit. Most commonly, progressive MS presents with a progressive myelopathy consisting of an upper motor neuron gait disorder with spasticity, neurogenic bladder and bowel impairment, and/or progressive weakness. Occasionally, patients with progressive MS have insidious cerebellar ataxia or dementia, in isolation or in association with the myelopathy. SPMS is diagnosed when a patient has had a prior history of at least one clinical attack (relapse) followed by more than 1 year of progressive neurologic disease. PPMS is diagnosed with progressive CNS disease consistent with MS and typical MRI brain or spinal lesions from onset without any prior relapse, often with cerebrospinal fluid (CSF) abnormalities that support the diagnosis.

Diagnosis

The diagnosis of MS is formalized by the continually revised McDonald criteria. Criteria must only be applied to individuals presenting with a syndrome typical for demyelination, and alternative diagnoses must be considered and excluded. A diagnosis of relapsing-remitting multiple sclerosis (RRMS) entails having two or more clinical attacks (relapses) in the accompaniment of objective clinical evidence of two or more lesions. The 2017 McDonald criteria allow some patients with a single clinical attack, clinically isolated syndrome (CIS), who meet additional criteria through MRI and/or CSF analysis, so-called dissemination in time and space, to be diagnosed with relapsing remitting multiple sclerosis.

Progressive MS is diagnosed when there is progressive CNS disease characteristic of MS for at least 1 year and at least two of the following: (1) one or more demyelinating MRI brain lesions typical for MS, (2) two or more demyelinating spinal cord lesions typical for MS, or (3) the presence of CSF-specific oligoclonal bands (Figure 1).

Occasionally, visual-evoked potentials and somatosensory-evoked potentials are used to further document dissemination of MS within the CNS. Serologic investigations are done primarily to rule out MS mimickers depending on and directed by any accompanying systemic symptoms and the clinical setting in individual patients. These may include antineuronal antibodies (aquaporin-4-IgG and myelin oligodendrocyte glycoprotein-IgG), antinuclear antibodies, erythrocyte sedimentation rate, anticardiolipin antibodies, vitamin B_{12}, Lyme serology, and/or chest imaging for sarcoidosis.

Differential Diagnosis

Other CNS demyelinating diseases can mimic relapsing or progressive MS. Acute disseminated encephalomyelitis is an acute, typically monophasic, and postinfectious CNS inflammatory demyelinating disease. It may be severe; however, if recurrent episodes are separated by at least 3 months, a diagnosis of RRMS should be considered.

Neuromyelitis optica is an autoimmune disease with severe acute attacks that are typically restricted to the optic nerves and spinal cord. However, other brainstem and deep cerebral structures, such as the area postrema, cerebral white matter, and hypothalamus, can also be involved. Brain MRI findings are usually not consistent with MS, at least early on in the disease, and a specific water channel autoantibody (aquaporin-4-IgG) is found in most cases.

Clinical syndromes of CNS demyelination with myelitis, optic neuritis, and acute disseminated encephalomyelitis with serologic presence of antibodies to myelin oligodendrocyte glycoprotein are increasingly recognized. Optic neuritis may be further mimicked by acute ischemic optic neuropathy. This condition is typically painless, occurs suddenly, and occurs in patients with advanced age and preexisting vascular risk factors.

Figure 1 Magnetic resonance image showing brain T_1 gadolinium-enhancing lesions (A) and T_2 thoracic spine (B) typical of multiple sclerosis.

Progressive myelopathies that mimic PPMS or SPMS include a compressive myelopathy (e.g., cervical spondylosis, disc disease, or neoplastic infiltration), nutritional deficiencies (e.g., vitamin B_{12} or copper deficiency), infectious causes (e.g., HTLV1), genetic causes (e.g., adrenoleukodystrophy), paraneoplastic disease (e.g., CRMP-5 auto-antibodies), systemic disorders (e.g., sarcoidosis), or a progressive vascular cause (e.g., dural arteriovenous fistula).

Treatment

Acute demyelinating MS attacks (relapses) may be treated with high doses of corticosteroids. These may be given orally or intravenously; however, high doses of corticosteroids are necessary and are superior to low doses. For example, a typical regimen is intravenous methylprednisolone (Solu-Medrol) 1000 mg once daily for 3 to 5 days without oral corticosteroid tapering doses. The oral equivalent to this intravenous regimen is prednisone 1000 to 1250 mg orally once daily for 3 to 5 days with no oral corticosteroid taper afterward. Gastrointestinal intolerance occurs in some patients, and concomitant use of stomach-protecting agents such as proton pump inhibitors may be recommended. Typical acute corticosteroid side effects include insomnia, irritability, and increased appetite. There are rare but well-known associations with avascular necrosis of the hip and acute psychosis. Chronic corticosteroid side effects such as diabetes mellitus, cataracts, osteoporosis, adrenal suppression, weight gain, and cushingoid habitus are more associated with chronic corticosteroid use and not short courses of steroids.

Generally, only MS attacks that are associated with functional impairment (vision loss, diplopia, motor weakness, and ataxia) are treated because clinical recovery is hastened, but final clinical recovery is not found to be altered by this therapy. Occasionally, patients have very severe acute attacks of MS or other demyelinating disease that does not improve with use of high-dose corticosteroids. In these patients, the use of plasma exchange (seven exchanges over approximately 14 days) is recommended. Approximately 45% of patients experience functional recovery within 1 month following plasma exchange. Side effects of plasma exchange therapy include paresthesias related to hypocalcemia, anemia, thrombocytopenia, or complications of central venous access that is required for many patients. Intravenous immunoglobulin (Gammagard)[1] has not yet been shown to improve severe clinical attacks of demyelinating disease.

Disease-modifying therapies (DMTs) are chronic immunomodulatory treatments used to reduce the number of clinical attacks of MS (somewhere between 30% and 70%, depending on the agent) and to reduce new inflammatory MRI lesions (somewhere between 40% and 95%, depending on the agent). The traditional approach to choosing a DMT is to start most patients on an agent that is relatively safe but of lower efficacy and only "escalating" if the disease is not controlled. This strategy is referred to as an "escalation approach." Newer therapies are more efficacious but have the potential for more side effects and have less known long-term risks. Starting with higher efficacy DMTs to minimize breakthrough disease that may leave permanent neurologic disability is known as an "induction approach" and is increasingly used by some MS experts. Trials are ongoing to compare long-term MS outcomes of these two treatment strategies. Either way, patients and healthcare professionals should realize that the medications are specifically for reduction in relapse-related disease and do not provide a cure or any symptomatic benefit.

Chronic parenteral therapy for RRMS includes the use of type 1 β interferons, glatiramer acetate (Copaxone), natalizumab (Tysabri), alemtuzumab (Lemtrada), ocrelizumab (Ocrevus), ofatumumab (Kesimpta), and ublituximab (Briumvi) (Table 1). Alternatively, oral therapies can be used and include teriflunomide

(Aubagio), sphingosine-1-phosphate (S1P) receptor modulators, and the fumarates. The S1P receptor modulators include fingolimod (Gilenya), siponimod (Mayzent), ozanimod (Zeposia), and ponesimod (Ponvory). Dimethyl fumarate (Tecfidera) was the first fumarate available. More recently, diroximel fumarate (Vumerity) and monomethyl fumarate (Bafiertam) have been approved. Cladribine (Mavenclad) is an oral medication for treatment-resistant disease as a second-line therapy. The FDA product labels for most of these parenteral and oral therapies have recently been updated to specifically include CIS and SPMS with activity (ongoing relapses and/or new MRI lesions co-occurring with progressive disease) as approved indications for their use. Cladribine is not recommended for CIS because of its side effect profile. Ocrelizumab is approved for treatment of all clinical courses of CNS demyelinating disease, including CIS, RRMS, SPMS with activity, and PPMS course.

The side effect profile is well known for traditional injectable agents such as interferons and glatiramer acetate (see Table 1), and they have been safely used for many years. The safety profile for oral therapies seems satisfactory, but their long-term side effect profile is still being assessed. For fingolimod, first-dose monitoring for 6 hours is required to assess heart rate and rhythm, and an eye exam is needed to screen for macular edema before initiating the medication and after several months. Serious infections including progressive multifocal leukoencephalopathy (PML) and disseminated varicella zoster have been reported. Additional S1P receptor modulators have been developed with similar but distinct receptor binding in an effort to improve the side effect profile. One such agent, siponimod, was studied and approved for use in individuals with secondary progressive MS with ongoing disease activity. As a result of more selective binding, siponimod has fewer cardiac side effects, requiring first-dose cardiac monitoring only in select circumstances. It does, however, require CYP genotyping before initiation because of genetic differences in drug metabolism. Ponesimod requires first-dose cardiac monitoring in some individuals but does not require genetic testing. Ozanimod does not require genetic screening or cardiac monitoring, although there is a theoretical risk of serotonin syndrome, and the concurrent use of monoamine oxidase inhibitors is not recommended.

Teriflunomide may be associated with liver disease, reactivation of tuberculosis, and teratogenicity. Dimethyl fumarate is associated with flushing and gastrointestinal discomfort, and rare patients have developed PML when taking this medication. Diroximel fumarate, a structurally similar drug, showed improved gastrointestinal tolerability compared with dimethyl fumarate in a clinical trial. Monomethyl fumarate, the active metabolite of dimethyl fumarate and diroximel fumarate, was not studied in a trial specific to patients with MS but was approved based on mechanism of action and safety data when studied in healthy individuals.

Highly active MS therapy may be indicated with natalizumab, alemtuzumab, or anti-CD20 agents (ocrelizumab, ofatumumab, and ublituximab) if first-line medications are intolerable, if therapeutic response is suboptimal (continued MS attacks or marked ongoing and new inflammatory disease on MRI despite therapy), or when a concerning clinical onset (severe attack with multiple lesions and incomplete recovery) occurs.

Natalizumab is clearly associated with the development of PML, a severely impairing and often fatal opportunistic brain infection caused by reactivation of the dormant JC virus. In North America, natalizumab is only available through the Tysabri Outreach: Unified Commitment to Health prescribing program. Risk factors for PML in natalizumab-treated patients include the presence and index value of JC virus serum antibody (JCV-Ab), duration of therapy of at least 2 years, and history of prior immunosuppressive medication therapy (e.g., methotrexate, azathioprine). Seropositivity of patients with MS for JC virus antibody is over 55%. The seroconversion rate from JC virus Ab negativity to positivity is approximately 2% to 5% per year, and false-negative results are rare (less than 3%). Currently, no cases

---

[1] Not FDA approved for this indication.

TABLE 1 Approved Immunomodulatory Therapy for Multiple Sclerosis

MEDICATION	DOSING	SIDE EFFECTS	MONITORING	ADDITIONAL INFORMATION
Interferon β1a (Avonex)	30 µg IM injection every week	Flulike symptoms (fever, chills, arthralgias, myalgias, and headaches), elevated LFTs, anemia, leukopenia, thrombocytopenia, depression, localized injection site rejections	CBC with differential, AST, ALT, ALP, and total bilirubin level at baseline, at 3 months, at 6 months × 2 years, and then annually Thyroid function cascade on initiation of therapy	Premedication with acetaminophen can ameliorate postinjection flulike symptoms
Interferon β1a (Rebif)	22-µg or 44-µg SC injection three times per week	Flulike symptoms (fever, chills, arthralgias, myalgias, headaches), elevated LFTs, anemia, leukopenia, thrombocytopenia, depression, localized injection site rejections	CBC with differential, AST, ALT, ALP, and total bilirubin level at baseline, at 3 months, at 6 months × 2 years, and then annually Thyroid function cascade on initiation of therapy	Premedication with acetaminophen can ameliorate postinjection flulike symptoms
Peginterferon β1a (Plegridy)	125 µg SC every 2 weeks	Flulike symptoms (fever, chills, arthralgias, myalgias, headaches), elevated LFTs, anemia, leukopenia, thrombocytopenia, depression, localized injection site rejections	CBC with differential, AST, ALT, ALP, and total bilirubin level at baseline, at 3 months, at 6 months × 2 years, and then annually Thyroid function cascade on initiation of therapy	Premedication with acetaminophen may ameliorate postinjection flulike symptoms
Interferon β1b (Betaseron, Extavia)	250-µg SC injection every other day	Flulike symptoms (fever, chills, arthralgias, myalgias, headaches), elevated LFTs, anemia, leukopenia, thrombocytopenia, depression, localized injection site rejections	CBC with differential, AST, ALT, ALP, and total bilirubin level at baseline, at 3 months, at 6 months × 2 years, and then annually Thyroid function cascade on initiation of therapy	Premedication with acetaminophen can ameliorate postinjection flulike symptoms
Glatiramer acetate (Copaxone)	20-mg SC injection daily or 40-mg SC injection three times per week	Injection site reactions (erythema, edema, pruritus, pain), transient chest pain, palpitations, facial flushing, anxiety, shortness of breath	None	
Fingolimod hydrochloride (Gilenya)	0.5 mg PO once daily	Headache, flulike symptoms, diarrhea, back pain, liver enzyme elevations, cough, hypertension, macular edema, and infections (disseminated varicella and herpes, rare cases of PML, opportunistic bacterial and fungal infections), increased risk of skin cancer; may cause a decrease in pulmonary function New FDA labeling required, investigating unexplained deaths occurring during treatment with fingolimod	CBC with differential, AST, ALT, and bilirubin at baseline and periodically thereafter Serology for VZV-IgG to determine immunity; if negative, vaccinate; if live-attenuated vaccine, give at least 4 weeks before initiation Latent infection screening (HIV, hepatitis, TB) in those at high risk Fundus examination at baseline and in 3–4 months for macular edema, repeated annually in those with diabetes mellitus or uveitis or if visual symptoms develop ECG, HR, and BP before first dose; first dose must be monitored for 6 hours for HR reduction and BP changes; 6-hour monitoring following oral dose must be repeated for patients who discontinue therapy for ≥2 weeks Periodic skin examinations	Should not be used in patients with recent MI, unstable angina, stroke, TIA, second- or third-degree AV block, CHF, SSS without cardiac pacing, or QTc >500 ms, or with class Ia or III antiarrhythmic drugs Overnight continuous ECG monitoring recommended for those with preexisting cardiac or cerebrovascular disease; recurrent syncope; severe, untreated OSA; use of β blockers; or prolonged QTc Caution for redemonstration of severe inflammatory disease on discontinuation

Drug	Dosing	Adverse Effects	Monitoring	Special Considerations
Siponimod (Mayzent)	Requires oral titration; the recommended maintenance dosage for most is 2 mg PO once daily. The recommended maintenance dosage in patients with a CYP2C9*1/*3 or CYP2C9*2/*3 genotype is 1 mg PO once daily. Contraindicated in CYP2C9*3/*3 genotype	Herpes infection, upper respiratory infection, fungal skin infection, hypertension, macular edema; may cause a decrease in pulmonary function	CYP2C9 genotype determination. CBC with differential, AST, ALT, and bilirubin at baseline and then periodically. Serology for VZV-IgG to determine immunity; if negative, vaccinate; give a live-attenuated vaccine at least 4 weeks before initiation. Latent infection screening (HIV, hepatitis, TB) in those at high risk. Fundus evaluation (OCT) at baseline and then annually for those with diabetes and uveitis or if visual symptoms develop. Recent ECG (within past 6 months) and baseline BP	Concomitant use of moderate or strong CYP3A4 inducers (e.g., modafinil, efavirenz [Sustiva]) is not recommended for patients with CYP2C9*1/*3 and CYP2C9*2/*3 genotype. Should not be used in patients with MI, unstable angina, stroke, TIA, or class III/IV CHF in the past 6 months or in patients with second- or third-degree AV block or in those with SSS unless the patient has a pacemaker. First-dose monitoring is recommended for patients with certain preexisting cardiac conditions; initial monitoring procedures must be repeated for interruption of treatment of ≥4 consecutive doses. Unknown whether rebound disease occurs with discontinuation, as seen in fingolimod
Ponesimod (Ponvory)	Requires oral titration; maintenance dose is 20 mg PO once daily	Herpes infection, upper respiratory infection, fungal skin infection, hypertension, macular edema, increased rate of cutaneous malignancies; may cause a decrease in pulmonary function	CBC with differential, AST, ALT, and bilirubin at baseline and then periodically. Serology for VZV-IgG to determine immunity; if negative, vaccinate; give a live-attenuated vaccine at least 4 weeks before initiation. Latent infection screening (HIV, hepatitis, TB) in those at high risk. Fundus evaluation (OCT) at baseline and then annually for those with diabetes and uveitis or if visual symptoms develop. Recent ECG (i.e., within past 6 months) and baseline BP. Periodic skin examinations	Should not be used in patients with MI, unstable angina, stroke, TIA, or class III/IV CHF in the past 6 months or in patients with second- or third-degree AV block or those with SSS unless the patient has a pacemaker. First-dose monitoring is recommended for patients with certain preexisting cardiac conditions; initial monitoring procedures must be repeated for interruption of treatment of ≥4 consecutive doses. Unknown whether rebound disease occurs with discontinuation, as seen in fingolimod
Ozanimod (Zeposia)	Requires oral titration; maintenance dose is 0.92 mg PO once daily	Herpes infection, upper respiratory infection, fungal skin infection, hypertension, macular edema; may cause a decrease in pulmonary function	CBC with differential, AST, ALT, and bilirubin at baseline and periodically thereafter. Serology for VZV-IgG to determine immunity; if negative, vaccinate; give a live-attenuated vaccine at least 4 weeks before initiation. Latent infection screening (HIV, hepatitis, TB) in those at high risk. Fundus evaluation (OCT) at baseline and then annually for those with diabetes and uveitis or if visual symptoms develop. Recent ECG (within past 6 months) and baseline BP	Should not be used in patients with MI, unstable angina, stroke, TIA, or class III/IV CHF in the past 6 months or in patients with second- or third-degree AV block or those with SSS unless the patient has a pacemaker. Do not use in severe untreated OSA or with concomitant use of an MAOI. Cardiac monitoring and genetic testing not needed. Unknown whether rebound disease occurs with discontinuation, as seen in fingolimod
Teriflunomide (Aubagio)	7 mg or 14 mg PO once daily	Diarrhea, abnormal LFTs, nausea, alopecia, hepatotoxicity, may cause significant birth defects if used during pregnancy, hypertension, peripheral neuropathy, can worsen psoriasis, TB reactivation, transient acute renal failure, hyperkalemia	CBC at baseline, 6 months, and then annually. AST, ALP, and bilirubin monthly for 6 months and then annually. Latent infection screening (HIV and hepatitis) in those at high risk. Tuberculin skin test and pregnancy test (women of childbearing potential) at baseline. BP at baseline and then periodically	Do not use in severe hepatotoxicity, pregnancy, or with concomitant leflunomide use. Prolonged half-life: recommend removal by activated charcoal or cholestyramine when required. Pregnancy: teratogenic, accelerated washout recommended before conception

Continued

TABLE 1 Approved Immunomodulatory Therapy for Multiple Sclerosis—cont'd

MEDICATION	DOSING	SIDE EFFECTS	MONITORING	ADDITIONAL INFORMATION
Dimethyl fumarate (Tecfidera)	120 mg PO twice daily for 1 week, then 240 mg PO twice daily	Flushing, abdominal pain, nausea, diarrhea, infection (rare cases of PML, disseminated herpes), lymphopenia, hepatotoxicity	CBC with differential at baseline and then every 6–12 months; if lymphopenia occurs, monitor more frequently; may need to discontinue AST, ALT, ALP, and bilirubin at baseline Latent infection screening (HIV, hepatitis, TB) in those at high risk	Discontinue in sustained lymphopenia ($<0.5 \times 10^9$/L) because increases risk of infections including PML or LFT elevation (>20x upper limit of normal or jaundice)
Monomethyl fumarate (Bafiertam)	95 mg PO twice daily for 1 week, then increase to 190 mg PO twice daily	Flushing, infection, lymphopenia, abdominal symptoms but generally less than dimethyl fumarate, hepatotoxicity	CBC with differential at baseline, at 6 months, and then annually AST, ALT, ALP, and bilirubin at baseline Latent infection screening (HIV, hepatitis, TB) in those at high risk	
Diroximel fumarate (Vumerity)	231 mg PO twice daily for 1 week, then increase to 462 mg PO twice daily	Flushing, infection, lymphopenia, abdominal symptoms but generally less than dimethyl fumarate	CBC with differential at baseline, at 6 months, and then every 6–12 months AST, ALT, ALP, and bilirubin at baseline Latent infection screening (HIV, hepatitis, TB) in those at high risk	Improved gastrointestinal intolerance
Ocrelizumab (Ocrevus)	300 mg IV once followed by a 300 mg dose 2 weeks later, then 600 mg IV every 24 weeks	Infusion reactions, respiratory tract infections, herpes infections, neutropenia, reduced immunoglobulins Possible increased risk of cancer including breast cancer; follow standard cancer screening	Rule out active hepatitis and latent TB before first dose; consult liver specialist if history of hepatitis before first dose Immunoglobulins at baseline and then annually	Do not administer if signs of infection; delay until infection resolves. If IgG <150 mg/dL or 150–500 mg/dL with recurrent infections, consider IVIg replacement Administer vaccines >6 weeks before ocrelizumab infusions; live and live-attenuated vaccines not recommended until B-cell counts recover after discontinuation
Ofatumumab (Kesimpta)	Initial dosing: 20 mg SC injection at weeks 0, 1, and 2 Subsequent dosing: 20 mg SC injection every 4 weeks starting at week 4	Injection reactions most common within 24 hours of the first injection Respiratory tract infections, herpes infections, neutropenia, reduced immunoglobulins	Rule out active hepatitis and latent TB before first dose Immunoglobulins at baseline and then annually	Do not administer if signs of infection; delay until infection resolves. If IgG <150 mg/dL or 150–500 mg/dL with recurrent infections, consider IVIg replacement Administer live and live-attenuated vaccines >4 weeks and inactivated vaccines >2 weeks before initiation; live and live-attenuated vaccines not recommended until B-cell counts recover after discontinuation
Ublituximab (Briumvi)	150 mg IV once followed by a 450-mg IV dose 2 weeks later, then 450 mg IV every 24 weeks	Infusion reactions possible, recommend patient monitoring for 1 hour after the first two infusions Respiratory tract infections, urinary tract infections, neutropenia, reduced immunoglobulins	Rule out active hepatitis before first dose Immunoglobulins at baseline and then annually	Do not administer if signs of infection; delay until infection resolves. If IgG <150 mg/dL or 150–500 mg/dL with recurrent infections, consider IVIg replacement Administer live and live-attenuated vaccines >4 weeks and inactivated vaccines >2 weeks before initiation; live and live-attenuated vaccines not recommended until B-cell counts recover after discontinuation

Drug	Dosing	Side effects	Monitoring	Considerations
Natalizumab (Tysabri)	300 mg IV once every 4 weeks	Urticaria and anaphylaxis, headache, arthralgias, nausea, depression, infections (urinary tract, pneumonia, herpes simplex or reactivation) Rare hypersensitivity reactions can occur and are often associated with antibodies against natalizumab; if occurs, DMT switch is required	Baseline JCV Ab serologic study every 6 months while JCV negative; if JCV seropositive, consider another DMT If conversion occurs while on drug, strong consideration should be given to switching DMT with interim close monitoring; extended dosing interval of 6–8 weeks can be considered, but long-term a switch is recommended If PML is suspected, discontinue immediately, PLEX to remove the drug, MRI head with and without gadolinium with diffusion-weighted imaging; CSF for JCV PCR	Risk of PML may be greater in patients with prolonged therapy and those previously treated with immunosuppressive medications; prescribing professional requires TOUCH enrollment Caution for redemonstration of severe inflammatory disease on discontinuation
Alemtuzumab (Lemtrada)	IV infusion over 4 h × two treatment courses First course: 12 mg/day on 5 consecutive days Second course: 12 mg/day on 3 consecutive days 12 months after the first treatment course	Infusion reactions with anaphylaxis; rarely MI, stroke, cervicocephalic artery dissections Autoimmune thyroid disorders, immune thrombocytopenia, antiglomerular basement membrane disease Malignancies including thyroid cancer, melanoma, lymphoproliferative disorders Opportunistic infections (PML, herpes, varicella, and other viral, bacterial, and fungal infections)	CBC with differential; serum creatinine; urinalysis with urine cell counts at baseline, then monthly; and TSH at baseline and then every 3 months until 48 months after last dose ALT, AST, bilirubin at baseline and then periodically until 48 months after last dose Serology for VZV-IgG to determine immunity; if negative, vaccinate, if live-attenuated vaccine, give at least 6 weeks before initiation Ensure no infections (HIV, hepatitis, TB) before treatment Baseline and yearly skin and cervical examinations	Contraindicated if HIV positive Premedicate with high-dose corticosteroids, and give herpetic prophylaxis at time of first dose, continuing for at least 2 months or until CD4+ lymphocyte count is >200 cells/μL, whichever occurs later Complete all necessary immunizations at least 6 weeks before initiation No live virus vaccines after a course of alemtuzumab
Cladribine (Mavenclad)	Two treatment courses (1.75 mg/kg per treatment course); one course per year for a total of 2 years Treatment course is divided into 2 treatment weeks separated by 4 weeks: each treatment week consists of 4–5 days on which a patient receives a single daily dose (dose depending on body weight)	Anemia, thrombocytopenia, lymphopenia, upper respiratory tract infection, headache, hypersensitivity reaction, may increase risk of malignancies	CBC 2 and 6 months after the start of each treatment course and then annually thereafter Ensure no infections (HIV, hepatitis, TB) before treatment Serology for VZV-IgG to determine immunity; if negative, vaccinate, if live-attenuated vaccine, give at least 4–6 weeks before initiation If lymphocyte count at month 2 is <200 cells/mL, hold cladribine, monitor monthly until month 6, and then administer herpes prophylaxis Follow standard cancer screening guidelines	Contraindicated in infections (HIV, active hepatitis, TB), current malignancy, pregnant women, and women and men of reproductive potential who do not plan to use contraception during dosing and for 6 months after the last dose in each treatment course Administer live-attenuated or live vaccines at least 4–6 weeks before starting; avoid vaccination with live-attenuated or live vaccines during and after treatment

Ab, Antibody; *ALP*, alkaline phosphatase; *ALT*, alanine aminotransferase; *AST*, aspartate aminotransferase; *AV*, atrioventricular; *BP*, blood pressure; *CBC*, complete blood count; *CHF*, congestive heart failure; *ECG*, electrocardiogram; *HR*, heart rate; *HIV*, human immunodeficiency virus; *IgG*, immunoglobulin G; *JCV*, JC virus; *LFT*, liver function test; *MI*, myocardial infarction; *MAOI*, monoamine oxidase inhibitor; *OCT*, optical coherence tomography; *OSA*, obstructive sleep apnea; *PCR*, polymerase chain reaction; *PLEX*, plasma exchange; *PML*, progressive multifocal leukoencephalopathy; *PO*, by mouth; *SC*, subcutaneously; *SSS*, sick sinus syndrome; *TB*, tuberculosis; *TIA*, transient ischemic attack; *TOUCH*, Tysabri Outreach: Unified Commitment to Health; *TSH*, thyroid-stimulating hormone; *VZV-IgG*, varicella zoster virus immunoglobulin G.

of PML have been found in patients persistently seronegative for JCV-Abs. Risk prevalence estimation after 2 years of treatment in JCV Ab–positive patients ranges from 1:250 for those without a history of immunosuppression to 1:90 in those with a history of prior immunosuppressive therapy. Evidence is emerging for extending the dosing interval to every 6 to 8 weeks in select individuals as a strategy to lower the risk of PML but maintain drug efficacy.

Ocrelizumab (anti-CD20 B cells; humanized form), an every-6-month infusion, is approved for relapsing MS and is the only therapy approved for PPMS. Initial clinical trials of ocrelizumab showed an increased rate of breast cancer in patients treated with ocrelizumab compared with those on placebo or interferons. As such, the FDA approval label recommends advising patients regarding a potential increased malignancy rate and that patients follow standard breast cancer screening guidelines. More recently, long-term follow-up safety data from several clinical trials, including open-label extension periods, were published and showed no increased risk of malignancy, including breast cancer, compared with matched reference MS and general populations. Ofatumumab is another anti-CD20 B-cell–depleting monoclonal antibody that has a similar risk profile to ocrelizumab but is given monthly through an autoinjector. The most recently FDA-approved anti-CD20 B-cell–depleting agent, ublituximab, is given every 6 months as an intravenous infusion and again shares a similar side effect profile.

Alemtuzumab is a monoclonal antibody (anti-CD52; T and B cells) for RRMS with major safety precautions that include potential for malignancy and the development of autoimmune thyroid disease, immune thrombocytopenia, and, rarely, antiglomerular basement membrane disease. More recently, serious and life-threatening infusion reactions including strokes and arterial dissections have been reported with alemtuzumab.

Mitoxantrone is a chemotherapy agent that is approved for SPMS, but given its severe side effect profile (acute and delayed cardiotoxicity, acute myelogenous leukemia), it is rarely used today. Daclizumab (Zinbryta) (anti-CD25, interleukin [IL]-2 receptor) was withdrawn voluntarily because of case reports of an association with presumably immune-mediated encephalitis.

Available, although limited, evidence suggests that autologous bone marrow transplantation with stem cell delivery is a promising therapy for select patients with MS. It appears that individuals most likely to benefit are young, are ambulatory, have recent disease onset, and have ongoing disease activity despite having tried first- and second-line agents. Risks are "front-loaded" and include the adverse effects resulting from cytotoxic agents (nausea, mucositis, and alopecia) and myelosuppression (infection and hemorrhage). Late toxicity includes engraftment syndrome, infertility, infection, myelodysplastic syndromes, and secondary autoimmune disorders. Several large randomized controlled trials are ongoing to supplement existing evidence.

The mechanism of action of most DMTs is to modulate the immune system. This can have important implications on timing of vaccine delivery (see Table 1) and vaccine response. Immunization status should be discussed early, and generally patients should be encouraged to update their vaccines as per public health guidelines. Administration of non-live vaccines is considered safe in patients with MS, including those taking a DMT, although response may be diminished with specific DMTs such as anti-CD20 B-cell–depleting agents and S1P receptor modulators. If a patient is experiencing an acute MS relapse, vaccination should be deferred until after symptoms resolve or plateau. If a patient has recently received a course of steroids, it is recommended to wait 6 weeks before vaccinating if possible. The inactivated seasonal influenza vaccine and non-live coronavirus disease 2019 (COVID-19) vaccines are recommended in all patients with MS. Guidelines regarding the number and timing of COVID-19 vaccinations are continuously changing as the understanding and epidemiology of COVID-19 evolve. Currently, consideration should be given to vaccination against COVID-19 before initiation of anti-CD20

B-cell–depleting agents and S1P receptor modulators because both have been shown to impair vaccine response. The Centers for Disease Control and Prevention recently recommended Shingrix, a recombinant non-live vaccine against herpes zoster, to individuals older than 18 years of age who are immunocompromised, such as those with MS on immunosuppressing DMTs. Live and live-attenuated vaccines should be avoided in persons with MS if possible. When needed, administration should be done before initiation of DMT, with timing dependent on the specific agent used (see Table 1). For instance, immunity against varicella zoster should be confirmed before initiating an S1P receptor modulator given reports of disseminated varicella on fingolimod. This requires a live vaccination series to be completed at least 1 month before beginning the S1P modulator to allow time for the vaccine to take effect.

Pregnancy and Lactation

Given the demographics of people diagnosed with multiple sclerosis, the use of DMTs around pregnancy and lactation is a commonly encountered scenario. Generally, DMTs are avoided during pregnancy because this is a time when new attacks and new lesions are less likely to occur, although an increase is often seen postpartum. No agent has FDA approval for use in pregnancy. Pregnancy registries show no clear or major safety risks regarding the use of interferons and glatiramer acetate during pregnancy, and these agents are occasionally continued on a case-by-case basis. Natalizumab has risk for severe MS rebound disease when stopped, and pregnancy does not appear to be protective against this. Therefore some clinicians will continue natalizumab off-label until 30 to 34 weeks of gestation with extended interval dosing (every 6–8 weeks) and then resume 1 to 2 weeks postpartum with screening of the newborn for hematologic abnormalities. FDA labels recommend a 6-month washout from last dose to time of conception for anti-CD20s, although based on pharmacokinetics, some clinicians will allow a shorter washout. It is recommended that the patient avoid becoming pregnant for at least 4 months following the last alemtuzumab infusion.

Oral agents are contraindicated during pregnancy. It is recommended that conception only be attempted 6 months after the last cladribine dose. A 2-month washout is recommended for fingolimod but risk for rebound of MS disease activity exists, so a switch to another agent is often entertained in advance of pregnancy planning. Teriflunomide is teratogenic and requires an accelerated washout or 24-month waiting period. Dimethyl fumarate can be stopped at the time of conception planning.

With respect to lactation, oral agents should again be avoided because they are small molecules and can pass into breast milk. Injectables and infusion-based monoclonal antibodies are sometimes used off-label on a case-by-case basis because breast milk transfer of these large molecules appears to be minimal and risk of exposure to the newborn is low.

Monitoring

Most, if not all, patients with MS should be followed by a neurologist at least occasionally. Recommendations for clinical assessment range from 6 to 18 months, depending on clinical activity of relapses and disability. The ideal scheduling of repeat brain MRI scans is controversial and varies depending on MS clinical activity and whether medications are initiated, changed, or discontinued, but general recommendations are every 1 to 2 years in stable patients.

Complications

MS is one of the main causes for impairment at a young age and trails only acute trauma. Often patients need gait assistance when impairment becomes more severe. This includes the use of a single gait aid, such as a cane or walking stick, or an ankle-foot orthosis for symptomatic foot drop. Dalfampridine (Ampyra) is a potassium channel blocker that has been shown to improve walking speed. Contraindications include a history of seizures and moderate to severe renal impairment.

Spasticity associated with upper motor neuron weakness in the lower extremities may be treated with an active daily exercise program directed by physical therapists and physiatrists. Judicious use of baclofen (Lioresal) is helpful (typically starting at 5 mg three times daily, with no more than a maximum of 80 mg per day). Baclofen side effects include drowsiness and liver enzyme elevations. Some patients with significant lower extremity weakness are assisted in their gait by the leg support provided by spasticity, and if spasticity is reduced pharmacologically, this can in fact worsen their gait. Alternatives to baclofen include tizanidine (Zanaflex) and clonidine (Catapres).[1] For focal spasticity, botulinum toxin (Botox) injection can be used. Gabapentin (Neurontin)[1] can be helpful as an adjuvant therapy, particularly in those with neuropathic pain or for monotherapy in those who failed first line agents. Oral cannabinoids (tetrahydrocannabinol and cannabidiol [Sativex][2]) have favorable evidence for patient-reported symptoms of spasticity, spasms, and central pain but may have cognitive side effects. Benzodiazepines have antispasticity properties but are not typically first line because of side effects and potential for dependency. Dantrolene (Dantrium) has been shown to be effective but is rarely used because of hepatoxicity.

Patients often experience symptoms of neurogenic bladder dysfunction. This includes symptoms of urinary urgency and urge-related incontinence. Bladder stimulants such as caffeine should be avoided. Patients with neurogenic bladder should be investigated for completeness of bladder emptying. If there is severe impairment in bladder emptying, urinary catheterization often is recommended. If bladder emptying is complete or only mildly impaired (<100 mL postvoid residual), use of medications such as oxybutynin (Ditropan), solifenacin (Vesicare), and tolterodine (Detrol) may be recommended for urge-related symptoms. These anticholinergic medications can cause confusion and should be used with caution in older adults or those with cognitive dysfunction. Mirabegron (Myrbetriq) may be preferable in such situations as it selectively acts as a beta-3 adrenergic receptor agonist to relax the detrusor smooth muscle but requires monitoring for hypertension. Regardless of drug choice, ongoing monitoring of bladder emptying is recommended. Some patients require formal urodynamic evaluation for complex bladder symptoms.

Constipation is a common symptom that may exacerbate neurogenic bladder symptoms. Treatment includes physical exercise, dietary fiber supplementation, and hydration. Stool softeners, promotility agents, bulking agents, or enemas may be required. Sexual dysfunction can occur in men and women, including reduced libido either with or without difficulty achieving erection and/or orgasm. Management may include nonpharmacologic and pharmacologic strategies similar to those used in non–MS-related sexual dysfunction.

Fatigue is a common MS-related symptom. A complete sleep history to ensure appropriate sleep hygiene is imperative. This includes initiating sleep promptly, maintaining sleep throughout the night, and awakening feeling refreshed. Encouragement of a formal exercise program to facilitate restful sleep and daytime vigor is important. Obstructive sleep apnea, restless leg syndrome, and other parasomnias must be ruled out as additional contributing factors to fatigue. If sleep hygiene is entirely normal and late afternoon fatigue remains a problem, pharmacologic therapy for MS-related fatigue can be considered. Medications that can be considered for debilitating MS fatigue that does not respond to nonpharmacologic management include amantadine hydrochloride (Symmetrel),[1] modafinil (Provigil),[1] armodafinil (Nuvigil),[1] amphetamines (including methylphenidate [Ritalin][1]), and fluoxetine (Prozac).[1] None of these medications have FDA approval specific to MS fatigue. The benefit of these medications remains unproven, and their use is often limited by their side effect profile.

Neuropathic pain and other uncomfortable sensations can occur in MS. Neuropathic pain agents such as gabapentin (Neurontin)[1] pregabalin (Lyrica),[1] duloxetine (Cymbalta),[1] and tricyclic antidepressants are frequently used. Paroxysmal attacks of sensory (Lhermitte phenomenon and trigeminal neuralgia) and motor (painful tonic spasms) symptoms can cause discomfort and interfere with function. Both sensory and motor symptoms are typically very sensitive to low-dose carbamazepine (Tegretol).[1]

Mood disorders such as anxiety and depression are prevalent in MS. Treatment includes nonpharmacologic management such as cognitive-behavioral therapy, and medications may be warranted in some patients. Pseudobulbar affect, uncontrollable episodes of laughter or crying, may occur. If this symptom is bothersome to the patient, dextromethorphan/quinidine (Nuedexta) is approved for this indication. Selective serotonin reuptake inhibitors, serotonin-norepinephrine reuptake inhibitors, and tricyclic antidepressants have been used off-label for pseudobulbar affect.

MS is a common CNS inflammatory demyelinating disease with heterogenous presentation and prognosis. CIS, RRMS, and active SPMS are treated with corticosteroids to hasten resolution of acute relapses and chronic immunomodulatory medications to reduce the number of future clinical attacks and new MRI lesions. Ocrelizumab is the only medication approved for PPMS. Symptomatic care is important in these patients, including the treatment of gait disorder, spasticity, neurogenic sphincter dysfunction, fatigue, paroxysmal symptoms, neuropathic pain, and mood disorders.

---

[1] Not FDA approved for this indication.

References

Ho PR, Koendgen H, Campbell N, et al: Risk of natalizumab-associated progressive multifocal leukoencephalopathy in patients with multiple sclerosis: a retrospective analysis of data from four clinical studies, *Lancet Neurol* 16:925–933, 2017.

Kjetil B, et al: Longitudinal analysis reveals high prevalence of Epstein-Barr virus associated with multiple sclerosis, *Science* 375(6578):296–301, 2022.

Langer-Gould A, Brara SM, Beaber BE, Zhang JL: Incidence of multiple sclerosis in multiple racial and ethnic groups, *Neurology* 80(19):1734–1739, 2013.

Montalban X, Belachew S, Wolinsky JS: Ocrelizumab in primary progressive and relapsing multiple sclerosis, *N Engl J Med* 376:1694, 2017.

Reich DS, Lucchinetti CF, Calabresi PA: Multiple sclerosis, *N Engl J Med* 378:169–180, 2018.

Sharrack B, Saccardi R, Alexander T, et al: Autologous haematopoietic stem cell transplantation and other cellular therapy in multiple sclerosis and immune-mediated neurological diseases: updated guidelines and recommendations from the EBMT Autoimmune Diseases Working Party (ADWP) and the Joint Accreditation Committee of EBMT and ISCT (JACIE), *Bone Marrow Transplant* 55:283–306, 2020.

Thompson AJ, Banwell BL, Barkhof F, et al: Diagnosis of multiple sclerosis: 2017 revisions of the McDonald criteria, *Lancet Neurol* 17(2):162–173, 2018.

Traboulsee AL, Knox KB, Machan L, et al: Prevalence of extracranial venous narrowing on catheter venography in people with multiple sclerosis, their siblings, and unrelated healthy controls: a blinded, case-control study, *Lancet* 383(9912):138–145, 2014.

van Kempen ZLE, Hoogervorst ELJ, Wattjes MP, et al: Personalized extended interval dosing of natalizumab in MS: a prospective multicenter trial, *Neurology* 95(6):e745–e754, 2020.

Wallin MT, Culpepper WJ, Campbell JD, et al: The prevalence of MS in the United States: a population-based estimate using health claims data, *Neurology* 92(10):e1029–e1040, 2019.

---

[1] Not FDA approved for this indication.
[2] Not available in the United States.

MYASTHENIA GRAVIS

Method of
Taylor B. Harrison, MD; and William P. Roche, MD

CURRENT DIAGNOSIS

- Myasthenia gravis (MG) is an autoimmune disorder that affects the neuromuscular junction, resulting in fatigable skeletal muscle weakness.
- Diagnosis may be based on clinical history and exam in combination with identification of autoantibodies (Ach-R Abs) or abnormalities on electrodiagnostic testing.
- Myasthenic crisis, defined by respiratory failure, can stem from respiratory or oropharyngeal weakness. It may develop abruptly and typically occurs in the setting of illness, change in medications, or early in the disease course.

CURRENT THERAPY

- Mild symptoms can respond well to anticholinestrase inhibitors such as pyridostigmine (Mestinon).
- A wide range of medications may be used to treat MG, including steroids, nonsteroidal immunosuppressants, as well as intravenous immunoglobulin[1] and plasmapheresis. Thymectomy may be considered in patients with acetylcholine receptor antibodies.
- It is important to recognize that certain medications may worsen MG.
- Myasthenic crisis is a medical emergency, and patients should be treated in the intensive care unit with close respiratory monitoring and possibly intubation. Intravenous immunoglobulin[1] and plasmapheresis are treatment options for myasthenic crisis.

[1]Not FDA approved for this indication.

Epidemiology

Myasthenia gravis (MG) is the most common acquired disorder of neuromuscular transmission, with an incidence of 8 to 10 per million annually. The prevalence is 150 to 250 per million, reflecting the disease's low mortality rate. An estimated 700,000 people are living with MG worldwide, with between 36,000 to 60,000 living in the United States.

There exists a bimodal age distribution with two peaks of incidence: the first peak in the second to third decades of life, and a second peak in the seventh to eighth decades. Women predominate in early-onset MG (defined by onset <50 years of age) whereas men predominate with late-onset disease (>50 years of age).

Risk Factors

MG is associated with thymoma: approximately one-third of patients with thymoma will develop myasthenia, and 10% of myasthenic patients have a thymoma. Certain HLA subtypes, which are known to predispose to autoimmune disorders in general, also increase the risk of MG. Other autoimmune disorders are present in about 15% of myasthenic patients, most commonly thyroiditis, followed by systemic lupus erythematosus and rheumatoid arthritis. A small percentage of patients may have a myasthenia-myositis overlap syndrome (Tables 1 and 2).

Pathophysiology

To understand the pathophysiology, a review of normal physiology is needed. In normal muscle contraction, an action

TABLE 1	Medications That May Exacerbate or Precipitate MG
Black box warnings:	
Telithromycin (Ketek)[2]	
Fluoroquinolones (ciprofloxacin [Cipro], moxifloxacin [Avelox], levofloxacin [Levaquin])	
Drugs to avoid:	
D-penicillamine (Cuprimine)	
Checkpoint inhibitors (ipilimumab [Yervoy], pembrolizumab [Keytruda], nivolumab [Opdivo])	
Quinine	
IV Magnesium	
Use only with caution:	
Macrolidess (erythromycin, azithromycin [Zithromax], clarithromycin [Biaxin])	
Aminoglycosides (gentamycin [Garamycin], neomycin, tobramycin)	
Procainamide (Pronestyl)	
Desferrioxamine (Desferal)	
Beta blockers (propranolol, metoprolol [Lopressor], carvedilol [Coreg])	
Statins (atorvastatin [Lipitor], pravastatin [Pravachol], rosuvastatin [Crestor], simvastatin [Zocor])	

[2]Not available in the United States.

TABLE 2	Suggested Medication Monitoring
MEDICATION	**SUGGESTED MONITORING**
Azathioprine (Imuran)	CBC, LFTs weekly for the first month then monthly to every 3 months
Cyclosporine (Sandimmune)	Monthly CBC, LFTs, renal function monthly for 3 months then quarterly Periodic trough level Blood pressure checks
Cyclophosphamide (Cytoxan)	CBC (attention to neutrophil count), electrolytes and renal function, LFTs, UA every 2–4 weeks
Eculizumab (Soliris)	CBC, renal function, LFTs
IVIG (Gammagard)	Renal function monthly, with repeated dosing maybe every 3 months
Methotrexate (Trexall)	CBC, LFTs monthly initially, then at stable dose at least every 3 months
Mycophenolate mofetil	CBC every 2 weeks for first month, then monthly to quarterly
Plasma exchange	Blood pressure and serum calcium
Prednisone	Weight and blood pressure Periodic potassium and HgbA1c Bone density test Periodic eye exam
Rituximab (Rituxan)	CD 20 counts may be considered but varies among providers
Efgartigimod (Vyvgart)	Evaluate the need to administer age-appropriate immunizations (live attenuated or live vaccines) according to immunization guidelines before initiation of a new treatment cycle

CBC, Complete blood count.

potential (AP) travels down a motor nerve to the presynaptic axon terminal. At the axon terminal, the AP triggers voltage-gated calcium channels to open, causing calcium influx. Calcium influx causes synaptic vesicles containing acetylcholine to fuse with the cell membrane, resulting in exocytosis of acetylcholine into the synaptic cleft. Acetylcholine diffuses across the synaptic cleft and binds with nicotinic acetylcholine receptors (AchRs) on the cell membrane of the muscle fiber. The AchRs are ligand-gated ion channels that, once opened, allow cation influx, generating an end plate potential (EPP). When the EPP reaches a threshold value, it triggers voltage-gated sodium channels in the postsynaptic membrane to open, resulting in further cation influx and membrane depolarization, resulting in a muscle fiber AP and muscle fiber contraction. Excess acetylcholine is then broken down by the enzyme acetylcholinesterase (AchE) in the synaptic cleft.

The safety factor is an important concept in understanding the muscle fatigability of MG. The safety factor is the ratio of postsynaptic EPP generated by a quantity of acetylcholine to the threshold required to generate an all-or-none muscle fiber AP and thus muscle fiber contraction. In the healthy state, more acetylcholine is released than is needed to generate a muscle fiber AP. In myasthenia the safety factor is lower, and sufficient acetylcholine may not be released to generate successive APs with repeated contractions. Exercise will result in insufficient neuromuscular transmission over time because of this reduction in safety factor, and as muscle fibers fail to reach threshold to generate an AP, fatigable weakness ensues.

MG is caused by antibodies targeting antigens of the postsynaptic membrane of the neuromuscular junction. In myasthenia gravis, the normal action of acetylcholine at the postsynaptic muscle cell membrane is disrupted by one of several antibody-mediated mechanisms. Most commonly, antibodies are formed against the AchR itself. These AchR antibodies interrupt normal transmission by cross-linking the receptors causing increased turnover or complement-mediated degradation or by inducing conformational changes in the channel, keeping acetylcholine from activating the channel. Other antibodies have been found to cause MG, including antibodies against muscle-specific kinase (MUSK), lipoprotein-related protein 4 (LRP4), or agrin. The postsynaptic cell membrane is folded into secondary synaptic folds, increasing the surface area of the cell membrane, and AchRs are organized in clusters at the peaks of these folds (adjacent to the nerve axon terminal). MUSK, LRP4, and agrin are proteins that participate in AchR clustering on these peaks. Antibody-mediated disruption of the function of these proteins causes reduced AchR concentration on the postsynaptic membrane with reduced safety factor, resulting in a myasthenia phenotype.

Some patients do not have antibodies that are detectable by current serologic testing. These patients are presumed to have antibodies against components of the postsynaptic membrane that have not yet been identified.

Prevention

Although there is no recognized prevention for developing myasthenia, exacerbations (myasthenic crises) are preventable by avoiding certain drugs. In particular, beta blockers, some antibiotics (aminoglycosides, fluoroquinolones, and macrolides), and chelating agents (penicillamine [Cuprimine]) should be avoided in myasthenic patients (see Box 1). Statins should be used cautiously and only at the lowest effective dose.

Clinical Manifestations

Patients with MG will present with weakness of the extraocular, bulbar, axial, or limb muscles. The most characteristic feature of the weakness seen in myasthenia is fatigability; that is, the tendency of a muscle to get weaker with repeated use. Thus, when thinking about weakness from MG, it is important to get a sense of whether the patient's symptoms are exacerbated by exercise, or demonstrate a diurnal fluctuation (with the most typical pattern being weakness that is worse at the end of the day).

Ocular symptoms (ptosis and diplopia) are the first symptoms of myasthenia in approximately 60% of patients, and in 15% to 20% of all myasthenic patients, weakness remains limited to the eye muscles (so-called "ocular myasthenia"). Patients will complain of a drooping eyelid or binocular double vision (that improves with closing one eye) that frequently fluctuates throughout the day or with activity. On physical examination, these patients have ptosis or limitations in extraocular movements that are triggered or exaggerated by sustained upgaze for 60 seconds (so-called "upgaze paresis"). The extraocular manifestations are rarely symmetric, and the ptosis is very often more significant on one side.

Weakness of the limbs tends to be symmetric and usually affects proximal more than distal muscles. Patients will frequently complain of reduced ability to perform repetitive actions of the proximal muscles, such as lifting an arm to comb hair or climbing stairs. On physical examination, fatigability can be demonstrated by having the patient activate the deltoids (arm abduction) or iliopsoas (hip flexion) either against gravity for 2 minutes or against examiner resistance for 5 repetitions of 5 seconds each. Typically, myasthenic patients with weakness of these muscle groups will have a significant decrement in strength between the first repetition and the last. Similar maneuvers can be performed using whichever muscle groups are affected, according to the patient's complaints.

Bulbar weakness manifests as difficulty with speech (dysarthria) or swallowing (dysphagia). These symptoms may also be fatigable; for example, patients may notice more difficulty enunciating toward the end of the day or at the end of a speech, or more trouble swallowing toward the end of a meal or when eating chewy foods such as steak. If shortness of breath is present, it typically improves moving from a supine to sitting position, which helps with diaphragm excursion. Strength of sniff and cough can be easily assessed at the bedside, and weakness of neck flexion may indicate risk for diaphragmatic weakness.

Sensation is not affected in MG. If a patient has sensory loss, static weakness that does not fluctuate with exercise, or other neurologic symptoms aside from weakness, this should prompt the examiner to consider an alternate diagnosis. Deep tendon reflexes are normal in myasthenia gravis.

Diagnosis

It is important to understand the proper diagnostic algorithm for MG, which is based on the combination of clinical history, examination findings, presence of autoantibodies, and results of electrodiagnostic testing. In the setting of a good clinical history and positive examination findings, the presence of pathologic autoantibodies is likely sufficient to confirm the diagnosis. When the clinical history or examination is suggestive but autoantibodies are not present, electrodiagnostic testing is important to confirm a suspected diagnosis, particularly if immunosuppressive or interventional therapies are considered.

Bedside tests to support a diagnosis include the ice pack test and edrophonium. Placement of ice over a ptotic eyelid may lead to clinical improvement, as cool temperature slows down the breakdown of Ach in the synapse due to slowed action of AchE. Edrophonium (Enlon, previously marketed as Tensilon) is a short-acting AchE inhibitor may be used to help confirm a clinical diagnosis. It is best used if the patient has ptosis or extraocular paresis because there is less subjectivity in assessing improvement. Edrophonium is given intravenously (IV) with 0.1 mL of a 10 mg/mL solution administered initially as a test to assess tolerance, and if no unwanted effects are noted, the remainder of the drug is injected and the patient is observed for a clinical response. If a cholinergic reaction occurs, which may include bradycardia or hypotension, then administer 0.5 mg atropine IV.

Laboratory evolution of autoantibodies is standard of care in patients with suspected MG. In generalized MG, Ach-R Abs are generally present in up to 85% of affected individuals with generalized MG. Ach-R Abs may include blocking, binding, as well as modulating antibodies. Of those patients with generalized MG who are seronegative for Ach-R Ab, approximately 30% to 40% are seropositive for MUSK antibodies. In ocular MG, where symptoms are limited to ptosis or binocular diplopia, only about 15% are seropositive for autoantibodies, and if present, those autoantibodies are Ach-R ab. The vast majority are seronegative and require further evaluation for confirmation of the diagnosis.

Electrodiagnostic testing for a disorder of neuromuscular transmission includes slow repetitive nerve stimulation (RNS). A stimulator is used to depolarize a motor nerve (resulting in an all-or-none nerve AP) and generate a muscle twitch recorded as a compound motor action potential (CMAP). A train of stimuli (between 4 to 6) are performed at a rate of 3 to 5 per second. In MG the dysfunction at the postsynaptic muscle membrane results in some muscle fibers not achieving depolarization sufficient to cause an all-or-none muscle fiber AP, and the size of the overall CMAP (from multiple muscle fibers) is reduced. The threshold for abnormality is a CMAP decrement of >10%, generally between the first and fourth stimuli. If a baseline study at rest is normal, the patient is asked to exercise the muscle for 1 minute, and the study is repeated at 1-minute intervals to assess for the development of decrement. It should be noted that the sensitivity of RNS is increased with the presence of fatigable weakness on examination, because the clinical correlate of a decrement is weakness. Aside from distal hand muscles, trapezius or facial muscles such as nasalis can be studied.

Single fiber electromyography looks for "jitter" or loss of synchronization of individual muscle fibers innervated by a single anterior horn cell in the spinal cord. This is the most sensitive electrodiagnostic test for MG.

Differential Diagnosis

The differential diagnosis for diplopia and ptosis includes cranial nerve palsies: oculomotor (cranial nerve III), trochlear (cranial nerve IV), and abducens (cranial nerve VI). Horner's syndrome may also cause ptosis due to weakness in Mueller's muscle, although other signs such as anisocoria (unequal pupils) that is worsened in the dark is present. Thyroid eye disease may cause any of these symptoms as well. The differential diagnosis for appendicular weakness without sensory loss includes myopathy, pure motor neuropathy, anterior horn cell disease, or a central nervous system pathology involving the motor pathways. These causes of weakness result in static rather than fluctuating weakness.

The main differential diagnosis for fatigable weakness as seen in MG is the Lambert-Eaton myasthenic syndrome (LEMS). LEMS is caused by antibodies against voltage-gated calcium channels on the presynaptic neuromuscular junction and may be paraneoplastic (small cell carcinoma of the lung) or autoimmune. MG and LEMS can be differentiated by the presence of postexercise facilitation of reflexes (after 10 seconds of sustained exercise), as well as antibody and electrodiagnostic testing.

Therapy

Overall, the treatment goal is to achieve freedom from symptoms or functional limitations, recognizing that patients may still have some weakness of some muscles (this is known as minimal manifestation status). Mainstays of treatment include anticholinesterase inhibitors, as well as oral steroids, and a variety of immunosuppressants, as well as intravenous immunoglobulin (IVIG),[1] and plasmapheresis may be used. Broadly, medical therapy can be classified as symptomatic or disease-modifying, the latter with

an immunomodulatory effect targeting the underlying disease pathophysiology.

It should be noted that there exists wide variation in therapeutic approaches, and there are limited head-to-head data comparing individual medications. Current treatments, as well as advances in clinical care, have significantly improved the mortality rate of MG and outcomes of myasthenic crisis.

Symptomatic Therapy

Pyridostigmine (Mestinon) is an AchE inhibitor that increases the amount of acetylcholine in the synaptic cleft by slowing its breakdown by AchE and should be considered as initial therapy. Onset of action is typically within 30 minutes, with benefit generally lasting 3 to 4 hours. As such it is initially dosed 60 mg 3 times daily by mouth and may be increased to 120 mg every 3 to 4 hours while awake, with the total dose typically not exceeding 480 mg/d. It does not penetrate the central nervous system, and most side effects are gastrointestinal. Side effects may include nausea, vomiting, abdominal cramping, diarrhea, sweating, blurred vision, or muscle twitching and cramps. Anticholinergic agents such as glycopyrrolate (Robinul) 1 mg or hyoscyamine sulfate (Levsin)[1] 0.125 mg with each pyridostigmine dose can usually treat these muscarinic side effects effectively. Data suggest that MUSK Ab–positive patients may have a lesser response to acetylcholinersterase therapy when compared with ACH-R–seropositive patients. In the setting of ocular myasthenia, there appears to be more of response in ptosis when compared with diplopia.

Corticosteroids

Corticosteroids, typically prednisone,[1] are a mainstay of immunotherapy and used when pyridostigmine alone does not achieve an adequate treatment response. Two general approaches exist, using either a low-dose or high-dose regimen. Decisions may be dictated by the severity of weakness, presence of significant bulbar dysfunction, or comorbid conditions (such as diabetes). A "low-dose" approach is used with milder disease and includes initiation of 10 to 20 mg daily, and increasing by 5 mg orally weekly to a lower target dose (generally 40–60 mg/d). Oral high-dose (1 mg/kg/d) steroid therapy may be used with moderate-severe weakness and generally has a latency of 2 to 4 weeks before onset of benefit with maximal benefit in 5 to 6 months. It is important to recognize that early clinical deterioration is possible (reported up to 50%) approximately 7 to 10 days after treatment initiation, generally when steroids are dosed at 1 mg/kg/d or higher. In those patients for whom high-dose therapy is introduced, concomitant treatment with either IVIG or plasma exchange (PLEX), discussed herein, may provide protection against early clinical deterioration.

For a patient who has achieved the treatment goal of minimal manifestation on a particular dose of steroids, it is important to consider weaning the dose to reduce side effects. A common approach is a slow taper decreasing 5 mg/d per month on alternate days, with a slower taper once a total dose of 10 mg daily is achieved. Many patients can be maintained on low doses of steroids.

Some patients have an inadequate response to steroids or intolerable side effects or are unable to taper because of recurrence of symptoms. These patients are typically treated with alternative, steroid-sparing, immunomodulatory therapies. Some patients with comorbidities that limit steroid dosing are started on steroids and nonsteroidal immunosuppressant medications concurrently.

Thymectomy

Thymectomy is considered standard of care for those with thymoma, which is present in approximately 15% of patients with generalized MG. A recent study supports thymectomy in Ach-R Ab–positive patients with at least moderately severe disease. Thymectomy patients demonstrated improved outcomes compared with placebo, required less steroids, fewer required

---

[1]Not FDA approved for this indication.

steroid-sparing immunosuppressants, and experienced fewer hospitalizations. Thymectomy is controversial for mild symptoms, purely ocular disease, older age (>60 years), and there exist various surgical approaches. It is considered standard of care to pretreat with IVIG or PLEX before surgery if patients are symptomatic.

Other Immunomodulatory Therapies

Azathioprine (Imuran)[1] is a purine analogue that inhibits nucleic acid synthesis, as well as T- and B-cell proliferation. It is a commonly used steroid-sparing immunosuppressant that is considered first-line and has shown efficacy in a randomized clinical trial. Azathioprine allows reduced steroid dose, reduces relapse rate, and prolongs duration of remission. Treatment is generally started at 50 mg daily, increasing by 50 mg every 1 to 2 weeks to approximately 150 to 200 daily (2–3 mg/kg/d), generally in split doses. Onset of action is estimated at 4 to 8 months, and therapy requires regular blood count and liver function monitoring. Side effects include a flulike illness at initiation (reported in up to 10% to 20%, requires cessation), leukopenia, and transaminitis. Thiopurine methyltransferase enzyme testing can be performed, if available, before starting to identify patients at high risk of bone marrow suppression (although monitoring of blood counts is favored by many practitioners).

Intravenous immunoglobulin (IVIG, Gammagard)[1] has been shown to improve weakness in MG. Its mechanism of action is unclear although presumed to stem from neutralizing circulating pathogenic autoantibodies. A dose of 2 g/kg spread over 5 days is a common algorithm for initial treatment, although in patients who previously tolerated it, IVIG could be given as 1 g/kg/d over 2 days. Onset of action is typically within the first week, and benefit may be sustained for 3 to 4 weeks after treatment. Side effects include headache (sometimes severe and related to aseptic meningitis), thrombosis because of increased serum viscosity, and renal failure. Avoidance of sucrose-containing products may decrease risk of renal failure. Slowed infusion rates may help avoid decompensation of heart failure. Patients on maintenance dosing may receive IVIG 1 g/kg every 3 to 4 weeks.

Mycophenolate mofetil (Cellcept)[1] inhibits guanosine nucleotide synthesis that is needed for B and T lymphocytes. Although there have been two negative randomized clinical trials, there are several retrospective reports supporting efficacy and consensus expert opinion is that it remains a treatment option. It is started at 500 mg twice daily and titrated to 1000 to 1500 mg twice daily. Side effects include nausea, vomiting, diarrhea, and leukopenia. It has teratogenic potential and should not be used in pregnancy.

Cyclosporine (Sandimmune)[1] is a calcineurin inhibitor that has suppressed inflammatory cytokines and has multiple effects on T-cell function. It is initiated at approximately 3 mg/kg daily as a twice-daily split dose and may be titrated up to 5 mg/kg/d with a target trough level <300 ng/mL. Onset of action is approximately 2 to 3 months. Side effects include hirsutism, hypertension, clinically significant nephrotoxicity, and increased cancer risk (including dermatologic cancers). Cyclosporine level may be affected by multiple drug interactions, and concomitant medications should be reviewed.

Methotrexate (Trexall)[1] is a folate antimetabolite that may be dosed orally or subcutaneously. A typical oral dose is initiated at 10 mg weekly and titrated to 15 to 25 mg orally once a week. It is recommended that the patient take folate[1] supplementation of approximately at least 1 mg daily. Side effects include stomatitis (folate supplementation may help prevent this), bone marrow suppression, as well as interstitial lung disease (rare). It is important to note that methotrexate is a known teratogen and should be avoided in women of childbearing potential.

Plasmapheresis or PLEX removes plasma from the circulation and replaces it, typically with albumin, with the net effect of removing pathologic autoantibodies and inflammatory cytokines. Typically five exchanges are performed over a period of 1 to 2 weeks, and benefit is typically observed by the third exchange. PLEX requires placement of a vascath or (if to be used as a maintenance therapy) a permacath. When used as a maintenance therapy, 1 to 2 exchanges are typically performed, at variable intervals, as frequently as weekly. There is a risk of deep venous thrombosis or line infection. Hypotension may occur because of citrate-induced hypovolemia, and it may be associated with hypocalcemia. ACE inhibitors need to be held 24 hours because of bradykinin-related vasodilation.

Rituximab (Rituxan)[1] is a CD20 antibody that has been evaluated in a randomized controlled trial, the results of which are pending. There exists retrospective data to support efficacy, particularly in MUSK Ab patients who have failed initial therapy. It is dosed 325 mg/m² weekly for 4 weeks, although it can also be dosed 1 g/m² with a second dose 2 weeks later. Dosing may be repeated at 6-month intervals. Side effects include infusion-related symptoms including pruritis, headache, hypotension, nausea, and chills. Rituximab may additionally result in leukopenia, anemia, or thrombocytopenia. Infusion-related symptoms can be pretreated with acetaminophen and diphenhydramine.

Eculizumab (Soliris) is a complement inhibitor that was FDA approved for AchR Ab generalized myasthenia gravis in 2017. It is dosed at 900 mg weekly for 4 weeks, followed by 1200 mg for the fifth week and thereafter 1200 mg every 2 weeks. Generally only mild infusion reactions are reported, typically managed by pretreatment acetaminophen and diphenhydramine, although there is risk for severe meningococcal infection. Meningococcal immunization is recommended before treatment initiation.

Cyclophosphamide (Cytoxan)[1] is typically reserved for treatment-refractory patients. It may be administered orally with a daily dose ranging from 1.5 to 5 mg daily. Potential side effects of oral cyclophosphamide include cystitis as well as bladder cancer, leading many treating physicians to use IV pulse dosing. A common approach for pulse dosing is 1 gm/m² monthly for 6 months (less toxic). Onset of action with pulse dosing is relatively quick, generally about 1 month.

Efgartigimod (Vyvgart) is a neonatal Fc receptor blocker, which was FDA-approved for AChR Ab generalized myasthenia gravis in 2022. It has a novel mechanism of action that effectively reduces IgG levels, including levels of pathogenic autoantibodies. As such, efgartigimod has been likened to "plasma exchange in a bottle." It is administered intravenously at a dose of 10 mg/kg weekly for a total of four treatments (a treatment cycle) and, depending on response, repeat cycles may be given after 8 weeks. Side effects include infusion reaction, headache, and respiratory and urinary tract infections. If a patient has an active infection at the time of a cycle, it is recommended that the treatment cycle be delayed.

Treatment Considerations in Pregnancy

Pregnancy and postpartum status have been reported to be triggers for worsening of myasthenia. Ideally, prepregnancy planning allows for optimization of clinical status to improve pregnancy outcomes. These patients require expert multidisciplinary care through the postpartum period. In pregnancy the treatment of choice is pyridostigmine, with steroids being the immunosuppressant of choice. Azathioprine[1] and cyclosporine[1] are relatively safe in expectant mothers who are not satisfactorily controlled or cannot tolerate corticosteroids. IVIG[1] and PLEX may also be treatment options.

Transient neonatal myasthenia may affect the newborn infant. This is difficult to predict and requires close attention for signs

---

[1]Not FDA approved for this indication.

[1]Not FDA approved for this indication.

Monitoring

After a diagnosis of MG is confirmed, additional testing or monitoring is indicated. The frequency of clinical assessment should be dictated by the severity and nature of the patient's symptoms, as well as the impact of the disease on function. Patients with MG should be managed in concert with a neurologist. Refractory MG is defined by symptoms that affect function and are unchanged or worse after corticosteroids and at least two other immunosuppressive agents used in adequate doses for adequate duration. Patients meeting criteria for refractory MG should be referred to a physician or medical center with expertise in MG.

Computed tomography of the chest should be performed to screen for thymoma. Assessment of thyroid function is important. If immunomodulatory medications are used for disease control, TB screening should be performed.

Pulmonary and swallowing dysfunction may be encountered. Pulmonary function testing should be performed for patients with symptomatic generalized MG, particularly if there are complaints of dyspnea. Speech therapy referral for a swallow evaluation should be performed if there is concern for dysphagia.

Periodic laboratory monitoring is required with use of immunomodulatory medications, which may vary depending on the specific medication used. Suggested tests and monitoring algorithms are detailed in Box 2.

Complications

The most severe complication of MG is myasthenic crisis, which is defined by worsening of weakness requiring intubation or noninvasive ventilation. Myasthenic crisis may be seen in up to 20% of patients at some point in disease course. Myasthenic crisis is most commonly encountered in the setting of concomitant illness, change in medications, or early in the disease course because maximum weakness occurs in the first year of the disease in 66% of patients. Respiratory failure can result from respiratory muscle weakness, oropharyngeal weakness, or a combination of both. It is important to recognize that new respiratory or swallowing complaints can quickly escalate, and patients with these complaints should be quickly assessed. One can assess diaphragm strength by the force of a strong sniff or cough; patients should be able to count to 20 after a deep breath. Staccato speech or dyspnea that precludes speaking in full sentences is of high concern for myasthenic crisis. Spirometry with forced vital capacity <2 L or negative inspiratory force of <40 cm H_2O should be sent to the hospital for further evaluation. Assessment of swallowing function by speech therapy and possible modified barium swallow should be considered in the context of dysphagia for solids and liquids.

IVIG and PLEX have comparable outcomes for the treatment of patients with moderate-to-severe weakness. The response to PLEX may be more predictable than IVIG in severe MG exacerbations, and retrospective data suggests PLEX may be more effective than IVIG in myasthenic crisis. PLEX, however, may be associated with more complications, as well as longer hospital stay and associated hospital costs.

References

Farmakidis C, Pasnoor M, Dimachkie M, Baron R: Treatment of myasthenia gravis, *Neurol Clin* 36:311–337, 2018.
Gilhus NE, Verschuuren JJ: Myasthenia gravis: subgroup classification and therapeutic strategies, *Lancet Neurol* 14:1023–1036, 2015.
Gilhus NE: Myasthenia gravis, *N Engl J Med* 375:2570–2581, 2016.
Myasthenia Gravis Foundation of America. Myasthenia Gravis: A Manual for the Healthcare Provider. Available at http://myasthenia.org/. [accessed April 1, 2018].
Sanders DB, Wilfe GI, Benatar M, et al: International consensus guidance for management of myasthenia gravis, *Neurology* 87:419–425, 2016.
Wilfe GI, Kaminski HJ, Aban IN, et al: Randomized trial of thymectomy in myasthenia gravis, *N Engl J Med* 375:511–522, 2016.

NEUROFIBROMATOSIS (TYPE 1)

Method of
Jason E. Marker, MD, MPA

CURRENT DIAGNOSIS

- Neurofibromatosis type 1 (NF1) can be diagnosed by physicians based on well-defined diagnostic criteria that can be met with a careful history and physical exam.
- Additional testing may be needed in some cases (including genetic testing) to confirm the diagnosis or to provide information that will be important for both short- and long-term management.
- NF1 has important genetic underpinnings, can have extremely variable expression within families, and will evolve in its need for medical intervention throughout the lifetime of the patient.

CURRENT THERAPY

- There is no treatment for NF1. However, there are many therapies for both the common and uncommon manifestations and complications of the condition.
- Many therapies are similar to those used for non-NF1 patients with the same symptoms. However, there are some manifestations where unique therapies are needed, and physicians need to know the difference between these.
- Proper monitoring of the patient aids in the identification of treatable symptoms and allows opportunities for anticipatory guidance and counseling.
- There are several emerging therapies related to the heritability of NF1 that are important for patients of childbearing age to be aware of.

Introduction and Epidemiology

Neurofibromatosis encompasses three distinct genetic entities: NF1, neurofibromatosis type 2 (NF2), and schwannomatosis. Because NF1 is so much more common (incidence of 1:1900 to 1:3000 livebirths) than NF2 (incidence of 1:25,000 to 1:33,000 livebirths) and schwannomatosis (incidence of 1:40,000 to 1:1.7M livebirths), when the word *neurofibromatosis* is used (or the older name, Von Recklinghausen disease), it is generally referring to NF1. NF1 is the primary topic of this chapter.

NF1 is an autosomal dominant genetic disorder and is progressive in that its clinical manifestations evolve over the lifespan. About half of the cases of NF1 are familial and the remainder are the result of new, spontaneous mutations. Life expectancy is reduced by 5 to 15 years and is related to the severity of the clinical manifestations, the emergence of malignant tumors, and excess hypertensive and vascular disease risk. There is no predilection based on race, ethnic origin, or country of birth.

Risk Factors

NF1 is an autosomal dominant condition and affects 50% of the offspring of parents where one parent is affected, making family history the primary predictable risk factor. Advanced paternal age increases the likelihood of a de novo mutation. Eighty percent of newly occurring mutations are believed to come from the paternally derived chromosome.

Pathophysiology

NF1 is the result of mutations in the *NF1* gene (chromosome 17q11.2) that codes for the protein neurofibromin. Neurofibromin is a protein in the GTPase-activating family that stimulates the Ras pathway for tumor suppression. Loss of neurofibromin results in "de-suppression" of tumor growth within susceptible tissues. Although genetic penetrance in NF1 is complete, NF1 is highly variable in its expression (even within families). This is because germline mutations must be coupled with somatic mutations in order for symptoms to manifest clinically.

Several thousand distinct *NF1* mutations have been identified. Many small mutations have demonstrated no genotype-phenotype correlation, while some individuals (1% to 5% of NF1 patients) will have complete loss of the 1.4 to 1.5 Mb of the *NF1* gene and are quite severely affected. Due to the large size of this gene, mutations in the *NF1* gene occur more often than in any other human gene.

Somatic and germline (rare) mosaicism occurs and can result in phenotypically unaffected offspring who could later transmit the mutated gene to their own children. Also, some individuals with neurocognitive symptoms have been found to have haploinsufficiency (heterozygous for a pathogenic variant with an intact second allele).

Prevention

There is no specific prevention for any of the clinical manifestations of NF1. Due to its variable expression, some individuals will simply be more or less affected. To the extent that having a diagnosis of NF1 *could* cause academic challenges, interpersonal hardships, and social isolation, robust anticipatory guidance throughout the lifespan can help these individuals develop proper support systems and personal resilience, preventing some of the morbidity of the disease.

Affected individuals of child-bearing age now have the option of genetic testing of fertilized eggs to select unaffected eggs for implantation. This is an emerging prevention strategy.

Clinical Manifestations

There are a number of clinical manifestations of NF1. Because of the variability of expression of the *NF1* gene, these manifestations may be variably present in any affected individual. The following section on diagnosis will discuss how these clinical manifestations fit into the diagnostic criteria for NF1.

Café-au-lait spots are flat, irregularly shaped, uniformly hyperpigmented macules that appear during the first year of life and then increase in number through childhood. These macules are present in 95% of adults with NF1 but tend to fade and become more indistinct later in life. Among the general population of individuals who do not have NF1, 15% will have one to three café-au-lait macules.

Freckling (primarily in areas of skin apposition like the axillae and inguinal folds) is distinct from café-au-lait macules as the freckles are smaller, more clustered, and generally appear later in childhood than the café-au-lait macules.

Lisch nodules are tan-colored hamartomas of the iris. Lisch nodules do not affect vision and may be seen with simple ophthalmoscopy (although the use of a slit lamp will help identify small nodules and distinguish them from iris nevi). These nodules are seen in up to 90% of adults with NF1, but fewer than 10% of children under 6 years old.

Neurofibromas present as several types of lesions with variable characteristics, risk of pathology, and symptomatology. Cutaneous peripheral neurofibromas are benign peripheral nerve sheath tumors that are generally soft, mobile, and fleshy. They may be dermal or epidermal on a broad or pedunculated base. These neurofibromas are nontender, are usually more common on the trunk, and can number from a few to thousands. Cutaneous peripheral neurofibromas do not degenerate into malignant peripheral nerve sheath tumors (MPNSTs). Plexiform peripheral neurofibromas can be superficial or deep inside the body. They tend to be more diffuse and involve plaques and tangles of abnormal tissues that can grow into a complex mass. On whole-body scanning, 50% of patients with NF1 will have at least one plexiform neurofibroma. Large plexiform neurofibromas can create symptoms by compressing nearby structures and, unlike cutaneous neurofibromas, they have the capacity to degenerate into MPNSTs. Nodular neurofibromas are firm and rubbery. Unlike the cutaneous neurofibromas, they

are sometimes tender, often deeper and usually less mobile. They are not as invasive as the plexiform neurofibromas but can undergo degeneration into MPNSTs.

Optic pathway gliomas (OPGs) occur in 15% of children younger than 6 (but rarely in older individuals) and can grow anywhere along the optic tracts. Most individuals are asymptomatic, but advanced tumors can affect vision or even upset the normal function of the hypothalamus with growth rate variations and premature or delayed puberty.

Orthopedic abnormalities are primarily long-bone dysplasias and pseudoarthroses. Anterolateral bowing of the tibia (usually unilateral) in infants and young children can easily go undetected until a pathologic fracture develops at the onset of ambulation. One half of fractures occur during the toddler years. Long-bone pseudoarthrosis has a male predisposition (1.7:1) and NF1 accounts for 50% to 70% of all long-bone pseudoarthroses. Other orthopedic findings in NF1 patients may include short stature (13% have a height less than 2 standard deviations below the mean), scoliosis (10% to 15% of NF1 patients are affected), sphenoid wing dysplasia (leading to facial asymmetry), osteoporosis, and macrocephaly.

Neurologic abnormalities encompass cognitive defects and learning disabilities as well as the risk of seizures. Although profound intellectual disability is rare (the likelihood of having an IQ <70 is similar to the general population), 81% of NF patients will have some impairment in one or more areas of cognitive functioning. While less than half of NF1 patients have a specific learning disability, more than half will have some amount of neuropsychological impairment, including speech articulation problems, AD/HD, or impairment of executive functioning. Seizures occur twice as often in patients with NF1 (prevalence 4% to 6%) as in the general population and can be of any type and occur at any age.

Other manifestations of concern: Rarely, other central nervous system (CNS) neoplasms develop. CNS astrocytomas usually arise during childhood and, when not an incidental finding on a scan being done for another purpose, may present with symptoms of increased intracranial pressure. Rare brainstem gliomas are usually symptomatic at presentation. Malignant peripheral nerve sheath tumors are highly malignant tumors that can arise from a preexisting plexiform or nodular neurofibromas. The lifetime risk of developing an MPNST in a patient with NF1 is 5% to 13% and most commonly occurs in teenagers and young adults. MPNSTs are usually diagnosed when a plexiform or nodular neurofibroma goes through a period of pain, change in consistency, and rapid growth. Hypertension, including hypertension as early as childhood, is common among NF1 patients. Although rare, renal neurovascular lesions can be the cause, and NF1 patients with hypertension should be evaluated for renal artery stenosis. Macrocephaly, congenital heart disease (primarily pulmonic stenosis and mitral valve defects), cerebrovascular dysplasia, and increased incidence of irritable bowel syndrome and constipation have been observed, more commonly in individuals with NF1, though not fully studied.

Diagnosis

The diagnosis of NF1 can be made reliably by a primary care team, but a multidisciplinary team of subspecialists is often involved in the long-term care of these individuals, including during the diagnostic phase. A comprehensive history (including a detailed family history) and examination should be undertaken. Additional testing or referral, as indicated by the initial evaluation, should be pursued to clarify the diagnosis, seek findings amenable to treatment, and facilitate proper anticipatory guidance and patient/family education.

The US National Institutes of Health (NIH) Consensus Conference in 1997 (with minor revisions in 2021) set forth the following diagnostic criteria for NF1:

At least two of the following clinical features must be present to make the diagnosis of NF1:

- Six or more café-au-lait macules greater than 5 mm (prepubertal) or greater than 15 mm (postpubertal) in longest diameter
- Two or more neurofibromas of any type (or a single plexiform neurofibroma)

- Freckling in the axillary or inguinal regions
- Optic pathway glioma
- Two or more Lisch nodules or two or more choroidal abnormalities (see below)
- A distinctive bony lesion (sphenoid dysplasia or a long-bone dysplasia with or without pseudoarthrosis)
- A heterozygous pathogenic NF1 variant allele fraction of 50% in apparently normal tissue (like WBCs)

A child with ONE of the above clinical findings AND a first-degree relative with NF1 based on these criteria meets diagnostic criteria for NF1.

These criteria are both sensitive and specific, and are met by 97% of NF1 patients by the age of 8 years (100% by the age of 20 years). Nearly half of individuals with a new sporadic mutation fail to meet these criteria by the age of 1 year. Therefore, in an infant with one clinical feature, close observation is needed to determine if other criteria will be met. If, by the age of 4 years, only one criterion is met, referral for a genetic diagnosis may be warranted if not already obtained.

Other specific testing may be needed to make the diagnosis, to determine the extent of involvement of the disorder, or to decide on treatment. These include the following:

- Dermatologic evaluation: If the identification of café-au-lait spots, whether café-au-lait spots meet diagnostic criteria, or the identification of criteria-meeting freckling is in question, referral to Dermatology may be needed. Likewise, the spectrum of neurofibromas is broad and a dermatologist may be needed to properly identify these lesions.
- Lisch nodules: Although occasionally seen with the naked eye or through an office ophthalmoscope, formal ophthalmologic consultation is recommended to look for small Lisch nodules and to assess for optic disk findings suggestive of OPGs or increased intracranial pressure. Choroidal abnormalities seen on optical coherence tomography/near infrared imaging (OCT/NIR) fall into this same diagnostic category.
- Optic pathway gliomas: Ophthalmologic evaluation is recommended as noted earlier. Brain MRI imaging is not recommended for asymptomatic patients with normal ophthalmologic evaluations.
- Orthopedic abnormalities: Plain radiographs of long bones or CT imaging of craniofacial bones may be needed to identify the diagnostic findings in these areas.
- Neurologic abnormalities: Because new focal seizures could be the result of a new intracranial neoplasm, neuroimaging is warranted with any new seizure activity.
- Other manifestations of concern: MPNSTs are best differentiated from benign plexiform or nodular neurofibromas by positron emission tomography (PET) scan. Evaluating for renal artery stenosis in individuals with new onset hypertension (including children) is indicated.
- Genetic counseling and testing: Genetic testing is usually reserved for cases where the diagnosis remains in question following a thorough history, examination, and nongenetic testing. Additionally, genetic testing may be indicated for family members of the affected individual. Knowing that expression is extremely variable, preconception, embryonic preimplantation, or prenatal (amniocentesis or chorionic villi sampling) testing for individuals in families with NF1 should be considered.

Differential Diagnosis

Because of the well-established diagnostic criteria and availability of genetic testing, the differential diagnosis of NF1 is limited. As noted at the outset, NF2 and schwannomatosis are lumped together with NF1 under the general diagnosis of neurofibromatosis. Schwannomatosis is a complex regional pain syndrome with some common underlying pathophysiology but no overlapping symptoms and unrelated genetics. NF2 will be discussed briefly in the discussion to come.

Legius syndrome includes café-au-lait macules, axillary freckling, and macrocephaly. It does *not* include neurofibromas or CNS tumors, however. Like NF1, Legius syndrome is an autosomal dominant disorder for loss of a tumor suppressor protein, but it affects an entirely different gene.

Constitutional mismatch repair-deficiency syndrome (CMMR-D) is a rare autosomal recessive condition that results in café-au-lait macules (and occasionally axillary freckling and Lisch nodules). Unlike in NF1, individuals with CMMR-D are at risk for hematologic malignancies in infancy and childhood, brain tumors (primarily glioblastomas) in mid-childhood, and colorectal cancer in adolescence and young adulthood. Rhabdomyosarcomas and optic pathway gliomas may occur rarely in CMMR-D.

NF2 is caused by the *NF2* gene on chromosome 22, which encodes for the tumor suppressor protein merlin (or schwannomin), which is a functionally different protein than that produced by *NF1*. Key differences between NF1 and NF2 include the following points about NF2:

- Few or nonexistent café-au-lait macules
- No Lisch nodules
- No risk of MPNSTs
- Spinal root tumors are schwannomas in NF2 (neurofibromas in NF1)
- No cognitive impairment
- High prevalence of bilateral acoustic schwannomas and resulting hearing loss in 90% to 95% of patients by the age of 30 years
- 60% to 80% have cataracts
- Presence of meningiomas

Noonan syndrome is characterized by short stature and may include café-au-lait macules that may meet the size and number criteria for NF1. Sometimes, the facial features of Noonan syndrome can overlap with the appearance of NF1. However, the webbed neck of Noonan syndrome and the association with pulmonic stenosis are not part of NF1. Although the Ras signaling pathway is involved in Noonan syndrome, the underlying genetics are entirely different.

Surveillance and Therapy

In 2020, the FDA approved oral selumetinib (Koselugo), a first-of-class kinase inhibitor, for pediatric patients 2 years of age and older with NF1 who have symptomatic, inoperable plexiform neurofibromas. The research that led to this approval showed statistically and clinically significant decreases in the size of these neurofibromas, as well as the pain and disability that often accompanies them. It remains unclear whether selumetinib treatment decreases the likelihood of malignant transformation of plexiform neurofibromas into MPNSTs. Similar medications are currently under study at this time..

The following areas of surveillance should be undertaken. Where research or expert opinion suggests a proper frequency, it is listed, although shared decision making with the patient/family as well as communication with your medical colleagues will be required to develop appropriate timelines. Therapeutic options are listed here for many of the common issues NF1 patients face, while the management of less common complications is outlined in the next section.

- Yearly examination of the skin for new neurofibromas and any signs of change within an existing neurofibroma should be done. Especially when nodular or plexiform neurofibromas exist (those at risk of malignant transformation), any history of rapid change or new pain should be evaluated thoroughly. A PET scan can distinguish between benign and malignant lesions. Referral to surgical and/or dermatologic colleagues should be made regarding these nodular or plexiform neurofibromas (for biopsy and management decisions) and should be strongly considered for all but the most clear and superficial cutaneous neurofibromas.
- Cutaneous neurofibromas that develop pruritus are often not responsive to antihistamines, although the itching is often improved by the use of gabapentin (Neurontin)[1].

---

[1] Not FDA approved for this indication.

- Yearly blood pressure measurement, even in children and young adults, should be done. Once the diagnosis of essential hypertension is made following testing that excludes the diagnosis of renal artery stenosis, blood pressure should be controlled following standard blood pressure goals and treatment algorithms. Hypertension that becomes hard to control may prompt an evaluation for pheochromocytoma, a rare finding in NF1.
- Growth tracking of weight, height, and head circumference should be done through childhood and adolescence in the usual manner. Additionally, any signs of premature or delayed puberty should be evaluated further. Growth and pubertal abnormalities should prompt an age-appropriate endocrinology referral for additional testing (serum, urine, and/or neuroimaging) and treatments based on these results.
- Neurodevelopmental and academic assessment should be undertaken, involving family members and school personnel when appropriate. Individuals who develop neuropsychiatric and academic problems should undergo formal neurodiagnostic testing, and any identified diagnoses should be treated. These treatments are no different than those used for non-NF1 individuals who carry the same neuropsychiatric diagnosis. Neuroimaging is not indicated in the evaluation of neuropsychiatric conditions unless neurologic deficits exist.
- NF1 patients who develop seizures are treated with the usual seizure management algorithms following neuroimaging to look for new intracranial pathologies. An electroencephalogram (EEG) is not indicated for asymptomatic individuals.
- Evaluation for skeletal changes including scoliosis, facial asymmetry, or long bone abnormalities should be performed yearly during childhood and adolescence, and then at the typical wellness visits into young adulthood (with prompting in these older ages to report any changes that are noticed between visits). Any abnormalities that are encountered should prompt additional imaging and referral to subspecialty care.
- Women with NF1 develop osteoporosis at an earlier age than their non-NF1 peers and should undergo earlier screening in accordance with this fact and with other standard risk factors they may have. When diagnosed, this osteoporosis is treated like it would be for any other patient.
- For unclear reasons, women with NF1 have an increased risk of breast cancer, especially women under the age of 40 (at the age of 70, the risk approximates that of the general population). These are usually invasive ductal carcinomas (the most common type overall) and are managed in the usual way, although these patients need both earlier education about, and screening for, breast cancer.
- Formal ophthalmologic evaluation for visual screening, slit lamp and intraocular examination should take place yearly at least through adolescence, usually in the context of a comprehensive examination. Lisch nodules are nonpathologic and no treatment is needed, but any signs of elevated intracranial pressure or optic disc pathology warrant further testing and management. The optimal frequency of MRI surveillance of an optic pathway glioma is unknown but should be based on symptomatology, size, and rate of progression.
- Brain MRI is not recommended as a routine screening test. It may be a part of the initial diagnostic workup but should not need to be repeated for asymptomatic patients who are otherwise receiving comprehensive surveillance. Of note, "NF-associated bright spots" may be seen on MRI imaging, and the data are inconclusive on the relationship between these spots and any pathologic process. These spots often resolve spontaneously by late childhood. Increased brain volume may be observed but is not definitively tied to any NF1 symptoms.
- Whole body MRI screening or MRI of nonbrain areas of potential concern (such as visible but stable and asymptomatic plexiform or nodular neurofibromas) is not recommended by most authorities. Likewise, screening PET scanning is not recommended.

Management of Complications

The previous section outlines the surveillance of and treatment for most of the common concerns for patients with NF1. Rarely, more significant complications present themselves. These are listed here along with their management plan.

- Symptomatic cutaneous neurofibromas that are cosmetically unacceptable, painful, itchy, or disfiguring will sometimes need to be managed. Once it is clear that the lesions in question are truly simple cutaneous neurofibromas, they may be removed in any manner, including by excision, cryotherapy, laser, or electrodessication.
- Symptomatic plexiform neurofibromas that have not degenerated into MPNSTs that are deemed in need of management or removal should be managed by a multidisciplinary team of surgeons and oncologists who are familiar with this type of tumor. These invasive tumors require nonstandard operative approaches and consideration of emerging chemotherapeutic agents.
- MPNSTs are often due to a co-mutated *SUZ12* gene (which lies contiguous to *NF1*). Individuals with large or complete deletions of the *NF1* gene (those who are generally more severely affected) are at an increased risk of this complication. MPNSTs are usually managed by surgeons and oncologists familiar with NF1 and often involve surgical excision with adjunctive radiation and possibly emerging chemotherapeutic agents.
- Optic pathway gliomas are most commonly found to be low-grade pilocystic astrocytomas. As such, they are often sensitive to the standard oncologic treatments for that type of tumor—but when to observe and when to proceed to treatment is controversial.
- Because the bony architecture of pathologic skeletal lesions is inherently abnormal in these patients, the risk of complications from corrective treatments is higher than in non-NF1 patients. Your local orthopedic colleagues need to be aware of this and obtain tertiary care backup when needed. Amputation is often the best long-term plan for long bone lesions.
- Refractory hypertension in the absence of renal artery stenosis that is ultimately found to be the result of pheochromocytoma should be managed by a multidisciplinary team experienced in the management of this diagnosis. It is managed in the same manner as non-NF1 patients with a pheochromocytoma.
- Short stature is often correctible with growth hormone therapy. However, this treatment is not often used because it compounds the inherent protumorgenic nature of NF1. In extreme cases of short stature when growth hormone is used, clinicians need to be alert to the evolution and potential malignant degeneration of new or existing tumors.
- NF1 patients are at a high risk of psychosocial issues arising from the symptoms they may experience from their NF1, its lack of treatability, and its genetic underpinnings. These symptoms may affect relationship building and reproductive decisions. Extra professional support may be needed, particularly during adolescence.

Although pregnancy is not a "complication" of NF1, its management can certainly be complicated by the diagnosis. Pregnant NF1 patients have increased morbidity (but not mortality) due to hypertensive and vascular complications. These complications should be anticipated and managed by an appropriately trained medical team. Genetic counseling should be recommended, ideally prior to conception, and steps taken to ensure proper evaluation and surveillance for the newborn.

References

Defendi GL: Genetics of neurofibromatosis type 1 and type 2. Available at https://emedicine.medscape.com/article/950151-overview. Accessed 15 November 2018.

Evans DG: Neurofibromatosis type 2. Available at https://www.uptodate.com/contents/neurofibromatosis-type-2. Accessed 15 November 2018.

Food and Drug Administration Package Insert for selumetinib (Koselugo). Available at: https://www.accessdata.fda.gov/drugsatfda-docs/label/2020/213756s000lbl.pdf. Accessed 15 November 2018.

Ferner RE, Huson SM, et al: Guidelines for the diagnosis and management of individuals with neurofibromatosis 1, *J Med Genet* 44:81–88, 2007.

Hart L: Primary care of patients with neurofibromatosis 1, *The Nurse Practitioner* 30(6), 2005.

Hersh JH: Committee on Genetics of the American Academy of Pediatrics: Health Supervision of Children with Neurofibromatosis, *Pediatrics* 121:633–645, 2008.

Human Genetics Society of Australia: *Choosing Wisely Australia: 5 Things Clinicians and Consumers Should Question*, October 2016. Available at http://www.choosingwisely.org.au/getmedia/bbc1ca07-7340-49ca-9e85-ad4c1a7bc197/GESA_Choosing_Wisely_Recommendations.pdf.aspx. Accessed 15 November 2018.

Korf BR: Neurofibromatosis type 1 (NF1): Management and prognosis. Available at https://www.uptodate.com/contents/neurofibromatosis-type-1-nf1-management-and-prognosis. Accessed 29 January 2022.

Korf BR: Neurofibromatosis type 1 (NF1): Pathogenesis, clinical features, and diagnosis. Available at https://www.uptodate.com/contents/neurofibromatosis-type-1-nf1-pathogenesis-clinical-features-and-diagnosis. Accessed 29 January 2022.

Legius E, Messiaen L, Wolkenstein P, et al. Revised diagnostic criteria for neurofibromatosis type 1 and Legius syndrome: an international consensus recommendation, *Genet Med* 23(8):1506–1513, 2021.

Selumetinib PPI Dec 2021: https://den8dhaj6zs0e.cloudfront.net/50fd68b9-106b-4550-b5d0-12b045f8b184/22c94947-0a99-4b03-9d06-866a301712bc/22c94947-0a99-4b03-9d06-866a301712bc_viewable_rendition__v.pdf.

Selumetinib PPI April 2020: https://www.accessdata.fda.gov/drugsatfda_docs/label/2020/213756s000lbl.pdf.

Stewart DR, Korf BR, et al: Care of adults with neurofibromatosis type 1: a clinical practice resource of the American College of Medical Genetics and Genomics (ACMG), *Genet Med* 20(7):671–682, 2018 Jul.

Tonsgard JH: Clinical manifestations and management of neurofibromatosis type 1, *Sem Pediatr Neurol, Elsevier* 13:2–7, 2006.

Williams VC, Lucas J, et al: Neurofibromatosis type 1 revisited, *Pediatrics* 123:124–133, 2009.

NONMIGRAINE HEADACHE

Method of
Sargun Walia, MD; and Stephen Ross, MD

CURRENT DIAGNOSIS

A more extensive diagnostic evaluation should be considered for any patient with headache who also has "red flags" (see Table 2).

CURRENT THERAPY

- Specific therapy for secondary cause of headache should be initiated when identified.
- Symptomatic therapy for headache should be selected based on the headache phenotype.

Evaluation and Diagnosis

Gathering of a thorough history and physical examination (Table 1) facilitates two principal goals of headache management:

1. The first is to determine the need for diagnostic studies to evaluate for potential secondary contributors. The more "red flags" (Table 2) the patient has, the more you must consider this. Depending on the differential diagnosis, evaluation may include brain and/or cervical spine imaging, spinal tap, and blood studies. Specific treatment can be initiated for some identified secondary contributors.

2. The second is to discern dominant headache phenotype (Figure 1) to guide symptomatic treatment. The two forms of secondary headache therapy include the specific treatment, which addresses underlying etiology and the symptomatic treatment, which is selected based on the dominant headache phenotype. Often headache phenotypes can be segregated into one or more of the following themes: migraine (covered in the chapter Migraine), tension-type headaches, trigeminal autonomic cephalalgias (TACs), and cranial neuralgias. The symptomatic treatment mirrors that used for the parallel primary headache disorders (see the following).

Headache Type and Therapy

For anyone with headache presentation, the first step in evaluation (history and physical) is to discern potential primary versus secondary source of the pain. If there is concern for possible secondary etiology, diagnostic studies should be considered. Symptomatic treatment is similar for primary and secondary etiologies but varies according to the pain phenotype (Table 3). General principles are to start low-dose treatment then titrate up if needed to control pain (understanding that often it can take 3 to 4 weeks before you see benefit of preventive treatments). If the pain is not adequately controlled despite maximum dose or treatment is not tolerated, then consider moving on to a second-line treatment. If there has been some (but not enough) improvement with the first treatment, then a second treatment can be added. If there has been no improvement with the first treatment, taper off the first while adding the second treatment.

Tension-type headache is experienced by almost everyone at some point in their lives. Most do not seek medical evaluation but rather self-manage. Diagnostic criteria are listed in Table 4. The presence or absence of "emotional tension" does not define this condition. Many individuals experience tension-type headache who are not "stressed" and do not have anxiety or depression. If a person is experiencing "stress" or is anxious, this can act as a trigger for tension-type headache, as well as the other primary headache conditions. Tension-type headache has both episodic and chronic forms. Chronic is defined as having symptoms at least 15 days/month for greater than 3 months.

Treatment of Tension-Type Headache

Generally, start with physical modalities/relaxation techniques (e.g., local heat, massage, analgesic cream) and/or as needed acetaminophen 325 mg or nonsteroidal antiinflammatory drugs (e.g., ibuprofen 200 mg, aspirin 325 mg, naproxen 220 mg, diclofenac 50 mg). If this is inadequate, titrate the dose (e.g., acetaminophen 325 mg up to 1000 mg, ibuprofen 200 mg up to 800 mg) and/or referral for additional physical/cognitive modalities (e.g., physical therapy, myofascial release therapy, biofeedback therapy, cognitive behavioral therapy). FDA-approved preventive treatments are lacking. If preventive treatment is needed, consider a tricyclic antidepressant (e.g., amitriptyline [Elavil][1] starting with 10 mg or 25 mg at bedtime, titrating up to 150 mg if needed/tolerated). Allow 3 to 4 weeks to assess efficacy before titration to the next dose. Prescreen with electrocardiogram (ECG) and monitor for side effects. Once you reach 100 mg, check amitriptyline blood level and repeat ECG. Alternatives could include venlafaxine [Effexor][1] starting 37.5 mg or 75 mg (two to three times per day or once per day if using the long-acting form) titrating if needed to 225 mg, tizanidine (Zanaflex)[1] starting with 4 mg ½ pill two to three times per day titrating if needed to 2 pills three times per day, baclofen (Lioresal)[1] starting with 5 mg or 10 mg tid titrating if needed up to 20 mg qid, mirtazapine (Remeron)[1] starting with 7.5 mg or 15 mg qhs titrating if needed up to 45 mg.

Trigeminal Autonomic Cephalalgias

TACs are syndromes characterized by intense pain and autonomic symptoms in a trigeminal distribution most commonly in the ophthalmic (V1) distribution. Common features among these types include (1) unilateral, side-locked location, typically in the V1 distribution, and (2) associated ipsilateral autonomic features like conjunctival injection, lacrimation, nasal congestion/rhinorrhea, eyelid edema, miosis and/or ptosis, and facial sweating. These disorders can be differentiated based on attack duration/frequency.

The most common TAC type is a cluster headache, but even this is 100 times less prevalent than migraine. Diagnostic criteria include (1) duration lasting 15 to 180 minutes, (2) more likely to have associated ipsilateral autonomic features, and (3) more likely to have agitation/activation during the attack (Box 1).

---

[1] Not FDA approved for this indication.

TABLE 1 — Headache Characteristics

Is there more than one type?	What is the location/radiation?	Is there any positional component?	Is there anything that triggers it?	Is there any pattern to occurrence (e.g., always 1 hour after going to bed, every spring)?
When was the onset?	What does it feel like (e.g., throbbing, pressure, burning)?	Are there any associated features (e.g., nausea, photophobia, ptosis, lacrimation)?	Is there anything that relieves it?	What treatments have been tried so far? What is the response to these?
What is the duration?	What is the frequency?	What is the intensity, along with ramp?	Is there any family history of this?	Is there any change with Valsalva?

TABLE 2 — Headache Red Flags

Onset after age 50 years	"Thunderclap" onset of pain	Positional exacerbation	Onset with recent malignancy, nontrivial head trauma, or seizures	Persistent or unexplained vomiting
Worst headache of life	Marked change in pain pattern	Precipitated by Valsalva maneuvers	Unexplained fever	Meningeal signs
First headache of life	Unusual associated features (blindness, diplopia, confusion, weakness)	Lack of response to abortive medications	Significant blood pressure elevation	Abnormal neurologic examination

Migraine

Throbbing
Unilateral
Mod-severe
Nausea
Photophobia
Phonophobia
Aura

Tension-type Headache

Pressing
Bilateral
Mild-moderate

Trigeminal Autonomic Cephalalgia

Unilateral
Orbital/temple
Severe
Ptosis, lacrimation, rhinorrhea, nasal congestion
Restlessness

Cranial Neuralgia

Electric/stabbing
Unilateral
Severe
Triggered by innocuous stimuli

Figure 1 Headache phenotypes.

Triptans or high-flow oxygen are first-line abortive treatments. Preference is given to faster acting agents (e.g., sumatriptan [Imitrex] 6 mg subcutaneous [SC] injection/20 mg nasal[1] or zolmitriptan [Zomig][1] 5 mg nasal; these may be repeated again in 1 to 2 hours if needed but have a maximum of two doses in a 24-hour period). Oxygen is best administered by nonrebreather face mask at 6 to 12 L/min for 7 to 15 minutes. An alternate abortive treatment is gammaCore, a noninvasive vagus nerve stimulator that may be administered to the anterior neck as a set of three 2-minute stimulations. Other options include intramuscular dihydroergotamine (D.H.E. 45) or 1 mL of 4% intranasal lidocaine[1]. Short-term preventives can include oral steroids or occipital nerve blocks.

First-line preventive treatment is short-acting verapamil[1] starting at 40 to 80 mg oral tid titrating if needed to 480 mg (total daily dose, although there are studies taking the dose up to 720 mg/day[3]). An effective alternative is galcanezumab (Emgality) given as three consecutive 100-mg SC shots (300 mg) each month while cluster headache is active. This is a monthly self-injection that blocks one of the neurotransmitters (calcitonin gene-related peptide) that propagates messages along the pain pathways. Third-line considerations are topiramate (Topamax)[1] or lithium[1]. For refractory cases consider referral to a specialty headache center for sphenopalatine ganglion stimulator.

A second type of TAC is paroxysmal hemicrania. This has the same diagnostic criteria as cluster headache with one exception, duration. Presents with severe, frequent, and brief (<30 minutes) attacks. These are usually more common in the female population. Diagnosed and treated with indomethacin (Indocin)[1]. Give 25 mg PO tid with meals; if no improvement after 1 week, titrate to 50 mg tid; if no improvement is seen in 1 week, can further titrate to 75 mg tid[3]; if no improvement is seen in 1 week after uptitration, consider an alternate etiology.

A third type of TAC is hemicrania continua. This is a unilateral, daily constant pain with exacerbations of pain intensity associated with autonomic/activation features similar to cluster headache. Diagnosis is mainly with indomethacin trial as above, often resulting in complete symptomatic relief. Sometimes

---

[1] Not FDA approved for this indication.

TABLE 3 Symptomatic Headache Treatment

MIGRAINOUS	TENSION-TYPE	CLUSTER-LIKE	NEURALGIFORM
Covered in chapter Migraine	Heat, massage, analgesic cream	Sumatriptan, zolmitriptan[1], oxygen	Carbamazepine, oxcarbazepine[1]
	Acetaminophen, NSAID	gammaCore	Topiramate[1], gabapentin, baclofen[1]
	Physical modalities	Verapamil[1]	Gamma-knife surgery
	Relaxation techniques	Galcanezumab	Microvascular decompression surgery
	Amitriptyline[1]	Topiramate[1], lithium[1]	
	Venlafaxine[1], tizanidine[1], baclofen[1]	For select types—indomethacin[1]	

[1]Not FDA approved for this indication.
NSAID, Nonsteroidal antiinflammatory drug.

TABLE 4 International Headache Society Criteria for Tension-Type Headache

AT LEAST TWO OF THESE FOUR CHARACTERISTICS	BOTH OF THE FOLLOWING
Bilateral location	No nausea or vomiting
Pressing or tightening (nonpulsating) quality	No more than one of photophobia or phonophobia
Mild or moderate intensity	
Not aggravated by routine physical activity, such as walking or climbing stairs	

BOX 1 International Headache Society Criteria for Cluster Headache

At least five attacks
Severe unilateral orbital, supraorbital, and/or temporal pain lasting 15–180 min
Either or both of the following:
- At least one of the following symptoms or signs, ipsilateral to the headache:
  - Conjunctival injection and/or lacrimation
  - Nasal congestion and/or rhinorrhea
  - Eyelid edema
  - Forehead and facial sweating
  - Miosis and/or ptosis
- A sense of restlessness or agitation

Occurring with a frequency between one every other day and eight per day
Not better accounted for by another diagnosis

patients continue the medication after a diagnostic trial and need to be weaned off very slowly.

A fourth type of TAC is short-lasting, unilateral, neuralgiform headache attack. The differentiating feature from other TAC types is very brief attacks (5 to 240 seconds) of stabbing orbital and temporal pain. Treatment is mainly done with lamotrigine[1]. Second-line agents include topiramate[1] and gabapentin[1].

Cranial Neuralgias

Most headache disorders are secondary to pathophysiology in the brain; however, individual nerves can be irritated in the peripheral nervous system that can lead to pain in the face and head. Common types include trigeminal neuralgia, glossopharyngeal neuralgia, and occipital neuralgia.

Trigeminal neuralgia is also known as *tic douloureux.* It presents as short paroxysmal attacks of severe unilateral shock like pain mostly in the V2 (maxillary)/V3 (mandibula) distribution of the trigeminal nerve. Triggers include eating, drinking, brushing teeth, touching the face, and even talking. First-line symptomatic treatment for trigeminal neuralgia includes carbamazepine (Tegretol) 100 mg bid titrating up to 1200 mg/day (monitoring level and metabolic panel) or oxcarbazepine (Trileptal)[1] 150 to 300 mg bid titrating up to 2400 mg/day. Second-line agents can include baclofen (Lioresal)[1], pregabalin (Lyrica)[1], gabapentin (Neurontin)[1], topiramate (Topamax)[1], and lamotrigine (Lamictal)[1]. For refractory cases consider referral for Gasserian ganglion percutaneous techniques, which are deep face injections typically performed by pain management. Other treatment options include gamma-knife treatment or microvascular decompression performed by neurosurgeons.

Glossopharyngeal neuralgia presents as stabbing pain in the ear, angle of jaw, tongue base, and tonsillar region. Triggers include chewing, swallowing, coughing, yawning, and talking. Treatment is similar to trigeminal neuralgia as detailed above.

Occipital neuralgia is an uncommon cause of headache in the occipital region. It presents as a paroxysmal stabbing pain in the greater, lesser, and third occipital nerve distribution. Examination can reveal local tenderness in the territory of the affected nerve. Treatment includes occipital nerve block using anesthetic along with glucocorticoid, targeting tender points palpated in the near greater and lesser divisions of the occipital nerve. Alternative treatment options include gabapentin[1], pregabalin[1], and amitriptyline[1].

[1] Not FDA approved for this indication.

References

Bendtsen L, Evers S, Linde M, et al: EFNS guideline on the treatment of tension-type headache - report of an EFNS task force, *Eur J Neurol* 17:1318–1325, 2010.

Bendtsen L, Zakrzewska JM, Abbott J, et al: European Academy of Neurology guideline on trigeminal neuralgia, *Eur J Neurol* 26(6):831–849, 2019.

Do TP, et al: Red and orange flags for secondary headaches in clinical practice: SNNOOP10 List, *Neurology* 92(3):134–144, 2019.

Gronseth G, Cruccu G, Alksne J, et al: Practice parameter: the diagnostic evaluation and treatment of trigeminal neuralgia (an evidence-based review): report of the quality standards subcommittee of the American Academy of Neurology and the European Federation of Neurological Societies, *Neurology* 71(15):1183–1190, 2008.

Headache Classification Committee of the International Headache Society (IHS): The international classification of headache disorders, 3rd edition, *Cephalalgia* 38(1):1–211, 2018.

Jensen RH: Tension-type headache - the normal and most prevalent headache, *Headache* 58(2):339–345, 2018.

Kahriman A, Zhu S: Migraine and tension-type headache, *Semin Neurol* 38(6):608–618, 2018.

Pareja JA, Caminero AB, Franco E, et al.: Dose, efficacy and tolerability of long-term indomethacin treatment of chronic paroxysmal hemicrania and hemicrania continua, *Cephalalgia* 21(9):906–910, 2001.

Robbins MS, Starling AJ, Pringsheim TM: Treatment of cluster headache: the American Headache Society evidence-based guidelines, *Headache* 56(7):1093–1106, 2016.

OPTIC NEURITIS

Method of
Heather E. Moss, MD, PhD; and Tanyatuth Padungkiatsagul, MD

CURRENT DIAGNOSIS

- Vision is impaired, including visual acuity, visual field, and/or color perception.
- Patients typically have eye pain that is worse with eye movement.
- Relative afferent pupillary defect (RAPD) can be observed if one eye is affected or both eyes are asymmetrically affected.
- The anterior optic nerve has a normal appearance in two-thirds of affected patients.

CURRENT THERAPY

- Consider IV methylprednisolone (Solu-Medrol, 1 g/day IV for 3 days) followed by oral steroids (1 mg/kg per day for 11 days).
- Avoid low-dose oral steroid monotherapy, as this is associated with a higher relapse rate.
- If brain MRI or blood testing suggest a high-risk, clinically isolated syndrome, consider disease-modifying therapy to delay progression to Multiple Sclerosis (MS) or Neuro-myelitis optica (NMO).
- If the clinical features suggest NMO spectrum disorder (NMOSD) optic neuritis, consider IV methylprednisolone and plasma exchange therapy.
- If the patient's history and testing suggest MS-, NMOSD-, or recurrent myelin oligodendrocyte glycoprotein (MOG)-IgG-associated disease, consider treatment for these conditions.

Epidemiology

The incidence of optic neuritis is approximately 1 to 5 in 100,000. Though it typically affects women in their fourth decade of life, 1 in 4 patients are male, and patients have been reported ranging from the first to seventh decades of life. Optic neuritis occurs worldwide in persons of various ethnicities.

Optic neuritis can be classified as a clinically isolated syndrome or in association with a disease such as multiple sclerosis (MS) or neuromyelitis optica spectrum disorder (NMOSD). NMOSD is clinically distinguished by more frequent involvement of the optic nerves and spinal cord and less involvement of the brain than MS and by distinct pathophysiology. A recently identified distinct classification is myelin oligodendrocyte glycoprotein (MOG)-immunoglobulin G (IgG)-associated optic neuritis. Approximately half of patients with optic neuritis as a clinically isolated syndrome develop MS. A small percentage develop NMOSD.

Risk Factors

A diagnosis of a disease associated with optic neuritis, such as MS or NMOSD, increases the risk of developing optic neuritis. In one study, more than 70% of patients with MS and 100% of patients with neuromyelitis optica (NMO) had unilateral optic neuritis at some point. Patients with recurrent MOG-IgG-associated disorder (MOGAD) flares or persistent elevated serum MOG-IgG may be at risk for recurrent optic neuritis.

Pathophysiology

Most optic neuritis occurs as a result of inflammation causing demyelination of the ganglion cell axons that compose the optic nerve. This is thought to be an immune-mediated process.

Prevention

Disease-modifying therapies have been shown to reduce risk of neurologic relapses in patients with MS or NMOSD. These therapies presumably also decrease the risk of MS-, NMOSD-, or recurrent MOG-IgG-associated optic neuritis because optic neuritis is a common relapse syndrome in these conditions.

Clinical Manifestations

A typical optic neuritis patient experiences acute or subacute loss of vision characterized by decreased visual acuity, visual field loss, and/or color vision loss, accompanied or preceded by pain in the affected eye that is worse with eye movements. However, 8% of patients do not have pain. Other symptoms include positive visual phenomena in 30% of patients. Other signs include a relative afferent papillary defect in cases where one eye is affected or both eyes are asymmetrically affected and a mildly swollen optic nerve head in approximately one-third of patients. Optic neuritis in NMOSD is more likely to have bilateral involvement and severe visual impairment. The spectrum of MOG-IgG-associated optic neuritis is being defined with initial case series describing a higher prevalence of and more severe optic nerve head swelling than MS- or NMOSD-associated optic neuritis.

The natural history of clinically isolated optic neuritis includes resolution of pain 3 to 5 days after onset and nadir of vision 7 to 14 days after onset. Spontaneous improvement in vision is typically evident within 3 weeks, and almost 70% of affected patients recover 20/20 visual acuity even in the absence of treatment. MOG-IgG associated optic neuritis also usually has a favorable final visual outcome. Optic neuritis associated with NMOSD tends to have less spontaneous recovery of vision and early recognition is important due to benefits of early treatment.

Diagnosis

The diagnosis is based on the clinical presentation. Where there is uncertainty, magnetic resonance imaging (MRI) of the orbits, including fat-saturated sequences (T2 and T1 with and without gadolinium contrast), can help visualize inflammation in the retrobulbar optic nerve. Changes on MRI involving the chiasm or more than 50% of the optic nerve are suggestive of NMOSD optic neuritis. MOGAD optic neuritis also has distinct imaging features, including perioptic nerve sheath enhancement.

Optic neuritis is often associated with other demyelinating syndromes, most commonly MS. Therefore it is important to screen for historical and current neurologic impairment through history and examination. MRI and/or and cerebrospinal fluid analysis documenting evidence of dissemination in time and space is diagnostic of MS in patients with clinically isolated optic neuritis. In addition, for patients not meeting criteria for MS at time of presentation with clinically isolated optic neuritis, MRI of the brain has been shown to be an important prognostic indicator for development of MS. MRI of the brain showing 0, 1, or more than 3 lesions typical for MS is associated, respectively, with a 25%, 60%, and 78% risk of progression to clinically definite MS.

Less commonly, optic neuritis is associated with other demyelinating syndromes such as NMOSD. This should be considered in patients with severe vision loss, bilateral involvement, or history of prior optic neuritis or transverse myelitis. A serum antibody, aquaporin-4 (AQP-4)-IgG, has been identified as a pathologic agent in this disorder. Testing for this is commercially available with a published sensitivity and specificity of 63% and 99%, respectively. Positive testing for AQP4-IgG in a patient with optic neuritis is diagnostic of NMOSD per published consensus criteria. A serum MOG-IgG is commercially available and aids in the identification of MOGAD optic neuritis.

Differential Diagnosis

Other diagnostic considerations in a patient with unilateral painful vision loss without explanatory pathology evident on ophthalmic examination include other optic neuropathies such as those due to sarcoidosis, lupus, vasculitis, neoplastic, vascular, and infectious causes. Atypical features for optic neuritis such as systemic symptoms, history of cancer, pain that persists beyond 2 weeks, progressive vision loss beyond 14 days, no spontaneous improvement in vision, retinal hemorrhages, cotton-wool spots, or macular exudates should prompt diagnostic evaluation for etiologies other than optic neuritis.

Treatment and Monitoring

The Optic Neuritis Treatment Trial (ONTT) was a randomized trial comparing placebo, oral prednisone, and IV methylprednisolone (1 g/day IV for 3 days) followed by oral prednisone (1 mg/kg per day for 11 days) for acute optic neuritis. IV steroids hastened recovery of vision without affecting final visual outcome compared with placebo treatment. Treatment with low-dose oral prednisone alone (1 mg/kg/day for 14 days) was associated with no improvement in vision and increased risk of relapse compared with placebo treatment. The 15-year follow-up results, published in 2008, demonstrated persistence of visual recovery. Studies have demonstrated non-inferiority of high-dose oral steroids (1250 mg prednisone/day for 3 days) to IV methylprednisolone with regards to vision recover following acute optic neuritis.

Many clinicians offer IV or high-dose oral steroid treatment to hasten visual recovery. Monotherapy with low-dose oral prednisone should be avoided. Regardless of the decision to treat or not with steroids, all patients should be monitored closely. Continued progression of vision loss, failure to spontaneously recover vision, or persistent pain should prompt additional diagnostic workup as well as consideration for additional IV steroid therapy for atypical optic neuritis. If this is not effective, plasma exchange has been reported as an effective acute therapy for atypical optic neuritis including NMOSD and MOGAD optic neuritis.

In patients with acute optic neuritis and NMOSD or acute optic neuritis on the NMO-spectrum, treatment with plasma exchange or rituxamab (Rituxan)[1] should be considered to improve functional visual outcome.

In patients with a clinically isolated syndrome, consideration should be given to institution of disease-modifying therapy for MS based on the type and number of lesions on brain MRI and oligoclonal bands in cerebrospinal fluid. Several clinical trials have shown an association between early treatment with MS therapies and decreased incidence of progression to clinically definite MS in patients with a recent clinically isolated syndrome and clinically silent lesions on brain MRI.

In patients who meet diagnostic criteria for either MS or NMOSD, consideration should be given to treating the underlying disease. Eculizumab (Soliris), Inebilizumab (Uplizna), and Satralizumab (Enspryng) have shown to reduced risk of relapse and increased remission rate in AQP-4-IgG-positive NMOSD. Decisions regarding chronic therapy following MOGAD optic neuritis are currently based on recurrence and persistently elevated serum antibody titers.

Complications

Though more than 70% of patients with optic neuritis recover objectively normal visual acuity, many have residual subjective visual disturbances. These often worsen or recur in heat, which is known as Uhtoff's phenomenon.

Complications of steroid therapy include insomnia, agitation, and stomach irritation. Long-term side effects of steroid treatment for this condition are rare owing to the brief period of treatment. Complications of disease-modifying therapies for MS-, NMOSD-, and MOG-IgG-associated disease are reviewed elsewhere.

References

Beck RQ, Cleary PA, Anderson MM, et al: A randomized, controlled trial of corticosteroids in the treatment of acute optic neuritis, *The Neuritis Study Group*, N Engl J Med 326:581–588, 1992.

Bonnan M, Valentino R, Debeugny S, et al: Short delay to initiate plasma exchange is the strongest predictor of outcome in severe attacks of NMO spectrum disorders, *J Neurol Neurosurg Psychiatry*. 89:346–351, 2018.

Cree BAC, Bennett JL, Kim HJ, et al. Inebilizumab for the treatment of neuromyelitis optica spectrum disorder (N-MOmentum): a double-blind, randomised placebo-controlled phase 2/3 trial, *Lancet* 394:1352–1363, 2019.

Chen JJ, Flanagan EP, Jitprapaikulsan J, et al: Myelin oligodendrocyte glycoprotein antibody-positive optic neuritis: clinical characteristics, radiologic clues, and outcome, *Am J Ophthalmol* 195:8–15, 2018.

Cobo-Calvo A, Sepúlveda M, Rollot F, et al: Evaluation of treatment response in adults with relapsing MOG-Ab-associated disease, *J Neuroinflammation* 16:134, 2019.

Hickman SJ, Ko M, Chaudhry F, et al: Optic neuritis: an update on typical and atypical optic neuritis, *Neuro-ophthalmology* 32:237–248, 2008.

Merle H, Olindo S, Bonnan M, et al: Natural history of the visual impairment of relapsing neuromyelitis optica, *Ophthalmology* 114:810–815, 2007.

Morrow SA, Fraser JA, Day C: Effect of treating acute optic neuritis with bioequivalent oral vs intravenous corticosteroids: a randomized clinical trial, *JAMA Neurol* 75(6):690-6, 2018.

Moss HE: Visual consequence of medications for multiple sclerosis: the good, the bad, the ugly and the unknown, *Eye Brain*. 29:13–21, 2017.

Optic Neuritis Study Group: The clinical profile of optic neuritis: experience of the optic neuritis treatment trial, *Arch Ophthalmol* 109:1673–1678, 1991.

Optic Neuritis Study Group: Multiple sclerosis risk after optic neuritis: final optic neuritis treatment trial follow-up, *Arch Neurol* 65:727–732, 2008.

Optic Neuritis Study Group: Visual function 15 years after optic neuritis, *Ophthalmology* 115:1079–1082, 2008.

Pittock SJ, Berthele A, Fujihara K, et al: Eculizumab in aquaporin-4-positive neuromyelitis optica spectrum disorder, *N Engl J Med* 381:614–625, 2019.

Roesner S, Appel R, Gbadamosi J, et al: Treatment of steroid-unresponsive optic neuritis with plasma exchange, *Acta Neurol Scand* 126(2):103–108, 2012.

Thompson AJ, Banwell BL, Carroll WM, et al: Diagnosis of multiple sclerosis: 2017 revisions of the McDonald criteria, *Lancet Neurol*. 17:162–173, 2018.

Vodopivec I, Matiello M, Prasad S: Treatment of neuromyelitis optica, *Curr Opin Ophthalmol* 26(6):476–483, 2015.

Winferchuk DM, Banwell B, Bennett JL, et al: International consensus diagnostic criteria for neuromyelitis optica spectrum disorders, *Neurology* 85:177–189, 2015.

Yamamura T, Kleiter I, Fujihara K, et al.: Trial of Satralizumab in neuromyelitis optica spectrum disorder, *N Engl J Med* 381:2114–2124, 2019.

PARKINSON DISEASE

Method of
Brian James Nagle, MD, MPH; and Kathleen Mary Shannon, MD

CURRENT DIAGNOSIS

- The cardinal features of Parkinson disease are "TRAP":
  - Tremor at rest
  - Rigidity
  - Akinesia or bradykinesia
  - Postural instability
- It is responsive to levodopa and has unilateral onset and a progressive course.
- Consider alternative diagnosis for rapid gait impairment or frequent falls at onset, cerebellar signs, symptoms symmetric or restricted to legs at onset, lack of progression in 5 years, early bulbar or respiratory dysfunction, severe autonomic failure, or lack of development of typical nonmotor symptoms.

---

[1] Not FDA approved for this indication.

CURRENT THERAPY

- There is no benefit to starting medication early given no evidence of disease-modifying benefits, but exercise may be neuroprotective.
- In early disease, levodopa, dopamine agonists (DAs), and monoamine oxidase-B (MAO-B) inhibitors are all efficacious.
  - Levodopa is superior for treating motor symptoms but carries risk of dyskinesias.
  - Avoid DAs and anticholinergics in those over 70 years because of side effect profile.
  - MAO-B inhibitors as monotherapy are beneficial for 2 to 3 years before additional medication is needed.
  - For patients under 60 years, anticholinergics (for tremor-predominant Parkinson disease) or amantadine (Symmetrel) can be considered.
- For motor fluctuations, MAO-B inhibitors, DAs, catechol-O-methyltransferase inhibitors, amantadine, and istradefylline (Nourianz) can be useful.
- Deep brain stimulation (DBS) is useful for treating levodopa-resistant tremor; reserve focused lesioning for nonsurgical candidates with limited life expectancy.
- DBS and continuous levodopa-carbidopa intestinal gel (Duopa enteral suspension) have the best efficacy for reducing motor fluctuations, but novel delivery options are under investigation.

Epidemiology

Parkinson disease (PD) is the second most common neurodegenerative disease, affecting about 1 million individuals in the United States, and is expected to increase to 1.2 million by the year 2030. Individuals with PD account for about 0.3% of the general population over the age of 40 years. Annual incidence is about 90,000 cases of PD each year. Males tend to be affected more than females, with lifetime risk of 2% and 1.3%, respectively, in those 40 years and older.

Pathophysiology

PD is a progressive neurodegenerative disease that results from loss of the dopaminergic neurons in the substantia nigra pars compacta (SNpc) of the midbrain, leading to an imbalance of motor pathways in the basal ganglia. The hallmark pathologic feature of PD is the presence of cytotoxic intracellular inclusions called Lewy bodies, which result from the misfolding and subsequent aggregation of the alpha-synuclein protein. The trigger of this misfolding is unknown, but most theories involve an environmental trigger in genetically susceptible individuals. Lewy bodies are also found outside of the SNpc with a preference for particular neuronal populations both centrally and peripherally, which correspond with symptoms seen at varying stages of PD, including the premotor stage. One theory suggests that misfolded proteins are transferred between these neuronal cell populations and induce alpha-synuclein misfolding in adjacent cells in a prion-like fashion. Current research is looking to uncover the pathologic mechanism for potential pharmacologic targets.

Risk Factors

Although age is the greatest risk factor with a mean age of onset of 60 years, 5% to 10% of cases occur before the age of 50 years. The majority of cases are sporadic or idiopathic. Having one first-degree relative increases the risk of PD by two to three times, and a pathogenic variant with known significance can be found in 10% to 15% of PD cases. Although genetic testing is not routinely done, there are commercially available panels that typically include the seven most common genes and can be considered with genetic counseling when there is a strong family history. One such pathogenic variant is a mutation in *GBA1*, which also causes Gaucher disease. Seen predominantly in those of Ashkenazi Jewish descent, its role in PD is likely related to the decreased activity of glucocerebrosidase, leading to lysosomal dysfunction that promotes accumulation of alpha-synuclein. Another common pathogenic variant involves mutations to leucine-rich repeat kinase 2 (*LRRK2*), which likely represents a distinct subset given it has been shown to have distinct pathologic findings and phenotype with slower progression and fewer nonmotor features. Inherited cases tend to have an earlier age of onset than idiopathic cases, and ongoing studies are looking for novel genetic and epigenetic variants because disease-modifying targets may vary for different genetic variants. Environmental factors that are associated with PD risk include pesticides, well water, heavy metals, traumatic brain injury, and some industrial chemicals. Conversely, caffeine, smoking, physical activity, and nonsteroidal antiinflammatory medications have been associated with decreased risk of PD.

Clinical Manifestations

Symptoms of PD can be divided into those that are either motor or nonmotor. Motor symptoms include the four cardinal symptoms: tremor at rest, rigidity, akinesia or bradykinesia, and postural instability. Tremor (an oscillating, rhythmic movement) is often the presenting symptom, though there are people who never develop tremor. The PD tremor typically occurs unilaterally at onset in one of the upper extremities but can also involve the legs and jaw. It is slower in frequency (4 to 6 Hz) and larger in amplitude than essential tremor and enhanced physiologic tremor, though early on amplitude may be small. It typically occurs at rest, though can occur after a few seconds with prolonged posture, known as a reemergent tremor. Although the tremor usually disappears or reduces during action, it can persist, though it should be more pronounced at rest. It often increases with stress and distraction, which can be observed during conversation or while distracted performing a motor task in another extremity or stating the days of the week backward. Another phenomenon patients may describe is an internal tremor or buzzing when no observable external tremor can be seen.

Bradykinesia (slowness of movements) is often seen with akinesia or hypokinesia (decreased amplitude of movements), and patients will describe difficulty with dexterity, changes in handwriting (micrographia), and slowing of reaction time. Additional signs are reduced arm swing during gait, decreased blink rate, and hypomimia (masked facies). Hypophonia (low or soft volume) is another common feature that may be noticed initially by the family. To test for bradykinesia, use rapid-alternating movements (RAMs) with emphasis on making big and fast movements, such as opening and closing the hand, finger tapping, supinating and pronating the hand, and tapping of toes and heels. When observing RAMs, it is important to note speed, amplitude, and rhythm, as patients may inadvertently gradually decrease the amplitude to maintain speed (decrement) or have brief pauses in the rhythm (hesitation). Gait changes due to bradykinesia are often noted by the family because of slowing with a quick, shortened stride often described as shuffling. It is important to listen to the patient's gait as scuffing of the soles on the floor can often be heard. Hesitation during gait is often referred to as "freezing of gait," occurring particularly at doorways and corners.

Rigidity is the resistance to passive movement that is independent of velocity ("lead pipe rigidity"), as opposed to spasticity, which is velocity dependent with resistance felt during rapid passive movements and absent when slow. The classic "cogwheel rigidity" is simply a tremor superimposed over the rigidity. Patients may describe stiffness with movements. Rigidity can be tested in the neck and all extremities with passive movements. Subtle rigidity can be enhanced via distraction such as contralateral activation by asking the patient to perform a RAM in the contralateral limb. This is distinct from dystonia, an abnormal sustained contraction of muscles that can lead to abnormal posturing, which can also be seen in PD. If dystonia occurs in the extremities they may describe cramping of muscles or gait difficulty due to curling of their toes or inversion of their foot. Cervical dystonia often causes neck stiffness and/or pain that limits activities like driving. Dystonia can also occur in the eyelids with difficulty opening the eyes (blepharospasm).

Postural instability is the lack of corrective movements to maintain balance and often presents as gait instability or imbalance. Patients will often develop stooped posture due to dysfunction of both motor and sensory pathways, including increased tone in axial flexors and paraspinal muscle weakness. This abnormal posturing can progress to camptocormia, but some may also lean to one side (Pisa syndrome). The abnormal axial posturing often does not persist in the supine position. Postural instability can be tested with the pull test, where patients are warned that the examiner will pull their shoulders from behind and instructed to protect themselves from falling by resisting the pull or taking a step backward. An abnormal response is when the examiner, who is standing close behind, needs to catch the patient because of lack of a protective response. This is best performed with the examiner standing in front of a wall to avoid falling backward with the patient. It is not necessary to test this in a patient who requires an assistive device to walk, as it can be implied that they are unable to stand unassisted.

Nonmotor symptoms can affect many other organ systems and may require multiple specialists for management. These can be broadly divided into those that are neuropsychiatric, autonomic, sleep, and sensory. Common nonmotor symptoms include depression and/or anxiety, constipation, rapid eye movement sleep behavior disorder, anosmia, orthostatic hypotension, and urinary urgency and frequency.

Diagnosis

The gold standard for diagnosis remains the histologic features noted above at autopsy. In 2015 the International Parkinson and Movement Disorder Society (MDS) published updated MDS Clinical Diagnostic Criteria for Parkinson Disease (MDS-PD Criteria), which first requires presence of clinical parkinsonism, defined as bradykinesia (both slowness *and* decrement in speed or amplitude) plus tremor and/or rigidity. Postural instability was not included as this is typically seen later in the disease course, and early onset of postural instability should indicate an alternative diagnosis. If parkinsonism is present, established PD diagnosis can be made with at least two supportive criteria, including clear and dramatic response to dopaminergic therapy (levodopa or dopamine agonist), levodopa-induced dyskinesias (involuntary writhing movements), marked motor fluctuations with end-of-dose wearing off, rest tremor of an extremity, anosmia, or evidence of cardiac sympathetic denervation with metaiodobenzylguanidine scintigraphy. Red flags that should warrant considering alternative diagnoses include rapid gait impairment or frequent falls, bilateral and symmetric symptoms at onset, lack of progression in 5 years, early bulbar or respiratory dysfunction, severe autonomic failure, or lack of development of typical nonmotor symptoms. The MDS-PD Criteria also define absolute exclusion criteria, which if present rule out PD, such as cerebellar signs, downward vertical gaze palsy, frontotemporal dementia, or parkinsonism restricted to the lower extremities. A thorough review of medication history is also important to evaluate for history of dopamine-blocking neuroleptics and time course that would suggest drug-induced parkinsonism. The most common associated drug classes are antipsychotics and antiemetics.

Ancillary testing can include magnetic resonance imaging of the brain to rule out vascular or other structural cause of secondary parkinsonism. Although dopamine transporter (DAT) positron emission tomography or single-photon emission computed tomography with reduced tracer uptake in the striatum can demonstrate nigrostriatal degeneration, making it suitable for distinguishing between neurodegenerative and nondegenerative etiologies (essential tremor, vascular, or drug-induced), it cannot distinguish PD from other neurodegenerative forms of parkinsonism, such as Lewy body dementia or multiple system atrophy (MSA).

Seeding amplification assay technologies that amplify minute amounts of misfolded alpha-synuclein to detect its presence in cerebrospinal fluid and tissue are under investigation and show promise as a future ancillary test, though this may not differentiate PD from other alpha-synucleinopathies. Skin biopsies with immunohistochemical staining for phosphorylated alpha-synuclein are another ancillary test undergoing investigation and have even been shown to differentiate PD from MSA.

The Unified Parkinson's Disease Rating Scale (UPDRS) was designed to rate severity of disease and should not be used to diagnose PD. Part III (Motor Examination) of the UPDRS is frequently used for tracking a patient's response to treatment and progression of disease. The Hoehn and Yahr Staging Scale is used to categorically stage progression (Table 1).

Current Therapy

The most recent guidelines for treatment were published in 2021 by the American Academy of Neurology for treatment in early PD. The MDS published more extensive guidelines in 2018 for both early and advanced PD.

Currently there are no disease-modifying therapies to slow or stop progression of PD, thus treatments are considered to be symptomatic for both motor and nonmotor symptoms. Nonpharmacologic therapies include physical, occupational, and speech therapies. In particular, the Lee Silverman Voice Treatment (LSVT) LOUD program focuses on voice projection to counter hypophonia, and the LSVT BIG program focuses on improving balance, posture, and gait. Studies using dietary supplements (e.g., coenzyme Q10 and creatine) to prevent or delay progression are either still investigational or have been shown not to be useful. Exercise is associated with decreased risk, but with regard to slowing progression, evidence is still insufficient and under investigation. There are also several PD-focused exercise programs, such as dance, tai chi, and boxing. There is no particular PD diet, but the Mediterranean diet is recommended.

In patients presenting with early stages of PD, that is mild symptoms that are either minimally or nondisabling, it is important to consider the impact of symptoms on their life, as physically nondisabling symptoms may still cause anxiety in social situations or interfere with their job. Other factors to consider are age, comorbidities, and the efficacy and side effect profiles of available treatments. For those that are nondisabling and do not affect the patient's life, it is reasonable to monitor symptoms clinically, as early initiation of treatment has not been shown to slow progression.

Pharmacologic treatments in early disease (Table 2) fall into two categories of medications: dopaminergic (levodopa, dopamine agonists [DAs], and monoamine oxidase-B [MAO-B] inhibitors) and nondopaminergic (anticholinergics and amantadine). There are benefits and risks with all three dopaminergic classes. Although levodopa is the most effective treatment for motor symptoms, it does carry a risk of developing dyskinesias. This typically occurs with daily doses greater than 400 mg, so it is important to use the lowest effective dose (150 to 300 mg/day). It is also important to note that there can be both short-term and long-term effects, so titration should be gradual with interval changes around every 3 to 4 months based on response to treatment, as rapid titration can lead to unnecessarily higher total daily doses that increase the risk of dyskinesias. Studies

TABLE 1	Hoehn and Yahr Staging Scale
STAGE	**DESCRIPTION**
1	Symptoms are unilateral only; minimal to no disability
2	Symptoms are bilateral, balance is intact; minimal disability
3	Mild to moderate bilateral symptoms, impaired balance; physically independent
4	Severe disability; able to walk and stand unassisted
5	Wheelchair or bedridden if unassisted

TABLE 2	Treatment of Motor Symptoms in Early Parkinson Disease			
DRUG CLASS	**DRUG NAMES**	**DOSING**	**SIDE EFFECTS**	**COMMENTS**
Levodopa	Carbidopa-levodopa IR (Sinemet)	25 mg/100 mg; 0.5–2 tabs TID	Dyskinesia, orthostatic hypotension, drowsiness, nausea, hallucinations	Titrating too quickly avoided, can take 2–3 months for benefit Higher risk of dyskinesia when levodopa >400 mg/day
Dopamine agonists (nonergot)	Pramipexole (Mirapex)	IR: 0.125–1.5 mg TID ER: 0.375–4.5 mg daily	Impulse control disorder, hallucinations, orthostatic hypotension	Avoided in elderly because of increased risk of side effects
	Ropinirole (Requip)	IR: 0.25–8 mg TID XL: 2–24 mg daily	TD: Skin irritation	Slow taper when discontinuing
	Rotigotine patch (Neupro)	TD: 2–8 mg/24 hr		
MAO-B inhibitors	Rasagiline (Azilect)	0.5–1 mg daily	Nausea, orthostatic hypotension, dyskinesia	Will likely need additional medication after 2–3 years of monotherapy
	Selegiline (Eldepryl)	5 mg daily or BID	Serotonin syndrome with SSRI, rare in PD	
Anticholinergics	Benztropine (Cogentin)	0.5–6 mg daily total; divided 2–4 doses	Nausea, dry mouth, blurred vision, constipation, urinary retention, confusion	Can reduce tremor in tremor-predominant PD Avoided in elderly
	Trihexyphenidyl (Artane)	1–15 mg daily total; divided 3–4 doses		
NMDA antagonist	Amantadine IR (Symmetrel)	50–100 mg BID or TID	Confusion, hallucinations, myoclonus, livedo reticularis, leg edema, insomnia, dry mouth	Discontinuation requires gradual taper Also used as adjunct to reduce dyskinesias

BID, Twice daily; *ER*, extended-release; *IR*, immediate-release; *MAO-B*, monoamine oxidase-B; *NMDA*, N-methyl-D-aspartate receptor; *PD*, Parkinson disease; *SSRI*, selective serotonin reuptake inhibitor; *TD*, transdermal; *TID*, three times daily; *XL*, extended-release.

comparing immediate release (IR) formulation with controlled-release formulation have not shown a difference in early disease, and no studies have compared extended-release (ER) formulation with IR in early disease. It is important to note that protein competes with levodopa in the gut for absorption. Early in the disease course, patients may be less affected clinically by taking levodopa too close to meals; to get the greatest bioavailability, it should be recommended to take levodopa 30 minutes before or after eating. Patients at higher risk of developing dyskinesias tend to be younger at onset, female, low weight, and have increased severity of disease. It is also important to note that tremor can be resistant to levodopa in some patients, which is important to keep in mind when assessing response to treatment.

Levodopa-sparing dopaminergic therapy for early disease includes the use of either DAs or MOA-B inhibitors, which can be considered for patients who are at higher risk of developing dyskinesias. Treatment with DA monotherapy can show improvement up to 5 years without needing the addition of levodopa. DAs should only be considered in patients under 60 years given the increased risk of side effects in the elderly. DAs should also be avoided in patients who have a history of impulse control disorder, cognitive impairment, hallucinations, or excessive daytime sleepiness. Patients should be warned about side effects and asked to involve a family member or caregiver in monitoring. Transdermal or ER formulations of DAs may also reduce the risk or severity of side effects. No specific DA has been shown to be superior, though the nonergot DAs (ropinirole, rotigotine, and pramipexole) are preferred over ergot DAs (bromocriptine [Parlodel], pergolide[2], cabergoline[1]) given the increased risk of cardiac fibrosis with the latter. Selection of DA should take cost and ease of use into consideration, and initiation should start with the lowest dose with a slow increase to the lowest dose of clinical efficacy. If side effects are seen, a slow, staged taper should be used to avoid DA withdrawal syndrome. MAO-B inhibitors rasagiline (Azilect) and selegiline (Eldepryl, Zelapar) have been shown to provide some benefit in early PD, though the response is not as robust as

levodopa or DAs, and most patients require another medication in 2 to 3 years. Concomitant use of MAO-B inhibitors and serotonin reuptake inhibitors carries a risk of serotonin syndrome, though they do not need to be avoided altogether as this is rarely seen in PD.

Nondopaminergic therapy for early PD with anticholinergics (benztropine [Cogentin] and trihexyphenidyl [Artane]) can be considered in young patients with tremor-predominant PD but should be avoided in the elderly because of risks of cognitive impairments and association with increased dementia risk. Amantadine IR (Symmetrel) can also be used as monotherapy in early disease with young patients.

As the disease progresses, most patients will need some formulation of levodopa (Table 3), and many will also require use of adjunct therapy (Table 4). In advanced PD, nigrostriatal dopaminergic presynaptic neurons are no longer able to store and release dopamine, which makes patients more susceptible to the pulsatile nature of oral medications, resulting in "wearing off," the reemergence of PD motor and nonmotor symptoms. This can take many forms and in some can be predominantly nonmotor, so asking patients if they feel *any* symptoms that indicate it is time for their next dose or if they miss a dose can be helpful to bring this to light. Dyskinesias can occur when levodopa peaks, and some may also experience them when wearing off (diphasic dyskinesia). It is important to distinguish whether the dyskinesias are bothersome, as most nonbothersome dyskinesias do not need to be treated. As mentioned previously, high-protein meals can affect absorption, as can constipation. It is also important to ask about dietary supplements, such as the bean *Mucuna pruriens* which contains naturally occurring levodopa, as supplements are not regulated as stringently, and the amount of levodopa has been shown to vary drastically and rarely corresponds with the label. Strategies to reduce motor fluctuations include switching carbidopa-levodopa from an IR formulation (Sinemet) to ER (Rytary) to minimize the pulsatility, or adding a catechol-O-methyltransferase inhibitor, MAO-B inhibitor, DA, or adenosine-A2A antagonist. When wearing off is unpredictable or sudden, use of on-demand therapies (levodopa or apomorphine [Apokyn]) can help reverse or lessen the symptoms (Tables 3 and 4). When dyskinesias are bothersome, amantadine is

[1] Not FDA approved for this indication.
[2] Not available in the United States.

commonly used. Clozapine (Clozaril)[1] can be used to treat dyskinesia and psychosis but is seldom used first-line because of the risk of agranulocytosis and need for frequent lab monitoring.

The most effective treatments currently for motor fluctuations and dyskinesias are deep brain stimulation (DBS) and continuous levodopa-carbidopa intestinal gel (CLIG; Duopa enteral suspension), which is delivered via a percutaneous gastrojejunostomy tube with a small battery-powered pump. DBS modulates pathways in the brain that reduce symptoms and allow reduction of dopaminergic therapy. CLIG reduces pulsatility with its continuous infusion. There is a continuous subcutaneous apomorphine infusion pump available in Europe (pending FDA approval) that can help reduce daily carbidopa-levodopa doses. There is also a continuous subcutaneous pump that delivers phosphorylated carbidopa-levodopa pending FDA approval. Focused lesioning can be done in a variety of ways, resulting in permanent destruction of a specific target in the brain to reduce tremor but does not reduce motor fluctuations or other PD features. Whereas prior lesioning techniques required surgery or radiation, focused ultrasound lesioning can be done nonsurgically, though it should be reserved for those who are not candidates for DBS and those with a limited life expectancy given the lack of long-term data.

Monitoring

PD is a neurologic disease that affects multiple systems in the body, thus a comprehensive review of systems at each visit should be completed. Table 5 highlights common nonmotor symptoms and management strategies. Management often requires a multidisciplinary approach.

Patients should undergo cognitive screening annually. The Montreal Cognitive Assessment is more sensitive than the Mini-Mental State Examination for identifying mild cognitive impairment. Cognitive decline can be treated with rivastigmine transdermal patch (Exelon), which is better tolerated than the oral formulation and is the only acetylcholinesterase inhibitor shown to improve cognition in PD. It was also shown to reduce falls. If rivastigmine is not tolerated, donepezil (Aricept),[1] galantamine (Razadyne),[1] or memantine (Namenda)[1] can be trialed.

Complications

When a patient is admitted to the hospital, great care should be taken to ensure they receive their PD medications in a timely fashion. Many formulations are not available in hospitals and require patients to bring their own medications, particularly in advanced disease. Patients should not have carbidopa-levodopa or DAs stopped acutely because of risk of dopamine withdrawal.

[1] Not FDA approved for this indication.

[1] Not FDA approved for this indication.

TABLE 3	Comparison of Carbidopa-Levodopa Formulations in Advanced Parkinson Disease			
FORMULATION	**DRUG NAMES**	**DOSAGE FORMS & IR EQUIVALENT***	**LEVODOPA PHARMACOKINETICS**	**COMMENTS**
C/L IR	Sinemet[†] C/L IR ODT (Parcopa)[†] C/L IR (Dhivy)[†]	Sinemet/Parcopa: 25 mg/100 mg tab (most common) 10 mg/100 mg tab 25 mg/250 mg tab Dhivy: 25 mg/100 mg tab (scored for ¼-tab dose increments)	Peak: 30–60 mins Half-life: 1.5–2 hr Frequency: every 2–3 hr, 4–8 times daily	Carbidopa prevents peripheral conversion, reducing side effects and increasing levodopa distribution in CNS Crush or chew for more rapid onset ODT useful with dysphagia
C/L CR	Sinemet CR	25 mg/100 mg ≈ 1 tab IR 50 mg/200 mg ≈ 2 tabs IR	Peak: 1.5–2 hr Half-life: 1.6 hr Frequency: every 4–8 hr (25–100 mg); every 6–8 hr (50–200 mg)	Wax matrix lowers bioavailability; variable, unpredictable response limits daytime use; primarily used overnight
C/L/entacapone	Stalevo	12.5 mg/50 mg/200 mg ≈ 0.5 tab IR 18.75 mg/75 mg/200 mg ≈ 0.75 tab IR 25 mg/100 mg/200 mg ≈ 1 tab IR 31.25 mg/125 mg/200 mg ≈ 1.25 tabs IR 37.5 mg/150 mg/200 mg ≈ 1.5 tabs IR 50 mg/200 mg/200 mg ≈ 2 tabs IR	Peak: 1–2 hr Half-life: 1.1–3.2 hr Frequency: every 2–8 hr, 3–8 times daily	Can combine dose with IR to increase C/L without increasing entacapone Can cause diarrhea and turn body fluids orange Increased risk of dyskinesias
C/L ER	Rytary	23.75 mg/95 mg ≈ 0.5 tab IR 36.25 mg/145 mg ≈ 0.75 tab IR 48.75 mg/195 mg ≈ 1 tab IR 61.25 mg/245 mg ≈ 1.25 tab IR	Peak: 1–4.5 hr Half-life: 1.9 hr Frequency: every 4–8 hr, 3–5 times daily	Can cause headaches Granule ratio: 1 IR:2 ER Sprinkle capsule contents into applesauce for more rapid onset
C/L intestinal gel	Duopa enteral suspension	Levodopa dose: Morning bolus: 100–200 mg over 10–30 min Daily maintenance: 20–120 mg/hr (max 2 g daily) Bolus: 10–40 mg every 1–2 hr as needed	Peak: 2.5–3 hr; therapeutic plasma levels 10–30 min after bolus Half-life: similar to IR Frequency: administered over 16 hr daily	Requires GJ-tube Some patients may need routine nighttime oral C/L after daily infusion
Levodopa oral inhalation	Inbrija[†]	INH: 84 mg per dose	Peak: 15–30 min Half-life: 1–2 hr Frequency: 1 dose per off-period, ≤5 doses daily	Used as needed for early wearing off

*Equivalent reference is carbidopa-levodopa IR 25 mg/100 mg tablet.
[†]Can be used as on-demand therapy.
C/L, Carbidopa-levodopa; *CNS*, central nervous system; *CR*, controlled-release; *ER*, extended-release; *GJ-tube*, gastrojejunostomy tube; *INH*, inhaled; *IR*, immediate-release; *ODT*, oral dissolving tablet.

Psychosis occurs in about half of patients and presents as visual illusions (misinterpretation of visual stimuli), hallucinations (visual or presence), and/or delusions. Visual hallucinations are generally well-formed and recurrent. Auditory hallucinations are less common and occur with visual hallucinations, rarely in isolation. When delusions are present, they are often paranoid in character with common themes of abandonment and spousal infidelity. PD psychosis diagnosis can be made when at least one of these occurs after the onset of PD and is recurrent or continuous for at least 1 month. The only FDA-approved treatment is pimavanserin (Nuplazid), a selective inverse agonist of serotonin receptor 2A, and evidence suggests it has a lower mortality than other antipsychotics. Clozapine (Clozaril)[1] is effective, though as noted earlier, requires frequent lab monitoring, so it is often reserved for refractory cases. Quetiapine (Seroquel)[1] is frequently used, though clinical studies have not shown benefit (Table 5).

Although PD clinical course is very heterogenous with varying rates of progression and symptomology, it generally follows a gradual and steady progression. When acute changes are seen, infections and metabolic derangements should be ruled out. Death is generally from another cause, complications from a fall, or related to failure to thrive or aspiration pneumonia in the setting of dysphagia.

---

[1] Not FDA approved for this indication.

TABLE 4 Adjunct Treatments of Motor Symptoms in Advanced Parkinson Disease

DRUG CLASS	DRUG NAMES	DOSING	SIDE EFFECTS	COMMENTS
Dopamine agonists*	Apomorphine (Apokyn)[†]	SC: 2–6 mg (0.2–0.6 mL), ≤5 doses daily	Nausea, orthostatic hypotension	Requires in-office or nurse-monitored titration
MAO-B inhibitors*	Safinamide (Xadago)	50–100 mg daily	Nausea, orthostatic hypotension, dyskinesia Serotonin syndrome with SSRI; rare in PD	
	Zonisamide (Zonegran)[1]	25–100 mg daily		
COMT inhibitors	Entacapone (Comtan)	200 mg with dose of C/L, up to 8 times daily	Potentiates levodopa; may worsen dyskinesias, hallucinations, hypotension, hyperhidrosis	Orange body secretions (urine, sweat, etc.)
	Tolcapone (Tasmar)	100–200 mg TID		Generally avoided because of hepatotoxicity, requiring monitoring
	Opicapone (Ongentys)	25–50 mg nightly		
NMDA antagonist*	Amantadine ER (Gocovri)	68.5–274 mg nightly	Confusion, hallucinations, myoclonus, livedo reticularis, leg edema, insomnia, dry mouth	Reduces dyskinesias; can also reduce off time
	Amantadine ER (Osmolex ER)	129–322 mg nightly		Gradual taper if discontinued
Adenosine A2A antagonist	Istradefylline (Nourianz)	20–40 mg daily	Dyskinesia	Reduces off time

[1] Not FDA approved for this indication.
*Refer to Table 2 for additional medications; dopamine agonists, MAO-B inhibitors, and amantadine used for early PD are also used as adjunct to levodopa.
[†] Used for on-demand therapy.
COMT, Catechol-O-methyltransferase; *ER,* extended-release; *MAO-B,* monoamine oxidase-B; *NMDA,* N-methyl-D-aspartate receptor; *PD,* Parkinson disease; *SC,* subcutaneous; *SL,* sublingual; *SSRI,* selective serotonin reuptake inhibitor; *TID,* three times daily.

TABLE 5 Treatment of Nonmotor Symptoms in Parkinson Disease

SYMPTOMS	MANAGEMENT	CONSIDERATIONS
Constipation*	Physical activity and hydration Stopping offending medications Nutrition: bran/wheat germ cereal, applesauce, and prune juice blended, 2 tablespoons 1–2 times daily Fiber: methylcellulose (Citrucel) daily Stool softener: docusate (Colace) Osmotic laxative: PEG (Miralax), milk of magnesia, or lactulose (Kristalose) Stimulant laxative: senna (Senokot) or bisacodyl (Dulcolax, oral or suppository) Enema	Avoid psyllium husk fiber supplements (Metamucil), which can worsen constipation with dehydration. Counsel on importance of prevention. Constipation often requires multiple agents with combination daily treatments for prevention and more aggressive, as needed, treatments. Constipation can decrease absorption and efficacy of oral medications.
Gastroparesis*	Diet modification (smaller frequent low-fat meals), H2 blockers, domperidone[2] For nausea, can consider ondansetron (Zofran)[1]	Avoid prochlorperazine (Compazine), promethazine (Phenergan), and metoclopramide (Reglan), which can worsen PD motor symptoms. Avoid PPIs, which may further slow gastric emptying.
Orthostatic hypotension*	Increased hydration, liberal salt intake, compression stockings +/– abdominal binders Droxidopa (Northera), fludrocortisone (Florinef)[1], or midodrine (Proamatine); can cause or worsen supine hypertension Pyridostigmine (Mestinon)[1]; does not cause supine hypertension	Degree of neurogenic orthostatic hypotension can be assessed with tilt table testing. If supine hypertension is present, instruct patient to sleep with head elevated 30 degrees; shorter-acting antihypertensive can be considered at bedtime. Orthostatic hypotension often requires comanagement with cardiology.

Continued

TABLE 5	Treatment of Nonmotor Symptoms in Parkinson Disease—cont'd	
SYMPTOMS	**MANAGEMENT**	**CONSIDERATIONS**
Pedal edema*	Compression stockings or elastic bandage wrap Lymphedema management clinic	Avoid diuretics, which can cause or worsen orthostatic hypotension.
Neurogenic bladder* (urinary retention, urgency, and frequency)	May be on-off fluctuations (especially if occurring primarily at night), optimize PD meds Mirabegron (Myrbetriq), vibegron (Gemtesa) Clean technique intermittent catheterization Referral to urologist or urogynecologist	Avoid anticholinergics given increased risk of confusion. BPH is frequent in older men, so urology referral can help rule out structural etiology.
Psychosis (hallucinations/ delusions)	Pimavanserin (Nuplazid) only FDA-approved treatment Quetiapine (Seroquel)[1] and clozapine (Clozaril),[1] lowest risk of worsening PD	Clozapine requires prescriber to be on registry and frequent CBC monitoring.
REM sleep behavior disorder (RBD)	Melatonin[7] Low-dose clonazepam (Klonopin)[1] if OSA ruled out or treated	Patients typically report vivid dreams; if no sleep partner, you can ask about falling out of bed, dramatic changes in position in bed, or noticing items knocked off nightstand upon waking.
Insomnia	Assessing timing of arousal; may be akathisia from wearing off; can use C/L CR or ER dose before bed or middle of night	Sleep study can be helpful as poor sleep quality or excessive daytime sleepiness may be due to OSA.
Restless legs syndrome	May be akathisia from wearing off, optimize meds If no response to dopaminergic changes, gabapentin (Neurontin)[1] or pregabalin (Lyrica)[1] can help In younger patients, can consider low-dose nonergot DA	
Mood disorders (anxiety, depression)	Episodic: likely on-off fluctuations, optimize PD meds Static: initiating antidepressant (SSRI, SNRI, bupropion [Wellbutrin], TCA); talk therapy, psychotherapy, transcranial magnetic stimulation	Bupropion (Wellbutrin) is least likely to worsen RBD.
Cognitive dysfunction	If due to on-off fluctuation, optimize meds Adding AChE inhibitor; rivastigmine patch (Exelon) preferred; if not tolerated, can use donepezil (Aricept)[1], galantamine (Razadyne)[1], or memantine (Namenda)[1]	Fluctuations in cognition are common. Transdermal patch is preferred over oral formulation because of fewer side effects; for skin irritation with patch, spray area with fluticasone (Flonase),[1] and dry it before applying patch.
Impulse control disorder	Reviewing medications Slow taper of DA, if taking	Impulse control disorder can manifest as gambling, excessive shopping or cleaning, hypersexuality, overeating, or excessive time and focus on a hobby.
Drooling	Hard, sour candy/lozenges RimabotulinumtoxinB (Myobloc) or incobotulinumtoxinA (Xeomin) injections in parotid +/– submandibular salivary glands	Complaints of dysphagia can be due to sialorrhea.
Dysphagia	Episodic: represents wearing off, consider on-demand therapy Speech-language pathology referral, modified barium swallow study, diet modification If severe, may require percutaneous gastrostomy tube	Dysphagia increases risk of aspiration pneumonia. C/L ODT (Parcopa) can be very useful when dysphagia occurs.
Weight loss	Monitoring, supplemental shakes, referral to nutritionist or dietician	Weight loss has a poorer prognosis; earlier dementia and death are possible.
Pain	Determining pain type For musculoskeletal, PT for stretching; if dystonia, stretching and botulinum toxin injections For neuropathic pain, gabapentin (Neurontin)[1], pregabalin (Lyrica)[1], or TCA For radicular pain, PT for core strengthening and treating for neuropathic pain; if severe, considering imaging and referral to surgeon	

*Symptom of dysautonomia.
[1]Not FDA approved for this indication.
[2]Not available in the United States.
[7]Available as dietary supplement.
AChE, Acetylcholinesterase; *BPH*, benign prostatic hypertrophy; *CBC*, complete blood count; *C/L*, carbidopa-levodopa; *CR*, controlled-release; *DA*, dopamine agonist; *ER*, extended-release; *H2*, histamine H2-receptor; *ODT*, oral dissolving tablet; *OSA*, obstructive sleep apnea; *PD*, Parkinson disease; *PEG*, polyethylene glycol; *PPI*, proton pump inhibitor; *PT*, physical therapy; *RBD*, REM sleep behavior disorder; *REM*, rapid eye movement; *SNRI*, serotonin and norepinephrine reuptake inhibitor; *SSRI*, selective serotonin reuptake inhibitor; *TCA*, tricyclic antidepressant.

References

Bisaglia M: Mediterranean diet and Parkinson's disease, *Int J Mol Sci* 24(1):42, 2022.

Brücke T, Brücke C: Dopamine transporter (DAT) imaging in Parkinson's disease and related disorders, *J Neural Transm (Vienna)* 129(5–6):581–594, 2022.

Calabresi P, Mechelli A, Natale G, et al: Alpha-synuclein in Parkinson's disease and other synucleinopathies: from overt neurodegeneration back to early synaptic dysfunction, *Cell Death Dis* 14(3):176, 2023.

Fox SH, Katzenschlager R, Lim SY, et al: International Parkinson and movement disorder society evidence-based medicine review: update on treatments for the motor symptoms of Parkinson's disease, *Mov Disord* 33(8):1248–1266, 2018.

Jan A, Gonçalves NP, Vaegter CB, et al: The prion-like spreading of alpha-synuclein in Parkinson's disease: update on models and hypotheses, *Int J Mol Sci* 22(15):8338, 2021.

Postuma RB, Berg D, Stern M, et al: MDS clinical diagnostic criteria for Parkinson's disease, *Mov Disord* 30(12):1591–1601, 2015.

Pringsheim T, Day GS, Smith DB, et al: Dopaminergic therapy for motor symptoms in early Parkinson disease practice guideline summary: a report of the AAN guideline subcommittee, *Neurology* 97(20):942–957, 2021.

Skrahina V, Gaber H, Vollstedt EJ, ROPAD Study Group, et al: The Rostock International Parkinson's Disease (ROPAD) study: protocol and initial findings, *Mov Disord* 36(4):1005–1010, 2021.

Thaler A, Alcalay RN: Diagnosis and medical management of Parkinson disease, *Continuum (Minneap Minn)* 28(5):1281–1300, 2022.

Yoo D, Bang JI, Ahn C, et al: Diagnostic value of α-synuclein seeding amplification assays in α-synucleinopathies: a systematic review and meta-analysis, *Parkinsonism Relat Disord* 104:99–109, 2022.

REHABILITATION OF THE STROKE PATIENT

Method of
Natalie Blonien, PT, DPT

CURRENT DIAGNOSIS

- The diagnosis of stroke will have been made before rehabilitation.

CURRENT THERAPY

- Individualized rehabilitation services in acute and postacute settings supplied by a multidisciplinary team provides the best outcome for stroke patients.
- Rehabilitation programs that are intensive, repetitive, and salient task-specific interventions performed in enriched environments promote neuroplasticity and functional recovery.
- Use of technology, such as functional electrical stimulation, virtual reality systems, and neuro-muscular electrical stimulation promote recovery.

According to the National Center for Chronic Disease Prevention and Health Promotion, stroke is the leading cause of serious long-term disability. Every year, more than 795,000 people in the United States have a stroke. Stroke reduces mobility in more than half of stroke survivors age 65 and older. There is wide diversity in stroke patients and stroke severity, but of those admitted to a hospital, about 65% of survivors receive rehabilitation services, and more than 30% have persistent deficits in autonomy, engagement, and participation in society.

The current guidelines for adult stroke rehabilitation and recovery include both medical and rehabilitation involvement. This includes prevention, medical management of comorbidities, and an individualized rehabilitation program that includes appropriate assessments and treatments based on the international classification of functioning, disability, and health. The goal of rehabilitation is to enable stroke survivors to reach and maintain their optimal functional levels by providing the skills and tools needed to attain independence and self-determination. The current treatment approach is based on the brain's ability to reorganize after an injury, known as neuroplasticity, and this continues well beyond the acute recovery phase. Best practice and research strongly support intensive, repetitive, and salient task-specific interventions to promote neuroplasticity and functional recovery.

Rehabilitation services are delivered by a multidisciplinary team of healthcare providers who can be involved at different points in the continuum of care. There is strong evidence that organized, interprofessional stroke care can reduce mortality rates, long-term disability, and institutional care. It can also enhance recovery and increase independence in activities of daily living (ADLs). Physiatrists and neurologists direct the healthcare team with the support of rehabilitation nurses, as well as physical therapists (PT), occupational therapists (OT), and speech and language pathologists (SLP). Other essential providers include neuropsychologists, social workers, case managers, vocational counselors, and pharmacists.

Rehabilitation services for stroke patients can be provided in acute hospitals, postacute care settings, and outpatient settings. In the acute care hospital, the primary goal is to medically stabilize the patient and deliver acute stroke treatments along with the implementation of preventative measures. Medical management focused on subsequent stroke prevention includes management of hypertension, dyslipidemia, diabetes, weight loss, physical activity, nutrition, and smoking cessation. Medical complications can occur poststroke that negatively affect recovery, including skin breakdown, joint contractures, deep venous thrombosis and pulmonary embolism, bowel and bladder incontinence, hemiplegic shoulder pain, central poststroke pain, falls, seizures, depression, and pneumonia. Rehabilitation therapies are initiated in this phase, but medical management is the priority. There is research to support the safety of administering early mobilization of stroke patients within 24 hours of onset, but the optimal timing and frequency are not clear. After the patient is medically stable, those with milder deficits could be discharged home with outpatient rehabilitation services. Patients with moderate to severe impairments are considered for postacute care settings for continued rehabilitation services (Figure 1).

In the postacute care setting, services can be provided in inpatient rehabilitation facilities (IRFs) or skilled nursing facilities (SNFs). IRFs provide hospital-level care for those who need intensive, 24-hour interdisciplinary rehabilitation that is provided under the direct supervision of a physician. These patients demonstrate the potential for improvement within a reasonable period and are likely to return to a community setting. Medicare regulations also generally dictate that patients participate in at least 3 hours of active therapy per day for at least 5 days per week. SNFs provide subacute rehabilitation to stroke survivors who need daily skilled nursing or rehabilitation care. These patients are recommended for an SNF over an IRF if the team feels they may not reach full or partial recovery of functional skills and they do not need daily physician supervision. The recommendation for IRF versus SNF requires collaborative decision-making involving the entire rehabilitation team to maximize the functional outcome of the patient while considering individual factors.

After postacute care, the rehabilitation team, the patient, and their support system determine the least restrictive environment for discharge. The goal is to return home with appropriate support services within the home or outpatient services. Assessment of patient goals and the home environment is critical. If discharge to the community is not feasible, a transition to a long-term residential facility may be necessary.

The role of therapy services becomes primary in the postacute and outpatient management of stroke survivors. These professionals evaluate and treat impairments, such as communication, comprehension, swallowing, cognition, motor function, muscle tone, vision, sensory perception, bowel and bladder function, balance, and weakness. These impairments impact gait, mobility, ADLs, and instrumental activities of daily living (IADLs). ADLs are the tasks needed for an individual to take care of their basic needs at home, such as bathing and toileting. IADLs are those activities that enable an individual to live independently within their home and community. The remainder of the chapter discusses clinical manifestations common in stroke patients with descriptions of evidence-based interventions.

Hemiplegia

Hemiplegia is the classic sign of neurovascular disease of the brain that involves paralysis or weakness of one side of the body. Hemiplegia is associated with changes in muscle activation, sensation, muscle tone, joint alignment, pain, and atypical movement patterns. Rehabilitation of motor functions involves physical and occupational therapies.

Electrical stimulation, such as functional electrical stimulation (FES) and neuromuscular electrical stimulation (NMES), delivers a current using transcutaneous electrodes applied to a muscle group to elicit a muscle contraction. FES and NMES are essentially the same, but FES is the term used when electrical stimulation is being used within a functional task. For example, FES is used as an orthotic to assist with drop foot during gait and to improve function (Figure 2). As a modality or as an orthotic, evidence supports that stroke patients show

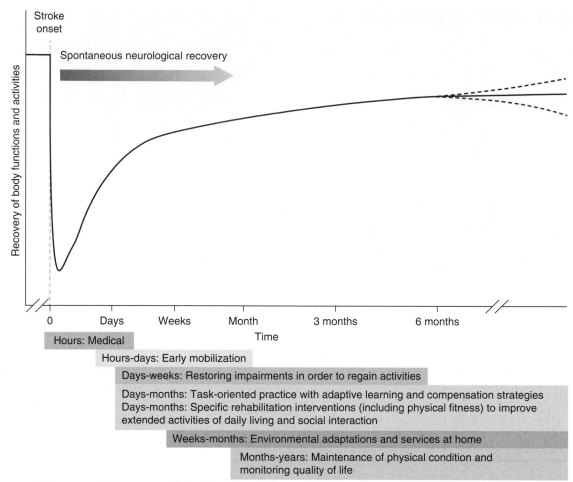

Figure 1 Framework for neurologic recovery of function after stroke. (Langhorne P, Bernhardt J, Kwakkel G. Stroke rehabilitation. *Lancet.* 2011;377(9778):1693-1702.)

Figure 2 Functional Electrical Stimulation (FES) used in gait. (Lazaro RT, Reina-Guerra SG, Quiben M, eds. *Umphred's Neurological Rehabilitation.* 7th ed. Elsevier Health Sciences; 2019:fig. 32.5.)

improvement in muscle activation of the muscles stimulated even when not wearing a device, thus promoting recovery. In upper limb recovery poststroke, there is a statistically significant benefit from FES when applied within 2 months of stroke on ADL participation.

Mirror therapy, where a stroke patient places a mirror in the midline and regards the image of the nonhemiparetic hand or leg as if it were the affected side while performing movement, has been found effective in improving motor impairments in patients with moderate to severe involvement. It is recommended as an adjunct to therapy in the clinic and is easily performed in the home with basic equipment and training.

Virtual reality (VR) is a promising intervention but has yet to be adapted to widespread clinical practice. VR is used to assist with both upper and lower limb recovery with evidence to support a correlation between neural plasticity changes and functional recovery; however, the underlying mechanism is unclear.

Stroke patients who demonstrate limited motor return can use equipment to compensate for hemiplegia. This can include adaptive equipment, orthotics, and mobility devices. OTs are primarily involved in the evaluation process for upper extremity orthotics and equipment related to adaptations for ADLs. This can include upper extremity slings, shower benches, dressing aids, and adaptive utensils (Figure 3). PTs are primarily involved in the evaluation of orthotics, assistive devices, and wheelchairs. Careful consideration and expertise are needed when recommending equipment to maximize function and minimize waste.

Joint Contracture

Development of a joint contracture on the affected side within the first year after stroke typically occurs at the elbow and wrist and

Figure 3 Adaptive equipment to assist with activities of daily living. (Gonzalez-Fernandez M, Feldman D. Rehabilitation of the stroke patient. In: Kellerman RD, Rakel DP, eds. *Conn's Current Therapy 2023*. Elsevier; 2023:780-784.)

is more likely with the presence of spasticity in patients with minimal functional hand use. Contractures can cause pain and make it difficult to perform ADLs. PTs and OTs commonly prescribe individualized daily stretching. Static positioning of the shoulder in maximal external shoulder rotation for 30 minutes a day in early stroke rehabilitation is effective in preventing shoulder contracture. Splints are commonly prescribed for both the upper and lower extremity joints at risk for developing contractures. Resting hand splints are often fabricated by OTs, and evidence supports splinting in conjunction with early spasticity treatments to minimize contracture development. PTs will recommend the use of ankle foot orthoses (AFO) to be worn for gait to remediate or prevent the development of ankle plantarflexion contractures and assist with foot positioning during the swing phase. In nonambulatory patients, resting ankle splints that position the foot at 90 degrees help minimize the development of plantarflexion contractures to improve sitting posture and participation in transfers.

Incontinence

Urinary and fecal incontinence are common after stroke with approximately 20% to 25% reporting problems at discharge from the acute hospital. Urinary incontinence is correlated with mortality and the need for nursing home care 3 months after stroke. Many factors contribute to incontinence, including impaired cognition, difficulty with mobility, communication difficulties, and impaired awareness of the need to void. It is recommended that appropriate management of bladder incontinence include urologic history before the stroke, assessment of urinary retention through bladder scanning or intermittent catheterizations, removal of Foley catheter within 24 hours of acute stroke admission, and assessment of cognitive awareness of the need to void. Treatments should be based on the contributing factors for impaired bladder management and can include the use of toileting schedules, pelvic floor muscle training, and addressing functional mobility. There are no specific stroke recommendations for fecal incontinence, and recommendations are based on the general population of adults.

Dysphagia

Dysphagia, difficulty swallowing, is found in approximately 15% of stroke survivors at 1 month poststroke and places the patient at risk for aspiration. It is recommended that stroke patients be evaluated for dysphagia with a valid screening tool first, followed by a clinical bedside evaluation and then a confirmatory study performed via instrumental evaluation (such as videofluoroscopy). Upon diagnosis of dysphagia, an effective treatment plan

can be administered. This can include swallow therapy and diet modifications. Common evidence-based swallow therapy behavioral interventions include swallowing exercises, environmental modifications that include proper body positioning, and safe swallow advice. Literature supports acupuncture as an adjunctive treatment for dysphagia.

Pain

Pain can affect the shoulder or the entire hemiplegic side, referred to as central poststroke pain. Hemiplegic shoulder pain primarily due to shoulder subluxation is correlated with changes in muscle tone, weakness, injury to shoulder tissues, glenohumeral joint restrictions, and altered somatosensory function. This results in functional impairments of the upper limb and negatively impacts rehabilitation, leading to depression and poor health-related quality of life. Noninvasive standard of care provided by PTs and OTs includes restoring scapular and humeral alignment, stretching within a pain-free range, strengthening the scapular and shoulder muscles, and thermal modalities such as ice or heat treatments. Effective medical interventions include botulinum toxin type A (BoNT-A [Botox, Dysport, Xeomin])[1] intramuscular injections, suprascapular nerve pulsed radiofrequency, anesthetic suprascapular nerve block, and trigger-point dry needling. These more invasive medical interventions can be used in conjunction with conventional therapy to improve outcomes.

Treatment for central poststroke pain has more limited evidence. A combination approach that includes pharmacotherapy, therapeutic exercise, and social support is common. Pharmacotherapy primarily consists of antidepressant medications and anticonvulsants, with amitriptyline[1] and lamotrigine (Lamictal)[1] commonly being used as first-line treatment.

Spasticity

Spasticity is a component of the upper motor neuron syndrome and is correlated with limitations in activity performance. Rehabilitation management includes both medications and therapist-led interventions. Botulinum toxins (Botox, Dysport, Myobloc[1], Xeomin) can be injected into specific muscles to temporarily reduce spasticity. It is commonly used for ankle plantar flexor spasticity in conjunction with serial casting to improve ankle range of motion. It is also used to treat upper limb spasticity and can improve impairments related to limitations in flexibility and

---

[1] Not FDA approved for this indication.

range of motion, but there is limited evidence that it will improve the functional use of the hand and limb.

Oral antispasticity medications, including baclofen (Lioresal), dantrolene sodium (Dantrium), and tizanidine (Zanaflex), have a marginal effect on tone management and cause additional systemic side effects.

Other modalities used in conjunction with therapy and pharmacologic treatments include NMES and vibration therapy. NMES was discussed in the section on hemiplegia and is used over the spastic muscles. Vibration therapy applies localized muscle vibration to either the spastic muscles or the antagonist muscle. Both NMES and vibration therapy are found to improve short-term management of spasticity in conjunction with conventional therapy but with limited long-term effect.

Depression

Depression is reported in up to 33% of stroke patients and is associated with a history of depression, severe disability, cognitive impairment, a history of previous stroke, and female sex. Depression can negatively affect participation in rehabilitation, so it is important to address symptoms early in recovery.

Medications commonly used and studied in treating depression in stroke patients include selective serotonin reuptake inhibitors (SSRIs) and tricyclic antidepressants. Patients should be closely monitored for effectiveness.

Exercise for depression has been well studied in the nonstroke population with good results. There seems to be a transient positive impact of exercise on depression symptoms in patients after a stroke who performed 1 month of exercise, but it does not appear this effect lasts beyond the termination of the exercise program.

Cognitive Dysfunction

Cognitive dysfunction is associated with mortality, increased disability, and increased skilled SNF placement. Deficits in cognitive domains can include attention, memory, executive functioning, and perceptual and visual-spatial abilities. Cognitive screening is recommended for all stroke patients. Brief tools such as the Neurobehavioral Cognitive Status Examination (https://www.sralab.org/rehabilitation-measures/cognistat-cognitive-assessment-neurobehavioral-cognitive-status-examination) provide a rapid and sensitive assessment. Formal neuropsychological examination may be useful after a screening tool.

Nonpharmacologic cognitive rehabilitation is performed by OTs and SLPs. The standard of practice recommends interventions should be actively applied to improve everyday function. Promoting recovery of cognitive impairments is positively correlated with time spent in enriched environments while participating in tasks that increase cognitive engagement. This can include books, games, VR, and music. Frequently, compensatory strategies are recommended to support cognitive deficits, like memory. This includes electronic and nonelectronic memory aids. Stroke patients with mild memory impairments can benefit from internalized strategies, such as visual imagery, along with external memory aids. The more severe a memory impairment, the less likely internal strategies are effective. Overall, cognitive rehabilitation has been found to improve attention, memory, visual neglect, and executive functioning.

Physical activity and exercise has a small positive effect on cognition, and studies suggest that exercise has a protective effect on cognitive decline in older adults without cognitive impairment. It is recommended as an adjunctive therapy to improve cognition and memory.

Pharmacologic management of cognition is studied less in stroke and effectiveness is unclear. Medications studied that specifically measured cognitive outcomes include donepezil (Aricept)[1], rivastigmine (Exelon)[1], and the antidepressants fluoxetine (Prozac)[1]

and nortriptyline (Pamelor, Aventyl)[1]. The usefulness of these medications is not well established.

Gait and Balance Impairment

Impairments related to gait and balance are common poststroke and contribute to falls. Multiple factors can contribute to falls, including low balance confidence, sensory impairments, impaired motor function, visual and perceptual issues, and cognitive factors. PTs are primarily involved in the assessment of gait, balance, and risk of falls. These factors need to be assessed to apply appropriate and individualized interventions.

A variety of interventions are available for stroke patients without a specific approach proving superior. Successful treatments are based on individualizing the intervention to specifically address the patient's impairments and functional limitations. The use of AFOs on the hemiplegic lower extremity along with an assistive device, such as a cane, are common compensation strategies that improve balance and gait. Strong evidence supports lower extremity strength training and is correlated with improvement in gait speed and functional outcomes. The use of intensive and repetitive task training to facilitate restoration of gait and gait-related activities is well supported in the literature. Interventions, such as treadmill training with or without body weight support and progressively more challenging tasks specific to gait, are necessary to promote recovery. There is promising evidence for the use of robotic assistive walking, which appears to be more beneficial than a treadmill for patients after acute stroke who are unable to walk even with the assistance of body weight support. Limitations in the clinical use of robotic devices include the cost of the equipment and availability in the clinic.

Communication

Communication and language impairments are common in stroke patients. This area of the deficit is primarily evaluated and treated by SLPs. These include aphasia, dysarthria, and apraxia. Aphasia can affect speaking, comprehension, reading, and writing with varying degrees of severity. Dysarthria is a group of motor speech disorders resulting from weakness or lack of coordination that impacts articulation. Apraxia is a disorder of motor planning where a person has difficulties with making correct speech sounds. All these communication disorders can negatively affect social participation and quality of life.

There is a variety of evidence-based treatment approaches for aphasia, and no treatment is the most effective. There is support for early daily aphasia therapy in the acute setting with overall improved long-term communication outcomes. Skilled interventions provided in the chronic phase of rehabilitation continue to prove effective. There is support for bouts of intensive speech and language therapy delivery, but dosing and timing are inconclusive.

Dysarthria and apraxia are considered disorders that affect the motor control of speech. Behavioral treatments include focus on supporting the physiology of respiration and sound production, strategies to address articulation, and rate of speech generation. They should be individually tailored to meet the patient's strengths and goals. There is evidence that patients may benefit from using augmentative communication devices to supplement speech, such as a simple communication board or a computerized device.

Visual and Perceptual Impairment

Visual impairments poststroke can involve impairments of eye movements, visual field loss, or deficits related to perceptual or visuospatial capabilities; these can affect mobility and ADLs. Assessments of visual impairments can be clinically performed primarily by neurologists, physiatrists, neuroophthalmologists, and OTs. A thorough evaluation to determine the type and severity of visual impairments is necessary to implement

---

[1] Not FDA approved for this indication.

[1] Not FDA approved for this indication.

appropriate treatments. Studies suggest that training in visual scanning strategies can improve scanning and reading but do not improve the degree of field loss. Also, increasing the sensory information during scanning tasks to include audio with visual input can enhance these effects. Targeted strengthening eye exercises, called *convergence,* are recommended for the treatment of impaired eye muscle strength and coordination. There is some support for the use of prism glasses to compensate for visual field loss. Computer-assisted training interventions demonstrate the ability to restore visual field deficits.

Upper Extremity Function and Activity

As discussed in the section on hemiplegia, upper limb paresis after stroke is very common with only a small percentage of patients regaining full hand function. Lack of bimanual use significantly limits ADLs and participation in occupations. Two interventions used frequently in the clinical setting are constraint-induced movement therapy (CIMT) and NMES. CIMT involves casting or immobilizing the uninvolved upper extremity to force the use of the hemiparetic side when the hemiparetic side demonstrates a baseline ability to have volitional control of finger and wrist extension. The protocol varies between 3 to 6 hours per day for 5 days a week for 2 weeks or modified dosing of 1 hour per day for 3 days a week for 10 weeks. Both demonstrate improvement in upper extremity participation in ADLs with similar efficacy. NMES is an effective intervention for stroke patients who have limited volitional control and was discussed in the hemiplegia section. It can be applied to the shoulder joint in the prevention or correction of shoulder subluxation or the wrist and hand during task-specific training.

Conclusions

Stroke rehabilitation requires a well-coordinated multidisciplinary team approach that systematically evaluates a stroke patient to identify impairments that affect activities and participation in daily life. Evidence-based interventions that are individualized for a patient and address specific needs are critical. Research demonstrates coordination between medical and rehabilitation interventions is important to optimize functional outcomes. Current evidence demonstrates that recovery continues years beyond the initial stroke, and advocacy for continued rehabilitation services beyond acute stroke management is vital.

References

Avvantaggiato C, Casale R, Cinone N, et al: Localized muscle vibration in the treatment of motor impairment and spasticity in post-stroke patients: a systematic review, *Eur J Phys Rehabil Med* 57(1):44–60, 2021.

Bath PM, Lee HS, Everton LF: Swallowing therapy for dysphagia in acute and subacute stroke, *Cochrane Database Syst Rev*, 2018. Issue 10.

Brady MC, Kelly H, Godwin J, et al: Speech and language therapy for aphasia following stroke, *Cochrane Database Syst Rev*, 2016. Issue 6.

Bruni MF, Melegari C, De Cola MC, et al: What does best evidence tell us about robotic gait rehabilitation in stroke patients: a systematic review and meta-analysis, *J Clin Neurosci* 48:11–17, 2018.

Centers for Disease Control and Prevention. Stroke. Available at. https://www.cdc.gov/stroke/facts.htm. [accessed 02/17/21]

Cicerone KD, Goldin Y, Ganci K, et al: Evidence-based cognitive rehabilitation: systematic review of literature from 2009 through 2014, *Arch Phys Med Rehabil* 100(8):1515–1533, 2019.

De Sire A, Moggio L, Demeco A, et al: Efficacy of rehabilitative techniques in reducing hemiplegic shoulder pain in stroke: systematic review and meta-analysis, *Ann Phys Rehabil* 65(5):101602, 2022.

Eraifej J, Clark W, France B, et al: Effectiveness of upper limb functional electrical stimulation after stroke for the improvement of activities of daily living and motor function: a systematic review and meta-analysis, *Syst Rev* 6(1):40, 2017.

Lazaro Rolando,T. et al: *Umphred's neurological rehabilitation*, ed 7, Elsevier Health Sciences (US), 2020.

Thieme H, Morkisch N, Mehrholz J, et al: Mirror therapy for improving motor function after stroke, *Cochrane Database Syst Rev*, 2018. Issue 7.

Winstein CW, Stein J, Arena R, et al: Guidelines for adult stroke rehabilitation and recovery, *Stroke* 47:98–169, 2016.

SEIZURES AND EPILEPSY IN ADOLESCENTS AND ADULTS

Method of
Jose A. Padin-Rosado, MD

CURRENT DIAGNOSIS

- Obtain a thorough clinical history, including a detailed description of the paroxysmal events from the patient and from witness accounts.
- Perform a complete physical and neurologic examination.
- Perform laboratory tests including electrolytes, blood glucose, liver function, and toxicology.
- Obtain a lumbar puncture if signs of infection are present.
- Neuroimaging is strongly recommended. Magnetic resonance imaging (MRI) is the preferred test because of its higher resolution. Head computed tomography (CT) is acceptable in the acute setting to rule out hemorrhage.
- Routine electroencephalography (EEG) with sleep deprivation and activation procedures should be performed as close to the time of occurrence of the paroxysmal event to increase the diagnostic yield.

CURRENT THERAPY

- Choose the right medication for the type of epilepsy and epilepsy syndrome.
- Consider the side-effect profile, cost, and drug dosing schedule, and adapt to the unique patient characteristics taking into consideration the patient's comorbidities.
- Aim for monotherapy whenever possible.
- Start low and increase slowly when initiating antiseizure drug (ASD) therapy to minimize side effects and increase compliance.
- An adequate ASD trial with titration of the medication until clinical effectiveness or side effects occur is recommended.
- When switching from one drug to another, consider overlapping medications to provide protection until the first drug is discontinued.
- If the patient fails two antiseizure drug trials either in monotherapy or polytherapy, refer the patient to an epilepsy center for evaluation.
- If the patient is seizure free after 2 years of treatment, consider withdrawing ASDs for epilepsies of unknown etiology or epilepsy syndromes known to resolve.

Epilepsy is a disease characterized by an enduring predisposition to generate seizures and by the neurobiologic, cognitive, psychological, and social consequences of this condition. Epilepsy is commonly defined as having two or more unprovoked seizures greater than 24 hours apart. However, as per the classification proposed by the International League Against Epilepsy (ILAE) in 2014, a single seizure can be classified as epilepsy if risk of seizure recurrence is high (see the "Classification" section later in this chapter).

A seizure is defined as transient signs or symptoms caused by abnormal excessive synchronous activity of brain neurons. Seizures can be classified as either acute symptomatic (provoked) or unprovoked. Acute symptomatic seizures are associated with a transient systemic or brain insult and will usually not require treatment with antiepileptic drugs because of the transient nature of the precipitant and the associated low risk for development of epilepsy. Unprovoked seizures, on the other hand, may represent the beginning of epilepsy.

ILAE 2017 Classification of Seizure Types Expanded Version[1]

Figure 1 Classification of seizure types. From Fisher RS, Cross JH, French JA, et al.: Operational classification of seizure types by the International League Against Epilepsy: Position Paper of the ILAE Commission for Classification and Terminology, *Epilepsia* 58(4):522–530, 2017.

Focal Onset

Aware — Impaired Awareness

Motor Onset
 automatisms
 atonic[2]
 clonic
 epileptic spasms[2]
 hyperkinetic
 myoclonic
 tonic
Non-Motor Onset
 autonomic
 behavior arrest
 cognitive
 emotional
 sensory

Focal to bilateral tonic-clonic

Generalized Onset

Motor
 tonic-clonic
 clonic
 tonic
 myoclonic
 myoclonic-tonic-clonic
 myoclonic-atonic
 atonic
 epileptic spasms[2]
Non-Motor (absence)
 typical
 atypical
 myoclonic
 eyelid myoclonia

Unknown Onset

Motor
 tonic-clonic
 epileptic spasms
Non-Motor
 behavior arrest

Unclassified[3]

1 Definitions, other seizure types and descriptors are listed in the accompanying paper and glossary of terms.

2 These could be focal or generalized, with or without alteration of awareness.

3 Due to inadequate information or inability to place in other categories.

Epidemiology

Epilepsy is one of the most common neurologic conditions, affecting more than 50 million people worldwide. The prevalence of epilepsy (number of people with active epilepsy) is approximately 1% in the United States, with 3.4 million people (3 million adults and 470,000 children) suffering from the disease. The incidence of epilepsy (number of new cases) is around 150,000 each year or 55 per 100,000 population. The incidence is higher in patients younger than 2 years of age and in those older than 65 years of age. The risk of developing epilepsy is slightly higher in men than in women. African Americans and disadvantaged populations are affected at a higher rate than Caucasians. The lifetime risk of developing a seizure is around 9% to 10%.

Classification

Definition of Epilepsy

In 2014, the ILAE published a practical definition of epilepsy. This definition classifies epilepsy as a disease of the brain characterized by any of the following criteria: at least two unprovoked or reflex seizures occurring more than 24 hours apart; one unprovoked or reflex seizure and a probability of recurrent seizures similar to the general recurrence risk (60%) after two unprovoked seizures, occurring over the next 10 years; or diagnosis of an epilepsy syndrome.

In 2017, the ILAE released a major revision of both the classification of the epilepsies and epilepsy syndromes and the classification of seizure types. The classification of the epilepsies and epilepsy syndromes has three levels: (1) classification of the seizure type, (2) classification of the epilepsy type, and (3) diagnosis of an epilepsy syndrome whenever possible. The cause and associated comorbidities are considered at each diagnostic step because these carry treatment implications.

The first step is to classify the type of seizure (Figure 1 and Box 1). It assumes that the patient has been diagnosed with an epileptic seizure and then organizes the seizures by where they originate in the brain into either a *focal-onset seizure*, formerly known as *partial-onset seizure* (emanating from networks in one lobe or hemisphere), *generalized-onset seizure* (engaging bilateral neural networks), and *unknown-onset seizures*. The term *secondary generalized seizure* is replaced by *focal to bilateral tonic-clonic seizure*, and it is placed in a special category. Then focal-onset seizures can be optionally classified into seizures with preserved awareness as *focal aware seizures*

BOX 1 Changes in Seizure Type Classification from 1981 to 2017

- Change of "partial" to "focal"
- Certain seizures types can be either of focal, generalized, or unknown onset.
- Seizures of unknown onset may have features that can still be classified.
- Awareness is used as a classifier of focal onset seizures.
- The terms *dyscognitive*, *simple partial*, *complex partial*, *psychic*, and *secondary generalized* were eliminated.
- New focal seizure types include automatisms, autonomic, behavioral arrest, cognitive, emotional, hyperkinetic, sensory, and focal to bilateral-tonic-clonic seizures. Atonic, clonic, epileptic spasms, myoclonic, and tonic seizures can be either focal or generalized.
- New generalized seizure types include absence with eyelid myoclonia, myoclonic absence, myoclonic-tonic-clonic, myoclonic atonic, and epileptic spasms.

From Fisher RS, Cross JH, French JA, et al.: Operational classification of seizure types by the International League Against Epilepsy: Position Paper of the ILAE Commission for Classification and Terminology, *Epilepsia* 58(4):522–530, 2017.

(formerly known as *simple partial seizures*) and seizures with impaired awareness as *focal impaired awareness seizures* (formerly known as *complex partial seizures*). Focal-onset seizures, generalized-onset seizures, and unknown-onset seizures can be optionally and further subdivided into whether they have associated motor symptoms or other nonmotor symptoms. In some settings, classification into seizure type will be the only attainable level possible for diagnosis because there may be no access to EEG, video, and imaging studies or too little information available to make a higher level of diagnosis.

The second step is to classify the type of epilepsy (Figure 2). This step in the classification assumes that the patient fulfills the diagnosis of epilepsy (according to the ILAE 2014 definition of epilepsy discussed earlier) and classifies the epilepsies into *focal* (focal clinical features and EEG with focal epileptiform abnormalities), *generalized* (bilateral clinical features and EEG with generalized epileptiform abnormalities), *combined generalized and focal* (features of both on

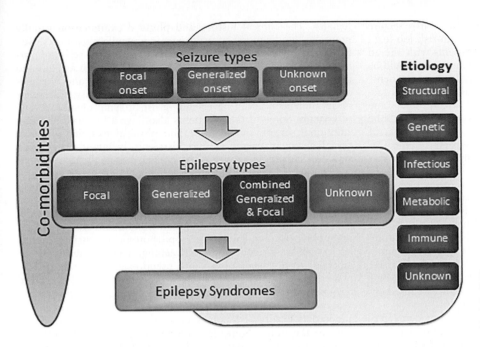

Figure 2 Classification of the epilepsies. From Scheffer IE, Berkovic S, Capovilla G, et al.: ILAE classification of the epilepsies: Position paper of the ILAE Commission for Classification and Terminology, *Epilepsia* 58(4):512–521, 2017.

clinical evaluation and on EEG), and *unknown* type (either no clinical information available and normal or no EEG available).

The third step is the diagnosis of an epilepsy syndrome whenever possible. A *syndrome* refers to a cluster of features such as seizure type, EEG findings, and imaging features that tend to occur together and may provide information regarding treatment implications and prognosis. Within the generalized epilepsies, a well-known subgroup, known as the *idiopathic primary generalized epilepsies*, exists and includes four distinct syndromes: *childhood absence epilepsy, juvenile absence epilepsy, juvenile myoclonic epilepsy,* and *generalized-tonic-clonic seizures.*

From the moment the patient is diagnosed with having an epileptic seizure, a cause should be sought. Etiologies include structural etiology (structural abnormality seen on brain MRI that is strongly associated with the development of seizures), such as temporal lobe seizures from mesiotemporal sclerosis; genetic etiology (epilepsies with a presumed genetic mutation), such as benign familial neonatal epilepsy with mutation in *KNCQ2* or *KNCQ3* (potassium channels); infectious etiology, such as neurocysticercosis; metabolic etiology, such as porphyria and pyridoxine-dependent seizures; immune etiology, such as anti-NMDA receptor encephalitis and anti-LG1 encephalitis; and unknown etiology.

Comorbidities should be considered for every patient with epilepsy at each stage of classification, just like etiology. Comorbidities include learning, psychological, and behavioral problems. The term *benign* is replaced by *self-limiting* (likely spontaneous resolution of a syndrome) and *pharmacoresponsive* (the epilepsy syndrome will be controlled with appropriate ASD treatment). This classification is aimed at providing tools for improved diagnosis and understanding of etiology and targeted therapies to the patient's disease.

Diagnosis

The diagnosis of a seizure and epilepsy is largely a clinical one and is highly dependent on the history and physical examination. The clinical history should be obtained from the patient and from a witness. After the aforementioned is obtained, the information is analyzed to determine whether indeed the paroxysmal event in question represents a true seizure or a seizure mimicker. If the event of concern represents a seizure, then it is further classified into *focal* or *generalized* and into *acute symptomatic,* a transient phenomena with lower seizure recurrence, or *unprovoked,* which confers a higher risk for seizure recurrence and development of epilepsy.

The clinical history is aimed at obtaining a clear description of the prodromal or premonitory state, the pre-ictal state, the ictal state, and the post-ictal state. The prodromal state occurs hours to days before the ictus and is most commonly seen in generalized seizures (but may also occur in focal onset seizures) and consists of behavioral changes, mood swings, fatigue, and changes in sleep patterns. Regarding the pre-ictal period, the patient should be questioned about the presence of warning signs immediately before the seizure onset, also known as *auras.* An aura is a simple partial seizure or a seizure without impaired awareness. An aura points to a focal seizure onset, and we can potentially determine the lobe of onset according to the description of the aura. For example, a rising gastric sensation and a sensation of déjà vu points to seizure onset in the temporal lobe, and visual hallucinations point to the occipital lobe.

The clinician then asks the patient what happened during the event (ictal period). Issues to consider include the level of awareness, the presence of ability to speak, the presence of automatisms (lip-smacking, ipsilateral hand automatisms, and contralateral dystonia points to ipsilateral temporal lobe seizures), other behavior, and the duration of the event (true seizures usually last less than 2 minutes, whereas nonepileptic events are usually of longer duration).

The next questions focus on what happened after the event (post-ictal period). These include whether there is any confusion or fatigue, how long it takes the patient to come back to baseline, the presence of tongue bites and muscle aches, and the presence of urinary incontinence (commonly seen with true seizures). The clinician also asks about triggers including sleep deprivation, stress, drug intake, and alcohol withdrawal.

Other information to obtain includes the presence of diurnal variations—for example, frontal lobe seizures usually occur at nighttime and generalized tonic-clonic and myoclonic seizures occur mostly during the morning. If more than one seizure occurs, the clinician then asks the patient about the maximum seizure-free period; seizure frequency to assess for disease severity and response to treatment; number of visits to the hospital or emergency department to assess for seizure severity; and the presence of falls or injuries during seizures to assess for risks and degree of seizure control.

Medical history should include questions regarding the patient's prenatal history and development to assess for remote symptomatic causes of seizures; history of febrile seizures; history of central nervous system (CNS) lesions (tumors, stroke) and infections; history of brain trauma, specifically with associated penetrating injuries with intraparenchymal blood, skull fractures, and prolonged loss of consciousness; and family history of epilepsy.

Social history should include questions about level of education and employment. Patients with a higher level of education usually will have a better understanding of their diagnosis and prognosis. Employment is important because patients at higher risk for development of subsequent seizures after a first seizure have a higher risk of injury if they work in a high-risk job (e.g., in construction handling heavy machinery). Patients with altered awareness during a seizure should not drive. Clinicians should be familiar with the specific state laws regarding driving in patients with seizures and epilepsy. Use of drugs and alcohol are risk factors for the development of a first provoked seizure, and some illegal drugs may exacerbate or cause seizures. Patients should be discouraged from using illegal drugs and from excessive intake of alcohol. Review of current medications or newly started medications should be performed to determine whether any can precipitate seizures (e.g., tramadol, bupropion).

After the medical history is obtained, a thorough physical and neurologic examination should be performed. The clinician should look for skin abnormalities such as neurocutaneous manifestations of diseases (tuberous sclerosis and neurofibromatosis). It is also important to test for muscle strength to rule out subtle weakness or post-ictal Todd paralysis; look for lateral tongue/cheek bites, which are commonly seen in true epileptic seizures; also look for bruises, scrapes from falls, burns, and muscle and back pain commonly seen in compression fractures caused by convulsive seizures.

The evaluation of a new-onset seizure should be aimed at determining whether the seizure represents an acute symptomatic seizure, usually a transient phenomenon or an unprovoked seizure.

If the history and physical examination points to a probable acute symptomatic seizure, then life-threatening conditions should be ruled out (e.g., hemorrhage, CNS infection, neoplasms) as soon as possible. Basic laboratory tests should be ordered including complete blood count, electrolytes (sodium), blood glucose, liver function tests, and toxicology to rule out drug use. If signs of CNS infection are present (fever, nuchal rigidity), consider performing a lumbar puncture. Emergency neuroimaging (usually head CT in an acute setting) should also be performed. If the patient continues to be altered or confused or to have focal deficits not explained by neuroimaging or is not at baseline 30 to 60 minutes after a seizure, emergency EEG or continuous video EEG monitoring should be performed to look for subclinical seizures. If there is evidence of provoking factors (sleep deprivation, alcohol or drug use), normal neuroimaging, and the patient is back to baseline, then the EEG can be delayed and performed in the outpatient setting. The EEG is important because some patients with symptomatic seizures can also have epileptiform abnormalities that may require ASD treatment, such as an alcohol withdrawal seizure with focal interictal epileptiform discharges (IEDs) originating from an area of encephalomalacia caused by a fall.

Unprovoked seizures are classified into seizures of unknown etiology and seizures with a preexistent brain lesion (remote symptomatic). If the initial workup points to a probable unprovoked seizure, an MRI with epilepsy protocol (3 Tesla MRI with 1- to 3-mm slices and coronal fluid–attenuated inversion recovery sequences) interpreted by a neuroradiologist should be performed to rule out subtle lesions such as cortical dysplasias and mesiotemporal sclerosis, which confer a higher risk for development of epilepsy. Also, the EEG is of paramount importance to stratify patients at risk for recurrent seizures. The EEG should be performed with sleep deprivation and with activating procedures and as close as possible to the seizure (within 24 hours) to increase the yield of detecting interictal epileptiform abnormalities. There is a 51% chance of recording epileptiform abnormalities if the EEG is performed 24 hours after a seizure.

Differential Diagnosis

The diagnosis of a seizure or epilepsy can be challenging. There are many paroxysmal conditions, both psychiatric and organic, that may mimic seizures. Of all the seizure mimickers, psychogenic nonepileptic attacks (also known as *psychogenic nonepileptic seizures*) are the condition most commonly misdiagnosed as epilepsy. The estimated prevalence of psychogenic nonepileptic attacks is 2 to 33 per 100,000, and most patients are younger

females. The clinical history and physical examination usually points to the diagnosis of psychogenic nonepileptic attacks. Red flags include poor control on multiple ASDs with a series of normal EEGs, psychiatric history, unusual triggers such as pain and getting upset, diagnosis of chronic pain syndrome and fibromyalgia, seizures in outpatient clinics or at doctor visits (presence of an audience), and a never-ending list of symptoms on review of systems. Some of these patients also have a history of sexual, emotional, or physical abuse. The physical examination may reveal give-way weakness and histrionic behavior. The "gold standard" for the diagnosis of psychogenic nonepileptic events is continuous video EEG monitoring. The combination of atypical semiology and lack of EEG findings during the paroxysmal event allows for a definitive diagnosis. Common behaviors seen during a nonepileptic paroxysmal event include position of convenience, ictal eye closure, retained awareness with bilateral motor features resembling a convulsive event, opisthotonic posturing (arched back), pelvic thrusting, crying/weeping, ictal stuttering, baby talk, side-to-side head movements, pseudo-sleep, irregular out-of-phase motor activity (like a fish out of water), gradual onset and termination, prolonged attacks, and stop-and-go phenomena.

Syncope is the second most common paroxysmal event misdiagnosed as seizures. Syncope represents a transient lack of blood flow to the brain. Some features are helpful in differentiating syncope from true seizures, and these include prodromal symptoms of general malaise, sweating, dizziness, nausea, palpitations and chest pain, and loss of consciousness with rapid recovery after hitting the ground as a result of rapid brain reperfusion. The challenging part is the fact that many syncopal events show "convulsive-like" behavior such as clonic phenomena, making the diagnosis more challenging. Syncopal events are usually shorter than typical convulsive seizures, and recovery is faster with no post-ictal state and usually no tongue-bites or urinary incontinence, a feature commonly seen in true convulsive seizures. The most common type of syncope is vasovagal and is precipitated by some situations such as pain and sight of blood. The other type is reflex syncope caused by micturition, cough, the Valsalva maneuver, and defecation. The EEG shows a typical progression of generalized slowing followed by suppression without any associated ictal features. Cardiac mechanisms should be explored because some could be life-threatening (e.g., Brugada syndrome or other arrhythmias) and require immediate intervention.

Migraines, especially complicated migraines, and migraine auras cause positive focal symptoms such as visual auras, sensorimotor phenomena, and weakness, which could potentially mimic partial seizures. However, the course of migraines is in the range of minutes, and the course of seizures is in the range of seconds. A complicated migraine may be misdiagnosed as Todd paralysis. Patients with migraines do have a history of headaches and retained awareness during the attack; these two features favor the diagnosis of migraine headaches.

Transient ischemic attacks (TIAs) should not be misdiagnosed as seizures because this entity has marked focal negative phenomena (weakness, numbness, aphasia), whereas seizures present mostly positive phenomena (movement, automatisms, jerking). Positive symptoms rarely occur during TIAs (limb-shaking TIA).

Other conditions that may mimic seizures include hypoglycemia, panic attacks, paroxysmal movement disorders, nonepileptic myoclonus, sleep disorders, parasomnias, cataplexia, and hypnic jerks. It is important therefore to obtain a detailed history, followed by continuous video-EEG monitoring to try to capture these events for final diagnostic purposes, because it is not uncommon to misdiagnose and mislabel these conditions as epilepsy.

Treatment

Treatment should be initiated only if the potential benefit from treatment exceeds the potential for harm. In general, if the patient has an acute symptomatic seizure, treatment with an antiseizure drug is usually not necessary because these seizures are caused by a transient and reversible precipitating factor. In these cases, it is best to treat the provoking factor (discontinue the offending drug or treat the electrolyte abnormality) or allow sufficient time for the acute provoking etiology to resolve.

If an acute symptomatic cause cannot be found, then it is possible that the patient's seizure represents the first unprovoked seizure of an underlying epileptic disorder. About 150,000 adults will have an unprovoked first seizure. Unprovoked seizures are classified into *remote symptomatic seizures* (preexistent brain lesion) or *seizures of unknown etiology*. The rate of seizure recurrence after an unprovoked single seizure ranges from 31% to 56% over 2 to 5 years, and most patients will experience a recurrence in the first year. Seizure recurrence rates are significantly higher if there is a prior brain insult (twofold increase), if the EEG shows epileptiform abnormalities, if there is an abnormality on neuroimaging, and if the seizure occurs out of sleep (nocturnal seizure). If any of the aforementioned factors are present, then ASD treatment may be warranted. If ASD treatment is recommended, then patients should be advised that the risk of side effects will range from 7% to 31%, and they are mild and reversible. Patients should be informed that immediate ASD therapy will reduce the risk of seizure recurrence in the first 2 years after the seizure but will not improve the long-term (>3 years) chance of attaining seizure remission. Also, a single seizure can potentially be treated if the consequences of a recurrent seizure will significantly affect quality of life such as driving, work, or general safety. If two or more unprovoked seizures separated by 24 hours occur or if seizure recurrence risk is equal to 60% or more after a single event, then epilepsy is diagnosed, and treatment with an ASD is strongly recommended.

The goal of therapy is complete seizure freedom with no side effects. Around 50% to 60% of patients become seizure free on a single drug. Unfortunately, this is not possible in 30% to 40% of patients, necessitating referral to epilepsy centers for evaluation to rule out seizure imitators, evaluate for the presence of possible surgically remediable syndromes, and to try other options including diets and/or devices (vagal nerve stimulator, responsive nerve stimulator).

When starting ASD treatment, it is important to choose the medication that is effective for the seizure type or epilepsy syndrome. Of all available ASDs, five have a "broad spectrum" of action (work for both focal and generalized seizures): valproate (Depakote), lamotrigine (Lamictal), levetiracetam (Keppra), topiramate (Topamax), and zonisamide (Zonegran).[1] Consider a broad-spectrum ASD if the type of seizure is unknown. All of the available ASDs are effective against focal seizures except ethosuximide (Zarontin); this medication is only effective for treatment of typical absence epilepsy.

Next, consider the side-effect profile, cost, and drug dosing schedule, and adapt to the unique patient characteristics taking into consideration the patient comorbidities (Tables 1 and 2). For example, drugs with a once-a-day dosing schedule are optimal for patients with a history of prior poor compliance and for older adults; in patients taking multiple drugs for other comorbidities, administration of liver enzyme inducers (phenytoin) should be avoided. If the patient suffers from obesity, topiramate should be considered. In patients with migraine, either valproate or topiramate should be considered because these drugs are also effective for migraine prophylaxis.

Aim for monotherapy whenever possible to decrease side effects and drug interactions. Begin titration with a low dose, and increase slowly to maximize compliance and decrease side effects. If mild side effects occur, reassure the patient because most are usually transient.

Increase the ASD dose until seizure freedom is achieved or until side effects occur. If side effects occur, decrease the dose to the maximum tolerated dose. When switching from one ASD to another, always overlap the medications. For example, if a new medication is added, consider titrating to the effective dose before decreasing the failed medication. This approach provides some protection against breakthrough seizures during medication transitions.

If polytherapy is needed, consider ASDs with different mechanisms of action (rational polytherapy) such as a sodium channel blocker with a GABA enhancer or synergistic mechanisms (e.g., valproate and lamotrigine). Consider medications with parenteral formulations and a rapid time to therapeutic onset for rapid control of seizures if you are planning to discharge the patient from the emergency department with an adequate therapeutic dose. Drug levels should be obtained when compliance is an issue. Medication drug levels are a guide and not a goal. Always follow the patient's clinical response to ASDs.

In general it is reasonable to consider ASD discontinuation in patients who have been seizure free for 2 years. The reported relapse rate after discontinuing ASDs is around 41% or less. Factors associated with higher relapse include symptomatic epilepsy, age of onset between 10 and 12 years, cognitive delay, abnormal neurologic examination, juvenile myoclonic epilepsy, symptomatic partial epilepsy, abnormal EEG, family history of seizures or epilepsy, poor initial response to a drug, and more than one drug before discontinuation. If epileptiform abnormalities are seen and there is worsening of the EEG (increased EEG abnormalities) during discontinuation, then relapse rates are higher. Therefore consider performing an EEG before and after AED discontinuation.

Characteristics of Specific Antiseizure Drugs
Phenytoin
Phenytoin (Dilantin) is one of the most used antiseizure medications. It is effective for treatment of focal seizures and generalized seizures, prophylaxis after neurosurgical procedures,[1] and status epilepticus that does not respond to benzodiazepines. It can exacerbate absence seizures and myoclonus. Phenytoin exerts its antiepileptic effect by blocking sodium channels, thereby preventing post-tetanic potentiation. It is metabolized by the cytochrome P450 enzyme system in the liver and follows zero-order or nonlinear kinetics, therefore very steep elevations in blood levels can occur with minimal drug increases when the blood level is close to 20 µg/mL. Idiosyncratic reactions include blood dyscrasias and hepatitis, but these are rare. Common cumulative side effects include gum hyperplasia, coarsening of facial features, hirsutism, ataxia caused by cerebellar degeneration, nystagmus, drowsiness, lethargy, rash, headaches, nausea, vomiting, bone marrow hypoplasia, vitamin K and folate deficiency, and osteoporosis. Phenytoin is a strong inducer of hepatic enzymes, and it alters the metabolism of other drugs.

Fosphenytoin sodium (Cerebyx) is a prodrug, with phenytoin as its active metabolite. This medication is intended for parenteral administration; it is better tolerated than parenteral phenytoin because it is an aqueous solution with a neutral pH and can be administered three times as fast as phenytoin (150 mg/min vs. 50 mg/min). It has fewer cardiovascular side effects, including less hypotension, because, unlike phenytoin, it is not mixed with polyethylene glycol and will not cause vein irritation or purple glove syndrome because of its neutral pH.

Carbamazepine
Carbamazepine (Tegretol) is one of the most used ASDs in the world. It has been used in the United States since 1974 for treatment of focal epilepsies and generalized tonic-clonic seizures. It is highly effective and usually well tolerated. Carbamazepine, like phenytoin, blocks sodium channels. This medication is metabolized in the liver, and the major metabolic pathway is epoxidation to CBZ 10-11-epoxide. This epoxide confers most of the toxicity associated with this drug. It undergoes autoinduction and therefore induces its own metabolism in the first 3 to 5 weeks, and it takes longer to reach steady-state blood levels. Usually

---

[1] Not FDA approved for this indication.

[1] Not FDA approved for this indication.

typical absence epilepsy. This medication will not work to control any other seizure types. Common side effects are minimal and include dyspepsia, nausea, loss of appetite, and tiredness.

Felbamate

Felbamate (Felbatol) is effective for treatment of multiple seizure types, but it was briefly withdrawn from the U.S. market in 1994 because of the occurrence of aplastic anemia and hepatic failure. It is now available only for patients with intractable seizures in whom other medications have failed and when the benefits outweigh the risks. Its mechanism of action is blockade of NMDA receptors, modulation of sodium channels, and blockade of calcium channels. The risk for hepatic failure is 14 in 110,000 patients and increases with polytherapy.

Gabapentin

Gabapentin (Neurontin) is similar to the structure of GABA but has no effect on the GABA receptor. It enhances GAD, thereby increasing levels of GABA. This medication has no drug interactions. It is excreted entirely unchanged in the kidneys. Gabapentin is used for treatment of focal seizures with or without secondary generalization. It is ineffective in myoclonus and primary generalized seizures, and it is ineffective at lower doses. The dose should be adjusted in patients with renal disease according to creatinine clearance.

Pregabalin

Pregabalin (Lyrica) is an analogue of GABA, but like gabapentin (Neurontin), it has no effect on the GABA receptor. It has no drug interactions, and it is usually well tolerated. It must be dose-adjusted in patients with renal failure, and it is 50% removed after hemodialysis. It is used as an adjunct in adult patients with focal epilepsies. Common side effects include dizziness, drowsiness, weight gain, dry mouth, and edema.

Lamotrigine

Lamotrigine (Lamictal) works by sodium channel blockade and inhibits release of glutamate. It is broad spectrum, and it is used for adjunctive treatment of focal-onset seizures with or without secondary generalization, for crossover to monotherapy, and in LGS. It is also effective for treatment of atypical absence seizures,[1] tonic/atonic seizures, and myoclonic seizures, although it may cause exacerbations in some patients with juvenile myoclonic epilepsy. It is one of the preferred drugs to treat older adult patients and pregnant women because of its favorable safety and pharmacokinetic profile. Lamotrigine levels should be closely watched and will increase significantly with coadministration of valproate; these two medications cause a synergistic therapeutic effect but could also increase adverse reactions (rash). It could cause a rash (5%) if the drug is titrated too quickly; this rash could progress into a life-threatening condition (Stevens-Johnson syndrome; 0.1%) and is more common in children with concomitant valproate use. If rash occurs, the medication should be discontinued immediately. Other common side effects include tremor, insomnia, headaches, ataxia, and somnolence. Pregnancy increases lamotrigine clearance by 50%, necessitating dose adjustments; therefore lamotrigine levels should be monitored before, during, and after pregnancy, and doses should be adjusted accordingly.

Levetiracetam

Levetiracetam (Keppra) is one of the most widely used ASDs because of its good pharmacokinetics, favorable side-effect profile, and multiple formulations, including parenteral and liquid (ease of administration). It is a broad-spectrum drug. It has a unique mechanism of action (binds to synaptic vesicle protein 2A-SV2A). It does not induce liver enzymes and therefore does not affect the metabolism of other drugs and does not bind to proteins in plasma. This medication must be dose-adjusted in patients with

renal disease and after hemodialysis (add an extra 500 mg). It is one of the only ASDs that decreases the interictal epileptic burden (the other one is Depakote). It is approved for adjunctive treatment of primary generalized tonic-clonic seizures in adults and children 6 years of age and older with idiopathic generalized epilepsy, adjunctive treatment of focal onset seizures in adults and children 4 years of age and older, and adjunctive treatment of myoclonic seizures in adults and adolescents 12 years of age and older with juvenile myoclonic epilepsy. It is also used off-label for prophylaxis in patients after traumatic brain injury and in status epilepticus. Common adverse effects include behavioral changes (avoid in patients with psychiatric conditions), somnolence, asthenia, headache, dizziness, and flulike symptoms. It does not have any serious idiosyncratic reactions and is safe for older adults and probably safe to take during pregnancy. Consider obtaining levels during pregnancy because clearance is increased during pregnancy, necessitating dose adjustments.

Brivaracetam

Brivaracetem (Briviact) is a chemical analogue of levetiracetam with a similar mechanism of action but a higher affinity (20-fold) for the SV2A receptor. Like levetiracetam, it exhibits linear kinetics with a favorable side-effect profile. It is indicated for adjunctive treatment of focal-onset seizures with or without secondary generalization in adults and children 16 years of age and older. It does not have added therapeutic benefit if coadministered with levetiracetam. It may increase serum concentrations of carbamazepine epoxide and phenytoin.

Oxcarbazepine

Oxcarbazepine (Trileptal) is an analogue of carbamazepine but without the toxic epoxide. Thus it is better tolerated than carbamazepine (Tegretol). It is metabolized to the 10 monohydroxy metabolite, which confers its pharmacologic effect. It is used as monotherapy or adjunctive therapy for focal epilepsies in adults, as monotherapy for focal epilepsies in children 4 years of age and older, and as adjunctive therapy in children 2 years of age and older. It may exacerbate myoclonic seizures and absence seizures. It interacts with oral contraceptives, thereby reducing its efficacy. Hyponatremia is rare in children but may be higher in older adult populations. Other side effects include dizziness, fatigue, and headache, and these are dose dependent. Patients who develop rash with carbamazepine (Tegretol) may develop rash if treated with oxcarbazepine (Trileptal) because of cross-reactivity.

Tiagabine

Tiagabine (Gabitril) works by reversible inhibition of the GABA-transporter-1, thereby increasing the availability of GABA in the synaptic cleft. It is approved as an adjunctive medication for treatment of refractory focal-onset seizures. It can worsen absence seizures and cause status epilepticus in patients with primary generalized epilepsy. Common side effects include tremor, nervousness, dizziness, abdominal pain, diarrhea, and emotional lability.

Topiramate

Topiramate (Topamax) is a broad-spectrum ASD with multiple mechanisms of action. It works by inhibiting sodium conductance and weakly inhibiting carbonic anhydrase, blocks the AMPA glutamate receptor, and enhances GABA. It is approved for adjunctive treatment of focal-onset seizures or primary generalized epilepsy and for treatment of LGS. Enzyme inducers (e.g., phenytoin) decrease topiramate levels by 50%. This medication will need dose adjustments in patients with renal failure. Topiramate (Topamax) reduces the levels of oral contraceptives, thereby decreasing its effectiveness. Common side effects include word-finding difficulties, weight loss (decreased appetite), paresthesias in the fingers and mouth, kidney stones, anhidrosis caused by the drug's carbonic-anhydrase effect, acute myopia in closed-angle glaucoma, ataxia, and tiredness. Usually doses >400 mg are poorly tolerated.

---

[1] Not FDA approved for this indication.

Zonisamide

Zonisamide (Zonegran) is a broad-spectrum ASD used for treatment of focal epilepsy with or without secondary generalization. It is also effective for treatment of myoclonus (juvenile myoclonic epilepsy)[1] and absence seizures (T-type calcium channel blockade). This ASD has a structure similar to the sulfonamides; therefore it is contraindicated in patients with allergies to these antibiotics. It has a long-half life (>60 hours); therefore it can be taken once a day, which increases compliance. The major mechanism of action is the blockade of sodium channels; it also works on T-type calcium channels and weak inhibition of carbonic anhydrase. Enzyme inducers and valproate (Depakote) decrease half-life. The most common adverse reactions include anorexia with associated weight loss, headache, mental slowing, confusion, ataxia, dizziness, kidney stones (1%), oligohidrosis, and paresthesias (carbonic anhydrase inhibition).

Vigabatrin

Vigabatrin (Sabril) is a structural analogue of GABA and binds irreversibly to the GABA-T (GABA transaminase), thereby increasing GABA concentrations in the brain. It is indicated for treatment of epileptic spasms in tuberous sclerosis and in refractory focal-onset epilepsies. It may exacerbate absence seizures and myoclonic seizures and, like tiagabine, may cause generalized spike-and-wave status epilepticus in patients with absence seizures or primary generalized epilepsy. This ASD causes visual field defects (nasal constriction and concentric constriction with preserved central vision), and these may be irreversible. Other side effects include fatigue, dizziness, headache, tremor, and double vision.

Rufinamide

Rufinamide's (Banzel) mechanism of action is probable modulation of sodium channels (prolongation of inactive state of the channel). It is indicated as adjunctive treatment of seizures associated with LGS in both children and adults.

Lacosamide

Lacosamide (Vimpat) has a novel mechanism of action by enhancing the slow inactivation of voltage-gated sodium channels. It is approved for the adjunctive treatment and conversion to monotherapy and monotherapy treatment of focal onset epilepsies. It is also used off label for treatment of status epilepticus in the intensive care unit because of availability of an IV formulation. This medication does not have significant drug interactions.

Clobazam

Clobazam (Onfi) is a benzodiazepine with a 1,5 substitution instead of the common 1,4 substitution; therefore it has less anxiolytic and sedative effects. It works by binding to the GABA-A receptor. It is approved for the adjunctive treatment of LGS. It may also be effective for treatment of primary or focal seizures with secondary generalized seizures[1] as well as catamenial epilepsy.[1] It has no significant clinical interactions. Side effects include sedation, dizziness, ataxia, and weakness. No idiosyncratic reactions have been identified.

Perampanel

Perampanel (Fycompa) is a noncompetitive AMPA receptor antagonist and is indicated in the adjunctive treatment of focal-onset seizures with or without secondary generalization and in primary generalized seizures in adults and adolescents 12 years of age and over. The recommended dose is 8 to 12 mg/day for focal seizures and 8 mg/day for primary generalized seizures. This medication has a black box warning because it can cause severe psychiatric and behavioral reactions (aggressiveness, suicidality, homicidal threats and ideation, and irritability). Common adverse effects include somnolence, headache, dizziness, and fatigue.

---

[1] Not FDA approved for this indication.

Eslicarbazepine

Eslicarbazepine (Aptiom) is a prodrug of S-licarbazepine with a mechanism of action similar to oxcarbazepine (Trileptal) sodium channel blockade. It is approved as monotherapy or adjunct therapy for treatment of focal-onset seizures. Common adverse effects include dizziness, nausea, diplopia, and headache.

Cannabidiol

Cannabidiol (EPIDIOLEX) is the first prescription pharmaceutical formulation of purified CBD oil approved by the FDA (in June 2018) for the treatment of seizures associated with LGS and Dravet syndrome in patients 1 year of age and older.

The most common side effects of this drug include increase in liver enzymes, especially when used in conjunction with valproate or valproate and clobazam, decreased appetite, diarrhea, rash, tiredness, sleepiness, and infections.

Fenfluramine

Fenfluramine (Fintepla) is a phenethylamine that is structurally similar to serotonin and exerts its antiepileptic effect by increasing the release of serotonin, which stimulates multiple 5-HT receptor subtypes, and by acting as a positive modulator of sigma receptors. This medication was approved by the FDA in June 2020 for treatment of seizures in Dravet syndrome and LGS in patients 2 years of age and older. The most common side effects include decreased appetite, weight loss, diarrhea, fatigue, lethargy, and pyrexia. It has few relative drug-drug interactions.

Everolimus

Everolimus (Afinitor) is a rapamycin derivative that inhibits mTOR (mammalian target of rapamycin). mTOR overactivation has been linked to the pathogenesis of tuberous sclerosis complex (TSC), therefore it can target the etiology of the disease. It was approved by the FDA as adjunctive treatment for TSC with partial onset seizures in patients 2 years of age and older. The most common adverse effects are stomatitis, pyrexia, pneumonia, diarrhea, and hypercholesterolemia.

Special Populations

Women

Epilepsy is one of the most common conditions occurring in women of reproductive age (1.1 million). Women of reproductive age who are taking ASDs for epilepsy should be counseled on the possibility of teratogenicity from ASD therapy and the potential interaction with contraception. Some ASDs (enzyme inducers) affect oral contraceptives (OCPs), leading to decreased effectiveness and unwanted pregnancies. These ASDs are phenobarbital, phenytoin, carbamazepine, oxcarbazepine, eslicarbazepine, felbamate, topiramate (doses >200 mg/day), lamotrigine (doses >300 mg/day), primidone, rufinamide, and clobazam. OCPs can reduce the levels of lamotrigine, leading to breakthrough seizures. In patients taking these ASDs, a second barrier method versus changing to a non–enzyme-inducing ASD is recommended. Seizures during pregnancy will remain the same or decrease, but around 15% to 30% will have an increase in seizure frequency. Most women (84% to 92%) with epilepsy who were seizure free 9 months before the pregnancy will remain free from seizures during the pregnancy. Blood levels of lamotrigine, phenytoin, carbamazepine (to a lesser extent), and possibly levetiracetam and the active oxcarbazepine metabolite, will decrease during pregnancy because of increased clearance; therefore these ASD levels should be monitored and medication dosages adjusted as needed. The risk to the fetus from seizures (especially convulsive seizures) is higher than the risk to the fetus from ASDs. More than 90% of female patients with epilepsy will deliver a normal baby. The rates of congenital malformations in women with epilepsy taking ASDs is around 4% to 6% (double that of the general population) but remain low. The risk of malformations increases with polytherapy and with higher dose of ASDs. Valproate/valproic acid is the ASD that carries the highest teratogenicity (6% to 10%), mostly associated with neural tube defects. It also produces long-term

TABLE 6 Clinical Pharmacology of Treatments for Restless Leg Syndrome

	MECHANISM OF ACTION	DOSAGE	TYPICAL ADVERSE EFFECTS	INTERACTIONS
Iron Replacement				
Ferrous sulfate[1]	Fe	324 mg, 1 tab every alternate day	Nausea, constipation	None
Ferrous fumarate+vit C[1]	Fe	200/125 mg, 1 tab every alternate day	Nausea, constipation	None
Carbidopa-Levodopa (Sinemet)[1]	DA	25/100 1–2 prn	Nausea, dizziness, ICD	None
Pramipexole (Mirapex)	DA	0.125–1.0 mg[2] qhs	Nausea, dizziness, ICD	None
Ropinirole (Requip)	DA	1–6 mg[2] qhs	Nausea, dizziness, ICD	None
Rotigotine (Neupro Transdermal Patch)	DA	1–3 mg qam	Nausea, dizziness, ICD	None
Gabapentin (Neurontin)[1]	Unknown	300–1200[2] mg qhs	Nausea, dizziness, pedal edema, weight gain	None
Gabapentin Enacarbil (Horizant)	Unknown	600 mg	Nausea, dizziness, pedal edema, weight gain	None
Pregabalin (Lyrica)[1]	Unknown	100–600 mg qhs	Nausea, dizziness, pedal edema, weight gain	None
Tramadol (Ultram)[1] Codeine	MRA MRA[1]	50 mg 400 mg qhs 30–60 mg	Nausea, dizziness Nausea, dizziness	None None
Oxycodone[1]	MRA	5–15 mg	Nausea, dizziness	None

[1]Not FDA approved for this indication.
[2]Exceeds dosage recommended by the manufacturer.
Abbreviations: mg=milligrams; Fe=iron replacement; DA=dopamine agonist; MOR=mu opiate receptor agonist.

Nonpharmacologic treatments including warm or cool baths, massage, stretching, or even the application of spontaneous compression devices have been reported to be effective anecdotally and in small case series, but an evidence base for these measures remains poor, and most patients seeking medical care for the symptom have severe enough symptoms to merit pharmacologic treatment.

Iron and pharmacologic treatments for RLS are outlined in Table 6. Iron deficiency, or even low normal body iron stores, may worsen or precipitate symptoms. Measuring a serum ferritin should be considered early in all RLS patients, with iron replacement therapy begun if serum ferritin values are less than 50 mcg/L. Iron therapy can be constipating or cause GI distress, and the formulation of iron with added vitamin C (Ferrex 150 Plus, Vitelle Irospan) is often better tolerated by those who cannot stomach ferrous sulfate.

Carbidopa-levedopa (Sinemet)[1] may be used for patients with only intermittently disturbing symptoms, but chronic nightly use of carbidopa-levodopa, especially above a dosage of 200 mg daily, may raise the risk of augmentation. For nightly use, the newer dopaminergic agonist medications pramipexole (Mirapex) or ropinirole (Requip) remain a mainstay of treatment. Pramipexole may be initiated at 0.125 to 0.25 mg nightly and titrated every few days to the 0.375 to 0.50 mg range or beyond if needed for symptom control. Doses beyond 1.0 mg[3] are typically not additionally effective and appear to raise augmentation risk. Ropinirole may be initiated at 0.5 to 1.0 mg with gradual upward titration to the 4 to 6 mg[3] range as needed and tolerated. Generally, dosing 1 hour prior to bedtime is sufficient, but if earlier evening or late afternoon symptoms emerge, cautious application of divided doses may be utilized, and some experts advice at least a low morning dosage administered daily to achieve a more chronic steady state of dopamine administration since this may be a sensible strategy to minimize augmentation risk. For either initial

first-line therapy, or particularly when patients are beginning to experience earlier symptom onset during the day and may have failed the other short-acting dopaminergic drugs pramipexole and ropinirole, a rotigotine (Neupro) patch has been an advent in RLS management and often may be substituted for those other agents to provide more day-long symptom relief and reduce a growing augmentation tendency. Rotigotine offers several other advantages, as its transdermal delivery system provides continuous day-long release of medication that may minimize peak/trough serum concentration variation and minimize the occurrence of other potential adverse effects. Rotigotine also appears to result in augmentation less frequently than other dopaminergic drugs. All patients receiving dopaminergic agents should be counseled upfront about the approximate 15% idiosyncratic risk of impulse control disorder symptoms (such as pathologic gambling, shopping, or hoarding/punding behaviors), and be forewarned that should such problems result, the medication must be withdrawn and another nondopaminergic drug substituted for symptom control. Typical dose-related adverse effects are also described further in Table 6.

Gabapentin (Neurontin)[1] is increasingly becoming an alternative first-line medication for RLS, dosed 300 to 1200[3] mg every night at bedtime as needed and tolerated. Gabapentin may be the agent of choice in patients with comorbid anxiety, pain and insomnia or in patients who are intolerant, resistant to, or have developed augmentation with dopamine agonist medications. On the other hand a dopamine agonist is still generally the first choice for pharmacologic treatment of RLS in severe cases and may be preferred over gabapentin in patients with comorbid depression, obesity, metabolic syndrome, OSA and history of falls. Gabapentin enacarbil (Horizant) is a prodrug of gabapentin that is better absorbed and carries an indication for RLS, but generic gabapentin is also frequently effective

---

[1]Not FDA approved for this indication.

[1]Not FDA approved for this indication.
[3]Exceeds dosage recommended by the manufacturer.

and well tolerated, and there has been no head-to-head trial showing superiority of the more expensive prodrug gabapentin encarbil over that of gabapentin. Other alternatives include clonazepam[1] and tramadol (Ultram).[1] For patients unresponsive to these measures, opiate treatment with oxycodone (Roxicodone)[1] 5 to 15 mg at bedtime, hydromorphone (Dilaudid),[1] or methadone (Dolophine)[1] are often effective. A large randomized trial showed that the combination oxycodone-naloxone (Targiniq ER)[1] resulted in substantial improvements in RLS symptoms in patients who had previously shown inadequate response to dopamine agonists. Small case series suggest other alternatives for refractory RLS such as carbamazepine (Tegretol),[1] oxcarbazepine (Trileptal),[1] and lamotrigine (Lamictal).[1] The impact of comorbid OSA should also be considered, as optimization of treatment for SDB may improve both subjective RLS symptoms as well as PLMD frequency in many patients.

Sleep-Related Leg Cramps

Sleep-related leg cramps are a common and enigmatic problem affecting 7% to 10% of children and up to 70% of elderly adults. Unfortunately, despite their extremely common occurrence and impact on the quality of life of cramp sufferers, little is known about the pathophysiology or treatment of this condition. Cramps are painful, involuntary sustained muscle contractions, lasting 2 to 10 minutes and affecting the unilateral or bilateral calves, thighs, or feet, with residual tenderness of the affected muscle lasting up to an hour or longer. The clinical approach to sleep-related leg cramps is to first determine whether they are also present during daytime in addition to sleep. If daytime cramping is prominent, exclusion of a precipitating neuromuscular disorder is paramount, including amyotrophic lateral sclerosis, peripheral neuropathy, myositis, or cramp-fasciculation syndrome. In elderly men, peripheral vascular disease and other systemic medical comorbidities are also common. (The reader is referred to the chapter on neuromuscular disorders for further advice on the diagnosis of these conditions.) A neurologic examination should be conducted on all cramp sufferers, and those having sensorimotor findings, fasciculations, or pathologic reflex findings should be referred for EMG, serum creatinine kinase, or additional blood and urine tests for exclusion of symptomatic causes of neuropathy as appropriate. While additional testing for electrolyte abnormalities such as hypomagnesemia, hypocalcemia, hyponatremia, and hypokalemia can be considered, they are of extremely low yield. When examination findings are normal and cramps are isolated to the sleep state, further diagnostic work-up can usually be avoided. Symptomatic treatment measures for sleep-related leg cramps include tonic water with lemon and advising adequate hydration and nightly stretching of the calves and thighs. Prescription quinine (Qualaquin)[1] carries a FDA black box warning for leg cramp treatment and is essentially no longer used for this indication. For refractory frequent cramp sufferers, a sodium-channel blocking anticonvulsant such as carbamazepine[1], oxcarbazepine[1], or lamotrigine[1] may also be considered.

Sleep-Related Bruxism

Sleep-related bruxism, rhythmic grinding of the teeth during sleep, may lead to significant tooth wear and dental or jaw pain. The condition is usually idiopathic, although it may be associated with psychiatric conditions such as mood or anxiety disorders, especially if it is also present during daytime. Treatment usually involves dental referral for consideration of a fitted mouth guard, although in extreme cases pharmacotherapy with clonazepam[1] or consideration of botulinum toxin (Botox)[1] may be necessary.

Other Sleep-Related Movement Disorders

Sleep-related rhythmic movement disorder usually occurs in patients with psychomotor maldevelopment and involves repetitive head and neck or axial body movements. This behavior is not strictly voluntary and often persists during PSG into deep drowsiness or light NREM sleep, so behavioral treatments alone are often ineffective. Head banging behavior, sometimes into the headboard of the bed, can be injurious at times: a protective helmet or treatment with clonazepam[1] is advisable in some cases. Most other movement disorders, such as organic tremors, myoclonus, or dyskinesias generated by the basal ganglia, are suppressed during sleep but may reemerge during drowsiness or nocturnal awakenings.

Propriospinal myoclonus at sleep onset is characterized by myoclonic jerks having their primary and earliest onset in abdominal and axial muscles prior to spreading to the limbs and may be associated with thoracic spinal cord pathology. Spinal imaging with MRI is advised. Treatment with clonazepam[1] is usual for this uncommon diagnosis, although it is unfortunately often ineffective, and many cases of propriospinal myoclonus are instead found to represent a functional movement disorder.

Isolated Symptoms and Normal Variants

These conditions are felt largely to represent either normal variants or otherwise largely benign disorders. The definition of long and short sleepers are somewhat arbitrary, but may be considered as greater than 10 hours or shorter than 5 hours of habitual sleep. Short or long sleep time are each assumed to be variants of normal behavior in the absence of hypersomnia or nighttime symptoms of insomnia.

Sleep talking, or somniloquy, in isolation is rarely of concern. History is often lifelong in such patients. When sleep talking is newly evolved in an elderly individual or a younger patient receiving antidepressant therapy, RBD should be considered in the differential diagnosis, and the patient should be questioned about other potential evidence for dream enactment behavior. A careful medication history and neurologic examination alone will usually dictate whether further evaluation with PSG may be indicated, but in most cases isolated sleep talking is not a cause for concern.

Sleep starts, hypnic jerks or physiologic myoclonus are near universal in their occurrence and often associated with recent excessive caffeine intake or emotional or physical stress. A history of occurrence of jerks limited to the arms, legs, or axial musculature causing arousal within the first 5 to 10 minutes of sleep, and lacking later recurrence during the night, is typical. Reassurance and avoidance of precipitating factors is advised; however, if hypnic jerks are excessive or recur later in the night, PSG is occasionally necessary to distinguish this benign diagnosis from PLMD or propriospinal myoclonus. Propriospinal myoclonus at sleep onset is characterized by myoclonic jerks having their primary and earliest onset in abdominal and axial muscles prior to spreading to the limbs and may be associated with thoracic spinal cord pathology. Spinal imaging with MRI is advised. Treatment with clonazepam[1] is usual for this uncommon diagnosis.

Other Sleep Disorders

Undesirable influences in the patient's sleep environment can serve to regularly distract or disturb him or her from initiating or maintaining sleep. Typical influences include a bed partner who snores loudly or who causes bed motion due to restless or disturbed sleep; pets who sleep in bed with the patient and cause awakening; environmental noise from neighborhood dogs, car alarms, or neighboring freeway or train way; too much outdoor ambient light; or undesirable household ambient temperature. There is considerable overlap in this category of environmental sleep disturbance with inadequate sleep hygiene, as activating stimuli in the environment may lead the patient toward chronic insomnia and adapting undesirable sleep-related behaviors that serve to further disrupt restful sleep.

---

[1]Not FDA approved for this indication.

[1]Not FDA approved for this indication.

Sleep-Related Medical and Neurologic Disorders

Fatal familial insomnia is an exceedingly rare, autosomal dominant variant form of familial Creutzfeldt-Jakob disease, a prion disorder that leads to progressive insomnia and progressive cognitive impairment, with death inevitably occurring within 3 years of onset. Aggregate prion protein accumulates in the thalamus and other brain regions, and relentlessly progressive insomnia, panic disorder, hallucinosis, and dementia ensue. Unfortunately, no treatments are currently known for this rare disorder.

Conclusions

Sleep disorders are common and result in significant patient morbidity, daytime dysfunction, and impaired quality of life. Untreated sleep disordered breathing (SDB) may also raise the risk for hypertension, vascular events, and mortality. The most common presenting symptoms of sleep disorders include insomnia, characterized by difficulty initiating and maintaining sleep with poor sleep quality, and hypersomnia, the symptom of excessive daytime sleepiness. Evaluation begins with a detailed history and physical examination, which in select cases may require support and clarification by polysomnography and multiple sleep-latency testing. Fortunately, effective therapies are available for the majority of sleep disorders. Insomnia typically requires behavioral or pharmacologic interventions, while SDB may be effectively treated in most cases with positive airway pressure (PAP) therapy. Primary CNS hypersomnias including narcolepsy require stimulant management in most cases, while most parasomnias benefit from clonazepam.[1] Circadian sleep disorders may require timed light and melatonin therapies. Patients having RLS and PLMD should be evaluated for iron deficiency and may enjoy symptom control through dopaminergic or other alternative symptomatic treatments. The majority of patients with sleep disorders benefit from a careful clinical evaluation and appropriately selected therapies.

[1]Not FDA approved for this indication.

References

American Academy of Sleep Medicine: *International Classification of Sleep Disorders: Diagnostic and Coding Manual*, ed 3, Darien, IL, 2014, American Academy of Sleep Medicine. 2014.

Auger RR, Burgess HJ, Emens JS, et al: Clinical practice guideline for the treatment of intrinsic circadian rhythm sleep-wake disorders: Advanced Sleep-Wake Phase Disorder (ASWPD), Delayed Sleep-Wake Phase Disorder (DSWPD), Non-24-Hour Sleep-Wake Rhythm Disorder (N24SWD), and Irregular Sleep-Wake Rhythm Disorder (ISWRD). An update for 2015. An American Academy of Sleep Medicine Clinical Practice Guideline, *J Clin Sleep Med* 11:1119–1236, 2015.

Chesson AL, Anderson WL, Pancer JP, Wise M: Practice parameters for the indications for polysomnography and related procedures: An update for 2005, *Sleep* 28:499–521, 2005.

Collop NA, Tracy SL, Kapur V, et al: Obstructive sleep apnea devices for out-of-center (OOC) testing: Technology evaluation, *J Clin Sleep Med* 7:531–548, 2011.

Costanzo MR, Ponikowski P, Javaheri S, et al: Sustained 12 month benefit of phrenic nerve stimulation for central sleep apnea, *Am J Cardiol* 121(11):1400–1408, 2018.

Johns MW: A new method for measuring daytime sleepiness: The Epworth sleepiness scale, *Sleep* 14:540–545, 1991. Also available online in a patient fillable version at http://www.stanford.edu/~dement/epworth.html.

Kushida CA, Littner MR, Morgenthaler T, et al: Indications for positive airway pressure treatment of adult obstructive sleep apnea patients: A consensus statement, *Chest* 115:863–866, 1999.

Luyster FS, Strollo Jr PJ, Zee PC, et al: Sleep: A health imperative, *Sleep* 35:727–734, 2012.

Morgenthaler TI, Lee-Chiong T, Alessi C, et al: Standards of Practice Committee of the American Academy of Sleep Medicine. Practice parameters for the clinical evaluation and treatment of circadian rhythm sleep disorders, *Sleep* 30:1445–1459, 2007.

Schutte-Rodin S, Broch L, Buysse D, et al: Clinical guideline for the evaluation and management of chronic insomnia in adults, *J Clin Sleep Med* 4:487–504, 2008.

Silber MH, Becker PM, Earley C, et al: Willis-Ekbom Disease Foundation revised consensus statement on the management of restless legs syndrome, *Mayo Clin Proc* 88:977–986, 2013.

St. Louis EK: Key sleep neurologic disorders: Narcolepsy, restless legs syndrome/Willis-Ekbom disease, and REM sleep behavior disorder, *Neurol Clin Pract* 4:16–25, 2014.

Wise MS, Arand DL, Auger RR, et al: American Academy of Sleep Medicine. Treatment of narcolepsy and other hypersomnias of central origin, *Sleep* 30:1712–1727, 2007.

Strollo Jr PJ, Soose RJ, Maurer JT, et al.: Upper-airway stimulation for obstructive sleep apnea, *N Engl J Med* 29;370(2):139–149, 2014.

SPORTS-RELATED HEAD INJURIES

Method of
Brandon Hockenberry, MD; Margaret Pusateri, MD; and Christopher McGrew, MD

CURRENT DIAGNOSIS

- Initial evaluation of any sports-related head injury should follow standard emergency medicine procedures.
- Presence of any "red flag" symptoms is concerning for a more serious head injury (skull fracture and intracranial hemorrhage) and requires emergency evaluation.
- If "red flag" symptoms are present and advanced imaging is indicated, a noncontrast computed tomography (CT) scan of the head is the initial study of choice.
- If no "red flag" symptoms are present, one of several validated neuropsychological tests should be administered to evaluate cognitive function (e.g., Sports Concussion Assessment Tool, version 5 [SCAT 5]; https://bjsm.bmj.com/content/bjsports/early/2017/04/26/bjsports-2017-097506SCAT5.full.pdf).
- Ultimately, concussion is still a clinical diagnosis.
- Advanced neuroimaging, fluid biomarkers, genetic testing, helmet sensors, and video surveillance have all been purported as possible prognostic indicators but require further validation.

CURRENT THERAPY

- Blood pressure control is critical for patients with intracranial hemorrhage.
- Small intracranial hemorrhages without midline shift or significant symptoms may be monitored, but surgical decompression is otherwise required.
- For patients requiring sedation, propofol (Diprivan)[1] is often preferred due to its short half-life, which makes it easier to monitor neurologic status.
- Mannitol can also be used to help lower intracranial pressure.
- For posttraumatic seizures, phenytoin (Dilantin)[1] is the preferred medication.
- If there is any concern for concussion, the athlete should immediately be removed from play.
- An athlete should never be allowed to return to play on the same day as the injury.
- After an initial rest period of 24–48 hours, an athlete should begin progressing through return-to-play and return-to-learn protocols (https://www.cdc.gov/headsup/providers/return_to_activities.html).
- In the first 24 hours after injury, acetaminophen is the treatment of choice for associated headaches; nonsteroidal antiinflammatory drugs (NSAIDs) and aspirin can worsen an undiagnosed intracranial hemorrhage.
- If headaches persist longer than 3–5 days, medications that do not pose a risk for rebound headaches (e.g., tricyclic antidepressants) can be used.
- Good sleep hygiene is important for recovery. If insomnia persists for more than 2–3 days after injury, medications can be considered.
- Typical recovery time is up to 2 weeks in adults and 4 weeks in children.
- Access to a multidisciplinary team including physical therapists, neurologists, and psychiatric providers is beneficial for athletes with complicated or prolonged recoveries.
- If an athlete has a history of a learning disability, depression, anxiety, or chronic headaches, recovery can be complicated by an exacerbation of the underlying disease.

[1]Not FDA approved for this indication.

Introduction and Epidemiology

Sports-related head injuries include a heterogenous group of insults to the brain caused by either a direct impact to the head or an impact to the body associated with energy transfer into the head.

In the United States, sports are among the leading causes of head injuries. Specifically between the ages of 15 and 24 years, athletic activities are the second leading cause of head injuries; only motor vehicle accidents have a higher incidence. Athletic and recreational activities vary widely in terms of biomechanics and kinetics, resulting in a wide range of associated risks. Many sports are limited by the speed at which an athlete can run (e.g., rugby or soccer), but others allow athletes to compete at much higher speeds, some nearly equivalent to those of motor vehicles (e.g., cycling or skiing). These sports potentially put athletes at a higher risk for more severe head injuries.

Sports- and recreation-related traumatic brain injuries (SRR-TBIs) are monitored by the National Electronic Injury Surveillance System—All Injury Program (NEISS-AIP). According to this program, there were more than 3.4 million visits to emergency departments (EDs) across the United States for SRR-TBIs between 2001 and 2012, or approximately 340,000 per year.

Concussion is by far the most common head injury associated with athletic activity. It is estimated that 1.7 to 3.0 million concussions per year are related to sports and recreational activities. The overall rate is 2.5 concussions per 10,000 athletic events, and concussions make up 5% to 18% of reported injuries in the National Collegiate Athletic Association. It is estimated that 50% of concussions go unreported or undiagnosed. The most common severe head injury is a subdural hematoma, which accounts for greater than 90% of all sport-related catastrophic head injuries. These are most often seen in American football, cheerleading, and skiing/snowboarding and occur in less than 1 per 100,000 athletic events. Fatalities from sports-related head injuries are very rare; however, subdural hematoma is a serious injury. In one study, it was reported that American football players with subdural hematoma had a fatality rate of 8.5% and a 48% rate of suffering permanent neurologic deficits.

Risk Factors

Every athlete is potentially at some risk for a head injury during activity. Many factors contribute to relative risk, with the type of activity being the largest contributing factor. In their younger years, males sustain the most head injuries playing football or wrestling, whereas bicycling and basketball take over top spots after the high school and college years. In females, bicycling and horseback riding contribute the most head injuries. It should be noted that some activities have higher incidence rates of head injuries than the aforementioned activities (e.g., men's/women's ice hockey) but are not as commonly played and therefore do not contribute to the sheer volume of injuries that other activities do. With respect to concussion specifically, men's ice hockey and football have the highest incidence rates (5.5 to 6.5 concussions per 10,000 athletic events) in the high school and college populations. On the women's side, soccer and lacrosse have the highest rates (3 to 3.5 concussions per 10,000 athletic events).

Children and teens are at increased risk for head injuries because they are developmentally immature and more frequently participate in activities that have a higher risk for head trauma. Overall, 70% of all SRR-TBIs are in the age group of 0 to 19 years. In the young athlete, a larger head-to-neck ratio, smaller amount of neck/shoulder musculature, and thinner cranial bones all contribute to an increased chance that a blow to the head will cause a head injury. The active elderly have better balance, fewer falls, and fewer TBIs than their more chronically ill counterparts. Therefore increased age is not an independent risk factor for SRR-TBIs.

At the high school and college levels, males have more concussions than do women in sheer numbers but a lower incidence rate overall. Females may have greater risk because of decreased neck musculature compared with males. Female sex has been associated more commonly with abnormal imaging, surgical intervention, complication, and death. A history of previous concussion increases risk for future concussions compared with nonconcussed athletes, and the greatest risk for repeat concussion is during the 10-day period after the most recent concussion.

Pathophysiology

The pathophysiology of SRR-TBIs and sports-related concussion (SRC) is multifactorial. Several mechanisms have been identified. Biomechanically, a combination of acceleration, deceleration, and rotational/translational forces directly applied or transmitted to the head affect change at the level of individual cells. Metabolic derangements, neurotransmitter dysfunction, changes in cerebral blood flood, neuroinflammation, microstructural damage, and diffuse axonal injury have all been implicated as potential pathways. Helmet-based measurement studies have attempted to quantify head impacts, providing information on force, frequency, and location. However, results vary widely among athletes diagnosed with concussions. In addition, the accuracy of the data detected by helmet sensors and video surveillance systems has been called into question; it does not necessarily reflect the impact on the brain itself, and there is no evidence to support the use of such systems to attempt to diagnose SRC.

Assessment and Diagnosis of Sports-Related Head Injury

The initial assessment of any sports-related head injury should follow standard emergency medicine procedures. Assessment of the "ABCs" (airway, breathing, and circulation) and evaluation for concomitant cervical spine injury should be the first steps in management. The presence of any red flag symptoms (Box 1) should raise concerns for a serious head injury, such as an intracranial hemorrhage or skull fracture, and requires immediate evaluation in the ED, likely advanced head or neck imaging, and possible specialist consultation. The appropriate emergency action plan should be initiated and the athlete stabilized and transported to the designated medical facility.

Once in the ED, the decision whether to obtain images needs to be made. Some assessment tools have been developed, such as the Pediatric Emergency Care Applied Research Network (PECARN; https://www.mdcalc.com/pecarn-pediatric-head-injury-trauma-algorithm) and Canadian CT Head Injury algorithms. A Glasgow Coma Scale score below 14, palpable skull fracture, or presence of red flag symptoms would all be reasons to image acutely. The initial imaging test of choice after head injury is a noncontrast head CT, which will show fractures, intracranial hemorrhage, midline shifts, and signs of edema. CT with angiography will show decreased blood flow into cerebral vessels because of increased intracranial pressure. However, if increased intracranial pressure due to malignant brain edema or an expanding hematoma is suspected, more invasive intracranial pressure monitoring is a more accurate measure and will be more useful to management (see Box 1).

If no red flag symptoms are present and the athlete does not require emergency medical treatment, he or she should be removed from the field of play if there is any suspicion for

---

BOX 1	Red Flag Symptoms

Persistent vomiting
Seizure
Severe "worst headache of my life"
Focal neurologic deficit
Blurred vision
Slurred speech
Significant drowsiness/poor awakening
Poor orientation to person/place/time
Declining mental status

The presence of any of these symptoms should prompt consideration of emergency department evaluation and head imaging. If no red flags are present, the clinician may be able to send the athlete home safely and follow up in the office the next day.

possible SRC. Several brief neuropsychological tests have been developed to evaluate cognitive function. Examples of practical and validated tests include the SCAT 5 and the Standardized Assessment of Concussion (SAC). The SCAT 5 is broken down into six steps: immediate or on-field assessment, symptom evaluation, cognitive screening, neurologic screening, delayed recall, and decision. In addition to an assessment of the aforementioned red flag symptoms, the immediate or on-field assessment section of the SCAT 5 also includes a review of observable signs (e.g., lying motionless on the playing field, facial injury after head trauma, and blank or vacant look), a memory assessment using the Maddocks Questions (Box 2), a measure of the Glasgow Coma Scale (Table 1), and a cervical spine assessment. It has been found that standard orientation questions (name, location, and year) are not reliable in the immediate assessment of SRC. The Maddocks questions, which focus on sport-specific memory assessment, provide better information to help the examiner determine whether there is a concern for an SRC. Once the initial assessment is complete, if there is any concern for an SRC, the athlete should be removed from the sporting environment and not allowed to return to play on the day of injury.

Diagnosis of SRC remains a clinical diagnosis. Over the past two decades, multiple investigations have focused on the use of advanced neuroimaging (e.g., functional magnetic resonance imaging [f-MRI] and electroencephalogram [EEG]) and body fluid analysis (blood, saliva, and cerebrospinal fluid) as potential tools to aid in the diagnosis of SRCs. (In addition, these modalities have been explored as potential prognostic indicators, attempting to predict clinical recovery or assess the cumulative risk of repetitive trauma.) At this time, advanced neuroimaging, fluid biomarkers, and genetic testing are important research tools but require further validation to determine their ultimate clinical utility in the evaluation and diagnosis of SRC.

Clinical Manifestations

Clinical manifestations after an SRR-TBI and SRC can be varied. The brain itself is a complex organ. Depending on which area is injured, different symptoms may present. With regard to the more serious diseases, such as intracranial hemorrhages or diffuse axonal injury, the athlete is often critically injured, again demonstrating red flag symptoms and signs of increased intracranial pressure. However, SRC is an evolving injury within the acute phase and can often have an initially subtle presentation. Signs and symptoms rapidly change, especially over the first 24 to 48 hours. Classically, symptoms fall into one of four categories: physical (headache, nausea, and dizziness), cognitive (difficulty concentrating and slowed reaction times), emotional (anxiety and irritability), and sleep disturbances (insomnia and hypersomnia). As part of the SCAT 5 and other concussion assessment tools, an in-depth symptom checklist is used to evaluate SRCs both initially and during follow-up. For example, Table 2 outlines the SCAT 5 symptom checklist. It is important to note that there are no specific scoring guidelines that are diagnostic of concussion. The scores are most commonly used to monitor an athlete's recovery, tracking improvement or decline over time. Of note, higher scores at the time of initial injury are associated with longer recoveries.

Treatment

Presence of red flag symptoms listed in Box 1 or a Glasgow Coma Scale score of less than 14 should raise suspicion for a more severe SSR-TBI, such as a skull fracture or intracranial hemorrhage, rather than a typical concussion. If an athlete sustains an SSR-TBI other than concussion, he or she should be evaluated in the ED. In the event of an intracranial hemorrhage of any kind, the largest concern is increasing intracranial pressure. Strict blood pressure control is incredibly important, because an increased blood pressure will increase the pressure in the bleeding vessel and thus the rate and severity of the bleed. Intracranial hemorrhages may be monitored if the bleed is small and not causing a midline shift or significant symptoms. However, definitive treatment with surgical decompression is preferred for subdural and epidural hemorrhages. Most patients will require intubation, sedation, and intracranial pressure monitoring. For sedation, propofol (Diprivan)[1] is the preferred agent at many institutions because it has a short half-life, making it easier to monitor the patient's neurologic status. In the presence of malignant brain edema, mannitol (Osmitrol) can be added to decrease intracranial pressure when strict blood pressure and pain control has failed. For a TBI causing posttraumatic seizure, phenytoin (Dilantin)[1] remains the preferred medication, although many institutions will use older antiepileptic drugs such as valproate (Depakote)[1] or carbamazepine (Tegretol)[1] as treatments of choice.

The current recommendation for the management of SRC is to remove the athlete from play and not allow a return on the same day. The athlete should avoid physical exertion and mental activities that make symptoms worse. After an initial rest

[1] Not FDA approved for this indication.

| BOX 2 | Memory Assessment: Maddocks Questions |

What venue are we at today?
What half is it now?
Who scored last in the game?
What team did you play last week?
Did your team win the last game?

Note: Can be adapted to specific sports as necessary.
These questions help make diagnosis of concussion. No official score cutoff is diagnostic; however, inability to answer them all correctly should raise suspicion for concussion or more severe head injury. Questions can be changed slightly if they are not relevant to a sport, such as swimming.

| TABLE 1 | Glasgow Coma Scale |

BEST EYE RESPONSE (E)	BEST VERBAL RESPONSE (V)	BEST MOTOR RESPONSE (M)
Eye opening spontaneously: 4	Oriented: 5	Obeys commands: 6
Eye opening to voice: 3	Confused: 4	Localizes to pain: 5
Eye opening to pain: 2	Inappropriate words: 3	Flexion/withdrawal from pain: 4
No eye opening: 1	Incomprehensible sounds: 2	Abnormal flexion to pain: 3
	No verbal response: 1	Abnormal extension to pain: 2
		No motor response: 1

Used to rate the severity of head injury. Scores in each category are added for a total of 15 points. Athletes with concussion typically have a Glasgow Coma Scale score of 14 (losing 1 point in the verbal response category) or 15. Scores less than 14 should prompt a visit to the emergency department for head imaging.

period of 24 to 48 hours, the patient should begin progressing to both physical (noncontact) and mental activities. The athlete should return to normal activities of daily living as much as is tolerated without symptom exacerbation. The newest consensus statement on concussion in sport outlines not only a return-to-play protocol but also a return-to-learn protocol. These are outlined in Tables 3 and 4. Children and adolescents should not return to sport until they have fully returned to school. It is important to note that there is no evidence to suggest that any medications or nutritional supplements will improve rate of recovery from concussion. Medications in concussion treatment are primarily used for symptomatic relief.

Monitoring Concussions

After concussion diagnosis, the clinically stable athlete can be sent home if a responsible adult is available to accompany him or her. Sleep is encouraged, and the athlete need not be awakened for evaluation. The athlete should be followed up in a qualified healthcare provider's office within 24 to 48 hours for reevaluation. Follow-up examination should include a symptom severity checklist (see Table 2), history, and neurologic examination at a minimum. Completing a full SCAT 5 evaluation is unnecessary if the athlete had one done at time of injury and still has symptoms. Advanced neuroimaging with MRI is not needed to monitor a concussion and by definition should be normal.

TABLE 2	SCAT 5 Symptoms Checklist
SYMPTOM	**SEVERITY**
Headache	0 1 2 3 4 5 6
"Pressure in head"	0 1 2 3 4 5 6
Neck pain	0 1 2 3 4 5 6
Nausea and/or vomiting	0 1 2 3 4 5 6
Dizziness	0 1 2 3 4 5 6
Blurred vision	0 1 2 3 4 5 6
Balance problems	0 1 2 3 4 5 6
Sensitivity to light	0 1 2 3 4 5 6
Sensitivity to noise	0 1 2 3 4 5 6
Feeling slowed down	0 1 2 3 4 5 6
Feeling like "in a fog"	0 1 2 3 4 5 6
"Don't feel right"	0 1 2 3 4 5 6
Difficulty concentrating	0 1 2 3 4 5 6
Difficulty remembering	0 1 2 3 4 5 6
Fatigue or low energy	0 1 2 3 4 5 6
Confusion	0 1 2 3 4 5 6
Drowsiness	0 1 2 3 4 5 6
More emotional	0 1 2 3 4 5 6
Irritability	0 1 2 3 4 5 6
Sadness	0 1 2 3 4 5 6
Nervous or anxious	0 1 2 3 4 5 6
Trouble falling asleep (if applicable)	0 1 2 3 4 5 6
Total number of symptoms	Of 22
Symptom severity score	Of 132

There is no score cutoff that is diagnostic of concussion; it is simply used to monitor a patient's improvement or decline over time. Higher scores at time of injury are associated with longer recovery times.
SCAT 5, Sports Concussion Assessment Tool version 5.

As the athlete returns to play, close supervision under a qualified healthcare provider such as a certified athletic trainer or physical therapist is ideal but not always possible. When an athlete has progressed through the return-to-play protocol (see Table 3), follow-up with an appropriate qualified healthcare provider should be arranged to obtain full medical clearance to return to full contact activity.

Management of Concussion Complications

Headaches are among the most common symptoms of a concussion and often the symptom that bothers the athlete the most. In the acute period after injury, medications have some potential to mask important symptoms. For the first 1 to 2 hours after the injury, it is important to be able to accurately monitor the patient for a changing clinical picture, which could suggest that the head injury is not a concussion but rather an evolving epidural or subdural hematoma. For the first 24 hours, NSAIDs and aspirin should be avoided because they can thin the blood and potentially make an undiagnosed hematoma become a more significant bleed. Acetaminophen (Tylenol) is the preferred medication for headache in the first 24 hours. After the first day, it is safe to switch to ibuprofen (Motrin), which may have more benefit. If headaches are not improving after 3 to 5 days, it is advisable to switch to another medication that does not pose the risk of creating rebound headaches. Tricyclic antidepressants are a good choice and work very well. Nortriptyline (Pamelor)[1] at a low dose (25 mg/d) is generally well tolerated in children as well as adults and may be stopped abruptly without withdrawal symptoms once the athlete is feeling well and ready to progress back to activities.

Sleep disturbances in athletes with concussion are also very common. Many will not sleep well the first night after injury and want to nap during the day. Other athletes may sleep much more than usual after initial injury. Although there are no clear studies proving the optimal amount of sleep, current trends are to try to return the athlete to normal sleep cycles and daily living as much as possible. An emphasis on sleep hygiene over the first few days is standard. If insomnia persists after 2 to 3 days, medications may be considered. Melatonin[7] is available over the counter, has very few side effects, and is generally well tolerated. The next step would be amitriptyline (Elavil)[1] at a low dose (10– 25 mg/d). This can be especially effective if the athlete has both headaches and poor sleep because it is more sedating than nortriptyline.

A concussion is expected to last no more than 14 days in an adult and less than 4 weeks in the pediatric population. Each individual physician will have a different comfort level treating concussion; however, it is reasonable to consider a referral to a specialty physician once an athlete has passed the normal expected recovery time and is not categorized as a "prolonged concussion." Each city or region will have a different culture about who takes care of the prolonged concussions. Neurologists, sports medicine physicians, and physical medicine and rehabilitation physicians are all well equipped to take care of these athletes. Physical therapists, particularly those who specialize in vestibular rehabilitation, can be very helpful to patients with continued balance problems, concentration difficulties, and other visual symptoms. Last, neuropsychologists can be extremely helpful in difficult cases. Some athletes have complicated clinical histories prior to the injury. Attention-deficit/hyperactivity disorder, depression, anxiety, and chronic headaches can all make the clinical picture very confusing when the athlete is having symptoms such as concentration difficulties, mood swings, insomnia, or headaches that are not improving as expected. It is important to remember that many athletes would not rate their symptom severity score as all

[1] Not FDA approved for this indication.
[7] Available as a dietary supplement.

TABLE 3 | Graduated Return-to-Play Protocol as Outlined by the Consensus Statement on Concussion in Sport

STAGE	AIM	ACTIVITY	GOAL OF EACH STEP
1	Symptom-limited activity	Daily activities that do not provoke symptoms	Gradual reintroduction of work/school activities
2	Light aerobic exercise	Walking or stationary cycling at slow to medium pace; no resistance training	Increase heart rate
3	Sport-specific exercise	Running or skating drills; no head impact activities	Add movement
4	Noncontact training drills	Harder training drills (e.g., passing drills); may start progressive resistance training	Exercise, coordination, and improved thinking
5	Full-contact practice	After medical clearance, participate in normal training activities	Restore confidence and assess functional skills by coaching staff
6	Return to sport	Normal game play	

Start step 1 after initial 24- to 48-hour period of rest. Each step should take a minimum 24 hours to progress through.

TABLE 4 | Example of a Graduated Return-to-Learn Protocol as Outlined by the Consensus Statement on Concussion in Sport

STAGE	AIM	ACTIVITY	GOAL OF EACH STEP
1	Daily activities that do not give the child symptoms	Typical activities of the child during the day as long as he or she does not increase symptoms (e.g., reading, texting, screen time). Start with 5–15 min at a time and build up	Gradual return to typical activities
2	School activities	Homework, reading, or other cognitive activities outside of the classroom	Increase tolerance to cognitive work
3	Return to school part time	Gradual introduction of schoolwork. May need to start with a partial school day or increased breaks during the day	Increase academic activities
4	Return to school full time	Gradually progress school activities until a full day can be tolerated	Return to full academic activities and catch up on missed work

Unlike the return-to-sport protocol, there is no minimum required time for each stage. Some children may be able to tolerate a full school day immediately after injury without difficulty, depending on symptom severity.

zeros at baseline, so expecting them to achieve this goal after injury is impractical. When this scenario is suspected, referral for neuropsychiatric testing can help to divide out which symptoms may be concussion related and which could be more chronic in nature.

Prevention

Helmets have been shown to reduce sports-related skull fractures and intracranial hemorrhages but have not been shown to decrease rates of concussion. Mouth guard use decreases the rate of dental injuries and lip lacerations but has not been definitively proven to decrease the rate of concussion or other brain injuries. Sport-specific rule changes have resulted in reduced rates of head injury. The most prominent and well-studied example is that of youth ice hockey. Introduction of the 2013 Canadian national body checking policy change disallowing body checking in Pee Wee hockey players below the age of 13 years resulted in a 50% relative reduction in injury rate and a 64% reduction in concussion rate in 11-year-old and 12-year-old hockey players in Alberta. Reduction of contact practices in certain team sports such as American football reduces exposure to head injury as well. Finally, epidemiologic evidence has demonstrated that the most likely period for repeat SRC is in the first 10 days after the most recent concussion, so disallowing contact activity during this interval has potential to reduce repeat concussions.

References

Black AM, Hagel BE, Palacios-Derflingher L, et al: The risk of injury associated with body checking among Pee Wee ice hockey players: an evaluation of Hockey Canada's national body checking policy change, *Br J Sports Med* 51:1767–1772, 2017.

Coronado VG, Haileyesus T, Cheng TA, et al: Trends in sports-and recreation-related traumatic brain injuries treated in US emergency departments: The National Electronic Injury Surveillance System—All Injury Program (NEISS-AIP), 2001- 2012, *J Head Trauma Rehabil* 30:185–197, 2015.

Gessel LM, Fields SK, Collins CL, et al: Concussions among United States high school and collegiate athletes, *J Athl Train* 42:495–503, 2007.

Harmon KG, Clugston JR, Dec K, et al: American Medical Society for Sports Medicine position statement on concussion in sport, *Br J Sports Med* 53:213–225, 2019.

Kerr ZY, Roos KG, Djoko A, et al: Epidemiologic measures for quantifying the incidence of concussion in national collegiate athletic association sports, *J Athl Train* 52:167–174, 2017.

Leddy J, Haider M, Ellis M, et al: Early subthreshold aerobic exercise for sports related concussion: a randomized clinical trial. *JAMA Pediatr,* 173(4):319–325, 2019.

McCrory P, Meeuwisse W, Dvorak J, et al: Consensus statement on concussion in sport—the 5th international conference on concussion in sport held in Berlin, October 2016, *Br J Sports Med* 51:838–847, 2017.

Munivenkatappa A, Agrawal A, Shukla DP, et al: Traumatic brain injury: Does gender influence outcomes? *Int J Crit Illn Inj Sci* 6(2):70–73, 2016.

Nagahiro S, Mizobuchi Y: Current topics in sports-related head injuries: a review, *Neurol Med Chir (Tokyo)* 54:878–886, 2014.

Sarmiento K, Thomas K, Daugherty J, et al: Emergency department visits for sports and recreation-related traumatic brain injuries among children—United States, 2010-2016, *MMWR* 68:237–242, 2019; number 10.

Steenerson K, Starling AJ: Pathophysiology of sports-related concussion, *Neurol Clin* 35:403–408, 2017.

TARGETED TEMPERATURE MANAGEMENT (THERAPEUTIC HYPOTHERMIA)

Scott Leikin, DO; Jennifer Wang, DO; and Adel Bassily-Marcus, MD

CURRENT THERAPY

- Targeted temperature management (therapeutic hypothermia) should be considered following resuscitation from cardiac arrest to reduce the risk of anoxic brain injury.
- There does not appear to be a benefit to cooling to a temperature of 33°C when compared to cooling to a temperature of 36°C (97°F).
- There is a paradigm shift of therapeutic hypothermia to preventing fever and instituting a targeted temperature.
- Cooling pads are the most commonly used method to induce hypothermia.

Introduction

Inducing patients to a targeted temperature to reduce anoxic brain injury post cardiac arrest has now become the standard of care at medical institutions around the world. Although the theory has multiple applications for multiple conditions, post cardiac arrest is the most common and studied indication and the focus of this chapter. Although each institution has their own protocol, there are common tenets that are included in each institution's protocols. Current nomenclature is Targeted Temperature Management (TTM) as the theories on ideal temperature for the post cardiac arrest patient have evolved from therapeutic hypothermia. The evolution of TTM is important to understand, as the current theory is fever prevention is where the benefit is and fever is what is associated with poor neurologic outcomes in the post cardiac arrest time period.

The first multicenter, randomized control study on post cardiac arrest care was conducted in Europe and published in the New England Journal of Medicine (NEJM) in 2002. A total of 3551 patients were deemed eligible, but only 275 were included. In the study, 137 were assigned to hypothermia (32 to 34°C as measured by bladder temperature for 24 hours) and 138 to normothermia. To qualify in the study, subjects must have had a witnessed cardiac arrest, with an initial rhythm of ventricular fibrillation (VF) with return of spontaneous circulation (ROSC). The results showed a favorable neurologic outcome in 75/136 patients (55%) in the hypothermia group compared to 54/137 patients (39%) in the normothermia group at 6 months as measured by the Pittsburgh cerebral-performance category. The mortality difference at 6 months was 41% in the hypothermia group and 55% in the normothermia group. This validated the utilization of mild therapeutic hypothermia to improve neurologic outcomes and decrease mortality for witnessed VF cardiac arrest.

In 2002, a NEJM study described survival with good neurologic outcome to hospital discharge in patients who were unconscious after ROSC in out-of-hospital cardiac arrest. In the study, 77 patients were assigned to normothermia or moderate hypothermia (core body temperature of 33°C within 2 hours of ROSC for 12 total hours). Usually, out-of-hospital cardiac arrests have survival rates of only 5% to 35%. The investigators found 21/43 (49%) patients in the hypothermia group survived and had a favorable neurologic outcome compared to 9/34 (26%) in the normothermia group with (P = .046). The authors concluded that moderate hypothermia improved outcomes in patients with coma after ROSC in out-of-hospital cardiac arrest patients.

In 2010, the American Heart Association (AHA) released a class I recommendation for post VF/VT TTM. Pulseless electrical activity/asystole was given a IIb recommendation. TTM is generally defined as a core temperature of 33 to 36°C. Since this recommendation, TTM has been adopted as common practice post cardiac arrest in comatose adult patients.

In May 2011, the Society of Critical Care Medicine published "Targeted temperature management in critical care: A report and recommendations from five professional societies" and determined that TTM with a core body temperature goal of 32 to 34°C be used for post out-of-hospital VF/VT arrest.

In December 2013, the NEJM published a study titled "Targeted Temperature Management at 33°C versus 36°C after Cardiac Arrest." This international multicenter study aimed to determine the optimal temperature associated with improved neurologic outcomes for out-of-hospital cardiac arrest patients. They found no significant 180-day neurologic outcome or mortality difference between the patients in the 33°C arm and the patients in the 36°C arm. There were no adverse effects or benefits to patients cooled to 33°C. The authors concluded that in patients who were unconscious after ROSC was obtained in out-of-hospital cardiac arrest, a temperature of 33°C did not confer a benefit compared to a temperature of 36°C. This shifted the paradigm of therapeutic hypothermia to preventing fever and instituting a targeted temperature.

The International Liaison Committee on Resuscitation and the AHA Emergency Cardiovascular Care Committee and the Council on Cardiopulmonary, Critical Care and Perioperative and Resuscitation reviewed 5045 studies, of which 6 were RCTs and 5 were observational. They recommended: target core temperatures between 32 and 36°C for at least 24 hours and against using pre-hospital cooling with cooled intravenous fluids.

The theoretical benefits of TTM are that it can reduce brain oxygen usage by 6% for every 1°C reduction while also preventing inflammation and cerebral edema. TTM is currently being studied for encephalopathy, bacterial meningitis, cardiogenic shock, traumatic brain injury, and organ donation.

Initiation

With few absolute contraindications, TTM should be considered in all patients who achieved ROSC post cardiac arrest regardless of the underlying rhythm during the cardiac arrest. Many post cardiac arrest patients with ROSC will go to the cardiac catheterization lab for an angiogram and this should not delay the initiation of TTM. Determining the etiology for the cardiac arrest is still extremely important and should not have a bearing on the initiation of TTM. The patient populations in whom TTM is considered a relative contraindication include intracranial hemorrhage, exsanguination, hypotension refractory to multiple vasopressors, severe sepsis, and pregnancy. At our tertiary care academic medical center, the only absolute contraindications are cryoglobulinemia, traumatic injury leading to cardiac arrest, and family refusal or advanced directives that preclude the use of TTM.

Eligibility requires a comatose patient; the patient should not be able to follow commands or respond to noxious stimuli. This is equivalent to a Richmond Agitation Sedation Score of –4 or –5 or Glasgow Coma Scale <8. The patient must have a sustained cardiac rhythm that results in adequate brain perfusion.

The most studied rhythms in cardiac arrest which benefited from TTM were VT or VF. It is uncertain whether pulseless electrical activity and a "nonshockable rhythm" would benefit from TTM but we would advocate that any patient regardless of the underlying rhythm have TTM utilized if ROSC is obtained. This is in line with the 2015 AHA guidelines on post cardiac arrest care and emergency cardiovascular care. The guideline committee came to this conclusion because cohorts who did not receive TTM had such significant neurologic morbidity that the benefits were considered to outweigh the risks. Significant head trauma should be ruled out in patients who present to an emergency department with a noncontrast head computed tomography (CT) scan. Ideally, TTM should be initiated as soon as ROSC is obtained but it is acceptable to initiate it within the first 6 hours, and even up to 12 hours post arrest. We strongly advocate initiating the process as soon as feasible. We would also recommend that pacer pads be applied to the patient's skin and kept in place. The target core temperature should be maintained at the desired temperature for 24 hours. Based on a review of the literature, initiating a core temperature between 32 and 36°C for these patients with external cooling pads is the target.

The most commonly used method to induce hypothermia is with external cooling pads. Once the process is started, the time to target temperature should be within 2 hours. Other less commonly used options include ice bags at the groin, chest, axilla, and neck, and infusing cold saline. Cooled intravenous saline will reduce core temperature by 1°C every 30 minutes. The 2015 AHA guidelines recommend against cooling patients in the prehospital setting with intravenous cooled saline, as survival and neurologic recovery were not shown to be improved in various trials. Urinary catheters with temperature probes are often used to measure core temperature. Other acceptable methods of temperature measurement include esophageal, rectal, central, tympanic, or nasal probes. Axillary and oral temperature measurements are not reliable in measuring core temperature. Potential complications of cooling include electrolyte abnormalities, hyperglycemia, coagulopathy, and arrhythmias.

Maintenance

In TTM, the targeted core temperature should be maintained within 0.5°C for 24 hours. Shivering should be avoided as it creates heat, thereby increasing oxygen demand. Bedside Shivering Assessment Scale (BSAS) should be utilized to help guide therapy for shivering. For sedation purposes, our recommended first-line treatment is propofol (Diprivan) 15 to 20 µg/kg/min. Midazolam (Versed) 1 to 2 mg/h is an alternative. Fentanyl 25 µg/h infusion can be used if adequate sedation is not achieved.

The BSAS treatment algorithm should be utilized to eliminate shivering. In the BSAS, neuromuscular blockade with an agent such as cisatracurium (Nimbex) 0.15 mg/kg IV bolus followed by an infusion of 1 µg/kg/min can be used, although this protocol may mask seizures. The lowest dose that eliminates shivering using agents with a short half life is recommended because hypothermia slows medication metabolism and elimination.

TTM may worsen or cause hemodynamic derangements and arrhythmias, such as hypotension and bradycardia, that are common post cardiac arrest. Maintenance of a mean arterial pressure (MAP) at or above 65 mm Hg will help ensure adequate brain perfusion.

TTM patients are mechanically ventilated, and some institutions use esophageal probes to track body temperature, although this is less common, as it is invasive. Oxygen saturation should be maintained at 94% to 96% to avoid hypoxia or hyperoxygenation. Hyperglycemia is common with TTM, so serum glucose should be checked at set intervals, with a goal <180 mg/dL. If serum glucose is persistently >200 mg/dL despite treatment, an insulin drip should be considered. Electrolyte abnormalities, especially hypokalemia, are common during TTM. Therefore, the serum potassium level should be checked every 4 to 6 hours and replenished if lower than 3.5 meq/L. Rewarming may increase potassium levels.

It has been reported in the literature that up to 66% of TTM patients will develop an infection. Fever and leukocytosis may be present in the absence of infection and are not reliable indicators of infection. A comprehensive plan needs to be developed for every patient when signs of infection are potentially present. Even if a high percentage of patients develop an infection, this has not been shown to affect mortality.

Rewarming

Rewarming should occur 24 hours after achieving the targeted temperature. Rewarming should not occur at a rate that is faster than 0.2°C/h until the patient reaches 37°C; this will likely take between 6 to 12 hours. Once at 37°C, this temperature should be maintained for 48 to 72 hours, as rebound hyperthermia is associated with poor neurologic outcomes. Electrolyte abnormalities such as hyperkalemia, hypoglycemia, and hypotension may occur. Blood pressure should be carefully monitored during the rewarming period.

Post-Therapeutic Hypothermia/Prognosis

The AHA recommends 72 hours before prognosticating neurologic recovery. Presence of at least two of the following: incomplete brain stem reflexes, presence of myoclonus, unreactive electroencephalography (EEG), and absent cortical somatosensory-evoked potentials suggest poor neurologic outcome. A full neurologic examination should be done daily. Involving neurology or neurocritical care is advised to help prognosticate neurologic recovery in post cardiac arrest TTM patients.

References

Badjatia N, Strongilis E, Gordon E: Metabolic impact of shivering during therapeutic temperature modulation the bedside shivering assessment scale, *Stroke* 39(12):3242–3247, 2008, https://doi.org/10.1161/STROKEAHA.108.523654.

Bernard, Gray, Buist: Treatment of comatose survivors of out-of-hospital cardiac arrest with induced hypothermia. *New England Journal of Medicine*, 346:557–563, 2002, https://doi.org/10.1056/NEJMoa003289.

Callaway Clifton W, et al: American heart association guidelines update for cardiopulmonary resuscitation and emergency cardiovascular care, *Circulation* 132(18):S315–S367, 2015, https://doi.org/10.1161/CIR.0000000000000252, 3 Nov. 2015.

Donnino MW, Anderson LW, Berg KM, Reynolds JC: Temperature management after cardiac arrest an advisory statement by the advanced life support task force of the international liaison committee on resuscitation and the american heart association emergency cardiovascular care committee and the council on cardiopulmonary, critical care, perioperative and resuscitation, *Circulation* 132(25):2448–2456, 2015. https://doi.org/10.1161/CIR.0000000000000313.

Friedman OA: *Critical care: targeted temperature management after cardiac arrest*, In JM Orpopello, V Kvetan, SM Pastores. Eds. New York, NY: McGraw Hill, Lange, 2017.

Moler MD, Silverstein FS, Hulubkov R, et al: Therapeutic hypothermia after out-of-hospital cardiac arrest in children, *New Eng Journal of Medicine*, 372:1898–1908, 2015, Available at: https://doi.org/10.1056/NEJMoa1411480.

Nielson MD, PhD, Wetterslev N, MD, PhD, J, & Cronberg, MD, PhD, T: Targeted temperature management at 33°c versus 36°c after cardiac arrest. *New England Journal of Medicine* 369:2197–2206, 2013, Available at: https://doi.org/10.1056/NEJMoa1310519.

Nunnally M, Jaeschke R, Bellingan G: Targeted temperature management in critical care: a report and recommendations from five professional societies, *Critical Care Medicine* 39(5):1113–1125, 2011, https://doi.org/10.1097/CCM.0b013e318206bab2.

T.: Mild therapeutic hypothermia to improve the neurologic outcome after cardiac arrest, *New England Journal of Medicine* 346:549–556, 2002, https://doi.org/10.1056/NEJMoa012689.

Scirica BM: Therapeutic hypothermia after cardiac arrest, *Circulation, Clinician update* 127(2):244–250, 2013, https://doi.org/10.1161/CIRCULATIONAHA.111.076851.

Yunen JR, Tolentino R: *Critical care: chapter: controversies in therapeutic hypothermia*, In JM Oropello, V. Kvetan, SM Pastores. Eds.). New York, NY: McGraw Hill Lange, 2017.

TRIGEMINAL NEURALGIA

Method of
Karlynn Sievers, MD; and Hugh Silk, MD, MPH

CURRENT DIAGNOSIS

The International Headache Society Diagnostic criteria (classic) are as follows:
- Recurrent paroxysms of unilateral facial pain in the distribution(s) of one or more divisions of the trigeminal nerve, with no radiation beyond, and fulfilling criteria B and C
- Characteristics of pain:
  - Last from a fraction of a second to 2 min
  - Severe intensity
  - Electric shock-like, shooting, stabbing, or sharp in quality
  - Precipitated by innocuous stimuli to the affected trigeminal distribution
- Demonstration on magnetic resonance imaging (MRI) or during surgery of neurovascular compression (not simply contact), with morphologic changes in the trigeminal nerve root
- Not better accounted for by another diagnosis
- International Headache Society Diagnostic criteria (secondary)
- Same as previous except
  - Secondary trigeminal neuralgia secondary to another disease process

CURRENT THERAPY

- Medications
  - Carbamazepine: start 100 mg twice daily and increase by 200 mg/day to a maximum of 1200 mg/day (number needed to treat = 2)
  - Alternative treatments are available but have not been proven to be as effective (Table 1).
  - For some patients with refractory or severe symptoms, surgical treatment (e.g., microvascular decompression, radiosurgery, alternative invasive procedures) can be helpful.

Epidemiology
The incidence of trigeminal neuralgia is estimated to be 5.9/100,000 women and 3.4/100,000 men. The peak incidence is in patients aged 60 to 70 years. It has also been called "tic douloureux" because of facial spasms that often accompany the disorder.

Risk Factors
Increasing age is a risk factor. Trigeminal neuralgia is rarely diagnosed in patients below 40 years of age. Other risk factors include multiple sclerosis (the incidence of trigeminal neuralgia in this population is 2% to 5%), stroke, and hypertension (especially in women). There is no racial predominance.

Pathophysiology
It is currently hypothesized that trigeminal neuralgia results from demyelination of the fifth cranial nerve, leading to electrical transmission of nerve impulses that are not mediated by neurotransmitters and that generate pain. Demyelination is most commonly caused by aberrant or tortuous blood vessels that cause nerve compression but can also be attributed to sources such as multiple sclerosis or amyloid deposition.

The most used classification system for trigeminal neuralgia has three categories: classical, secondary, and idiopathic. With classical trigeminal neuralgia, there is no underlying cause for the demyelination other than vascular compression, as described previously. With secondary trigeminal neuralgia, an alternate cause

TABLE 1	Treatment Options for Trigeminal Neuralgia With Evidence of Effectiveness
TREATMENT TYPE	**EVIDENCE OF EFFECTIVENESS**
Medical therapy	
Carbamazepine (Tegretol)	Likely to be beneficial (gold standard)
Oxcarbazepine (Trileptal)[1]	Likely to be beneficial*
Baclofen (Lioresal)[1]	Likely to be beneficial,* particularly in patients with TN caused by MS
Gabapentin (Neurontin)[1]	Unknown effectiveness
Lamotrigine (Lamictal)[1]	Unknown effectiveness
Surgical therapy	
Microvascular decompression	Trade-off between benefits and harms*
Stereotactic radiosurgery	Trade-off between benefits and harms*
Percutaneous destructive radiosurgical techniques	Trade-off between benefits and harms*

*Based on observational studies and/or consensus.
[1]Not FDA approved for this indication.
MS, Multiple sclerosis; *TN*, trigeminal neuralgia.

such as multiple sclerosis or tumor is responsible for the demyelination. A third category would include idiopathic trigeminal neuralgia, where there are no radiologic findings that account for the patient's symptoms.

Prevention
There is no known method for the prevention of trigeminal neuralgia.

Clinical Manifestations
Trigeminal neuralgia is a clinical diagnosis made based on recurrent attacks of unilateral facial pain. The pain is intense and is usually described as sharp, shock-like, or stabbing. Any of the branches of the trigeminal nerve can be affected, but the maxillary branch is the most common and the ophthalmic branch the least common. The pain lasts for seconds, and most patients are asymptomatic between attacks (though some will have a mild, dull, persistent ache around the affected nerve). Attacks can recur infrequently or hundreds of times per day.

Often, patients have trigger zones that will set off paroxysms of pain with minimal stimulation. Activities such as chewing, teeth brushing, or touching a trigger area can set off attacks; sometimes even minimal stimulation such as a light breeze can trigger an episode. Not all patients have trigger zones; however, the presence of these is nearly pathognomonic for trigeminal neuralgia.

Diagnosis
The diagnosis is clinical, based on the commonly described symptoms listed earlier. Diagnosis of trigeminal neuralgia should be considered in all patients who describe unilateral intense paroxysmal facial pain on three or more occasions. Careful examination of the head and neck and thorough neurologic examination should be performed in all patients. Exam findings are typically normal in patients with trigeminal neuralgia; therefore exam abnormalities should prompt reconsideration of the diagnosis. Sensory abnormalities (including vision or hearing loss), facial muscle weakness, or loss of the corneal reflex are not associated with trigeminal neuralgia and warrant further workup.

Laboratory studies are typically not helpful in making the diagnosis. Temporal mandibular joint or dental radiographs may be helpful to rule out other pathology for those who present with mid or lower face symptoms. Magnetic resonance imaging ([MRI] with and without contrast) of the brain can be helpful in distinguishing between classic and symptomatic trigeminal neuralgia and should be considered in all patients

TABLE 1 Clinical and Laboratory Characteristics of Viral Meningitis

VIRUS	TRANSMISSION	KEY CLINICAL FEATURES	DIAGNOSIS	COMMENTS
Enterovirus	Fecal-oral	May have rash on exam (e.g., Coxsackie, hand–foot–mouth) Patients with impaired humoral immunity or those <2 wk old can present with a sepsis-like syndrome with multiorgan dysfunction, DIC, cardiovascular collapse	CSF enterovirus PCR	More prevalent in summer and fall
Parechovirus	Fecal-oral, less commonly respiratory	Can cause sepsis-like illness in neonates <3 mo CSF will often have few to no WBCs	CSF parechovirus PCR	More prevalent in the summer and fall
Herpes simplex viruses 1 and 2	Vertical transmission during birth (HSV2), horizontal transmission via contact (HSV1 or HSV2)	10%–30% of adults have symptoms of meningitis with primary HSV2 infection; look for genital vesicular lesions on exam Mollarets meningitis: >3 episodes of fever and meningismus lasting 2–5 d, with spontaneous resolution; episodes may be months to years apart often due to chronic HSV2 CNS infection	CSF HSV1/HSV2 PCR	Meningitis is uncommon with nonprimary HSV2 infection
Arboviruses	Subcutaneous inoculation via mosquito or tick and rarely through ingestion of unpasteurized milk from infected livestock Prevention: Minimize tick and mosquito exposure with personal protection measures including insect repellents and covering exposed skin	Zika virus associated with Guillan-Barré syndrome and in newborn infants microcephaly; sexual transmission is possible	CSF arboviral PCR Zika RT-PCR (performed at CDC Arbovirus laboratory on CSF or serum within first 5–7 days of symptoms); Zika IgM cross reacts with other flaviviruses (e.g., Dengue)	More prevalent in summer and fall Geographic distribution within the U.S.: Eastern equine encephalitis: Eastern U.S. Western equine encephalitis: Western U.S. St. Louis encephalitis: Across the U.S. (majority of cases in Central and Eastern U.S.) West Nile virus: Across the U.S. California encephalitis (LaCrosse): Midwestern, mid-Atlantic, and Southeastern U.S. Zika virus: Small epidemics occurred in Southeastern U.S. and Gulf Coast states. Currently, there is no local transmission of zika virus in the continental U.S.
Lymphocytic choriomeningitis virus	Virus is present in rodent secretions, feces, and urine Ingestion of contaminated food, exposure of open wounds, or inhalation of aerosolized virus Lab workers, pet owners, and those living in impoverished conditions are highest risk for illness	Accompanied by a flulike illness	Serum LCMV titers (acute and convalescent) CSF findings: May have decreased glucose and WBC count >1000/mL	More prevalent in winter and spring
Cytomegalovirus	Exposure to infected body fluids (e.g., saliva, blood)		CSF CMV PCR	Reactivation of prior infection typically only occurs in the immunosuppressed

VIRUS	TRANSMISSION	KEY CLINICAL FEATURES	DIAGNOSIS	COMMENTS
Epstein–Barr virus	Exposure to infected body fluids (e.g., saliva, blood)	Alice in Wonderland syndrome: altered body image and distortion of visual perception	CSF EBV PCR	Most common neurologic complication with primary infection
HIV	Exposure to contaminated blood or other body fluids (e.g., transfusion, sexual contact, percutaneous blood exposure)	During primary infection, a subset have meningitis or meningoencephalitis May expect thrush and cervical lymphadenopathy	HIV studies	Treatment with HAART
Human herpesvirus 6	Respiratory	Roseola: febrile illness followed by viral exanthem	CSF HHV6 PCR	HHV6 has been demonstrated in the CSF of asymptomatic persons Immunosuppressed persons at risk for symptomatic infection and reactivation
Varicella	Respiratory	Typical vesicular skin lesions of chickenpox on exam CSF pleocytosis has also been demonstrated with reactivation; can also occur in the absence of cutaneous findings of herpes zoster ("zoster sine herpete")	CSF VZV PCR	Rarely diagnosed during acute chickenpox infection; usually a postinfectious complication Other neurologic sequelae of varicella infection are more common than aseptic meningitis; most common is cerebellar ataxia
Mumps	Respiratory	Parotitis on exam is the most prominent sign of infection Aseptic meningitis can precede or follow clinical exam findings CSF profile can demonstrate an unusually high protein with a mild pleocytosis and normal glucose	Serum titers	More common in winter and spring
Measles	Respiratory	CSF pleocytosis in ≤30% of patients with measles; patients are usually without clinical meningitis	Serum titers	In the U.S., most cases are imported (e.g., occur in returning travelers), but in recent years there have been outbreaks of measles in the U.S. associated with pockets of unvaccinated people
Influenza	Respiratory	Aseptic meningitis is a less common neurologic complication of influenza infection (encephalopathy is more common)	CSF influenza PCR	More prevalent in winter Increased risk of neurologic complication in young patients and in those with pre-existing medical disease
COVID-19	Respiratory	CSF profile can demonstrate pleoyctosis and elevated protein	CSF SARS-CoV-2 RT PCR	Rare complication of COVID-19 infection

Abbreviations: CMV = cytomegalovirus; CNS = central nervous system; CSF = cerebrospinal fluid; DIC = disseminated intravascular coagulopathy; HHV = human herpesvirus; HSV = herpes simplex virus; LCMV = lymphocytic choriomeningitis virus; PCR = polymerase chain reaction; VZV = varicella zoster virus; WBC = white blood cell.

Differential Diagnosis

The major item on the differential diagnosis for viral meningitis is bacterial meningitis. The bacterial meningitis score, validated in children 29 days to 19 years, is a clinical prediction rule that identifies patients as at very low risk (0.1%) for bacterial meningitis if they lack all of the following: positive CSF Gram stain, CSF absolute neutrophil count (ANC) of at least 1000 cells/μL, CSF protein of at least 80 mg/dL, peripheral blood ANC of at least 10,000 cells/μL, and a history of seizure before or at the time of presentation. While C-reactive protein (CRP) is not generally useful because it can be high in viral meningitis and low in the initial stages of bacterial disease, elevated serum procalcitonin levels (>0.5 μg/mL in children and >0.2 μg/mL in adults) are more sensitive and specific for distinguishing viral from bacterial meningitis.

Other diagnoses to consider include parameningeal infections (i.e., subdural or epidural empyema, brain abscess), meningitis due to fungi, mycobacteria, rickettsia, mycoplasma, parasites, and other CNS infectious or inflammatory processes including

BOX 1 The Alcohol-Use Continuum

Low Risk Use, Including No Use
Consumption of alcohol below amounts identified as hazardous; and use in circumstances not defined as hazardous (context)
Example: One glass of wine with dinner several days per week

Hazardous Use
Alcohol use that increases the risk for health consequences

Hazardous Consumption
Females; males ≥65 years of age: >3 drinks/day and/or >7 drinks/week
Males <65 years of age: >4 drinks/day and/or >7 drinks/week

Hazardous Context
Example: Alcohol use during pregnancy

Harmful Use
Alcohol use with health consequences in the absence of addiction
Example: College student who sustains a forehead laceration secondary to falling down while intoxicated

Alcohol Use Disorder
Addiction to alcohol per the *Diagnostic and Statistical Manual of Mental Disorders (DSM-5-TR)*
- Mild: 2–3 criteria
- Moderate: 4–5 criteria
- Severe: ≥6 criteria

The shaded portion represents unhealthy alcohol use (UAU).

BOX 2 Two-Step Process for Screening for Unhealthy Alcohol Use (UAU) and Associated Management

Step 1: Single-Question Screener (SQS)
How many times in the past year have you had X or more drinks in a day?
where X = 4 for females and males ≥65 years of age; and X = 5 for males <65 years of age

Management
0 times: None/done (negative screen)
≥1 times: Proceed to Step 2

Step 2: Alcohol Use Disorders Identification Test (AUDIT)
Administer full-scale AUDIT (10 items) (https://auditscreen.org/check-your-drinking/)

Management
<8 points: None/done (negative screen)
8–15 points: Brief intervention
16–19 points: Brief intervention and continued monitoring
>19 points: Assess for Alcohol Use Disorder (AUD), initiate treatment if present

TABLE 1 U.S. Standard Drinks: By Definition, One Standard Drink Contains 14 Grams of Ethonol

BEVERAGE	ALCOHOL BY VOLUME	DRINK SIZE
Beer (regular)	5%	12 fl oz
Wine	12%	5 fl oz
Distilled spirits*	40%†	1.5 fl oz

*Examples include vodka, gin, whiskey, rum, and tequila
†80 proof
Data from U.S. Department of Agriculture and U.S. Department of Health and Human Services. Dietary Guidelines for Americans, 2020–2025 (9th ed). Washington, DC: U.S. Department of Agriculture, 2020, p. 49

period than was intended" and "recurrent alcohol use resulting in a failure to fulfill major role obligations at work, school, or home." Consumption (frequency and quantity), the defining features of hazardous use, has never been part of the construct.

Harmful use exists when alcohol-related harm has occurred but the "problematic pattern" and/or criterion threshold for AUD have not been satisfied.

Epidemiology

Large, population-based surveys have found that 17.1% to 24.4% of Americans binge drink, with considerable regional variability. This translates into healthcare settings. For example, a cross-sectional study of 2.7 million primary care patients determined that 6.1% exceeded recommended daily consumption limits (male: 8.7%; female: 3.8%).

A similar pattern exists for AUD. The third wave of the National Epidemiologic Survey on Alcohol and Related Conditions (NESARC-III), a cross-sectional survey of American adults, found that 13.9% and 29.1% of the population met criteria for AUD in the preceding year and on a lifetime basis, respectively. Coincidentally, the corresponding prevalence is 13.9% in primary care settings.

Diagnosis

In light of its prevalence and considerable harms, the USPSTF recommends "screening for UAU in primary care settings in adults 18 years or older, including pregnant women, and providing persons engaged in risky or hazardous drinking with brief behavioral counseling interventions to reduce unhealthy alcohol use."

Various screening instruments exist. The author prefers a two-step process beginning with a single-question screener (SQS)[a] to reduce the testing burden for both patients and clinicians (Box 2). Positive screens are then clarified with the AUDIT (https://bit.ly/3JjuVSA). Both instruments are in the public domain and may be used without formal permission or licensing.

Although patients with UAU can engage in malingering and deception, the reported sensitivity of the SQS ranges from 0.73 to 0.88. Its negative predictive value (NPV), which depends on prevalence, is 0.94 to 0.98 when 5% to 15% of those screened have UAU. Said differently, this corresponds to a 2% to 6% false-negative classification ("miss rate") at typical base rates in primary care.

Patients with significantly elevated AUDIT scores (>19 points) require careful assessment for AUD. This can be accomplished through structured clinical interviews ("checklists" based on *DSM-5-TR* criteria) or referral to a mental health professional for diagnostic assessment. Suggested checklists include the Structured Clinical Interview for DSM-5 Disorders (SCID-5-CV; Module E) and the Mini International Neuropsychiatric Interview (MINI; Module I).

Treatment

Management of UAU depends on patient classification (see Box 1). Most patients, including those with AUD, are appropriate for initial treatment in primary care settings.

Goals

Total abstinence from alcohol has traditionally been the treatment goal; however, this disease-oriented outcome is difficult to achieve and maintain in both clinical trials and "real-world" settings. The author prefers pragmatic, patient-oriented treatment goals ("progress not perfection") that are consistent with the trend toward non-abstinent recovery.[b] This is analogous to

[a]Also known as the NIAAA single-item question or one of the AUDIT-C (consumption) questions.
[b]Sometimes referred to as "harm reduction." The author considers the term confusing as all of medicine is ultimately harm reduction. Of greater concern, the term is potentially pejorative and can interfere with the therapeutic alliance.

other chronic diseases in which improvement is celebrated (e.g., reduction in hemoglobin A_{1c}), even if the ideal state has not been achieved.

For patients who meet *DSM-5-TR* criteria for AUD, a reduction in severity represents clinical progress, for example, when a patient who fulfilled seven criteria ("severe") at baseline now fulfills three criteria ("mild"). Remission is achieved when no criteria for AUD have been satisfied for at least 3 months, except for the criterion for craving. As noted previously, consumption is not part of the *DSM-5-TR* construct: abstinence is not required for remission.

Relapse is a nonclinical term that generally means that drinking has interrupted a period of continuous abstinence. The author suggests using more clinically accurate categories in the UAU spectrum.

Counseling

The USPSTF recommends behavioral counseling interventions for patients with UAU. This generally begins with simple advice about drink sizes, daily and weekly drinking limits, pacing and spacing, and avoiding and managing triggers. The NIAAA offers a variety of free patient materials to facilitate these discussions and serve as behavioral prescriptions (https://bit.ly/3Jb6mHh).

MI is a person-centered style of counseling that is used to address ambivalence about changing one's behaviors. Systematic reviews have consistently demonstrated its effectiveness for various alcohol-related outcomes, although a recent meta-analysis questioned its efficacy in maintaining abstinence in primary care settings. The method involves open questions, reflective listening, and other communication techniques (Box 3). The goal is to lead patients to recognize that their current choices and behaviors are ultimately inconsistent with their stated goals and values. This discrepancy, when recognized and felt, provides the psychic energy or motivation for the patient to change. Self-help books can provide structure and cadence for office visits and can serve as out-of-session "homework" between visits (https://amzn.to/3usxUD0).

Chain analysis helps patients recognize the many intermediate steps between a stimulus to drink alcohol and eventually consuming it. Patients can "break the chain" by developing and following action plans for each link in the chain. Patient worksheets can be used to analyze their behaviors and serve as tools that they can use in the community (https://bit.ly/38z4rPb, General Worksheet 2).

CBT helps patients recognize how their distorted (irrational) beliefs cause unhealthy negative emotions and behaviors, including drinking. Irrational beliefs take four general forms:
- Rigid demands: Must, should, ought
- Awfulizing: "It's awful … Terrible … End of the world"
- Frustration intolerance: "I can't stand it"
- Depreciation beliefs: "I'm no good," "She's no good," "It's no good"

For example, a patient may experience family conflicts or financial adversities. Frustration intolerance may lead them to use alcohol to numb, avoid, or chemically cope with the situation.

CBT helps patients transform their irrational beliefs into flexible preferences (e.g., "My financial situation is challenging, but I've had money problems before and can tolerate it). These new rational beliefs tend to reduce alcohol use. Patient worksheets (https://bit.ly/3i4QF8A) and inexpensive self-help books (https://bit.ly/35Y2zyD) can support these efforts.

Medications

Addiction pharmacotherapy, sometimes described as *medication-assisted treatment* (MAT),[c] is generally reserved for patients with AUD (Box 4). Disulfiram (Antabuse), which was approved by the U.S. Food and Drug Administration in 1951, has generally fallen into disuse secondary to lack of efficacy, medication interactions, and potential for various harms.

---

[c] The author prefers to describe addiction pharmacotherapy as *disease-modifying therapy* (DMT) because medications are often the primary or sole treatment for addiction, especially for other substance use disorders such as opioid addiction.

| BOX 3 | Motivational Interviewing |

The patient completed the SQS (positive) and AUDIT (score = 17) as part of a well-adult examination. This exchange demonstrates Open questions, Affirming, Reflecting and Summarizing (OARS), the core motivational interviewing skills.

Provider: Thanks for filling out that paperwork before our visit. [A]
Patient: No problem.

Provider: Would it be okay to discuss some of your answers?
Patient: Sure.

Provider: It looks like you're drinking alcohol on most days. [S]
Patient: Yeah, I have a few glasses of wine with dinner.

Provider: Seems like that might be a change from last year. [O]
Patient: Probably. Work has been stressful.

Provider: Say more. [O]
Patient: We're short-staffed, so I've been working a ton of hours. And customers have been tough to deal with—they want everything yesterday.

Provider: How do you think that's connected to wine? [O]
Patient: I'm pretty wound up after work. I guess wine helps me relax and chill out.

Provider: What else? [O]
Patient: Well, work is always on my mind. Wine takes that down a few notches. It also helps me sleep.

Provider: Work has been stressful, and alcohol helps you with tension and worry. [S]
Patient: Yeah; it calms me down.

Provider: And getting good sleep is important to you. [R]
Patient: Totally—I need energy and have to be mentally sharp for my job.

Provider: You're stuck in a vicious cycle at work, and alcohol helps you cope with that—so it's helpful from that standpoint. [R]
Patient: [Nods in agreement]
The patient's AUDIT score suggests alcohol-related problems. The provider might segue to problem items in the following way.

Provider: But it seems like alcohol might have some downsides, too. [S]
Patient: Maybe.

Naltrexone (ReVia [oral], Vivitrol [IM]) and acamprosate (Campral) both improve drinking outcomes, although with various nuances depending on trial design and type of data analysis. In placebo-controlled trials, acamprosate but not naltrexone increased abstinence, while naltrexone but not acamprosate reduced heavy drinking. Head-to-head trials found differences between the medications; however, they were ultimately equivalent when these data were subject to meta-analysis. Overall, the author selects one medication over the other based on patient preference and factors such as medication compliance and end-organ function.

The literature continues to evolve on the off-label use of medications including baclofen (Lioresal), gabapentin (Neurontin), and topiramate (Topamax). In the author's opinion, these should generally be prescribed in consultation with an addiction medicine specialist after patients have tried and failed adequate therapeutic trials of acamprosate and naltrexone despite robust psychosocial treatments.

Historically, medically managed withdrawal ("detoxication") has occurred in supervised settings. Reliable, carefully selected patients can safely be withdrawn on an ambulatory basis. The author uses the Short Alcohol Withdrawal Scale (SAWS), a patient self-rating scale, to trigger benzodiazepine administration.

BOX 4 Addiction Pharmacotherapy

Acamprosate
Brand name: Campral
Usual maintenance dosing: 666 mg by mouth three times per day
Mechanism of action: Postulated to be a gamma-amino butyric acid (GABA) agonist, glutamate antagonist, or both
Elimination: Excreted unchanged in urine
Adverse effects: Principally gastrointestinal, especially diarrhea
Prescribing pearls:

- Obtain baseline renal function test. Moderate impairment does not preclude therapy but requires monitoring. Do not use if eGFR <30 mL/min
- Initiate therapy at usual maintenance dose. Reduce dose to 666 mg two times per day for patients <60 kg. Reduce dose to 333 mg three times per day for eGFR 30–60 mL/min
- Gastrointestinal symptoms, if they develop, generally occur with initiation of treatment and are dose-related and transient. Consider temporary dose reduction (e.g., 333 mg three times per day for 7 days) for severe symptoms that threaten ongoing therapy
- Can be safely used with benzodiazepines and alcohol. May be started during medically managed withdrawal. Patients who resume drinking should be encouraged to continue taking acamprosate

Naltrexone
Brand names: ReVia (oral), Vivitrol (injectable)
Usual maintenance dosing: ReVia 50 mg by mouth daily; Vivitrol 380 mg intramuscularly every 4 weeks
Mechanism of action: Opioid antagonist
Elimination: Extensively metabolized by the liver, primarily excreted in urine

Adverse reactions: Opioid withdrawal syndrome, including precipitated withdrawal if opioid tolerant; hepatotoxicity; injection site reactions
Prescribing pearls:

- Patient must be opioid-free for ≥7 days before initiating therapy. Consider urine toxicology if abstinence cannot be reliably established by history
- Obtain baseline liver function tests. Alcohol-related transaminase elevations are common at baseline and should improve as alcohol consumption decreases. Do not use if transaminases are >5 times normal
- Obtain baseline renal function test. Moderate impairment does not preclude therapy but requires monitoring. Do not use if eGFR <30 mL/min
- Initiate oral therapy at 25 mg per day, titrating to usual maintenance dose over 7–14 days
- Mild opioid withdrawal symptoms, if they develop, generally occur with initiation of treatment, are dose-related and transient (they are likely caused by antagonism of endogenous opioids, e.g., endorphins). Consider temporary oral dose reduction (e.g., 12.5 mg per day for 7 days) for severe symptoms that threaten ongoing therapy
- Repeat liver function tests at 1 month and periodically thereafter
- Can be safely used with benzodiazepines and alcohol. May be started during medically managed withdrawal. Patients who resume drinking should be encouraged to continue taking naltrexone
- Always establish tolerability with the oral formulation before switching to injectable

Data from Center for Substance Abuse Treatment. Incorporating alcohol pharmacotherapies into medical practice. Treatment Improvement Protocol (TIP) Series 49. HHS Publication No. (SMA) 09-4380. Rockville, MD: Substance Abuse and Mental Health Services Administration, 2009.

Comorbidities

Other mental disorders frequently co-occur[d] with AUD and often precede its onset. In this context, AUD may represent a maladaptive coping mechanism for affective and anxious symptoms and for psychological trauma. Nascent evidence is mixed on treatment priorities and modalities. In the absence of firm guidance, management is empiric and should likely occur in consultation with local mental health experts.

Similarly, medical conditions such as chronic pain syndromes often co-occur with AUD and portend poorer drinking outcomes. Here, too, the literature is incipient, and management should occur in consultation with local experts (e.g., addiction medicine, pain medicine).

Uncertainties and Controversies

Alcoholic Anonymous (AA) formed in the 1930s and continues to play a central role in the recovery community. Its effectiveness has long been debated secondary to defects in trial design such as standardization of interventions, selection bias, blinding, and patient attrition. A recent systematic review focused primarily on manualized Twelve-Step Facilitation (TSF), a standardized, professionally delivered treatment that facilitates involvement in AA. It found that TSF improved complete abstinence compared with MI and CBT, and it was equivalent for six remaining outcomes such as drinking intensity and alcohol-related consequences. The certainty of evidence was variable and ranged from very low to high, depending on the outcome. None of the studies included a true control condition (e.g., wait list control) or compared TSF to addiction

pharmacotherapy. The author takes a "might help, can't hurt" posture but does not consider community-based (peer-led) AA a substitute for treatments for which there is stronger evidence.

The American Society of Addiction Medicine (ASAM) maintains a comprehensive guideline (The ASAM Criteria) for assessing patients and matching them to the most appropriate level of care (e.g., outpatient vs. residential treatment) based on their clinical characteristics (https://bit.ly/3joihWN). It first appeared in 1991 and is widely used by treatment providers and funders (health plans, government agencies). The framework represents expert opinion for which outcome data are sparse. Some have more bluntly noted that matching patients to treatment options based on expert opinion is little better than assigning patients by chance. The author considers The ASAM Criteria helpful for risk stratification but gives considerable weight to patient preferences in terms of treatment setting. A carefully supervised trial of office-based addiction treatment is reasonable if a patient is unwilling or unable to pursue a higher level of care, provided imminent danger[e] is absent.

---

[e]ASAM's doctrine of imminent danger consists of three components: (1) a strong probability that certain behaviors will occur; (2) the likelihood that such behaviors will present a significant risk of serious adverse consequences to the individual and/or others; and (3) the likelihood that such adverse events will occur in the very near future, within hours and days, rather than weeks or months.

---

[d]There is an old, ungrammatical saw in addiction medicine: "Which came first and which came worse?" Did generalized anxiety disorder (GAD), for example, develop first and then chemical coping and AUD followed? Or, did AUD develop first and anxious symptoms instead represent a substance-induced anxiety disorder? This is often difficult to establish by history and only becomes evident on a post hoc basis.

References

The ASAM Clinical Practice Guideline on Alcohol Withdrawal Management, *J Addict Med* 14(3S Suppl 1):1–72, 2020. PMID: 32511109.

American Psychiatric Association: *Diagnostic and statistical manual of mental disorders*, ed 5, text revision, Arlington, VA, 2022, American Psychiatric Association, p 553ff.

Gossip M, Keaney F, Stewart D, et al: A Short Alcohol Withdrawal Scale (SAWS): development and psychometric properties, *Addict Biol* 7(1):37–43, 2002.

Hall K, Gibbie T, Lubman DI: Motivational interviewing techniques—facilitating behaviour change in the general practice setting, *Aust Fam Physician* 41(9):660–667, 2012. PMID: 22962639.

Miller WR, Rollnick S: *Motivational interviewing*, ed 3, New York, 2013, Guilford Press, pp 62–73, p 25–36.

Saitz R: Unhealthy alcohol use, *N Engl J Med* 352(6):596–607, 2005. PMID: 15703424.

Saitz R, Miller SC, Fiellin DA, Rosenthal RN: Recommended use of terminology in addiction medicine, *J Addict Med* 15(1):3–7, 2021. PMID: 32482955.

Searight HR: Counseling patients in primary care: evidence-based strategies, *Am Fam Physician* 98(12):719–728, 2018. PMID: 30525356.

Sim MG, Wain T, Khong E: Influencing behaviour change in general practice. Part 1—brief intervention and motivational interviewing, *Aust Fam Physician* 38(11):885–888, 2009. PMID: 19893835.

Sim MG, Wain T, Khong E: Influencing behaviour change in general practice. Part 2—motivational interviewing approaches, *Aust Fam Physician* 38(12):986–989, 2009. PMID: 20369152.

Spithoff S, Kahan M: Primary care management of alcohol use disorder and at-risk drinking. Part 1: screening and assessment, *Can Fam Physician* 61(6):509–514, 2015. PMID: 26071154.

Spithoff S, Kahan M: Primary care management of alcohol use disorder and at-risk drinking. Part 2: counsel, prescribe, connect, *Can Fam Physician* 61(6):515–521, 2015. PMID: 26071155.

Stuart MR, Lieberman JA: *The fifteen minute hour: efficient and effective patient-centered consultation skills*, ed 6, Boca Raton, FL, 2019, CRC Press.

Tiglao SM, Meisenheimer ES, Oh RC: Alcohol withdrawal syndrome: outpatient management, *Am Fam Physician* 104(3):253–262, 2021. PMID: 34523874.

US Preventive Services Task Force: Screening and behavioral counseling interventions to reduce unhealthy alcohol use in adolescents and adults: US Preventive Services Task Force recommendation statement, *J Am Med Assoc* 320(18):1899–1909, 2018. PMID: 30422199.

AUTISM

Method of
Rachel Brown, MBBS

CURRENT DIAGNOSIS

- Autism spectrum disorder (ASD) is characterized by the presence of persistent deficits in social communication and social interaction as well as by restricted,repetitive patterns of behavior, interests, or activities
- Symptoms must be present in the early developmental period, cause clinically significant impairment in important areas of functioning, and not be better explained by intellectual disability or global developmental delay.
- ASD may co-occur with intellectual disability, language impairment, with another medical, genetic, environmental, neurodevelopmental, mental or behavioral disorder, or with catatonia.
- Patients with ASD require different levels of support.

CURRENT TREATMENT

- Early identification and intensive intervention is associated with improved outcomes.
- Intervention should start in early childhood and may need to be lifelong. It should focus on improving functional independence through structured education, supported employment and daily living, therapy focused on social skills and communication, and behavioral therapy, especially applied behavioral analysis (ABA).
- Ongoing surveillance and the management of co-occurring medical (sleep, constipation, etc.) and psychiatric (ADHD, anxiety, etc.) conditions is important.
- No biomedical agent reliably improves the core symptoms.
- Stimulants, guanfacine (Intuniv), and atomoxetine (Strattera) have shown benefit for co-occurring ADHD. Treatment of anxiety and depression should follow practice guidelines for those conditions. Antipsychotic agents, such as risperidone (Risperdal) and aripiprazole (Abilify), reduce symptomatic challenging behaviors. However, potential adverse effects include weight gain, sedation, and extrapyramidal symptoms.

Epidemiology

Older epidemiologic studies suggested that autism spectrum disorder (ASD) was a rare disorder, with a prevalence of only 4 in every 10,000 population. With time, estimates of prevalence have steadily increased, and current estimates are 0.6% to 0.7%, with some as high as 1% to 2%. The reasons for the increase are not completely known. Improved awareness of the disorder, especially in those less severely affected, and broader diagnostic criteria have played a significant role. However, a real increase in prevalence remains a possibility. Approximately 45% of individuals with ASD also have intellectual disability.

Studies have consistently shown that males with ASD outnumber females by a factor of at least 2–3 to 1. Older studies placed the male predominance even higher, and there is a suggestion that females have been historically under-recognized. Girls are diagnosed somewhat later in life, and studies suggest that more concurrent behavioral or cognitive problems need to be present in girls for the disorder to be recognized. Around a third of individuals with ASD have a pattern of regression (loss of previously acquired skill) occurring in the second year of life.

Risk Factors, Etiology, and Pathophysiology

The theory that ASD is the consequence of maternal mistreatment has been disproven, and there is no evidence that ASD is caused by vaccination. Both genetic and environmental factors probably play a role. Studies have consistently shown a familial pattern for ASD. Twin studies demonstrate a much higher concordance for monozygotic twins (between 80% and 90%), compared to dizygotic and other siblings, where the risk ranges from around 7% to as high as 20%. The data is somewhat complicated because of the recognition of a so-called "broader autism phenotype" that includes milder but qualitatively similar features to the defining features of autism. Some conditions with known genetic etiology are associated with high rates of ASD. Those include fragile X, Rett, tuberose sclerosis, Down, Angelman, and a variety of others. For the majority of patients with ASD, however, specific syndromes are not present, and the search for a single "autism gene" has been fruitless. Instead, a wide variety of genes are probably associated with ASD susceptibility. Many of the genes are related to transcriptional control, chromatin remodeling, protein synthesis and cellular metabolism, and synapse development and function. Although the estimated heritability of ASD is relatively high, environmental factors also play a part. Recognized risk factors include older maternal and paternal age, gestational hypertension and diabetes, prematurity, and maternal immune activation. Studies of the neurobiology of autism suggest that autism is associated with atypical neural connectivity, and is a problem of neural networks, rather than a structurally discrete abnormality. One commonly reported feature is generalized brain overgrowth in the first 2 years of life, manifested by a larger than average head circumference in a portion of patients with ASD. Studies have also shown some consistent neurologic abnormalities of both white and grey matter in a variety of brain regions, as well as evidence of cortical dysgenesis. Alterations in serotonin and γ-aminobutyric-acid (GABA) systems, as well as oxytocin, vasopressin, and androgens/estrogens are under active investigation. Information about the genetics and neurobiology of this condition are rapidly evolving. It is likely that, in time, ASD may be sub-classified into a number of related conditions, each of which may be diagnosed and treated differently, according to the underlying etiology.

Clinical Manifestations

For the diagnosis of ASD to be made, patients must have both persistent deficits in social communication and interaction as well as repetitive, restrictive behaviors emerging in early childhood (Table 1). Human beings, including children and young babies, are inherently social and interaction seeking. However, in patients with ASD, social approach and interaction is either absent or qualitatively abnormal. In some patients, the onset of abnormality important to screen for drug or alcohol withdrawal, as this can present with delirium.

Differential Diagnosis

Many other diseases may closely resemble delirium. Cognitive impairment and mood disorders may be confused with delirium, including dementia or depression. See Table 2 for a comparison of characteristics of these diseases. In the elderly and those with postoperative side effects, it is important to consider urinary and fecal retention. The Critical Illness, Brain Dysfunction and Survivorship (CIBS) Center website (http://www.icudelirium.org) has many mnemonics that can be useful when one is considering other circumstances that mimic delirium. One such mnemonic is "I WATCH DEATH."

Infection	Sepsis, urinary tract infection, pneumonia, HIV, SARS-CoV-2
Withdrawal	Alcohol, barbiturates, sedative-hypnotics, opiates
Acute metabolic	Acidosis, alkalosis, electrolyte disturbance, renal or hepatic failure
Trauma	Head injury, heat stroke, postoperative, burns
Cenral nervous system pathology	Abscess, hemorrhage, subdural hematoma, seizures, encephalitis, meningitis, stroke, tumors, hydrocephalus, syphilis
Hypoxia	Anemia, hypotension, respiratory failure, congestive heart failure, carbon monoxide poisoning
Deficiencies	Vitamin B12, folate, thiamine, niacin
Endocrinopathies	Hypo/hyperthyroid, hypo/hyperglycemia, hyperparathyroidism, adrenal disease
Acute vascular	Hypertensive emergency, pulmonary embolism, arrythmia, myocardial infarction
Toxins/drugs	Anticholinergics, benzodiazepines, alcohol, illicit drugs, pesticides, solvents
Heavy metals	Lead, mercury, manganese

Monitoring

Although many assessment tools exist, the Confusion Assessment Method (CAM) is the most effective screening tool, with a sensitivity of 94% to 100% and a specificity of 90% to 95%. Screening should be performed by a trained health professional and done at least once per shift in patients at moderate to high risk. One should routinely monitor for precipitating factors, including changes in medications, laboratory values, clinical symptoms, and physical examination findings.

Prevention

Prevention is the key to decreasing delirium incidence, hospital costs, and complications. Delirium may be preventable up to 40% of the time. Efforts should involve a multidisciplinary and multi-component approach. This includes early mobilization, cognitive reorientation activities using calendars and clocks, promotion of normal sleep-wake cycles using protocols that control light and noise stimuli, clustering of patient activities, and improving access to sensory equipment like glasses or hearing aids. Other key interventions include nutrition and fluid replacement, adequate pain management, and the prevention of constipation. Although antipsychotic medications should not be used for the prevention of delirium, home psychiatric medications should be restarted when possible so as to lower the risk for delirium.

Treatment

Treatment of delirium includes the identification and management of the underlying etiologies, assessment of risk factors, and review of the medication list. Delays to initiation of treatment may result in the prolongation of symptoms, the possibility of long-term cognitive impairment, and higher mortality. Treatment is primarily aimed at prevention utilizing the nonpharmacologic measures described earlier. The Hospital Elder Life Program (HELP) is a widely used evidence-based model that uses this approach and involves physicians, nurses, caregivers, family members, and patients. Research has shown that support of family and caregiver involvement can further increase the effectiveness of this model and can contribute to shorter length of hospitalization, reduced healthcare costs, and a decreased incidence of delirium. Pharmacologic therapies are used when nonpharmacologic strategies are not effective. There are currently no antipsychotic medications that are approved by the US Food and Drug Administration for the treatment of delirium. Antipsychotics should be reserved for patients in whom behavioral interventions have failed or are not possible or in those who have a potential for harm to themselves or others. Antipsychotic medications should be used at the lowest effective dose for the shortest possible duration. Haloperidol (Haldol)[1] is the antipsychotic medication used most often for delirium management; however, atypical antipsychotic medications have been shown to be as effective. Haloperidol, risperidone (Risperdal)[1], and quetiapine (Seroquel)[1]

---

[1]Not FDA approved for this indication.

TABLE 2	Differential Diagnosis of Delirium		
	DELIRIUM	**DEMENTIA**	**DEPRESSION**
Features	Confusion and inattention	Memory loss	Sadness, anhedonia
Onset	Acute	Insidious	Slow
Course	Fluctuating, worse at night	Chronic, progressive, stable over course of a day	Single episode or recurrent
Duration	Hours to months	Months to years	—
Consciousness	Altered	Normal	Normal
Attention	Impaired	Normal, except in late stages	May be impaired
Orientation	Fluctuates	Poor	Normal
Speech	Incoherent	Mild errors	Normal or slow
Thought	Disorganized	Impoverished	Normal
Illusions	Common (visual hallucinations)	Rare, except in late stages	Not usually
Psychomotor changes	Yes	No	Yes
Reversible	Usually	Rarely	Possibly

TABLE 3	Prevention and Treatment of Delirium
NONPHARMACOLOGIC	**PHARMACOLOGIC**
Identify underlying etiology	**Typical Antipsychotics**
Medication review	Haloperidol (Haldol)[1] 0.5–2.0 mg PO q4h or IM q30–60min prn; maximum dose 20 mg q24h
Early mobilization	**Atypical Antipsychotics**
Cognitive reorientation	Risperidone (Risperdal)[1] 0.25–2 mg PO qd–bid
Sensory enhancement	Quetiapine (Seroquel)[1] 25–200 mg PO bid
Pain management	Olanzapine (Zyprexa)[1] 2.5–10 mg PO qd
Cluster activities	Ziprasidone (Geodon)[1] 20–80 mg PO bid
Sleep-wake cycle enhancement	Aripiprazole (Abilify)[1] 10–30 mg PO qd
Family and caregiver support	**Benzodiazepines**
Nutritional and fluid replacement	Lorazepam (Ativan)[1] 0.5–1 mg orally q4h prn
Prevention of constipation	
Restart home psychiatric medications	
Routine use of the Confusion Assessment Method	

[1]Not FDA approved for this indication.

are considered the safest when used for delirium. Benzodiazepines should not be used for delirium unrelated to alcohol or benzodiazepine withdrawal. Nonopiate medications should be used initially to treat pain in patients diagnosed with delirium. If sedation is required in ICU patients with delirium, studies suggest the use of dexmedetomidine (Precedex) rather than benzodiazepines. See Table 3 for delirium prevention and treatment strategies.

Complications

Delirium is associated with significant long-term complications. Although cognitive impairment following a diagnosis of delirium may improve with time, lasting effects are possible. A longer duration of delirium in critically ill patients has been associated with worse long-term executive function and global cognition. The severity of lasting cognitive impairment has been compared to mild Alzheimer disease or moderate traumatic brain injury. Other complications include the development of mood disorders, loss of function in activities of daily living (ADLs), hospital readmission, longer duration of mechanical ventilation, and increased lengths of stay in the ICU and in hospital. Family members and caregivers may also experience stress in caring for their loved ones with cognitive impairment. Adverse effects of medications used in the treatment of delirium are also impactful and can include extrapyramidal symptoms, QT interval prolongation, insulin resistance, sedation, increased risk of falls, and hypotension. Mortality in patients suffering from delirium is as high as 37% during hospitalization, with a 10% increased risk of death per hospital day. Patients diagnosed with delirium are also up to three times more likely to die at 6 months after discharge. Mortality is greater in those with hypoactive delirium.

References

American Geriatric Society Abstracted Clinical Practice Guideline for Postoperative Delirium in Older Adults. *J Am Geriatr Soc* 63:142-150, 2015.
Critical Illness, Brain Dysfunction, and Survivorship (CIBS) Center. Available at http://www.icudelirium.org. Accessed January 22, 2020.
Delirium. In: American Psychiatric Association: *Diagnostic and Statistical Manual of Mental Disorders*, 5th ed, Arlington, VA, 2013, American Psychiatric Association, pp 596–602.
Downing LJ, Caprio TV, Lyness JM: Geriatric Psychiatry Review: Differential Diagnosis and Treatment of the 3 D's - Delirium, Dementia, and Depression, *Curr Psychiatry Rep* 15:365, 2013, Available at: https://doi.org/10.1007/s11920-013-0365-4, Accessed 27 April 2020.
Hospital Elder Life Program (HELP) for Prevention of Delirium. Available at http://www.hospitalelderlifeprogram.org. Accessed January 29, 2020.
Kalish VB, Gillham JE, Unwin BK: Delirium in older persons: Evaluation and management, *Am Fam Physician* 90(3):150–158, 2014.
Pandharipande PP, Girard TD, Jackson JC, et al: Long-term cognitive impairment after critical illness, *New Engl J Med* 369(14):1306–1316, 2013.
Salluh JIF, Wang H, Schneider EB, et al: Outcome of delirium in critically ill patients: systematic review and meta-analysis, *BMJ* 350:h2538, 2015, Available at: https://doi.org/10.1136/bmj.h2538, Accessed 29 January 2020.
Tyson B, Shahein A, Erdodi L, et al: Delirium as a presenting symptom of COVID-19. *Cogn Behav Neurol*, 1;35(2):123–129, 2022.
Wang YY, Yu JR, Xie DM, et al: Effect of the tailored, family-involved hospital elder life program on postoperative delirium and function in older adults, *JAMA Internal Medicine* 180(1):17–25, 2019.

DEPRESSIVE, BIPOLAR, AND RELATED MOOD DISORDERS

Method of
Alice M. Ing, MD, MA; and Andrei Novac, MD

CURRENT DIAGNOSIS

- Clinical evaluation of mood disorders starts with a thorough psychosocial and medical history.
- Identify symptoms and patterns of the appearance of mood changes.
- Differentiate between unipolar and bipolar symptom patterns.
- Use collateral history, if possible.
- For recent-onset disorder, rule out new medical disorders. Always check thyroid function.

CURRENT THERAPY

- Any underlying medical conditions must be treated simultaneously.
- The mainstay of treatment for all mood disorders remains the combination of pharmacology and psychotherapy.
- Monitor frequently for suicidality.
- Allow at least 2 to 4 weeks for response before a medication switch.
- Switch medication early in cases of intense side effects.
- Monitor for hypomanic switch on medications in undiagnosed bipolarity.

Introduction

Unipolar and bipolar mood disorders are part of a large group of psychiatric conditions referred to as *mood disorders* or *affective disorders*. They are among the medical conditions that are most commonly encountered in everyday clinical practice. Although current psychiatric texts classify mood disorders in two broad categories (unipolar and bipolar), the clinician must keep in mind that many mood disorders are mixed and manifest in many comorbid and atypical forms. Thus, mood disorders and related mood dysregulation encompass a broad range of human experiences: (1) psychiatric disorders, which are well defined and described in medical texts; (2) a variety of mood syndromes, often comorbid and less well classified and often undiagnosed, which coexist with medical and other psychiatric disorders alike; and (3) mood dysregulation, an aggregate of dispositional traits, at times

TABLE 5 Medications Used for the Treatment of Unipolar and Bipolar Depression

MEDICATION GROUP	MEDICATION	USUAL DAILY DOSE	CAUTIONS
SSRI	Fluoxetine (Prozac) Sertraline (Zoloft) Paroxetine (Paxil) Citalopram (Celexa) Escitalopram (Lexapro) Fluvoxamine (Luvox)[1]	10–80 mg 25–200 mg 5–60 mg 10–40 mg 5–20 mg 50–300 mg	All can cause sedation, agitation, insomnia, GI side effects, and sexual dysfunction
SSRIs with combined action	Vilazodone (Viibryd) Functions of SSRI and a 5-HT$_{1A}$ receptor agonist Vortioxetine (Trintellix) Functions of SSRI and multiple serotonin receptor agonists and antagonists	10–40 mg 5–20 mg	Same as above
SNRI	Venlafaxine XR (Effexor XR) Desvenlafaxine (Pristiq) Levomilnacipran ER (Fetzima)	37.5–225 mg 50–100 mg 40–120 mg	Insomnia, sedation, possible HTN, mydriasis, and urinary hesitation
Dopamine/norepinephrine agonist	Bupropion SR, XL (Wellbutrin SR, XL)	100–450 mg	Agitation, GI side effects, and possible HTN
Stimulants (usually used to enhance effects of other antidepressants)	Methylphenidate (Ritalin)[1] Dextroamphetamine (Dexedrine)[1] Amphetamine/dextroamphetamine mixed (Adderall)[1]	10–60 mg 5–60 mg 5–60 mg	Agitation, insomnia, psychosis, HTN, and seizures
Second-generation neuroleptics	Olanzapine (Zyprexa)[1] Quetiapine (Seroquel) Aripiprazole (Abilify) Risperidone (Risperdal)[1] Lurasidone (Latuda) mainly for bipolar disorder Cariprazine (Vraylar)[1]	2.5–20 mg (in unipolar depression, olanzapine 5 mg, plus fluoxetine 20 mg [Symbyax]) 50–300 mg (up to 800 mg in bipolar disorder) 2–30 mg 0.5–6 mg 20–120 mg 1.5–6 mg	Metabolic syndrome, sedation Oversedation, metabolic syndrome, and cardiovascular complications in older adults Oversedation, metabolic syndrome, and hyperprolactinemia Somnolence or agitation from akathisia and extrapyramidal symptoms
Tricyclic antidepressants	Amitriptyline (Elavil) Imipramine (Tofranil) Doxepin (Sinequan) Desipramine (Norpramin) Nortriptyline (Pamelor) Maprotiline (Ludiomil) Protriptyline (Vivactil)	50–300 mg 50–300 mg 50–300 mg 50–300 mg 20–200 mg[3] 100–225 mg 20–60 mg	All can cause anticholinergic effects and sedation; occasional agitation and weight gain
Mixed-action (presynaptic and postsynaptic, multiple neurotransmitter action)	Mirtazapine (Remeron) Trazodone (Desyrel) Clomipramine (Anafranil)[1]	15–30 mg 150–600 mg 50–300 mg[3]	Sedation, weight gain
MAOI (dietary restrictions are obligatory)	Phenelzine (Nardil) Tranylcypromine (Parnate)	15–90 mg 30–60 mg	Hypertensive crisis, occasional sedation/activation
Mood stabilizers	Lithium carbonate/citrate/ER[1] Valproate (valproic acid, Depakote ER)[1] Lamotrigine (Lamictal)/XR[1] Carbamazepine (Tegretol)*[1]	600–1800 mg (attaining blood level from 0.6 to 1.2 mEq/L) 250–1500 mg (attaining blood level from 50 to 100 mcg/mL) 50–400 mg 200–1000 mg (attaining blood level from 5 to 12 mg/mL)	Signs of toxicity: tremor, nausea, vomiting, and staggering gait; monitor kidney and thyroid function Oversedation, GI side effects, may affect blood levels of other medications, and weight gain A variety of severe skin rashes, Stevens-Johnson syndrome Monitor blood count for aplastic anemia/agranulocytosis, possible Stevens-Johnson syndrome, and sedation

[1]Not FDA approved for this indication.
[3]Exceeds dosage recommended by the manufacturer.
ER, Extended release; *GI*, gastrointestinal; *HTN*, hypertension; *MAOI*, monoamine oxidase inhibitor; *SNRI*, serotonin-norepinephrine reuptake inhibitor; *SSRI*, selective serotonin reuptake inhibitor.

declared. However, clinical judgment in assessing each circumstance, especially regarding suicide risk, is crucial. Often in the initial phase of response, the physical symptom of low energy remits first while cognitive symptoms of depression (persistent thoughts of death) persist. The coexistence of higher energy and thoughts of death may constitute a temporary suicide risk in the initial phase of antidepressant treatment. Currently, biological markers for the prediction of treatment response and side effects

TABLE 6	Biological Treatments for Medication-Resistant Mood Disorders		
TYPE OF INTERVENTION	**REPORTED RESPONSE**	**CURRENT AVAILABILITY**	
Electroconvulsive therapy (ECT)	50.9%–53.2% remission rate	Common	
Transcranial magnetic stimulation (TMS)	41.5%–56.4% response rate, 26.5%–28.7% remission rate	Accepted by several insurance plans	
Vagal nerve stimulation (VNS)	53% response rate, 33% remission rate after 1 year	Rare (neurosurgical)	
Deep brain stimulation (DBS)	29% response rate after 1 year	Rare (neurosurgical)	
Ketamine (Ketalar) infusion[1]	79% response rate	Very rare (only in selective institutions)	
Anterior cingulotomy	33.3% response rate after 30 months	Very rare (only in selective institutions, neurosurgical)	

[1]Not FDA approved for this indication.

are being considered. The Psychiatric EEG Evaluation Registry (PEER) uses quantitative EEG technology to compare variations of normal awake EEG readings with a large database of medication responders. Results are available for antidepressants, mood stabilizers, stimulants, second-generation antipsychotics, and so forth. The validity of PEER has been supported by a wealth of published literature; however, more recently the usefulness of PEER has been disputed. The AmpliChip CYP450 test (Roche Molecular Diagnostics, Alameda, CA) is a method that predicts side effects by measuring the activity of genes that control the cytochrome P450 hepatic enzyme system and, implicitly, the ability to metabolize a specific drug. Both methods are promising, but high cost and questions about large individual response variability have so far prevented general use.

Given the risk of suicide, close monitoring during the treatment of MDD is required. The choice of medication and adjustment must be tailored according to the most dominant initial presentation. For patients with severe insomnia, an SSRI is indicated. If the initial choice (e.g., citalopram [Celexa], escitalopram [Lexapro], or sertraline [Zoloft]) shows little impact in improving sleep, the temporary addition of a sleep aid is a reasonable choice. Alternatively, some clinicians prefer to avoid hypnotics, which may allow close monitoring of the natural improvement in sleep during the first 2 weeks of SSRI treatment. This in turn may predict a favorable response. In geriatric patients, long-term SSRI treatment has been found to delay progression from mild cognitive impairment to dementia. For many years, in patients with hypersomnia and hyperphagia—a variant known as *atypical depression*—the first choice was a monoamine oxidase inhibitor (MAOI). Currently, for atypical depression, clinicians prefer as a first choice a norepinephrine/serotonin reuptake inhibitor (venlafaxine [Effexor], desvenlafaxine [Pristiq]), or a norepinephrine/dopamine-active medication (bupropion [Wellbutrin]). Response to medications is often difficult to predict. Again, early in treatment, a thorough medical workup, which should always include a thyroid panel, should be the norm. Sometimes, switches to other classes of antidepressants (dopamine enhancers, tricyclics) are necessary before a result is obtained. Pharmacologic augmentation with mood stabilizers, neuroleptics, and thyroid hormone has been used in cases of treatment-resistant depression. In cases in which severe anxiety, insomnia, and poor appetite dominate the picture, the early addition of a second-generation neuroleptic (olanzapine [Zyprexa][1], quetiapine [Seroquel XR], risperidone [Risperdal][1], aripiprazole [Abilify], and, more recently, cariprazine [Vraylar][1]) is recommended (see Table 5). Medication resistance (after several failed trials) dictates the reassessment of diagnosis to further rule out psychiatric and medical comorbidity. Table 6 presents a list of further biological treatments for medication-resistant mood disorders. Some of these treatments are promising but have yet to be included as routine choices in some of the most difficult-to-treat patients.

[1]Not FDA approved for this indication.

Psychotherapy

For mood disorders, CBT, interpersonal therapy, and more recently, mindfulness-focused psychotherapy have been considered therapies of choice. CBT and mindfulness therapy directly address the negative, pessimistic bias of the depressive thinking, which is a maintenance factor of depressed mood. The latter addresses social and interpersonal functioning by enhancing coping abilities. Their popularity has been increasing; however, they require special training and supervision. In clinical practice, though, the most readily available therapies remain supportive and insight-oriented psychotherapy. They too complement the effect of pharmacology. Brain-imaging studies have revealed that the activity of the subgenual anterior cingulate cortex (Brodmann area 25) predicts the outcome of response to CBT in depression. As a general rule, therapies should have specific goals that must be discussed with patients at the onset of treatment. This must be part of an overall "informed consent" approach to treatment. Given the availability of a variety of clinicians with different levels of expertise that provide psychotherapy, it is important to monitor results and coordinate care. If "split" treatment (pharmacology and psychotherapy provided by different clinicians) is chosen, communication between parties of the treatment team remains a crucial requirement for rapid response and recovery. Other therapeutic measures, such as an increase in physical activity, normalization of sleep, and improvement of social support, are particularly important in promoting recovery.

Neurostimulation

TMS was approved by the U.S. Food and Drug Administration (FDA) in 2008. Over the past 2 years, the majority of insurance plans and Medicare have approved TMS treatment for MDD. It is the treatment modality approved by the FDA that has made the greatest strides in providing neuromodulation treatment for patients with MDD in over 1000 centers nationwide. Table 6 includes other neuromodulation treatments that must be considered when TMS remains ineffective.

Treatment of Bipolar Disorders (Bipolar Type I, Type II, Mixed Type, and Cyclothymia)

The treatment of bipolar disorder has been well refined over the years by a large body of literature. For acute mania, treatment with mood stabilizers and/or antipsychotics has remained the main approach for the past several decades. Severe forms of mania and psychosis usually require hospitalization. Table 7 indicates intervention options for different phases of bipolar disorder.

As indicated in the Table 7, some of the medication choices overlap between different clinical presentations. For chronic forms of bipolarity, such as mixed bipolar and cyclothymic disorder, a variety of new approaches has been developed, including social rhythm therapy. The latter includes monitoring and optimization of social interactions, sleep, and circadian rhythms that seem to benefit bipolar patients. Chronic bipolarity, with its significant impairment and suicide risk, remains a major problem, often requiring multidisciplinary consultations and referral to a tertiary institution. In treatment-resistant cases, employment of electroconvulsive therapy and other novel biological approaches can be lifesaving. Even with partial treatment response, maintenance is paramount. Lifelong maintenance treatment is likely to prevent suicide and further functional deterioration. More recently, suicide prevention both in chronic mood disorders and in personality disorders has been reported with maintenance treatment of lithium carbonate and clozapine (Clozaril).[1] Among bipolar patients, chronic depression is one of the most treatment-resistant conditions in psychiatry. In any patient with treatment-resistant, undiagnosed bipolar depression, the addition of mood stabilizers may result in the conversion of a treatment nonresponder to a responder. In addition, the value of treatment with lithium carbonate has been recently reiterated in a Finnish study. Lithium carbonate, besides an effective antimanic treatment, can prevent rehospitalization for bipolar disorder. One 2018 study revealed a significant response when 7000-lux bright white light was administered daily for 4 to 6 weeks in conjunction with mood stabilizers. The response rate was 68.2% compared with 22.2% in the placebo group. Among the treatment cases, no mood polarity switches occurred. This improvement occurs even in patients who are not diagnosed with SAD. Further replication of these findings may reveal bright light to be a new modality of treatment for bipolar depression, which is readily available and free from significant side effects.

Mood Dysregulation

Mood dysregulation is a broad phenomenon encountered both in clinical and nonclinical settings. For clinicians, a variety of difficult-to-classify syndromes remain relevant (referred to here as *mood syndrome variants*). These mood syndrome variants present anecdotal but clinically pertinent manifestations collected from the medical literature of the past century. Psychiatric and medical disorders often coexist with different degrees of mood dysregulation. Table 8 provides examples of mood syndrome variants with different degrees of mood dysregulation as encountered in the literature over the past century. A more detailed description of each clinical entity in Table 8 is beyond the scope of this chapter. As shown in Table 8, different forms of mood dysregulation can occur both within and outside the *DSM-V* diagnoses. For instance, atypical depression has been included in the *DSM-V*, whereas other syndromes, such as neurasthenia, remain unclassified. When encountered, any of the listed syndromes should raise suspicion of an underlying mood disorder. A diagnosis of *unspecified depressive disorder* (F32.9) can be made, and the entire mood disorder treatment armamentarium should be considered.

Clinical Course and Prognosis of Mood Disorders

Given the heterogeneity of mood disorders, there is great variation in clinical outcome. Clinical course and outcome depend on whether treatment is available, whether an individual is sensitive or resistant to the treatment, and the degree of compliance. Many individuals with mild and subsyndromal disorders remain undiagnosed, whereas others with severe forms of mood disorders refuse treatment. As a general rule, most untreated mood disorders tend to become chronic. Episodic disorders, such as bipolar I and II and depression, recurrent type, may show more frequent recurrences with advancement in age. Other patients with hyposymptomatic presentations and infrequent episodes may show long-term remissions. Such remissions are favored by stable, low-stress lifestyles. Dyslipidemia, hypertension, type 2 diabetes, coronary vascular disease, and stroke are among the numerous medical complications of chronic mood disorders. Some of these complications are direct side effects of long-term use of psychotropic medications, in particular second-generation antipsychotics. They all contribute to shortened life expectancy of individuals with mood disorders. Table 9 demonstrates the severe impact on life expectancy of bipolar disorder. Mortality comes from suicide, cardiovascular disease, and respiratory disorders. However, treatment can at least partially reverse these trends.

TABLE 7	Intervention Options for Phases of Bipolar Disorder	
PHASE OF DISORDER	**INTERVENTIONS**	
Acute	Hospitalization if necessary Antipsychotics, tranquilization, and start mood stabilizers	
Subacute	Antipsychotics/neuroleptics, mood stabilizers If already medicated, adjust dose	
Rapid cycling/mixed	As in acute phase; check thyroid; and medical workup Rule out substance abuse May require treatment indefinitely	
Cyclothymia	Mood stabilizers, long term, with or without antidepressants based on history Close initial monitoring May need treatment indefinitely	

TABLE 8	Examples of Mood Syndrome Variants with Different Degrees of Mood Dysregulation as Encountered in the Literature Over the Past Century		
I MSV WITH MANIFESTATIONS OF OTHER PSYCHIATRIC DISORDERS	**II MSV WITH UNUSUAL SYMPTOMS (MASKED DEPRESSION)**	**III MSV AS PART OF OTHER CONDITIONS**
Atypical depression Subaffective dysthymia Hysteroid dysphoria Pseudodementia Pseudoborderline Somatic depression Underground depression Neurasthenia Mood syndrome as part of personality disorders Mood syndromes and depression in schizophrenia	Mood dysregulation and thrill-seeking behavior (gambling, racing, substance abuse, hypersexuality) Reactive overeating Isolated sleep disturbance and mood dysregulation Atypical facial pain Dysphagia Monosymptomatic hypochondriasis Monosymptomatic delusions	Postpartum depression Depression secondary to chronic pain Substance- and medication-induced mood dysregulation* "Organic" mood disorders (due to central nervous system disorders) Vicarious traumatization†

*Medications more often associated with depression are, among others, reserpine, α-methyldopa (Aldomet), some α- and β-blockers, sedative hypnotics, cimetidine (Tagamet), indomethacin (Indocin), anticancer medications, oral contraceptives, and corticosteroids.
†It has been described as a form of secondary trauma in mental health professionals who treat victims of trauma.
MSV, Mood syndrome variant.
From Novac and Djenderedjian, unpublished data.

TABLE 9	Causes of Mortality in Patients With Bipolar Disease: Index Group Compared with the General Population		
CAUSE OF DEATH	OBSERVED DEATHS (% STUDY GROUP)	EXPECTED DEATHS (% REGISTRAR GENERAL'S FIGURES)*	MORTALITY RATIO (ACTUAL STUDY)
Suicide	15.7	0.67	23.4
Cardiovascular system	42.1	14	3.0
Respiratory system	33.3	1.08	30.8

*Edinburgh Registrar General's Office.
Data from Sharma R, Markar HR: Mortality in affective disorder. *J Affect Disord* 31(2):91–96, 1994.

Prevention

Primary prevention of mood disorders requires a concerted effort to educate the public and policymakers for funding of prevention. Depression Awareness Week and other community efforts enhance awareness and decrease stigma. Primary prevention may also include promoting general health and healthy work environments and addressing major social problems, including avoiding early trauma and family problems and preventing excessive stress and trauma in adults. These are all known to be associated with mental illness. Populations at risk must be identified in primary care settings. Secondary prevention requires the availability of mental health services, including early detection, education about the need for adequate treatment, and continuity of care to prevent impairment. Tertiary prevention would include the continuation of treatment to prevent comorbidity of other psychiatric disorders and catastrophic complications, including suicide. Finally, in the case of mood disorders, quaternary prevention would include long-term follow-up, monitoring of recurrences, and medical comorbidity (accidents; cardiovascular, respiratory, and other medical conditions) to avoid overburdening the healthcare system.

The high medical comorbidity rate recently found among patients with mood disorders varies by medical diagnosis and socioeconomic background. Chronic pain, neurologic conditions, gastrointestinal disorders, cardiovascular disorders, and metabolic syndrome are the most common medical conditions associated with mood disorders. Except for thyroid disorders, the seriousness of the comorbid condition seems to be even higher among patients of lower socioeconomic background. This poses a significant medical and socioeconomic burden of untreated mood disorders.

References

Amare AT, Schubert KO, Klingler-Hoffman M, et al: The genetic overlap between mood disorders and cardiometabolic diseases: A systematic review of genome wide and candidate gene studies, *Transl Psychiatry* 7, 2017, Available at: https://doi.org/10.1038/tp.2016.261.

American Psychiatric Association: *Diagnostic and Statistical Manual of Mental Disorders (DSM-5)*, ed 5, Washington, DC, 2013, American Psychiatric Publishing.

Bartels C, Wagner M, Wolfsgruber S, et al: Impact of SSRI therapy on risk of conversion from mild cognitive impairment to Alzheimer dementia in individuals with previous depression, *Am J Psychiatry* 175:232, 2018.

Binzer S: Multiple Sclerosis. Presented at European Committee for Treatment and Research in Multiple Sclerosis, *Abstract 99* 24(Suppl 2):41, 2018.

Cepeda MS, Stang P, Makadia R: Depression is associated with high levels of C-reactive protein and low levels of fractional exhaled nitric oxide: Results from the 2007-2012 National Health and Nutrition Examination Surveys, J Clin Psychiatry 77(12), 2016 December.

Connolly KR, Thase ME: If at first you don't succeed: A review of the evidence for antidepressant augmentation, combination and switching strategies, *Drugs* 71:43–64, 2011, Available at: https://doi.org/10.2165/11587620-000000000-00000.

Dobson KS, Dozois DJA, editors: *Risk Factors in Depression*, San Diego, CA, 2008, Academic Press (Elsevier).

Fogel J, Eaton WW, Ford DE: Minor depression as a predictor of the first onset of major depressive disorder over a 15-year follow-up, *Acta Psychiatr Scand* 113(1):36–43, 2006.

Frank E, Kupfer DJ, Thase ME, et al: Two-year outcomes for interpersonal and social rhythm therapy in individuals with bipolar I disorder, *Arch Gen Psychiatry* 62:996, 2005.

Griffiths R, Johnson M, Carducci M, et al: Psilocybin produces substantial and sustained decreases in depression and anxiety in patients with life-threatening cancer: A randomized double-blind trial, *J Psychopharmacol* 30(12):1181–1197, 2016.

Hasin DS, Sarvet AL, Meyers JL, et al: Epidemiology of adult DSM-5 major depressive disorder and its specifiers in the United States, *JAMA Psychiatry* 75(4):336–346, 2018, https://doi.org/10.1001/jamapsychiatry.2017.4602.

Iosifescu DV, Neborsky RJ, Valuck RJ: The use of the Psychiatric Electroencephalography Evaluation Registry (PEER) to personalize pharmacotherapy, *Neuropsychiatric Dis Treat* 12:2131–2142, 2016, Available at: https://doi.org/10.2147/NDT. S113712.

Janicakk PG. What's new in transcranial magnetic stimulation: Recent developments have enhanced the benefits of this treatment. *Current Psychiatry* 18(3):11-16.

Lahteenvulo M, Tanskanen A, Taipale H, et al: Real-world effectiveness of pharmacologic treatments for the prevention of rehospitalization in a Finnish nationwide cohort of patients with bipolar disorder, *JAMA Psychiatry* 75:347–355, 2018.

Lamers F, van Oppen P, Comijs HC, et al: Comorbidity patterns of anxiety and depressive disorders in a large cohort study: The Netherlands Study of Depression and Anxiety (NESDA), *J Clin Psychiatry* 72:341–348, 2011, Available at: https://doi.org/10.4088/JCP.10m06176blu.

Laursen TM, Musliner KL, Benros ME, et al: Mortality and life expectancy in persons with severe unipolar depression, *J Affect Disord* 193:203–207, 2016.

Merikangas KR, Akiskal HS, Angst J, et al: Lifetime and 12-month prevalence of bipolar spectrum disorder in the national comorbidity survey replication, *Arch Gen Psychiatry* 64:543–552, 2007, Available at: https://doi.org/10.1001/archpsyc.64.5.543.

Metcalf CA, Gold AK, Davis BJ, Sylvia LG, Battle CL: Mindfulness as an intervention for depression, *Psychiatric Annals* 49(1), 2019.

Comorbidity Survey-Replication National: *Appendix Tables: Table 1 and 2*. Available at: http://www.hcp.med.harvard.edu/ncs/publications.php, 2011.

Qato DM, Ozenberger K, Olfson M: Prevalence of prescription medications with depression as a potential adverse effect among adults in the United States, *JAMA* 319(22):2289–2298, 2018, https://doi.org/10.1001/jama.2018.6741.

Sachs GS, Dupuy JM, Wittmann CW: The pharmacologic treatment of bipolar disorder, *J Clin Psychiatry* 72:704–715, 2011.

Sharma R, Markar HR: Mortality in affective disorder, *J Affect Disord* 31:91–96, 1994.

Siegle GJ, Thompson WK, Collier A, et al: Toward clinically useful neuroimaging in depression treatment: Prognostic utility of subgenual cingulate activity for determining depression outcome in cognitive therapy across studies, scanners, and patient characteristics, *Arch Gen Psychiatry* 69:913–924, 2012, Available at: https://doi.org/10.1001/archgenpsychiatry.2012.65.

Sit DK, McGowan J, Wiltrout C, et al: Adjunctive bright light therapy for bipolar depression: A randomized double-blind placebo-controlled trial, *Am J Psychiatry* 175:131–139, 2018, https://doi.org/10.1176/appi.ajp.2017.16101200.

Smith D, Court H, McLean G, et al: Depression and multimorbidity in psychiatry and primary care, *J Clin Psychiatry* 75(11):1202–1208, 2014.

Tohen M, Frank E, Bowden CL, et al: The International Society for Bipolar Disorders (ISBD) Task Force report on the nomenclature of course and outcome in bipolar disorders, *Bipolar Disord* 11:453–473, 2009.

Weissman M: The psychological treatment of depression, *Arch Gen Psychiatry* 36:1261–1269, 1979.

DRUG USE DISORDERS

Method of
William M. Greene, MD; and Mark S. Gold, MD

CURRENT DIAGNOSIS

- Screen for substance use in all primary care and emergency settings.
- The clinical interview remains the mainstay of diagnosis.
- Clinicians should have a low threshold for ordering a urine drug test.
- Collateral information should be obtained from family or other sources.
- DSM-5 offers current diagnostic criteria for substance use disorders (Box 1).

CURRENT THERAPY

- Effective pharmacologic and psychosocial treatments exist.
- Formal detoxification is indicated for dangerous withdrawal states or in patients with serious medical comorbidity.
- Pharmacologic relapse prevention options are substance specific, and particularly useful options exist for nicotine and opioids.
- Psychosocial treatments remain the mainstay of substance treatment, and these range along a continuum of intensity from outpatient counseling to long-term residential treatment.
- Patients should be referred to self-help groups (e.g., Narcotics Anonymous) to complement other therapies.
- Indefinite remission is an attainable goal for many—a relapse does not constitute total failure but provides an opportunity to reevaluate the treatment approach.

Epidemiology

Widespread pathologic use of intoxicating substances, both legal and illegal, remains one of the greatest public health concerns facing our nation. According to the 2018 National Survey on Drug Use and Health, 53.2 million Americans (19.4% of the population) aged 12 years and older used an illicit drug within the preceding year. By order of frequency, these drugs included marijuana, prescription pain relievers, prescription sedatives, hallucinogens, cocaine, prescription stimulants, methamphetamine, and heroin. In addition, 58.8 million Americans (21.5%) aged 12 years and older used tobacco within the previous month, mostly in the form of cigarettes. Each year in the United States, approximately 480,000 people die of an illness attributable to cigarette smoking, making this the foremost cause of preventable death. Overdose deaths have remained a matter of pressing national concern in the United States; opioids were involved in 67.8% of the estimated 70,237 overdose deaths in 2017. Synthetic opioids such as fentanyl accounted for approximately 3000 deaths in 2013; in 2018, they accounted for over 30,000. US life expectancy increases ended in 2010 and started falling in 2014, with fatal overdoses playing a key role in this shift. They rose by almost 387% between 1999 and 2017. Overall, the estimated annual economic cost of tobacco, alcohol, and illicit drugs in the United States is a staggering $740 billion, including costs related to crime, lost work productivity, and health care.

From 1997 to 2019, the rate of past-month cigarette use among 12- to 17-year-olds has steadily dropped from 28.3% to 3.7%. The 2019 Monitoring the Future survey data confirm that cigarette smoking has continued to fall to the lowest rate in the survey's history (i.e., past month use among 12th graders is now at only 5.7%, compared with 36.5% in 1997). Encouraging though these trends may be, they are counterbalanced by the explosive growth of vaping. Among 12- to 17-year-olds, past-month vaping of nicotine has increased from 7.5% in 2017 to 18.1% in 2019. Similarly, past-month vaping of marijuana among 12- to 17-year-olds has increased from 3.6% in 2017 to 10.1% in 2019. Between 2011 and 2019, the number of 12th graders who reported having used any illicit drug at some point in their lives has been holding steady between 47% and 50%. Despite advances in our understanding and treatment of substance use disorders, drug use remains an epidemic, especially in the areas of drugged driving and drug use (including tobacco) in pregnancy.

Diagnosis

The fifth edition of the *Diagnostic and Statistical Manual of Mental Disorders* (DSM-5), published in 2013, eliminated the diagnostic categories of substance abuse and substance dependence. In the interest of consistency and clarity and based on large-population data, they were replaced by a new diagnostic entity: "substance use disorder" (Box 1). It is no longer necessary for the clinician to decide between two different diagnoses. Those familiar with

the terminology of DSM-IV will find the new criteria quite familiar, as they essentially represent a combination of the old abuse and dependence criteria with two notable exceptions: one, the legal problem has been eliminated; and two, a craving criterion has been added. When one is diagnosing a substance use disorder, the specific substance for which criteria are met must be listed. In addition, it is also important to document the severity of the disorder based on the number of symptoms present. Examples of specific diagnoses using the new nomenclature would be "alcohol use disorder, moderate" or "alprazolam use disorder, severe." This simpler evidence-based diagnostic schema should eliminate some of the confusion previously surrounding the term "dependence," which was often mistaken to be synonymous with "physiological dependence." It has long been understood, in the context of certain prescribed drugs, that the presence of tolerance and withdrawal is not pathologic in nature; rather, these represent an expected state of neuroadaptation. This fact is reflected in the new criteria for use disorders involving opioids, stimulants, and sedatives. For these three categories, the tolerance and withdrawal criteria are not considered to be met if present when the substance is taken solely under appropriate medical supervision. It should be noted this exception does not apply to cannabis, even if it is "prescribed."

Despite the importance and usefulness of the DSM-5, many patients (and clinicians) may still be left wondering if the problem at hand would appropriately be characterized as "addiction." In a 2011 public policy statement, the American Society of Addiction Medicine offered the following short definition of addiction, which has been well received:

Addiction is a primary, chronic disease of brain reward, motivation, memory and related circuitry. Dysfunction in these circuits leads to characteristic biological, psychological, social and spiritual manifestations. This is reflected in an individual pathologically pursuing reward and/or relief

TABLE 1 Pharmacotherapy for Nicotine Dependence

DRUG	MECHANISM OF ACTION	DOSAGE	INSTRUCTIONS	COMMENTS
Nicotine patch (Nicoderm CQ)	NRT	7 mg, 14 mg, 21 mg	1 patch daily	Tapering of doses recommended to discontinue
Nicotine gum (Nicorette)	NRT	2 mg, 4 mg	Chew slightly then "park" on oral mucosa	Tapering of doses recommended to discontinue
Nicotine lozenge (Commit)	NRT	2 mg, 4 mg	Absorbed through oral mucosa; minimize swallowing	Tapering of doses recommended to discontinue
Nicotine inhaler (Nicotrol Inhaler)	NRT	4 mg/cartridge	6–16 cartridges/day	By prescription only; tedious administration
Nicotine nasal spray (Nicotrol NS)	NRT	0.5-mg/spray	1–2 sprays in each nostril q1h; max 80 sprays/day	By prescription only
Bupropion HCl (Wellbutrin[1], Zyban)	Inhibits reuptake of NE and DA	150-mg SR tab, 300-mg XL tab	300 mg PO (divided qd [XL tab]-bid [SR tab]) daily for 7–12 weeks	Helps with comorbid depression; can help prevent weight gain
Varenicline (Chantix)	Partial agonist at $\alpha_4\beta_2$ nicotinic acetylcholine receptor	0.5 mg, 1 mg	0.5 mg PO qd for 3 days, then 0.5 mg PO bid for 4 days, then 1 mg PO bid for 11weeks	May smoke during first week; may continue for an additional 12 weeks
Nicotine vaccine (NicVAX)[5]	Antibody sequestration of nicotine	N/A	N/A	In clinical trials

DA, Dopamine; *max,* maximum; *N/A,* not applicable; *NE,* norepinephrine; *NRT,* nicotine replacement therapy; *SR,* sustained release; *XL,* extended release.
[1]Not FDA approved for this indication.
[5]Investigational drug in the United States.

by substance use and other behaviors. Addiction is characterized by inability to consistently abstain, impairment in behavioral control, craving, diminished recognition of significant problems with one's behaviors and interpersonal relationships, and a dysfunctional emotional response. Like other chronic diseases, addiction often involves cycles of relapse and remission. Without treatment or engagement in recovery activities, addiction is progressive and can result in disability or premature death.

Tobacco and Nicotine

Nicotine is the main addictive component in tobacco. It is administered via smoking (e.g., cigarettes, cigars, pipes, bidis, hookah) or in smokeless formulations (e.g., dip, snuff, snus, chew) and now also via vaporization (e.g. electronic cigarettes, vaping devices). Adverse health effects are not equivalent among the different routes of administration; cigarette smoking causes nicotine, affects brain monoamine oxidase (MAO), and other effects in the smoker, some resulting from the smoke and some from the nicotine.

Following administration, nicotine rapidly binds to nicotinic acetylcholine receptors in the central nervous system (CNS), where it acts as a mild psychostimulant and mood modulator in a nonimpairing yet profoundly addictive manner. When the user is tired, smoking has a stimulating effect. When the user is anxious or stressed, smoking exerts a calming effect. Smoking is like an injection without a needle and, given its short half-life, repeated self-administration serves to effectively relieve unpleasant withdrawal symptoms from the nicotine itself. Repeated use quickly leads to both physiologic and psychological dependence.

As with other drugs of abuse, cue-induced cravings play an important role in maintaining the addiction. For example, the smell of the smoke, the sound of a lighter, and the feel of a cigarette on the lips all contribute to an overall process addiction beyond just addiction to the nicotine itself. Tobacco use is also strongly associated with alcohol use, with which it has synergistic toxic effects.

Toxicities from tobacco use are well described and include severe pulmonary disease, cardiovascular disease, and carcinomas of the upper aerodigestive tract and of the bladder. Even second-hand smoke, previously considered harmless, is now correctly regarded as a serious health risk to the nonsmoker and a "drug" itself. Cigarette smoke contains more than nicotine (up to 4700 components, all of which affect the smoker). Additionally, secondhand tobacco exposure in utero can cause serious adverse health effects in the fetus.

Although quitting remains difficult for even the most motivated tobacco users, effective treatments for tobacco use disorder now exist. Clinical trials indicate that a combination of counseling and medications offers the best chance for success and should be offered to patients who are willing to make an attempt to quit. A wide range of nicotine replacement therapies that have been approved by the US Food and Drug Administration (FDA) are readily available and have similar rates of efficacy (Table 1). Patches (Nicoderm CQ), gums (Nicorette), and lozenges (Commit) are available over the counter, but the nasal spray (Nicotrol NS) and inhaler (Nicotrol Inhaler) are available by prescription only. Recently "electronic cigarettes" have gained in popularity, but unlike other nicotine products, they are not yet regulated as drugs by the FDA.

Nonnicotine prescription medications with proven efficacy are available. Bupropion HCl (Wellbutrin) is an antidepressant that was serendipitously noted to dramatically reduce nicotine cravings in some patients; it is now widely used for this purpose (as Zyban). Varenicline (Chantix) was specifically developed to treat tobacco use disorder and represents a considerable advancement, with improved smoking cessation rates. It acts as a partial agonist at the nicotine receptor and effectively serves to satisfy cravings while simultaneously blocking the effects of exogenously administered nicotine. Although probably the most effective agent, varenicline carries a significant risk of psychiatric side effects. The "nicotine vaccine" (NicVAX)[5], a novel approach, failed phase III clinical trials in 2011 and currently does not appear to hold much promise.

---

[5]Investigational drug in the United States.

Nicotine replacement, bupropion, and varenicline are all considered first-line pharmacotherapy. Bupropion but not varenicline may also be used in combination with nicotine replacement therapies. All pharmacotherapy options are enhanced with the coadministration of counseling or behavioral therapies. Helpful resources for patients interested in quitting include www.smokefree.gov (a government website dedicated to helping people quit smoking), 1-800-QUIT-NOW (a free phone-based services with coaches and educational materials), and a variety of resources available through the American Cancer Society and American Heart Association.

Cannabis

Cannabis (marijuana, pot, weed, grass, ganja, hash) remains the most used illicit drug in the world. As of 2018, 43.5 million Americans aged 12 or older have reported using marijuana during the preceding year (15.9% of the US population). Cannabis is readily harvested from *Cannabis sativa*; typically it is smoked, although it may also be ingested or vaporized. Despite a recent trend whereby states have legalized the use of marijuana for medicinal and recreational purposes, it is still listed as a Schedule I drug by the Drug Enforcement Agency (DEA), which implies a high potential for abuse and no currently accepted medical use. Delta-9-tetrahydrocannabinol (THC) is the active ingredient, which exerts its desired psychoactive effects at CB_1 receptors diffusely throughout the CNS. Marijuana's THC concentration has been steadily increasing as a result of the selective breeding of plants. Annual analysis of the DEA's record of seizures indicates that the average concentration of TCH increased from approximately 1% in 1975 to approximately 10% in 2008. To what extent this makes the drug more dangerous or more addictive remains unclear.

Acute psychoactive effects of cannabis include euphoria, relaxation, heightened sensations, increased appetite, distorted sense of time, slowed reaction time, illusions and hallucinations, paranoia, and anxiety. Acute somatic effects include conjunctival injection, xerostomia, increased heart rate and blood pressure, muscle relaxation, and reduced intraocular pressure. There is no known risk of dangerous overdose, and withdrawal symptoms are generally mild; however, they include irritability, cravings, diminished appetite, and insomnia. Cannabis is now recognized as unequivocally addictive. Users of this drug commonly develop tolerance and demonstrate loss of control and continued use despite negative consequences—the hallmarks of addiction. It is estimated that 1 million Americans sought treatment for cannabis as their primary drug of choice in 2010.

Not surprisingly, with more than 400 chemicals identified in its smoke, cannabis is dangerous with respect to long-term health. Chronic cannabis use is associated with lung cancer, chronic obstructive pulmonary disease, cardiovascular disease, impaired immunity, persistent disruption of memory and attention, and various psychiatric disorders, most commonly anxiety disorders and depressive disorders. There is a growing body of evidence that cannabis abuse can lead to lasting psychosis (i.e., schizophrenia) in predisposed persons.

Currently, treatment of cannabis use disorder remains entirely psychosocial. Various existing drugs (including fluoxetine [Prozac][1], lithium, and buspirone [Buspar][1]) have been investigated. However, well-controlled clinical trials to support their use are lacking. Preliminary data suggest that dronabinol (Marinol)[1] may be of some utility in relieving cravings and withdrawal symptoms without causing intoxication. Rimonabant (Acomplia)[2], a CB_1 antagonist previously prescribed for weight loss in Europe, showed promise but has failed to achieve FDA approval because of psychiatric side effects.

Cocaine, Methamphetamine, and Other Stimulants

As a class, cocaine and other stimulants work primarily by enhancing dopamine transmission in a dose-dependent fashion, either directly (amphetamines) or by blocking reuptake (cocaine). Cocaine and a variety of amphetamines (e.g., amphetamine/dextroamphetamine [Adderall], dextroamphetamine [Dexedrine], methamphetamine [Desoxyn], methylphenidate [Methylin, Ritalin]) are available for legitimate medical use as Schedule II drugs. Cocaine (in solution) is still used as a topical anesthetic, and amphetamine derivatives are used to treat attention-deficit/hyperactivity disorder (ADHD), narcolepsy, obesity, and binge-eating disorder[1], Any of these agents may be misused and all carry significant potential for addiction. Even newer "safer" agents such as modafinil (Provigil) and armodafinil (Nuvigil) are associated with use disorders, albeit less commonly than the traditional stimulants.

Prescription stimulant misuse can involve the ingestion of excessive doses to achieve a euphoric high or nonmedical use or diversion of prescriptions (e.g., students sharing medication to facilitate studying). When taken at prescribed doses for an appropriate condition, even methamphetamine is generally safe and effective. In contrast, when it is synthesized in clandestine laboratories and smoked or injected in extremely large quantities, methamphetamine (crystal meth, ice, crank, speed) is alarmingly dangerous. No other commonly abused drug is so strongly associated with permanent brain damage, resembling that seen in victims of traumatic brain injury. As ADHD becomes more recognized and treated, physicians must be aware of the potential for misuse of their well-intentioned prescriptions. To this end, several recent pharmacologic developments have introduced improved options for treatment. Extended-release formulations of methylphenidate (e.g., Concerta) and amphetamine/dextroamphetamine (Adderall XR) are considered to have less abuse potential than the short-acting formulations. Better still, the formulation of lisdexamfetamine (Vyvanse) includes the amino acid lysine coupled with the amphetamine molecule, consequently acting as a prodrug with the least abuse potential of all ADHD stimulants.

Cocaine and other stimulants induce sympathomimetic effects including tachycardia, hypertension, mydriasis, and diaphoresis. These drugs are commonly associated with seizures, myocardial infarction, hemorrhagic stroke, dyskinesias and dystonias, and psychosis when taken at the doses typically used to achieve euphoria. Withdrawal is generally experienced as a crash and includes fatigue, depressed mood, increased appetite, and cravings. Considered nonaddictive until about 1980, cocaine is now widely recognized as one of the most addictive drugs, particularly in the base form (crack or freebase). MDMA (methylenedioxymethamphetamine), or ecstasy, shares the pharmacodynamic properties of the stimulants combined with serotoninergic effects of the hallucinogens.

Currently no medication has demonstrated efficacy in treating cocaine or stimulant use disorders. Pharmacologic treatment remains symptomatic during the acute withdrawal phase. Stimulant-induced psychosis and mania respond well to traditional psychotropics when warranted; however, to date, no medications have reliably demonstrated efficacy in preventing relapse. A "cocaine vaccine,"[5] which enlists the immune system to develop antibodies rendering cocaine useless, has been studied in humans in a phase III trial that unfortunately has not been successful. In the meantime, traditional psychosocial treatments remain the mainstay of clinical care.

Opioids

Opioids are categorized as endogenous (endorphins, enkephalins, dynorphins), opium alkaloids (morphine, codeine), semisynthetic (heroin, oxycodone [Roxicodone, OxyContin]), or synthetic (methadone [Dolophine], fentanyl [Sublimaze, Duragesic]). The last three categories have a wide range of clinical uses including analgesia, anesthesia, antidiarrhea, cough suppression, detoxification, and maintenance therapy.

Opioids exert their clinical effect at mu, delta, and kappa opioid receptors. The effect on mu receptors is considered the most important, with its activation directly linked to both analgesic

---

[1]Not FDA approved for this indication.
[2]Not available in the United States.

[5]Investigational drug in the United States.

TABLE 2	Useful Medications in Treating Opioid Use Disorders				
DRUG	**UTILITY**	**FORMS**	**ADMINISTRATION**	**NOTES**
Naloxone (Narcan)	Overdose; additive to prevent abuse[1]	SC, IM, IV	0.4–2 mg q2–3 min prn	$T_{1/2}$ = 1 h; wears off quickly
Naltrexone (ReVia, Vivitrol)	Prevention of relapse	PO, IM	ReVia: 50–100 mg PO daily; Vivitrol: 380 mg IM q4wk	Potential for hepatotoxicity; precipitates withdrawal; useful for ETOH as well
Clonidine (Catapres, Catapres-TTS patch)[1]	Withdrawal	PO, transdermal	0.1–0.2 mg PO tid prn; 0.1–0.3 mg q24h transdermal via weekly patch	Monitor for hypotension
Methadone (Dolophine)	Withdrawal; maintenance	PO	Start 20–30 mg PO qd Target 80–120 mg PO qd	Restricted to methadone clinics
Buprenorphine (Subutex, Suboxone [with naloxone], Buprenex injection[1])	Withdrawal; maintenance	SL, IM, IV	Start 2–4 mg SL qd-bid Target 4–32 mg SL daily divided qd-tid	Requires special DEA certification

DEA, Drug Enforcement Administration; *ETOH,* ethanol.
[1]Not FDA approved for this indication.

and euphoric effects. Most humans subjectively experience opioids with a neutral to aversive response. However, when used in sufficient quantities by genetically vulnerable persons, some users experience energy, relief of emotional pain, and a euphoria many describe as a "total body orgasm." Intoxication manifests with miosis, impaired consciousness, slurred speech, bradycardia, and depressed respiration. Overdose is potentially fatal via respiratory depression, but it is quite amenable to treatment with repeated doses of naloxone (Narcan). The withdrawal syndrome is characterized by a constellation of miserable but not life-threatening symptoms including mydriasis, piloerection, muscle cramps, diaphoresis, vomiting, lacrimation, rhinorrhea, chills, insomnia, cravings, and autonomic hyperactivity.

Since pain was recognized as "the fifth vital sign" in the 1990s, concurrent with heavy marketing campaigns from pharmaceutical companies, the United States experienced a veritable explosion of widespread opioid prescribing for nonmalignant pain. An industry of pain management developed, with the unfortunate side effect of having a sizable proportion of its output being used nonmedically. It is important for prescribers to recognize that the abuse potential of prescription opioids matches—or in some cases even exceeds—that of heroin. Today, oxycodone has a street value of approximately $1.00 per milligram.

The most common method of misuse involves simply taking more than prescribed, usually by the appropriate route of administration. Alternatively, individuals with opioid use disorders commonly take their medications via nasal insufflation or inject them intravenously. The extended-release property of certain medications, such as oxycodone (OxyContin), can easily be circumvented by crushing the pills, which greatly enhances the euphoric effect. Even transdermal fentanyl patches (Duragesic) can be misused by any number of methods, such as applying heat to a worn patch, employing complex extraction techniques described online, or simply sucking on the patch itself. If the prescription is used up before its renewal date, the user must either supplement the supply or face the unpleasant effects of withdrawal.

There is no shortage of methods to obtain opioids illicitly. These include seeing multiple prescribers (doctor shopping), purchasing online at foreign "pharmacies," and general trade or purchase on the black market. Also alarming is the growing problem of diversion from hospitals and pharmacies by health care professionals, who are not immune to the disease of addiction. Almost all states have now implemented controlled substance databases (i.e., prescription drug monitoring programs [PDMPs]) aimed at curbing the problem of use disorders involving opioids and other prescription drugs.

Acute detoxification from opioids is achieved by one of two basic strategies: symptomatic treatment with unrelated medications or substitution with a cross-tolerant (opioid) drug with less potential for abuse (Table 2). The first strategy may employ the use of clonidine (Catapres)[1], an α_2-adrenergic agonist, to help with the autonomic component of withdrawal. This is commonly done in combination with other symptomatic treatments on an as-needed basis, using agents such as diazepam (Valium) for anxiety, loperamide (Imodium) for diarrhea, and promethazine (Phenergan)[1] or ondansetron (Zofran)[1] for nausea.

The second strategy typically involves either methadone or buprenorphine (Subutex, with naloxone [Suboxone]). Methadone, a pure mu agonist with a half-life of about 36 hours, is usually started in the 20- to 30-mg range and titrated cautiously by 10 mg every 4 to 7 days. Maintenance therapy with methadone occurs only in the setting of a highly regulated methadone clinic. Buprenorphine, a partial agonist (and kappa antagonist) at the mu receptor, is administered sublingually and has a half-life similar to that of methadone. It was approved in 2002 for office-based treatment of opioid addiction, making pharmacotherapy much more widely available. Caution should be used to avoid administering buprenorphine too soon (before the onset of withdrawal syndrome); otherwise acute withdrawal can actually be precipitated. Buprenorphine is available either alone or in combination with naloxone (Suboxone, Zubsolv, Bunavail). Here, the role of naloxone is primarily to deter intravenous use, because naloxone has negligible bioavailability when taken sublingually as prescribed. The FDA has recently approved longer-acting formulations of buprenorphine, including a monthly subcutaneous injection (Sublocade) and a 6-month subdermal implant (Probuphine). These hold promise and give patients more options.

Buprenorphine and methadone are useful in managing acute withdrawal as well as in long-term (months to years) maintenance therapy for preventing relapse to heroin or the opioid of choice. As maintenance therapy, these agents serve to block euphoria, satisfy cravings, and reduce illicit use, with consequent verifiable harm reduction. Buprenorphine, with a built-in ceiling effect because of its unique pharmacology, is much safer than methadone, which is often fatal in overdose. Recent evidence supports the benefit of continuing long-term maintenance therapy indefinitely, as discontinuation is often associated with relapse and other adverse outcomes. Buprenorphine is increasingly being initiated in emergency department settings, and this trend is associated with improved patient outcomes. Increasingly, buprenorphine is being used as an analgesic as well (Butrans Transdermal Patch), and it may be the ideal choice in patients with comorbid pain and addiction who have demonstrated an inability to use other opioids safely.

Also approved for the prevention of opioid relapse is naltrexone, an opioid antagonist, which is available in oral (ReVia) and intramuscular depot formulations (Vivitrol).

---

[1]Not FDA approved for this indication.

TABLE 3	Common Sedative-Hypnotics, Equivalent Dose Conversions	
GENERIC NAME	**TRADE NAME**	**DOSE (mg)**
Benzodiazepines		
Diazepam	Valium	10
Alprazolam	Xanax, Niravam	0.5–1
Lorazepam	Ativan	2
Clonazepam	Klonopin	1–2
Chlordiazepoxide	Librium	25
Clorazepate	Tranxene	7.5
Oxazepam	Serax	10–15
Temazepam	Restoril	15
Triazolam	Halcion	0.25
Flurazepam	Dalmane	15
Barbiturates		
Phenobarbital	N/A	30
Pentobarbital	Nembutal	100
Secobarbital	Seconal	100
Butalbital (with caffeine and aspirin or acetaminophen)	Fiorinal, Fioricet	100
Amobarbital	Amytal	100
Related compounds		
Carisoprodol	Soma	700
Meprobamate	Miltown, Equanil	1200
Chloral hydrate	Noctec	500
Methaqualone[2]	Quaalude	300
Ethchlorvynol[2]	Placidyl	500
Zolpidem	Ambien	20
Zaleplon	Sonata	20
Eszopiclone	Lunesta	3

N/A, Not applicable.
[2]Not available in the United States.

Sedative-Hypnotics

This class of drugs includes a wide array of compounds (benzodiazepines, barbiturates, and various related compounds) (Table 3), most of which have at least some potential for abuse. Overall, these medications do much more good than harm and are useful in treating anxiety disorders, insomnia, seizures, and muscle spasms. They are also important in managing withdrawal states and as a component of surgical anesthesia. These drugs act as CNS depressants, and their primary mechanism of action is to enhance inhibitory GABA neurotransmission. The risk of toxicity is by respiratory depression, which is magnified by concomitant use of opioids or other CNS depressants, such as alcohol.

Sedative-hypnotic intoxication and withdrawal states closely resemble those of alcohol except for the more protracted time course of withdrawal. Anxiety, restlessness, insomnia, tremor, nystagmus, tachycardia, and hypertension usually appear 2 to 12 hours after the last dose, and symptoms gradually resolve over 1 to 2 weeks. Withdrawal seizures, psychosis, and delirium are fairly common. Detoxification is best accomplished on an inpatient basis and typically involves tapering doses of a long-acting benzodiazepine (e.g., clonazepam [Klonopin], diazepam, clorazepate [Tranxene]) at a rate of about 10% of the initial daily requirement per day. Acute sedative overdose is managed primarily with supportive care and airway management. Flumazenil (Romazicon) 0.2 to 0.5 mg/min IV may be used for acute benzodiazepine overdose, but only with caution because it can precipitate severe acute withdrawal symptoms.

Since their introduction in the 1960s, benzodiazepines, given their enhanced safety profile, have largely replaced barbiturates. However, barbiturates still in common use include phenobarbital and butalbital. Phenobarbital, used mainly for treating seizures, is considered to have a low potential for abuse. Butalbital, compounded with caffeine plus acetaminophen or aspirin (Fioricet, Fiorinal), has moderate abuse potential, typically in combination with other drugs. Carisoprodol (Soma), though not a barbiturate, is metabolized into meprobamate, a barbiturate-like drug. Commonly taken in combination with opioids and other sedatives, carisoprodol is highly abused.

Alprazolam (Xanax) stands out among its peers as the single most abused, most addictive, and yet currently most prescribed sedative-hypnotic. Its rapid onset (T_{max} 1 to 2 hours) and relatively short half-life (6 to 14 hours) contribute to its abuse liability and propensity for withdrawal seizures. Diazepam, historically the most prescribed sedative, also has a relatively rapid onset and significant addictive potential, but its long half-life makes it an ideal agent for use in treating withdrawal from other sedatives. Flunitrazepam (Rohypnol, "roofies") is a benzodiazepine that causes anterograde amnesia. It is now illegal in the United States because of its use in drug-facilitated sexual assaults.

γ-Hydroxybutyric acid (GHB) and baclofen (Lioresal) also act as GABAergic CNS depressants, with intoxication and withdrawal states consistent with the class. Oddly, GHB is considered a Schedule I drug with high abuse potential and no accepted medical use, but when marketed as sodium oxybate (Xyrem), GHB is available as a Schedule III drug (with special restrictions) for use in treating narcolepsy. Baclofen, on the other hand, appears to have rather low addictive potential and may actually play a role in the treatment of alcoholism.[1]

Relatively new drugs—such as zolpidem (Ambien), zaleplon (Sonata), and eszopiclone (Lunesta)—are benzodiazepine-like drugs with CNS depressant activity; they are approved for the short-term treatment of insomnia and have at least some potential for abuse and dependence. Clonazepam (Klonopin) is generally considered to have the lowest potential for euphoria and addiction and is thus the agent of choice if a benzodiazepine must be given to patients with a relative contraindication, such as a history of any drug use disorder.

Conclusion

Despite intensive supply-reduction strategies, improved primary prevention efforts, and the many recent pharmacotherapy advances, drug use disorders remain largely unchanged in their overall scale with the notable exceptions of the increased use of dangerous opioids and increased vaping of nicotine and cannabis. Another notable exception is the significant reduction in tobacco use since the turn of the century. It is estimated that 25% of patients seen in office settings and 50% of those seen in emergency departments have active problems related to substance use. All patients in primary care settings must be screened for tobacco, alcohol, and illicit drug use. Patients should be asked directly about substance use at the initial point of contact (e.g., emergency departments, primary care offices), and clinicians should maintain a healthy degree of skepticism toward patients' responses, remembering that many patients minimize substance use. When any suspicion exists, urine drug screens should be readily utilized without hesitation or fear of communicating mistrust. A variety of affordable quick screen kits are available, which can be sent out for laboratory confirmation of positive results if necessary.

Physicians and other health care professionals are in a unique position to intervene with drug use disorders at the individual level because these disorders are commonly encountered in clinical practice. The problem must first be identified and, depending on the skill set of the primary provider, patients should be treated

[1]Not FDA approved for this indication.

episodes occur at a mini
3-month period. Binge
feelings of guilt and emb
hide eating. Furthermor
rapid and results in feel
with BED have at least
of respondents in one st

Epidemiology
Lifetime prevalence of B
in two separate studies
rates across ethnic and
later adolescence or ea
children and is often as
well as psychological s
sity, an estimated 1%
experience BE/loss of c
dates dieting and subse
onset of both dieting a
than in other eating di
similar to BN.

Etiology
The etiology of BED is
dissatisfaction, pressur
symptoms, and limite
onset of adolescent BE
there may be a genetic
.39 and .45. Potential
Kleine-Levin syndrome
drome, and gastrointe
be ruled out during as
are common among a
anxiety disorders, and
ders and personality
among individuals wit
linked to the severity

Treatment
Treatment for adults
tion in RCTs compa
Most treatments targe
and weight loss for th
BMI categories. CBT
GSH, CD-ROM deliv
and appears to have
CBT outperformed g
was more effective ii
(BWL). CBT target
behaviors that main
personal psychothera
therapy targeting int
order. IPT is helpful
and motivational int
cognitive restraint, d
thought to maintain

DBT is another tre
geting affected regula
ing mechanism of B
DBT to a waitlist
BE and related eating
half abstinent from
supportive psychoth
more quickly in the
at follow-up. Pilot
group, and skills coz

Pharmacologic tr
been tested alone an
may be improvemer
therapy. The combi

---

or referred appropriately. There is an initiative to incorporate formal SBIRT (screening, brief intervention, and referral to treatment) into routine clinical practice. Current procedural terminology (CPT) codes and a reimbursement schedule for screening and brief intervention may be located online at https://www.samhsa.gov/sbirt/coding-reimbursement. Screening may involve the written or verbal assessment of substance use to determine whether the patient exhibits a problematic level of use. The brief intervention aspect of SBIRT targets those with milder substance use disorders and provides effective strategies for intervention before the need for more extensive or specialized treatment arises. Referral to specialized treatment is recommended for patients with moderate-to-severe substance use disorders. Data suggest that this approach can be successful in modifying problematic substance use behavior. In addition to formal treatment, physician referral to local 12-step recovery programs (Alcoholics Anonymous, Narcotics Anonymous) has proved beneficial. Ample scientific evidence supports the effectiveness of these programs. Local chapters readily provide physicians with the names and telephone numbers of members willing to welcome newcomers (www.aa.org; na.org).

Physicians are usually well equipped to treat the sequelae of drug use disorders, but they often forget that addiction itself is a treatable disease entity. Treatment ranges in intensity along a continuum that includes medically managed inpatient detoxification, partial hospitalization, intensive outpatient treatment, and outpatient care. The American Society of Addiction Medicine provides patient placement criteria that dictate the appropriate level of treatment based on a multidimensional assessment. Health care professionals should be familiar with the treatment centers in their area; these can place the patient in the appropriate level of care.

It is important to remember that relapse is a characteristic of addiction and does not equate to treatment failure but rather indicates a need for an adjustment in the level of treatment or that of monitoring. Other chronic diseases, such as diabetes and hypertension, necessitate ongoing monitoring and adjustment of treatment interventions as needed, and the same is true of addiction. Recently published data on the treatment and monitoring of recovering physicians (a subgroup of addicts that boasts a 5-year success rate >78%) teach us the lesson that adequate initial treatment coupled with ongoing monitoring is critical. Sustained recovery from a substance use disorder is readily attainable and is characterized by voluntary sobriety, improved personal health, and improved citizenship.

References
American Psychiatric Association: *Diagnostic and Statistical Manual of Mental Disorders*, 5th ed., Washington, DC, 2013, American Psychiatric Publishing.
American Society of Addiction Medicine: Public policy statement: Definition of addiction. August 15, Available at http://www.asam.org/docs/publicy-policy-statements/1definition_of_addiction_long_4-11.pdf, 2011.
Bailey JA, Hurley RW, Gold MS: Crossroads of pain and addiction, *Pain Med* 11:1803–1818, 2010.
DuPont RL, McLellan AT, White WL, et al: Setting the standard for recovery: physicians health programs, *J Subst Abuse Treat* 36:159–171, 2009.
Gold MS, Kobeissy FH, Wang KK, et al: Methamphetamine- and trauma-induced brain injuries: comparative cellular and molecular neurobiological substrates, *Biol Psychiatry* 66:118–127, 2009.
Johnston LD, Miech RA, O'Malley PM, et al: *Monitoring the Future national survey results on drug use 1975-2019: Overview, key findings on adolescent drug use,* Ann Arbor, 2020, Institute for Social Research, University of Michigan.
Kelly JF, Humphreys K, Ferri M: Alcoholics Anonymous and other 12–step programs for alcohol use disorder, *Cochrane Database Syst Rev* (Issue 3):Art. No.: CD012880 2020. https://doi.org/10.1002/14651858.CD012880.pub2.
Office of National Drug Control Policy: *The Economic Costs of Drug Abuse in the United States: 1992–2002,* Washington, DC, 2004, Executive Office of the President, [Publication No. 207303].
Pardo B, Taylor J, Caulkins J P, et al: *The Future of Fentanyl and Other Synthetic Opioids,* Santa Monica, CA, 2019, RAND Corporation, Also available in print form https://www.rand.org/pubs/research_reports/RR3117.html.
Scholl L, Seth P, Kariisa M, et al: Drug and opioid-involved overdose deaths — United States, 2013–2017, *MMWR Morb Mortal Wkly Rep* 67:1419–1427, 2019, https://doi.org/10.15585/mmwr.mm675152e1.
Substance Abuse and Mental Health Services Administration: *Key substance use and mental health indicators in the United States: Results from the 2018 National Survey on Drug Use and Health (HHS Publication No. PEP19-5068, NSDUH Series H-54),* Rockville, MD, 2019, Center for Behavioral Health Statistics and Quality, Substance Abuse and Mental Health Services Administration. Retrieved from https://www.samhsa.gov/data/.

EATING DISORDERS

Method of
Nandini Datta, PhD; and James Lock, MD, PhD

Bulimia Nervosa

CURRENT DIAGNOSIS

- Binge-eating episodes occur at least once per week for 3 months (eating objectively large quantities of food in a discrete period of time accompanied by a loss of control while eating).
- Compensatory purging episodes occur at least once per week for a period of 3 months (e.g., self-induced vomiting, laxatives, diuretics, excessive and compulsive exercise, enemas) to prevent weight gain.
- Shape and weight are overvalued and impact self-worth and self-esteem.
- Weight is at or above expected range given age, height, and historical growth curves.

CURRENT TREATMENT

- Cognitive behavioral therapy (CBT) is the most evidence-based treatment for bulimia nervosa (BN).
- Interpersonal psychotherapy (IPT) is an appropriate alternative.
- Family-based treatment (FBT) is useful for adolescents with BN.
- Antidepressant treatment (selective serotonin reuptake inhibitors [SSRIs]) may be useful in augmenting psychotherapy or as an alternative in the event that psychotherapy is not effective, refused, or unavailable. It is not as effective as CBT and thus not a front-line approach.

Diagnosis
To diagnose bulimia nervosa (BN), an individual must engage in recurrent binge episodes with compensatory behaviors (e.g., self-induced vomiting, diuretic or laxative use, excessive and compulsive exercise). A binge is a discrete episode of eating a quantity of food that is more than the average person would eat in the same setting, accompanied by a loss of control or feeling as though one cannot stop eating. Nonpurging forms of bulimia occur when an individual uses extreme dietary restriction/fasting and/or exercise as a means of compensating for binge episodes. A disproportionate emphasis on weight and shape in one's self-evaluation is also required in diagnosing BN. DSM-5 criteria require that these episodes occur at a minimum of once weekly for 3 months. Unlike individuals with anorexia nervosa (AN), who may binge and purge, individuals with BN are within range of or above the median body mass index (BMI).

Significant health consequences may accompany BN. Laboratory studies often reveal electrolyte abnormalities, which can lead to cardiac arrhythmias and cardiac arrest in severe cases. Physical examination may detect enamel decay and parotid gland enlargement as a consequence of recurrent vomiting. When ipecac[1] is used to induce vomiting, severe cardiac and skeletal myopathies may develop. Laxative abuse is associated with metabolic acidosis and elevated serum amylase levels. BN has an elevated risk for mortality (crude mortality of 3.9%–6% in an inpatient sample), with many dying by suicide. Most common comorbid psychiatric

diagnoses are r
borderline perso

Epidemiology
BN behaviors t
14–16), with c
and early adult
mate of DSM-5
known about n
for between 10
number of years
of existing treat
patients fully re
remaining 23%

Etiology
BN can be exp
psychological, a
BN aggregates i
ance in heritabi
levels may be re
tonergic circuit
of cultural idea
for women, wh
lar with low bo
appearance are
may increase ri
mon precipitan
teasing. Person
include perfecti
relationships. C
risk for BN.

Treatment
Given the signifi
associated with
ranging difficul
trials (RCTs) e
adolescents. M
medications, or
treatment of ch
a large number
that bulimic bel
about shape, w
lead to an overe
sive dieting typi
logical deprivat
Feelings of guilt
engaging in pu
the use of self-n
behaviors, thou
CBT is found
cebo, nondirecti
ing, stress mana
Response to CB
20% with signi
ment. CBT is a
a more recent R
previous rates c
help (GSH) ver
alternative inter
demonstrates a
symptoms at th
ences appear to
while less effici
for BN to target
development an
studied with ad
More recently
taining features
difficulties, clin

prescription. Regular use of vitamin C supplements[1,7] (at least 200 mg/d) may decrease duration of cold symptoms, but they are not effective if started after cold symptoms start. Oral zinc sulfate[1,7] may decrease URI symptom duration and severity, but it is not routinely recommended because of adverse effects (bad taste and nausea).

Croup
Croup affects children with a peak incidence between 6 and 36 months of age, annually affecting 3% of those in this age range. Parainfluenza virus types 1 to 3 constitute 75% of all cases, but infection with many different viruses can produce this illness. Although some cases of croup can be caused by bacteria, it does not change how it is managed.

Croup is diagnosed clinically. Initially, patients experience cold-like symptoms: low-grade fevers and coryza. Inspiratory stridor, hoarseness, and a barking cough are typical findings that follow, peaking between 24 to 48 hours after onset. These symptoms are caused by mucosal inflammatory swelling of the larynx, trachea, and bronchi. Symptoms are often worse at night and can be exacerbated by emotional distress. Most (85%) cases are considered mild, but nasal flaring and retractions, increased respiratory rate, hypoxia, and tachycardia are indicators of more severe croup. Routine radiologic imaging is not encouraged, because the steeple sign that is often associated with croup is actually nonspecific and can be seen in other causes of glottic and subglottic narrowing such as epiglottitis and bacterial tracheitis.

Management of croup is dependent on the severity of the disease. Administration of corticosteroids (single dose of dexamethasone [Decadron][1] 0.6 mg/kg) are recommended for croup of any severity because it reduces return visits and hospitalization rates. Oxygen should be given to children with hypoxia or respiratory distress. Nebulized epinephrine[1] (0.05 mL/kg of racemic epinephrine 2.25% [max dose = 0.5 mL] or 0.5 mL per kg of L-epinephrine 1:1,000 via nebulizer [max dose = 5 mL]) is recommended for moderate or severe croup. It takes effect by vasoconstriction of the upper airway mucosa, leading to decreased edema. It has a quick onset of action, but efficacy wanes after 1 to 2 hours, so monitoring patients beyond 2 hours is recommended.

Humidified air has been commonly used for croup, but it has not been shown to be effective in decreasing croup symptoms or hospital admissions in moderate croup.

Pertussis
Pertussis should be suspected when patients have more than 2 weeks of a characteristic paroxysmal, whooping cough and post-tussive emesis, or recent pertussis exposure. Most pertussis is caused by the bacteria B pertussis. The number of outbreaks and pertussis incidence has increased in recent years. In the early catarrhal stage (1–2 weeks), it is difficult to discern from a common cold. The cough becomes more frequent, and severe bouts characterize the following paroxysmal stage (1–6 weeks, maximum of 10 weeks). Paroxysms of cough can be debilitating and cause post-tussive emesis, weight loss, and other conditions related to severe cough, but there are few symptoms otherwise. After this stage, the cough gradually improves over the course of a few weeks.

Atypical presentations are not uncommon, because those who have acquired immunity can present with a lesser degree of paroxysm. Thus pertussis should be suspected if cough symptoms last more than 3 weeks. Infants may also have atypical presentation of cough without paroxysmal whooping.

Diagnosis can be confirmed with either culture, polymerase chain reaction (both better for early stages), or serology (accurate in later stage). Efficacy of antibiotics is questionable because treatment does not improve symptoms. However, antibiotics

---

[1]Not FDA approved for this indication.
[7]Available as a dietary supplement.

(Azithromycin [Zithromax][1] is first line—Children: 10 mg/kg/d for 3 days, or 10 mg/kg on day 1, then 5 mg/kg/d on days 2-5; Adults: 500 mg/d for 3 days, or 500 mg on day 1, then 250 mg/d on days 2–5) are still recommended because they eradicate B pertussis from the nasopharynx and may decrease transmission. Immunization is critical to prevent further outbreaks of pertussis.

Bronchiolitis
Bronchiolitis is the most common cause for infant hospitalization of infants. Respiratory syncytial virus is the most common cause of bronchiolitis. Bronchioles become plugged with detached epithelium and inflammatory cells. Onset of upper respiratory symptoms is often soon followed by rapid development of wheezing and labored breathing. Infants with bronchiolitis typically do not have a marked response to asthma treatment with bronchodilators and corticosteroids, despite similar presenting symptoms. Treatment primarily consists of supplemental oxygen and intravenous fluids as needed to prevent dehydration. Palivizumab (Synagis) is used to prevent hospitalization rate for high-risk infants, such as those with premature birth, chronic lung disease, and hemodynamically significant congenital heart disease.

Therapy (or Treatment)
Decreasing Antibiotic Use
Antibiotic use in the treatment of bronchitis is strongly discouraged in all major guidelines, but they are often prescribed regardless of the recommendations. The strongest predictor of whether a patient will receive antibiotics is whether the clinician perceives the patient desires them. Patient education such as setting the expectation that cough from acute bronchitis can last 3 weeks, that antibiotics would not effectively aid in shortening the duration of symptoms, and explaining the undesired consequences of inappropriate antibiotic use such as antibiotic resistance and adverse effects is important. One in five patients treated with antibiotics will experience side effects such as headache, nausea, skin rash, diarrhea, and vaginitis. Patients are more likely to respond to this sort of education if they feel their concerns have been heard and addressed. In some cases, using a delayed prescription strategy wherein patients would need to call for a prescription or agree to pick up antibiotics after a certain number of days may be effective in decreasing antibiotic use. Providing methods for symptomatic management is also important for patients who desire treatment.

Recommended Cough Treatment
Dextromethorphan, guaifenesin, and honey may be considered to relieve cough symptoms. Dextromethorphan (30 mg orally every 6 to 8 hours) is a central-acting antitussive that reduces the cough reflex. In placebo-controlled studies, it was shown to decrease coughs by 19% to 36% (8 to 10 fewer coughs per 30 minutes) compared with placebo. Guaifenesin ([immediate-release] 200 to 400 mg orally every 4 hours) is an expectorant that increases respiratory tract secretions, hence decreasing mucus thickness. Study results vary, but it has been shown to decrease cough frequency and severity compared with placebo. Honey (2.5–10 mL [0.5–2 teaspoons]) has been compared with dextromethorphan, diphenhydramine, and no treatment in children. It was found to be better than no treatment in its effectiveness in decreasing cough severity and frequency and improving sleep quality. Honey would be an option for children older than 1 year, because antitussive use is not recommended in small children.

Cough Treatments that are not Recommended
There is no evidence that centrally acting antitussive codeine[1] has any effect to decrease cough symptoms, and benzonatate (Tessalon Perles), a peripherally acting antitussive has only been shown to be effective in conjunction with guaifenesin. Unfortunately, many over-the-counter therapies do not significantly

impact acute bronchitis symptoms. Clinical trials have shown that ibuprofen (Motrin)[1] and antihistamines are not effective in reducing symptoms of cough. The FDA warns against using cough medications that have antihistamines and antitussives in children younger than 4 years of age because of the high risk for potential harm. Use of beta-agonists is also not recommended, unless the patient presents with wheezing at the time of presentation.

---

[1]Not FDA approved for this indication.

References

Altunaiji S, Kukuruzovic R, Curtis N, et al: Antibiotics for whooping cough (pertussis), *Cochrane Database Syst Rev* 2007 (3):CD004404.

Barnett ML, Linder JA: Antibiotic prescribing for adults with acute bronchitis in the United States, 1996-2010, *JAMA* 311:2020–2022, 2014.

Ebell MH, Lundgren J, Youngpairoj S: How long does a cough last? Comparing patients' expectations with data from a systematic review of the literature, *Ann Fam Med* 11:5–13, 2013.

Kinkade S, Long N: Acute bronchitis, *Am Fam Physician* 94:560–565, 2016.

Oduwole O, Meremikwu MM, Oyo-Ita A, et al: Honey for acute cough in children, *Cochrane Database Syst Rev*, 2014. Rev (12):CD007094.

Petrocheilou A, Tanou K, Kalampouka E, et al: Viral croup: diagnosis and a treatment algorithm, *Pediatr Pulmonol* 49:421–429, 2014.

Russell KF, Liang Y, O'Gorman K, et al: Glucocorticoids for croup, *Cochrane Database Syst Rev*, 2011. Rev (1):CD001955.

Smith D, McDermott A, Sullivan J: Croup: diagnosis and management, *Am Fam Physician* 97:575–580, 2018.

Smith SM, Fahey T, Smucny J, et al: Antibiotics for acute bronchitis, *Cochrane Database Syst Rev*, 2014. Rev (3):CD000245.

Smith SM, Schroeder K, Fahey T: Over-The-Counter (OTC) medications for acute cough in children and adults in community settings, *Cochrane Database Syst Rev*, 2014. Rev (11):CD001831.

ACUTE RESPIRATORY FAILURE

Method of
Anthony J. Faugno III, MD; and Scott K. Epstein, MD

CURRENT DIAGNOSIS

- History and physical examination can give insight into the etiology of hypoxic and hypercapneic respiratory failure but may be insufficient to make a definitive diagnosis and guide therapy.
- An arterial blood gas is mandatory to define severity and whether hypoxic or hypercapneic (or both) respiratory failure is present.
- Additional diagnostic modalities, including chest radiograph, electrocardiogram, cardiac laboratory tests (troponin, brain natriuretic peptide), echocardiography, and selected use of a pulmonary artery catheter, can help identify a specific etiology.

CURRENT THERAPY

- Treatment of acute respiratory failure often begins with non-specific approaches such as oxygen and mechanical ventilation (noninvasive or invasive).
- The goal of mechanical ventilation is to improve gas exchange and rest the respiratory muscles while waiting for the beneficial effects of specific therapy aimed at the underlying cause (e.g., bronchodilators, antibiotics, and corticosteroids in acute exacerbations of chronic obstructive pulmonary disease [COPD]).
- Noninvasive ventilation avoids many complications associated with invasive ventilation and improves outcomes for patients with acute cardiogenic pulmonary edema and acute exacerbations of COPD.

- High-flow nasal cannula is emerging as the preferred therapy for hypoxic respiratory failure in patients with non-cardiogenic pulmonary edema who do not require urgent intubation.
- Invasive mechanical ventilation can be lifesaving but can cause clinical deterioration if not properly administered.
- Using low tidal volumes (6 mL/kg ideal body weight) can help avoid dangerous dynamic hyperinflation in acute exacerbations of COPD and further lung injury in acute lung injury (e.g., volutrauma, barotrauma).
- Once signs of improvement are evident, focus rapidly shifts to liberating the patient from the ventilator using spontaneous breathing trials to assess the need for ventilatory support followed by airway assessment to determine readiness for extubation.

The respiratory system serves many complex physiologic functions, the most important of which is gas exchange. Using the interface between the alveolar space and capillaries, O_2 is taken up and CO_2 is eliminated. Acute respiratory failure, a life-threatening entity, is present when this system fails, over the course of minutes to hours, resulting in hypoxemia (type I) or hypercapnia (type II), or both. Most patients with acute respiratory failure present with dyspnea, although the correlation with disease severity is poor. Indeed, dyspnea might seem mild in those with baseline chronic respiratory failure, and it might be absent in those with an underlying neurologic process (e.g., drug overdose). Other symptoms and signs such as cough, chest pain, orthopnea, fever, tachypnea, rales, and wheezing are insensitive and nonspecific.

This chapter outlines the general pathophysiology and therapeutic approach to acute respiratory failure by using the examples of three common entities: acute respiratory distress syndrome (ARDS), cardiogenic pulmonary edema (congestive heart failure [CHF]), and acute exacerbation of chronic obstructive pulmonary disease (AECOPD).

Definitions and Pathophysiology

Acute Hypoxic Respiratory Failure

Hypoxic respiratory failure is conventionally defined as an arterial oxygen tension (PaO_2) of less than 60 mm Hg. Because this definition ignores the inspired fraction of oxygen (FiO_2), some favor a PaO_2/FiO_2 ratio of less than 300. To account for the arterial CO_2 tension ($PaCO_2$), others favor an alveolar–arterial (A–a) O_2 gradient greater than 250 mm Hg, using the equation

$$A\text{–a } O_2 \text{ gradient} = PAO_2 - PaO_2$$
$$= (713 \times FiO_2) - (PaO_2 + PaCO_2/0.8)$$

where 713 is the barometric pressure (760) minus the water vapor pressure. A normal A–a O_2 is less than 10 mm Hg, but this threshold value increases with age. The determination of PaO_2 requires an invasive test, an arterial blood gas. Oxygenation can be continuously monitored noninvasively by pulse oximetry, which provides an estimate of arterial oxygen saturation (SaO_2). In general, an SaO_2 of 0.90 corresponds to a PaO_2 of 60 mm Hg, but the relation depends on temperature, pH, $PaCO_2$, and 2,3-diphosphoglycerate (2,3-DPG). Accuracy is adversely affected by low perfusion states, dark skin pigmentation, nail polish, dyshemoglobins (e.g., carboxyhemoglobin, methemoglobin), intravascular dyes, motion, and ambient light.

Clinicians tend to focus on PaO_2 and SaO_2, but the real parameter of interest is O_2 delivery (DO_2) to organs and tissues. DO_2 depends on cardiac output and O_2 carrying capacity of arterialized blood (CaO_2):

$$DO_2 = CO \times CaO_2$$

where

$$CaO_2 = k (Hb \times SaO_2) + 0.003 \ PaO_2$$

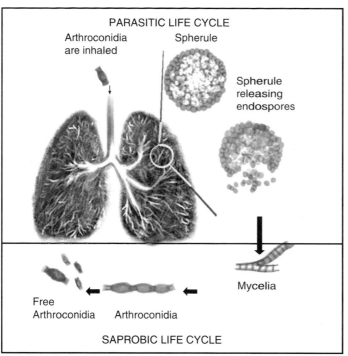

Figure 1 Life cycle of *Coccidioides* sp. indicating parasitic phase in the host and the saprobic phase present in environment.

in nonendemic areas because of travel or reactivation of prior infection. In the United States an estimated 150,000 cases of CM occur annually, with the clinical presentation ranging from a self-limited respiratory infection to devastating disseminated disease. The incidence of CM is increasing in the United States because of rising populations and the resulting construction in the endemic areas. Risk factors for increased severity of CM include receiving immunosuppressive medications (corticosteroids, transplant drugs, and tumor necrosis factor–α antagonists); pregnancy (esp. the third trimester); genetic factors (i.e., defects in the interleukin-12/interferon-γ axis and STAT3 pathways, certain ABO blood group and human leukocyte antigen types); and specific races/ethnicities (African Americans, Asian–Pacific Islanders, and Native Americans). Outbreaks may occur after dust storms, earthquakes, droughts, and activities causing soil disruption, such as construction and archeological digs. Persons with occupations involving exposure to soil are also at risk for acquiring CM.

Coccidioides is dimorphic; in the soil, the organism exists in its mycelial form, which produces barrel-shaped arthroconidia. The usual means of infection is the inhalation of arthroconidia; uncommon routes include direct cutaneous inoculation and organ transplantation. Arthroconidia germinate to produce spherules filled with endospores, the characteristic tissue phase. Spherules rupture to release endospores, which form additional spherules (Figure 1). The spherules become surrounded by neutrophils and macrophages, which leads to granuloma formation. Both B and T lymphocytes are essential for host defense against this pathogen.

Clinical Manifestations

CM is asymptomatic in 60% of infected individuals. In the remaining 40% a self-limited, flu-like illness with dry cough, pleuritic chest pain, myalgias, arthralgia, fever, sweats, anorexia, and weakness develops 1 to 3 weeks after exposure. Primary infection may be accompanied by immune complex–mediated complications including an erythematous macular rash, erythema multiforme, and erythema nodosum. Acute infection usually resolves without therapy, although symptoms may persist for weeks. In 5% of these patients, asymptomatic pulmonary residua persist, including pulmonary nodules and cavitation.

Immunocompromised patients may develop chronic progressive pulmonary infection, with the evolution of thin-walled cavities that may rupture, leading to bronchopleural fistula and empyema formation.

Extrapulmonary disease develops in 1 of every 200 patients and can involve the skin, soft tissues, bones, joints, and meninges. The most common cutaneous lesions are verrucous papules, ulcers, or plaques. The spine is the most frequent site of osseous dissemination, although the typical lytic lesions may also occur in the skull, hands, feet, and tibia. Joint involvement is usually monoarticular and most commonly involves the ankle or knee. Fungemia may occur in immunocompromised patients and carries a poor prognosis.

In coccidioidal meningitis, the basilar meninges are usually affected. Cerebrospinal fluid findings include lymphocytic pleocytosis (often with eosinophilia), hypoglycorrhachia, and elevated protein levels. The mortality rate is greater than 90% at 1 year without therapy, and chronic infection is the rule. Hydrocephalus or hydrocephalus coexisting with brain infarction is associated with a higher mortality rate. CM is a great imitator and has many diverse clinical presentations, including immune thrombocytopenia, ocular involvement, massive cervical lymphadenopathy, laryngeal and retropharyngeal abscesses, endocarditis, pericarditis, peritonitis, hepatitis, and lesions of the male and female genitals and urogenital tracts.

Diagnosis

CM may be diagnosed by direct observation of spherules in tissues or in wet mounts of sputa or exudates. The growth of *Coccidioides* in culture usually occurs in 3 to 5 days, with sporulation after 5 to 10 days. Definitive identification is made by DNA probe or exoantigen testing. Laboratory personnel should exercise extreme caution when handling cultures of *Coccidioides*.

Serologic methods are useful in establishing the diagnosis and for monitoring the course of CM. Immunoglobulin M (IgM) antibodies are present soon after infection or relapse but then wane; quantification does not correlate with disease severity. The immunoglobulin G (IgG) antibody appears later and remains positive for months. Rising titers of IgG are associated with progressive disease, and declining titers are associated with resolution. The IgG antibodies can fix complement when combined with coccidioidal antigen and can be detected by immunodiffusion (immunodiffusion complement fixation [IDCF]); titers of 1:16 or greater suggest disseminated disease. In the cerebrospinal fluid, a positive IDCF of any titer is considered diagnostic of meningitis and is much more sensitive than culture in making the diagnosis. An enzyme immunoassay (EIA) is also available for the detection of IgM and IgG antibodies, but it is less specific. The sensitivity and specificity of serologic testing is high for pleuropulmonary disease. Polymerase chain reaction testing on pleural fluid is not as sensitive and is comparable to pleural fluid culture. Adenosine deaminase levels in pleural fluid are inconsistently elevated. According to Infectious Diseases Society of America guidelines, an indeterminate EIA IgM and IgG test result should be considered nonreactive. If only the EIA IgM assay is reactive, this could be a false-positive result, and IgM/IgG testing should be repeated at a later time. A specific urinary antigen test is also available for the diagnosis of CM; this assay has a sensitivity of 71% in moderate to severe disease, compared with 84% for culture, 29% for histopathologic examination, and 75% for serologic testing. The majority of cases with disseminated or meningeal CM have elevated serum 1,3-β-D-glucan levels. However, 1,3-β-D-glucan values correlate poorly with coccidioidal complement fixation antibody titers.

Treatment

In most patients, primary pulmonary infection resolves spontaneously without treatment. However, all patients require observation for at least 2 years to document resolution of infection and to identify any complications as soon as possible. For patients who have risk factors for disseminated disease (listed earlier), treatment is necessary. Other indications for treatment are severe disease (infiltrates involving both lungs or more than half of one lung; significant hilar or mediastinal lymphadenopathy; complement fixation titers >1:16) and highly symptomatic disease (weight loss >10%; night sweats present for >3 weeks; symptoms present for >2 months).

For diffuse or severe pneumonia, therapy with amphotericin B deoxycholate (Fungizone) 0.5 to 1.5 mg/kg/day or a lipid formulation of amphotericin B (Abelcet or AmBisome)[1] 2 to 5 mg/kg/day should be given for several weeks, followed by an oral azole, such as itraconazole (Sporanox)[1] 200 mg twice daily or fluconazole (Diflucan)[1] 400 to 800 mg/day. The total duration of therapy should be at least 1 year; for immunosuppressed patients, oral azole therapy should be maintained as secondary prophylaxis. In HIV patients with CD4-positive T-cell counts greater than 250 cells/mm[3] who had focal pneumonias that responded to azoles, antifungals may be discontinued. Azole therapy may be used initially for less severe disease. During pregnancy, amphotericin B is the preferred drug, because of the teratogenicity of azoles.

An asymptomatic patient with a solitary nodule or pulmonary cavitation due to *Coccidioides* does not require specific antifungal therapy or resection. However, the development of complications from the cavitation, such as hemoptysis or bacterial or fungal superinfection, necessitates initiation of azole therapy. Resection of the cavities is an alternative to antifungal therapy. Rupture of a cavity into the pleural space requires surgical intervention with closure by lobectomy with decortication, in addition to antifungal therapy. For chronic pneumonia, the initial treatment should be an oral azole for at least 1 year. If the disease persists, one may switch to another oral azole, increase the dose if fluconazole was initially selected, or switch to amphotericin B. Resection should be performed for patients with refractory focal lesions or severe hemoptysis.

The treatment of disseminated infection without central nervous system involvement is based on oral azole therapy, such as itraconazole[1] or fluconazole[1] (400 mg/day, or higher in case of fluconazole). If there is little or no improvement or if there is vertebral involvement, treatment with amphotericin B is recommended (dosage as for diffuse pneumonia). Concomitant surgical débridement or stabilization is also recommended. In patients with refractory CM that has failed to respond to fluconazole, itraconazole, and amphotericin B and its lipid formulations, treatment with posaconazole (Noxafil)[1] suspension 200 mg four times daily with a fatty meal or voriconazole (Vfend)[1], at doses of 400 to 600 mg/day, has been successful. A posaconazole tablet with improved oral bioavailability and an intravenous preparation are now available, and likely these new forms of posaconazole are more efficacious. The posaconazole tablet has been dosed at 300 mg/day[2]. Clinical experience with voriconazole is limited.

For coccidioidal meningitis, lifetime treatment with azoles is indicated. Fluconazole[1] at doses of 800 mg/day or higher[2] is recommended. There have been several reports of successful treatment of coccidioidal meningitis with voriconazole (Vfend)[1] 200 mg orally twice daily after a loading dose. Itraconazole is not recommended because of its irregular oral absorption. Limited studies exist for the use of isavuconazole (Cresemba)[1] in the treatment of CM, including coccidioidal meningitis. For patients with increased intracranial pressure at the time of meningitis diagnosis, repeated lumbar punctures are recommended. Obstructive hydrocephalus requires shunting. Intrathecal amphotericin B[1] is now strictly reserved for meningitis refractory to high-dose azoles or coccidioidal meningitis in the first trimester of pregnancy. In patients with CNS vasculitis with cerebrovascular accident due to

CM, those that received corticosteroids were less likely to develop additional infarcts compared with those who did not. Reduction of immunosuppression is an important adjunct to antifungal therapy, including the initiation of antiretroviral therapy if the patient has HIV infection. In patients with AIDS and nonmeningeal coccidioidomycosis, antifungal therapy can be discontinued when the CD4 count exceeds 250 cells/mm[3].

References

Ampel NM: Coccidioidomycosis: changing concepts and knowledge gaps, *J Fungi (Basel)* 6:354, 2020.

Bays DJ, Thompson 3rd GR: Coccidioidomycosis, *Infect Dis Clin North Am* 35:453–469, 2021.

Bays DJ, Thompson GR, Reef S, et al: Natural history of disseminated coccidioidomycosis: examination of the VA-armed forces database, *Clin Infect Dis* 73:e3814–e3819, 2020.

Diep AL, Hoyer KK: Host response to *Coccidioides* infection: fungal immunity, *Front Cell Infect Microbio* 10:581101, 2020.

Donovan FM, Zangeneh TT, Malo J, Galgiani JN: Top questions in the diagnosis and treatment of coccidioidomycosis, *Open Forum Infect Dis* 4:ofx197, 2017.

Gabe LM, Malo J, Knox KS: Diagnosis and management of coccidioidomycosis, *Clin Chest Med* 38:417–433, 2017.

Galgiani JN, Ampel NM, Blair JE, et al: Infectious Diseases Society of America (IDSA) clinical practice guideline for the treatment of coccidioidomycosis, *Clin Infect Dis* 63:e112–e146, 2016.

Gorris ME, Ardon-Dryer K, Campuzano A, et al: Advocating for coccidioidomycosis to be a reportable disease nationwide in the United States and encouraging disease surveillance across North and South America, *J Fungi (Basel)* 9:83, 2023.

Hartmann CA, Aye WT, Blair JE: Treatment considerations in pulmonary coccidioidomycosis, *Expert Rev Respir Med* 10:1079–1091, 2016.

Heidari A, Quinlan M, Benjamin DJ, et al: Isavuconazole in the treatment of coccidioidal meningitis, *Antimicrob Agents Chemother* 63:e02232-18, 2019.

Kassis C, Durkin M, Holbrook E, et al: Advances in diagnosis of progressive pulmonary and disseminated coccidioidomycosis, *Clin Infect Dis* 72:968–975, 2021.

Kim MM, Vikram HR, Kusne S, Seville MT, Blair JE: Treatment of refractory coccidioidomycosis with voriconazole or posaconazole, *Clin Infect Dis* 53:1060–1066, 2011.

McCotter OZ, Benedict K, Engelthaler DM, et al: Update on the epidemiology of coccidioidomycosis in the United States, *Med Mycol* 57(Suppl 1):S30–S40, 2019.

Odio CD, Marciano BE, Galgiani JN, Holland SM: Risk factors for disseminated coccidioidomycosis, United States, *Emerg Infect Dis* 23:308–311, 2017.

Stockamp NW, Thompson 3rd GR: Coccidioidomycosis, *Infect Dis Clin North Am* 30:229–246, 2016.

Thompson 3rd GR, Blair JE, Wang S, et al: Adjunctive corticosteroid therapy in the treatment of coccidioidal meningitis, *Clin Infect Dis* 65:338–341, 2017.

Thompson 3rd GR, Lewis 2nd JS, Nix DE, Patterson TF: Current concepts and future directions in the pharmacology and treatment of coccidioidomycosis, *Med Mycol* 157(Suppl 1):S76–S84, 2019.

Thompson 3rd GR, Sharma S, Bays DJ, et al: Coccidioidomycosis, *Chest* 143(3):776–781, 2013, https://doi.org/10.1378/chest.12-1312.

Van Dyke MCC, Thompson GR, Galgiani JN, Barker BM: The rise of *Coccidioides*: forces against the dust devil unleashed, *Front Immunol* 10:2188, 2019.

CYSTIC FIBROSIS

Method of
Hanna Phan, PharmD; and Cori L. Daines, MD

CURRENT DIAGNOSIS

- Cystic fibrosis (CF) is an autosomal recessive genetic disorder that causes dysfunction of the cystic fibrosis transmembrane conductance regulator (CFTR) on the apical surface of epithelial cells, leading to the inability to move adequate ions, specifically chloride, out of the cell.
- This defect leads to thick, dehydrated mucus in the respiratory tract that manifests as chronic cough and recurrent infections.
- Diagnosis is made via a sweat chloride test using quantitative pilocarpine iontophoresis.
- Close to 2000 *CFTR* mutations are known, leading to a multitude of clinical phenotypes and disease severity.

CURRENT THERAPY

- A given patient's overall treatment regimen is often based on various factors, including age, clinical presentation, organ systems involved, disease progression/severity, *CFTR* genotype, and comorbidities.
- Primary treatment includes augmented airway clearance with bronchodilators, mucolytics, or mucus hydrators along with mechanical airway vibration.
- For the vast majority of patients, secondary treatment includes use of a cystic fibrosis transmembrane conductance regulator modulator.
- Nutritional therapy consists of enzymes and vitamin replacement for those who are pancreatic insufficient.

Epidemiology

Cystic fibrosis (CF) is an autosomal recessive, inherited multisystem disease caused by mutations of the *CFTR* gene on chromosome 7. There are currently close to 2000 known *CFTR* mutations. Carriage of the gene is highest in individuals of Northern European descent, leading to an incidence of 1 in 3000 non-Hispanic White people in the United States. The incidence is lower in Hispanic White people and those of African descent. There are more than 32,000 individuals with CF in the United States, more than 100,000 individuals worldwide, and approximately 1000 new diagnoses each year. The average life expectancy is increasing with new therapies but still varies among countries. In the United States and Canada, the life expectancy is currently 56.6 years, with estimates of nearly 65 years in babies born today.

Pathophysiology
Cystic Fibrosis Transmembrane Regulator
Genotypes–Genotype/Phenotype

The cystic fibrosis transmembrane conductance regulator (CFTR) is a protein in the adenosine triphosphate–binding cassette transporter family that has two transmembrane domains, two nucleotide-binding domains, and a regulatory domain. It shares structural elements with other membrane pumps. Mutations in the gene coding the CFTR fall broadly into six categories. The first category includes premature truncation mutations, leading to no full-length protein. The second category includes the *Phe508del* (i.e., *F508del*) mutation, which is the most common mutation and accounts for 75% of all mutations in the United States. Class II mutations result in the cell degrading the CFTR before full maturation and function. Class III mutations result in a chloride channel at the cell surface that does not function (also called a *gating mutation*). Class IV mutations result in a chloride channel embedded at the cell surface that has decreased and ineffective chloride movement function, and class V mutations are promoter or splicing abnormalities that result in a reduced number of functional chloride channels at the cell surface. Class VI mutations result in a chloride channel that is not stable on the cell surface and, like class V mutations, insufficient quantities of chloride channel at the cell surface.

Understanding the genetics of any given individual with cystic fibrosis (CF) is vital in understanding the pathophysiology. Disease manifestation is directly related to the amount of chloride moved at the cell surface. Class I, II, and III mutations result in minimal chloride movement, less than 5% of normal, and "classic" or severe disease phenotype. The presence of one mutation in the class IV, V, or VI categories results in greater chloride movement at the surface, typically 10% or more, and a "mild" or "nonclassic" phenotype. Approximately 15% of individuals with CF fall into this latter category and have some preserved chloride channel activity and milder disease phenotype.

Mechanism

CF affects all organs with epithelial cells expressing CFTR, which typically means the cells lining a ductal system and the fluid outside that system are affected. In the lungs, the respiratory epithelium is lined with cells that express CFTR. When CFTR does not move appropriate amounts of chloride, the chloride is trapped inside the cell, which leads to the epithelial sodium channel pumping additional sodium into the cell to balance. The resulting salt inside the cell creates an osmotic gradient across the cell surface, and water enters the cell. The water first comes from the periciliary fluid layer, dehydrating the fluid around the cilia, making it difficult for them to beat. Next, the water is removed from the outer mucus layer, also dehydrating it, making it thick and viscous. In the sinopulmonary tract, this inspissation of the mucus limits natural mucociliary clearance and leads to inflammation and an advantageous environment for bacterial colonization. Damage to the airways becomes irreversible and leads to a loss of lung function.

A similar process occurs in other organs with any epithelial cell lining a ductal system. In the pancreas, for instance, epithelial cells line the ducts of the exocrine pancreas. The cells pull water from the normal pancreatic excretion, dehydrating it and clogging the ducts. The enzymes then autodigest the exocrine pancreas, rendering it nonfunctional. The same is true in the biliary ducts of the liver. In the sweat glands, salt and water are trapped in the ducts, making the sweat very salty and leading to the diagnostic result of the sweat chloride test.

Clinical Manifestations
Pulmonary

The tracheobronchial tree in CF has poor mucociliary clearance, as noted previously. Patients with CF have excessive cough, make mucus, and might wheeze. They have periodic episodes of exacerbation in which excessive mucus builds up and bacterial infection occurs. The thick mucus becomes a source of persistent infection with bacteria that are unable to be cleared. Often, the infections are caused by bacteria that are not present in the normal undamaged airway, especially *Staphylococcus aureus* and *Pseudomonas aeruginosa*. When the bacteria become active and the patient experiences an exacerbation, the cough and sputum production will worsen. Exacerbations in children are often triggered by viruses and typical childhood illnesses, and in adults, exacerbations may also be triggered by other environmental factors. With exacerbation, there may be shortness of breath, chest pain, wheezing, dyspnea on exertion or at rest, and fatigue. Other symptoms of a pulmonary exacerbation include weight loss, poor appetite, and fever. Over time, there is progressive loss of lung function resulting from infections, mucus, and inflammation. Symptoms become more persistent and bothersome over time, and exacerbations become more common. Additionally, more than 30% of individuals with CF also have asthma.

Sinuses

The sinuses in CF have the same mucostasis that occurs in the lungs. The mucus impaction leads to chronic sinus congestion and obstruction, persistent infections, and persistent inflammation. More than 50% of adults with CF have chronic sinusitis. Patients with CF are more likely to develop polyps as well. Symptoms include nasal congestion or drainage, sinus headache, and inability to smell.

Pancreas

Poor growth occurs because of insufficient nutrient breakdown and absorption, resulting in malabsorptive, greasy stools. Fat-soluble vitamins in the diet are also poorly absorbed because of the malabsorption of fat. Individuals with CF can develop significant deficiencies in vitamins A, D, E, and K. In general, the endocrine pancreas that makes insulin is not initially affected in CF. Over time, individuals with CF often develop CF-related diabetes (CFRD) caused by global inflammation of the pancreas. More than 40% of adults with CF will develop CFRD.

Liver

In the liver, there is inspissation of the bile in the bile duct caused by excessive reabsorption of water from the bile. The resulting blockage of the bile ducts leads to hepatic inflammation. In general, this is asymptomatic for the patient with CF and is found by checking laboratory levels of liver function tests. Occasionally, this bile blockage is severe and leads to chronic inflammation and biliary cirrhosis of the liver. A small percentage of individuals with CF, typically less than 5%, have cirrhosis with portal hypertension, esophageal varices, and splenomegaly and would need a liver transplant.

Intestines

Excessive reabsorption of fluid in the gut can lead to constipation and even small bowel obstruction. This can also occur when stools are malabsorptive. Some people with CF will have rectal prolapse caused by straining, with either malabsorptive or constipated stools. Other manifestations of CF in the intestines can be a result of medication side effects.

Sweat Glands

Excessive salt is trapped in the sweat, leading to excessive salt loss in the sweat and electrolyte imbalance and dehydration.

Genitourinary

Men with CF generally all have congenital absence of the vas deferens, rendering them naturally infertile. Men still produce sperm but do not have the other structures. Women with CF may have decreased fertility as a result of poor nutritional status, but they typically can have children.

Other

CF causes clubbing of the fingers, which is usually more prominent as lung disease progresses. CF-related arthropathies occur in a small percentage of individuals with CF, usually caused by inflammatory markers in circulation that deposit in the joints. Mental health issues, such as depression and anxiety, are common in teenagers and adults with CF, with an incidence of approximately 30%.

Diagnosis

Because CF is an insidiously progressive disease, it is important to make an early diagnosis and begin therapies as soon as possible. In the United States the majority of diagnoses are made via newborn screening. Depending on the state, testing involves immunoreactive trypsinogen levels with possible genetic panels of mutations. When the state reports a positive newborn screen, the care provider must order/obtain a sweat chloride test on the infant. Diagnoses are then based on the results of the screens. The Cystic Fibrosis Foundation guidelines state that a positive sweat diagnosis of CF is greater than 30 mmol/L chloride, with 30 to 60 mmol/L chloride being the intermediate zone. Consensus remains that if a child has two mutations, symptoms, and an abnormal sweat chloride (30 to 60 mmol/L), this is consistent with a diagnosis of CF. Children with symptoms and a sweat chloride greater than 60 mmol/L have CF as well. A secondary diagnosis of CF-related metabolic disorder (CRMS) designates those individuals whose diagnoses are unclear. Those with one mutation and an intermediate sweat (30 to 60 mmol/L) or those with two mutations and a negative sweat (<30 mmol/L) are followed prospectively for the development of symptoms and should have periodic sweat tests and periodic evaluations for the evolution of symptoms at a certified CF center, where the testing methodology is certified by the national Cystic Fibrosis Foundation.

As newborn screening has only been widely available for the past 10 to 20 years, children and adults who did not receive newborn screening are still being diagnosed the traditional way, which is the presence of symptoms and a positive sweat test. Here again, a positive sweat means a value of 60 mmol/L, whereas a value of 30 mmol/L or greater deserves further investigation, such as genetic testing. Sweat tests should be done at a certified

CF center. Traditional symptomatology per the Cystic Fibrosis Foundation is represented in the following:

- Very salty-tasting skin
- Persistent coughing, at times with phlegm
- Frequent lung infections, such as pneumonia or bronchitis
- Wheezing or shortness of breath
- Poor growth or poor weight gain in spite of a good appetite
- Frequent greasy, bulky stools, or difficulty with bowel movements
- Nasal polyps
- Chronic sinus infections
- Clubbing or enlargement of the fingertips and toes
- Rectal prolapse
- Male infertility

If a diagnosis of CF is suspected because of symptomatology, a sweat test for a definitive diagnosis should be performed regardless of the patient's age or newborn screening status.

Treatment

Pulmonary Treatment

Nonpharmacologic Therapy

Because of the increased viscosity of airway secretions and the subsequent obstruction and even mucus plugging in CF, there is a fundamental need for airway clearance or chest physiotherapy as part of chronic care. As a core component of therapy in the pulmonary management of CF, airway clearance or chest physiotherapy helps loosen this mucus, and help with expectoration should be done routinely two to three times per day as part of chronic management for patients of all ages; increased frequency may be necessary during periods of pulmonary exacerbation. Manual physiotherapy or percussion and postural drainage is often the first technique introduced into care. Other airway clearance techniques can be used, depending on age and access to devices. These techniques include the use of autogenic drainage, the active cycle of breathing technique, high-frequency chest compression (e.g., vest), the use of oscillatory positive expiratory pressure (e.g., MetaNeb) devices, and exercise.

Chronic Pharmacologic Therapy

The selection of medications used in the pulmonary management of chronic CF is currently based on age and clinical need. This is based on current guidelines, U.S. Food and Drug Administration (FDA)-approved indications for newer agents (e.g., CFTR modulators), and current evidence in cases of off-label medication use. Such pharmacotherapy consists of various medication classes, including bronchodilators, mucolytics, inhaled antibiotics, anti-inflammatory agents, and CFTR modulators.

Inhaled medications are used in conjunction with chest physiotherapy to facilitate airway clearance, helping loosen mucus and expectoration, and suppress bacterial growth of pathogens in the airways. The use of a short-acting β-agonist, such as albuterol (Proventil, Ventolin),[1] in either meter dose inhaler or aerosolized or nebulizer form, facilitates mucociliary clearance through bronchodilation and decreases occurrence of bronchospasm from subsequent inhaled therapies such as mucolytics (e.g., hypertonic saline (sodium chloride 7% [HyperSal, PulmoSal]), dornase alfa (Pulmozyme), mannitol inhalation powder (Bronchitol), and antibiotics. Mucolytics are also fundamental in mucociliary clearance. Nebulized hypertonic saline, most commonly sodium chloride 7% and administered twice a day, increases hydration of sputum through osmotic action, thinning sputum for airway clearance. Dornase alfa breaks down extracellular DNA in sputum, thereby decreasing its viscosity. This nebulized mucolytic is most commonly administered daily, usually after the use of nebulized hypertonic saline in sequence. The use of hypertonic saline and dornase alfa is recommended to help improve lung function and reduce exacerbations. Recently approved as a possible add-on maintenance therapy for persons with CF ages 18 years and older, mannitol inhalation powder (Bronchitol) is a dry

---

[1] Not FDA approved for this indication.

powder formulation and thus does not require use of a nebulizer for administration and is dosed twice daily. Because of its acute bronchospasm risk, it should only be used in those who have passed the Bronchitol Tolerance Test, which is administered and performed under supervision. Inhaled corticosteroids with or without a long-acting β-agonist are not used to treat CF itself but are appropriate in cases of concurrent asthma.

Some patients with CF may require the use of an inhaled antibiotic to help suppress bacterial burden in the airways and improve patient outcomes, such as lung function and exacerbation frequency. Currently, the only FDA-approved inhaled antibiotics are tobramycin inhalation solution (Bethkis, Tobi), tobramycin inhalation powder (Tobi Podhaler), and aztreonam inhalation solution (Cayston) for patients with CF with *P. aeruginosa*. For patients who newly acquire *P. aeruginosa*, it is recommended to treat with an inhaled antibiotic for 28 days, with the preferred agent being tobramycin-inhaled solution, in an attempt to eradicate the pathogen. The use of an inhaled antibiotic to prevent acquisition of *P. aeruginosa* is not recommended. For patients with CF with the persistent presence of *P. aeruginosa* from respiratory cultures, the chronic use of inhaled antibiotics, such as tobramycin or aztreonam, is recommended to improve lung function and reduce exacerbations. For chronic use, cycling (e.g., on 28 days, off 28 days) of an inhaled antibiotic is common. The use of continuous inhaled antibiotic therapy in which two different inhaled antibiotics (e.g., tobramycin and aztreonam) are used rotationally is not routine but has been used by specialists in cases of multidrug-resistant pathogens, advanced or severe lung disease, or frequent acute exacerbations.

Antiinflammatory agents—specifically oral azithromycin and/or high-dose ibuprofen—are also noted in the current guidelines. Azithromycin (Zithromax), a macrolide antibiotic, is not used in chronic CF for its antiinfective properties but for its antiinflammatory and immunomodulatory properties. For patients with CF with the persistent presence of *P. aeruginosa* from respiratory cultures, the use of chronic azithromycin[1] is recommended to improve lung function and reduce exacerbations. Use in patients with CF who lack the persistent presence of *P. aeruginosa* can be considered to help reduce the frequency of exacerbations. Monitoring for the presence of nontuberculosis mycobacterium in respiratory cultures and the potential for drug interactions with azithromycin (e.g., medications that may prolong the QT interval) is recommended with the use of chronic azithromycin. A less commonly used antiinflammatory agent used among certified CF centers is high-dose ibuprofen[1]. The therapeutic benefit of slowing the loss of lung function is greatest in children 6 to 17 years of age. This therapy requires therapeutic drug monitoring (i.e., pharmacokinetic assessment of serum ibuprofen levels) and dose adjustment. Subtherapeutic levels can have negative effects on lung function because of an increase in inflammatory mediators, and supratherapeutic levels increase the risk for toxicities (e.g., bleeding, nephrotoxicity). This therapy is less commonly used because of its potential for adverse effects, the need for laboratory monitoring, and the need for pharmacokinetic-based dosing. Routine, chronic use of systemic steroids such as prednisone is not recommended in the chronic management of CF.

CFTR modulators, a newer class of medications, are available for patients with CF with certain CF genotypes. The initial consideration for use and dosing of CFTR modulators is based on age, CF genotype, weight, concurrent therapy, ability to swallow tablets or capsules, and available dosage forms. There are three main types: potentiators, correctors, and amplifiers; however, the latter type is not currently available and is being developed and studied. Ivacaftor (Kalydeco) is a potentiator, increasing chloride movement through the CFTR protein channel. Ivacaftor is currently approved for patients aged 1 month or older who have the approved genotypes with gating and conducting mutations. Lumacaftor is a corrector, facilitating correct formation and stabilization of the CFTR protein. Lumacaftor is combined with ivacaftor as Orkambi for the treatment of CF and is currently approved for

patients aged 1 year or older whose genotype is homozygous *Phe-508del*. Tezacaftor is also a corrector but is longer acting and has some differences compared with lumacaftor with regard to drug interactions and side effects. Like lumacaftor, tezacaftor is a corrector combined with ivacaftor as Symdeko for chronic treatment of CF. Symdeko is currently approved for patients aged 6 years or older whose genotype is homozygous *Phe508del* and a number of residual function mutations. Elexacaftor is also a corrector; however, it binds to a different site on the CFTR protein than tezacaftor. Elexacaftor provides an additive effect in improving cellular processing and trafficking of CFTR, resulting in improved outcomes, including lung function, symptoms (cough, sputum production), exacerbation rate, and nutritional status. Elexacaftor is combined with tezacaftor and ivacaftor as Trikafta and is currently approved for patients aged 2 years or older who have at least one *Phe508del* mutation or other approved genotypes. Patients on lumacaftor-ivacaftor or tezacaftor-lumacaftor should be considered for transition to elexacaftor-tezacaftor-ivacaftor when of appropriate age. Currently, tezacaftor-lumacaftor and elexacaftor-tezacaftor-ivacaftor are available in tablet blister packs with combination tablets (morning doses) and ivacaftor (evening doses). It is important to make patients/caregivers aware of the different-appearing packaging, prescribed dosing, and administration. With the availability of highly effective CFTR modulator therapy, such as elexacaftor-tezacaftor-ivacaftor, studies about possibly "stepping down" chronic therapy (i.e., discontinuing inhaled mucolytic therapy such as hypertonic saline and/or dornase alfa) in adolescents and adults with CF are ongoing.

All of the mentioned CFTR modulators have similar administration and monitoring considerations. Liver function tests for aspartate aminotransferase (AST), alanine aminotransferase (ALT), and total bilirubin should be done before starting therapy, followed by every 3 months for the first year of therapy and annually thereafter. More frequent monitoring may be indicated if AST and/or ALT elevations are identified. As noncongenital lens opacities or cataracts have been reported in pediatric patients with ivacaftor, a baseline ophthalmologic examination (e.g., slit lamp exam) is also recommended in patients who are younger than 18 years of age. Follow-up ophthalmologic examinations are recommended, but the frequency is not well defined. Doses should be taken with a fatty meal and with pancreatic enzymes (for those who require the use of pancreatic enzymes as part of CF management). All of the listed CFTR modulators are substrates and/or inducers of CYP3A4 and other CYP450 isoenzymes (e.g., CYP2C9), so screening for and managing drug interactions are essential. In addition, dosing modifications or discontinuation may be necessary for moderate or severe hepatic dysfunction. FDA-approved age and CF genotype indications for each of the CFTR modulators may be updated with ongoing clinical trials in young ages and other CF genotypes; thus it is recommended to check the latest FDA-approved indications when considering use.

Acute Pharmacologic Therapy

Many patients with CF, despite the use of chronic therapies, experience pulmonary exacerbations requiring treatment. In addition to increased frequency of airway clearance or chest physiotherapy, acute pulmonary exacerbations may require the use of systemic antimicrobials. Whenever possible, the selection of systemic antimicrobial agents should be guided by a patient-specific history of respiratory cultures and patient clinical response to past regimens.

When a systemic antimicrobial is required for outpatient management, an oral antibiotic is commonly used, with the duration of most agents being 10 to 14 days. For example, if a given patient has a history of *P. aeruginosa*, use of oral ciprofloxacin (Cipro)[1] or levofloxacin (Levaquin)[1] for 14 to 21 days may be appropriate. Patients who have inhaled antibiotics as part of their chronic regimen may continue treatment cycles during outpatient

---

[1] Not FDA approved for this indication.

[1] Not FDA approved for this indication.

treatment for acute pulmonary exacerbation. Some CF centers may use home infusion services for intravenous (IV) antimicrobials; however, this requires additional logistic considerations, including nursing support, infusion equipment, and laboratory monitoring. In addition, factors related to adherence to airway clearance, social support system at home, and appropriateness of home IV access should be considered.

For inpatient management, the use of IV antibiotics is more common, and the use of oral antibiotic(s) may also be part of the regimen. *P. aeruginosa* is often "double-covered" when possible, specifically when hospitalized and/or requiring IV antimicrobials. "Double-coverage" involves the use of two agents active against *P. aeruginosa* from two different antibiotic classes (e.g., beta-lactam and aminoglycoside). The use of both inhaled and systemic (e.g., IV) antibiotics of the same class (e.g., aminoglycosides) simultaneously is not common. Another approach is starting IV antimicrobials in the inpatient setting, with transition and completion of the therapy course with home infusion services.

There are special instances in which longer courses of medications such as antibiotics or antifungal therapy may be necessary. For example, in the treatment of nontuberculosis mycobacterium (e.g., *Mycobacterium abscessus*), multiple types of antibiotics (e.g., inhaled and oral) may be used for extended durations (e.g., months). In the treatment of allergic bronchopulmonary aspergillosis, antifungal therapy may be used in addition to systemic corticosteroids (e.g., prednisone) for extensive periods (e.g., weeks or months). These more complex antimicrobial treatment courses are often managed by specialists (e.g., pulmonary and/or infectious disease specialists).

Nutritional/Gastrointestinal Treatment
Nonpharmacologic Therapy
Persons with CF often have greater dietary energy intake needs. Consistent, high-calorie dietary intake can be a challenge because of several physiologic factors, including loss of taste or smell caused by chronic sinusitis and chronic gastroesophageal reflux. Behavioral factors may affect nutritional intake, necessitating behavioral intervention by dietitians and/or psychologists. For patients of all ages with continued suboptimal growth, the use of enteral feeding modes may also be necessary. For patients who have chronic constipation or a history of distal intestinal obstructive syndrome (DIOS), appropriate hydration and increased fiber content in the diet are recommended.

Infant formulas and breast milk do not provide adequate sodium for infants with CF. Because of excessive sodium loss through insensible loss, infants are at risk for developing hyponatremic, hypochloremia dehydration. It is recommended that ⅛ teaspoon of table salt be provided from birth and increased with time to ¼ teaspoon by 6 months through 1 year of age, divided throughout the day by feedings. Additional supplementation may be necessary for children and adults living in high-temperature climates and/or involved in considerable physical activities (e.g., sports).

Chronic Pharmacologic Therapy
For patients with pancreatic insufficiency, the use of pancreatic enzyme replacement therapy (PERT) is needed. There are various brands of PERT that contain various amounts of lipase, protease, and amylase. Pancreatic enzymes should be taken at meal times and snack times and in coordination with enteral feeds (when applicable). The dosing of PERT is based on the lipase component. Typical pancreatic enzyme initial dosing ranges from 500 to 1500 units of lipase per kilogram of body weight per meal, with a maximum of either 10,000 units of lipase per kilogram per day or 2500 units of lipase per kilogram per meal. Enzyme preparations come in a range of concentrations to accommodate all patient needs and minimize the number of capsules required. Given the number of medications a person with CF may require for chronic management, clinicians should be mindful about how many capsules are required per meal or snack when selecting a brand and strength of pancreatic enzyme. When maximal PERT dosing is reached and

the patient continues to present with symptoms of malabsorption (e.g., steatorrhea), other etiologies should be investigated. Some clinicians may add an acid suppression agent (e.g., a proton pump inhibitor or H2 receptor antagonist) to help enhance the activity of pancreatic enzymes through decreasing duodenal acidity; however, the potential risks of long-term acid suppression (e.g., small intestinal bacterial overgrowth [SIBO]) should be considered. A proton pump inhibitor or H2 receptor antagonist may also be used to treat concurrent gastroesophageal reflux disease.

Supplementation of fat-soluble vitamins (i.e., A, D, E, K) should be provided via specially formulated multivitamins, available in various dosage forms with dosing based on age. Monitoring of vitamin levels is often done at least annually, with adjustments in supplementation of individual vitamins (e.g., vitamin D, cholecalciferol) based on adherence to current treatment, age, and level of deficiency.

For those with chronic constipation or history of DIOS, chronic use of an osmotic laxative such as over-the-counter polyethylene glycol 3350 (MiraLAX)[1] may be helpful. Oral N-acetylcysteine (Mucomyst)[1] has also been used for the prevention of mucus accumulation in the gastrointestinal (GI) tract of some individuals with DIOS.

Acute Pharmacologic Therapy
Patients presenting with DIOS often require more aggressive treatment than that for chronic constipation related to CF. Treatment of DIOS may include laxatives at higher doses or the use of electrolyte intestinal lavage solution (e.g., GoLYTELY)[1] or hyperosmolar enemas. Oral and/or rectal administration[1] of N-acetylcysteine solution has also been used for the treatment of mucus accumulation in the GI tract of some individuals with DIOS.

Monitoring
Monitoring of pulmonary symptoms should be done at each encounter. Spirometry to assess lung function is recommended as part of CF clinic visits to assess changes in forced expiratory volume in 1 second (FEV1) relative to baseline. In addition, routine respiratory cultures including screening for acid-fast bacilli and fungi to monitor for pathogens and susceptibilities are recommended. Nutritional status (e.g., weight, height, weight for length, body mass index) should also be monitored regularly. Annual routine laboratory testing is also done through CF centers and screenings for complications (e.g., CFRD). Recommended monitoring for the various chronic therapies is discussed in the previous section.

Management of Other Complications
In addition to the general manifestation of CF (e.g., pulmonary, growth, and nutrition), complications may appear with age and disease progression. The following are examples and general management approaches. Referral to other specialists, such as endocrinology, gastroenterology, otorhinolaryngology, or transplant (when appropriate for advanced disease), may be necessary.

Sinusitis
Treatment of the acute exacerbations of sinusitis can include systemic (e.g., oral) antibiotics, which are also used in pulmonary exacerbations. The use of intranasal irrigations of antimicrobials (e.g., gentamicin)[1] may also be considered, although guidelines defining and comparing intranasal irrigation agent selection, formulation, dosing, and monitoring are currently lacking.

Small Intestinal Bacterial Overgrowth
Treatment of SIBO in persons with CF is similar to treatment of those without CF, including the use of oral antibiotics (e.g., rifaximin [Xifaxan][1]). Nonpharmacologic treatment may include dietary manipulation, such as reducing carbohydrate consumption, resulting in a high-fat, low-carbohydrate diet.

---

[1] Not FDA approved for this indication.

BOX 1 Etiologies of Transudative and Exudative Effusions

Transudative
Congestive heart failure
Cirrhosis
Pulmonary emboli
Peritoneal dialysis
Renal disorders
Myxedema
Sarcoidosis

Exudative
Malignancy
Infection
Drugs (e.g., nitrofurantoin [Marcodantin, Macrobid],
    methotrexate [Trexall])
Chylothorax
Pulmonary emboli
Gastrointestinal diseases (e.g., pancreatitis)
Collagen vascular disease (e.g., rheumatoid arthritis)
Asbestos exposure
Trauma (e.g., hemothorax, chest surgery)
Postpericardiectomy or postmyocardial infarction syndrome
Pleuropericarditis

effusions. The causes are varied, but the most common causes are malignancy, infection, and pulmonary emboli.

Diagnosis

Imaging

Approximately 200 to 500 mL of pleural fluid is necessary before it can be visualized on a posteroanterior upright chest x-ray, usually as blunting of the costophrenic angle. A lateral decubitus chest x-ray is more sensitive, often discerning fluid with as little as 100 mL present; layering of the fluid confirms that it is free flowing. Loculations can be seen on x-ray but may be mistaken for lung or pleural masses. Large effusion can completely opacify the hemithorax where the effusion is located. Distinguishing pleural fluid from atelectatic lung due to airway occlusion can be challenging and, in such cases, drainage should not be attempted until ambiguity is resolved by additional imaging studies.

Ultrasound is useful in defining the location and extent of an effusion and can also identify loculated effusions, pleural thickening, and masses. When used to help guide thoracentesis, it can increase diagnostic accuracy and yield and decrease complications.

Chest computed tomography (CT) has distinct advantages over x-ray and ultrasound, although without intravenous contrast it may still be difficult to differentiate pleural fluid from consolidated lung. The utility of chest CT to detect masses is significantly decreased when there is a large effusion associated with compressive atelectasis. Imaging with CT after initial drainage of a large effusion is recommended to obtain the most information regarding the possible etiologies of the effusion and aid in operative planning for treatment of an empyema. It also delineates pleural masses and helps differentiate pleural disease from lung pathology (e.g., loculated effusion vs. lung abscess).

Thoracentesis

It is often difficult to discern the cause of an effusion solely based on the patient's clinical presentation and image studies. Also, when concerned about a malignant process or an infected effusion, these studies do not give enough information to make a definitive diagnosis. Thoracentesis is the diagnostic procedure of choice, allowing drainage of the fluid to relieve symptoms for the patient and provide a specimen for evaluation. Ultrasound should be employed to help guide thoracentesis, especially if the effusion is small or loculated. Care must be taken when draining a large amount of fluid in one setting due to the risk of reexpansion pulmonary edema. If a patient becomes symptomatic during the procedure (persistent cough, significant pleuritic pain, or shortness of breath), no more fluid should be removed at that time. Coagulopathy is a contraindication to thoracentesis due to the risk of intrathoracic bleeding. If the fluid appears cloudy, bloody, or milky then leaving a drainage catheter in place following thoracentesis should be strongly considered. Imaging should be obtained after all drainage procedures to document resolution and ensure that no pneumothorax is present. Pneumothorax after thoracentesis may be iatrogenic but may also reflect inability of a trapped lung to fully expand (ex vacuo pneumothorax) and warrants additional work-up.

Pleural Fluid

The initial evaluation of pleural fluid is done at the bedside by inspecting the fluid for color, viscosity, and odor. These simple steps can point the clinician toward the correct diagnosis. In addition to bedside evaluation, the fluid should be sent for the following laboratory studies: pH, glucose, lactate dehydrogenase (LDH), protein, cytology, Gram stain, and culture (including fungal and viral). Serum pH, protein, LDH and glucose should be sent at the same time.

Light's criteria are helpful in differentiating between an exudative and transudative effusion (Box 2). The sensitivity and specificity of Light's criteria is 82% to 90%.

Transudative effusions rarely need any further intervention, and the goal of treatment is directed at the underlying condition (see Box 1). For exudative effusions, the cause of the effusion dictates the treatment. Incorporating the clinical picture and radiographs with the pleural fluid chemistry studies, cytology, and cultures, the diagnosis is often obtained. Malignant effusions can have positive cytology, but they are more likely to have a pleural fluid glucose level less than 60 mg/dL and to be bloody. An elevated amylase level is seen in esophageal perforation, pancreatitis, and malignant effusions. Chylothorax can be definitively diagnosed if the triglyceride level is more than 110 mg/dL within the pleural fluid. Finally, pH, glucose, and cultures are useful in the treatment of patients with a presumed infected pleural effusion (empyema).

Up to 25% of patients will not have a definitive diagnosis based on the clinical scenario and pleural fluid evaluation. These patients can require further diagnostic testing, including repeat thoracentesis or evaluation of the chest cavity via video-assisted thoracoscopic surgery (VATS) with pleural biopsies.

Treatment

After initial evacuation of pleural fluid effusion, treatment is directed at preventing reaccumulation. In the case of hepatic hydrothorax, cardiogenic effusion or effusion related to renal insufficiency, the effusion should resolve with appropriate medical treatment of the underlying disease. Esophageal perforation and chylothorax generally require addressing the primary process with endoscopic, interventional, or surgical approaches. Special cases in which surgical management may be indicated include malignant and infectious effusions.

Malignant Pleural Effusion

Palliation of malignant pleural effusions is accomplished either by pleurodesis or palliative indwelling catheter. Both strategies are more likely be successful in patients being treated with appropriate chemotherapy.

The most effective strategy for chemical pleurodesis is thoracoscopically directed spray talc pleurodesis, which will achieve resolution in about 85% of cases. A VATS approach has the added advantage that directed pleural biopsies may be obtained, with a significantly higher sensitivity for diagnosing pleural metastatic disease than fluid cytology alone. Bedside pleurodesis via tube thoracostomy can be attempted but is less likely to be successful.

Pleural fluid-to-serum ratio of protein >0.5
Pleural fluid-to-serum ration of LDH >0.6
Absolute pleural fluid LDH >2/3 of upper limit of normal
   serum levels

LDH, Lactate dehydrogenase.

For very high output malignant effusions or if incompletely lung expansion occurs, a tunneled indwelling long-term silicone-elastic catheter (PleurX) may be placed either operatively or percutaneously. This tube may be drained with a closed suction canister either on a regular schedule or as needed for symptoms. Regular drainage of malignant effusion achieves spontaneous pleurodesis in the majority of cases in about 6 weeks.

Infected Pleural Space and Empyema

A parapneumonic effusion (exudative effusion in the setting of pulmonary infection) is seen in 20% to 40% of patients admitted for pneumonia, of whom 10% to 20% will develop a complicated parapneumonic effusion or empyema (pus in the pleural space). Progression to empyema is most often due to delay in treatment and leads to longer hospital stays and increased morbidity and mortality. Other causes of infected effusions are trauma, thoracic surgical procedures, perforated esophagus, systemic infection, and transdiaphragmatic spread.

Parapneumonic effusions can be separated into three stages: exudative (stage I), fibropurulent (stage II), and organizational (stage III). Stage I effusions are free flowing, sterile reactive exudates and often do not reaccumulate after initial drainage. Although small, minimally symptomatic stage I effusions may resolve with appropriate antibiotics, it is difficult to determine the stage of an effusion clinically and at a minimum thoracentesis is indicated in most cases. Careful consideration should always be given to leaving a drainage tube in case a more advanced parapneumonic effusion is diagnosed.

Stage II effusions, or complicated parapneumonic effusions, are more viscous with lower glucose level and pH. Multiple pockets of loculated fluid with proteinaceous septations may be present. Complete drainage of all loculations is required to prevent progression to empyema or organized effusion and a chest drain (image-guided percutaneous catheter or thoracostomy tube) should be left behind in all cases. Early surgical intervention with thoracoscopic adhesiolysis may be considered if loculations are present. Alternatively, combination therapy with intrapleural tissue plasminogen activator (t-PA) and deoxyribonuclease (DNase) improves fluid drainage and reduces the need for surgical intervention. Complete drainage of all loculated pockets is of paramount importance and surgery may still be necessary after treatment with fibrinolytics.

Complicated parapneumonic effusions may go unrecognized and be treated late, particularly in patients with other medical or social comorbidities such as diabetes mellitus, dementia, developmental delay, and intravenous drug use. The result is progression to frank intrapleural pus, or empyema. Complete evacuation of the effusion is now required, and initial tube thoracostomy is indicated although often insufficient. If the patient does not improve promptly or the space is not completely drained, then surgery is recommended. The initial attempt at drainage should be thoracoscopic although conversion to thoracotomy may be required. Multiple large-bore chest tubes should be left in place until drainage has resolved. In the presence of frank pus, fibrinolytic therapy is less likely to be of benefit, although it may be considered in patients who are medically unable to tolerate surgery.

If infected fluid is evacuated but a residual cavity remains, then chronic infection is likely. This risk is greatly increased by the presence of a bronchopleural fistula, either arising from a lung abscess or due to surgical complication. In these situations, long-term drainage with an open thoracostomy or Eloesser flap, may be required to eradicate the infection. Ultimate obliteration of the space may require a rotational muscle flap.

If the pleural space is incompletely drained but adequately sterilized with antibiotics, the effusion may progress to the organizational stage. This is characterized by heavy fibrin deposit with the formation of a thick peel throughout the pleura with loculations and trapping of the lung, preventing re-expansion. Patients may report significant dyspnea and pulmonary function tests will show a restrictive pattern. Classic CT findings include thickened pleura with multiple loculations. Decortication, either via VATS or thoracotomy, is required to completely remove the peel off the parietal and visceral pleura. A robotic-assisted approach increases the likelihood of successful minimally invasive decortication.

References

Davies Helen E, et al: Effect of an indwelling pleural catheter vs chest tube and talc pleurodesis for relieving dyspnea in patients with malignant pleural effusion: the TIME2 randomized controlled trial, *JAMA* 307(22):2383–2389, 2012.

de Campos JR, Vargas FS, de Campos Werebe E, et al: Thoracoscopy talc poudrage: A 15- year experience, *Chest* 119:801–806, 2001.

Feller-Kopman David, Light Richard: Pleural disease, *N Engl J Med* 378(8):740–751, 2018.

Luh SP, Chen CY, Tzao CY: Malignant pleural effusion treatment outcomes: Pleurodesis via Video- Assisted Thoracic Surgery (VATS) versus tube thoracostomy, *Thorac Cardiovasc Surg* 54:332–336, 2006.

Luh SP, Hsu GJ, Cheng- Ren C: Complicated parapneumonic effusion and empyema: Pleural decortication and video- assisted thoracic surgery, *Curr Infect Dis Rep* 10:236–240, 2008.

Rahman NM, Chapman SJ, Davies RJ: Diagnosis and management of infectious pleural effusion, *Treat Respir Med* 5:295–304, 2006.

Rahman Najib M, et al: Intrapleural use of tissue plasminogen activator and DNase in pleural infection, *N Engl J Med* 365(6):518–526, 2011.

PNEUMOCONIOSIS: ASBESTOSIS AND SILICOSIS

Method of
David N. Weissman, MD

CURRENT DIAGNOSIS

- History of inhalation of mineral or metal dust
- Respiratory symptoms such as cough and dyspnea
- Spirometry and lung volumes show restriction or mixed obstruction/restriction in advanced disease
- Interstitial lung disease can usually be demonstrated by chest imaging. Biopsy is usually unnecessary in the setting of good exposure history and typical findings on chest imaging.
- No other likely cause of interstitial lung disease is present

CURRENT THERAPY

- Treatment is symptomatic and similar to that for other patients with chronic lung disease
- Give pneumococcal and influenza vaccinations.
- Provide empiric treatment with short- and long-acting inhaled bronchodilators and inhaled corticosteroids when they are found to provide symptomatic relief.
- Give supplemental oxygen therapy if pulmonary hypertension is present or to prevent pulmonary hypertension if O_2 saturation is less than 88% at rest, with exercise, or with sleep.
- Consider lung transplantation in the setting of end-stage lung disease.

TABLE 1   Representative Pneumoconioses

SOURCE	MAIN CLINICAL FEATURES	OCCUPATION	DUST
Crystalline silica	Silicosis, COPD, increased susceptibility to TB, lung cancer, autoimmune diseases	Mining, stone cutting, pottery, foundry work, artificial stone countertop work	Free crystalline silica (SiO_2)
Asbestiform fibers	Asbestosis, bronchogenic carcinoma, mesothelioma, various forms of benign pleural disease	Insulation, shipbuilding, construction, some mining (e.g., vermiculite mining in Libby, MT)	Various asbestiform fibers
Coal	Coal workers' pneumoconiosis, COPD	Coal mining	Coal mine dust
Hard metal	Hard metal lung disease (cobalt lung), asthma	Machinists, metal workers	Hard metal, composed primarily of tungsten carbide and cobalt

COPD, chronic obstructive pulmonary disease; *TB*, tuberculosis.

The pneumoconioses are a group of interstitial fibrotic lung diseases predominantly associated with occupational exposures. They are caused by inhalation of mineral or metallic dust particles small enough to penetrate into the deep lung (respirable size range) (Table 1). These agents interact with pulmonary target cells, including alveolar macrophages and alveolar epithelial cells, to activate a cascade of inflammatory mediators including growth factors. Although exposure to these dusts can induce other types of respiratory disease as well, the final common pathway leading to pneumoconiosis is alveolar epithelial cell damage and interstitial fibrosis. This chapter focuses on silicosis and asbestosis, two common forms of pneumoconiosis.

Asbestosis

Asbestos is composed of strong, heat-resistant fibers of hydrated magnesium silicate classified morphologically as serpentine (chrysotile) or amphibole (crocidolite [riebeckite asbestos], amosite [cummingtonite-grunerite asbestos], anthophyllite asbestos, actinolite asbestos, and tremolite asbestos). In addition, certain asbestiform fibers (winchite, richterite, erionite) can cause adverse health effects identical to those of asbestos. Fiber dimensions and persistence in tissues are key determinants of toxicity. There is a dose–response effect between the quantity of asbestos inhaled and the severity of fibrotic lung disease. Asbestos is also a carcinogen, and increasing exposure is associated with increased risk for lung cancer, mesothelioma, ovarian cancer, and laryngeal cancer.

Although asbestos is no longer mined in the United States, importation of asbestos-containing products continues. Exposures also continue to occur, especially in construction and renovation (due to reservoirs of asbestos that are still present in many older buildings), the heating trades (where asbestos is often encountered), and with exposure to older or imported asbestos-containing automotive friction products such as brake linings and clutch facings. Workers exposed to asbestos can carry it home on their clothing, resulting in exposure of family members. Living near geological formations prone to asbestos formation in California has been implicated as a risk factor for mesothelioma.

The Occupational Safety and Health Administration (OSHA) permissible exposure limit (PEL) for asbestos is 0.1 fiber per cc air. This limit was based in part on the limits of the analytical methodology used in exposure assessment. Exposure to the PEL every day over a 45-year working lifetime has been estimated to be associated with an increased risk of cancer (lung, mesothelioma, and gastrointestinal) of 336 cases per 100,000 exposed persons and an increased risk of asbestosis of 250 cases per 100,000 exposed persons.

Asbestosis causes symptoms of dyspnea and cough. Latency between initial exposure and disease onset is related to exposure intensity. In the United States, this period is generally about two or more decades. The disease can lead to chronic respiratory failure. Effects of smoking add to the severity of the disease and can cause obstructive findings in addition to the expected decreased lung volume and diffusion capacity associated with fibrotic lung diseases. Bibasilar inspiratory crackles on auscultation, finger clubbing, and bibasilar small, irregular parenchymal opacities on chest x-ray with extension to mid- and upper-zones with advancing disease are characteristic.

The International Labour Organization (ILO) has established a system for classification (grading) of radiographs for the presence of radiographic abnormalities in lung parenchyma and pleura that are associated with pneumoconiosis, as well as their severity. The ILO classification system is widely used in epidemiology, surveillance, administrative, and legal settings. The small opacity profusion grades of 0/1 and 1/0 are often considered as defining the boundary between normal and abnormal lung parenchyma.

High-resolution computed tomography (CT) is the most sensitive imaging method for suspected asbestosis. Findings associated with asbestos exposure include lower lobe or diffuse irregular opacities, bronchial wall thickening, rounded atelectasis, and pleural abnormalities such as pleural plaques and diffuse pleural thickening. The presence of pleural plaques on radiography (particularly bilateral calcified pleural plaques); or uncoated asbestos fibers or fibers coated with an iron-rich proteinaceous material (asbestos bodies) in sputum, bronchoalveolar lavage, or lung biopsy help differentiate asbestosis from idiopathic pulmonary fibrosis.

Criteria for Diagnosis

Diagnosis is supported by radiographic chest imaging or lung biopsy findings of interstitial lung disease compatible with asbestosis; documentation of exposure to asbestos by history, the presence of pleural plaques (bilateral pleural plaques are essentially pathognomonic for asbestos exposure), or the presence of asbestos bodies or an excessive burden of uncoated asbestos fibers in lung biopsy tissue or possibly via bronchoalveolar lavage or sputum; and no other likely explanation for the diffuse fibrotic lung disease.

Asbestos-Related Benign Pleural Disease

Pleural plaques are characteristic forms of localized parietal pleural thickening that are usually bilateral and asymmetrical, involve the lower lung fields or the diaphragm, and spare the costophrenic angles and apices. Pleural plaques are a marker for exposure to asbestos and are often associated with other asbestos-related conditions. Pleural plaques generally result in minimal reductions in forced vital capacity and do not degenerate into malignant lesions.

In contrast, diffuse visceral pleural thickening can result in adhesions between the visceral and parietal pleura with major decreases in forced vital capacity and respiratory insufficiency sufficient for considerathon of decortication.

Benign pleural effusions can occur in the first decade after asbestos exposure and contain erythrocytes and a mixed inflammatory cell infiltrate of lymphocytes, neutrophils, and eosinophils. The thickened visceral pleura and adjacent atelectatic lung tissue can result in a pleural-based area of rounded atelectasis, simulating a lung mass on chest radiography. CT can reveal the comet sign, a pleural band connecting the apparent mass to an area of thickened pleura.

Lung Cancer and Malignant Mesothelioma

Exposure to all forms of asbestos increases the risk of lung cancer. The peak risk occurs at about 30 to 35 years after the onset of exposure. Tobacco smoking increases this risk in a supra-additive fashion, increasing risk to a level greater than for asbestos or smoking alone. In contrast, smoking does not further increase the asbestos-associated risk for malignant mesothelioma. Asbestos-associated malignant mesothelioma can also affect the peritoneum (and sometimes the pericardium), but when it affects the pleura, this disease manifests with dyspnea, chest pain, and bloody pleural effusion (most often unilateral). A latency period of 30 years or longer after initial exposure is common. Biopsy and specialized immunohistochemical stains are typically required to distinguish malignant mesothelioma from benign mesothelial proliferations and various carcinomas such as adenocarcinomas. It is currently unclear when to screen asbestos-exposed individuals at increased risk for lung cancer with low-dose chest computed tomography.

Treatment

Treatment of asbestosis is primarily symptomatic and similar to that for other patients with chronic lung disease (Box 1). The U.S. Food and Drug Administration (FDA) recently approved the anti-fibrotic drug nintedanib (Ofev) to slow the rate of decline of pulmonary function in chronic fibrosing interstitial lung diseases with a progressive phenotype. However, the safety and effectiveness of treating progressive asbestosis with nintedanib[1] has not yet been documented in the literature and hence, remains unknown. Lung transplantation should be considered in the setting of end-stage lung disease. Treatment of benign pleural disease is also symptomatic; as already noted, decortication is an option for managing severe cases of diffuse visceral pleural thickening. Depending on extent of disease, mesothelioma may be treated with surgery, radiation, chemotherapy, or some combination of these. In general, prognosis is poor. Mesothelioma-associated malignant pleural effusion can require palliation through procedures such as pleurodesis, pleurectomy, and decortication. Asbestos-associated lung cancer is managed in the same fashion as lung cancer occurring without a history of exposure to asbestos.

Silicosis

Silicosis is a fibrosing interstitial lung disease resulting from the inhalation of crystalline silicon dioxide (silica) in dust of respirable size. The commonest form of crystalline silica is quartz, which is the main component of sand and is present in most rocks. Noncrystalline (amorphous) silica, like that in diatomaceous earth or glass, does not cause silicosis. However, heating amorphous silica, as occurs in foundries when molten metal is poured into clay castings, can convert amorphous silica into cristobalite, a hazardous form of crystalline silica. Mining, stone cutting, sandblasting, and foundry work are all examples of trades associated with exposure to respirable dust containing crystalline silica. The International Agency for Research on Cancer (IARC) has designated crystalline silica as a Group 1 human lung carcinogen.

In 2016, OSHA established a new PEL for respirable crystalline silica of $0.05 \, mg/m^3$. It also established requirements for engineering and administrative controls, personal protective equipment, and medical surveillance including periodic chest radiography and spirometry obtained at least every 3 years. Reporting of silicosis cases to public health authorities is required in some states.

[1]Not FDA approved for this indication.

Radiographic Patterns of Silicosis

Three main radiographic patterns of silicosis have been described. Two are nodular interstitial patterns and one is an alveolar-filling pattern. The *simple* pattern is associated with nodules that are smaller than 10 mm and that are predominantly rounded and in the upper lung zones. *Progressive massive fibrosis* (PMF) is found in more advanced interstitial disease. It is associated with multiple coalescent larger nodules, upper lobe fibrosis, upward retraction of the hila, and compensatory hyperinflation of the lower lobes. The large upper-zone opacities can cavitate, sometimes in the setting of superimposed mycobacterial infection. Hilar adenopathy can occur in association with either pattern, sometimes with an egg-shell pattern of hilar node calcification. A third radiographic pattern is an alveolar-filling process. Overwhelming silica exposure over a short period can cause a pathologic response called *silicoproteinosis*, in which alveoli become flooded with proteinaceous fluid. The condition resembles idiopathic pulmonary alveolar proteinosis. The radiographic alveolar filling pattern favors the lower lung zones and is not necessarily associated with the changes of simple silicosis or PMF.

Silicosis Syndromes

Three syndromes of silicosis can be defined based on clinical course and radiographic pattern. Chronic silicosis develops slowly, usually 10 to 30 years after first exposure. It most often has the simple radiographic pattern, but it can be associated with PMF.

Accelerated silicosis develops more rapidly, within 10 years after first exposure. It is associated with higher intensity exposures and can be associated with either the simple or PMF radiographic patterns. Accelerated silicosis is differentiated from chronic silicosis by its more rapid course. Patients with accelerated courses are at greater risk for developing PMF. The clinical presentations of chronic and accelerated silicosis are variable but include cough, dyspnea, and a variety of chest findings ranging from a normal chest examination to crackles, rhonchi, or wheezing. PMF is associated with more severe symptoms and respiratory impairment. Findings compatible with both restrictive and obstructive lung disease (decreased forced vital capacity [FVC], forced expiratory volume at 1 sec [FEV$_1$], FEV$_1$/FVC, diffusion capacity) can occur, potentially leading to cor pulmonale and respiratory failure.

Acute silicosis is associated with very intense exposures to silica, leading to symptoms within a few weeks to a few years after exposure. Intense exposure results in lung injury caused by flooding of alveoli with proteinaceous material, or silicoproteinosis. As already noted, the radiographic appearance is that of an alveolar-filling pattern favoring the lower lung zones. Patients present weeks to a few years after exposure with cough, weight loss, fatigue, and occasional pleuritic chest pain, crackles on auscultation, and progression to respiratory failure often complicated by mycobacterial infection.

Criteria for Diagnosis

The diagnosis of silicosis is predicated on a history of exposure to respirable crystalline silica, typical chest x-ray findings, and the lack of a more likely diagnosis. High-resolution CT detects changes of silicosis with greater sensitivity than chest radiography. Lung biopsy is seldom required for diagnosis in the setting of a good exposure history and typical findings on chest imaging.

Treatment

Treatment is primarily symptomatic and similar to that for other patients with chronic lung disease (see Box 1). Experimental therapies such as oral corticosteroid therapy and whole-lung lavage have been reported, but clinical benefit is unclear. Similarly, as noted for asbestosis, the clinical benefit of treating progressive silicosis with the antifibrotic drug nintedanib is also currently unclear. Lung transplantation should be considered for patients with end-stage lung disease.

All forms of silicosis, as well as substantial exposure to crystalline silica in the absence of silicosis, are associated with an increased risk of pulmonary tuberculosis and fungal infections. Patients should be evaluated for latent tuberculosis infection by tuberculin skin testing or with an interferon gamma release assay. A positive tuberculin skin test in a patient with a history of substantial silica exposure of at least 10 mm of induration should be considered evidence of tuberculosis infection, regardless of previous immunization with bacille Calmette-Guérin. If testing for latent tuberculosis infection is positive, an evaluation for active tuberculosis should be performed and active disease treated. If active tuberculosis is not present, treat for latent infection. As in other settings, treatment for active or latent infection should be provided using one of the drug treatment protocols recommended by the Centers for Disease Control and Prevention. Vaccination for influenza should be provided annually. In addition, adults with silicosis should be vaccinated with 15-valent pneumococcal conjugate vaccine (PCV 15, Vaxneuvance) and 23-valent pneumococcal polysaccharide vaccine (PPSV23, Pneumovax 23) or with PCV 20 (Prevnar 20) alone, according to current Centers for Disease Control and Prevention recommendations.

Disclaimer

The findings and conclusions in this report are those of the authors and do not necessarily represent the views of the National Institute for Occupational Safety and Health or the Centers for Disease Control and Prevention.

References

American Thoracic Society: Diagnosis and initial management of nonmalignant diseases related to asbestos, *Am J Respir Crit Care Med* 170(6):691–715, 2004.
CDC (Centers for Disease Control and Prevention). 2016. Recommended vaccines by age. Available at: https://www.cdc.gov/vaccines/vpd/vaccines-age.html, accessed 3/14/2017.
Department of Labor: Mine Safety and Health Administration: 30 CFR Parts 56, 57, and 71. Asbestos exposure limit; proposed rule, *Fed Reg* 70:43950–43989, 2005.
Leung CC, Yu IT, Chen W: Silicosis, *Lancet* 379(9830):2008–2018, 2012.
Miller A: Radiographic readings for asbestosis: misuse of science—validation of the ILO classification, *Am J Ind Med* 50:63–67, 2007.
Oksa P, Wolff H, Vehmas T, Pallasaho P, Frilander H, editors: *Asbestos, Asbestosis, and Cancer—Helsinki Criteria for Diagnosis and Attribution 2014*, Tampere, 2014. (Juvenes Print.
Petsonk EL, Rose C, Cohen R: Coal mine dust lung disease. New lessons from old exposure, *Am J Respir Crit Care Med* 187(11):1178–1185, 2013.

PULMONARY HYPERTENSION

Method of
Dan Schuller, MD; and Anthony Peter Catinella, MD, MPH

CURRENT DIAGNOSIS

- Pulmonary arterial hypertension (PAH) is a type of pulmonary hypertension (PH) based on restricted flow because of vascular wall remodeling and increased pulmonary vascular resistance. PH does not equal PAH.
- The clinical presentation of PH is subtle and nonspecific with dyspnea, fatigue, and exercise limitation. A high index of suspicion is required.
- Echocardiography is the recommended initial screening test.
- Right heart catheterization, preferably at an expert center, should be obtained before initiation of specific PAH treatments.
- PAH is a diagnosis of exclusion.
- Multimodality risk stratification with combination of functional class assessment, echocardiography, exercise testing (6-minute walk test), B-type natriuretic peptide, and hemodynamic parameters are required at the time of initial diagnosis and for longitudinal monitoring.

CURRENT THERAPY

- Early referral to a PH expert center is recommended.
- General measures and supportive care include avoiding pregnancy and high-altitude travel, influenza, coronavirus disease 2019 (COVID-19), and pneumococcal immunizations; supplemental oxygen for hypoxemia; diuretics and electrolyte replacement when needed; correction of anemia and optimal evaluation; and management of associated comorbidities.
- There are now 13 U.S. Food and Drug Administration (FDA)-approved drugs for the treatment of PAH.
- With a few exceptions, patients with PAH at low or intermediate risk should be treated with upfront combination therapy with endothelin receptor antagonists (ERAs) and phosphodiesterase-5 inhibitors (PDE5i).
- In high-risk patients with PAH, combination therapy including intravenous prostanoid and referral for lung transplantation is recommended.
- PAH requires a multidimensional approach to care that includes rehabilitation, psychosocial and spiritual support, and palliative care.

Definition and Classification

Pulmonary hypertension (PH) is defined by a mean pulmonary arterial pressure (mPAP) greater than 20 mm Hg at rest. The definition of pulmonary arterial hypertension (PAH) also implies a pulmonary vascular resistance (PVR) >2 Wood units and pulmonary capillary wedge pressure (PCWP) ≤15 mm Hg. Based on Ohm's law, resistance is directly proportional to a pressure gradient and inversely proportional to flow. Thus the PVR is calculated by dividing the pressure gradient (mPAP minus venous pressure as measured by the PCWP) by the cardiac flow rate using the cardiac output or CO:

$$PVR = (mPAP - PCWP)/CO$$

Rearranging the equation to calculate the mPAP yields mPAP = (PVR × CO) + PCWP. From this simple equation, different hemodynamic profiles leading to PH can be distinguished (Figure 1). PH can occur because there is an increase in PVR (or precapillary PH), an increase in PCWP (or postcapillary PH), an increase in

HEMODYNAMIC PROFILES IN PULMONARY HYPERTENSION

Pulmonary Arterial Pressure = (Pulmonary Vascular Resistance) (Cardiac Output) + Wedge Pressure

PRE-CAPILLARY PH

mPAP > 20 mmHg, PCWP < 15 mmHg, PVR > 2 Wood Units)

- PH Group 1 – PAH ➔ vasculopathy (endothelial dysfunction, cellular proliferation, in situ thrombosis)
- PH Group 3 – due to chronic lung disease
- PH Group 4 – CTEPH
- PH Group 5

POST-CAPILLARY PH

mPAP > 20 mmHg, PCWP > 15 mmHg, PVR < 2 Wood Units

- PH Group 2
  - ○ Left ventricular dysfunction
  - ○ Mitral valvular disease
  - ○ Aortic valvular disease
  - ○ Others
- PH Group 5

HIGH CARDIAC OUTPUT / INCREASED FLOW

- Left to right cardiac shunts: congenital heart diseases
- Portopulmonary hypertension
- Hyperthyroidism
- Anemia
- Systemic shunts
- Pregnancy
- Fever

Figure 1 Hemodynamic profiles in pulmonary hypertension.

flow (high cardiac output state), or any combination of these. Isolated precapillary PH occurs when the mPAP is greater than 20 mm Hg to define the PH state, and the PVR is elevated (>2 Woods units) while the PCWP is normal (≤15 mm Hg). Likewise, isolated postcapillary PH occurs when the mPAP is greater than 20 mm Hg and the PCWP is greater than 15 mm Hg while the PVR is normal at less than 2 Woods units. Commonly, one finds combined pre- and postcapillary PH with all values abnormally elevated.

Understanding these equations permits appropriate classification, which has therapeutic implications, and insight into sudden clinical worsening with progression of the natural history of the underlying conditions. For instance, a patient with idiopathic PAH can have an increase in pulmonary pressures caused by progression of the disease (precapillary) or from interval development of a high output state such as fever, anemia, or pregnancy or from interval development of fluid overload or left ventricular dysfunction (postcapillary).

PH has a prevalence of 1% globally and is classified into five groups (Box 1) based on common underlying mechanisms or pathophysiology. Only PH group 1 is designated as PAH with restricted flow caused by vascular wall remodeling and increased PVR. PH group 2 is caused by left heart disease, a common condition that elevates pulmonary venous pressures; this group represents the highest proportion of patients with PH in the United States. PH group 3 is caused by chronic intrinsic lung diseases with chronic hypoxia and/or hypercapnia as a common mechanism; in patients with mild to moderate chronic obstructive pulmonary disease, the prevalence of PH is about 20% and increases to 50% in more advanced cases of the disease. PH group 4 is predominantly caused by chronic thromboembolic disease, which

causes obliteration of the pulmonary vascular bed by chronic organized thrombus leading to increased PVR. PH group 5 consists of heterogeneous conditions with multifactorial mechanisms that affect PH.

PAH is a rare, progressive, incurable disease of the small pulmonary arteries characterized by precapillary PH, vascular cell proliferation, aberrant remodeling, and thrombosis in situ (Figure 2). This group is amenable to specific PAH therapies. PAH is further subdivided into categories because of various etiologies and risk factors linked to a common pathogenesis but with significant variability in presentation, natural history, and response to treatment.

Recent registry data from economically developed countries indicate a PAH incidence and prevalence of ~6 and 48 to 55 cases/million adults, respectively. In the United States, almost half of the cases of PAH are idiopathic, whereas approximately 25% are associated with connective tissue disease (predominantly scleroderma), nearly 10% with congenital heart disease, 5% with liver disease (porto-pulmonary hypertension), and 5% with drugs or toxins (e.g., methamphetamine [Desoxyn], dasatinib [Sprycel], or appetite suppressants). Schistosomiasis is a rare parasitic infection in the United States, but it is endemic in 74 countries. Worldwide, 85% of persons infected with schistosomiasis are in sub-Saharan Africa, and the disease represents the most common cause of PAH worldwide.

Heritable PAH has been associated with a number of genetic mutations (predominantly the bone morphogenetic protein receptor type 2 [*BMPR2*] gene, activin receptor-like kinase type 1 [*ALK1*], and endoglin) and accounts for almost 3% of cases in the United States. It is transmitted as an autosomal dominant trait, with incomplete penetrance estimated to be approximately

BOX 1 Clinical Classification of Pulmonary Hypertension

Group 1: Pulmonary Arterial Hypertension
- Idiopathic PAH
  - Nonresponders at vasoreactivity testing
  - Acute responders at vasoreactivity testing
- Heritable PAH
- Associated with drugs and toxins
- PAH associated with:
  - Connective tissue disease
  - HIV infection
  - Portal hypertension
  - Congenital heart disease
  - Schistosomiasis
- PAH with overt features of venous/capillaries pulmonary veno-occlusive disease/pulmonary capillary hemangiomatosis involvement
- Persistent PH of the newborn

Group 2: Pulmonary Hypertension Associated With Left Heart Disease
- Heart failure
  - with preserved left ventricular ejection fraction
  - with reduced or mildly reduced ejection fraction
- Valvular heart disease
- Congenital/acquired cardiovascular conditions leading to postcapillary PH

Group 3: Pulmonary Hypertension Associated With Lung Diseases and/or Hypoxia
- Obstructive lung disease
- Restrictive lung disease
- Lung disease with mixed restrictive/obstructive pattern
- Hypoventilation syndromes
- Hypoxia without lung disease (e.g., high altitude)
- Development lung disorders

Group 4: Pulmonary Hypertension Associated With Pulmonary Artery Obstructions
- Chronic thromboembolic PH
- Other pulmonary artery obstruction

Group 5: Pulmonary Hypertension With Unclear and/or Multi-factorial Mechanism
- Hematologic disorders (including chronic hemolysis and myeloproliferative disorders)
- Systemic disorders (including sarcoidosis)
- Metabolic disorders
- Chronic renal failure with or without hemodialysis
- Pulmonary tumor thrombotic microangiopathy
- Fibrosing mediastinitis

Figure 2 Typical advanced pulmonary arteriopathy in idiopathic pulmonary arterial hypertension. Note the proliferative changes in all three vessel layers, including intimal hyperplasia, medial hypertrophy, and adventitial fibrosis. From Broaddus VC, Mason RJ, Ernst JD, et al. *Murray & Nadel's Textbook of Respiratory Medicine.* 6th ed. Philadelphia: Elsevier; 2016.

Early physical findings of PH may be nonspecific and include an accentuated pulmonary component of the second heart sound (P2) and a midsystolic ejection murmur. Physical findings in more advanced cases that involve right ventricular failure include a right parasternal lift, right ventricular gallop, diastolic murmur of pulmonary regurgitation, jugular venous distention, lower extremity edema, ascites, and signs of low cardiac output, including cool extremities. A murmur of tricuspid regurgitation may be audible, and this murmur intensifies with inspiration, unlike that of mitral regurgitation. Patients with suspected PH may also exhibit signs of associated conditions, such as telangiectasias, Raynaud's phenomenon, sclerodactyly, calcinosis, or malar erythema in connective tissue diseases; evidence of liver cirrhosis or portal hypertension; venous insufficiency or varicosities suggestive of possible thromboembolic disease; and obvious signs of underlying cardiac or respiratory diseases, including obstructive sleep apnea. Suggestive electrocardiographic findings include right axis deviation greater than 110 degrees, which has a positive predictive value between 72% and 93% and a negative predictive value between 26% and 65%. Other associated findings include right atrial enlargement and right ventricular hypertrophy.

Diagnosis

The diagnostic evaluation is aimed at screening high-risk individuals, excluding secondary causes of PH, and evaluating possible associated conditions. In addition, various elements of the comprehensive examination are useful for subsequent risk stratification, which is required to select the best therapeutic option and assess prognosis. PAH is always a diagnosis of exclusion.

After reviewing pertinent previous medical records and performing a complete history and physical examination, the pivotal test in the diagnostic algorithm by the primary care provider or non-PH expert center is a transthoracic echocardiogram (TTE) to assess the probability of PH. An echocardiogram has an intermediate or high risk for PH based on a peak tricuspid regurgitation velocity 2.8 m/s or greater or right ventricular systolic pressure ≥35 mm Hg. In one series, TTE had a sensitivity of 87% (95% confidence interval, 84.8%, 90.0%) and specificity of 66% (95% confidence interval, 60.7%, 71.6%). After a positive screen, a decision has to be made as to whether to fast track the referral of the patient to a PH expert center or to advance locally the diagnostic evaluation with additional testing aimed at diagnosing common causes of PH and ruling out chronic thromboembolic pulmonary hypertension (CTEPH). A comprehensive evaluation may include

10% to 20%. Genetic anticipation, distinguished by decreasing age of disease onset, has been reported in families affected with heritable PAH.

Clinical Manifestations

The initial symptoms of PAH are often subtle and nonspecific; mean time between symptom onset and PAH diagnosis is approximately 2 years. Patients often report progressive or exertional breathlessness, fatigue, and exercise limitation. With progression, patients may present with near syncope or syncope, palpitations, or anginal chest pain. Early detection requires a high index of suspicion because attribution to conditions such as asthma or "being out of shape" is a common error that can contribute to delay in diagnosis. Failure to respond to typical treatments for heart failure or asthma may be an important clue. Dysphonia or hoarseness caused by compression of the recurrent laryngeal nerve (Ortner's syndrome), which is caused by an enlarged pulmonary artery, occurs in less than 1% of patients.

References

Humbert M, Kovacs G, Hoeper MM, et al: 2022 ESC/ERS Guidelines for the diagnosis and treatment of pulmonary hypertension, *Eur Heart J* 43:3618–3731, 2022.

Leber L, Beaudet A, Muller A: Epidemiology of pulmonary arterial hypertension and chronic thromboembolic pulmonary hypertension: identification of the most accurate estimates from a systemic literature review, *Pulm Circ* 11:2045894020977300, 2021.

Al-Naamani K, Hijal T, Nguyen V, Andrew S, Nguyen T, Huynh T: Predictive values of the electrocardiogram in diagnosing pulmonary hypertension, *Int J Cardiol* 127(2):214–218, 2008.

Arunachalam A, Chaisson NF, Tonelli AR: Methods to improve the yield of right heart catheterization in pulmonary hypertension, *Respir Med*, 2020. https://doi.org/10.1016/j.yrmex.2020.100015.

Aryal SR, Moussa H, Sinkey R, et al: Management of reproductive health in patients with pulmonary hypertension, *Am J Obstet Gynecol MFM* 2:100087, 2020.

Barnes H, Yeoh HL, Fothergill T, et al: Prostacyclin for pulmonary arterial hypertension, *Cochrane Database Syst Rev* 5(5):CD012785, 2019.

Benza RL, Gomberg-MaitandM, Elliot G, et al: Predicting survival in patients with pulmonary arterial hypertension. The reveal risk score calculator 2.0 and comparison with ESC/ERS- based risk assessment strategies, *Chest* 156(2):323–333, 2019.

Boucly A, Weatherald J, Savale L, et al: Risk assessment, prognosis and guideline implementation in pulmonary arterial hypertension, *Eur Respir J* 50(2):1700889, 2017.

Broderick-Forsgren K, et al: Improving on the diagnostic characteristics of echocardiography for pulmonary hypertension, *Int J Cardiovasc Imaging* 33(9):1341–1349, 2017.

Farha S: COVID-19 and pulmonary hypertension, *Cleve Clin J Med*, 2020.

Frost A, Badesch D, Gibbs JSR, et al: Diagnosis of pulmonary hypertension, *Eur Respir J* 53(1):1801904, 2019.

Galiè N, Barberà JA, Frost AE, et al: Initial use of ambrisentan plus tadalafil in pulmonary arterial hypertension, *N Engl J Med* 373(9):834–844, 2015.

Galie N, Humbert M, Vachiery JL, et al: 2015 ESC/ERS guidelines for the diagnosis and treatment of pulmonary hypertension, *Eur Heart J* 37(1):67–119, 2016.

Ghofrani HA, Galiè N, Grimminger F, et al: Riociguat for the treatment of pulmonary arterial hypertension, *N Engl J Med* 369(4):330–340, 2013.

Jha N, Jha AK, Mishra SK, Sagili H: Pulmonary hypertension and pregnancy outcomes: systemic review and meta-analysis, *Eur J Obstet Gynecol Reprod Biol* 253:108–116, 2020.

HoeperMM, Bogaard HJ, Condliffe R, et al: Definitions and diagnosis of pulmonary hypertension, *J Am Coll Cardiol* 62(25 Suppl), 2013. D42–50.

Klinger JR, Elliot CG, Levine DJ, et al: Therapy of pulmonary arterial hypertension in adults: update of the chest guidelines and expert panel report, *Chest* 155(3):565–586, 2019.

Konstantinides SV: Trends in pregnancy outcomes in patients with pulmonary hypertension: still a long way to go, *Eur J Heart Fail* 18:1129–1131, 2016.

Kovacs G, Avian A, Foris V, et al: Use of ECG and other simple non-invasive tools to assess pulmonary hypertension, *PLoS One* 11(12):e0168706, 2016.

McLaughlin V, Channick RN, Ghofrani HA, et al: Bosentan added to sildenafil in patients with pulmonary arterial hypertension, *Eur Respir J* 46(2):405–413, 2015 Aug.

McGoon MD, Ferrari P, Armstrong I, et al: The importance of patient perspectives in pulmonary hypertension, *Eur Respir J* 53(1):1801919, 2019.

McLaughlin VV, Benza RL, Rubin LJ, et al: Addition of inhaled treprostinil to oral therapy for pulmonary arterial hypertension: a randomized controlled clinical trial, *J Am Coll Cardiol* 55(18):1915, 1922. 2010.

McLaughlin VV, Channick RN, Ghofrani HA, et al: Bosentan added to sildenafil in patients with pulmonary arterial hypertension, *Eur Respir J* 46(2):405–413, 2015.

Pulido T, Adzerikho I, Channick RN, et al: Macitentan and morbidity and mortality in pulmonary arterial hypertension, *N Engl J Med* 369(9):809–818, 2013.

Raina A, Humbert M: Risk assessment in pulmonary arterial hypertension, *Eur Respir Rev* 25(142):390–398, 2016.

Rich S, Kaufmann E: High dose titration of calcium channel blocking agents for primary pulmonary hypertension: guidelines for short-term drug testing, *J Am Coll Cardiol* 18:1323–1327, 1991.

Ryan JJ, Melendres-Groves L, Zamanian RT, et al: Care of patients with pulmonary arterial hypertension during the coronavirus (COVID19) pandemic, *Pulm Circ* 10(2):1–7, 2020.

Sahay S, Farber HW: Management of hospitalized patients with pulmonary arterial hypertension and COVID-19 infection, *Pulm Circ* 10(3):1–5, 2020.

Simonneau G, Montani D, Clermajer DS, et al: Haemodynamic definitions and updated clinical classification of pulmonary hypertension, *Eur Respir J* 53(1):1801913, 2019.

Sitbon O, Channick R, Chin KM, et al: Selexipag for the treatment of pulmonary arterial hypertension, *N Engl J Med* 373(26):2522–2533, 2015.

Sliwa K, van Hagen IM, Budts W, et al: Pulmonary hypertension and pregnancy outcomes: data from the registry of pregnancy and cardiac disease (ROPAC) of the European society of cardiology, *Eur J Heart Fail* 18:1119–1128, 2016.

Tapson VF, Jing ZC, Xu KF, et al: Oral treprostinil for the treatment of pulmonary arterial hypertension in patients receiving background endothelin receptor antagonist and phosphodiesterase type 5 inhibitor therapy (the FREEDOM-C2 study): a randomized controlled trial, *Chest* 144(3):952–958, 2013.

SARCOIDOSIS

Method of
W. Ennis James, MD

CURRENT DIAGNOSIS

- The diagnosis of sarcoidosis is one of exclusion.
- Tissue biopsy, confirming noncaseating granulomatous inflammation, is required in most cases.
- Initial evaluation should include screening for dangerous organ involvement.

CURRENT THERAPY

- Many cases of sarcoidosis do not require treatment.
- Treatment is typically indicated when sarcoidosis results in impaired quality of life or involves potentially dangerous organs.
- Corticosteroids are the most commonly used initial therapy but are associated with significant side effects.

Sarcoidosis is a multisystem granulomatous disease of unknown cause. The lung is most commonly affected, but any organ may be involved. The natural course of sarcoidosis is variable, ranging from an asymptomatic state to a progressive disease causing significant organ dysfunction that may be life-threatening. This variability in organ involvement and disease presentation often makes the diagnosis of sarcoidosis problematic.

Epidemiology

Sarcoidosis occurs worldwide and affects all races and ages. The disease is most common between ages 20 and 40, although analyses from large databases have revealed that the incidence and prevalence of the disease is bimodal, with a second peak between ages 45 and 65. Onset of disease tends to occur at an earlier age in Black people and males. A large analysis from an American national healthcare database found an incidence of 17.8 per 100,000 in African Americans and 8.1 per 100,000 in American White people, and a prevalence of 141 per 100,000 in African Americans and 50 per 100,000 in American White people. Incidence and prevalence rates were lower in Hispanic Americans than in White people and lower still in Asian Americans. The highest prevalence of sarcoidosis is found in White people in Scandinavia and in Black Americans. Sarcoidosis appears to affect more women than men across all racial/ethnic groups. In the United States, Black women have the highest prevalence of sarcoidosis, almost twice that of Black American men. The relative risk for having sarcoidosis increases significantly if a family member has it as well. In the United States nearly 20% of African Americans with sarcoidosis have an affected first-degree relative, compared with 5% in White people.

The clinical presentation and severity of sarcoidosis vary among racial and ethnic groups. The disease tends to be more severe in African Americans, whereas White people are more likely to be asymptomatic at report. Extrathoracic manifestations are more common in certain populations, such as ocular and cardiac sarcoidosis in Japanese populations, chronic uveitis and lupus pernio in African Americans, and erythema nodosum in Europeans. There is increasing evidence that genetic polymorphisms affect the risks and manifestations of the disease. This is consistent with the current theory that sarcoidosis does not have a single cause but is the result of an abnormal granulomatous host response to one of many potential antigens in a genetically susceptible person.

Immunopathogenesis

The exact immunopathogenesis of sarcoidosis is unknown, but it is thought to be similar to that of other granulomatous diseases. That is, antigen-presenting cells (APCs), usually either macrophages or dendritic cells, process and present an antigen via a human leukocyte antigen (HLA) class II molecule to T lymphocytes and their receptors. These T lymphocytes are usually of the CD4 T-helper 1 (T_H1) class. The antigen involved in this reaction is unknown, and there may be many antigens that are each associated with a specific HLA class II molecule and T-cell receptor. This could explain the inability to determine one specific cause of sarcoidosis and the varied phenotypic expressions of the disease.

The interaction of APCs and T lymphocytes activates the APCs to produce tumor necrosis factor α (TNF-α) and other cytokines. A proliferation of CD4 T_H1 lymphocytes also ensues, which results in the secretion of interferon-γ, interleukin (IL)-2, IL-12, and other cytokines. These cytokines activate and recruit monocytes and macrophages and transform them into giant cells, which are important building blocks of the granuloma. Additional factors may also lead to this series of immunologic events, such as the persistence of antigens like soluble AA amyloid fibrils that prevent antigen degradation.

The typical sarcoidosis lesion is a noncaseating (nonnecrotic) granuloma. The sarcoid granuloma consists of a compact core of macrophage-derived epithelioid and multinucleated giant cells surrounded by a perimeter of monocytes, lymphocytes, and fibroblasts. Granulomas can resolve spontaneously or with therapy; however, they can also persist and lead to persistent hyalinization and fibrosis. The development of such fibrosis can cause permanent organ dysfunction and in large part determines the prognosis.

Clinical Features and Clinical Course

Pulmonary Sarcoidosis

Between 30% and 60% of patients with pulmonary sarcoidosis are asymptomatic, and the disease is detected incidentally on chest x-ray. Some patients report with nonspecific pulmonary symptoms, such as dyspnea, cough, wheezing, and chest pain. Respiratory failure from sarcoidosis is extremely rare at report. Unlike in many other interstitial lung diseases, crackles are rarely heard on chest auscultation. Abnormalities on the chest radiograph occur in more than 90% of patients with pulmonary sarcoidosis. Bilateral hilar adenopathy occurs in 50% to 85% at disease report, and 25% to 50% have parenchymal infiltrates. On computed tomography, small nodules from granulomatous inflammation most commonly occur in the mid- and upper-lung zones and have a predilection for the bronchovascular bundles, subpleural locations, intralobular septa, and the airways.

A radiographic staging system was developed several decades ago (Table 1). Groups of patients with higher radiographic stages have more severe pulmonary dysfunction, lower remission rates, and greater mortality. However, there is significant overlap

among these groups, and stages are highly inaccurate predictors of outcomes for individual patients.

Advanced pulmonary stage IV (fibrocystic) sarcoidosis displays destruction of the lung architecture, with upward traction of the hila, lung distortion, upper-lobe volume loss, fibrocystic disease, honeycombed cysts, and decreased lung volumes. Aspergillomas can develop in these large cystic lesions and may be associated with life-threatening hemoptysis. Bronchiectasis from airway distortion also can occur and is an additional potential cause of hemoptysis.

The cause of dyspnea in pulmonary sarcoidosis is multifactorial. It may be the result of abnormalities of gas exchange, lung mechanics, weakness of the respiratory muscles, obesity from corticosteroid therapy, pulmonary hypertension, or sarcoidosis involvement of the heart. Pulmonary function and the chest radiographic findings are often discordant and often do not correlate with symptom severity. In patients with pulmonary sarcoidosis with a normal lung parenchyma (stage I), the vital capacity, diffusing capacity, partial pressure of arterial oxygen (PaO_2) at rest, PaO_2 with exercise, and lung compliance are abnormal in 20% to 40% of cases. The majority of patients with pulmonary sarcoidosis have a vital capacity of greater than 70% of that predicted at diagnosis; however, those with abnormal lung parenchyma have abnormal pulmonary function tests 50% to 70% of the time.

Patients with stage IV fibrocystic sarcoidosis tend to have the most severe pulmonary dysfunction and often have a restrictive ventilatory defect found on spirometry. It is underappreciated, however, that endobronchial involvement and airway distortion from fibrosis may cause airflow obstruction to be the major abnormality found on pulmonary function testing. Wheezing may be the prominent reporting symptom of sarcoidosis, and many cases of sarcoidosis are misdiagnosed as asthma.

Only 3% to 5% of patients die of sarcoidosis. In the United States 75% of these deaths are the result of complications of advanced pulmonary fibrosis, including pulmonary hypertension, infection, and life-threatening hemoptysis, which may result from the development of aspergillomas. Despite these potential complications, the overall prognosis is favorable in patients with stage IV sarcoidosis, with a 10-year survival of over 80%. Staging systems, including one that incorporates the lung function, pulmonary artery to ascending aorta diameter ratio greater than 1, and the presence of greater than 20% fibrosis on imaging, can be useful predictors of mortality. Other organs that result in fatalities from sarcoidosis are the heart and the central nervous system (CNS). In Japan, death from sarcoidosis is more commonly caused by cardiac than pulmonary involvement.

Patients who report with Löfgren syndrome (described in the next section) or with asymptomatic bilateral hilar adenopathy on chest radiograph have a good prognosis. African Americans tend to have a lower forced vital capacity and worse prognosis compared with White people and are more likely to develop new organ involvement within 2 years of diagnosis. Box 1 lists risk factors associated with a poor prognosis.

Extrapulmonary Sarcoidosis

The extrapulmonary manifestations of sarcoidosis are present in up to 67% of patients, can be the presenting manifestation of systemic sarcoidosis, and can affect the prognosis and treatment options for sarcoidosis.

The eyes and skin are the most common extrapulmonary organs involved with sarcoidosis. Ocular manifestations occur in 25% to 50% of patients; anterior uveitis is the most common manifestation. Symptoms of anterior uveitis may include red eyes, painful eyes, and photophobia. However, one-third of patients with anterior uveitis from sarcoidosis have no ocular symptoms. In addition, an intermediate or posterior uveitis can cause vision problems or can be asymptomatic. For these reasons, all patients with sarcoidosis should undergo an eye examination by an ophthalmologist. Other ocular manifestations of sarcoidosis include conjunctivitis, keratoconjunctivitis sicca (dry eyes), scleritis, and optic neuritis.

TABLE 1	Chest Radiograph Stages of Sarcoidosis	
RADIOGRAPHIC STAGE	BILATERAL HILAR LYMPH NODE ENLARGEMENT	PARENCHYMAL DISEASE
I	Yes	No
II	Yes	Nonfibrotic
III	No	Nonfibrotic
IV	No or yes	Fibrotic

Adapted from Judson MA, Baughman RP. Sarcoidosis. In: Baughman RP, du Bois RM, Lynch JP, Wells AU, eds. *Diffuse Lung Disease: A Practical Approach*. Arnold; 2004:109-129.

<table>
<tr><td>BOX 1</td><td>Factors Associated With a Poor Prognosis in Sarcoidosis</td></tr>
</table>

- Symptomatic at report
- African American race
- Extrathoracic disease
- Stage II to III versus stage I on chest x-ray
- Age greater than 40 years
- Splenic involvement
- Lupus pernio
- Disease duration greater than 2 years
- Forced vital capacity less than 1.5 L
- Stage IV chest x-ray or aspergilloma
- Pulmonary hypertension

Data from Judson MA, Baughman RP. Sarcoidosis. In: Baughman RP, du Bois RM, Lynch JP, Wells AU, eds. *Diffuse Lung Disease: A Practical Approach.* Arnold; 2004:109-129.

Figure 1 Skin lesions of sarcoidosis. (A) Sarcoid lesions may occur at any site, and they may take nodular, papular, or plaque forms. Biopsy is often necessary for diagnosis. (B) *Lupus pernio* is the term used to describe a dusky-purple infiltration of the skin of the nose, cheeks, or ears in chronic sarcoidosis. (From Forbes CD, Jackson WF. *Color Atlas and Text of Clinical Medicine.* 3rd ed. Mosby; 2003, with permission.)

Skin lesions in sarcoidosis can be classified into two categories: specific lesions that demonstrate noncaseating granulomas on biopsy and nonspecific lesions that do not (Figure 1). The specific skin lesions are often papular and commonly occur around the nose, eyes, and nape of the neck. They also have a predilection for areas of previous scars and tattoos, which is often referred to as "scar sarcoidosis" and is highly specific to sarcoidosis. Lupus pernio is a type of specific skin lesion causing disfiguring lesions on the face, often with erythema and significant induration. These lesions have a tendency to appear on the nose, cheeks, medial and lateral sides of the eyes, and lateral sides of the mouth. Lupus pernio lesions are relatively recalcitrant to therapy and often respond only partially to corticosteroids. The most common nonspecific skin lesion is erythema nodosum, which is often seen with an acute sarcoidosis presentation of fever, arthritis (especially in the ankles), pulmonary symptoms, and bilateral hilar adenopathy on chest radiograph. This syndrome is known as *Löfgren syndrome* and tends to have a good long-term prognosis.

Cardiac and neurologic sarcoidosis can be life-threatening and is therefore important to recognize. Cardiac involvement is detected clinically in 5% to 10% of patients with sarcoidosis during life but has been found in up to 25% at autopsy. Cardiac sarcoidosis can cause left ventricular dysfunction, cardiac arrhythmias, and sudden cardiac death. All patients with sarcoidosis should be screened for cardiac sarcoidosis, which, at a minimum, should include an electrocardiogram (ECG), as well as eliciting symptoms of left ventricular dysfunction (e.g.,

orthopnea, peripheral edema) and cardiac arrhythmias (e.g., palpitations, sensation of skipped heartbeats, syncope). Transthoracic echocardiography (TTE) and Holter monitoring have been recommended by some as appropriate additional screening tests. Patients with either significant symptoms or abnormal ECG or TTE should undergo more definitive testing for the diagnosis of cardiac sarcoidosis. Cardiac magnetic resonance imaging (MRI) provides both diagnostic and prognostic data and is recommended over cardiac positron emission tomography (PET) as the initial test of choice; however, this may vary depending on local expertise and availability. The diagnosis of cardiac sarcoidosis is typically made noninvasively, based on a combination of a typical clinical presentation coupled with the detection of characteristic findings on advanced imaging after other possible etiologies have been excluded. Because myocardial involvement is patchy, endomyocardial biopsy is diagnostic in less than 25% and is not commonly performed to make the diagnosis of cardiac sarcoidosis.

Clinically apparent neurosarcoidosis occurs in less than 10% of patients with sarcoidosis. Palsy of the seventh cranial nerve is the most common manifestation of neurosarcoidosis, and it often predates the diagnosis of the disease. Sarcoidosis can affect any part of the peripheral nervous system and CNS and can cause a cranial nerve palsy, mononeuropathy or polyneuropathy, aseptic meningitis, seizures, mass lesions in the brain and spinal cord, hydrocephalus, and encephalopathy. Brain and spinal cord MRI with contrast is the imaging test of choice to evaluate for potential CNS sarcoidosis in patients with a compatible clinical presentation.

Sarcoidosis causes clinically apparent extrathoracic lymphadenopathy in more than 10% of patients. The spleen may be involved in up to 50% of patients, but it is usually asymptomatic and rarely causes hypersplenism. Histologic evidence of hepatic sarcoidosis is present in 50% to 80% of patients with sarcoidosis, although most of these patients are asymptomatic and have normal liver function tests. Hepatomegaly, abdominal pain, and pruritus are the most common symptoms associated with hepatic sarcoidosis but are present only in 15% to 25% of patients with hepatic involvement. Elevation of the serum alkaline phosphatase is the most common liver function test abnormality. Sarcoidosis rarely involves the thyroid, kidney, breast, genitourinary tract, and gastrointestinal tract.

Bone involvement is occasional, usually occurring as small cysts or cortical defects found in the small bones of the hands and feet, but can also be found incidentally on imaging of the long bones and axial skeleton. An acute sarcoid arthritis often is present at disease onset and has a good prognosis. This is commonly found in the ankles of patients who report with Löfgren syndrome. Chronic sarcoid arthritis is rare. It is usually a nondestructive arthropathy of the shoulders, wrists, knees, ankles, and small joints of the hands and feet.

Sarcoidosis of the upper respiratory tract is underappreciated and can occur in the nasopharynx, hypopharynx, larynx, or any of the sinuses. Sarcoidosis of the upper respiratory tract is often relatively recalcitrant to therapy, and sinus involvement is more common in those with lupus pernio.

Hypercalcemia or hypercalciuria leading to nephrolithiasis can occur with sarcoidosis and may result in renal dysfunction. These phenomena are the result of the enzyme 1α-hydroxylase in activated macrophages that convert 25-hydroxyvitamin D to 1,25-dihydroxyvitamin D, the active form of the vitamin, which results in increased gut absorption and increased renal excretion of calcium that can cause nephrolithiasis. Patients with sarcoidosis-associated hypercalcemia typically have low 25-hydroxyvitamin D levels with 1,25-dihydroxyvitamin D levels that are elevated or at the upper limits of normal in combination with a low or low-normal parathyroid hormone.

Patients can have constitutional symptoms such as fever, night sweats, weight loss, malaise, and fatigue at report. These symptoms may be associated with hepatic sarcoid involvement but also may be a sign of the systemic nature of the disease, presumably from cytokine release, rather than specific organ involvement. A small fiber neuropathy may occur with sarcoidosis and cause pain or autonomic dysfunction.

Diagnosis and Initial Workup

The diagnosis of sarcoidosis requires a compatible clinical picture, histologic demonstration of noncaseating granulomas, and exclusion of other diseases capable of producing a similar histologic and clinical picture. It is prudent to bear a healthy degree of skepticism in the diagnosis, and patients should be evaluated closely for additional clues supporting an alternative diagnosis. Mycobacterial and fungal diseases must always be considered as alternative causes of granulomatous inflammation. Therefore stains and cultures of tissue specimens for mycobacteria and fungi should always be obtained when the diagnosis of sarcoidosis is considered. Hypersensitivity pneumonitis, a granulomatous lung disease from inhalation of bioaerosols, may also mimic sarcoidosis. Bioaerosols from hot tubs and birds are the most common causes of hypersensitivity pneumonitis, and clinicians should specifically inquire about these two exposures in individuals who are being evaluated for sarcoidosis. Sarcoidosis is a systemic disease, so signs or symptoms of extrathoracic disease should be sought. All patients should be evaluated for "dangerous" extrapulmonary manifestations, including cardiac, CNS, renal, and ocular involvement, as well as sarcoidosis-associated hypercalcemia.

It is prudent to select a biopsy site associated with less morbidity, such as the skin, if a lesion is present. Transthoracic needle aspiration of mediastinal lymph nodes under ultrasound guidance (EBUS-TBNA) via bronchoscopy has a high yield for the diagnosis of pulmonary sarcoidosis and was recommended over mediastinoscopy on recently published guidelines. Transbronchial lung biopsy has a diagnostic yield of 40% to more than 90% in pulmonary sarcoidosis. Endobronchial biopsy has a 40% to 60% sensitivity and adds to the yield of transbronchial biopsy.

Bronchoalveolar lavage (BAL) with examination of lymphocyte populations has been used in the evaluation of possible pulmonary sarcoidosis. In sarcoidosis, there is an increased number of BAL lymphocytes, and these are predominantly CD4+. It has been proposed that an increase in BAL lymphocytes and a BAL CD4/CD8 ratio greater than 3.5 makes the diagnosis of sarcoidosis highly likely.

Although serum angiotensin-converting enzyme (ACE) often is elevated in active sarcoidosis, the specificity and sensitivity of this test are inadequate for it to be used diagnostically. Serum ACE may be used as supportive evidence for the diagnosis, and it also may be used in some instances to follow disease activity.

Gallium-67 (^{67}Ga) scanning is cumbersome because it takes several days to complete and is infrequently used as a diagnostic test. However, bilateral hilar uptake and right paratracheal uptake (lambda sign) coupled with lacrimal and parotid uptake (panda sign) with ^{67}Ga strongly suggest a diagnosis of sarcoidosis. Fluorodeoxyglucose PET scanning (outside the CNS) and MRI studies using contrast (CNS and cardiac) have essentially replaced ^{67}Ga scanning for detecting sarcoidosis activity.

Ideally, the diagnosis of sarcoidosis requires a demonstration of noncaseating granulomas in at least one organ. However, according to recently published guidelines, certain clinical presentations are so specific for the diagnosis of sarcoidosis that biopsy may not be necessary. Extreme caution must be used in these situations to ensure that there is no clinical information that would suggest an alternative diagnosis that should prompt a tissue biopsy. Clinical or laboratory findings that strongly support the diagnosis of sarcoidosis without a tissue biopsy are listed in Box 2.

In addition to screening for neurologic (symptoms) and cardiac (symptoms, ECG) involvement, all patients should undergo evaluation by an ophthalmologist (even in the absence of ocular symptoms). Laboratory testing to evaluate for other organ involvement at the time of diagnosis should include serum calcium, creatinine, alkaline phosphatase, and a complete blood count with differential.

BOX 2 Clinical or Laboratory Findings That Strongly Support a Diagnosis of Sarcoidosis Without a Tissue Biopsy

- Löfgren syndrome
- Heerfordt syndrome (uveoparotid fever)
- Asymptomatic bilateral hilar adenopathy on chest x-ray
- Lupus pernio

Treatment

Therapy is often not mandatory for sarcoidosis because the disease can remit spontaneously. Systemic antisarcoidosis therapy is indicated for dangerous organ involvement and for disease causing significant quality-of-life impairment. Potentially dangerous disease includes neurosarcoidosis, cardiac sarcoidosis, renal sarcoidosis, hypercalcemia that does not respond to dietary measures, and ocular sarcoidosis that does not respond to topical (eye drop) therapy. Therapy should also be considered when the disease is progressive and at risk of resulting in long-term morbidity. In general, treatment is discouraged for asymptomatic stage I pulmonary sarcoidosis, elevations of serum liver function tests, or specific levels of ACE.

The decision to treat sarcoidosis can be problematic because the disease has a variable prognosis that must be weighed against the potential side effects of therapy. It is often most prudent to monitor patients without therapy if they are asymptomatic or have only mild organ dysfunction. For pulmonary sarcoidosis, patients who are asymptomatic and those with mild disease that might spontaneously remit usually are not treated. For patients with clinical findings that predict spontaneous remission (e.g., erythema nodosum), the benefits of treatment often are offset by the toxicity of therapy. Often these patients can be managed with supportive therapy such as nonsteroidal antiinflammatory drugs for arthralgias and fever or bronchodilators and inhaled corticosteroids for wheezing and cough.

It is recommended that patients with mild to moderate pulmonary sarcoidosis be observed for 2 to 6 months, if possible. Patients who improve will have avoided the toxicity of corticosteroids, and patients who deteriorate over this period should be considered for treatment. Patients with pulmonary dysfunction who neither improve nor deteriorate during the observation period may be given a corticosteroid trial, or they may be observed further. Patients with severe pulmonary dysfunction or pulmonary symptoms causing significant impairment should be treated.

Corticosteroids are considered first-line therapy for the treatment of sarcoidosis, but the dose, duration of therapy, and methods by which one can assess effectiveness have not been standardized. Topical corticosteroid therapy should be used whenever possible in an attempt to minimize systemic complications. This includes corticosteroid eye drops for anterior sarcoid uveitis and corticosteroid creams and injections for localized skin lesions. Prolonged use of topical steroids for ocular and cutaneous sarcoidosis is associated with an increased risk of side effects (glaucoma, cataracts, skin discoloration and thinning). Recent guidelines published by the European Respiratory Society provide some guidance to the dosing of oral steroid regimens. Pulmonary sarcoidosis usually is treated initially with 20 mg/day of prednisone or its equivalent. Higher doses may be required for neurosarcoidosis and cardiac sarcoidosis. Some advocate for doses as high as 1 mg/kg/day for cardiac and neurologic involvement, although this should not be considered standard practice for all presentations because studies have not consistently shown a clear benefit. Regardless of the starting dose, the patient should be evaluated within 2 to 12 weeks for a response, with the goal of tapering corticosteroids down to the lowest effective dose (ideally <10 mg/day) as quickly as possible. This dose is usually continued for at least 6 months. Patients failing to respond to therapy within

3 months are unlikely to respond to a more protracted course of therapy or a higher dose.

The relapse rate after corticosteroid therapy is withdrawn may be as high as 70%, and therefore patients need to be followed closely as the corticosteroid dose is tapered and discontinued. In some patients, there may be recurrent relapses requiring long-term, low-dose therapy. On occasion, the chronic prednisone dose needed to prevent relapse is less than 5 mg/day. Patients who relapse after corticosteroids have been withdrawn can be retreated with corticosteroids. However, corticosteroid-sparing agents should be considered in patients who are unable to taper the corticosteroids to less than 10 mg/day to control the disease.

Methotrexate (Trexall)[1] is the most studied alternative sarcoidosis medication and is usually used as a corticosteroid-sparing agent but at times can be used as replacement therapy. Methotrexate is most useful for pulmonary, skin, joint, and eye sarcoidosis. The goal weekly dose is 10 to 15 mg. Hydroxychloroquine (Plaquenil)[1] given once or twice daily may be used for sarcoidosis of the skin, joints, nerves, and for hypercalcemia from sarcoidosis, but it has not been shown to be beneficial for pulmonary sarcoidosis. Because of the risk of retinal toxicity, most patients should not receive a daily dose greater than 5 mg/kg/day or greater than 400 mg, whichever is lower. Azathioprine (Imuran)[1] is also useful as a second-line therapy for sarcoidosis. The initial dose is typically 50 mg once a day, which can be increased by 50 mg every 2 to 4 weeks as tolerated to a maximum dose of 2 mg/kg once daily. Leflunomide (Arava)[1] has also been shown to be useful in the treatment of pulmonary and extrapulmonary sarcoidosis. Monoclonal antibodies against TNF-α, such as infliximab (Remicade)[1] and adalimumab (Humira)[1], are useful agents in patients with severe sarcoidosis and/or who fail to respond to the aforementioned treatments. Minocycline (Minocin)[1] and doxycycline (Vibramycin)[1] (100 mg twice daily) may be useful for skin sarcoidosis. Cyclosporine is ineffective for pulmonary sarcoidosis. Nintedanib (Ofev)[1], an antifibrotic tyrosine kinase inhibitor used in treatment of fibrotic interstitial lung diseases, has recently been under investigation as a treatment for progressive fibrotic pulmonary sarcoidosis. At this point, however, its efficacy in sarcoidosis remains unclear and its role (if any) in the treatment of fibrotic sarcoidosis requires further investigation. Therapy should also be considered for the nongranulomatous aspects of the disease. Sarcoidosis-associated small fiber neuropathy may respond to medications for neuropathic pain, monoclonal antibodies against TNF-α, or intravenous immunoglobulin[1]. Sarcoidosis-associated fatigue may benefit from a physical training program, neurostimulants, or monoclonal antibodies against TNF-α.

---

[1] Not FDA approved for this indication.

References

Baughman RP, Culver DA, Judson MA: A concise review of pulmonary sarcoidosis, *Am J Respir Crit Care Med* 183:573–589, 2011.

Baughman RP, Field S, Costabel U: Sarcoidosis in America: analysis based on health care use, *Ann Am Thorac Soc* 13:244–252, 2016.

Baughman RP, Nunes H, Sweiss NJ, et al: Established and experimental medical therapy of pulmonary sarcoidosis, *Eur Respir J* 41(6):1424–1438, 2013.

Baughman RP, Teirstein AS, Judson MA, et al: Clinical characteristics of patients in a case control study of sarcoidosis, *Am J Respir Crit Care Med* 164:1885–1889, 2001.

Baughman RP, Valeyre D, Korsten P, et al: ERS clinical practice guidelines on treatment of sarcoidosis, *Eur Respir J* 58(6):2004079, 2021. 16.

Belperio JA, Shaikh F, Abtin FG, et al: Diagnosis and treatment of pulmonary sarcoidosis: a review, *JAMA* 327(9):856–867, 2022.

Birnie DH, Sauer WH, Bogun F, et al: HRS expert consensus statement on the diagnosis and management of arrythmias associated with cardiac sarcoidosis, *Heart Rhythm* 11:1304–1323, 2014.

Chen ES, Song Z, Willett MH, et al: Serum amyloid A regulates granulomatous inflammation in sarcoidosis through Toll-like receptor-2, *Am J Respir Crit Care Med* 181:360–373, 2010.

Elliot CD, Maier LA, Wilson KC, et al: Diagnosis and detection of sarcoidosis: an official American Thoracic Society clinical practice guideline, *Am J Respir Crit Care Med* 201(8):e26–e51, 2020.

Hamzeh N, Steckman D, Sauer W, Judson MA: Pathophysiology and clinical management of cardiac sarcoidosis, *Nat Rev Cardiol* 12:278–288, 2015.

Judson MA: The clinical features of sarcoidosis: a comprehensive review, *Clinic Rev Allerg Immunol* 49:63–78, 2015.

Judson MA: The diagnosis of sarcoidosis, *Clin Chest Med* 29:415–427, 2008.

Judson MA, Costabel U, Drent M, et al: The WASOG sarcoidosis organ assessment Investigators. The WASOG sarcoidosis organ assessment instrument: an update of a previous clinical tool, *Sarcoidosis Vasc Diff Lung Dis* 31:19–27, 2014.

Lower EE, Baughman RP: Prolonged use of methotrexate in refractory sarcoidosis, *Arch Intern Med* 155:846–851, 1995.

Nardi A, Brillet P, Letoumelin P, et al: Stage IV sarcoidosis: comparison of survival with the general population and cause of death, *Eur Respir J* 38:1368–1373, 2011.

Tavee JO, Karwa K, Ahmed Z, et al: Sarcoidosis-associated small fiber neuropathy in a large cohort: clinical aspects and response to IVIG and anti-TNF alpha treatment, *Respir Med* 126:135–138, 2017.

Thillai M, Atkins CP, Crawshaw A, et al: BTS clinical statement on pulmonary sarcoidosis, *Thorax* 76(1):4–20, 2021.

TUBERCULOSIS AND OTHER MYCOBACTERIAL DISEASES

Method of
Laura Elyse Shevy, MD; and Parisa Mortaji, MD

CURRENT DIAGNOSIS

- Latent tuberculosis (TB) infection is diagnosed in an asymptomatic person previously exposed to TB who has a positive tuberculin skin test or interferon-γ release assay.
- A positive tuberculin skin test (TST) or interferon-γ release assay (IGRA) does not distinguish latent tuberculosis infection (LTBI) from TB disease.
- The gold standard for diagnosing active pulmonary TB disease is acid fast bacilli (AFB) culture on respiratory specimens; AFB smear and nucleic acid amplification testing are also useful in diagnosis.
- All patients with LTBI or TB disease should undergo HIV testing.

CURRENT THERAPY

- LTBI: rifamycin-based regimen for 3 to 4 months.
- Treatment of TB disease should be done in conjunction with the local public health department.
- Drug-susceptible pulmonary TB disease: isoniazid (INH) + rifampin (RIF) + pyrazinamide (PZA) + ethambutol (EMB) for 2 months, followed by 4 months of INH + RIF.
- Drug-susceptible extrapulmonary TB disease is typically treated as per pulmonary TB disease but treatment and duration vary based on anatomic site(s) involved.
- Treatment of drug-resistant TB disease should be done in consultation with a TB expert.

Overview

Mycobacterial diseases occur worldwide and cause significant morbidity and mortality. These organisms comprise *Mycobacterium tuberculosis* complex, the causative pathogen in tuberculosis disease and latent tuberculosis infection; *Mycobacterium leprae* complex, the etiologic agent of Hansen's disease (leprosy); and around 80 pathogenic species of nontuberculous mycobacteria. This chapter mainly focuses on the diagnosis and management of tuberculosis, with a brief overview of Hansen's disease, and some infections caused by nontuberculous mycobacteria.

Tuberculosis

Mycobacterium tuberculosis, the bacteria responsible for tuberculosis (TB) disease and latent tuberculosis infection (LTBI), affects people in every country. It is the leading cause of infectious diseases mortality by a single pathogen worldwide, and it is the ninth leading cause of death overall. An estimated 2 billion people, or 25% of the global population, are thought to be infected with *M. tuberculosis*. The majority of individuals who become infected remain asymptomatic and develop LTBI. Risk factors for TB infection include overcrowding, congregate healthcare and incarceration facilities, poverty, human immunodeficiency virus (HIV) and AIDS, malnutrition, excessive alcohol use, tobacco use, drug use, silicosis, end-stage renal disease, diabetes mellitus, malignancy, and other immunosuppressive disorders and medications. TB disproportionately affects racial and ethnic minorities and people experiencing homelessness.

Pathophysiology

M. tuberculosis is an aerobic, non–spore forming, acid-fast staining, slow-growing bacillus. There are at least nine species in the genus *Mycobacterium* that comprise *M. tuberculosis* complex, although not all are pathogenic to humans. The majority of TB infections worldwide are caused by *M. tuberculosis* sensu stricto; in West Africa, up to 50% of cases are caused by *M. africanum*. Humans are the only known reservoir of *M. tuberculosis*. Transmission occurs from person to person via aerosolized droplets, which can remain suspended in the air for several hours. For this reason, the proximity, frequency, and duration of exposure are some of the most important factors in infection transmission. Other general factors include immune status of the exposed individual, infectiousness of the person with TB disease, and environmental factors.

Primary infection occurs after inhalation of the tubercle bacilli, which establish in the midlung zone terminal air spaces and are engulfed by alveolar macrophages. When the tubercle bacilli destroy the macrophages, pneumonitis develops. The bacilli are released and travel via lymphatics to regional lymph nodes and can then spread hematogenously throughout the body. The most commonly affected sites that uptake infected cells and allow for bacilli multiplication include the apical posterior lung, lymph nodes, kidneys, long bones, vertebrae, and brain/eyes/meninges. These sites may become nidi of infection either during the acute infection or after a latent period.

The majority of infections are contained through the host's cell-mediated immune response 3 to 9 weeks after transmission. The initial immunologic cascade encapsulates the bacilli and creates granulomas—protective shells that keep the tubercle bacilli in check. This leads to infection latency. Such people with latent TB infection are not symptomatic of TB disease and are not contagious to others.

A minority of people may develop significant infection in the area of initial pulmonary transmission (the Ghon complex) and necrosis and radiographically visible calcification of draining regional lymph nodes (the Ranke complex). This may progress to pneumonia, also known as "progressive primary disease," and occurs most often in children, older adults, and patients living with HIV.

Progression from LTBI to TB disease occurs in about 5% to 10% of immune competent patients, usually within the first 2 years after infection or under certain medical conditions. Tubercle bacilli multiply rapidly and when no longer contained by the immune response cause TB disease. Pulmonary TB disease is most commonly seen in the lung apices (Figure 1). Reactivation of infection can occur throughout the body, with common extrapulmonary infections including pleural empyema, lymphadenitis, genitourinary infection, vertebral osteomyelitis, meningitis, uveitis, and pericarditis.

Prevention

Prevention of TB disease transmission is mainly through rapid identification and airborne isolation of patients with suspected or confirmed disease and prompt initiation of treatment. In countries with a high prevalence of TB, the bacille Calmette-Guerin (BCG) vaccine is often administered. This live, attenuated vaccine is derived from *Mycobacterium bovis* and has shown to be effective at preventing severe infection, mainly in children.

Clinical Manifestations

TB can cause two conditions: latent TB infection and active TB disease. By definition, a person with LTBI has no symptoms of TB disease. TB disease may be pulmonary or extrapulmonary. Clinical features of pulmonary TB disease may include fever, drenching night sweats, weight loss, anorexia, malaise, pleuritic chest pain, productive cough, and hemoptysis, typically with several weeks of symptoms. Clinical manifestations of extrapulmonary TB disease are myriad and are manifestations of the involved organ systems as outlined above.

Principles of Diagnosis

Of utmost importance, latent TB must be distinguished from active TB disease. Treatment for latent TB infection and TB disease differ greatly. Treating for LTBI when active TB disease is present can induce drug resistance, lead to increased morbidity

Figure 1 Posteroanterior (A) and left lateral (B) chest x-rays showing typical reactivation (postprimary) tuberculosis in the adult. Bilateral upper lobe fibrocavitary disease affects predominantly the apical and posterior segments of the right upper lobe. From Weller PF, Guerrant RL, Walker DH: *Tropical Infectious Diseases: Principles, Pathogens and Practice*, 3rd ed., Elsevier; 2011.

and mortality, and potentially increase risk of transmission. Typically a test for previous TB exposure is performed—the tuberculin skin test (TST) and/or an interferon-γ-release assay (IGRAs). The following must be performed: a full history and physical to evaluate current symptoms and signs of disease; past medical and social history to evaluate for risk factors for infection and progression from infection to TB disease if infection is present; medications for possible drug–drug interactions if treatment is warranted; and so on. A chest radiograph should be performed to evaluate for active pulmonary involvement (i.e., airspace opacities, pleural effusions, parenchymal cavitary lesions). Sputum for other respiratory specimens, and/or sampling of other infected sites, is performed for diagnostic testing as outlined in the following.

Diagnosis

Latent Tuberculosis Infection

There are two methods to diagnose LTBI: the TST (Tubersol) and IGRAs. TST is an intradermally injected protein precipitate of heat-inactivated tubercle bacilli—purified protein derivative (PPD)—or tuberculin. In people with previous TB infection and cell-mediated immunity, intradermal PPD induces a delayed-type hypersensitivity reaction characterized by induration. The test is interpreted via transverse diameter measurement of the induration (not erythema) after 48 to 72 hours. The TST therefore requires two clinical visits for TST placement and subsequent interpretation. Table 1 outlines interpretation of the TST based on risk group. False positive results can occur in people who have received BCG vaccination or who have infections with nontuberculous mycobacteria (NTM).

IGRAs are blood tests and measure T-cell release of interferon-γ in response to stimulation with highly TB-specific antigens. False positive results do not occur from previous BCG vaccination and are much less likely to occur in setting of NTM infections, which make them more specific than TST. Two commercially available IGRAs include the QuantiFERON-TB Gold Plus (QFT-Plus) and the T-SPOT®TB test (T-Spot). If available and feasible, the IGRA should be used over TST, especially if the patient has a history of receiving the BCG vaccine, is unlikely to return to have the TST interpreted, or has a high likelihood of TB infection.

Due to limited data on IGRA testing reliability in children, TST is the recommended method of testing for children under 5 years old. The American Academy of Pediatrics (AAP) recommends that either a TST or an IGRA be used in children 2 years of age and older. For children previously vaccinated with BCG—regardless of age—IGRA is preferred to avoid a false-positive TST result caused by the previous BCG vaccination.

Of extreme importance to recognize is that neither TST nor IGRA can distinguish TB disease from LTBI. A true positive TST or IGRA only indicates the person has, at some point, been exposed to and developed some cell-mediated immunity against *M. tuberculosis*. TST and IGRAs cannot be used alone to diagnose active TB disease.

Active Tuberculosis Disease

Active pulmonary TB disease is diagnosed in the presence of symptoms and/or signs of TB disease and by obtaining three sputum specimens 8 to 24 hours apart for acid-fast bacilli (AFB) smears, cultures, and nucleic acid amplification testing when available. Rapid molecular rifampin (Rifadin, Rimactane)/INH susceptibility testing should be performed, when available, for specific patient populations. *M. tuberculosis* typically takes about 3 to 8 weeks for visible growth on solid media and 10 to 20 days for liquid broth culture growth. Nucleic acid amplification testing (NAAT) uses real-time polymerase chain reaction (PCR) amplification to aid in detection of *M. tuberculosis* genetic material. However, culture remains the gold standard for diagnosis, and susceptibility testing should be performed on the initial positive culture. If a person cannot produce sputum, hypertonic saline can be used to induce sputum production. As a last resort, flexible bronchoscopy can be pursued to obtain respiratory specimens. If a respiratory specimen is positive by AFB smear but negative by NAAT, it is unlikely that the positive smear result represents active TB disease. In a patient in whom suspicion for TB disease is intermediate-high, if a respiratory specimen AFB smear is negative but NAAT is positive, a presumptive diagnosis of TB disease can be given. However, a negative NAAT is not sufficient to exclude pulmonary TB disease.

Active extrapulmonary disease requires sampling of potentially affected fluid or tissues. Cell counts and chemistries should be measured on amenable fluid specimens including pleural, cerebrospinal (CSF), ascitic, and synovial fluids. Adenosine deaminase can be measured on pleural, CSF, ascitic, and pericardial fluids. AFB smear microscopy, culture, NAAT, and histopathology should be performed on available specimens. False negative AFB smears and NAAT are not uncommon and should not be used to exclude diagnosis of active TB disease.

Principles of Treatment

Treatment of both LTBI and TB disease should be patient-centered, with care tailored to the patient's social situation, medical comorbidities, and clinical condition. Directly observed therapy (DOT), the practice of observing the patient physically

TABLE 1	Interpreting Tuberculin Skin Testing (TST) Results	
RISK OF INFECTION **DEGREE OF INDURATION**		**POSITIVITY BY RISK GROUP**
	≥5 mm	• People living with HIV • Recent contacts of people with infectious TB disease • People who have fibrotic changes on chest radiograph • Recipients of solid organ transplants • Other immunosuppressed patients (e.g., patients on prolonged therapy with corticosteroids >15 mg per day of prednisone, patients on TNF-α antagonists)
	≥10 mm	• People born in countries where TB disease is common, including Mexico, the Philippines, Vietnam, India, China, Haiti, Guatemala, and other countries with high rates of TB • People who inject or use drugs • Mycobacteriology laboratory workers • People who live or work in high-risk congregate settings (e.g., nursing homes, homeless shelters, or correctional facilities) • People with certain medical conditions that place them at high risk for TB (e.g., silicosis, diabetes mellitus, severe kidney disease, certain types of cancer, and certain intestinal conditions) • People who are <90% of ideal body weight • Children <5 years of age • Infants, children, and adolescents exposed to adults in high-risk categories
	≥15 mm	• Individuals without known TB risk factors

Adapted from American Thoracic Society: Targeted tuberculin testing and treatment of latent tuberculosis infection. *MMWR Recomm Rep* 49:1–51, 2000.

TABLE 2	Preferred Treatment Regimens for Latent Tuberculosis Infection		
PREFERRED REGIMENS	**DURATION OF THERAPY**	**DOSAGES**	**FREQUENCY OF ADMINISTRATION**
INH* + RPT	3 months	Adults and children aged >12 years: INH: 15 mg/kg; 900 mg maximum dose RPT: 10–14 kg: 300 mg 14–25 kg: 450 mg 25–32 kg: 600 mg 32–49.9 kg: 750 mg ≥50 kg: 900 mg maximum dose Children ages 2–11 years: INH: 25 mg/kg; maximum dose 900 mg RPT: as above	Once weekly
RIF	4 months	Adults: 10 mg/kg, maximum dose 600 mg Children: 15–20 mg/kg, maximum dose 600 mg	Daily
INH + RIF	3 months	Adults: INH: 5 mg/kg, maximum dose 300 mg RIF: 10 mg/kg, maximum dose 600 mg Children: INH: 10–20 mg/kg, maximum dose 300 mg RIF: 15–20 mg/kg, maximum dose 600 mg	Daily

INH, Isoniazid (Nydrazid); *RIF,* rifampin (Rifadin, Rimactane); *RPT,* rifapentine (Priftin)
*Vitamin B6 (pyridoxine)[1] is given in conjunction with INH for those at risk for developing—or already suffering from—peripheral neuropathy per text above.
[1]Not FDA approved for this indication.
Adapted from Sterling TR, Njie G, Zenner D, et al: Guidelines for the treatment of latent tuberculosis infection: Recommendations from the National Tuberculosis Controllers Association and CDC, 2020. *MMWR Recomm Rep* 69(No. RR-1):1–11, 2020.

ingest antituberculous medications, is a widely implemented standard of practice in TB programs in the United States and has been shown to significantly improve treatment success compared with self-administered therapy. Thus DOT is recommended for routine treatment of patients with all forms of TB as feasible.

The purpose of treating LTBI is to prevent progression to TB disease in those individuals at high risk for infection and progression to disease.

The objectives of treating TB disease are to cure the individual patient, decrease risk of morbidity and mortality from disease, reduce transmission of *M. tuberculosis* to other people, and prevent development of drug resistance during antituberculous therapy.

The treatment of multidrug resistant (MDR) TB disease (defined as resistance to INH and rifampin [Rifadin, Rimactane]) and extensively drug resistant (XDR) TB disease (resistance to INH, rifampin [Rifadin, Rimactane], levofloxacin [Levaquin[1]], and at least one second-line injectable agent) is complicated, and therapy should be pursued in consultation with a TB expert.

Treatment

Latent Tuberculosis Infection
The decision to initiate prophylactic therapy for latent TB infection is a risk-benefit decision based on the patient's likelihood of infection and likelihood of progression from LTBI to TB disease. The risk of progression from LTBI to TB disease in an immunocompetent host is 5% to 10% over a lifetime. People with diabetes have a 30% lifetime risk. People living with HIV have a 7% to 10% risk per year of progressing from LTBI to TB disease. Studies have demonstrated benefit in decreasing incidence of TB disease by treating LTBI in people who are under 5 years old, living with HIV, otherwise immunosuppressed (e.g., corticosteroid use >15 mg/prednisone or equivalent/day, use of immunosuppressive drugs such as tumor necrosis factor (TNF)-α inhibitors), household contacts of or have had recent exposure to a person with active TB disease, residents of high-risk congregate health facilities, persons with abnormal chest radiographs consistent with previous TB, and people with silicosis, among other conditions.

Treatment regimens are outlined below. It is advisable to consult a TB expert if the patient is a contact of an individual with known drug-resistant TB disease.

In 2020, the National Tuberculosis Controllers Association (NTCA) and Centers for Disease Control and Prevention (CDC) updated guidelines for treatment of LTBI for persons living in the United States. There are now three preferred regimens, all rifamycin-based, of 3 to 4 months' duration. These regimens are preferred due to their effectiveness, safety profile, and high treatment success rate. Some potential downsides of these regimens include increased cost over alternatives, adverse drug effects and potential for significant drug-drug interactions (including warfarin, oral contraceptives, antifungals, HIV antiretroviral therapy, among others). If drug–drug interactions preclude use of a preferred regimen, alternative regimens of daily isoniazid (Nydrazid) (INH) monotherapy for 6 or 9 months' duration can be used. Daily INH regimens are effective, but caution should be used due to the increased risk of hepatotoxicity, and the potential to induce drug resistance from the longer treatment duration. From 25 to 50 mg of pyridoxine (vitamin B6)[1] should be added for those people at risk of developing peripheral neuropathy such as pregnant women or people with diabetes mellitus, chronic kidney disease, malnutrition, HIV, alcohol use disorder, or other conditions; 100 mg dose is recommended for people who already have peripheral neuropathy. If daily INH cannot be used, rifabutin (Mycobutin)[1] may substitute for rifampin (Rifadin, Rimactane) in one of the three preferred regimens, as the former has fewer drug interactions (Table 2).

Drug-Susceptible Pulmonary Tuberculosis Disease
The preferred treatment regimen for drug-susceptible pulmonary TB disease includes an intensive treatment phase with 2 months of isoniazid (Nydrazid) (INH), rifampin (Rifadin, Rimactane) (RIF), pyrazinamide (Zinamide) (PZA), and ethambutol (Myambutol) (EMB), followed by a continuation phase of 4 months of INH and RIF. If drug susceptibilities are available prior to starting treatment, EMB can be omitted; as soon as susceptibility to

[1]Not FDA approved for this indication.

[1]Not FDA approved for this indication.

INH and RIF are confirmed, ethambutol (Myambutol) can be discontinued. The CDC recommends continuous daily dosing of the above agents rather than intermittent dosing for both the intensive and continuation phase of treatment. Pyridoxine,[1] or vitamin B6, should be given throughout the duration of INH administration as discussed above. It is highly advised these regimens are given by DOT. If this frequency of DOT is difficult to achieve, alternative regimens can be used as outlined in the Official American Thoracic Society/Centers for Disease Control and Prevention/Infectious Diseases Society of America Clinical Practice Guidelines: Treatment of Drug-Susceptible Tuberculosis.

Drug-Susceptible Extrapulmonary Tuberculosis Disease

The treatment regimens for drug-susceptible extrapulmonary TB disease largely follow that of pulmonary TB disease with 2 months of intensive phase INH, RIF, PZA, EMB, followed by a continuation phase with INH and RIF. The duration of the continuation phase, however, depends on anatomic site involved. Disease that is treated with a standard 6-month regimen, as for pulmonary TB disease above, include tuberculous pericarditis, lymphadenitis, pleural, genitourinary, peritoneal, military, and other disseminated disease.

There has been some controversy in the literature about adjunctive corticosteroid use for TB pericarditis to prevent development of constrictive pericarditis: current ATS/CDC/IDSA guidelines do not recommend routine use of steroids in TB pericarditis, but consideration to steroid use can be given to patients with large pericardial effusion, high levels of inflammatory cells/markers in the pericardial fluid, or those with early signs of constriction.

TB meningitis is treated for 2 months with the standard four-drug regimen (INH, RIF, PZA, EMB) in adults, followed by 7 to 10 months of INH and RIF for drug-susceptible disease. In pediatric patients, the American Academy of Pediatrics recommends initial 2 months of treatment with INH, RIF, PZA, and either ethionamide (Trecator), if possible, or an aminoglycoside, followed by INH and RIF for the 7 to 10 month consolidation phase. Optimal treatment duration of TB meningitis is not well known. Serial lumbar punctures may be of utility to help define total duration. Adjunctive steroids are recommended in the acute illness as they have been demonstrated to provide mortality benefit in clinical trials; steroids should be tapered over 6 to 8 weeks.

Bone and joint infection is typically treated with 9 months total duration, up to 12 months in setting of extensive hardware. Spinal TB disease with TB meningitis is treated as for meningitis above.

Multidrug-Resistant TB

Resistance in *M. tuberculosis* develops through spontaneous point mutations. MDR TB is defined as that which is resistant to both INH and RIF. XDR TB is a subset of MDR TB with additional resistance to a fluoroquinolone and a second-line injectable agent. MDR and XDR TB can be acquired as the primary infection, or resistance can develop while on therapy for a previously susceptible TB isolate. Acquisition of primary drug-resistant TB is influenced by geographic area where infection was acquired. Risk factors for development drug resistance while on therapy include incomplete medication adherence, inadequate drug absorption or dosing, and single-drug treatment. Consultation with a TB expert is advised if MDR or XDR TB is suspected or confirmed.

Tuberculosis Disease in Special Circumstances

Sputum/Culture-Negative Tuberculosis

Sputum/culture-negative pulmonary TB is defined as failure to isolate organisms in the setting of high clinical suspicion of disease. Potential etiologies for negative cultures include low bacillary populations, inadequate sputum specimens, or overgrowth of cultures with other microorganisms. If clinical suspicion is high, treatment should be initiated with reevaluation every 2 to 3 months.

---

[1] Not FDA approved for this indication.

Tumor Necrosis Factor-α Inhibitors

Patients being treated with TNF-α inhibitors are at increased risk for reactivation of latent TB and death from disseminated TB disease. Patients who are being considered for initiation of these drugs should have clinical evaluation for TB exposure/disease, IGRA testing (or TST if IGRA is not available), and radiographic chest imaging prior to initiation of anti-TNF-α therapy. All patients should receive treatment for LTBI if identified, and if no absolute contraindications exist, TNF-α inhibitor initiation delayed at least a month into the start of LTBI treatment if feasible.

Patients Living With HIV

Patients living with HIV are at high risk for developing TB infection; with a 20- to 40-fold increased risk compared with the general population. TB infection can occur at any CD4 T lymphocyte cell count, and a direct correlation between degree of immunodeficiency and TB infection risk exists. There are many potential complications of treating TB in patients living with HIV, and it is highly advised that treatment be done in conjunction with a specialist in treating HIV and TB. There are numerous drug–drug interactions between rifamycins and many classes of HIV antiretroviral therapy (ART). Patients with HIV-related TB disease are at risk for immune reconstitution inflammatory syndrome (IRIS), a paradoxical worsening of signs and symptoms of infection after initiation of ART. Finally, even with treatment, these patients are at increased risk for reinfection with TB compared with the general population.

The timing of ART initiation for HIV in setting of TB infection is complicated and beyond the scope of this text, and management by an HIV/TB treatment expert is highly advised. At all CD4 counts, people with HIV without active TB disease have significantly improved outcomes with early initiation of ART. However, there are some opportunistic infections for which early initiation of ART is potentially injurious, including patients with both HIV and TB meningitis.

When TB occurs in patients already on ART, treatment for TB should be started immediately and ART modified to prevent any drug interactions while still working toward virologic suppression.

In patients who have already been on ART, the standard 6-month TB treatment regimen should be used for drug-susceptible TB (Table 3). If ART has not yet been initiated, the continuation phase of TB therapy should be extended by 3 months, for a total of 7 months. ART should be initiated in the first 2 weeks if the CD4 count is <50 cells/uL and by 8 to 12 weeks if the CD4 count is 50 or greater, the exception being in the setting of TB meningitis as above, in which case ART should be held until 8 weeks of TB treatment have been completed.

The most up-to-date TB treatment recommendations for persons living with HIV infection can be found in the AIDSinfo guidelines "Guidelines for the Prevention and Treatment of Opportunistic Infections in Adults and Adolescents with HIV." Consultation with, and evaluation and management by, an expert in HIV and TB treatment is highly advised for patients with these complicated clinical presentations.

Monitoring and Complications

All patients diagnosed with LTBI or TB disease should have baseline HIV testing. If the patient has risk factors for hepatitis B and/or C, baseline serologies should be checked as well.

All patients should be advised of the potential minor and serious adverse effects of their medication regimens (Table 4). Patients taking rifampin (Rifadin, Rimactane) should be warned about the innocuous orange/rust-colored staining of body fluids (urine, sweat, tears). The most common adverse effects of the first-line agents are outlined below.

Rash is a major adverse effect of all four of the first-line agents and can be due to various mechanisms and of various severities. A pruritic rash without associated symptoms can be

TABLE 3 Preferred Regimens for Drug-Susceptible Pulmonary TB Disease

INTENSIVE PHASE	DURATION	ADULT DOSAGE FOR DAILY ADMINISTRATION
INH* RIF PZA EMB	7 days per week for 8 weeks OR 5 days per week for 8 weeks	INH: 5 mg/kg (typically 300 mg) RIF: 10 mg/kg (typically 600 mg) PZA: 30–40 mg/kg EMB: 15–25 mg/kg

CONTINUATION PHASE	DURATION	ADULT DOSAGE FOR DAILY ADMINISTRATION
INH RIF	7 days per week for 18 weeks OR 5 days a week for 18 weeks	INH: 5 mg/kg (typically 300 mg) RIF: 10 mg/kg (typically 600 mg)

DOT, Directly observed therapy; *EMB*, ethambutol (Myambutol); *HIV*, human immunodeficiency virus; *INH*, isoniazid (Nydrazid); *PZA*, pyrazinamide (Zinamide); *RIF*, rifampin (Rifadin, Rimactane).
*Vitamin B6 (pyridoxine)[1] is given in conjunction with INH for those at risk for developing—or already suffering from—peripheral neuropathy per text above.
[1]Not FDA approved for this indication.

TABLE 4 Major Adverse Effects of First-Line Medications for the Treatment of Tuberculosis Disease

FIRST-LINE MEDICATIONS	MOST COMMON ADVERSE SIDE EFFECTS
INH	Hepatotoxicity Rash Drug-induced lupus Peripheral neuropathy
Rifamycins (RIF, RPT, RFB)	Hepatotoxicity Rash GI upset Thrombocytopenia Hypersensitivity reactions
PZA	Hepatotoxicity Rash GI upset Gout
EMB	Optic neuritis Rash

EMB, Ethambutol (Myambutol); *INH*, isoniazid (Nydrazid); *PZA*, pyrazinamide (Zinamide); *RFB*, rifabutin (Mycobutin); *RIF*, rifampin (Rifadin, Rimactane); *RPT*, rifapentine (Priftin).

managed symptomatically with antihistamines. A petechial rash may indicate thrombocytopenia from rifamycin hypersensitivity and warrants permanent discontinuation of the rifamycin. Rash associated with fever, mucus membrane involvement, or generalized erythema is more likely to suggest Steven-Johnson syndrome or toxic epidermal necrolysis and warrants prompt discontinuation of all medications and consultation with a dermatologist.

The most serious adverse drug event associated with isoniazid (Nydrazid), pyrazinamide (Zinamide), and rifampin (Rifadin, Rimactane) is drug-induced liver injury (DILI). DILI should be suspected if the ALT level is at least three times the upper limit of normal in the presence of hepatitis symptoms or at least five times the upper limit of normal in the absence of symptoms. An asymptomatic increase in ALT concentration occurs in nearly 20% of patients, and in this case therapy should be continued.

Latent Tuberculosis Infection

For routine LTBI treatment in an otherwise healthy patient, apart from HIV and viral hepatitis serologies as above, no other baseline or serial laboratory monitoring is necessary. Patients who have/are at risk to have chronic liver disease, use alcohol regularly, are pregnant, are within 3 months postpartum, or have HIV should have baseline alanine aminotransferase (ALT), aspartate aminotransferase (AST), bilirubin, and alkaline phosphatase checked. Liver tests as above should be considered for patients of advanced age, those with chronic medical conditions, and those taking multiple chronic medications. Active viral hepatitis and end-stage liver disease are relative contraindications to the use of INH, RIF, or RPT in LTBI treatment.

While on LTBI treatment, the patient should have a minimum of once monthly medical assessments. During visits, the patient should be evaluated for development of symptoms/signs of TB disease, adherence to LTBI treatment regimen, and symptoms/signs of adverse effects. Serial liver tests, as above, should be monitored in those who have baseline abnormal LFTs, are at risk for hepatitis, or who develop symptoms/signs of hepatitis while on therapy. Treatment should be discontinued if any of the liver enzymes are greater than three times the upper limit of normal in presence of hepatitis symptoms or five times the upper limit of normal in an asymptomatic individual. For liver enzyme elevations less than three times the upper limit of normal in a symptomatic patient, treatment continuation can be considered provided there is close clinical and laboratory monitoring.

At completion of therapy, patients should be provided documentation of their initial TST or IGRA, treatment regimen and duration, and date of treatment completion. They should be advised to present such documentation if TB testing is required in the future, as IGRAs and TSTs are likely to remain positive despite successful LTBI treatment. Patients should be reminded that treatment for LTBI greatly decreases the risk of progression to TB disease but does not eliminate it 100%, and counseling on the symptoms/signs of TB disease and when/how to seek further care should be provided.

Active Tuberculosis Disease

Within a week of diagnosis, a treatment and monitoring plan specific to the patient should be developed in collaboration with the local department of health. As previously mentioned, all patients should have baseline HIV testing and viral hepatitis testing as indicated. All patients should have a baseline assessment of platelets, creatinine, ALT, AST, bilirubin, alkaline phosphatase, and a diabetes screen as recommended by the American Diabetes Association. Those patients for whom ethambutol (Myambutol) is included in treatment regimen should have a baseline Snellen test for visual acuity as well as color discrimination tests.

While on therapy, patients should be seen monthly and evaluated for treatment response and any adverse medication effects. Repeat laboratory testing should be done periodically if laboratory abnormalities were present at baseline, or if the patient develops symptoms/signs of adverse drug effects. Patients taking ethambutol (Myambutol) should be asked at each visit about vision changes and undergo monthly color discrimination tests.

During treatment of pulmonary TB disease, sputum, or other specimens for AFB/culture should be obtained at least monthly until cultures convert from positive to negative. If treatment has been continued for at least 2 months and the patient remains culture-positive, repeat drug susceptibility testing should be performed. Repeat chest radiographs can be pursued if there is clinical worsening or failure of symptoms to improve.

Treatment failure can occur for a number of reasons including medication nonadherence, unrecognized drug resistance, malabsorption, drug–drug interactions, or laboratory error (erroneously positive culture in a patient who is otherwise clinically well). The standard of care should be to add two to three new drugs. A single new agent should never be added to a failing regimen as it can lead to amplification of drug resistance as well as acquired resistance to the newly added drug.

The treatment of TB disease can be complicated, especially in patients who have HIV, are pregnant, have chronic liver disease and other comorbid conditions, have or develop drug-resistant TB, or develop serious adverse reactions to therapy. Clinicians who do not have experience with such complicated circumstances should consult a TB expert.

Nontuberculous Mycobacteria

NTM are a diverse group of environmental bacteria found worldwide. NTM are species other than *M. tuberculosis* and *M. leprae* complex. Not all NTM species are pathogenic to humans. *Mycobacterium avium* complex (MAC) is the most prevalent NTM causing human infection, and pulmonary disease is its most common presentation. NTM infections most often present as pulmonary infections in hosts with altered local or systemic immune function. Extrapulmonary infections can occur in both immune competent and immune suppressed hosts and include infections of lymph nodes, skin/soft tissue, bone, and prosthetic devices and catheters; disseminated infections occur almost exclusively in patients with advanced immunosuppression (e.g., patients with stage III HIV). Diagnosis of NTM infections requires a clinical syndrome supported by imaging and microbiologic data. Treatment varies by species and susceptibility patterns and typically requires a multidrug regimen to prevent development of drug resistance. Management of these complicated infections should be undertaken in conjunction with an expert in nontuberculous infection diagnosis and treatment.

Pathophysiology

As above, nontuberculous mycobacterial infections are typically acquired through contact with contaminated soil, water, dust, vegetable matter, or less commonly through zoonotic spread. NTM are not part of normal human flora. Pulmonary infections have been associated with inhalation or microaspiration from contaminated recirculating water systems, as have some skin and soft tissue infections been directly correlated to such aqueous sources. However, the ubiquitous presence of these organisms in nature makes it difficult to determine where a specific person's infection was acquired. Human-to-human transmission does not occur with the rare exception of pulmonary infections transmitted between persons with cystic fibrosis.

Host risk factors for infections include immunosuppression, especially corticosteroid use, uncontrolled HIV, TNF-α antagonist use, certain inherited disorders of immune suppression, and other systemic immunosuppressive states and medications; gastroesophageal reflux disease (GERD); and chronic pulmonary disease such as cystic fibrosis, bronchiectasis, and chronic obstructive pulmonary disease. Some activities that have been associated with NTM infections include use of hot tubs, saunas, steam rooms, and prolonged showers; cleaning swimming pools and fish tanks; waxing hair removal and pedicures at nail salons; and tattooing and other cosmetic procedures.

Prevention

When possible, reversing/treating causes of immunosuppression can help prevent nontuberculous mycobacterial infections. Prompt initiation of effective ART for patients with HIV and CD4 T lymphocytes $<50/mm^3$, for example, can help prevent MAC and other NTM infections, without need for prophylaxis with macrolides. Previous practice guidelines for people with HIV and CD4 T lymphocytes $<50/mm^3$ included initiation of azithromycin (Zithromax) for MAC prophylaxis. Due to the rapid viral suppression observed with current HIV ART, such patients who are starting effective ART no longer require MAC prophylaxis. For patients with chronic lung disease, it is reasonable to avoid exposure to potentially aerosolized NTM such as with recirculating water systems (hot tubs, steam rooms, prolonged showers, swimming pools) and aerosolized soil exposure. For patients with chronic lung disease and known NTM pulmonary colonization or disease, it is advisable to limit systemic and inhaled steroids as much as feasible. Like with *M. tuberculosis*, TNF-α inhibitors increase risk for NTM infection, and more aggressive disease progression and should be avoided when possible for susceptible patients. Avoiding nonsterile and nonregulated tattooing, cosmetic procedures, etc., can also help prevent some NTM infections.

Clinical Manifestations

Infections have a wide variety of presentations and largely depend on anatomic site of infection, host immune response, and infecting NTM species. Pulmonary infections comprise 80% of NTM infections. Pulmonary infections typically occur in people with underlying lung disease or immunosuppression and in some with chest wall deformities. Presentation is usually subacute or chronic and includes cough; other symptoms may include cough, shortness of breath, low-grade fevers, night sweats, weight loss, anorexia, and fatigue.

Cervicofacial lymphadenitis ("scrofula") is the most common extrapulmonary manifestation of MAC and is typically seen in children. This presents with typically painless, unilateral, firm lymph node swelling in the mandibular or jugular regions. Systemic symptoms are uncommon in the immune-competent host. Notably when seen in adults, cervicofacial lymphadenitis is more likely to be due to *M. tuberculosis* than NTM.

Various NTM different species cause skin and soft tissue infections, usually due to direct inoculation after traumatic wound, injections, and cosmetic procedures; rarely cutaneous manifestations of systemic disease can be seen. Lesions can appear as ulcers, papules, nodules, eschars, sporotrichoid lesions, or plaques with local swelling. Tenderness, erythema, swelling may be present and systemic symptoms are often absent.

Multiple species of NTM have been found to cause bone and joint infection. Injuries and implanted prosthetic devices (e.g., prosthetic joints) are risk factors for such infections. Patients may present with pain, swelling, erythema, purulent drainage, and pathologic fractures, with or without systemic symptoms.

Disseminated NTM infections occur in immunocompromised hosts and may present with fevers, chills, sweats, weight loss, and fatigue. Pancytopenia due to bone marrow and splenic involvement can lead to shortness of breath and pallor, easy bleeding/bruising, and superimposed infections due to neutropenia. Gastrointestinal involvement may cause diarrhea, abdominal pain, and hepatosplenomegaly.

Healthcare-associated infections also occur, especially in the setting of implanted prosthetic devices/material and intravascular catheters and after cosmetic procedures including mammoplasty and tattooing.

Diagnosis

The diagnosis of pulmonary NTM disease requires pulmonary symptoms, radiographic evidence of disease, exclusion of other diagnoses, and microbiologic criteria: Positive culture results from at least two sputum specimens or positive culture from at least one bronchial wash or lavage or lung tissue with granulomatous inflammation and >1 positive sputum or bronchial wash culture. AFB smears are notoriously insensitive. Colonization of the airways can occur with NTM, so a single positive sputum culture is not diagnostic of disease. Patients who don't meet all of the criteria should be followed closely over time, as NTM pulmonary disease may still develop.

Diagnosis of extrapulmonary NTM infections is typically through AFB culture(s) performed on the involved tissue or body fluid in the setting of a compatible clinical syndrome. NTM can colonize nonsterile areas in the body, so the presence of a positive AFB culture without an associated clinical syndrome must be interpreted cautiously. NTM lymphadenitis is best diagnosed by excisional lymph node biopsy for AFB culture and histopathology, as aspiration of NTM infected lymph nodes can lead to fistula formation. Explanted prosthetic devices can be sonicated and AFB culture performed on fluid. Tissue biopsies of affected areas may demonstrate noncaseating granulomatous changes on histopathology, with or without AFB seen on smear, and AFB culture is still necessary for diagnosis and treatment.

Disseminated MAC is diagnosed by isolation of the organism in AFB blood culture or other sterile site such as bone marrow, liver, or spleen. When available, direct detection of MAC in blood by PCR may be as sensitive and specific as culture, with results available in hours as opposed to weeks.

Drug susceptibility testing done on the mycobacterial species isolated is necessary to help guide treatment decisions.

Treatment

Treatment of NTM infections is, with few exceptions, complicated and requires input or management by specialists in NTM infections. NTM have intrinsic resistance to many antibiotics and can develop resistance on therapy. Treatment therefore typically requires two or three antimicrobial agents for a prolonged period of time, often 6 months to a year. If underlying immune suppression can be mitigated (e.g., holding or decreasing doses of immunosuppressive agents), such modifications should be made. Specific treatments vary for the different anatomic sites affected, species of NTM involved, antibiotic susceptibility patterns, host immune status, and the patient's tolerance for specific antimicrobials, prolonged duration, and the potential adverse effects. For pulmonary NTM disease, not all patients who meet diagnostic criteria need to be treated: Some people will have spontaneous resolution without antimicrobial therapy; when treated, duration is quite prolonged; treatment requires multiple drugs with various side effect profiles; treatment may require months of intravenous antibiotics; and pulmonary infection has a significant rate of relapse/recurrence.

Mycobacterium leprae *Complex*

Hansen's disease, also known as leprosy, is an indolent mycobacterial infection largely affecting skin and nerves caused by *Mycobacterium leprae* complex (*Mycobacterium leprae* and lepromatosis). It is an underdiagnosed disease due to its insidious onset of symptoms, the stigma associated with diagnosis and the healthcare system, and misrecognition of symptoms especially in areas of low prevalence. According to the World Health Organization (WHO), in 2019 there were 202,256 new cases diagnosed globally, with prevalence of 22.9 per million people. The majority of cases are reported from India, Brazil, and Indonesia. Untreated, Hansen's disease leads to significant morbidity and very impaired quality of life. The psychosocial stigma associated with the disease, however, is often felt by patients to be worse than the physical symptoms and must be addressed from time of initial evaluation through and beyond treatment.

Pathophysiology

Hansen's disease is a granulomatous infection caused by *Mycobacterium leprae* and *lepromatosis*, which comprise M. *leprae* complex. These organisms are gram-positive AFB that cannot be grown in culture. They replicate slowly, and average disease incubation period is 5 years. Though incompletely understood, transmission is felt to be person-to-person through nasal and respiratory secretions. Nine-banded armadillos in the southeastern United States, red squirrels in Scotland and England, chimpanzees, and macaques have all been found to carry M. *leprae* or M. *lepromatosis*, so zoonotic transmission is also implicated, though less frequently.

More than 95% of people worldwide are felt to have immunity to M. *leprae* complex, so in actuality, Hansen's disease is not very transmissible. Clinical and histopathologic disease occurs on a continuum, classified into five types by the Ridley-Jopling schema, depending on degree of host cell-mediated immune response to M. *leprae* complex. Disease types range from polar tuberculoid form (TT) with a strong immune response including well-formed granulomas, few bacilli, and more classic clinical manifestations, to the polar lepromatous type (LL) with minimal cell-mediated immune response, foamy macrophages without granulomas, and many bacilli seen on histopathology. LL clinical manifestations are less commonly recognized and are described below. Borderline tuberculoid (BT), mid-borderline (BB), and borderline lepromatous (BL) types have various degrees of both cell-mediated and humoral response.

Prevention

As with TB, the mainstay of prevention of Hansen's disease is early diagnosis and treatment of infected patients. There is currently no FDA approved vaccine to prevent infection with M.

leprae complex. BCG vaccine[1]—that given in endemic regions to prevent severe TB disease in children—when given to household contacts of people with Hansen's disease may decrease risk of transmission of M. *leprae* complex. Additionally, in household contacts of infected patients, BCG vaccination decreases likelihood of developing multibacillary disease.

Patients with Hansen's disease who have hypoesthetic lesions are at risk to develop injuries, such as burns and ulcers, in the insensate areas. Daily checks for foot wounds, avoiding walking barefoot, use of protective silicone gloves when cooking, and so on are important in the prevention and early detection and management of injury.

Clinical Manifestations

As M. *leprae* complex cannot be grown in culture, a high degree of clinical suspicion is necessary to pursue diagnosis. M. *leprae* complex requires cooler temperatures for growth and therefore has a predilection for cooler areas of the body including skin, cutaneous nerves, ears, and nose, including septum, eyes, larynx, and testes. Presentations vary according to degree of immune response to the bacilli. Cutaneous manifestations can include macules, patches, papules, or nodules. Lesions can be hypopigmented or reddish. The skin may be thick, scaly, or dry appearing. The hypopigmented areas are often hypoesthetic. Injuries to hypoesthetic areas are common and cause painless ulcers, burn wounds, lacerations, etc. Wounds may become infected. There may be madarosis: loss of the eyebrows and/or eyelashes. Thickening and nodularity of skin on the face can lead to a "leonine facies" appearance. Involvement of the nasal bridge can cause a "saddle nose" deformity. Perforation of the nasal septum can occur. Laryngeal involvement can lead to hoarseness. Eye involvement can include episcleritis and iridocyclitis. Lagophthalmos can occur leading to keratitis, corneal opacities, ectropion, entropion, and trichiasis. Neural involvement can lead to not only anesthetic areas but also thickened peripheral nerves, peripheral neuropathy, claw hand, foot drop, or paralysis of an extremity.

A particular area of concern that significantly affects patients living with Hansen's disease is the associated stigma and negative beliefs surrounding Hansen's disease, due to historic, religious, and social implications. Thus one must consider psychological burden associated with this infection when relaying diagnosis and throughout the patient's care.

Diagnosis

There are two main schema used for diagnosis: a binary clinical classification schema devised by the WHO for use where histopathology is not readily available and the histopathologic and clinical spectrum of the Ridley-Jopling classification. The WHO schema divides disease into multibacillary and paucibacillary, depending on number of skin lesions visible. The Ridley-Jopling schema classifies disease on a spectrum as outlined above and is based on skin biopsy for histopathology and Fite stain. Additional methods of identification of M. *leprae* complex include identification of the bacilli DNA in tissue biopsies by nucleic acid amplification techniques such as PCR.

Treatment

Using multidrug regimens, Hansen's disease is curable. Early recognition and treatment are key to preventing disability. The most active antimicrobial agents used to treat Hansen's disease include dapsone, rifampin (Rifadin, Rimactane),[1] and clofazimine (Lamprene). Other agents with efficacy include some fluoroquinolones, minocycline (Cleeravue-M, Dynacin, Minocin, Myrac, Solodyn, Ximino),[1] and clarithromycin (Biaxin).[1] As in other mycobacterial infections, multidrug regimens are imperative to prevent emergence of drug resistance and increase cure rates. Glucose-6-phosphate dehydrogenase (G6PD) deficiency testing should be performed prior to starting dapsone and the drug avoided if deficiency is present. Clofazimine (Lamprene) can only be obtained in the United States through the National

---

[1]Not FDA approved for this indication.

Hansen's Disease Program (NHDP) in Louisiana. The NHPD is the sole facility in the United States dedicated to Hansen's disease diagnosis, treatment, and research. Consultation with their expert physicians and pharmacists is highly recommended. There are many resources available to patients and healthcare providers alike through the NHDP, including review of histopathology specimens, consultation regarding molecular diagnosis of *M. leprae* complex, antimicrobial therapy free of costs for patients, and educational materials for physicians and patients to improve understanding of the disease and help prevent injury and disability. Finally, resources are available through NHDP for surgical care and rehabilitation of patients referred for digit or limb threatening wounds. Contact information can be found at https://www.hrsa.gov/hansens-disease/index.html.

Monitoring

G6PD deficiency testing should be performed prior to starting dapsone, and the drug avoided if deficiency is present. Patients should be monitored frequently while on therapy for potential adverse effects of various medications including anemia, QTc prolongation (clofazimine [Lamprene] and clarithromycin [Biaxin]), and skin discoloration (minocycline). Treatment efficacy is indicated by resolution of skin lesions and lack of new skin or nerve lesions. Patients should be monitored closely and educated about the signs and symptoms of reversal reactions, which can occur before, during, and even after therapy. At every visit, examination of all extremities should be performed to evaluate new and existing wounds.

Complications

Complications of Hansen's disease itself stem from injuries to hypoesthetic areas as above (largely hands and feet) and complications of peripheral neuropathy such as claw hand and foot drop. Evaluation and management by occupational and physical therapists and appropriate surgical referrals are often indicated.

As mentioned above, G6PD levels should be checked prior to initiation of dapsone and the drug avoided if patient is deficient in the enzyme, otherwise hemolytic anemia may develop. CBC with differential and ECG for QTc should be evaluated at baseline and periodically while on clofazimine (Lamprene) therapy.

Before, during, or even after therapy, pathologic immune reactions including reversal reactions and erythema nodosum leprosum can occur. Rarely, specific reversal reactions can be life threatening. Reversal reactions are inflammatory states, and measurement of biomarkers of inflammation can be helpful for evaluation and monitoring. Reversal reactions are treated with various immunosuppressing agents and consultation with the experts at NHDP is recommended.

References

American Thoracic Society: Targeted tuberculin testing and treatment of latent tuberculosis infection, *MMWR Recomm Rep (Morb Mortal Wkly Rep)* 49:1–51, 2000.

Bennett J, Dolin R, Blaser M: Infections cause by nontuberculous mycobacteria other than Mycobacterium avium complex. In Bennett J, Dolin R, Blaser M, editors: *Mandell, Douglas, and Bennett's Principles and practice of infectious diseases*, 9 ed, Elsevier, pp 3049–3058, 2020.

Bennett J, Dolin R, Blaser M: *Mycobacterium avium* complex. In Bennett J, Dolin R, Blaser M, editors: *Mandell, Douglas, and Bennett's Principles and practice of infectious diseases*, 9 ed, Elsevier, pp 3035–3048, 2020.

Bennett J, Dolin R, Blaser M. *Mycobacterium leprae* (leprosy). In Bennett J, Dolin R, and Blaser M, editors: Mandell, *Douglas, and Bennett's Principles and practice of infectious diseases*, 9 ed, Elsevier, pp. 3022-3034, 2020.

Bennett J, Dolin R, Blaser M: Mycobacterium tuberculosis. In Bennett J, Dolin R, Blaser M, editors: *Mandell, Douglas, and Bennett's Principles and practice of infectious diseases*, 9 ed, Elsevier, pp 2985–3021, 2020.

Daley CL, Iaccarino JM, Lange C, et al: Treatment of nontuberculous mycobacterial pulmonary disease: an Official ATS/ERS/ESCMID/IDSA clinical practice guideline, *Clin Infect Dis* 71(4):e1–e36, 2020.

Daley CL, Winthrop KL: *Mycobacterium avium* complex: Addressing Gaps in diagnosis and management, *J Infect Dis* 222(S4):S199–S211, 2020.

Dheda K, Barry 3rd CE, Maartens G: Tuberculosis, *Lancet* 387(10024):1211–1226, 2016 (Erratum in: Lancet 2016; 387(10024):1162).

Lewinsohn DM, Leonard MK, LoBue PA, et al: Official American Thoracic Society/ Infectious Diseases Society of America/Centers for Disease Control and Prevention clinical practice guidelines: diagnosis of tuberculosis in adults and children, *Clin Infect Dis* 64(2):e1–e33, 2017.

Leon KE, Jacob JT, Franco-Paredes C, et al: Delayed diagnosis, leprosy reactions, and nerve injury among individuals with Hansen's disease seen at a United States clinic, *Open Forum Infect Dis* 3(2):ofw063, 2016. Available at: https://academic.oup.com/ofid/article/3/2/ofw063/2399323. [Accessed 17 May 2021].

Nahid P, Dorman SE, Alipanah N, et al: Official American Thoracic Society/Centers for Disease Control and Prevention/Infectious Diseases Society of America clinical practice guidelines: treatment of drug-susceptible tuberculosis, *Clin Infect Dis* 63(7):e147–e195, 2016.

Nahid P, Mase SR, Migliori GB, et al: Treatment of drug-resistant tuberculosis. An Official ATS/CDC/ERS/IDSA clinical practice guideline [published correction appears in Am J Respir Crit care med. 2020 Feb 15;201(4):500-501], *Am J Respir Crit Care Med* 200(10):e93–e142, 2019.

National Hansen's Disease (Leprosy) Program Caring and Curing Since 1894. Available at: https://www.hrsa.gov/hansens-disease/index.html. [Accessed 06/17/2021].

Office of AIDS Research Advisory Council, Centers for Disease Control and Prevention, National Institute of Health, HIV Medicine Association (HIV-MA) of the Infectious Diseases Society of America (IDSA). Guidelines for the Prevention and Treatment of Opportunistic Infections in Adults and Adolescents with HIV. Available at: https://clinicalinfo.hiv.gov/en/guidelines/adult-and-adolescent-opportunistic-infection/whats-new-guidelines [accessed 06/18/2021].

Sterling TR, Njie G, Zenner D, et al: Guidelines for the treatment of latent tuberculosis infection: recommendations from the National Tuberculosis Controllers Association and CDC, 2020, *MMWR Recomm Rep (Morb Mortal Wkly Rep)* 69(No. RR-1):1–11, 2020.

World Health Organization. Leprosy (Hansen's Disease). Available at: https://www.who.int/news-room/fact-sheets/detail/leprosy [accessed 06/19/2021].

VENOUS THROMBOEMBOLISM

Method of
Moniba Nazeef, MD; and John P. Sheehan, MD

CURRENT DIAGNOSIS

- A comprehensive history is the most important diagnostic tool to assess risk factors including recent surgery, bedridden state, trauma, orthopedic procedure, or active cancer.
- Moderately high–sensitivity D-dimer assays (>85% sensitivity) can be used to exclude venous thromboembolism if there is low clinical probability but should be combined with imaging in all other cases.
- Venous compression ultrasonography is a noninvasive, affordable, and widely available test for the diagnosis of deep venous thrombosis. Computed tomography pulmonary angiography is the current gold standard for the diagnosis of pulmonary embolism.

CURRENT THERAPY

- The choice of initial therapy is frequently guided by the clinical scenario. Initial therapy includes unfractionated heparin, low-molecular-weight heparin, fondaparinux (Arixtra), or the direct oral anticoagulants—rivaroxaban (Xarelto) or apixaban (Eliquis).
- The traditional heparin-warfarin regimen has been increasingly supplanted by the use of direct oral anticoagulants.
- Standard treatment for a new episode of deep venous thrombosis or pulmonary embolism is 3 to 6 months of therapeutic anticoagulation. The recommended duration of anticoagulation for venous thromboembolism requires individualized analysis of the clinical presentation and patient specific factors that weigh both recurrence and bleeding risk.

Venous thromboembolism (VTE) is a significant health problem, with surveillance data suggesting that 60,000 to 100,000 people die of VTE each year in the United States. Approximately 50% to 60% of this disease burden is associated with a recent hospitalization, underscoring the importance of VTE prophylaxis. VTE comprises superficial vein thrombosis (SVT), deep venous thrombosis (DVT), and pulmonary embolism (PE). DVT typically starts in the deep veins of the lower extremities and progresses proximally. If untreated, a clot can break off and travel to the lungs where it is trapped in the pulmonary circulation, resulting in PE. DVT confined to the deep veins of the calf is termed *isolated distal DVT*, whereas involvement of the popliteal or more proximal veins is termed *proximal DVT*. SVT represents thrombosis in the superficial veins of the legs or arms and rarely progresses to DVT. The focus of this chapter is to understand the risk factors, diagnosis, treatment, and prevention of DVT and PE.

Pathophysiology/Risk Factors

Venous blood flow is maintained by a delicate homeostatic balance of prothrombotic and antithrombotic factors. Virchow's triad describes the major factors leading to VTE from a pathophysiologic standpoint: (1) intrinsic hypercoagulability, (2) endothelial damage, and (3) venous stasis. Most often, a combination of these factors leads to the development of VTE. Based on the presence or absence of typical clinical risk factors, VTE occurrences can be considered either provoked (e.g., postsurgical) or unprovoked (spontaneous). Furthermore, provoking risk factors may be transient/reversible (e.g., estrogen use) or nontransient/irreversible (e.g., lower extremity paresis), which has implications for decisions regarding duration of anticoagulant therapy (Table 1).

Acquired Risk Factors

Certain clinical conditions shift the balance between procoagulant and anticoagulant factors to promote thrombosis. These conditions include surgery, pregnancy and puerperium, inflammation, active cancer, major trauma, specific medications, and a variety of conditions that lead to immobility. A more comprehensive list is provided in Table 1. Many of these clinical conditions cause multiple changes relevant to VTE risk. For example, surgical interventions may induce endothelial damage, immobilization leading to venous stasis, platelet activation, and trigger inflammatory responses that increase fibrinogen, factor VIII, and von Willebrand factor levels. Orthopedic procedures involving the lower limbs and abdominopelvic surgeries in cancer patients are especially high risk from a VTE standpoint. Active cancer is associated with 20% of all VTE and involves a variety of mechanisms leading to hypercoagulability, including increased tissue factor expression, venous obstruction, indwelling catheters, reduced mobility, and chemotherapy.

Pregnancy and the puerperium, oral contraceptives (OC), and hormone replacement therapy (HRT) are important VTE risk factors in women. OC and HRT are associated with a number of changes in hemostatic protein levels and platelet function that appear globally prothrombotic. Higher estrogen content is associated with increased thrombotic risk and is modulated by a combination with specific progestins. Additionally, there is a higher risk of VTE in OC users with a positive family history, suggesting an underlying genetic predisposition.

A variety of conditions that involve prolonged immobilization enhance VTE risk. Cast immobilization of the lower extremity, paresis after neurologic events, multiple trauma, orthopedic surgeries, travel-associated immobility (>4 to 6 hours), or a bedridden state due to a variety of medical or surgical conditions result in stasis that promotes venous thrombosis. Many of these clinical situations are also associated with an inflammatory state that concomitantly increases intrinsic hypercoagulability of the blood. Venous wall injury may occur via a variety of mechanisms, including surgical interventions, indwelling intravenous catheters, trauma, and vasculitis.

Genetics of Venous Thromboembolism

Although acquired clinical risk factors are critical to assessing risk, the genetic contribution to VTE is also substantial, with heritability of VTE estimated at 40% to 47%. Like many complex phenotypes, VTE has a multigenic basis in which most individual alleles make relatively small contributions to overall risk. Factor V Leiden and the prothrombin G20210A polymorphism are examples of such alleles (two- to fourfold relative risk). At least 17 genes have been identified that harbor VTE-associated variants. Importantly, family history remains an independent risk factor even after excluding known gene variants associated with thrombophilia, suggesting that unidentified genes also contribute to VTE risk. Deficiencies of the coagulation inhibitors antithrombin, protein C, and protein S are rare conditions with a more substantial effect on the relative risk of VTE (10- to 20-fold increase) but tend to be diagnosed erroneously in the setting of acute thrombosis. The multigenic basis of VTE has implications for thrombophilia testing that include: (1) identification of minor alleles (e.g., factor V Leiden) is not helpful for prediction of VTE recurrence risk, (2) a careful family history is generally more valuable than a thrombophilia evaluation, and (3) the *absolute* risk for carriers of thrombophilic alleles is generally quite small and does not justify indefinite anticoagulation. A robust estimate of individual genetic risk requires systematic screening of all known VTE risk genes or whole genome/exome sequencing approaches that are not routinely available. Thus current thrombophilia testing rarely contributes to clinical decision making in patients with VTE. Testing should never be pursued for provoked events and is best limited to selected situations such as presentations at a young age (<30 years) or known thrombophilic traits occurring in the context of a family history of VTE. A thorough personal and family history is generally sufficient to determine the likelihood of an underlying inherited hypercoagulable state.

Epidemiology and Natural History

The exact incidence of VTE is unknown, but it is estimated that about 300,000 to 600,000 Americans are affected by VTE each year. VTE incidence appears approximately 30% higher in African Americans and approximately 70% lower in Asian and Native American populations relative to Whites. Importantly, the incidence of VTE increases with age, particularly after age 50. Whereas overall VTE is slightly more common in men, women have an increased incidence before age 40 based on the influence

---

TABLE 1	Risk Factors for Venous Thromboembolism

Transient/Reversible

Surgery (esp. lower limb orthopedic surgery)
General anesthesia > 30 min
Immobility due to surgical or medical condition
Oral contraceptives/hormone replacement therapy
Pregnancy, puerperium
Major trauma
Acute inflammation
Indwelling venous catheters
Heparin-induced thrombocytopenia
May-Thurner syndrome
Travel-associated thrombosis
Medications including tamoxifen, L-asparaginase, immunomodulatory agents (lenalidomide [Revlimid]), erythropoietin

Permanent/Nonreversible

Active cancer
Antiphospholipid syndrome
Myeloproliferative neoplasms
Paroxysmal nocturnal hemoglobinuria
Lower extremity paresis from neurologic disease
Sickle cell disease
Nephrotic syndrome
Active autoimmune conditions (SLE, IBD, ITP, TTP)
Chronic infection/inflammation
Morbid obesity (BMI > 40)

BMI, Body mass index; *IBD,* inflammatory bowel disease; *ITP,* immune thrombocytopenic purpura; *SLE,* systemic lupus erythematosus; *TTP,* thrombotic thrombocytopenic purpura.

of pregnancy and contraceptives. In older age groups, the frequency of PE is increased relative to DVT. Finally, the incidence of VTE has been increasing steadily since the mid-1980s, which may, in large part, represent the increased use and enhanced sensitivity of computed tomography (CT) scans and magnetic resonance (MR) imaging.

The natural history of VTE is affected by the underlying clinical risk factors, provoked versus unprovoked nature of the event, reversibility of risk factors, and location/nature of the thrombotic event. In general, untreated thrombi tend to extend proximally, break off, and embolize to the pulmonary circulation, where they may result in infarction and pulmonary hypertension. The risk of PE is increased for proximal versus distal involvement with DVT. More than 75% of VTE starts in the calf veins, and 20% to 30% of these cases progress to involve proximal veins in the leg or pelvis. Approximately 50% of patients with untreated symptomatic proximal DVT develop symptomatic PE, whereas the incidence of asymptomatic PE is even higher. Importantly, 10% of symptomatic PE is rapidly fatal, and 30% of patients with untreated symptomatic nonfatal PE will have a fatal recurrence. Thus recognition of PE is of the utmost clinical importance. Anticoagulant therapy inhibits thrombus growth and largely prevents interval recurrence, whereas endogenous thrombolysis may result in partial or complete resolution of the thrombus. Uncommonly, progressive thrombosis in the presence of anticoagulation may occur in high-risk situations such as metastatic malignancy or the antiphospholipid syndrome.

The risk of VTE recurrence after stopping anticoagulation varies significantly based on clinical presentation. About 20% to 40% of VTE episodes are unprovoked in nature, which is associated with a substantially higher recurrence rate. For unprovoked clots, recurrence rate is estimated to be approximately 10% in 1 year, approximately 30% in 5 years, and approaches approximately 40% in 10 years. In contrast, the recurrence risk of VTE associated with surgery (a transient risk factor) is less than 3% per year. Recurrences tend to occur in a similar site to the initial event, which is particularly important in the case of PE, as 25% of PE presents as sudden death. In contrast, the risk of recurrent VTE is much smaller in isolated distal (calf) DVT compared with proximal DVT and PE.

Long-Term Complications of Venous Thromboembolism
Postthrombotic Syndrome
About 20% to 50% patients with DVT develop some degree of postthrombotic syndrome (PTS) within the subsequent 1 to 2 years. Chronic venous obstruction, inflammation, endofibrosis, and valvular dysfunction contribute to the chronic venous insufficiency of PTS. Risk factors for PTS include persistent DVT symptoms after 1 month, extensive or recurrent DVT, inadequate anticoagulation, and advanced age. Manifestations include chronic leg edema, pain, heaviness, erythema, and venous ulcers that may result in significant disability. PTS is largely nonreversible, emphasizing the importance of DVT prevention. Graduated compression stockings provide symptomatic relief by preventing pooling of blood in the lower extremities but do not prevent PTS. In the 5% to 10% of patients with severe PTS, active supportive care and consultation with vascular surgery, dermatology, or vein specialists should be sought early to avoid development of debilitating venous ulcers.

Chronic Thromboembolic Pulmonary Hypertension
Chronic thromboembolic pulmonary hypertension (CTEPH) is a long-term complication of PE affecting 3% to 4% patients despite adequate anticoagulation. CTEPH is characterized by progressive pulmonary hypertension and right-side heart failure due to remodeling of pulmonary vasculature by thrombotic material. Patients with large central or extensive pulmonary emboli, hemodynamic compromise, and right heart dysfunction at diagnosis are at highest risk. Chronic progressive dyspnea with exertion is the most common symptom, and the clinician must have a high clinical suspicion based on the patient's history of PE. An

CLINICAL VARIABLE	POINTS
Active cancer (treatment ongoing or within previous 6 months or palliative)	1
Recently bedridden >3 days or major surgery within 4 weeks	1
Pitting edema confined to the symptomatic leg	1
Dilated superficial veins (nonvaricose)	1
Previous documented DVT	1
Paralysis, paresis, or recent plaster immobilization of the lower extremities	1
Localized tenderness along the distribution of the deep venous system	1
Calf swelling 3 cm greater than asymptomatic side measured 10 cm below tibial tuberosity	1
Alternative diagnosis at least as likely as DVT	–2

Clinical probability by interpretation of total score: >2, high; 1 or 2, moderate; <1, low.
DVT, Deep venous thrombosis.

echocardiogram revealing elevated pulmonary arterial hypertension should trigger evaluation with a ventilation/perfusion (V/Q) scan. The presence of chronic mismatched segmental perfusion defects on the V/Q scan is diagnostic of CTEPH. If anatomically feasible, treatment of choice is pulmonary endarterectomy, which can reverse the hemodynamic and functional abnormalities. Early recognition and referral to a specialized surgical treatment center are critical to patient outcomes. Lifelong anticoagulation is recommended for all patients with CTEPH.

Diagnosis of Deep Venous Thrombosis
The diagnosis of DVT proceeds via determination of clinical probability, D-dimer screening, and confirmatory imaging.

Clinical Features
Diagnosis begins with evaluation of the clinical scenario for VTE risk factors and suspicious physical exam findings. Suggestive features in the patient's recent history include recent surgery or bedridden state, trauma or orthopedic procedure, active cancer, and other typical risk factors (Table 1). Classic symptoms of DVT include limb swelling, pain, and erythema. On exam, unilateral calf swelling, pitting edema, dilated veins, and tenderness on palpation can be seen. The clinical probability becomes stronger when more of these findings are present. Risk stratification systems such as the Wells model (Table 2) use these clinical features to rapidly classify patients as high (~60% thrombosis), moderate (~25%), or low (~5%) risk for DVT. Differential diagnosis of DVT includes trauma, cellulitis, osteomyelitis, chronic venous insufficiency, arterial ischemia, ruptured Baker cyst, hematoma, and superficial thrombophlebitis. Because neither history nor physical examination findings are specific for DVT, D-dimer screening and objective imaging must be pursued if sufficient clinical suspicion exists. A simplified algorithm for diagnosis of DVT is provided (Figure 1).

D-dimer Screening
D-dimer is a specific fibrin degradation product generated by plasmin cleavage of cross-linked fibrin clot, formed by thrombin and factor XIII activity. D-dimer represents a useful screening tool based on excellent sensitivity and a high negative predictive value for VTE. However, D-dimer lacks specificity, as it is increased in a variety of conditions, including acute inflammation, recent surgery or trauma, pregnancy, disseminated intravascular

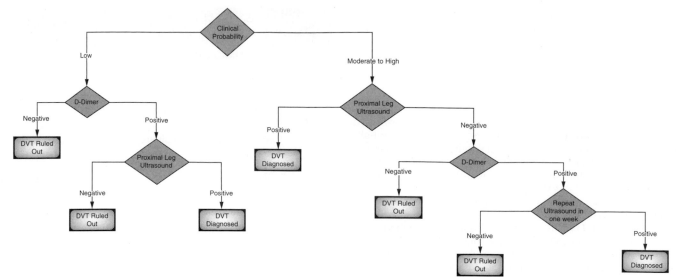

Figure 1 Suggested diagnostic algorithm for diagnosis of deep venous thrombosis *(DVT)*.

coagulation, advanced age, or cancer. The level of clinical suspicion also impacts interpretation of D-dimer results. Specific D-dimer assays vary in sensitivity and specificity, although qualitative testing has largely been replaced by enzyme-linked immunosorbent assay–based quantitative assays. More recently, highly sensitive assays (>95% sensitivity) using latex-enhanced immunoturbidimetric immunoassays provide rapid quantitation for use in the diagnosis of VTE. Point-of-care testing with specified cutoff values are also available. Thus the clinician should be familiar with the type of D-dimer testing available locally. Highly sensitive assays have a good negative predictive value to rule out VTE without further testing. Moderately high–sensitivity assays (>85% sensitivity) can be used to exclude VTE if there is low clinical probability but should be combined with imaging in all other cases. Qualitative or semiquantitative assays are generally not reliable for excluding thrombosis. Finally, if clinical suspicion for DVT or PE is high, a negative D-dimer should not be used to rule out VTE, and appropriate imaging should be pursued to confirm the diagnosis.

Imaging

Ultrasonography

Venous compression ultrasonography (CUS) is a noninvasive, affordable, and widely available test for the diagnosis of DVT. The deep veins are assessed by use of a compression probe with lack of compressibility in a venous segment indicative of thrombus. Duplex technology or color-coded Doppler scanning visualizes blood flow to allow accurate identification of deep veins. Lack of flow plus noncompressibility increases diagnostic accuracy and also facilitates diagnosis in veins that cannot be compressed (e.g., pelvic and subclavian veins). Venous ultrasonography has an excellent sensitivity and specificity (~94%) for diagnosis of proximal limb DVT. The common femoral, femoral, and trifurcation of calf veins are readily visualized. In most cases, a negative test is sufficient to rule out proximal VTE. Currently two methods for CUS are used: (1) the two-point compression technique, which only evaluates the proximal veins in the groin and popliteal fossa; and (2) whole-leg ultrasound scanning evaluating both proximal and distal veins. The sensitivity and specificity of CUS for calf vein DVT is significantly lower and highly operator dependent. Therefore many centers only perform the proximal vein assessment, which is reliable, reproducible, and efficient. If clinical suspicion remains high after a negative proximal vein ultrasound scan, repeat ultrasound scanning should be performed in about a week to assess for proximal extension in the deep venous system. If negative, no further testing is needed. A negative whole-leg CUS test result essentially rules out DVT and does not need follow-up testing. However, this approach is time-consuming and may

lead to increased diagnosis of calf vein thromboses and potential overtreatment. The 3-month incidence of symptomatic proximal venous thrombosis in patients with a normal initial test are comparable at approximately 1% for both approaches. For upper extremities, compression ultrasonography is about 86% sensitive and specific.

Contrast Venography

Once the gold standard for diagnosis of DVT, contrast venography is rarely used because it is invasive and requires contrast exposure. CT and MR venography have a sensitivity and specificity of greater than 90% for DVT in lower extremities. However, these studies are also not widely used for diagnosis because of increased cost, radiation, and contrast exposure. CT and MR venography are useful to define anatomy in patients with multiple recurrent DVT (evaluation by CUS is problematic), an indeterminate abnormality on ultrasound scanning, or a thrombus diagnosed in the setting of very low clinical suspicion.

Diagnosis of Pulmonary Embolism

Similar to DVT, the diagnosis of PE requires determination of clinical probability, consideration of D-dimer testing, and confirmatory imaging.

Clinical Features

A patient presenting with risk factors for VTE and antecedent history of DVT should raise the suspicion for PE. The most common symptoms of PE are shortness of breath and chest pain. Pleuritic chest pain is typical, but PE may also present with substernal pressure or be confused with musculoskeletal pain. Other symptoms may include cough and hemoptysis. Clinical signs include tachypnea, tachycardia, and hypoxia. The findings of DVT in the lower extremities increase the probability of PE. The Wells model for PE provides a useful framework to estimate the pretest probability using these variables (Table 3).

Chest X-ray, Electrocardiography, and Troponin

Chest x-ray should be performed in all suspected cases. The classic Hampton hump or peripheral wedge-shaped opacity corresponding to a large pulmonary infarct is seldom appreciated and not very sensitive or specific. However, a chest x-ray is useful in assessing for other conditions such as pneumonia, pneumothorax, and pulmonary edema that can present in similar fashion. Electrocardiography (ECG) should be performed in anyone presenting with chest pain to rule out myocardial infarction. Evidence of right heart strain on ECG has predictive and prognostic value in assessment of PE. Similarly, a troponin level is usually obtained in evaluation for myocardial ischemia. An elevated troponin level in the absence of ECG evidence of ischemia can be suggestive of myocardial injury in the setting of massive or submassive PE.

Ventilation/Perfusion Scanning

V/Q scans have largely been replaced by computed tomography pulmonary angiography (CTPA). However, V/Q scans remain useful in selected patients with significant renal insufficiency (to avoid contrast dye) and young or pregnant females (to avoid radiation exposure). This technique uses inhaled and intravenous radioisotopes to evaluate ventilation and circulation in the pulmonary parenchyma and vasculature, respectively. A normal perfusion scan in the setting of a normal chest x-ray excludes PE. The addition of a ventilation scan increases specificity by accounting for other pulmonary disorders. A normal chest x-ray and ventilation scan in areas with multiple large perfusion defects that involve greater than 75% of a segment (V/Q mismatch) is associated with greater than 80% probability of PE and considered a high-probability V/Q scan. An intermediate-probability scan usually requires further diagnostic evaluation because it is considered nondiagnostic in most situations. Three-dimensional single-photon emission CT (SPECT) is now used by many centers in place of planar V/Q scans. SPECT may be more accurate than planar V/Q scanning, resulting in fewer nondiagnostic studies.

Computed Tomography Pulmonary Angiography

CTPA is the modality of choice for diagnosis of PE. It is a relatively noninvasive procedure that can provide prompt diagnosis of PE. With recent advancements, the availability of thin-slice scans provides a detailed analysis of pulmonary vasculature that increases the sensitivity for detecting thrombi at the subsegmental and peripheral arterial level. In contrast to V/Q scanning, CTPA provides detailed visualization of the lung parenchyma, which can detect peripheral pulmonary infarctions and alternative diagnoses. When required, the CTPA examination can be extended to include the iliac veins, providing a detailed view with a single contrast exposure. CTPA has excellent sensitivity and specificity for diagnosis of lobar and segmental PE. Diagnostic accuracy is lower at the subsegmental level, and results should be interpreted in the context of clinical probability, proximal lower extremity ultrasound results, and D-dimer level. A simplified algorithmic approach to diagnosis of PE is provided (Figure 2). CTPA use is limited by costs, exposure to potentially nephrotoxic contrast dye, and chest radiation. It should be avoided in younger women because of the associated increased risk of breast cancer.

Pulmonary Angiography

Once the gold standard for the diagnosis of PE, pulmonary angiography is an invasive procedure that has been replaced by CTPA and is now very rarely performed.

Magnetic Resonance Angiography

Pulmonary contrast-enhanced magnetic resonance angiography (CE-MRA) is emerging as a useful alternative to CTPA in select patients such as younger females and those with severe iodinated contrast allergy. Currently, CE-MRA has limited availability and usefulness that is dependent on the expertise and experience of the available radiologist.

Diagnosis of Recurrent Deep Vein Thrombosis

The diagnosis of recurrent DVT can be challenging because signs and symptoms of PTS in the affected extremity can obscure the diagnosis. Clinical assessment of the probability for recurrent DVT is less well standardized than initial episodes; however, many predictive factors are expected to be shared. The clinician should assess for the presence of ongoing clinical risk factors, attempt to discern between chronic and acute signs and symptoms, and

TABLE 3	Wells Model for Predicting Pretest Probability of Pulmonary Embolism	
CLINICAL VARIABLE		**POINTS**
Clinical signs and symptoms of DVT (minimum leg swelling and pain with palpation of the deep veins)		3
An alternative diagnosis is less likely than PE		3
Heart rate > 100 beats/min		1.5
Immobilization or surgery in the previous 4 weeks		1.5
Previous DVT/PE		1.5
Hemoptysis		1
Active cancer (treatment ongoing or within previous 6 months or palliative)		1

Clinical probability by interpretation of total score: >6, high; 4–6, moderate; <4, low.
DVT, Deep venous thrombosis; *PE,* pulmonary embolism.

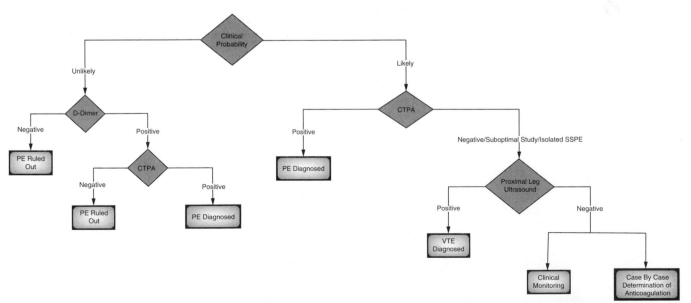

Figure 2 Suggested diagnostic algorithm for diagnosis of pulmonary embolism *(PE). CTPA,* Computed tomography pulmonary angiography; *SSPE,* subsegmental pulmonary embolism.

consider D-dimer testing. A negative D-dimer test can be used to exclude recurrent DVT, although the accuracy of this approach has not been well studied. If D-dimer testing is positive or has not been done, CUS is performed. The finding of noncompressibility of an ipsilateral femoral or popliteal vein segment, which was previously unaffected, can be considered diagnostic. For diagnosing recurrent DVT in a previously affected vein segment, an increase in thrombus diameter of at least 4 mm on serial CUS in combination with a D-dimer measurement can serve as helpful criteria. This diagnosis requires the expertise of an experienced radiologist with the previous ultrasound available for comparison. In practice, comparison with previous CUS is difficult, given the operator-dependent characteristics of the test. If comparison with the previous examination is equivocal or unavailable, CT or MR venography may be considered. An intraluminal filling defect suggests acute rather than remote thrombosis. Alternatively, a patient with initially equivocal CUS findings can undergo serial repeat examinations to detect DVT extension.

Treatment of Venous Thromboembolism

Anticoagulation Therapy for Venous Thromboembolism

Patients with newly diagnosed VTE should be promptly initiated on therapeutic anticoagulation. In the absence of a severely symptomatic lower extremity, high thrombus burden PE with right ventricular dysfunction or significant cardiovascular comorbidity, management is predominantly outpatient. In the presence of PE, a simplified PE severity index (sPESI; https://www.mdcalc.com/calc/1247/simplified-pesi-pulmonary-embolism-severity-index) is often used to assess appropriateness for outpatient therapy. The sPESI score includes the following factors (1 point each): age greater than 80 years, history of cancer, chronic cardiopulmonary disease, pulse greater than 110 beats/min, systolic blood pressure less than 100 mm Hg, and arterial oxygen saturation less than 90%. Patients with a sPESI score greater than or equal to 1 are considered high risk and should be considered for initial inpatient management.

Choice of Initial Anticoagulant Therapy

The choice of initial therapy is frequently guided by the clinical scenario. Initial therapy includes unfractionated heparin (UFH), low-molecular-weight heparin (LWMH), fondaparinux (Arixtra), or the direct oral anticoagulants—rivaroxaban (Xarelto) or apixaban (Eliquis) (Table 4). Therapeutic UFH is administered intravenously (IV) and demonstrates complex pharmacokinetics (both hepatic and renal clearance) that requires laboratory monitoring of drug effect (activated partial thromboplastin time [aPTT] or anti–factor Xa activity). Thus UFH therapy requires hospital admission and has largely been replaced by other options. UFH may still be appropriate for patients experiencing inpatient VTE events, especially if a need for invasive procedures is anticipated (half-life, 1 to 2 hours). The therapeutic target range for UFH is a 1.5- to 2.5-fold increase over the baseline aPTT or 0.3 to 0.7 U/mL anti–factor Xa activity. In contrast, LMWH is administered subcutaneously and primarily cleared by the kidneys, resulting in predictable pharmacokinetics. Subcutaneous administration facilitates outpatient treatment, and predictable pharmacokinetics allow weight-based dosing without laboratory monitoring. Fondaparinux, a synthetic pentasaccharide, is exclusively cleared by the kidneys with a long half-life (17 to 21 hours) that allows for once-daily, weight-adjusted subcutaneous dosing. Fondaparinux similarly does not require routine laboratory monitoring, but caution is warranted in patients with mild renal insufficiency where drug accumulation may increase bleeding risk. Heparin therapy (UFH, LMWH, or fondaparinux) for VTE is administered for a *minimum* of 5 days followed by transition to longer-term oral anticoagulation with an oral vitamin K antagonist (VKA) or a direct oral anticoagulant (DOAC). Alternatively, rivaroxaban or apixaban can be initiated immediately after VTE diagnosis and bypass the need for heparin therapy (see later).

Historically, VKAs are the primary oral anticoagulants for the long-term treatment of VTE. Warfarin (Coumadin) is the VKA used almost exclusively in the United States. Warfarin and other VKAs inhibit vitamin K-dependent γ-carboxylation of the

TABLE 4	Drugs for the Treatment of Venous Thromboembolism			
DRUG	**DOSING**	**ELIMINATION**	**HALF-LIFE**	**MONITORING**
UFH	80 units/kg IV bolus, then 18 U/kg/hour initial infusion rate	Complex, hepatic/renal metabolism	1–2 hours	aPTT Anti–factor Xa activity
LMWH	Dalteparin (Fragmin): 200 U/kg SQ QD Enoxaparin (Lovenox): 1 mg/kg SQ BID	Predominantly renal	3–5 hours	None required*
Fondaparinux (Arixtra)	5.0 mg SQ QD (<50 kg) 7.5 mg SQ QD (50–100 kg) 10 mg SQ QD (>100 kg)	Renal	17–21 hours	None required*
Warfarin (VKA) (Coumadin)	Initially 5 mg PO QD, broad range (2.5–10 mg)	Extensive hepatic metabolism Renal excretion for metabolites	Pharmacokinetics: 20–60 hours, variable Pharmacodynamics: 42–72 hours†	PT/INR (2.0–3.0)
Dabigatran (Pradaxa)	Parenteral anticoagulant × 5–10 days, then dabigatran 150 mg PO BID	>80% renal, 20% biliary Prodrug	12–17 hours 14–17 hours (elderly)	None required
Rivaroxaban (Xarelto)	15 mg PO BID × 21 days; then 20 mg PO QD	66% renal, 33% biliary CYP450 substrate	5–9 hours 9–12 hours (elderly)	None required
Apixaban (Eliquis)	10 mg PO BID × 7 days, then 5 mg PO BID	25% renal, 75% biliary CYP450 substrate	8–15 hours	None required
Edoxaban (Savaysa)	Parenteral anticoagulant × 5–10 days, then edoxaban 60 mg PO QD (30 mg QD for ≤60 kg)	35% renal, 60% biliary	10–14 hours	None required

*Anti–factor Xa activity can be used in selected circumstances such as extremes of body weight (<45 kg or >100 kg).
†Pharmacodynamics of coagulation protein recovery most relevant to in vivo effect of VKA.
aPTT, Activated partial thromboplastin time; *BID*, twice daily; *INR*, international normalized ratio; *IV*, intravenous; *LMWH*, low-molecular-weight heparin; *PO*, orally; *PT*, prothrombin time; *QD*, once daily; *SQ*, subcutaneous; *UFH*, unfractionated heparin; *VKA*, vitamin K antagonist.

TABLE 5	Reversal Agents		
DRUG	**REVERSAL AGENT**	**DOSING**	**COMMENTS**
Heparin	Protamine*	1–1.5 mg/100 U UFH IV	Hypersensitivity reactions, less effective vs. LMWH
Warfarin	Four-factor PCC (Kcentra) FFP Vitamin K	25–50 U/kg IV 2–4 L 1–10 mg PO or IV	Dose depends on INR, PCC favored over FFP Volume overload, transfusion reaction Reversal takes 6–24 hours
Dabigatran	Idarucizumab (Praxbind)	2.5 g IV for 2 doses (within 15 min)	Drug specific monoclonal Fab fragment
Rivaroxaban Apixaban Edoxaban	Andexanet alfa (Andexxa) (approved for reversal of rivaroxaban or apixaban only) Four-factor PCC†	800 mg IV bolus at 30 mg/min, then 960 mg infusion at 8 mg/min 50 U/kg IV	Reverses factor Xa active site inhibitors

*FDA approved for treatment of heparin overdose. Off-label uses: heparin neutralization (adults); intracranial hemorrhage associated with heparin or LMWH; LMWH overdose (adults).

†Evidence for reversal of factor Xa inhibitors by PCC is low quality.

Fab, Fragment antigen-binding; *FDA*, U.S. Food and Drug Administration; *FFP*, fresh frozen plasma; *INR*, international normalized ratio; *IV*, intravenous; *LMWH*, low-molecular-weight heparin; *PCC*, prothrombin complex concentrate; *PO*, orally; *UFH*, unfractionated heparin.

coagulation zymogens (proenzymes). This posttranslational modification is required for both efficient protein secretion and function (membrane binding) of coagulation factors VII, IX, X, and II. Vitamin K is oxidized during γ-carboxylation of these coagulation factors, and warfarin inhibits enzymatic regeneration of the reduced form of vitamin K, creating a functional deficiency. This mechanism of action is the basis for (1) the reversibility of the warfarin by administration of the reduced form of vitamin K, (2) the reduction in warfarin effect by dietary vitamin K, and (3) the enhancement of the warfarin effect by many antibiotics, as bacterial flora are a major source of vitamin K. Warfarin also undergoes extensive metabolism by the liver, which provides multiple opportunities for drug interactions. Thus genetic variation in liver metabolism, variable dietary vitamin K intake, and numerous potential drug interactions generate substantial individual variation in warfarin dose requirements.

Warfarin (2.5- to 10-mg initial dose) is usually started the same day as heparin, overlapped with parenteral heparin therapy for a *minimum* of 5 days and discontinued once a therapeutic warfarin level is obtained on two consecutive days. The warfarin effect is monitored by the international normalized ratio (INR), which represents a prothrombin time that has been corrected for specific reagent sensitivity. The target INR for VTE treatment is 2.0 to 3.0. The pharmacodynamic effects of warfarin on the INR are primarily determined by the in vivo half-lives of the relevant coagulation factors. Thus the full effect of a warfarin dose change on the INR is usually not seen for 48 to 72 hours, correlating with the half-life of factors IX, X, and prothrombin (factor II). This delayed effect necessitates overlap with heparin therapy for at least 5 days, or longer if further warfarin dose titration is required to reach a therapeutic INR. Initial warfarin dosing should be conservative (2.5 mg daily) if enhanced sensitivity is expected, including patients that are elderly (>65 years old), low body weight (<45 kg), hypoalbuminemic (<2 g/dL), on antibiotic therapy, or have poor oral intake.

The traditional heparin-warfarin regimen has been increasingly supplanted by the use of DOACs. DOACs are orally available, low-molecular-weight compounds that directly inhibit the active site of either factor Xa (rivaroxaban, apixaban, edoxaban [Savaysa]), or thrombin (dabigatran [Pradaxa]). In general, these drugs possess predictable pharmacokinetics and relatively short half-lives, allowing fixed once- or twice-daily oral dosing without routine monitoring. Both rivaroxaban and apixaban are approved for initial use after the VTE diagnosis with a more intensive dose regimen that tapers to the standard maintenance dose after 21 days for rivaroxaban or 7 days for apixaban (Table 4). Edoxaban and dabigatran are approved for continued treatment of VTE at their standard maintenance dose after 5 to 10 days of a parenteral anticoagulant (usually LWMH). Differences in clearance mechanisms have implications for clinical usage. For instance, dabigatran is heavily dependent on renal clearance and can accumulate with increased bleeding risk in patients with significant renal insufficiency (CrCl < 30 mL/min). In contrast, apixaban dosing is less affected by renal insufficiency but should not be used in patients with significant liver dysfunction or biliary stasis.

Comparison of Warfarin Versus DOACs

DOACs demonstrate equivalent efficacy to the traditional combination of LMWH and warfarin in the treatment of VTE. Advantages of the DOACs include rapid onset of action, predictable dose response, no monitoring requirement, elimination of parenteral therapy (rivaroxaban and apixaban), no significant diet interactions, limited drug interactions, and an overall safety signal equivalent to or better than warfarin. Metaanalyses of DOAC trials demonstrate that fatal bleeding, intracranial hemorrhage (ICH), and clinically relevant, nonmajor bleeding are reduced with DOACs compared with warfarin. The rate of gastrointestinal (GI) bleeding was similar. Given the potentially life-changing nature of ICH, the lower rate with DOACs is particularly significant. Disadvantages of DOACs include cost, inability to monitor compliance with routine coagulation testing, the effect of renal function on drug clearance, and lack of widely available reversal agents. The relatively short half-lives of DOACs and recent development of reversal agents (Table 5) partially overcome the reversibility advantage for warfarin. Largely based on safety profile and ease of use, recent guidelines provide a weak recommendation for DOACs over warfarin in patients without cancer.

Cancer-Associated Thrombosis

VTE associated with cancer accounts for approximately 20% of all cases and clearly is a heterogeneous patient population. Treatment of cancer-associated thrombosis is problematic in that patients are at increased risk for both VTE recurrence and bleeding complications. In addition to the multiple drug interactions that complicate VKA use in cancer patients, LMWH demonstrates significantly lower rates of recurrent VTE relative to VKA therapy. Thus LMWH for the first 6 months after the event has been the standard recommendation. The role of DOACs in cancer-associated thrombosis continues to evolve. Metaanalysis of subgroups from the large DOAC VTE trials demonstrates no difference in VTE recurrence or major bleeding compared with LMWH for primarily low-risk cancer patients. Subsequent comparison of edoxaban[1] and dalteparin (Fragmin) (Hokusai trial)

---

[1] Not FDA approved for this indication.

in a broader population of active cancer patients demonstrated a lower rate of VTE recurrence but higher rate of major bleeding. A randomized study comparing rivaroxaban[1] to dalteparin (SELECT-D) demonstrated similar findings with reduced VTE rate and increased nonmajor bleeding in the DOAC arm. The increased bleeding was primarily observed in patients with upper GI or urothelial cancers in both studies. Ongoing studies will further address the role of DOACs in this setting. Duration of therapy is generally at least 6 months but may be modified based on disease response, bleeding risk, and prognosis.

Special Considerations in the Acute Management of Venous Thromboembolism

Although the vast majority of patients diagnosed with VTE should be promptly initiated on therapeutic anticoagulation, a limited number of acute presentations may require a modified approach as described in the following sections.

Massive Pulmonary Embolism With Hemodynamic Instability

Patients presenting with hemodynamically unstable PE (systolic blood pressure < 90 mm Hg for 15 minutes, requiring vasopressors or overt shock) are at high risk for right heart failure and death. The focus for these patients should be resuscitation (IV fluids, pressors, oxygenation, and airway control) and rapid confirmation of diagnosis (perfusion scan or CTPA). If highly unstable, then bedside echocardiogram may be used for a presumptive diagnosis based on right ventricular findings. Prompt thrombolytic therapy (tPA [Activase][1] 100 mg IV) or consideration of emergency endovascular therapy should be pursued, with the former being more readily available.

Patients who present with worsening right heart failure, preresuscitation cardiopulmonary arrest, free-floating thrombus, or high thrombus burden in the absence of systemic hypotension may also be considered for thrombolytic therapy. Many institutions have a PE response team to facilitate decision making and institution of therapy. However, for the majority of patients presenting with evidence of right ventricular dysfunction (by echocardiogram or CT) without systemic hypotension (i.e., submassive or intermediate risk PE), the use of thrombolytic therapy remains controversial. This controversy stems from both heterogeneity in patient selection for these trials and the inability to demonstrate long-term benefits over anticoagulation alone.

Broader use of thrombolytic therapy is primarily limited by the increased risk of major bleeding (9.2%) versus anticoagulation (3.4%), which includes a 1.5% incidence of intracranial bleeding. Contraindications include previous ICH, known intracranial vascular lesion or malignancy, ischemic stroke within 3 months, suspected aortic dissection, active bleeding or bleeding diathesis, and closed head/facial trauma within 3 months. Relative contraindications include poorly controlled hypertension, recent surgery (14 days), and pregnancy. The use of combined modalities (catheter-based fibrinolysis, pharmacomechanical clot dissolution) and lower doses of tissue plasminogen activator (tPA[1] 50 mg IV) may modulate the bleeding risk, but currently, broader application of thrombolytic therapy remains controversial.

Extensive Proximal Vein Lower Extremity Thrombosis

Proximal iliac vein thrombosis is often highly symptomatic and may result in severe PTS. Rarely, compromise of the arterial supply may occur, as described for phlegmasia alba dolens ("milk leg") and phlegmasia cerulea dolens. The former describes a swollen, white extremity with early compromise of arterial flow secondary to extensive DVT. The latter is an advanced stage characterized by severe swelling, cyanosis, and blue discoloration of the extremity—a precursor of venous gangrene. These entities are emergencies that require prompt anticoagulation, elevation, and consideration of endovascular intervention. The presence of bilateral proximal iliac vein thrombosis should prompt evaluation for inferior vena cava (IVC) thrombus or agenesis, particularly in younger patients. Catheter-directed thrombolysis and endovascular approaches have been pursued in proximal iliofemoral venous thrombosis in an attempt to reduce the risk of severe PTS. Recent studies have been unable to demonstrate that the desired benefit in PTS reduction outweighs the increased risk of bleeding. Thus the routine use of thrombolytic therapy for proximal iliofemoral venous thrombosis cannot be recommended, and patient selection for this approach remains controversial.

Spontaneous Proximal Upper Extremity Thrombosis

The majority of upper extremity DVT is related to intravenous catheters, malignancy, or thrombophilia. Spontaneous upper extremity DVT in the absence of provocation is rare. This entity (Paget-Schroetter syndrome) tends to occur in a younger, often adolescent population with a recent history of exercise or strenuous activity usually involving the dominant upper extremity. This presentation in the absence of usual VTE risk factors should prompt an evaluation for venous thoracic outlet syndrome (TOS). Because of the younger age of these patients and significant disability associated with PTS in the upper extremity (particularly the dominant hand), the initial approach has included thrombolysis (within 14 days), anticoagulation, and evaluation for venous TOS. However, no rigorous comparison of these approaches or combinations of approaches has been undertaken. If evidence for venous TOS is demonstrated, first rib resection on the affected side is often recommended. In the absence of a predisposing anatomic abnormality, an underlying thrombophilic state or occult malignancy should be considered.

Venous Thromboembolism Presenting With Paradoxical Embolism

The occurrence of arterial embolism, most commonly cryptogenic stroke, in the presence of DVT and a right-to-left shunt (i.e., patent foramen ovale [PFO]) suggests the diagnosis of paradoxical embolus. Standard anticoagulation for VTE is recommended, followed by PFO closure when complete. If indefinite anticoagulation is planned, the additional benefit of PFO closure is unclear.

DOACs in End-Stage Renal Disease

Warfarin has been the mainstay for treatment of VTE in patients with end-stage renal disease (ESRD). Most DOACs cannot be used in patients with creatinine clearance less than 30 mL/min because of the lack of randomized trial data in this population. However, apixaban is FDA approved for use even in patients with ESRD without dose adjustment based on its predominantly hepatic clearance and pharmacokinetic data.

Apixaban has been increasingly used in these patients because of its convenient dosing and lack of UFH bridging that typically requires hospitalization. Several small-center studies and a large retrospective study of patients with ESRD and newly diagnosed VTE who received either apixaban or warfarin suggest apixaban is associated with lower incidence of major bleeding with comparable incidence of recurrent VTE and all-cause mortality. It must be borne in mind that bleeding rates in ESRD patients on anticoagulation are overall higher than the general population. At this time, an individualized approach is recommended based on patient risk factors for bleeding and recurrent thrombosis, as well as treatment duration and cost, in determining appropriateness of apixaban in such cases.

DOACs in Obesity

There is a lack of consensus regarding direct oral anticoagulant dosing for the management of VTE in obese patients, particularly morbidly obese patients, given the relative scarcity of randomized clinical trial data in patients with a body mass index greater than 40 kg/m[2] or weight greater than 120 kg. This stems from concern that fixed dosing in obese patients might lead to decreased drug exposure and lower efficacy.

---

[1] Not FDA approved for this indication.

Retrospective and prospective studies, as well as metaanalyses comparing DOAC with VKA in VTE, have shown similar efficacy and bleeding signal in obese patients. As a result, in patients with BMI greater than 40 kg/m^2 or weight greater than 120 kg, the 2021 International Society on Thrombosis and Hemostasis (ISTH) guidelines suggest that standard doses of apixaban or rivaroxaban and weight-based LMWH are appropriate for the treatment of VTE and VTE prophylaxis. Data on other DOACs are not sufficient at this time.

Moreover, ISTH no longer recommends regularly monitoring peak or trough drug-specific DOAC levels because there are insufficient data to influence management decisions. It is therefore reasonable to consider using standard doses of apixaban or rivaroxaban in obese patients after weighing the risks and benefits.

In obese patients receiving LMWH for acute VTE, the initial LMWH dose is recommended according to *actual body weight* rather than a fixed maximum daily dose by American Society of Hematology guidelines. Routine monitoring of LMWH is no longer recommended because of the unclear effect of anti–factor Xa levels with bleeding and lack of standardization.

Acute Venous Thromboembolism With Contraindication to Anticoagulation

Occasionally patients diagnosed with acute VTE will have an absolute contraindication to anticoagulation. Placement of a temporary IVC filter may be considered in these patients to provide short-term protection from PE. However, the vast majority of contraindications to anticoagulation are temporary, and definitive anticoagulation therapy should be instituted as soon as feasible. IVC filter use is associated with increased risk of lower extremity DVT. Evaluation for IVC filter removal should be planned within 3 to 6 months, depending on the clinical scenario.

Isolated Subsegmental Pulmonary Embolism and Incidental Venous Thromboembolism

The enhanced sensitivity of current CT scanners and extensive use of CT angiography has led to an increased diagnosis of isolated subsegmental PE. Treatment of isolated subsegmental PE (where proximal DVT has been excluded) is controversial as the natural history and benefit of anticoagulation is unclear. If an isolated subsegmental defect occurs in a clinical context that is high risk for recurrent VTE (e.g., malignancy), therapeutic anticoagulation is preferred. Alternatively, for an isolated subsegmental PE occurring in a patient that is otherwise low risk for VTE recurrence, clinical surveillance is preferred. Based on the frequency of diagnostic and staging CT scans in cancer patients, an incidental diagnosis of VTE is not an uncommon finding. Although outcome data are limited in this setting, incidental VTE appears to have similar effects on mortality and risk of VTE recurrence. Because the outcomes for incidental and symptomatic VTE in cancer patients appear similar, most cases of incidental VTE should be treated similar to symptomatic VTE.

Special Circumstances for Anticoagulant Monitoring

The predictable dose responses for LMWH, fondaparinux, and the DOACs allow use without monitoring. However, select circumstances exist where monitoring may be desirable. LMWH is the preferred anticoagulant in pregnancy, but weight-based dosing may not be as accurate during pregnancy. Periodic confirmation of therapeutic target levels (0.5 to 1.2 U/mL anti–factor Xa activity) 4 hours after subcutaneous injection is often recommended. Likewise, the accuracy of weight-based LMWH dosing with a body weight less than 45 kg or greater than 100 kg is not extensively validated. Confirmation of therapeutic peak levels in these individuals is recommended. Similarly, a need for DOAC drug levels may arise when assessing compliance, bleeding with potential drug overdose, or for an emergent procedure. DOACs directed against factor Xa (rivaroxaban, apixaban, and edoxaban) are monitored with an anti–factor Xa activity assay using a drug-specific standard curve. Significant dabigatran drug effect

is excluded with a normal thrombin time. Alternatively, dabigatran drug effect can be detected by prolongation of the aPTT or more specialized coagulation tests. The INR is not sensitive to dabigatran.

Reversal Agents

Acute reversal of anticoagulation may be required for drug overdose with clinically significant bleeding or emergent procedures. If the situation is nonemergent, holding warfarin (4 to 5 days depending on INR) or DOACs (2 to 3 days depending on renal function) is preferable. If urgent reversal is required, specific agents exist for UFH, warfarin, and, more recently, DOACs (Table 5). Although UFH overdose may be reversed with dose-adjusted protamine, the short half-life of UFH and potential toxicity of protamine often mitigate against use. Protamine is most commonly used to reverse high-dose UFH after cardiopulmonary bypass. LMWH overdose may also be treated with protamine,[1] but significantly less effectively. Warfarin is fully reversed by administration of four-factor prothrombin complex concentrate (PCC) or fresh frozen plasma (FFP). The four-factor PCC dose is modified based on the INR and favored over FFP, which may be complicated by volume overload and transfusion reactions. Immediate reversal with PCC or FFP should be followed with 5 to 10 mg vitamin K by the oral or IV route. Vitamin K takes 6 to 24 hours to act but is critical to maintaining anticoagulant reversal because the PCC or FFP effect will wane based on plasma half-life of the coagulation factors. Notably, high doses of vitamin K can result in relative warfarin resistance for the ensuing 1 to 2 weeks. Lower doses of vitamin K (1 to 2 mg) may be appropriate for less serious bleeding where early reinitiation of warfarin is anticipated. Highly specific agents for the reversal of DOACs are now available. Dabigatran is rapidly reversed by administration of idarucizumab (Praxbind), a humanized monoclonal fragment antigen-binding (Fab) fragment that neutralizes the parent drug and major metabolites. DOACs targeting factor Xa (rivaroxaban, apixaban, edoxaban) may be rapidly reversed with andexanet alfa (Andexxa), a truncated, inactive form of recombinant factor Xa that acts as a decoy for small molecules targeting the factor Xa active site. Andexanet alfa was approved for life-threatening bleeding in patients treated with rivaroxaban and apixaban based on an open-label, single-group study (ANNEXA-4). Given the relatively short half-lives of the DOACs, high cost, and association with increased risk of thromboembolic events for andexanet alfa, it should be reserved for truly emergent procedures or life-threatening anticoagulant-related bleeding. Use of andexanet alfa in patients treated with edoxaban or betrixaban is off-label.

Duration of Anticoagulation

Standard treatment for a new episode of DVT or PE has traditionally been 3 to 6 months of therapeutic anticoagulation. The recommended duration of anticoagulation for VTE requires individualized analysis of the clinical presentation and patient-specific factors that weigh both recurrence and bleeding risk (Figure 3).

Clinical Presentation

Recurrence risk varies widely based on clinical presentation (see Epidemiology and Natural History). The key distinction is between events that occur in the absence (unprovoked) versus the presence (provoked) of established VTE risk factors (Table 1). The majority of cases with clinical risk factors present may be categorized as transient/reversible (e.g., surgery, estrogen) or permanent/nonreversible (e.g., dense hemiplegia secondary to stroke). Surgery is a major transient risk factor for VTE with a low recurrence risk (3% at 5 years). Three months of anticoagulation is sufficient for this population, whereas shorter durations are associated with increased risk of recurrence. Estrogen-related events have a similarly low risk of recurrence if reexposure is avoided. A second category of VTE events occurs in association with a

---

[1] Not FDA approved for this indication.

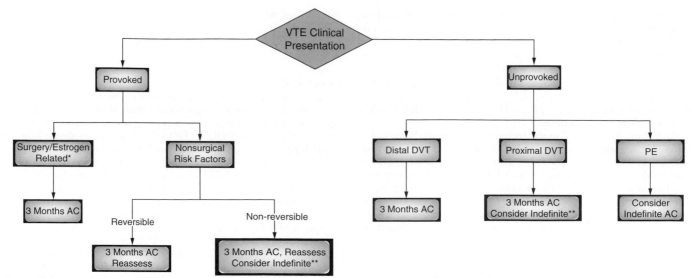

Figure 3 Suggested algorithm for treatment of venous thromboembolism *(VTE)*. *Estrogen-related includes oral contraceptives, hormone replacement therapy, pregnancy, and puerperium. **Indefinite anticoagulation *(AC)* includes reduced-dose direct oral anticoagulant options after initial 3 months therapeutic AC. *DVT*, Deep venous thrombosis; *PE*, pulmonary embolism.

nonsurgical transient risk factor (leg injury, significant medical illness, travel association) and demonstrates an intermediate recurrence risk (15% at 5 years). This subgroup is substantially more heterogeneous than the surgical group, with a variety of triggering factors and broader recurrence risk estimates. VTE events associated with nonreversible clinical risk factors may require extended anticoagulation with periodic reassessment of risks and benefits. Unprovoked VTE demonstrates a high risk of recurrence (30% at 5 years) and, in many respects, behaves as a chronic disease. Finally, patients with an underlying malignancy represent approximately 20% of VTE cases but are usually excluded from natural history studies. Cancer-associated thrombosis demonstrates a 15% annualized recurrence risk with longer-term risk more difficult to estimate based on competing mortality from the underlying cancer. These patients have concomitant increased bleeding risk, complicating the risk-benefit analysis for anticoagulation.

Thrombus Site

Thrombus location significantly influences recurrence risk, with more proximal events demonstrating higher rates of recurrence. Patients with isolated distal or calf vein DVT are half as likely to have recurrent events compared with proximal DVT or PE. Patients presenting with proximal DVT have similar recurrence risk to patients with PE. However, patients initially presenting with PE are substantially more likely to have a PE recurrence relative to patients presenting with DVT only. This finding takes on particular importance when one considers the cause-specific mortality rate associated with PE is greater than 10%. Thus patients presenting with unprovoked PE deserve particular attention with regard to consideration of indefinite anticoagulation.

Standard Versus Indefinite Anticoagulation

Clinical presentation categorizes patients with regard to recurrence risk, which is critical to the decision between standard (3 months) and indefinite anticoagulation (Figure 3). This decision is also influenced by bleeding risk and requires clinical judgment. As mentioned earlier, VTE associated with surgical or estrogen-related provoking factors and distal DVT (provoked or unprovoked) should be treated with therapeutic anticoagulation for 3 months. Conversely, most patients with unprovoked proximal DVT or PE should be considered for indefinite therapy based on their substantial recurrence risk unless they also have high bleeding risk. There is little rationale for arbitrary extended periods of anticoagulation beyond the standard 3 to 6 months, unless awaiting resolution of a risk factor (e.g., extended immobilization). Prolongation

of anticoagulation beyond 6 months in patients with unprovoked VTE delays but clearly does not prevent recurrence. A number of strategies, including postanticoagulation D-dimer testing (3 to 5 weeks) and risk stratification models, have attempted to identify patients with unprovoked VTE for which anticoagulation may be safely stopped. Postanticoagulation D-dimer testing is the most established strategy, further stratifying these patients into high (8.8%) and low (3.0%) first-year recurrence rates. Conversely, the presence of persistent or multiple antiphospholipid antibodies increases recurrence risk (1.8- to 4.5-fold) for patients presenting with unprovoked VTE. Alternative approaches to risk reduction in unprovoked VTE include indefinite anticoagulation with reduced-intensity DOACs or daily acetylsalicylic acid (ASA). ASA reduces recurrence risk by approximately one-third in unprovoked VTE but is inferior to reduced-dose rivaroxaban and apixaban (EINSTEIN CHOICE, AMPLIFY-EXT).

VTE associated with nonsurgical risk factors is more problematic with regard to definitive assessment of recurrence risk. Patients who suffer VTE with minor provocations may have a recurrence rate that approaches unprovoked VTE. These patients should be treated for at least 3 months and reassessed. Clinical factors that may impact a decision for indefinite anticoagulation include underlying cardiopulmonary disease (decreased ability to tolerate recurrence), ongoing inflammation (inflammatory bowel disease, autoimmune disease, chronic infections), prolonged immobilization (stroke), and male sex. For patients with a prolonged but ultimately reversible risk factor (i.e., stroke immobility improving with physical therapy), prolongation of anticoagulation until resolution of the underlying risk factor is reasonable. Similarly, travel-associated thrombosis may be a recurring risk that requires an intermittent prophylaxis plan. Bleeding risk assessment is important to decisions regarding recommended duration of therapy. Major risk factors for bleeding on anticoagulation include advanced age, previous bleeding history, cancer, renal or liver failure, previous stroke, diabetes mellitus, nonsteroidal inflammatory drugs or antiplatelet therapy, comorbidity and reduced functional capacity, recent surgery, frequent falls, and alcohol (Table 6). Additional risk assessment tools (e.g., HAS-BLED score) exist, primarily validated for warfarin therapy.

Clinical Decision Making

Particularly for clinical situations with modest evidence, shared decision making between physician and patient is desirable in determining the duration of anticoagulant therapy. Medical comorbidities affecting bleeding or fall risk in the elderly, patient anxiety about recurrent VTE events, and occupational/lifestyle risks for trauma may substantially affect anticoagulation

| **TABLE 6** | Risk Factors for Bleeding With Anticoagulant Therapy and Estimated Risk of Major Bleeding in Low-, Moderate-, and High-Risk Categories |

Risk Factors

Age > 65 y

Previous bleeding

Cancer

Metastatic cancer

Renal failure

Liver failure

Thrombocytopenia

Previous stroke

Diabetes

Anemia

Antiplatelet therapy

Poor anticoagulant control

Comorbidity and reduced functional capacity

Recent surgery

Frequent falls

Alcohol abuse

Nonsteroidal antiinflammatory drug

Categorization of Risk of Bleeding

	ESTIMATED ABSOLUTE RISK OF MAJOR BLEEDING		
	LOW RISK (0 RISK FACTORS)	**MODERATE RISK (1 RISK FACTOR)**	**HIGH RISK (≥2 RISK FACTORS)**
Anticoagulation 0–3 mo			
Baseline risk (%)	0.6	1.2	4.8
Increased risk (%)	1.0	2.0	8.0
Total risk (%)	1.6	3.2	12.8
Anticoagulation after first 3 mo			
Baseline risk (%/y)	0.3	0.6	≥2.5
Increased risk (%/y)	0.5	1.0	≥4.0
Total risk (%/y)	0.8	1.6	≥6.5

Data from the Ninth Edition of the Antithrombotic Guideline (AT9).

decisions. Family history should be obtained with particular attention to first-degree relatives affected by VTE, including unprovoked events and age of presentation. Questions regarding the underlying cause for a VTE event often drive requests for thrombophilia evaluations. These requests generally fail to acknowledge the complex, multigenic basis for VTE and rarely contribute to clinical decision making (see Genetics of Venous Thromboembolism). The clinical presentation and family history are substantially more useful than identification of minor thrombophilia traits, which are poor predictors of VTE recurrence. Finally, when a decision is made to pursue indefinite anticoagulation, periodic reassessment of this decision is important. The risk-to-benefit ratio of anticoagulation may change as the patient's medical history evolves. The hematology consultant serves an important role in facilitating difficult anticoagulation decisions.

Prevention of Venous Thromboembolism

About 60% of VTE events are associated with recent hospitalization or surgery, and up to 70% of these cases are preventable. However, less than half of hospitalized patients receive appropriate prophylactic measures. Given the significant morbidity and mortality associated with VTE, primary prophylaxis strategies in high-risk situations are of great medical importance and may provide a cost savings. Risk stratification of patients based on surgery or medical illness, patient characteristics (e.g., previous VTE, active cancer, duration of immobility), and bleeding risk impact recommendations for pharmacologic and mechanical prophylaxis. Pharmacologic agents include LMWH, fondaparinux, low-dose UFH, VKA, and DOACs. The focus in this section is primarily on heparin and DOACs given the available evidence. Mechanical prophylaxis includes graduated compression stockings (GCS) that are greater than 15 mm Hg at the ankle or intermittent pneumatic compression devices (IPCs). IPCs enhance lower extremity deep vein blood flow and may increase fibrinolytic activity. These modalities can be used alone or in combination for patients with high bleeding risk who cannot use pharmacologic prophylaxis. IPCs are considered more effective than GCS alone, particularly after orthopedic surgery.

General Surgery

For general surgery patients, well-established risk assessment tools such as the Caprini or Rogers scores stratify patients by VTE risk to identify those who would benefit from pharmacologic prophylaxis. In general, if the risk of VTE is moderate to high and bleeding risk is low, pharmacologic prophylaxis with LMWH or low-dose UFH should be given. If the bleeding risk is high, intermittent pneumatic compression with or without GCS should be used. Ideally, the minimal duration of prophylaxis is 5 to 10 days but varies widely based on duration of bed rest, inpatient stay, and comorbid conditions. In patients with active cancer undergoing abdominopelvic surgery, prophylaxis should be extended to 4 weeks after surgery.

Orthopedic Surgery

Orthopedic procedures are associated with high risk of VTE, especially those involving the lower extremities and pelvic region. For patients undergoing total hip or total knee arthroplasty, pharmacologic prophylaxis using LMWH, UFH, DOACs, or adjusted-dose warfarin should be used if no contraindication exists. LMWH is quite effective and safe with the benefit of long-term experience with these agents. Low-dose DOACs have shown comparable efficacy to enoxaparin in this population with a similar low absolute risk of bleeding. Low-dose apixaban (2.5 mg twice daily), rivaroxaban (10 mg daily), and dabigatran (220 mg daily) appear safer than higher doses. Prophylaxis should continue at least 10 to 14 days, and prolongation up to a month should be considered for major orthopedic surgery. Low-dose aspirin[1] has been shown to be effective for extended prophylaxis after initial acute phase of therapy (~5 days) with standard anticoagulants in patients undergoing total hip or knee arthroplasty; however, anticoagulants are generally favored for high-risk patients. IPCs should be used during the inpatient stay in addition to pharmacologic prophylaxis. If bleeding risk is high, IPCs should be used until pharmacologic agents can be safely administered. For arthroscopic procedures of the knee and other low-risk procedures, prophylaxis is generally not indicated unless other risk factors exist. A summary of available agents and recommendations for prophylaxis is provided (Table 7).

Acute Medical Illness

For hospitalized patients with medical illnesses, the risk of VTE is approximately eightfold higher than the general population.

---

[1] Not FDA approved for this indication.

TABLE 7 Risk Factor Stratification and Prophylaxis Options

RISK STRATIFICATION	RECOMMENDED PROPHYLAXIS	DURATION
Low Risk		
Same-day surgery Medical illness in a fully mobile patient	Early mobilization	–
Moderate Risk		
Most general surgery procedures	LMWH UFH IPC/GCS with or without pharmacologic prophylaxis as appropriate	5–14 days

Most acute medical illnesses	LMWH
	UFH
	Betrixaban*[2]
		Duration of inpatient stay
		Extended duration beyond hospitalization may
		  be appropriate for very high-risk patients in
		  whom bleeding risk is low

High Risk		
Hip or knee replacement surgery	LMWH UFH Fondaparinux Rivaroxaban Apixaban Dabigatran[†] Adjusted dose warfarin	At least 10–14 days Extended duration up to 4 weeks preferred ASA[1] may be used subsequently for extended duration of therapy

General surgery with active cancer, previous
  VTE
	LMWH‡
	UFH
	Adjusted dose warfarin
		Extended duration (4 weeks) for
		  abdominopelvic surgeries in cancer patients

Major trauma, spinal cord injury	IPC with or without GCS, use pharmacologic prophylaxis when appropriate	

*FDA approved for patients hospitalized for acute medical illness at high risk of VTE.
†FDA approved for VTE prevention after hip replacement surgery.
‡Off-label use in cancer patients.
[1]Not FDA approved for this indication.
[2]Not available in the United States.
ASA, Acetylsalicylic acid; *DVT,* deep venous thrombosis; *FDA,* U.S. Food and Drug Administration; *GCS,* graduated compression stockings; *IPC,* intermittent pneumatic compression; *LMWH,* low-molecular-weight heparin; *UFH,* unfractionated heparin; *VTE,* venous thromboembolism.

Patients expected to be hospitalized with reduced mobility for more than 3 days, a previous history of VTE, active infection or malignancy, recent surgery or trauma, heart failure, or respiratory failure should be considered for prophylaxis. The Padua score is a prospectively validated risk assessment model that stratifies patients into groups with high (~11%) or low (0.3%) incidence of VTE. Current prophylaxis options for medical patients include LMWH, low-dose UFH, and fondaparinux.[1] When bleeding risk is considered moderate to high, mechanical prophylaxis using IPCs or GCS should be used until it is safe to add anticoagulants. For low-risk patients admitted for short duration or remaining ambulatory, withholding prophylaxis may be appropriate. Clinical context and bleeding risk assessment should also impact these decisions.

Although pharmacologic prophylaxis is typically limited to the acute illness during the inpatient stay, analysis of population-based data suggests that approximately 75% of VTE events occur well after discharge, at a median of almost 3 weeks. Furthermore, increased compliance with inpatient prophylaxis over time has not resulted in the expected decrease in the rate of VTE. The effect of extended DOAC prophylaxis (35 to 42 days) has been examined in medical patients for apixaban[1] and rivaroxaban. Reduced-dose apixaban and rivaroxaban demonstrated similar VTE prevention to standard enoxaparin prophylaxis but increased bleeding events. Extended prophylaxis is an area of ongoing investigation with unresolved issues that include appropriate patient selection and discerning the effects of specific anticoagulants versus prophylaxis duration on outcomes.

[1] Not FDA approved for this indication.

References

Chatterjee S, Chakraborty A, Weinberg I, et al: Thrombolysis for pulmonary embolism and risk of all-cause mortality, major bleeding, and intracranial hemorrhage: a meta-analysis, *JAMA* 311(23):2414–2421, 2014.

Connors JM: Thrombophilia testing and venous thrombosis, *N Engl J Med* 377:1177–1187, 2017.

Ellenbogen MI, Ardeshirrouhanifard S, Segal JB, Streiff MB, Deitelzweig SB, Brotman DJ: Safety and effectiveness of apixaban versus warfarin for acute venous thromboembolism in patients with end-stage kidney disease: a national cohort study, *J Hosp Med* 17:809–818, 2022, https://doi.org/10.1002/jhm.12926.

Heit JA, Crusan DJ, Ashrani AA, Petterson TM, Bailey KR: Effect of a near-universal hospitalization-based prophylaxis regimen on annual number of venous thromboembolism events in the US, *Blood* 130:109–114, 2017.

Kearon C, Akl EA, Ornelas J, et al: Antithrombotic therapy for VTE disease: CHEST guideline and expert panel report, *Chest* 149:315–352, 2016.

Kearon C, Parpia S, Spencer FA, et al: Antiphospholipid antibodies and recurrent thrombosis after a first unprovoked venous thromboembolism, *Blood* 131:2151–2160, 2018.

Konstantinides SV, Vicaut E, Danays T, et al: Impact of thrombolytic therapy on the long-term outcome of intermediate-risk pulmonary embolism, *J Am Coll Cardiol* 69:1536–1544, 2017.

Martin KA, Beyer-Westendorf J, Davidson BL, Huisman MV, Sandset PM, Moll S: Use of direct oral anticoagulants in patients with obesity for treatment and prevention of venous thrombo- embolism: updated communication from the ISTH SSC Sub- committee on Control of Anticoagulation, *J Thromb Haemost* 19(8):1874–1882, 2021.

Raskob GE, van Es N, Verhamme P, et al: Edoxaban for the treatment of cancer-associated venous thromboembolism, *N Engl J Med* 378:615–624, 2018.

Ortel TL: American Society of Hematology 2020 guidelines for management of venous thromboembolism: treatment of deep vein thrombosis and pulmonary embolism, *Blood Adv* 4(19):4693–4738, 2020.

Vedantham S, Goldhaber SZ, Julian JA, et al: Pharmacomechanical catheter-directed thrombolysis for deep-vein thrombosis, *N Engl J Med* 377:2240–2252, 2017.

Weitz JI, Lensing AWA, Prins MH, et al: Rivaroxaban or aspirin for extended treatment of venous thromboembolism, *N Engl J Med* 376:1211–1222, 2017.

Zoller B, Ohlsson H, Sundquist J, Sundquist K: A sibling based design to quantify genetic and shared environmental effects of venous thromboembolism in Sweden, *Thromb Res* 149:82–87, 2017.

VIRAL AND MYCOPLASMAL PNEUMONIAS

Method of
Cheston B. Cunha, MD; and Burke A. Cunha, MD

CURRENT DIAGNOSIS

Influenza (human, avian, swine)

- Mild influenza A or B presents acutely with headache, fever, sore throat, plus/minus rhinorrhea.
- Severe influenza A presents with an acute onset (patients often able to name the hour the influenza began) and rapidly become bed bound.
- Headache, myalgias, and prostration may be severe.
- With swine influenza, gastrointestinal symptoms (e.g., nausea/vomiting or diarrhea) may be prominent.
- Auscultation of the lungs is quiet, disproportionate to the degree of respiratory distress. Influenza is an interstitial process and not alveolar, which explains the absence of rales.
- With severe influenza, patients rapidly become hypoxemic. Hypoxemia is accompanied by an A-a gradient >35, which indicates a interstitial oxygen diffusing defect.
- Severe tracheobronchitis is common and manifested by hemoptysis.
- Relative lymphopenia with monocytosis occurs early followed by thrombocytopenia and later leukopenia. Low titer elevations of cold agglutinins are not infrequent (≥1:18).
- Patients may have chest pain exacerbated by breathing mimicking pleuritic chest pain. This is the result of direct intracostal muscle involvement with the influenza virus, which results in myositis and pain on inspiration.
- The chest radiograph in early influenza in mild to moderate cases is normal or near normal, with minimal, if any, increase in interstitial markings. The chest radiograph in fulminant cases shows symmetrical bilateral patchy infiltrates without pleural effusion in 48 hours.
- Severe influenza A is accompanied by severe hypoxemia cyanosis, and may be followed by an early fatal outcome.
- Influenza pneumonia most often presents alone without bacterial superinfection, but bacterial infection may accompany (e.g., MSSA/CA-MRSA) or follow influenza (e.g., *S. pneumoniae* or *H. influenzae*).
- Purulent sputum with influenza indicates concurrent bacterial pneumonia usually caused by *S. aureus* (methicillin-susceptible *Staphylococcus aureus* [MSSA]/methicillin-resistant *Staphylococcus aureus* [MRSA]). Bacterial pneumonia following influenza (after 1–2 weeks), is suggested by leukocytosis, focal or segmental pulmonary infiltrates, and purulent sputum; the pathogens are not *S. aureus,* but most commonly are *S. pneumoniae* or *H. influenzae*.
- A laboratory diagnosis may be made by multiplex polymerase chain reaction (PCR) of respiratory secretions.

COVID-19

- COVID-19 is caused by a novel β-coronavirus (different than the novel β-coronaviruses causing severe acute respiratory syndrome [SARS] and Middle East respiratory syndrome [MERS]) identified as SARS-CoV-2.
- Common nonspecific laboratory abnormalities include leukopenia, relative lymphopenia, thrombocytopenia, and mildly elevated serum transaminases.
- Chest x-ray (CXR) early resembles that of influenza pneumonia (i.e., essentially unremarkable, without definite/discreet infiltrates).
- As COVID-19 pneumonia progresses, the CXR shows bilateral interstitial fuzzy/fluffy peripheral infiltrates.

- Chest computed tomography (CT) scans may show bilateral peripheral infiltrates with or without consolidation.
- Diagnosis of COVID-19 is by reverse transcription PCR (RT-PCR) of respiratory tract specimens or antigen testing. RT-PCR usually becomes positive early in the disease course (days).
- COVID-19 seems to preferentially affect adults, with relative sparing of young children. Elderly patients with advanced lung/cardiac disease are particularly predisposed to severe disease/complications.

Mycoplasma pneumoniae

- In a patient with community-acquired pneumonia (CAP) who has a dry, nonproductive cough without severe headache or myalgias, the most likely diagnosis is *M. pneumoniae*. *M. pneumoniae* CAP is commonly accompanied by nonexudative pharyngitis and/or loose stools or watery diarrhea.
- The temperature is usually less than 102°F (38.9°C) and is not accompanied by frank rigors or pleuritic chest pain.
- Relative bradycardia and elevations in the serum transaminases are not features of *M. pneumoniae* CAP.
- Respiratory viruses are often associated with mild elevations of cold agglutinins (≤1:16) but *M. pneumoniae* is the only pathogen causing CAP associated with highly elevated cold agglutinin titers (≥1:64). Elevated cold agglutinin titers occur in up to 75% of patients with *M. pneumoniae*, and occur early and transiently.
- In a patient with CAP, elevated cold agglutinin titers (>1:8) effectively rule out the typical pathogens, as well as *Legionella* species and *C. pneumoniae*.
- Elevated *M. pneumoniae* ELISA IgG titers indicate past exposure/infection and not current infection or co-infection with another pathogen.
- In the absence of an antecedent respiratory tract infection (e.g., nonexudative pharyngitis, otitis, etc., in the preceding 3 months), the presence of an increased *M. pneumoniae* ELISA IgM titer is diagnostic of acute infection.

CURRENT THERAPY

Viral Influenza

- The aim of therapy is to inhibit the influenza virus and prevent its attachment/spread to uninfected respiratory epithelial cells.
- The neuramidase inhibitors shorten the course of influenza by 1 to 2 days and have antiviral activity. These agents are active against both influenza A and B.
- Most strains of human and avian flu, but not swine flu, are resistant to amantadine (Symmetrel) or rimantadine (Flumadine).
- Amantadine and rimantadine may have an important therapeutic effect in severe influenza A by increasing distal airway dilation and increasing oxygen action.
- Peramivir (Rapivab) may be useful in those unable to take oral neuraminase inhibitors.

COVID-19

- Oral agents are now available to treat outpatient COVID-19 patients: Nirmatrelvir/ritonavir (Paxlovid, approved for Emergency Use Authorization by the FDA) is more effective than molnupiravir (Lagevrio, approved for Emergency Use Authorization by the FDA) in preventing disease progression.
- Effective therapy for hospitalized patients with COVID-19 pneumonia is with remdesivir (Veklury) 200 mg (IV) for the first dose, then 100 mg (IV) q24h for 5 to 10 days.
- Dexamethasone[1] 6 mg IV/ PO daily for 10 days should be considered in patients who are hospitalized and require supplemental oxygen.

Mycoplasma pneumoniae

- Monoclonal antibodies have been shown to be effective in limiting severity of disease and preventing progression/need for hospitalization if given early.
- The agents active against *M. pneumoniae* are macrolides, tetracyclines, quinolones, and ketolides. β-Lactam antibiotics are not active against *M. pneumoniae* because it does not contain a bacterial cell wall.
- Goals of therapy of *M. pneumoniae* CAP are to eradicate the infection, decrease the shedding of *M. pneumoniae* in respiratory secretions posttherapy, and to prevent post-treatment asthma.
- Therapy is equally efficacious with macrolides, doxycycline (Vibramycin), or a respiratory quinolone intravenously, orally, or in combination for 1 to 2 weeks.
- The mode of administration is determined by the severity of the CAP and the setting. Outpatients are usually treated orally. Patients hospitalized with severe CAP are initially treated intravenously and then changed to an oral agent.
- Macrolide resistance to *M. pneumoniae* has been described in children and reported in adults.

[1]Not FDA approved for this indication.

Influenza pneumonia is the most important cause of viral pneumonia in adults. Influenza A is the predominant type of influenza found in adults, and influenza B is more common in children. Influenza A has the potential for severe disease, occurs seasonally, and is the predominant type involved in influenza pandemics. *M. pneumoniae* CAP was first recognized decades ago as distinctive from bacterial and viral pneumonias. It was originally described by Eaton as "Eaton agent" pneumonia caused by a pleuropneumonia-like organism (PPLO), later shown to be caused by *M. pneumoniae*. *M. pneumoniae* is a common cause of pneumonia in all age groups, but the peak incidence of *M. pneumoniae* CAP is in young adults. *M. pneumoniae* CAP is a common cause of ambulatory CAP.

The term *atypical pneumonia* was first applied to viral pneumonias because the clinical laboratory and radiologic findings were different from those caused by typical bacterial pulmonary pathogens. In influenza pneumonia, the clinical findings are confined to the trachea, bronchi, lung parenchyma, and central nervous system. *M. pneumoniae* CAP is a systemic infection with a pulmonary component. Over the years, atypical pneumonia has come to refer to pneumonia caused by systemic nonviral/nonbacterial pathogen agents that have a pulmonary component. Viral pneumonias are no longer considered atypical pneumonias. Atypical pneumonias may be divided into nonzoonotic and zoonotic atypical CAPs. Nonzoonotic CAPs are most commonly caused by *M. pneumoniae*, *Chlamydia pneumoniae*, or *Legionella* species, whereas the three most common zoonotic atypical pneumonias are caused by *Chlamydia psittaci* (psittacosis), *Francisella tularensis* (tularemia), or *Coxiella burnetii* (Q fever). All of the atypical pneumonias are distinct clinical entities that may be differentiated on the basis of their characteristic pattern of extrapulmonary organ involvement. Although some viruses may occasionally have extrapulmonary manifestations (i.e., influenza, adenovirus with viral pneumonias), the primary clinical features are confined to the lungs. *M. pneumoniae* is a critical cause of nonzoonotic atypical CAP, particularly in the ambulatory setting. *M. pneumoniae* CAP may be severe in patients with impaired host defenses or those with severe, preexisting cardiopulmonary disease.

Influenza (Human, Avian, and Swine)

Viral influenza pneumonia affects children and adults. Influenza B is the primary cause of mild influenza in children and adults. Influenza A is primarily an infection of adults that may be mild to severe. Influenza A has the potential for pandemic spread (e.g., swine influenza [H_1N_1]).

Influenza occurs during the winter months, usually peaking in February. Influenza is spread by aerosolized droplet infection from person to person and via fomites. Influenza A is classified into subtypes based on hemagglutinin (H) and neuramidase (N) surface proteins. An important characteristic of the influenza A virus is antigenic drift, which refers to minor changes in surface protein shift in the neuramidase or hemagglutinin receptors. With influenza A, these surface receptor proteins are important in cellular adherence of the influenza virus and spread of influenza from respiratory epithelial cells. The vaccine for the flu season most often includes the influenza hemagglutinin and neuramidase types seen at the end of the preceding year's season. Prevention of attachment and spread of the virus is helpful in controlling the spread of influenza; vaccine protection conferred by specific antibody response to influenza A is highly protective (approximately 80% in noncompromised hosts).

During the years when influenza B has been prevalent, vaccines for the subsequent year contain an influenza B component.

Clinical manifestations of influenza A in adults varies considerably from mild to fatal infection. Mild infection is usually manifested as an acute febrile illness characterized by headache and myalgias with dry, unproductive cough and rhinorrhea. Mild influenza may be caused by influenza A or B and usually resolves in a few days without complications in normal hosts who have good cardiopulmonary function.

Severe influenza A (human, avian, swine) occurs in normal healthy adults and may be fatal. The onset of severe influenza A (human, avian, swine) is sudden, and the patient often recalls the exact hour of onset. The patient is febrile, with early/extreme prostration rendering the patient bedridden. Fever rapidly rises and may be accompanied by chills. Neck soreness, severe headache, and myalgias are typical. Sore throat, eye pain, conjunctival injection, and hemoptysis are frequently present. Chest pain worsened by deep inspiration is not truly pleuritic but rather reflects influenza A myositis of the intracostal muscles. Shortness of breath is related to the degree of hypoxemia. Severe influenza A causes an oxygen diffusion defect as manifested by an increased A-a gradient (>35). Profound hypoxemia may be accompanied by cyanosis. Hypotension caused by hypoxemia and vascular collapse may follow. The course of fulminant viral influenza A is of short duration.

Physical findings are few in viral influenza (i.e., conjunctival suffusion). Auscultation reveals absolutely quiet lungs because the infectious process is interstitial and not alveolar. Routine blood tests are usually unremarkable except for leukopenia, relative lymphopenia, and thrombocytopenia. Atypical lymphocytes are not present, but low titers of cold agglutinins may be present. Cold agglutinins (if present) have titers less than or equal to 1:18. In fatal cases, a pale blue hue of the skin may be noted, and there may be bleeding from multiple orifices before death. The chest radiograph in uncomplicated influenza A is unremarkable, with minimal perihilar bilateral increased prominence of interstitial markings possible. In severe influenza A pneumonia, the chest radiograph shows bilateral symmetrical perihilar infiltrates without pleural effusions in <48 hours.

Patients may die from severe influenza A without superimposed bacterial pneumonia. Most deaths during the 1918–1919 pandemic were young military recruits who died of influenza A pneumonia without bacterial pneumonia. Influenza may be complicated by bacterial pneumonia. Bacterial pneumonias complicating influenza may occur concurrently at presentation or may occur after an interval of improvement 1 to 2 weeks after the presentation of influenza. Influenza A presenting concurrently with bacterial pneumonia is caused by *Staphylococcus aureus*. In contrast to influenza alone, MSSA/CA-MRSA is manifested by an increase in fever, shaking chills, leukocytosis, purulent sputum, localized rales on auscultation, bacteremia, and focal/segmental infiltrates on chest radiograph that rapidly cavitate in less than 72 hours. Alternatively, patients with influenza A may develop a secondary bacterial infection 1 to 2 weeks later. Secondary bacterial pneumonia is less severe and is usually caused by *Streptococcus pneumoniae* or *Haemophilus influenzae*.

Viral influenza-like illnesses (ILIs) most often present during the winter months or influenza season. For clinical and therapeutic purposes, it is important to differentiate influenza A from viral ILIs in hospitalized adults. Some clinical features may point to a specific ILI viral etiology, but a specific viral diagnosis can be made by viral respiratory PCR of nasopharyngeal swab specimens. The only viral ILI likely to mimic influenza A presenting with a fulminant severe viral CAP is MERS. The mimics of ILIs are presented (Table 1). The main nonviral mimic of influenza A in hospitalized adults is Legionnaire's disease (LD). LD may be differentiated from influenza A and other viral ILIs by CXR findings and characteristic nonspecific laboratory tests. With LD CAP, the CXR shows one or more nonfocal infiltrates. Fever, usually greater than 102° F, is accompanied by relative bradycardia. With LD, the ESR is highly elevated (>90 mm/h), the ferritin is highly elevated (>2 times normal), and the serum phosphorus is decreased early, as is serum sodium. Although an elevated CPK and mild transaminitis often accompany LD, these findings are not uncommon in influenza A and some viral ILIs. There are few infections that may mimic the dry, productive cough of

TABLE 1 Mimics of Influenza A in Hospitalized Adults Presenting with Influenza-like Illnesses (ILIs)

INFLUENZA-LIKE ILLNESSES (ILIS)	CHEST FILM FEATURES	CLINICAL CLUES
MERS	Ill-defined infiltrates (early) Bilateral dense interstitial nodular infiltrates (late) Severe cases often develop ARDS	Recent travel to Middle East or contact with MERS case Dry cough and sore throat Hemoptysis (in some) Diarrhea (common) WBC count normal, thrombocytopenia Elevated LDH
COVID-19	CXR: Ill-defined infiltrates (early) Bilateral, peripheral dense interstitial infiltrates Severe cases often develop ARDS	Fever and dry cough Diarrhea (common) Myocarditis (late, in some) ARDS (in some) Leukopenia Relative lymphopenia Thrombocytopenia Mildly elevated serum Transaminases (early) Elevated CPK (in some) Elevated D-dimer may herald coagulopathy
RSV	Clear CXR (early) Bilateral ill-defined infiltrates on CXR (late) Chest CT: GGO (non-specific)	Antecedent/concurrent rhinorrhea Hoarseness Lymphocyte/monocyte ratio >2
HPIV-3	Clear CXR (early) Bilateral ill-defined infiltrates on CXR (late)	Hoarseness Prolonged lymphocyte/monocyte ratio <2 Monocytosis
EV-D86	Clear CXR (early) Bilateral ill-defined infiltrates on CXR (late)	Diarrhea (common) Flaccid paralysis
Legionnaire's disease	Rapidly progressive, asymmetric, ill-defined infiltrates on CXR Consolidation and small pleural effusions (common) Cavitation (rare)	High fevers (>102 °F) Highly elevated ESR (>90 mm/h) Ferritin (>2 xn) Leukocytosis with relative lymphopenia Elevated CPK (in some) Mild transient elevated transaminases common (early) Microscopic hematuria (early)

Abbreviations: MERS = Middle East respiratory syndrome; COVID-19: Coronavirus disease; RSV = respiratory syncytial virus; HPIV = human parainfluenza virus; EV = enterovirus; GGO = ground gloss opacity; CXR = chest x-ray; ARDS = acute respiratory distress syndrome.

TABLE 2 Mimics of Mycoplasma pneumoniae in Community Acquired Pneumonia (CAP) Hospitalized Adults

MYCOPLASMA CAP MIMICS	CHEST FILM FEATURES	CLINICAL CLUES
C. pneumoniae	Ill-defined lower lobe infiltrates (often ovoid) No consolidation, cavitation or effusion	No seasonal predisposition Hoarseness Protracted dry cough Mycoplasma-like illness that doesn't respond to erythromycin Wheezing (in some) No diarrhea No cold agglutinins Rhinorrhea proceeds dry cough (1–2 weeks)
Pertussis	Perihilar illdefined infiltrates ("shaggy heart" sign) No consolidation, cavitation or effusions	Protracted dry cough Persistent cough (without typical "whoop" of children) Afebrile or minimal fevers Marked lymphocytes (> 60%) No cold agglutinins

M. pneumoniae CAP. Pertussis is most likely to mimic myco-plasma. Pertussis, unlike mycoplasma, is not accompanied by watery diarrhea. The distinguishing laboratory feature of *M. pneumoniae* CAP is elevated cold agglutinins not found with pertussis. The key non-specific laboratory finding in pertussis is marked lymphocytosis (Table 2).

COVID-19 emerged from Wuhan, China in 2019 and spread worldwide early in 2020, resulting in a pandemic. COVID-19 is caused by a novel β-coronavirus (different than the novel β-coronaviruses causing SARS and MERS) identified as SARS-CoV-2. SARS-CoV-2 is thought to have been contracted from wild animals in food markets. COVID-19 spreads rapidly via airborne transmission, and may be spread from asymptomatic individuals.

Patients most commonly present with fever, headache, sore throat, dry cough, shortness of breath, and diarrhea (in some).

Clinically, the spectrum of COVID-19 ranges from asymptomatic cases to symptomatic cases. Symptomatic COVID-19 most often presents as a mild ILI; in more severe cases, it presents as a viral pneumonia (not unlike influenza pneumonia). Severe COVID-19 pneumonias have severe hypoxemia caused by an oxygen diffusion defect (high A-a gradient). Fatal cases are due to ARDS and/or myocarditis. Common nonspecific laboratory abnormalities include leukopenia, relative lymphopenia, thrombocytopenia, and mildly elevated serum transaminases. Serum LDH or CPK are often elevated. Elevated D-dimers also present frequently and may herald a subsequent coagulopathy.

Early CXR resembles that of influenza pneumonia (i.e., essentially unremarkable without definite/discrete infiltrates). As COVID-19 pneumonia progresses, the CXR shows bilateral interstitial peripheral infiltrates. CXR demonstrates no/small bibasilar effusions. Chest CT scans may show bilateral nodular infiltrates with or without consolidation. Cavitation is not a feature of COVID-19 pneumonia. Co-infection or superinfection is a rare occurrence in COVID-19.

Diagnosis of COVID-19 is by RT-PCR of respiratory tract specimens. A positive RT-PCR result may be present early in the disease course, although it may not become positive for a few days. If clinical suspicion is high, serial testing may reveal RT-PCR + after 2 to 3 repeat tests. The RT-PCR should not be used as a test of cure. RT-PCR + may persist for 1 to 2 weeks after clinical recovery, although transmission should not occur during this time period. Antibody testing may become positive after several weeks.

COVID-19 seems to preferentially affect adults, with relative sparing of young children. Elderly patients with advanced lung/cardiac disease are particularly predisposed to severe disease/complications.

Anti-Influenza Therapy

Therapy of viral influenza is directed at inhibiting viral replication and preventing further infection of respiratory epithelial cells. The neuramidase inhibitors zanamivir (Relenza), oseltamivir (Tamiflu), and peramivir (Rapivab) have anti-influenza A and B activity. Neuramidase inhibitors decrease the severity and duration of influenza symptoms by 1 to 2 days. Current flu strains are resistant to amantadine and rimantadine, but these drugs may still be useful to increase peripheral airway dilation and oxygenation, which may be of critical importance in severe influenza A with severe hypoxemia. Mild influenza A/B may be treated with neuramidase inhibitors. Mild cases of influenza A should be treated at the onset of the illness. For severe influenza A, neuramidase inhibitors provide optimal anti-influenza therapy (Table 3). For human and avian influenza (H_5N_1), these antiviral drugs may be ineffective, but are effective against swine influenza.

COVID-19 Therapy

At the time of writing, optimal therapy of COVID-19 continues to evolve. Effective therapy for hospitalized patients with COVID-19 pneumonia who require oxygen is remdesivir (Veklury) 200 mg (IV) for the first does, then 100 mg (IV) q24h for 5 to 10 days.

TABLE 3	Adult Anti-Influenza Antivirals	
ANTIVIRAL	**TREATMENT DOSE**	**PROPHYLACTIC DOSE**
Mild Influenza A/B		
Zanamivir (Relenza)*	2 inhalations (5 mg per inhalation) q12h × 5 d	2 inhalations (5 mg per inhalation) q24h × 5 d
Influenza		
Baloxavir (Xofluza)	80 mg (PO) × 1 dose	80 mg (PO) × 1 dose
Oseltamivir (Tamiflu)*	75 mg (PO) q12h × 5 d†	75 mg (PO) q24h × 7 d
Peramivir (Rapivab)	600 mg (IV) over 30 min × 1 d	None

*Currently most human and avian influenza strains are resistant.
†For avian (H5N1) influenza, 150 mg (PO) q12h may be effective.

A 3-day course of IV remdesivir can be considered for high risk patients with mild disease. This can be administered as an outpatient treatment if an infusion center is able to offer this therapy. Oral therapy for COVID-19 is now available for high-risk patients. Nirmatrelvir with ritonavir (Paxlovid, approved for Emergency Use Authorization by the FDA) is currently the most effective PO agent available. Due to the ritonavir component, drug-drug interactions need to be considered when prescribing this medication. Molnupiravir (Lagevrio, approved for Emergency Use Authorization by the FDA) is an alternate PO option but has lower efficacy than Paxlovid in preventing serious disease in high risk patients. Monoclonal antibodies are no longer recommended due to lack of activity against current circulating variants. Dexamethasone[1] has a role in limiting mortality in patients admitted with COVID-19 who require supplemental oxygen. Interlukin inhibitors (IL-6 in particular) have a role in select patients with COVID-19. Vaccines play a critical role in prevention of COVID-19, although the increasing number of genetic variants may blunt the effectiveness of existing vaccines.

Mycoplasma Pneumoniae

M. pneumoniae is a common cause of ambulatory CAP. It affects all age groups, and in normal hosts with intact cardiopulmonary function, *M. pneumoniae* CAP is usually a mild, self-limiting infection. However, *M. pneumoniae* derives its importance from difficulty in diagnosis, the necessity for non–β-lactam therapy, and because of its effect on peripheral airways.

M. pneumoniae CAP is one of the nonzoonotic causes of CAP (the others being *Legionella* and *Chlamydia pneumoniae*). *M. pneumoniae* is an atypical pneumonia that is a systemic infectious disease with a pulmonary component. It may be distinguished from other atypical pneumonias by its characteristic pattern of extrapulmonary organ involvement. *M. pneumoniae* CAP most closely resembles *C. pneumoniae* CAP clinically, but is very different from LD in terms of its epidemiology, age distribution, pattern of extrapulmonary organ involvement, and severity.

Clinically, *M. pneumoniae* presents as a subacute febrile illness. Temperatures rarely exceed 102°F (38.9°C). Rigors are not a feature of *M. pneumoniae* CAP, but patients may complain of chilly sensations. Mild headache and/or myalgias are not uncommon. The most common presenting symptom in *M. pneumoniae* CAP is the prolonged, nonproductive, dry cough. Patients with *M. pneumoniae* CAP often complain of or have mild nonexudative pharyngitis. Rhinorrhea and conjunctivitis are not features of *M. pneumoniae* CAP. Watery diarrhea is commonly

---

[1]Not FDA approved for this indication.

present in *M. pneumoniae* CAP, but abdominal pain is not a clinical finding. Other extrapulmonary manifestations are uncommon or rare (e.g., meningoencephalitis, pericarditis, hemolytic anemia, glomerular nephritis, Guillain-Barré syndrome, erythema multiforme). *M. pneumoniae* has a distinctive pattern of extrapulmonary organ involvement that does not include cardiac involvement (relative bradycardia) or hepatic involvement, including normal serum glutamate-oxaloacetate transaminase (SGOT) or serum glutamate-pyruvate transaminase (SGPT). The distinguishing laboratory feature of *M. pneumoniae* CAP is elevated cold agglutinin titers. Although a variety of infectious and noninfectious diseases are associated with cold agglutinin elevations, they are usually of low titer (i.e., <1:16). There are no pulmonary infections presenting as CAP that are associated with high elevations of cold agglutinin titers (i.e., ≥1:64). Although elevated cold agglutinins occur early in up to 75% of patients with *M. pneumoniae* CAP, they are still diagnostically important when present. In a patient with CAP and a cold agglutinin titer greater than or equal to 1:64, the diagnosis of *M. pneumoniae* CAP is very likely.

M. pneumoniae may be differentiated from the typical bacterial pneumonias because of the presence of extrapulmonary findings, including nonexudative pharyngitis, loose stools or watery diarrhea, erythema multiforme, and high cold agglutinin. Patients with typical bacterial CAP usually have a more acute onset of presentation, a productive cough, and temperatures that may exceed 102°F (38.9°C), often accompanied by chills. Patients with typical pneumonia often have pleuritic chest pain, which is not a feature of *M. pneumoniae* CAP. Among the atypical pneumonias, the zoonotic pneumonias (i.e., tularemia, psittacosis, Q fever) may be eliminated from consideration if there is a recent zoonotic contact history with the appropriate vector.

C. pneumoniae CAP resembles closely *M. pneumoniae* CAP. *C. pneumoniae* may be distinguished by the absence of cold agglutinins and the presence of hoarseness, which is a feature of *C. pneumoniae* CAP but not *M. pneumoniae* CAP. Loose stools or watery diarrhea are not usual features of *C. pneumoniae* CAP. The most common clinical problem is differentiating *Legionella* from *Mycoplasma* CAP; this may be done by appreciating the differences in the pattern of extrapulmonary organ involvement with each of these pathogens. *Legionella* may be clinically differentiated from *Mycoplasma* by acuteness of onset or severity, the presence of relative bradycardia, temperatures greater than 102°F (38.9°C), and the presence of abdominal pain. From a laboratory standpoint, highly elevated cold agglutinin titers argue strongly against the diagnosis of *Legionella* and point to *M. pneumoniae*. Nonspecific laboratory tests in a patient with CAP that suggest *Legionella* and argue against *M. pneumoniae* include otherwise unexplained hypophosphatemia, hyponatremia, microscopic hematuria, and increased creatinine. *Legionella* does not affect the upper respiratory tract as does *Mycoplasma* (e.g., nonexudative pharyngitis). Ear findings are not a feature of Legionnaires' disease but are common in *M. pneumoniae* CAP. The finding most likely to cause confusion between *M. pneumoniae* and *Legionella pneumophila* is the presence of loose stools or watery diarrhea, which is found in both.

M. pneumoniae may be cultured from the throat in viral culture media, but the diagnosis is usually made serologically. An elevated enzyme-linked immunosorbent assay (ELISA) or enzyme immuno-assay (EIA) IgM titer suggests acute or recent infection, but an elevated IgG titer indicates past exposure but not acute infection. Elevated IgG titers regardless of degree of elevation are not diagnostic of current infection with *M. pneumoniae* and only indicate previous antigenic exposure. *M. pneumoniae* ELISA IgM levels may take up to 3 months to decrease. Therefore, clinicians should take into account recent antecedent respiratory illness to properly interpret elevated IgM titers, including patients with nonexudative pharyngitis within 3 months prior to the presentation of CAP. The combination of an increased *M. pneumoniae* IgM titer and highly elevated cold agglutinin titers is virtually diagnostic of acute infection. Cold agglutinin titers are elevated transiently early and rapidly fall; the simultaneously elevated cold

agglutinins and IgM titers of *M. pneumoniae* indicate active or current infection. In patients with CAP caused by another organism (e.g., *S. pneumoniae*), the presence of elevated *Mycoplasma* IgG titers does not indicate co-infection but only preexisting serologic exposure to *M. pneumoniae*.

M. pneumoniae Therapy

M. pneumoniae has a predilection for the respiratory epithelial cells and resides on their surface. Mycoplasmas have no definite cell wall like the typical pathogens causing CAP. Their position on the surface of the respiratory epithelium and their absence of a cell wall necessitates the therapeutic approach, which includes non–β-lactam antibiotics with the capacity to penetrate into the *Mycoplasma* organisms. Traditionally, macrolides and tetracyclines have been used successfully to treat *M. pneumoniae*. Both tetracyclines and macrolides are effective against *Mycoplasma* because they interfere with intracellular protein synthesis at the ribosomal level. Tetracyclines penetrate intracellularly better than macrolides, with the exception of penetration into the alveolar macrophage, which is relevant in *Legionella* but not *M. pneumoniae* infections. Macrolides and tetracyclines are both active against *Mycoplasma*. Patients treated with macrolides or tetracyclines defervesce rapidly over 24 to 48 hours. Clinical defervescence manifests by an increased feeling of well-being and a decrease in fever. The dry cough persists during and after therapy regardless of the anti-*Mycoplasma* antimicrobial used.

There are important differences in the shedding rates of *Mycoplasma* from respiratory epithelial cells posttherapy when using tetracyclines instead of macrolides. Tetracycline therapy is associated with a more rapid decrease in shedding. Tetracyclines with better ability to penetrate intracellularly, such as doxycycline (Vibramycin), are the most rapid at decreasing *Mycoplasma* shedding, which is an important public health consideration. Mycoplasmas are transmitted by aerosolized droplet infection. Because patients with *Mycoplasma* have a prolonged cough, organisms not eliminated from respiratory epithelial cells may be aerosolized during coughing for weeks following the acute infection, spreading the infection to susceptible individuals via aerosolized droplets. The aim of therapy is to rapidly treat the patient's pneumonia and extrapulmonary sites of involvement. The secondary goal is to rapidly decrease shedding and aerosolization to prevent the spread of *Mycoplasma* to other individuals. An additional therapeutic goal is to decrease the incidence of post-*Mycoplasma* asthma seen in some patients. *M. pneumoniae* CAP may exacerbate preexisting asthma, but may also cause permanent post-CAP asthma in some individuals.

Until recently, doxycycline was the most active antimicrobial to use against *M. pneumoniae*. Currently, the "respiratory quinolones," levofloxacin (Levaquin) and moxifloxacin (Avelox), are highly active anti–*M. pneumoniae* antimicrobials. The respiratory quinolones and doxycycline penetrate cells efficiently and interfere with intracellular enzymes or protein synthesis of intracellular organisms. Respiratory quinolones and doxycycline are highly effective anti-*Mycoplasma* agents and rapidly decrease shedding of *M. pneumoniae* in respiratory secretions.

Therapy for *M. pneumoniae* is ordinarily 1 to 2 weeks. Patients who have impaired cardiopulmonary disease or are immunocompromised may require 2 full weeks of therapy. In patients with borderline cardiopulmonary function, *M. pneumoniae* as with other relatively low virulence pathogens may present as severe CAP. Antimicrobial therapy for typical or atypical CAP should be directed against the presumed pathogen and not based on co-morbidities. Normal healthy hosts are treated with the same antimicrobial as patients hospitalized with severe CAP. Patients hospitalized with compromised cardiopulmonary function caused by severe *M. pneumoniae* CAP are most often initially treated intravenously with doxycycline (Vibramycin), a macrolide, or a respiratory quinolone. Most patients with *M. pneumoniae* CAP present in the ambulatory setting, which permits therapy with oral doxycycline, a macrolide, or a respiratory quinolone (Table 4).

TABLE 4	Antibiotics Effective Against *M. pneumoniae*
ANTIBIOTIC	**DOSE (ADULT)**
Mild/Moderate CAP	
Doxycycline	100 mg (IV/PO) q12h
Erythromycin	500 mg (base, estolate, stearate) (PO) q6h
Erythromycin lactobionate	1 g (IV) q6h
Clarithromycin (Biaxin)	500 mg (PO) q12h
Azithromycin (Zithromax)	500 mg (IV) q24h x 2 doses, followed by 500 mg (PO) q24h
Severe CAP	
Levofloxacin (Levaquin)	500 mg (IV/PO) q24h, or 750 mg IV/PO q24h (may allow for shorter duration of therapy)
Moxifloxacin (Avelox)	400 mg (IV/PO) q24h

CAP, Community-acquired pneumonia.

References

Ali NJ, Sillis M, Andrews BE, et al: The clinical spectrum and diagnosis of *Mycoplasma pneumoniae* infection, *Q J Med* 58:241–251, 1986.

Cunha BA: Hepatic involvement in *Mycoplasma pneumoniae* community-acquired pneumonia, *J Clin Microbiol* 3:385–386, 2003.

Cunha BA: Influenza: Historical aspects of epidemics and pandemics, *Infect Dis Clin North Am* 18:141–155, 2004.

Cunha BA: The atypical pneumonia: Clinical diagnosis and importance, *Clin Microbiol Infect* 12(12–24), 2006.

Cunha BA: *Pneumonia essentials*, ed 3, Sudbury, MA, 2010, Jones & Bartlett.

Cunha BA, Corbett M, Mickail N: Human parainfluenza virus type 3 (HPIV-3) viral community-acquired pneumonia (CAP) mimicking swine influenza (H1N1) during the swine flu pandemic, *Heart Lung* 40:76–80, 2011.

Cunha BA, Pherez FM, Strollo S, Syed U, Laguerre M: Severe swine influenza A (H1N1) versus severe human seasonal influenza A (H3N2): clinical comparisons, *Heart Lung* 40:257–261, 2011.

Cunha BA, Raza M: During influenza season: all influenza-like illnesses are not due to influenza: dengue mimicking influenza. *J Emerg Med* 2015;48:e117–20.

Cunha CB, Cunha, BA: *Antibiotic Essentials*, ed 17. New Delhi, 2020, Jaypee Medical Publishers.

Cunha CB, Opal SM. Middle East respiratory syndrome (MERS): a new zoonotic viral pneumonia, *Virulence* 5:650–654, 2014.

Cunha CB: The first atypical pneumonia: the history of the discovery of Mycoplasma pneumoniae, *Infect Dis Clin North Am* 24:1–5, 2010.

Debré R, Couvreur J: Influenza: Clinical features. In Debré R, Celers J, editors: *Clinical Virology: the evaluation and management of human viral infections*, Philadelphia, 1970, WB Saunders, pp 507–515.

File TM, Tan JS: *Mycoplasma pneumoniae* pneumonia. In Marrié TJ, editor: *Community-acquired pneumonia*, New York, 2001, Kluwer Academic/Plenum Publishers, pp 487–500.

Foster CB, Friedman N, Carl J, Piedimonte G: Enterovirus D68: a clinically important respiratory enterovirus, *Cleve Clin J Med* 82:26–31, 2015.

Gottlieb RL, Vaca CE, Paredes R, et al: GS-US-540-9012 (PINETREE) Investigators. Early remdesivir to prevent progression to severe Covid-19 in outpatients, *N Engl J Med* 2022 27;386(4):305–315.

Hammerschlag MR: *Mycoplasma pneumoniae* infections, *Curr Opin Infect Dis* 14:181–186, 2001.

Hurt AC, Selleck P, Komadina N, et al: Susceptibility of highly pathogenic A(H5N1) avian influenza viruses to the neuraminidase inhibitors and adamantanes, *Antiviral Res* 73:228–231, 2007.

Louria DB, Blumenfield HL, Ellis JT: Studies on influenza in the pandemic of 1957–1958. II. Pulmonary complications of influenza, *J Clin Invest* 38:213–265, 1959.

Lu QB, Wo Y, Wang HY, Wei MT, Zhang L, Yang H, et al: Detection of enterovirus 68 as one of the commonest types of enterovirus found in patients with acute respiratory tract infection in China, *J Med Microbiol* 63:408–414, 2014.

Marrie TJ: Empiric treatment of ambulatory community-acquired pneumonia: always include treatment for atypical agents, *Infect Dis Clin North Am* 18:829–841, 2004.

Murray HW, Masur H, Senterfit LS, Roberts RB: The protean manifestations of *Mycoplasma pneumoniae* infection in adults, *Am J Med* 58:229–242, 1975.

Nisar N, Guleria R, Kumar S, et al: Mycoplasma pneumoniae and its role in asthma, *Postgrad Med J* 83:100–104, 2007.

Recovery Collaborative Group, Horby P, Lim WS, et al: Dexamethasone in hospitalized patients with COVID-19 - preliminary report, *N Engl J Med*, 2020.

Yang Y, Guo F, Zhao W, Gu X, Huang M, Cao Q, et al: Novel avian-origin influenza A (H7N9) in critically ill patients in China, *Crit Care Med* 43:339–345, 2015.

VIRAL RESPIRATORY INFECTIONS

Method of
Robert C. Welliver Sr., MD

CURRENT DIAGNOSIS

- Rapid diagnostic kits are available for many common respiratory viruses. These tests are used increasingly to establish that antibiotic therapy is not necessary in many patients with febrile respiratory illnesses or with lower respiratory tract infections.
- The presence of wheezing on physical examination virtually excludes bacterial infection from consideration in subjects with lower respiratory disease.

CURRENT THERAPY

- The management of most viral respiratory infections consists of rest, adequate caloric and fluid intake, and management of fever and malaise.
- Corticosteroids are essential in the management of croup.
- Specific antiviral therapy is available for influenza virus and SARS-CoV-2 infections, and beneficial effects have been more readily achieved in prevention rather than treatment.

Viral infections of the respiratory tract are among the most common infections in humans, and they account for significant morbidity at all ages. Infants and young children can sustain six to eight such infections annually, and adults have an average of nearly two such infections per year.

Rhinoviruses are the most commonly identified etiologic agents and cause illness year-round. Other common causative agents during winter months include influenza viruses and respiratory syncytial virus (RSV), and enteroviruses predominate in summer months. The parainfluenza viruses also commonly cause respiratory infection, particularly in autumn (type 1) and late spring or summer (type 3). Coronaviruses, metapneumoviruses, adenoviruses, and other agents are identified less often.

Although each of these agents can cause a common cold, some viral infections are associated with characteristic patterns of respiratory disease. Most of these viruses can also exacerbate asthma, cystic fibrosis, and chronic obstructive pulmonary disease.

Common Colds

Colds are the most common of the viral respiratory illnesses. Pharyngitis is usually the earliest sign of a cold, beginning a few days after infection has taken place. Nasal congestion and clear or slightly cloudy rhinorrhea usually follow within 24 to 48 hours. Cough occurs in approximately 30% to 40% of those infected, and fluid can accumulate in middle ear or sinus cavities that have become blocked as a result of mucosal swelling. Ear and sinus cavity infections occur when this fluid is trapped for a week or more. Treatment with antibiotics is ineffective before this time, and they are ineffective especially in the absence of other clinical signs of ear and sinus infections.

Colds are a frequent cause of missed school and work, and even of mild morbidity, but they are rarely serious in otherwise healthy persons. The most appropriate approach to treatment therefore entails rest, with adequate nutrition and hydration. Agents that inhibit the activity of cyclooxygenase probably represent the most effective form of pharmacologic intervention. These compounds include acetaminophen (Tylenol) and the nonsteroidal antiinflammatory agents such as ibuprofen (Motrin). They are effective in reducing fever and, perhaps more importantly in most colds, reducing malaise, headache, and pharyngitis.

Nasal congestion and some rhinorrhea during colds are related to dilation of blood vessels in the nose and sinuses. Therefore vasoconstrictors have been used extensively to attempt to reverse these symptoms. Oral decongestants such as pseudoephedrine (Sudafed) have minimal effect on nasal congestion and can result in systemic hypertension, anxiety, and difficulty sleeping. The propensity for these compounds to cause cardiac arrhythmias in the very young child has led to recommendations against their use in the first year or two of life. Nasal sprays containing vasoconstricting agents such as oxymetazoline (Afrin) can result in mild temporary relief of nasal obstruction. However, the use of these compounds for more than 3 or 4 days can result in rebound vasodilation and paradoxically increased rhinorrhea.

Numerous investigations have evaluated the role of antihistamines in colds. The release of histamine itself is not associated with fever, cough, or malaise, so effects on these symptoms would not be expected. Furthermore, nasal congestion and discharge may be more related to the release of kinins and not histamine. Indeed, the administration of antihistamines in adults and, particularly, in children has not demonstrated strikingly positive results. As many as 40% of subjects treated with placebo report beneficial effects. Side effects of histamine use, primarily sedation and dry mouth, are commonly encountered.

Cough can be one of the most irritating symptoms during colds. Cough during colds is principally caused by secretions entering the airway (postnasal drip) and not by inflammation of the airway itself. Therefore it is not surprising that cough suppressants, especially codeine, have little effect on cough induced by colds. Antihistamines have also been found to be ineffective in relief of cough during colds.

Influenza-Like Illness

The influenza syndrome is defined as the abrupt onset of fever, headache, and striking degrees of malaise and prostration, often with intense myalgia. Respiratory symptoms can occur concurrently, but they might not be prominent features. The principal cause is, of course, influenza virus, although infection with many other viruses can cause similar (although not as intense) symptoms. The illness is generally self-limited, and most symptoms resolve over 4 or 5 days. Lassitude can persist for up to 2 weeks.

Influenza virus infection and influenza-like illness are best treated symptomatically, relying on rest, adequate intake of fluids and calories, and appropriate analgesic therapy. Compounds referred to as *M2 inhibitors* such as amantadine (Symmetrel) and rimantadine (Flumadine) have been approved for therapy. Positive outcomes from therapy with these agents are observed only when therapy is instituted within 48 hours after the onset of symptoms, and benefits are not striking. In recent years, resistance to M2 inhibitors has been commonly observed among circulating epidemic strains of influenza virus.

Inhibitors of the activity of influenza viral neuraminidase have been used in treatment and prevention of influenza virus infection in adults and children. Oseltamivir (Tamiflu) has been used to prevent and to treat influenza virus infection. As with M2 inhibitors, it is believed that treatment should be started within the first 48 hours of symptoms and that prophylaxis should be instituted within 48 hours of exposure. Treatment with oseltamivir shortens the duration of subsequent illness by only about 24 hours. Treatment can prevent some of the complications of influenza infection, including pneumonia. The drug may be more effective as a therapeutic agent because it may be up to 90% effective in preventing culture-positive symptomatic influenza illness. The recommended dose for adults is 75 mg orally every 12 hours for 5 days. In children, the appropriate dose based on body weight is 30 mg twice daily for children weighing less than 15 kg, 45 mg twice daily for children weighing 15 to 23 kg, 60 mg twice daily for children weighing 23 to 40 kg, and 75 mg twice daily for children weighing more than 40 kg. The principal side effect is nausea, which can be reduced by taking the drug with food.

A new type of antiviral (baloxavir marboxil [Xofluza]) was released for treatment of influenza infections in 2018. This drug acts by a different mechanism than previous antivirals used to treat influenza infections. The advantages are that it is given as a single dose for the entire course of treatment and reduces the duration of influenza illness by approximately 24 hours. It does not seem more effective than oseltamivir in reducing influenza-related symptoms. The appropriate doses are 40 mg for individuals age 12 years or older and weighing less than 40 kg to less than 80 kg, and 80 mg for individuals weighing at least 80 kg.

In 2009, a novel H1N1 strain of influenza caused a worldwide pandemic. At the time of this writing, both this epidemic H1N1 strain and the seasonal influenza A/H3N2 and type B strains continue to circulate in the world. The considerable majority of these epidemic and seasonal strains continue to show sensitivity to oseltamivir, whereas most are resistant to M2 inhibitors. All strains continue to show sensitivity to zanamivir.

TABLE 1 Use of Antiviral Agents for Treatment of COVID-19 Infection

DRUG	PROPHYLAXIS	AMBULATORY, MILD-MODERATE DISEASE	HOSPITALIZED, MILD-MODERATE DISEASE, NO OXYGEN REQUIREMENT	HOSPITALIZED, MORE SEVERE DISEASE, SPO$_2$ ≤ 94%	HOSPITALIZED, CRITICAL ILLNESS (ICU, MECHANICAL VENTILATION, ECMO, SEPTIC SHOCK)
Remdesivir (Veklury)*	No recommendation	**Adults:** 200 mg on day 1, 100 mg on days 2 and 3 **Pediatrics:** 5 mg/kg on day 1, 2.5 mg/kg days 2 and 3	**Adults:** 200 mg on day 1, 100 mg on days 2 and 3 **Pediatrics:** 5 mg/kg on day 1, 2.5 mg/kg days 2 and 3	5 days recommended (10 days optional)	Suggest against use
Nirmatrelvir/ ritonavir (Paxlovid)†	No recommendation	**Adults:** Recommended for use within 5 days of disease onset, if patients have high risk of progression to severe disease **Children:** >12 years and ≥40 kg body mass	**Adults:** Recommended for use within 5 days of disease onset, if patients have high risk of progression to severe disease **Children:** >12 years and ≥40 kg body mass	No recommendation	No recommendation

*Remdesivir should not be used if patient alanine transaminase is >10 times the upper limit of normal.

†Paxlovid therapy pack contains 150 mg nirmatrelvir and 100 mg ritonavir tablets. The recommended dose for adults and children >12 years and ≥40 kg body mass is two nirmatrelvir tablets (300 mg) and one ritonavir tablet (100 mg) taken together every 12 hours for 5 days. If the glomerular filtration rate (GFR) is >30 to <60 mL/min, the dose should be reduced to one nirmatrelvir tablet (150 mg) and one ritonavir tablet (100 mg) every 12 hours. The drug should not be administered if the GFR is <30 mL/min.

Nirmatrelvir/ritonavir has numerous interactions with other drugs, which may seriously affect the activity of other drugs, as well nirmatrelvir/ritonavir itself. For important information about drug interactions, check https://www.fda.gov/media/155050/download.

ECMO, Extracorporeal membrane oxygenation; *ICU,* intensive care unit; *SpO₂,* oxygen saturation.

Croup

Croup is defined by the occurrence of hoarseness or laryngitis, a deep, brassy, or barking cough, and inspiratory stridor. Airway obstruction in croup is caused by constriction in the subglottic area, often noted on radiographs by a steeple-shaped narrowing of the air column in this region. Affected children are usually afebrile and nontoxic in appearance.

Parainfluenza virus type 1 is the primary cause of croup, although infection with many different viruses can produce this illness, and influenza virus can cause a particularly severe form of croup. Bacterial secondary infection occurs uncommonly, but it can result in fever and severe obstruction of the airway. Administration of dexamethasone (Decadron)[1] at 0.6 mg/kg either orally or intramuscularly markedly reduces the rate of hospitalization, admission to the intensive care unit (ICU), and intubation for croup.

Bronchiolitis

Bronchiolitis represents the most common cause for hospitalization of infants in developed countries. Infants present with a history of several days of upper respiratory symptoms, followed by the rapid onset of wheezing and labored breathing. RSV is the most common cause and is the agent found in the most severe cases that result in respiratory failure. Contrasting with asthma, obstruction of the airway in bronchiolitis is a result of plugging of bronchioles with detached epithelium and inflammatory cells. Mucus plugging and constriction of smooth muscle are not prominent. Also in contrast with asthma is the absence of a sustained response to bronchodilators and corticosteroids among infants with bronchiolitis.

Therapy of bronchiolitis primarily consists of administration of supplemental oxygen and replacement of fluid deficits as needed. Ribavirin (Virazole)[1] is a compound with antiviral activity against RSV, but controlled studies have not demonstrated meaningful differences in outcomes between treated and untreated subjects. The compound is quite expensive and must be delivered via a special aerosol generator.

Palivizumab (Synagis), a preparation consisting of a monoclonal antibody against the fusion protein of RSV, has proved to be effective in reducing the rate of hospitalization for RSV infection by approximately 50% when given to high-risk infants. Infants who may be considered candidates for therapy include those with chronic lung disease, those born prematurely, and those with hemodynamically significant congenital heart disease. Doses of palivizumab (15 mg/kg) are given on a monthly basis throughout the local RSV season, usually November through March.

The U.S. Food and Drug Administration (FDA) has recently given approval for the use of two recombinant RSV vaccines (Arexvy by GlaxoSmithKline, and Abrysvo by Pfizer). These vaccines are approved for prevention of RSV infection in adults 60 years or older. No RSV vaccine has been approved for individuals younger than 60 years old.

---

[1] Not FDA approved for this indication.

Severe Acute Respiratory Syndrome Coronavirus-2 (SARS-CoV-2)

The appearance of SARS-CoV-2 has profoundly affected healthcare worldwide. Although symptoms are generally milder in children, respiratory illness can, at times, be severe or even fatal. Symptoms are not readily distinguishable from other respiratory viral infections early on but may become severe as the illness progresses. Numerous antivirals and antibody formulations have been developed, but the use of antibodies has essentially been eliminated as variants of the parent virus have become resistant to antibody preparations, including convalescent plasma. A summary of the use of currently FDA-recommended antiviral preparations that can be used in adults and children is presented in Table 1.

The use of corticosteroids, particularly dexamethasone, is not supported by the Infectious Diseases Society of America for outpatients and those inpatients with no need for supplemental oxygen. The use of dexamethasone[1] is *suggested* in patients hospitalized and with oxygen saturation values of 94% or less and recommended in subjects with critical illnesses (ICU admission, use of mechanically assisted ventilation or extracorporeal membrane oxygenation). In these patients, the appropriate dexamethasone dose is 6 mg intravenously (IV) or orally for 10 days, or until the patient is discharged home. In children, the dose for dexamethasone is 0.15 mg/kg IV or intramuscularly every day for a maximum of 10 days.

---

[1] Not FDA approved for this indication.

References

Akerlund A, Klint T, Olen L, Runderantz H: Nasal decongestant effect of oxymetazoline in the common cold: an objective dose-response study in 106 patients, *J Laryngol Otol* 103:743–746, 1989.

Buckingham SC, Jafri HS, Bush AN, et al: A randomized, double-blind, placebo-controlled trial of dexamethasone in severe respiratory syncytial virus (RSV) infection: effects on RSV quantity and clinical outcome, *J Infect Dis* 185:1222–1228, 2002.

Curley FJ, Irwin RS, Pratter MR, et al: Cough and the common cold, *Am J Respir Crit Care Med* 138:305–311, 1988.

Flores G, Horwitz RI: Efficacy of β_2-agonists in bronchiolitis: a reappraisal and meta-analysis, *Pediatrics* 100:233–239, 1997.

IDSA Guidelines on the Treatment and Management of Patients with COVID-19. Available at: https://www.idsociety.org/practice-guideline/covid-19-guideline-treatment-and-management.

Johnson DW, Jacobson S, Edney PC, et al: A comparison of nebulized budesonide, intramuscular dexamethasone, and placebo for moderately severe croup, *N Engl J Med* 339:498–503, 1998.

Muether PS, Gwaltney Jr JM: Variant effect of first- and second-generation antihistamines as clues to their mechanism of action on the sneeze reflex in the common cold, *Clin Infect Dis* 33:1483–1488, 2001.

Randolph AG, Wang EL: Ribavirin for respiratory syncytial virus lower respiratory tract infection, *Arch Pediatr Adolesc Med* 150:942–947, 1996.

Tavorner D, Danz C, Economos D: The effects of oral pseudoephedrine on nasal patency in the common cold: a double-blind single-dose placebo-controlled trial, *Clin Otolaryngol* 24:47–51, 1999.

Treanor JJ, Hayden FG, Vrooman PS, et al: Efficacy and safety of the oral neuraminidase inhibitor oseltamivir in treating acute influenza: a randomized controlled trial. US Oral Neuraminidase Study Group, *JAMA* 283:1016–1024, 2000.

Van Voris LP, Betts RF, Hayden FG, et al: Successful treatment of naturally occurring influenza A/USSR/77 H1N1, *JAMA* 245:1128–1131, 1981.

12 Rheumatology and the Musculoskeletal System

AXIAL SPONDYLOARTHRITIS

Method of
Atul A. Deodhar, MD, MRCP; and Sonam R. Kiwalkar, MD

CURRENT DIAGNOSIS

- *Axial spondyloarthritis* (axSpA) is an umbrella term that includes ankylosing spondylitis (AS) and nonradiographic axial spondyloarthritis (nr-axSpA). The presence or absence of definitive sacroiliitis on radiographs differentiates AS (also called *radiographic axSpA*) from nr-axSpA. The latter is a condition with the same clinical features and similar disease burden, except that definitive radiographic features of sacroiliitis are lacking.
- In the absence of diagnostic criteria, the diagnosis of AS is made by the presence of definitive sacroiliitis on sacroiliac (SI) joint radiographic imaging plus either chronic (>3 months) inflammatory back pain or restriction in spinal movements or chest expansion (Modified New York Criteria for Classification of AS).
- Because definitive sacroiliitis may take up to 10 years to appear on a radiograph from the start of chronic inflammatory back pain (the most common first symptom), early or mild disease can be missed.
- When AS is suspected with features of inflammatory back pain (usually starting before 45 years of age) along with other clinical features of spondyloarthritis—such as uveitis, psoriasis, enthesitis, asymmetric peripheral inflammatory arthritis, family history of spondyloarthritis, high C-reactive protein (CRP), inflammatory bowel disease, favorable response to nonsteroidal antiinflammatory drugs (NSAIDs)—but a radiograph of the SI joints is negative or uncertain for definitive sacroiliitis, magnetic resonance imaging (MRI) of the SI joints and/or human leukocyte antigen (HLA)-B27 typing may help in making the diagnosis of axSpA.

CURRENT THERAPY

- Nonpharmacologic interventions include active physical therapy, self-directed physical exercise, patient education, and smoking cessation.
- NSAIDs are the first line of pharmacologic treatment.
- In patients who do not respond adequately to NSAIDs, treatment with a tumor necrosis factor-α inhibitor (TNFi), interleukin-17 inhibitor (IL-17i), or Janus kinase inhibitor (JAKi) is recommended.
- Retrospective analysis in cohorts of patients with AS using long-term TNFi therapy has shown a reduced rate of new bone formation in the spine, although no pharmaceutical agents have shown "disease-modifying" ability in placebo-controlled prospective studies to date.
- Conventional synthetic antirheumatic drugs, such as sulfasalazine or methotrexate,[1] or methotrexate,[1] can be used to treat peripheral arthritis in patients with axSpA, but they do not have efficacy in axial disease.

[1]Not FDA approved for this indication.

Definition and Spectrum of the Disease

Axial spondyloarthritis (axSpA) is an umbrella term that includes ankylosing spondylitis (AS) and nonradiographic axial spondyloarthritis (nr-axSpA). The presence or absence of definitive sacroiliitis on radiographic imaging differentiates AS (also called *radiographic axSpA*) from nr-axSpA.

AxSpA is a chronic, immune-mediated inflammatory disorder involving the sacroiliac (SI) joints, the spine, and often the hips. In some, spinal bony fusion develops gradually over several years and may lead to reduced spine and neck flexibility. The axial skeleton is always involved, and involvement of the peripheral joints occurs in approximately 30% of patients. Enthesitis is a common occurrence. Extraarticular manifestations (EAMs) include osteoporosis, psoriasis, acute anterior uveitis, and inflammatory bowel disease (IBD) (i.e., Crohn disease or ulcerative colitis).

Epidemiology

Based on the 2009 to 2010 National Health and Nutritional Examination Survey (NHANES), the estimated prevalence of axSpA in the U.S. population is about 1.0%, of which 0.5% of patients are reported to have AS. The prevalence of nr-axSpA is thus assumed to be the other 0.5% because pelvic radiographs and SI magnetic resonance imaging (MRI) examinations were not carried out in this population-based study. Based on 2006 to 2014 data from the U.S. Medicare Fee-for-Service and IBM MarketScan databases, a retrospective observational cohort study showed an increase in the diagnostic prevalence of AS and axSpA, which could possibly be attributed to increased disease awareness.

The prevalence of axSpA varies with geographic region and, in general, depends on the prevalence of human leukocyte antigen (HLA)-B27. Prevalence of HLA-B27 is less than 1% in Japanese populations, is 3% in African Americans, and is more than 20% in some native populations of eastern Siberia and Alaska. It is 8% in Western Europe and 10% to 16% in Scandinavian countries. AxSpA is thus rare in Japanese and African American populations. The prevalence of axSpA is about 0.5% in persons of European descent and 1.4% in those of Scandinavian ancestry, whereas it increases to 2% to 3% in natives of eastern Siberia and Alaska. The risk of axSpA is increased among those with an affected first-degree relative. The male-to-female ratio is 2:1 for the diagnosis of AS. In contrast, there is hardly any difference in the prevalence of nr-axSpA among males and females, suggesting that male sex is a prognostic indicator for progression from nonradiographic to radiographic axSpA.

Pathogenesis

Genetics plays a major role in the pathogenesis of spondyloarthritis, and the *HLA-B27* gene has a major association with AS. *HLA-B27* is present in about 70% to 90% of patients with AS in most ethnic groups. The risk of disease in family members of patients with AS is 63% in monozygotic twins, 20% in dizygotic twins, 8.2% in first-degree relatives, 1% in second-degree relatives, and 0.7% in third-degree relatives. The overall contribution to AS heritability by *HLA-B27* is estimated to be approximately 20%. Some other genes associated with AS—such as endoplasmic reticulum aminopeptidases (ERAP-1 and ERAP-2) and interleukin-23 receptor (IL-23R)—have been implicated to play a role in the pathogenesis.

The following hypotheses have been put forth to explain the role of *HLA-B27* in the pathogenesis of AS:

1. **Arthritogenic peptide presentation.** Certain antimicrobial peptides have molecular mimicry to self-peptides found in the joints, and it is hypothesized that *HLA-B27* presents these to cytotoxic T cells. The activated T-cell lymphocytes then lead to autoreactivity, arthritis, and spondylitis.
2. **HLA-B27 heavy chain homodimer.** The heavy chains of the HLA-B27 molecule can form homodimers when they are expressed on the cell surface, resulting in their recognition by natural killer cell receptors. This can enhance the survival and proliferation of CD-4 T cells and increase the production of IL-17 in vivo.
3. **HLA-B27 misfolding and unfolded protein response.** HLA-B27 assembly takes place in the endoplasmic reticulum (ER) before it is expressed on the cell surface. The misfolded HLA-B27 molecules accumulate in the ER, leading to cellular stress secondary to the unfolded protein response. This then activates the IL-23/IL-17 pathway of inflammation.
4. **HLA-B27 shaping of the human gut microbiome.** The human body contains a large community of commensals and symbiotic bacteria, fungi, and viruses called *microbiota*. The term *microbiome* refers to the genomes of these microorganisms. The composition of the gut microbiome is influenced by genes and other environmental factors. It is postulated that HLA-B27 predisposes to AS by influencing the gut microbiome. Studies have shown that the microbiota composition of patients with AS differs from that of patients with rheumatoid arthritis as well as healthy controls. Further, *HLA-B27*–positive healthy individuals have a microbiome that differs from that of HLA-B27–negative subjects.

In animal models of spondyloarthritis, *HLA-B27* transgenic rats and mice did not develop spondyloarthritis when raised in a germ-free environment, but they developed spondyloarthritis-like disease when they were housed in a typical laboratory environment, suggesting a role for microbes in the pathogenesis of spondyloarthritis. More than 60% of patients with AS have subclinical acute or chronic intestinal inflammation. This loss of architectural and functional integrity in the intestinal epithelium enables the passage of microbial products into the submucosa and then into the systemic circulation. Innate and adaptive immune cells recognize these microbial products and produce proinflammatory cytokines. These microbial products and the immune cells travel from the gut to distant sites, such as peripheral joints and entheses, causing inflammation.

Clinical Manifestations

The most common manifestations of axSpA include chronic inflammatory low back, hip, and/or buttock pain. The typical characteristics of inflammatory back pain include age of onset before 40 years, insidious onset without any identifiable cause, improvement with exercise or activity and no improvement with rest, and pain in the second half of the night. Neck pain is rarely the presenting feature due to involvement of the cervical spine; when this is present, it is more commonly seen in women.

The limitation of spinal motion is initially the result of axial inflammation and later is secondary to the ossification of ligamentous structures, bony fusion of apophyseal joints, and outer fibers of the annulus fibrosus of the intervertebral disks, leading to the development of syndesmophytes.

Hip involvement is seen in up to 40% of patients. The typical symptoms are pain in the groin or radiation of pain to the medial thigh or the knee. Hip involvement is associated with significant functional impairment. Other peripheral joints—such as the ankles, knees, shoulders, and, to a lesser extent, the sternoclavicular joint, the temporomandibular joint, and small joints of the hands and feet—may also be involved.

Enthesitis is a classic feature of axSpA. Enthesitis presents as pain, stiffness, and tenderness at the sites of insertions of ligaments, muscles, or tendons to a bone. Typical areas of enthesitis include the Achilles tendon, plantar fascia attachment to the calcaneus, costochondral junctions, and the paraspinal muscle attachment to the pelvic rim. Diffuse swelling of the toes or fingers, called *dactylitis* ("sausage digits"), is occasionally seen in axSpA.

EAMs associated with axSpA include psoriasis, IBD, uveitis, and osteoporosis. A large epidemiologic study found that 42% of patients with axSpA had one or more EAMs; uveitis was present in 27%, IBD in 10%, and psoriasis in 11%. Uveitis seen in association with axSpA presents as eye discomfort during the prodromal phase followed by an acute onset of eye redness, pain, photophobia, and miosis. The usual characteristics of uveitis associated with axSpA are acute in onset, unilateral, and involve the anterior part of the uvea. Even though overt IBD is seen in only 10% of patients with axSpA, more than 60% have subclinical mucosal inflammation in the gut.

Diagnosis

Within the United States, there is a significant delay of 10 to 14 years in the diagnosis of axSpA from symptom onset. There are many reasons for this, including the commonality of back pain in the general population and the rarity of axSpA as a cause of back pain. There are no specific physical findings or laboratory tests to diagnose axSpA; the diagnosis is based on pattern recognition and clinical reasoning. Patients with back pain are generally seen by nonrheumatologists who may not be familiar with features of inflammatory back pain and may not suspect axSpA. In the optimal clinical setting with a patient complaining of onset of chronic (>3 months) inflammatory back pain starting before 45 years of age, the presence of other features of spondyloarthritis (as described earlier), a positive *HLA B-27* test, and a plain radiograph of the SI joint showing sacroiliitis, the diagnosis of AS would be straightforward. Radiographic findings, such as sclerosis, joint erosions, or widening, narrowing, or ankylosis of the SI joint, suggest sacroiliitis.

During this early stage of disease (also known as *nr-axSpA*), MRI (without contrast) of the SI joints may show evidence of active inflammation and may also show structural changes such as sclerosis, fatty metaplasia, or erosions that aid in making the diagnosis. The required sequence of MRI and the features that suggest a diagnosis of nr-axSpA include the following:
1. T1-weighted sequence. Structural changes such as erosions and ankylosis can be seen. Fat metaplasia appears hyperintense.
2. Fat-suppressed T2-weighted (short-TI inversion recovery [STIR]) sequence, osteitis, representing active inflammation and reported as bone marrow edema; appears hyperintense.

When the clinical suspicion of axSpA is high but radiographic imaging of the SI joints is negative or inconclusive for sacroiliitis, the presence of the features previously noted on MRI of the SI joints may help in confirming a diagnosis of nr-axSpA.

The changes of inflammation on STIR imaging (i.e., "osteitis") can be seen in professional athletes, military recruits, and even in normal individuals because of mechanical stress ("false-positive MRI"). It is therefore important to emphasize that ruling out common causes of back pain, pattern recognition, and clinical reasoning is the key to a diagnosis of axSpA.

Plain radiographs of the spine may show characteristic changes in AS. Romanus lesions or the *shiny corner sign* and squaring of the vertebral body are seen as a result of erosions at the attachments of the spinal ligaments at the vertebral corners in early disease. This is followed by ossification of the outer layer of annulus fibrosus, leading to syndesmophyte formation on plain radiographs. In the late stages, ankylosis of the spine, also known as *bamboo spine,* may be seen in a small percentage of patients with AS. The role of low-dose computed tomography (CT) in the diagnosis of axSpA is currently being researched.

An elevated erythrocyte sedimentation rate (ESR) or C-reactive protein (CRP) is seen in only 30% to 40% of patients with active AS.

Differential Diagnosis

Chronic nonspecific back pain is common in the general population (19% according to the NHANES study); hence mechanical causes of back pain should be considered first.

Diffuse idiopathic skeletal hyperostosis (DISH) is sometimes mistaken for "bamboo spine of AS." DISH is a noninflammatory condition affecting the spine. It is more commonly seen in males with obesity and diabetes, often older than 50 years of age. Radiographically, DISH is characterized by calcification of the anterior longitudinal ligament involving at least four contiguous vertebral bodies, sometimes referred to as *flowing osteophytes*. The flowing osteophytes are bulky and typically appear on the right side of the spine. SI joints are not involved in patients with DISH.

Osteitis condensans ilii (OCI) can be mistaken for sacroiliitis but is usually an asymptomatic benign disorder of multiparous women. OCI is characterized by radiographic findings of a triangular area of dense sclerosis on the lower and inferior part of iliac side of the SI joint. OCI is not associated with erosions or ankylosis of the SI joints.

Inflammatory back pain with sclerotic changes on SI joint radiographs can also be seen in conditions such as (1) postpartum insufficiency fracture of the sacrum; (2) septic sacroiliitis from tuberculosis, brucellosis, fungi, and other infectious agents; and (3) rarely, malignancies such as acute lymphoblastic leukemia.

Treatment

The goals of treatment of axSpA are to reduce symptoms, improve and maintain spinal flexibility and normal posture, reduce functional limitations, and decrease complications of the disease. The mainstay of treatment has been NSAIDs, exercise and physical therapy, biologics such as tumor necrosis factor-α inhibitors (TNFi) and interleukin-17 inhibitors (IL-17i), and small-molecule drugs such as Janus kinase inhibitors (JAKi).

Treatment of axSpA can be divided into nonpharmacologic, pharmacologic, and surgical interventions.

Nonpharmacologic Interventions

Nonpharmacologic interventions include active physical therapy (on land or aquatic), self-directed physical exercise, patient education, and smoking cessation. These are recommended during all stages of the disease.

Pharmacologic Interventions

Box 1 outlines pharmacologic interventions for the treatment of axSpA.

The use of biologics and small molecules has been associated with an increased risk of serious infections. Though bacterial infections are seen in both classes of drugs, herpes zoster is seen mostly with JAKi, and reactivation of latent tuberculosis is mostly seen with TNFi. Therefore screening for latent tuberculosis should be performed before these therapies are initiated.

Some of the side effects of TNFi and IL-17 therapy include injection site reactions with subcutaneous preparations or infusion reactions with infliximab (Remicade) or golimumab (Simponi). Some of the other adverse effects of TNFi are the development of demyelinating disease, worsening of heart failure, recurrence of lymphoma or malignant melanoma, and paradoxical development of psoriasis-like skin lesions. Adverse events associated with IL-17i therapy include leukopenia, candidiasis, and the development or worsening of IBD. The ORAL Surveillance Study, a postmarketing safety trial ordered by the FDA, showed a higher risk of major adverse cardiac events (fatal and nonfatal myocardial infarctions and nonfatal strokes) and a higher risk of cancers (excluding nonmelanoma skin cancers) in those on JAKi therapy compared with those on TNFi therapy. As a result, the FDA placed a black box warning on tofacitinib (Xeljanz) and extended the warning to upadacitinib (Rinvoq) because it is in the same class of drugs.

Surgical Interventions

Total hip arthroplasty should be considered in patients with refractory hip pain or functional decline in the presence of radiographic evidence of structural damage. Spinal corrective osteotomies are occasionally necessary for fixed kyphotic deformities seen in advanced AS but should be undertaken only in centers of expertise.

Monitoring

Patients should be monitored regularly for disease activity, functional impairment, and medication safety. The frequency of monitoring is individualized. Assessment of disease activity can be performed by the following methods:

1. Use of the Bath Ankylosing Spondylitis Disease Activity Index (BASDAI): This is a patient-administered questionnaire with six questions answered on a visual analog scale of 0 to 10.

BOX 1   Pharmacologic Interventions for the Treatment of Axial Spondyloarthritis

1. Nonsteroidal antiinflammatory drugs (NSAIDs) are used in full doses either continuously or on an as-needed basis, depending on the severity of symptoms, comorbidities, and patient preferences. No particular NSAID is preferred over any other.
2. If patients continue to have symptoms despite a 4-week trial of full-dose NSAIDs, therapy is escalated to TNFi or IL-17i.
   a. Though certolizumab is the only TNFi approved for nr-axSpA, all five TNFi agents are FDA approved for the treatment of AS.
   b. Soluble receptor of TNF—Etanercept (Enbrel) 50 mg, SC injection once weekly.
   c. TNFi monoclonal antibodies:
      i. Adalimumab (Humira) 40 mg SC every 2 weeks
      ii. Golimumab (Simponi) 50 mg SC once a month or (Simponi Aria) 2 mg/kg intravenous (IV) at weeks 0, 4, and then every 8 weeks thereafter
      iii. Certolizumab pegol (Cimzia) 200 mg SC twice a month or 400 mg SC once a month
      iv. Infliximab (Remicade) 5 mg/kg IV infusion every 6 weeks
   d. No TNFi is preferred over any other, except in patients with concomitant uveitis or IBD, in whom monoclonal antibodies are preferred over soluble receptor TNFi therapy.
3. In case of primary failure of TNFi, treatment can be switched to IL-17i or JAKi. In case of secondary failure of TNFi therapy (failing after initial benefit), either an alternative TNFi or IL-17i or JAKi can be used.

   a. Secukinumab (Cosentyx), an IL-17i, is given SC as 150 mg at weeks 0, 1, 2, 3, and 4, followed by 150 mg or 300 mg every 4 weeks. Ixekizumab (Taltz), another IL-17i, can also be used. It is given subcutaneously as 160 mg once, followed by 80 mg every 4 weeks. Both are approved for the treatment of AS and nr-axSpA. In case of primary failure of IL-17i, treatment can be switched to TNFi or JAKi. In case of secondary failure of IL-17i therapy (failing after initial benefit), either an alternative IL-17i or TNFi or JAKi can be used.
   b. Though both JAKi tofacitinib (Xeljanz) 5 mg two times a day and upadacitinib (Rinvoq) 15 mg once a day are approved for the treatment of AS, only upadacitinib is approved for nr-axSpA.
   c. Bimekizumab (Bimzelx),[2] an IL-17A and IL-17F inhibitor, has shown promising results in phase III trials.
4. Conventional synthetic DMARDs like sulfasalazine (Azulfidine),[1] up to 3 g/day, and methotrexate,[1] up to 25 mg/week, are effective in the treatment of peripheral joint involvement but not of axial disease in axSpA.
5. Local glucocorticoid injections for enthesitis or intraarticular injections for active peripheral arthritis can provide relief for flareups. However, injection of inflamed weight-bearing tendons such as the Achilles tendon is not recommended because of the risk of rupture.
6. Systemic glucocorticoids do not have any benefit in axSpA and should be avoided.

---

[1] Not FDA approved for this indication.
[2] Not available in the United States.

A BASDAI score of ≥4 is indicative of active disease. Clinically significant improvement is defined as an absolute change ≥2.

2. Use of the Ankylosing Spondylitis Disease Activity Score (AS-DAS): This incorporates three questions used in the BASDAI, a patient global assessment of disease activity, and CRP. An ASDAS score <1.3 is defined as inactive disease, a score of 1.3 to 2.1 is low disease activity, 2.1 to 3.5 is high disease activity, and >3.5 is very high disease activity. A reduction of ≥1.1 in ASDAS is considered a significant improvement.

Structural damage resulting from axSpA can be measured using the modified Stoke Ankylosing Spondylitis Spine Score. This score correlates with disease activity as measured with the ASDAS.

Functional impairment can be measured by the Bath Ankylosing Spondylitis Functional Index. This is a patient-administered questionnaire that includes 10 activities of daily living. The Bath Ankylosing Spondylitis Metrology Index is an index of spinal and hip mobility in patients with AS. It includes lateral lumbar flexion, tragus-to-wall distance, modified Schober test, maximal intermalleolar distance, and cervical rotation.

The ESR and CRP may be useful in monitoring disease activity. MRI of the SI joints or spine is expensive and is not indicated to monitor disease activity of AS. Spine radiographs are not used for monitoring purposes in daily practice, although they may be used to counsel patients about lifestyle changes (such as stopping smoking) or to start biologic therapy.

Complications

The prevalence of osteoporosis is approximately 25% after 10 years of axSpA. Vertebral fractures are seen in about 10% of patients with AS. The lower cervical spine is the most commonly involved area, where there is often also neurologic compromise. One should consider vertebral fractures in patients with neck and back pain that has changed in intensity or character from baseline. Another rare complication is the cauda equine syndrome from long-standing AS resulting from inflammation of the lumbosacral nerve roots caused by arachnoiditis. Cardiac manifestations include aortic valve insufficiency and conduction abnormalities. Pulmonary manifestations are rare and include chest expansion restriction from ossification of costovertebral joints and upper lobe–predominant interstitial lung disease. Patients with AS can have IgA nephropathy or, in late stages, renal amyloidosis if the disease is left untreated. Cardiovascular disease is being recognized as a common comorbidity in patients with AS and is linked to chronic inflammation. All patients with AS should be counseled about the traditional risk factors for cardiovascular disease, and appropriate treatment should be instituted if necessary.

References

Bennett AN, McGonagle D, O'Connor P, et al: Severity of baseline magnetic resonance imaging-evident sacroiliitis and HLA-B27 status in early inflammatory back pain predict radiographically evident ankylosing spondylitis at eight years, *Arthritis Rheum* 58(11):3413–3418, 2008, https://dx.doi.org/10.1002/art.24024.

Braun J, Sieper J: Ankylosing spondylitis, *Lancet (London, England)* 369(9570):1379–1390, 2007, https://dx.doi.org/10.1016/S0140-6736(07)60635-7.

Brophy S, MacKay K, Al-Saidi A: The natural history of ankylosing spondylitis as defined by radiological progression, *J Rheumatol* 29(6):1236–1243, 2002.

Curtis JR, Winthrop K, Bohn RL, et al: The annual diagnostic prevalence of ankylosing spondylitis and axial spondyloarthritis in the United States using Medicare and MarketScan databases, *ACR Open Rheumatology* 3(11):743–752, 2021, https://dx.doi.org/10.1002/acr2.11316.

de Winter JJ, van Mens LJ, van der Heijde D: Prevalence of peripheral and extra-articular disease in ankylosing spondylitis versus non-radiographic axial spondyloarthritis: a meta-analysis, *Arthritis Res Ther* 18(1), 2016, https://dx.doi.org/10.1186/s13075-016-1093-z.

Deodhar A, Mease PJ, Reveille JD, et al: Frequency of axial spondyloarthritis diagnosis among patients seen by US rheumatologists for evaluation of chronic back pain, *Arthritis Rheum* 68(7):1669–1676, 2016, https://dx.doi.org/10.1002/art.39612.

Reveille JD: Genetics of spondyloarthritis - beyond the MHC, *Nat Rev Rheumatol* 8(5):296–304, 2012, https://dx.doi.org/10.1038/nrrheum.2012.41.

Reveille JD, Witter JP, Weisman MH: Prevalence of axial spondylarthritis in the United States: estimates from a cross-sectional survey, *Arthritis Care Res* 64(6):905–910, 2012, https://dx.doi.org/10.1002/acr.21621.

Rudwaleit M, Khan MA, Sieper J, et al: Commentary: the challenge of diagnosis and classification in early ankylosing spondylitis: do we need new criteria? *Arthritis Rheum* 52(4):1000–1008, 2005, https://dx.doi.org/10.1002/art.20990.

Ward MM, Deodhar A, Gensler LS, et al: Update of the American College of Rheumatology/Spondylitis Association of America/Spondyloarthritis Research and Treatment Network recommendations for the treatment of ankylosing spondylitis and nonradiographic axial spondyloarthritis, *Arthritis Care Res*, 2019, https://dx.doi.org/10.1002/acr.24025.

Ytterberg SR, Bhatt DL, Mikuls TR, et al: ORAL surveillance investigators: cardiovascular and cancer risk with tofacitinib in rheumatoid arthritis, *N Engl J Med* 386(4):316–326, 2022, https://dx.doi.org/10.1056/NEJMoa2109927.

Baraliakos X, Østergaard M, Poddubnyy D, et al: effect of secukinumab versus adalimumab biosimilar on radiographic progression in patients with radiographic axial spondyloarthritis: a randomized phase IIIb Study [abstract], *Arthritis Rheumatol* 74(suppl 9), 2022. https://acrabstracts.org/abstract/effect-of-secukinumab-versus-adalimumab-biosimilar-on-radiographic-progression-in-patients-with-radiographic-axial-spondyloarthritis-a-randomized-phase-iiib-study/. Accessed February 4, 2023.

Ramiro S, Nikiphorou E, Sepriano A, et al: ASAS-EULAR recommendations for the management of axial spondyloarthritis: 2022 update, *Ann Rheum Dis* 82:19–34, 2023.

▮ BURSITIS AND TENDINOPATHY

Method of
Kyle Goerl, MD

CURRENT DIAGNOSIS

Tendinopathy
- Tendinitis is an inflammatory condition only present within the first weeks of a tendon injury.
- Tendinosis is a degenerative condition usually developing weeks after the initial injury.
- The diagnosis is typically made clinically with a thorough history and physical examination.
- Most tendinopathies occur secondary to overuse, and can be acute, chronic, or recurrent.
- Tendinopathies are usually characterized by pain, possible swelling, and dysfunction of the affected tendon.
- If the diagnosis is in question, magnetic resonance imaging and ultrasound are helpful diagnostic aides.

Bursitis
- Bursitis is an inflammatory reaction of a bursa.
- Bursitis is typically the result of overuse or trauma, but systemic illnesses can also cause bursitis.
- The olecranon, prepatellar, and trochanteric bursa are particularly susceptible to traumatic bursitis because of their location immediately under the skin with minimal subcutaneous fat for protection.
- Bursitis rarely occurs alone, so a search should be conducted for an associated condition such as tendinopathy or a tendon tear.
- Imaging studies demonstrate that lateral hip pain is usually tendinopathy, not "trochanteric bursitis," a term that should be reserved for image-proven bursitis.
- Septic bursitis usually only affects the olecranon and prepatellar bursa, and care must be taken to distinguish it from aseptic bursitis.
- Common pathogens in septic arthritis include *Staphylococcus aureus* and β-hemolytic *Streptococcus.*
- If the diagnosis of septic bursitis is in question, aspiration should be performed, and the aspirate sent for Gram stain, cell count and differential, culture and crystal analysis, and blood should be sent for culture, complete blood count, C-reactive protein, and erythrocyte sedimentation rate.

CURRENT THERAPY

Tendinopathy

- Given that tendonitis is an inflammatory condition, NSAIDs should be considered. Ice, activity modification, and rest are also effective.
- Tendinosis is not an inflammatory condition, so NSAIDs are not usually a part of the treatment regimen.
- Tendinosis responds well to physical therapy and, in particular, eccentric exercises. Deep tissue massage with tools is also an effective treatment modality.
- Steroid injections can be effective for short term pain relief, but not for long-term healing, and should not be a routine part of the treatment plan. Steroid injections can be considered if the patient is in too much pain to perform physical therapy.
- Injections of blood products such as whole blood and platelet-rich-plasma, prolotherapy and sclerotherapy have varying levels of evidence supporting their effectiveness, but are reasonable alternatives to surgery.
- When conservative measures fail, more invasive procedures such as teno tomy, tendon scraping, and open débridement should be considered, but are rarely needed.

Bursitis

- Early treatment should include NSAIDs, ice, activity modification, and rest.
- If an associated condition like tendinopathy is discovered, appropriate treatment should target that condition as well, and typically involves physical therapy.
- In the event of septic bursitis, antibiotic treatment should be initiated. Parenteral medication should be heavily considered, given the high failure rate of oral antibiotics.
- Surgery is rarely needed for bursitis.

Tendinopathy

Background

Tendon is a connective tissue used to attach muscle to bone. Normal tendon tissue is dense and has a highly regular and fibrillar pattern. Tendinopathy is the term used to describe a clinical syndrome typically resulting from overuse of a tendon. Traditionally the term tendonitis has been used to describe all tendon injuries, but the suffix "–itis" indicates the presence of inflammation, and inflammation is only present early on in the tendinopathy disease process. Inflammation may have resolved and inflammatory cells may no longer be present, but the patient may still have pain. At that point the disease process has changed from one of inflammation to a degenerative problem more appropriately termed tendinosis (Table 1).

Tendinopathies are characterized by pain, swelling, and impairment of functional activities of the affected region. They can be acute, chronic, or recurrent. The diagnosis is usually clinical based on history and physical examination. Typically, there is a history of repetitive motion, which can be anything from painting a wall

to playing a sport like tennis. If this historical information is lacking, then a systemic medical condition should be considered.

With repetitive activities and inadequate recovery time tenocytes will begin producing inflammatory substances, and the load-bearing matrix of the tendon will begin to breakdown and become fibrotic. The collagen matrix becomes disorganized with fibers separating and healing in an erratic, disorganized manner. There is an increase in mucoid ground substance, hypercellularity, and pathologic vessel and sensory afferent nerve formation. The abnormal nerve formation likely contributes to the sensation of pain. This histopathological degenerative process is more appropriately called tendinosis. The degenerative mechanism appears to be multifactorial, with contributions from:

1. Classic inflammatory mediators like interleukins, prostaglandins, and substance P.
2. Altered load bearing on a tendon as in shoulder impingement.
3. Systemic influences such as aging.

Tendinopathy is occurring at higher rates in the developed world secondary to an increase in recreational sport participation. Lower extremity tendons, like the Achilles and patellar tendons, bear a large amount of tensile force (Table 2). Thirty percent of runners will suffer Achilles tendinopathy in their lifetime, with an odds ratio of 31:2 when compared with age matched controls, and repetitive exposure is a risk factor. One in 3 patients with Achilles tendinopathy do not participate in sports. With respect to patellar tendinopathy, jumping sports like volleyball and basketball are risk factors. Historically, most lateral hip pain was labeled "trochanteric bursitis." Research using imaging techniques, including magnetic resonance imaging (MRI) and ultrasound (), has concluded that lateral hip pain around the greater trochanter is more likely caused by tendon tears or tendinopathy of the gluteus medius and gluteus minimus muscle-tendon complex than inflammation of the trochanteric bursa. Rarely is there an actual bursitis present, so the diagnosis "trochanteric bursitis" should no longer be used regularly unless there is documented bursitis on an imaging study. This is important because the patient is more likely to benefit long-term from physical therapy (PT) as opposed to nonsteroidal antiinflammatory drugs (NSAIDs), or steroid injections, attributable to the underlying pathology being more likely tendon related than bursa related. Without an imaging study, the better term for lateral hip pain at this time is greater trochanteric pain syndrome (GTPS).

Many upper extremity tendons, such as those of the wrist, are adapted to gliding through synovial sheaths. The most commonly affected tendons in the upper extremity are the rotator cuff, specifically the supraspinatus tendon, and the common extensor tendon (more precisely the extensor carpi radialis brevis) involved in lateral epicondylopathy, commonly known as *tennis elbow*. Despite names like tennis elbow and golfer's elbow, upper extremity tendinopathies (see Table 2) are more likely the result of repetitive motion from work or hobby related activities. When sports are a cause of upper extremity tendinopathy, they are typically sports

TABLE 1	Tendinopathy Progression	
	TENDONITIS	**TENDINOSIS**
Pathology	Inflammatory	Degenerative
Timing	Days to weeks	Weeks to years
Imaging	Typically unnecessary	Radiographs initially Ultrasound or magnetic resonance imaging for persistent symptoms

TABLE 2	Common Tendinopathy Sites

Upper Extremity

- Rotator cuff (especially supraspinatus)
- Medial epicondyle
- Lateral epicondyle (especially extensor carpi radialis brevis)
- First dorsal compartment of the wrist (De Quervain)

Lower Extremity

- Gluteus medius and gluteus minimus
- Iliopsoas
- Patellar
- Achilles

requiring overhead motion like baseball, volleyball, and tennis. Up to 35% to 50% of adult tennis players will develop an elbow tendinopathy during their lifetime. A common cause of tendinopathy in the wrist is De Quervain tenosynovitis. De Quervain tenosynovitis affects the first dorsal compartment of the wrist containing the abductor pollicis longus and extensor pollicis brevis tendons. As the term "tenosynovitis" suggests, this condition results in irritation and swelling of not only the tendons themselves, but also of the synovial sheath encapsulating those tendons.

Some patients will develop tendinopathies without repetitive activity. Diseases of glucose metabolism and atherosclerosis are associated with a higher incidence of tendinopathy. Some common medications are also associated with tendinopathy including statins, fluoroquinolone antibiotics, and steroids, especially when steroids are injected intratendinously, which should be avoided.

Evaluation

On physical examination the affected tendon will sometimes appear swollen, and it is typically tender to palpation. The affected tendon-muscle complex may exhibit restricted flexibility, and stretching it or activating it against resistance may reproduce the patient's pain.

When the diagnosis of a tendinopathy is in question, imaging can be helpful. Radiographs of the affected area should be considered, to look for abnormalities such as large calcifications within tendons (Figure 1, A). When the diagnosis is in question or the patient has failed a course of physical therapy, advanced imaging should be considered. This is usually accomplished by either ultrasound or MRI. Ultrasound can reveal thickening or structural changes within the tendon consistent with degeneration and other abnormalities such as calcification. As tendinopathies are commonly associated with bursitis, bursal thickening consistent with bursitis may also be seen (Figures 1, B-C, 2, and 3). Similar findings may be demonstrated on MRI (Figure 4).

Determining which imaging modality to use can be challenging. MRI is considered the gold-standard for diagnosing tendinopathies and has the advantage of demonstrating an anatomic overview of the affected area, in addition to providing soft tissue contrast. However, in trained hands, the advantages of ultrasound include ease of use, point-of-care examination, dynamic evaluation of the tendon and muscles, better resolution than MRI, and guidance for injections and procedures.

Prevention

Prevention is always the best option. Tendons do not respond well to acute changes in routine or long periods of rest. This should be kept in mind by athletes during the off-season, someone taking on a new labor job on an assembly line, or a secretary with a new work space. These "potential patients" should be eased into their new routines, because all of these scenarios are classic setups for the development of a tendinopathy. Maintaining activity during the offseason and preparing one's self for changes in the workplace will help to mitigate the risk of tendinopathy development.

Treatment

Medications are rarely employed in the treatment of tendinosis because the patient usually does not present to the clinician's office until long after the disease process has begun. If the patient is caught early enough, for example within a week or two of the offending event (eg, lateral epicondylitis a week after painting a house), then the disease process is still likely an inflammatory one, and appropriately termed a tendonitis. In this case, NSAIDs are appropriate to try to stop the inflammatory process and ultimately try to prevent it from progressing to a degenerative process. Other effective treatments for tendonitis include activity modification, rest, and ice. However, if the patient has had pain for months, the process has likely progressed to tendinosis. The use of NSAIDs has been shown to negatively affect the repair mechanism involved in tendinosis, thus they should be used cautiously in this situation.

Expectations about healing tendinosis should be addressed early. To begin with, tendon healing takes significant time and

Figure 1 A, AP of the patients shoulder demonstrating a calcific lesion near the humeral head. B, Long axis view; C, short axis view both by ultrasound of the same patient's supraspinatus tendon *(outline)* near its attachment at the humeral head. The humeral cortex shows as hyperechoic on the bottom of the tendon. The calcification is noted to be within the tendon near the attachment. Acoustic shadowing is noted underneath the calcification, which prevents viewing the entire calcific structure and the underlying humeral cortex. *Abbreviations:* CALC=calcification, SS=supraspinatus.

effort on the part of the patient. Additionally, many of the treatment modalities used to heal tendons will produce a reasonable amount of pain in and of themselves. This is actually a good thing as it indicates the patient is working hard enough to heal and that the healing process is occurring. It is not uncommon to have minor setbacks during the rehabilitation process. There should be an overall trend from a state of disease to health, but the path to recovery is not typically linear. The initial management of tendinopathy should be rehabilitation through PT. The patient should be informed that the "work" of PT is not done at the therapist's office, but it is done at home on their own. Failing to adhere to the treatment program will almost ensure a lack of recovery.

The exercises performed in PT aim to reorganize the degenerative matrix, reduce tenocyte activity, improve tendon compliance,

Figure 2 A, Long axis view; B, short axis view both by ultrasound of a patellar tendon (outline) demonstrating tendinosis as evidence by the hypoechoic heterogeneous region outline, which represents the degeneration and irregularity of tendinosis. Abbreviations: DIST=distal, HFP=Hoffa's fat pad, MED=medial, LAT=lateral, LAX=long axis, P=patella, PROX=proximal, SAX=short axis.

Figure 4 MRI appearance of tendinopathy. Sagittal T1-weighted image of the knee in a professional basketball player demonstrates abnormal signal and increased size in the patellar tendon, consistent with severe tendinopathy (arrow). The tendon is normally devoid of signal. (From Grainger RG, Allison DJ, Adam A, Dixon AK. Grainger and Allison's Diagnostic Radiology, 4th ed. Philadelphia: Churchill Livingstone; 2001.)

and provide analgesia. Specifically, eccentric exercises have proven to be an effective treatment. An eccentric exercise is one that strengthens the muscle-tendon complex while lengthening the complex. For example, if a patient is being treated for lateral epicondylosis, the eccentric exercise would be to move the wrist from extension to flexion against resistance, lengthening the common extensor tendon. Strengthening exercises also work to hypertrophy the muscle, which is commonly atrophied after long periods of abnormal use from compensatory movement by the patient to try to reduce pain. The time needed for the exercises to work well is 3 months, which correlates with the time needed to form new fibroblasts, the presumed mechanism by which eccentric exercises work.

PT exercises should be done bilaterally as there is a proven crossover effect for tendinopathies, whereby exercising the non-affected side actually improves the affected side. Adding static stretching to eccentric exercises has been shown to improve outcomes over eccentric exercises alone in patellar tendinopathy, and should be included in an effective rehabilitation program. Before releasing an athlete back to sports activity, the final components of an optimal rehabilitation program includes explosive concentric movements (e.g., weightlifting or box jumps), higher eccentric loading exercises (e.g., jumping from an elevated surface like a box and landing on the ground), and sports-specific movements like sprinting and cutting.

The other treatment modality commonly employed by a physical therapist in tendinosis is deep soft tissue massage with tools. These tools are used to scrape along the pathologic tendon, which promotes blood flow and inflammation leading to the breakdown of the degenerative tissue and ultimately healing of that tissue.

When these conservative measures fail, more aggressive treatment methods should be considered. It is important to point out that the following treatment options are supported by limited high quality evidence, but are nonetheless reasonable alternatives to a surgical procedure. Less invasive methods include extracorporeal shockwave therapy and low-intensity pulsed

Figure 3 A, long axis view; B, short axis view both by ultrasound of a supraspinatus tendon with a subacromial-subdeltoid bursitis. The tendon is hyperechoic and fibrillar, which is in contrast to the overlying hypoechoic bursa. Abbreviations: ANT=anterior, GT=greater tuberosity, HH=humeral head, LAX=long axis, POST=posterior, SAX=short axis, SUPRA T=supraspinatus tendon.

ultrasound. Glyceryl trinitrate patches are sometimes used to promote blood flow, and have been shown to provide some pain relief. Injections are common treatment modalities in tendinopathies. Steroid injections are commonly used, but usually provide short-term pain relief at best. There is evidence for long-term negative effects of steroids, so they should be used judiciously. A reasonable time to try a steroid injection is when the patient is experiencing so much pain that they are unable to perform therapy. Ultrasound guidance in the hands of a trained physician can help ensure that the injection is placed properly, and specifically not intratendinously. Other treatment options requiring a more trained physician, such as a sports medicine specialist, include prolotherapy, sclerotherapy, and biological blood product injections. Prolotherapy, the injection of hypertonic glucose, is thought to work by inducing a local inflammation-repair mechanism. In sclerotherapy, a sclerotic agent, typically polidocanol, is injected to degrade the tendinopathy pain generators, namely the abnormal vessels and sensory nerves within the tendinopathic tissue. Blood products, including whole blood and platelet-rich-plasma, are used with the intent to deliver a high concentration of growth factors to the tendinopathic tissue, where blood flow is typically low.

If the tendinopathy does not respond to these treatment options, then more invasive measures are typically considered. A tenotomy procedure uses a sharp object, typically a large bore needle, to repetitively fenestrate the degenerated portion of tendon tissue, as noted on ultrasound guidance, to cause bleeding, and stimulate tissue healing. There is a newer technique, whereby the outside of tendon is scraped with a needle or scalpel. The procedure is guided by increased color Doppler signal on ultrasound indicating high vascularity and presumed nerve formation. The recovery from these techniques is usually a minimum of 6 weeks, so they should be reserved for recalcitrant cases. Finally, an open procedure can be performed to remove macroscopically abnormal tissue through an incision in the tendon; unfortunately the recovery for this sort of a procedure is in the time frame of 4 to 12 months.

Bursitis

Background

Bursas are fluid filled sacs designed to reduce friction between various tissues including bones, skin, tendons, and muscles. Typically, there is little fluid within a bursa, but with irritation from overuse or trauma, the bursa may swell with fluid leading to pain and dysfunction. This is referred to as bursitis because of the inflammatory nature of the condition.

There are multiple locations in the body where bursitis more commonly occurs, including the shoulder, elbow, hip, and knee. Bursitis usually develops from either trauma or overuse, but systemic illnesses like rheumatoid arthritis, diabetes mellitus, gout or pseudogout, and immunosuppression may also lead to bursitis. Bursas that are more susceptible to traumatic bursitis include the prepatellar, olecranon, and trochanteric bursas; they are closer to the skin and have little subcutaneous fat over them, thus they are more likely to sustain a direct impact. Both the olecranon and prepatellar bursa are also at risk for chronic irritation and trauma. Olecranon bursitis is seen in patients who frequently rest on their elbows, as in desk workers and truck drivers. Prepatellar bursitis is seen in patients who kneel for work like carpet layers and house cleaners.

Septic bursitis is rare, and it most commonly affects the olecranon and prepatellar bursa. This occurs via direct inoculation from the traumatic event. The most common organisms isolated are *Staphylococcus aureus* followed by β-hemolytic *Streptococcus*, with about 10% being polymicrobial infections.

The other bursas in the body are more susceptible to overuse injuries. The bursas around the shoulder most commonly affected include the subacromial-subdeltoid bursa, and the scapulothoracic bursa. Athletes who perform overhead movements in sports like baseball, softball, tennis, volleyball, and swimming are at greater risk for irritating these bursas. Of course, athletes are not the only people at risk for bursitis. Manual laborers working with

their arms, especially when flexed or abducted regularly can also develop bursitis around the shoulder.

The hip and pelvis have multiple bursas, but the more commonly affected include the bursas around the greater trochanter and iliopsoas. As stated in the tendinopathy section, lateral hip pain is rarely caused by "trochanteric bursitis," but there are bursa present under the gluteus maximus, gluteus medius, and gluteus minimus muscle-tendon complexes. Bursitis in this region is rarely found without an associated problem like gluteal tendinopathy, or iliotibial (IT) band syndrome. In fact, it is likely that one of these underlying problems led to the bursitis. There is also a bursa under the iliopsoas muscle as it crosses the iliopectineal eminence and anterior hip joint.

Rare causes of knee bursitis include irritation of the suprapatellar bursa, deep infrapatellar bursa, pes anserine bursa, semimembranosus bursa, and medial collateral ligament bursa (Voshell bursa). Bursitis at these locations is almost always from chronic overuse. In the ankle, the retrocalcaneal bursa may also be irritated from overuse.

Evaluation

Evaluation of a patient with suspected bursitis should always begin with a thorough history. Usually the clinician will discover a history of either trauma or overuse, but the patient should also be questioned about the presence of systemic illness. Physical exam of the affected region should include inspection for erythema and swelling. Warmth may be noted on palpation. Range of motion may be limited, but is not a consistent finding. Strength is rarely affected. The appearance of decreased strength may only reflect pain, not true weakness. True weakness would suggest an associated concern like tendinopathy or a tendon tear.

Patients with the presenting symptom of shoulder pain should be evaluated for rotator cuff tendinopathy and scapulothoracic dysfunction and winging, which predispose the athlete to impingement and bursitis. For patients complaining of hip pain, another symptom they may complain of is snapping. The patient should be questioned if the snap is reliably reproducible. If so, then have the patient demonstrate the snap. Snapping laterally is typically the gluteus maximus muscle or the iliotibial band snapping over the greater trochanter, and this is a risk factor for bursitis. If the snapping is anterior in the hip, it is likely the iliopsoas tendon snapping over the iliopectineal eminence or anterior femoral head, which can lead to iliopsoas bursitis.

For the olecranon and prepatellar bursas, special attention must be given to the fact that they are more likely to develop into a septic bursitis from a bacterial infection. If there is evidence of an abrasion in these particular areas, the physician needs to ensure there is not an associated infection. Erythema, progressive swelling, and painful range of motion may point towards the presence of an infection, but these symptoms are often present in aseptic bursitis as well, making the diagnosis difficult. Fever may be present, but its absence does not rule out infection. If there is any concern for infection, the bursa needs to be aspirated and fluid sent for cell count and differential, crystal analysis, gram stain, and culture before starting antibiotics. Blood should also be sent for a complete blood count, C-reactive protein, erythrocyte sedimentation rate, and cultures.

Imaging is not always necessary to diagnose bursitis. Swelling and erythema over a known bursa may be enough to make a diagnosis, but if the diagnosis is in question, then imaging typically begins with radiographs. Radiographs can evaluate for bony abnormalities that may suggest an underlying reason for bursitis. For example, spurring on the undersurface of the acromion can be a risk factor for subacromial-subdeltoid bursitis. Radiographs can also be used to rule out fracture or to evaluate for a foreign body, especially in the setting of olecranon or prepatellar bursitis.

Further evaluation is typically done with either MRI or ultrasound. MRI offers the advantage of global assessment of the affected region, in addition to allowing enhancement of soft tissues. In skilled hands, ultrasound is an effective tool to demonstrate bursitis throughout the body (see Figure 3). Ultrasound also has the distinct advantage of real-time imaging during a dynamic examination of the affected tissue. If aspiration or injection is needed, ultrasound can help guide the procedure. Both MRI and ultrasound modalities are useful in assessing for associated diagnoses like tendinopathy.

Treatment

Bursitis treatment usually begins with conservative measures like rest or activity modification, NSAIDs, compression, padded splinting, and ice. If the bursitis is acute, it is typically responsive to these basic treatments. As stated previously in this chapter, it is common to find associated problems with the bursitis. These include rotator cuff tendinopathy, gluteal tendinopathy, and iliotibial band syndrome. It is imperative that these issues be treated as well or the bursitis will likely reoccur. This typically requires a home exercise plan usually best directed by a physical therapist.

If these problems fail to respond to this conservative approach, including rehabilitation, then a steroid injection can be considered. There is reasonable evidence that doing the injection under ultrasound guidance will lead to better outcomes, especially for the subacromial-subdeltoid bursa, but blind injections are certainly reasonable if ultrasound is not available. Research reveals that steroid injections for greater trochanteric pain syndrome demonstrate clinically relevant relief at 3 months postinjection when compared with usual care, but that difference disappears by 12 months. This is a common finding with steroid injections. Thus, it is reasonable to consider a steroid injection for pain relief, especially if the patient is unable to participate in PT, but it is unlikely to "fix" the patient's problem long-term.

For olecranon and prepatellar bursitis, the clinician must first differentiate between septic and aseptic bursitis. If the bursa is infected, following aspiration and lab collection, antibiotics must be initiated. The decision about whether to use oral versus parenteral antibiotics and whether admission is warranted depends upon the severity of the infection and the reliability of the patient. Oral therapy should be used cautiously, as treatment failure has been seen in up to 39% to 50% of patients. The duration of antibiotic treatment is usually 10 to 14 days. Surgical intervention is rarely necessary, but should be considered in patients who fail to respond to incision and drainage and appropriate antibiotics, if there is suspicion of a foreign body, or there is an inability to adequately drain the bursa.

With aseptic bursitis of the prepatellar and olecranon bursas, the clinician should resist the urge to aspirate and inject with steroids. Aspiration and injection is a possible treatment option, but should only follow a failed conservative approach. The reason for this is that once drained, the bursa is likely to fill with fluid again quickly, and there is a risk for an iatrogenic infection. Steroids are also known to cause skin atrophy. A 6- to 8-week trial of the conservative approach is reasonable.

References

Ackermann PW, Renstrom P: Tendinopathy in sport, *Sports Health* 4:193–201, 2012.
Chang A, Miller TT: Imaging of tendons, *Sports Health* 1:293–300, 2009.
Long SS, Surrey DE, Nazarian LN: Sonography of greater trochanteric pain syndrome and the rarity of primary bursitis, *Am J Roentgenol* 201:1083–1086, 2013.
Reilly D, Kamineni S: Olecranon bursitis, *J Shoulder Elbow Surg* 25:158–167, 2016.
Scott A, Docking S, Vicenzino B, et al: Sports and exercise-related tendinopathies: a review of selected topical issues by participants of the second International Scientific Tendinopathy Symposium (ISTS) Vancouver 2012, *Br J Sports Med* 47:536–544, 2013.
Seroyer ST, Nho SJ, Bach BR, et al: Shoulder pain in the overhead throwing athlete, *Sports Health* 1:108–120, 2009.
Williams BS, Cohen SP: Greater trochanteric pain syndrome: a review of anatomy, diagnosis and treatment, *Anesth Analg* 108:1662–1670, 2009.
Wu T, Song HX, Dong Y, Li JH: Ultrasound-guided versus blind subacromial-subdeltoid bursa injection in adults with shoulder pain: A systematic review and meta-analysis, *Semin Arthritis Rheum* 45:374–378, 2015.

COMMON SPORTS INJURIES

Method of
Andrew S.T. Porter, DO

CURRENT DIAGNOSIS

- **Lateral Ankle Sprain**—Pain over lateral ankle ligament(s) with localized swelling. Often associated with laxity and pain with anterior drawer and/or talar tilt test. Obtain x-rays based on the Ottawa ankle and foot rules.
- **Medial Ankle Sprain**—Less common than lateral ankle sprain. Pain in the deltoid ligament with localized swelling. Obtain x-rays based on Ottawa ankle and foot rules.
- **High Ankle Sprain**—Syndesmotic injury. Pain with squeeze test and/or dorsiflexion with external rotation.
- **Osteochondral Ankle Injuries**—Most commonly seen in the talar dome. Associated with an ankle inversion injury and ankle pain. Often have a joint effusion and soft tissue swelling and can have mechanical symptoms (catching, locking, crepitus, and a feeling of giving way). Obtain x-rays initially and then magnetic resonance imaging (MRI) to grade degree of injury.
- **Anterior Cruciate Ligament (ACL) Injuries**—Most common after noncontact injuries. Physical examination reveals a diffuse knee effusion, positive Lachman, and/or anterior drawer test. Obtain x-rays then MRI for further evaluation.
- **Posterior Cruciate Ligament (PCL) Injuries**—Occur with varus/valgus stress with the knee in full extension. Physical examination reveals a positive posterior drawer and sag sign. Obtain x-rays then MRI for further evaluation.
- **Medial Collateral Ligament (MCL) Injuries**—Occur with valgus stress or twisting with or without contact. Physical examination reveals localized effusion and a positive valgus stress testing and tenderness to palpation along the MCL. Graded 1 to 3.
- **Osteochondral Knee Injuries**—Most commonly seen in the femoral condyle. Associated with a knee injury. Knee pain and, often, mechanical symptoms of the knee. Palpation of the femoral condyles with the knee in flexion reproduces pain. Obtain x-rays initially and then MRI to grade degree of injury.
- **Mallet Finger**—Disruption of the extensor mechanism insertion into the distal phalanx.
- **Jersey Finger**—Occurs after avulsion of the flexor digitorum profundus tendon from its insertion on the distal phalanx.
- **Proximal Interphalangeal (PIP) Joint Dorsal Dislocation**—Injury to the volar plate with or without an avulsion fracture.
- **Scaphoid Fracture**—Pain over the scaphoid with or without a fall on an outstretched hand injury is a scaphoid fracture until proven otherwise. Obtain wrist x-rays with a scaphoid view.
- **Tendinosis**—Repetitive chronic tendon injuries result in scarring, disorganization of fibers, degeneration, and are without an inflammatory component.
- **Stress Fractures**—Most often seen in active patients as a result of excessive stress on normal bone from overactivity or normal stress on a bone that is deficient (osteoporotic, poor nutrition, or in female athlete triad). History is positive for bone pain, and physical examination reveals tenderness to palpation in the affected bone and often a positive tuning fork test, hop test, and fulcrum test. Obtain x-rays first, then MRI or bone scan if needed.
- **Spondylolysis/Spondylolisthesis**—Most often seen in young athletes with insidious onset low back pain and history of repetitive extension. Positive stork test. X-rays initially, and if negative, may proceed with limited CT and SPECT scan or MRI.

CURRENT THERAPY

- Lateral Ankle Sprain—Treat with RICE (rest, ice, compression, elevation) and early rehab. Return to play (RTP) is generally 1 to 4 weeks and is based on functional progression. RTP with ankle brace.
- Medial Ankle Sprain—Treat with RICE and early rehab. RTP with ankle brace.
- High Ankle Sprain—Treat with RICE and boot for 1 to 3 weeks and then rehab. RTP takes a longer time compared with lateral ankle sprain.
- Osteochondral Ankle Injuries—Degree of injury is graded via MRI, and this guides treatment and RTP.
- ACL Injuries—ACL tears often need reconstruction that is individualized in active patients who require knee stability.
- PCL Injuries—Isolated PCL injuries often heal conservatively with protected weight bearing in an extension brace and knee rehab.
- MCL Injuries—Often heal conservatively with bilateral hinged knee brace and knee rehab. Generally, RTP in 2 to 6 weeks.
- Osteochondral Knee Injuries—Degree of injury is graded via MRI, and this guides treatment and RTP.
- Mallet Finger—Treat with continuous full-extension stack splinting of the distal interphalangeal joint for 6 weeks and then nighttime splinting and activity splinting for 6 weeks.
- Jersey Finger—Treatment is referral to orthopedic surgeon for surgical intervention.
- PIP joint dorsal dislocation—Reduce dislocation and obtain x-rays. Treat with progressive extension blocking splint with 30° to 40° of flexion and decrease by 10° per week.
- Scaphoid Fracture—If x-rays with scaphoid view are negative, place in a short-arm thumb spica cast and follow up in 2 weeks. If x-rays remain negative but pain persists, obtain a CT or MRI. Treat nondisplaced scaphoid fractures with short-arm thumb spica cast: proximal-third fractures 12 to 20 weeks, middle-third fractures 10 to 12 weeks, and distal-third fractures 4 to 6 weeks.
- Tendinosis—Treat by creating inflammation to facilitate healing.
- Stress Fractures—Treat with general treatment for stress fractures plus specific treatment based on stress fracture site.
- Spondylolysis/Spondylolisthesis—Treat with extension blocking brace, rest, rehabilitation with core strengthening and lower extremity flexibility, and gradual RTP.

Ankle Injuries

The ankle is the most common joint injured in athletes. Ankle sprains are common, as they represent 25% of all sports-related injuries. The Ottawa ankle and foot rules help in the decision to obtain x-rays (Box 1). In general, treatment will consist of RICE (rest, ice, compression, elevation), early mobilization, and rehab. Prevention of ankle injuries is important and consists of ankle braces, ankle taping, neuromuscular training program, and regular sport-specific warm-up exercises.

Lateral Ankle Sprain

The most common ankle sprain is a lateral inversion sprain that results from landing on an inverted foot with or without plantarflexion. The lateral ankle ligaments are the anterior talofibular ligament (ATFL), calcaneofibular ligament, and the posterior talofibular ligament. The ATFL is the most commonly sprained ligament. Lateral ankle sprains are most commonly treated with RICE initially, then early ambulation, range of motion, progression into strengthening, and then proprioception rehabilitation. Proprioception rehabilitation includes balancing on one leg and performing balancing exercises on a wobble board. For example, patients can balance on one leg when brushing their teeth.

| BOX 1 | Ottawa Ankle and Foot Rules |

- An ankle x-ray series is indicated if there is pain in the malleolar zone and any of these findings are made:
  - Tenderness over the lateral malleolus
  - Tenderness over the medial malleolus
  - Inability to bear weight four steps immediately after the injury or in the emergency department or physician's office
- A foot x-ray series is indicated if there is pain in the midfoot zone and any of these findings are made:
  - Tenderness over the base of fifth metatarsal
  - Tenderness over the navicular bone
  - Inability to bear weight four steps immediately after the injury and in the emergency department or physician's office

---

*X-rays are indicated if any of these criteria are met.
Data from Bachmann and colleagues (2003) and Tiemstra (2012).

Athletes should return to play (RTP) with a lace-up/velcro ankle brace after injury with or without taping. This added stability will help prevent future ankle injuries and also decrease the severity of ankle injuries. Most athletes will RTP in a few days to 4 weeks; this return is based on pain, obtaining full active range of motion and full strength, and functional stability.

Medial Ankle Sprain

Medial ankle ligament sprains are rare, account for < 10% of ankle injuries, and are often accompanied with a lateral malleolar fracture or syndesmotic injury. The medial ankle ligament is the deltoid ligament and is injured via external rotation or eversion. These ankle sprains are treated similarly to lateral ankle sprains.

High Ankle Sprain

High ankle sprains, also known as syndesmotic ankle sprains, occur through forced external rotation of a dorsiflexed foot most commonly but also occur by forced internal rotation of a fixed plantar flexed foot. The syndesmotic ligaments connect and stabilize the distal tibia to the distal fibula. The syndesmotic ligaments are the anterior tibiofibular ligament, posterior tibiofibular ligament, transverse tibiofibular ligament, interosseous ligament, and the interosseous membrane. Palpate the fibular head for pain. Pain on palpation of the fibular head might indicate a maisonneuve fracture, a fracture of the proximal third of the fibula associated with syndesmotic disruption. A high ankle sprain has a longer healing time compared to a lateral ankle sprain. Often these need immobilization with a boot or cast for 1 to 4 weeks to help with healing before beginning rehab. RTP after a high ankle sprain depends on pain, achieving a full active range of motion, full strength, and functional stability. Incomplete healing of a high ankle sprain can result in distal tibia and fibula instability.

Osteochondral Ankle Injuries

Osteochondral injuries are injuries to the articular surface of a joint. These injuries range from small undisplaced depressions and cracks in the osteochondral surface to small pieces of articular cartilage and bone that break off of the articular surface and float within the joint. Osteochondral injuries occur most commonly on weight-bearing articular surfaces. In osteochondral injuries, osteonecrosis of subchondral bone occurs, resulting in separation of cartilage and subchondral bone from underlying, well-vascularized bone. The term *osteochondral lesion* (OCL) is favored over the previously used term *osteochondritis dessicans* because there might not be an inflammatory component of the injury. OCLs are often associated with repeated trauma or overuse in athletes. OCLs typically present with pain in the affected joint and can develop with a specific injury or over several months in highly active athletes. OCLs are more

Figure 1 X-rays of the left ankle, AP and mortise views, which demonstrate a grade 2 osteochondral lesion (OCL) along the medial talar dome.

Figure 3 CT scan without contrast. Sagittal image of ankle, which demonstrates a grade 4 OCL of the talar dome.

Figure 2 X-ray of the left ankle, mortise view, which demonstrates a grade 4 OCL along the lateral talar dome.

common in younger patients with open physes (growth plates) and are referred to as juvenile OCLs. Adult OCLs describe this condition in skeletally mature patients.

Osteochondral injuries are a cause for pain in up to 25% of ankle injuries and need to be considered when a patient presents with ankle pain. Acute osteochondral injuries in the ankle most commonly affect the talar dome (Figures 1–3) but can also be found in the distal tibia (Figure 4). OCLs are first evaluated by x-rays (see Figures 1 and 2) and then graded by magnetic resonance imaging (MRI) (Table 1). CT scan (see Figure 3) is sometimes utilized as well. Grade 1 to 3 juvenile OCLs and grade 1 to 2 adult OCLs are treated conservatively. Conservative treatment consists of no weight bearing (NWB) in a cast or boot for 6 to 10 weeks followed by partial weight bearing (PWB) to full weight bearing (FWB) over 2 to 6 weeks, followed with an ankle brace for 3 months, and ensuring adequate calcium and vitamin D intake to facilitate healing. Nonsteroidal antiinflammatory drugs (NSAIDs) should be avoided because they can slow bone healing, and OCLs are probably not an inflammatory process. For grade 4 juvenile OCLs, grade 3 and 4 adult OCLs, and those that have not clinically healed with conservative care operative treatment is required. Operative treatment options depend on OCL size and type and include removal of the OCL followed by transchondral drilling and microfracture to stimulate fibrocartilage

Figure 4 CT scan without contrast. Coronal image of ankle, which demonstrates a grade 1 OCL of the distal lateral tibia.

TABLE 1	Classification of Osteochondral Lesions	
STAGE	PLAIN X-RAY FINDINGS	MRI FINDINGS
1	Depressed osteochondral fragment	Articular cartilage thickening and low signal changes in subchondral bone
2	Osteochondral fragment attached by bone	Articular cartilage breached, no synovial fluid around fragment
3	Detached nondisplaced fragment	Articular cartilage breached, synovial fluid around fragment
4	Displaced fragment	Loose foreign body

formation, fixation of the OCL with an osteochondral allograft, osteochondral autograft transfer, and autologous chondrocyte implantation.

Knee injuries—The knee joint lacks intrinsic bone stability, so most stability is from the major knee ligaments.

Anterior Cruciate Ligament Injuries

The anterior cruciate ligament (ACL) is the key stabilizer of the knee and is one of two major intraarticular knee ligaments, the other being the posterior cruciate ligament (PCL). Most ACL tears occur from noncontact injuries. Women experience ACL tears up to nine times more often than men do. The main function of the ACL is to prevent excessive anterior tibial translation relative to the femur. Patients who sustain an injury to their ACL often describe hearing a pop, feeling instability in their knee, experiencing pain immediately after the injury, and develop an associated knee effusion. On-the-field evaluation is ideal in an ACL injury, as the hamstrings will often start to tighten up shortly after the injury, preventing anterior tibial translation. This will prevent an isolated test of the ACL and give the false impression that an ACL endpoint is present when in fact the ACL is completely torn. The anterior drawer (Figure 5) and Lachman test (Figure 6) are the main physical examination tests to evaluate the ACL. Obtain x-rays and then MRI if an ACL tear is suspected. The blood supply to the ACL is poor and is provided by the middle geniculate artery off of the popliteal artery. Because of the poor blood supply, ACL tears often need reconstruction if

Figure 5 Anterior drawer test for ACL laxity. Patient's knee is flexed 90°. Examiner applies anterior force to the tibia in relation to the patient's femur to evaluate for laxity.

Figure 6 Lachman test for ACL laxity. Patient's knee is flexed 20°–30°. Examiner grasps the distal femur and proximal tibia and applies anterior force to the tibia and posterior force to the femur to evaluate for ACL laxity.

athletes want to return to a high level of activity and knee stability is needed. ACL reconstruction timing is important and often will occur 3 to 4 weeks after injury to allow for swelling to decrease, ROM and strength to improve, and inflammation to decrease. Also during this presurgical time, it is important to have patients perform pre-hab (presurgical rehabilitation), focusing on AROM and knee strengthening. A knee effusion will cause the quadriceps muscles to weaken and atrophy. Hamstring tendon autograft, patella tendon autograft, quadriceps tendon autograft, and allograft are all used for ACL reconstruction. Each graft has advantages and disadvantages and should be discussed with the orthopaedic surgeon before reconstruction and individualized for each patient. Continuing to participate in high-level activity after an ACL tear if undiagnosed can lead to a knee dislocation and further intraarticular knee injury.

PCL Injuries

The PCL is the other major intraarticular knee ligament. Isolated PCL injuries are much less common than ACL injuries and make up only 3.5% of ligamentous knee injuries in sports, with the remaining 96.5% of PCL injuries associated with multiligamentous knee injuries. PCL injuries, unlike ACL injuries, are the result of external forces (e.g., a soccer player sliding into the goal post and tearing his or her PCL). The main function of the PCL is to resist posterior tibial translation. Posterior drawer testing (Figure 7) and a sag sign test (Figure 8) are the physical examination tests used to evaluate the PCL. Obtain x-rays then MRI if a PCL tear is suspected. The blood supply to the PCL is better than the blood supply to the ACL. Isolated PCL injuries (grades 1 and 2) are treated conservatively because surgical reconstruction has not been shown to be helpful. Conservative treatment consists of protected weight bearing in an extension brace followed by quadriceps rehabilitation and ROM exercises. RTP is generally 4 to 6 weeks after a PCL injury. Surgical intervention is recommended for associated injuries to the ACL, medial collateral ligament (MCL), and posterior lateral corner (grade 3 PCL injury).

Figure 7 Posterior drawer test for PCL laxity. Patient's knee is flexed 90°. Examiner applies posterior force to the tibia in relation to the patient's femur to evaluate for laxity.

Figure 8 Sag sign test for PCL laxity. Examiner views the tibia condyles from the lateral side to evaluate for a posterior sag (displacement) in the appearance that would indicate a PCL injury.

Figure 9 X-ray of the bilateral knees, AP view, which demonstrates a grade 1 OCL along the right knee medial femoral condyle.

Figure 10 Magnetic resonance imaging (MRI) of the right knee, without contrast. Coronal T2 fat saturation image, which demonstrates a grade 4 OCL of the medial femoral condyle.

MCL Injuries

The MCL is an extraarticular ligament that resists knee valgus forces. An MCL sprain results from a valgus stress to a partially flexed knee. Athletes will present with localized pain and swelling along the medial aspect of the knee. Most MCL injuries are isolated ligament injuries, but more severe MCL injuries can involve tears of the medial meniscus and ACL, commonly referred to as the "terrible triad." The MCL is examined by palpation and valgus stress testing at 0° and 30° of knee flexion. MCL injuries are graded 1, 2, or 3 depending on severity of injury. A patient with a grade 1 MCL sprain has pain in the MCL but no valgus stress testing laxity. A grade 2 MCL sprain has valgus stress testing laxity but a solid endpoint. A grade 3 MCL sprain has no endpoint with valgus stress testing. Thankfully, the MCL has a rich vascular supply and can often heal conservatively. Treatment consists of RICE for the first 1 to 2 weeks and a bilateral hinged knee brace to facilitate healing. Weight bearing and ROM and strengthening exercises are started when they are tolerable. RTP after an MCL injury depends on the grade and generally takes 2 to 6 weeks.

Osteochondral Knee Injuries

Osteochondral injuries occur in the knee as well as in the ankle. Osteochondral injuries of the knee most commonly affect the lateral aspect of the medial femoral condyle but can be found anywhere along the medial or lateral femoral condyle, patella, or trochlea. History is significant for knee pain, with or without swelling and mechanical symptoms (catching, locking, crepitus, and feeling of giving way). On palpation, patients can have pain in the affected area with knee flexion with or without crepitus. Obtain x-rays initially (Figure 9) and then grade the OCL severity by MRI (Figure 10). CT scans are also utilized sometimes. Grade 1 to 3 juvenile knee OCLs and grade 1 to 2 adult knee OCLs are

Figure 11 X-ray of the left hand, lateral view, which demonstrates a mallet finger of the fifth finger. Note the flexion of the DIP joint and avulsion fracture of the distal phalanx that involves about 30% of the joint space.

Figure 12 Stack splint with Coban wrap added for stability that immobilizes the DIP joint at neutral to 5° of hyperextension.

Figure 13 X-ray of the left hand, oblique view, which demonstrates a proximal interphalangeal (PIP) joint dorsal and lateral dislocation.

treated conservatively. Grade 4 juvenile OCLs, grade 3 to 4 adult OCLs and all OCLs that have failed conservative care are treated operatively.

Hand Injuries
Mallet Finger
A mallet finger occurs after forced flexion of an actively extended distal interphalangeal (DIP) joint, resulting in disruption of the extensor mechanism insertion into the distal phalanx. Patients with a mallet finger are unable to actively extend the DIP joint. This injury can be associated with an avulsion fracture (Figure 11). For acute injuries, general treatment consists of continuous extension splinting of the DIP joint (0° to 10° of hyperextension) for at least 6 weeks. The 6-week clock starts over if the DIP joint is allowed to flex at all during the initial 6 weeks of treatment or if, at the end of the 6 weeks, the mallet finger is not completely healed. After the initial 6 weeks, it is recommended to continue with nighttime splinting and activity splinting for another 6 weeks to ensure adequate healing and avoidance of surgery. To perform this splinting, a stack splint is well tolerated and is protective (Figure 12). Orthopaedic referral is indicated if the patient is unable to obtain full passive extension of the DIP joint or if the avulsion fracture involves over 30% of the joint space.

Jersey Finger
A jersey finger results from the avulsion of the flexor digitorum profundus tendon from its insertion on the distal phalanx. This commonly occurs in football and rugby players when the tip of their flexed finger is caught in a jersey and the DIP joint of the finger is then forcefully extended. After this injury occurs, the patient is unable to actively flex the DIP joint. Treatment is urgent referral to an orthopaedic surgeon for surgical intervention.

Proximal Interphalangeal Joint Dorsal Dislocation
Proximal interphalangeal (PIP) joint injuries are the most common joint injuries in sports. Most PIP dislocations are dorsal and

result from hyperextension with an axial load. Dislocations are described by the position of the distal fragment in relation to the proximal fragment. PIP dorsal dislocations cause injury to the volar plate with or without avulsion fracture. Pre-reduction x-rays are preferred if they can be obtained promptly (Figure 13). X-rays of the finger with at least one view being a true lateral view should be obtained to rule out fracture. However, many PIP dorsal dislocations occur on the playing field and it is reasonable to reduce these dislocations, buddy tape the affected finger, and allow the patient to RTP with x-rays obtained after the athletic competition. Reduction is usually uncomplicated and is performed urgently via hyperextending the joint, applying traction in plane with the finger, then flexing the joint. Post reduction films are a necessity (Figure 14). Stability testing of the collateral ligaments should be performed after the reduction. Full flexion and extension of the PIP joint will be possible if the joint is stable. A stable joint without a large avulsion fragment should be treated with a progressive extension blocking splint (Figures 15 and 16). Start with 30° to 40° of flexion and decrease by 10° per week over 3 to 4 weeks, then buddy tape the injured finger with activity PRN (8). Some PIP dorsal dislocations have a lateral component to them and these are treated similar to pure dorsal dislocations (see Figure 13). Orthopaedic surgeon referral is indicated if there is a large avulsion fracture or the joint is unstable.

Scaphoid Fracture
The scaphoid bone is the most common carpal bone that is fractured and is a common injury that is encountered in primary care. Interestingly, scaphoid fractures occur most commonly in young men. Scaphoid fractures occur less commonly in young children and the elderly because of the relative weakness of the distal radius compared with the scaphoid in these age groups. Often a scaphoid fracture is caused by a FOOSH (fall on an outstretched hand) injury. On physical examination, if the patient has pain over the scaphoid tubercle or in the anatomical snuffbox with or without a history of a FOOSH injury, the clinician needs to have a high index of suspicion for a scaphoid fracture when evaluating the wrist

Figure 14 X-ray of the left hand, lateral status postreduction view, which demonstrates a relocated proximal interphalangeal (PIP) joint. Note the avulsion fracture of the middle phalanx.

Figure 15 Dorsal extension blocking splint at 30°–40° of flexion at the PIP joint. Note that there is no pressure over the PIP joint volar plate and that flexion and extension at the DIP joint is possible.

x-rays. Obtain the standard wrist x-rays (AP, lateral, and oblique views) plus a dedicated scaphoid view (AP with ulnar deviation) and be aware that early imaging with x-rays is often unrevealing for a scaphoid fracture (Figure 17). If a fracture is not seen on x-rays, the clinician needs to have a high index of suspicion for a scaphoid fracture, place the patient in a short-arm thumb spica cast, and have the patient follow up in 2 weeks. If repeat x-rays remain negative and the patient continues to have scaphoid pain, proceed with an MRI of the wrist with T2 fat saturation views or a CT scan. If a scaphoid fracture is noted on imaging, the location

Figure 16 Dorsal extension blocking splint at 30°–40° of flexion at the PIP joint. This figure illustrates the freedom of motion that is possible at the PIP joint (full flexion and limited extension) and the DIP joint (full flexion and extension).

of the scaphoid fracture will guide treatment. Because the blood supply to the scaphoid is distal to proximal, scaphoid fractures are harder to heal than other carpal fractures. Nondisplaced middle-third or proximal-third scaphoid fractures are treated with a long- or short-arm thumb spica cast with the wrist at 20° to 30° of extension and the thumb in slight extension and abduction for 10 to 20 weeks. Middle-third fractures should be immobilized for 10 to 12 weeks. Proximal-third fractures should be immobilized from 12 to 20 weeks. It is much easier to regain flexion in the wrist after casting than it is to regain extension. If the elbow is incorporated in the cast, it should be casted at 90° of flexion. A long-arm cast may decrease healing time, but it does not improve nonunion rates. A nondisplaced distal-third fracture should be treated in a short-arm thumb spica cast for 4 to 6 weeks. For displaced fractures or non-healing fractures, a referral to an orthopedic surgeon is recommended. Use acetaminophen for pain control and avoid nonsteroidal antiinflammatory drugs (NSAIDs) because NSAIDs can impair bone healing. Ensure adequate energy availability via diet and adequate calcium and vitamin D intake, and avoid tobacco exposure to help heal the fracture. Bone health and bone nutrition are a part of the big picture in fracture healing.

Overuse Injuries

Tendinosis

The paradigm and management of tendon overuse injuries is changing. The term *tendinitis* is generally used to refer to painful overuse tendon conditions and implies that inflammation is present. However, the most common pathology in chronic painful tendons is tendinosis. Tendinosis occurs after repetitive injuries to a tendon results in intertendinous scarring, disorganization of tendon fibers, and degeneration. Tendinosis does not have an inflammatory component. Early on in a tendon injury, there is inflammation resulting in tendinitis, but after about 6 weeks this generally evolves into tendinosis. Early activity modification and treatment of tendinitis with NSAIDs and rehabilitation may prevent the development of tendinosis. Tendinosis is a problematic condition that affects many active people, young and old. To address these more chronic tendon injuries, healing is facilitated by creating an inflammatory response. To create inflammation, treatments such as eccentric strengthening (Figure 18), deep soft tissue massage with tools (e.g., gua sha or Graston, or ASTYM) (Figure 19), nitroglycerin patches (Nitro-Dur),[1] and musculoskeletal ultrasound-guided percutaneous needle tenotomy (with or without injection of autologous blood, prolotherapy, or platelet-rich plasma) have all been utilized and have been shown to be effective (Table 2). It is important to avoid NSAIDs when trying to create inflammation because NSAIDs will prevent the

---

[1] Not FDA approved for this indication.

inflammatory response. This concept of tendinosis diagnosis and treatment can be utilized for tendons throughout the body and is most commonly applied to the Achilles tendon, patella tendon, iliotibial (IT) band, piriformis, gluteus medius, hamstrings, biceps, common elbow flexor tendon, and common elbow extensor tendon.

Stress Fractures

Stress fractures occur when osteoclastic activity overwhelms osteoblastic activity. Bone injury unfolds over a continuum of time, starting with normal bone that progresses to stress reaction, then stress fracture, and finally fracture if the bone continues to be injured. This can occur as a result of excessive stress on normal bone from overactivity or normal stress on a bone that is deficient (osteoporotic, poor nutrition, or in female athlete triad).

Figure 17 Scaphoid view x-ray (AP view with ulnar deviation) is important to obtain in addition to your standard wrist views (AP, lateral, and oblique) when scaphoid fracture is suspected. This scaphoid fracture was not seen on the x-rays on the day of the injury. Patient continued to have wrist pain and then presented 10 weeks later, and x-rays were obtained demonstrating the scaphoid fracture.

Stress fractures are common injuries in athletes and occur most often in the lower extremities. Running sports account for 69% of stress fractures. Stress fractures should be considered in someone who is active, presents with bone pain, and who performs repetitive activities with limited rest or with a recent increase in activity. Physical examination tests to perform in the area of interest are palpation, the tuning fork test, the fulcrum test, and the hop test (Table 3). If a stress fracture is suspected, x-rays should be obtained, keeping in mind that it takes 2 to 3 weeks for signs of stress fracture (i.e., periosteal reaction, callus formation, fracture line) to show up on an x-ray, and often stress fractures do not show up on x-rays. If x-rays are negative and a diagnosis is needed to help guide care and RTP, a bone scan or MRI with T2 fat saturation views (Figures 20 and 21) should be obtained. The bone scan and MRI are equally sensitive, but an MRI is more specific and avoids patient radiation exposure. An MRI is more expensive. Because a bone scan can stay positive for up to 18 months, clinical progress should not be monitored with a bone scan.

To prevent stress fractures, athletes should distribute loading forces on the bone with cross training and biomechanical adjustments (i.e., orthotics, proper shoes, stretches, strengthening, running mechanics), consume sufficient calories to maintain adequate energy availability, and ensure appropriate intake of calcium and vitamin D. A study by Lappe of female Navy recruits showed reductions in stress fractures in those consuming 2000 mg of calcium[1] and 800 IU vitamin D[1] daily, either as a supplement or through consumption of dairy products. Tobacco should be avoided. Additionally, women of child bearing age should try to maintain regular menses by consuming adequate calories and avoiding a negative energy balance.

General treatment for stress fractures can be grouped into nutrition, medication, and biomechanical recommendations. Nutrition recommendations include optimizing energy availability in the diet, ensuring adequate calcium and vitamin D intake, and avoidance of tobacco exposure. Medication recommendations include using acetaminophen as needed for pain control and avoidance of NSAIDs. Biomechanical recommendations are to offload the affected bone and reduce activity to pain-free functioning and pain-free cross-training. Crutches may be needed to offload the injured area even more than a walking boot/cast or steal shank. The patient may require complete non-weight bearing (NWB) with the overall goal being to obtain pain-free ambulation during the initial treatment. Tables 4 and 5 outline recommended guidelines for protected weight bearing for specific stress fracture sites. Additional recommendations are to begin a rehabilitation program when tolerated and to stretch and strengthen supporting

---

[1] Not FDA approved for this indication.

Figure 18 Eccentric exercises for Achilles tendinosis. (**A**) Patient begins with the injured leg straight and the ankle in flexion. The assistance of the uninjured leg was utilized to get in this starting position. (**B**) The ankle of the injured leg (right leg, in this case) is slowly lowered in a controlled fashion to full dorsiflexion to eccentrically strengthen (while lengthening the calf muscles) the right Achilles tendon. The left leg is then brought back down, and full plantarflexion in both ankles is performed, recruiting the uninjured leg to assist with getting back to position (**A**). (**C**) The eccentric exercise from (**B**) is repeated with the knee bent at 45°.

Figure 24 SPECT scan lumbar spine, PA view, w[...] acute bilateral L3 and L4 spondylolysis.

Figure 25 CT scan without contrast. Axial image[...] pars interarticularis fractures that appear acute wi[...] rotic fracture edges.

MRI or with SPECT scan. If the SPECT sca[...] 24), then proceed with limited CT scan (I[...] If radiation exposure is a concern, or if hig[...] readily accessible, thinly sliced stacked ax[...] saturation views in all planes using a high-d[...] test of choice (Figure 27). A spectrum of r[...] ments and conservative approaches that [...] and safe RTP are reasonable. For acute sp[...] ommended treatment consists of a warm [...] blocking back brace worn all day except [...] bathing (23–24 hours per day) for the fi[...] ment in conjunction with rest from activ[...] ond month, use of the brace during the day[...] is suggested. Rehabilitation consists of

structures. Start a gradual increase in activity when the patient is pain-free.

Because of their propensity for delayed healing and nonunion, certain stress fractures are considered high risk, necessitate prompt treatment, and may ultimately require surgical fixation.

Figure 19 ASTYM® tools.

TABLE 2	Treatment of Tendinosis
TREATMENT MODALITY	**DESCRIPTION**
Deep soft tissue massage with tools (gua sha, Graston, ASTYM) (Figure 19)	One to three times per week for 4–6 wk; most common with athletic trainer certified or physical therapist
Nitroglycerin patches (Nitro-Dur)[1]	0.1 mg/h patch, apply Q24 h to a different location on tendon for at least 6 wk
Eccentric strengthening (Figure 18)	3 sets of 15 exercises, twice daily, for 12 wk
Musculoskeletal ultrasound-guided percutaneous needle tenotomy with or without autologous blood injection, prolotherapy, or platelet-rich plasma	Referral to primary care sports medicine physician

[1]Not FDA approved for this indication.

TABLE 3	Stress Fracture Physical Exam Tests
PHYSICAL EXAM TEST	**POSITIVE TEST**
Palpation	Pain over affected bone with palpation
Stork test (Figure 22)	Back extension with rotation while standing on one leg increases pain in the pars interarticularis region
Fulcrum test	Pain in fracture site while applying a bending force (e.g., over the exam table) to distal extremity while proximal extremity is kept relatively immobilized
Hop test	Hopping 10 times on affected leg reproduces pain at fracture site
Tuning fork test	Vibrating tuning fork over fracture site results in pain at site

Low-risk stress fractures have a lower incidence of delayed healing and nonunion. High-risk stress fractures that appear stable and nondisplaced can be treated nonoperatively with close follow-up. Consider referral to an orthopaedic surgeon for failed

Figure 20 MRI of the right hip without contrast. Coronal T2 fat saturation image demonstrates a compression-sided femoral neck stress fracture (note surrounding bone edema in white).

Figure 21 MRI of the right hip without contrast. Axial T2 fat saturation image that demonstrates a compression sided femoral neck stress fracture (note edema in white and probable fracture line in black that measures up to 11 mm).

TABLE 4 High-Risk Stress Fractu

HIGH-RISK STRESS FRACTURE	INITI
Femoral neck (compression side) (Figures 20 and 21)	NWB FW
Anterior tibia (tension side)	NWB FW
Medial malleolus	Pneun
Navicular	NWB RT
Base of fifth metatarsal (Jones)	NWB
May consider surgery for quicker RTP	
Sesamoids	NWB

Abbreviations: NWB = non-weight bearing; PV full weight bearing.

TABLE 5 Low-Risk Stress Fractur

LOW-RISK STRESS FRACTURE	
Sacrum/pelvis	WB
Femoral shaft	WB
Posterior medial tibia (compression side)	WB ti tr b
Fibula	WB
Metatarsal (2nd–5th)	Stee

Abbreviations: WBAT = weight bearing as toler

conservative treatment. Biomechan
with activity are used to classify ti
tures. For example, during running
different forces exerted on different
compresses posteriorly, so there is n
posterior tibia and more tension alor
tibia. The femoral neck compresses i
running, so there is more compressic
aspect of the femoral neck and more
lateral aspect of the femoral neck. T
ferent parts of the bone affect the p
and nonunion.

Spondylolysis and Spondylolisthesi

Spondylolysis is a nondisplaced stress
ticularis. Spondylolisthesis occurs whe
ysis with listhesis (slippage) of the vert
is graded 1 to 4 depending on how m
each grade, accounting for 25% (i.e.,

When a young athlete presents
dylolysis needs to be considered: th
pain up to 47% of the time. Spondy
caused by repetitive hyperextensio
increased incidence in ballet dancer
players, and football linemen. L5
for a spondylolysis. The history i
onset of deep pain in the low back
Physical examination shows a positi
often with reproduction of pain on
(Figure 22). If history and physical ex
interarticularis injury, x-rays of th

TABLE 1 American College of Rheumatology 2016 Revised Fibromyalgia

Criteria

A patient satisfies modified 2016 fibromyalgia criteria if the following three conditions are met:

(1) Widespread pain index (WPI) ≥ 7 and symptom severity scale (SSS) score ≥ 5 OR WPI of 4–6 and SSS score ≥ 9.
(2) Generalized pain, defined as pain in at least 4 of 5 regions, must be present. Jaw, chest, and abdominal pain are not included in generalized pain definition.
(3) Symptoms have been generally present for at least 3 months.

Ascertainment

(1) WPI: note the number of areas in which the patient has had pain over the last week. In how many areas has the patient had pain? Score will be between 0 and 19.
Left upper region (Region 1)
  Jaw, left
  Shoulder girdle, left
  Upper arm, left
  Lower arm, left
Right upper region (Region 2)
  Jaw, right
  Shoulder girdle, right
  Upper arm, right
  Lower arm, right
Left lower region (Region 3)
  Hip (buttock, trochanter), left
  Upper leg, left
  Lower leg, left
Right lower region (Region 4)
  Hip (buttock, trochanter), right
  Upper leg, right
  Lower leg, right
Axial region (Region 5)
  Neck
  Upper back
  Lower back
  Chest
  Abdomen
(2) SSS score
  Fatigue
  Waking unrefreshed
  Cognitive symptoms
For the each of the 3 symptoms above, indicate the level of severity over the past week using the following scale:
  0 = No problem
  1 = Slight or mild problems, generally mild or intermittent
  2 = Moderate, considerable problems, often present and/or at a moderate level
  3 = Severe: pervasive, continuous, life-disturbing problems
  The SSS score: is the sum of the severity scores of the 3 symptoms (fatigue, waking unrefreshed, and cognitive symptoms) (0–9) plus the sum (0–3) of the number of the following symptoms the patient has been bothered by that occurred during the previous 6 months:
(1) Headaches (0–1)
(2) Pain or cramps in lower abdomen (0–1)
(3) And depression (0–1)

The final symptom severity score is between 0 and 12

The fibromyalgia severity (FS) scale is the sum of the WPI and SSS

A diagnosis of fibromyalgia is valid irrespective of other diagnoses. A diagnosis of fibromyalgia does not exclude the presence of other clinically important illnesses.

considered as variables and optimally treated when attempting to diagnose this complex syndrome.

Treatment

FM is best approached by using an integrated, multidisciplinary approach where pharmacologic and nonpharmacologic treatments are provided in parallel. Engaging and motivating the patient toward their treatment goals as an active participant in their care is vital for success. As stated before, FM can be diagnosed and treated in the primary care setting. Referral to specialists should only be necessary when pain is refractory to therapy (e.g., comprehensive pain management clinic), those in whom the diagnosis is uncertain (e.g., to a rheumatologist or neurologist depending on symptoms), or those with significant comorbid mood or psychiatric disturbances. Forming treatment teams can be very useful and should include clinicians with expertise in exercise/physical activity (e.g., physical therapists), patient education, and pain psychology.

Most comprehensive guidelines on treatment of FM generally recommend that all patients should receive education on their condition, the importance of being an active participant in their care, and that setting reasonable and attainable goals and expectations for treatment. Patients need to be informed that instead of searching for treatments to cure the condition, that management of the condition should focus on pain reduction (not complete pain relief), increased physical functioning, and improved quality of life. This management should rely heavily on stress reduction, exercise and physical activity, adequate sleep, and improving function through cognitive restructuring (e.g., reducing catastrophizing, increasing self-efficacy). Pharmacologic treatments can be effective in alleviating some of the symptoms of FM, but rarely will patients achieve significant improvements without embracing these essential self-management strategies.

In the United States, there are three drugs currently approved by the US Food and Drug Association (FDA) for the treatment of FM: (1) pregabalin (Lyrica), (2) milnacipran (Savella), and (3) duloxetine (Cymbalta). These drugs mechanistically treat FM through either increasing the activity of inhibitory neurotransmitters (milnacipran and duloxetine) or to decrease the activity of excitatory neurotransmitters (pregabalin). Table 2 highlights the FDA-approved medications in the pharmacologic treatment of FM. Careful initiation and titration are recommended to improve patient compliance and response, given the incidence of side effects or drug-drug interactions. There are a variety of commonly utilized drugs other than those listed previously, although none of them have an FDA approval for the FM indication. These other medications have been shown in a variety of research studies to provide pain and symptom relief in FM and include gabapentin (Neurontin)[1], tricyclic antidepressants (e.g., nortriptyline [Pamelor][1], amitriptyline [Elavil][1]), cyclobenzaprine (Flexeril)[1], and venlafaxine (Effexor)[1]. Basic analgesics such as acetaminophen and nonsteroidal antiinflammatories (NSAIDs) have little evidence supporting effectiveness for FM. Other emerging therapies such as low-dose naltrexone (ReVia, Vivitrol)[1] warrant further investigation and should only be used in refractory cases by those who are familiar with its use. There exists no evidence that mu-opioid agonists are helpful in the long-term treatment of FM and ultimately increase central amplification overtime, thereby increasing the potential for worsening pain and functioning whilst placing the patient at risk for dependence and addiction. Clinicians and patients should recognize that in many cases, treatment with pharmacologic agents may

TABLE 2 — Comparison of FDA-approved Pharmacologic Therapies for Fibromyalgia

DRUG	DATE OF FDA APPROVAL	MECHANISM OF ACTION	AVAILABLE STRENGTHS	DOSING	COMMON SIDE EFFECTS
Duloxetine (Cymbalta)	June 16, 2008	Serotonin norepinephrine reuptake inhibition	20 mg; 30 mg; 60 mg	• 60 mg/day recommended total dose (doses higher than 60 mg rarely helpful for pain) • Start 30 mg/day for 1 week or longer and then may increase to 60 mg/day	Dry mouth, somnolence, nausea, constipation, decreased appetite, hyperhidrosis
Milnacipran (Savella)	January 14, 2009	Serotonin norepinephrine reuptake inhibition	12.5 mg; 25 mg; 50 mg; 100 mg; convenience starter pack	• Convenience starter pack dosing: Start 12.5 mg daily × 1 day, then 12.5 mg bid × 2 days, then 25 mg bid × 4 days, then 50 mg bid • Max dose 100 mg bid (200 mg/day)	Nausea, constipation, hot flush, hyperhidrosis, vomiting, palpitations, increased heart rate, dry mouth, hypertension
Pregabalin (Lyrica)	June 21, 2007	Non-selective alpha-2-delta calcium channel blocker	25 mg; 50 mg; 75 mg; 100 mg; 150 mg; 200 mg; 225 mg; 300 mg	• Start at 75 mg bid (can start much lower in sensitive or older patient population) • May increase to 150 mg bid within 1 week • Max dose 225 mg bid (450 mg/day)	Dizziness, somnolence, dry mouth, peripheral edema, blurred vision, weight gain, abnormal thinking/cognitive difficulties

be ineffective. The choice of drug should always be discussed with the patient and should focus on targeting the most bothersome symptoms. Oftentimes multiple types of drugs/drug combinations are needed. If a drug is trialed and does not lead to clinically meaningful relief after four weeks at the full recommended dose, it should be tapered or stopped, and an alternative drug trialed.

Nonpharmacologic treatment for FM consists of psychological and educational interventions, in addition to physical modalities and should be an integral part of a comprehensive FM treatment plan. Education should be a foundational intervention applied immediately with diagnosis or early in the patient's treatment plan, and should consist of information on the underlying pain mechanisms causing clinical pain and associated symptoms (e.g., central nervous system pain and sensory amplification) and information on the nature of the condition (e.g., nonprogressive, chronic, and lifelong with episodic flares, risk of other comorbid conditions). This will provide a strong foundation to then add psychological therapies, which are typically behavioral based and focused on acceptance theories. Cognitive behavioral therapy has been shown to be effective for the treatment of FM and focuses on the link between pain, mood, thoughts, and behavior, and trying to unravel negative coping mechanisms such as catastrophizing and poor self-efficacy. Mind-body therapies, including stress reduction, biofeedback, and mindfulness, have also shown good benefit for FM.

Physical activity, including active and passive modalities, is perhaps the most important nonpharmacologic treatment for FM. Physical therapy, including warm-water aquatherapy, can be utilized initially to help patients improve their conditioning and obtain education on how to incorporate movement and activity into their daily lives. Among different exercise interventions, aerobic exercise has been shown to be the most beneficial. Patients should start with low-to-moderate intensity activities (such as walking, stationary cycling, or swimming).

Over time, patients can increase their intensity and duration over time to a goal of at least 20 min/day at least two to three times weekly. It is important to counsel patients on pacing themselves and that initially they may have more soreness or pain as they gradually build their physical conditioning and strength. Continuation of the exercise regimen is of paramount value as ongoing exercise has been associated with maintenance of improvements in FM. Passive forms of physical activity such as balneotherapy (heated spa treatments), manipulation, massage, transcutaneous electrical stimulation, and ultrasound have only weak evidence to support their use. Complementary and alternative medicine options that may be considered include acupuncture, yoga, tai chi, and qi gong meditation, but there are few high-quality evidence studies to support their use as first-line therapy.

Monitoring

No laboratory or imaging monitoring is required in the treatment of FM. Regular/frequent outpatient engagement with patients is recommended—to discuss the comprehensive care plan and focus on patient goals for treatment, as increased outpatient engagement has been shown to reduce morbidity and mortality (including risk of suicide) in patients with FM.

References

Arnold LM, Gebke KB, Choi EHS: Fibromyalgia: management strategies for primary care providers, *Int J Clin Pract* 70(2):99–112, 2016.

Borchers AT, Gershwin ME: Fibromyalgia: A critical and comprehensive review, *Clinic Rev Allerg Immunol* 49:100–151, 2015.

Clauw DJ: Fibromyalgia: A clinical review, *JAMA* 311(15):1547–1555, 2014.

Perrot S: Fibromyalgia: A misconnection in a multi-connected world?, *Eur J Pain*, 2019. https://doi.org/10.1002/ejp.1367. Available at: [Epub ahead of print].

Rahman A, Underwood M, Carnes D: Fibromyalgia. *BMJ* 348:g1224, 2014.

Talotta R, Bazzichi L, Di Franco M, et al: One year in review 2017: fibromyalgia, *Clin Exp Rheumatol* 35(Suppl. 105):S6–S12, 2017.

Wolfe F, Clauw DJ, Fitzcharles M, et al: 2016 Revisions to the 2010/2011 fibromyalgia diagnostic criteria, *Semin Arthritis Rheum* 46(3):319–329, 2016.

JUVENILE IDIOPATHIC ARTHRITIS

Method of
Ashley Cooper, MD

CURRENT DIAGNOSIS

- Juvenile idiopathic arthritis (JIA) is a clinical diagnosis. JIA is diagnosed when objective signs of arthritis persist in a child for at least 6 weeks in the absence of another identifiable cause.
- Children who present with musculoskeletal pain without accompanying objective signs of joint inflammation (swelling or painful, limited range of motion) are unlikely to have arthritis. In many children with JIA, swelling and joint limitation are more prominent than pain.
- Laboratory testing has limited value in diagnosing JIA. In some cases, no laboratory tests are needed to make the diagnosis. When clinically indicated, laboratory tests are used to exclude other causes of arthritis such as infection (including Lyme disease in endemic areas), malignancy, or underlying systemic autoimmune disease.
- The antinuclear antibody (ANA), rheumatoid factor (RF), and anticitric citrullinated peptide (anti-CCP) have prognostic but *not* diagnostic value in JIA. These tests should not be drawn to evaluate musculoskeletal pain in children in the absence of objective signs of arthritis.

CURRENT THERAPY

- Medical therapy is individualized for each child based on severity and number of affected joints and comorbidities. The goal of treatment is to completely control joint inflammation to minimize symptoms and prevent damage.
- Many rheumatologists use a step-up treatment approach, titrating medication until inactive disease is achieved. In children with severe arthritis, early combination therapy is sometimes used. With appropriate use of currently available medications, most children with JIA can achieve clinically inactive disease.
- Current treatment options include scheduled nonsteroidal antiinflammatory drugs (NSAIDs), intraarticular corticosteroid injections, disease-modifying antirheumatic drugs (DMARDs, most commonly methotrexate), and biologic response modifiers (such as antitumor necrosis factor alpha, anti-interleukin-1, or anti-interleukin-6 therapy).
- With the currently available medications, many children with JIA do not require systemic corticosteroids. Steroids should not be prescribed to a child presenting with joint pain or swelling of unclear etiology.
- Optimal timing and approach to medication discontinuation in patients who have achieved inactive disease are unclear. Relapse rates are high after medication discontinuation in most JIA subtypes.
- A partnership between the child's rheumatologist and primary care provider is key to safe use of immune-modulating medications. Optimal management includes:
  - Medication toxicity monitoring with periodic laboratory studies;
  - Prompt evaluation of infectious symptoms in immunosuppressed patients;
  - Administration of age-appropriate vaccines (with avoidance of live virus vaccines in patients on immunosuppression);
  - Counseling of adolescents to avoid alcohol while on methotrexate and pregnancy while on teratogenic medications.

- Children with JIA should remain physically active and be allowed to continue participating in sports and leisure activities as tolerated. Physical and/or occupational therapy is indicated for patients with limited mobility, deconditioning, or compromised activities of daily living.
- Regular screening for uveitis is an essential part of JIA management to allow prompt treatment of this sight-threatening complication.

Juvenile idiopathic arthritis (JIA) is an umbrella term that encompasses multiple forms of chronic, immune-mediated arthritis that begin in childhood. The classification system currently used for JIA was established in 1995 by the International League of Associations for Rheumatology (ILAR). By replacing the term *juvenile rheumatoid arthritis* with *juvenile idiopathic arthritis* and defining additional subtypes, the ILAR criteria better reflect the clinical heterogeneity among children with arthritis. Absence of the term "rheumatoid" from the current nomenclature appropriately highlights that most cases of juvenile arthritis are not simply early onset rheumatoid arthritis (RA), as only 5% of all children with JIA have rheumatoid factor (RF) positive polyarticular disease.

The subtypes of JIA are summarized in Table 1 and include oligoarticular, polyarticular (RF negative and RF positive), enthesitis-related (a childhood-onset spondyloarthropathy closely related to ankylosing spondylitis), psoriatic, and systemic arthritis.

Although each of these conditions has a distinct phenotype, the presence of chronic inflammatory arthritis is the unifying feature and sine qua non of JIA. A careful history and physical exam are the most important tools in diagnosis. A complete exam of all joints should be performed in children with possible JIA as the pattern of affected joints impacts disease classification. Additional affected joints are often identified on exam that have not been apparent to patients and parents. Common pitfalls in diagnosis of arthritis in children include the following:

- *Diagnosing JIA in the absence of objective clinical signs of arthritis (joint inflammation).* Most children who present to the primary care office with joint pain (even chronic pain) do not have JIA. Isolated pain in the absence of objective findings of arthritis such as swelling predicts against JIA or other chronic rheumatic disease.
- *Attempting to rule in JIA with laboratory studies.* ANA tests can be positive in up to 30% of healthy children, and the most common cause of a positive RF in children is recent viral infection. Due to the high frequency of positive results in children without rheumatic disease, these tests should not be drawn to evaluate for arthritis in the setting of normal exam findings.
- *Attempting to rule out JIA with laboratory studies.* Arthritis is a clinical diagnosis. If a child presents with chronic joint swelling, limited range of motion or contractures, one should not be falsely reassured by normal labs. Many children with arthritis have completely normal inflammatory markers and a negative ANA, and 95% of children with JIA are RF negative.

Risk Factors/Prevention

All JIA subtypes are generally thought to result from an aberrant immune response to an environmental trigger in a genetically predisposed person. A monozygotic twin concordance of 25% to 40% and increased autoimmunity in family members of children with JIA suggest a significant genetic contribution to disease development. Recent genome-wide association studies have revealed susceptibility loci for JIA, though differences in genetic factors exist between clinical JIA subtypes. Strong genetic associations are rare for most JIA subtypes and many identified risk loci are associated with multiple autoimmune diseases. The exception is that 80% to 90% of children with enthesitis-related arthritis (ERA) are human leukocyte antigen (HLA) B27 positive. Testing for specific HLA alleles currently has no diagnostic utility in JIA. For the interested reader, Hersh and Prahalad recently

XII Rheumatology and the Musculoskeletal System

TABLE 1	International League of Associations for Rheumatology Classification Criteria for Juvenile Idiopathic Arthritis

JIA CLASSIFICATION CRITERIA

JIA Definition:
Inflammatory arthritis in at least one joint that begins before age 16, persists at least 6 weeks, and has no other identifiable cause.

JIA SUBTYPE	DESCRIPTION
Oligoarthritis	Arthritis affects 1–4 joints in the first 6 months
• Persistent	Never extends beyond 4 joints
• Extended	Extends to affect 5 or more joints after first 6 months
Polyarthritis	Arthritis affects 5 or more joints in the first 6 months
• RF negative	
• RF positive	
Enthesitis-Related Arthritis	Arthritis and enthesitis, OR Arthritis or enthesitis with at least 2 of the following: • Signs of sacroiliitis, • Positive HLA-B27, • Onset in a boy age 6 or older, • Acute anterior uveitis, • HLA-B27-related disease in a first-degree relative.
Psoriatic Arthritis	Arthritis and psoriasis, OR Arthritis and at least 2 of the following: • Dactylitis, • Nail pitting or onycholysis, • Psoriasis in a first-degree relative.
Systemic JIA	Arthritis in at least 1 joint with at least 2 weeks of fever that is daily for at least 3 days, with at least one of the following: • Evanescent erythematous rash, • Generalized lymphadenopathy, • Hepatomegaly and/or splenomegaly, • Serositis.
Undifferentiated	Fulfills criteria for no category or 2 or more categories

JIA, Juvenile idiopathic arthritis.
Data from Petty RE, Southwood TR, Manners P, et al. International League of Associations for Rheumatology classification of juvenile idiopathic arthritis: second revision, Edmonton, 2001. *J Rheumatol.* 2004;31(2):390–392.

reviewed the genetics of JIA, and Yasin and Schulert published a detailed review of the genetics and pathophysiology of systemic JIA (SJIA).

There is no known prevention for JIA.

Pathophysiology

Synovitis in JIA is characterized by synovial hypertrophy, edema, and hypervascularity. A mixed inflammatory infiltrate of T and B lymphocytes, plasma cells, macrophages, and dendritic cells is found in the synovial lining of affected joints. Infiltrating mononuclear cells produce proinflammatory cytokines and chemokines that contribute to bone and cartilage erosion and perpetuate recruitment of inflammatory cells.

SJIA is uniquely characterized by significant innate immune activation, including increased production of the proinflammatory cytokines interleukin-1 (IL-1) and 6 (IL-6). Some experts suggest that SJIA may be better classified as an autoinflammatory disease.

Given their unique clinical phenotypes, the epidemiology, clinical manifestations, diagnosis, and management of the JIA subtypes will each be discussed separately. Some general principles of diagnosis and management reviewed in "Current Diagnosis and Therapy", previously discussed, and introduced in the oligoarticular JIA section are applicable to all JIA subtypes.

Oligoarticular Juvenile Idiopathic Arthritis
Epidemiology
Oligoarticular JIA is the most common JIA subtype, comprising 40% to 50% of all cases, with an incidence of approximately 1 in 10,000 children per year. Peak age of onset is 1 to 4 years, with a female predominance. It is most commonly seen in children of Northern European descent.

Clinical Manifestations
Children with oligoarticular JIA present with arthritis in one to four joints, without spread to more than four joints in the first 6 months of disease. Oligoarthritis typically affects large joints in an asymmetrical pattern. The most common presentation is arthritis of a single knee. Swelling is the predominant symptom, often with little or no apparent pain early in the disease course. Affected joints may have a limited range of motion or contractures. A relatively painless limp is common, and is sometimes the first symptom apparent to parents. Stiffness is worse in the morning or after inactivity, though may be difficult for children to describe. Children with oligoarthritis may experience a persistent oligoarticular course (limited to four or fewer affected joints throughout the child's life) or an extended articular course (spread to five or more joints after the first 6 months of disease).

Diagnosis
A careful history and exam are key to diagnosis. Persistent joint swelling for more than 6 weeks, joint contracture, and/or gait disturbance are the most common presenting symptoms of oligoarticular JIA. Physical exam reveals joint effusion or thickened synovium indicating joint inflammation. Some children may also have warmth, decreased range of motion, contracture, or pain with range of motion on exam. Atrophy of adjacent muscles can be seen in chronic arthritis. Children with oligoarticular JIA are otherwise well-appearing. Severe pain (especially with nighttime waking), extremely red or hot joints, *migratory* swelling, fevers, rash, pallor, or a generally ill-appearing child suggest an alternative diagnosis.

All forms of JIA are diagnosed on the basis of objective signs of arthritis, a history of at least 6 weeks of persistent symptoms, and exclusion of alternative diagnoses *as appropriate based on the patient's clinical picture.* As there is no single test that can confirm the diagnosis of JIA, the value of lab testing is limited to excluding other diagnoses and for prognostic purposes in confirmed cases of JIA (see "Complications"). Radiographs have limited diagnostic value with the exception of detecting other conditions such as malignancy. MRI or musculoskeletal ultrasound can be useful in cases of equivocal or challenging physical exam (such as in obese patients).

Differential Diagnosis
In some patients with a classic clinical picture, no specific workup for other diagnoses is needed. Prompt evaluation by a pediatric rheumatologist is key to confirming the presence of arthritis, determining an appropriate individualized workup, and rapidly initiating treatment if a diagnosis of JIA is established.

Features that suggest the need to evaluate for alternative diagnoses include the following:
- Atypical demographics (age, ethnicity)—may suggest a different JIA subtype such as ERA in older children (see "Enthesitis-Related Arthritis").
- Travel history—may suggest the need to evaluate for Lyme arthritis or tuberculosis in patients residing in or traveling to endemic areas.
- Atypical clinical features—severe pain, constitutional symptoms such as weight loss, fevers, fatigue, or an ill appearance should prompt consideration of infection, malignancy, inflammatory bowel disease, or systemic collagen vascular disease such as lupus in a child with arthritis. Acute, subacute, or migratory arthritis suggests an infectious or postinfectious cause (including rheumatic fever). Episodic joint swelling, especially after trauma, may suggest a bleeding disorder or intra-articular vascular malformation.

Treatment

Treatment of JIA aims to completely control joint inflammation to control symptoms and mitigate the risk of joint damage. In oligoarticular JIA, either scheduled nonsteroidal antiinflammatory drugs (NSAIDs) or intraarticular corticosteroid injections are used as first line therapy. NSAIDs must be administered at antiinflammatory doses on a scheduled basis to control inflammation, and may take 6 to 8 weeks to be effective. Naproxen (Naprosyn) is often preferred due to twice daily dosing and available liquid formulation. Steroid joint injections can control inflammation rapidly and are often used for patients with contractures or severe arthritis to more rapidly restore physical function. Intraarticular steroid injections should not be repeated more frequently than every 3 months. In patients with arthritis refractory to NSAIDs or steroid injections, traditional or biologic disease modifying antirheumatic drugs (DMARDs), such as methotrexate (Trexall) and tumor necrosis factor (TNF) inhibitors, can be used (some are off-label) in a stepwise fashion until disease control is achieved. DMARDs should be prescribed and monitored by a rheumatologist.

Monitoring

JIA disease control is monitored by a rheumatologist on the basis of history and physical exam. The frequency of follow-up visits varies depending on the patient's disease course and medications. Assessments of functional status should be performed to identify patients who would benefit from physical and occupational therapy service or school accommodations. Eye screening for uveitis is a critical part of JIA monitoring (see "Complications"). Medication toxicity monitoring depends on the medication used:

- Daily NSAIDs: complete blood count (CBC), comprehensive metabolic panel (CMP), and urinalysis every 6 to 12 months.
- Methotrexate: CBC and CMP at baseline, 1 month after starting or dose escalation, and then every 3 months on stable doses. Urine pregnancy screening should be considered in girls of reproductive age.
- Biologic DMARDS: Similar lab screening to methotrexate, with some variation depending on medication. Testing for tuberculosis should be performed prior to starting biologic medications.

Patients on immunosuppressive medications should be evaluated promptly for symptoms of infection. They should avoid live virus vaccines, but receive all other age-appropriate vaccinations including an annual flu vaccine.

Complications

Articular complications include joint limitation, contractures, and muscle atrophy, leading to chronic disability and pain, though these complications are less common with currently available treatments. A complication of arthritis unique to the growing child is local growth disturbance, most commonly seen as leg length discrepancy as a result of knee arthritis. Inflammation near the open growth plate can cause overgrowth of the affected limb in young children or premature growth plate closure leading to a shorter limb in adolescents.

Chronic anterior uveitis is a common complication of JIA, particularly oligoarticular and RF negative polyarticular JIA. Chronic uveitis is treatable but carries a high risk of morbidity including cataract, glaucoma, synechiae (adhesions leading to an irregular pupil), band keratopathy (corneal calcium deposits), and blindness. Chronic uveitis is often completely asymptomatic until damage has occurred. Because it can only be detected by slit lamp exam performed by an eye doctor, regular screening is critical to early detection, treatment, and prevention of permanent damage. Uveitis is more likely to occur early in the course of disease, in patients who are ANA positive, and who have an early age of arthritis onset. Well-established screening recommendations guide the frequency of eye exams, ranging from every 3 to 12 months, depending on risk factors. Risk stratification for uveitis is the only use of ANA testing in patients with JIA. Uveitis may occur independent of active arthritis, so eye screening is a critical

part of health maintenance for people with JIA throughout their lives. All children diagnosed with uveitis should see an ophthalmologist with experience treating uveitis. Topical corticosteroids are first-line therapy for anterior uveitis, though long-term use is not advisable given the risk of cataracts and glaucoma. Methotrexate[1] and the TNF inhibitors adalimumab (Humira) and infliximab (Remicade)[1] are used widely in children with refractory uveitis. Some patients require more aggressive treatment for uveitis than for arthritis.

Polyarticular Juvenile Idiopathic Arthritis
Epidemiology

Polyarticular arthritis has two subtypes. RF negative polyarthritis has two peaks of onset (at 1 to 4 years and in adolescence) and comprises 20% of all JIA. It is more common in girls and occurs in all ethnicities. RF positive polyarthritis makes up only 5% of JIA, has a peak onset of 9 to 11 years, and is more common in girls and in nonwhites.

Clinical Manifestations

Children with polyarthritis present with evidence of arthritis (swelling, morning stiffness, pain, limited range of motion) in five of more joints. Young children may present with gait disturbance or loss of milestones, while older children may present with prolonged morning stiffness or difficulty with activities of daily living and fine motor tasks. Large and small joints in the extremities are affected (often symmetrically). Long-standing disease can produce bony overgrowth of the small joints in the hands or joint deformities including wrist subluxation and boutonniere deformities of the fingers. Arthritis of the cervical spine (presenting with limited extension) and temporomandibular joint (TMJ; presenting with decreased mouth opening, jaw deviation, or micrognathia) are common and cause significant morbidity. Mild to moderate systemic symptoms, including fatigue and weight loss, may be present; however, high grade fevers should not occur.

Diagnosis

Diagnosis hinges on the presence of arthritis in five or more joints on physical exam (typically with some degree of wrist and hand involvement), at least 6 weeks of symptoms, and exclusion of other causes. There are no confirmatory tests; however, in patients with polyarticular JIA diagnosed clinically, the RF and anticitric citrullinated peptide (anti-CCP) have prognostic value. RF and anti-CCP positivity are associated with a more severe, erosive course. Some children with polyarticular JIA have normal inflammatory markers, while others have a moderately elevated erythrocyte sedimentation rate (ESR) and anemia of chronic disease. These findings are more useful for assessing overall health and monitoring response to therapy than in establishing an initial diagnosis, as they are nonspecific.

Differential Diagnosis

Reactive arthritis may present with polyarticular joint swelling, but is typically acute in onset and characterized by more pain than is seen in JIA. The arthritis of acute rheumatic fever is typically exquisitely painful and has a unique migratory pattern. While patients with polyarticular JIA may experience an *additive* arthritis pattern early in the disease course, *migratory* arthritis (i.e., swelling resolving completely in one joint and moving to another) is not seen in JIA. In patients with extreme pain, bone pain, pallor, or severe fatigue, malignancy such as leukemia or neuroblastoma should be considered.

Polyarthritis can occur as a manifestation of other underlying autoimmune diseases, including systemic lupus erythematosus, mixed connective tissue disease, or inflammatory bowel disease. The best approach to evaluating for these conditions is a thorough history and physical exam. Oral ulcers, Raynaud phenomenon, or malar or discoid rashes raise concern for lupus. Because ANA tests are nonspecific and have a high positive rate in both the healthy and JIA populations, an ANA test in isolation is not helpful in evaluating for lupus unless it is negative (which essentially excludes lupus). In cases in which the history or physical raises concern for lupus, using a combination of several laboratory studies is more helpful. A reasonable initial workup for lupus when clinical suspicion is high includes an ANA, specific lupus antibodies (Smith, double-stranded DNA), ESR, C3 and C4 levels, CBC to evaluate for cytopenias, a urinalysis, creatinine, and blood pressure measurement.

Inflammatory bowel disease can present with inflammatory arthritis. Inflammatory bowel disease (IBD) should be considered in patients with significant oral ulcers, chronic abdominal pain and/or diarrhea, weight loss, significantly elevated ESR, or anemia.

Treatment

The goals of treatment are the same as for oligoarticular disease, although children with polyarticular JIA often require more aggressive medical therapy to attain inactive disease. Scheduled NSAIDs are often started first line or in conjunction with other medications for pain relief, but rarely are effective as monotherapy. Intraarticular steroid injections may be used in combination with systemic therapy for severely affected or critical joints, but monotherapy with steroid injections is not a viable approach to treating this disease.

Most children with polyarticular JIA require treatment with DMARDs for disease control. There are two general approaches to initiation of medications: step-up therapy and early aggressive (combination) therapy. The choice of approach may be driven by provider and/or patient preference or severity of disease. In a step-up approach, methotrexate is most commonly used as the first DMARD. Methotrexate (10 to 15 mg/m^2 or 0.4 to 1 mg/kg) once weekly is administered orally or subcutaneously, with subcutaneous dosing preferred by many pediatric rheumatologists on the basis of possible improved absorption and mitigation of side effects.

Biologic medications shown to be effective in JIA refractory to methotrexate include TNF inhibitors (etanercept [Enbrel], adalimumab [Humira], golimumab [Symponi], and infliximab [Remicade][1]), the IL-6 inhibitor tocilizumab (Actemra), the T cell costimulation inhibitor abatacept (Orencia) and the Janus kinase inhibitor tofacitinib [Xeljanz]. Selection of an initial biologic medication can be driven by a variety of factors including patient/parent preference, logistics of administration, side effects, comorbid medical conditions, and (in our current health system) insurance restrictions. The anti-CD20 medication rituximab (Rituxan)[1] is sometimes used in patients with RF positive disease, usually after failure of other medications.

Early aggressive approach, such as first-line combination therapy with methotrexate and a TNF inhibitor with or without adjunctive NSAIDs, intraarticular steroid injections, or a short oral steroid bridge, is sometimes used. With earlier aggressive use of DMARDs, treatment with systemic corticosteroids can now be limited to short courses or avoided altogether in most children. While systemic steroids can produce rapid improvements in pain, symptoms return quickly after discontinuation and their side effect profile makes long-term use unacceptable. Systemic steroids should *never* be initiated in a child presenting with musculoskeletal pain of unknown etiology, given the danger of corticosteroids in undiagnosed infection or malignancy.

Monitoring

Monitoring of clinical disease and medications (NSAIDs, methotrexate, TNF inhibitors) is the same as described for oligoarthritis. Other biologic medications have similar monitoring requirements, including testing for latent tuberculosis (TB) prior to initiation. Some biologics have additional recommended laboratory monitoring parameters. Given the expertise needed to safely prescribe and monitor DMARDs, these medications should only be prescribed to children with JIA by a rheumatologist. In patients with systemic inflammation or anemia at presentation, these labs should be followed as adjunctive markers of disease activity, but normalization should not falsely reassure that arthritis is well controlled if the joint exam indicates otherwise. Children with polyarticular JIA who develop fever while on immunosuppression should be assessed promptly for infection.

Complications

Articular complications in polyarticular JIA include joint contractures, deformities, growth disturbances, and progressive, erosive disease. Cervical spine, TMJ, hip, and wrist involvement are associated with higher morbidity. Fortunately, with earlier aggressive treatment, severe joint destruction and severe physical disability are now less common. Surgical interventions are sometimes required for patients with severe micrognathia (mandibular distraction or reconstruction techniques), joint destruction (joint replacements), or severe growth disturbances (limb inequality procedures).

Children with polyarticular JIA can also develop chronic uveitis. Similar to oligoarticular JIA, age of onset, duration of disease, and ANA status are risk factors for development of uveitis and direct frequency of eye screening. The exception is that uveitis is rare in RF positive polyarticular JIA; thus eye screening is needed only once yearly in this subtype.

Enthesitis-Related Arthritis

Epidemiology

ERA is the only JIA subtype more common in boys, makes up 9% to 19% of all JIA, and has a peak age of onset of 10 to 13 years.

Clinical Manifestations

ERA is a childhood form of spondyloarthropathy and closely related to ankylosing spondylitis. Spondyloarthropathies are characterized by axial arthritis, although in children peripheral arthritis precedes axial disease, sometimes by years. Peripheral arthritis in ERA preferentially affects the lower extremities, often asymmetrically. Arthritis of the hips and sacroiliac joints, tenosynovitis (inflammation of tendon sheaths), and *enthesitis* (inflammation at the bony insertions of tendons, ligaments, or fascia) are common findings. *Tarsitis,* diffuse swelling of the dorsum of the foot, is relatively unique to ERA. Pain is more prominent in ERA than other JIA subtypes. Axial arthritis develops in some patients in late adolescence or adulthood. Uveitis in ERA is acute and symptomatic (with a red, photophobic eye), distinct from uveitis in other forms of JIA.

Diagnosis

ERA usually presents as monoarthritis or oligoarthritis in the lower extremities (hips, knees, ankles). Diagnosis is made on the basis of arthritis on exam with a history supporting a chronic course. HLA-B27 positivity can support the diagnosis, though the HLA-B27 is not a diagnostic test (as some ERA patients are B27 negative and many B27 positive individuals are healthy). Though most children do not have sacroiliitis or spinal arthritis at presentation, findings of inflammatory spinal arthritis on radiographs or magnetic resonance imaging strongly suggest this diagnosis.

Differential Diagnosis

School-aged children with ERA often present with arthritis of a single knee or ankle. In addition to the diagnostic considerations outlined above for oligoarthritis, ERA must be distinguished from oligoarticular JIA itself. Clues to diagnosis in this clinical scenario are older age (recall that the peak age of onset of oligoarticular JIA is age 1 to 4), male gender, and supporting clinical features if present (tenosynovitis, enthesitis, acute uveitis).

In children presenting with hip symptoms, infectious and orthopedic conditions (including slipped capital femoral epiphysis or Perthes) should be considered. Rarely, older adolescents present with sacroiliitis. Low back stiffness, worse in the morning, helps distinguish from infectious and orthopedic conditions, though imaging is usually required to make this distinction with confidence. The vast majority of children with chronic low back pain have mechanical rather than inflammatory pain.

Treatment

The general approach to treatment of ERA is similar to polyarticular JIA, though for patients with sacroiliitis or spinal arthritis, TNF inhibition should be considered early in the disease course.

Monitoring

Monitoring is very similar to polyarticular JIA with a few exceptions:

1. Children with ERA should be monitored closely for development of axial arthritis. This may include a combination of the following approaches: querying symptoms of inflammatory back pain, eliciting sacroiliac pain on exam, measuring spine mobility (with a modified Schober test), and/or imaging sacroiliac joints with x-ray or magnetic resonance imaging (MRI).
2. Eye exams are only required once yearly and as indicated based on symptoms as uveitis in ERA is usually symptomatic.

Complications

Acute uveitis occurs in some patients with ERA, and often responds to topical corticosteroids. Patients who develop a red or photophobic eye should be evaluated promptly by an eye doctor. Arthritis of the spine, sacroiliac joints, and hips can be difficult to control, sometimes leading to joint destruction, even in the setting of prompt and aggressive therapy. In adulthood, these patients are at risk for progressive, ascending ankylosis of the spine.

Juvenile Psoriatic Arthritis

Epidemiology

Juvenile psoriatic arthritis comprises approximately 10% of JIA, is more common in girls, and has two peaks of onset: preschool and late childhood.

Clinical Manifestations

Psoriatic arthritis usually presents with peripheral joint involvement and can occur in a monoarticular, oligoarticular, or polyarticular pattern. Both small and large joints can be affected, often in an asymmetrical pattern. *Dactylitis,* or a sausage digit, is a unique feature of psoriatic arthritis not seen in other forms of JIA. Dactylitic fingers and toes exhibit diffuse swelling that extends beyond individual joints. Arthritis of the distal interphalangeal (DIP) joints is also unique to psoriatic arthritis among children with JIA. There is some clinical overlap between psoriatic arthritis and ERA. Enthesitis and tenosynovitis are prevalent features and sacroiliitis can occur in up to 30% of adolescents. Nail changes, including pitting, horizontal ridges, and onycholysis, are common, and overt psoriasis occurs in about half of children. Both chronic uveitis (with risk factors similar to patients with oligo- and polyarticular JIA) and acute uveitis (in HLA-B27 positive patients) can occur.

Diagnosis

Unlike adults, children with psoriatic arthritis often present with arthritis prior to skin disease. In patients with chronic arthritis and psoriasis, the diagnosis is relatively straightforward. In those with chronic arthritis without psoriasis, clinical clues to diagnosis include dactylitis, psoriatic nail changes (pitting or onycholysis), or a first-degree relative with psoriasis.

Differential Diagnosis

Depending on the pattern of joint involvement, differential diagnosis includes other forms of JIA (oligoarticular, polyarticular, ERA) and other conditions listed previously in the differential of these JIA subtypes. Small joint involvement or dactylitis help distinguish psoriatic from oligoarticular JIA in young children with less than five affected joints.

Treatment

The treatment approach is similar to polyarticular JIA, though for patients with sacroiliitis, enthesitis, or dactylitis, TNF inhibition has the most well-established efficacy.

Monitoring

Monitoring is similar to other forms of JIA including eye screening for chronic uveitis described for oligo- and polyarthritis and monitoring for axial arthritis described for ERA. In addition, patients who have not developed skin manifestations should be monitored for development of psoriasis.

Complications

Articular and ocular complications are similar to other JIA subtypes, though children with psoriatic arthritis often have poorer functional outcomes and lower rates of remission off medication than those with oligo- or polyarticular JIA.

Systemic Juvenile Idiopathic Arthritis

Epidemiology

SJIA occurs in children of all ages and into adulthood (Still disease in adults). It is the only form of JIA that affects boys and girls equally. SJIA makes up 10% to 20% of JIA. It occurs in all ethnicities, with increased prevalence in some Asian countries including Japan.

Clinical Manifestations

SJIA is characterized by fever, rash, and arthritis. Fevers in SJIA are high grade, typically spiking once (quotidian) or twice (double quotidian) daily with return to normal temperature between fevers. The rash seen in SJIA is salmon-colored or erythematous, macular or urticarial, sometimes with associated Koebner phenomenon. A unique feature of the SJIA rash is its *evanescent* nature: it appears with fever and resolves or fades during afebrile periods. The arthritis in SJIA can affect any number of joints, in any pattern, and is not always present at disease onset. In some patients, the latent period between onset of systemic features and arthritis is weeks or months. Many patients exhibit nonspecific symptoms, including fatigue, irritability, and myalgia during fevers.

Children with SJIA have significant systemic inflammation during periods of disease activity. Profoundly elevated white blood count, platelet count, ESR, CRP, and anemia are common.

SJIA is truly a systemic disease, with some patients exhibiting lymphadenopathy, hepatosplenomegaly, and serositis (pleural or pericardial effusions). The most feared complication of SJIA is macrophage activation syndrome (MAS; see "Complications").

Diagnosis

SJIA is diagnosed based on the presence of quotidian fevers, evanescent Stills rash, arthritis, and systemic inflammation, with exclusion of similar conditions. SJIA often leads to inpatient evaluation, given patients' high grade fevers and ill appearance. Children who lack arthritis at the time of presentation are challenging to diagnose. In practice, SJIA is often presumptively diagnosed before arthritis has been present for 6 weeks (and sometimes in the absence of arthritis), as the severity of this disease can necessitate urgent treatment.

Differential Diagnosis

SJIA has a broad differential diagnosis that includes infectious (viral, bacterial), oncologic (leukemia, neuroblastoma), and inflammatory conditions (Kawasaki, polyarteritis nodosa, inflammatory bowel disease, among others). Involvement of infectious disease and oncology consultants can help exclude these mimics, particularly if treatment with corticosteroids is being considered. Additional workup, including infectious studies and bone marrow biopsy, is appropriate in cases of diagnostic uncertainty.

Treatment

The treatment paradigms have evolved more for SJIA than any other JIA subtype over the last decade. Traditionally, children with SJIA were treated with systemic corticosteroids, resulting in the full spectrum of anticipated morbidities (growth delay, infections, osteoporosis, etc.). Traditional DMARDs and TNF inhibitors are significantly less effective than for other JIA subtypes. Targeted therapy with inhibition of IL-1 (with anakinra [Kineret][1] or canakinumab [Ilaris]) or IL-6 (with tocilizumab [Actemra]) is the emerging standard of care, though optimal timing of these medications is unclear. Many pediatric rheumatologists are now using IL-1 or IL-6 blockade first line or after a failed NSAID trial to avoid or minimize corticosteroids. Systemic corticosteroids continue to have a role in severe disease or MAS. Other treatments for MAS include cyclosporine (Neoral)[1] and etoposide (Toposar)[1].

Monitoring

Monitoring is similar to polyarticular JIA, with a few exceptions. As uveitis is rare in SJIA, eye exams are needed only annually. Laboratory markers of systemic inflammation are useful in monitoring disease activity and evaluating for impending MAS, which can develop even when disease otherwise appears well controlled. Given the serious and life-threatening nature of this disease, all children with SJIA should be followed closely by a pediatric rheumatologist or an adult rheumatologist with experience managing SJIA.

Complications

Articular complications of SJIA are similar to polyarticular JIA, though the arthritis of SJIA is often aggressive and destructive. There is emerging evidence that earlier treatment with targeted biologics may prevent progression to chronic polyarthritis.

MAS is a serious complication of SJIA, characterized by unregulated production of proinflammatory cytokines, macrophage proliferation, and hemophagocytic activity in the bone marrow and other organs. MAS is a potentially fatal rheumatologic emergency. It is often suspected on the basis of rapidly worsening clinical status and the development of continuous fever. Laboratory findings include a profoundly elevated ferritin, elevated lactate dehydrogenase and transaminases, falling blood cell counts, and paradoxically low or falling ESR and fibrinogen in the setting of other signs of systemic inflammation. MAS is currently considered a secondary form of hemophagocytic lymphohistiocytosis (HLH).

---

[1] Not FDA approved for this indication.

References

Aeschlimann FA, Chong S, Lyons TW, et al: Risk of serious infections associated with biologic agents in juvenile idiopathic arthritis: a systematic review and meta-analyses, *J Pediatr* 204:162–171, 2019.

Clarke SLN, Sen ES, Ramanan AV: Juvenile Idiopathic arthritis-associated uveitis, *Pediatric Rheumatol Online J* 14:27, 2016.

Crayne CB, Beukelman T: Juvenile idiopathic arthritis: oligoarthritis and polyarthritis, *Pediatr Clin N Am* 65:657–674, 2018.

Hersh AO, Prahalad S: Genetics of juvenile idiopathic arthritis, *Rheum Dis Clin N Am* 43:435–448, 2017.

Lee JJL, Schneider R: Systemic juvenile idiopathic arthritis, *Pediatr Clin N Am* 65:691–709, 2018.

Petty RE, Southwood TR, Manners P, et al: International League of Associations for Rheumatology classification of juvenile idiopathic arthritis: second revision, Edmonton, 2001, *J Rheumatol* 31(2):390–392, 2004.

Shoop-Worrall SJW, Kearsley-Fleet L, Thomson W, Verstappen SMM, Hyrich KL: How common is remission in juvenile idiopathic arthritis: a systematic review, *Semin Arthritis Rheum* 47:331–337, 2017.

Wong KO, Bond K, Homik J, Ellsworth JE, Karkhaneh M, Ha C, Dryden DM: Antinuclear antibody, rheumatoid factor, and cyclic-citrullinated peptide tests for evaluating musculoskeletal complaints in children: Comparative Effectiveness Review No. 50, *Agency for Healthcare Research and Quality*, 2012. Available at https://effectivehealthcare.ahrq.gov/sites/default/files/pdf/musculoskeletal-complaints-tests-children_research.pdf. Accessed 1 January 2019.

Yasin S, Schulert GS: Systemic juvenile idiopathic arthritis and macrophage activation syndrome: update on pathogenesis and treatment, *Curr Opin Rheumatol* 30:514–520, 2018.

OSTEOARTHRITIS

Method of
Rachel Chamberlain, MD; Jacob Christensen, DO; and Christopher Bossart, MD

CURRENT DIAGNOSIS

- Risk factors for osteoarthritis (OA) include age, gender, genetics, and anatomic factors, which are nonmodifiable; modifiable risk factors include body mass index (BMI), tobacco use, trauma, physical activity, and muscle strength.
- OA is diagnosed using both clinical and radiologic information.
- Clinical signs and symptoms include joint pain, crepitus, mild swelling, and joint line tenderness to palpation. Symptoms wax and wane and may be related to activity but can be present at varying times of day.
- The Kellgren-Lawrence Classification system can help determine the grade of OA, but the ultimate determination of the severity is based on clinical factors.

CURRENT THERAPY

- First-line therapy for OA includes exercise, physical therapy, and weight loss (if the patient is overweight or obese).
- Nonsteroidal antiinflammatory drugs (NSAIDs) are the best studied pharmacologic treatment for OA pain. Their use must be balanced by their side effects and the patient's comorbid conditions.
- Injections of corticosteroids may be used for OA pain management, but their pain relief effects are not long term.
- Hyaluronic acid injections can be considered in patients with mild to moderate OA of the knee, but this is an expensive therapy and evidence of effectiveness is mixed.
- No current treatment either in systemic medications or injections alters the course of OA. Research in the long-term benefits of biologic agents is ongoing.
- Total joint replacement is an expensive but definitive treatment for many patients with OA. The referring clinician should consider the patient's overall health and help optimize the patient's health for a successful outcome when referring for a total joint replacement.

Osteoarthritis (OA), also known as degenerative joint disease, is the most common form of arthritis worldwide. OA is a significant cause of morbidity, disability, and decreased quality of life. It is one of the leading contributors to global years lived with disability (YLDs) by Global Disease Burden studies. It is the leading cause of lower extremity disability. OA affects about one in eight people in the United States, or 27 to 31 million, and about 250 million people worldwide, with the most commonly affected joints being the knees, hips, hands, feet, and spine. As the age of the population and the rates of obesity increase, the economic impact of OA also increases. It is estimated that OA costs 1% to 2.5% of GDP in developed countries, with the majority of cost for treatment (85%) coming from joint replacement surgeries.

OA has been previously characterized pathologically by varying levels of cartilage involvement. One may find fissures and microfibrillations in mild or early disease, and erosive destruction of the joint surfaces may be seen in more advanced disease. However, it is recognized that the effects of OA can be seen throughout the entire joint including the bone, synovium, menisci, and ligaments.

(FDA)–approved on urine in the above scenarios but is used off-label in laboratories that have met all regulatory requirements.

Patients who screen positive for *C. trachomatis* need to be screened for other STIs, including gonorrhea, syphilis, and HIV.

Abstinence and monogamous relationships are ideal to help prevent the transmission of *C. trachomatis*. Safer sex practices to limit the spread of *C. trachomatis* include the consistent use of condoms. Epidemiologic studies show that people often base their decision to use condoms on their perception of their partner's risk. Given the high prevalence of asymptomatic *C. trachomatis* infections in certain American populations, selective condom use is not an effective strategy.

Clinical Manifestations

Most infections are asymptomatic. However, some women will report vaginal discharge, postcoital or intermenstrual bleeding, or lower abdominal pain. Men are more commonly symptomatic than women and may report dysuria or urethral discharge.

Untreated *C. trachomatis* in women has significant health sequelae. Approximately 40% of women with untreated *Chlamydia* go on to develop pelvic inflammatory disease (PID). Women with PID may become infertile (20%), develop debilitating chronic pelvic pain (18%), or suffer ectopic pregnancy (9%).

Men do not tend to experience as severe sequelae from *C. trachomatis*. The most common illness is urethritis, but men may also experience epididymitis, proctitis, and conjunctivitis. Reactive arthritis is also more common in men.

Diagnosis

Tests used for detection of *C. trachomatis* can be divided into molecular (NAAT, DNA probing, and hybrid capture), antigen detection (direct immunofluorescence and enzyme immunoassay), and cell culture.

The most reliable method of testing for *C. trachomatis* is NAAT. It is FDA-approved for use on vaginal/endocervical secretions, male intraurethral swabs, and first-catch urine. It is not FDA-approved for rectal or oropharyngeal use but is used off-label in laboratories as described above. The primary benefit of NAAT is the lack of a need for viable organisms to induce a positive test result; this increases its sensitivity to more than 95% because of the ability to detect *C. trachomatis* even if only one copy of the targeted RNA or DNA is present. Its specificity is also desirable at 99%.

C. trachomatis cell culture is used as the reference standard for all testing but has many limitations, including expense, long turnaround time (72 hours), and transport and specimen storage requirements. Its sensitivity is 80% to 85%. It is not readily available.

Limiting barriers to screening is important. If testing in the clinic is difficult to arrange, self-collected vaginal swab specimens perform at least as well as other approved specimens using NAAT. First-catch urine NAAT testing is also more acceptable to many patients, particularly asymptomatic men and women who do not otherwise need a pelvic examination.

Differential Diagnosis

Infection with *Chlamydia* is often asymptomatic but is included in the differential diagnosis of various organ system complaints. It should be ruled out in any sexually active patient presenting with urethritis, mucopurulent cervicitis, epididymitis, and proctitis. There is significant overlap in the symptoms caused by *C. trachomatis* with *N. gonorrhoeae,* so testing for both bacteria with NAAT is preferred. Other agents that are included in the differential diagnosis after *C. trachomatis* and *N. gonorrhoeae* have been ruled out include *Trichomonas vaginalis,* HSV, adenovirus, *Mycoplasma* species, and *Ureaplasma.* More specifically, persistent urethritis after treatment with doxycycline can be caused by infection with *T. vaginalis* or doxycycline-resistant *Urea urealyticum* or *Mycoplasma genitalium.*

C. trachomatis should be ruled out in newborn infants with conjunctivitis in the first 30 days of life or pneumonia at 1 to

---

BOX 1 *Chlamydia trachomatis:* Recommended Treatment Regimens by Clinical Syndrome

Recommended Regimen for Non-Pregnant Adolescents and Adults With Chlamydial Infection
- Doxycycline (Vibramycin) 100 mg orally twice daily for 7 days

Alternative Regimens
- Azithromycin (Zithromycin) 1 g orally in a single dose
- Levofloxacin (Levaquin)[1] 500 mg orally once daily for 7 days

Recommended Regimen for Pregnant Patient With Chlamydial Infections
- Azithromycin 1 g orally in a single dose

Alternative Regimens
- Amoxicilin[1] 500 mg orally three times/day for 7 days

Recommended Regimen for Neonates With Chlamydial Infection
- Erythromycin base or ethyl succinate 50 mg/kg body weight/day orally divided into four doses daily for 14 days*

Recommended Regimen for Infants and Children Who Weigh <45 kg With Chlamydial Infection
- Erythromycin base or ethylsuccinate 50 mg/kg/day orally divided into 4 doses daily for 14 days*

Alternative Regimen
- Azithromycin suspension 20 mg/kg/day orally, one dose daily for 3 days**

Recommended Regimen for Children Who Weigh ≥45 kg but Who Are <8 Years Old
- Azithromycin 1 g orally in a single dose

Recommended Regimens for Children Aged ≥8 Years
- Azithromycin 1 g orally in a single dose
  or
- Doxycycline 100 mg orally twice a day for 7 days

Inpatient and Outpatient PID
- Please refer to PID chapter for treatment regimens

---

* Infants <6 weeks of age who are treated with erythromycin should be followed for signs and symptoms of infantile hypertrophic pyloric stenosis.
** There are limited data about the effectiveness and optimal dosing of azithromycin for treating chlamydial infection among infants and children weighing <45 kg.
[1] Not FDA approved for this indication.
Providers should consult the Centers for Disease Control and Prevention's website at http://cdc.gov/std/treatment for up-to-date treatment recommendations.

---

3 months of life, especially if they were born to mothers with untreated chlamydial infections.

Treatment

Recommendations for treatment regimens are summarized in Box 1. Doxycycline (Vibramycin) has become the preferred antibiotic for *C. trachomatis* in nonpregnant patients. It has demonstrated effectiveness not only for urogenital infection but also for rectal and oropharyngeal infection. Azithromycin (Zithromycin) is the treatment of choice for pregnant patients and has shown efficacy for urogenital infection. It can also be considered as a suitable alternative if nonadherence to doxycycline arises. Presumptive treatment for *C. trachomatis* should be considered for high-risk patients with cervicitis. High-risk patients include women up to 25 years old; those with new or multiple sexual partners; those who engage in unprotected sex, especially if follow-up cannot be ensured; and those for whom a relatively insensitive diagnostic test is used in place of NAAT.

The CDC only recommends presumptive treatment for *C. trachomatis* for patients being treated for *N. gonorrhoeae* when coinfection is not excluded. Coinfection is common, as illustrated in a study that found 20% of men with *N. gonorrhoeae* and 42% of women with N. *gonorrhoeae* were also infected with *C. trachomatis*. Cotreatment is also recommended in the hope that it will impede the development of antimicrobial-resistant N. *gonorrhoeae*.

Chlamydia trachomatis is a reportable infectious disease. The patient is instructed to refer all of his or her sexual partners for testing and treatment if they have had sexual contact during the previous 60 days. If the patient has not been sexually active for the last 60 days, then the patient is to refer his or her most recent sexual contact for treatment. The patient's recent sexual partners should be treated empirically even if their personal STI evaluation returns negative results. The patient and his or her sexual partners should be counseled to abstain from sexual activity until after the final dose of the 7-day regimen or for 7 days posttreatment following a one-dose therapy. Reinfection, rather than recurrence, is the more common etiology of repeat *C. trachomatis* infection.

Expedited partner therapy is an option in certain cases. This entails the patient delivering the antibiotic to his or her partner(s) without a physician first seeing the patient. Patients are to give their partners written materials on the importance of following up with a physician if any signs of complications occur (e.g., pelvic pain in women or testicular pain in men). It can be used effectively in certain situations but is not routinely recommended in men who have sex with men because of the high risk for coexisting infections, especially undiagnosed HIV infection, in their partners. Please refer to the CDC website (www.cdc.gov/std/ept) to check on legality in individual states. In general, using the traditional patient-physician model is preferred.

Infants born to women with untreated *C. trachomatis* infection are at increased risk for vertical transmission. Prophylactic treatment with oral erythromycin for *C. trachomatis* is not recommended. The state-mandated standard erythromycin eye ointment that all newborns receive is still indicated but is not adequate treatment if the infant ultimately develops conjunctivitis. Overall, infants born to infected mothers need to be closely monitored for any signs and symptoms of infection and treated appropriately.

Intrauterine devices (IUDs) have regained popularity in the United States after they were implicated in causing PID in the 1970s. The IUD has evolved and now the risk of PID appears increased only in the first 3 weeks postinsertion. If *C. trachomatis* or PID is contracted with an IUD in place, practitioners must decide whether the IUD should be removed. Research has found insufficient evidence to mandate removal, but close follow-up is mandatory.

Monitoring

Repeat testing is recommended for all patients, including pregnant women, treated for *C. trachomatis* at 3 months regardless of the treatment status of the patient's partner(s) because reinfection is so common. If the patient does not follow up at 3 months, he or she should be retested upon presentation for medical care within the first 12 months posttreatment.

Test of cure, which is testing at 4 weeks posttreatment, is recommended only for pregnant patients. Testing for cure earlier than 3 to 4 weeks increases the rate of false positive results. Pregnant women who are at high risk for STI's include those who were treated for *C. trachomatis* during the pregnancy; these women also qualify to be rescreened in the third trimester for N. *gonorrhoeae*, HIV, and syphilis in addition to *C. trachomatis*.

Complications

C. trachomatis is a major public health concern because it results in serious health complications and sequelae. In women it can cause PID, endometritis, ectopic pregnancy, infertility, salpingitis, and perihepatitis (Fitz-Hugh-Curtis syndrome). In men it is associated with postgonococcal or nongonococcal urethritis and epididymitis. Reactive arthritis can occur in both men and women.

C. trachomatis is especially problematic in pregnancy because it is associated with an increased risk of preterm labor and preterm premature rupture of membranes. Infants born to women infected with C. trachomatis risk experiencing pneumonia and conjunctivitis.

C. trachomatis pneumonia can present as an afebrile pneumonia often with a staccato cough without wheezing between 1 and 3 months of life. *C. trachomatis* conjunctivitis, also known as ophthalmia neonatorum, is uncommon in the United States, but worldwide it is the number one cause of blindness. It usually presents within the 5th and 12th day of life but can present at up to 1 month of age. State-mandated prophylactic eye ointment given to babies at birth mainly helps prevent gonococcal ophthalmia; it does not prevent perinatal transmission of C. trachomatis from mother to infant. Therefore the screening of pregnant women and ultimate treatment of their *C. trachomatis* during pregnancy is the best method of preventing complications in newborn infants.

References

Bebear C, de Barbeyrac B: Genital *Chlamydia trachomatis* infections, *Clin Microbiol Infect* 15:4–10, 2009.
Blas MM, Canchihuaman FA, Alva IE, et al: Pregnancy outcomes in women infected with *Chlamydia trachomatis*: a population-based cohort study in Washington State, *Sex Transm Infect* 83:314–318, 2007.
Centers for Disease Control and Prevention (CDC). Sexually Transmitted Disease Surveillance 2021. Available at: https://www.cdc.gov/std/statistics/2021/default .htm. Accessed April 24, 2023.
Centers for Disease Control and Prevention (CDC): Sexually transmitted infections treatment guidelines, 2021, *MMWR Recomm Rep (Morb Mortal Wkly Rep)* 70(No.4):65–82, 2021.
Honey E, Augood C, Templeton A, et al: Cost effectiveness of screening for *Chlamydia trachomatis*: a review of published studies, *Sex Transm Infect* 78:406–412, 2002.
Johnson RE, Newhall WJ, Papp JR, et al: Screening tests to detect *Chlamydia trachomaitis* and *Neisseria gonorrhoeae* infections—2002, *MMWR Recomm Rep (Morb Mortal Wkly Rep)* 51(RR-15):1–38, 2002.
Kramer A, Schewebke I, Kampf G: How long do nosocomial pathogens persist on inanimate surfaces? A systematic review, *BMC Infect Dis* 6:130, 2006.
LeFevre ML, U.S. Preventive Services Task Force: Screening for chlamydia and gonorrhea: U.S. Preventive services Task Force recommendation statement, *Ann Intern Med* 161(12):902–910, 2014.
Lyss SB, Kamb ML, Peterman TA, et al: *Chlamydia trachomatis* among patients infected with and treated for *Neisseria gonorrhoeae* in sexually transmitted clinics in the United States, *Ann Intern Med* 139:178–185, 2003.

CONDYLOMATA ACUMINATA

Method of
M. Chantel Long, MD

CURRENT DIAGNOSIS

- Condylomata acuminata are usually flesh-colored, brown, or gray and can be flat, plaquelike, or exophytic papules, giving them the classic "cauliflower" appearance.
- The lesions may be single or multiple and can range in size from minute to several centimeters in diameter.
- When the appearance of the lesion is typical, confirmatory tests are usually unnecessary.
- Suspicious lesions or uncertain diagnoses warrant biopsy to rule out malignancy.

CURRENT THERAPY

- In the absence of dysplasia, treatment of subclinical human papilloma virus infection is not recommended.
- The goal of therapy is to eliminate symptoms, namely clinically apparent warts, rather than address the underlying HPV infection.
- Common treatment options include podofilox (Condylox), imiquimod (Aldara, Zyclara), sinecatechins (Veregen), trichloroacetic acid (Tri-Chlor), cryotherapy, and surgery.

Epidemiology

Condylomata acuminata, commonly known as genital warts, is a sexually transmitted disease caused by the human papilloma virus (HPV). It is estimated that 43 million people are infected with HPV in the United States, with the highest prevalence in adolescents and young adults. Lifetime incidence of HPV infection is greater than 50% and appears to be increasing, making it the most common sexually transmitted disease.

Risk Factors

Risk factors associated with HPV infection include sex with an infected partner, early age at first sexual intercourse, multiple sexual partners, history of sexually transmitted infections, cigarette smoking, and lack of condom use. The majority of patients whose sexual partner has condyloma will themselves develop condyloma within 3 months. An even larger percentage of people are believed to develop subclinical infection.

Pathophysiology

About 90% of warts are caused by HPV types 6 and 11; condyloma can be coinfected with types 16, 18, 31, 33, 35, and 45, which have oncogenic potential, especially in patients with HIV infection. Genital skin appears to be less susceptible to the oncogenic potential of HPV compared to the transformation zones of the cervix and anal canal.

The virus is easily transmitted via sexual contact. Vertical transmission and autoinoculation are possible. The average incubation period between infection and appearance of condyloma ranges from 3 months to several years. Condyloma can persist or recur after therapy, undergo malignant transformation, or spontaneously regress.

Prevention

Prevention options include HPV vaccination, abstinence, routine condom use, and limiting sexual partners. Once patients have condyloma, they should be encouraged to use condoms consistently. Educate patients that condoms can decrease transmission but might not completely prevent infection.

One HPV vaccine series is currently available in the United States. Gardasil 9 is a 9-valent HPV vaccine indicated for male and female patients aged 9 to 26 years for prevention of cervical cancer and genital warts. It may also be given to patients age 27 to 45 years based on shared clinical decision-making between the patient and clinician.

Clinical Manifestations

Most genital warts are asymptomatic on presentation, although patients can present with complaints of a "bump." Localized irritation, pruritus, pain, or bleeding can occur, and symptoms may vary based on the location and size of the lesions. Usually, the warts appear flesh-colored, brown, or gray and can be flat, plaquelike, or exophytic papules, giving them the classic "cauliflower" appearance. The lesions may be single or multiple and range in size from minute to several centimeters in diameter. Flat HPV lesions might not be grossly visible.

The majority of HPV infections are either subclinical or unrecognized. Clinically apparent disease might represent only a small portion of the actual infected area.

Diagnosis

When the clinical appearance of the lesion is typical, confirmatory tests are usually unnecessary. The entire anogenital tract should be examined because of the widespread nature of HPV. A magnifying glass and anoscopy may be helpful for thorough detection and examination. Application of dilute 3% to 5% acetic acid solution to the skin surface can help detect subtle HPV lesions by producing an acetowhitening of the condyloma; however, this is not a specific test and is not routinely recommended. Pap smears or tissue biopsy can provide histopathologic confirmation of the diagnosis. Biopsy is recommended to rule out malignancy in any suspicious lesions, such as large or rapidly growing condyloma; pigmented, atypical, friable, bleeding, or ulcerated lesions; sites of previous treatment failure; areas of recurrence; acetowhite lesions; or lesions in immunocompromised patients. Although costly and not recommended, HPV identification via DNA testing can be performed.

Differential Diagnosis

Table 1 outlines the differential diagnosis for condylomata acuminata.

Treatment

In the absence of dysplasia, the Centers for Disease Control and Prevention recommends no treatment of subclinical HPV infection. The goal of treatment is to eliminate symptoms, namely clinically apparent warts, rather than address the underlying HPV infection. Current treatments do not eradicate the virus.

Ideally, treatment of condyloma should continue until all warts are gone. A repeated course of therapy is often required to achieve a wart-free state. Recurrence may be due to latent HPV in the surrounding normal tissue, HPV reinfection, or improper selection or use of a therapy modality. Nearly all treatment regimens have similar efficacy and rates of intolerance and toxicity. All are known to cause local pain and irritation. Any given treatment has a 40% to 80% rate of wart clearance and up to a 50% recurrence rate. It is unknown whether eliminating warts will decrease infectivity of current or future sexual partners.

The factors to consider when deciding on treatment include location and size of the warts, the patient's tolerance and preference, cost, convenience, and the clinician's preference. Patient-applied options allow the patient greater control; however, this requires good compliance, and the warts must be accessible by the patient or caregiver. Provider-applied treatments are good choices for large treatment areas. Data regarding the efficacy of using more than one modality at a time are lacking. It is common practice for health care providers to combine treatment modalities. Table 2 outlines current therapy regimens. Podophyllin resin (Podocon-25) is no longer recommended. Failure to respond after four treatments or failure to clear within 3 months warrants a change in therapy modality and possible reevaluation of the diagnosis.

Advise patients to abstain from sexual activity while undergoing treatment for genital warts.

Monitoring

Counseling of patients regarding prevention and recognition of condyloma as well as screening and treatment of sexual partners should be part of the comprehensive management plan. One should consider testing for other sexually transmitted diseases because

TABLE 1	Differential Diagnosis	
LESION	**APPEARANCE**
Verruca vulgaris	Occurs anywhere Tends to be thicker, drier, and hyperkeratotic
Molluscum contagiosum	Occurs anywhere Smooth, round papules with central umbilication
Seborrheic keratoses	Occurs anywhere Multiple waxy, rough, hyperpigmented papules
Condyloma latum	Moist, rounded, white papules of syphilis
Pearly penile papules	Smooth, uniform, small, 1–2mm at corona, benign
Vestibular papillae	Both sides of vulva, female equivalent of pearly penile papules
Lichen planus	Purplish, pruritic rash or flat-topped polygonal papules
Nonpigmented nevi	Occurs anywhere Flat or raised, reddish or flesh colored

TABLE 2	Treatment Regimens			
DRUG	**USE ON**	**ADVANTAGES**	**DISADVANTAGES**	**INSTRUCTIONS**
Patient Applied				
Podofilox 0.5% gel or solution (Condylox)	Moist warts	Relatively inexpensive	Avoid in pregnancy Avoid on mucous membranes Do not exceed 10cm² area Do not exceed 0.5mL daily; can have systemic side effects	Apply bid × 3d, then 4d off Repeat weekly May use for 4–6 cycles[3]
Imiquimod 5% cream (Aldara)	Dry or moist warts		Avoid with large warts >10cm² Requires compliance Hypo- or hyperpigmentation of treated skin can occur Local inflammatory skin reaction	Apply nightly, 3 times per week Use up to 16 weeks Wash off after 6–10h
Sinecatechins 15% ointment (Veregen)	Dry warts		Avoid in pregnancy and genital herpes Avoid in immunocompromised patients	Apply tid Use up to 16wk Do not wash off
Provider Applied				
Trichloroacetic acid (TCA) (Tri-Chlor) or bichloroacetic acid (BCA)[2] 80%–90% solution	Small, few Moist warts	May use on vagina, cervix May use on anal warts May use in pregnancy	Avoid with dry and large warts	Apply sparingly with cotton tip Air dry Repeat weekly to every other week Do not allow to "run" on normal skin Neutralize with soap or sodium bicarbonate
Cryotherapy	Small, few, flat Dry or moist	May use in pregnancy May use liquid nitrogen in vagina, meatus, anus	Avoid with large warts Avoid cryoprobe use in vagina or anus	Freeze q1–2wk Freeze 1–2mm border May offer/need local anesthesia
Surgery	Small or large Dry or moist	May use on anal warts Use on large warts and large treatment areas	Avoid in patients with bleeding disorder	Scissors, shave biopsy, punch excision, curettage, cautery, laser
Interferon-α-2b injections (Intron A)	Refractory warts		Expensive Flulike side effects	Multiple intralesional injections Several times a week Often requires specialty referral
Laser vaporization	Refractory warts	May use on intraurethral and large warts as well as large treatment areas	Expensive	Requires specialty referral

[2]Not available in the United States.
[3]Exceeds dosage recommended by the manufacturer.

they often coexist with HPV. Encourage patients to discuss their HPV diagnosis with sexual partners. Asymptomatic partners likely harbor a subclinical infection, and examination for genital warts is appropriate if lesions are suspected. Discuss the need for smoking cessation and regular physician examinations, including Pap smears, as ways to prevent early HPV-related neoplasm.

Complications
Anogenital HPV infection with high-risk genotypes is associated with squamous cell carcinoma of the cervix, vagina, vulva, penis, and anus. Persistent HPV infection is the most important risk factor for development of cervical intraepithelial neoplasia and cancer.

References
American Academy of Pediatrics. Human papillomavirus. In: Pickering LK, Baker CJ, Kimberlin DW, Long SS, editors. Red Book: 2009 Report of the Committee on Infectious Diseases. 28th ed. Elk Grove Village, IL: American Academy of Pediatrics; 2009. p. 477–483.
Centers for Disease Control and Prevention: *Epidemiology and Prevention of Vaccine-Preventable Diseases. The Pink Book*, ed 12, Washington, DC, 2011, Public Health Foundation.
Centers for Disease Control and Prevention: 2010 Sexually transmitted diseases treatment guidelines, *MMWR* 59:1–5, 2010. 69–78.
Centers for Disease Control and Prevention. Anogenital warts and human papillomavirus (HPV) infection HPV information for clinicians. Available at www.cdc.gov/std/treatment-guiedlines/toc.htm [accessed December 28, 2021].
Gilbert SM, Lambert SM, Weiner D: Extensive condylomata acuminata of the penis: Medical and surgical management, *Infect Urol* 16:65–76, 2003.
Kodner CM, Nasrat S: Management of genital warts, *Am Fam Physician* 70:2335–2342, 2004.

GENITAL ULCER DISEASE: CHANCROID, GRANULOMA INGUINALE, AND LYMPHOGRANULOMA

Method of
Todd Stephens, MD

Chancroid, granuloma inguinale, and lymphogranuloma venereum (LGV) are important genital ulcer diseases that should be included in the differential diagnosis of patients presenting with anal or genital ulcers with or without inguinal adenopathy. Syphilis and herpes simplex virus testing should be considered on all such patients because of similarities in clinical presentation. Testing or treatment for other potential sexually transmitted infections (STIs), including HIV, should be considered given the high risk for concomitant infection.

Chancroid
History
Chancroid, also called soft sore, was first distinguished from the hard chancre of syphilis by Ricord in 1838. Ducrey, in Naples, demonstrated that inoculation of material from the chancroid ulcer into the skin of the forearm could reproduce the ulcer, and he went on to identify the causative organism, which bears his name.

Epidemiology

Chancroid is an important cause of genital ulceration in most countries of the developing world, accounting for about 10 million cases annually. Chancroid was diagnosed in 60% of patients who had genital ulcers and who presented to STI clinics in Africa before the HIV epidemic. Now, herpes simplex lesions represent a higher percentage. The prevalence of this disease is highest among commercial sex workers, and the presence of chancroid lesions significantly increases the risk of transmission of HIV. Although generally rare in industrialized countries, there have been several well-documented outbreaks in urban centers of North America, particularly among men who have sex with men.

Etiology

Chancroid is caused by *Haemophilus ducreyi*, a small anaerobic Gram-negative bacillus that forms streptobacillary chains on Gram stain and grows only on enriched media.

Clinical Features

After an incubation of 3 to 7 days, a papule appears that soon ulcerates, leaving a soft ulcer with an undermined edge and a purulent base. Vesicles are not seen. About half of patients develop unilateral inguinal adenopathy (Figure 1). Both the adenopathy and the lesions are very painful. Lesions can be single or multiple, and atypical presentations occur. Kissing lesions often occur on adjacent cutaneous surfaces. Not infrequently, a giant ulcer develops with several smaller satellite ulcers around the periphery, which can mimic the ulcerative phase of herpes simplex. More than half of the lesions occur on the prepuce, particularly in uncircumcised men. In women, the majority of lesions are on the fourchette, labia, and perianal area. Adenopathy can progress to bubo formation with tender, overlying erythema. These buboes can rupture and produce inguinal abscesses.

Diagnosis

Gram stain of smears obtained from the ulcer base has been advocated in the past for diagnosis, but this lacks both sensitivity and specificity. The preferred diagnostic modality is swabs for culture from the ulcer base or undermined edge. These are plated directly on enriched media (GC agar and Mueller-Hinton agar base) and

Figure 1 Chancroid. This photo shows an early chancroid ulcer on the penis along with accompanying regional inguinal adenopathy. (Courtesy of Dr. Pirozzi, Centers for Disease Control and Prevention.)

incubated for 72 hours in an atmosphere of 5% carbon dioxide at 33°C. Polymerase chain reaction (PCR) and immunochromatography tests are also available.

However, clinically, a probable diagnosis of chancroid can be made if all of the following four criteria are met: (1) the patient has one or more painful genital ulcers; (2) the clinical presentation, appearance of genital ulcers and, if present, regional lymphadenopathy are typical for chancroid; (3) the patient has no evidence of T. pallidum infection by darkfield examination or NAAT (i.e., ulcer exudate or serous fluid) or by serologic tests for syphilis performed at least 7–14 days after onset of ulcers; and (4) HSV-1 or HSV-2 NAAT or HSV culture performed on the ulcer exudate or fluid are negative.

Treatment

The Centers for Disease Control and Prevention (CDC) recommend a syndromal management approach in which a positive diagnosis is suggested if the patient has one or more painful ulcers and no evidence of syphilis or herpes simplex virus. Ulcers with painful adenopathy are pathognomonic (Table 1 lists antimicrobial

TABLE 1 Clinical Features and Treatment Summary of Chancroid, Granuloma Inguinale, and Lymphogranuloma Venereum

FEATURES AND TREATMENT	CHANCROID	GRANULOMA INGUINALE	LYMPHOGRANULOMA VENEREUM
Clinical Features			
Incubation period	3–7 days	3–40 days	1–28 days
Primary lesion	Papule	Papule	Papule or vesicle
Ulcerative lesion painful	Yes	No	No
Lymphadenopathy	Yes (unilateral)	No	Yes (unilateral or bilateral)
Base	Purulent	Raised, easily bleeds	Nonvascular
Border	Round, raised, undermined edges	Irregular, expansion along skin folds	Irregular, ragged
Treatment			
Treatment of choice (any of the options listed)	Azithromycin (Zithromycin) 1g Ciprofloxacin (Cipro)[1] 500mg bid × 3d Ceftriaxone (Rocephin)[1] 250mg IM once	Azithromycin[1] 1g PO once a week or 500 mg qd for >3 weeks until all lesions have completely healed Doxycycline (Vibramycin) 100mg bid × 3 wks	Azithromycin[1] 1g weekly × 3wk Doxycycline 100mg bid × 3wk
Alternative treatment (any of the options listed)	Erythromycin (Ery-Tab)[1] 500mg qid × 7d	Azithromycin[1] 1g PO qwk × 3 wk Erythromycin[1] 500mg qid × 3 wk Ciprofloxacin[1] 750mg bid × 3 wk Ceftriaxone[1] 1 gm IM daily for at least 3 weeks and until all lesions have completely healed.	Erythromycin[1] 500mg qid × 3wk

[1]Not FDA approved for this indication.

treatment). The safety and efficacy of azithromycin (Zithromax) for pregnant and lactating women have not been established. Ciprofloxacin (Cipro)[1] is contraindicated during pregnancy and lactation. No adverse effects of chancroid on pregnancy outcome have been reported. Serologic testing for syphilis, HIV, and other appropriate STIs should be performed. Chancroidal ulcers should be kept clean with regular washing in soapy water and kept dry. Fluctuant buboes might require incision and drainage, which is preferable over needle aspiration. Treatment of all sexual partners within 60 days should be pursued, and treatment is similar to that for the source patient. Patients should not engage in sexual activity until the ulcers are healed.

Granuloma Inguinale (Donovanosis)

History
Granuloma inguinale was first recognized in India, where Donovan observed, in an oral lesion of the disease, the bodies that bear his name. There is considerable confusion about terminology between this disease and LGV, because various similar synonyms have been used inconsistently. Adding to the confusion, Donovan's name is associated with two tropical diseases that he discovered: leishmaniasis, with the discovery of intracellular protozoan inclusions that bear his name (Leishman-Donovan bodies), and granuloma inguinale (whose intracellular inclusions were believed to be caused by protozoa but are now known to be caused by bacteria).

Epidemiology
Endemic areas are localized to a few specific areas of the tropics, particularly India, Papua New Guinea, Brazil, and the eastern part of South Africa, particularly Durban. Commercial sex workers and men are primarily involved.

Etiology
The disease is caused by an encapsulated Gram-negative coccobacillus *Klebsiella granulomatis* (previously known as *Calymmatobacterium* or *Donovania granulomatis*).

Clinical Features
A firm, painless papule or nodule is the presenting sign of granuloma inguinale. The incubation period is variable from 3 to 40 days from inoculation. This nodule quickly ulcerates, and the base is highly vascular, is beefy red, and bleeds easily. Lymphadenopathy is not part of the clinical presentation of this disease, distinguishing granuloma inguinale from chancroid and LGV. However, the ulcer can be easily confused with chancroid, condyloma lata, ulcerated verrucous warts, and squamous carcinoma. Untreated, the ulcers slowly expand, particularly along skin folds toward the inguinal region or anus (Figure 2). The ulcers are flat

---

[1]Not FDA approved for this indication.

Figure 2 Granuloma inguinale. (Source: NEHC http://www.nhec.med.navy.mil/hp/sharp/std_pictures.htm)

and raised and have slightly hypertrophic margins, but the bases are typically free of pus and necrotic debris. Less-common presentations include extragenital lesions involving the neck and mouth; cervical lesions that resemble carcinoma; and involvement of the uterus, tubes, and ovaries, producing hard masses, abscesses, or frozen pelvis.

Diagnosis
Diagnosis requires the demonstration of intracellular Donovan bodies from Giemsa or Wright staining of smears taken from a swab of the ulcer base or from biopsy material.

Treatment
See Table 1 for antimicrobial treatment. Treatment should be continued until lesions are resolved and, if possible, a little longer to reduce the risk of relapse.

Lymphogranuloma Venereum

History
LGV was first differentiated from syphilis in 1906 by Wasserman, though the first full description of the disease was given by Durand, Nicolas, and Favre in 1913. In 1925, Frei developed an intradermal skin test that gave positive responses in most LGV patients. The term "tropical bubo" was associated with the disease later.

Epidemiology
LGV is largely confined to the tropics and is not a common STI. The global overall incidence is in a decline. It is seen more commonly in men, but since 2004, there has been a resurgence manifesting as proctitis in North America and Europe among HIV-positive men who have sex with men.

Etiology
LGV is a chlamydial infection caused by the invasive L1, L2, and L3 serovars of *Chlamydia trachomatis*, an intracellular gram-negative bacterium.

Clinical Features
LGV is essentially a systemic disease whose natural course is divided into three distinct phases. The initial phase of LGV is normally an inconspicuous genital lesion beginning as a typically small, painless papule or vesicle occurring 1 to 28 days after inoculation. This papule or vesicle quickly ulcerates and heals without a scar, and it often goes unrecognized by the patient (Figure 3). However, the second phase of LGV is the development of increasingly painful lymphadenopathy, often with fever and malaise. The lymphadenopathy progresses to bubo formation over 1 to 2 weeks. When a sexually active adult patient presents with an inguinal bubo not associated with genital ulcers, LGV is an important diagnosis to consider. The infected nodes are usually unilateral (bilateral in a third of cases) and often coalesce into a matted mass that can project outwards above or below the inguinal ligament, producing the pathognomonic groove sign present in 20% of patients with LGV. The buboes are likely to rupture, forming multiple sinuses. Untreated, LGV can cause extensive lymphatic damage, resulting in elephantiasis of the genitalia. Anal involvement, likewise, can lead to perirectal abscesses, fistulas, and rectal strictures. These complications represent the late phase of LGV.

Diagnosis
The diagnosis of LGV can only be confirmed using PCR methods of smears, scrapings, or aspirated material. Alternatively, the ability to perform micro-immunofluorescence serology testing using a fluorescein-conjugated monoclonal antibody and viewing the slide with a fluorescence microscope can demonstrate the inclusion bodies within the cytoplasm of macrophages. Gram staining by itself lacks appropriate sensitivity or specificity. Additional laboratory findings include leukocytosis, elevated erythrocyte sedimentation rate, and increases in immunoglobulin G and cryoglobulins.

Differential Diagnosis

Differential diagnosis should include drug-induced acne (especially from steroids), which can be identified by seeing all lesions at nearly the same stage of development. Rosacea should also be considered in the differential diagnosis of AV, though the age of onset and symptomatology are usually distinguishing.

Treatment

The topical therapy of AV includes the use of agents that are available over the counter or via prescription. Therapy choice may be influenced by age of the patient, site of involvement, extent and severity of disease, cost, and patient preference. Topical therapies may be used as monotherapy in combination with other topical agents or in combination with oral agents in both initial control and maintenance.

Additionally, it is key to set realistic expectations about how acne can be controlled with the regular use of a variety of agents and how it can take 6 to 8 weeks to see improvement. If these issues are not addressed, the likelihood of adherence and long-term improvement are low.

Commonly used topical acne therapies include benzoyl peroxide, salicylic acid, antibiotics, combination antibiotics with benzoyl peroxide, retinoids, retinoid with benzoyl peroxide (BP), retinoid with antibiotic, azelaic acid, and sulfone agents.

BP is an antibacterial agent that kills *P. acne* through the release of free oxygen radicals and is also mildly comedolytic. No resistance to this agent has been reported, and the addition of BP to regimens of antibiotic therapy enhances results and may reduce development of drug resistance. BP is available as topical washes, foams, creams, or gels and can be used as leave-on or wash-off agents. Strengths available for acne therapy range from 2.5% to 10% in prescription and over-the-counter products. Benzoyl peroxide therapy is limited by skin irritation, staining and bleaching of fabric, and uncommon contact allergy. Total skin contact time and formulation can also affect efficacy. Lower concentrations (e.g., 2.5–5%), water-based, and wash-off agents may be better tolerated in patients with more sensitive skin. Results may be noted in as soon as 5 days.

Topical antibiotics for acne accumulate in the follicle and have been postulated to work through antiinflammatory mechanisms and via antibacterial effects. These agents are best used in combination with BP, which increases efficacy and decreases the development of resistant bacterial strains. Monotherapy with topical antibiotics in the management of acne is not recommended because of the development of antibiotic resistance.

Clindamycin 1% solution or gel is currently the preferred topical antibiotic for acne therapy. Topical erythromycin in 2% concentration is available as a cream, gel, lotion, or pledget but has reduced efficacy in comparison with clindamycin because of resistance of cutaneous *Staphylococci* and *P. acnes*.

Topical retinoids (tretinoin [Retin-A, Altreno, Avita], adapalene [Differin], tazarotene [Tazorac, Arazlo], and trifarotene [Aklief]) are all extremely effective for abnormal keratinization and comedone development and thus treat existing lesions and prevent the development of new lesions. These can be irritating and come in a variety of strengths. Patients might need to start at the lowest strength with every-other-day dosing and work up to the highest strength needed and tolerated. Some formulations of tretinoin (primarily generic products) are not photo stable and should be applied in the evening. All are contraindicated in pregnancy.

Topical retinoids enhance other topical acne regimens and allow for maintenance of clearance after discontinuation of oral therapy. Retinoids are ideal for comedonal acne and, when used in combination with other agents, for all acne variants. Four topical products are available that combine a retinoid with other product: adapalene 0.1%/BP 2.5% gel (Epiduo) and tretinoin 0.1%/BP 3% cream (Twyneo) are approved for use in patients 9 years of age or older, while adapalene 0.3%/BP 2.5% gel (Epiduo Forte) and tretinoin 0.025%/clindamycin 1.2% (Veltin, Ziana) are approved for patients 12 years of age or older.

Salicylic acid preparations are comedolytic and can be used for patients who cannot tolerate either benzoyl peroxide or topical retinoids, although salicylic acid preparations have not been shown to be as effective. Azelaic acid 20% cream (Azelex) is mildly effective as a comedolytic, antibacterial, and antiinflammatory agent; it is also a category B in pregnancy.

The sulfone agent, dapsone 5% gel (Aczone), is available as a twice-daily agent for the therapy of AV. In clinical trials, topical dapsone showed modest to moderate efficacy, primarily in the reduction of inflammatory lesions. Combination with topical retinoids may be indicated if comedonal components are present. Topical dapsone may be oxidized by the coapplication of BP, causing orange-brown coloration of the skin, which can be brushed or washed off.

Topical dapsone 5% gel is pregnancy category C and has efficacy and safety data down to patients 12 years of age. Clascoterone cream 1% (Winlevi), an androgen receptor inhibitor, was approved by the FDA in 2021 for treatment of acne vulgaris in patients 12 years of age or older. Aluminum chloride[1] possesses antibacterial activity and therefore has been investigated in the treatment of acne. There is some evidence to suggest the efficacy of sodium sulfacetamide (Klaron, Ovace Plus[1]). Only Klaron lotion and topical suspension are indicated for treatment of acne vulgaris. Topical niacinamide (nicotinamide)[7] 2% to 4% gel is available over the counter.

For patients with moderate inflammatory and comedonal lesions, it can be appropriate to start both BP and topical retinoids at the initial visit; however, the applications should be separated in time because the BP will inactivate the retinoid. An effective regimen (if tolerated) is a BP wash in the morning and topical retinoid at bedtime.

Antibiotics should be added if response to topical BP and retinoids is inadequate at the 6- to 8-week follow-up visit. Topical clindamycin (Cleocin-T) and erythromycin (Akne-Mycin) have demonstrated efficacy and can be used twice a day at the same time as the BP. There are also combination agents that conveniently add the two agents into a single preparation: clindamycin 1%/BP 5% gel (BenzaClin), clindamycin 1.2%/BP 2.5% gel (Acanya), clindamycin 1.2%/BP 5% gel (Duac) and erythromycin 3%/BP 5% gel (Benzamycin). They are more expensive, however.

Oral antibiotics should be started if the acne is moderate to severe, if it is too widespread to reasonably cover with topical antibiotics, or if there is an inadequate response after 6 to 8 weeks of topical antibiotics. The tetracycline class of antibiotics should be considered first-line therapy in moderate to severe acne, except when contraindicated because of other circumstances (i.e., pregnancy, <8 years of age, or allergy).

Minocycline in an extended-release form (Ximino) appears safest (at 1 mg/kg once daily), but no dose response was found for efficacy. Doxycycline appears effective in the 1.7 to 2.4 mg/kg dose range. Subantimicrobial dosing of doxycycline (i.e., 20 mg twice daily [immediate release] to 40 mg daily [delayed release][3]) has also shown efficacy in patients with moderate inflammatory acne. Adverse events with the tetracycline class vary with each medication. Photosensitivity can be seen with the tetracycline class, doxycycline being more photosensitizing than minocycline. Doxycycline is more frequently associated with gastrointestinal disturbances. Doxycycline is primarily metabolized by the liver and can be used safely in most patients with renal impairment. Minocycline has been associated with tinnitus, dizziness, and pigment deposition of the skin, mucous membranes, and teeth. Minocycline-induced skin pigmentation is more common in patients taking higher doses for longer periods of time. The rare serious events associated with minocycline include autoimmune disorders, such as drug reaction with eosinophilia and systemic symptoms (DRESS), drug-induced lupus, and other hypersensitivity reactions. Finally, pseudo tumor cerebri is a rare phenomenon associated with the tetracycline class of antibiotics.

Erythromycin[1] and azithromycin[1] have also been used in the treatment of acne. Azithromycin has been primarily studied in the treatment of acne with different pulse dosing regimens ranging from 3 times a week to 4 days a month, with azithromycin being an effective treatment in the time span of usually 2 to 3 months.

---

[1] Not FDA approved for this indication.
[3] Dosage exceeds recommendation by the manufacturer.
[7] Available as dietary supplement

However, a recent study compared using azithromycin 3 times per month to daily doxycycline use and showed that doxycycline had superior results. The macrolide class of antibiotics is most commonly associated with gastrointestinal disturbances. Erythromycin is associated with a higher incidence of diarrhea, nausea, and abdominal discomfort than azithromycin.

TMP-SMX (trimethoprim-sulfamethoxazole [Bactrim, Septra DS])[1] taken twice daily also has side effects to consider but can be useful when other agents are not tolerated. The adverse events of TMP/SMX include gastrointestinal upset, photosensitivity, and drug eruptions. Multiple skin reactions have been observed with patients on this medication, the most severe eruptions being Stevens-Johnson syndrome and toxic epidermal necrolysis. Other adverse effects can include blood dyscrasias, such as neutropenia, agranulocytosis, aplastic anemia, and thrombocytopenia. Although these are rare adverse events, patients on long-term therapy with this medication should be periodically monitored with a complete blood cell count.

Penicillins and cephalosporins are sometimes used in the treatment of acne and can be used as an alternative treatment when circumstances dictate. In particular, these medications represent a useful option in patients who may be pregnant or who have allergies to the other classes of antibiotics.

Sarecycline (Seysara), a tetracycline antibiotic, has recently been approved for inflammatory lesions of nonnodular moderate to severe acne vulgaris in patients 9 years of age or older. The dose is weight based (33 to 54 kg: 60 mg QD, 55 to 84 kg: 100 mg QD, 85 to 136 kg: 150 mg QD). Adverse effects include photosensitivity and gastrointestinal distress. It is contraindicated in pregnancy and young children.

All oral agents should be used in combination with BP and/or a topical retinoid but not in combination with topical antibiotics. If significant improvement is noted, oral agents should be decreased after 3 to 4 months or stopped in order to attempt maintenance control with topical agents. Limiting systemic antibiotic use is urged because of the reported associations of inflammatory bowel disease, pharyngitis, C. difficile infection, and the induction of Candida vulvovaginitis.

Combined oral contraceptives can be very helpful in female patients with moderate acne because of their antiandrogenic effects, which decrease sebum production. There are currently four combined oral contraceptives (COCs) approved by the FDA for the treatment of acne. They are ethinyl estradiol/norgestimate (Ortho Tricyclen), ethinyl estradiol/norethindrone acetate/ferrous fumarate (Estrostep Fe, Tilia Fe, Tri-Legest Fe), ethinyl estradiol/drospirenone (Yasmin, Yaz), and ethinyl estradiol/drospirenone/levomefolate (Beyaz, Rajani).

COC use is associated with cardiovascular risks. Venous thromboembolic events (VTEs) have been the center of an ongoing debate regarding COCs. Traditionally, higher doses of ethinyl estradiol have been linked to increased risks of VTE. However, in recent years, some progestins have been implicated as risk factors for VTE. A recent Cochrane meta-analysis evaluated 25 publications reporting on 26 studies focused on oral contraceptives and venous thrombosis. The analysis concluded that all COC use increases the risk of VTE compared with nonusers. The relative risk of venous thrombosis for COCs with 30 to 35 micrograms of ethinyl estradiol and gestodene desogestrel, cyproterone acetate, or drospirenone was similar and about 50% to 80% higher than for COCs with levonorgestrel. To put this increased risk into perspective, it is important to note that the baseline risk of VTE in nonpregnant, nonusers of COCs is 1 to 5 per 10,000 woman-years. Users of COCs have a VTE risk of 3 to 9 per 10,000 woman-years. Users of drospirenone containing COCs have a VTE risk of about 10 per 10,000 woman-years. Pregnant women have a VTE risk between 5 and 20 per 10,000 woman-years, and women within 12 weeks postpartum have a VTE risk of between 40 and 65 per 10,000 woman-years.

Oral isotretinoin (Accutane, Claravis) has demonstrated marked benefit for patients with severe recalcitrant acne, even inducing a full remission. It is a potent teratogen; therefore every woman of child-bearing potential taking isotretinoin should be carefully counseled regarding various contraceptive methods (including long-acting reversible contraception) that are available. Isotretinoin has a host of other significant side effects, including cheilitis, epistaxis, photosensitivity, and many others. Prescribed at 0.5 to 2 mg/kg per day over 20 weeks, it is like chemotherapy for acne. It is extremely tightly regulated, and both prescribers and patients must register with the iPledge program to write for the medicine and to receive the prescriptions. See www.ipledgeprogram.com. When all the precautions are managed, it can be an extremely effective option for the patients with the worst cases of acne.

References

Gannon M, Underhill M, Wellik KE: Which oral antibiotics are best for acne? J Fam Pract 60:290–292, 2011.

Knutsen-Larson S, Dawson AL, Dunnick CA, et al: Acne vulgaris: pathogenesis, treatment, and needs assessment, Dermatol Clin 30:99–106, 2012.

Strauss JS, Krowchuk DP, Leyden JJ, et al: Guidelines of care for acne vulgaris management, J Am Acad Dermatol 56:651–663, 2007.

Titus S, Hodge J: Diagnosis and treatment of acne, Am Fam Physician 86:734–740, 2012.

Zaenglein AL, Pathy AL, Schlosser BJ, et al: Guidelines of care for the management of acne vulgaris, J Am Acad Dermatol 74(Issue 5):945–973, 2016. e33.

ATOPIC DERMATITIS

Method of
Peck Y. Ong, MD

CURRENT DIAGNOSIS

- Itch must be present for the diagnosis of atopic dermatitis. In addition, the diagnosis must include three or more of the following criteria (U.K. Working Party's Diagnostic Criteria for Atopic Dermatitis):
  - History of generalized dry skin
  - Visible flexural dermatitis
  - Onset of the skin condition before 2 years (not used for patients younger than 4 years)
  - History of itchy skin involving the following areas: elbows, behind knees, front of ankles, or around the neck
  - History of asthma or allergic rhinitis (or for children younger than 4 years, history of atopic disease in a first-degree relative)

CURRENT THERAPY

- Bathe or shower for 10 to 20 minutes daily and pat dry gently.
- Follow immediately by applying an emollient on unaffected areas and an antiinflammatory medication on affected areas.
- Use topical corticosteroids as a first-line antiinflammatory medication. Alternative medications are topical calcineurin inhibitors, topical phosphodiesterase 4 inhibitor topical or oral janus kinase (JAK) inhibitors andmonoclonal antibodies targetting IL-13 or IL-4/IL-13.
- Avoid environmental triggers such as extreme heat, humidity, or dryness.
- Avoid food allergens that may cause anaphylaxis. Consult an allergist regarding the interpretation of serum-specific IgE tests or food challenge.
- Treat skin infection only when clinical signs are present (e.g., oozing, impetigo).
- Severe, generalized infection or vesicular lesions may indicate herpes simplex virus infection; persistent fever may indicate invasive S. aureus infection.

Atopic Dermatitis

---

[1] Not FDA approved for this indication.

Skin tests and serum specific IgE are useful in the context of negative or undetectable test results because they have a negative predictive value of more than 95%. The level of a positive test result (i.e., skin test wheal size or serum-specific IgE level), which correlates with the chance of a reaction, should be interpreted in the context of a clinical reaction. Consider consultation with an allergist regarding food challenge if there are still concerns regarding positive serum-specific IgE. More accurate epitope-specific IgE assays may be available to clinicians in the near future.

Patients with confirmed food allergy should avoid any amount of the food allergen. Parents or patients should be instructed to read food allergen labels carefully. All packaged foods in the United States are required to label the contents of milk, eggs, peanuts, wheat, soybeans, fish, shellfish, or tree nuts. Organizations, such as the Food Allergy Research & Education, can provide patients and parents with useful information on potential hidden food allergens and alternative food sources.

AD children often have multiple food allergies, including cow's milk and soy, and the use of a hydrolyzed or amino acid–based formula can provide an alternative source of nutrition. For these patients, consultation with a dietitian can be helpful in managing food avoidance and nutrition needs.

Patients or parents of children with anaphylactic reactions should be prescribed and instructed on the use of an epinephrine autoinjector (EpiPen or Auvi-Q 0.15 mg for patients who weigh more than 15 kg but less than 30 kg; 0.3 mg for patients who weigh 30 kg or more, while Auvi-Q 0.1 mg for patients who weigh 7.5–15 kg).

Infants with severe AD who consume peanut products early have a 86% relative risk reduction in the development of peanut allergy. For any infants with AD under a year, clinicians should consider introducing peanut products early in their diet according to the guidelines of National Institute of Allergy and Infectious Disease, or consult an allergist.

Infections
Most AD patients are colonized by *S. aureus* on their skin lesions or in their nostrils. The frequency of colonization increases with AD severity. Exacerbation of AD is frequently associated with secondary *S. aureus* skin infections. Other common skin pathogens in AD include group A β-hemolytic *Streptococcus* and herpes simplex virus (HSV), which causes eczema herpeticum (Figure 2). Many reports have documented invasive *S. aureus* infections such as bacteremia, septic arthritis, osteomyelitis, and endocarditis in AD patients. Persistent fever or focal limb pain should alert the physician to the possibility of these infections.

The reasons for the high rate of bacterial colonization and skin infections in AD are not completely understood. A defective skin barrier and decreased cutaneous innate immunity (i.e., deficiency in natural skin antibiotics) likely contribute to the frequency of skin infections in patients with AD.

Because of the concern about increasing bacterial resistance, antibiotics are not recommended unless clinical infection is confirmed. The use of dilute bleach in treating AD remains controversial.

Inhalant Allergies and Asthma
Eighty-five percent of AD infants have concurrent respiratory allergies or are at risk for allergic rhinitis or asthma. However, whether inhalant allergens lead to a worsening of AD remains controversial. Randomized, double-blind, placebo-controlled studies have shown positive and negative effects of house dust mites (HDM) as a trigger for AD symptoms. Because there is no serious side effect associated with the use of HDM-proof bed and pillow encasings, unless cost is an issue, these encasings are recommended for AD patients with HDM sensitization. Further research is needed to confirm the

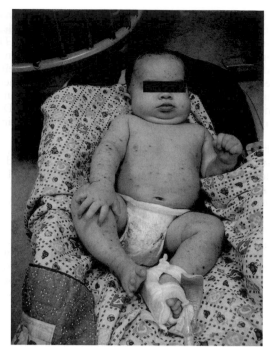

Figure 2 Eczema herpeticum.

role of inhalant allergens, including furry pets and pollens, as triggers for AD.

Referral to Specialists
Patients who have failed topical treatments or who have been limited by their eczema in daily activities should be considered for referral to specialists in allergy/immunology or dermatology for systemic treatments.

References
Beattie PE, Lewis-Jones MS: A comparative study of impairment of quality of life in children with skin disease and children with other chronic childhood diseases, *Br J Dermatol* 155:145–151, 2006.

Beck LA, Thaçi D, Hamilton JD, et al: Dupilumab treatment in adults with moderate-to-severe atopic dermatitis, *N Engl J Med* 371:130–139, 2014.

Chopra R, Vakharia PP, Sacotte R, Silverberg JI: Efficacy of bleach baths in reducing severity of atopic dermatitis: a systematic review and meta-analysis, *Ann Allergy Asthma Immunol* 119(5):435–440, 2017.

Du Toit G, Roberts G, Sayre PH, et al: Randomized trial of peanut consumption in infants at risk for peanut allergy, *N Engl J Med* 372:803–813, 2015.

Eichenfield LF, Basu S, Calvarese B, et al: Effect of desonide hydrogel 0.05% on the hypothalamic-pituitary-adrenal axis in pediatric subjects with moderate to severe atopic dermatitis, *Pediatr Dermatol* 24:289–295, 2007.

Elias PM: Barrier-repair therapy for atopic dermatitis: corrective lipid biochemical therapy, *Expert Rev Dermatol* 3:441–452, 2008.

Faught J, Bierl C, Barton B, Kemp A: Stress in mothers of young children with eczema, *Arch Dis Child* 92:683–686, 2007.

Friedlander SF, Hebert AA, Allen DB: for the Fluticasone Pediatrics Safety Study Group: Safety of fluticasone propionate cream 0.05% for the treatment of severe and extensive atopic dermatitis in children as young as 3 months, *J Am Acad Dermatol* 46:387–393, 2002.

Leung DYM, Paller AS, Guttman-Yassky E. New therapies for atopic dermatitis: How will they impact skin care? *Ann Allergy Asthma Immunol* 31:S1081-1206(22)00044-8, 2022. https://doi.org/10.1016/j.anai.2022.01.023. Epub ahead of print. PMID: 35093553.

Paller AS, Fölster-Holst R, Chen SC, et al: No evidence of increased cancer incidence in children using topical tacrolimus for atopic dermatitis, *J Am Acad Dermatol* 83(2):375–381, 2020. Aug.

Suprun M, Sicherer SH, Wood RA, et al: Early epitope-specific IgE antibodies are predictive of childhood peanut allergy, *J Allergy Clin Immunol* 146(5):1080–1088, 2020.

Togias A, Cooper SF, Acebal ML, et al: Addendum guidelines for the prevention of peanut allergy in the United States: report of the National Institute of Allergy and Infectious Diseases-sponsored expert panel, *J Allergy Clin Immunol* 139:29–44, 2017.

Wang V, Boguniewicz J, Boguniewicz M, Ong PY: The infectious complications of atopic dermatitis, *Ann Allergy Asthma Immunol* 126(1):3–12, 2021.

AUTOIMMUNE BULLOUS DISEASES

Method of
Dominic J. Wu, MD; and Anand Rajpara, MD

CURRENT DIAGNOSIS

- There is a significant overlap between the major autoimmune bullous diseases, which include pemphigus vulgaris, bullous pemphigoid, dermatitis herpetiformis, linear IgA bullous disease, and more.
- Biopsy is usually required for diagnosis, including routine hematoxylin and eosin stain (H&E) histology and other special tests including direct immunofluorescence (DIF), indirect immunofluorescence (IIF), and ELISA.
- Preferred biopsy sites include edge or entire intact blister/bulla (H&E), perilesional "normal" appearing skin (DIF).
- Different staining patterns on DIF, salt-split skin, and IIF can help differentiate between diseases that appear similar on routine histology.
- It is important to evaluate for other causes of blistering disease, including infectious causes such as bullous impetigo, herpes simplex virus, varicella zoster virus, and noninfectious causes such as severe contact allergic dermatitis, poison ivy dermatitis, and others.

CURRENT THERAPY

- Immunosuppressive medications are the mainstay treatment for autoimmune bullous diseases.
- Specific treatments for each diagnosis are listed under each section. Many of the treatment regimens are not Food and Drug Administration (FDA)–approved treatments and should only be attempted by experienced clinicians familiar with each medication and their side effect profiles and monitoring parameters.
- Traditional first-line therapy is with oral corticosteroids to induce remission, with or without adjunctive steroid-sparing therapy.
- Topical corticosteroids should be attempted for milder cases of bullous pemphigoid prior to initiation of systemic corticosteroids because of side effects and risks for systemic steroids and efficacy of topicals.
- Adjunctive steroid-sparing therapy may help clinicians lower and eventually taper the doses of corticosteroids.
- Patients on higher doses of corticosteroids and/or longer courses of treatment with corticosteroids may require prophylaxis or treatment of osteoporosis and peptic ulcer disease.
- Early involvement of relevant specialties is critical given the complex nature of the disease and treatment options.

Epidemiology

The autoimmune bullous diseases are a heterogenous group of diseases, mostly occurring in the elderly. Please see each section for specific epidemiologic comments.

Pathophysiology

Specific antibodies and pathophysiology will be discussed under specific diseases discussed in this chapter.

Diagnosis

There is significant clinical overlap between the major autoimmune bullous diseases. In addition to obtaining a detailed clinical history, biopsies are usually required for diagnosis. Ideal sample sites for routine histology (H&E) are of the blister/bullae (intact if possible, or the edge of the bulla), and normal-appearing perilesional skin for direct immunofluorescence (DIF). Punch biopsies (usually 4 mm punch tool) or deeper shave biopsies are common biopsy methods. Specific staining patterns are noted under each individual disease entity below. Indirect immunofluorescence (IIF) may also be helpful, although it is beyond the scope of this chapter and will not be discussed in detail.

Pemphigus

Pathophysiology

In normal skin tissue, epithelial cells are held together by adherens and desmosome protein junctions. In pemphigus diseases, different desmosomal proteins are targeted by autoantibodies, causing a loss of connection between adjacent cells, resulting in splitting of skin layers. The causes of pemphigus diseases vary, including idiopathic, drug-induced cases (traditionally penicillamine and ACE inhibitors such as captopril), underlying conditions such as thymoma, myasthenia gravis, autoimmune thyroiditis, and more. Epidemiologic studies have shown higher incidence in people of Jewish ancestry. Certain genetic predispositions have also been identified, including HLA-DRB1, HLA-DR4, and HLA-DR6.

The pemphigus group of bullous diseases includes (1) pemphigus vulgaris and pemphigus vegetans, (2) pemphigus foliaceus and pemphigus erythematosus, and (3) paraneoplastic pemphigus. Pemphigus vulgaris and pemphigus vegetans are caused by circulating IgG autoantibodies, primarily against desmoglein 3 (Dsg3), which is mostly found on the lower portion of the epidermis. Desmogleins are desmosomal cadherin proteins that form desmosomes, which join cells together. Patients with pemphigus foliaceus have autoantibodies directed against desmoglein 1 (Dsg1). As its name denotes, paraneoplastic pemphigus is a paraneoplastic syndrome associated with an underlying neoplastic disorder (most frequently non-Hodgkin's lymphoma, CLL, Castleman's disease, thymoma, sarcoma, and Waldenström's macroglobulinemia). In paraneoplastic pemphigus, patients may have circulating autoantibodies against nearly all the different components of the desmosome junction including plakin family proteins and both Dsg1 and Dsg3.

Clinical Manifestations

Pemphigus vulgaris presents with painful flaccid skin blisters/bullae and erosions in the oral cavity. Oral involvement is typically seen in cases of pemphigus vulgaris, which can be quite helpful in distinguishing between pemphigus foliaceus (typically no oral involvement) and other autoimmune bullous diseases such as bullous pemphigoid, in which a smaller subset of patients have oral mucosal involvement. Nikolsky sign (shearing of skin with slight pressure or rubbing of perilesional skin) and Asboe-Hansen (pressure placed on intact bulla results in spreading of bulla to surrounding skin) are both found in cases of pemphigus vulgaris.

Pemphigus foliaceus (including the Brazilian endemic variant Fogo Selvagem and pemphigus erythematosus) typically present with impetigo-like crusted erosions involving the face, scalp, and upper trunk. Blisters tend to be more superficial and fragile, creating what is frequently described as a cornflake-like scale and crust. Nikolsky sign also is typically positive. Pemphigus foliaceus typically spares mucosal surfaces, differentiating it from pemphigus vulgaris.

Paraneoplastic pemphigus presents as a more severe-appearing form of pemphigus. In addition to pemphigus vulgaris-like skin findings, paraneoplastic pemphigus typically presents with severe mucosal involvement with extensive crusted stomatitis extending onto the vermillion lip and scarring conjunctivitis. There may also be erosions in the esophagus, genitalia, and nasopharynx. Palms and soles may also be affected, distinguishing this entity from pemphigus vulgaris.

Diagnosis

In addition to classic clinical findings, biopsy is usually required to confirm diagnosis with routine H&E histology, DIF, and other workup as indicated (including IIF, ELISA, and immunoprecipitation/immunoblotting).

Pemphigus vulgaris biopsies initially show eosinophilic spongiosis, followed by suprabasilar acantholysis without keratinocyte necrosis. Classically, one would also expect to find a tombstoning pattern of vertically oriented keratinocytes of the basal layer attached to the basement membrane zone (BMZ). DIF shows intercellular IgG deposition (with or without C3) in a chicken-wire appearance, with greater concentration in the lower epidermis.

Pemphigus foliaceus and its variants appear similarly to pemphigus vulgaris on histology, but on DIF one would expect to find higher concentration of IgG +/- C3 deposition in the upper epidermis. Pemphigus erythematosus may also have granular to linear IgG and C3 deposition along the BMZ.

Paraneoplastic pemphigus histology demonstrates intercellular IgG and C3 deposition, in addition to linear IgG and C3 deposition along the BMZ. Gold standard of diagnosis of paraneoplastic pemphigus is immunoprecipitation or immunoblotting for antibodies against plakin proteins, and ELISA detection of anti-DsG antibodies.

Treatment and Monitoring

Pemphigus can be a severe and deadly disease requiring immunosuppressive treatment. Because of the complex nature of the disease and treatment, early involvement of relevant specialists including but not limited to dermatology, rheumatology, gastroenterology, otolaryngology, oral medicine, and ophthalmology is critical. Clinicians prescribing immunosuppressive medications must be comfortable and familiar with the medications, including their side effect profile and monitoring parameters.

First-line treatment of pemphigus diseases is systemic corticosteroids for rapid disease control in conjunction with steroid-sparing immunosuppressive medications such as azathioprine (Imuran),[1] mycophenolate mofetil (CellCept),[1] or rituximab (Rituxan only for pemphigus vulgaris). Although numerous systemic steroids may be used, most frequently clinicians use prednisone 1 mg/kg/day. Higher doses of prednisone (100–150 mg daily) may sometimes be needed for more severe diseases, but prolonged use of higher doses may result in greater morbidity and mortality. In our practice, we aim to taper patients completely off of corticosteroids within 3 to 6 months. However, low-dose regimens such as prednisone 5 mg daily may be required for several years. For patients on long-term corticosteroid therapy vitamin D, calcium supplementation, and especially bisphosphonate therapy can help prevent or treat osteoporosis, while H_2 blockers (e.g., famotidine [Pepcid][1], ranitidine [Zactac][2]) or PPIs (e.g., omeprazole [Prilosec][1]) are recommended to prevent or treat peptic ulcer disease in patients taking concomitant nonsteroidal antiinflammatory drugs (NSAIDs).

Corticosteroid therapy should be initiated in combination with a steroid sparing agent because these agents typically take 3 to 6 months to take full effect. First-line steroid sparing agents include azathioprine[1] (2–3 mg/kg/day based on the patient's thiopurine methyltransferase [TPMT] levels), mycophenolate mofetil[1] (1–1.5 g twice daily), and rituximab (Rituxan only for pemphigus vulgaris). In our practice we dose rituximab IV 1000 mg once every 2 weeks for 2 doses, followed by maintenance dose of 500 mg at months 12 and 18, and every 6 months thereafter based on clinical response. Milder cases may be treated with dapsone[1] (25 mg daily for 1 week, then increase dose in 25 mg increments weekly based on clinical response up to maximum 100 mg daily), niacinamide[1] (nicotinamide), and tetracycline.[1] Topical corticosteroids such as triamcinolone 0.1% ointment or clobetasol. 0.05% ointment twice daily may be helpful in milder cases for pruritic

or painful skin lesions. Second-line steroid-sparing agents with varying levels of efficacy described include methotrexate[1] (10–25 mg once weekly with folic acid supplementation[1] on days not taking methotrexate), cyclophosphamide,[1] and TNF-a inhibitors.[1] Severe refractory cases may be treated with IV immunoglobulin (IVIG)[1] therapy, or with rituximab or cyclophosphamide,[1] with or without plasmapheresis.

Treatment response should be monitored with IIF or ELISA levels, which can help detect quantitative levels of circulating antibodies.

Patients with paraneoplastic pemphigus may also have improvement in cutaneous lesions with systemic steroids, with or without adjunctive steroid-sparing agents. Excision of benign neoplasms such as thymomas and localized Castleman's disease may lead to resolution within months. Cases of paraneoplastic pemphigus from underlying malignancies are highly recalcitrant to treatment and carry a poor prognosis of up to a 90% mortality rate.

Bullous Pemphigoid
Pathophysiology

Bullous pemphigoid (BP) is the most common autoimmune blistering disorder and typically affects elderly patients. Patients with BP have circulating autoantibodies against different proteins, along the BMZ. The most common and important antigenic targets in BP include IgG autoantibodies targeted against the hemidesmosomal proteins BP180 (also referred to as BPAG2 and type XVII collagen) and BP230 (also referred to as BPAG1). BP180 is the primary mediator of BP. Complement activation causes eosinophilic and neutrophilic infiltration to the tissues, release of mediators and degradatory enzymes resulting in subepidermal blisters. Drug-induced cases of BP are most frequently because of furosemide, ACE inhibitors, NSAIDs, and antibiotics including cephalosporins, beta-lactams, and D-penicillamine.

Clinical Manifestations

BP initially presents as pruritic urticarial papules and plaques on the trunk, abdomen, and flexures of extremities. This progresses to tense fluid-filled blisters and bullae on a urticarial base. Patients often complain of intense pruritus. After the bullae and blisters rupture, denuded areas of erosions and crusted areas remain.

Diagnosis

In addition to clinical findings and history, biopsy is required for diagnosis. On histology, lesions of the urticarial phase demonstrate eosinophilic spongiosis with eosinophils lining up at the dermoepidermal junction (DEJ). During the bullous phase, lesions demonstrate subepidermal split with numerous eosinophils in the blister cavity and dense inflammation in the dermis. DIF is the most sensitive test for BP and shows linear IgG and C3 deposition along the DEJ. Salt-split skin DIF is a special type of modified DIF study that uses NaCl solution to split the biopsy specimen at the lamina lucida, allowing for localization of the bound antibodies. BP antibodies classically show staining on the top of the blister cavity. Unlike in pemphigus vulgaris, IIF levels do not correlate well with BP disease activity and are not useful for determining treatment response.

Treatment

Although BP carries lower mortality risk compared with pemphigus vulgaris, treatment is indicated for its significant morbidity.

There have not been many controlled trials performed for BP therapies, and recommendations tend to be based on consensus opinion and clinician experience. Most frequently used first-line therapy includes high-potency topical corticosteroids or systemic corticosteroids and steroid-sparing immunosuppressive medications. Some studies have shown that topical clobetasol propionate (Temovate, Clobex) 0.05% may have better response than oral prednisone 0.5–1 mg/kg/day, with

---

[1] Not FDA approved for this indication.
[2] Not available in the United States.

fewer side effects. Although prednisone has traditionally been the standard approach to oral therapy, side effects should be weighed highly, and topical steroids should be attempted first in mild to moderate cases. Dapsone[1] (see pemphigus vulgaris section on treatment) or tetracycline[1] (500 mg four times daily) given with niacinamide[1] (500 mg three times daily) may also be efficacious as first-line treatment. There have been increasing reports of successful treatment with dupilumab (Dupixent)[1] (600 mg subcutaneous injection loading dose, followed by 300 mg every other week) and prednisone. We have implemented this successfully in patients with BP in our institution.

Immunosuppressive medications may be necessary in severe or recalcitrant cases. Azathioprine[1] and mycophenolate mofetil[1] have shown similar efficacy. Rituximab,[1] methotrexate,[1] cyclophosphamide,[1] IVIG,[1] and cyclosporine[1] (4–5 mg/kg/day) are potentially effective second-line options. IVIG may be especially helpful in steroid-resistant cases. Dosing regimens for these medications are similar to those of pemphigus. There have been several case reports of omalizumab (Xolair)[1] (monoclonal anti-IgE antibody) showing good response in some patients.

In our practice, for patients with severe bullous pemphigoid and no contraindications, we start prednisone at 0.5 mg/kg/day along with mycophenolate mofetil. We aim to taper the patient off of steroids in 3 to 6 months while increasing mycophenolate mofetil to a max dose of 1.5 gm twice daily if needed. For patients with mild to moderate disease, or in patients with severe disease but contraindications to corticosteroids and/or immunosuppressants, we treat with topical steroids in conjunction with doxycycline/nicotinamide, IVIG, and/or dapsone.

Denuded, eroded areas tend to heal spontaneously and may not require further treatment other than appropriate wound care. BP is considered a chronic condition, although some cases may be self-limited over a period of about 5 years. High levels of BP180 at the time of discontinuing therapy are associated with a higher risk of relapse.

Mucous Membrane Pemphigoid
Pathophysiology
Mucous membrane pemphigoid (MMP), also referred to as *cicatricial pemphigoid*, is a rare autoimmune bullous disease with numerous targets in the anchoring filament zone including epiligrin (also referred to as laminin 332), $\alpha_6\beta_4$ integrin (specifically the β_4 subunit), and c-terminus of BP180. Antiepiligrin MMP has a strong association with underlying malignancy, most frequently adenocarcinoma. Patients with antibodies against the $\alpha_6\beta_4$ integrin may have exclusive ocular involvement. MMP most frequently affects the elderly, with a female predominance.

Clinical Manifestations
As its name denotes, MMP mostly involves the mucosa, most commonly the oral and conjunctival mucosa. Patients with oral involvement present with numerous painful chronic erosions of the oral mucosa including the gingiva, buccal mucosa, palate, and lips. Eye involvement is typically bilateral, initially presenting as a relatively nonspecific conjunctivitis, which progresses to fibrosis and eventual formation of adhesions of the bulbar and palpebral conjunctiva (symblepharon), ectropion, dry eyes, and inward facing eyelashes (trichiasis). Skin involvement is less common and tends to be more limited. The most common extramucosal sites include the scalp, face, neck, and upper trunk. Skin lesions may heal with atrophic scars, which may help distinguish this entity from BP.

[1] Not FDA approved for this indication.

Diagnosis
In addition to clinical history[1] and examination findings, biopsy is required for diagnosis including routine histology, DIF, and salt-split skin. IIF may also be helpful. Routine histology findings are similar to BP with fewer eosinophils. DIF staining shows linear IgG, IgA, +/- C3 deposition along the BMZ. Salt-split skin testing shows an epidermal staining pattern, except for antiepiligrin, which shows dermal staining pattern.

Treatment
For patients with mild, limited oral disease, treatment with topical triamcinolone acetonide (Oralone) 0.1% dental paste twice daily to oral lesions can be quite effective. Dapsone[1] (start 25 mg daily and titrate slowly based on response after 1 week) is our first-line systemic treatment for mild-moderate oral mucosal disease. Limited cutaneous disease can be treated with topical corticosteroids such as triamcinolone 0.1% ointment or clobetasol 0.05% ointment twice daily to affected areas on the body. Tetracycline[1] (500 mg four times daily) with niacinamide[1] (500 mg three times daily) may also be effective.

In patients with more severe oral disease and/or ocular disease, treatment with systemic steroids and cyclophosphamide is often needed. Most frequently oral prednisone 1 mg/kg/day is started with cyclophosphamide[1] (1–2 mg/kg/day), and therapy may continue after clinical remission for maintenance. Clinicians should attempt to taper prednisone after remission is achieved if possible, although some patients may continue to require low doses of prednisone to prevent recurrence. Ocular disease may result in scarring, and early involvement of an experienced ophthalmologist is essential.

MMP is a chronic condition which may result in scarring, disfigurement, and even blindness.

Linear IgA Bullous Dermatosis/Chronic Bullous Disease of Childhood
Pathophysiology
Adult-onset linear IgA bullous dermatosis (LABD) is a rare autoimmune subepidermal bullous disease affecting elderly patients greater than 60 years old. Chronic bullous disease of childhood (CBDC) is typically a self-limited bullous disease affecting young children beginning around 2 or 3 years old and may remit by teenage years. Patients with LABD/CBDC have circulating IgA autoantibodies targeting antigens derived from BPAG2, and some patients may have both IgA and IgG autoantibodies. Medication-induced LABD/CBDC is most frequently caused by vancomycin, followed by penicillin and cephalosporin antibiotics, captopril, NSAIDs, phenytoin, and many more offending medications.

Clinical Manifestations
Both adult-onset LABD and CBDC present with tense blisters/bullae and urticarial plaques that may be arranged in an annular or polycyclic formation, often described as *crown of jewels arrangement*. Individual lesions may appear quite similar to that of bullous pemphigoid and dermatitis herpetiformis. The most frequently affected sites include the trunk, flexures of extremities, groin, buttocks, and the face (in children). Patients may or may not have mucosal involvement.

Diagnosis
Biopsies of early urticarial lesions may show diffuse neutrophilic infiltrate along the BMZ. Biopsies of bullous lesions show subepidermal blisters/bullae filled with neutrophils and a neutrophil-predominant infiltrate in the papillary dermis. DIF of perilesional skin is the gold standard for diagnosis and shows linear IgA deposition along the BMZ. Salt-split skin testing may show epidermal staining.

Treatment

Dapsone[1] is considered first-line therapy for cases of LABD and CBDC. We recommend starting at 25 mg daily, which may be increased weekly by increments of 25 mg based on clinical response (maximum dose varies by age). Second-line agents for those who cannot tolerate dapsone include colchicine[1] (up to 0.6 mg two times daily in pediatric patients and up to three times daily in adult patients) and sulfapyridine[2] (500 mg twice daily starting dose, titrated appropriately based on clinical response).

In cases of drug-induced LABD/CBDC, the offending medication should be discontinued. Lesions are expected to resolve within a few weeks of stopping the medication.

Epidermolysis Bullosa Acquisita

Pathophysiology

Epidermolysis bullosa acquisita (EBA) is a very rare acquired bullous disease, most commonly found in adults of East Asian and African American descent. It is frequently associated with inflammatory bowel disease (especially Crohn's disease), multiple myeloma, systemic lupus erythematosus, diabetes mellitus, hepatitis C infection, and other underlying diseases.

Patients may have IgG autoantibodies targeting type VII collagen, which is a major component of anchoring fibrils in the basement membrane zone.

Clinical Manifestations

The noninflammatory, or mechanobullous, variant of EBA is the most commonly recognized subtype. Patients present with hemorrhagic bullae and erosions on trauma-prone sites including the dorsal hands and feet, elbows, and knees. Lesions may heal with scarring, milia, and nail dystrophy. Inflammatory EBA clinically is indistinguishable to BP. Lesions of inflammatory EBA may also heal with scarring and milia. Patients may also have oral and ocular erosions which may appear similarly to MMP.

Diagnosis

In addition to clinical findings, biopsy is required for diagnosis of EBA to distinguish it from other subepidermal bullous diseases. Routine histology shows subepidermal blisters with varying degrees of neutrophilic and eosinophilic infiltrates. DIF of perilesional skin shows linear IgG and C3 deposition along the BMZ. Unlike BP, DIF of EBA lesions tend to show more linear IgG deposition rather than C3. Salt-split skin technique shows dermal staining.

Treatment Options

Some patients may have good response to prednisone (0.5–1 mg/kg/day), with or without dapsone. Dapsone[1] monotherapy may also be effective for patients (initiated at 25 mg daily and increased appropriately based on clinical response). This dose should be maintained for several months prior to tapering attempts. Colchicine[1] (0.6 mg twice to thrice daily) may be effective. Patients with resistant or severe disease may have more rapid relief with cyclosporine[1] (4–5 mg/kg/day). Other agents with reported success include rituximab,[1] IVIG,[1] infliximab (Remicade),[1] minocycline,[1] plasmapheresis, and PDE-4 inhibitors.[1]

Unfortunately, cases of EBA tend to be quite resistant to treatment relative to BP and other subepidermal bullous diseases. The disease is usually chronic and waxes and wanes. Patients should avoid trauma as much as possible because it may contribute to further blister formation. The inflammatory subtype of EBA may have better response to therapy compared with the mechanobullous noninflammatory subtype.

---

[1] Not FDA approved for this indication.
[2] Not available in the United States.

Dermatitis Herpetiformis

Pathophysiology

Dermatitis herpetiformis (DH) is a chronic and relapsing bullous disease which is strongly associated with celiac disease. People of Northern European descent are most commonly affected, and it is quite rare in patients of Asian and African American descent. More than 97% of patients with DH and celiac disease have one or both HLA-DQ2 and HLA-DQ8 alleles. In addition to celiac disease, DH is also associated with other autoimmune conditions including Hashimoto's thyroiditis, type 1 diabetes mellitus, and pernicious anemia.

Gluten is a grain protein found in many foods containing wheat, rye, and barley. Gluten is broken down into gliadin during digestion, which is then transported across the gastrointestinal (GI) mucosa to the lamina propria, where it binds with tissue transglutaminase 2 (TTG2). This complex is recognized by HLA-DQ2 or HLA-DQ8 on antigen presenting cells (APCs) and activating the T-cell and B-cell activated autoinflammatory cascade to form IgA autoantibodies against TTG2 or the TTG2-gliadin complex. These bound IgA antibodies lead to neutrophil recruitment, resulting in damage to intestinal villi. Epitope spreading (diversification of epitope specificity) results in production of IgA autoantibodies against epidermal transglutaminase (TTG3), which then binds to TTG3 within dermal papillae. Neutrophils recruited by this process release elastase and other proteolytic enzymes, resulting in the formation of subepidermal blisters seen in DH.

Clinical Manifestations

Patients with DH classically present with extremely pruritic herpetiform vesicles on an urticarial base. The vesicles can be ruptured very easily, so excoriations, rather than intact vesicles, are more frequently seen on examination. Lesions are typically distributed on the symmetric extensor extremities (elbows and knees), buttocks, back, neck, face, and scalp. A minority of approximately 20% of patients with DH have symptomatic gastrointestinal disease; however, the majority of patients have evidence of gluten-sensitive enteropathy on gastrointestinal biopsy samples.

Diagnosis

Clinical history can be particularly helpful in cases of DH. A history of worsening of disease with gluten-containing diets is a useful clue, although patients are not always aware of their specific dietary habits unless they keep a careful food diary.

Biopsy samples should be obtained on early blisters if possible. Routine histology shows subepidermal bullae most pronounced above the dermal papillae, and neutrophilic infiltrates in the dermal papillae. These findings can be quite similar to LABD, so DIF testing and serologic testing can be helpful. DIF of perilesional skin shows granular IgA deposits with or without C3 deposition in the dermal papillae. Serologic testing for DH and celiac disease can be helpful, including serum antitissue transglutaminase or antiendomysial antibodies (present in approximately 80% of patients with DH and greater than 95% of patients with celiac disease); however, it is important to keep in mind that tests can also be falsely negative if the patient has been keeping a gluten-free diet. Patients with IgA deficiency may also have falsely negative testing for anti-TTG antibodies, so IgA levels should be assessed concurrently.

Treatment Options

Dapsone is the treatment of choice in patients with DH. Patients tend to have a rapid response to dapsone (within 2–3 days) with improvement in cutaneous disease. The usual dose of dapsone in DH is to start at 50 mg daily and increase in increments of 25 mg based on clinical response to a maximum of to a maximum of 100–200 mg daily. Typically, patients are well controlled on

50–100 mg daily. Patients do not typically see an effect on their GI disease, if present. Prior to initiating dapsone, it is important to evaluate for G6PD deficiency. Sulfapyridine[2] is an effective second-line therapy with less risk of hemolysis.

Gluten-free diets (avoiding wheat, rye, and barley) can be effective to control both cutaneous and gastrointestinal disease. It may also reduce the risk of development of GI lymphomas associated with celiac disease. DH is typically a lifelong, chronic, relapsing disease. It is important to involve relevant specialties including dermatology, nutrition, and gastroenterology to help manage patients with DH.

---

[2] Not available in the United States.

References

Abdat R, Waldman RA, et al: Dupilumab as a novel therapy for bullous pemphigoid: a multicenter case series, *J Am Acad Dermatol* 83(1):46–52, 2020.

Bolotin D, Petronic-Rosic V: Dermatitis herpetiformis, *J Am Acad Dermatol* 64(6):1017–1033, 2011.

Cizenski JD, Michel P, et al: Spectrum of orocutaneous disease associations: immune-mediated conditions, *J Am Acad Dermatol* 77(5):795–806, 2017.

Feliciani C, Joly P, et al: Management of bullous pemphigoid: the European Dermatology Forum consensus in collaboration with the European Academy of Dermatology and Venereology, *Br J Dermatol* 172(4):867–877, 2015.

Gouveia A, Teixeira A, et al: Linear immunoglobulin A bullous dermatosis, *J Pediatr* 170:338, 2016. e1.

Kirtschig G, Murrell D, et al: Interventions for mucous membrane pemphigoid/cicatricial pemphigoid and epidermolysis bullosa acquisita: a systematic literature review, *Arch Dermatol* 138(3):380–384, 2002.

Murrell DF, Peña S, et al: Diagnosis and management of pemphigus: recommendations of an international panel of experts, *J Am Acad Dermatol* 82(3):575–585, 2020.

Mutasim DF: Management of autoimmune bullous diseases: pharmacology and therapeutics, *J Am Acad Dermatol* 51:859–877, 2004.

Wojnarowska F, Kirtschig G, et al: Guidelines for the management of bullous pemphigoid, *Br J Dermatol* 147:214–221, 2002.

BACTERIAL DISEASES OF THE SKIN

Method of
Karissa Gilchrist, MD

CURRENT DIAGNOSIS

- The large variety of bacterial skin infections can usually be distinguished by history, physical exam, and clinical presentation.
- Bacterial infections can range from those affecting the superficial layers of skin to the deep layers and soft tissue.
- Many infections are precipitated by a breach in the normal skin barrier.
- Infection can vary in severity depending on how extensive and invasive it is.
- Deep infection can lead to systemic toxicity.
- Necrotizing infection can rapidly progress and cause extensive tissue damage and even death.

CURRENT THERAPY

- Antibiotic therapy is selected based on knowledge of the most likely causative pathogen or based on culture results.
- When a loculated abscess is identified, procedural incision and drainage should be performed.
- Broad-spectrum empiric antibiotic coverage should be initiated when a rapidly progressing necrotizing infection is suspected.
- Delay in surgical consultation and debridement of necrotizing infection may result in tissue damage, limb loss, and/or death.
- Tissue culture of necrotizing infection can guide antibiotic choice.

TABLE 1	Primary Pathogen for Common Bacterial Skin Infections
DIAGNOSIS	**ORGANISM**
Cellulitis	Streptococci (*Staphylococcus aureus* less common)
Impetigo	*S. aureus* Group A beta-hemolytic streptococci
Folliculitis	*S. aureus* Gram-negative bacteria
Abscess	*S. aureus*, predominantly MRSA

MRSA, Methicillin-resistant *S. aureus*.

Bacterial infections of the skin can manifest in a broad range of clinical presentations. Bacterial skin diseases can occur both superficially and in the deep layers. They can also range from mild to aggressive and life-threatening infection. Skin infections have increased in prevalence and severity in part due to the development of resistant bacterial organisms. For this reason, it is critical for clinicians to be able to promptly recognize and manage bacterial infections of the skin.

Common Infections

Cellulitis

Cellulitis is an acute bacterial skin infection that causes poorly demarcated areas of erythema, warmth, tenderness, and edema of the skin involving the deep dermal and subcutaneous layers. Depending on the extent of edema and inflammation, the affected skin may develop bullae, ecchymosis, or maceration. Cellulitis may occur on any area of the skin but is typically found on the lower extremities and is almost always unilateral. Cellulitis develops when there is a break in the skin and pathogens are able to breach the surface. It most commonly arises from infection with streptococci. *Staphylococcus aureus* is a less common cause of cellulitis but should be considered in special circumstances such as bite wounds, penetrating trauma, intravenous drug use, or in immunocompromised patients (Table 1).

Culture or biopsy of the affected skin is not routinely recommended for the diagnosis of cellulitis. Cultures often yield negative or unhelpful results as the rapidly spreading skin manifestations may be more likely related to a strong inflammatory response to the inciting pathogen and may not be representative of the bacterial load. Blood cultures may be considered if there are systemic signs of infection. Diagnosis of cellulitis should be made clinically. Labs and imaging may be obtained to help distinguish cellulitis from other diagnoses and rule out complications such as underlying abscess, deep venous thrombosis, osteomyelitis, or necrotizing fasciitis. Stasis dermatitis is commonly mistaken for cellulitis and can be differentiated by its bilateral appearance and lack of skin trauma.

In the treatment of mild cases of uncomplicated nonpurulent cellulitis without systemic signs of infection, an oral antibiotic agent that is active against streptococci—such as cephalexin (Keflex), dicloxacillin[1], or amoxicillin/clavulanate (Augmentin)—should be used. If the patient has a penicillin allergy, clindamycin can be used as an alternative. The typical treatment duration is 5 days, but this may be extended in the case of residual symptoms. In patients who fail oral antimicrobial treatment or in those with systemic signs of infection, an intravenous regimen with an agent such as cefazolin (Ancef), ceftriaxone (Rocephin), or clindamycin should be considered. In cases where there is increased risk of methicillin-resistant *S. aureus* (MRSA) infection, such as

---

[1] Not FDA approved for this indication.
[2] Not available in the United States.

TABLE 2	Suggested Antibiotic Agents for Common Bacterial Skin Infections
DIAGNOSIS	**ANTIBIOTIC**
Cellulitis	• Cephalexin (Keflex) • Dicloxacillin[1] • Amoxicillin/clavulanate (Augmentin) Alternative: • Clindamycin Severe infection: • Cefazolin (Ancef) • Ceftriaxone (Rocephin) MRSA risk factors: • Vancomycin
Impetigo	Mild cases: • Topical mupirocin (Bactroban) Severe or extensive cases: • Cephalexin (Keflex) • Dicloxacillin[1] MRSA risk factors: • Doxycycline • Clindamycin • Trimethoprim/sulfamethoxazole (Bactrim DS)[1]
Folliculitis	Suspected *S. aureus*: • Topical mupirocin (Bactroban)[1] or clindamycin[1] • Cephalexin (Keflex) • Dicloxacillin Suspected *Pseudomonas*: • No treatment • Ciprofloxacin (Cipro)[1]
Abscess	• Trimethoprim/sulfamethoxazole (Bactrim DS)[1] • Clindamycin

MRSA, Methicillin-resistant *S. aureus*.
[1]Not FDA approved for this indication.

penetrating trauma or intravenous drug use, intravenous vancomycin should be added (Table 2).

Erysipelas

For some, the term *erysipelas* is synonymous with cellulitis. However, erysipelas refers to infection that is limited to the upper dermis; cellulitis extends into the deeper dermis. The borders of the erysipelas rash are more clearly demarcated than those of cellulitis. Erysipelas is always nonpurulent. The treatment outlined earlier for cellulitis can be applied to erysipelas with antibiotics targeted against streptococci and, if systemic signs or symptoms are present, parental agents can be used.

Impetigo

Impetigo is a common bacterial skin infection that can occur at any age but is most commonly seen in children. It is most prevalent in hot, humid conditions and is highly contagious. It is transmitted by direct contact and may develop secondarily after a disruption of the skin occurs from an insect bite or other underlying disease such as eczema or psoriasis.

Impetigo can be classified into two major categories: bullous and nonbullous. Bullous impetigo is a result of *S. aureus* infection. Strains of this organism produce a factor that cleaves the junction between the epidermal and dermal skin layers. This causes a delicate vesicle to form, which may break open, leaving behind a crusted erosion. Nonbullous impetigo is most commonly caused by *S. aureus*, group A beta-hemolytic streptococci, or a combination of both (see Table 1). This form of impetigo typically begins as erythematous papules or pustules. These lesions develop a discharge that dries and forms a classic honey-colored crust.

Treatment for both bullous and nonbullous impetigo consists of antibiotic therapy aimed at both staphylococcal and streptococcal organisms (see Table 2). Either topical or oral antibiotics can be used for treatment of impetigo depending on the severity and extent of infection. Topical treatment with mupirocin (Bactroban) ointment 2% three times daily for 5 days can be effective for mild cases of impetigo. Over-the-counter topical bacitracin[1] or triple antibiotic ointments are not as effective as mupirocin in the treatment of impetigo. If an oral agent is desired for more severe or extensive cases, therapy should consist of an antibiotic medication that is active against *S. aureus*, such as cephalexin (Keflex) or dicloxacillin[1] for 7 days. *S. aureus* isolates from impetigo are typically methicillin-susceptible *S. aureus* (MSSA); however, if MRSA is suspected or confirmed with direct culture of an impetiginous lesion or its drainage, treatment with doxycycline, clindamycin, or sulfamethoxazole-trimethoprim (Bactrim DS)[1] for 7 days is recommended.

Ecthyma

Ecthyma is a form of impetigo that infects deeper layers of the skin into the dermis. Lesions appear as "punched out" ulcerations with an overlying crust and surrounding erythematous edema. Ecthyma differs from impetigo in that it heals with scarring due to the deep skin involvement. The principal pathogen causing ecthyma is group A streptococcus (GAS). Treatment of ecthyma differs from that of impetigo and always requires oral antibiotic therapy. Penicillin is the first-line choice of antibiotic agent. With both impetigo and ecthyma, care should be taken to use contact precautions and frequent handwashing to prevent spread.

Ecthyma Gangrenosum

Ecthyma gangrenosum is a skin eruption that classically arises in immunocompromised patients with *Pseudomonas aeruginosa* bacteremia. An ecthyma gangrenosum lesion typically begins as an erythematous macule or pustule and quickly develops into a gangrenous ulcer. This lesion results from bacterial invasion of the vascular wall and subsequent tissue ischemia and necrosis. There may be one single eruption or several. Lesions can occur in any location, with the axilla and genital regions most commonly affected. Although it is possible for lesions to occur in an immunocompetent patient without any signs of systemic illness, the presence of ecthyma gangrenosum should definitely raise the clinician's suspicion for bacteremia, especially with *P. aeruginosa*. Treatment involves empiric antibiotic therapy with an antipseudomonal agent. Blood cultures should be obtained, and lesions can be swabbed for culture to help guide antibiotic narrowing.

Folliculitis

Folliculitis is the infection and inflammation of hair follicles. It typically presents as erythematous papules or pustules in hair follicles. As with most inflammatory skin diseases, pruritus is the most frequent symptom. Lesions may be painful. Folliculitis is typically infectious, with the most common etiology being bacterial. It can also be caused by viral, fungal, or parasitic infection. Bacterial folliculitis is most frequently caused by *S. aureus* but may also result from infection with gram-negative bacteria (see Table 1). Multiple factors may predispose a patient to develop folliculitis; these include underlying immunodeficiency, frequent scratching (from underlying eczema or other pruritic skin disease), nasal colonization with *S. aureus*, shaving in the opposite direction of hair growth, hyperhidrosis, or prolonged use of topical corticosteroids. Exposure to underchlorinated heated water is the classic risk factor for developing "hot tub folliculitis," which is caused by *P. aeruginosa* infection. In this example of gram-negative folliculitis, pustules appear on the areas of hair-bearing skin that were exposed to the contaminated water. Onset may occur up to 48 hours after exposure.

Diagnosis is typically made clinically, and the distribution of lesions may be suggestive of a pathogenic etiology. Folliculitis occurring primarily on the face or scalp is most likely due to *S. aureus*. Culture of pustule contents may be considered if the diagnosis is unclear. Pseudomonal folliculitis is often self-limiting but

[1]Not FDA approved for this indication.

may necessitate treatment with oral ciprofloxacin (Cipro)[1] in the setting of immunodeficiency or in severe cases. Topical mupirocin (Bactroban)[1] or topical clindamycin[1] is an effective treatment for cases of superficial folliculitis thought to be caused by *S. aureus*. In very mild and localized cases of *S. aureus*, lesions may even resolve spontaneously. If the disease is extensive, refractory to topical treatment, or appears to involve the deep areas of the follicles, an oral antibiotic should be used for treatment. First-line agents include cephalexin (Keflex) or dicloxacillin treatment for 7 to 10 days. If MRSA is suspected or confirmed on culture, oral trimethoprim/sulfamethoxazole (Bactrim DS)[1], clindamycin, or doxycycline should be used for treatment (see Table 2). It is important to try to minimize or eliminate any predisposing factors identified in order to prevent recurrence.

Abscess

An abscess is a collection of pus within the skin or soft tissue. It presents as an erythematous, painful nodule that is fluctuant, sometimes with an overlying pustule. *S. aureus* is responsible for the majority of abscesses (see Table 1), with a large portion being due to methicillin-resistant strains (MRSA). Immunosuppression or any disruption of the normal skin barrier may predispose a patient to develop one or multiple abscesses. Procedural incision and evacuation of the abscess debris should be performed for treatment. Care should be taken to probe the cavity and release loculated areas within the abscess. Proper wound care should follow with application of a dry gauze dressing with or without packing of the wound space. Systemic antibiotics should be used in addition to incision and drainage in cases of multiple lesions, abscesses larger than 2 cm, immunosuppression, signs of systemic toxicity, refractory lesions, extensive surrounding cellulitis, or presence of implanted medical devices. It is reasonable to forgo antibiotic therapy in an otherwise healthy patient with a single small abscess, especially in the setting of numerous antibiotic allergies. However, there is now evidence to suggest that treatment with trimethoprim/sulfamethoxazole (Bactrim DS)[1] or clindamycin for any patient who has undergone incision and drainage may improve cure rates and decrease the risk of recurrence (see Table 2).

Furuncle and Carbuncle

When an abscess forms at the base of a hair follicle, it is referred to as a furuncle. This is different from folliculitis, where infection does not extend deeper than the epidermis. A carbuncle develops when several furuncles occur in multiple adjacent follicles and the infection coalesces into a larger mass of pus. Carbuncles commonly occur on the back of the neck and in the axilla. As in the case of cutaneous abscesses, the principal pathogen for furuncles and carbuncles is *S. aureus*. Many furuncles will rupture spontaneously, allowing the pus to drain. The application of moist heat may also help to encourage spontaneous drainage. Carbuncles and larger furuncles should be treated with incision and drainage.

Invasive Infections

Necrotizing Soft Tissue Infection

Necrotizing cellulitis is an aggressive, rapidly spreading life-threatening bacterial infection of the skin. When there is involvement of the fascia or muscle, the descriptive term becomes *necrotizing fasciitis* or *necrotizing myositis*, accordingly. These infections result in significant tissue destruction and have a high mortality rate. Necrotizing infections may be precipitated by varying degrees of disruption of the skin barrier due to anything from insect bites to intravenous drug use or major penetrating trauma. Diabetes increases the risk of developing a necrotizing soft tissue infection.

Necrotizing infection presents as skin erythema, edema, and warmth with underlying crepitus that develops quickly over the course of hours and progresses rapidly. Skin findings are usually

---

| TABLE 3 | Suggested Antibiotic Agents for Invasive Bacterial Skin Infections |

DIAGNOSIS	ANTIBIOTIC
Necrotizing soft tissue infection Group A streptococcal infection with toxic shock syndrome	1. Vancomycin, linezolid (Zyvox), or daptomycin (Cubicin) plus 2. Piperacillin-tazobactam (Zosyn) or a carbapenem or Ceftriaxone (Rocephin) plus metronidazole (Flagyl) or Fluoroquinolone plus metronidazole (Flagyl)
Invasive	1. Clindamycin plus 2. Penicillin
Staphylococcal scalded skin syndrome	Intravenous oxacillin, nafcillin, cefazolin (Ancef), or vancomycin
Tularemia	Mild or moderate disease: • Oral fluoroquinolone or doxycycline Severe disease: • IV/IM gentamicin[1] or IM streptomycin

[1]Not FDA approved for this indication.

associated with severe pain, which may be out of proportion to findings on examination. Signs of systemic toxicity, such as fever or hemodynamic instability, may also appear. Delayed clinical recognition can result in extensive tissue damage, limb loss, or death. Prompt surgical consultation should be made if a necrotizing soft tissue infection is suspected. If the diagnosis is unclear, a computed tomography scan may be helpful in revealing the presence of gas in the soft tissues, but it should not delay surgical intervention. Treatment should include emergent surgical debridement as well as empiric antibiotic administration. Care should be taken to provide hemodynamic support as needed. Blood cultures would ideally be obtained prior to the administration of antibiotics. Empiric therapy should consist of a polymicrobial approach with a combination of agents aimed at treating MRSA, aerobes, and anaerobes (Table 3). Antibiotic therapy can be tailored according to culture results from tissue obtained during surgical debridement.

Fournier Gangrene

Fournier gangrene is a form of necrotizing soft tissue infection involving the perineal region. It is typically seen in middle-aged adults, particularly those who have diabetes mellitus. Potential predisposing factors may include recent urologic procedures, chronic use of an indwelling urinary catheter, or urethral trauma. However, this condition can develop without these risk factors. Cutaneous and systemic findings are similar to those of other necrotizing soft tissue infections, and prompt surgical debridement with broad-spectrum empiric antibiotic coverage is critical.

Invasive Group A Streptococcal Infection with Toxic Shock Syndrome

GAS is a common cause of superficial skin infections, as outlined earlier in this chapter. However, this pathogen can sometimes lead to invasive disease and result in necrotizing infection. Toxic shock syndrome is a complication that may arise when invasive GAS produces a toxin that induces the subsequent release of inflammatory cytokines. Skin manifestations include induration and erythema of the affected areas, eventually giving rise to hemorrhagic skin sloughing. It is often associated with signs of systemic toxicity and multiorgan failure. Toxic shock syndrome may also develop as a result of invasive postpartum endometritis. It is a rapidly progressive disease and prompt treatment should be provided along with hemodynamic support. Antibiotic treatment includes coverage with both clindamycin and penicillin (see Table 3). Clindamycin has the

---

[1]Not FDA approved for this indication.
[3]Exceeds dosage recommended by the manufacturer.

additional benefit of helping to suppress the toxin-mediated inflammatory response. Dual coverage with penicillin is important due to potential clindamycin resistance.

Staphylococcal Scalded Skin Syndrome

Staphylococcal scalded skin syndrome is a complication that can arise from any infection caused by *S. aureus*, such as impetigo, for example. It typically occurs in children and develops as a result of exotoxins produced by the bacteria. Skin findings include painful erythema and desquamation; the mucous membranes are spared. Fever and generalized malaise usually accompany the cutaneous findings. Diagnosis can usually be made clinically; however, culture of the suspected primary infection can be collected for confirmation. One should keep in mind that areas of desquamation or bullae in scalded skin syndrome will be sterile, as these lesions are a result of the exotoxins and not direct bacterial infection. Therefore culture of these areas is unlikely to be helpful.

Patients with staphylococcal scalded skin syndrome are typically treated in an inpatient setting with intravenous antibiotics and supportive care. First-line antibiotic agents include oxacillin, nafcillin, cefazolin (Ancef), and vancomycin (see Table 3). Clindamycin is not a recommended first-choice agent due to high rates of resistance.

Tularemia

Tularemia is an uncommon infection caused by *Francisella tularensis*; it occurs after exposure to an infected insect or animal, most commonly a tick or rabbit. Clinical manifestations vary in severity. The most common form of tularemia is ulceroglandular disease. Symptom onset typically occurs within 3 to 5 days following exposure and begins with nonspecific constitutional symptoms such as fever, headache, myalgias, and generalized malaise. Cutaneous manifestations commonly begin with a single erythematous ulceration with or without a central eschar. Location of the skin lesion is based on the site of inoculation, and the anatomic distribution of findings is regional. Rarely, there may be multiple skin lesions. Ulceroglandular tularemia is associated with localized tender lymphadenopathy. Glandular tularemia has the same characteristics as ulceroglandular tularemia without the ulcerations.

When tularemia is suspected clinically, serology should be sent for diagnosis. It generally takes 2 weeks for antibodies to *Francisella* to reach diagnostic levels, and serology may need to be repeated if clinical suspicion is high. Polymerase chain reaction (PCR) testing can be completed more rapidly depending on lab availability of the test. Blood or tissue cultures are rarely positive; if such specimens are collected, laboratory staff should be notified in advance of tularemia suspicion in order to optimize conditions for culture growth as well as for infection control precautions. Treatment consists of selecting an effective antibiotic regimen. In general, an oral fluoroquinolone or doxycycline would be a reasonable initial treatment for patients with mild or moderate disease. If the infection is severe, intravenous or intramuscular gentamicin[1] or intramuscular streptomycin is recommended (see Table 3). Of note, *F. tularensis* has the potential to be used as a bioterrorism agent, as it is easily disseminated and infection can occur at low exposure. In such a case, recognition and reporting are critical.

---

[1]Not FDA approved for this indication.

References

Daum RS, Miller LG, Immergluck L, et al: A placebo-controlled trial of antibiotics for smaller skin abscesses, *N Engl J Med* 376:2545–2555, 2017.

Handler MZ, Schwartz RA: Staphylococcal scalded skin syndrome: diagnosis and management in children and adults, *J Eur Acad Dermatol Venereol* 28:1418–1423, 2014.

Jeng A, Beheshti M, Li J, Nathan R: The role of beta-hemolytic streptococci in causing diffuse, nonculturable cellulitis: a prospective investigation, *Medicine (Baltimore)* 89:217–226, 2010.

Luelmo-Aguilar J, Santandreu MS: Folliculitis: recognition and management, *Am J Clin Dermatol* 5:301–310, 2004.

Pereira LB: Impetigo – review, *An Bras Dermatol* 89:293–299, 2014.

Raff AB, Kroshinsky D: Cellulitis: a review, *JAMA* 316:325–337, 2016.

Snowden J, Simonsen KA: Tularemia. In *StatPearls*. Treasure Island (FL), StatPearls Publishing, 2020.

Stevens DL, Bisno AL, Chambers HF, et al: Practice guidelines for the diagnosis and management of skin and soft tissue infections: 2014 update by the Infectious Diseases Society of America, *Clin Infect Dis* 59:e10–52, 2014.

CONTACT DERMATITIS

Method of
Yul W. Yang, MD, PhD; and James A. Yiannias, MD

CURRENT DIAGNOSIS

- Gather a detailed history on skin exposures, including use of the following items:
  - Irritants
  - Alkalis: soaps, detergents, cleansers
  - Acids
  - Hydrocarbons: petroleum, oils
  - Solvents
  - Potential allergens including:
    - Metals: nickel sulfate; cobalt chloride (e.g., jewelry, makeup, personal products)
    - Fragrances: balsam of Peru (Myroxylon pereirae; fragrance); fragrance mix
    - Methylisothiazolinone, methylchloroisothiazolinone (preservatives)
    - Benzalkonium chloride (preservative)
    - Formaldehyde and formaldehyde-releasing preservatives such as quaternium-15
    - Topical antibiotics such as neomycin, bacitracin
- Examine the skin for the location and pattern of eruption:
  - Eyelid: nail polish
  - Postauricular scalp: perfume
  - Perioral area: chewing gum, toothpaste
  - Trunk: dyes, clothing finish
  - Wrist: nickel, chrome
  - Waistline: rubber
  - Feet: shoes
  - Wounds: topical antibiotic ointment
- Perform patch testing:
  - T.R.U.E. TEST with 35 allergens (note: two common allergens, benzalkonium chloride and propolis, are not included in this panel)
  - Customized series with 70 or more allergens

CURRENT THERAPY

- Avoid irritants and allergens, using the prepared patient handout.
- Consult the SkinSAFE shopping list of skin care products free from the top 10 most common allergens (if patch testing is not performed).
- Consult a customized SkinSAFE shopping list of skin care products free from the patient's contact allergens, based on patch test results.
- Topical corticosteroids can be applied.
- Hydrocortisone 2.5% (Hytone) can be applied twice daily on the face, neck, axillae, groin, and intertriginous areas.
- Triamcinolone 0.1% (Kenalog) can be applied twice daily on the body.
- For severe reactions, short-term, higher-potency steroids can be applied (e.g., clobetasol [Clobex] 0.05% twice daily).
- Sedating antihistamines can be taken: doxepin (Sinequan)[1] 10 to 20 mg qhs.
- Steroid-sparing topical agents can be applied twice daily to any skin surface (but may be more expensive than topical corticosteroids): tacrolimus 0.1% (Protopic),[1] pimecrolimus 1% (Elidel),[1] crisaborole 2% (Eucrisa),[1] ruxolitinib 1.5% (Opzelura)[1]
- For severe, acute episodes, systemic corticosteroids can be taken in a several-week tapering course (e.g., prednisone 60 mg for 5 days, 40 mg for 5 days, and 20 mg for 5 days).

- Longer-term systemic therapy is possible for severe or recalcitrant disease.
- Phototherapy with narrow-band ultraviolet B[1] is suggested.
- Azathioprine (Imuran)[1] can be taken 1 to 3 mg/kg qd.
- Mycophenolate mofetil (CellCept)[1] can be taken 2 to 3 g qd.
- Methotrexate[1] can be taken 10 to 25 mg per week.
- Cyclosporine (Neoral)[1] can be taken 2.5 to 5 mg/kg qd short term.
- Dupilumab (Dupixent)[1] can be taken by injection at 600 mg initially and then 300 mg every other week.
- Tralokinumab (Adbry)[1] can be taken by SQ injection at 600 mg initially and then 300 mg every other week.
- Upadacitinib (Rinvoq)[1] can be taken 15 to 30 mg qd.
- Abrocitinib (Cibinqo)[1] can be taken 100 to 200 mg qd.

[1]Not FDA approved for this indication.

BOX 1 | **Top 10 Most Common Allergens**

North American Contact Dermatitis Group
- Nickel sulfate
- Methylisothiazolinone (MI)
- Fragrance mix
- Formaldehyde 2%
- Methylisothiazolinone/methylchloroisothiazolinone (MI/MCI)
- Balsam of Peru
- Neomycin
- Bacitracin
- Formaldehyde 1%
- *p*-Phenylenediamine

Mayo Clinic Contact Dermatitis Group
- Nickel sulfate
- MI
- Balsam of Peru
- Neomycin
- Cobalt chloride
- Benzalkonium chloride
- Fragrance mix I
- Potassium dichromate
- Bacitracin
- MI/MCI

Data from DeKoven JG, Warshaw EM, Zug KA, et al. North American Contact Dermatitis Group Patch Test Results: 2015–2016. *Dermatitis.* 2018;29(6):297–309; Veverka KK, Hall MR, Yiannias JA, et al. Trends in patch testing with the Mayo Clinic standard series, 2011–2015. *Dermatitis.* 2018;29(6):310–315.

Dermatitis typically manifests as papules and vesicles with weeping and oozing that can become lichenified and scaly when chronic. When this clinical picture is secondary to an exogenous substance coming into contact with the skin, it is termed *contact dermatitis*. Further delineation leads to irritant versus allergic contact dermatitis, although in practice these often overlap.

Irritant contact dermatitis is not an allergic process. It represents damage to the skin from repeated and cumulative exposure to an agent. Irritants do not require prior sensitization. A decreased barrier function of the skin (e.g., with frequent handwashing) can predispose to the condition or exacerbate it. Examples include alkalis (in soaps, detergents, and cleansers), acids (in germicides, dyes, and pigments), hydrocarbons (in petroleum and oils), and solvents.

Allergic contact dermatitis is an immunologic process classified as a type IV cell-mediated delayed hypersensitivity reaction. Poison ivy is a classic example. It requires an initial exposure to the contactant in which sensitization occurs but without outward physical effect. Subsequent exposure can elicit a striking response that is independent of the amount of the contactant.

From 1994 to 2016, the most common contact allergens have changed little. Based on studies performed by the North American Contact Dermatitis Group (NACDG) and the Mayo Clinic Contact Dermatitis Group (MCCDG), the allergens most consistently in the top 10 were nickel sulfate, balsam of Peru, fragrance mix, quaternium-15, neomycin, bacitracin, formaldehyde, and cobalt chloride (Box 1). However, in the past few years, two additional preservatives have gained prominence: methylisothiazolinone (MI) and benzalkonium chloride. Common sources of exposure to nickel include costume jewelry, snaps, zippers, and other metal objects. Balsam of Peru and fragrance mix are markers for fragrance sensitivity. Sources of exposure to formaldehyde include skin care products, household products, and the resins in plastics and clothing. Quaternium-15 is a formaldehyde-releasing preservative and may be found in items such as skin care products, paper, inks, and photocopier toner. Neomycin and bacitracin are topical antibiotics available alone and in combination with polymyxin (Neosporin), antifungals, and corticosteroids. Cobalt is found with other metals, including zinc, and in items such as jewelry, crayons, hair dye, and antiperspirants. MI is a common preservative found in personal care products and may be used in combination with another preservative, methylchloroisothiazolinone (MCI). Benzalkonium chloride is commonly used in the healthcare field as a cleanser, antiseptic, and preservative, but it is also found in personal care products such as wipes and an increasing number of skin care products.

Others less consistently in the top 10 during that period were methyldibromo glutaronitrile, gold sodium thiosulfate, potassium dichromate, *p*-phenylenediamine, thiuram mix, MI/MCI, and propolis. Methyldibromo glutaronitrile is a preservative and can be found in healthcare and personal products. Clinically relevant sources of gold may be found in jewelry and dental appliances. Potassium dichromate is used in cement, leather, and steel surfaces. Permanent hair dyes are the usual source of *p*-phenylenediamine. Thiuram mix is in rubber and some personal products. Propolis is another marker of fragrance sensitivity.

Each year since 2000, the American Contact Dermatitis Society has designated an allergen of the year, designed to spotlight allergens, common or not, that are increasing in significance. For 2023, lanolin was chosen, which is a complex wax mixture of chemicals, historically derived from wool. Lanolin is used extensively in personal care products such as an emulsifiers and emollients/moisturizers but is also applied in various industrial products, including metallic surfaces, ink, and furniture/leather/shoe polish.

Other designated allergens of the year have been alkyl glucosides, cobalt chloride, benzophenones, MI, acrylates, dimethyl fumarate, neomycin, mixed dialkyl thioureas, nickel, fragrance, *p*-phenylenediamine, corticosteroids, cocamidopropyl betaine, bacitracin, thimerosal, gold, disperse blue, propylene glycol, non-allergen parabens, isobornyl acrylate, acetophenone azine, and aluminum. Alkyl glucosides are surfactants that are pervasive in consumer products, including cosmetics. Benzophenones, such as oxybenzone, are chemical ultraviolet light filters that are found in sunscreens and personal care products. Artificial nails, dentures, and bone cement contain acrylates, but these substances are only allergenic when in the liquid, powder, or paste forms. Dimethyl fumarate is a biocide in furniture, shoes, and textiles. It is often placed in little paper packets with these items. Rubber products and shoe glue are common sources of mixed dialkyl thioureas. Shampoos often contain cocamidopropyl betaine as a lathering agent. Thimerosal is a preservative for medications and personal care products, including contact lens solution. Disperse blue is a fabric dye. Patients with an allergy to disperse dyes may also react to *p*-phenylenediamine. Propylene glycol is a common ingredient in personal care products, topical corticosteroids and other medications, and foods. Parabens are preservatives commonly found in cosmetics, foods, pharmaceuticals, dentifrices, and suppositories. Isobornyl acrylate, an adhesive, is often used in medical

Introduction

Eczema, also known as dermatitis, is an inflammation of the skin due to dryness, irritation, or possible external allergy. Eczema/dermatitis is not contagious.

Some skin care products contain fragrance even though the package says "fragrance free" or "unscented." Therefore, please choose the skin care products as listed below by their *exact brand name*.

Suggestions

Soaps/cleansing
- Vanicream cleansing bar
- Free and clear liquid cleanser
- Aveeno moisturizing bar for dry skin fragrance free or aveeno advanced care body wash
- Oilatum unscented soap
- Neutrogena original formula fragrance-free (bar or liquid)

Any of the shampoos listed in this brochure may be used as your hand or body soap.
- Vanicream shave cream for sensitive skin

Moisturizers
- Vanicream, vanicream lite
- Aveeno daily moisturizing lotion fragrance free
- Plain vaseline, vaniply
- DML unscented
- Use moisturizers twice daily.
- All of the above are OK to use on the face.
- After showering, blot excess water with hands and apply cream. Do not use a towel to dry.
- Robathol bath oil

Deodorants
- Almay unscented antiperspirants
- Plain cornstarch from the grocer can be used.

Avoid

Soaps/cleansing
- No hot water (use lukewarm).
- Avoid hot tubs.
- No rubbing alcohol.

Moisturizers
- No creams, lotions, oils or powders other than those recommended in this brochure.
- No neosporin, triple antibiotic, or bacitracin antibiotic ointments.

Fragrances
- No perfumes, colognes, after shave, or pre-shave on any part of body/clothing.

Shampoo
- Free and clear shampoo and conditioner
- DHS clear shampoo and DHS conditioner
- If you have dandruff, use DHS sal shampoo or neutrogena T-SAL shampoo (not T-Gel).
- Conditioners can be used as "leave on" hair gel.

Hairspray
- Fragrance-free hairspray such as free and clear hairspray
- Caution: Hairsprays labeled as "unscented" may not be fragrance free.

Laundry and home care
- Unscented laundry detergents (tide free, cheer free and gentle, all free clear, arm and hammer unscented, wisk free, purex unscented)
- Wash all new clothes and linens five times before using.
- Old clothes and fabrics are preferred.
- Use white vinegar in rinse cycle to help remove soap.

Hand, nail, and general skin care tips
- Wear cotton gloves under rubber/vinyl gloves for any activities where hand-wetting is expected.
- Trim nails short. Long nails are dangerous to skin, especially when sleeping.

Sunscreens
- Vanicream sunscreen #30 or #60

Make-ups/cosmetics
- If you would like a list of make-ups and cosmetics that are free of the most common allergy-causing ingredients, ask your provider about "virtual patch testing" using the Mayo SkinSAFE program, www.SkinSafeProducts.com

Laundry and home care
- No fabric softener in washer.
- Bounce unscented fabric softener sheets in dryer if desired.
- No washing machine water softener such as calgon (in-house water softeners are acceptable).
- White vinegar may be used as a general household cleaner.

Hand, nail, and general skin care tips
- No wetting of hands more than five times a day.
- Avoid tight-fitting clothes unless your doctor has advised you to wear a pressure garment such as support hose.
- No scrubbing! No loofah! No pumice stone!
- Do not pull off dead skin. Snip with scissors instead.

Figure 1 Sample of prepared handout (used at the Mayo Clinic Arizona) with recommendations for the patient on hypoallergenic skin care products.

devices, such as insulin pumps, and can also be found in acrylic nails. Acetophenone azine is found in shin pads and footwear that contain cushioning foam made of ethyl vinyl acetate. Aluminum is a common metal used both as a metal in industry and everyday life and also as a salt in cosmetics, sunscreen, food, tattoos, medicine, and water purification.

Diagnosis

The evaluation of a patient with suspected contact dermatitis begins with the history. Specific questions directed at the patient's occupation, hobbies, and home routine will be helpful. Examination should note the location and pattern of the eruption. Although eyelid dermatitis may be seen in the atopic patient, nail polish may be the source of the offending allergen. Dyshidrotic eczema occurs as vesicles along the lateral aspects of the fingers, whereas eczematous changes along the dorsal hands are more commonly caused by an allergen. Other distributions as clues include postauricular scalp (perfume), perioral area (chewing gum, toothpaste), trunk (dyes or clothing finish), wrist (nickel or chrome), waistline (rubber), feet (shoes), and history or presence of wounds (topical antibiotic ointment).

Patch testing can confirm or reveal a contact allergy. It involves placement of allergens against the skin of the patient's back for 48 hours. An initial reading is then done, with follow-up readings typically at 96 hours. Prepared series include the thin-layer, rapid-use epicutaneous (TRUE) test, which consists of 35 allergens and 1 negative control (https://mytruetest.com/). Customized series, such as the NACDG Standard Series with 70 allergens and the Mayo Clinic's Standard Series with 80 allergens, must be manually assembled. The majority of dermatologists performing patch testing use the TRUE test. Note that benzalkonium chloride, MI, and propolis are not included in this panel. Overall, the NACDG estimates that 25% to approximately 40% of allergic reactions would have been missed by the TRUE test based on their data for 2015 to 2016.

In addition to ascertaining degree of positivity, relevance must be determined. This involves collaborating with patients to assess the likelihood that they are currently exposed to the positive antigen.

Treatment

Ideally, the allergen or allergens will be identified and avoided. Realistically, compliance is a challenge. To assist patients in avoiding antigens in skin care products, SkinSAFE was created in 1999. It includes 15,627 ingredients and 90,402 individual over-the-counter and prescription skin care products as of January 31, 2023. Once the patient's allergens have been identified with patch testing, they can be entered into the database, and a list of products free from those substances is generated. The patient should be reminded that even small and infrequent exposures can perpetuate the eczema.

Topical corticosteroids applied twice daily are helpful in hastening resolution and may also be used for disease control when the allergen is unknown. Low-potency corticosteroids such as 2.5% hydrocortisone (Hytone) are recommended for the thinner skin of the face, neck, axillae, groin, and intertriginous areas. Midpotency steroids such as triamcinolone 0.1% (Kenalog, Kenonel) are appropriate for the thicker skin of the body. Short-term use of higher-potency steroids may be necessary if the reaction is severe. If there is significant pruritus, sedating antihistamines such as doxepin (Sinequan)[1] 10 to 20 mg taken nightly 2 hours before bedtime can provide relief. Steroid-sparing topical immunomodulators such as tacrolimus (Protopic),[1] pimecrolimus (Elidel),[1] crisaborole (Eucrisa)[1] and ruxolitinib 1.5% (Opzelura)[1] may be helpful adjuncts, but they may be more expensive. Treatment for severe acute episodes can entail a several-week tapering course of systemic corticosteroids, especially if the eruption is widespread. Other longer-term systemic therapies for severe or

resistant disease include phototherapy or systemic immunosuppressants such as azathioprine (Imuran),[1] mycophenolate mofetil (CellCept),[1] methotrexate,[1] cyclosporine (Neoral),[1] or dupilumab (Dupixent).[1] Newer agents include tralokinumab (Adbry),[1] upadacitinib (Rinvoq),[1] and abrocitinib (Cibinqo).[1]

It may take many weeks before the skin reverts to a normal appearance despite successful avoidance of antigens. A prepared handout with concrete recommendations for the patient on truly hypoallergenic skin care is beneficial. A sample of that used at Mayo Clinic Arizona is shown in Figure 1.

If patch testing is not performed, an initial approach may be to instruct the patient on avoiding the most common contact allergens via a handout and prescribing symptomatic treatment including topical and oral therapies. SkinSAFE can generate a shopping list of products free from the top 10 allergens as identified by the NACDG and the MCCDG. Patients may access SkinSAFE independently (at https://www.skinsafeproducts.com, the Apple App Store, or the Google Play Store under SkinSAFE) to generate this list or build customized lists free from fragrances, common preservatives, parabens, nickel, lanolin, coconut, and topical antibiotics. In 35% of patients, simply using products free from the top 10 allergens can prompt clearance. Some physicians follow these measures for several months, especially if the eruption is mild, before pursuing formal patch testing.

An excellent primer for the physician interested in learning more about contact allergy diagnosis and management is *Contact and Occupational Dermatology*.

---

[1] Not FDA approved for this indication.

References

Aerts O, Herman A, Mowitz M, et al: Isobornyl acrylate, *Dermatitis*, 2020, https://doi.org/10.1097/DER.0000000000000549. [Epub ahead of print].

Bruze M, Zimerson E: Dimethyl fumarate, *Dermatitis* 22:3–7, 2011.

Castanedo-Tardana MP, Zug KA: Methylisothiazolinone, *Dermatitis* 24:2–6, 2013, https://doi.org/10.1097/DER.0b013e31827edc73.

DeKoven JG, Warshaw EM, Belsito, et al: North American contact dermatitis group patch test results 2013-2014, *Dermatitis* 28:33–46, 2017, https://doi.org/10.1097/DER.0000000000000225.

DeKoven JG, Warshaw EM, Zug KA, et al: North American contact dermatitis group patch test results: 2015-2016, *Dermatitis* 29:297–309, 2018, https://doi.org/10.1097/DER.0000000000000417.

Heurung AR, Raju SI, Warshaw EM: Benzophenones, *Dermatitis* 25:3–10, 2014, https://doi.org/10.1097/DER.0000000000000025.

Jacob SE, Scheman A, McGowan MA: Allergen of the year: propylene glycol, *Dermatitis*, 2017, https://doi.org/10.1097/DER.0000000000000315.

Macneil JS: Henna tattoo ingredient is allergen of the year, *Skin & Allergy News*, 2006. Available at http://www.skinandallergynews.com/index.php?id=372&cHash=071010&tx_ttnews%5Btt_news%5D=559.

Marks JG, Elsner P, DeLeo VA: *In Contact and occupational dermatology*, Mosby, 2002.

Nelson SA, Yiannias JA: Relevance and avoidance of skin care product allergens: pearls and pitfalls, *Dermatol Clin* 27:329–336, 2009.

Raison-Peyron N, Sasseville D: Acetophenone azine, *Dermatitis* 32:5–9, 2021.

Sasseville D: Acrylates, *Dermatitis* 23(3–5), 2012, https://doi.org/10.1097/DER.0b013e31823d5cd8.

Splete H: Dermatologists name isobornyl acrylate contact allergen of the year, *Dermatology News*, 2019. Available at https://www.mdedge.com/dermatology/article/195656/contact-dermatitis/dermatologists-name-isobornyl-acrylate-contact.

Thin-layer rapid-use epicutaneous test (T.R.U.E. TEST), https://www.smartpractice.com/shop/wa/category?cn=Products-T.R.U.E.-TEST&id=508222&m=SPA, 2021.

Veverka KK, Hall MR, Yiannias JA, et al: Trends in patch testing with the Mayo Clinic standard series, 2011-2015, *Dermatitis* 29(6):310–315, 2018, https://doi.org/10.1097/DER.0000000000000411.

Warshaw EM, Belsito DV, Taylor JS, et al: North American contact dermatitis group patch test results: 2009 to 2010, *Dermatitis* 24:50–59, 2013.

Warshaw EM, Maibach HI, Taylor JS, et al: North American contact dermatitis group patch test results: 2011-2012, *Dermatitis* 26(1):49–59, 2015, https://doi.org/10.1097/DER.0000000000000097.

Wentworth AB, Yiannias JA, Keeling JH, et al: Trends in patch test results and allergen changes in the standard series: a Mayo Clinic 5-year retrospective review. January 1, 2006, through December 31, 2010, *J Am Acad Dermatol* 70:269–275.e4, 2014. https://doi.org/10.1016/j.jaad.2013.09.047.

Yiannias J: *Virtual patch testing: data driven empiric contact allergen avoidance*, Baltimore, MD, 2013, American College of Allergy, Asthma and Immunology Annual Scientific Meeting, November 11, 2013.

---

[1] Not FDA approved for this indication.

CUTANEOUS T-CELL LYMPHOMAS, INCLUDING MYCOSIS FUNGOIDES AND SÉZARY SYNDROME

Method of
Gary S. Wood, MD

CURRENT DIAGNOSIS

For cutaneous T-cell lymphomas, obtain the following:
- History: duration and pace of lesion development
- Skin examination: extent of patches, plaques, tumors, and ulcers
- Extracutaneous examination: status of lymph nodes, liver, and spleen
- Laboratory: complete blood cell count, differential, and lesional biopsy results
- Imaging: CT or fused PET/CT scans of the chest, abdomen, and pelvis (not needed for early-stage mycosis fungoides)

CURRENT THERAPY

Guidelines are primarily for mycosis fungoides and Sézary syndrome:
- Stages IA–IIA: skin-directed therapy with potent topical corticosteroids, topical mechlorethamine (Valchlor), or phototherapy; radiation therapy or topical bexarotene (Targretin) in selected cases
- Stages IIB–IVB: skin-directed therapy plus one or more systemic therapies, such as pegylated interferon alfa-2a (Pegasys),[1] bexarotene (Targretin), romidepsin (Istodax), targeted antibodies, or methotrexate; photopheresis for erythrodermic cases
- Combination therapies are often used in intermediate- and advanced-stage disease.
- Multiagent chemotherapy is usually not an effective long-term treatment strategy.

[1]Not FDA approved for this indication.

Cutaneous T-Cell Lymphomas
Classification

Virtually every subtype of T-cell lymphoma involves the skin primarily or secondarily. The principal types of primary cutaneous T-cell lymphomas (CTCLs) recognized in the World Health Organization and European Organization for Research and Treatment of Cancer classification include mycosis fungoides (MF) and its leukemic variant, the Sézary syndrome (SS); CD30+ large cell lymphoma and lymphomatoid papulosis (LyP); CD30− large cell lymphoma; and pleomorphic CD4+ small or medium cell variants (Table 1). All other primary CTCLs comprise only a few percent of the total. This discussion focuses on MF and SS because they account for up to 75% of primary cutaneous cases.

Standard Diagnosis and Staging Methods

The evaluation of patients with CTCL begins with a thorough clinical history and physical examination. Key elements of the history include the pace and nature of disease development, the presence or absence of spontaneous regression of lesions, prior therapy, and ingestion of drugs (e.g., anticonvulsants, antihistamines, other agents with antihistaminic properties) that have been associated with pseudolymphomatous skin eruptions that can mimic CTCLs. The review of systems should establish

CTCL TYPE	PROPORTION OF PRIMARY CTCL (%)	5-YEAR SURVIVAL RATE (%)
TABLE 1 Simplified Classification of Primary Cutaneous T-Cell Lymphomas		
MF and variants	60	85
SS	3	35*
CD30+ large cell/LyP	25	<95
Pleomorphic small/medium cell†	8	99
Miscellaneous	<1	Variable

Complete classification in Willemze R, Cerroni L, Kempf W, et al. The 2018 update of the WHO-EORTC classification for primary cutaneous lymphomas. *Blood* 2019;133(16):1703–1714.
CTCL, Cutaneous T-cell lymphoma; *MF,* mycosis fungoides; *SS,* Sézary syndrome.
*The 5-year survival rate depends on the criteria used to define SS, and it may be as low as 10%.
†Now regarded as a lymphoproliferative disorder, not lymphoma.

the presence of lymphoma-associated constitutional symptoms (e.g., fever of unknown origin, night sweats, weight loss, fatigue). In addition to general aspects, the physical examination should document the type and distribution of skin lesions and whether there is lymphadenopathy, hepatosplenomegaly, or edema of extremities (i.e., potential sign of lymphatic obstruction).

Histopathologic analysis of representative lesional skin biopsy specimens is the primary means of confirming the clinical diagnosis. Biopsy specimens should be deep enough to include the deepest portions of the cutaneous lymphoid infiltrates because these areas often exhibit the most diagnostic features. Putative extracutaneous involvement should be confirmed by biopsy if it is relevant to clinical management.

Routine blood tests include a complete blood cell count, differential review, and general chemistry panel. A "Sézary prep" is used to assess peripheral blood involvement.

Internal nodal and visceral involvement by lymphoma usually is assessed with chest radiography, computed tomography (CT), or combined positron emission tomography and CT (PET/CT) scans of the chest, abdomen, and pelvis. These radiologic studies usually are not needed for patients with early forms of MF (i.e., nontumorous skin lesions without evidence of extracutaneous involvement assessed by physical examination); however, they are usually obtained during the workup of other types of CTCLs. The role of immunopathologic and molecular biologic assays in the diagnosis and staging of CTCLs is discussed later.

An algorithm for the diagnosis of early MF has been proposed by the International Society for Cutaneous Lymphomas (ISCL). It relies on a combination of clinical, histopathologic, immunopathologic, and clonality criteria. This differs from former approaches that have been based primarily on histopathologic criteria.

Mycosis Fungoides, Sézary Syndrome, and Variants
Clinical Features

MF classically manifests as erythematous, scaly, variably pruritic, flat patches or indurated plaques, often favoring the most sun-protected areas. The patches or plaques may progress to cutaneous tumors and involvement of lymph nodes or viscera, although this usually does not occur as long as the skin lesions are reasonably well controlled by therapy. SS manifests as total-body erythema and scaling (i.e., erythroderma), generalized lymphadenopathy, hepatosplenomegaly, and leukemia. Large-plaque parapsoriasis is essentially the prediagnostic patch phase of MF. Lesions may exhibit poikiloderma (i.e., atrophy, telangiectasia, and mottled hyperpigmentation and hypopigmentation) and have then been referred to as *poikiloderma atrophicans vasculare*.

Follicular mucinosis refers to a papulonodular eruption in which hair follicles are infiltrated by T cells and contain pools of mucin. In hairy areas, this may result in alopecia. Follicular mucinosis may exist as a lesional variant of MF (i.e., follicular MF) or as a clinically benign entity (i.e., alone or associated with other lymphomas). Clinicopathological criteria can distinguish between indolent and aggressive forms of follicular MF. Granulomatous slack skin is a variant of MF that manifests with pendulous skin folds in intertriginous areas. Lesional skin biopsy specimens contain atypical T cells in a granulomatous background.

Pagetoid reticulosis manifests as a solitary or localized, often hyperkeratotic plaque containing atypical T cells that are frequently confined to a hyperplastic epidermis. Some authorities regard it as a variant of unilesional MF, whereas others think it is a distinct entity.

Other variants of MF include hypopigmented, palmoplantar, bullous, and pigmented purpuric forms. The latter form shows clinicopathologic overlap with the pigmented purpuric dermatoses. *Tumor d'emblee* MF is an outmoded concept used in the past to refer to supposed cases of MF that manifested as cutaneous tumors in the absence of patches or plaques. Most experts now prefer to classify such cases as other forms of CTCL, depending on their histopathologic features.

Histopathologic and Cytologic Features

A well-developed plaque of MF contains a bandlike, cytologically atypical lymphoid infiltrate in the upper dermis that infiltrates the epidermis as single cells and cell clusters known as Pautrier's microabscesses. The atypical lymphoid cells exhibit dense, hyperchromatic nuclei with convoluted, cerebriform nuclear contours and scant cytoplasm. The term *cerebriform* comes from the brainlike ultrastructural appearance of these nuclei. In more advanced cutaneous tumors, the infiltrate extends diffusely throughout the upper and lower dermis and may lose its epidermotropism. In the earlier patch phase of the disease, the infiltrate is sparser, and lymphoid atypia may be less pronounced. In some cases, it may be difficult to distinguish early patch-type MF from various types of chronic dermatitis. The presence of lymphoid atypia and absence of significant epidermal intercellular edema (i.e., spongiosis) help establish the diagnosis of early MF.

Involvement of lymph nodes by MF begins in the paracortical T-cell domain and may progress to complete effacement of nodal architecture by the same types of atypical lymphoid cells that infiltrate the skin. These cells can be seen in low numbers in the peripheral blood of many MF patients; however, those with SS develop gross leukemic involvement, usually defined as at least 1000 tumor cells/mm³. These cells are known as Sézary cells, and they are traditionally detected by manual review of the peripheral blood smear (the so-called Sézary prep). They may also be defined by various immunophenotypic criteria.

Immunophenotyping

Cellular antigen expression is usually assessed by immunoperoxidase methods for tissue biopsy specimens and by flow cytometry for blood specimens. Almost all cases of MF or SS begin as phenotypically and functionally mature CD4+ T-cell neoplasms of skin-associated lymphoid tissue (SALT). MF and SS express homing markers consistent with "effector memory" and "central memory" T cells, respectively. They express the SALT-associated homing molecule cutaneous lymphocyte antigen (CLA) and most mature T-cell surface antigens, with the exceptions of CD7 and CD26, which are often absent. As disease progresses, the tumor cells often dedifferentiate and lose one or more mature T-cell markers, such as CD2, CD3, or CD5.

Cases typically express the α/β form of the T-cell receptor. At least in advanced cases, the cytokine profile is consistent with the T_H2 subset of CD4+ T cells (i.e., production of interleukin [IL]-4, IL-5, and IL-10 rather than T_H1 cytokines such as IL-2 and interferon-γ). Expression of the high-affinity IL-2 receptor (CD25, TAC) ranges widely, with most cases showing a variable minority of lesional CD25+ cells. Tumor cells can be induced to express a regulatory T-cell phenotype (Treg) in vitro. MF cases that express CD8+ or other aberrant phenotypes occur occasionally but behave like conventional cases. They should not be confused with rare aggressive CTCLs exhibiting cytotoxic T-cell differentiation.

In addition to tumor cells, MF and SS lesions contain a minor component of immune accessory cells (i.e., Langerhans cells and macrophages) and CD8+ T cells with a cytolytic phenotype. This presumed host response correlates positively with survival and tends to decrease as lesions progress. A favorable response to therapy such as photopheresis appears to correlate with normal levels of circulating CD8+ cells.

Molecular Biology

Well-developed MF or SS is a monoclonal T-cell lymphoproliferative disorder. Southern blotting or polymerase chain reaction (PCR) assays demonstrate monoclonal T-cell receptor gene rearrangements. The greater sensitivity of PCR assays allows the demonstration of dominant clonality in many early patch-type lesions of MF. These assays sometimes detect dominant clonality in lesional skin showing only chronic dermatitis histopathologically. These cases are called *clonal dermatitis* and may represent the earliest manifestation of MF because several have progressed to histologically recognizable MF within a few years. However, some cases of clinicopathologically defined early-phase MF lack a detectable monoclonal T-cell population until later in their clinical course. Next generation high throughput T-cell receptor sequencing is emerging as a more sensitive and quantitative alternative to other molecular assays of T-cell clonality.

In addition to aiding initial diagnosis, gene rearrangement analysis has facilitated staging and prognosis. Because some patients without MF or SS can have low levels of circulating Sézary-like cells and because not all cases of peripheral blood involvement in MF or SS exhibit morphologically recognizable tumor cells, the demonstration of dominant clonality that matches the clone in lesional skin has proved to be a useful diagnostic adjunct. The same holds true for assessing lymph node involvement. T-cell receptor gene rearrangement analysis of MF and SS lymph nodes is more sensitive than histopathology and possesses at least some prognostic relevance. Mutations in more than 80 genes can occur in MF/SS, including those involving T-cell receptor–related pathways *TP53* and *PD1*. In addition to providing insights into pathogenesis and prognosis, these mutations will form the basis of future precision medicine–based treatments.

TNMB Staging

Although several proposed methods have used a weighted extent approach to more accurately determine the MF or SS tumor burden, the preferred approach is the tumor–node–metastasis–blood (TNMB) system, which is detailed in Tables 2 and 3. The original tumor (skin), lymph nodes, and metastasis (visceral organs) version of this system has been modified by the ISCL to incorporate the extent of blood involvement (B classification) into the staging process. Table 2 shows the TNMB classification relevant to MF and SS, and Table 3 shows how this information is used to determine the stage of disease. The prognostic relevance of this staging system has been supported by numerous studies, and use of the TNMB helps to guide the selection of therapies. For example, early-stage MF is the most amenable to control with topically directed

TABLE 2	TNMB Classification of Mycosis Fungoides and Sézary Syndrome

Skin (T)

T1	Patches and/or plaques; <10% body surface area
T2	Patches and/or plaques; ≥10% body surface area
T3	Tumors with/without other skin lesions
T4	Generalized erythroderma

Lymph Nodes (N)

N0	Not clinically enlarged; histopathology not required
N1	Clinically enlarged; histopathologically negative
N2	Clinically enlarged; histopathologically equivocal
N3	Clinically enlarged; histopathologically positive

Visceral Organs (M)

M0	No involvement
M1	Involvement

Peripheral Blood (B)

B0	Atypical cells ≤5% of lymphocytes
B1	Atypical cells >5% of lymphocytes
B2	Atypical cells ≥1000/mm^3

T1 and T2 can be subclassified as patch only vs. plaque +/− patch. N and B categories can be subclassified as clone positive or negative. For updates, see www.nccn.org.

Treatment

Treatment guidelines for CTCL published by the National Comprehensive Cancer Network can be found at www.nccn.org. Rather than cure, which is attained in less than 10% of cases, the goal of MF and SS therapy is to reduce the effect of the skin disease on quality of life. For most patients, this is achieved by reducing pain, itch, and infection and improving clinical appearance. Appearance is affected by the disfigurement of the eruption and by the profound degree of scale shedding in some patients. Because the natural history of early-stage MF predicts a virtually normal life span, the goal of treatment must be directed at quality of life. For more advanced stages, prolongation of life expectancy may be a reasonable treatment goal.

Regardless of presentation, relief of symptoms should be addressed early. For dryness and scaling, the use of emollient ointments is indicated. These include petrolatum, Aquaphor, and commercially available shortening such as Crisco (an inexpensive alternative).[1] For modest dryness, creams (e.g., Nivea, Cetaphil, Eucerin) can be adequate and more acceptable to patients. Mild superfatted soaps such as Dove and Oil of Olay are recommended. Soap substitutes such as Cetaphil are also acceptable. Pruritus can be addressed with oral agents such as hydroxyzine (Atarax) or diphenhydramine (Benadryl)[1] 2 to 4 mg/kg/day and divided into four daily doses. Antipruritics work better when used on a regular basis rather

[1] Not FDA approved for this indication.

TABLE 3	TNMB Staging System for Mycosis Fungoides and Sézary Syndrome

STAGE	SKIN	LYMPH NODES	VISCERA	BLOOD
IA	T1	N0	M0	B0–1
IB	T2	N0	M0	B0–1
IIA	T1–2	N1–2	M0	B0–1
IIB	T3	N0–2	M0	B0–1
IIIA	T4	N0–2	M0	B0
IIIB	T4	N0–2	M0	B1
IVA-1	T1–4	N0–2	M0	B2
IVA-2	T1–4	N3	M0	B0–2
IVB	T1–4	N0–3	M1	B0–2

Modified from Olsen E, Vonderheid E, et al: Revisions to the staging and classification of mycosis fungoides and Sézary syndrome: A proposal of the International Society for Cutaneous Lymphomas (ISCL) and the cutaneous lymphoma task force of the European Organization of Research and Treatment of Cancer (EORTC). *Blood* 2007;110(6):1713–1722. For updates, see www.nccn.org.

than on an as-needed basis. Nonsedating antihistamines tend to be less effective. Measures to reduce dryness also help reduce pruritus. Secondary infection needs to be treated with appropriate antibiotics. Their selection is guided by results of skin cultures but usually involves coverage of gram-positive organisms.

Phototherapy

Two main phototherapeutic regimens are used to treat CTCLs. Ultraviolet B radiation (290–320-nm broad band or 311-nm narrow band) can be used for patients with patches but not those with well-developed plaques or tumors. Seventy percent of patients achieve total clinical remission, usually within about 3 to 5 months. Another 15% achieve partial remission. Narrowband UVB usually is more effective than broadband UVB and achieves maximal responses more rapidly. A synthetic form of hypericin (HyBryte)[5] applied topically and activated by visible fluorescent light has undergone clinical trials and is currently being evaluated by the FDA.

Psoralen–ultraviolet A (PUVA) photochemotherapy uses oral 8-methoxypsoralen (8-MOP)[1] 0.6 mg/kg as a photosensitizer before UVA (320–400 nm) exposure. Sixty-five percent of patients with patch or plaque disease achieve complete remissions, and 30% have partial responses to this modality. For most patients, maximal responses are achieved within 3 months, and after 5 months, it is unlikely that further improvement will be gained. Limitations of these modalities include actinic damage, photocarcinogenesis, retinal damage (if eyes are not protected), and the inconvenience of getting to phototherapy centers. PUVA also has the risk of nausea and a theoretical risk of cataract induction without proper eye protection.

During the clearing phase of treatment, phototherapy treatments usually are administered three times per week. After resolution of skin lesions, treatment frequency is usually tapered gradually to once weekly for UVB and once every 4 to 6 weeks for PUVA. These maintenance regimens are often continued for months to years because abrupt cessation of phototherapy is commonly associated with rapid relapse, which is probably related to the persistence of microscopic disease after clinical clearing.

[1] Not FDA approved for this indication.
[5] Investigational drug in the United States.

Topical Therapy

Like phototherapeutic regimens, topical therapies are appropriate for disease confined to the skin (stage I). Topical corticosteroids are frequently used for CTCLs, often before diagnosis. Low-potency formulations are useful on the face and skin folds. Medium-potency preparations are appropriate for the trunk and extremities. High-potency formulations are useful for recalcitrant lesions; however, prolonged use of such potent agents can cause local atrophy and adrenal suppression. Roughly half of patients achieve complete remissions, and most others have partial remissions. Response duration varies widely with the individual pace of disease and patient compliance. Topical corticosteroids are particularly useful as a means to relatively quickly ameliorate severe signs and symptoms and as an adjuvant therapy in combination with other primary treatments.

Mechlorethamine (nitrogen mustard, HN_2, Mustargen) is applied topically in an aqueous solution or in an ointment, such as Aquaphor. Although these forms are not FDA approved for this indication, a 0.016% gel formulation (Valchlor) is now commercially available and FDA approved. The aqueous form is prepared at home and involves a daily dose totaling 10 mg in 60 mL water. The ointment form is prepared by a pharmacist in 1-pound lots at a concentration of 10 mg mechlorethamine per 100 g ointment. Only the amount of ointment needed to apply a thin layer is used. Either formulation is usually applied at bedtime to lesional skin for limited disease or to the entire skin surface (excluding the head unless it is also involved) for more extensive disease. It is then showered off every morning using soap and water. Results are similar to those from PUVA. Advantages include therapy at home and availability in all regions of the country. Disadvantages are daily preparation (aqueous form only), daily application, and possible allergic contact dermatitis (more common with the aqueous preparation). Maximal efficacy is expected within 6 months. Mild flare-ups of disease may occur during the first few months of treatment and probably represent inflammation of subclinical skin lesions, analogous to the clinical accentuation of actinic damage during topical therapy with 5-fluorouracil (Efudex). As with phototherapy, topical mechlorethamine is tapered gradually after remission is achieved in an effort to delay clinical relapse.

Carmustine (BCNU, BiCNU)[1] is applied to the total skin surface as an alcohol/aqueous solution (10–20 mg in 60 mL).[6] Complete responses are seen in 85% of patients with stage IA disease (<10% involvement) and 50% of patients with stage IB disease (>10% involvement). Another 10% of patients obtain partial responses. Advantages include those described for nitrogen mustard and reports of success with application only to lesional skin. Disadvantages include skin irritation followed by telangiectasia formation and possible bone marrow suppression necessitating blood monitoring.

A topical gel formulation of the retinoid X receptor (RXR)–specific retinoid, bexarotene (Targretin), is useful for localized or limited skin lesions. The principal side effect is local irritation.

Radiotherapy

Conventional radiotherapy for MF therapy has been used for approximately 100 years. It is useful in the treatment of isolated, particularly problematic lesions such as recalcitrant tumors or ulcerated plaques. In addition to benefit from the photons delivered by radiotherapy, electron beam therapy (0.4 Gy per week for 8–9 weeks) is useful for CTCL therapy. An approximately 85% complete response rate of skin disease with a median duration of 16 months is expected with electron beam therapy. An advantage is an excellent rate of complete response. Disadvantages include limited access to required equipment and expertise and cutaneous toxic effects, such as alopecia, sweat gland loss, radiation dermatitis, and skin cancers. As with other skin-directed therapy, the benefit for internal disease is limited. Cumulative toxicity also limits the number of courses a patient may receive. Localized electron beam therapy is also useful for treating cases of limited-extent MF and in treating selected problematic MF lesions in patients who are otherwise responding to therapy. After completion of total-skin electron beam therapy, patients require maintenance therapy such as topical mechlorethamine[6] or phototherapy to prolong remission. Low dose radiotherapy is emerging as an effective alternative to conventional regimens.

Apheresis-Based Therapy

Leukapheresis and particularly lymphocytapheresis (6000–7000 mL of blood treated three times per week initially, then according to response) have been used in the treatment of patients with SS. Benefit has been reported in several case reports and small case series; however, response rates are not possible to determine. Photopheresis (i.e., extracorporeal photochemotherapy) describes an apheresis-based therapy in which circulating lymphocytes are first exposed to a psoralen (orally or extracorporeally) and then exposed to UVA extracorporeally. In contrast to leukapheresis, in which leukocytes are discarded, all cells are returned to the patient's circulation during photopheresis. Response rates in erythrodermic patients are 33% to 50%, and median survival for patients with SS is prolonged from 30 months to more than 60 months. In recent years, extracorporeal photochemotherapy has been used increasingly in conjunction with one or more systemic therapies to enhance efficacy. The toxicity of the systemic agents is diminished because they are often used in combination at reduced doses.

Cytokine Therapy

Pegylated interferon alfa-2a (Pegasys)[1] has replaced interferon alfa-2a and alfa-2b, both of which have been discontinued. Ninety to 180 μg is given subcutaneously or intralesionally once weekly. Response rates are approximately 55%, with complete responses occurring in 10% of patients. Advantages include the relative ease of delivery. Disadvantages include anorexia, fever, malaise, leukopenia, and risk of cardiac dysrhythmia. An alternative treatment is interferon gamma-1b (Actimmune)[1] (1-2 MU) injected three times weekly. Interferon combined with narrowband UVB or PUVA is effective for many patients with generalized skin lesions unresponsive to phototherapy alone.

Tumor-Associated Antigen-Directed Therapies

Various specific tumor-associated antigens have been targeted with antibody-based therapy. Less specific targets are CD4, CD5, and IL-2 receptors. Of this class of agent, an improved version of the now discontinued denileukin diftitox (Ontak, DAB389 IL2, known as E7777 [I/ONTAK][2]) is approved for CTCL in Japan. Additional approvals are pending. This agent is a fusion protein combining IL-2 and diphtheria toxin. Cells bearing the IL-2 receptor (in the lesions of at least one half of MF patients) bind and internalize the drug. The drug also may destroy Treg cells that are CD25+ and suppress immune responses. Inside the cell, the toxin portion of the molecule disrupts protein synthesis, leading to cell death. Total response rates of about 33% have been reported. Adverse events include capillary leak syndrome, flulike symptoms, and allergic reactions. Alemtuzumab (Campath)[1] is an antibody directed against CD52. It has shown benefit in advanced-stage disease. This agent can be used alone or in conjunction with multiagent chemotherapy. Brentuximab vedotin (Adcetris)[1] is an anti-CD30 antibody linked to the microtubule toxin monomethyl auristatin E. It can be effective in those cases of MF

---

[1] Not FDA approved for this indication.
[6] May be compounded by pharmacists.

[1] Not FDA approved for this indication.
[2] Not available in the United States.
[6] May be compounded by pharmacists.

that express sufficient CD30. Mogamulizumab (Poteligeo) is an antibody directed against CCR4. It is approved for relapsed or refractory MF or SS after at least one other systemic therapy. Pembrolizumab (Keytruda)[1] is an antibody directed against PD1. It can be of benefit for relapsed or refractory MF or SS.

Systemic Chemotherapy

Various regimens of single-agent and multiagent chemotherapy have been used in the treatment of MF and SS. Oral methotrexate, chlorambucil (Leukeran)[1] with or without prednisone,[1] and etoposide (VePesid)[1] have shown therapeutic activity. The best response has been in erythrodermic patients treated with methotrexate (5 to 125 mg weekly),[3] who have shown a 58% response rate. The combination of low-dose methotrexate and interferon alfa has been reported to yield a high response rate in advanced-stage MF and SS.

The use of multiagent regimens is controversial because of the small number of patients treated with any given regimen. There is even some evidence that, for some populations of patients with CTCL, survival may be reduced. For individual patients with advanced disease, however, cyclophosphamide (Cytoxan),[1] doxorubicin (Adriamycin),[1] vincristine (Oncovin),[1] and prednisone[1] (CHOP regimen) can provide some short-term palliation. In some cases, CHOP has successfully eradicated large cell transformation of MF and returned patients to their more clinically indolent patch or plaque baseline disease. Idarubicin (Idamycin)[1] in association with etoposide, cyclophosphamide, vincristine, prednisone, and bleomycin (Blenoxane)[1] (VICOP-B regimen) has demonstrated response rates of 80% (36% complete response rate) for patients with stage II through IV disease and 84% for patients with MF, with a median duration of response longer than 8 months. Other regimens have been used with more modest success.

Several purine nucleoside analogs have been used for CTCL treatment, including erythrodermic variants. These include 2-chlorodeoxyadenosine (cladribine [Leustatin],[1] with a response rate of 28%), 2-deoxycoformycin (pentostatin [Nipent],[1] with a response rate of 39%), and fludarabine (Fludara).[1] Toxicities include pulmonary edema, bone marrow and immune suppression, and neurotoxicity.

Retinoids

Retinoids have therapeutic activity against MF and SS alone and in combination with other therapies, such as interferon alfa or PUVA (the latter combination is called Re-PUVA). Arotinoid,[5] acitretin (Soriatane),[1] and 13-*cis*-retinoic acid (isotretinoin [Accutane])[1] have various degrees of efficacy, and they typically are used in conjunction with other modalities. A newer RXR-specific retinoid, bexarotene, has an overall response rate of about 40% and can be used alone or in combination with phototherapy and other systemic agents such as interferon alfa-2. Disadvantages of bexarotene therapy include signs of hypothyroidism and vitamin A toxicity, particularly hyperlipidemia.

Enzyme Inhibitors

Vorinostat (Zolinza) is the first histone deacetylase inhibitor to be FDA approved for MF and SS. The overall response rate approaches 40% using a standard oral dose of 400 mg/day. Side effects include gastrointestinal symptoms, thrombocytopenia, and cardiac conduction abnormalities. Romidepsin (Istodax) is an intravenously administered histone deacetylase inhibitor approved by the FDA for MF and SS. Preclinical studies show that treatment of CTCL cells with romidepsin and birabresib[5] (a BET inhibitor) suppresses oncogenic p73 isoforms and kills CTCL cells. Forodesine[5] is a purine nucleoside phosphorylase inhibitor that preferentially affects T cells because they contain relatively high concentrations of this enzyme. Forodesine has undergone clinical trials for MF and SS in the United States and appears to have a response rate of about 40%.

Miscellaneous Therapies

Various other therapies have been tried for MF and SS with modest success. Nonmyeloablative allogeneic stem cell transplantation has led to favorable responses in some patients; however, the total number treated is small. Cyclosporine (Sandimmune)[1] has been used for MF and SS. Transient improvement is followed by worsened survival due to immunosuppression, and it is not a recommended therapy. Thymopentin[5] has given excellent results in SS patients (i.e., 40% complete response rate and 35% partial response rate, with a median duration of response of 22 months). The lack of follow-up reports in recent decades leaves the status of this therapy in question. Inhibitors of Janus kinase/signal transducers and activators of transcription (JAK/STAT) and other signal transduction pathways may be useful in patients bearing relevant activating mutations.

Selection of Therapy

Initial choices among conventional treatments for MF and SS depend on the types of lesions and the stage of disease. Disease subsets are followed by recommended initial treatments in parentheses: unilesional or localized MF (local radiation therapy), patch MF (broad- and narrowband UVB, PUVA, mechlorethamine), patch/plaque MF (PUVA, mechlorethamine), thick plaque/tumor MF (electron beam radiation therapy, interferon alfa-2, bexarotene, histone deacetylase inhibitors), erythrodermic MF/SS (photopheresis), and nodal or visceral MF or SS (interferon alfa-2, bexarotene, histone deacetylase inhibitors, experimental systemic therapies, systemic chemotherapy). Targeted monoclonal antibodies are also indicated for patients with stage IIB or greater disease.

Second-line therapeutic choices often involve interferons, retinoids, or histone deacetylase inhibitors, usually in combination with primary modalities. Multimodality combinations, often at reduced doses, are used commonly to treat patients with stage IIB or more advanced disease. Medium-potency topical corticosteroids, such as 0.1% triamcinolone cream or ointment (Kenalog),[1] are useful adjuncts to many different therapies. The optimal use of newer therapeutic agents in various subtypes and stages of MF and SS is still being established. Evidence-based guidelines for MF and SS therapy have been developed by the National Comprehensive Cancer Network (NCCN) (www.nccn.org).

Lymphoproliferative Disorders Associated With Mycosis Fungoides and Sézary Syndrome

Types and Clinical Features

Patients with MF or SS are at increased risk for large T-cell lymphomas, lymphomatoid papulosis, and Hodgkin's disease. Molecular biologic analysis has shown that these disorders and MF often share the same clonal T-cell receptor gene rearrangement when they arise in the same individual. As a consequence, they are considered to be subclones of the original MF tumor clone. The development of large T-cell lymphoma in a patient with MF or SS is referred to as *large cell transformation of MF*. This occurs in up to 20% of cases in some series and is associated with a median survival of only 1 to 2 years. One half of these large T-cell lymphomas are CD30+; however, the generally favorable prognosis of primary cutaneous CD30+ anaplastic large cell lymphoma may not extend to these secondary forms of CD30+ lymphoma. These patients

---

[1] Not FDA approved for this indication.
[3] Exceeds dosage recommended by the manufacturer.
[5] Investigational drug in the United States.

---

[1] Not FDA approved for this indication.
[5] Investigational drug in the United States.

may need to be treated with systemic chemotherapy such as CHOP or with experimental systemic therapies appropriate for advanced-stage CTCL.

Lymphomatoid papulosis manifests as recurrent, usually generalized crops of spontaneously regressing, erythematous papules that can exhibit crusting or vesiculation before resolution. It is the clinically benign end of a disease continuum that has primary cutaneous CD30+ anaplastic large cell lymphoma at its other extreme. Intermediate forms of disease can occur. Histopathologically, lesions contain a mixed-cell infiltrate, including large, atypical T cells that resemble Reed-Sternberg cells and their mononuclear variants (so-called type A) or large MF-type cells (so-called type B). Type A cells are CD30+. A type C form is also recognized. It has sheets of type A cells histologically mimicking CD30+ large T-cell lymphoma but is different from it clinically. A type D variant containing CD8+ CD30+ large, atypical cells has also been described recently, as well as a few other rare subtypes. All types of lymphomatoid papulosis behave similarly. Patients with lymphomatoid papulosis sometimes respond to tetracycline[1] or erythromycin[1] (500 mg PO bid), presumably on the basis of antiinflammatory activity. Most cases improve within 1 month with low-dose methotrexate (10–20 mg PO every week). PUVA and narrow-band UVB given three times per week are other therapeutic options.

Treatment

In most cases, non-MF/SS CTCLs are treated with radiation therapy (with or without complete surgical excision) if they are localized or with various multiagent systemic chemotherapy regimens if they are generalized. The roles of other agents remain to be defined, except that studies have proved that methotrexate (10–40 mg PO every week) is effective therapy for most cases of primary cutaneous CD30+ anaplastic large cell lymphoma. Therapies being investigated for this lymphoma include anti-CD30 antibodies, alone or conjugated to toxins. One of these antibody conjugates (brentuximab vedotin [Adcetris]) is FDA approved for primary cutaneous anaplastic large cell lymphomas and CD30+ MF. Denileukin diftitox (now discontinued) and histone deacetylase inhibitors have been reported to be effective against some subcutaneous panniculitic T-cell lymphomas. The recent discovery of JAK fusion mutations in aggressive epidermotropic cytotoxic CTCL (Berti's lymphoma) suggests that JAK inhibitors might be beneficial in this rare disorder.

---

[1] Not FDA approved for this indication.

References

Olsen E, Vonderheid E, et al: Revisions to the staging and classification of mycosis fungoides and Sézary syndrome: a proposal of the International Society for Cutaneous Lymphomas (ISCL) and the cutaneous lymphoma task force of the European Organization of Research and Treatment of Cancer (EORTC), *Blood* 110(6):1713–1722, 2007.

Park J, Daniels J, Wartewig T, et al: Integrated genomic analyses of cutaneous T-cell lymphomas reveal the molecular bases for disease heterogeneity, *Blood* 138(14):1225–1236, 2021.

Pimpinelli N, Olsen EA, Santucci M, et al: Defining early mycosis fungoides, *J Am Acad Dermatol* 53(6):1053–1063, 2005.

Richardson SK, Lin JH, Vittorio CC, et al: High clinical response rate with multimodality immunomodulatory therapy for Sézary syndrome, *Clin Lymphoma Myeloma* 7(3):226–232, 2006.

Vonderheid EC, Bernengo MG, Burg G, et al: Update on erythrodermic cutaneous T-cell lymphoma: report of the international society for cutaneous lymphomas, *J Am Acad Dermatol* 46(1):95–106, 2002.

Willemze R, Cerroni L, Kempf W, et al: The 2018 update of the WHO-EORTC classification for primary cutaneous lymphomas, *Blood* 133(16):1703–1714, 2019.

Wood GS, Greenberg HL: Diagnosis, staging, and monitoring of cutaneous T-cell lymphoma, *Dermatol Ther* 16(4):269–275, 2003.

Zhao L, Xiao T, Stonesifer C, Daniels J, et al: The robust tumoricidal effects of combined BET and HDAC inhibition in CTCL can Be reproduced by ΔNp73 depletion, *J Invest Dermatol* 142:3253–3261, 2022.

CUTANEOUS VASCULITIS

Method of
Molly A. Hinshaw, MD; and Susan Lawrence-Hylland, MD

CURRENT DIAGNOSIS

- Cutaneous vasculitis can be limited to skin (leukocytoclastic vasculitis) or associated with systemic disease.
- Perform punch biopsy of intact, nonulcerated skin lesion.
- "Vasculitis" on skin biopsy describes vessel appearance and is not a clinical diagnosis.
- Thorough review of systems and physical examination are necessary to evaluate for systemic vasculitis.

CURRENT THERAPY

Leukocytoclastic Vasculitis
- First identify instigating factors: infection, medications.
- Care is symptomatic. Lesions typically remit without treatment.
- If needed, short course of prednisone may be given and tapered over 3 to 6 weeks.

All Forms of Vasculitis
- Treat underlying systemic vasculitis.

Vasculitis is an inflammatory-mediated destruction of blood vessels. The systemic vasculitides have historically been differentiated by their involvement of small, medium, or large blood vessels. Names used to describe isolated cutaneous vasculitis have included hypersensitivity vasculitis and leukocytoclastic vasculitis (LCV). In 1990, the American College of Rheumatology proposed five criteria for the classification of hypersensitivity vasculitis: age older than 16 years, possible drug trigger, palpable purpura, maculopapular rash, and skin biopsy showing neutrophils around vessel. At least three out of five criteria yield a sensitivity of 71% and specificity of 84%. In 1994, a new nomenclature proposed at the Chapel Hill International Consensus Conference in North Carolina further classified vasculitis (Box 1). The term "hypersensitivity vasculitis" was not used, because most vasculitides that would have previously been in this category fall into either microscopic polyangiitis or cutaneous LCV. LCV is vasculitis restricted to the skin without involvement of vessels in other organs. Cutaneous vasculitis may be a clue to systemic vasculitis and guides the clinician to a comprehensive evaluation (Table 1).

Vasculitis can affect almost any organ, and once affected, end organs can become dysfunctional. Such dysfunction may be as innocuous as cutaneous, tender, transient papules or as devastating as a stroke. A thorough evaluation of the patient with a complete review of systems, physical examination, laboratory evaluation, and clinical follow-up allows a distinction to be made between the different forms of vasculitis.

Leukocytoclastic Vasculitis

Epidemiology

LCV is common. The incidence and prevalence are unknown. Mean age of onset ranges from 34 to 49 years of age. The female-to-male ratio ranges from approximately 2:1 to 3:1.

Risk Factors

LCV is often secondary to a known trigger including infection, drug ingestion, or malignancy. LCV can also be a presenting feature of autoimmune disease.

BOX 1 Chapel Hill Consensus 1994 Classification of Vasculitis

Large-Vessel Vasculitis
Giant cell arteritis
  Takayasu's arteritis

Medium-Vessel Vasculitis
Classic polyarteritis nodosa
  Kawasaki's disease

Small-Vessel Vasculitis
Churg-Strauss syndrome
  Cutaneous leukocytoclastic vasculitis
  Essential cryoglobulinemia
  Henoch-Schönlein purpura
  Microscopic polyangiitis (polyarteritis)
  Wegener's granulomatosis

Pathophysiology

LCV is best characterized as immune complex–mediated inflammatory destruction of the postcapillary venules of any organ. The exact mechanisms of vascular destruction is unknown.

Clinical Manifestations

LCV typically manifests as nonblanchable macules that evolve to papules or, less commonly, pustules and ulcers (Figure 1). Clues to the diagnosis include a monomorphous, ruddy-brown appearance owing to leakage of hemosiderin pigment from vessels. Lesions measure a few millimeters to a few centimeters in diameter. LCV is often localized to the lower extremities but may be diffuse. Pruritus, pain, or burning of the skin lesions are indicators that the patient might have a vasculitis extending beyond LCV.

Diagnosis

To confirm a clinical impression of LCV, perform a punch biopsy in the center of a nonulcerated cutaneous lesion that is less than 24 to 48 hours old and submit the sample in 10% formalin (standard medium). It is important to biopsy an intact, nonulcerated active lesion (Figure 2) because ulcers can show histologic features simulating vasculitis regardless of whether the patient has true vasculitis or not.

Pathology reveals a mononuclear or polymorphonuclear inflammation of the small blood vessels (called LCV), most prominent in the postcapillary venules. The appearance may be necrotizing or non-necrotizing.

Differential Diagnosis

LCV manifests as erythematous papules or occasionally as papulopustules that can simulate a variety of entities (see Table 1). The review of systems and physical examination should be directed to evaluate for diseases that have cutaneous vasculitis as a component of their presentation (see Table 1). All patients with LCV should have a urinalysis to evaluate for hematuria as a sign of kidney involvement, with subsequent evaluation and management if identified.

Treatment

The primary goal in the management of LCV is to identify and treat instigating factors, including infection and medications. Supportive treatment includes resting, elevating legs, and wearing support hose. When review of systems, physical examination, and urinalysis do not reveal associated systemic diseases, treatment of LCV is generally not necessary. Lesions typically remit without treatment. In rare patients with symptomatic, extensively pustular, or progressive lesions, a short course of prednisone[1] dosed at 1 mg/kg/day initially and tapered over 3 to 6 weeks may be used,

---

[1]Not FDA approved for this indication.

TABLE 1 Diseases with Cutaneous Vasculitis as a Component of Their Presentation

DISEASE	SKIN LESIONS	CLUES AND CONFIRMATION
Urticarial vasculitis	Individual lesions look like urticaria but last >24 h; typical urticaria last a few hours, always <24 h Pruritus, burning of skin lesions	May be associated with connective tissue disease, medications, low complement, viral infections (e.g., hep B, hep C, EBV) Skin biopsy
Henoch-Schönlein purpura	Wheals progress to petechia, ecchymoses and palpable purpura Lesions are in gravity-dependent or pressure-dependent areas such as legs or the buttocks in toddlers	Arthralgia or arthritis, hematuria, abdominal pain, melena Skin biopsy and DIF for IgA
Essential mixed cryoglobulinemia	Palpable purpura	Peripheral neuropathy, GN Hep C positive Serum cryoglobulins
Wegener's granulomatosis	Palpable purpura, hemorrhagic lesions, petechiae, skin ulcers	c-ANCA >80% Pulmonary hemorrhage, GN Biopsy affected organ
Churg-Strauss syndrome	Maculopapular rash, palpable purpura, hemorrhagic lesions, subcutaneous nodules, livedo reticularis or Raynaud's disease	ANCA (50%) Asthma, allergic rhinitis Eosinophilia >1.5 × 10^9/L Pulmonary infiltrates, pulmonary neuropathy Biopsy affected organ
Microscopic polyangiitis	Palpable purpura, hemorrhagic lesions, petechiae, skin ulcers, splinter hemorrhages	p-ANCA >60% Pulmonary hemorrhage, GN Biopsy affected organ
Polyarteritis nodosa	Livedo reticularis, tender nodules, skin ulcers, bullae or vesicles	Hypertension, elevated creatinine, abdominal pain, constitutional symptoms (fever) Abnormal angiogram Biopsy affected organ

Abbreviations: c-ANCA = classic antineutrophil cytoplasmic antibody; DIF = direct immunofluorescence; EBV = Epstein-Barr virus; GN = glomerulonephritis; hep = hepatitis; Ig = immunoglobulin; p-ANCA = protoplasmic-staining antineutrophil cytoplasmic antibody.

Figure 1 Leukocytoclastic vasculitis: palpable, purpuric, nonblanching, erythematous to ruddy-brown thin papules. Additional secondary changes include small pustules (pustular vasculitis) or shallow, small ulcerations.

Figure 2 Biopsy of intact clinical lesion of leukocytoclastic vasculitis. Histology shows destruction of postcapillary venules with fibrin deposition, degenerate inflammatory cells, and extravasated erythrocytes.

although no controlled trials have been performed using oral corticosteroids for isolated LCV. Rapid steroid taper can lead to rebound. Systematic evaluation of the use of other medications, such as colchicine[1] or dapsone,[1] to treat isolated LCV has not been performed.

Monitoring
Patients with LCV are at risk for recurrent or chronic vasculitis. In addition, apparent LCV can occur as a systemic disease that is not recognizable at the first episode. Patients with persistent or recurrent LCV require follow-up to ensure disease clearance, to monitor for medication side effects, and to evaluate for evolving disorders known to be associated with cutaneous vasculitis (see Table 1).

Complications
Isolated LCV generally resolves without sequelae. However, pustular or ulcerative LCV may be complicated by local sequelae such as cutaneous ulcerations and scars.

Cutaneous Vasculitis Associated with Systemic Vasculitis
Cutaneous vasculitis may be a component of the presentation of multiple diseases (see Table 1). When a clinician reads a pathology report from a biopsy of a skin lesion that states "vasculitis," it is important to realize that this term is a descriptor of the histopathology. It is the clinician's challenge to determine whether "vasculitis" is as potentially innocuous as LCV or part of a more severe systemic disease. Symptoms that are clues to a systemic process can include fever, arthralgias, myalgias,

anorexia, abdominal pain, pulmonary abnormalities, or neurologic symptoms.

Skin biopsy may aid in the diagnosis of a systemic vasculitis (Henoch-Schönlein purpura), but biopsy of an affected end organ may be necessary to confirm a diagnosis. Pathology focuses on the confirmation of vasculitis in a small, medium, or large vessel.

Aside from Henoch-Schönlein purpura, treatment of systemic vasculitis is typically much more aggressive than treatment of LCV and should be pursued in conjunction with involvement of a rheumatologist, nephrologist, or pulmonologist. Systemic disease leads to severe complications including renal failure, pulmonary damage, permanent vascular disease, or neurologic insult depending on the viscera affected.

References
Gayraud M, Guillevin L, le Toumelin P, et al: Long-term followup of polyarteritis nodosa, microscopic polyangiitis, and Churg-Strauss syndrome: Analysis of four prospective trials including 278 patients, *Arthritis Rheum* 44:666–675, 2001.

Hannon CW, Swerlick RA: Vasculitis. In Bolognia J, Jorizzo J, Rapini R, editors: Dermatology, vol 1. St Louis, 2003, Mosby, pp 381–402.

Hoffman GS, Kerr GS, Leavitt RY, et al: Wegener granulomatosis: An analysis of 158 patients, *Ann Intern Med* 116:488–498, 1992.

Jennette JC, Thomas DB, Falk RJ: Microscopic polyangiitis (microscopic polyarteritis), *Semin Diagn Pathol* 18:3–13, 2001.

Jenette JC, Falk RF, Andrassy K, et al: Nomenclature of systemic vasculitides. Proposal of an international consensus conference, *Arthritis Rheum* 37(2):187–192, 1994.

DISEASES OF THE HAIR
Method of
Dirk M. Elston, MD

CURRENT DIAGNOSIS

- A sudden increase in shedding most commonly represents telogen effluvium.
- Hair thinning is more likely to represent pattern alopecia.
- Scarring alopecia generally requires a biopsy for diagnosis.
- Most medically significant hirsutism results from polycystic ovarian syndrome.
- New-onset virilization suggests the possibility of a tumor.

CURRENT THERAPY

- Pattern alopecia in men is treated with oral finasteride (Propecia), low dose oral minoxidil[1] or topical minoxidil (Rogaine), or both.
- Pattern alopecia in women is treated with antiandrogens (such as spironolactone [Aldactone][1]) and oral[1] or topical minoxidil. Platelet-rich plasma injections may be of benefit in both men and women.
- Alopecia areata can require intralesional corticosteroid injections, topical immunotherapy, or therapy with agents such as methotrexate (Trexall)[1] or Janus kinase (JAK) inhibitors.
- A scalp biopsy is critical to guide therapy in scarring alopecia.
- Hirsutism may be treated with laser epilation or systemic antiandrogens. Topical eflornithine (Vaniqa) can slow regrowth of hair.

[1]Not FDA approved for this indication.

Epidemiology
Hair disorders are common, with more than half of the population affected by pattern alopecia and the prevalence of hirsutism varying significantly by ethnicity.

Risk Factors
Most causes of alopecia and hirsutism are genetically determined.

Pathophysiology

Pattern alopecia relates to increased sensitivity to dihydrotestosterone. Telogen effluvium relates to an alteration in the normal hair cycle, with many hairs shedding synchronously. Alopecia areata represents an inflammatory insult directed against melanocytes in the hair bulb. There is strong evidence that the disease is mediated by Th1 lymphocytes. Polycystic ovarian syndrome is an insulin-resistance syndrome resulting in excess production of androgens.

Prevention

Little can be done to prevent hair disorders, so the focus is generally on diagnosis and treatment.

Clinical Manifestations

Pattern alopecia manifests with apical scalp thinning. In men, receding of the hairline at the temples is typical, whereas women demonstrate widening of the part but retain the anterior hairline. Telogen effluvium manifests with diffuse shedding of telogen hairs (hairs with a nonpigmented bulb). Alopecia areata typically occurs with patchy hair loss. Shed hairs demonstrate tapered fracture at the base. Syphilitic alopecia resembles alopecia areata but often affects smaller areas, with only partial hair loss, resulting in a moth-eaten appearance. Scarring alopecia shows permanent areas of smooth alopecia lacking follicular openings.

Polycystic ovarian syndrome manifests with evidence of anovulation and excess androgen production. Signs of virilization suggesting a possible tumor include new onset of hirsutism, deepening of the voice, change in body habitus, and clitoromegaly.

Diagnosis

Alopecia

The first step is to determine whether a hair shaft abnormality exists (Box 1). This is particularly important in Black patients, in whom trichorrhexis nodosa is a common cause of hair loss. Trichorrhexis nodosa results from overprocessing of the hair. Hair density is normal at the level of the scalp, but hairs break off, leaving patches of short hair.

The next step is to determine whether telogen effluvium exists. Telogen effluvium manifests with increased shedding of hairs with a blunt nonpigmented bulb (Figure 1), and it commonly follows an illness, surgery, delivery, or crash diet by 3 to 5 months. Hairs can often be easily extracted with a gentle hair pull or 1 minute of combing. The presence of tapered fracture suggests alopecia areata, syphilis, or heavy metal poisoning. Alopecia areata can result in diffuse hair loss, but it more commonly manifests with well-defined round patches of hair loss. The skin is either normal or salmon pink. Syphilis more often shows a moth-eaten pattern of alopecia (Figure 2).

Most patients with hair loss need only limited laboratory testing or none at all. Thyroid disorders and iron deficiency are common, and testing for them is relatively inexpensive. I recommend them when telogen effluvium is present. Their presence can also accelerate the course of pattern alopecia, and it is reasonable to test for them in women with this disorder. Thyroid-stimulating hormone is the best screen for thyroid disorders. The role of iron deficiency in telogen hair loss is controversial, but iron deficiency is common, easily established, and inexpensive to correct. Iron status also serves as an indicator of overall nutritional status. Although a low ferritin level proves iron deficiency, ferritin behaves as an acute phase reactant and a normal level does not rule out iron deficiency. Therefore, I recommend measurement of ferritin, serum iron, iron binding capacity, and saturation.

A scalp biopsy is required in any patient with scarring alopecia. It may also be necessary in other patients if history and physical examination do not establish a diagnosis and the alopecia is progressive. The scalp biopsy should be performed with a 4-mm biopsy punch oriented parallel to the direction

---

BOX 1 Diagnosis of Alopecia

Trichodystrophy
Types
- Trichorrhexis nodosa
- Inherited trichodystrophies
- Fractures

Causes
- Alopecia areata
- Chemotherapy
- Heavy metal

Determine Type
Anagen Effluvium
Tapered fractures can be caused by
- Alopecia areata
- Chemotherapy
- Heavy metal

Loose anagen can be caused by
- Loose anagen syndrome
- Easily extractable anagen in scarring alopecia

Telogen Effluvium
Increased shedding of club hairs can be caused by
- Diet, illness
- Pregnancy
- Medication
- Papulosquamous disorders
- Pattern alopecia

Diagnosis
Laboratory Studies
- Iron
- Thyroid-stimulating hormone
- Endocrine studies in virilized women

Biopsy
Nonscarring types
- Telogen effluvium
- Pattern alopecia
- Alopecia areata

Scarring types
- Lupus erythematosus
- Lichen planopilaris
- Folliculitis decalvans

Other Permanent Alopecia
- Idiopathic pseudopelade
- Morphea

---

of hair growth. Collagen hemostatic sponge (Gelfoam and others) can be placed into the resulting hole to stop bleeding and eliminate the need for sutures. The biopsy should be done in a well-established but still active area of inflammation if one can be identified. A combination of vertical and transverse sections increases the diagnostic yield and is usually recommended. In patients with scarring alopecia, half of the vertically bisected specimen should be sent for direct immunofluorescence. An additional biopsy of an end-stage scarred area can demonstrate characteristic patterns of scarring with an elastic tissue stain. This can help distinguish among causes of scarring alopecia such as lupus erythematosus (Figure 3), lichen planopilaris, pseudopelade, and folliculitis decalvans.

Hirsutism

Patients with *new-onset* virilization should be evaluated to rule out an ovarian or adrenal tumor. Ovarian and adrenal imaging

Figure 1 Telogen hair on *left*, anagen hair on *right* for comparison.

Figure 2 Moth-eaten syphilitic alopecia.

studies and a total testosterone level are the best screens. A total testosterone more than 200 ng/dL or dehydroepiandrostenedione sulfate (DHEAS) more than 8000 ng/dL suggests tumor. In patients with physical signs of Cushing disease, a 24-hour urine cortisol should be obtained. Most patients with *chronic* medically significant hirsutism have polycystic ovarian syndrome (PCOS). The diagnosis is established by means of history and physical examination, and the most important laboratory tests are serum lipids and fasting glucose to establish associated cardiac risk factors. A clinical diagnosis of PCOS requires the presence of hirsutism, acne or pattern alopecia, and evidence of anovulation (fewer than nine periods per year or cycles longer than 40 days). Ratios of luteinizing hormone (LH) to follicle-stimulating hormone (FSH) have poor sensitivity and specificity for diagnosing PCOS. Imaging for ovarian cysts seldom affects management.

Figure 3 Scarring alopecia secondary to chronic cutaneous lupus erythematosus.

Differential Diagnosis

Syphilis can mimic alopecia areata, and serologic testing should be performed in any sexually active patient with a new diagnosis of alopecia areata. Correct diagnosis of scarring alopecia depends of a thorough examination for other cutaneous signs of lupus erythematosus or lichen planus as well as the results of a skin biopsy.

Tinea capitis can occur as inflammatory boggy areas with hair loss (kerion) or with subtle seborrheic-type scale and black-dot areas of hair loss. A potassium hydroxide (KOH) examination can be performed by rubbing the affected area with moist gauze and examining broken hairs that cling to the gauze.

Hirsutism should be distinguished from hypertrichosis. Hirsutism is a male pattern of hair growth occurring in a woman and is hormonal in nature. Hypertrichosis is excess hair growth that occurs outside of an androgen-dependent distribution. It can be found in metabolic disorders such as porphyria or may be a sign of internal malignancy (Figure 4).

Nonclassic 21-hydroxylase deficiency accounts for up to 10% of patients with medically significant hirsutism. Screening with a baseline morning 17-OH-progesterone is associated with many false positive results. A stimulated 17-OH-progesterone is more specific, but the results of testing seldom affect management because outcomes with dexamethasone (Decadron)[1] are no better than with spironolactone (Aldactone).[1]

Treatment

Alopecia

Telogen effluvium commonly resolves spontaneously once the cause has been eliminated. Poor diet and papulosquamous diseases of the scalp such as seborrheic dermatitis and psoriasis can perpetuate a telogen effluvium and should be treated. The importance of a diet containing adequate protein and trace minerals should be emphasized. Deficiencies and thyroid abnormalities should be addressed. Seborrheic dermatitis responds to topical corticosteroids. Medicated shampoos containing selenium sulfide (Selsun Blue) or zinc pyrithione (T-gel Daily Control) can be helpful. Scalp psoriasis can require more potent topical steroids such as fluocinonide solution (Lidex) and calcipotriene (Dovonex) applied on weekends or daily. Systemic agents such as methotrexate (Trexall)[1] at doses of 7.5 to 20 mg once weekly may be required to control severe scalp psoriasis.

Pattern alopecia in men is mediated by dihydrotestosterone (DHT). Men with pattern alopecia may be treated with daily topical minoxidil 2% to 5% (Rogaine), oral minoxidil (Loniten)[1] in doses from 0.5 to 5 mg daily, and oral finasteride (Propecia) at a dose of 1 mg daily. In women, the pathogenesis

---

[1]Not FDA approved for this indication.

Figure 4 Malignant hypertrichosis secondary to ovarian cancer.

TABLE 1	Treatment of Tinea Capitis	
ANTIFUNGAL AGENT	**DOSAGE**	**USUAL DURATION OF THERAPY**
Griseofulvin (Fulvicin U/F)	Required dosages are often higher than reflected in the product label; 4–10 mg/kg/day is a good starting dosage	1 month or more
Fluconazole (Diflucan)[1]	5–6 mg/kg/day; adult: 200 mg/day	1 month or more
Itraconazole (Sporanox)[1]	3–5 mg/kg/day; adult: 200 mg/day	1 week, repeated monthly until cured
Terbinafine (Lamisil)	Patient <20 kg: 62.5 mg/day Patient 20–40 kg: 125 mg/day Patient >40 kg: 250 mg/day	1 month or more

[1]Not FDA approved for this indication.

is complex, and adrenal androgens may play a larger role. Finasteride[1] is of less benefit in the majority of women with pattern alopecia. Spironolactone[1] 100 mg twice daily can be helpful and may be combined with oral minoxidil.[1] In women of childbearing potential, spironolactone should always be used in conjunction with an oral contraceptive. Side effects are uncommon but can include urinary frequency, irregular periods, dyspareunia, and nausea. Most patients demonstrate a minor increase in serum potassium. Those with kidney failure are at risk for life-threatening potassium retention. Topical 2% minoxidil can also be of benefit, and some women derive added benefit from the 5% formulation. All patients with pattern alopecia should be evaluated for superimposed causes of telogen effluvium such as inadequate diet and seborrheic dermatitis.

Tinea capitis is often overlooked in adults and Black children, in whom the manifestations of inflammation can be subtle. Black dot and seborrheic tinea are common in Black children. Patchy hair loss is an important clue to the diagnosis. Treatment is summarized in Table 1.

Localized patches of alopecia areata respond to intralesional injections of triamcinolone hexacetonide (Aristospan) (2.5–5 mg/mL) given once per month. Approximately 0.1 mL/cm² is injected to a maximum of 3 mL during any one session. Minoxidil solution produces slow regrowth in some patients who cannot tolerate other treatments. Anthralin (Dritho-Scalp 0.5%)[1] is sometimes used in children. It is applied 30 minutes before showering. It can stain skin and anything else it touches.

Topical immunotherapy with dinitrochlorobenzene (DNCB)[1], squaric acid dibutylester (SADBE),[1] or diphenylcyclopropenone (DPCP)[1] is more effective than either minoxidil or anthralin. DNCB is mutagenic in the Ames assay and none of the topical immunotherapies are currently approved for human use. A 2% solution of the sensitizer is applied to the arm in acetone to induce initial sensitization. Subsequently, diluted solutions, starting at about 0.001%, are applied weekly to the scalp with a cotton-tipped applicator. Roughly 20% to 60% of patients have responded to this regimen in various studies.

Baricitinib (Olumiant), tofacitinib (Xeljanz)[1] and other JAK inhibitors are often effective in patients with refractory alopecia areata. Biologic agents have shown mixed results. Methotrexate[1] in psoriatic doses (7.5–20 mg weekly for an adult) can be effective. Sulfasalazine (Azulfidine)[1] is sometimes effective in doses ranging from 500 to 1500 mg three times a day.[3] Patients should be encouraged to read about new therapies on the National Alopecia Areata Foundation website (https://www.naaf.org).

Early, aggressive therapy for discoid lupus erythematosus is recommended to prevent permanent scarring. Topical corticosteroids are rarely sufficient. Intralesional injections are performed in a manner similar to that described above. Initial control of severe disease can be achieved with a single 3-week tapered course of oral prednisone at a dose of 60 mg daily for the first week, 40 mg daily for the second week, and 20 mg daily for the third week. Intralesional steroid injections or a systemic steroid-sparing agent are required for maintenance therapy. Systemic agents that can be effective include antimalarials, dapsone,[1] methotrexate,[1] mycophenolate mofetil (CellCept),[1] and thalidomide (Thalomid).[1] I generally begin treatment with hydroxychloroquine (Plaquenil)[1] at a dose of 400 mg daily for an adult. Dapsone is used at a dose of 100 mg daily for an adult. Thalidomide has been used effectively at doses of 50 to 100 mg daily, but peripheral neuropathy and teratogenicity limit its use. Mycophenolate mofetil is used at a dose of 1 g twice daily, and methotrexate is used at doses of 7.5 to 20 mg weekly. Background pattern (androgenetic) alopecia should be treated as well.

End-stage cicatricial alopecia is best treated by scalp reduction and hair transplantation. The disease can flare up in response to surgery, and it is best to plan a 3-week tapered course of prednisone[1] or a month of cyclosporine (Neoral)[1] to help prevent the flare.

Lichen planopilaris is treated in a manner similar to lupus, except that hydroxychloroquine[1] is of less benefit and oral retinoids (acitretin [Soriatane][1] at doses of 25 to 50 mg daily) are more likely to be successful. Topical calcineurin inhibitors can be effective in achieving and maintaining remission. A few months of pioglitazone (Actos)[1] can induce remission in a subset of patients and the frontal fibrosing alopecia variant can respond to dutasteride (Avodart).[1] Patients should be aware of the risks associated with each of these treatments, including bladder cancer and hypospadias in a male fetus. Mycophenolate mofetil (CellCept)[1] 1 g twice daily or a JAK inhibitor may be effective when other treatments fail, and excimer laser can also be effective for lichen planopilaris. It is contraindicated in lupus erythematosus.

Folliculitis decalvans manifests with crops of pustules that result in permanent scarring. Patients respond to weekend applications of clobetasol (Clobex, Olux) together with prolonged use of antistaphylococcal antibiotics such as doxycycline (Doryx)[1] 100 mg twice daily.

[1]Not FDA approved for this indication.
[3]Exceeds dosage recommended by the manufacturer.

[1]Not FDA approved for this indication.

Hirsutism

Treatment options include laser epilation, eflornithine (Vaniqa) cream to reduce the rate of hair growth, or spironolactone[1] at a starting dose of 100 mg twice daily as described for pattern alopecia. Cyproterone acetate is used in some countries but is not available in the United States. Other options that are less commonly used include insulin sensitizers, flutamide (Eulexin),[1] metformin (Glucophage),[1] and leuprolide (Lupron)[1] plus estrogen.[1]

Monitoring

Patients treated with topical or intralesional corticosteroids should be monitored for cutaneous atrophy. Patients on JAK inhibitors should have quarterly evaluations of blood count, chemistries, and lipids. Those on hydroxychloroquine should be monitored for ocular toxicity, including corneal deposits and retinal damage, although these are very rare at usual doses. They should also be monitored periodically for thrombocytopenia, agranulocytosis, and hepatitis. Patients beginning dapsone therapy should be screened for G6PD deficiency. Potential side effects include hemolysis, methemoglobinemia, and neuropathy. Monitoring includes periodic blood count assessment and measurement of strength and sensation. Mycophenolate mofetil can produce pancytopenia, and blood counts should be monitored. Methotrexate is cleared by the kidneys, and kidney function should be assessed at baseline. Periodic assessment of liver-function tests and blood count is warranted, as is a yearly chest radiograph. I also monitor procollagen 3 terminal peptide levels quarterly to assess the risk of hepatic fibrosis. Patients on antiandrogen therapy should be monitored for dyspareunia resulting from vulvar atrophy.

Complications

Patients with pattern alopecia and PCOS have a greater risk of metabolic syndrome with cardiac complications. They should be evaluated for lipid abnormalities and glucose intolerance and treated appropriately.

[1]Not FDA approved for this indication.

References

Brown J, Farquhar C, Lee O, et al: Spironolactone versus placebo or in combination with steroids for hirsutism and/or acne, *Cochrane Database Syst Rev* (2)CD000194, 2009.

Buzney E, Sheu J, Buzney C, Reynolds RV: Polycystic ovary syndrome: a review for dermatologists: Part II. Treatment, *J Am Acad Dermatol* 71(5):859.e1–859.e15, 2014.

Durdu M, Ozcan D, Baba M, Sec̦kin D: Efficacy and safety of diphenylcyclopropenone alone or in combination with anthralin in the treatment of chronic extensive alopecia areata: a retrospective case series, *J Am Acad Dermatol* 72:640–650, 2015.

Elston DM, Ferringer T, Dalton S, et al: A comparison of vertical versus transverse sections in the evaluation of alopecia biopsy specimens, *J Am Acad Dermatol* 53(2):267–272, 2005.

Fukumoto T, Fukumoto R, Magno E, Oka M, Nishigori C, Horita N: Treatments for alopecia areata: a systematic review and network meta-analysis, *Dermatol Ther* 25:e14916, 2021, https://doi.org/10.1111/dth.14916. Epub ahead of print 33631058.

Gentile P, Garcovich S, Scioli MG, et al: Mechanical and controlled prp injections in patients affected by androgenetic alopecia, *J Vis Exp* 27(131), 2018.

Giordano S, Romeo M, di Summa P, et al: A meta-analysis on evidence of platelet-rich plasma for androgenetic alopecia, *Int J Trichology* 10(1):1–10, 2018.

Ramadan WM, Hassan AM, Ismail MA, El Attar YA: Evaluation of adding platelet-rich plasma to combined medical therapy in androgenetic alopecia, *J Cosmet Dermatol* 12, 2021, https://doi.org/10.1111/jocd.13935. Epub ahead of print 33438346.

Somani N, Turvy D: Hirsutism: an evidence-based treatment update, *Am J Clin Dermatol* 15(3):247–266, 2014.

Vano-Galvan S, Pirmez R, Hermosa-Gelbard A, et al: Safety of low-dose oral minoxidil for hair loss: a multicenter study of 1404 patients, 00418-7 *J Am Acad Dermatol* S0190-9622(21)00418-7, 2021, https://doi.org/10.1016/j.jaad.2021.02.054. Epub ahead of print 33639244.

Waśkiel-Burnat A, Kołodziejak M, Sikora M, et al: Therapeutic management in pediatric alopecia areata: a systematic review, *J Eur Acad Dermatol Venereol* 25, 2021, https://doi.org/10.1111/jdv.17187. Epub ahead of print 33630354.

DISEASES OF THE MOUTH

Method of
Lisa Simon, MD, DMD; and Hugh Silk, MD, MPH

CURRENT DIAGNOSIS

High-risk conditions
- Ludwig angina: Spread of infection most commonly from a mandibular molar into the sublingual and submaxillary spaces that surround the airway, causing urgent respiratory compromise.
- Cavernous sinus thrombosis: Ascending infection and thrombosis of intracranial vessels that can be caused by a maxillary dental infection. Requires urgent neurologic and neurosurgical evaluation.
- Lesions concerning for oral cancer: Most commonly squamous cell carcinoma (SCC) may present as sessile or fungating, with red or white shading. Usually asymptomatic, may feature fixed, painless lymph nodes. Associated with alcohol and tobacco use.

Common conditions
- Dental caries: Most common infectious disease globally, near 100% prevalence. Dental pain indicates that the tooth will require root canal therapy or extraction to resolve the infection.
- Periodontal disease: Inflammatory loss of the tooth's attachment structure, which can cause pain, tooth mobility, and eventual tooth loss.

Oral ulcers
- Acute ulcers most likely infectious (herpes simplex virus [HSV], Coxsackie) or aphthous ulcers, tend to resolve within 7 to 10 days.
- Chronic ulcers will appear more desquamative and widespread within the oral cavity. They are more likely to be due to a dermatologic condition (pemphigus vulgaris, mucous membrane pemphigoid, lichen planus) and should prompt investigation of other dermatologic findings.

Oral lesions and masses
- Cessation of triggering activity (e.g., use of chewing tobacco) and evaluate for resolution.
- Refer for biopsy if lesions persist for more than 14 days.

Xerostomia
- Perception of dry mouth, which can make speaking and swallowing more difficult and predisposes patients to rampant dental decay.
- Associated with polypharmacy, especially drugs with known anticholinergic properties.
- Can also be due to autoimmune destruction of salivary glands from SICCA syndrome.

Osteonecrosis of the jaw
- Antibiotics for purulent exudate.
- Refer to oral surgeon or oral medicine specialist for monitoring and possible resection of necrotic bone.

Antibiotic prophylaxis for dental procedures
- For infective endocarditis prevention, this is necessary only in individuals with prosthetic valves or implants, unrepaired cyanotic congenital heart disease or repair with residual defect, history of cardiac transplant with valvular regurgitation, or history of infective endocarditis.
- No prophylaxis necessary for individuals with prosthetic joints.
- Prophylaxis necessary only for procedures that involve manipulating the gingiva.
- Prophylaxis can be taken up to 2 h after a procedure with equivalent efficacy.

2 years without further surgery or adjuvant systemic therapy. The use of neoadjuvant immunotherapies is now being integrated into multidisciplinary patient care.

Metastatic melanoma is an aggressive, immunogenic, and molecularly heterogeneous disease. In the last decade, treatment of melanoma took a dramatic turn with the discovery of targeted therapy aimed at the *BRAF* mutations in the mitogen-activated protein kinase (MAPK) pathway and immune checkpoint inhibitors. In 2011 the FDA approved ipilimumab, an anti–CTLA-4 antibody for metastatic melanoma therapy. Since then, novel monoclonal antibody agents that inhibit PD-1—pembrolizumab and nivolumab—were approved in 2014, followed by the nivolumab plus ipilimumab combination therapy in 2015 and, more recently, the nivolumab plus relatlimab combination therapy (anti-PD-1 plus anti-LAG-3 antibodies; Opdualag) in 2022. Two additional classes of immunotherapy have been FDA approved, including the intralesional oncolytic viral therapy T-VEC (Imlygic) in 2015 for patients with palpable metastatic melanoma and the bispecific gp100 peptide-HLA–directed CD3 T cell engager tebentafusp (Kimmtrak) for HLA-A*02:01-positive patients with metastatic uveal melanoma. The selective *BRAF* inhibitor vemurafenib (Zelboraf) was also approved in 2011 for the treatment of patients with advanced *BRAF* V600 mutant melanoma. Additional *BRAF* targeted regimens were subsequently approved, with the combination *BRAF* plus MEK inhibitors now the standard approach based on improvement in survival over monotherapy. The three approved *BRAF* plus MEK inhibitor regimens include dabrafenib (Tafinlar) plus trametinib (Mekinist), vemurafenib (Zelboral) plus cobimetinib (Cotellic), and encorafenib (Braftovi) plus binimetinib (Mektovi). Long-term survival of patients has dramatically improved with the new classes of *BRAF* targeted and anti-PD-1 therapies. Historically, approximately 10% of patients with advanced unresectable melanoma were alive at 5 years. Recent prospective studies with dabrafenib plus trametinib, pembrolizumab, nivolumab, and nivolumab plus ipilimumab have shown 5-year survival rates of 34%, 43%, 44%, and 52%, respectively.

Although melanoma has traditionally been regarded as a near-uniformly fatal malignancy, personalized treatment of this cancer relies on the recognition of its genetic heterogeneity and our ability to pharmacologically target these specific and recurrent changes. Recent advances in the treatment of melanoma have come from the understanding that melanoma is a large family of molecularly distinct diseases. Emerging evidence suggests that different melanoma subtypes may each be driven by diverse mechanisms of progression, associated with differing mechanisms of tumor escape and specific immunosuppression, innate immune cell activation, and altered T-cell trafficking into tumor sites that in turn modulate response to immunotherapies.

Monitoring

Most metastases occur in the first 1 to 3 years after treatment of the primary tumor, and an estimated 4% to 8% of patients with a history of melanoma develop another primary melanoma, usually within the first 3 to 5 years following diagnosis. The risk of new primary melanoma increases in the presence of multiple dysplastic nevi and family history of melanoma. Consider cancer genetics consultation in patients with three or more melanomas in aggregate in first-degree or second-degree relatives on the same side of the family, families with three or more cases of melanoma or pancreatic cancer on the same side of the family, and (in low-incidence countries) patients with three or more primary melanomas.

The frequency of dermatologic monitoring is as follows:
- For patients with stage IA to IIA: every 6 to 12 months for 5 years, then every year as needed
- For patients with stage IIB to IV every 3 to 6 months for 2 years, then every 3 to 12 months for 3 years, then every year as neeod

Follow-up visits for all patients should include a thorough medical history, review of systems, complete skin examination, and examination of lymph nodes. In patients at high risk for recurrent metastatic disease (resected stages IIB–IV) or with abnormal examination/symptoms, appropriate imaging studies, laboratory studies, or biopsies may be indicated. Evidence to support the use of routine imaging and laboratory studies in patients who are asymptomatic with low-risk resected stage I to IIA melanoma is limited and so they are not recommended by the NCCN guidelines.

Complications

Metastasis may occur locally in the regional lymph node basins, or it can occur distally in the skin (away from the melanoma scar), the remote lymph node(s), the viscera, and skeletal and central nervous system sites. In patients treated with immune checkpoint inhibitor therapies, immune-related adverse events can occur even after therapy discontinuation.

References

Abbasi NR, Shaw HM, Rigel DS, et al: Early diagnosis of cutaneous melanoma: revisiting the ABCD criteria, *JAMA* 292:2771–2776, 2004.

Cancer Genome Atlas N: Genomic classification of cutaneous melanoma, *Cell* 161:1681–1696, 2015.

Gershenwald JE, Scolyer RA, Hess KR, et al: Melanoma staging: evidence-based changes in the American Joint Committee on Cancer eighth edition cancer staging manual, *CA Cancer J clin* 67:472–492, 2017.

Guy Jr GP, Thomas CC, Thompson T, et al: Vital signs: melanoma incidence and mortality trends and projections - United States, 1982-2030, *MMWR Morb Mortal Wkly Rep* 64:591–596, 2015.

Kwak M, Farrow NE, Salama AKS, et al: Updates in adjuvant systemic therapy for melanoma, *J Surg Oncol* 119:222–231, 2019.

Larkin J, Chiarion-Sileni V, Gonzalez R, et al: Five-year survival with combined nivolumab and ipilimumab in advanced melanoma, *N Engl J Med* 381:1535–1546, 2019.

Luke JJ: *Lancet.* 399(10336):1718–1729, 2022 https://doi: 10.1016/S0140-6736(22)00562-1. Epub 2022 Apr 1.

National Comprehensive cancer Network (NCCN) clinical practice guidelines in Oncology. Cutaneous melanoma. Version 3.2023. nccn.org.

Patel SP: *N Engl J Med.* 388(9):813–823, 2023 https://doi: 10.1056/NEJMoa2211437.

Robert C, Grob JJ, Stroyakovskiy D, et al: Five-year outcomes with dabrafenib plus trametinib in metastatic melanoma, *N Engl J Med* 381:626–636, 2019.

Siegel RL, et al: *CA Cancer J Clin.* 73:17–48, 2023.

Sladden MJ, Balch C, Barzilai DA, et al: Surgical excision margins for primary cutaneous melanoma, *Cochrane Database Syst Rev* CD004835, 2009.

Soura E, Eliades PJ, Shannon K, Stratigos AJ, Tsao H: Hereditary melanoma: update on syndromes and management: genetics of familial atypical multiple mole melanoma syndrome, *J Am Acad Dermatol* 74:395–407, 2016; quiz 408-310.

Wong SL, Faries MB, Kennedy EB, et al: Sentinel lymph node biopsy and management of regional lymph nodes in melanoma: American Society of Clinical Oncology and Society of Surgical Oncology clinical practice guideline update, *J Clin Oncol* 36:399–413, 2018.

Yeh I, Jorgenson E, Shen L, et al: Targeted genomic profiling of acral melanoma, *J Natl Cancer Inst* 111:1068–1077, 2019.

NEVI

Jane M. Grant-Kels, MD; and Michael Murphy, MD

CURRENT DIAGNOSIS

Benign Melanocytic Lesions
- Symmetric
- Sharply demarcated border
- Uniform color
- Diameter usually 6 mm or less and stable

Malignant Melanocytic Lesions
- Asymmetric
- Poorly circumscribed border
- Variegated in color
- Diameter often >6 mm and increasing (changing or evolving)

traumatically) and have recurred weeks to months later. Irregular brown pigmentation is clinically noted within the scar site. If the original biopsy demonstrated a benign melanocytic nevus, retreatment is unnecessary unless there is suspicion for a malignancy, such as from an extension of pigment clinically beyond the scar. However, these nevi can demonstrate pseudomelanomatous histologic features. Therefore if the repigmented area is excised, the dermatopathologist should be notified of the clinical history and, if possible, the slides from the original biopsy should be obtained and reviewed to ensure that the lesion is not histologically misdiagnosed.

Halo (Melanocytic) Nevi

Halo (melanocytic) nevi are melanocytic nevi in which a white rim or halo has developed. This phenomenon most commonly occurs around compound or intradermal nevi and is histologically associated with a dense, bandlike inflammatory infiltrate. The white halo area is histologically characterized by diminished or absent melanocytes and melanin. Approximately 20% of patients with halo nevi also exhibit vitiligo.

Although a halo can develop around many lesions in the skin, the most important differential diagnosis is between a halo nevus and melanoma with a halo. The halo and the central melanocytic proliferation of halo nevi are symmetric, round or oval, and sharply demarcated. Halo nevi most commonly occur in adolescence as an isolated event, but approximately 25% to 50% of affected persons have two or more.

The clinical course of halo nevi is variable. With time, the halo can repigment while the central nevus persists. Alternatively, the melanocytic nevus can regress completely and leave a depigmented macule that can persist or repigment over months or years.

Halo nevi do not require surgical excision unless atypical features clinically and dermoscopically suggest the possibility of an atypical melanocytic lesion. It is advisable (particularly in adults, in whom halo nevi are less common) to perform a complete cutaneous examination with and without the aid of a Wood's lamp to rule out any associated atypical pigmented or regressed lesions. It is recommended that, if a middle-aged or older adult reports with a sudden appearance of halo nevi and there is no obvious melanoma or history of melanoma, the patient should be referred to an ophthalmologist for an ocular exam to exclude a choroidal halo nevus. All patients should be advised to use sunscreen or protective clothing because of the increased risk of sunburn in the depigmented halo region.

Congenital Melanocytic Nevi

By definition, congenital melanocytic nevi (CMN) are present at birth. CMN can be classified by their clinical features, including size, location, number of satellite lesions, and morphologic characteristics (such as color, rugosity, nodularity, hypertrichosis). This classification can help stratify patients according to their risk for adverse outcomes, including neurocutaneous melanosis and progression to melanoma. Arbitrarily, they have been classified into small (<1.5 cm), medium (1.5 to 20 cm), large (>20 to 40 cm), and giant (>40 cm) lesions. Terms such as *bathing trunk* or *garment-type* nevi refer to CMN that cover a significant portion of the cutaneous surface. The spectrum of initiating mutations typically correlates with the size of the nevus. The majority of large CMN harbor NRAS mutations, with a minority harboring kinase fusions or BRAF mutation. Most small CMN harbor BRAF mutations. Recent studies suggest that pathogenesis of large/giant CMN is associated with deficient mismatch repair (MMR) mechanisms and linked to lesion size and presence of multiple lesions.

The approximate incidence of small congenital nevi is 1% of all live births. Large congenital nevi are rare and reported in only 1 in 20,000 births. Histologically, some congenital nevi have distinguishing histologic features (melanocytic nevus cells that extend into the deeper dermis as well as the subcutis and melanocytic nevus cells arranged periadnexally, angiocentrically, within nerves, and interposed between collagen bundles). However, these features have been identified in some acquired melanocytic nevi and are absent in some congenital nevi (especially small ones). In addition, the history obtained from the patient or their parents is often inaccurate. Consequently, it can be very difficult in some cases to distinguish a small congenital nevus from an acquired nevus.

Congenital nevi can give rise to dermal or subcutaneous nodular melanocytic proliferations. Most of these lesions, particularly in the neonatal period, are biologically benign, despite a worrisome clinical presentation and atypical histologic features. Genetic analysis has shown that benign melanocytic proliferations within congenital nevi harbor aberrations that are qualitatively and quantitatively different from those seen in melanoma.

Patients with multiple CMN (two or more, of any site or size) are at risk for extracutaneous (i.e., endocrine, metabolic, neurologic) manifestations, termed *CMN syndrome*. The primary significance of congenital nevi is related to the potential risk for progression to melanoma. Essentially, the larger the nevus, particularly if accompanied by multiple small CMN, the greater the risk of progression to melanoma. Historically, even small nevi were estimated to exhibit a lifetime melanoma risk of 5%. However, recent prospective studies suggest that small and medium congenital nevi are associated with a low risk that may approximate the risk of acquired nevi. Conversely, large congenital nevi have a lifetime risk of melanomatous progression of approximately 6.3%. Up to two-thirds of melanomas that arise within these giant congenital nevi have a nonepidermal origin (arising mainly in the deep dermis and subcutis with high Breslow thickness on report), thus making clinical observation for malignant change difficult. Approximately 50% of these melanomas occur in the first 5 years of life, 60% in the first decade, and 70% before 20 years of age. Patients with large congenital nevi, especially those that involve posterior axial locations (head, neck, back, or buttocks) and are associated with satellite congenital nevi, are at increased risk for neurocutaneous melanosis (melanosis of the leptomeninges) and primary central nervous system (CNS) melanoma. Recent data suggest that in up to one-third of these patients, the primary melanoma develops within the CNS rather than the skin. The risk of melanoma appears to be higher in those with congenital abnormalities of the CNS (12% vs. 1% to 2% without CNS changes).

For large congenital nevi that involve a posterior axial location, screening magnetic resonance imaging (MRI) is indicated to characterize congenital disease, if any, and act as a baseline should the child report with new neurologic symptoms at a later stage. If clinical symptoms or MRI indicate neurocutaneous melanosis, excision of the large nevus should be postponed until 2 years of age (the median age of neurologic symptoms). Patients with neurocutaneous melanosis have a greater than 50% mortality rate within 3 years. Due to the risk and morbidity of multiple, staged excisions of a large CMN, it is not appropriate in patients with symptomatic neurocutaneous melanosis. All other large CMN are candidates for excision as soon as general anesthesia is considered a relatively safe risk. Other issues that need to be considered before undertaking staged excisions include cosmetic issues, functional outcome, and psychosocial issues. The staged excisions are usually started after 6 months of age for nevi on the trunk and extremities and later for those on the scalp to allow closure of the fontanelle. If removal is not undertaken, follow-up with monthly self-examination, as well as routine follow-up using photography, serial dermoscopy, and reflectance confocal microscopy, is recommended.

For small congenital nevi, routine excision is not always recommended because the risk of melanoma is lower, and if it occurs, it usually arises within the epidermis after puberty. If the lesions are not excised, follow-up by alternating visits to a dermatologist and primary care physician, along with serial photography, is indicated. Inasmuch as small congenital nevi typically enlarge with the growth of the child and can change in appearance with time, educating families on benign, predictable changes in contradistinction to potentially alarming changes is extremely important. If a lesion enlarges or changes suddenly or if parental anxiety or cosmetic issues arise, excision should then be contemplated for even small congenital nevi. Elective excision is best done when the patient is approximately 8 years old. With the use of topical anesthetic cream EMLA (eutectic mixture of local anesthetics: 2.5% lidocaine plus 2.5% prilocaine) or topical 4% lidocaine (ELA-Max), children of this age are usually cooperative and unscathed by the procedure.

Blue Nevi

Blue nevi occur primarily on the face and scalp, in addition to the dorsal surfaces of the hands and feet, as well-circumscribed, slightly raised or dome-shaped bluish papules that are usually less than 1 cm in diameter. Although these lesions are usually acquired in childhood and adolescence, rare congenital lesions have been reported. Histologically, the majority of blue nevi demonstrate a combination of intradermal spindle or dendritic melanin-pigmented melanocytes and melanophages with dermal fibrosis. Hypopigmented variants have also been described. The cellular subtype contains central fascicles of spindled melanocytes with ovoid nuclei. The blue appearance of these lesions is a function of both the depth of the melanin in the dermis and the Tyndall phenomenon: longer wavelengths of light penetrate the deep dermis and are absorbed by the lesional melanin, and shorter wavelengths (e.g., blue) are reflected back. Blue nevi that are clinically stable and that do not demonstrate atypical features do not require removal.

Blue nevi are initiated by activating mutations of the Gαq pathway, typically point mutations in GNAQ or GNA11 (shared with uveal and leptomeningeal melanocytic proliferations). Less commonly, hotspot mutations in CYSLTR2, PLB4, or protein kinase C (PKC) fusions are reported and associated with unique histopathological features. BAP1 inactivation in blue nevus–type lesions suggests malignant transformation and portends a poor prognosis.

Spitz Nevi

According to the 4th WHO Classification of Skin Tumors, the Spitz group of melanocytic proliferations is defined by a combination of distinctive morphologic features and driver molecular genetic events. This group includes benign Spitz nevi, in addition to atypical Spitz tumors and spitzoid melanomas. Morphologically, all of these neoplasms are characterized by large, oval, polygonal, epithelioid, and/or spindled melanocytes with abundant eosinophilic cytoplasm and vesicular nuclei with prominent nucleoli, often in association with epidermal hyperplasia. A lack of interobserver agreement in histopathological classification of skin tumors with spitzoid morphology is well reported.

Spitz nevi are relatively uncommon. In Australia, an annual incidence of 1.4 per 100,000 people has been recorded. Most Spitz nevi are noted in children and adolescents: One-third occur before the age of 10 years, one-third between the ages 10 to 20 years, and one-third past the age of 20 years. Rarely, lesions can occur in patients older than 40 years. Seven percent of Spitz nevi have been reported as congenital.

Four clinical types of Spitz nevi are recognized: light-colored soft Spitz nevi that can resemble a pyogenic granuloma; light-colored hard Spitz nevi that can resemble a dermatofibroma; dark Spitz nevi that must be distinguished from other melanocytic

lesions, including melanoma; and disseminated or agminated Spitz nevi. Spitz nevi are typically smaller than 6 mm in diameter and dome shaped, with a smooth pink or tan surface and sharp borders. Although they can occur anywhere on the cutaneous surface except mucosal or palmoplantar areas, they are mostly seen on the face (especially in children) and legs (especially in women). Spitz nevi in adults are usually more heavily melanized than those in children. A Reed nevus or pigmented spindle cell nevus of Reed, a variant of a Spitz nevus, generally presents as an acquired 2- to 8-mm dark-brown to black macule or papule on the leg of a young adult.

Dermoscopy can assist in establishing the clinical diagnosis of some Spitz nevi. Histologically, the lesion can demonstrate features similar to those of melanoma, which earned the lesion its original designation by Sophie Spitz as a melanoma of childhood. Because Spitz nevi can be histologically difficult to distinguish from melanoma in some cases, if a biopsy is performed on a lesion because of parental, cosmetic, transitional, or clinical/dermoscopic concern, complete excision with clear margins is recommended.

Based on the underlying driver genetic aberrations, Spitz melanocytic proliferations can be divided into distinct groups: (1) 11p amplified/HRAS mutated proliferations (20% of cases), (2) proliferations with tyrosine kinase or serine/threonine kinase fusions (50% of cases), and (3) proliferations with Spitz morphology but no driver genetic changes characteristic of other defined melanocytic subgroups. Immunohistochemistry can be used for screening purposes to detect specific fusion proteins. Specific driver aberrations are often associated with distinctive histopathological changes and tumor aggressiveness—11p amplification/HRAS mutation and tyrosine kinase fusions correlate with indolent behavior—whereas serine-threonine kinase (MAP3K8, BRAF) fusions are more frequent in the atypical/malignant spectrum of Spitz melanocytic proliferations with a potential for aggressive biologic behavior. Additional genetic events (biallelic inactivation of CDKN2A and TERT promoter mutations) are often necessary for the development of overt Spitz malignancy.

Dysplastic Melanocytic Nevi

Dysplastic melanocytic nevi, or Clark's nevi, or nevi with architectural disorder and cytologic atypia, can occur sporadically as an isolated lesion or lesions or as part of a familial autosomal dominant syndrome. When such lesions occur sporadically, they are considered a marker for a patient who is at increased risk of melanoma (6% risk vs. an approximate 0.6% risk in the normal White population in the United States). In association with a family history or personal past medical history of melanoma, patients with dysplastic melanocytic nevi should be considered to have a significant risk of melanoma. One first-degree family member with melanoma is associated with a lifetime risk of melanoma of 15% for the patient with dysplastic melanocytic nevi. Two or more first-degree family members with melanoma place a patient with dysplastic melanocytic nevi at a lifetime risk of developing melanoma that approaches 100%. Less commonly, dysplastic melanocytic nevi can progress to melanoma. Such progression has been documented by serial photography. However, these data are confounded by the fact that, clinically and histologically, dysplastic melanocytic nevi may be difficult to distinguish from an early melanoma.

Dysplastic melanocytic nevi are clinically distinguished from common AMN by a diameter usually larger than 6 mm, an irregular border, asymmetry, and variable color with possible shades of brown, red, pink, and black; dysplastic melanocytic nevi can be flat, with or without a raised center (fried egg appearance). The lesions begin to appear in mid-childhood and early adolescence. New lesions can appear throughout the patient's life. In addition to the back and extremities, these lesions can occur on sun-protected areas, including the scalp, buttocks, and female breasts. Dysplastic melanocytic nevi can be few or numerous, with hundreds of lesions. Dysplastic nevi show significant upregulation of follicular keratinocyte–related genes compared with AMN.

Histologically, dysplastic melanocytic nevi show architectural disorder: extension of the junctional component beyond the dermal component (shouldering), bridging of nests between adjacent rete ridges, papillary dermal concentric and lamellar fibroplasia, and a variable lymphocytic infiltrate with vascular ectasias. They also show cytologic atypia of melanocytes: increased nuclear size, hyperchromasia, dispersion, or variation of nuclear chromatin patterns and the presence of nucleoli. There are no set and universally accepted criteria on the spectrum of melanocytic dysplasia, and cytologic atypia is often reported as mild, moderate, or severe. However, discordance exists in the histologic grading of dysplastic nevi among dermatopathologists. According to the revised MPATH-Dx reporting system and 2018 WHO Classification of Skin Tumors, there is evidence to support the use in clinical practice of a simplified two-tier grading system: low-grade dysplasia and high-grade dysplasia. The probability of having a personal history of melanoma in any given patient with dysplastic melanocytic nevi correlates with the grade of cytologic atypia in melanocytic nevi cells. In addition, the presence of severe cytologic atypia in dysplastic melanocytic nevi correlates with a significantly greater risk of melanoma development (19.7%) compared with moderate (8.1%) or mild (5.7%) cytologic atypia.

Management of these patients is difficult. Dysplastic melanocytic nevi are not uncommon. Reportedly, as many as 4.6 million people in the United States have one or more sporadic dysplastic melanocytic nevi. Familial dysplastic melanocytic nevi are estimated to involve 50,000 patients in the United States. The risk of melanoma for these patients is probably on a continuum and correlated with their family history of melanoma or dysplastic melanocytic nevi, personal history of melanoma, number of acquired and dysplastic melanocytic lesions, and history of sun exposure. Removal of all dysplastic melanocytic nevi is inappropriate inasmuch as the chance of any single lesion becoming malignant is small, and, in addition, most melanomas arise de novo.

In cases of mild and moderate dysplastic nevi with microscopically positive margins and no concerning residual clinical lesion, observation, rather than reexcision, is the recommended form of management. All severely dysplastic nevi should be reexcised. Partial biopsy of any pigmented lesion that is clinically or pathologically suspicious for melanoma can lead to delayed melanoma diagnosis and is discouraged.

Management includes patient education and total body photography for comparison at future skin examinations and sequential dermoscopy. Patients should avoid the sun and use sunscreens and protective clothing. These patients should have regular biannual or quarterly examinations of the entire integument, including the scalp and the oral, genital, and perianal mucosa, and an ophthalmologic examination. Comparison with the previous total body photographs and use of the dermatoscope can be helpful. Any lesions that are suspicious for melanoma should be excised. Examination of first-degree family members (parents, siblings, and children) of patients with melanoma or dysplastic melanocytic nevi is recommended to identify other persons at high risk.

References

Andea AA: Molecular testing for melanocytic tumors: a practical update, *Histopathology* 80:150–156, 2022.

Argenziano G, Catricala C, Ardigo M, et al: Dermoscopy of patients with multiple nevi, *Arch Dermatol* 147:46–49, 2011.

Arumi-Uria M, McNutt NS, Finnerty B: Grading of atypia in nevi: correlation with melanoma risk, *Mod Pathol* 16:764–771, 2003.

Barnhill RL, Elder DE, Piepkorn MW, et al: Revision of the Melanocytic Pathology Assessment Tool and Hierarchy for Diagnosis classification schema for melanocytic lesions: a consensus statement, *JAMA Netw Open* 6:e2250613, 2023.

Bauer J, Bastian BC: Distinguishing melanocytic nevi from melanomas by DNA copy number changes: comparative genomic hybridization as a research and diagnostic tool, *Dermatol Ther* 19:40–49, 2006.

Burian EA, Jemec GBE: Eruptive melanocytic nevi: A review, *Am J Clin Dermatol* 20(5):669–682, 2019.

de Snoo FA, Kroon HP, Bergman W, et al: From sporadic atypical nevi to familial melanoma: risk analysis for melanoma in sporadic atypical nevus patients, *J Am Acad Dermatol* 56:748–752, 2007.

Drozdowski R, Spaccarelli N, Peters MS, Grant-Kels JM: Dysplastic nevus part I: Historical perspective, classification, and epidemiology, *J Am Acad Dermatol* 88:1–10, 2023.

Elder DE, Massi D, Scolyer RA: *WHO classification of skin tumours*, vol 11, ed 4, International Agency for Research on Cancer, 2018.

Ferrara G, Soyer HP, Malvehy J, et al: The many faces of blue nevus: a clinicopathologic study, *J Cutan Pathol* 34:543–551, 2007.

Gelbard AN, Tripp JM, Marghoob AA, et al: Management of Spitz nevi: a survey of dermatologists in the United States, *J Am Acad Dermatol* 47:224–330, 2002.

Goodson AG, Florell SR, Boucher KM, et al: Low rates of clinical recurrence after biopsy of benign to moderately dysplastic melanocytic nevi, *J Am Acad Dermatol* 62:591–596, 2010.

King R, Hayzen BA, Page RN, et al: Recurrent nevus phenomenon: a clinicopathologic study of 357 cases and histologic comparison with melanoma with regression, *Mod Pathol* 22:611–619, 2009.

Kinsler VA, O'Hare P, Bulstrode N, et al: Melanoma in congenital melanocytic naevi, *Br J Dermatol* 176:1131–1143, 2017.

Maher NG, Scolyer RA, Colebatch AJ: Biology and genetics of acquired and congenital melanocytic naevi, *Pathology* S0031-3025(22):00683-3, 2022.

Naeyaert JM, Brochez L: Dysplastic nevi, *N Engl J Med* 349:2233–2240, 2003.

Price HN, Schaffer JV: Congenital melanocytic nevi: when to worry and how to treat: facts and controversies, *Clin Dermatol* 28:283–302, 2010.

Que K, Grant-Kels JM, Longo C, Pellacani G: Basics of confocal microscopy and the complexity of diagnosing skin tumors: new imaging tools in clinical practice, diagnostic workflows, cost-estimate and new trends, *Dermatol Clinics* 34:367–375, 2016.

Roh MR, Eliades P, Gupta S, Tsao H: Genetics of melanocytic nevi, *Pigment Cell Melanoma Res* 28:661–672, 2015.

Šekoranja D, Pižem J, Luzar B: An update on molecular genetic aberrations in spitz melanocytic proliferations: correlation with morphological features and biological behavior, *Acta Med Acad* 50:157–174, 2021.

Sommer LL, Barcia SM, Clarke LE, Helm KF: Persistent melanocytic nevi: a review and analysis of 205 cases, *J Cutan Pathol* 38:503–507, 2011.

Spaccarelli N, Drozdowski R, Peters MS, Grant-Kels JM: Dysplastic nevus part II: Dysplastic nevi: Molecular/genetic profiles and management, *J Am Acad Dermatol* 88:13–20, 2023.

Tetzlaff MT, Reuben A, Billings SD, et al: Toward a molecular-genetic classification of spitzoid neoplasms, *Clin Lab Med* 37:431–448, 2017.

Wei B, Gu J, Gao B, et al: Deficient mismatch repair is detected in large-to-giant congenital melanocytic naevi: providing new insight into aetiology and diagnosis, *Br J Dermatol* 188:64–74, 2023.

Yeh I: Melanocytic naevi, melanocytomas and emerging concepts, *Pathology* S0031-3025(22):00679-1, 2022.

NONMELANOMA CANCER OF THE SKIN

Method of
Jake Lazaroff, MD; and Diana Bolotin, MD, PhD

CURRENT DIAGNOSIS

- Skin cancers are polymorphous in appearance, ranging from small papules and plaques to nodules and tumors of different colors, sizes, and consistencies.
- The surface may be smooth, scaly, ulcerated, or crusted.
- A common feature is that all of these skin neoplasms grow continuously and relapse when superficially treated.
- The distinction between skin cancers and benign neoplasms or inflammatory dermatoses may be difficult for the nondermatologist to make.

with slow taper over weeks to months. Colchicine[1] 0.6 mg PO three times a day has shown success as monotherapy or used in conjunction with corticosteroids. Cyclosporine (Neoral, Sandimmune)[1] 2.5 to 5 mg/kg/day divided twice a day has been demonstrated to lead to rapid improvement in pain and improvement in ulceration. Combination therapy with systemic corticosteroids and cyclosporine has also demonstrated success. Milder localized disease can be treated with intralesional corticosteroid injections such as with triamcinolone acetonide (Kenalog) 10 mg/mL into the ulcer edge or high-potency topical corticosteroids.

Alternative therapies utilized with success for moderate to severe disease include infliximab (Remicade)[1] 5 mg/kg IV at weeks 0, 2, and 6; adalimumab (Humira)[1] 80 mg SC loading dose, followed by 40 mg SC weekly or every other week; mycophenolate mofetil (Cellcept)[1] 750 mg to 1.5 g PO twice a day; dapsone[1] 50 to 150 mg daily; sulfasalazine (Azulfidine) 0.5 to 6 g PO daily divided in 3 to 4 doses, methotrexate[1] 2.5 to 25 mg PO, SC, or IM weekly, and more. The authors have also seen success with intravenous immunoglobulin (IVIG)[1] 1.5 to 3 g/kg IV monthly given over 2 to 5 days, although this can be incredibly expensive and is generally used as adjuvant therapy. IVIG is also an option for treatment if there is secondary infection and immunosuppressive therapies with TNF-α inhibitors are contraindicated.

Tetracycline antibiotics such as minocycline (Minocin)[1] 200 to 300 mg/day divided in 2 doses have also been reported to show success in treatment of PG, thought to be related to their antiinflammatory properties by reducing chemotaxis of neutrophils.

Appropriate wound care for PG ulcers is essential, depending on the clinical appearance of the lesion. Wound care specialists should be utilized if possible. Occlusive dressings are often utilized to increase the rate of healing by promoting angiogenesis, promoting collagen synthesis, and acting as a barrier against secondary infection. Hydrogels and films such as Tegaderm may be used in lesions with minimal exudate. In more exudative lesions, more absorptive dressings such as hydrocolloids, foams, and alginates would be more appropriate. Examples of these dressings that are frequently utilized for ulcer management include DuoDERM and SeaSorb. It is important to note that these dressings, especially alginates, may be associated with foul odor due to their reaction with healing tissue and may not actually be an indicator of secondary infection. Avoid wet-to-dry dressings, as this debridement may incite pathergy and cause aggravation of the wound.

Monitoring

PG tends to be a chronic and recurrent disease. Ulcers may take many months to heal, and it is essential to monitor for any signs of developing infection. Patients and clinicians should monitor for increased pain, increased purulence, fevers, increased erythema and/or streaking—all of which can be indicators for secondary infection. Topical and oral antimicrobials may be helpful; however, this may lead to antibiotic resistance and should be utilized only if secondary infection is confirmed.

Adequate control of any contributing underlying conditions is essential, and patients should be advised that trauma and elective surgical procedures may trigger the development of future PG lesions.

Many of the treatments utilized in the management of PG also have their large range of adverse side effects, and it is important to monitor patients closely when they are taking these medications. For example, systemic corticosteroids are the most commonly employed agents in PG. More severe or resistant lesions may require prolonged therapy and at higher doses, which can lead to increased adverse side effects. These patients should be closely monitored, and consider recommending supplemental calcium, vitamin D, proton pump inhibitors if indicated, and even bisphosphonates. The duration of treatment is case-dependent and should be determined based on clinical response and any concerning side effects.

[1]Not FDA approved for this indication.

References

Ahronowitz I, Harp J, Shinkai K: Etiology and management of pyoderma gangrenosum: a comprehensive review, *Am J Clin Dermatol* 13(3):191–211, 2012.

Braswell SF, Kostopoulos TC, Ortega-Loayza AG: Pathophysiology of pyoderma gangrenosum (PG): an updated review, *J Am Acad Dermatol* 73(4):691–698, 2015.

Brooklyn T, Dunnill G, Probert C: Diagnosis and treatment of pyoderma gangrenosum, *BMJ* 333(7560):181–184, 2006.

Cummins DL, Anhalt GJ, et al: Treatment of pyoderma gangrenosum with intravenous immunoglobulin, *Br J Dermatol* 157(6):1235–1239, 2007.

Davis MDP, Moschella SL: Neutrophilic Dermatoses: pyoderma gangrenosum. In Bolognia JL, et al: *Dermatology 2018*, ed 4, Philadelphia, 2018, Elsevier, pp 459–463.

Maverakis E, Ma C, et al: Diagnostic criteria of ulcerative pyoderma gangrenosum: a Delphi consensus of international experts, *JAMA Dermatol* 154(4):461–466, 2018.

Neill BC, Seger EW, et al: The 5 P's of pyoderma gangrenosum, *J of Drugs in Dermatol* 18(12):1283, 2019.

Patel F, Fitzmaurice S, et al: Effective strategies for the management of pyoderma gangrenosum: a comprehensive review, *Acta Derm Venereol* 95(5):525–531, 2015.

■ ROSACEA

Method of
Lisa M. Johnson, MD; and Daniel J. Van Durme, MD, MPH

CURRENT DIAGNOSIS

- Rosacea is a chronic inflammatory disease of the skin that predominantly affects the convexities of the central face (cheeks, chin, nose, and central part of forehead). It most commonly occurs in adults aged 30 to 50 years.
- Rosacea is a clinical diagnosis.
- Transition to a phenotype-based approach to the diagnosis, classification, and management of rosacea from the traditional subtype-based approach is occurring, allowing more individualized management of symptoms that most concern a patient.
- Two cutaneous phenotypes may be considered independently diagnostic of rosacea: (1) fixed centrofacial erythema in a characteristic pattern that may periodically intensify, or (2) phymatous changes.
- The presence of two or more major phenotypes (flushing, telangiectasia, inflammatory lesions, and ocular manifestations) may be considered diagnostic of rosacea.
- Common exacerbating factors that intensify signs and symptoms include alcohol, heat, spicy foods, and sunlight.

CURRENT THERAPY

- Therapy is best chosen based on severity and predominant manifestation(s).
- Avoidance of known triggers is key for all types,
- Brimonidine tartrate 0.33% gel (Mirvaso, Onreltea) and oxymetazoline hydrochloride 1% cream (Rhofade) are useful for facial flushing. Ivermectin cream (Soolantra) and metronidazole gel (Metrogel, Rosadan) can be effective for papules and pustules. Isotretinoin (Accutane, Claravis)[1] can be effective in treating very severe and refractory rosacea.
- Ocular rosacea can be treated with increased eyelid hygiene, adding topical or oral antibiotics if needed.
- Rhinophyma (sebaceous gland hypertrophy and fibrosis) needs surgical management.

[1]Not FDA approved for this indication.

Rosacea is well established as a chronic cutaneous syndrome, encompassing various combinations of potential signs and symptoms that manifest primarily on the convexities of the central face (cheeks, chin, nose, and central part of forehead). Signs and symptoms are often characterized by repeated remissions and exacerbations. Rosacea is commonly diagnosed in certain demographic groups, and in epidemiologic studies of Whites, its prevalence has been 10% or higher. Although it has been most frequently observed in patients with fair skin, rosacea has also been diagnosed in Asians, Latin Americans, African Americans, and Africans. The disorder is identified more often in women than in men, and although it may occur at any age, the onset typically occurs at any time after age 30.

Diagnosis

The classification of rosacea was updated in 2016 and modified in 2019 by the global ROSacea COnsensus panel (ROSCO). This panel recommended transitioning to an individualized phenotype-based approach to the diagnosis, classification and management of rosacea rather than the traditional subtype-based approach. By focusing on individual lesions rather than a group of dermatologic characteristics constituting a subtype, treatment can be tailored to the signs and symptoms that most concern an individual patient.

Diagnostic Phenotypes

The panel identified two phenotypes as independently diagnostic of rosacea: (1) centrofacial erythema associated with periodic intensification, and (2) phymatous changes. Phymatous changes include patulous follicles, skin thickening or fibrosis, glandular hyperplasia, and a bulbous appearance of the nose. Rhinophyma is the most common form, but other phymas may occur.

Major Phenotypes

Flushing transient erythema, telangiectasia, inflammatory lesions, and ocular manifestations were major phenotypes commonly identified in patients with rosacea but were not considered individually diagnostic. In the absence of one of the two diagnostic phenotypes, the presence of two or more of these major phenotypes may be considered diagnostic.

Secondary Phenotypes

Secondary signs and symptoms of rosacea may appear with one or more diagnostic or major phenotypes and include burning or stinging, edema, and a dry appearance.

Ocular Rosacea

Ocular rosacea can occur in the context of mild, moderate, or severe dermatologic disease and may also appear in the absence of diagnostic skin manifestations. Ocular signs strongly suggestive of ocular rosacea include lid margin telangiectases, interpalpebral conjunctival injection, spade-shaped infiltrates in the cornea, and scleritis and sclerokeratitis.

Treatment

One key aspect of management is to have the patient maintain a careful diary for the purpose of determining and then avoiding his or her own triggers. Common triggers include alcohol, heat, certain foods, sunlight, stress, and menstruation, among others. Broad-spectrum sunblock (UVA and UVB) should be used daily, along with application of moisturizers for dry skin and drying applications for oily skin, and gentle cleansing of the whole face. Cosmetics with a red-neutralizing green pigment can help appearance.

Brimonidine tartrate 0.33% gel (Mirvaso, Onreltea) is a selective alpha2-adrenergic receptor agonist with vasoconstrictive activity and has been approved for the treatment of persistent (nontransient) facial erythema in adults 18 years and older with rosacea, along with oxymetazoline hydrochloride 1% cream ([Rhofade] an alpha1A-adrenoreceptor agonist that also activates alpha2-receptors at higher concentration).

Patients with mild to moderate papules and pustules benefit from topical 1% ivermectin cream (Soolantra), which is applied to the face once daily, and topical antibiotics such as metronidazole 0.75% to 1% cream, lotion, or gel (Metro-Cream 0.75%, Noritate 1% cream, MetroLotion 0.75%, Rosadan 0.75% gel, Metrogel 1%) or azelaic acid 20% cream

[Azelex][1] or 15% gel [Finacea]) applied once or twice daily. Persistent telangiectasias can be effectively treated with laser therapy and intravascular aethoxysklerol ([Asclera] 0.5%–1%)[1] injections.

Patients affected by mild phymata benefit from tetracycline[1] therapy. Standard therapies for advanced phymata are ablative (destructive) laser and dermato-surgery. Low-dose isotretinoin (Accutane, Claravis)[1] appears to reduce phymata by its antiinflammatory capacity and by lessening the number of sebaceous glands and inhibiting their proliferation.

There is no US Food and Drug Administration (FDA)–approved therapy for facial edema. Immunomodulators such as isotretinoin[1] and dapsone (oral or topical [Aczone gel])[1] or combination therapies with doxycycline (Oracea)/prednisolone[1] have been tried, but the therapeutic value is unclear.

Both prescribers and patients must register with the iPledge program to prescribe and to receive the prescriptions for isotretinoin. See www.ipledgeprogram.com.

Ocular rosacea can often be controlled with increased eyelid hygiene, washing with warm water and baby (no-tears) shampoo twice a day along with artificial tears. Long-term consumption of omega-3 fatty acids[7] may improve meibomian-gland dysfunction. Topical ophthalmic cyclosporine drops (Restasis)[1] applied as one drop to the eye twice daily (12 hours apart) demonstrate statistically significant improvement in common signs and symptoms compared with artificial tears. If severe, it can be treated with systemic tetracycline.[1] If it persists, ophthalmology referral is necessary.

---

[1]Not FDA approved for this indication.
[7]Available as a dietary supplement.

References

Buddenkotte J, Steinhoff M: Recent advances in understanding and managing rosacea, *F1000Res* 7:F1000 Faculty Rev-1885, 2018, https://doi.org/10.12688/f1000research.16537.1. Published 2018 Dec 3.

Gallo RL, Granstein RD, Kang S, Mannis M, Martin S, Tan J, Thiboutot D: Standard classification and pathophysiology of rosacea: the 2017 update by the National Rosacea Society Expert Committee, *J Am Acad Dermatol* 78(1):148–155, 2018.

Goldgar C, Keahey DJ, Houchins J: Treatment options for acne rosacea, *Am Fam Physician* 80:461–468, 2009.

Powell FC: Clinical practice: rosacea, *N Engl J Med* 352:793–803, 2005.

Schaller M, Almeida LMC, Bewley A, et al: Recommendations for rosacea diagnosis, classification and management: update from the global ROSacea COnsensus 2019 panel, 182(5):1269–1276, 2020.

Tan J, Almeida LMC, Bewley A, et al: Updating the diagnosis, classification and assessment of rosacea: recommendations from the global ROSacea COnsensus (ROSCO) panel, *Br J Dermatol* 176:431–438, 2017.

Wollina U: Rosacea and rhinophyma in the elderly, *Clin Dermatol* 29:61–68, 2011.

STEVENS-JOHNSON SYNDROME AND TOXIC EPIDERMAL NECROLYSIS

Method of
Scott Worswick, MD

CURRENT DIAGNOSIS

- A diagnosis of toxic epidermal necrolysis (TEN) can be rendered when the body surface area (BSA) involved contains more than 30% denuded skin.
- A diagnosis of Stevens-Johnson Syndrome (SJS) can be rendered when less than 10% of the BSA involves denuded skin.
- SJS-TEN overlap is diagnosed when the involved BSA is between 10% and 30% BSA.
- Patients with SJS, SJS-TEN overlap, and TEN should have involvement of not only the cutaneous surface but also at least one mucosal region (most commonly the oral mucosa). Cases do exist with no mucosal involvement but this is rare and should prompt consideration of an alternate diagnosis.
- A thorough drug history and skin biopsy (ideally using the fresh-frozen technique) are essential when considering a diagnosis of SJS or TEN.

- Conservative therapy is a cornerstone of therapy for all patients. This includes appropriate wound care, monitoring for fluid loss and electrolyte imbalance, thorough daily skin exams, and monitoring of vital signs to rule out concurrent infection.
- A dermatologist should be involved in the care of all hospitalized patients with Stevens-Johnson Syndrome and toxic epidermal necrolysis. In the appropriate clinical context, ophthalmology and OBGYN should also be involved. Depending on hospital resources, ICU and/or plastic surgery and the burn unit should be involved early in the care of these patients.
- Classically, systemic corticosteroids and intravenous immunoglobulin (IVIG)[1] were utilized in the management of these patients. New data suggest either cyclosporine (Neoral, Sandimmune)[1] or etanercept (Embrel)[1] may improve overall outcomes.

[1]Not FDA approved for this indication.

Epidemiology

Toxic epidermal necrolysis (TEN) is a rare diagnosis, only afflicting approximately one patient per million per year (most studies cite this incidence rate, though one study from the United States did cite an incidence rate as high as 12.7 per year). Stevens-Johnson Syndrome (SJS) and SJS-TEN overlap affect approximately five per million patients per year. The overall mortality varies greatly among different studies but is currently estimated to be ~25% for TEN. It can affect patients of any age, and most data regarding therapy are stratified by age into pediatric and adult cohorts. There are some experts who feel there may be a viral trigger or co-factor for the disease because prevalence increases in the spring.

Risk Factors

Common implicated agents include sulfonamide antibiotics as well as more recently described penicillin and cephalosporin antibiotics, aromatic anticonvulsants, allopurinol (Zyloprim), and nonsteroidal antiinflammatory drugs (NSAIDs). Numerous other medications have been reported to trigger the disease and some other common offending agents include the anti-programmed death-1 and anti-cytotoxic T-lymphocyte-associated protein 4 chemotherapeutic agents, dapsone and nevirapine (Viramune). The most important intervention is to determine and remove the offending agent as some studies cite an increase in mortality of 34% per day if the offending agent is not removed from the patient's regimen.

Certain tests can be performed after hospitalization in selected cases to determine the most likely offending agent if unknown. For example, patch testing can be done, and in the case of carbamazepine-induced SJS-TEN, has a sensitivity greater than 70%. Likewise, if multiple drugs are suspected as potential inciting agents, it may be worth checking the patient's human leukocyte antigen (HLA) types and correlating this with his/her ethnicity to make an educated guess about likely agent (if a patient has three potential inciting agents including allopurinol, the patient is of Asian descent, and HLA-typing reveals positive HLA-B5801, it could be concluded with a higher level of certainty that allopurinol is the most likely agent).

Less common triggers include vaccines such as MMR and less commonly the meningococcal, varicella and influenza vaccines, herpes, and ultraviolet light. These are more likely to be implicated in patients with target lesions or low body surface area (BSA) involvement and are exceedingly rare in patients diagnosed with full-blown TEN. An important trigger to consider in the work-up is mycoplasma, which can be responsible for causing mycoplasma-induced rash and mucositis (MIRM). MIRM is a clinical mimicker common in pediatric patients, which is characterized by lower BSA but worse mucosal involvement (typically involving two sites and usually including the ocular mucosa in dramatic fashion).

In addition to the causes of SJS and TEN described previously, there are risk factors that seem to predispose patients to the disease. These include: HIV (some studies cite a thousand-times increased chance of developing TEN among HIV-positive patients, even when controlled for the number and type of medications these patients were exposed to), lupus, female gender, Asian or African ethnicity, patients undergoing brain cancer treatment with corticosteroids and radiation, and certain HLA types. For example, one recent meta-analysis found that certain HLA-B subtypes predispose Asian patients to the development of carbamazepine-induced TEN, including HLA-B1502, HLA-B4001, HLA-B4601, and HLA-B5801. Other studies have identified HLA-B1502 as a risk factor for aromatic anticonvulsant-induced TEN among various Asian populations, HLA-B5801 as a risk factor for allopurinol-induced TEN among Asians, HLA-C0401 for nevirapine-induced TEN among patients in Malawi, and HLA type B3802, A29, B12, and DR7 as a risk factor among Europeans for sulfonamide-induced TEN.

Pathophysiology

As described previously, an immunologic basis for the development SJS and TEN is hypothesized given the fact that certain HLA types among certain groups predispose them to development of the disease. There currently exist four theories to explain how small drugs might interact with HLA and T-cell receptors (TCRs) to initiate a chain of events leading to SJS/TEN.

In the hapten theory (which has been validated in the case of penicillin-induced drug reactions), it is presumed that the drug molecule combines with an endogenous peptide and this is presented to the HLA molecule and recognized by the TCR. In the p-i model (pharmacologic interaction with the immune receptors), which has been validated in carbamazepine-HLA-B1502 interactions, the drug itself binds directly, reversibly, and noncovalently to HLA and/or TCR. In the altered peptide repertoire model, it is proposed that the drug binds to the peptide-binding groove of the HLA molecule thereby altering the overall binding ability of the HLA molecule. Lastly, in the altered TCR repertoire model, it is suggested that some drugs (such as sulfamethoxazole) can bind directly to the TCR (but not with the HLA molecule) and thereby alter the conformation of the TCR giving them the ability to bind to self-HLA.

Regardless of the type of interaction that allows a drug to alter the way HLA and TCR react to self, patients with TEN exhibit increased activity of natural killer (NK) cells and specific T lymphocytes (NK T-cells and CD* + cytotoxic T-cells). These cells mediate keratinocyte cell death via a cascade of events including Fas–FasL binding and procaspase-8 activation, increased tumor necrosis factor-α and interferon-γ levels, and activation of the perforin-granzyme-granulysin apoptosis pathway.

Differential Diagnosis

Patients with SJS and TEN typically complain of skin pain before the eruption begins. A prodrome consisting of low-grade fever, malaise, and/or flu-like symptoms is not uncommon. Within days some degree of mucosal involvement (which can take the form of dusky erythema, bullae/vesicles, denuded mucosal surface(s), dysuria, ocular erythema, pain with defecation, or pain with swallowing) is almost universal, while the extent of cutaneous involvement can vary dramatically but should include either a dusky erythema with eventual vesicles, bullae, or denuded skin, or less commonly targetoid lesions. The majority of patients with SJS and TEN present with painful red-purple (dusky) patches or macules that progress over the span of a few days. Areas that began with dusky erythema develop superimposed bullae, vesicles, or denuded skin.

Most patients with SJS and TEN do not present with typical targets on cutaneous exam. Such lesions are characterized by a small red central papule surrounded by a white ring and finally most peripherally by another ring of erythema. These lesions characterize erythema multiforme, which is much more commonly the result of herpes rather than drug allergy. However, there are rare reported cases of SJS and TEN that do include or are even dominated by cutaneous typical or atypical targets.

The main differential diagnosis for patients with classic dusky erythema, mucosal involvement, and skin pain includes acute graft-versus-host disease (GVHD), bullous lupus, generalized fixed drug eruption (FDE), cutaneous burns, paraneoplastic pemphigus (PNP), in pediatric patients MIRM, and in infants infection with the Chikungunya virus. The majority of these entities can be ruled out by clinical history alone, as patients with acute GVHD should have had a recent transplant and patients with PNP a concurrent malignancy. Dramatic mucosal involvement, in any age group, should prompt work-up for mycoplasma; when MIRM is suspected it should be treated with empiric antibiotics and in severe cases IVIG[1]. Patients with a known malignancy (particularly chronic lymphocytic leukemia [CLL], lymphoma, Castleman disease, sarcoma, or thymoma) and/or of older age and with significant mucosal disease should have, in addition to a biopsy, a direct immunofluorescence (DIF) performed and serum drawn for indirect immunofluorescence and ELISA performed to rule out PNP. It is important to check a DIF as well in any patients with joint pain or other symptoms suggestive of systemic lupus erythematosus (SLE), as well as antinuclear antibody (ANA), anti-Sjogren's syndrome–related antigen (SSA), and anti-Sjogren's Syndrome Type B (SSB), anti-dsDNA and anti-Smith. Likewise, if you are evaluating an infant who has no medication exposure and is from an endemic area, it is important to check serum titers for the Chikungunya virus.

Diagnosis

Determining the inciting agent is as important as making a quick diagnosis of TEN. A thorough drug history is essential including prn medication usage (frequently patients do not report their NSAID use or a recent antibiotic exposure). If SJS or TEN is suspected and the inciting agent is known, it is important to immediately inform the patient and his/her family of the suspected allergy and add it to the patient's medication allergy list. Dermatology should be consulted and when possible/necessary will ideally perform a skin biopsy to be processed emergently using the fresh-frozen technique (results can be ready within 30 minutes). Hematoxylin and eosin staining will also be done on permanent sections (and these results are available 1 to 3 days later depending on the site/lab).

After making a diagnosis of SJS or TEN, a practitioner can employ a scoring system called SCORTEN to estimate the patient's mortality. In this system a patient receives one point if he/she is aged above 40 years, BSA greater than 10%, history of concurrent malignancy within 2 years, serum blood urea nitrogen greater than 28 mg/dL, glucose greater than 252 mg/dL, bicarbonate level less than 20 mEq/L, and heart rate more than 120 beats per minute during the first 24 hours. With each increasing point, mortality increases such that a score of 2 confers an expected mortality of 12%; a score of 3 equates to a 35% mortality; a score of 4 with a 58% mortality; and a score of 5 or higher with an expected 90% chance of mortality.

Therapy
Medical Therapy

Classic therapy for SJS and TEN was with systemic corticosteroids but this has fallen out of favor in the United States due to recent meta-analyses suggesting no improvement in outcomes. Likewise, IVIG[1] was a mainstay of therapy in the early 21st century, but a large review from Europe found a worsened mortality in patients given IVIG compared with those given steroids or supportive care alone. Other data are conflicting with some studies suggesting that a 4-day dose of daily 1 g/kg IV[1] provides a mortality benefit, with other studies finding no improvement.

More recent success seems to have come from the utilization of etanercept (Enbrel)[1] or cyclosporine (Neoral, Sandimmune)[1] in the treatment of this disease. In 2014 a group from Italy treated 10 patients with one 50 mg subcutaneous dose and found not only a 0% mortality despite an expected mortality of 47%, but also decreased time to re-epithelialization. Likewise, in 2018 a

Taiwanese group found an improved mortality benefit of etanercept over corticosteroids among 96 patients.

Similarly, data emerging in the last decade have suggested that cyclosporine also confers a mortality benefit. In 2010 a British case series found a 0% mortality in patients receiving 3 mg/kg per day orally despite a predicated ~30% mortality based on SCORTEN. Another study cites a significantly decreased time to re-epithelialization (3.67 days) among patients who survived after receiving cyclosporine at a dose of 3 to 4 mg/kg per day.

Adjuvant Mucosal Therapies

Patients with SJS/TEN can suffer from long-term skin/hair/nail complications including post-inflammatory hyperpigmentation, photosensitivity (70% of patients according to one study), chronic pruritus, eruptive nevi, nail changes, hypertrophic scars, and telogen effluvium. They also have a significant morbidity when their mucosal surfaces are severely involved with disease. Ocular complications can include ectropion, trichiasis, ankyloblepharon, corneal scarring, and even blindness. To some extent these complications are minimized by a choice of systemic therapy to mediate disease (i.e., either etanercept or cyclosporine). However, other measures can also be employed including amniotic membrane grafting by ophthalmology (which has been shown in a randomized controlled trial to improve multiple ocular outcome measures), topical steroid application, oxygen therapy, and bronchodilators. Likewise, urogenital sequelae occur in about one in four patients and can include adhesions leading to dyspareunia or even total vaginal fusion. Therefore involvement of gynecology or urology in the care of any patient with genital SJS/TEN is essential.

Monitoring

It is important to remember that the cutaneous examination of a patient with TEN differs greatly depending on the time of exam relative to the onset of eruption. With onset it is possible the patient will only complain of pain and have no skin lesions whatsoever. Within days a typical exam would include florid oral mucosal involvement with areas of skin showing dusky erythematous macules or patches. Over the next few days, most of the cutaneous lesions will evolve and become vesicles, bullae, or entire surfaces will denude. Monitoring for efficacy of chosen therapy means being aware of what is expected in terms of progression (that some or all areas that were dusky will denude), and ensuring that no new dusky areas develop.

The most common cause of death in patients with TEN is infection, so checking daily white blood cell counts and following vitals every 2 to 4 hours if not more frequently is essential. Fevers can occur simply as the result of the disease process itself, but any fever should prompt blood, urine, and sputum cultures. Prophylactic antibiotics have not been shown to improve outcomes but when an infection is suspected it must be treated immediately.

References

Canavan TN, Mathes EF, Friedan I, et al: Mycoplasma pneumonia-induced rash and mucositis as a syndrome distinct from Stevens-Johnson syndrome and erythema multiforme: A systematic review, *JAAD* 72(2):239–245, 2015.

Chahal D, Aleshin M, Turegano M, et al: Vaccine-induced TEN: A case and systematic review, *Dermatology, Online Journal* 24(1), 2018.

Chen CB, Abe R, Pan RY, et al: An updated review of the molecular mechanisms in drug hypersensitivity, *Journal of Immunology Research*, 2018.

Conner C, McKenzie E, Owen C: The use of cyclosporine for SJS-TEN spectrum at the University of Louisville: A case series and literature review, *Dermatology Online Journal* 24(1), 2018.

Lee HY, Walsh SA, Creamer D: Long-term complications of SJS/TEN: The spectrum of chronic problems in patients who survive an episode of SJS/TEN necessitates multidisciplinary follow-up, *British Journal of Dermatology* 177:924–935, 2017.

Paradisi A, et al: Etanercept therapy for TEN, *JAAD* 71(2):278–283, 2014.

Schneck J, et al: Effects of treatment on the mortality of SJS and TEN: A retrospective study on patients included in the prospective EuroSCAR Study, *JAAD* 58(1):33–40, 2008.

Valeyrie-Allanore L, Wolkenstein P, Brochard L, et al: Open trial of ciclosporin treatment for SJS and TEN, *British Journal of Dermatology* 163(4):847–853, 2010.

Wang CW, Yang LY, Chen CB, et al: Randomized, controlled trial of TNF-alpha antagonist in CTL-mediated severe cutaneous adverse reactions, *J Clin Invest* 128(3):985–996, 2018.

Wang Q, Sun S, Xie M, et al: Association between the HLA-B alleles and carbamazepine-induced SJS/TEN: A meta-analysis, *Epilepsy Research* 135:19–28, 2017.

---

[1]Not FDA approved for this indication.

Urticaria, or hives, is a common cutaneous eruption that occurs in up to 25% of the general population sometime during their lives (Bailey, 2008). It is characterized by transient, circumscribed, pruritic, erythematous papules or plaques, often with central pallor. Individual lesions often coalesce into large wheals on the trunk and extremities that may resolve over a few hours without leaving any residual skin changes. The process is mediated by mast cells in the superficial dermis, and skin changes often resolve within 30 min to 24 hr.

Angioedema is a similar process occurring in deep dermis or subcutaneous tissue. Angioedema may occur independently, accompanied by urticaria, or as a component of anaphylaxis. It is characterized by localized swelling that develops over minutes to hours and resolution may take up to 72 hours. Common locations of angioedema include the mucosa and areas with loose connective tissue, such as the face, eyes, lips, tongue, and genitalia. Patients usually do not have pruritus, but they may have pain and a sensation of warmth. Angioedema is usually a benign process that resolves without sequelae unless it involves the larynx. African Americans are disproportionately affected, representing up to 40% of the hospital admissions for angioedema.

Classification

Urticaria can be classified as acute or chronic, depending on the duration. Acute urticaria usually lasts for less than 6 weeks and can be spontaneous or triggered by infection, medication, insect bite, and food (Table 1). The chronic form, lasting more than 6 weeks, accounts for approximately 30% of cases of urticaria, and no clear causes can be identified in more than 80% of these cases. Stress however has been identified as a trigger in some of the cases. Depending on the triggers, chronic urticaria can be classified as cold, heat, solar, delayed pressure, vibratory, cholinergic, contact, or aquagenic urticaria. A significant number of patients with chronic urticaria may have persistent symptoms for more than 10 years. Approximately 40% of patients with chronic urticaria have associated angioedema, although the incidence of laryngeal edema is low.

Diagnosis

Urticaria is diagnosed clinically in most cases. A detailed history, physical examination, and complete review of systems are essential for diagnosing patients with urticaria and angioedema. The history should include the distribution and characteristics of lesions (e.g., pain, pruritus), duration of skin eruption, accompanying angioedema, airway involvement and other associated systemic symptoms (e.g., fever, arthralgia, swelling joints, refusal to walk by children). Patients should also be questioned about changes in dietary habits, stress, recent exposures, infection, and newly administered medications, including antibiotics, over-the-counter analgesia, and hormones. Patients who suffer from recurrent angioedema should be asked about their use of angiotensin-converting enzyme (ACE) inhibitor medications.

Laboratory assessment is usually not helpful in diagnosing patients with acute urticaria who lack any history or clinical findings to suggest an underlying disease process. A limited number of diagnostic tests are indicated in the evaluation of patients with chronic urticaria when there is sign of systemic disease associated, such as a complete blood cell count with differential white blood cell count, an erythrocyte sedimentation rate (ESR) or C-reactive protein (CRP) determination, a thyroid-stimulating hormone (TSH) level, antithyroglobulin and antimicrosomal antibodies, antinuclear antibodies (ANA), folate, B12, ferritin, liver function test, and hepatitis B and C serologies. A detailed review of systems may help to narrow the focus of the screening test.

A skin biopsy of an early lesion should be performed to rule out urticarial vasculitis if the affected individual has skin lesions that are painful and last for more than 2 to 3 days with residual ecchymosis or petechiae. In patients with angioedema, prominent edema of the interstitial tissue may be demonstrated by biopsy. It is associated with antibodies against C1q, which leads to persistent complement activation and low serum C3, C4. Serum measurements of C4 and C1-esterase inhibitor are recommended initial tests if hereditary or acquired angioedema is suspected. Hereditary angioedema is caused by deficiency (type I) or dysfunction (type II) of C1-esterase inhibitor protein. A C1q level should be obtained to screen for the acquired form of angioedema if the affected individual is middle-aged. Additional constitutional symptoms and extracutaneous manifestations are often present in patients with autoinflammatory syndromes such as Schnitzler's syndrome, cryopyrin-associated periodic syndrome (CAPS), Muckle-Wells syndrome (MWS), neonatal-onset multisystem inflammatory disease (NOMID) and, rarely, hyper-IgD syndrome (HIDS) and tumor necrosis factor receptor alpha-associated periodic syndrome (TRAPS).

Treatment

More than two thirds of cases of urticaria are self-limited. Spontaneous remission of chronic urticaria and angioedema is also common. The primary objective of management is to identify and discontinue the offending trigger. A patient presenting with angioedema must first be assessed for signs of airway compromise. Medical therapy is indicated for those who are symptomatic.

Antihistamines remain the first-line therapy for most patients with urticaria, because the primary complaint of pruritus is predominantly mediated by histamine released from mast cells. First-generation antihistamines such as hydroxyzine (Atarax or Vistaril 1 mg/kg (max 25 mg/dose) for children and 25–50 mg every 6 hours in adults), diphenhydramine (Benadryl 25–50 mg every 6 hours), cyproheptadine (Periactin 4 mg three times daily), and chlorpheniramine[1] (Chlor-Trimeton 4 mg every 6 hours) are potent and have the quickest onset of action. However, the treatments are often limited by their sedating and anticholinergic side effects. Many first-generation antihistamines are available over the counter, providing accessible first-line therapy for patients. Patients with urticaria that lasts for several days should be considered for treatment using second-generation antihistamines such as loratadine (Claritin[1] 10 mg twice daily[3]), desloratadine[1] (Clarinex 5 mg twice daily[3]), cetirizine[1] (Zyrtec 10 mg twice daily[3]), levocetirizine[1] (Xyzal 5 mg daily), and fexofenadine[1] (Allegra 180 mg twice daily[3]). If urticaria is not adequately controlled, the second generation antihistamine dosage can be at least doubled. Doxepin (Sinequan),[1] an H_1- and H_2-receptor antagonist, is seven times more potent than hydroxyzine in suppression of wheal and flare responses. Because of its central nervous system side effects, combined use of doxepin with a first-generation antihistamine should be restricted. Topical 5% doxepin cream (Zonalon)[1] may help to suppress pruritus in patients with localized urticaria. Anti-IgE

TABLE 1 Mechanisms in Urticaria and Angioedema

DISORDER	CAUSES
Immunoglobulin-mediated urticaria	Ig-E mediated: food, medication, insect bites, contact allergen, aeroallergens, other causes Urticaria associated with autoimmunity: antinuclear antibodies (ANAs), thyroid autoantibodies, other causes
Direct activation of mast cell degranulation	Physical stimuli: exercise, heat, cold, pressure, aquagenic, solar radiation, etc. Other agents: opiates, antibiotics (e.g., vancomycin [Vancocin]), radiocontrast, ACTH (Cortrosyn), muscle relaxants
Complement-mediated	Viral infections, parasites, blood transfusion
C1-esterase inhibitor deficiency	Genetic and acquired angioedema, paraproteinemia
Reduced kinin metabolism	Angiotensin-converting enzyme (ACE) inhibitors
Reduced arachidonic acid metabolism	Aspirin

[1]Not FDA approved for this indication.
[3]Exceeds dosage recommended by the manufacturer.

treatment using omalizumab (150–300 mg per month) for chronic urticaria refractory to high-dose antihistamine therapy has been approved by the FDA for patients over 12 years of age in US. While the treatment is highly effective, safe, and suitable for long-term use, it has a high cost.

Systemic prednisone at 30 to 40 mg in a single morning dose is sufficient to suppress acute urticaria in adults. Tapering should be gradual over a 3- to 4-week period by decreasing the dosage 5 mg every 3 to 5 days to minimize rebound. Alternate-morning dosing when reaching 20 mg daily may help to minimize the steroid side effects. Methylprednisolone (Solu-Medrol 40 mg) should be given intravenously as initial therapy to patients with angioedema. This may be followed by a tapering oral course. Chronic therapy with systemic steroids is to be avoided. Three months of off-label treatment with cyclosporine (Neoral)[1] at 3 to 5 mg/kg can be given safely to patients who are refractory to corticosteroid or omalizumab therapy. Close monitoring for hypertension and renal insufficiency is necessary during the treatment.

Leukotriene inhibitors such as zileuton (Zyflo[1] 600 mg four times daily), zafirlukast (Accolate[1] 20 mg twice daily), and montelukast (Singulair[1] 10 mg once daily) may be effective for patients with autoimmune urticaria.

Proper management of underlying autoimmune thyroid disease or autoimmune collagen vascular diseases has been beneficial for patients with associated urticaria. Life-threatening angioedema triggered by angiotensin-converting enzyme (ACE) inhibitors has been successfully treated with infusion of fresh-frozen plasma. Hereditary angioedema can be prevented with tranexamic acid[1] or modified androgens. Intravenous C1-esterase inhibitor (Cinryze) or icatibant (Firazyr), a bradykinin B2 antagonist, can be administered to prevent acute attacks. Subcutaneous injection of C1-esterase inhibitor (Haegarda) has been approved by FDA in 2017 to prevent hereditary angioedema attacks. Treatments with methotrexate[1], warfarin (Coumadin),[1] plasmapheresis, colchicine,[1] hydroxychloroquine (Plaquenil),[1] anti-TNF-alpha,[1] interferon,[1] and intravenous immunoglobulin (Baygam)[1] have been reported for severe, refractory[1] urticaria. Vitamin D[1] supplementation can also be beneficial in reducing symptoms in patients with a deficiency. These treatments are administered only by specialists on an individual basis. Non-pharmacotherapeutic means such as frequent use of skin emollients, avoidance of hot shower, scrubbing, and excessive sun exposure should also be recommended as part of management plans.

[1]Not FDA approved for this indication.

References

American Academy of Allergy, Asthma and Immunology response to the EAACI/GA 2 LEN/EDF/WAO guideline for the definition, classification, diagnosis, and management of Urticaria 2017 revision, 74(2):411–413, 2019.

Bailey E, Shaker M: An update on childhood urticaria and angioedema, *Curr Opin Pediatr* 20(4):425–430, 2008.

Champion RH, Roberts SO, Carpenter RG, Roger JH: Urticaria and angio-oedema. A review of 554 patients, *Br J Dermatol* 81(8):588–597, 1969.

Joint Task Force on Practice Parameters: The diagnosis and management of urticaria: A practice parameter. Part II. Chronic urticaria/angioedema, *Ann Allergy Asthma Immunol* 85(2):521–544, 2000.

Kaplan AP, Joseph K, Maykut RJ, et al: Treatment of chronic autoimmune urticaria with omalizumab, *J Allergy Clin Immunol* 122(3):569–573, 2008.

Lin RY, Cannon AG, Teitel AD: Pattern of hospitalizations for angioedema in New York between 1990 and 2003, *Ann Allergy Asthma Immunol* 95(2):159–166, 2005.

Longhurst H, Cicardi M, Craig T, et al: Prevention of hereditary angioedema attacks with a subcutaneous C1 inhibitor, *N Engl J Med* 376(12):1131–1140, 2017 Mar 23.

Maurer M, Rosen K, Shieh HJ: Omalizumab for chronic urticaria, *N Engl J Med* 386:2530, 2013, https://doi.org/10.1056/JEJMc1305687.

Maurer M, Rosen K, Hsieh HJ, et al: Omalizumab for the treatment of chronic idiopathic or spontaneous urticaria, *N Engl J Med* 368:924–935, 2013.

Nizami RM, Baboo MT: Office management of patients with urticaria: An analysis of 215 patients, *Ann Allergy* 33(2):78–85, 1974.

Powell RJ, Du Toit GL, Siddique N, et al: BSACI guidelines for the management of chronic urticaria and angio-oedema, *Clin Exp Allergy* 37(5):631–650, 2007.

Saini SS, Bindslev-Jensen C, Maurer M, et al: Efficacy and safety of omalizumab in patients with chronic idiopathic/spontaneous urticaria who remain symptomatic on H1 antihistamines: a randomized, placebo-controlled study, *J Invest Dermatol* 135:67–75, 115, 2015.

VENOUS ULCERS

Method of
Marita Yaghi, MD; Jose A. Jaller, MD; and Robert S. Kirsner, MD, PhD

CURRENT DIAGNOSIS

- Venous ulcers are the most common cause of lower-extremity ulceration.
- Valvular incompetence, vein distention, muscular weakness, and/or a decrease in the range of motion of the ankle may lead to venous insufficiency.
- The mechanism of cutaneous ulceration resulting from venous insufficiency remains unclear.
- The typical location for a venous ulcer is on the medial malleolus.
- Complications of chronic venous ulcers are cellulitis and less often squamous cell carcinoma.
- Compression is the gold standard of treatment of venous disease.

CURRENT THERAPY

- Compression therapy is used to deliver a graded compression of 30 to 40 mm Hg at the ankle. Arterial disease should be excluded prior to full compression.
- Systemic medications as adjuvant therapy to compression bandages include aspirin,[1] pentoxifylline (Trental),[1] or micronized purified flavonoid fraction (Daflon 500 mg).[2]
- Other treatments, along with compression, include debridement, engineered skin, placental or skin grafting, electrical stimulation, locally derived growth factors, and venous surgery.
- The lifelong use of elastic compression stockings (30–40 mm Hg) is the mainstay of prevention.

[1]Not FDA approved for this indication.
[2]Not available in the United States.

Ulcers resulting from venous insufficiency are the most common cause of leg ulceration. The Wound Healing Society classifies wounds as *acute* if they sustain restoration of anatomic and functional integrity in an orderly and timely process and *chronic* if they do not. Venous leg ulcers (VLUs) are more frequently seen in the elderly population; however, about one in five primary VLUs occur in patients under 40 years of age. Personal or family history of venous disease, obesity, smoking, advanced age, female sex, hypertension, and leg injuries are strong risk factors to the development of VLUs.

Epidemiology

Venous insufficiency affects approximately 5% of the world's population and about 2% of the American population. VLUs affect 1% to 2% of adults in the United States, accounting for over 2 million lost workdays annually. The associated pain, inability to perform daily activities, and social stigma due to the appearance and odor of the wounds drastically diminish patients' quality of life. Moreover, the high cost of treatment, time off work, and hospital admissions forge a massive economic burden in the healthcare system. Seventy percent of all leg ulcers result solely from venous disease, and an additional 20% of patients have mixed arterial and venous disease. A recent report that used claims data from 2013 private and governmental insurance companies revealed that wounds and ulcers had the highest direct U.S. healthcare cost of all skin diseases, $12 billion, a considerable increase from the $1 billion estimate in 1990, and caused

Primary prevention focuses on BP, diet, exercise, and, in some cases, aspirin and/or statins. Furthermore, SGLT2i have demonstrated significant benefits with regard to cardiovascular events and mortality in this high-risk group that are driven, in large part, by a reduction in congestive heart failure events. Similarly, but specific to patients with diabetic kidney disease, finerenone also reduces the frequency of adverse cardiovascular events. The data available for cardiovascular risk management in CKD are limited in part because of the exclusion of patients with significant CKD in many large cardiovascular studies. Hence the utility of aspirin and statins (if any) in this setting is not well established. CKD patients often present with atypical symptoms of CVD; therefore a high index of suspicion is important.

References

Agarwal R, Sinha AD, Cramer AE, et al: Chlorthalidone for hypertension in advanced chronic kidney disease, *N Engl J Med* 385(27):2507–2519, 2021.

Bakris GL, Agarwal R, Anker SD, et al: Effect of finerenone on chronic kidney disease outcomes in type 2 diabetes, *N Engl J Med* 383(23):2219–2229, 2020.

Chebib FT, Perrone RD, Chapman AB, et al: A practical guide for treatment of rapidly progressive ADPKD with tolvaptan, *J Am Soc Nephrol* 10:2458–2470, 2018.

Cheung AK, Chang TI, Cushman WC, et al: Executive summary of the KDIGO 2021 clinical practice guideline for the management of blood pressure in chronic kidney disease, *Kidney Int* 99(3):559–569, 2021.

Herrington WG, Staplin N, Wanner C, et al: Empagliflozin in patients with chronic kidney disease, *N Engl J Med* 388(2):117–127, 2023.

Inker LA, Eneanya ND, Coresh J, et al: New creatinine- and cystatin C-based equations to estimate GFR without race, *N Engl J Med* 385(19):1737–1749, 2021.

Joshi S, McMacken M, Kalantar-Zadeh K: Plant-based diets for kidney disease: a guide for clinicians, *Am J Kidney Dis* 77(2):287–296, 2021.

KDIGO: Clinical practice guideline update for the diagnosis, evaluation, prevention, and treatment of chronic kidney disease–mineral and bone disorder (CKD-MBD), *Kidney Int Suppl (2011)* 7(1):1–59, 2017.

Kidney Disease: Improving Global Outcomes (KDIGO) Diabetes Work Group: KDIGO 2020 clinical practice guideline for diabetes management in chronic kidney disease, *Kidney Int* (4S) S1–S115, 2020.

Mottl AK, Alicic R, Argyropoulos C, et al: KDOQI US Commentary on the KDIGO 2020 clinical practice guideline for diabetes management in CKD, *Am J Kidney Dis* 79:457–479, 2022.

Pitt B, Filippatos G, Agarwal R, et al: Cardiovascular events with finerenone in kidney disease and type 2 diabetes, *N Engl J Med* 385(24):2252–2263, 2021.

Raphael K: Metabolic acidosis in CKD: core curriculum 2019, *Am J Kidney Dis* 74(2):263–275, 2019.

Tangri N, Grams ME, Levey AS, et al: Multinational assessment of accuracy of equations for predicting risk of kidney failure: a meta-analysis, *JAMA* 315(2):164–174, 2016.

Toyama T, Neuen BL, Jun M, et al: Effect of SGLT2 inhibitors on cardiovascular, renal and safety outcomes in patients with type 2 diabetes mellitus and chronic kidney disease: a systematic review and meta-analysis, *Diabetes Obes Metab* 21(5):1237–1250, 2019.

Wright Jr JT, Williamson JD, Whelton PK, et al: A randomized trial of intensive versus standard blood pressure control, *N Engl J Med* 374(23):2284, 2016.

MALIGNANT TUMORS OF THE UROGENITAL TRACT

Method of
Danica May, MD; and Moben Mirza, MD

CURRENT DIAGNOSIS

Prostate cancer

- Prostate cancer is the most common cancer diagnosis for men in the United States.
- Screening with prostate-specific antigen (PSA) should be offered starting at age 45 to 50 and ending at age 70 for the average risk patient. For higher risk patients (African American patients or strong family history of prostate cancer), screening should be discussed starting between 40 and 45.
- Prostate cancer risk factors include African ancestry, family history, as well as Lynch syndrome and other genetic mutations.
- Transrectal ultrasound (TRUS)-guided biopsy is the diagnostic test for prostate cancer and may be indicated for patients with elevated PSA or abnormal DRE.

- Staging involves cross-sectional abdominal and pelvic imaging as well as bone scan for patients with high risk cancer.

Benign and malignant renal tumors

- Most patients with renal cell carcinoma (RCC) are diagnosed incidentally on imaging work-up for other symptoms or complaints. The classic triad of a palpable mass, hematuria, and flank pain is a relatively rare presentation.
- Risk factors for RCC are smoking, obesity, hypertension, and genetic syndromes such as von Hippel-Lindau disease, Birt-Hogg-Dube syndrome, and tuberous sclerosis complex.
- Most malignant renal masses are renal cell carcinoma, but lymphoma, metastases from other malignancies, and other renal malignancies should be considered in the differential as treatment options will vary.
- Benign masses include oncocytoma, angiomyolipoma (AML), renal cysts, and adenomas among others.
- Staging of renal masses involves abdominal imaging with CT scan or MRI. Chest imaging should be obtained. Laboratory analysis should include a CBC, CMP, and urinalysis. CT-guided core renal mass biopsy may be obtained after urologic consultation.

Urothelial cell carcinoma

- Urothelial cell carcinoma can affect the renal pelvis, ureter, bladder, or urethra, though most cases occur in the bladder.
- The average patient is older than age 60 and may have significant medical comorbidities.
- Risk factors include smoking, radiation, certain chemical exposures, and Lynch syndrome.
- Microscopic or gross hematuria is the most common presentation. Patients may also present with urgency, frequency, dysuria, flank pain, or have hydronephrosis discovered on imaging.
- Work-up involves a CT urogram for patients with adequate renal function and cystoscopy.
- Tumors discovered in the bladder should be resected endoscopically for diagnosis and staging. Tumors in the renal pelvis or ureters can be biopsied ureteroscopically.

Primary carcinoma of the prostate and urethra

- Primary urethral malignancies typically consist of urethral or squamous cell carcinoma.
- Patients often present with hematuria, and overall survival remains poor.
- Studies are lacking on this rare disease state, but treatment depends on stage, disease location, and histology.

Penile cancer

- Penile cancer is a rare malignancy with poor prognosis for men with advanced stage disease.
- Presentation often involves an ulceration or palpable mass, and biopsy is the key to diagnosis.
- The vast majority of penile lesions are squamous cell carcinomas.
- Risk factors for penile cancer involve chronic inflammation, tobacco use, lack of neonatal circumcision, STDs, HPV infection specifically with subtypes 6, 16, and 18, and phimosis.
- Staging scans involve chest, abdomen, and pelvis imaging with attention paid to the inguinal lymph nodes.

Testicular cancer

- Testicular cancer is diagnosed in men with a median age of 33 years and has excellent outcomes at 5 years.
- Risk factors for testicular cancer include undescended testis and a personal or family history of testicular cancer.
- The majority of testicular cancers are germ cell tumors, which include seminoma and non-seminoma.
- Germ cell tumors can also present in extra-testicular locations such as the retroperitoneum or mediastinum.
- Men with a testicular mass should undergo an ultrasound and intratesticular masses that are concerning for malignancy should be removed via radical orchiectomy. Sperm banking should be offered.
- Serum tumor markers include beta-hCG, AFP, and LDH. Staging, pathology, and tumor markers dictate next management steps.

CURRENT THERAPY

Prostate cancer
- Treatment options depend on PSA, Gleason grade, clinical stage, and the patient's overall health and life expectancy. Men with limited life expectancy may be good candidates for watchful waiting. Active surveillance is an option for men with low-risk and some men with favorable intermediate risk prostate cancer.
- Treatment options for clinically localized prostate cancer include radical (typically robotic) prostatectomy and radiation therapy in the form of external beam or brachytherapy with or without androgen deprivation therapy.
- The cornerstone of treatment for men with nodal or metastatic disease involves androgen deprivation therapy.
- Other treatment options include chemotherapy, immunotherapy, or newer secondary hormone therapies.
- Following definitive therapy, follow up for men treated for prostate cancer involves regular PSA monitoring every few months for 5 years and then yearly after that.

Benign and malignant renal tumors
- Surgery remains a mainstay of treatment for localized renal cell carcinoma. Partial or radical nephrectomy can be performed taking into consideration the clinical stage, tumor location, patient's overall health, renal function, presence or absence or a contralateral kidney, and genetic syndromes predisposing the patient to future malignancies.
- Ablative therapy and active surveillance are options for small renal masses.
- Simple renal cysts do not require treatment. Complex or enhancing cysts should be treated based on their risk of malignancy.
- Follow up for patients treated for renal cell carcinoma involves periodic laboratory analysis as well as cross-sectional abdominal and chest imaging.
- Systemic therapy options for patients with metastatic renal cell carcinoma have increased drastically with the newest treatments including immune checkpoint inhibitors.
- The treatment of angiomyolipomas (AMLs) is often based on size and is directed toward prevention of the complication of retroperitoneal hemorrhage. Embolization or surgical removal has traditionally been proposed at a 4-cm size, although larger AMLs can be safely observed.

Urothelial cell carcinoma
- Treatment options depend on stage, grade, and tumor location.
- Superficial low-grade bladder tumors can be managed with resection and periodic surveillance cystoscopy.
- Patients with superficial high-grade cancer or cancers invasive into the lamina propria (T1) diagnosed on initial resection may be offered a repeat resection. Treatment following this often involves induction and maintenance intravesical Bacillus Calmette-Guérin (BCG) therapy. Patients with high-grade T1 bladder cancer should be counseled and offered radical cystectomy. These patients should have periodic cystoscopy and upper tract imaging as indicated.
- The standard of care for patients with muscle invasive (T2) bladder cancer is cisplatin-based neoadjuvant chemotherapy followed by radical cystectomy. Patients ineligible for cisplatin-based chemotherapy should undergo immediate radical cystectomy.
- For patients who are unwilling or unfit for radical cystectomy, chemoradiation therapy can be offered.
- Upper tract tumors of the renal pelvis or ureter are managed by grade as well as clinical stage. The pathologic stage may not be accurately established prior to definitive treatment.
- Nephroureterectomy should be offered for patients with upper tract urothelial cell carcinoma. Other options can include endoscopic management with tumor ablation or partial resection of the ureter if tumor location is amenable. Cisplatin-based neoadjuvant or adjuvant chemotherapy should be considered.

Primary urothelial carcinoma of the prostate and urethra
- Superficial urothelial tumors (Tis, Ta, T1) of the urethra can be resected or biopsied followed by intravesical BCG therapy.
- The surgical treatment for men with T2 proximal urethral cancer involves removal of the bladder and prostate with urethrectomy. More distal disease involving the pendulous urethra can be managed with a distal urethrectomy or partial penectomy.
- Women are often treated with cystectomy and urethrectomy.
- Patients with higher stage urethral cancer may be offered neoadjuvant or adjuvant chemotherapy or radiation therapy.

Penile cancer
- Organ sparing approaches include topical therapy, laser therapy, Mohs surgery, glansectomy, radiation therapy, or wide local excision and are most utilized in patients with superficial or properly selected penile cancer patient with T1 disease.
- More aggressive tumors should be treated with partial or total penectomy.
- Higher risk patients need to undergo inguinal node dissection and pelvic node dissection should be considered for highly selected patients.
- Neoadjuvant chemotherapy should be considered for bulky, bilateral, or fixed inguinal lymphadenopathy.

Testicular cancer
- Following radical orchiectomy, imaging of the chest, abdomen, and pelvis is key for staging. Repeat tumor markers should also be collected as persistent tumor marker elevation after orchiectomy changes treatment.
- Patients with localized seminoma with normal tumor markers can undergo surveillance, chemotherapy, or radiation therapy.
- For patients with more advanced disease, treatment options should include chemotherapy or radiation therapy.
- In patients with pure seminoma and a residual retroperitoneal mass, further work-up with a PET/CT scan can aid in characterization of residual disease.
- Radiation therapy is not a standard treatment for men with non-seminoma testicular cancer.
- Patients with localized non-seminoma with normal tumor markers can undergo observation, chemotherapy, or retroperitoneal lymph node dissection (RPLND).
- For patients with more advanced disease, treatment options should include chemotherapy and/or surgical resection.
- Residual retroperitoneal masses in the patient treated for non-seminoma testicular cancer should be removed via RPLND.
- Follow up for all patients with testicular cancer includes surveillance with chest, abdominal, and pelvic imaging as well as periodic tumor markers.

Prostate Cancer
Background
Prostate cancer is the most common cancer diagnosis among men in the United States. It accounts for over 268,490 new cases in 2022 and is the second most common overall malignancy after breast cancer. It is a relatively indolent cancer with 96.8% 5-year relative survival. Family history of prostate cancer, particularly among first-degree relatives, is a well-known risk factor for developing prostate cancer. Known genetic alterations include both germline as well as somatic mutations. Common mutations include BRCA1/2, ATM,

MLH1, MSH2, MSH6, and PMS2, among many others. Syndromes linked to prostate cancer include Lynch syndrome and hereditary breast and ovarian cancer (HBOC) syndrome. Other risk factors for development of prostate cancer include increasing age, African American ancestry, smoking, and Ashkenazi Jewish heritage.

Diagnosis

Prostate cancer is most often diagnosed in a localized and asymptomatic state via screening. Rarely, prostate cancer is detected at a locally advanced state with symptoms of pelvic pain, urinary retention, or ureteral obstruction with hydronephrosis. The minority of men are diagnosed in the metastatic state, with the most frequent complaint being bone pain from metastases. The utilization of prostate-specific antigen (PSA) blood testing has drastically changed the diagnosis of prostate cancer from a historically predominantly metastatic state to a localized and potentially curable state in the current era. In 2012, the US Preventive Services Task Force released a grade D recommendation against the use of PSA-based screening for any man. This recommendation was modified in 2018 to allow for informed decision making for prostate cancer screening in men aged 55 to 69. The American Urological Association recommends individualized prostate cancer screening for men aged 40 to 54 who are at higher risk, shared decision-making for men aged 45 to 69, and cessation of screening for men aged 70 or older or those men with life expectancy less than 10 to 15 years. Screening of prostate cancer with PSA should not be dismissed with the assumption that prostate cancer is an indolent cancer. Screening can lead to diagnosis and appropriate risk stratification.

The basis of prostate cancer screening is serum PSA. While PSA is only produced by the prostate, it is not specific to malignant versus benign cells, and there are a variety of causes of elevated PSA. Benign causes of elevated PSA include benign prostate hypertrophy, prostatitis, instrumentation of the urethra such as catheterization or utilization of cystoscopy, and urinary tract infections. One of the difficulties of PSA utilization is that there is no cutoff normal level. In fact, 6.6% of men with a PSA of 0.5 ng/mL or less were found to have prostate cancer with rates increasing to 26.9% in men with PSA of 3.1 to 4.0 ng/mL. In general, PSA increases with age. Some men may have an abnormal DRE, which can prompt further work-up. Worrisome findings include induration or nodules palpable within the prostate.

Following screening with PSA, further work-up includes prostate biopsy. The vast majority of prostate biopsies are performed with transrectal ultrasound (TRUS) to help with volumetric and anatomical surveys. The majority of prostate cancer is detected in the peripheral zone, so the standard 12-core biopsy template targets this area in a systematic fashion. Prostatic volume as well as anatomy such as large intravesical lobes should be noted as this information can be helpful in surgical planning.

Prostate MRI is an increasingly utilized tool in men with various clinical situations including elevated PSA with a prior negative biopsy, performance of active surveillance (AS; further discussed below), staging, and surgical planning, as well as in men whose pathology appears discordant with their rectal examination or PSA level. Multiparametric MRI gives not only detailed anatomic information, but also functional assessment of various tumor regions. This information can then be used for an MRI-guided biopsy or more commonly fusion biopsy via platforms that fuse concerning MRI findings with real-time TRUS biopsy for improved lesion targeting.

The vast majority of prostate cancers are adenocarcinomas. Prostate biopsy pathology is based on Gleason grading system 1 to 5, with 5 reflecting poorly differentiated and most aggressive cells. The grading system is translated into a score that adds the most common and second most common grading pattern to yield a score between 2 and 10. Further classification into a Gleason group between 1 and 5 informs appropriate risk classification. In general, low-risk prostate cancer consists of Gleason 6 prostate cancer (Gleason group 1), while intermediate risk prostate cancer consists of Gleason 7 prostate cancer (Gleason group 2 and 3). High-risk prostate cancer includes Gleason sums 8, 9,

and 10 prostate cancer (Gleason groups 4 and 5). Risk groups also take into account clinical stage, PSA levels, and biopsy core positivity. TNM staging is used for prostate cancer. Prostate cancer diagnosed either surgically via a transurethral resection of the prostate or via TRUS biopsy is stage T1. T2 is organ-confined prostate cancer, while T3 is defined as extra-prostatic extension. Finally, T4 involves invasion of surrounding structures including the bladder, pelvic floor or sidewall, or rectum (Table 1). Grade, stage, and risk group are instrumental in treatment decisions.

Current recommendations include germline testing for patients with positive family history of prostate cancer; high-risk, regional, or metastatic prostate cancer; Ashkenazi Jewish ancestry; or intraductal histology. Various genetic alterations necessitate genetic counseling as well as change some treatment options. Staging imaging should be carried out for certain men diagnosed with prostate cancer. Current recommendations include pelvic imaging with or without abdominal imaging via CT or MRI as well as a radionuclide bone scan in men with unfavorable intermediate, high risk, and very high-risk disease.

Treatment

Treatment decisions for men diagnosed with prostate cancer depend on a series of factors including risk group, staging, and clinical node status on imaging, as well as the patient's overall health and life expectancy. In patients with limited life expectancy, observation may be utilized. Observation of known prostate cancer involves monitoring the patient with eventual initiation of palliative androgen deprivation therapy (ADT) for symptomatic or imminently symptomatic disease. On the other hand, AS may be utilized for patients with very low risk or low risk disease, and the properly selected favorable intermediate risk disease patient with adequate life expectancy. AS involves periodic assessment of PSA, DRE, and surveillance biopsies. Prostate MRI may also be utilized in an AS algorithm. AS aims to allow for early disease reclassification with ability to perform definitive treatment at that point. Approximately two-thirds of men on AS will be able to avoid treatment and the associated side effects. Another effect of AS is less overtreatment of small, indolent prostate cancers.

The preferred treatment for very low risk and low risk prostate cancer patients with adequate life expectancy is AS. Other options in the properly selected patient population include external beam radiation therapy (EBRT) or brachytherapy, radical prostatectomy (RP), or observation. As previously mentioned, AS remains an option for patients diagnosed with favorable intermediate risk prostate cancer. This cohort of men may also be treated with EBRT or brachytherapy as well as RP. Treatment recommendations for men with unfavorable intermediate risk prostate cancer include RP, EBRT combined with ADT, or EBRT and brachytherapy boost with ADT. For men with high risk or very high risk prostate cancer, treatment recommendations include EBRT and ADT with or without abiraterone (Zytiga), EBRT with brachytherapy and ADT, or RP. In men with regional lymphadenopathy, the cornerstone of treatment is ADT. This may be combined with EBRT or abiraterone (Zytiga).

Following definitive treatment, patients should be monitored with PSA and DRE every 3 to 6 months. Following RP, PSA should be undetectable as all prostate and prostate cancer tissue has theoretically been surgically removed. Men treated with EBRT or brachytherapy should have a decline in PSA to a low, steady level. In men with detectable or rising PSA after RP, repeat imaging including bone imaging, CT, MRI, C-11 choline, F-18 fluciclovine PET/CT, or PET/MRI may be utilized to assess for sites of disease recurrence. If no metastases are detected, observation or EBRT with or without ADT are treatment options. When metastases are detected, ADT combined with apalutamide (Erleada), docetaxel (Taxotere), abiraterone (Zytiga), enzalutamide (Xtandi), darolutamide (Nubeqa), or EBRT to the primary tumor in the setting of low volume metastases are treatment options. Most men with metastatic prostate cancer initially have castration-naïve prostate cancer and respond to medical or surgical (orchiectomy) castration. A rising PSA in the setting of castrate

TABLE 1 Risk Stratification and Staging Workup

NCCN RISK GROUP	CLINICAL/PATHOLOGIC FEATURES	IMAGING
Very low	T1c AND Gleason score ≤6/grade group 1 AND PSA <10 ng/mL AND Fewer than 3 prostate biopsy fragments/cores positive, ≤50% cancer in each fragment/core AND PSA density <0.15 ng/mL/g	Not indicated
Low	T1–T2a AND Gleason score ≤6/grade group 1 AND PSA <10 ng/mL	Not indicated
Favorable intermediate	T2b–T2c OR Gleason score 3 + 4 = 7/grade group 2 OR PSA 10–20 ng/mL AND Percentage of positive biopsy cores <50%	Bone imaging: not recommended for staging Pelvic ± abdominal imaging: recommended if nomogram predicts >10% probability of pelvic lymph node involvement
Unfavorable intermediate	T2b–T2c OR Gleason score 3 + 4 = 7/grade group 2 or Gleason score 4 + 3 = 7/grade group 3 OR PSA 10–20 ng/mL	Bone imaging: recommended if T2 and PSA >10 ng/mL Pelvic ± abdominal imaging: recommended if nomogram predicts >10% probability of pelvic lymph node involvement
High	T3a OR Gleason score 8/grade group 4 or Gleason score 4 + 5 = 9/grade group 5 OR PSA >20 ng/mL	Bone imaging: recommended Pelvic ± abdominal imaging: recommended if nomogram predicts >10% probability of pelvic lymph node involvement
Very high	T3b–T4 OR Primary Gleason pattern 5 OR >4 cores with Gleason score 8–10/grade group 4 or 5	Bone imaging: recommended Pelvic ± abdominal imaging: recommended if nomogram predicts >10% probability of pelvic lymph node involvement

NCCN, National Comprehensive Cancer Network; PSA, prostate-specific antigen.
From Partin AW: *Campbell-Walsh-Wein Urology*, ed 12, Elsevier, 2021.

level testosterone indicates the advent of castration-resistant prostate cancer (CRPC), and ADT should be continued indefinitely. Once castration resistance has been identified, bone health should be prioritized with utilization of denosumab (Xgeva) or zoledronic acid (Zometa) in the setting of bone metastases. Therapy options include abiraterone (Zytiga), docetaxel (Taxotere), enzalutamide (Xtandi), sipuleucel-T (Provenge), radium Ra 223 dichloride (Xofigo) for symptomatic bone metastases, or mitoxantrone (Novantrone) for palliation in men who cannot tolerate other therapies. Painful bony metastases can be palliated with EBRT.

Benign and Malignant Renal Tumors

Background
Kidney and renal pelvis cancers account for 4.1% of all new cancer cases at more than 79,000 cases in the United States in 2022 leading to 13,920 deaths. The 5-year relative survival from 2010 to 2016 is approximately 76.5%. The majority of kidney masses are detected incidentally on cross-sectional imaging for other chief complaints, and the median age at diagnosis is 65 years. These tumors can be primary renal cell carcinoma (RCC), metastases from second primaries such as breast, lung, ovarian, or melanoma as well as lymphoma deposits, or benign renal tumors such as oncocytoma, angiomyolipoma (AML), renal cysts, leiomyoma, and adenomas. RCC subtypes include clear cell, chromophobe, papillary, collecting duct, translocation, and medullary carcinoma. The majority of tumors are clear cell RCC, which comprise 70% of RCC subtypes.

Hereditary syndromes predisposing patients to RCC include von Hippel-Lindau (VHL) disease, hereditary papillary renal carcinoma (HPRC), hereditary leiomyomatosis and renal cell carcinoma (HLRCC), tuberous sclerosis complex (TSC), and Birt-Hogg-Dube (BHD) syndrome, among others. Other risk factors include smoking, obesity, and hypertension.

Diagnosis
Rarely patients with RCC present with a triad of symptoms including hematuria, a flank mass, and flank pain. More commonly, patients are found to have a renal mass on imaging performed for other indications and the frequency of incidental detection has increased with widespread abdominal imaging. In the patient with a renal mass, laboratory analysis should include a CBC, CMP, and urinalysis. Cross-sectional abdominal imaging with CT or MRI with contrast should be obtained if not already performed. A chest x-ray is required to complete staging but chest CT, bone scan, brain MRI, and core-needle biopsy may also be obtained. Patients who present with multiple renal masses or young age (<46 years old) may be referred for genetic evaluation. Core-needle biopsy of renal masses may be indicated in patients with unclear etiology of their renal mass such as concern for an infiltrating mass like lymphoma, AS guidance, or in combination with ablation strategies.

TNM stage and histologic grade are important for prognosis and treatment guidance in the patient with RCC. Stage T1 tumors are tumors ≤7 cm in greatest dimension and are limited to the kidney. T2 tumors are greater than 7 cm but ≤10 cm and are limited to the kidney. T3 disease involves invasion into major veins including the renal vein or vena cava or invasion into perinephric tissue, while T4 disease is invasion beyond Gerota's fascia. Histologic grade is graded as G1 through G4 with increasing dedifferentiation.

Renal cysts are a very common benign finding and are graded via Bosniak classification with scores ranging from I to IV. Simple cysts are defined as thin-walled cysts without septa, calcifications, or solid component and lack enhancement. As the Bosniak score increases, so does the complexity and malignancy risk of the cyst with Bosniak IV cysts defined as cysts with enhancing soft tissue components and thick or irregular walls or septa. Oncocytomas are the most common benign, enhancing mass and are associated with BHD syndrome. They are often diagnosed on pathology as diagnosis via imaging characteristics can include hypervascularity with a central scar but are not definitive findings. AMLs are common manifestations in patients with TSC but are often easily diagnosed on CT or MRI due to the presence of macroscopic fat, which has negative Hounsfield units. While benign, AMLs are the leading cause of spontaneous retroperitoneal hemorrhage and intervention is targeted toward prevention of this outcome. A cutoff size of 4 cm

ERECTILE DYSFUNCTION

Method of
Aleksandr Belakovskiy, MD; Joel J. Heidelbaugh, MD; and Karl T. Rew, MD

CURRENT DIAGNOSIS

- Questionnaire
- Sexual Health Inventory for Men (SHIM) [also called International Index of Erectile Function (IIEF-5)] https://www.baus.org.uk/_userfiles/pages/files/Patients/Leaflets/SHIM.pdf
- Assessment of risk factors
- Tobacco use
- Diabetes
- Hypertension
- Hyperlipidemia
- Obesity
- Iatrogenic causes
- Psychogenic causes
- Physical exam including vitals, body mass index (BMI), genital exam, and assessment for secondary sex characteristics
- Relationship between erectile dysfunction, endothelial dysfunction, and coronary heart disease

CURRENT THERAPY

- Lifestyle modifications including tobacco cessation, weight-loss, increased exercise
- Sexual health counseling
- Medication modification if taking medications knownto contribute to erectile dysfunction
- Pharmacotherapy (Table 1)
- Oral phosphodiesterase type 5 (PDE-5) inhibitors:avanafil (Stendra), sildenafil (Viagra), tadalafil (Cialis), and vardenafil (Levitra, Staxyn)
- Prostaglandin: alprostadil; either by intracavernosal injection(Caverject, Edex) or as an intraurethral suppository (Muse)
- Requires a test dose in the office and instruction ontechnique for proper administration
- Vacuum erectile devices
- Penile implants

Erectile dysfunction is the inability to attain or maintain a penile erection sufficient for sexual satisfaction.

Epidemiology

Numerous studies have investigated the prevalence of erectile dysfunction in men of various ages. Based on the most recent studies, worldwide prevalence increases with age. For men under age 40 the prevalence is 1% to 10%; for ages 40 to 49 it is 2% to 15%; for men ages 50 to 59 it is mixed, ranging from 15% to 40%; for ages 60 to 69 it is 20% to 40%; and for men 70 and older it is 50% to 100%. Among men in the United States the prevalence is 22% overall. This is higher than the 16% prevalence for seven other countries found in a study comparing the United States to Brazil, Mexico, United Kingdom, Germany, France, Italy, and Spain. Accurate diagnosis of erectile dysfunction has varied over time, with current literature favoring the use of validated questionnaires such as the Sexual Health Inventory for Men (SHIM; https://www.baus.org.uk/_userfiles/pages/files/Patients/Leaflets/SHIM.pdf).

Risk Factors

A number of medical conditions can predispose to erectile dysfunction. Numerous studies have demonstrated the correlation between cardiovascular disease and the incidence of erectile dysfunction. Risk factors that predispose to cardiovascular disease also play similar roles in erectile dysfunction, including increasing age, diabetes, hypertension, hyperlipidemia, tobacco use, and obesity.

Certain classes of medications can contribute to the development of erectile dysfunction. One of the most common is the antidepressants, specifically selective serotonin reuptake inhibitors (SSRIs) and serotonin norepinephrine reuptake inhibitors (SNRIs). Common antihypertensive medications can also contribute to or exacerbate erectile dysfunction, including beta blockers, alpha blockers, calcium channel blockers, and thiazides. Other medication classes that should be considered in patients with erectile dysfunction include opiates, first-generation antihistamines, and benzodiazepines.

Risk factors for psychogenic erectile dysfunction should also be evaluated. Psychogenic erectile dysfunction can occur at any age, but it is frequently seen in men under age 40, and it often occurs in men with anxiety, stress, depression, or a history of sexual abuse. Assess for healthy sexual partnerships by asking about performance anxiety and sexual desire discrepancy, both of which are common contributors to erectile dysfunction. Clues that erectile dysfunction may have a psychogenic component include the ability to have normal erections with masturbation, and the continued presence of nocturnal erections. If needed for evaluation, nocturnal tumescence testing can be performed.

Tobacco, alcohol, opioids, and substances such as marijuana and cocaine can cause erectile dysfunction. All substance use should be assessed. Many other health issues can contribute to erectile dysfunction, including a history of prostate or pelvic surgery, radiation therapy, or trauma; gonadal, thyroid, or other diseases that affect hormone levels; testicular pain; and chronic diseases that affect general health and well-being.

Pathophysiology

The pathophysiology of erectile dysfunction depends on the etiology of the condition. Many men have multiple potential causes. Psychogenic erectile dysfunction is due to nonorganic causes, while individuals with risk factors for cardiovascular disease primarily have etiologies stemming from vascular disease. Iatrogenic erectile dysfunction due to medication use or prior surgery may be caused by inhibition of the parasympathetic nervous system or other mechanisms of action.

Erectile dysfunction can be a warning sign of silent cardiovascular disease. The relationship between erectile dysfunction and the risk factors for coronary heart disease was noted in the Massachusetts Male Aging Study. The endothelial dysfunction that can precede the clinical stage of atherosclerotic disease is recognized as an additional risk factor for erectile dysfunction in men without symptoms of cardiovascular disease. Endothelial function is mediated by nitric oxide, which is also the mechanism responsible for the vascular dilatation required to obtain and maintain an erection. A man with erectile dysfunction should be considered at risk for cardiovascular disease until proven otherwise.

Prevention

Erectile dysfunction prevention is centered around treating modifiable risk factors. Treatment of overweight and obesity with dietary changes and increased aerobic exercise can aid in the prevention of erectile dysfunction. For tobacco users, cessation should be strongly encouraged. Bupropion (Zyban) and varenicline (Chantix) can be used for smoking cessation with limited risk of exacerbating erectile dysfunction. Nicotine replacement therapy can be used as a bridge to help with tobacco cessation. Appropriate treatment of comorbid diseases, including diabetes, hypertension, and hyperlipidemia can also aid in prevention. Sexual health counseling that focuses on good partner communication and healthy relationship dynamics can help prevent psychogenic erectile dysfunction.

Clinical Manifestations

Many men are uncomfortable mentioning problems of sexual function. Some men will report erectile dysfunction without providing information on the specifics of their concern. It is important for physicians to proactively ask about sexual function, and to clarify if a patient's concern is with achieving or maintaining an erection, or if it may be related to ejaculation or low libido. Low libido can be secondary to stress, mood disorders, hypogonadism, or other causes. The evaluation and potential treatments will differ based on the specific concern. Questionnaires such as the SHIM (https://www.baus.org.uk/_userfiles/pages/files/Patients/Leaflets/SHIM.pdf) can provide additional information to help distinguish the specific clinical manifestation.

Diagnosis

The history provides the majority of information needed for the diagnostic evaluation, including a review of known medical and surgical history, use of medications and substances, an assessment of current relationship satisfaction, and a questionnaire such as the SHIM. The history should include risk factor evaluation, assessment for any history of cardiovascular disease, diabetes, hypertension, hyperlipidemia, or mood disorders, as well as a review of medications that might contribute to erectile dysfunction. A physical exam should also be performed, including evaluation of blood pressure, body mass index, secondary sex characteristics, and a genital exam.

The role of laboratory studies is limited. In individuals who lack secondary sex characteristics, as well as those with refractory symptoms despite PDE-5 inhibitor use, check a morning total testosterone to assess for hypogonadism. Limited evidence supports obtaining a morning total testosterone in all men with erectile dysfunction. If the initial morning total testosterone is low, it should be repeated at least once in several months to confirm the diagnosis. If morning testosterone levels are normal in a patient with high likelihood of hypogonadism, a free testosterone or bioavailable testosterone can be checked to help account for the effects of sex hormone–binding globulin. If evidence of hypogonadism is found, additional testing to distinguish primary versus secondary hypogonadism should be done. Hemoglobin A1c and a lipid panel may be helpful if there is a suspicion for underlying diabetes, hyperlipidemia, or cardiovascular disease contributing to erectile dysfunction. If a review of symptoms elicits a suspicion for hypothyroidism, checking a thyroid stimulating hormone level may be indicated. Consultation with a urologist, endocrinologist, or men's health specialist may be helpful when the etiology is unclear.

Differential Diagnosis

In men presenting with concern for erectile dysfunction, the differential diagnosis is geared toward deciphering the underlying cause. As previously mentioned, there are numerous potential contributing factors to erectile dysfunction. It is important to assess for both organic and psychogenic causes. The history should include asking about nocturnal tumescence, as well as the ability to achieve and maintain an erection with and without a partner. If erectile dysfunction occurs regardless of situation, this is more likely to indicate an organic etiology. If it occurs primarily with a partner, further evaluation of the relationship is indicated. As mentioned above, numerous factors can predispose to erectile dysfunction, and related diagnoses may include cardiovascular disease, tobacco use, diabetes, hypertension, hyperlipidemia, obesity, and metabolic syndrome. Medications should also be reviewed, because they can cause iatrogenic erectile dysfunction in some patients.

Therapy (or Treatment)

Lifestyle modifications play an important role in both the prevention and treatment of erectile dysfunction. Weight reduction for overweight or obese men (BMI >25 kg/m^2) and increased exercise for all men can improve SHIM scores. Underlying illnesses such as hyperlipidemia, hypertension, and diabetes should be adequately controlled in order to decrease their potential impact on erectile dysfunction. Another important consideration is tobacco cessation; current or former smoking increases the risk of erectile dysfunction. Sexual health counseling is often helpful for individuals and couples dealing with erectile dysfunction, no matter what the etiology is. Referral to a mental health professional or sexuality expert may be beneficial.

Pharmacologic treatment begins with oral PDE-5 inhibitors. They prevent the breakdown of cyclic guanosine monophosphate (cGMP) and allow increased nitric oxide levels, causing smooth muscle relaxation of the corpora cavernosa, and helping to sustain an erection. This requires a functional libido as well as intact vasculature in order to achieve an erection. There are four PDE-5 inhibitors currently approved in the United States for treatment of erectile dysfunction: avanafil (Stendra), sildenafil (Viagra), tadalafil (Cialis), and vardenafil (Levitra, Staxyn) (see Table 1). There are no significant differences in safety or benefit among these medications. Tadalafil has a longer duration of action than the others.

PDE-5 inhibitors are usually taken on an as-needed basis, with onset of effects typically within about 1 hour of ingestion. The lowest effective dose should be used to reduce the risk of adverse reactions. Higher doses do not lead to a linear increase in beneficial effect, but can increase the risk of adverse reactions. Tadalafil, because of its longer duration of action, can be taken daily at a lower dose with similar efficacy to as-needed dosing. The duration of adverse effects may be longer with daily use.

The most common adverse reactions to PDE-5 inhibitors include headache, flushing, dyspepsia, dizziness, nasal congestion, visual disturbance, and myalgias. Overall, these adverse reactions tend to be mild to moderate in nature and are similar across all four medications. Special consideration should be given to individuals who take nitrate-containing medications; the combination of a PDE-5 inhibitor with nitrates can cause severe hypotension that may be life threatening.

Testosterone is not an effective monotherapy for erectile dysfunction. However, for men with confirmed hypogonadism, the combination of a PDE-5 inhibitor with testosterone replacement may be effective.

If patients do not have adequate symptom relief with lifestyle modification, sexual health counseling, and oral PDE-5 inhibitor use, the prostaglandin alprostadil (Caverject, Edex, Muse) can be considered. Alprostadil works by relaxing arterial smooth muscle and is available in intraurethral and injectable preparations (see Table 1). The intraurethral formulation (Muse) is a dissolvable suppository placed in the urethra with an applicator. The injectable form (Caverject, Edex) is injected directly into one side of the corpora cavernosa. Alprostadil can be used as a single agent or in combination with a PDE-5 inhibitor. If the patient is amenable to a trial of alprostadil, an in-office test dose should be administered to find the lowest effective dose and to teach proper administration technique. Some patients may not be suitable candidates if they are not comfortable with injections or intraurethral insertion. Alprostadil should be avoided in patients who have sickle cell anemia or other risk factors for priapism.

If pharmacological therapies are ineffective or contraindicated, patients may elect to use a vacuum erectile device. These prescription devices are placed over the penis and a vacuum pump removes air from inside the device, creating an influx of blood into the penis and leading to an erection. A ring is then slid from the base of the vacuum tube onto the penis to constrict the outflow of blood and maintain the erection. To avoid ischemic injury, the ring should only be used for up to 30 minutes. Adverse effects of vacuum erectile devices may include the erect penis feeling cool or cold to the touch due to the restricted blood flow, and bending at the base of the penis due to the application of the constricting ring. Overall, these devices have a fairly high satisfaction rate. Caution should be used when considering a vacuum erectile device for patients who are taking anticoagulants or have bleeding disorders.

For patients with erectile dysfunction refractory to the above treatments, surgical implantation of a penile prosthesis can be offered. Penile prostheses come in several forms, including inflatable devices and persistently semirigid implants. Patients and

TABLE 1 Pharmacotherapy for Erectile Dysfunction

GENERIC NAMES	BRAND NAMES	SIZES	TYPICAL DOSING	COMMENTS
Oral Phosphodiesterase Type 5 (PDE-5) Inhibitors				
avanafil	Stendra	50-, 100-, 200-mg tablet	50–200 mg by mouth once daily as needed, 1 h before sexual activity	Use lowest effective dose. Contraindicated with nitrates.
sildenafil	Viagra	25-, 50-, 100-mg tablet	25–100 mg by mouth once daily as needed, 1 h before sexual activity	Use lowest effective dose. Contraindicated with nitrates.
tadalafil	Cialis	2.5-, 5-, 10-, 20-mg tablet	5–20 mg by mouth once daily as needed, 1 h before sexual activity OR 2.5–5 mg by mouth once daily without regard to sexual activity	Use lowest effective dose. Contraindicated with nitrates. Has a longer duration of action than other PDE-5 inhibitors.
vardenafil	Levitra Staxyn	5-, 10-, 20-mg tablet 10-mg oral dissolving tablet	5–20 mg by mouth once daily as needed, 1 h before sexual activity	Use lowest effective dose. Contraindicated with nitrates. Available as a 10 mg oral dissolving tablet (Staxyn)
Prostaglandin				
alprostadil injectable	Caverject20 mcg/mL, 40 mcg/mL vials	Caverject Impulse10 mcg/0.5 mL, 20 mcg/0.5 mL prefilled syringesEdex 10 mcg/mL, 20 mcg/mL, 40 mcg/mL cartridges	Initiate dose at 1.25 or 2.5 mcg intracavernosally and titrate does with no more than 2 doses per 24 hours (maximum dose: 40 mcg [Edex], 60 mcg [Caverject]). Self administration: maximum 3 times/week with 24 hours between doses	Provide an in-office test dose and instruction in proper technique for administration. Use lowest effective dose.
alprostadil intraurethral	Muse	125-, 250-, 500-, 1000-mcg urethral suppositories	Initiate dose at 125 or 250 mcg intraurethrally and titrate dose on separate occasions in physician's office. Maximum 2 suppositories per 24 hours for self-administration	Provide an in-office test dose and instruction in proper technique for administration. Use lowest effective dose.

their partners should be counseled regarding risks and benefits to ensure realistic postsurgical expectations. Risks include scarring, penile shortening, recurrent infections, and mechanical failure requiring removal.

Monitoring

A validated questionnaire such as the SHIM (https://www.baus.org.uk/_userfiles/pages/files/Patients/Leaflets/SHIM.pdf) is a simple and reliable tool for monitoring ongoing symptoms. A periodic clinical evaluation, including a review of all supplements and medications, can be helpful to identify potential causes of symptoms and any adverse reactions.

Management of Complications

The majority of adverse reactions with PDE-5 inhibitors are mild to moderate in nature and can be limited by using the lowest effective dose. PDE-5 inhibitors are contraindicated in patients taking nitrates because of the significant risk of life-threatening hypotension. If accidentally ingested, the patient should be monitored by healthcare professionals. The risk also depends on which specific agent was ingested, as the duration of action differs between medications. While the risk of prolonged erection (priapism) is low with PDE-5 inhibitors, men with erections lasting greater than 4 hours should seek emergency attention.

The major potential complication of alprostadil is a prolonged erection lasting greater than 4 hours, which will require emergent urological treatment. Penile fibrosis is also a risk that has been reported in 4.9% of patients using alprostadil at 4 years.

Treatment with exogenous testosterone impairs spermatogenesis and should be avoided in men who are trying to conceive or are interested in future fertility.

The major complication of vacuum erectile devices is ischemic injury, generally when the constricting ring is left in place for greater than 30 minutes at a time. Any suspicion for ischemic injury should also prompt emergent urologic intervention.

Patients with penile implants are prone to recurrent infections or mechanical failure, potentially requiring removal of the device.

References

Burnett AL, Nehra A, Breau RH, et al: Erectile dysfunction: AUA Guideline, *J Urol* 200(3):633–641, 2018 Sep, https://doi.org/10.1016/j.juro.2018.05.004. Epub 2018 May 7.

Buvat J, Büttner H, Hatzimouratidis K, et al: Adherence to initial PDE-5 inhibitor treatment: randomized open-label study comparing tadalafil once a day, tadalafil on demand, and sildenafil on demand in patients with erectile dysfunction, *J Sex Med* 10(6):1592–1602, 2013.

Costa P, Grandmottet G, Mai HD, Droupy S: Impact of a first treatment with phosphodiesterase inhibitors on men and partners' quality of sexual life: results of a prospective study in primary care, *J Sex Med* 10(7):1850–1860, 2013.

Ghanem HM, Salonia A, Martin-Morales A: SOP: physical examination and laboratory testing for men with erectile dysfunction, *J Sex Med* 10(1):108–110, 2013.

Khayyamfar F, Forootan SK, Ghasemi H, Miri SR, Farhadi E: Evaluating the efficacy of vacuum constrictive device and causes of its failure in impotent patients, *Urol J* 10(4):1072–1078, 2014.

Martin-Morales A, Haro JM, Beardsworth A, Bertsch J, Kontodimas S: Therapeutic effectiveness and patient satisfaction after 6 months of treatment with tadalafil, sildenafil, and vardenafil: results from the erectile dysfunction observational study (EDOS), *Eur Urol* 51(2):541–550, 2007.

Mccabe MP, Sharlip ID, Lewis R, et al: Incidence and prevalence of sexual dysfunction in women and men: a consensus statement from the Fourth International Consultation on Sexual Medicine 2015, *J Sex Med* 13(2):144–152, 2016.

Mulhall JP, Trost LW, Brannigan RE, et al: Evaluation and management of testosterone deficiency: AUA Guideline, *J Urol* 200(2):423–432, 2018 Aug, https://doi.org/10.1016/j.juro.2018.03.115. Epub 2018 Mar 28.

Rosen RC, Fisher WA, Eardley I, et al: The multinational Men's Attitudes to Life Events and Sexuality (MALES) study: I. Prevalence of erectile dysfunction and related health concerns in the general population, *Curr Med Res Opin* 20(5):607–617, 2004.

Selvin E, Burnett AL, Platz EA: Prevalence and risk factors for erectile dysfunction in the US, *Am J Med* 120(2):151–157, 2007.

PROSTATE CANCER

Method of
William G. Nelson, MD, PhD

CURRENT DIAGNOSIS

- Serum prostate-specific antigen (PSA) testing, with or without digital rectal examination (DRE), can be used for prostate cancer screening for men beginning at 50 years of age until 70 years of age.
- Prostate cancer screening carries significant risks of overdiagnosis and overtreatment of clinically insignificant prostate cancers.
- The diagnosis of prostate cancer is usually made via ultrasound-guided transrectal core needle biopsies that sample the prostate; magnetic resonance imaging (MRI) is increasingly used to direct core biopsies to regions of the prostate suspicious for harboring aggressive prostate cancers.
- Histologic grade (Gleason score) and anatomic stage provide the prognosis needed for treatment decision making. Several different tumor-based molecular biomarker tests can add further prognostic information.
- Metastatic prostate cancer can be evaluated using ^{99m}Tc-methylene diphosphonate (MDP) or ^{18}F-sodium fluoride (NaF) bone scans, abdominopelvic computed tomography (CT) or MRI scan, and ^{11}C-choline, ^{18}F-fluciclovine, ^{68}Ga-PSMA, or ^{18}F-piflufolastat positron emission tomography (PET) studies.
- Germline genetic testing for DNA repair gene variants along with tumor testing for DNA repair gene defects tends to accompany diagnosis of high-risk localized, locoregionally advanced, and metastatic prostate cancer.

CURRENT THERAPY

- Options for management of localized prostate cancer include active surveillance, radical prostatectomy, external-beam radiotherapy (EBRT), brachy therapy, and proton-beam radiotherapy.
- Androgen-deprivation therapy (ADT) using gonadotrophic hormone-releasing hormone analogues is a mainstay of systemic prostate cancer treatment.
- CYP17 inhibitors and androgen receptor antagonists can be added to further ablate androgen signaling.
- CYP17 inhibitors, androgen receptor antagonists, and taxane chemotherapy can improve survival when given along with ADT for hormone-sensitive metastatic prostate cancer or upon progression to castration-resistant prostate cancer (CRPC).
- Stereotactic bone radiation therapy (SBRT) can be directed at metastatic lesions in the setting of oligometastatic disease progression to prolong progression-free survival.
- The α-particle–emitting calcium mimetic ^{223}Ra can palliate painful bony metastases.
- Poly(ADP-ribose) polymerase (PARP) inhibitors may be effective in up to 20% of men with CRPC who carry germline and/or somatic mutations in homologous recombination repair genes (BRCA1, BRCA2, ATM, and others).
- Immune checkpoint blockade may be of benefit for patients with mismatch repair–deficient prostate cancer.
- Platinum-based chemotherapy can be used to treat small cell/neuroendocrine prostate cancer.

Prostate cancer comprises the most commonly diagnosed cancer among men in the United States, with an estimated 268,490 new cases and 34,500 deaths expected for 2022. At some point during life, 1 in 8 men can expect to be diagnosed with prostate cancer, though the risk of dying from the disease is only about 1 in 41. African-American men suffer disproportionately with the disease, exhibiting more than twice the age-adjusted mortality as Caucasians.

The prostate gland itself is a male sex accessory gland located adjacent to the rectum in the pelvis and surrounding the urethra to supply secretions to the ejaculate. Why it should spawn so many cancers has proven enigmatic. The prostate can be divided into three zones: a *peripheral zone*, where most prostate cancers arise; a *transition zone* near the urethra that is prone to benign enlargement (benign prostatic hyperplasia/hypertrophy [BPH]); and a *central zone*. Under the influence of the male androgenic hormones testosterone (T) and dihydrotestosterone (DHT), normal epithelial cells produce the serine protease prostate-specific antigen (PSA; encoded by the *KLK3* gene). The appearance of PSA in the bloodstream tends to indicate epithelial barrier dysfunction within the prostate gland, attributable to three highly prevalent conditions in aging men in the United States: inflammation (prostatitis), BPH, or prostate cancer. Blood testing for PSA has emerged as a common screening tactic for prostate cancer, necessarily confounded by the near-ubiquitous coexistence of prostatitis and BPH.

Most patients present with prostate cancer apparently confined to the prostate gland, often detected by PSA screening. Though usually indolent, when aggressive, prostate cancer tends to spread to bony sites, causing pain by undermining bone architecture through stimulating osteoblastic activity, a phenomenon readily evident via NaF bone scanning. Patients dying of prostate cancer also manifest metastasis to lymph nodes, liver, the dura, and elsewhere.

Patients who are diagnosed with prostate cancer today confront a large and often confusing array of treatment options. The typical patient diagnosed with the disease is at least 65 years of age or older; the risks and benefits associated with different treatment choices in this age range are relevant not only for prostate cancer specialty care, but for general medical care as well. The 5-year survival for a man with localized prostate cancer is >95%, underscoring the need for balancing prostate cancer treatment selection with other health priorities.

Epidemiology

Heredity plays as significant a role in prostate cancer development as for any other common cancer. Analyses of concordance for prostate cancer between monozygotic (identical) versus dizygotic (fraternal) twins have consistently found excess prostate cancers among the identical twins despite similar environmental exposures, leading to the estimate that as many as 42% of prostate cancer cases may be attributable to inheritance. Two sets of inherited susceptibility genes merit special attention for prostate cancer treatment. Germline defects in DNA double-strand break repair genes, such as *BRCA1*, *BRCA2*, *ATM*, *PALB2*, *FANCA*, *RAD51D*, and *CHEK2*, or in DNA mismatch repair genes, such as *MSH2*, *MLH1*, *MSH6*, and *PMS2*, may increase the risk of developing prostate cancer or of exhibiting metastatic prostate cancer progression. Defective DNA repair in prostate cells has important treatment implications. When germline DNA repair gene defects are accompanied by somatic alterations at the remaining allele, crippling of DNA double-strand break repair can serve as an indication for treatment with poly(ADP-ribose) polymerase (PARP) inhibitors, while loss of DNA mismatch repair constitutes an indication for treatment with immune checkpoint inhibitors. With a growing role in prostate cancer treatment decision making, both germline testing and tumor tissue testing for DNA repair gene defects has become increasingly common for patients with the disease. Of course, the detection of defective DNA repair genes in the germline of a patient with prostate cancer should also alert his physician to consider cascade genetic testing of relatives as abnormal repair gene carriers could be at risk for breast, ovarian, colorectal, or other cancers.

for recurrence, stage II to IV cancers, and all serous and clear cell carcinomas often require adjuvant therapy in the form of radiation, chemotherapy, or a combination of both.

Early-Stage Disease

Surgery alone is usually curative for women with early-stage, low-risk disease. Women with early-stage, high-risk or high-intermediate-risk factors are often recommended adjuvant radiation. The treatment can be in the form of external beam radiation therapy or vaginal brachytherapy. All serous and clear cell carcinomas of the uterus are recommended to receive adjuvant platinum-based combination chemotherapy regardless of stage. Adjuvant systemic therapy in patients with high-risk early-stage endometrioid carcinoma remains controversial and is an active area of research.

Advanced-Stage Disease

Approximately 10% to 15% of patients will present with metastatic disease at presentation. Surgical cytoreduction is the preferred treatment approach if complete resection is achievable because it is associated with improved progression-free and overall survival. This would be followed by adjuvant therapy because of the increased risk for recurrence. The optimal form of adjuvant therapy is controversial. Extrauterine disease confined to lymph nodes may be treated with pelvic radiation therapy alone or with combination chemotherapy. Platinum-based combination chemotherapy is regarded as the foundation for systemic therapy of extrauterine disease. The most common regimens are carboplatin (Paraplatin)[1] plus paclitaxel (Taxol)[1] or the triple drug combination of cisplatin (Platinl),[1] doxorubicin (Adriamycin),[1] plus paclitaxel[1].

Recently, National Comprehensive Cancer Network guidelines added immune-checkpoint inhibitors (pembrolizumab [Keytruda] and dostarlimab [Jemperli]) up front as preferred, primary therapy options in combination with chemotherapy based on data from two large phase III randomized placebo-controlled trials. Both trials significantly improved progression-free survival in patients with primary advanced or recurrent endometrial cancer.

Patients who are not candidates for surgical cytoreduction either because of grossly metastatic disease or too poor a surgical candidate have a poor prognosis, with 5-year relative survival of <20%. These patients should be offered systemic chemotherapy generally with palliative intent. Radiation therapy to achieve local control in the pelvis to palliate bleeding, discharge, and pain is often performed.

Recurrent Disease

Local recurrences, distance metastases, and simultaneous local and distant metastases are found in 50%, 29%, and 21%, respectively. Isolated vaginal recurrences are often salvaged with either surgery or radiation. Distant recurrent endometrial cancer portends a poor prognosis. Systemic chemotherapy with immunotherapy is offered with a palliative intent.

Hormone Therapy

Prior to development of endometrial cancer, the risk of endometrial hyperplasia and the development into carcinoma can be significantly reduced with administration of a progestin. After the development of carcinoma, tumors that test positive for estrogen receptor and progesterone receptor are associated with longer survival, with progesterone receptor being a stronger predictor than estrogen receptor. However, the role of adjuvant progestins in stage I or II endometrial cancer has not been demonstrated to be of value and may worsen cardiovascular disease. Progestins

are commonly used in advanced or recurrent, well-differentiated endometrial cancers. Oral megestrol acetate (Megace) and medroxyprogesterone acetate (Provera)[1] are two of the most commonly used progestins.

The selective estrogen receptor modulator tamoxifen has been used to treat patients with recurrent endometrial cancer. The response rate is approximately 22%. The aromatase inhibitors anastrozole (Arimidex)[1] and letrozole (Femara)[1] were investigated in the treatment of recurrent and metastatic endometrial cancer and demonstrated minimal activity.

Targeted Therapy

Multiple novel agents are being evaluated in clinical trials for use in treatment against endometrial cancer. Bevacizumab (Avastin)[1] is a monoclonal antibody directed against vascular endothelial growth factor that is active in endometrial cancer. Pembrolizumab (Keytruda) and dostarlimab (Jemperli) are immune checkpoint inhibitors that are often used for treatment of disease progression after platinum-based chemotherapy in women with mismatch repair gene or microsatellite instability tumors. However, immunotherapy is now the preferred option for primary systemic therapy in advanced-stage or recurrent endometrial cancer. Trastuzumab (Herceptin)[1] and lapatinib (Tykerb)[1] are anti–human epidermal growth factor 2 agents being tested as single agents and in combination with chemotherapy in some endometrial cancers. Chemotherapy with the addition of trastuzumab is now the preferred regimen for advanced-stage human epidermal growth factor 2–positive uterine serous tumors or carcinosarcomas. The mammalian target of rapamycin inhibitors everolimus (Afinitor)[1] and ridaforolimus[5] have been used to treat advanced-stage and recurrent endometrial cancers with mixed response.

Monitoring

Surveillance recommendations for endometrial cancer are stratified by risk of recurrence, and most women diagnosed and treated for endometrial cancer will fall into the low-risk category. High risk for recurrence is defined as advanced-stage or grade 3 endometrioid, serous, or clear cell histology. Follow-up recommendations for low-risk women involve a history and physical examination, including a speculum and pelvic examination, scheduled every 6 months for the first 2 years and then yearly. Women with high risk of recurrence should have the same follow-up at intervals of 3 months for the first 2 years, every 6 months in years 2 to 5, and then yearly. Pap test/cytology, CA 125 testing, and routine radiographic imaging are not recommended. Women suspected of recurrence should have imaging performed.

---

[1] Not FDA approved for this indication.
[5] Investigational drug in the United States.

References

Eskander RN, Sill MW, Beffa L, et al: Pembrolizumab plus chemotherapy in advanced endometrial cancer, *N Engl J Med* 10, 2023.

Kandoth C, et al: Integrated genomic characterization of endometrial carcinoma, *Nature* 497(7447):67–73, 2013.

Mirza MR, Chase DM, Slomovitz BM, et al: Dostarlimab for primary advanced or recurrent endometrial cancer, *N Engl J Med* 10, 2023.

Pecorelli S: Revised FIGO staging for carcinoma of the vulva, cervix, and endometrium, *Int J Gynaecol Obstet* 105(2):103–104, 2009.

Salani R, et al: An update on posttreatment surveillance and diagnosis of recurrence in women with gynecologic malignancies: Society of Gynecologic Oncology (SGO) recommendations, *Gynecol Oncol* 146(1):3–10, 2017.

Siegel RL, Miller KD, Wagle NS, Jemal A: Cancer statistics, 2023, *CA Cancer J Clin* 73(1):17–48, 2023, https://doi.org/10.3322/caac.21763.

The American College of Obstetricians and Gynecologists Committee Opinion no. 631: Endometrial intraepithelial neoplasia, *Obstet Gynecol* 125(5):1272–1278, 2015.

---

[1] Not FDA approved for this indication.

CANCER OF THE UTERINE CERVIX

Method of
Lucybeth Nieves-Arriba, MD; and Peter G. Rose, MD

CURRENT DIAGNOSIS

- New recommendations for cytology screening recommend starting screening at 21 years of age.
- Initial workup must include a biopsy.
- Imaging techniques including magnetic resonance imaging and positron emission tomography–computed tomography can assist in treatment planning.

CURRENT THERAPY

- Despite recent availability of human papillomavirus (HPV) vaccination (Gardasil[2], Gardasil 9, Cervarix[2]) and advances in screening, cervical cancer remains a significant global health problem, especially in underserved populations.
- Improved understanding of the disease has allowed more conservative treatment of selected patients with early-stage disease.
- For advanced and high-risk cervical cancer, chemoradiation has had a significant impact on survival.

[2]Not available in the United States.

Epidemiology

Worldwide, cervical cancer is the fourth most common cancer in women. It is the greatest cancer killer of young women and the most common cause of death from cancer in women in the developing world. Worldwide in 2020, among the 604,237 new cases of cervical cancer, the highest incidence rates were in Africa, Central and South America, and Asia. In the United States, it is estimated that approximately 14,100 new cases were diagnosed and 4280 patients died from cervical cancer in 2022. Significant disparities in incidence and stage at time of diagnosis have been identified among different ethnic groups—African Americans, Asian Americans, European Americans, and Latin Americans—in the United States. Factors that increase the risk of cervical cancer include early age at first coitus, multiple sexual partners, history of sexually transmitted diseases, low socioeconomic status, cigarette smoking, immunosuppression, and Fanconi syndrome.

Pathophysiology

Cervical cancer occurs secondary to viral transformation of the surface (epithelial) cells by high-risk types of the human papillomavirus (HPV), and it is the only gynecologic cancer that can be prevented by regular screening. Persistent infection with high-risk HPV has been identified as the essential factor in the pathogenesis of the majority of cervical cancers. The virus's ability to transform human epithelium has been associated with the expression of two viral gene products, E6 and E7, which interact with p53 (a tumor-suppressor protein) and retinoblastoma protein (pRB), respectively, and affect control mechanisms of the cell cycle.

The prevalence of genital HPV infection in the world is estimated to be 400 million. Data from the National Health and Nutrition Examination Survey (NHANES) estimate the prevalence of HPV infection among girls and women in the United States aged 14 to 59 years is 26.8%. In about 90% of cases, the high-risk HPV infection is cleared by the immune system within 16 months. HPV infections in girls and younger women are more likely transient and therefore less likely to be associated with significant cervical lesions.

Prevention and Screening

Advances in molecular biology have allowed the development of viral-like particles using the L1 protein (major immunogenic capsid protein) of the HPV virus. Currently approved HPV vaccines include: Gardasil (2006)[2], Cervarix (2009)[2], and Gardasil 9 (2014). These vaccines are approved to use in girls/boys and women/men between the ages of 9 and 26 years. The FDA expanded its approval in 2018 to include men and women between 27 and 45 years old. Awareness of the importance of HPV vaccination has increased but vaccination rates for US adolescents are still not at goal with only 58.6% completed vaccination series as of 2021.

The current standard screening algorithm in the United States for preventing cervical cancer is presented in Table 1. Women with abnormal cytology are referred for a colposcopic examination. The colposcopic examination is used to guide biopsies of the exocervix, and in most cases an endocervical biopsy is also performed. The biopsy results then determine the type of follow-up and or therapy required.

Staging

The International Federation of Gynecology and Obstetrics (FIGO) defined the most commonly accepted staging of cervical cancer. This staging is based on a careful clinical examination and the results of specific radiologic studies and procedures. FIGO's latest update (2018) is summarized in Table 2.

In cervical cancer, primary lesions initially progress to lymphatics in the parametrium and pelvic nodes and then extend laterally to the pelvic side wall, bladder, and rectum. The two major spread patterns identified in cervical cancer include direct extension and lymphatic spread.

Diagnosis

The initial workup for cervical cancer depends on whether a cervical lesion is visible. Patients without a visible cervical lesion require a cone biopsy to diagnose stage IA1 or IA2 tumor. Patients with a cervical lesion are assessed by history and physical examination and possibly by examination under anesthesia for biopsy, cystoscopy, sigmoidoscopy, and conventional imaging (chest x-ray, intravenous pyelogram). Other imaging modalities including computed tomography (CT), magnetic resonance imaging (MRI), and fluorodeoxyglucose positron emission tomography (FDG-PET) are useful in evaluating nodal or other metastatic sites. MRI performed significantly better than CT in detecting parametrial invasion, presence of bladder or rectal invasion, and identification of women suitable for fertility-preserving surgery. PET-CT is the most sensitive modality in identifying nodal metastasis or metastatic disease assisting with radiotherapy planning and evaluation of metabolic response to therapy. A 3-month posttherapy PET scan is highly predictive of long-term survival outcome.

Treatment

Multiple factors including tumor stage, size, histologic features (lymphovascular space invasion [LVSI], nonsquamous components, and depth of cervical stromal invasion), and evidence of lymph node metastasis influence the choice of treatment for cervical cancer. Patients with stage IA1 cervical cancer have undergone a cone biopsy, and pathology demonstrates stromal invasion greater than 3 mm in depth, no LVSI, and negative margins. Patients with this extent of disease can safely be treated with a less-radical hysterectomy, an extrafascial hysterectomy.

[1]Not available in the United States.

tion in stages IB2, IIA, IIB, IIIB and IVA cervical carcinoma limited to the pelvis: a Gynecologic Oncology Group study, *J Clin Oncol* 32(5):458–464, 2014.

Dunne EF, Unger ER, Sternberg M, et al: Prevalence of HPV infection among females in the United States, *JAMA* 297(8):813–819, 2007.

Finan MA, Decesare S, Fiorica JV, et al: Radical hysterectomy for stage IB1 vs IB2 carcinoma of the cervix: does the new staging system predict morbidity and survival? *Gynecol Oncol* 62(2):139–147, 1996.

Keys HM, Bundy BN, Stehman FB, et al: Cisplatin, radiation, and adjuvant hysterectomy compared with radiation and adjuvant hysterectomy for bulky stage IB cervical carcinoma, *N Engl J Med* 340(15):1154–1161, 1999. Erratum in N Engl J Med 1999;341(9):708.

Long 3rd HJ, Bundy BN, Grendys EC, et al: Randomized phase III trial of cisplatin with or without topotecan in carcinoma of the uterine cervix: A Gynecologic Oncology Group study, *J Clin Oncol* 23(21):4626–4633, 2005.

Monk BJ, Sill MW, McMeekin DS, et al: Phase III trial of four cisplatin-containing doublet combinations in stage IVB, recurrent, or persistent cervical carcinoma: A Gynecologic Oncology Group study, *J Clin Oncol* 27(28):4649–4655, 2009.

Moore DH, Blessing JA, McQuellon RP, et al: Phase III study of cisplatin with or without paclitaxel in stage IVB, recurrent, or persistent squamous cell carcinoma of the cervix: A Gynecologic Oncology Group study, *J Clin Oncol* 22(15):3113–3119, 2004.

Morris M, Eifel PJ, Lu J, et al: Pelvic radiation with concurrent chemotherapy compared with pelvic and para-aortic radiation for high-risk cervical cancer, *N Engl J Med* 340(15):1137–1143, 1999.

National Cancer Institute: Cervical cancer. Available at: http://www.cancer.gov/cancertopics/types/cervical. [Accessed 27 May 2019].

Omura GA, Blessing JA, Vaccarello L, et al: Randomized trial of cisplatin versus cisplatin plus mitolactol versus cisplatin plus ifosfamide in advanced squamous carcinoma of the cervix: A Gynecologic Oncology Group study, *J Clin Oncol* 15(1):165–171, 1997.

Pearcey R, Brundage M, Drouin P, et al: Phase III trial comparing radical radiotherapy with and without cisplatin chemotherapy in patients with advanced squamous cell cancer of the cervix, *J Clin Oncol* 20(4):966–972, 2002.

Peters 3rd WA, Liu PY, Barrett 3rd RJ, et al: Concurrent chemotherapy and pelvic radiation therapy compared with pelvic radiation therapy alone as adjuvant therapy after radical surgery in high-risk early-stage cancer of the cervix, *J Clin Oncol* 18(8):1606–1613, 2000.

Rose PG, Bundy BN, Watkins EB, et al: Concurrent cisplatin-based radiotherapy and chemotherapy for locally advanced cervical cancer, *N Engl J Med* 340(15):1144–1153, 1999.

Tewari KS, Sill MW, Long HR, et al: Improved survival with bevacizumab in advance cervical cancer, *N Engl J Med* 370(8):734–743, 2014.

Whitney CW, Sause W, Bundy BN, et al: Randomized comparison of fluorouracil plus cisplatin versus hydroxyurea as an adjunct to radiation therapy in stage IIB-IVA carcinoma of the cervix with negative para-aortic lymph nodes: A Gynecologic Oncology Group and Southwest Oncology Group study, *J Clin Oncol* 17(5):1339–1348, 1999.

Wright JD, Nathavithrana R, Lewin SN, et al: Fertility-conserving surgery for young women with stage IA1 cervical cancer: Safety and access, *Obstet Gynecol* 115(3):585–590, 2010.

CONTRACEPTION

Method of
Rachel A. Bonnema, MD, MS

CURRENT THERAPY

- Long-acting reversible contraception (LARC) such as an implant or intrauterine device (IUD) is safe and extremely effective and should be considered in all women, including nulliparous women.
- Combined estrogen and progesterone methods (e.g., pills, patch, ring) are effective and commonly used. They provide excellent cycle control and decreased rates of ectopic pregnancy, pelvic inflammatory disease, and endometrial and ovarian cancer, and they can be used in extended-cycle methods for patients who desire fewer than 12 periods per year.
- The use of estrogen has been associated, albeit rarely, with the development of deep venous thrombosis, myocardial infarction, and stroke; estrogen should not be used in smokers older than 35 years of age and in patients with diabetes with end organ damage, coronary artery disease, migraines with aura, or a known hypercoagulable condition.
- For women with a contraindication to estrogen, progestin-only methods are safe to use.

Nearly one-half of all pregnancies in the United States are unplanned, a rate higher than the rate in other developed countries. Primary care physicians need up-to-date knowledge on contraceptive counseling for women to provide the best match between patient and contraceptive method, in part because providers frequently need to supply contraceptives to women who have particular medical comorbidities. Newer contraceptive preparations are now available, including a vaginal ring that can be reused for up to 1 year and a progestin-only pill (POP) with a wider window for missed doses.

Nonhormonal Methods

Nonhormonal methods of contraception include barrier methods and the copper intrauterine device (IUD). These methods are safe, easily available, inexpensive, and reversible. Common barrier methods include male and female condoms, spermicides, vaginal sponges, diaphragms, and cervical caps (Table 1). Only condom use has been consistently found to protect against sexually transmitted infections (STIs) including HIV, and condom use may reduce the risk of cervical cancer as well. Of note is a novel pH-buffering spermicide, Phexxi, that is available by prescription only. Although it is not more effective than non-oxynol-9 spermicides, further studies are planned to evaluate Phexxi as a novel STI prevention method. Barrier methods have the lowest efficacy rates of all contraceptive methods, and users should also be counseled about emergency contraception (EC). The copper IUD is an extremely effective form of long-acting reversible contraception (LARC) and is a particularly attractive option for women who have contraindications to hormone use and desire effective contraception.

Combined Hormonal Contraception

Combined hormonal contraception (CHC) contains estrogen and a progestin and work primarily by preventing the surge of luteinizing hormone and thereby preventing ovulation. The majority of CHCs contain ethinyl estradiol (EE), though a new contraceptive has been approved with a novel endogenous estrogen, estetrol (E4). CHC can be delivered as an oral contraceptive pill (OCP), as a vaginal ring (NuvaRing, Annovera), or as a transdermal patch (Xulane, Twirla). Risks, benefits, side effects, and contraindications of CHC are thought to be largely similar across delivery methods.

There are many noncontraceptive benefits to CHC, including first-line treatment for dysfunctional uterine bleeding, dysmenorrhea, and menorrhagia. Benefits in addition to menstrual control include reduction in the risk for and symptoms of endometriosis, ovulatory pain, ovarian cysts, benign breast disease, premenstrual syndrome, and premenstrual dysphoric disorder. CHCs also reduce the risk of ovarian and endometrial cancers; these risk reductions extend for years after discontinuing CHC. The most common side effects of CHC are outlined in Table 2. The risk of venous thromboembolism (VTE) may be higher in obese patients, smokers, and those who use certain progestins such as desogestrel or drospirenone. This risk is lower, however, than the risk of VTE associated with pregnancy, and the absolute risk of VTE among CHC users remains small. The novel OCP with E4 (E4 plus drospirenone [Nextstellis]) has demonstrated more neutral effects on the liver, with preliminary findings suggesting lower VTE risk compared with other CHC.

CHCs can be used safely by those with a range of medical conditions, including well-controlled hypertension, uncomplicated diabetes, migraines *without* aura when younger than 35 years of age, and a family history of breast cancer, to name a few. CHC use is contraindicated in patients who have a history of migraine headache with aura at any age or in those older than 35 years of age with any migraine because of an elevated risk for stroke. CHC is also contraindicated in patients with diabetes with end organ damage, those with known cardiovascular disease, and individuals who smoke after 35 years of age because of an elevated risk for cardiovascular disease. Other contraindications include a personal history of breast cancer, an estrogen-dependent tumor, unexplained vaginal bleeding, stroke, known thromboembolic disorder, or known VTE. Elevated risk of VTE

TABLE 1 Nonhormonal Contraception

| | BARRIER METHODS | | | | INTRAUTERINE DEVICE |
	CONDOM (MALE/FEMALE)	DIAPHRAGM OR CERVICAL CAP	SPONGE	SPERMICIDE	COPPER IUD
Duration	Female condom can be inserted up to 8 h before intercourse; male condoms must be changed with each act of intercourse	Can be placed up to 6 h before intercourse and should be removed within 6 h after	Can be left in for 30 h and through multiple acts of intercourse	Placed 30–60 min before intercourse; proper instructions should be followed according to product directions	Approved for up to 10 years
Typical-use failure rate*	15%	15%	15%	10%–22%†	Less than 0.1%
Side effects and considerations	High failure rates: condom can break or slip Acceptability by partner may be limited	Requires expert fitting Must be refitted after childbirth Requires dexterity and self-placement by patient Use with spermicide increases efficacy but can lead to risk of UTIs, increased risk of toxic shock syndrome, and potential increased risk of HIV transmission	May increase risk of UTIs Use with spermicide increases efficacy but can lead to risk of UTIs, increased risk of toxic shock syndrome, and potential increased risk of HIV transmission	Vulvovaginal burning/ itching can occur Phexxi is a novel spermicide available only with prescription; nonoxynol-9 formulations are commonly available over the counter	Bleeding and cramping with menses initially Low risk of ectopic pregnancy, premature delivery, perforation, or expulsion Avoid with active infection, undiagnosed genital bleeding, cervical cancer, or Wilson disease
Consider in:	Patients at risk for STIs Patients without access to medical care and who are looking for nonhormonal, reversible, and convenient methods of contraception	Women who are looking for nonhormonal, reversible, and convenient methods of contraception	Women who are looking for nonhormonal, reversible, and convenient methods of contraception Patients without access to medical care	Women using other barrier methods or looking for moderately effective contraception	Women with contraindication to hormones or who desire hormone-free, long-acting, reversible contraception Women in need of EC followed by long-term effective contraception

*Trussell J. Contraceptive failure in the United States. *Contraception.* 2011;83(5):397–404.
†Varies according to product, Wong JC, Creinin MD. 2021 update on contraception. *OBG Manag.* 2021;33(10):23–25, 30–32, 34, e1.
EC, Emergency contraception; *HIV,* human immunodeficiency virus; *IUD,* intrauterine device; *UTI,* urinary tract infection.

and negative effect on lactation restrict the use of CHC in the first 6 weeks after delivery.

Combined Oral Contraceptive Pills

There are dozens of formulations of OCPs that differ by their estrogen type and dosage, progestin type and dosage, and hormone delivery schedule. OCPs can be monophasic in which each pill contains the same amount of hormones, or multiphasic in which pills contain different amounts of hormones throughout the monthly cycle. The different formulations offer patients options in cycle length, hormone levels, duration of withdrawal bleeding, and side-effect profile. Education should include taking the pill at the same time each day. If a pill is missed, it should be taken as soon as remembered. If 2 days of pills are missed, the regimen includes two pills daily for 2 days in a row with a backup method utilized. If 3 days of pills are missed, the pill pack should be discarded and a backup method utilized. At that point, it should be discussed whether to start a new pack or to change contraceptive methods.

For those who desire fewer days of menses or fewer than 12 menses per year, extended-cycle OCP regimens can be offered that offer a placebo week every 4 months or eliminate the placebo week altogether. Extended-cycle regimens have other benefits, including decreased hormone withdrawal symptoms such as headaches, tiredness, bloating, excessive bleeding, or menstrual pain. In addition to estrogen dose and scheduling, it is also important to consider the progestin component, which theoretically may affect libido, weight gain, acne, and hirsutism.

Contraceptive Patch

Norelgestromin/EE (Xulane) is a thin transdermal patch delivering a daily dose of 35 µg/day EE and 150 µg/day norelgestromin. Levonorgestrel/EE (Twirla) is a newly approved patch delivering a daily dose of 30 µg/day EE and 120 µg/day levonorgestrel. Both patches are administered similarly: changed weekly for 3 weeks on "patch change day" followed by a patch-free week during which menses occur. Only one patch should be worn at a time, and no more than 7 days should pass during the patch-free week. Both have decreased efficacy in obese women and are contraindicated in patients with a BMI >30 kg/m². Most of the noncontraceptive benefits, side effects, cardiovascular risks, and contraindications are similar to those of other forms of CHC, but there may be an increased risk of VTE in patch users compared with OCP users, though studies are controversial as to the actual

BOX 1 Uterine Fibroid Risk Factors

African American descent
First-degree relative with uterine fibroid
Early menarche
Less than three obstetric deliveries
Five years since last birth
Obesity
Metabolic syndrome
Decreased physical activity
Childhood trauma
Beef, red meat, ham
Vitamin D deficiency
Alcoholic beverages (especially beer)
Caffeine intake (younger women)
Hormone replacement therapy

Prevention

There are currently no proven therapies that prevent uterine fibroid formation. Identification of the genes responsible for fibroid growth in patients genetically predisposed to fibroids could possibly lead to genomic-mediated prevention of fibroids.

Clinical Manifestations

About 50% to 80% of uterine fibroids are asymptomatic. Heavy menstrual bleeding and pelvic pain are the most common symptoms associated with uterine fibroids. Additional symptoms include secondary dysmenorrhea, abdominal distention, pelvic pressure, urinary symptoms (urgency, frequency, incontinence, hydronephrosis), bowel dysfunction including constipation, back pain, dyspareunia, and infertility.

Diagnosis

Physical examination of the abdomen and pelvis may elucidate an enlarged uterus secondary to uterine fibroids. Transvaginal ultrasonography is 90% to 99% sensitive in the detection of uterine fibroids but may miss small or subserosal fibroids. Hysteroscopy or sonohysterography increase diagnostic sensitivity for subserosal myomas.

Differential Diagnosis

Diagnostic possibilities in patients presenting with symptoms of uterine fibroids include adenomyosis, ectopic pregnancy, endometrial polyp, endometriosis, pregnancy, endometrial carcinoma, uterine carcinosarcoma, uterine sarcoma, and metastatic disease.

Treatment of Myomas

Myomas are benign lesions, hence, there is no a priori requirement for treatment. Management is based on symptoms and patient's wishes. Three parameters control recommendations: uterine size, severity of symptoms, and the patient's interest in childbearing.

There are a limited number of options for management:
- Definitive surgery
  - Hysterectomy (various methods)
- Palliative/uterine conserving surgery
  - Myomectomy (open or laparoscopic)
  - Hysteroscopic myomectomy
  - Uterine artery embolization
  - Radiofrequency focused ablation
- Symptomatic treatment
  - Nonsteroidal antiinflammatory drugs (NSAIDs)
  - Oral contraceptives
  - Progestational agents
  - Gonadotropin-releasing hormone (GnRH) agonists
  - Endometrial ablation

The indicators for surgical intervention include the following:
- Uterine size >12 weeks (>14 weeks for some insurers to cover)
- Anemia from menometrorrhagia
- Soiling of clothing or bedding from menometrorrhagia
- Intractable dysmenorrhea or dyspareunia
- Urinary or bowel obstruction

The choice of procedure is strongly constrained by a patient's desire for future childbearing. This precludes hysterectomy and procedures that destroy the endometrial cavity to stop bleeding, such as endometrial ablations. Uterine conservation may prove impossible or have marked complications if the number of myomas is large. Of note, surgical intervention for subfertility is indicated in selected cases but the data related to optimal methods of management is limited and inconclusive.

Hysterectomy

While multiple newer treatments have been introduced, hysterectomy remains the single most common management. It is definitive, ending mass impingement symptoms, bleeding, pain, urinary frequency, and constipation with a single intervention. Recurrence of myomas is extremely rare after hysterectomy.

The route of hysterectomy remains under debate. When possible, a vaginal hysterectomy is the preferred route, as it has the lowest morbidity of all types. More than two-thirds of hysterectomies for myomas are still done by open abdominal route, despite laparoscopy and robotic surgery having been repeatedly demonstrated as equivalent or superior for blood loss and complications.

Surgical complications of hysterectomy are common, but significant complications are rare. The most common problems are urinary tract infection (~25%) and superficial wound disruptions. More serious complications include deep venous thrombosis and pulmonary embolism, anaerobic pelvic cellulitis, and pneumonia. Organ injury to bowel, bladder, blood vessel, or ureter occurs in approximately 1/500 cases, 1/1000 for vaginal procedures. Bleeding sufficient to require transfusion occurs in about 1% of hysterectomies.

Myomectomy

Myomectomy is the procedure of choice for symptomatic myomas in women desiring fertility preservation. Myomas may be removed abdominally, vaginally, laparoscopically, or via hysteroscopy, depending on their size and location. Myomectomy does not necessarily lead to future cesarean delivery, but if cavity integrity is violated or there is an extensive dissection it then becomes mandatory.

Laparoscopic procedures are much less invasive but require significant skill. Closure of myomectomy defects is also difficult and time consuming. Hystereoscopic resection is an elegant technique applicable only to intracavitary myomas.

Between 40% and 75% of patients undergoing myomectomy will have a future hysterectomy. Complication rates from open myomectomy are significantly higher than for hysterectomy, accounted for by fever and blood loss.

Uterine Artery Embolization

Uterine artery embolization (UAE) now accounts for approximately 3% of myomectomies. The method uses injectable microspheres placed under fluoroscopic guidance. It is effective for isolated myomas of moderate size (up to 5 cm), although lesions up to 9 cm have been treated by UAE. It is an outpatient procedure done in interventional radiology suites without entering the abdominal cavity.

There are several significant problems with UAE that have limited its broad application. Inflammatory mediators released by myoma necrosis can cause substantial cramping and bowel symptoms. Lesion defects cannot be closed, leading to uterine wall defects with secondary placental implantation abnormalities and uterine rupture in pregnancy. Vascular anatomy is quite variable, and microspheres can be injected into any of the branches of the internal iliac. This can lead to necrosis of bladder, buttock, or vulva. Limitations in available facilities as well as trained and experienced operators, combined with the significant complications, has limited usage of UAE.

TABLE 2 Incidence of Regional Node Metastases by Tumor Diameter

TUMOR DIAMETER (CM)	% POSITIVE INGUINAL NODES
<1	1–15
5–20	
25–35	
35–50	
≥50	≥50

TABLE 3 Incidence of Regional Node Metastases by Depth of Tumor Invasion

DEPTH OF INVASION (MM)	% POSITIVE INGUINAL NODES
<1	1–5
1–3	10–15
3–5	15–30
5–10	30–45

but occasionally an invasive Paget's. In addition, up to 30% of patients have a synchronous adenocarcinoma of the breast, colon, rectum, or upper genital tract. Screening for these cancers is therefore recommended. To assess for invasion, the lesion should be excised via wide local excision or simple vulvectomy with at least 5 mm of the adjacent subcutaneous tissue. Achieving negative margin status is frequently difficult. However, the risk of recurrence is approximately 30% whether margins are negative or positive. Thus expectant management, reserving treatment for symptomatic recurrences, is usually recommended.

Invasive Vulvar Lesions

Less than 5% of gynecologic cancers arise on the vulva. Over 90% are squamous cell carcinomas. The etiology of this type appears mixed. The differentiated type is more common, occurs in older women (age 60–69, mean age 65) and is associated with vulvar dystrophies. The classic or usual type is predominantly associated with HPV-16. These women are slightly younger (age 45–52 years) and present with earlier stage disease. Other histologic types are melanomas (5%–10%), basal cell carcinomas (2%–3%), adenocarcinomas (1%), and sarcomas (1%–2%). Most patients present with a combination of symptoms, including pruritus, discomfort, and complaints of a mass. Examination frequently reveals a suspicious lesion, which should be biopsied for diagnosis. Vulvar cancers typically spread by local extension and lymphatic dissemination. Factors that influence dissemination include tumor size (Table 2), depth of invasion (Table 3), lymphovascular space invasion, and tumor grade. Staging is surgical and classified using the tumor, nodes, and metastasis (TNM) system as well as the International Federation of Gynecology and Obstetrics (FIGO) system (Table 4).

Squamous Cell Carcinomas and Adenocarcinomas

Surgical management of squamous cell carcinomas and adenocarcinomas depends on the size, depth of invasion, and location of the lesion. The vulvar lesion is managed with a radical excision. Management of the groins is based on depth of invasion. Lesions with invasion of less than 1 mm (Stage IA) have minimal risk of lymphatic spread (<1%) and do not require lymphadenectomy. All others require surgical assessment of the lymph nodes. Lesions less than 2 cm in size of the primary tumor, greater than 2 cm from the vulvar midline and are of squamous histology require only unilateral lymphadenectomy. Those without these characteristics or have palpable lymph nodes of the contralateral side require bilateral assessment. This surgical approach is associated

TABLE 4 Staging Vulvar Carcinoma

TNM CATEGORIES	FIGO STAGES	
T Primary tumor		
T0		No evidence of primary tumor
Tis		Carcinoma in situ
T1	I	Confined to vulva
T1a	IA	Lesions ≤2 cm in size, confined to the vulva or perineum and with stromal invasion ≤1 mm
T1b	IB	Lesions >2 cm in size OR any size with stromal invasion >1.0 mm, confined to the vulva or perineum
T2	II	Tumor of any size with extension to adjacent perineal structures (lower/distal 1/3 urethra, lower/distal 1/3 vagina, anal involvement)
T2	III	Tumor of any size with or without extension to adjacent perineal structures (lower/distal 1/3 urethra, lower/distal 1/3 vagina, anal involvement) with positive inguino-femoral lymph nodes
T3	IVA	Tumor of any size with extension to any of the following: upper/proximal 2/3 of urethra, upper/proximal 2/3 vagina, bladder mucosa, rectal mucosa, or fixed to pelvic bone
T3	IVB	Any distant metases including pelvic lymph nodes

TNM CATEGORIES	FIGO STAGES	
N Regional lymph nodes		
N0		No lymph node metastases
N1		One or two regional lymph nodes with the following features:
N1b	IIIAi	One lymph node metastasis, ≥ 5 mm
N1a	IIIAii	One to two lymph node metastases, < 5 mm
N2	IIIB	Regional lymph node metastasis with the following features:
N2b	IIIBi	Two or more lymph node metastases, ≥ 5 mm
N2a	IIIBii	Three or more lymph node metastases, <5 mm
N2c	IIIC	Lymph node metastasis with extracapsular spread
N3	IVA	Fixed or ulcerated regional lymph node metastasis

TNM CATEGORIES	FIGO STAGES	
M Distant metastases		
M0		No distant metastases
M1	IVB	Distant metastasis (including pelvic lymph node metastasis)

Abbreviations: TNM = tumor, node, metastasis; FIGO = International Federation of Gynecology and Obstetrics.

TABLE 5	Survival Rate by FIGO Stage for Patients With Invasive Squamous Cell Vulvar Cancer		
FIGO STAGE	**OVERALL SURVIVAL (PERCENT)**		
	One year	Two years	Five years
I	96.4	90.4	78.5
II	87.6	73.2	58.8
III	74.7	53.8	43.2
IV	35.3	16.9	13.0

Abbreviation: FIGO = International Federation of Gynecology and Obstetrics.

Modesitt SC, Waters AB, Walton L, et al: Vulvar intraepithelial neoplasia III: Occult cancer and the impact of margin status on recurrence, *Obstet Gynecol* 92(6):962–966, 1998.
Phillips GL, Bundy BN, Okagaki T, et al: Malignant melanoma of the vulva treated by radical hemivulvectomy, a prospective study of the Gynecologic Oncology Group, *Cancer* 73:2626–2632, 1994.
Tebes S, Cardosi R, Hoffman M: Paget's disease of the vulva, *Am J Obstet Gynecol* 187:281–284, 2002.
Trimble CL, Trimble EL, Woodruff JD: Diseases of the vulva. In Hernandez E, Atkinson BE, editors: *Clinical Gynecologic Pathology*, Philadelphia, 1995, WB Saunders, pp 1–90.
Van de Nieuwenhof, et al. Vulvar squamous cell carcinoma development after diagnosis of VIN increases with age. *Eur J Canc* 45:851, 2009.
Wright VC, Chapman WB: Colposcopy of intraepithelial neoplasia of the vulva and adjacent sites, *Obstet Gynecol Clin North Am* 20(1):231–255, 1993.

with significant morbidity including disfigurement, wound breakdown, and problems with lymphocysts and chronic lymphedema. For patients with very large lesions or lesions in sensitive areas such as the clitoris, preoperative radiation, followed by less radical excision of residual disease, may minimize problems with the vulvar wound. Current investigations are ongoing in the use of sentinel lymph node dissections as a method of minimizing the groin morbidity without sacrificing survival. Positive vulvar margins or metastases to lymph nodes are managed with postoperative radiation. Survival depends on stage at diagnosis (Table 5).

Verrucous Carcinoma

Verrucous carcinoma is a large exophytic tumor that resembles giant condyloma acuminatum. It is a variant of squamous carcinomas but has an excellent prognosis because of the lack of metastases. Verrucous carcinomas have a high tendency to recur and should be managed with radical local excision.

Malignant Melanoma

Malignant melanoma is the second most common vulvar malignancy. Most patients have disease on the mucosal surfaces of the vulvar introitus, clitoris, and labia minora. The vulvar lesion is treated by radical excision, but management of the groins is controversial. The risk of spread is significant with a tumor thickness greater than 0.75 mm, but survival at 5 years is only approximately 10% with groin node metastases. Some argue against node dissection for this reason. However, given some long-term survivors with modern melanoma therapy, either lymphadenectomy or sentinel lymph node dissection, as is done for other cutaneous melanomas, appears indicated.

Basal Cell Carcinoma

Basal cell carcinomas typically occur in elderly white women, are commonly located on the labia majora, and have characteristics similar to basal cell carcinomas at other sites. Treatment is wide local excision only because metastases are rare. Basal cell carcinomas are prone to local recurrence, however. A malignant squamous component must be ruled out because it should be managed as a squamous cell carcinoma.

Sarcomas

Leiomyosarcoma is the most common vulvar sarcoma and usually arises in the labia majora. Malignant fibrous histiocytoma is the second most common. Management of these lesions is radical vulvar excision.

References

Beller U, Quinn MA, Benedet JL, et al: Carcinoma of the vulva, *Int J Gynaecol Obstet* 95:S7, 2006.
Garland SM: Imiquimod, *Curr Opin Infect Dis* 16:85–89, 2003.
Homesley HD, Bundy BN, Sedlis A, et al: Prognostic factors for groin node metastasis in squamous cell carcinoma of the vulva (a Gynecologic Oncology Group study), *Gynecol Oncol* 49:279–283, 1993.
Hording U, Junge J, Lundvall F: Vulvar intraepithelial neoplasia III: a viral disease of undetermined progressive potential, *Gynecol Oncol* 56(2):276, 1995.
Krebs HB: The use of topical 5-fluorouracil in the treatment of genital condylomas, *Obstet Gynecol Clin North Am* 14(2):559–568, 1987.

VULVOVAGINITIS

Heather L. Paladine, MD, MEd; and Urmi Desai, MD, MS

CURRENT DIAGNOSIS

- The most common causes of vulvovaginitis are bacterial vaginosis (BV), candidal vulvovaginitis, and *Trichomonas* infection.
- Vulvovaginitis should be diagnosed by a combination of patient history, physical examination findings, and office-based or laboratory testing. Patients should not be treated presumptively based on history and physical examination.
- BV is diagnosed based on at least three of four of the Amsel criteria: fishy vaginal odor spontaneously or with potassium hydroxide (KOH) testing; vaginal pH above 4.5; thin, homogeneous vaginal discharge; and clue cells on saline microscopy.
- Vulvovaginal candidiasis is diagnosed based on symptoms of a thick whitish discharge, itching, and/or discomfort together with budding or pseudohyphae on KOH microscopy or positive fungal culture.
- The gold standard for *Trichomonas* diagnosis is nucleic acid amplification testing.

CURRENT TREATMENT

- Treatment of bacterial vaginosis (BV) is recommended for patients who are symptomatic, and both oral and topical metronidazole (Flagyl tablet 500 mg[1] as well as MetroGel [0.75%]) or topical clindamycin (Cleocin 2%) are first-line treatments for both pregnant and nonpregnant people.
- First-line treatment for symptomatic people with vulvovaginal candidiasis includes either oral fluconazole (Diflucan) or topical azole therapy for nonpregnant individuals; for pregnant people, topical azole therapy is preferred.
- First-line therapy for *Trichomonas* vaginal infection includes a 1-week course of metronidazole.
- Patients should be adequately counseled about treatment regimens for vaginitis, including potential weakening of condoms by oil-based topical therapies, and the importance of avoidance of sexual intercourse until treatment of BV or *Trichomonas* is complete. The Centers for Disease Control and Prevention no longer recommends that patients abstain from drinking alcohol while taking oral metronidazole.

[1]Not FDA approved for this indication.

Epidemiology

The term *vulvovaginitis* includes conditions that result in irritation of the vagina or vulva, causing symptoms of itching, burning,

TABLE 1 Diagnosis of Vulvovaginitis

CONDITION	SYMPTOMS	EXAMINATION FINDINGS	pH	MICROSCOPY FINDINGS
Normal	Discharge changes with menstrual cycle	Thin, clear or whitish discharge	Normal (4–4.5)	Epithelial cells, lactobacilli
Bacterial vaginosis	Fishy odor, vaginal discharge, vaginal discomfort/dyspareunia	Homogenous gray/white discharge	Elevated (≥4.6)	Clue cells on wet mount
Vulvovaginal candidiasis	Vulvar irritation or itching, vaginal discharge	Vulvar excoriations or erythema Thick, clumpy white discharge	Normal (4–4.5)	Pseudohyphae or budding yeast on potassium hydroxide examination
Trichomonas	Foul-smelling discharge, vaginal pain or discomfort	Cervical inflammation with "strawberry cervix," yellow-green frothy vaginal discharge	Elevated (≥4.6)	Mobile trichomonads on wet mount, white blood cells
Genitourinary syndrome of menopause (formerly *atrophic vaginitis*)	Vulvar itching, vaginal pain or discomfort, dyspareunia, vaginal dryness	Vulvar excoriations, clear vaginal discharge, thin friable mucosa with loss of vaginal rugae	Elevated (≥4.6)	May have white blood cells, parabasal cells, decreased lactobacilli
Irritant/allergic vaginitis	Vulvar or vaginal discomfort or pain	Vulvar or vaginal erythema, fissures, lichenification	Elevated (≥4.6)	May have white blood cells, parabasal cells, decreased lactobacilli
Inflammatory vaginitis	Vulvar or vaginal discomfort, pain, or burning Vaginal discharge	Purulent vaginal discharge Vaginal erythema or rash	Elevated (≥4.6)	Many white blood cells, parabasal cells, decreased lactobacilli

pain, odor, or discharge. Vulvovaginitis is a common condition in primary care, accounting for about 10% of office visits each year and affecting almost every person with a vagina at some point in their life. The three most common causes of vulvovaginitis are bacterial vaginosis (BV, accounting for up to 50% of cases in which a diagnosis is made), vulvovaginal candidiasis (VVC, accounting for 30% of cases), and *Trichomonas* (accounting for 15% to 20% of cases). The remaining diagnoses include genitourinary syndrome of menopause (GSM, formerly called *atrophic vaginitis*), inflammatory vaginitis, and allergic/irritant vaginitis. A specific cause is not found in up to 30% of patients.

Risk Factors

Risk factors for vulvovaginitis vary by condition. Although BV is not a sexually transmitted infection, it occurs almost exclusively in people of reproductive age with vaginas who are sexually active and more commonly in individuals with new or multiple sexual partners. BV is found more often in people with vaginas who smoke cigarettes or douche.

VVC is more common in patients who are immunosuppressed, such as those who have HIV or diabetes or are pregnant. Recent antibiotic use is also a risk factor.

Trichomonas is a sexually transmitted infection and is more likely to occur in people who have other sexually transmitted infections, who have multiple sexual partners, or who have had unprotected intercourse. As with many sexually transmitted infections, disparities exist in the prevalence of *Trichomonas,* with infections more commonly occurring in non-White, low-income, and formerly incarcerated people.

Pathophysiology

In people of reproductive age, the normal vaginal environment is acidic, with a pH of less than 4.6. This is thought to be caused by the prevalence of lactobacilli, which produce lactic acid, as part of the normal vaginal flora; however, the exact mechanism is unclear. BV represents a shift in the normal vaginal flora to anaerobic bacteria. The mechanism of this shift is also not entirely clear but is associated with risk factors such as douching and intercourse, which may change the vaginal pH.

VVC is caused by infection with species of candidal fungi, most commonly *Candida albicans*. Some 10% to 30% of individuals may have candida organisms among their normal vaginal flora. Candidal infections result from an interaction among biologic, genetic, and environmental factors leading to differences in the host immune response, host susceptibility, and the virulence of different strains of *Candida*.

Trichomonas is a protozoan infection. The risk factors as already described are similar to those for other sexually transmitted infections.

Prevention

Although previous studies have defined risk factors for BV, it is not known whether avoiding these risk factors (e.g., douching, unprotected intercourse) will reduce the risk. Studies that have looked at the prevention of recurrent BV through treatment with probiotics such as lactobacilli or other methods to maintain an acidic vaginal pH have not been conclusive.

Routine testing for conditions such as HIV or diabetes is not recommended in people with VVC unless they have other risk factors. Patients who are prone to develop VVC after taking antibiotics can use topical or oral antifungal medications during their treatment with antibiotics. Although probiotics are commonly used for the prevention and treatment of VVC, they have not been well studied.

Trichomonas is a sexually transmitted infection; therefore prevention includes condom use or being in a monogamous relationship.

Clinical Manifestations

Table 1 includes symptoms and physical examination findings for the common causes of vulvovaginitis. These symptoms can cause significant feelings of shame, distress, and decreased quality of life, especially in people with recurrent infections.

Diagnosis

The diagnosis of vulvovaginitis is unreliable based on history and physical examination findings alone and should include office-based or laboratory testing to confirm. There is a risk of

TABLE 2	Amsel Criteria	
CRITERION	**POSITIVE RESULT**
Vaginal discharge	Thin homogeneous discharge
Odor of discharge	Fishy odor on testing with potassium hydroxide
Vaginal pH	pH ≥4.6
Microscopy	Clue cells on saline microscopy

Three positive criteria are needed for a diagnosis of bacterial vaginosis.

Figure 1 Clue cells on saline microscopy. (From Brunzel NA. *Fundamentals of Urine & Body Fluid Analysis*. 4th ed. Elsevier; 2018.)

misdiagnosis or delay in diagnosis with presumptive treatment, as patients may get temporary relief of vulvovaginal symptoms with topical antifungals even if they do not have a fungal infection. Although newer laboratory tests have become available for the diagnosis of BV and VVC, the American College of Obstetricians and Gynecologists continues to recommend testing with history, examination, microscopy, and pH testing unless microscopy is not available. The newer tests include DNA testing for *Gardnerella vaginalis* or for the presence of vaginal sialidase activity for the diagnosis of BV, as well as DNA testing for *Candida* species. The newer tests are also less cost-effective. Table 1 also includes pH and microscopy findings for causes of vulvovaginitis.

BV is traditionally diagnosed via the Amsel criteria (Table 2), although Gram stain is considered the gold standard. A positive diagnosis requires three out of four criteria: fishy vaginal odor or positive odor on testing of vaginal discharge with 10% potassium hydroxide (KOH); vaginal pH above 4.5; a thin, homogeneous vaginal discharge; and clue cells (epithelial cells with adherent bacteria (Figure 1) on microscopic examination of vaginal discharge with normal saline (wet mount).

VVC is diagnosed based on the combination of clinical signs and symptoms and either microscopy or fungal culture of vaginal discharge. Microscopy has a sensitivity of 50% to 70% for candidal vulvovaginitis; therefore fungal culture is recommended when microscopy is negative in a patient with typical symptoms. Figure 2 demonstrates microscopy results with KOH that are positive for yeast. Fungal culture can also identify non*albicans* species of *Candida*, which may be more difficult to treat.

Nucleic acid amplification testing is recommended for the diagnosis of *Trichomonas* as microscopy is only 50% to 60% sensitive. Commercial DNA probe tests and a point-of-care antigen detection test are also available. Sensitivities may be lower with the newer tests, although this varies by test. Figure 3 shows positive saline microscopy for *Trichomonas*.

Differential Diagnosis

In addition to BV, VVC, and *Trichomonas*, other less common conditions can result in vulvovaginal symptoms. GSM was formerly known as *atrophic vaginitis* and results from a decrease in estrogen levels after menopause. People who are breast-feeding or using progestin-only contraception also have a relative estrogen deficiency and may experience similar symptoms. GSM is characterized by vaginal dryness and discomfort and may also include urinary tract symptoms and clear vaginal discharge. GSM is a presumptive diagnosis made on characteristic examination findings in a postmenopausal woman once other causes of vaginitis have been excluded.

Vulvovaginitis may be caused by a reaction to irritant or allergen exposure. Triggers can include latex (used in condoms), spermicides, and chemicals in sanitary pads or toilet paper. This is also a diagnosis of exclusion. In unclear cases, referral to an allergist for patch testing may be helpful.

Inflammatory conditions are thought to be underdiagnosed and may be responsible for many of the cases of vulvovaginitis that were not previously given a diagnosis. They occur more commonly in individuals who are perimenopausal. The patient has a purulent vaginal discharge with vulvovaginal erythema or rash, and microscopy characteristically demonstrates many white blood cells. The etiology is thought to be autoimmune.

Figure 2 Candidal pseudohyphae on potassium hydroxide microscopy. (From Herran CP, Nucci MR. Gynecologic Pathology: A Volume in the Series Foundations in Diagnostic Pathology. 2nd ed. Elsevier; 2021.)

Figure 3 *Trichomonas* on saline microscopy. (From Mandell GL, Bennett JE, Dolin R. *Principles and Practice of Infectious Diseases*. 7th ed. Churchill Livingstone Elsevier; 2010.)

TABLE 3	Treatment of Bacterial Vaginosis
Initial regimens	Metronidazole (Flagyl)[1] 500 mg PO twice daily for 7 days OR metronidazole 0.75% gel (MetroGel), one full applicator (5 g) intravaginally daily for 5 days OR clindamycin 2% cream (Cleocin), one full applicator (5 g) intravaginally at bedtime for 7 days
Alternative regimens	Secnidazole (Solosec) 2 g PO once Tinidazole (Tindamax) 2 g PO daily for 2 days OR Tinidazole 1 g PO once daily for 5 days OR clindamycin[1] 300 mg PO bid for 7 days OR clindamycin ovules 100 mg intravaginally at bedtime for 3 days
Pregnancy	Either oral or vaginal regimens suggested in initial treatment section
Treatment of recurrence	First recurrence: retrial of same regimen or trial of alternative initial regimen Multiple recurrences: metronidazole 0.75% gel, intravaginally twice weekly for 4–6 months[3]

[1]Not FDA approved for this indication.
[3]Exceeds dosage recommended by the manufacturer.
PO, Orally.

Treatment

Bacterial Vaginosis

Treatment of BV is recommended to alleviate symptoms but may also be helpful in reducing susceptibility to other sexually transmitted diseases including HIV and those caused by *Chlamydia trachomatis, Neisseria gonorrhoeae,* and *Trichomonas vaginalis.* Treatment also reduces the risk of recurrence. Additionally, in pregnant people, treatment has been associated with potential decreases in adverse outcomes including late miscarriages and poor neonatal outcomes, although it may not have a significant effect on the prevention of preterm labor, as may have been thought in the past. Treatment is recommended for all people who are symptomatic. Both initial oral and topical therapies are acceptable treatments in pregnancy.

Initial and alternative treatment regimens are presented in Table 3; considerations in choosing regimens include patient preference and cost. Of note, secnidazole (Solosec) is a newer oral agent that provides for one-time dosing; however, it may be cost-prohibitive for patients. The Centers for Disease Control and Prevention (CDC) no longer recommends avoidance of alcohol while patients are taking oral metronidazole. The previous warning was based on laboratory experiments and not on clinical data. Patients should also be counseled that oil-based topical therapies including clindamycin may weaken latex condoms or diaphragms. Additionally, to prevent recurrent infection, patients should be counseled to avoid sexual intercourse until after completion of therapy and to avoid douching.

Vulvovaginal Candidiasis

The rationale for the treatment of VVC is relief of symptoms. Treatment regimens for VVC are listed in Table 4 for initial treatment and treatment of recurrence. In nonpregnant patients, the choice between oral and topical azoles can be based on patient preference. Those patients who are prescribed topical therapies should be counseled that topical azole preparations may be oil based and can weaken latex condoms. Topical therapies may cause local irritation or hypersensitivity reactions, although systemic effects are not of concern. Oral azoles can cause nausea, abdominal pain, headache, and rarely elevations in liver function tests. For pregnant patients, only topical therapies should be prescribed.

TABLE 4	Treatment of Vulvovaginal Candidiasis
Initial regimens	*Topical azole therapy:* clotrimazole (Gyne-Lotrimin) 1% cream 5 g intravaginally daily for 7–14 days OR clotrimazole 2% cream 5 g intravaginally daily for 3 days OR miconazole 2% cream 5 g intravaginally daily for 7 days OR miconazole 4% cream 5 g intravaginally daily for 3 days OR miconazole 100 mg vaginal suppository, one suppository daily for 7 days OR miconazole 200 mg vaginal suppository, one suppository for 3 days OR miconazole 1200 mg vaginal suppository, one suppository for 1 day OR tioconazole (Monistat 1-Day) 6.5% ointment 5 g intravaginally in a single application *Prescription intravaginal agents:* Butoconazole (Gynazole–1) 2% cream (single-dose bioadhesive product), 5 g intravaginally in a single application OR terconazole (Terazol 7) 0.4% cream 5 g intravaginally daily for 7 days OR terconazole (Terazol 3) 0.8% cream 5 g intravaginally daily for 3 days OR terconazole 80 mg vaginal suppository, one suppository daily for 3 days OR fluconazole (Diflucan) 150 mg PO once
Alternative regimens	N/A
Pregnancy	Topical azole therapy applied intravaginally for 7 days
Treatment of recurrence	Topical azole therapy for 7–14 days OR fluconazole 150 mg every 3 day for three doses[3] *For maintenance:* oral fluconazole (100, 150, or 200 mg) weekly for 6 months[3]; consider topical treatment if oral is not feasible

[3]Exceeds dosage recommended by the manufacturer.

For those with severe VVC or with immunocompromise, longer treatment may be necessary, such as a 7- to 14-day course.

For recurrent VVC (four or more episodes within a year), longer duration of initial therapy followed by maintenance therapy is recommended. Non*albicans* VVC should also be considered and appropriate diagnostic testing performed to guide treatment, which may include a 7- to 14-day course of an azole topical or oral regimen (other than fluconazole [Diflucan]) and potentially a 2-week course of treatment with boric acid[1] if recurrent.

Trichomonas

The rationale for the treatment of *Trichomonas* infection includes a decrease of symptoms and reduced transmission to sexual partners. *Trichomonas* infection in pregnant patients is associated with adverse outcomes including preterm birth and low-birth-weight infants; however, treatment has not shown a definite reduction in these outcomes. For patients with HIV, *Trichomonas* infection is associated with pelvic inflammatory disease; thus screening and treatment can help prevent this complication. Regimens for initial therapy and treatment of recurrence are listed in Table 5. The CDC no longer recommends single-dose treatment for *Trichomonas* infection for vaginitis; a 7-day course has been shown to be more effective.

Persistent or recurrent *Trichomonas* infection is often caused by reinfection. When patients are being counseled about treatment, they should be advised to avoid intercourse until treatment is completed, symptoms have resolved, and partners have

[1]Not FDA approved for this indication.

TABLE 5 Treatment of Trichomonas Infection

Initial regimens	For vaginitis: metronidazole (Flagyl) 500 mg PO twice daily for 7 days For urethritis: metronidazole 2 g PO in a single dose
Alternative regimens	Tinidazole 2 g PO in a single dose
Pregnancy	Metronidazole 500 mg PO twice daily for 7 days
Treatment of recurrence	Trial of metronidazole, 500 mg twice daily for 7 days *If metronidazole 500 mg twice daily for 7 days fails:* trial of metronidazole, 2 g daily for 7 days *If above regimens fail:* susceptibility testing considered (contact Centers for Disease Control and Prevention)

PO, Orally.

been treated. All patients diagnosed with *Trichomonas* should be asked to inform partners of the need for presumptive treatment. Additionally, patients should be retested within 3 months of diagnosis to ensure adequate treatment and address potential reinfection. In cases in which treatment-resistant infection is suspected, a 1-week regimen should be attempted. If the infection still persists, further testing should be implemented according to guidance from the CDC.

Noninfectious Vaginitis

Treatment of GSM includes low-dose vaginal estrogen therapy or topical lubricant therapy for less severe symptoms. Inflammatory vaginitis is still not well understood, although long-term maintenance therapy with topical clindamycin[1] or steroids may be helpful.

---

[1]Not FDA approved for this indication.

References

American College of Obstetricians and Gynecologists: Vaginitis in nonpregnant patients. ACOG Practice Bulletin No. 215, *Obstet Gynecol* 135:e1–e17, 2020.

Anderson MR, Klink K, Cohrssen A: Evaluation of vaginal complaints, *JAMA* 291(11):1368–1379, 2004.

Centers for Disease Control and Prevention: Sexually Transmitted Diseases Treatment Guidelines, *MMWR Recomm Rep* 70(4):1–187, 2021.

Rahn DD, Carberry C, Sanses TV, et al: Vaginal estrogen for genitourinary syndrome of menopause: a systematic review, *Obstetr Gynecol* 124(6):1147, 2014.

Reichman O: Sobel J: Desquamative inflammatory vaginitis, *Best Prac Res Clin Obstetr Gynaecol* 28(7):1042–1050, 2014.

Sobel JD: Recurrent vulvovaginal candidiasis, *AJOG* 214(1):15–21, 2016.

18 Pregnancy and Antepartum Care

ANTEPARTUM CARE

Method of
Matthew K. Cline, MD; and Natawadee Young, MD

CURRENT DIAGNOSIS

- Pregnancy evaluation should begin 3 to 6 months before conception with optimization of underlying medical conditions, update of immunizations, and commencement of prenatal vitamins with 400 μg of folic acid.[1]
- Preconception counseling with a specialist in high-risk pregnancies should be considered in all patients with underlying medical conditions, such as diabetes and hypertension.
- Early ultrasound (< 13 weeks) assists with establishment of accurate estimated date of confinement and is an essential task in the first prenatal visit.
- The first prenatal visit should include a review of the medical and obstetric histories, current medications, allergies, herbal remedies, supplements, and tobacco, alcohol, and drug use.
- Prenatal laboratory studies should be done at the first visit after a pregnancy is confirmed with a urine pregnancy test. These studies include hemoglobin, platelet count, blood and Rh type and antibody screening, rubella status, hepatitis B and C screening, syphilis screen, and a urine culture. All women should be screened for HIV. High-risk patients should be screened for gonorrhea and chlamydia.
- Genetic screening should be offered based on ethnic history.
- Offer aneuploidy screening to all women in the first trimester along with counseling about risks and benefits. These tests aid in diagnosis of chromosome abnormalities. If a patient opts for a first-trimester screen, it is important to perform an alpha-fetoprotein (AFP) screen in the second trimester to screen for neural tube defects. All women should be offered amniocentesis or chorionic villous sampling for genetic testing with appropriate counseling.
- Appropriate weight gain in pregnancy depends on maternal body mass index (BMI) before pregnancy. In patients with a normal BMI, a 25- to 30-pound weight gain is recommended. Underweight patients are encouraged to gain 30 to 35 pounds, and overweight patients are encouraged to gain no more than 20 pounds.
- Prenatal visits should begin at 8 to 12 weeks' gestation and continue monthly until 28 weeks. Visits should then be every 2 weeks until 36 weeks and then weekly. Each visit should include assessment of maternal weight, blood pressure (BP), fundal height measurement, documentation of fetal heart tones, and review of symptoms of preterm labor and preeclampsia.
- All patients should undergo a glucose challenge test at 24 to 28 weeks. This is done nonfasting by administering a 50-g load of glucose and obtaining a serum sample 1 hour after administration. A level greater than 140 mg/dL is considered abnormal, and a 3-hour glucose tolerance test is indicated (which is done after a 12-hour fast with a 100-g oral glucose load). If a woman demonstrates abnormalities in two of the four values, gestational diabetes is diagnosed.

[1]Not FDA approved for this indication.

CURRENT THERAPY

- Administration of the inactivated influenza vaccine (Fluzone, FluLaval, Fluarix) is recommended in all pregnant patients, regardless of trimester, who will be pregnant (or up to 3 months postpartum) during the flu season.
- Additionally, administer Tdap vaccine (Adacel, Boostrix) in each pregnancy given between 27 and 36 weeks or immediately postpartum in order to decrease rates of pertussis in this age group.
- Vaccination during pregnancy for protection against Covid-19 is a rapidly changing area of preventive therapy. The most updated recommendations can be accessed at the CDC website at https://www.cdc.gov/coronavirus/2019-ncov/vaccines/recommendations/pregnancy.html.
- Folic acid supplementation[1] should begin before conception. The recommended dose is 400 μg daily and is usually given as a prenatal vitamin. In patients with a previous pregnancy complicated by a neural tube defect, 4 mg daily[3] is recommended to decrease the chance of recurrence of a neural tube defect.
- All patients with HIV should be treated with appropriate HAART (highly active anti-retroviral therapy) for the patient and her HIV viral type throughout the pregnancy.
- Intrapartum zidovudine (Retrovir) is recommended for all patients with HIV whose HIV RNA load is ≥ 50 copies/ml or who have concerns with adherence to HAART therapy. Consideration of cesarean delivery is appropriate based on viral load evaluation.

[1]Not FDA approved for this indication.
[3]Exceeds dosage recommended by the manufacturer.

Antepartum Care

Ideally, antepartum care commences 3 to 6 months before conception with the recommendation that women who are sexually active and not using contraception should begin taking daily multivitamin or folic acid supplements. The most convincing trials of this were performed in Europe and China when it was concluded that women of reproductive age should take multivitamin supplements containing 0.4 mg of folate daily to reduce the incidence of neural tube defects. Women with histories of children with neural tube defects or other anomalies should increase this dose to 4 mg[3] of folate in the periconceptional period to reduce risks of recurrence.

Preconception counseling should also include an accurate assessment of preexisting maternal medical conditions. This is the ideal time to stress changes in factors that respond to early intervention: quitting smoking, refraining from alcohol or drug abuse, treating gum disease, and avoiding teratogens. Alcohol is a known teratogen. Immunization status should be reviewed and vaccines should be administered as appropriate. Special consideration is given to patients with thyroid disease. Concern focuses on associations with low intelligence quotients (IQs) in children conceived by hypothyroid mothers. Patients with diabetes should

[3]Exceeds dosage recommended by the manufacturer.

False-positive nonreactive tracings are more common before 28 weeks' gestation.

Biophysical Profile

The biophysical profile (BPP) consists of an NST with ultrasound observations. A total of 10 points is given for the following elements (2 points each):
- Reactive NST
- Presence of fetal breathing movements of 30 seconds or more in 30 minutes
- Fetal movement defined as three or more discrete body or limb movements within 30 minutes
- Fetal tone defined as one or more episodes of fetal extremity extension and return to flexion
- Quantification of amniotic fluid volume, defined as a pocket of fluid that measures at least 2 cm by 2 cm

The results of a BPP are usually reported out of 8 points if done without the NST, and out of 10 points if done with an NST. Scores of 8 or 10 points (out of 10) are considered reassuring, with retesting indicated in 4 to 7 days depending on the original indication for the testing. A score of 6 points is borderline; testing should be repeated in 24 hours. Scores of 4 or 2 points are nonreassuring and should prompt additional testing, treatment, or planning for delivery depending on the setting.

References

ACOG Committee Opinion No: 743. Low-dose aspirin use during pregnancy, *Obstet Gynecol* 132(1):44–52, 2018.

ACOG Committee Opinion No: 797. Prevention of group B streptococcal early-onset disease in newborns, *Obstet Gynecol* 35(2):51–72, 2020.

ACOG Practice Advisory: COVID-19 Vaccination Considerations for Obstetric-Gynecologic Care. Last updated Jan. 26, 2023 [Accessed March 3, 2023]

American College of Obstetricians and Gynecologists: *Compendium of selected publications*, Atlanta, 2012, American College of Obstetricians and Gynecologists.

American College of Obstetricians and Gynecologists: Screening for fetal aneuploidy. Practice Bulletin 163, *Obstet Gynecol* 127(5):e123–e137, 2016.

Centers for Disease Control and Prevention: Guidelines for Vaccination Pregnant Women. Available at: https://www.cdc.gov/vaccines/pregnancy/hcp-toolkit/guidelines.html. [accessed March 3, 2023].

Centers for Disease Control and Prevention: COVID-19 Vaccines While Pregnant or Breastfeeding. Available at: https://www.cdc.gov/coronavirus/2019-ncov/vaccines/recommendations/pregnancy.html. [accessed March. 3, 2023].

Centers for Disease Control and Prevention: Sexually Transmitted Infections Treatment Guidelines 2021. Available at: https://www.cdc.gov/std/treatment-guidelines/toc.htm. [accessed March 3, 2023].

Committee Opinion No: 711. Opioid use and opioid use disorder in pregnancy, *Obstet Gynecol* 130(2):81–94, 2017.

McParlin C, O'Donnell A, Robson SC, et al: Treatments for hyperemesis gravidarum and nausea and vomiting in pregnancy: a systematic review, *JAMA* 316(13):1392–1401, 2016.

Middleton P, Shepherd E, Crowther CA: Induction of labour for improving birth outcomes for women at or beyond term, *Cochrane Database of Systematic Reviews* 5:CD004945, 2017, https://doi.org/10.1002/14651858, CD004945.pub4.

Nelson HD, Bougatsos C, Blazina I: Screening women for intimate partner violence: a systematic review to update the U.S. Preventive Services Task Force Recommendation, *Ann Intern Med* 156:796–808, 2012, W279–82.

Zolotor A, Carlough M: Update on prenatal care, *Am Fam Physician* 89(3):199–208, 2014.

ECTOPIC PREGNANCY

Method of
Christina M. Kelly, MD

CURRENT DIAGNOSIS

- Vaginal bleeding and abdominal pain in the first trimester of pregnancy raise concern for ectopic pregnancy, but a normal intrauterine pregnancy (IUP) or early pregnancy loss (EPL) could exist.
- High-resolution transvaginal ultrasound (TVUS) and measurement of serum β–human chorionic gonadotropin (hCG) are the best initial steps in determining whether a pregnancy is ectopic.

- A single hCG value is not diagnostic of pregnancy location, viability, or gestational age. It can determine whether the level is in the discriminatory zone.
- If the hCG is above the discriminatory zone (3000–3500 mIU/mL), absence of a gestational sac with a yolk sac or embryo visualized in the uterus is highly suggestive of a nonviable gestation, either an early pregnancy loss or an ectopic pregnancy.
- If the initial hCG is below the discriminatory zone and there is no ultrasound evidence of ectopic pregnancy, patients should be followed up with repeat hCG levels every 48 hours. There is no universal method to predict an expected minimal rise for serial hCG levels for a viable IUP. Rather, it is dependent on the initial hCG level. Updated guidelines about the appropriate hCG patterns help guide decision making and determine whether additional diagnostic interventions are needed.
- If definitive findings of an intrauterine or ectopic pregnancy are not present on TVUS in a pregnant patient with a positive hCG level, a pregnancy of unknown location exists. Serial monitoring is needed to either establish a definitive diagnosis or reasonably exclude an IUP before an ectopic pregnancy is diagnosed and treated. Uterine aspiration can be considered to confirm the diagnosis of early pregnancy loss or ectopic pregnancy based on the presence or absence of chorionic villi.

CURRENT THERAPY

- Surgical management of ectopic pregnancy is indicated when a patient is hemodynamically unstable, exhibits signs of intraperitoneal bleeding, reports symptoms concerning for a ruptured ectopic mass, or has a contraindication to methotrexate.
- For a patient who is clinically stable and has a nonruptured ectopic pregnancy, either surgical or medical management of ectopic pregnancy are safe and effective options. A shared decision-making model can be used to help patients make informed decisions, which reviews the risks and benefits of both approaches and considers the clinical features of the ectopic pregnancy, stability of the patient, future fertility plans, and additional patient characteristics that would preclude one approach or the other.
- Medical management with systemic methotrexate (not approved by the Food and Drug Administration) requires regular patient follow-up for laboratory and office visits until hCG levels are undetectable.
- Medical management with methotrexate is most effective when ectopic pregnancies are less than 4 cm on TVUS, pretreatment hCG levels are less than 5000 mIU/mL, and fetal cardiac activity is not detected on TVUS.
- Expectant management of ectopic pregnancy may be considered in special circumstances, such as an asymptomatic and informed patient with reliable social resources in the setting of decreasing hCG levels that indicate pregnancy resolution.

An ectopic pregnancy is a potentially serious threat to the general and reproductive health of a pregnant person. Despite vast improvements in the clinical care of patients with ectopic pregnancy over recent years, diagnostic challenges and therapeutic controversies regarding this condition still exist. The objective of this chapter is to provide an overview of the epidemiology, diagnosis, and contemporary management of ectopic pregnancy. The chapter focuses on ectopic pregnancies that implant in the fallopian tube, which represent greater than 95% of all ectopic pregnancies.

Epidemiology

Of all pregnancies in the United States, approximately 1% to 2% are diagnosed as ectopic. Ectopic pregnancy incidence is difficult to calculate accurately due to insufficient hospital and outpatient data tracking, but recent studies estimate that over the last 25 years, it has increased sixfold. This rise may be the result of enhanced diagnostic capabilities, increased incidence of sexually transmitted infections and other risk factors, expanded use of infertility treatments, and heightened awareness of health professionals.

Ectopic pregnancy is the leading cause of maternal mortality in the first trimester of pregnancy in the United States, accounting for 2.7% of pregnancy-related deaths, and there should be continued high suspicion for at risk patients. However, the ectopic-related mortality rate is declining despite the increase in incidence. Between 1980 and 2007, 876 deaths were attributed to ectopic pregnancy, which represented a 56.6% decline in mortality rate between 1980 to 1984 and 2003 to 2007. However, age and racial disparities still persist. The ectopic pregnancy mortality ratio was 6.8 times higher for Black people compared with whites and 3.5 times higher for patients over 35 years old compared with those younger than 25 years old.

Pathophysiology
Damage to the fallopian tube and fallopian tube dysfunction are the primary factors associated with development of ectopic pregnancy. Normal embryo transport can be disrupted by damage to the structural integrity of the mucosal portion of the fallopian tube. Intratubal scarring secondary to infection or trauma could lead to trapping of a conceptus within intratubal adhesions or diverticula. Alteration of the hormonally mediated events leading to implantation, which can occur during infertility treatments, offers another mechanism for consideration. A change in the estrogen-to-progesterone ratio could theoretically affect smooth muscle activity in the fallopian tube, immobilizing ciliary activity.

Risk Factors
Half of all patients with ectopic pregnancy will not report any known risk factors; therefore the absence of risk factors should not decrease clinical suspicion. However, identification of clinical and historical risk factors for ectopic pregnancy could aid in early diagnosis. The most significant historical risk factors include prior ectopic pregnancy, prior fallopian tube surgery, infertility treatment, and hospitalization for pelvic inflammatory disease (PID). History of prior ectopic pregnancy is the strongest of these. Major clinical risk factors include pain or moderate-to-severe vaginal bleeding at presentation. Less significant risk factors are tobacco use and age >35 years old. Up to 53% of pregnancies that occur with a copper or progestin-releasing intrauterine device (IUD) in place are ectopic; however, the overall failure rate of IUDs is less than 1%.

Diagnosis and Clinical Manifestations
Although some patients present acutely with a ruptured ectopic pregnancy and hemoperitoneum, the vast majority (up to 80%) of ectopic pregnancies are diagnosed in stable patients who can be managed in the outpatient setting. Therefore reproductive-age people who present with symptoms of vaginal bleeding or abdominal discomfort need to be tested for pregnancy. If a patient is found to be pregnant, then their pregnancy needs to be differentiated as an ectopic pregnancy, an intrauterine gestation at risk for EPL, or a normally developing IUP. The use of TVUS and hCG assays represent the current standard for this differentiation and for accurate and timely diagnosis of ectopic pregnancy.

Transvaginal Ultrasonography
Proper evaluation of a patient with suspected ectopic pregnancy with TVUS requires an understanding of the typical findings for normal and abnormal pregnancies. The earliest ultrasonographic finding of a normal IUP is the gestational sac surrounded by a thick echogenic ring, located eccentrically within the endometrial cavity. On average, the gestational sac is seen on TVUS 5 weeks after the first day of the last menstrual period. The gestational sac grows and follows an approximate developmental timeline, which is represented by the following findings on TVUS: a yolk sac seen within the

gestational sac at 5.5 weeks of gestation, an embryonic (fetal) pole at 6 weeks gestation, and cardiac activity at 6.5 weeks gestation.

A definitive IUP can be diagnosed by TVUS when a gestational sac with a yolk sac or embryo with or without cardiac activity is seen. A normal-appearing gestational sac should not solely be used to diagnose an IUP because it can be simulated by a pseudo- gestational sac, which occurs in 8% to 29% of patients with ectopic pregnancy. The pseudogestational sac likely represents bleeding into the endometrial cavity by the decidual cast. The presence of an adnexal gestational sac with a fetal pole and cardiac activity is the most specific but least sensitive sign of ectopic pregnancy, occurring in only 10% to 17% of cases. Adnexal rings (fluid sacs with thick echogenic rings) that have a yolk sac or nonliving embryo are accepted as specific signs of ectopic pregnancy and are visualized in ectopic pregnancies 33% to 50% of the time.

A critical concept in the evaluation of early pregnancy by TVUS is that of the hCG discriminatory zone—the level at or above which an examiner should see a normal intrauterine gestation, if present. In the setting of an hCG level above the discriminatory zone and no IUP on ultrasound, an ectopic pregnancy or an abnormal intrauterine pregnancy is highly likely. The exact hCG discriminatory value varies based on the institution, ultrasound machine, ultrasonographer's experience, and hCG assay used. The value used should be conservatively high—at least 3000 mIU/mL and up to 3500 mIU/mL—to minimize the risk of misdiagnosing a desired IUP as an ectopic pregnancy and treating it as such.

Hormonal Assays
Many patients with suspected ectopic pregnancy will present with a pregnancy of unknown location (PUL), where a hCG is below the discriminatory zone and a TVUS does not definitively diagnosis an intrauterine or extrauterine gestation (7%–20%). Serial monitoring is needed for PUL to establish a definitive diagnosis. Repeat hCG measurements are indicated at least every 48 hours to evaluate the appropriateness of hormonal trends along with serial TVUS studies. Comparing serial measurements of hCG from an individual patient to accepted patterns of hCG trends in early pregnancy helps distinguish an ectopic pregnancy from a viable IUP or a spontaneous EPL.

When evaluating serial hCG levels and predicting an expected minimal rise between values for a viable IUP, current evidence demonstrates there is not a universal trend that applies to all pregnancies at all gestations. Rather, it depends on the initial hCG level. Previous data showed that approximately 99% of viable intrauterine pregnancies are associated with a ≥53% increase in β-hCG values every 2 days. For pregnancies with an initial hCG value below 1500 mIU/mL, this calculation could apply. However, for pregnancies with higher initial hCG values, a laxer calculation should be used. One study suggests the following for an expected minimal rise for different initial hCG levels: 49% for levels <1500 mIU/mL, 40% for levels 1500 to 3000 mIU/mL, and 33% for levels >3000 mIU/mL. This represents a more conservative approach to incorporating invasive diagnostic procedures when following hCG values and preventing the interruption of normal IUPs.

Patients with symptomatic first-trimester pregnancies, nondiagnostic ultrasound, and a hCG level that is declining (when the initial value is below the discriminatory zone) should also be followed with serial hCG levels until resolution to distinguish a resolving EPL from an ectopic pregnancy. Fifty percent of patients with ectopic pregnancies will present with declining hCG levels. Research describing the expected elimination of hCG in spontaneous EPL indicate that the minimum rate of decline ranges from 12% to 35% at 2 days to 34% to 84% at 7 days. Faster rates of decline occur with higher initial hCG levels. When the serial decline in hCG is in the range associated with spontaneous EPL, continued surveillance is indicated. If the hCG decline is slower than expected for an EPL, an ectopic pregnancy must be highly suspected.

Uterine Aspiration
The patient presenting with either (1) initial hCG below the discriminatory zone followed by an abnormal rise or decline or (2)

initial hCG value at or above the discriminatory zone with no detectable IUP has an abnormal pregnancy. The only exception to the rule for the second scenario would be if a multiple gestation had been conceived. The challenge for the clinician is then to determine whether the pregnancy is nonviable IUP or an ectopic pregnancy. Office uterine vacuum aspiration or dilation and curettage in the operating room can help confirm the diagnosis of EPL or ectopic pregnancy based on the presence or absence of chorionic villi. However, before this is considered, a progressing IUP must be reasonably excluded through serial monitoring with TVUS and hCG levels.

Uterine aspiration may spare some patients from receiving methotrexate[1]. If chorionic villi are present in the uterine aspiration specimen, then a failed IUP is confirmed. No further treatment is indicated. If chorionic villi are absent, hCG levels need to be monitored starting at 12 to 24 hours after the procedure to determine whether they increase, plateau, or decrease appropriately. The hCG trend after uterine aspiration determines whether medical management of ectopic pregnancy with methotrexate should be implemented. The patient's preference, presence of symptoms, and level of clinical suspicion for ectopic pregnancy also play an important role in whether methotrexate is indicated.

There is debate in the literature on whether uterine aspiration is needed before methotrexate is given to treat ectopic pregnancy. Empiric treatment of suspected ectopic pregnancy without the performance of uterine vacuum aspiration or dilation and curettage could result in inappropriate treatment of up to 40% of patients. Performing uterine aspiration could delay treatment of an ectopic pregnancy; however, the risk of tubal rupture for these patients is low (1.7%).

Treatment and Therapeutic Monitoring

Surgery has long been the mainstay of treatment for ectopic pregnancy, but medical management is a widely used alternative. Both are safe and effective treatment options for patients who are clinically stable. The choice of any treatment depends on factors such as clinical presentation, the risks of either surgery or medical management to the patient, and future fertility plans.

Surgical Management

Patients with hemodynamic instability caused by a ruptured ectopic pregnancy require laparotomy and salpingectomy of the involved fallopian tube due to extensive tubal damage. Most patients with ectopic pregnancy who are stable can be safely treated with laparoscopy. For patients with an unruptured ectopic pregnancy, surgical options include tube-sparing salpingostomy or removal of the fallopian tube (salpingectomy).

The decision between salpingostomy and salpingectomy depends on the location of the ectopic pregnancy within the fallopian tube, the extent of the damage to the fallopian tube, and the patient's desire for future fertility. Ideal candidates for salpingostomy include patients who have an ectopic pregnancy in the ampulla or infundibulum of the fallopian tube. Salpingectomy is reserved for patients with isthmic ectopic pregnancies, tubal rupture, or an ipsilateral recurrent ectopic pregnancy. Patients who have completed childbearing might be better candidates for salpingectomy than salpingostomy.

With respect to future fertility, subsequent IUP, and repeat ectopic pregnancy, a systematic review and meta-analysis of two randomized controlled trials (RCT) and 16 cohort studies showed that for the RCTs, there was no difference between salpingectomy and salpingostomy. For the cohort studies, salpingectomy was associated with a lower likelihood of subsequent IUP. The cohort studies also found a higher risk for repeat ectopic pregnancy among pregnant people treated by salpingectomy with risk factors for future infertility (previous ectopic pregnancy, endometriosis, history of infertility, history of tubal surgery, pregnancy conceived with in-vitro fertilization, known hydrosalpinx or

tubal occlusion, or intraoperative identification of contralateral tubal pathology).

Medical Management

Methotrexate (MTX) is a folic acid antagonist that impairs DNA synthesis and cellular replication targeting rapidly proliferating cells such as trophoblasts. It can be used for medical management of ectopic pregnancy[1] in patients who have a confirmed or high clinical suspicion of ectopic pregnancy, an unruptured mass, and no contraindication to the medication.

Absolute contraindications to medical management of ectopic pregnancy are listed in Table 1. Among the most important of these is the inability of the patient to comply with follow-up after initiation of therapy. Without the ability to monitor the response to MTX and provide additional doses if deemed appropriate, opportunities to prevent ectopic rupture could be missed. To ascertain whether a patient is eligible for MTX therapy, a comprehensive laboratory and medical evaluation should first be performed, including a complete blood count and renal and liver function tests. Treatment failure occurs when the hCG level decline is deemed inadequate and surgery is required. In some cases, medication failure presents as tubal rupture requiring emergent surgery.

Relative contraindications in Table 1 pertain to patient characteristics that reduce the odds of successful treatment. The strongest predictor for the efficacy of MTX treatment is an initial hCG concentration >5000 mIU/mL, and it is associated with a failure rate of at least 14.3%.

Three methotrexate treatment regimens exist: single-dose, two-dose, and multidose regimens (Table 2). These designations refer more to the number of intended doses in the protocol rather than the actual number of doses received by all patients. For any of the protocols, once hCG levels have declined by at least 15% between interval assessments, no additional doses of medication are required, but hCG must still be followed until complete resolution to ensure treatment efficacy. A systematic review and meta-analysis of six RCTs demonstrated that the single-dose and multiple-dose regimens have similar success rates, and the difference between the single-dose and double-dose regimens was not statistically significant. More side effects occurred with the multiple-dose regimen compared with single-dose and double-dose. The definition of successful treatment with MTX is resolution of the ectopic pregnancy without surgery, and the success rate ranges from 70% to 95% depending on the initial hCG level and treatment protocol.

TABLE 1	Contraindications to Medical Management of Ectopic Pregnancy With Methotrexate
Absolute contraindications	Intrauterine pregnancy; breastfeeding; laboratory evidence of immunodeficiency; preexisting blood dyscrasias (bone marrow hypoplasia, leukopenia, thrombocytopenia, or clinically significant anemia); known sensitivity to methotrexate; active pulmonary disease; peptic ulcer disease; clinically significant hepatic, renal, or hematologic dysfunction; hemodynamically unstable patient; inability to participate in follow-up*
Relative contraindications	Ectopic mass >4 cm by TVUS; embryonic cardiac activity by TVUS; high initial hCG concentration (>5,000 mIU/mL); refusal to accept blood transfusion

TVUS, transvaginal ultrasound; hCG, β–human chorionic gonadotropin.
Data are from the American College of Obstetricians and Gynecologists (ACOG).
*A committee opinion published by the American Society for Reproductive Medicine (ASRM) has the same contraindications listed, but the inability to participate in follow-up is listed as a relative contraindication.

---

[1] Not FDA approved for this indication.

[1] Not FDA approved for this indication.

	SINGLE DOSE	TWO DOSE	MULTIDOSE
Day 1	Check hCG value. Administer first dose of MTX 50 mg/m² IM.	Check hCG value. Administer first dose of MTX 50 mg/m² IM.	Check hCG value. Administer first dose of MTX 1 mg/kg IM followed by folinic acid (leucovorin)[1] 0.1 mg/kg IM on day 2. Check hCG on day 2.
Day 4	Check hCG value.	Check hCG value. Administer second dose of MTX 50 mg/m² IM.	Administer second dose of MTX (day 3) and folinic acid (day 4). Administer third dose of MTX (day 5). Check hCG on day 3 and 5.
Day 7	Check hCG value looking for 15% decrease between days 4 and 7. If >15% fall, check hCG weekly until undetectable. If <15% fall, administer second dose of MTX 50 mg/m² IM.	Check hCG value for 15% decrease between days 4 and 7. If >15% fall, check hCG weekly until undetectable. If <15% fall, administer third dose of MTX 50 mg/m² IM.	Continue administering alternating doses of MTX and folinic acid until hCG values decline by 15%. Do not exceed 4 doses. If >15% decline, check hCG weekly until undetectable.
Day 11		Check hCG value for 15% decrease between days 7 and 11. If >15% decline, check hCG weekly until not detectable in serum. If <15%, administer fourth dose of MTX 50 mg/m² IM.	
Weekly surveillance	If follow-up hCG value plateau or rise, consider surgical intervention or repeat dose of MTX as additional therapy.	If follow-up hCG value plateau or rise, consider surgical intervention or repeat dose of MTX as additional therapy.	If follow-up hCG value plateau or rise, consider surgical intervention or repeat dose of MTX as additional therapy.

hCG, β–Human chorionic gonadotropin; IM, intramuscular; MTX, methotrexate.
[1]Not FDA approved for this indication.

The biggest risk of medical management with MTX is ectopic pregnancy rupture. Additional risks include fetal death or teratogenic effects if an IUP occurs shortly after treatment, and patients should be counseled to wait one ovulatory cycle after hCG levels are undetectable before attempting pregnancy again.

Side effects of MTX therapy occur in up to 30% of patients; however, most resolve rapidly and are mild. Abdominal pain is common early in treatment, possibly due to tubal miscarriage, but it can also be a sign of tubal rupture. Additional potential side effects include nausea, vomiting, diarrhea, gastritis, stomatitis, and liver transaminitis. Serious side effects such as alopecia and neutropenia can occur but are extremely rare.

Reproductive success after successful MTX therapy appears similar to that after salpingostomy. The most critical predictors of fertility after ectopic pregnancy treated by any conservative means are the condition of the contralateral fallopian tube and the presence of additional ectopic risk factors.

Expectant Management

Because numerous ectopic pregnancies resolve spontaneously, there has been great interest in considering expectant management in patients who are asymptomatic, have a plateau or decreasing hCG level, and are willing to accept the risks (spontaneous rupture, hemorrhage, and need for emergency surgery). A systematic review and meta-analysis of four RCTs showed no statistically significant difference between expectant management and MTX for these selected patients when the hCG level is less than 2000 IU/L. Expectant management includes close monitoring of symptoms, determination of hCG levels every 48 hours, serial TVUS. Medical or surgical management is indicated if hCG levels do not sufficiently decrease.

Trauma-Informed Care

Being diagnosed with and treated for an ectopic pregnancy is a traumatic event for many patients, and the psychological implications can be overlooked. A multicenter prospective cohort study found patients with an ectopic pregnancy met criteria for posttraumatic stress (23%), moderate to severe anxiety (21%), and moderate to severe depression (7%) one month after their experience. These psychological sequelae declined over time but were still clinically significant at 9 months. A trauma-informed approach can help clinicians be intentional in supporting patients with an ectopic pregnancy during treatment, posttreatment, and with any future pregnancies.

References

ACOG: Practice bulletin No. 193 interim update: tubal ectopic pregnancy, *Obstet Gynecol* 131:e91–e103, 2018.

Barnhart KT, Guo W, Cary MS, et al: Differences in serum human chorionic gonadotropin rise in early pregnancy by race and value at presentation, *Obstet Gynecol* 128:504–511, 2016.

Barnhart K, van Mello NM, Bourne T, et al: Pregnancy of unknown location: a consensus statement of nomenclature, definitions, and outcome, *Fertil Steril* 95:857–866, 2011.

Connolly A, Ryan DH, Stuebe AM, Wolfe HM: Reevaluation of discriminatory and threshold levels for serum beta-hCG in early pregnancy, *Obstet Gynecol* 121:65–70, 2013.

Farren J, Jalmbrant M, Falconieri N, et al: Posttraumatic stress, anxiety and depression following miscarriage and ectopic pregnancy: a multicenter, prospective, cohort study, *Am J Obstet Gynecol* 222(4):367.e1–367.e22, 2020.

Hendriks E, Rosenberg R, Prine L: Ectopic pregnancy: diagnosis and management, *Am Fam Physician* 101(10):599–606, 2020. PMID: 32412215.

Insogna IG, Farland LV, Missmer SA, Ginsburg ES, Brady PC: Outpatient endometrial aspiration: an alternative to methotrexate for pregnancy of unknown location, *Am J Obstet Gynecol* 217:185.e1–185.e9, 2017.

Naveed AK, Anjum MU, Hassan, A, et al: Methotrexate versus expectant management in ectopic pregnancy: a meta-analysis, *Arch Gynecol Obstet* 305(3):547–553, 2022.

Ozcan MCH, Wilson JR, Frishman GN: A systematic review and meta-analysis of surgical treatment of ectopic pregnancy with salpingectomy versus salpingostomy, *J Minim Invasive Gynecol* 28(3):656–667, 2021. https://doi.org/10.1016/j.jmig.2020.10.014. Epub 2020 Oct 24. PMID: 33198948.

Yang C, Cai J, Geng Y, Gao Y: Multiple-dose and double-dose versus single-dose administration of methotrexate for the treatment of ectopic pregnancy: a systematic review and meta-analysis, *Reprod Biomed Online* 34(4):383–391, 2017. https://doi.org/10.1016/j.rbmo.2017.01.004.

HYPERTENSIVE DISORDERS IN PREGNANCY

Method of

Marc Parrish, DO; and Juliana Bakk, MD

CURRENT DIAGNOSIS

- Hypertensive disorders in pregnancy complicate 2% to 8% of pregnancies and are among the leading causes of maternal and perinatal death worldwide.
- Hypertensive disorders are divided into four categories:
  - Chronic hypertension
  - Chronic hypertension with superimposed preeclampsia (with and without severe features)
  - Gestational hypertension
  - Preeclampsia (with and without severe features)
- Preeclampsia can be diagnosed without proteinuria in the presence of end organ damage.

CURRENT THERAPY

- The only current method for prevention of preeclampsia is administration of aspirin[1] (81 mg/day) to patients who are at risk, optimally prior to 16 weeks' gestation.
- The definition for an elevated blood pressure (BP) during pregnancy is either systolic greater than 140 mm Hg or diastolic greater than 90 mm Hg on two occasions more than 4 hours apart. New-onset hypertensive disease of pregnancy requires these elevations occur after 20 weeks' gestation. If they are prior to 20 weeks' gestation, the patient meets the diagnosis of chronic hypertension.
- Two severe-range BP values (≥160/110 mm Hg), taken 15 to 60 minutes apart, constitute a hypertensive emergency and require intravenous (IV) treatment if the patient has new-onset hypertension in pregnancy.
- Patients with chronic hypertension should receive pharmacologic therapy to keep BP less than 140/90 mm/Hg during pregnancy to decrease adverse events, as reported in the Chronic Hypertension and Pregnancy trial.
- Nifedipine and labetalol are the preferred agents for use during pregnancy. Methyldopa can be used but is typically the second-line because of side effects and lower efficacy.
- Patients diagnosed with gestational hypertension or preeclampsia without severe features can be managed closely as outpatients. They require frequent BP and symptom assessments in addition to laboratory monitoring and fetal testing.
- Delivery is the definitive treatment for preeclampsia, but preeclampsia and eclampsia can present after delivery.
- Hypertensive disorders necessitate earlier delivery. Delivery timing is based off of severity of maternal disease and fetal monitoring.
- IV or intramuscular magnesium sulfate is used for treatment of eclampsia and for prevention of eclampsia in patients diagnosed with preeclampsia with severe features.
- Patients with preeclampsia are at risk for developing hypertension and cardiovascular or renal disease later in life.

[1]Not FDA approved for this indication.

Epidemiology

In the United States, 84% of all maternal deaths have been determined to be preventable. In high-income countries, 16% of maternal deaths are attributed to hypertensive disorders. Chronic hypertension complicates approximately 2% of pregnancies, with the incidence increasing each year because of increasing rates

TABLE 1	Risk Factors for Development of Preeclampsia*
High Risk (incidence ≥8%)	
Chronic hypertension	
History of preeclampsia, especially with adverse outcome	
Autoimmune disease (systemic lupus erythematous, antiphospholipid antibody syndrome)	
Kidney disease	
Pregestational type 1 or 2 diabetes	
Multifetal gestation	
Moderate Risk Factors	
Nulliparity	
Obesity (body mass index > 31)	
First-degree family history of preeclampsia	
Black race	
Low socioeconomic status	
Age ≥ 35 years	
In vitro fertilization	
Personal history factors (low birth weight or small for gestational age, previous adverse pregnancy outcome, >10-year pregnancy interval)	

*Low birth weight or small for gestational age, previous adverse pregnancy outcome, >10-year pregnancy interval.

Data from American College of Obstetricians and Gynecologists. Low-dose aspirin use for the prevention of preeclampsia and related morbidity and mortality. Practice Advisory. ACOG; 2021. Accessed August 22, 2023. https://www.acog.org/clinical/clinical-guidance/practice-advisory/articles/2021/12/low-dose-aspirin-use-for-the-prevention-of-preeclampsia-and-related-morbidity-and-mortality

of advanced maternal age pregnancies and obesity. Approximately 20% to 50% of patients with chronic hypertension will develop superimposed preeclampsia, and 75% of patients with end organ disease prior to pregnancy will develop it. Between 2017 and 2019, the rates of hypertensive disorders of pregnancy among delivery hospitalizations increased from 13.3% to 15.9%, according to the Centers for Disease Control and Prevention. Prevalence is highest among non-Hispanic Black women and women 35 years and older.

Pathophysiology

There are many theories about the development of preeclampsia, but the precise mechanism is still unknown. It is believed that uteroplacental ischemia and inappropriate remodeling of the spiral arterioles within the placenta lead to increased circulating concentrations of antiangiogenic factors and angiogenic imbalances. The complex interaction of vasoactive agents, such as prostacyclin, thromboxane A2, nitric oxide, and endothelins, with opposing effects ultimately results in intense vasospasm. Decreased colloid oncotic pressure causes capillary leak, resulting in increased edema and risk of flash pulmonary edema that is often exacerbated by intravenous (IV) fluid therapy.

Prevention

Low-dose aspirin[1] (81 mg/day) is recommended in women with one high risk factor or more than one moderate risk factor. Table 1 highlights these risk factors. This should be initiated between 12 and 28 weeks' gestation, with the best outcomes resulting from initiation prior to 16 weeks. It should be continued daily until delivery. There is currently no consensus on the optimal dosing of aspirin for the prevention of preeclampsia because some trials have demonstrated a larger impact on prevention with higher doses (100–150 mg/day). No trials have evaluated the efficacy of doses greater than 150 mg, but the higher dose

[1]Not FDA approved for this indication.

TABLE 2	Diagnostic Criteria for Preeclampsia
Blood pressure	Systolic BP ≥140 mm Hg or diastolic BP ≥90 mm Hg on two occasions at least 4 hours apart after 20 weeks' gestation with previously normal blood pressures Systolic BP ≥160 mm Hg or diastolic BP ≥110 mm Hg (severe hypertension can be confirmed within minutes to ensure timely treatment)
and	
Proteinuria	≥300 mg per 24-h urine collection Protein/creatinine ratio ≥ 0.3 Dipstick reading of 2+ (used only if other methods are not available)

Or in the absence of proteinuria, new-onset hypertension with new onset of any of the following:

Thrombocytopenia (platelet count < 100 × 10⁹/L)	Pulmonary edema
Elevated transaminases more than twice upper limit of normal	Severe headache unresponsive to medication and not accounted for by other diagnoses
Renal insufficiency (creatinine > 1.1 mg/dL or doubling of baseline concentration)	Visual disturbances

Adapted from *ACOG Practice Bulletin #222: Gestational Hypertension and Preeclampsia.*

TABLE 3	Diagnostic Criteria for Preeclampsia With Severe Features*

Only one criteria is required for diagnosis of severe features as long as it cannot be explained by another cause or diagnosis.

Symptoms	Severe and persistent right upper quadrant pain or epigastric pain unresponsive to medication Severe headache unresponsive to medication Visual disturbances
Laboratory	Thrombocytopenia (platelet count < 100 × 10⁹/L) Elevated transaminases more than twice upper limit of normal Renal insufficiency (creatinine > 1.1 mg/dL or doubling of baseline concentration)
Vitals/Physical Exam	Systolic blood pressure ≥160 mm Hg or diastolic blood pressure ≥110 mm Hg on two occasions 4 hours apart Pulmonary edema

*Of note, fetal growth restriction and significant proteinuria (>5 g/24 h) are no longer considered severe features.

in North America can be achieved by taking two 81-mg tablets daily. The mechanism by which aspirin prevents preeclampsia is not completely understood but is speculated to be due to improvement in the placentation process and antithrombotic/antiinflammatory effect.

A United States Preventive Services Task Force report on low-dose aspirin identified no increased risk of placental abruption, postpartum hemorrhage, mean blood loss, or congenital anomalies. Aspirin should be avoided in patients with known nasal polyps (use may result in life-threatening bronchoconstriction), aspirin-induced bronchospasm, gastrointestinal bleed, active peptic ulcer disease, or hypersensitivity to nonsteroidal antiinflammatory drugs. Bed rest, dietary modification, and salt restriction have been proven not to assist in the prevention of preeclampsia and are therefore not recommended for this purpose.

Diagnosis

Hypertensive disease prior to 20 weeks' gestation or outside of pregnancy is considered *chronic hypertension*. Patients without this diagnosis who present after 20 weeks' gestation with new-onset hypertension, either systolic blood pressure (BP) of 140 mm Hg or greater or diastolic of 90 mm Hg or greater on two occasions more than 4 hours apart, are considered to have *gestational hypertension*.

In 2017, the American College of Cardiology/American Heart Association Hypertension Clinical Practice Guidelines lowered the threshold for diagnosis of stage 1 hypertension outside of pregnancy from 140/90 mm Hg to 130/80 mm Hg. Patients who meet this new definition of hypertension outside of pregnancy should be managed as having chronic hypertension during pregnancy. Observational studies have shown increased risk of adverse pregnancy outcomes with BPs greater than 130/80 mm Hg in early pregnancy with no previous diagnosis of hypertension, but further studies are necessary to lower the threshold for diagnosis of hypertension during pregnancy. A workup for secondary hypertension should be considered when chronic hypertension is refractory to treatment, if it is diagnosed at a young age, or in patients with features favoring secondary hypertension.

Preeclampsia is a disorder that can affect multiple organ systems and can present any time after 20 weeks' gestation, including during the immediate postpartum period. The traditional diagnosis involves new-onset hypertension (as with gestational hypertension), with the additional finding of proteinuria. Clinically significant proteinuria is 300 mg or greater on a 24-hour urine protein collection or a ratio of 0.3 or greater for spot protein/creatinine. The use of a dipstick for diagnosis is discouraged but can be used if neither of the preferred options is available; concerns for preeclampsia are raised if 3+ protein on dipstick is observed. Severity of proteinuria does not typically correlate with worse disease, and serial measurements of proteinuria are therefore not necessary after the diagnosis is made.

It is important to note that some patients can present with signs of end organ damage *without proteinuria* and would thus still meet the diagnosis of preeclampsia. The presence of any severe feature is concerning for severe disease and impending eclampsia. These features include thrombocytopenia, renal insufficiency (serum creatinine > 1.1 mg/dL), impaired liver function (serum aspartate transaminase [AST] and alanine aminotransferase [ALT] double the institutional upper limits of normal), persistent right upper quadrant pain, pulmonary edema, headache unresponsive to medication, or new visual disturbances.

Women with new-onset hypertension in pregnancy who develop severe-range BPs (two BP values ≥160/110 mm Hg taken ≥4 hours apart) should be diagnosed with preeclampsia with severe features. Other criteria for severe features are listed in Table 3. Patients with preeclampsia superimposed on chronic hypertension will meet criteria for severe features with any of these findings as well.

Management
Chronic Hypertension

Chronic hypertension is associated with many complications of pregnancy (fetal growth restriction, placental abruption, medically indicated preterm birth, perinatal death) and is the greatest risk factor for the development of preeclampsia. Patients with chronic hypertension are also at an increased risk for gestational diabetes, pulmonary edema, acute kidney injury, cardiomyopathy or cardiac events, stroke, and maternal mortality. Prior to 2022 treatment of chronic hypertension of pregnancy aimed to keep the blood pressure below 160/100 mm Hg. Studies using lower target blood pressure levels with higher doses and more frequent dosing of antihypertensive medications showed increased rates of fetal growth restriction and a lack of improved maternal outcomes.

The Chronic Hypertension and Pregnancy trial published in 2022 resulted in Society of Maternal-Fetal Medicine and American Congress of Obstetricians and Gynecologists recommending targeting BPs below 140/90 mm Hg during pregnancy. This study

| | | TABLE 4 | Common Dosages for Oral Antihypertensive Agents During Pregnancy | | |

DRUG	DOSE	TYPICAL INITIAL DOSE	TYPICAL MAXIMUM DOSE	CAUTION
Labetalol	200–2,400 mg/d PO, 2–3 times daily	100–200 mg twice daily	800 mg three times daily	Avoid labetalol with history of asthma or heart dysfunction
Nifedipine (extended-release)	30–120 mg/d PO	30 mg once daily	60 mg twice daily[3]	Avoid nifedipine with tachycardia. Sublingual and immediate-release formulations are reserved for treatment of acute elevations
Methyldopa	500–3000 mg/d PO, 2–4 times daily	250 mg twice daily	3 g/d in 2–4 divided doses	Side effects are sedation, depression, and dizziness.

[3]Exceeds dosage recommended by the manufacturer.
Not recommended during pregnancy: angiotensin-converting enzyme inhibitors, angiotensin receptor blockers, renin inhibitors, and mineralocorticoid receptor antagonists.
PO, Orally.
Adapted from American College of Obstetricians and Gynecologists (ACOG): *Chronic Hypertension in Pregnancy. Practice Bulletin #223*, January 2019.

found that patients in this treatment group compared with standard treatment had a lower composite incidence of preeclampsia with severe features, medically indicated preterm birth at less than 35 weeks' gestation, placental abruption, or fetal or neonatal death, (30.2% vs. 37.0% for adjusted risk ratio of 0.82 [95% CI 0.74 to 0.92, *P* < 0.001]) without an increase in the incidence of small-for-gestational-age birth weights or other neonatal morbidity. Patients with underlying renal dysfunction or comorbidities may benefit from a lower threshold for treatment. However, it is recommended to maintain BPs at or above 120/80 mm Hg during pregnancy.

Preferred treatment of hypertension during pregnancy includes nifedipine and labetalol. Methyldopa is less effective and has more adverse side effects. Hydrochlorothiazide can be used but is typically second-line and administered in consultation with maternal fetal medicine (see Table 4 for dosage information). The use of angiotensin-converting enzyme inhibitors, angiotensin receptor blockers, renin inhibitors, and mineralocorticoid receptor antagonists is generally not recommended for use during pregnancy. Nonpregnant women taking these medications who are of childbearing age should be counseled about effective birth control methods or transitioned to a different regimen. Atenolol (Tenormin) is also not recommended because of the increased risk of fetal growth restriction.

Patients with chronic hypertension should have baseline laboratory testing (complete blood count, serum liver function levels, electrolyte levels, creatinine levels, blood urea nitrogen levels, and urine protein/creatinine ratio with 24-hour urine protein if the protein/creatinine ratio is abnormal or borderline) in the first trimester. If there is concern about heart disease or the patient has long-standing hypertension, electrocardiogram with or without transthoracic echocardiogram should be obtained. The fetus should be monitored with serial growth ultrasounds every 4 weeks after 20 weeks' gestation and with weekly antenatal testing after 32 weeks, with nonstress testing or a biophysical profile; the choice is typically institution-dependent because of the lack of definitive data.

Gestational Hypertension

Gestational hypertension is managed expectantly with delivery scheduled no later than 37 weeks' gestation or at diagnosis if after 37 weeks' gestation. Prior to 37 weeks, patients can be monitored as outpatients twice weekly with BP and symptom assessments, laboratory monitoring, and antenatal testing. Fetal growth should be monitored at least every 4 weeks. Patients should be closely monitored for worsening disease, with a low threshold for inpatient observation and administration of corticosteroids (12 mg betamethasone [Celestone Soluspan][1] intramuscularly [IM] every

24 hours for 2 doses OR 6 mg betamethasone every 12 hours for 4 doses) to prompt fetal lung maturity if preterm.

Preeclampsia With and Without Severe Features

Preeclampsia without severe features should be managed similarly to gestational hypertension. If severe features develop (see Table 3) before 34 weeks' gestation, the patient should be managed as an inpatient until delivery at 34 weeks' gestation. If prior to 34 weeks' gestation, the patient should be given corticosteroids to prompt fetal lung maturity, and delivery should be delayed for 48 hours unless there are contraindications to expectant management. The contraindications to expectant management include uncontrolled severe-range BPs not responsive to antihypertensive medication, persistent headache refractory to repeat treatment without other cause, epigastric or right upper quadrant pain without other cause unresponsive to repeat analgesics, stroke, myocardial infarction, HELLP (*h*emolysis, *e*levated *l*iver enzymes, and *l*ow *p*latelet count) syndrome, worsening renal dysfunction, eclampsia, pulmonary edema, suspected acute placental abruption, abnormal fetal testing, fetal death, or lethal anomaly/extreme prematurity. If severe features develop later than 34 weeks' gestation, the patient should be delivered without waiting for the corticosteroid window to be complete.

If the patient is able to be expectantly managed until delivery at 34 weeks' gestation, oral antihypertensives can be initiated to increase the time before delivery is necessary (see Table 5 for agents used for acute BP control). It is recommended to start magnesium sulfate (MgSO4) to prevent eclampsia, and this can be discontinued once stability is proven and if the patient is not being delivered. MgSO4 is initiated with a 4 to 6 g IV loading dose given over 15 to 30 minutes, followed by 1 to 2 g/h maintenance infusion. Patients less than 32 weeks' gestation have the added benefit of fetal neuroprotection from magnesium and should be treated with the higher dose if tolerated. Patients on magnesium should be monitored with hourly neurologic exam, vitals and intake/output (see Table 6 for signs and symptoms of magnesium toxicity). If this is suspected, magnesium should be immediately discontinued, and the magnesium level should be obtained. Patients at risk of impending respiratory depression may require intubation and treatment with 10 mL of 10% calcium gluconate IV along with IV furosemide. Patients undergoing inpatient expectant management should have MgSO4 reinitiated prior to anticipated delivery and continued for 24 hours postpartum.

Patients should be counseled on mode of delivery by usual obstetric indications. However, the likelihood of cesarean delivery ranges from 65% to 97% if delivery is occurring at less than 32 weeks' gestation. The decision for mode of delivery should be individualized in these circumstances, as well as in patients with associated fetal morbidities.

Preeclampsia may begin or worsen in the postpartum period, so serum labs (liver function, electrolyte levels, creatinine levels, blood urea nitrogen), symptoms, and BP should be monitored

[1] Not FDA approved for this indication.

TABLE 5 Antihypertensive Agents Used for Acute Blood Pressure Management

The trigger is severe-range BP (SBP ≥160 mm Hg or DBP ≥110 mm Hg) that persists for 15 minutes or more; continue treatment algorithm if BP continues to be severe range on rechecks

DRUG ALGORITHM	CAUTION	FIRST DOSE	SECOND DOSE	THIRD DOSE/ ACTION	FOURTH ACTION
Labetalol (maximum daily dose 300 mg, administer each dose over 2 minutes)	Avoid labetalol with active asthma and heart disease/CHF. It may cause fetal bradycardia.	20 mg IV, BP repeated in 10 minutes	40 mg IV, BP repeated in 10 minutes	80 mg IV, BP repeated in 10 minutes	Move to hydralazine algorithm, and consult.*
Hydralazine[1] (maximum daily dose 20 mg)	Risk of maternal hypotension is higher with frequent dosing.	5–10 mg IV, BP repeated in 20 minutes	10 mg IV, BP repeated in 20 minutes	Move to labetalol algorithm.	Consult.*
Nifedipine[1] (immediate-release, maximum daily dose 180 mg)	Nifedipine may cause reflex tachycardia and headaches.	10 mg PO, BP repeated in 20 minutes	20 mg PO, BP repeated in 20 minutes	20 mg PO, BP repeated in 20 minutes	Move to labetalol algorithm, and consult.*

BP, Blood pressure; *CHF,* congestive heart failure; *DBP,* diastolic blood pressure; *IV,* intravenously; *PO,* orally; *SBP,* systolic blood pressure.
*Consult should be placed emergently to MFM, internal medicine, anesthesia, or critical care.
[1]Not FDA approved for this indication.

closely before discharge. Patients with elevated BP around the time of delivery should have a clinic visit to check for vital signs and undergo a limited physical exam no later than 1 week postpartum. Preeclampsia is a risk factor for the future development of hypertension, cardiovascular disease, and renal disease; the risk is twofold higher in women with preeclampsia and eightfold higher for early-onset preeclampsia requiring delivery earlier than 34 weeks' gestation. Two- to five-year follow-up rates of chronic hypertension can be as high as 50%. Patients should be counseled and encouraged to undergo yearly follow-up with their primary care physician, with the workup including, at a minimum, weight monitoring and assessments of BP, lipids, and fasting glucose.

Complications

HELLP Syndrome

HELLP syndrome is a severe form of preeclampsia because of the increased rate of morbidity and mortality. There is debate about the specific criteria for diagnosis, but many clinicians use lactate dehydrogenase (LDH) of 600 IU/L or greater, AST and ALT greater than twice the upper limit of normal, and platelets less than 100×10^9/L as a threshold guide. Other markers for hemolysis besides LDH can be used (peripheral smear, bilirubin > 1.2 mg/dL). HELLP syndrome can have an atypical or slow onset, with 15% of patients lacking hypertension or proteinuria. Thirty percent can present postpartum. Patients can present with generalized malaise, nausea and vomiting, and right upper quadrant pain.

Patients with HELLP syndrome should have serum lab testing for coagulopathy (prothrombin time, partial thromboplastin time, platelet count and fibrinogen) because patients can progress to disseminated intravascular coagulopathy very quickly. Neuraxial anesthesia is typically contraindicated in patients with platelets less than 70×10^9/L because of the risk of epidural hematoma. Platelet transfusion is indicated for platelet counts less than 20 $\times 10^9$/L before vaginal delivery and less than 50×10^9/L before cesarean delivery or with active bleeding.

Patients with stable serum labs can be expectantly managed on MgSO4 through the corticosteroid window (48 hours after the first dose) if they are diagnosed prior to 34 weeks' gestation. Management and delivery timing in this situation should occur with consultation of a maternal-fetal medicine specialist.

Eclampsia

Eclampsia is a life-threatening complication of hypertensive disorders of pregnancy involving new-onset tonic-clonic, focal, or

TABLE 6 Signs and Symptoms of Magnesium Toxicity

SERUM MAGNESIUM CONCENTRATION (mg/dL)	EFFECT
5–9	Typical therapeutic range
>9	Loss of patellar reflex, double vision
10–12	Somnolence, slurred speech
>12	Respiratory paralysis
>30	Cardiac arrest

Contraindications to magnesium: myasthenia gravis; avoid with pulmonary edema and use caution in renal insufficiency (magnesium sulfate is renally cleared).

multifocal seizures in the absence of other causative conditions. A small proportion of patients with preeclampsia without severe features (1.9%) or preeclampsia with severe features (3.2%) developed eclampsia in the placebo arm of two randomized controlled trials evaluating seizure prophylaxis. Eclampsia is a significant cause of maternal death, especially in low-resource settings, and should be treated as an obstetric emergency. Eclampsia can occur before, during, or after delivery and is typically preceded by neurologic symptoms, such as severe headache or visual changes, suggesting cerebral irritation. As with HELLP syndrome, eclampsia can occur in the absence of hypertension or proteinuria. Seizures are typically shorter than 90 seconds, self-limited, and followed by a postictal state. Patients without an IV can have 5 g of MgSO4 administered IM in each buttock. For those with IV access, a loading dose of 6 g of MgSO4 should be given over a period of 15 to 30 minutes and then the maintenance infusion should be 2 g/h and continued for 24 hours after the last seizure. If seizures persist, the patient should be evaluated for other causes and treated with lorazepam (Ativan) 2 to 4 mg IV (repeated after 10–15 minutes if necessary) or diazepam 5 to 10 mg IV every 5 to 10 minutes (maximum dose of 30 mg). Care should be taken during the seizure to protect the patient's airway, reduce risk of aspiration, and prevent maternal injury. Fetal monitoring should be accomplished when feasible, but delivery should not be undertaken until the mother is stable. If the patient lacks refractory seizures or other factors necessitating emergent delivery, the patient can undergo an induction of labor and have cesarean delivery reserved for usual obstetric circumstances.

References

ACOG Committee Opinion No. 743: Low-dose aspirin use during pregnancy, *Obstet Gynecol* 132:e44–e52, 2018.

American College of Obstetricians and Gynecologists (ACOG): Gestational Hypertension and Preeclampsia, *Practice Bulletin* 222, 2020.

American College of Obstetricians and Gynecologists (ACOG): Chronic Hypertension in Pregnancy, *Practice Bulletin* 223, 2019.

CDC Pregnancy-Related Deaths: Data from Maternal Mortality Review Committees in 36 US States, 2017–2019. Susanna Trost, MPH; Jennifer Beauregard, MPH, PhD; Gyan Chandra, MS, MBA; Fanny Njie, MPH; Jasmine Berry, MPH; Alyssa Harvey, BS; David A. Goodman, MS, PhD

CDC Morbidiy and Mortality Weekly Report. Hypertensive Disorders in Pregnancy and Mortality at Delivery Hospitalization — United States, 2017–2019. Weekly / April 29, 2022 / 71(17);585–591. Nicole D. Ford, PhD[1]; Shanna Cox, MSPH[1]; Jean Y. Ko, PhD[1]; Lijing Ouyang, PhD[1]; Lisa Romero, DrPh[1]; Tiffany Colarusso, MD[1]; Cynthia D. Ferre, MA[1]; Charlan D. Kroelinger, PhD[1]; Donald K. Hayes, MD[2]; Wanda D. Barfield, MD[1]

Creasy & Resnik's Maternal-Fetal Medicine: Chapter 72: Pregnancy as a Window to Future Health; and Chapter 48: Pregnancy-Related Hypertension

Davidson KW, Barry MJ, Mangione CM, et al: Aspirin use to prevent preeclampsia and related morbidity and mortality: US Preventive Services Task Force Recommendation Statement. US Preventive Services Task Force, *JAMA* 326:1186–1191, 2021.

Roberge S, Nicolaides K, Demers S, Hyett J, Chaillet N, Bujold E: The role of aspirin dose on the prevention of preeclampsia and fetal growth restriction: systematic review and meta-analysis, *Am J Obstet Gynecol* 216(2):110–120, 2017.

(The RCT ASPRE Trial), Rolnik DL, Wright D, Poon LC, et al: Aspirin versus Placebo in Pregnancies at High Risk for Preterm Preeclampsia, *N Engl J Med* 377(7):613–622, 2017.

Tita AT, Szychowski JM, Boggess K, et al: Chronic Hypertension and Pregnancy (CHAP) Trial Consortium. Treatment for Mild Chronic Hypertension during Pregnancy, *N Engl J Med* 386(19):1781–1792, 2022.

Whelton PK, Carey RM, Aronow WS, et al: 2017 ACC/AHA/AAPA/ABC/ACPM/AGS/APhA/ASH/ASPC/NMA/PCNA Guideline for the Prevention, Detection, Evaluation, and Management of High Blood Pressure in Adults: A Report of the American College of Cardiology/American Heart Association Task Force on Clinical Practice Guidelines, *Hypertension* 71(6):e13–e115, 2018, https://doi.org/10.1161/HYP.0000000000000065. Epub 2017 Nov 13. Erratum in: Hypertension. 2018 Jun;71(6):e140-e144.

POSTPARTUM CARE

Tara J. Neil, MD

CURRENT DIAGNOSIS

- The postpartum period consists of the period from delivery of the infant until 6 to 8 weeks postpartum.
- Postpartum hemorrhage is a medical emergency and is usually caused by uterine atony.
- Fever during the postpartum period is typically caused by endometritis or mastitis.

CURRENT THERAPY

- Continue to monitor and check for resolution of any complications or medical conditions that arise during pregnancy.
- Uterine atony responds to massage and medications. Providers should be familiar with the medications and their dosages.
- Postpartum contraception counseling should be started immediately and all forms can be used by 6 weeks postpartum.
- Breastfeeding is the preferred nutrition for newborns and success is dependent on provider counseling and encouragement.

Postpartum care encompasses the period after delivery of infant and placenta until 6 to 8 weeks after delivery. The hormonal and physiologic systems that underwent changes during pregnancy return to normal during this time. During the initial 24 to 48 hours, most patients are monitored in the hospital for possible complications after delivery.

BOX 1	**Causes of Postpartum Hemorrhage**

- Uterine atony
- Vaginal or cervical laceration
- Coagulation disorder
- Uterine inversion
- Retained placenta/products

Postpartum Hemorrhage

Postpartum hemorrhage is defined as blood loss greater than 500 mL after vaginal delivery or greater than 1000 mL after cesarean section. It is the major cause of maternal morbidity and mortality worldwide. Practitioners should be prepared to diagnose and treat the cause.

Some common causes of hemorrhage are identified in Box 1, including the most common cause: uterine atony. Once abnormal bleeding is identified, resuscitation measures should be started, including intravenous (IV) access, nursing assistance, starting fluid resuscitation with crystalloids or blood products, and anesthesia if needed. In addition, administration of tranexamic acid (Cyklokapron)[1] 1000 mg IV has been shown to decrease mortality regardless of the cause of bleeding. The uterus should be examined using a bimanual examination and vigorous massage. If the uterus is boggy, the medications listed in Table 1 can be used to improve uterine tone and decrease bleeding. If the bladder is full, a catheter should be placed. Careful inspection of the cervix, vaginal walls, and perineum should be performed to identify other sources of hemorrhage. If bleeding is not slowed or the cause of hemorrhage not identified, manual exploration of the uterus can be performed with proper anesthesia to check for retained products. Surgical treatment with dilation and curettage and hysterectomy can also be used if manual exploration and medical management do not control bleeding. If the patient is hemodynamically stable and the resources are available, embolization of the uterine arteries can also control bleeding.

Postpartum Care After Hospital Dismissal

Clinical care in the postpartum period should be focused on continued care of the mom and baby and not as a single visit. To better facilitate this, the patient should have clinical contact by phone or at appointment with the provider or clinical team in the first 3 weeks. Ongoing care should be provided on an as-needed basis. Ultimately, the postpartum period ends with a comprehensive visit and exam occurring by 12 weeks. This visit should include full physical and psychosocial assessment as well as discussion of interpregnancy spacing and management of any chronic health conditions.

Fever and Infection

Fever greater than 38°C (100.4°F) should be evaluated and a source identified. Box 2 lists the most common causes of postpartum fever. Evaluation should include a physical examination to include the uterus and breasts, with attention to any lacerations or incisions. Laboratory testing should include urinalysis, complete blood count (CBC), and blood cultures if appropriate.

Endometritis, a polymicrobial infection of the endometrium of the uterus, typically causes fever in the first 1 to 2 weeks postpartum. Diagnostic criteria include fever and uterine pain with palpation. Endometritis is treated with IV broad-spectrum antibiotics until fever and uterine pain resolve. If there is no clinical improvement after several days of treatment, imaging with computed tomography (CT) or ultrasound of the pelvis can be used to look for complications, including pelvic abscess and septic pelvic thrombophlebitis.

---

[1]Available as dietary supplement.

TABLE 1 Medications Used to Treat Uterine Atony

MEDICATION	ADMINISTRATION	FREQUENCY	SPECIAL CONSIDERATIONS
Oxytocin (Pitocin)	10 units IM 10–40 units in 1000 mL of IV solution	Once Continuous to maintain uterine tone	Should not be given directly in IV
Methylergonovine maleate (Methergine)	0.2 mg IM/IV 0.2 mg PO	Repeat every 2–4 h as needed 3–4 times daily for maximum of 7 days	Contraindicated in hypertension
Carboprost tromethamine (Hemabate)	0.25 mg IM	Repeat every 15–90 min. Maximum dose 2 mg	Contraindicated in active cardiac, renal, pulmonary, and liver disease. Use cautiously in asthmatics.
Misoprostol (Cytotec)[1]	800–1000 µg rectally[3]	One-time dose	

[1]Not FDA approved for this indication.
[3]Exceeds dosage recommended by the manufacturer.

BOX 2 Causes of Postpartum Fever

- Mastitis
- Endometritis
- Urinary tract infection
- Wound infection (perineal or abdominal)
- Septic thrombophlebitis
- Deep vein thrombosis

Mastitis causes fever in breastfeeding mothers. It is caused by the introduction of skin flora through cracks in the nipple and skin and infects milk ducts and surrounding soft tissues in areas of stasis. Treatment includes frequent feeding or pumping to alleviate the stasis. There is inadequate evidence to support antibiotic use, but if symptoms persist after effectively emptying breasts, most practitioners treat with a 10- to 14-day course of oral narrow-spectrum antibiotics. Complications can include breast abscesses, which are usually diagnosed by ultrasound.

Immunization

Immunizations should be updated during the postpartum period. Rubella status is routinely checked during the prenatal period and immunization should be given if indicated. Tdap (tetanus toxoid, reduced diphtheria toxoid, and acellular pertussis vaccine [Adacel, Boostrix]) should be given to the patient and offered to other members of the family if they have not received a pertussis booster to help protect the infant from contracting pertussis. Influenza vaccine should be given if it was not given during pregnancy. Rh(D)-negative mothers should receive anti-D immune globulin if their infants are Rh(D) positive.

Breastfeeding

Breast milk is universally recognized as the best nutrition for newborns. Infants who are breastfed have fewer ear, lower respiratory, and gastrointestinal infections. They are also less likely to develop asthma, diabetes, and obesity. Contraindications to breastfeeding include human immunodeficiency virus (HIV), active herpetic lesions on breasts, maternal drug abuse, and certain medications. Any medications prescribed during breastfeeding should be checked for safety. It is currently recommended, when possible, for infants to be exclusively breastfed until 6 months and supplemented with foods between the ages of 6 months and 1 year. Clinicians play a crucial role in educating mothers about the importance of breastfeeding and supporting them during breastfeeding.

Contraception

Discussing contraception after delivery is important for healthy birth spacing. Ovulation can occur as early as 3 weeks after delivery. Breastfeeding mothers can use lactational amenorrhea during this period if they are exclusively breastfeeding. They can also use progesterone-only contraception (Micronor, Depo-Provera, Nexplanon) or intrauterine device starting 6 weeks postpartum. Combined estrogen-progesterone formulations can be started as early as 3 weeks postpartum in nonbreastfeeding mothers. Starting estrogen-containing formulations before this can increase the risk for thromboembolism. Intrauterine devices and diaphragms are typically placed at 6 weeks after the uterus has returned to its normal size. Medroxyprogesterone intramuscular (IM) injection (Depo-Provera) and etonogestrel subcutaneous (SC) implant (Nexplanon) may be given in the first 5 days postpartum if a patient is not breastfeeding.

Other Considerations

Close evaluation and continued management of medical conditions that develop during pregnancy, including thyroid disease, gestational diabetes, and preeclampsia, should be continued.

The postpartum period is an important time for new mothers. Open communication with their providers during this time helps support them and helps them to recognize conditions that are important for their health and the health of their newborn.

References

American College of Obstetricians and Gynecologists: *Compendium of selected publications*, Atlanta, 2007, American College of Obstetricians and Gynecologists.

Breastfeeding, Family Physicians Supporting. Available at. http://www.aafp.org/online/en/home/policy/policies/b/breastfeedingpositionpaper.html (accessed February 25, 2020).

Centers for Disease Control: Pertussis (whooping cough) vaccination. Available at http://www.cdc.gov/vaccines/vpd-vac/pertussis/default.htm (accessed February 25, 2020).

French LM, Smaill FM: Antibiotic regimens for endometritis after delivery, *Cochrane Database Syst Rev* (4):CD001067, 2004.

Jahanfar S, Ng C-J, Teng CL: Antibiotics for mastitis in breastfeeding women, *Cochrane Database Syst Rev* 1:CD005458, 2009.

Optimizing postpartum care. ACOG Committee Opinion No. 736: American College of Obstetricians and Gynecologists, *Obstet Gynecol* 131:e140–e150, 2018.

Truitt ST, Fraser AB, Gallo MFet al, et al: Combined hormonal versus nonhormonal versus progestin-only contraception in lactation, *Cochrane Database Syst Rev* (2):CD003988, 2003.

WOMAN Trial Collaborators: Effect of early tranexamic acid administration on mortality, hysterectomy, and other morbidities in women with post-partum haemorrhage (WOMAN): an international, randomised, double-blind, placebo-controlled trial, *Lancet* 389(10084):2105–2116, 2017.

TABLE 2 Selected Antidepressant Characteristics for Postpartum Depression

CLASS	MEDICATION	RCT SUPPORTING USE?	PREGNANCY CONSIDERATIONS	BREAST-MILK LEVELS	POSSIBLE INFANT ADVERSE EFFECTS?	CLINICAL COMMENTS
SSRIs	Sertraline (Zoloft)[1]	Yes	Preferred SSRI	Very low	None known	Most studied; preferred SSRI during breastfeeding
	Paroxetine (Paxil)[1]	Yes	Possibly higher risk of neonatal symptoms, cardiac malformations	Very low	None known	Well-studied in breastfeeding. Avoid in pregnancy. High risk for maternal withdrawal symptoms
	Fluoxetine (Prozac)[1]	Yes	Delayed infant clearance (long half-life)	Low-medium	Possible: poor weight gain. Case reports: colic, sleep disturbance, GI disturbance.	Metabolite with long half-life may dose-accumulate in infant
	Citalopram (Celexa)[1]/ escitalopram (Lexapro)[1]	No*	Preferred SSRI	Low	Case reports: sleep disturbance, irritability.	Escitalopram is less well-studied than citalopram in breastfeeding, although clinical experience supports a similar safety profile
SNRIs	Venlafaxine (Effexor)[1]	No	Less well-studied than SSRIs	Low	None known	Case reports of higher infant levels of active metabolite. High risk for maternal withdrawal symptoms
	Duloxetine (Cymbalta)[1]	No	Minimal data	Low	None known	Less-studied in breastfeeding. Case reports of galactorrhea
Tricyclics	Nortriptyline (Pamelor)[1]	Yes	Less well-studied than SSRIs	Low	None known	Well-studied in breastfeeding
	Amitriptyline (Elavil)[1]	No		Low	Case report: Oversedation.	
Allopregnanolone analogues	Zuranolone (Zurzuvae)	Yes	May cause fetal harm	Low	Unknown; pregnancy registry available	Administer orally
	Brexanolone (Zulresso)	Yes	May cause fetal harm	Low	Unknown; pregnancy registry available	Administer IV
Other	Bupropion (Wellbutrin)[1]	No	Minimal data	Low	Case report: seizure	Case report of galactorrhea
	Mirtazapine (Remeron)[1]	No	Minimal data	Low	None known	Less-studied in breastfeeding. Case reports of galactorrhea

GI, Gastrointestinal; *RCT*, randomized controlled trial; *SNRIs*, serotonin/norepinephrine reuptake inhibitors; *SSRIs*, selective serotonin reuptake inhibitors.
[1]Not FDA approved for this indication.
*Citalopram (Celexa) and escitalopram (Lexapro) were among medications used in a naturalistic open-label RCT.

References

Association AP: *Diagnostic and statistical manual of mental disorders (DSM-5®)*, American Psychiatric Pub, 20132013.

Dennis CL, Dowswell T: Psychosocial and psychological interventions for preventing postpartum depression, *The Cochrane Database of Systematic Reviews*(2), 2013. Cd001134.

Field T: Postpartum depression effects on early interactions, parenting, and safety practices: a review, *Infant Behavior & Development* 33(1):1–6, 2010.

Larsen ER, Damkier P, Pedersen LH, et al: Use of psychotropic drugs during pregnancy and breast-feeding, *Acta Psychiatrica Scandinavica Supplementum*(445)1–28, 2015.

Lindahl V, Pearson JL, Colpe L: Prevalence of suicidality during pregnancy and the postpartum, *Archives of Women's Mental Health* 8(2):77–87, 2005.

Meltzer-Brody S, Colquhoun H, Riesenberg R, et al: Brexanolone injection in post-partum depression: two multicentre, double-blind, randomised, placebo-controlled, phase 3 trials, *The Lancet* 392(10152):1058–1070, 2018.

Molyneaux E, Howard LM, McGeown HR, Karia AM, Trevillion K: Antidepressant treatment for postnatal depression, *Cochrane Database of Systematic Reviews* (9), 2014.

Molyneaux E, Telesia LA, Henshaw C, Boath E, Bradley E, Howard LM: Antidepressants for preventing postnatal depression, *The Cochrane database of systematic reviews* 4, 2018:Cd004363.

Nillni YI, Mehralizade A, Mayer L, Milanovic S: Treatment of depression, anxiety, and trauma-related disorders during the perinatal period: A systematic review, *Clinical Psychology Review* 66:136–148, 2018.

Norhayati MN, Hazlina NH, Asrenee AR, Emilin WM: Magnitude and risk factors for postpartum symptoms: a literature review, *Journal of Affective Disorders* 175:34–52, 2015.

O'Connor E, Rossom RC, Henninger M, Groom HC, Burda BU: Primary Care Screening for and Treatment of Depression in Pregnant and Postpartum Women: Evidence Report and Systematic Review for the US Preventive Services Task Force, *JAMA* 315(4):388–406, 2016.

Rundgren S, Brus O, Bave U, et al: Improvement of postpartum depression and psychosis after electroconvulsive therapy: A population-based study with a matched comparison group, *Journal of Affective Disorders* 235:258–264, 2018.

Sharma V, Doobay M, Baczynski C: Bipolar postpartum depression: An update and recommendations, *Journal of Affective Disorders* 219:105–111, 2017.

US Food and Drug Administration. FDA Approves First Oral Treatment for Postpartum Depression. August 4 2023. Available at: https://www.fda.gov/news-events/press-announcements/fda-approves-first-oral-treatment-postpartum-depression. Accessed August 20, 2023.

Venkatesh KK, Zlotnick C, Triche EW, Ware C, Phipps MG: Accuracy of brief screening tools for identifying postpartum depression among adolescent mothers, *Pediatrics* 133(1):e45–53, 2014.

VAGINAL BLEEDING IN PREGNANCY

Method of
Zachary J. Baeseman, MD, MPH

CURRENT DIAGNOSIS

- There are several diagnoses in the differential of dangerous late pregnancy bleeding and management varies based on the etiology.
- Avoid digital vaginal examination in a patient with late pregnancy bleeding until placenta previa has been excluded by ultrasound.
- Uterine tenderness with vaginal bleeding is consistent with a clinical diagnosis of placental abruption.
- Vaginal bleeding with a rupture of membranes should prompt consideration of vasa previa.
- Early pregnancy bleeding in a hemodynamically stable patient is worked up with a complete history and physical, complete blood count, human chorionic gonadotropin, and a transvaginal ultrasound.

CURRENT THERAPY

- Placenta previa requires cesarean delivery; however, with a placental edge of more than 2 cm from the cervical os, a vaginal delivery may be attempted in a stable patient.
- Antenatal diagnosis of vasa previa by ultrasound, appropriate administration of antenatal steroids, and a planned cesarean delivery between 34 and 36 weeks gestation is associated with significantly reduced perinatal morbidity and mortality.
- Definitive management of a patient with late-pregnancy bleeding who is hemodynamically unstable should not be delayed in order to obtain an ultrasound or other diagnostic testing.
- In early and late pregnancy bleeding, attention must be directed to the Rh status of the pregnant woman.

Vaginal Bleeding in Late Pregnancy

Epidemiology

Bleeding in the second half of pregnancy complicates 2% to 5% of pregnancies. Placental previa, placental insertion into the lower uterine segment covering all or part of the internal cervical os, causes 30% of late-pregnancy bleeds and occurs in 0.5% of all pregnancies. Placental abruption, premature separation of the placenta from the uterine wall, causes 20% of antepartum hemorrhages and occurs in 1% of all pregnancies. The diagnosis of placental abruption is typically clinical; ultrasound can be useful to rule in the diagnosis, but notably, it can miss >50% of diagnoses. Other serious causes include uterine rupture (occurs in approximately 0.7% of women with a history of previous low-transverse cesarean section) and vasa previa (0.5% of late-pregnancy bleeding and approximately 0.0002% to 0.0008% of all pregnancies). Vasa previa occurs when fetal blood vessels are present in the membranes, traversing the cervix beneath the fetal presenting part.

Risk Factors

Higher parity and maternal age, smoking or cocaine use, a prior history of placenta previa or placental abruption, and multifetal gestation are risk factors for both placenta previa and abruption. Risk factors for placenta previa also include uterine abnormalities, assisted reproductive technology (ART), and history of uterine surgery, including cesarean section. Additional risk factors for abruption include blunt abdominal trauma, polyhydramnios,

hypertensive disorders in pregnancy, and external cephalic version. The greatest risk factor for uterine rupture is a trial of labor after cesarean section (TOLAC), particularly with induction and the use of prostaglandins, which are contraindicated in TOLAC. A uterine scar increases risk; spontaneous uterine rupture is rare on an unscarred uterus. Other risk factors include uterine abnormalities, maternal connective tissue disease, abnormal placentation, and uterine hyperstimulation during labor. Shortened interpregnancy interval (less than 18 to 24 months between pregnancies) can also increase risk. Risk factors for vasa previa include artificial reproductive techniques, bilobed or succenturiate lobed placenta (odds ratio [OR] = 22.11), placenta previa (OR = 22.86), certain fetal anomalies, and a velamentous cord insertion.

Pathophysiology

The cause of placenta previa is unknown but may be related to impaired placental attachment in a uterus with a previous scar. Placental abruption, defined as premature separation of the placenta from the uterus, is caused by hemorrhage where the placenta and decidua meet. Abruption is often preceded by vasospasm (such as that induced by cocaine), thrombosis, or shearing forces. Some cases are acute, but many cases could present a chronic process in which abruption is the end result. Uterine rupture most often occurs in a uterus with a previous scar and is a dehiscence of that scar; often the presenting sign is an abnormal fetal heart rate or a regression of fetal station in labor. The pathophysiology of vasa previa is unknown, although it is theorized to be caused by abnormal development or growth of the umbilical cord secondary to a velamentous insertion or reduced intrauterine space.

Prevention

Previous cesarean section is a risk factor for both placenta previa and uterine rupture, therefore reducing unnecessary cesarean sections can prevent these conditions. Patients who have had a cesarean section should be advised to space out their next pregnancy by 18 to 24 months to mitigate the risk of uterine rupture. Uterine rupture may also be prevented by limiting or avoiding certain agents to induce or augment labor. In women undergoing TOLAC, spontaneous labor is preferred due to the lower risk of uterine rupture. Although vasa previa cannot be prevented, fetal morbidity and mortality are significantly reduced by early diagnosis and delivery. Placental abruption is associated with smoking and cocaine use; counseling directed to cessation theoretically reduces risk. Seat belts are recommended for all pregnant women; trauma sustained during a motor vehicle accident is a potential cause of abruption due to shearing forces. Control of hypertension and treatment of thrombophilia have not been proved to prevent abruption, although both interventions are recommended. Magnesium sulfate given intrapartum to women with preeclampsia can reduce the risk of placental abruption.

Clinical Manifestations

Placenta previa classically manifests with painless vaginal bleeding, whereas placental abruption and uterine rupture are typically associated with pain and bleeding. Because these conditions are not mutually exclusive, it is important to consider the possibility of more than one serious cause of antepartum hemorrhage. Bleeding secondary to placenta previa may be heavy or light, can recur, and is not associated with the degree of previa or prognosis. Thirty percent of women with placental abruption may not present with vaginal bleeding and have a retroplacental clot concealing an abruption. Approximately one half of women with placental abruption present in labor, and 30% of cases are complicated by fetal death. Monitoring can reveal uterine irritability or hypertonicity. Uterine rupture can manifest with abnormal fetal heart tracing, loss of fetal station, or palpable uterine defect. Pain and bleeding might not occur until after uterine rupture, when both maternal and fetal status are compromised. Vasa previa is detectable on ultrasound and color Doppler imaging, but it most commonly presents as vaginal bleeding with rupture ofmembranes. Placental abruption, uterine rupture, and vasa previa can manifest with concerning fetal heart tracings.

Diagnosis

Ultrasound can reliably detect placenta previa and vasa previa. Transvaginal ultrasonography (TVU) is recommended to establish placental location because transabdominal ultrasonography has a false-positive rate for placenta previa up to 25%. TVU has a sensitivity of 87.5% and a specificity of 98.8% for placenta previa and is safe in the presence of vaginal bleeding. Vasa previa can be diagnosed using TVU and color Doppler. High-risk women may be screened in order to plan for cesarean delivery at 34 to 36 weeks of gestation. Vasa previa may also be detected on magnetic resonance imaging (MRI; rarely used), amnioscopy, palpitation of vessels during reginal examination, or identifying fetal blood cells in vaginal blood, although tests to detect fetal hemoglobin cannot be performed quickly enough to be clinically useful. Placental abruption is primarily a clinical diagnosis; it can be ruled in by ultrasound, but notably >50% of cases of placental abruption are missed on ultrasound. The diagnosis is made clinically in a patient with bleeding and a hard or tender uterus, uterine irritability, and often a nonreassuring fetal heart tracing; bleeding may be absent in 20% to 30% of presentations.

Differential Diagnosis

In addition to placenta previa, placental abruption, uterine rupture, and vasa previa, diagnostic considerations include bloody show, cervical trauma, cervical polyp, cervical cancer, or infection.

Therapy

Women with placenta previa and active bleeding are managed expectantly in the hospital, although outpatient management may be a reasonable approach in women who are not bleeding, have adequate support at home, and are able to get to the hospital quickly. Women with any degree of placental overlap with the cervical os should be delivered by cesarean section.

Treatment of women with placental abruption depends on multiple factors including severity of clinical presentation, gestational age, fetal status, and maternal status. In the most severe cases in which there has been fetal death, vaginal delivery is acceptable if the maternal status is reassuring. Because of risk for disseminated intravascular coagulopathy (DIC) and blood loss, women should be carefully monitored, proceeding to cesarean section for worsening maternal status or failed vaginal delivery. In mild cases of placental abruption before term, steroids should be administered between 24 and up to 36 6/7 weeks of gestation; preterm birth is the leading reason for perinatal death. With a stable abruption in a preterm patient with reassuring fetal and maternal status, outpatient management may be reasonable after a period of inpatient observation. Antenatal magnesium sulfate in women <32 weeks gestation can reliably decrease cerebral palsy and neonatal gross motor dysfunction, however, tocolysis is not routinely recommended in placental abruption. Labor may progress toward a goal of vaginal delivery if both maternal and fetal status are reassuring, although cesarean section should be performed expeditiously for any fetal or maternal compromise. Longer decision-to-incision intervals are associated with worse perinatal outcomes. When placental abruption is known or suspected in a term patient, delivery should proceed.

Vasa previa is managed with immediate cesarean section if diagnosed during labor and with a planned cesarean section if diagnosed antenatally. Administration of steroids is recommended at 28 to 34 weeks of gestation depending on the timing of planned delivery, and hospitalization should be considered at around 30 to 32 weeks of gestation because approximately 10% of women have premature rupture of membranes and could need an urgent cesarean section. Certain patients are appropriate candidates for outpatient management. Optimal time for planned cesarean section is not definitely established and has been recommended between 34 and 36 weeks gestation. Neonatal resuscitation,

including fluid resuscitation or transfusion, may be required and should be anticipated.

Uterine rupture is associated with high perinatal morbidity and mortality. When rupture is clinically recognized or suspected, cesarean delivery should proceed rapidly. Occasionally a uterine window can be seen antenatally within the previous uterine scar on ultrasound. Scheduled cesarean delivery at 37 weeks is recommended for these patients and labor is contraindicated due to the risk of uterine rupture during labor.

Monitoring

In placenta previa, the distance between the placental edge and cervical os is monitored during pregnancy by ultrasound because the placental location can change with advancing pregnancy. After 35 weeks' gestation, women with a placental edge more than 20 mm from the internal cervical os may be offered a trial of labor because they are likely to achieve vaginal delivery. When the placental edge is greater than 0 mm but less than 20 mm from the internal cervical os, vaginal delivery might still be possible, although the likelihood of cesarean section and intrapartum complications are much higher. Women at increased risk of vasa previa should be screened with TVU and color Doppler. When vasa previa is identified, serial ultrasound is indicated because abnormal vessels regress in up to 15% of women. If a woman has an Rh negative blood type and experiences bleeding in pregnancy, she should receive a standard dose of 300 µg Rho(D) human immune globulin to prevent maternal Rh alloimmunization. For massive maternal-fetal hemorrhage a Kleihauer-Betke test should be performed in Rh negative mothers to assist in confirming maternal-fetal hemorrhage and Rho(D) human immune globulin dosing.

Complications

Maternal risks associated with placenta previa include need for cesarean section, postpartum hemorrhage, and blood transfusion. Women who have history of cesarean section and who have placenta previa are at increased risk for placenta accreta. Fetal risks are primarily associated with prematurity. Placental abruption can cause hypovolemic shock, postpartum hemorrhage, and DIC. Perinatal complications include prematurity, intrauterine growth restriction, anemia, coagulopathy, and death. Uterine rupture can be catastrophic for both mother and baby. Maternal risks include surgical risk associated with cesarean section, hypovolemic shock and hemorrhage, and hysterectomy. Perinatal morbidity can include hypoxic-ischemic encephalopathy. Stillbirth and neonatal death are possible as well. When undiagnosed prior to labor vasa previa carries a fetal mortality rate of greater than 60%. Antenatal diagnosis with planned cesarean section decreases fetal mortality to 2% to 3% and reduces the need for transfusion from 60% to 3%. Because the hemorrhage is fetal blood, maternal risk from vasa previa is primarily associated with complications related to cesarean section.

Vaginal Bleeding in Early Pregnancy
Epidemiology

Vaginal bleeding in early pregnancy is common and has been reported in 20% to 40% of pregnant women. A viable intrauterine pregnancy is the most common diagnosis. The two most common complicating diagnoses of early pregnancy bleeding are threatened abortion and ectopic pregnancy. Threatened abortion, an intrauterine pregnancy with bleeding and pain before 20 weeks gestation that has cardiac activity and a closed cervix, is the cause of 12% to 57% of early pregnancy bleeding. The incidence of ectopic pregnancy is 19.7 cases per 1000 pregnancies and is increasing worldwide. Ectopic pregnancy is the leading cause of morbidity and maternal mortality in the first trimester of pregnancy.

It has been suggested that the rate of miscarriage can be as high as 30% to 50% of all fertilized eggs and often goes undetected. The incidence of miscarriage in an intrauterine pregnancy with confirmed fetal cardiac activity is 2.1% in women under 35 years of age and 16.1% in women greater than 35 years of age. Other common causes of early pregnancy bleeding include intercourse, cervicitis, pelvic inflammatory disease, functional placenta hormonal changes, fertilized egg implantation into the uterine wall, and gestational trophoblastic disease.

Pathophysiology

The most common diagnosis of bleeding in early pregnancy is a normal and viable intrauterine pregnancy. Vaginal spotting can commonly occur after implantation of a fertilized egg into the intrauterine wall, usually occurring a few days prior to the expected onset of menstruation (8 to 9 days after ovulation and fertilization). Early pregnancy bleeding may also be caused by the commencement of a hormonally functional placenta, usually at 6 to 7 weeks of gestation. Concerning causes of early pregnancy bleeding are maternal hormonal deficiency, placental dysfunction, subchorionic hemorrhage, extrauterine implantation of the embryo, and nonviability of the pregnancy. The amount of hemorrhage in early pregnancy may be associated with the risk of pregnancy loss.

Management

Early pregnancy bleeding is worked up with a complete set of vital signs, a complete history and physical examination including visualization of the cervix with a speculum, a complete blood count, β-hCG (human chorionic gonadotropin), and a transvaginal ultrasound (TVU) to determine fetal viability and exclude an ectopic pregnancy. Concern for ectopic or early pregnancy loss should be raised if the β-hCG level is greater than the discriminatory level (1500 to 3000 mIU/mL) without intrauterine contents seen on TVU. If the patient is hemodynamically unstable, urgent surgical consultation is paramount as it is possible to have intra-abdominal exsanguination from a ruptured ectopic pregnancy. If the patient is hemodynamically stable and the pregnancy is viable, bleeding is most often managed expectantly, provided the fetus has not reached extrauterine viability of 23 to 24 weeks gestation.

If the patient is hemodynamically stable, a miscarriage can be managed expectantly, inducing medical expulsion of the nonviable fetal tissue with a combination of mifepristone and misoprostol, or surgical management with dilation and suction curettage depending on the risk of infection, maternal hemorrhage and anemia, maternal preference, and medical necessity. Medical management has been proven to increase the effectiveness and decrease the time of complete expulsion compared to expectant management. Due to the risk of alloimmunization, it is recommended that women who are Rh negative blood type have surgical management and receive prophylactic Rho(D) human immune globulin to reduce the risk of alloimmunization. Alloimmunization is a devastating complication where an Rh negative mother can develop antibodies to Rh positive fetal blood, placing future pregnancies at risk.

If a woman has an Rh negative blood type and experiences bleeding in pregnancy, she should receive Rho(D) human immune globulin to prevent maternal Rh alloimmunization. Failure to receive Rho(D) human immune globulin can complicate all subsequent pregnancies and ultimately lead to future severe fetal anemia and hydrops fetalis (severe and life-threatening fetal edema secondary to profound fetal anemia). For early pregnancy bleeding in an Rh negative mother of less than 12 weeks of gestation, 150 µg of Rho(D) is sufficient; greater than 12 weeks of gestation, a standard dose of 300 µg should be given. These dosages provide maternal protection from up to 30 mL of fetal whole blood. For massive maternal-fetal hemorrhage a Kleihauer-Betke test should be performed in Rh negative mothers to assist in confirming maternal-fetal hemorrhage and Rho(D) human immune globulin dosing.

If there is recurrent pregnancy loss, defined as greater than 3 total pregnancy losses, two consecutive pregnancy losses, or a pregnancy loss greater than 20 weeks of gestation, secondary causes should be sought including a workup for antiphospholipid antibody disorder, clotting disorders, and maternal or fetal chromosomal testing. The products of conceptions resulting from gestational trophoblastic disease should undergo chromosomal analysis.

References

Antenatal corticosteroid therapy for fetal maturation. Committee Opinion No. 677. American College of Obstetricians and Gynecologists, *Obstet Gynecol* 128:e187–194, 2016.

Deutchman M, Tubay AT, Turok D: First trimester bleeding, *Am Fam Physician* 79(11):985–994, 2009 Jun 1.

Duley L, Guelmezoglu AM, Henderson-Smart DJ, Chou D: Magnesium sulphate and other anticonvulsants for women with pre-eclampsia, *Cochrane Database Syst Rev* 11, 2010.

Early Pregnancy Loss: Practice Bulletin No. 200. American College of Obstetricians and Gynecologists, *Obstet Gynecol*, August 29, 2018. Interim Update.

Gagnon R, Morin L, Bly S, et al: Guidelines for the management of vasa previa, *J Obstet Gynaecol Can* 31:748–760, 2009.

Hasan R, Baird DD, Herring AH, et al: Patterns and predictors of vaginal bleeding in the first trimester of pregnancy, *Ann Epidemiol* 20(7):524–531, 2010, Available at: https://doi.org/10.1016/j.annepidem.2010.02.006.

Hendricks E, et al: First trimester bleeding: evaluation and management, *Am Fam Physician* 99(3):166–174, 2019 Feb 1.

Krywko DM, Shunkwiler SM: Kleihauer Betke Test. [Updated 2019 Jan 27]. In: StatPearls [Internet]. Treasure Island (FL): StatPearls Publishing; 2019 Jan-. Available from: https://www.ncbi.nlm.nih.gov/books/NBK430876/.

Magann EF, Cummings JE, Niderhauser A: Antepartum bleeding of unknown origin in the second half of pregnancy: A review, *Obstet Gynecol Surv* 60:741–745, 2005.

Management of preterm labor. Practice Bulletin No. 171. American College of Obstetricians and Gynecologists, *Obstet Gynecol* 128:e155–164, 2016.

Oppenheimer L, Armson A, Farine D, et al: Diagnosis and management of placenta previa, *J Obstet Gynaecol Can* 29:261–266, 2007.

Oyelese Y, Ananth C: Placental abruption, *Obstet Gynecol* 108:1005–1016, 2006.

Royal College of Obstetricians and Gynaecologists (RCOG): *Antepartum hemorrhage*, London (UK), November 2011, Royal College of Obstetricians and Gynaecologists (RCOG) November 2011.

Sinha P, Kuruba N: Ante-partum hemorrhage: An update, *J Obstet Gynaecol* 28:377–381, 2008.

Smith JG, Mertz HL, Merrill DC: Identifying risk factors for uterine rupture, *Clin Perinatol* 35:85–99, 2008.

Smith KE, Buyalos RP: The profound impact of patient age on pregnancy outcome after early detection of fetal cardiac activity, *Fertil Steril* 65:35–40, 1996.

Tenore J: *Am Fam Physician* 61(4):1080–1088, 2000 Feb 15.

Zlatnik MG, Cheng YW, Norton ME, et al: Placenta previa and the risk of preterm delivery, *J Matern Fetal Neonatal Med* 20:719–723, 2007.

19 Children's Health

ACUTE LEUKEMIA IN CHILDREN

Method of
Stacy Cooper, MD; and Rachel E. Rau, MD

Leukemias are characterized by a marked proliferation of abnormal blood cells in the bone marrow and blood that may be associated with widespread infiltration in extramedullary sites including the central nervous system (CNS), testes, thymus, liver, spleen, and lymph nodes.

Classification

The first level of classification of leukemia is *acute* versus *chronic*. Acute leukemia is characterized by the predominance of very immature white blood cell precursors, or blasts, and is an aggressive, rapidly fatal disease if left untreated. Conversely, chronic leukemia is characterized by proliferation of relatively mature white blood cells and is typically a more indolent disease. Chronic leukemias are uncommon in pediatrics.

The second level of classification is *lymphoid* versus *myeloid*, depending on whether the leukemic cells display characteristics of lymphocyte precursors or myelocyte (granulocyte, erythrocyte, monocyte, or megakaryocyte) precursors. Acute lymphoblastic leukemia (ALL) and acute myeloid leukemia (AML) account for the overwhelming majority of pediatric leukemias.

ALL and AML are further subclassified by morphology and expression of cell surface antigens using flow cytometry. For ALL, classification is largely based on cell surface and cytoplasmic marker expression (Table 1). AML cases are classified by characteristic chromosomal abnormalities (if present) or by light microscopic morphology in cases where these specific chromosomal changes are absent (Box 1).

Epidemiology

Leukemia accounts for approximately 30% of childhood cancers, making it the most common form of childhood cancer. The distribution of the major forms of leukemia is vastly different in children than in adults (Figure 1). In general, children are far more likely to have acute leukemia, and ALL is much more common than AML. In adults, most cases of leukemia are chronic, and AML is more common than ALL. Specifically, there are approximately 3100 children and adolescents diagnosed with ALL in the United States each year and approximately 700 children and adolescents diagnosed with AML in the United States each year.

The incidence of the various forms of leukemia varies by age in both children and adults (Figure 2). This is especially true for childhood ALL, for which there is a marked incidence peak in the 2- to 4-year-old age group. This ALL age peak is primarily found in children living in industrialized nations, leading to speculation that a common environmental exposure, coupled with age-related immunologic susceptibility, is at least partially responsible for many cases of ALL. Except for a small peak in infants, the incidence of AML is fairly constant in childhood but rises quickly in later adulthood.

Prognosis

One of the most dramatic success stories in modern medicine is the improvement in survival of children with ALL over the past four decades. Leukemia was once a uniformly fatal diagnosis, with less than a 5% to 10% cure rate until the mid- to late 1960s. Today, approximately 90% of children with ALL are cured. The improved prognosis has been built on pioneering observations on the efficacy of multiagent systemic therapy and the importance of CNS treatment in the late 1960s and early 1970s. Further successive, incremental improvements in outcome have been achieved due to clinical trials conducted by large single centers and national and international cooperative groups that have successfully enrolled a high percentage of eligible children.

Similar approaches have unfortunately not been quite so successful in improving the prognosis of children with AML. Although approximately one half of children with AML are cured today, this has been accomplished by intensifying therapy to the point that the toxic death rate in the early phases of therapy is about 10%. Current research in AML is therefore focusing on developing novel molecularly targeted agents that hold the promise of improving efficacy and limiting toxicity.

TABLE 1	Classification of Childhood Acute Lymphoblastic Leukemia					
	PHENOTYPIC MARKER					
ALL SUBTYPE	CD19	CD10	CLG	SLG	%	**COMMENT**
Pre-pre B	+	–	–	–	5	Mostly infants, poor prognosis, frequent *KMT2A* 11q23 rearrangements
Early pre-B	+	+	–	–	63	Common ALL, young children, good prognosis
Pre-B	+	+	+	–	16	Older children, good prognosis with intense therapy
B-cell	+	+	+	+	4	Burkitt leukemia, *MYC/Ig* fusion genes, good prognosis with lymphoma-type therapy
T-cell	–	–	–	–	12	Adolescents, anterior mediastinal mass, CNS involvement, good prognosis with intense therapy

ALL, Acute myeloid leukemia; *clg,* cytoplasmic immunoglobulin; *CNS,* central nervous system; *slg,* surface immunoglobulin.

Acute Myeloid Leukemia With Recurrent Genetic Abnormalities

Acute myeloid leukemia with t(8;21)(q22;q22), *(RUNX1/RUNX1T1)*

Acute myeloid leukemia with abnormal bone marrow eosinophils and inv(16)(p13q22) or t(16;16)(p13;q22), *(CBFβ/MYH11)*

Acute promyelocytic leukemia with t(15;17)(q22;q12), *(PML/RARA),* and variants

Acute myeloid leukemia with 11q23 *(KMT2A)* abnormalities

Acute Myeloid Leukemia, Not Otherwise Categorized

Acute myeloid leukemia, minimally differentiated (FAB M0)

Acute myeloid leukemia without maturation (FAB M1)

Acute myeloid leukemia with maturation (FAB M2)

Acute myelomonocytic leukemia (FAB M4)

Acute monoblastic/acute monocytic leukemia (FAB M5)

Acute erythroid leukemia (FAB M6)

Acute megakaryoblastic leukemia (FAB M7)

FAB, French–American–British classification.

Etiology

The question "What is the cause of leukemia?" can be considered on a few different levels. First, what is wrong with *this child* that caused the child to develop leukemia? Second, what is wrong with *the leukemia cell* that causes it to behave so badly? Third, what is wrong with *the leukemia cell's genes* that cause the cell to behave that way?

Predispositions

The answer to the first question is unknown in the vast majority of cases. Attempts to correlate various genetic features or environmental or infectious exposures with risk of childhood leukemia have been largely uninformative. It is presumed that children are particularly susceptible to ALL because of the marked expansion and genetic rearrangement of lymphocytes that occurs during early childhood as the result of exposure to a multitude of immunogenic antigens for the first time. The proliferation required to meet the constant demand for granulocytes, erythrocytes, and platelets is likely a setup for the development of AML in children.

Although a number of constitutional and single-gene disorders confer an increased risk of childhood leukemia (Table 2), in total, these are known to be involved in only a minority of cases. However, with a growing list of recognized genetic disorders predisposing to myeloid malignancies in particular, a careful

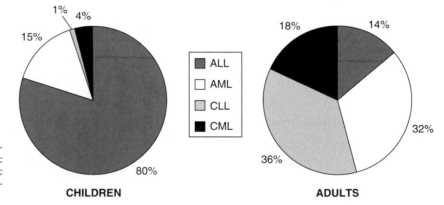

Figure 1 Relative incidence of four major leukemia subtypes in children and adults. *ALL,* Acute lymphoblastic leukemia; *AML,* acute myeloid leukemia; *CLL,* chronic lymphoblastic leukemia; *CML,* chronic myeloid leukemia.

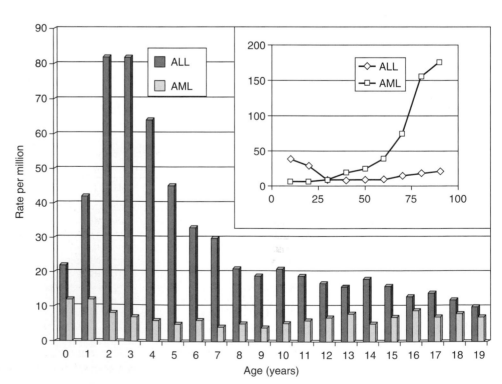

Figure 2 Age-specific incidence of acute lymphoblastic leukemia *(ALL)* and acute myeloid leukemia *(AML)* in children and in adults *(inset).*

TABLE 2	Summary of Known Constitutional and Heritable Childhood Leukemia Predispositions		
DISORDER	INHERITANCE	MALIGNANCY TYPE	COMMENTS
Ataxia-telangiectasia	AR	ALL, NHL	*ATM* gene mutations lead to defective DNA repair
Bloom's syndrome	AR	AML, ALL	Chromosomal instability, sister chromatid exchanges
Down syndrome	Sporadic	AML, ALL	See text
Li-Fraumeni syndrome	AD	AML, ALL, many others	*p53* mutations; leukemias less common than solid tumors
Fanconi's anemia	AR	AML	Chromosomal instability, increased sensitivity to DNA damage
Kostmann's syndrome	AR	AML	G-CSF receptor mutations lead to agranulocytosis
Neurofibromatosis type 1	AD	AML, JMML, MPNST	*NF1* gene mutations lead to enhanced *RAS* signaling
Familial platelet disorder with associated myeloid malignancy	AD	MDS, AML, ALL	Loss of function mutations of the myeloid transcription factor RUNX1 lead to abnormal myeloid development. Individuals have platelet defects and ~35% risk of myeloid malignancy development
Germline CEBPA mutations	AD	AML	Estimated penetrance of AML development ~90% in affected individuals. Approximately 10% of patients with biallelic *CEBPA* mutant AML have a germline *CEBPA* mutation. AML in those with germline CEBPA mutations are chemosensitive, but individuals have high rates of second primary AMLs.
MonoMAC syndrome; germline *GATA2* mutations	AD	MDS, AML	MonoMAC is an immunodeficiency with risk for mycobacterial, fungal, and human papilloma virus infections with monocytopenia and risk for MDS/AML, often with monosomy of chromosome 7
MIRAGE syndrome, ATXPC/MLSM7 syndrome; Germline mutation of *SAMD9* and *SAMD9L*	Mostly de novo		MIRAGE syndrome (myelodysplasia, infection, restriction of growth, adrenal hypoplasia, genital phenotypes, enteropathy); ATXPC, ataxia-pancytopenia syndrome and MLSM7, myelodysplasia and leukemia syndrome with monosomy 7 caused by gain of function mutation of *SAMD9* or *SAMD9L*
CBL syndrome	AD	JMML	Impaired growth, developmental delay, cryptorchidism, deafness, and predisposition to JMML caused by loss of function mutation of rumor suppressor gene *CBL*. JMML that develops can be self-resolving. Vasculitis risk later in life after JMML resolution.

AD, Autosomal dominant; *ALL*, acute lymphoblastic leukemia; *AML*, acute myeloid leukemia; *AR*, autosomal recessive; *G-CSF*, granulocyte colony-stimulating factor; *JMML*, juvenile myelomonocytic leukemia; *MPNST*, malignant peripheral nerve sheath tumor; *NHL*, non-Hodgkin lymphoma.

past medical history, family history, and examination for dysmorphisms and low threshold for genetic referral is warranted for any child with a myeloid malignancy. The most common of these is Down syndrome. Children with Down syndrome have a 10- to 20-fold increased risk of leukemia, with an approximately equal incidence of ALL and AML. The peak age at onset of leukemia for children with Down syndrome is earlier than for other children. In the newborn period, patients with Down syndrome can present with transient myeloproliferative disease (also known as transient abnormal myelopoiesis), which can manifest with hepatomegaly and peripheral blasts, that appears indistinguishable from congenital AML but usually resolves spontaneously within 3 to 6 months. These children have an increased risk of megakaryoblastic leukemia (AMKL, FAB classification M7) within the first 4 years of life. Children with Down syndrome tend to present with leukemia that is particularly susceptible to chemotherapy agents (e.g., cytarabine [Cytosar], methotrexate), but they also suffer increased toxicity from therapy. On balance, the prognosis of leukemia in Down syndrome patients with ALL is inferior to those without Down syndrome, whereas in AML, children with

Down syndrome have favorable outcomes compared with children without Down syndrome.

The only environmental exposures that are known to predispose to leukemia are ionizing radiation (such as was seen with atomic bomb survivors) and prior exposure to certain chemotherapy drugs (e.g., cyclophosphamide [Cytoxan], etoposide [Toposar, VePesid]). There is also evidence that in utero exposure to maternal diagnostic radiation also increases the risk of childhood cancer (including leukemia), particularly if the exposure is in the first trimester. Other environmental or infectious exposures remain unproven as risk factors for childhood leukemia, including electromagnetic fields from power lines.

Cellular Pathogenesis

Three major characteristics of leukemia cells distinguish them from normal hematopoietic cells. They proliferate rapidly, they do not differentiate, and they have defects in apoptosis. This results in a growth advantage for leukemia cells, leading to progressive replacement of the normal bone marrow with a massive clonal population of poorly differentiated leukemic blasts.

TABLE 5   Summary of Late Effects of Leukemia Treatment

LATE EFFECT	TREATMENT-RELATED RISK FACTORS	DIAGNOSTIC APPROACH
Bone	Avascular necrosis, osteonecrosis	X-ray and/or MRI of major joints for persistent pain
Cardiac dysfunction	Anthracyclines: cardiomyopathy (risk related to cumulative dose, higher risk in AML)	ECG or echocardiogram every 3–5 years (cardiomyopathy can occur decades after treatment)
Cataracts	CNS RT	Yearly eye examination
CNS and psychosocial	CNS RT, IT chemotherapy: learning problems, neurocognitive dysfunction	Yearly educational assessment, neurocognitive testing
Dental abnormalities	CNS RT	Yearly dental examinations
Endocrine and reproductive	CNS RT: pituitary dysfunction Alkylators: primary gonadal failure	Yearly growth curves, TSH, LH, FSH LH, FSH, estradiol or testosterone, semen analysis
Hepatic dysfunction	Methotrexate, 6-mercaptopurine, 6-thioguanine: late hepatic fibrosis	Yearly LFTs
Secondary neoplasms	CNS RT: brain tumors Alkylators or epipodophyllotoxins: secondary AML	MRI for symptoms CBC in symptomatic patients

ALL, Acute lymphoblastic leukemia; *AML,* acute myeloid leukemia; *FSH,* follicle-stimulating hormone; *IT,* intrathecal; *LFT,* liver function test; *LH,* luteinizing hormone; *MRI,* magnetic resonance imaging; *RT,* radiation therapy; *TSH,* thyroid-stimulating hormone.

oncology centers have developed late-effects programs to conduct surveillance for the development of these problems and provide follow-up care to patients who develop late complications of therapy.

References

Special section: cancer in children and adolescents. In: American Cancer Society: cancer Facts and Figures 2014. American Cancer Society, 2014, pp 25-42.

Bolouri H, Farrar JE, Triche T, et al: The molecular landscape of pediatric acute myeloid leukemia reveals recurrent structural alterations and age-specific mutational interactions, *Nat Med* 24(1):103–112, 01 2018, https://doi.org/10.1038/nm.4439.

Brown AL, Arts P, Carmichael CL, et al: RUNX1-mutated families show phenotype heterogeneity and a somatic mutation profile unique to germline predisposed AML, *Blood Adv* 4(6):1131–1144, 03 2020, https://doi.org/10.1182/bloodadvances.2019000901.

Brown PA, Ji L, Xu X, et al: Effect of postreduction therapy consolidation with blinatumomab vs chemotherapy on disease-free survival in children, adolescents, and young adults with first relapse of B-cell acute lymphoblastic leukemia: a randomized clinical trial, *J Am Med Assoc* 325(9):833–842, 03 2021, https://doi.org/10.1001/jama.2021.0669.

Buitenkamp TD, Izraeli S, Zimmermann M, et al: Acute lymphoblastic leukemia in children with Down syndrome: a retrospective analysis from the Ponte di Legno study group, *Blood* 123(1):70–77, Jan 2, 2014, https://doi.org/10.1182/blood-2013-06-509463.

Creutzig U, Zimmermann M, Reinhardt D, et al: Changes in cytogenetics and molecular genetics in acute myeloid leukemia from childhood to adult age groups, *Cancer* 122(24):3821–3830, Dec 2016, https://doi.org/10.1002/cncr.30220.

Davidsson J, Puschmann A, Tedgård U, Bryder D, Nilsson L, Cammenga J: SAMD9 and SAMD9L in inherited predisposition to ataxia, pancytopenia, and myeloid malignancies, *Leukemia* 32(5):1106–1115, 05 2018, https://doi.org/10.1038/s41375-018-0074-4.

Gaynon PS, Qu RP, Chappell RJ, et al: Survival after relapse in childhood acute lymphoblastic leukemia: Impact of site and time to first relapse—the Children's Cancer Group Experience, *Cancer* 82:1387–1395, 1998.

Gibson BE, Wheatley K, Hann IM, et al: Treatment strategy and long-term results in paediatric patients treated in consecutive UK AML trials, *Leukemia* 19:2130–2138, 2005.

Greaves MF, Wiemels J: Origins of chromosome translocations in childhood leukaemia, *Nat Rev Cancer* 3:639–649, 2003.

Hunger SP, Mullighan CG: Acute lymphoblastic leukemia in children, *N Engl J Med* 373(16):1541–1552, Oct 15, 2015, https://doi.org/10.1056/NEJMra1400972.

Locatelli F, Zugmaier G, Rizzari C, et al: Effect of blinatumomab vs chemotherapy on event-free survival among children with high-risk first-relapse B-cell acute lymphoblastic leukemia: a randomized clinical trial, *J Am Med Assoc* 325(9):843–854, 03 2021, https://doi.org/10.1001/jama.2021.0987.

Loh ML, Sakai DS, Flotho C, et al: Mutations in CBL occur frequently in juvenile myelomonocytic leukemia, *Blood* 114(9):1859–1863, Aug 27, 2009.

Maude SL, Laetsch TW, Buechner J, et al: Tisagenlecleucel in children and young adults with B-cell lymphoblastic leukemia, *N Engl J Med* 378(5):439–448, 02 2018, https://doi.org/10.1056/NEJMoa1709866.

Möricke A, Zimmermann M, Reiter A, et al: Long-term results of five consecutive trials in childhood acute lymphoblastic leukemia performed by the ALL-BFM study group from 1981 to 2000, *Leukemia* 24(2):265–284, Feb 2010, https://doi.org/10.1038/leu.2009.257.

Pui CH, Campana D, Pei D, et al: Treating childhood acute lymphoblastic leukemia without cranial irradiation, *N Engl J Med* 360(26):2730–2741, Jun 2009, https://doi.org/10.1056/NEJMoa0900386.

Pui CH, Cheng C, Leung W, et al: Extended follow-up of long-term survivors of childhood acute lymphoblastic leukemia, *N Engl J Med* 349:640–649, 2003.

Pui CH, Pei D, Sandlund JT, et al: Long-term results of St Jude total therapy studies 11, 12, 13A, 13B, and 14 for childhood acute lymphoblastic leukemia, *Leukemia* 24(2):371–382, Feb 2010, https://doi.org/10.1038/leu.2009.252.

Ries LAG, Melbert D, Krapcho M, et al: *SEER cancer statistics review, 1975–2004,* Bethesda, Md, 2007, National Cancer Institute2007.

Silverman LB, Stevenson KE, O'Brien JE, et al: Long-term results of Dana-Farber Cancer Institute ALL Consortium protocols for children with newly diagnosed acute lymphoblastic leukemia (1985-2000), *Leukemia* 24(2):320–334, Feb 2010, https://doi.org/10.1038/leu.2009.253.

Stahnke K, Boos J, Bender-Gotze C, et al: Duration of first remission predicts remission rates and long-term survival in children with relapsed acute myelogenous leukemia, *Leukemia* 12:1534–1538, 1998.

Uffmann M, Rasche M, Zimmermann M, et al: Therapy reduction in patients with Down syndrome and myeloid leukemia: the international ML-DS 2006 trial, *Blood* 129(25):3314–3321, 06 2017, https://doi.org/10.1182/blood-2017-01-765057.

Wakeford R, Little MP: Risk coefficients for childhood cancer after intrauterine irradiation: a review, *Int J Radiat Biol* 79:293–309, 2003.

Wlodarski MW, Hirabayashi S, Pastor V, et al: Prevalence, clinical characteristics, and prognosis of GATA2-related myelodysplastic syndromes in children and adolescents, *Blood* 127(11):1387–1397, Mar 2016, https://doi.org/10.1182/blood-2015-09-669937. quiz 1518.

Woods WG, Neudorf S, Gold S, et al: A comparison of allogeneic bone marrow transplantation, autologous bone marrow transplantation, and aggressive chemotherapy in children with acute myeloid leukemia in remission, *Blood* 97:56–62, 2001.

ADOLESCENT HEALTH

Kari R. Harris, MD

CURRENT DIAGNOSIS

- In addition to general medical care, it is important to identify psychosocial health concerns at all adolescent visits.
- The key components of a psychosocial history are addressed in the HEADS private and confidential interview.
- Conducting a Home/Education/Employment/Activities/ Accident Prevention/Diet/Disordered Eating/Drugs/ Depression/Suicide/Self-harm/Sex/Sleep/Social Media (HEADS) interview is standard practice for adolescent care: it should be part of all adolescent well-checks and used, as time permits, in acute visits for teens who have high-risk behaviors or have no regular health care.
- High-acuity areas identified from the HEADS interview include substance use, disordered eating, sexual activity, and mental health.
- Anxiety and depression screening should be part of well visits for all adolescents.
- Substance use screening should be included in all adolescent well visits.
- HIV universal screening should be completed initially between 15 and 18 years of age and the need for rescreening reassessed annually.
- Immunization status should be assessed at every visit, with routine and catch-up vaccines provided.

CURRENT THERAPY

- Long-acting reversible contraception (LARC) provides safe and effective contraception for teenagers.
- Emergency contraception should be offered within 5 days of unprotected sexual activity.
- Treatment for teens is often multidisciplinary, involving subspecialists, mental health providers, medical or psychiatric inpatient units, and county welfare or health departments.

Setting the Stage for the Adolescent Visit

Comprehensive care for adolescents includes screening for high-risk behaviors in addition to routine medical care. To facilitate open communication, providers should be clear about consent and confidentiality policies in their practices. This can be achieved by discussing policies with patients and parents/ caretakers during young adolescent visits (11 to 14 years) and by providing materials documenting the policies and practices, such as a standard letter to parents. Policies can also be displayed in the office, provided in practice newsletters and materials, and made available through patient access portals.

Adolescent visits differ from early childhood visits in several important respects. At the beginning of the visit, time should be spent with both the teen and parent or caregiver clarifying medical history and current concerns. The adolescent should then be offered time without the parent or caregiver present to discuss sensitive issues, including reproductive and mental health. At the end of the visit, the parent/caregiver should be provided with a summary of the visit, limited to the nonconfidential portion, and including recommendations and arrangements for follow-up appointments.

Consent and Confidentiality Laws—Consent Does Not Equal Confidential

Consent and confidentiality laws vary by state. Most states allow minors to consent for reproductive health care, including testing and treatment for sexually transmitted infections (STIs). Most states also allow providers to prescribe contraceptives to minors. Many states have a "mature minor" statute that allows physicians to provide care if they deem the adolescent patient mature and capable of understanding the medical care. These laws give teens autonomy to consent to their own health care and they also enable care to be provided when a parent is unable to attend the appointment.

While consent and confidentiality laws are related, they are separate entities. Many states allow minors to consent for specific health services but do not prohibit a provider from informing the teen's parent/caretaker about that service. Even if allowed by law, expert consensus holds that such disclosures should only be made when in the best interest of the minor patient. The disclosure should not compromise future health care. Many teens will not seek reproductive health care if they have to involve a parent, making confidentiality necessary for comprehensive adolescent health care.

Confidentiality is limited when a minor patient is in direct harm, such as intimate partner violence, sexual coercion or rape, certain pregnancy, suicidality, or self-harm. In such instances, a parent/caretaker should become involved, unless he/she is the perpetrator or some other extraordinary circumstances exist. Local authorities or social welfare agencies may also need to be contacted. These necessary breaches in confidentiality to protect safety must be explained beforehand to the patient and be included in written policies. Any breach of confidentiality must be carried out in a professional manner, explained sensitively to the patient and others, and be well documented. Every attempt must be made not to compromise future care.

Information on consent and confidentiality laws for each state is available at the Guttmacher Institute website (guttmacher.org).

The HEADS Interview

The HEADS acronym provides a structured psychosocial history-taking tool that also screens for high-risk behaviors (Table 1). Although several variations of HEADS have been described, they all cover the most common risk categories for adolescents. Progressing from the least invasive topics to the most sensitive issues, HEADS covers all essential categories (see Table 1).

When using the HEADS interview tool, it is important to build rapport with the patient. The teen deserves explanation of why they are being asked personal questions and every attempt should be made to increase patient comfort and trust. The interview begins with questions regarding hobbies, school, and home life. Once rapport is established, questions proceed to more sensitive issues. Questioning should be open-ended, nonassuming, and nonjudgmental. This allows for honest answers and does not discriminate among patients.

Home/Education/Employment/Activities/Accident Prevention

These topics begin the confidential interview with the least risky activities for adolescents. Although grouped together in this text, each category deserves its own time and questions (see Table 1). All adolescents should have a trusted adult with whom they can discuss concerns. Safety at home and school safety, including any bullying or coercion regardless of site or circumstances, should be discussed and addressed. Current school performance, concerns, grades and post graduation goals should be discussed. After-school employment has benefits but can also negatively impact academic performance, mood, or family dynamics. These should be screened for and addressed if present. Healthy after-school activities should be encouraged. Predictably, adolescent illegal activity, drug use, and sexual activity peak during after-school

Patient Example 2

- 8 y.o. boy—2 week history of polydipsia, polyuria and vomiting for for the past 24 hours.
- In doctors office: glucose 380 mg/dl and urine ketones are large.
- In emergency room serum HCO3 9, anion gap 25.
- Admitted to ICU for insulin drip, IV fluids, and frequent monitoring.
- At 7 am the following morning: glucose 120, HCO3 20.
- Weight: 25
- Family would like to avoid insulin at lunch as school nurse not available.

- Total daily dose 0.6 X 25 kg = 15 units
- 2/3 am = 10 units
  - 2/3 NPH ~ 6.5 units
  - 1/3 rapid acting 3.5 units
- 1/3 pm = 5 units
  - 1/3 rapid acting ~ 1.5 units before dinner
  - 2/3 NPH 3.5 units at bedtime
- Supplement with sliding scale: 0.5 unit rapid-acting insulin per 50 mg/dl above 200 mg/dl.

Figure 2 An 8-year-old boy who presented in diabetic ketoacidosis. He was treated with an insulin drip overnight and his acidosis had resolved by morning. The parents requested a regimen that would not require insulin at lunch time. The total daily insulin dose is shown in Table 1.

Patient Example 3

- 14 y.o. boy with cognitive delays presents with 3-week history of polydipsia and polyuria and 10 lb weight loss.
- Glucose 625 mg/dl in ER
- Bicarbonate 19 meq/l.
- Tanner 4 on exam
- Weight 44 kg
- Parents also have cognitive impairments

- Total daily dose: 44 kg X 0.6 u/kg/d = 26.4 units per day.
- Medical team decides fixed mixed 75/25 insulin regimen may be best.
- 2/3 TDD given before breakfast = 17 units
- 1/3 before dinner = 9 units
- Sliding scale rapid acting: 1 unit per 50 mg/dl over 200 mg/dl.

Figure 3 A 14-year-old boy with intellectual impairments presents with new-onset type 1 diabetes without diabetic ketoacidosis. Because of cognitive delays in both the patient and his parents, a simplified two-injection regimen was derived using the previously described calculations. This regimen may be supplemented with a sliding scale of rapid-acting insulin.

lunchtime. Typically, two-thirds of the daily dose is given in the morning; then two-thirds NPH, one-third rapid-acting insulin, and one-third of the daily dose is given in evening. The evening dose is divided, with one-third rapid-acting before dinner and two-thirds NPH at bedtime. The patient should, however, consume a relatively fixed amount of carbohydrate at each meal. Consistency in meal content and portion size is very important in overall glycemic control. A simplified sliding scale of rapid-acting insulin may be added to the NPH and rapid-acting insulin regimen.

In certain challenging cases where there are significant compliance or cognitive deficits, fixed doses of premixed intermediate- and rapid- or short-acting insulin such as Humalog mix (75/25) can be used before breakfast and before dinner (Fig. 3). Premixed 75/25 insulin preparations come in vials or pens and consist of 75% intermediate-acting neutral protamine hagedorn; (NPH) and 25% rapid-acting (lispro) insulins. Insulin pens are a very convenient way to give insulin, but in some cases, because of patient preference or insurer restrictions, dosing by syringe is preferred or required.

Treatment of Diabetic Ketoacidosis

There are critical differences in the treatment of DKA between children and adults. A major complication of the treatment of DKA in children is cerebral edema, a complication rarely seen in adults. Although a relatively infrequent complication (<1% of DKA episodes), cerebral edema can be associated with serious morbidity and mortality.

Risk factors for the development of cerebral edema include new-onset diabetes, younger age at diagnosis, longer duration of symptoms before diagnosis, and severity of acidosis—manifested as DKA with hypocapnia, high blood urea nitrogen, bicarbonate boluses, and failure for the corrected serum sodium to rise as treatment for DKA progresses. For these reasons, overly aggressive fluid resuscitation and boluses of bicarbonate are avoided in the treatment of pediatric DKA.

TABLE 2	Formulas for the Calculation of Maintenance Fluids for Infants and Children
For infants 3.5–10 kg, daily fluid requirement = 100 mL/kg	
For children 11–20 kg, daily fluid requirement = 1000 mL + 50 mL/kg for every kg over 10 years of age	
For children >20 kg, daily fluid requirement = 1500 mL + 20 mL/kg for every kg over 20, up to a maximum of 2400 mL daily	

Judicious fluid replacement with a bolus of normal saline—initially 10 mL/kg and, if necessary, a second 10-mL/kg bolus of saline solution—may be given in the first hour of treatment. Thereafter half normal saline with 40 mEq/L of potassium acetate or potassium phosphate at a fluid rate of no more than 1.5 to 2.0 times maintenance is administered (Table 2). Potassium should not be added to intravenous fluid until the K is <5 meq/L. The two-bag system for fluid management of DKA—in which two bags contain identical electrolytes but differ in that one bag contains no dextrose and the second bag contains 10% dextrose—can be useful. The relative contribution of each bag is then titrated depending on the blood glucose level. Although estimates of fluid deficit in DKA are between 5% and 10% of body weight, intravascular volume is often preserved in the hyperosmolar state; hence hypovolemic shock is uncommon in DKA. The goal is to replace the fluid deficit slowly over 24 to 48 hours. Frequent neurologic checks are highly recommended in the first 24 hours of treatment. Altered mental status or the development of a severe headache during treatment for DKA is a potentially serious sign of cerebral edema.

Insulin plays a critical role in the treatment of DKA, not only in lowering serum glucose levels but also in the paramount role of shutting down ketogenesis in the liver. The standard insulin drip for pediatric DKA is 0.1 U/kg per hour; however, treatment with 0.05 U/kg per hour has also been effective. Human regular insulin remains the standard insulin in the intravenous treatment of DKA.

Once the acidosis has resolved, as reflected by a normal anion gap and serum bicarbonate greater than 15 mmol/L and pH greater than 7.35, the insulin drip can be discontinued. Hyperchloremic non–anion gap acidosis (HCO$_3$ <15 but normal anion gap <12) can occur during the recovery phase of DKA. Hyperchloremic metabolic acidosis is likely due to a large amount of chloride administered in intravenous fluids as both NaCl and KCL supplementation. For this reason many centers typically give 50% of the potassium replacement as potassium phosphate. Once the acidosis is resolved and the patient can tolerate oral intake, subcutaneous insulin can be started per the section, Treatment of Type 1 Diabetes Mellitus, earlier in this chapter. The most convenient time to do so is just before a meal.

Importantly, treatment of pediatric DKA should ideally occur in centers with experienced pediatric intensivists, endocrinologists, and nursing staff. If referral to a pediatric center is not practical, then early contact with a pediatric endocrinologist for treatment guidance is highly recommended.

Finally, the most common causes of pediatric DKA are (1) new-onset diabetes presenting in DKA and (2) infusion site failure in a patient on an insulin pump or missed long-acting insulin injections in a patient on insulin injections. Infections including gastroenteritis and febrile illnesses are infrequently the exclusive cause of DKA in pediatrics.

Diabetes Self-Management Education

Children and adolescents with type 1 diabetes should receive outpatient care by multidisciplinary teams including an endocrinologist, certified diabetes educator, nurse, registered dietician, and licensed clinical social worker. Provision of comprehensive education at the time of diagnosis is essential because this is the time when the patient and family are most receptive and impressionable. Patients who do not receive proper early education often fall into habits of suboptimal diabetes care, which can be hard to undo once established.

Important educational topics that must be rapidly learned by the family and patient (in addition to glucose monitoring and insulin administration) include diet and carbohydrate counting, prevention and treatment of hypoglycemia, emergency glucagon, exercise and hypoglycemia, prevention of ketoacidosis, and sick day management. Learning to count carbohydrates accurately can be a particular challenge.

Mental Health Considerations in Type 1 Diabetes Mellitus

Diabetes "burnout" issues are common in the treatment of youth with diabetes, particularly during the adolescent years. Conflicts between parents and teens can often arise during this time. It is important for the parents to maintain a healthy supporting role with their child or teenager in a manner appropriate to the child's age and level of development. Recognition of relatively common mental health comorbidities—such as depression, anxiety, and eating disorders—is essential to the overall well-being of the pediatric patient with T1DM.

Goals of Therapy for Patients With Type 1 Diabetes Mellitus

The number-one goal of the diabetes health care team is to prevent readmission to the hospital for severe hypoglycemia or ketoacidosis. Resumption of the full range of daily activities, including returning to school and work as well as engaging in essentially all meaningful activities that preceded the diagnosis of diabetes, is to be expected.

Although the goal in the pediatric age group is to reduce hemoglobin A1c to below 7.5%, less than 25% of pediatric patients in the United States are able to achieve that goal. The average hemoglobin A1c in the pediatric population is approximately 8.2%, whereas in 19-year-olds the average hemoglobin A1c is 9.2%.

The Diabetes Control and Complications Trial (DCCT) in 1993 showed convincingly that lowering the hemoglobin A1c from 9% to 7.1% resulted in significantly less diabetes-related retinopathy, nephropathy, and neuropathy. Most patients in the DCCT trial who were randomized to the intensively treated group used insulin pumps to achieve tighter control, but tight control was achieved with injectable insulin regimens as well.

Sick Day Management

Patients with T1DM who have intercurrent infectious illnesses are prone to develop hyperglycemia with ketosis and also hypoglycemia, depending on the nature of the illness. Blood glucose levels should be monitored every 1 to 3 hours during illnesses. Rapid-acting insulin may need to be administered every 2 to 4 hours for hyperglycemia, especially in the presence of serum or urine ketones. Rapid-acting insulin can be dosed at 0.1 to 0.2 U/kg per dose in this setting. Improvement in hyperglycemia and particularly in ketosis using this treatment regimen can be invaluable in preventing ketoacidosis or hospitalization. Patients with persistent vomiting who are unable to keep fluids down need to be referred to the emergency department for intravenous hydration and assessment for DKA.

For patients on an insulin pump, ketosis with nausea and vomiting is often a sign that the insulin infusion set is not properly functioning. Insulin therefore should be given by syringe or pen device until the ketones have cleared and a new infusion set has been placed.

Poor oral intake during a gastrointestinal illness may result in hypoglycemia. Frequent small volumes of sugar-containing fluids such as juice or sports drinks may be necessary to keep the blood glucose above 70 mg/dL, and basal insulin requirements may need to be decreased by 10% to 50%. Low-dose glucagon may be used in the setting of recurrent hypoglycemia and poor oral intake. Glucagon can be dosed at 1 unit on an insulin syringe for every year of age, using a standard 1-mg/mL glucagon preparation. The dose may be repeated every 15 minutes as needed. In some cases, persistent low glucose levels (<70 mg/dL) in the setting of recurrent vomiting may be best managed in an emergency department or hospital setting where intravenous dextrose-containing fluids are readily available.

Risk for Additional Autoimmune Disorders

Patients with one autoimmune disorder are at increased risk for the development of one or more additional autoimmune conditions. Children and adolescents with T1DM are particularly at risk for thyroid and celiac disorders. Screening for thyroid disorders with serum TSH and free T_4 should occur in the first 6 months after the T1DM diagnosis and every 1 to 2 years thereafter. Celiac disorder should also be screened in the first year after the T1DM diagnosis. Most cases of celiac disorder are detected within the first 5 years after the diagnosis of T1DM, and the majority of cases are asymptomatic. Recent American Diabetes Association recommendations include screening for celiac disorder at diagnosis and again at 2 and 5 years after diagnosis. Elevated serum tissue transglutaminase levels should be referred to a pediatric gastroenterologist. Because celiac disorder is a lifelong condition, it is advised to obtain a small bowel biopsy. Autoimmune adrenal (Addison) disease rarely occurs with T1DM but has the unique presentation of recurrent hypoglycemia, necessitating significant reductions in daily insulin requirements. Sending simultaneous adrenocorticotropic hormone and cortisol levels on a morning blood specimen will usually render the diagnosis of Addison disease.

Screening for Complications of Type 1 Diabetes Mellitus

Microvascular complications of T1DM are infrequent in the pediatric age group, although background retinopathy and microalbuminuria become more prevalent in the late-adolescent and young-adult age ranges. Proactive early screening regimens are advocated to detect diabetes complications early so that medical interventions can prevent more serious diabetes-related complications such as proliferative retinopathy and end-stage renal disease.

Annual screening for microalbuminuria with a random urine specimen should be performed at puberty or at age 10 years and above once the child has had diabetes for 5 years. Elevated urine albumin/urine creatinine (>30 mg/g creatinine) ratios should be repeated two to three times over a 6-month period to confirm the diagnosis because transient microalbuminuria is a common finding. Variables such as exercise or recent illness can lead to microalbuminuria; therefore a repeat study after recovery and on a first morning specimen will often yield a normal result. In addition, individuals with the benign condition of orthostatic albuminuria can be identified by finding completely normal albumin excretion on a first morning voided specimen, whereas a random specimen will often be frankly proteinuric. When urinary albumin/creatinine ratios are found to be consistently elevated, treatment with an angiotensin converting enzyme inhibitor is recommended. Referral to a pediatric nephrologist should be arranged in complex cases.

Annual dilated eye examinations are recommended after age 10 or at pubertal onset (whichever comes first) once the patient has had diabetes for 3 to 5 years. Referral to an eye care professional with expertise in diabetic retinopathy is recommended.

Cardiovascular risk factors including blood pressure and lipid profiles should be monitored in patients with T1DM. Blood pressure should be obtained at each visit.

High blood pressure is defined as systolic or diastolic blood pressure above the 90th percentile, and hypertension is defined as above the 95th percentile for age, sex, and height. Blood pressure measurements should be obtained using an appropriate cuff size, particularly in the overweight patient. White-coat hypertension can be problematic in the adolescent population. Such patients will often demonstrate an elevated heart rate as a clue to stress-induced hypertension. Monitoring blood pressure in a nonthreatening environment, such as at home, using an accurate home blood pressure monitor, may be helpful. When white-coat hypertension is suspected, 24–hour home blood pressure monitoring can be very useful.

Initial management of high blood pressure includes salt restriction and weight-control measures. For persistent hypertension, treatment with an antihypertensive medication (lisinopril) may be necessary.

Shortly after diagnosis and once glucose control has been established, it is important to obtain nonfasting total and high-density lipoprotein cholesterol readings. If total cholesterol is high, a fasting morning lipid panel should be obtained. If low-density lipoprotein (LDL) cholesterol is below 100, it would be reasonable to repeat it in 5 years. For LDL cholesterol above 100, dietary measures are taken, along with efforts to improve metabolic control. For patients beyond 10 years of age with an LDL cholesterol above 130 to 160 in whom lifestyle changes have resulted in inadequate control, statin therapy may be considered. Referral to a pediatric preventive cardiology program would also be appropriate.

Technologic Changes in the Care for Patients With Type 1 Diabetes Mellitus

Technological changes have revolutionized the care of patients with T1DM. Unheralded changes such as the emergence of ultra-fine lancet technology coupled with glucose test strips requiring less than 10 μL of blood resulted in rapid, essentially painless fingerstick glucose monitoring. Ultrafine insulin syringes and pen needles helped usher in widespread adoption of intensive insulin regimens with rapid-acting insulin taken before all meals and snacks.

The insulin pump further advanced diabetes care in making insulin dosing before meals and snacks even less challenging, especially for children. The development of a tubeless insulin pump (Omnipod) led to an even wider array of choices.

Continuous glucose monitoring (CGM) has evolved into a very powerful and widely used technology in T1DM. Subcutaneous fluid glucose levels are determined every 1 to 5 minutes and the user is provided with meaningful feedback to influence diabetes self-management decisions in real time. Particularly useful are alarm functions for impending low glucose levels; these can be invaluable in the prevention of hypoglycemia. Alarms for hyperglycemia are also used with this technology. The accuracy of glucose determinations by CGM technology is now approaching subcutaneous blood glucose technology, and the improved accuracy has led the US Food and Drug Administration (FDA) to approve insulin-dosing decisions based on CGM data (e.g., the Dexcom G6 products). It is important to remember, however, that subcutaneous glucose levels lag behind whole blood glucose levels by about 15 minutes. This fact is particularly important when glucose levels are changing rapidly, so the user is advised to pay attention to the glucose trend. Alarms for predicting hypoglycemia are very important in this regard.

A historic drawback to CGM technology had been the need to calibrate the device accurately with periodic fingerstick glucose checks. However, the Dexcom G6, which was released to market in 2018, and the Abbot Libre, are factory-calibrated and do not require consumer calibration. Remarkably, patients using calibration-free CGM devices may no longer be required to check fingerstick glucose levels! A CGM sensor placed on the arm or abdomen will last for 10 to 14 days before having to be changed.

The most remarkable technologic change emerging in the care of patients with T1DM is the coupling of CGM and real-time adjustments in insulin delivery via insulin pump therapy. Thus insulin delivery is suspended when hypoglycemia has occurred or is likely to occur, and basal insulin can be significantly increased when hyperglycemia is predicted to occur or has occurred. *Hybrid closed-loop* refers to the fact that some aspects of management, such as carbohydrate counting and manual bolusing for meals, are still required. The first hybrid closed-loop insulin pump was FDA approved in 2016 (Medtronic 670G). Prevention of postprandial hyperglycemia is particularly problematic, but prebolusing rapid-acting insulin 10 to 30 minutes before eating will help to limit postprandial hyperglycemia. Prebolusing of insulin is often difficult in view of modern lifestyles. Use of the Medtronic 670G insulin pump has proven to be challenging in the real-world setting due to frequent calibration requirements and forced exits from the automatic insulin delivery mode. The Tandem insulin pump with Control IQ technology was FDA approved in 2019. This hybrid closed-loop system is user friendly, with no calibration requirements or forced exits from automated insulin delivery. Hybrid closed-loop technology can be particularly useful for optimizing glycemic control overnight, the time when many patients and families are most fearful of hypoglycemia. The very popular Omnipod 5 tubeless hybrid closed-loop insulin pump was FDA approved in 2022, giving individuals with T1DM even more choices to improve glycemic control.

Type 2 Diabetes in Children

Since the 1990s, type 2 diabetes mellitus (T2DM) in patients below 18 years of age has risen dramatically. The increased incidence of type 2 diabetes has coincided with the obesity epidemic. Children from minority populations (non-Hispanic blacks, Hispanics, and Native Americans) and those patients with a positive family history of T2DM are at the greatest risk. The majority of pediatric T2DM is found in adolescents and children above 10 years of age.

Diagnosis of T2DM can be made with a fasting glucose above 126 mg/dL, random glucose above 200 mg/dL, and the 2-hour glucose from an oral glucose tolerance test above 200 mg/dL. A hemoglobin A1c greater than 6.5% is indicative of diabetes as well and is a particularly convenient test in the outpatient setting. An elevated fasting or random glucose and an elevated hemoglobin A1c are diagnostic of T2DM in high-risk patients.

Pediatric patients with T2DM are often symptom free at diagnosis but can present acutely with classic diabetes symptoms and even ketosis or mild ketoacidosis. Distinguishing the latter group from T1DM can be difficult initially, but the absence of β cell antibodies and very stable glycemic control after diagnosis are often telltale signs of T2DM.

In individuals who present with marked hyperglycemia (hemoglobin A1c >8.5%), ketosis, or both, stabilization with insulin initially may be required. Basal bolus regimens using a combination of long- and short-acting insulins can be instituted. Insulin resistance may be quite significant at the time of diagnosis, and relatively high doses of insulin can be required to achieve target glucose levels.

Metformin (Glucophage) is the mainstay of treatment for T2DM in those below 18 years of age. Maximal dosing is 1000 mg bid or 2000 mg/day of the extended-release preparation. Gastrointestinal side effects are relatively common, and metformin should be taken with meals. Initial dosing can be 500 mg bid or 1000 mg extended-release daily; the dose can be titrated upward as needed and tolerated. **Dietary modifications such as weight control and exercise are of fundamental importance in the treatment of T2DM.** Liraglutide (Victoza), a glucagon-like peptide (GLP-1) agonist, was FDA approved in 2019 for the treatment of T2DM for patients above 10 years of age. GLP-1 agonists are associated with early satiety, weight loss, and improved glycemic control in T2DM. GLP-1 agonist have become increasingly popular in the treatment of T2DM as they promote weight loss, while insulin may facilitate weight gain. Side effects of GLP-1 agents include nausea, vomiting, and, less commonly, pancreatitis. Therefore patients with T2DM need to be as vigilant as patients with T1DM, in monitoring their glucose levels regularly and following up every 3 to 6 months with their healthcare teams.

Monogenic or Maturity-Onset Diabetes of Youth

Single gene mutations leading to diabetes are referred to as *maturity onset diabetes of youth (MODY) diabetes* or *monogenic diabetes*. More than 30 different genes have been identified that are associated with MODY, although some 80% of cases are due to glucokinase and *HNF1A* and *HNF1B* gene mutations. Patients can be diagnosed at any age but are usually diagnosed before age 35 years. Routine laboratory testing or laboratory testing during an illness may lead to the detection of MODY diabetes incidentally. Patients with MODY are often lean, and the family history may reveal two to three affected generations. Testing for islet cell antibodies is universally negative.

Glucokinase diabetes is a very mild form of MODY diabetes that is nonprogressive and does not require treatment, whereas *HNF1A* and *HNF1B* forms of MODY diabetes are progressive; these patients can develop long-term complications of diabetes. HNF diabetes is uniquely sensitive to sulfonylureas, and hence the diagnosis can be life changing in an individual who has been treated with insulin prior to definitive diagnosis.

Genetic panels for MODY diabetes are available commercially. It is important to test for both mutations and deletions of the most common forms of MODY. A full list of laboratories that offer MODY testing is available at the NCBI Genetic Testing Registry (http://www.ncbi.nlm.nih.gov/gtr/).

Neonatal diabetes can also be due to monogenic forms of diabetes, and these infants are usually diagnosed before 6 to 9 months of age. Testing for monogenetic forms of diabetes should be considered in infants below 9 to 12 months of age whose islet cell autoantibodies are negative. Single gene mutations in the K-ATP channel of the β cell leading to neonatal diabetes can be remarkably responsive to oral sulfonylureas. Transient forms of neonatal diabetes in an infant born with intrauterine growth retardation and macroglossia are often associated with imprinting abnormalities on chromosome region 6q24. This type of diabetes usually resolves by 18 months but can recur at adolescence.

References

American Diabetes Association: Children and adolescents: Standards of medical care in diabetes—2018, *Diabetes Care* 41(Suppl 1):S126–S136, 2018.

Copeland KC, Zeiter P, Geffner M, et al: Characteristics of adolescents and youth with recent-onset type 2 diabetes: the TODAY cohort at baseline, *J Clin Endocrinol Metab* 96:159–167, 2011.

Delli AJ, Lernmark A: Type 1 (insulin-dependent) diabetes mellitus: Etiology, pathogenesis, prediction, and prevention. In *Endocrinology: Adult and Pediatric*, Saunders, 2016.

Levitsky L, Misra M: Epidemiology, presentation and diagnosis of type 1 diabetes in children and adolescents. Up To Date. Available at Up To Date. Accessed March 3, 2020.

Miller KM, Foster NC, Beck RW, et al: Current state of type 1 diabetes treatment in the US: updated data from the T1D Exchange Clinic Registry, *Diabetes Care* 38:971–978, 2015.

Sperling MA, Tamborlane WR, et al: In *Pediatric Endocrinology*, Philadelphia, 2014, Elsevier, pp 847–900.

The Environmental Determinants of Diabetes Study: Available at: https://teddy.epi.usf.edu/. Accessed 9/3/20.

The National Center for Monogenic Diabetes at the University of Chicago Monogenic Diabetes Registry. Available at Monogenic https://monogenicdiabetes.uchicago.edu/. Accessed 9/3/20.

White NH: Long-term outcomes in youth with diabetes mellitus, *Pediatr Clin North Am* 62:889–909, 2015.

Wolfsdorf JI: The International Society of Pediatric and Adolescent Diabetes guidelines for management of ketoacidosis: do the guidelines need to be modified? *Pediatric Diabetes* 15:277–286, 2014.

Wolfsdorf JI, Garvey K: Diabetes mellitus in children. In Jameson L, DeGroot L, editors: *Endocrinology adult and pediatric*, ed 7, Philadelphia, 2016, Saunders, pp 854–882.

Writing Group for the TRIGR Study Group: Effect of hydrolyzed infant formula vs conventional formula on the risk of type 1 diabetes, *JAMA* 319:38, 2018.

Yeung W, Rawlinson W, Craig M: Enterovirus infection and type 1 diabetes mellitus: Systematic review and meta-analysis of observational molecular studies, *BMJ* 342(7794):421, 2011.

■ ENCOPRESIS

Method of
Sarah Houssayni, MD

CURRENT DIAGNOSIS

- Voluntary or involuntary passage of stools into inappropriate places at least once a month for 3 consecutive months once a chronologic or developmental age of 4 years has been reached.
- Encopresis can be primary when it persists from infancy onward or secondary when it appears after toilet training.
- The behavior is not due to the direct effects of a substance such as a laxative or a general medical condition except those associated with constipation.
- Distinguishing subtypes is essential because treatment differs:
  - Retentive encopresis: occurs as a result of involuntary leakage of liquid stools due to severe constipation and impaction.
  - Nonretentive encopresis: children pass bowel movements into their underwear due to their refusal to use the toilet.
  - Children occasionally fail to wipe after bowel movements and the secondary soiling should be distinguished from encopresis.

CURRENT THERAPY

Retentive Encopresis
Initial Disimpaction
- Hyperphosphate enemas (Pedia-Lax Enema) (one daily for 2 or 3 days):
  - Less than 1 year old: 60mL.[3]
  - Greater than 1 year old: 6mL/kg, up to 135mL twice.[3]
- Glycerin suppositories (Glycerin Pediatric Suppositories) for infants and toddlers.

Older Children—Slow Disimpaction
- Polyethylene glycol with electrolytes (Golytely, Colyte)[1] ingested over 2–3 days: 25mL/kg/hr up to 1L/hr until stooling clear bowel movements. (This is not approved for bowel cleansing for children.)
- Over 5–7 days:
  - Mineral oil[1] 3mL/kg twice a day for 1 week. (Mineral oil is not approved for use in children younger than 6 years of age.)
  - Lactulose[1] 2mL/kg twice a day for 1 week.
  - Magnesium hydroxide (Milk of Magnesia) 2mL/kg twice a day for 1 week.
  - Polyethylene glycol without electrolyte (MiraLax)[1] 1.5g/kg/day for 3 days.

Maintenance Therapy
- Polyethylene glycol 3350 (MiraLax)[1] age greater than 1 month: 0.7g/kg divided into 1–2 doses daily.
- Lactulose or sorbitol 70% solution age greater than 1 month: 1–3mL/kg/day divided into 1–2 doses daily for 1–3 months.
- Sennosides (Senna, Senna-GRX, Senexon) are habit forming, doses vary greatly in the different available formulations, and they can only be used for short-term treatment. Give at bedtime for a morning bowel movement. Dose is 5mL (1 tablet) for 1–[1] 5-year-olds and 2 tablets for 5- to 15-year-olds for a maximum of three tablets daily. (Sennosides are not approved for use in children younger than 2 years of age.)
- Glycerin enemas and bisacodyl suppositories (Dulcolax) can be used for short-term constipation treatment.

Randomized controlled trials have demonstrated that the enuretic alarm has greater efficacy than other forms of treatment. The enuretic alarm is triggered when a sensor in the sheets or night clothes gets wet; a bell or buzzer is thereby activated. Presumably, alarm therapy startles the child and improves arousal from sleep either by classical conditioning or avoidance conditioning. A disadvantage of alarm therapy is that it takes a couple of weeks to take effect. As such, alarms should be used for at least 6 weeks in children who do not respond before discontinuing their use. Because success depends on a cooperative, motivated child, conditioning therapy with an alarm device is generally used in children over 6 years of age.

It has been shown that combination of alarm and desmopressin works better than either treatment alone. Such treatment may be considered for children with refractory nocturnal enuresis.

When an anatomic abnormality or defect in urinary concentration ability is present, the underlying problem may require specific dietary, pharmacologic, or surgical treatment. Any underlying constipation should also be treated.

References

Brown ML, Pope AW, Brown EJ: Treatment of primary nocturnal enuresis in children: a review, *Child Care Health Dev* 37:153–160, 2011.
Glazener CM, Evans JH: Desmopressin for nocturnal enuresis in children, *Cochrane Database Syst Rev* 3:CD002112, 2002.
Glazener CM, Evans JH, Pero RE: Alarm interventions for nocturnal enuresis in children, *Cochrane Database Syst Rev* 2:CD002911, 2005.
Kamperis K, Hagstroem S, Rittig S, et al: Combination of the enuresis alarm and desmopressin: Second line treatment for nocturnal enuresis, *J Urol* 179:1128–1131, 2008.
Leung AK: Nocturnal enuresis. In Leung AK, editor: Common Problems in Ambulatory Pediatrics: Specific Clinical Problems, vol 1. New York, 2011, Nova Science Publishers, pp 161–171.
Lottmann H, Froeling F, Alloussi S, et al: A randomized comparison of oral desmopressin lyophilisate (MELT) and tablet formulations in children and adolescents with primary nocturnal enuresis, *Int J Clin Pract* 61:1454–1460, 2007.
Nevéus T: Nocturnal enuresis—theoretic background and practical guidelines, *Pediatr. Nephrol* 26:1207–1214, 2011.
Robson WL: Evaluation and management of enuresis, *N Engl J Med* 360:1429–1436, 2009.
Robson WL, Leung AK, van Howe R: Primary and secondary nocturnal enuresis: similarities in presentation, *Pediatrics* 115:956–959, 2005.
Robson WL, Leung AK, Norgaard JP: The comparative safety of oral versus intranasal desmopressin in the treatment of children with nocturnal enuresis, *J Urol* 178:24–30, 2007.
Van de Walle J, Rittig S, Bauer S, et al: Practical consensus guidelines for the management of enuresis, *Eur J Pediatr* 171:971–983, 2012.

INFANT AND CHILDREN FEEDING PROBLEMS

Method of
Sarah Edwards, DO; and Dana M. Bakula, PhD

CURRENT DIAGNOSIS

- As of 2021, the primary diagnostic code used to describe feeding problems in infants and children is *pediatric feeding disorder (PFD)*.
- PFD is defined as impairments in oral intake that are not age appropriate.
- PFD is caused by medical, nutritional, psychosocial, and/or feeding skill problems.
- As a result of both the broad criteria and the complex multifactorial nature of the condition, the presentation of PFD can vary significantly from child to child, as can treatments.

CURRENT THERAPY

- A thorough assessment of medical, nutritional, psychosocial, and feeding skills issues is needed to optimize treatment planning.
- It is imperative to treat underlying medical conditions that may be contributing to pediatric feeding disorder.
- Nutritional monitoring is necessary to ensure patient safety and guide clinical decision-making.
- If adequate nutrition cannot be achieved orally, enteral nutrition should be considered.
- Feeding therapy is often necessary to treat feeding skill issues that prevent safe or efficient oral feeding.
- Behavioral treatment is often needed to treat parent and/or child factors that prevent oral feeding.

Pathophysiology

As of 2021, pediatric feeding disorder (PFD) is the primary diagnosis used to describe feeding problems of infants and children. PFD is often multifactorial, including medical, nutritional, psychosocial, and skill-based issues, and typically involves concerns in one or more of these domains. The progression of feeding from breastmilk or formula at birth to table foods is a typical pattern of development that occurs without issue for many children. However, when this typical pattern of development is interrupted, PFD can develop.

Medical etiologies: Cow's milk protein allergy, gastroesophageal reflux disease, and eosinophilic esophagitis are the most common gastrointestinal (GI) etiologies of PFD. They can lead to discomfort with feeding that can contribute to the development of a feeding aversion. Although less common, physiologic processes that increase metabolic demand can lead to PFD, as they make it difficult for the infant or child to keep up with their caloric needs. This is most common in children with congenital heart disease. Medical conditions, such as cardiorespiratory compromise during oral feeding and aspiration and recurrent aspiration pneumonitis, may be causes of feeding problems. Underlying syndromes, neuromuscular disabilities, and genetic differences can interrupt the typical progression of feeding, contributing to feeding intolerance, poor oral intake, or oral aversion. Premature infants who spent time in the neonatal intensive care unit have an increased incidence of feeding difficulties that can be, in part, due to delay of development and multiple painful procedures around their mouth and face that can contribute to oral aversion.

Nutritional etiologies: A nutritional deficit may result from inadequate caloric intake, increased metabolic demand, or excessive GI losses. Inadequate caloric intake can be caused by a decreased hunger drive, often from a grazing pattern of eating, which effectively alleviates the child's sensation of hunger. Therefore the child does not eat an adequately sized meal. Increased metabolic demand results from a medical condition that causes the patient to be unable to gain weight even with usually adequate caloric intake as their nutritional needs are greater than typical for age. This can include such etiologies as congenital heart disease, cystic fibrosis, metabolic disorders, or neuromuscular disorders. Excessive GI losses may occur with vomiting or diarrhea, where calories that are taken in are not effectively used. Malnutrition and nutrient deficiencies may result from a lack of dietary diversity.

Psychosocial etiologies: Infants and children can develop aversions to feeding for several reasons. Psychosocial etiologies may interact with medical or feeding skill concerns. For instance, a child may begin refusing all foods because of a cow's milk allergy as they fear that all foods may result in discomfort, or a child may refuse to drink any liquid because they typically choke on thin liquids. Environmental factors, such as distractions present at meals (e.g., iPad) or a lack of mealtime structure can prevent a child from having sufficient time and opportunity to feed. Further, parents and caregivers for children with feeding challenges can feel anxious or stressed at meals. Parental stress or cultural expectations surrounding feeding may impact how parents interact with their child at meals. Some parents may engage in maladaptive strategies, attempting to get their child to eat more by force-feeding or yelling, which only worsens the problem. Underlying psychosocial conditions, such as autism, attention-deficit/hyperactivity disorder, and oppositional defiant disorder can result in behavioral challenges at mealtimes that prevent sufficient oral intake. Even among infants, these psychosocial factors can manifest. For instance, postpartum depression can impact how mothers interact with their infants during feeding.

Feeding skill etiologies: Oral motor skills are a common contributor to feeding problems. Oral motor problems can be secondary to an anatomic cause, such as a laryngeal cleft or underlying muscle weakness due to a neurologic disorder, or may be idiopathic. Oral motor difficulties may result from inefficient and ineffective chewing and swallowing mechanics. When a child struggles to eat effectively, this can result in the child struggling to eat age-appropriate foods or to consume a sufficient volume of food and to have unsafe swallows, which may lead to aspiration and risk of respiratory infections. Oral motor skill problems can also cause a child to eat less efficiently, resulting in fatigue and longer mealtimes, which may exacerbate child frustrations with mealtimes. In addition, the experiences of discomfort and fear that may come with a child struggling to effectively control the food or liquid in their mouth may result in oral aversion.

Prevention

The key to prevention is in identifying feeding concerns early and providing proactive education and treatment. One common pitfall is to assume that a child who is of normal weight does not have PFD; these are not mutually exclusive. Although a significant proportion of patients with PFD have malnutrition, this is not seen in every case and malnutrition is not typically the first symptom of feeding problems. For instance, well before weight loss is identified, the clinician might hear from a parent that they are having to feed their baby around the clock, that each feeding lasts well over 30 minutes, or that a parent is "having to force-feed" their child to make sure they eat enough. In older children the clinician may hear that parents are only giving the child a few preferred foods because the parent has learned that this is the only way the child will eat. These situations can lead to severe micronutrient deficiencies. For infants, key red flags the clinician should be attuned to listen for include infants who are primarily "dream-feeding" (feeding during sleep), falling asleep during all feedings, not waking to feed on their own, sweating with feedings, choking with feedings, and exhibiting fussiness with feedings. With older children, key red flags the clinician should be attuned to identify are the child being unwilling to eat foods they were once eating, choking on food, fearing feeding, cutting foods into very small pieces, vomiting after every feed, or eating only a few foods until they burn out on that food and then move to another food (food jags). Early identification and evaluations are the key to prevention.

Clinical Manifestations

Patients can present with a wide spectrum of symptoms. Oral motor concerns can manifest as coughing or choking with feeds, feeling fatigued during feeds, or refusing to eat due to insufficient skills. It is important to understand the timing of when the feeding problems began. If the child ate well for the first 2 years of life but then started to lose interest in foods they were once readily taking without the development of any GI symptoms, this can incite concern for an autism spectrum disorder or sensory sensitivity.

Evaluation of weight and linear growth or height is important. Assessment for malnutrition on the age-appropriate growth chart (World Health Organization growth chart for 0 to 2 years of age and Centers for Disease Control and Prevention growth chart for patients older than 2 years) should be routine. Not all patients with PFD present with malnutrition. Some patients may eat a narrow range of foods, yet they eat enough calories that they gain appropriate weight, and it is not until further investigation that micronutrient deficiencies are identified. Additionally, poor linear growth that precedes difficulty with weight gain can indicate a metabolic etiology for malnutrition.

A thorough history, physical examination, and observation of a feeding are key parts of the evaluation. A history of prematurity or chronic medical conditions can increase the risk of PFD. Attention should be given to the respiratory history and any report of recurrent lower respiratory tract infections or chronic congestion. Timing, volume, and length of feeds, as well as how formula is mixed, are key questions for understanding the total amount of calories a patient is ingesting. Children who demonstrate a grazing pattern of eating typically have less hunger drive and subsequently less oral intake than those patients who eat three meals and two snacks with no food in between. Children taking a long time to feed may be fatigued during the feed or averse to feeding. Questions about a history of vomiting, concerns for pain with feeding and stooling pattern can help identify feeding intolerances. The physical exam should include an oral exam to evaluate for dental caries, palatal abnormalities, or oral lesions; a lung exam to evaluate for aspiration pneumonia or respiratory findings; an abdominal exam to listen for bowel sounds and palpate for masses, distension, or any areas of tenderness; and an evaluation of muscle strength for any signs of hypotonia or hypertonia.

Diagnosis

PFD is the primary diagnostic code used for infants and children with feeding problems. PFD involves impairments in oral intake that are not age appropriate. PFD is a multifactorial condition and is associated with medical, nutritional, psychosocial, and/or feeding skills. As a result of both the broad criteria and the complex multifactorial nature of the condition, the presentation of PFD can vary significantly from child to child, as can the necessary treatments. You may also find it helpful to have families answer the Infant and Child Feeding Questionnaire (a six-question screener), which is freely available and distributed by Feeding Matters, an advocacy organization for children with PFD (https://www.feedingmatters.org/what-is-pfd/is-it-pfd/).

Treatment

Treatment depends on the cause and severity of the feeding impairment. For children who are otherwise healthy but are having difficulty gaining weight, starting with a mealtime structure including three meals with two to three snacks is key. Meals and snacks should be separated by 2 to 3 hours, without any grazing in between. Children may have water between meals, but no other foods or caloric beverages because grazing can lead to an overall decrease in oral intake. The clinician should also seek to increase the caloric density of the child's foods. For infants, this typically means concentrating their feeds from 20 calories an ounce to 22 to 24 calories an ounce. In a child who drinks cow's milk, add 1 tablespoon of heavy whipping cream to 4 ounces of whole milk or add in an oral nutrition supplement. Parents can also add oils or other foods that are high in fats to a child's meal to help supplement their caloric intake. Consultation with a dietitian will help determine optimal next steps for supporting a child's weight gain and growth. Dieticians are specially trained to evaluate a child's current diet and how that diet compares to one that would best meet the child's health needs and to make tailored recommendations to the family.

For patients with symptoms concerning for aspiration or oral motor difficulties, a feeding and swallowing evaluation should be considered. A videofluoroscopic swallow study may be indicated. The child may benefit from consultation with a feeding therapist to improve their feeding skills and may need eating modifications to allow them to eat safely. For instance, a swallow study may identify that the patient is aspirating thin liquids. If this is the case, the feeding therapist may recommend a thickener be added to the child's thin liquids. There may also be special feeding utensils or equipment, feeding position modification, or other strategies recommended to help the child eat safely while the therapist works with the child on progressing their oral motor skills.

Medical interventions should be employed to target any underlying conditions that are impacting the child's feeding problems. This can include upper endoscopy to evaluate for eosinophilic esophagitis, upper GI x-ray to evaluate for anatomic abnormalities such as esophageal stricture, tracheoesophageal fistula or pH study to evaluate for gastroesophageal reflux. Special consideration should be taken to use the North American Society for Gastroenterology, Hepatology and Nutrition guidelines on treatment of gastroesophageal reflux. For example, a formula change may help a child with milk protein allergy before performing a trial of acid suppression. It is also essential to treat constipation for children with PFD as poor feeding puts the child at higher risk for constipation, and constipation may increase abdominal discomfort and/or decrease appetite and therefore increase aversion to feeding. Cyproheptadine[1] can be used for appetite stimulation, but we would caution its use in patients with aversion who may have an undiagnosed underlying, painful condition.

Behavioral interventions may be needed to support children with feeding issues, as psychosocial factors play a significant role in the development of PFD. The paramount recommendation is that mealtimes are positive and that parents do not engage in any force-feeding. When children feel pressured to eat, they can feel stressed and eat even less, or act out during the meal. Parents should be encouraged to make mealtimes pleasant and avoid pressuring or forcing their child to eat. Families can be taught to use the feeding "division of responsibility," which is the concept that parents decide what goes on the child's plate at a meal, when the meal starts and ends, and where the child is during the meal, but the child ultimately decides what they eat or do not eat during the meal. Parents should be encouraged to limit distractions present at mealtimes, such as the television or other screens. Families should be encouraged to have a consistent and predictable schedule of meals and snacks, with clear expectations for how long children must stay seated for meals and snacks. When children do not have a predictable and consistent structure at meals, they are much less likely to engage in the meal and notice their internal hunger cues. Finally, parents should be encouraged to offer the child a variety of foods on their plate, including at least one or two items that are foods the child prefers or enjoys. Sometimes families can be tempted to help a child expand the variety of foods they eat by offering a plate full of new foods at a meal. This can lead to more behavioral challenges, so it is important that children have "preferred foods" on their plate in addition to options that are new or "nonpreferred." Children with significant behavioral concerns at meals, underlying behavioral problems, developmental disabilities, or significant anxiety around feeding may benefit from consultation with a psychologist or other behavioral specialist, such as an applied behavioral analysis specialist. If a psychologist or behavioral specialist is not readily accessible in the clinician's setting, consider consulting a social worker who may help the family identify behavioral treatment options.

In sum, a multidisciplinary approach is paramount to the success of treatment of children with complex or severe PFD. This may include involvement of a medical professional, feeding therapist (occupational therapist or speech pathologist), psychologist, dietitian, and nurse. It is optimal for these specialists to work together as a team, but, when the development of a team is not possible, we recommend developing strong channels of communication between the various healthcare professionals involved to support the treatment of a child's PFD. Further, the treatment approach should always be tailored to the needs of the child and guided by a clear understanding of the etiology of the feeding issues.

Monitoring

Children with feeding issues should be monitored for ongoing medical, developmental, and behavioral concerns. Micronutrient deficiencies should be evaluated regularly. This includes analyzing the child's dietary intake through patient interviews and checking labs, such as complete blood count and ferritin and vitamin D levels. The clinician may consider running labs that are specific to the child's diet, such as checking a B_{12} level if the child is not consuming much meat, fish, or dairy. The child's weight should be checked at regular intervals, with special attention to the trends of their weight and where they fall on the growth curve, to ensure they are gaining weight adequately for their age. For infants who were born prematurely, age-corrected growth charts should be used. Changes to a child's diet, such as a child no longer being willing to eat a food they used to enjoy, should be monitored regularly This is particularly concerning when children eat very few foods and/or begin "dropping" multiple preferred foods.

The clinician should monitor any changes to the child's GI tolerance, paying special attention to any vomiting, changes in stooling pattern, abdominal pain, or discomfort. These symptoms may indicate a concern about an underlying medical condition that may warrant treatment so that the child does not begin to associate eating with painful or uncomfortable experiences. The child's feeding skills should be monitored over time, with special attention to whether the child has an age-appropriate progression of feeding skills. Difficulties meeting age-appropriate benchmarks may warrant treatment and intervention from a feeding therapist.

Behavioral concerns at meals should be monitored regularly. The clinician should ask if the child is coming to meals willingly most of the time, is able to stay seated or stay at the table for the full meal, and is willing to engage during mealtime. The caregiver should not engage in any force-feeding (i.e., putting food into the child's mouth against their will). This can have adverse iatrogenic side effects.

Enteral Feeding

For children who are receiving enteral nutrition, there should be continuous monitoring of their need for tube feeding. Enteral nutrition may be necessary for only a few months for some children or a lifetime for others. Enteral nutrition can be taxing on a child and family's quality of life, so signs of tube-weaning readiness should be regularly monitored. Signs of tube-weaning readiness include improvement in oral motor skills, treatment of the underlying etiology, and improvement in oral aversion. Next steps include a decrease of enteral nutrition to promote improvement in hunger. It is important that these patients are in weekly feeding therapy as studies show that multidisciplinary tube-weaning interventions are most effective.

Complications

Children with feeding problems may begin to lose weight or have insufficient weight gain for their age. This may result in the need for hospitalization or use of enteral nutrition. In general, the least invasive methods for addressing feeding problems should be attempted first (e.g., feeding therapy, behavioral changes, treatment of underlying medical conditions), but hospitalization and enteral nutrition may be required when a child is experiencing significant difficulties with feeding and it is not possible for them to sustain adequate nutrition by mouth. Dehydration may also be a concern when children struggle with feeding, and

---

[1] Not FDA approved for this indication.

every attempt should be made to encourage oral intake with feeding therapy and behavior modification. In situations where this is not possible, hospitalization and/or enteral nutrition are sometimes needed, especially when children with feeding issues experience acute illness, causing their oral intake to worsen from their baseline. Micronutrient deficiencies may occur in children who eat a limited variety of foods; thus it is critical to monitor for these complications in addition to monitoring the child's weight. Finally, behavioral escalations and general behavioral challenges may emerge as a result of pediatric feeding issues. Children who struggle with feeding may find mealtime to be a difficult and stressful experience. Parents of these children are also experiencing notable stress, and this can result in additional behavioral challenges, especially at meals. Encouraging parents to follow behavioral mealtime strategies and consult with a behavioral specialist if concerns persist will be helpful in managing this complication.

References

Berlin KS, Davies WH, Lobato DJ, Silverman AH: A biopsychosocial model of normative and problematic pediatric feeding, *Child Health Care* 38(4):263–282, 2009.

Chen TL, Chen YY, Lin CL, Peng FS, Chien LY: Responsive feeding, infant growth, and postpartum depressive symptoms during 3 months postpartum, *Nutrients* 12(6):1766, 2020.

Davies W, Satter E, Berlin KS, et al: Reconceptualizing feeding and feeding disorders in interpersonal context: the case for a relational disorder, *J Fam Psychol* 20(3):409, 2006.

Edwards ST, Glynn EF, Slogic M, et al: Demographics of children with feeding difficulties from a large electronic health record database, *J Parenter Enteral Nutr* 46:1022–1030, 2022, https://doi.org/10.1002/jpen.2379.

Feeding Matters. Feeding Matters.org. Is it Pediatric Feeding Disorder (PFD)? Accessed February 14, 2023. https://www.feedingmatters.org/what-is-pfd/is-it-pfd/. Accessed May 29, 2023.

Goday PS, Huh SY, Silverman A, et al: Pediatric feeding disorder: consensus definition and conceptual framework, *J Pediatr Gastroenterol Nutr* 68(1):124–129, 2019, https://doi.org/10.1097/MPG.0000000000002188.

Kovacic K, Rein LE, Szabo A, Kommareddy S, Bhagavatula P, Goday PS: Pediatric feeding disorder: a nationwide prevalence study, *J Pediatr* 228:126–131.e3,ISSN 0022–3476, 2021, https://doi.org/10.1016/j.jpeds.2020.07.047.

Killian, H. J., Bakula, D. M., Wallisch, A., et al. (in press). Pediatric tube weaning: a meta-analysis of factors contributing to success. *J Clin Psychol Med Settings*.

Milano K, Chatoor I, Kerzner B: A functional approach to feeding difficulties in children, *Curr Gastroenterol Rep* 21:51, 2019, https://doi.org/10.1007/s11894-019-0719-0.

OBESITY IN CHILDREN

Salama Mostafa, MBBCh; and Seema Kumar, MD

CURRENT DIAGNOSIS

- Obesity is a serious health problem affecting a large number of children and adolescents in the United States and worldwide. Body mass index (BMI) derived from weight and height is used to classify overweight and obesity. It is calculated as weight in kilograms divided by height (or length) in meters squared (kg/m²).
- A child 2 years of age or older is diagnosed as having overweight if the BMI is at or above the 85th percentile and below the 95th percentile for age and sex, as having obesity if the BMI is at or above the 95th percentile, and as having severe obesity if the BMI is at or above 120% of the 95th percentile or at or above 35 kg/m² (whichever is lower).
- The Centers for Disease Control and Prevention (CDC) recommends using growth curves based on the World Health Organization reference standards for infants and toddlers younger than 2 years of age and using the CDC/National Center for Health Statistics growth reference standards for children 2 years of age or older.

CURRENT THERAPY

- Lifestyle modifications including dietary changes, increased physical activity, and decreased sedentary time are crucial for prevention and treatment of childhood obesity.
- Family-based lifestyle interventions and a multidisciplinary team approach are key components to implement healthy lifestyle changes.
- Pharmacotherapy is recommended as an adjunct to health behavior and lifestyle modification for adolescents aged 12 and older with obesity (BMI ≥ 95th percentile).
- Bariatric surgery has been shown to result in significant weight loss and should be considered for adolescents with severe obesity and those who have significant obesity-related comorbidities.

Introduction

Childhood obesity has emerged as an important public health problem in the United States and across the globe. The increasing prevalence of childhood obesity, severe obesity, and weight-related comorbidities places great risk on affected individuals, societies, and healthcare infrastructure. Moreover, childhood obesity tracks closely with obesity in adulthood, especially those with severe obesity and/or a strong family history of obesity, a relationship that foreshadows bigger problems for future generations. Childhood obesity and evidence-based treatment guidelines are discussed in this chapter.

Diagnosis

Childhood obesity is marked by excess accumulation of body fat. Body mass index (BMI) is considered the most practical method for evaluation of obesity. BMI is calculated from weight in kilograms and the square of the height (or length) in meters, as shown:

$$BMI = \frac{Weight\ (kg)}{Height\ (m^2)}$$

Normal growth and development during childhood results in dynamic changes in weight and height, which vary based on age and sex. Childhood growth parameters, including BMI, may then be plotted against growth curves created from standardized reference populations, normalized by age and sex. The World Health Organization (WHO) has developed growth standards for infants and children up to 5 years of age, and the Centers for Disease Control and Prevention (CDC) has similarly published reference standards for individuals between ages 2 and 20 years. The CDC recommends using the WHO standards from infancy until a child's second birthday and the CDC/National Center for Health Statistics standards for children 2 years of age and older.

Weight status categories for children are generally segregated by BMI percentile by age and sex. Weight status in childhood is categorized as follows: underweight, normal weight, overweight, obese, and severe obesity. Obesity can be further classified as follows: class I obesity, defined as BMI at or above the 95th percentile to less than 120% of the 95th percentile; class II obesity, defined as BMI at or above 120% to less than 140% of the 95th percentile or BMI at or above 35 kg/m² and below 40 kg/m² (whichever is lower); and class III obesity, defined as BMI at or above 140% of the 95th percentile or BMI at or above 40 kg/m² (whichever is lower).

Epidemiology

The prevalence of obesity among children has more than tripled over the last 4 decades. However, it has stabilized in recent years (Figure 1). The prevalence of severe obesity in childhood, on the other hand, continues to increase. According to the

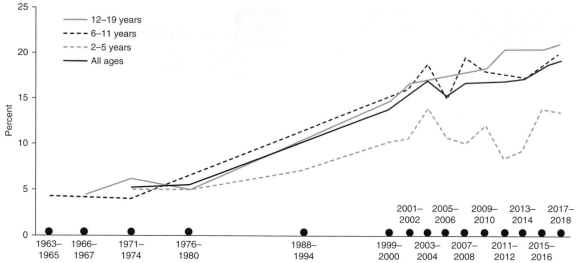

Figure 1 Trends in obesity among children and adolescents aged 2 to 19 years, by age: United States, 1963 to 1965 through 2017 to 2018. National Center for Health Statistics, National Health Examination Surveys II [ages 6–11], III [ages 12–17]; and National Health and Nutrition Examination Surveys [NHANES] I–III, and NHANES 1999–2000, 2001–2002, 2003–2004, 2005–2006, 2007–2008, 2009–2010, 2011–2012, 2013–2014, 2015–2016, and 2017–2018.

2017 to 2018 National Health and Nutrition Examination Survey, 16.1% of U.S. children have overweight, and 19.3% have obesity. Overweight affects 12.3% of preschool-aged children, 15.4% of school-aged children, and 19.4% of adolescents. Obesity affects 13.4% of preschool-aged children, 20.3% of school-aged children, and 21.2% of adolescents. The overall prevalence of severe obesity in this survey was 6.1%. Childhood obesity is more common among Black populations, Mexican Americans, and American Indians than in non-Hispanic White populations and Asians. The presence of parental obesity increases the risk of obesity in children. Additionally, higher prevalence of obesity is associated with lower socioeconomic status.

Pathophysiology

Childhood obesity develops as a result of a complex interaction between genetic, metabolic, environmental, and behavioral factors. As such, our historical understanding of "weight equals calories in minus calories out" is an oversimplification of obesity and its pathophysiology. Environmental factors such as family socioeconomic status, wealth, and access to food; neighborhood safety and available community activities; and family dietary patterns are all critical components. Approximately 40% to 85% of variability in adipose tissue deposition may be contributed to heritable factors (polygenic and largely unidentified genetic changes). Having one obese parent increases the risk of childhood obesity by two- to threefold; having two obese parents increases that risk by up to 15-fold. Obesity can rarely (<1% of childhood obesity) result from single gene mutations (e.g., melanocortin 4 receptor deficiency, leptin deficiency, leptin receptor deficiency) and congenital syndromes (e.g., Prader-Willi, Bardet-Biedel, Cohen) (Table 1). As children age and gain more control over their surroundings, individual factors such as lifestyle and dietary choices may also play a role. A host of other etiologic factors include endocrine disorders, neurologic and hypothalamic disorders, and medications.

Environmental factors affecting childhood obesity are diverse and complex. Specific dietary factors that portend risk of childhood obesity include sugar-sweetened beverages, sweet snacks, fast foods, large portion sizes, and maladaptive coping strategies such as eating to suppress negative emotions. Adverse childhood events and emotion and psychological distress increase the risk of childhood obesity. Intrauterine growth restriction and birth size, as well as antibiotic use, may also be predictive factors. Children, adolescents, and adults are also now spending less time being physically active. Time is increasingly spent in sedentary

TABLE 1	Secondary Causes of Pediatric Obesity
Monogenic Disorders	
Leptin deficiency	
Leptin dysfunction	**Endocrine**
Leptin receptor deficiency	Hypothyroidism
Proopiomelanocortin deficiency	Glucocorticoid excess (Cushing syndrome)
Melanocortin 4 receptor haploinsufficiency	Growth hormone deficiency
Melanocortin receptor accessory protein 2	Pseudohypoparathyroidism
Proconvertase 1 deficiency	**Drug Induced**
Syndromes	Tricyclic antidepressants
Prader-Willi	Steroid hormones (e.g., glucocorticoids, birth control pills)
Bardet-Biedl	Antipsychotic drugs
Cohen	Antiepileptic drugs
Alström	Diabetic medications (e.g., sulfonylureas, insulin, thiazolidinediones)
Albright hereditary osteodystrophy	Antidepressants (e.g., tricyclic antidepressants, selective serotonin reuptake inhibitors)
Beckwith-Wiedemann	Beta blockers
Carpenter	**Hypothalamic Causes**
Neurologic	Tumor
Brain injury	After brain surgery/radiation (craniopharyngioma)
Brain tumor	ROHHAD/ROHHADNET syndrome

ROHHAD, Rapid-onset obesity with hypoventilation, hypothalamic, and autonomic dysregulation; *ROHHADNET*, rapid-onset obesity with hypoventilation, hypothalamic, autonomic dysregulation, neuroendocrine tumor.
Adapted from Kumar S, Kelly AS. Review of childhood obesity: from epidemiology, etiology, and comorbidities to clinical assessment and treatment. *Mayo Clin Proc.* 2017;92(2):251-265.

activities such as use of electronic devices: cellular phones, television, tablets, and computers. Evidence suggests that shortened sleep duration and/or decreased quality of sleep also contribute to development of obesity.

Clinical Manifestations and Associated Comorbidities

Obesity is categorized as a complex chronic disease by the American Medical Association. Obesity affects essentially every organ system, most notably the endocrine, gastrointestinal, pulmonary, cardiovascular, musculoskeletal, and psychological systems. Importantly, comorbid conditions once thought to be "adult onset"—type 2 diabetes mellitus (T2DM), dyslipidemia, obstructive sleep apnea (OSA), and steatohepatitis—are now commonly encountered in children with obesity.

Cardiometabolic and Cardiovascular

Children with obesity have increased risk of developing prediabetes and T2DM, an association that varies with age and ethnicity. Children with T2DM tend to have higher rates of poor response to metformin therapy and more rapid progression of complications of diabetes, compared with those who present with T2DM later in life. Children with obesity also have a high prevalence of cardiometabolic risk factors, including hypertension (approximately 50% of obese children and adolescents) and associated echocardiographic left ventricular hypertrophy, low levels of high-density lipoprotein cholesterol, and elevated triglycerides. Obesity during childhood is associated with an increased risk for cardiovascular disease during adult life, even after adjusting for BMI during adulthood.

Endocrine

Children with obesity may experience accelerated linear growth and skeletal maturation. Postpubertal females with obesity are also at greater risk of developing hyperandrogenism and polycystic ovarian syndrome, commonly associated with menstrual irregularities, hirsutism, acne, and acanthosis nigricans.

Pulmonary

Obesity during childhood is a significant risk factor for OSA. The severity of OSA and its prevalence are directly related to the severity of obesity. Children with obesity are also at risk for alveolar hypoventilation syndrome, which can result in significant blood-oxygen desaturation and carbon dioxide retention. Childhood obesity is also associated with asthma.

Gastrointestinal

Childhood obesity is associated with a spectrum of liver abnormalities known as nonalcoholic fatty liver disease. This disease spectrum—progressing from nonalcoholic fatty liver to nonalcoholic steatohepatitis to cirrhosis—is the most common cause of liver disease in children in the United States. Children with obesity also are at increased risk for gastroesophageal reflux disease.

Musculoskeletal

Limited mobility, lower extremity joint pain and back pain, genu valgum, lower extremity malalignment, and fractures are more common among obese children than nonobese children. Obesity during childhood is also a predisposing factor to unilateral or bilateral slipped capital femoral epiphysis and tibia vara (Blount disease).

Psychosocial

Psychosocial consequences of childhood obesity are numerous and include poor self-esteem, depression, anxiety, alienation, distorted body image, and low self-reported quality of life. Psychosocial disturbances increase in prevalence and severity with age and are more common in females. Children with obesity are more likely to experience bullying and discrimination. Adult women who were obese during childhood years completed fewer years of advanced education and had greater rates of poverty and lower rates of marriage compared with normal-weight peers. Obesity has also been associated with disordered eating patterns. Overweight or obese adolescents are more likely to engage in self-induced vomiting or laxative use. Weight talk by family members and healthcare providers, and especially weight teasing, is related to disordered eating patterns.

Dermatologic

Obesity is associated with several dermatologic conditions, including acanthosis nigricans, intertrigo, hidradenitis suppurativa, furunculosis, and stretch marks.

Neurologic

Idiopathic intracranial hypertension (pseudotumor cerebri) is rare in childhood but more prevalent among obese children. This risk is further increased among children with severe obesity. Symptoms include headache, vomiting, visual disturbances, and retroocular eye pain. Retinal examination is significant for papilledema.

Clinical Evaluation of the Child With Obesity

Initial evaluation of a pediatric patient with obesity should include a thorough history and physical examination. These components are generally sufficient to determine the cause of the obesity and help the clinician in selecting the children that need further evaluation with laboratory and radiologic testing.

Obtaining an effective history requires identifying factors contributing to obesity and screening for obesity-related comorbid conditions. Dietary history should detail eating habits including frequency, content, and location of meals and snacks. Identifying intake of both calorie-dense foods, such as fruit juices and soda, as well as healthy foods such as fresh vegetables and fruits, is helpful with dietary recommendations and with motivational interviewing. Physical activity assessment should detail time spent in unstructured play, organized sports, school recess, physical education, and recreational screen time. Identifying interest in specific physical activities, regardless of current participation, can be incorporated into motivational interviewing techniques. Medical history should include height, weight, and BMI growth trajectories and use of medications that may cause weight gain such as steroids, antipsychotic drugs, and antiepileptic drugs. Identification of developmental delay during a careful developmental history may suggest genetic or chromosomal causes for obesity. A complete review of systems may be helpful in determining secondary causes of obesity (Table 1) and screening for obesity-related comorbidities such as OSA, musculoskeletal problems, and idiopathic intracranial hypertension. Psychosocial screening should evaluate for bullying, depression, disordered eating habits, and family support and other social support.

Physical examination should include accurate measurement of weight and height and evaluation for dysmorphic features that could represent monogenic or syndromal obesity. Children with obesity and short stature are more likely to have a genetic or syndromic form of obesity. Weight gain in a child with poor linear growth can be indicative of an endocrine cause for obesity such as Cushing syndrome. Physical examination should include evaluation for comorbid features of obesity. A few examples include skin examination for acanthosis nigricans, funduscopic examination to evaluate for papilledema, and musculoskeletal examination for bowing of the legs. Laboratory evaluation is recommended to identify comorbid conditions in children with obesity. These specific recommendations include obtaining fasting lipid profile for all children who have overweight or obesity, and the frequency of follow-up testing should be every 1 to 3 years depending on the child's risk profile. Measurement of serum alanine aminotransferase (ALT) is recommended for screening for fatty liver disease in children who have obesity, with retesting every 2 to 3 years if initial ALT is normal. Screening for T2DM with fasting glucose or hemoglobin A1c is recommended in children with overweight or obesity with one or more risk factors for T2DM. These risk factors include family history of T2DM in a first- or second-degree relative; high-risk race/ethnicity (Native American, African American, Hispanic, Asian American, Pacific Islander); maternal history of diabetes or gestational diabetes mellitus during the child's gestation; small for gestational age; signs of insulin resistance on physical examination such as acanthosis nigricans; and conditions associated with insulin resistance (hypertension, polycystic ovary syndrome, dyslipidemia). Screening for T2DM is recommended starting at 10 years of age or sooner if onset of puberty occurs before age 10. Rescreening should occur every 1 to 3 years depending on the weight trajectory and risk factor profile.

Children in whom a genetic, syndromic, or endocrine cause of obesity is suspected need to undergo specific testing. Children with signs and symptoms of OSA should be evaluated with overnight polysomnography. Children with features suggestive of idiopathic intracranial hypertension require head imaging and referral to appropriate experts.

Treatment

Managing childhood overweight and obesity is challenging but, when conducted properly, can be both effective and rewarding. It is crucial to treat obesity as a chronic disease. Therefore long-term care strategies should be considered. These include ongoing monitoring of obesity and associated comorbidities and ensuring access to treatment. Obesity management requires a primary healthcare team approach. A patient-centered, nonstigmatizing approach should be offered to every child with obesity.

Weight Management Goals

The goals for weight management are dependent on the child's age, the severity of the obesity, and the presence of obesity-related comorbidities. In children with mild obesity who are continuing to grow, maintenance of weight or slower rate of weight gain compared with previous is sufficient as that itself will lead to a decrease in BMI percentile. On the other hand, weight loss is recommended for children with severe obesity. A weight loss of up to 1 lb per month is safe for children between 2 and 11 years of age with obesity and comorbid conditions. More weight loss (up to 1–2 lbs per week) is safe in adolescents with obesity and comorbidities, although this degree of weight loss may not be feasible with lifestyle interventions only. Very modest reductions in BMI z score have been associated with improvement in cardiometabolic risk factors.

Lifestyle Interventions

Management of obesity should start with identifying the child's and family's motivations to change, which can be achieved by using a motivational interviewing model. This is a nonjudgmental method of interviewing that helps people resolve feelings of ambivalence about wanting to change and not wanting to change and to find the inner motivation to make lifestyle changes. The process involves reflective listening and helps children/families realize their own strengths, values, and motivation to change. This tool has been shown to be useful in treatment of childhood obesity. This can be reinforced by engaging families to change selected behaviors such as increasing physical activity, choosing healthier dietary options, and improving sleep hygiene.

The ongoing relationship between the patient/family and healthcare team should identify challenges that can predispose to treatment failure. Underlying health conditions, mental health issues, and socioeconomic barriers may challenge the achievement of weight loss. Children and their families should identify appropriate behavioral changes and strategies to improve weight status. These strategies include encouraging healthy nutrition, increasing physical activity, and decreasing sedentary behavior. The treatment team should emphasize realistic expectations and develop plans to deal with relapse.

Intensive health behavior and lifestyle change are preferred and recommended for children and adolescents with obesity. This can be facilitated by a multidisciplinary team with dieticians, behavioral counselors (e.g., social workers, psychologists, other mental health practitioners or trained nurse practitioners), an exercise specialist, and a primary care provider who oversees the intervention and manages medical issues. Evidence suggests that delivering 26 hours or more of face-to-face family-based counseling over at least a 3- to-12-month period is effective for weight management for children. Unfortunately, programs with this level of intensity may not be available to each family due to limited resources and financial or transportation challenges. The primary care team can support families by connecting them with community resources to support nutrition and address food insecurity (e.g., food provision programs) and physical activity (e.g., local parks, recreation programs). There is no evidence that intensive lifestyle and behavior interventions cause any serious adverse effects in children or adolescents with overweight or obesity. Evidence-based pediatric obesity treatment has also been shown to reduce the risk for disordered eating.

Specific health behaviors should be recommended to improve energy balance and quality of life. A family-centered approach has been shown to be more effective than a child-centered approach to achieve sustainable weight reduction.

Physical Activity

Enhancing physical activity is an important component of lifestyle change for weight management. Sixty minutes of moderate to vigorous physical activity per day is associated with improved BMI status and cardiometabolic profile. Activities that are fun for children, such as water-based and other non–weight-bearing activities are frequently preferred. Another important component of lifestyle change is reduction in sedentary behavior, including a limitation on screen time. The American Academy of Pediatrics (AAP) recommends no screen time for children younger than 18 months and only 1 hour per day for children ages 2 to 5 years. For older children, parents should have a monitoring plan for media use with a goal of appropriate, non excessive use but without a defined upper limit. Alternative options that are widely accepted by children and adolescents include video "exergames" that require light to moderate physical activity.

Nutrition

Adequate nutrition is a fundamental aspect of lifestyle change for weight management. Consumption of sugar-containing beverages and energy drinks has been associated with increased weight gain in children. Limiting the intake of food made with simple sugar or with a high fat or caloric content is recommended. As nutrition is crucial for children's growth and development, it is important to ensure a balanced meal composition, without caloric restriction, including nutrient-dense but not caloric-dense meals with an adequate mixture of protein and carbohydrates. Some weight management programs use a "traffic light" dietary format, labeling foods as red, yellow, or green on the basis of energy density (red foods indicate high calorie density, green foods indicate low calorie density). Children are encouraged to eat green foods frequently and red foods more sparingly, such as on special occasions. Behavioral modifications, including avoidance of breakfast skipping and maintenance of good sleep hygiene, are associated with better weight reduction outcomes. There is no evidence suggesting greater short-term or long-term efficacy of a specific type of diet for weight loss in children with obesity.

The 5–2–1–0 model includes multiple aspects of lifestyle modification such as nutrition, screen time and physical activity.

DRUG NAME	MECHANISM OF ACTION	FDA INDICATION	SIDE EFFECTS	ADOLESCENT WEIGHT-LOSS OUTCOMES DATA
FDA Approved				
Phentermine (Adipex-P)	Sympathomimetic amine	Obesity >16 years of age for short-term treatment	Dry mouth, insomnia, irritability, increased heart rate, blood pressure, constipation, anxiety	Decreased BMI by 4.1% at 6 months
Phentermine/ topiramate (Qsymia)	Sympathomimetic/ Modulation of various neurotransmitters	Obesity in ≥12 years	Phentermine: Insomnia, dry mouth, palpitation, anxiety, increased blood pressure. Topiramate: cognitive dysfunction, metabolic acidosis, teratogenicity, and kidney stones	Randomized double-blind clinical trial: 15 mg of phentermine and 92 mg of extended-release topiramate associated with decrease in BMI of 10.44%, whereas 7.5 mg of phentermine and 46 mg of extended-release topiramate associated with an 8.11% BMI reduction
Liraglutide (Saxenda)	GLP-1 receptor agonist	Obesity in ≥12 years	Nausea, vomiting, abdominal pain, diarrhea, potential hypoglycemia	Placebo subtracted BMI reduction of −0.22 kg/m^2 at 56 weeks
Semaglutide (Wegovy)	GLP-1 receptor agonist	Obesity in ≥12 years	Nausea, vomiting, abdominal pain, diarrhea, potential hypoglycemia	Double blind randomized placebo controlled trial: BMI reduction of 16.1% from baseline relative to 0.6% in placebo-treated group
Setmelanotide (Imcivree)	Melanocortin 4 receptor agonist	Obesity at age ≥6 years due to genetically confirmed POMC, PCSK1, or LEPR deficiency	Injection site reaction, skin hyperpigmentation, nausea, vomiting, skin discoloration	BMI reduction of at least 5% achieved by 43% of subjects; At least 10% weight loss at approximately 1 year achieved by 80% of participants with POMC deficiency and 45% of participants with LEPR deficiency
Orlistat (Xenical)	Pancreatic and gastric lipase inhibitor	Obesity ≥12 years	Flatulence, diarrhea, oily spotting, fatty stools, micronutrient deficiencies	Weight loss of 2.6 kg more than placebo at 1 year; Placebo subtracted BMI reduction of −0.7 kg/m^2 at 1 year
Not FDA Approved for Obesity				
Metformin	Activation of protein kinase pathway	≥10 years of age for type 2 diabetes mellitus	Epigastric discomfort, diarrhea, flatulence	Decreased BMI z score by 0.10 and BMI by 0.86
Topiramate	Modulation of various neurotransmitters	Treatment of epilepsy ≥2 years and migraines prevention ≥12 years of age	Cognitive dysfunction, metabolic acidosis, kidney stones, teratogenicity	Decreased BMI by 4.9% on topiramate 75 mg daily for at least 3 months

BMI, Body mass index; *FDA*, U.S. Food and Drug Administration; *GLP-1*, glucagon-like peptide-1; *LEPR*, leptin receptor; *PCSK1*, proprotein convertase subtilisin/kexin type 1; *POMC*, proopiomelanocortin.
Adapted from Srivastava G, Fox CK, Kelly AS, et al. Clinical considerations regarding the use of obesity pharmacotherapy in adolescents with obesity. *Obesity*. 2019;27(2):190-204.

The model entails five servings of fruits and vegetables a day in addition to a balanced diet, 2 hours or less of screen time per day, 1 hour or more of moderate to vigorous physical activity per day, and no (or nearly no) sugar-sweetened beverages.

Pharmacologic Therapy

Use of medications for weight loss in children should be done under the care of a physician with expertise in use of these medications. Regular monitoring for efficacy and side effects is essential (Table 2). Pharmacotherapy can be considered as an adjunct to lifestyle interventions, especially in adolescents with severe obesity and associated comorbidities. Continuation of pharmacotherapy is recommended if the medication is felt to be effective, as demonstrated by a 5% or greater BMI reduction from baseline within 12 weeks on the optimal dose, or if slowing down/arrest

of weight gain is considered satisfactory due to linear growth in adolescence. Weight-loss medications should be discontinued in the presence of side effects that persist despite adjustment of the dose. Adolescence is defined as ages 10 to 19 years by the WHO and ages 11 to 21 years by the AAP.

Orlistat (Xenical) is approved by the U.S. Food and Drug Administration (FDA) for treatment of obesity in children 12 years of age and older. It is a lipase inhibitor that, when taken at the recommended dose of 120 mg three times a day with meals, blocks absorption of about one-third of fat digested in a meal. Lower doses of 60 mg three times per day with meals are available over the counter (Alli).[1] Side effects include flatulence, oily spotting, fatty stools, diarrhea, and potential for

---

[1]Not FDA approved for this indication.

micronutrient deficiencies. Long-term safety data are lacking. The efficacy of orlistat over placebo for treatment of childhood obesity is modest, decreasing BMI by less than 1 kg/m² after 1 year of therapy.

Liraglutide (Saxenda) is a glucagon-like 1 (GLP-1) receptor agonist that is FDA approved for weight management in children and adolescents 12 years and older. It is given subcutaneously at a maximum dose of 3 mg daily. A recent randomized, double-blind, controlled trial in adolescents 12 to less than 18 years of age showed placebo-subtracted BMI reduction of –0.22 kg/m² at 56 weeks; 43% of subjects achieved a BMI reduction of at least 5%. Adverse effects include nausea, vomiting, abdominal pain, diarrhea, and potential hypoglycemia. Semaglutide (Wegovy) is another GLP-1 receptor agonist that is given subcutaneously once weekly and is approved by the FDA for weight management in children at least 12 years of age. In a double-blind, randomized, placebo-controlled trial including 180 adolescents aged from 12 to less than 18 years, semaglutide was associated with a change in mean BMI of –16.1% relative to 0.6% in the placebo group. GLP-1 receptor agonists are contraindicated in patients with a personal or family history of medullary thyroid cancer or multiple endocrine neoplasia 2A or 2B.

Phentermine (Adipex-P) is a sympathomimetic drug (Schedule IV controlled substance) that potentiates the release of norepinephrine in the hypothalamus, causing decreased appetite. It is approved by the FDA for short-term use in individuals 17 years of age or older. In one study, phentermine was associated with greater reduction in BMI by –1.6% at 1 month of treatment (95% confidence interval [CI] –2.6, –0.6%; $P = 0.001$), –2.9% at 3 months of treatment (CI –4.5, –1.4%, $P < 0.001$), and –4.1% at 6 months (95% CI –7.1, –1%, $P = 0.009$) of treatment compared with standard care consisting of lifestyle interventions only. Adverse effects of phentermine include insomnia, restlessness, dry mouth, anxiety, euphoria, palpitations, hypertension, cardiac arrhythmias, headache, dizziness, visual disturbances, and ocular irritation. Phentermine is contraindicated in patients with hyperthyroidism, glaucoma, cardiovascular disease, or history of drug abuse.

Topiramate (Topamax) is a medication that is used off-label for treatment of obesity in children. The weight-loss effect is likely mediated through modulation of various neurotransmitters. This drug is FDA approved for treatment of epilepsy in children aged 2 years and older and for migraine prophylaxis in children 12 years of age and older. Adverse effects include cognitive dysfunction, paresthesias, metabolic acidosis, kidney stones, and teratogenicity. Adolescents must be counseled about pregnancy because of decreased efficacy of oral contraceptives with treatment. Topiramate has modest efficacy for treatment of obesity. In a small, randomized, placebo-controlled, clinical pilot trial of 30 adolescents, a 2% reduction in BMI at 6 months was noted on topiramate 75 mg daily.

A combination of both topiramate and phentermine (Qsymia) is approved by the FDA for treatment of children with obesity at least 12 years of age. A dose of 15 mg of phentermine and 92 mg of extended-release topiramate was associated with a decrease in BMI of 10.44%, whereas 7.5 mg of phentermine and 46 mg of extended-release topiramate was associated with an 8.11% BMI reduction.

Setmelanotide (Imcivree), a melanocortin 4 receptor agonist, is approved for adults and children at least 6 years of age with obesity due to genetically confirmed proopiomelanocortin (POMC), proprotein convertase subtilisin/kexin type 1, or leptin receptor (LEPR) deficiency. In a single-arm, open-label, multicenter phase III trial, 80% (8/10) of participants with POMC deficiency and 45% (5/11) of participants with LEPR deficiency achieved at least 10% weight loss at approximately 1 year. Adverse events include injection site reaction, skin hyperpigmentation, nausea, vomiting, and skin discoloration.

TABLE 3	Indications for Bariatric Surgery in Adolescents	
WEIGHT CRITERIA	**COMORBID CONDITIONS PRESENT**
BMI ≥120% to <140% of the 95th percentile or BMI ≥35 kg/m² and <40 kg/m²	Moderate to severe obstructive sleep apnea, T2DM, idiopathic intracranial hypertension, NASH, Blount disease, slipped capital femoral epiphysis, hypertension, gastroesophageal reflux disease
BMI ≥140% of the 95th percentile or BMI ≥40 kg/m²	None required, though commonly present

BMI, Body mass index; *NASH,* nonalcoholic steatohepatitis; *T2DM,* type 2 diabetes mellitus.
Adapted from Armstrong SC, Bolling CF, Michalsky MP, Reichard KW. Pediatric metabolic and bariatric surgery: evidence, barriers, and best practices. *Pediatrics* 144(6), 2019.

Metformin (Glucophage, Glumetza, Riomet) is approved by the FDA for treatment of T2DM in children 10 years of age and older. Use of metformin for weight loss is considered off-label. It may be particularly useful in adolescents with prediabetes,[1] metabolic syndrome,[1] polycystic ovary syndrome,[1] and insulin resistance.[1] Metformin also may be helpful in children with weight gain secondary to treatment with antipsychotic drugs.[1] The dose may be gradually increased as tolerated to a maximum of 2000 mg/day. Improvements in BMI have been modest, with a metaanalysis finding BMI z-score reduction of 0.10 and BMI reduction of 0.86 mg/kg². Adverse effects include abdominal discomfort, diarrhea, flatulence, vitamin B_2 deficiency, and lactic acidosis.

Bariatric Procedures

Bariatric procedures, including bariatric surgery, should be considered for adolescents (≥13 years) with severe obesity and, often, with significant health comorbidities (Table 3). Severe obesity in childhood is a unique subset that has outpaced less severe forms of childhood obesity in prevalence. Importantly, lifestyle modifications alone have not demonstrated significant and lasting weight loss in children with severe obesity.

Eligibility criteria for bariatric surgery include:
1. BMI at least 120% of the 95th percentile for age and gender or BMI at least 35 kg/m², whichever is lower, and a severe comorbidity having significant effects on health (e.g., moderate to severe OSA; apnea-hypopnea index >15), T2DM, idiopathic intracranial hypertension, or severe and progressive steatohepatitis
or
BMI at least 140% of the 95th percentile for age and gender or BMI at least 40 kg/m², whichever is lower (obesity-related comorbid conditions are not required);
2. History of previous sustained efforts to lose weight through changes in diet and physical activity;
3. Commitment from the patient and family to adhere to recommended pre- and postoperative treatments, including vitamin and mineral supplementation; and
4. Patient and family understanding of the risks and benefits of bariatric surgery.

The most recent expert guidelines do not recommend withholding surgery in those that have not completed puberty or physical maturity as determined by Tanner stage or skeletal maturation. Contraindications for bariatric surgery include:
1. Medically correctable cause of obesity;

---

[1]Not FDA approved for this indication.

Common bariatric procedures

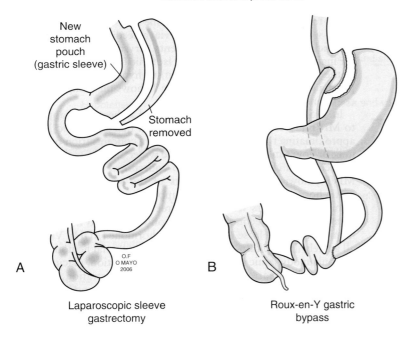

Laparoscopic sleeve gastrectomy

Roux-en-Y gastric bypass

Figure 2 Bariatric surgical procedures commonly used for the surgical treatment of childhood obesity. (A) Laparoscopic sleeve gastrectomy. (B) Roux-en-Y gastric bypass.

2. An ongoing substance abuse problem (within the preceding year);
3. A medical, psychiatric, psychosocial, or cognitive condition that prevents adherence to postoperative dietary and medication regimens or impairs decisional capacity;
4. Current or planned pregnancy within 12 to 18 months of the procedure; and
5. Inability on the part of the patient or parent to comprehend the risks and benefits of the surgical procedure.

Types of Bariatric Procedures

The sleeve gastrectomy (SG; Figure 2A) is the most commonly performed procedure among adolescents with obesity. SG involves resecting the majority of the greater curvature of the stomach, leaving a tubular structure that serves as the new stomach. SG was initially performed as the first stage of a two-stage procedure in high-risk adults with extreme obesity. The SG procedure is attractive during adolescence and particularly for adolescents with cognitive deficits. The procedure is less complex and can be converted to gastric bypass in the future if there is weight regain. The risk of micronutrient deficiencies is theoretically lower, as it is a purely restrictive procedure.

Roux-en-Y gastric bypass (RYGB; Figure 2B) was previously considered the gold standard of bariatric procedures among adolescents with severe obesity but is now performed less frequently than the SG. The surgery involves creation of a small proximal gastric pouch (<30 mL) and separation of the pouch from the distal stomach and anastomosis to a Roux limb of small bowel that measures 75 to 150 cm in length. Though it is primarily considered a restrictive surgery, some degree of malabsorption does occur that leads to weight loss and places patients at risk for micronutrient deficiencies.

Both bariatric procedures have been shown to result in significant decreases in body weight and BMI in most adolescents undergoing those procedures. In the largest prospective study of bariatric surgery in adolescents (Teen-LABS), 26% reduction in BMI after SG and 28% reduction after RYGB was noted at 3 years. BMI reduction of 29.2% was noted at 5 years in 58 individuals undergoing RYGB. Both procedures have been shown to result in improvement of various comorbid conditions including T2DM, prediabetes, hypertension, dyslipidemia, and renal disease.

Long-term adverse effects include deficiencies of iron, vitamin D, thiamine, and vitamin B_{12}. Adolescents undergoing bariatric surgery need long-term monitoring as long-term safety and efficacy data in this age group are limited.

Conclusion

Childhood obesity presents a growing public health concern in the United States and globally. Weight-related comorbid conditions are common among children with obesity, conferring significant health risks. Treatment of obesity in childhood should be initiated in a timely manner and should begin with lifestyle and behavior change. The list of antiobesity medications for children is increasing, and these medications should be considered as an adjunct to lifestyle changes. Bariatric surgery in adolescents has been associated with significant weight loss and improvement in weight-related comorbid conditions in the short and intermediate term.

References

Armstrong SC, Bolling CF, Michalsky MP, et al: Pediatric metabolic and bariatric surgery: evidence, barriers, and best practices, *Pediatrics* 144, 2019.

Hampl SE, Hassink SG, Armstrong SC, et al: Clinical practice guideline for the evaluation and treatment of children and adolescents with obesity, *Pediatrics* 151, 2023.

Inge TH, Courcoulas AP, Jenkins TM, et al: Weight loss and health status 3 years after bariatric surgery in adolescents, *N Engl J Med* 374:113, 2016.

Kelly AS, Barlow SE, Rao G, et al: Severe obesity in children and adolescents: identification, associated health risks, and treatment approaches: a scientific statement from the American Heart Association, *Circulation* 128:1689, 2013.

Kumar S, Kelly AS: Review of childhood obesity: from epidemiology, etiology, and comorbidities to clinical assessment and treatment, *Mayo Clin Proc* 92:251, 2017.

Srivastava G, Fox CK, Kelly AS, et al: Clinical considerations regarding the use of obesity pharmacotherapy in adolescents with obesity, *Obesity* 27:190, 2019.

TABLE 2 BEARS Mnemonic: A Screening Tool for Sleep Disorders in Children

	PRESCHOOL (2–5 YEARS)	SCHOOL-AGE (6–12 YEARS)	ADOLESCENT (13–18 YEARS)
Bedtime problems	Does your child have any problems going to bed? Falling asleep?	Does your child have any problems at bedtime? (P) Do you have any problems going to bed? (C)	Do you have any problems falling asleep at bedtime? (C)
Excessive daytime sleepiness	Does your child seem overly tired or sleepy during the day? Does your child still take naps?	Does your child have difficulty waking in the morning, seem sleepy during the day, or take naps? (P) Do you feel tired a lot? (C)	Do you feel sleepy a lot during the day? In school? While driving? (C)
Awakenings during the night	Does your child wake up a lot at night?	Does your child seem to wake up a lot at night? Any sleepwalking or nightmares? (P) Do you wake up a lot at night? Have trouble getting back to sleep? (C)	Do you wake up a lot at night? Have trouble getting back to sleep? (C)
Regularity and duration of sleep	Does your child have a regular bedtime and wake time? What are they?	What time does your child go to bed and get up on school days? Weekends? Do you think your child is getting enough sleep? (P)	What time do you usually go to bed on school nights? Weekends? How much sleep do you usually get? (C)
Sleep-disordered breathing	Does your child snore a lot or have difficulty breathing at night?	Does your child have loud or nightly snoring or any breathing difficulties at night? (P)	Does your teenager snore loudly or nightly? (P)

Abbreviations: C = child; P = parent.
From Owens JA, Dalzell V: Use of the "BEARS" sleep screening tool in a pediatric residents' continuity clinic: A pilot study. Sleep Med 2005;6:63–69.

TABLE 3 Principles of Sleep Hygiene in Children

The child's bedroom should be dark and quiet.

Bedtime routines should be strictly enforced. Routines should be relaxing and only 20 to 30 minutes in length.

The time of morning awakening should be firmly and consistently structured.

Bedroom temperatures should be kept comfortably cool (< 75 °F).

Environmental noise should be minimized as much as possible. Background music and/or white noise may inhibit extraneous noise.

Children should not go to bed hungry and may have a snack before bedtime.

Excessive fluids before bedtime may result in bladder distention and arousal and disrupt sleep.

Children should learn to fall asleep alone (i.e., without their parents' presence in the room).

Vigorous activity should be avoided before bedtime.

A bath is often a stimulating activity for children. If bedtime struggles are present after a child's bath, it may be moved to the morning or separated from the child's bedtime by at least 2 hours.

Methylxanthine-containing beverages and food (e.g., caffeinated beverages/colas, tea, chocolate) should be avoided several hours before bedtime.

Parents should read labels on all over-the-counter and prescription medications. Some may contain alcohol or caffeine and may disrupt sleep.

Naps should be developmentally appropriate. Brief naps may be refreshing, but prolonged naps or napping too frequently may result in significant accumulation of sleep during the day and make it more difficult to fall asleep at night.

Modified from Sheldon SH, Ferber R, Kryger M (eds): Principles and Practice of Pediatric Sleep Medicine. Philadelphia: Elsevier Saunders, 2005.

excessive napping, or napping after age 5 years (intentionally or unintentionally). School-age children often display symptoms of behavioral problems or inattentiveness rather than sleepiness. Sleep-wake patterns on school days, weekends, and vacations need to be detailed. Often the child's most natural sleep pattern will emerge over the summer months.

Determining the child's sleep hygiene or good sleep practices is important in diagnosing and treating sleep disorders. Principles of good sleep hygiene are listed in Table 3.

Past Medical History/Family History

A history of prematurity, trisomy 21, velopharyngeal cleft palate repair, or hypotonia is each associated with an increased risk of sleep-disordered breathing. A past history of adenotonsillectomy for snoring is important information to obtain. Chronic nasal obstruction can cause maxillary hypoplasia. Arnold-Chiari malformation, myelomeningocele, or a brainstem lesion can predispose to central sleep apnea due to impaired central respiratory drive. Chronic health issues can also be associated with sleep disruption and consequently with behavioral problems associated with sleep.

A family history of obstructive sleep apnea (OSA), insomnia, or restless legs syndrome (RLS) is important; a family history of RLS can be used to support a diagnosis of RLS in the child. In particular, questioning the mother if she had symptoms of RLS during any of her pregnancies can be helpful because this is a common time for RLS to present or worsen. Morning or evening preferences (i.e., "night-owl" or "lark" tendencies) can also have a familial element. In addition, sleepwalking can be found to occur in families.

Focused Physical Examination

The physical examination in a child presenting with a sleep complaint should include a general assessment. Presence/absence of sleepiness, fatigue, and irritability/hyperactivity are all important. Height, weight, and body mass index (BMI) should be recorded. Children with OSA can have poor growth and even failure to thrive. Obesity is a risk factor for OSA. Special attention to a child's craniofacial features is important because these may make a child more at risk for sleep-disordered breathing.

Assessment of tonsil size, oropharyngeal crowding (using the Mallampati or Friedman classification systems can be useful), and presence of maxillary/mandibular hypoplasia can all offer clues to an airway that may predispose to OSA. The practitioner should evaluate for evidence of nasal obstruction by noting mouth breathing and signs of allergy (i.e., allergic shiners, nasal crease).

Diagnostic Tools

Polysomnography

The AASM has published practice parameters on both the respiratory and nonrespiratory indications for polysomnography (PSG) in pediatric patients. In this chapter, a sleep study or PSG will refer only to an in-laboratory attended study, because home monitoring currently has not been sufficiently evaluated in the pediatric population. PSG in children entails spending the night at a sleep center. A parent or caregiver must also spend the night. During the night, the child's sleep characteristics, respiratory function, and movement are analyzed. This is done by the following measures: electroencephalography (EEG), electromyography (EMG) of chin and limbs, airflow by thermistor and nasal pressure, end-tidal or transcutaneous carbon dioxide measurements, and induction plethysmography to measure respiratory effort. Scoring of a PSG performed on a child is done using pediatric scoring rules set forth by the AASM.

The most common indication for a sleep study in children is OSA. PSG can be used to both diagnose OSA and treat sleep apnea with continuous positive airway pressure (CPAP). PSG can also be used to evaluate for elevated periodic limb movements of sleep, and in rare cases to characterize abnormal nocturnal behavior such as evaluation of parasomnias or nocturnal seizures.

Overnight Oximetry

The gold standard for diagnosis of pediatric OSA is PSG. Overnight oximetry has been suggested as an alternative screening tool for pediatric sleep-disordered OSA. Although an abnormal oximetry will suggest OSA, a normal oximetry does not rule out OSA. Children can have sleep apnea that is severe and still maintain normal oxygenation. In a study by Brouillette and colleagues (2000), when a positive oximetry graph was present (defined by three or more desaturation clusters and at least three desaturations < 90%) in a referred population, the positive predictive value for OSA on PSG was 97%. A negative or inconclusive oximetry by this definition did not rule out OSA and there was still a 47% chance OSA was present on PSG.

Sleep Logs/Actigraphy

Sleep logs can be effective in demonstrating a child's sleep-wake patterns. Actigraphy is often done in conjunction with a sleep log. Actigraphy is a portable wristband that measures movement. The absence of movement over a certain time period is used as a surrogate marker of sleep, and the presence of movement over a certain time period is used as a surrogate for wakefulness. Some devices also measure ambient light exposure. Used in conjunction with actigraphy sleep logs can be extremely helpful in demonstrating discrepancies between perceived and actual sleep, and are helpful in demonstrating insufficient sleep and circadian rhythm disorders. Those that measure light as well can aid in uncovering sleep hygiene issues.

Multiple Sleep Latency Test

The multiple sleep latency test (MSLT) is a daytime study used to objectively measure sleepiness. It is often used to aid in the diagnosis of narcolepsy or hypersomnia. It is a set of four to five scheduled naps that typically occur the day after an overnight sleep study. Often 2 weeks of actigraphy are done before the MSLT to determine sleep-wake patterns.

Common Pediatric Sleep Diagnoses and Treatment

Obstructive Sleep Apnea

Epidemiology

Up to one-fifth of children can have intermittent snoring. Prevalence rates of OSA range from 1.2% to 5.7%. OSA is most common in children 2 to 8 years of age corresponding to the peak age of adenotonsillar hypertrophy. Due to the rise in childhood obesity there is now a corresponding rise in older children diagnosed with OSA.

Pathophysiology

The pharynx has many roles, including swallowing, speaking, and maintaining airway patency. Pharyngeal size is determined by the bones and soft tissue. The soft tissue is affected by the size of the tonsils and adenoids, as well as adipose tissue. Airway patency is maintained during wakefulness; a small airway can become vulnerable during sleep resulting in partial or total closure of the airway, hypoxemia, hypercapnia, and an arousal that results in opening of the airway and termination of the obstructive event. This leads to sleep disruption and daytime consequences. OSA in children likely results from a combination of narrowing of the upper airway, abnormal upper airway tone, and genetic factors.

Clinical Manifestation

OSA in adults is typically associated with daytime sleepiness. Associations have been made with hypertension, stroke, and metabolic syndrome. In children, OSA may not present with daytime sleepiness. Children may present with daytime inattention and/or neurocognitive and behavioral issues. Symptoms include snoring with or without apneic pauses or gasps. Restless sleep or secondary enuresis may also be noted. Parents may comment on increased work of breathing while sleeping. Other associations include poor growth, obesity, hypertension, and systemic inflammation.

Diagnosis

The gold standard for diagnosis of pediatric OSA is an in-laboratory attended PSG by an accredited sleep laboratory. History and physical examination lack sensitivity and specificity in predicting which children with snoring have OSA. However, a history of loud snoring, tonsillar hypertrophy, and abnormal oximetry is strongly suggestive of the diagnosis of OSA (see above). History alone cannot distinguish children with OSA from those with primary snoring. Criteria for the diagnosis of OSA in children are met when there is one or more apnea or hypopnea events per hour identified using scoring criteria by the AASM.

Differential Diagnosis

Other forms of sleep-disordered breathing are not as common as OSA. Sleep-related hypoventilation can occur in patients with neuromuscular weakness. Central hypoventilation syndromes are rare, but should be considered in children with persistent gas exchange abnormalities without additional explanation. Sleep-related hypoxemia can be present in pediatric patients with chronic lung disease. Central sleep apnea should be thought of in patients with brainstem abnormalities or Arnold-Chiari malformation. Sleep-related seizures may be difficult to differentiate from OSA in infants and an extended EEG montage may be necessary during their sleep study. Normal breathing patterns of infants and children should also be identified; brief (less than 10 seconds), central respiratory pauses that are self-resolving (and without significant desaturation) are common in normal children in either REM sleep or post-arousal/post-sigh.

Treatment

Treatment of OSA in most children is adenotonsillectomy. Recent guidelines from the AAP recommend an overnight sleep study in children where the practitioner had a clinical suspicion of OSA before adenotonsillectomy. Children with mild OSA preoperative can be monitored clinically postoperatively. Children with moderate to severe OSA, as well as children with craniofacial abnormalities, neurologic disorders, and obesity, should have a follow-up PSG to demonstrate resolution of OSA after surgery. Recent randomized controlled trials have shown that some children may outgrow their OSA, particularly if it is mild. Children who are not candidates for adenotonsillectomy may be treated with CPAP and use may have an impact on neurobehavioral outcomes. Treatment with CPAP therapy in children requires close follow-up because pressure needs may change with growth. In certain children, treatment with intranasal corticosteroids and/or montelukast may be considered with close follow-up.

Difficulty with Sleep Initiation and Night Wakings
Epidemiology
Bedtime problems and night wakings occur in up to 30% of children.

Clinical Manifestations
The diagnosis of insomnia includes difficulty going to sleep and/or staying asleep, the complaint that sleep is not of good quality, and the report of poor daytime functioning. The sleep complaints of infants and young children are often in the words of their parent or caregiver.

In preschool-age children both bedtime problems and night wakings are common and characterized by two types of behavioral insomnia of childhood: sleep-onset association type and limit-setting type. The definition of the *sleep-onset association type*, as defined in the ICSD-3, includes the following: sleep initiation is an extended process, associations are demanding, if the associations are not present sleep onset is delayed, and awakenings require caregiver intervention. The *limit-setting type* involves difficulty initiating or maintaining sleep, there is bedtime stalling or refusal, and the caregiver does not set sufficient and appropriate limits around this behavior. Children with frequent and prolonged night wakings have the sleep-onset association type. They often require an intervention by the caretaker to reinitiate sleep. Both problems can be present at once. Children who have difficulty going to sleep and provide resistance to bedtime have the limit-setting type. Parents of these children may complain of daytime behavioral issues due to the parent's inability to set limits during the day as well.

Diagnosis
Diagnosis is made from the history in the majority of cases. An overnight sleep study may be indicated in cases where another sleep disorder is suspected.

Differential Diagnosis
The differential diagnosis of insomnia or behavioral insomnia of childhood includes sleep disorders such as OSA, RLS, or nocturnal seizures. These disorders can prompt nocturnal awakenings or make sleep initiation difficult. If there is clinical suspicion of one of these disorders, an overnight sleep study may be indicated.

Treatment
Behavioral interventions have been shown to be effective in treating all forms of insomnia. In older children, primary and secondary insomnia can be effectively treated with cognitive-behavioral therapy. This often includes stimulus control and sleep restriction. Stimulus control includes maintaining a regular sleep-wake pattern and using the bed and bedroom only for sleeping. It involves getting out of bed if sleep is not initiated within about 20 minutes. Sleep restriction includes minimizing the time in bed to be only sleeping. It often includes delaying bedtime to the child's actual sleep onset, and then over time gradually advancing the bedtime. Sleep hygiene should be effectively addressed, including development of a relaxing bedtime routine, maintaining a regular sleep-wake pattern, and eliminating electronic use before bedtime.

There are several treatments of behavioral insomnia of childhood sleep-onset association type. No one treatment has been found to be superior. The goal of all of these methods is for the child to fall asleep in his or her crib or bed on the child's own. These include extinction (i.e., "cry it out"), which is often not palatable to caregivers. There is the graduated extinction method, which has parents ignoring crying or protests for specified periods of increasingly longer intervals. Some prefer an even more gradual approach of sitting next to the child's bed in a chair and over several days to weeks moving that chair across the room and out of the room. A consistent bedtime routine should also be implemented. Use of a transitional object can be helpful. Treatment of the limit-setting type includes firm limit setting. Positive reinforcement and limiting negative reinforcement should be used. The use of a reward system can be helpful. Effectively addressing behavioral treatment of sleep issues can be challenging for the primary care provider because of time constraints.

Restless Legs Syndrome/Willis Ekbom Disease
Epidemiology
Prevalence rates for pediatric RLS/WED have ranged from 1% to 6%.

Risk Factors
Risk factors include a family history and a history of anemia or iron deficiency. Attention-deficit/hyperactivity disorder (ADHD) is associated with RLS.

Pathophysiology
Decreased dopamine has been suggested in the pathophysiology of RLS/WED. Iron is a cofactor in the synthesis of dopamine and treatment of iron deficiency or low ferritin, if present, may improve symptoms.

Diagnosis
Diagnosis of pediatric RLS/WED is a clinical diagnosis. It is made using the adult criteria set forth in the ICSD-3 but with some modification for children due to developmental issues. It consists of the child reporting an urge to move the legs, usually accompanied by an uncomfortable sensation; this urge or sensation worsens during rest or inactivity; the sensations are improved or resolved by movement; the sensations are present or worsen in the evening or night. If a child cannot express a description in his or her own words, diagnosis can be made using two out of the following three criteria: a sleep disturbance for age, a family history of RLS, and a periodic limb movement index on PSG of > 5 per hour. Because of this last criterion, a sleep study can be helpful in children to make this diagnosis. There can be an association with sleep initiation and maintenance difficulties.

Differential Diagnosis
Differential diagnosis of RLS should include insomnia, sleep-disordered breathing, or neurologic or musculoskeletal etiologies for the discomfort.

Treatment
Nonpharmacologic treatment of RLS includes good sleep hygiene, moderate exercise a few hours before bedtime, and

avoidance of substances that are associated with worsening of RLS symptoms, including caffeine, alcohol, antihistamines, and antiemetics. A serum ferritin should be drawn in all children with RLS and if < 50 ng/mL, treatment with 6 mg/kg/day of oral elemental iron should be considered. Oral iron absorption is enhanced by vitamin C and impaired by calcium. Gastrointestinal upset and constipation can be common side effects. Compliance can be difficult. A serum ferritin should be rechecked at 3 months to evaluate therapy. Referral to a sleep medicine specialist should be made if lifestyle and oral iron therapy have been unsuccessful. There are no FDA-approved medications for the treatment of RLS in children. Dopamine agonists, gabapentin (Neurontin),[1] clonazepam (Klonopin)[1], and clonidine (Catapres)[1] have been used to treat pediatric RLS.

Delayed Sleep Phase Syndrome
Epidemiology
Delayed sleep phase syndrome (DSPS) occurs most commonly in adolescents and young adults.

Clinical Manifestations
Symptoms usually present in adolescents but can occur in younger children. Adolescents with DSPS consistently have sleep onset at a later time, typically after midnight. They have difficulty initiating sleep earlier. They do not have difficulty maintaining sleep. They have difficulty waking in the morning unless able to sleep until their preferred time, which is typically after 10 AM. They may have sleepiness during the daytime if forced to rise early (i.e., for school); however, during long vacations or summer breaks when allowed to sleep to preferred wake time they feel refreshed. Children who already have a preferred evening preference may find this exacerbated in adolescence. Poor school performance can be present.

Diagnosis
Diagnosis is made from history; actigraphy and sleep logs are also useful. An overnight sleep study may be indicated if another sleep disorder is suspected (e.g., OSA).

Differential Diagnosis
The differential diagnosis includes insomnia, poor sleep hygiene, insufficient sleep, mood disorder, OSA, and RLS.

Treatment
Treatment is typically behavioral and includes good sleep hygiene. Typically either the patient's sleep-wake schedule is advanced (if there is less than 3 hours between actual and desired bedtime) by 15 minutes every 2 to 3 days until the goal bedtime is achieved. Rise time is advanced as well and if set at the desired wake time initially it should facilitate the advancement of the bedtime by increasing sleep drive. If the desired bedtime of the adolescent is greater than 3 hours from the current bedtime, phase delay can be considered. Bedtime is delayed by 2 to 3 hours each day until the target bedtime is reached. Timing of this therapy should be considered, because it will interfere with school or other daytime activities. Parental or caregiver support is necessary, as well as commitment by the adolescent.

Once the new pattern is established weekends must not differ from weekdays by more than 1 to 2 hours. This is particularly important for the rise time. Relapse is common if strict sleep-wake patterns are not adhered to, a problem common on vacations.

Both bright light exposure and melatonin have been used to help reset the circadian rhythm. Exposure to bright light in the morning is encouraged and can be as simple as increasing sun exposure in the morning. Light boxes using 2500 to 10,000 lux can be used in the morning for 20 to 30 minutes. Exposure to light in the evening should be limited. A small dose of melatonin[7] (0.5 mg) can be used in the early evening (about 5 hours before desired bedtime) to attempt to physiologically advance sleep onset. If the timing is not optimal for both light and melatonin, the phase delay can be worsened; consultation with a sleep physician should be considered.

Parasomnias
Parasomnias can occur out of both non-REM (NREM) and REM sleep. Those occurring out of NREM sleep include sleepwalking, sleep terrors, and confusional arousals. They typically occur in the first one-third of the night, when NREM-3 sleep is most prevalent, and are not recalled the next day. They can be part of normal development, but depending on their nature, they can be distressing to caregiver and child. Parasomnias occurring out of REM sleep include nightmares and REM-sleep behavior disorder (RBD). Nightmares are commonly recalled and have been associated with anxiety in children. Nightmares typically peak in the school-age child. RBD is rare in children but has been reported; it involves the loss of atonia that occurs in REM sleep and consequently dreams are "acted out."

Risk Factors
Poor sleep hygiene, insufficient sleep, irregular sleep-wake patterns, and a positive family history are all risk factors. Sleep disruption from sleep-disordered breathing or periodic limb movements of sleep can exacerbate parasomnias.

Differential Diagnosis
The differential diagnosis should include nocturnal seizures. In addition, if another sleep disorder is present, parasomnias can be exacerbated.

Treatment
Safety is most important in children with parasomnias, and it is important that the child's sleep environment is kept clear of things that could cause injury. Door alarms can be effective. The child should not be awakened during the episode. The event should not be referred to the next morning because this can cause distress for the child. Maintaining good sleep hygiene and regular sleep-wake patterns is important. If the events occur at a predictable time each night, the caregiver can do planned awakenings 30 minutes before the event typically occurs for several weeks. This may abolish the episodes. It can also have the effect of pushing the episode to later in the night. Pharmacologic treatment with a small dose of a benzodiazepine (e.g., 0.5 mg of clonazepam [Klonopin][1] at bedtime) may be indicated in severe cases with the drug tapered slowly after episodes are suppressed.

Hypersomnias
A full discussion of primary hypersomnias (including narcolepsy) in children is beyond the scope of this chapter. Consideration for a primary hypersomnia should be made in a child who is sleepy after common causes of sleepiness such as insufficient sleep and obstructive sleep apnea have been ruled out. Symptoms of narcolepsy include disrupted nocturnal sleep, hallucinations on going to sleep or waking up, and sleep paralysis. Daytime sleepiness is present with "sleep attacks" both during quiet activities and while active. Cataplexy may

---

[1]Not FDA approved for this indication.

[1]Not FDA approved for this indication.
[7]Available as dietary supplement.

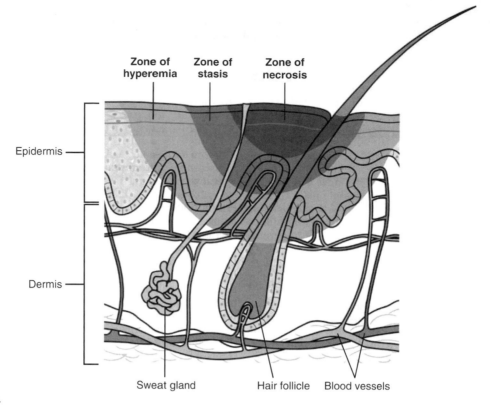

Figure 1 Burn injury.

TABLE 1	Types of Burns				
DEPTH	**ANATOMY**	**APPEARANCE**	**SENSATION**	**TIME**	**TREATMENT**
Superficial	Epidermis only	Pink or red and dry, blanches	Painful	Days	Topical
Superficial partial thickness	Epidermis and upper papillary dermis	Pink, clear blisters, moist surface, blanches	Painful	14–21 days	Debride and topical medication
Deep partial thickness	Epidermis, papillary dermis, and lower reticular dermis	Pink or red, moist surface, blisters, may be hemorrhagic, does not blanch	Painful, may have decreased sensation	Weeks or may progress to full thickness	Debride, topical medication, possible surgery
Full thickness	Epidermis, dermis, and into underlying tissue	White or brown, dry, leathery, does not blanch	Insensate	Weeks, and heals by contraction and scarring	Surgical

which is further characterized as superficial partial or deep partial, and full thickness (Table 1). Superficial burns involve the epidermis alone. These injuries are typically painful and erythematous, and they will heal without scarring. These injuries are not included in calculations of the percentage total body surface area (TBSA) burned. Superficial partial thickness burns involve the entire epidermis and extend down to the papillary region of the upper dermis. These injuries are painful, erythematous, and moist, and they form blisters. Deep partial thickness burns involve the entire epidermis and extend deeper into the lower reticular dermis. These wounds are typically painful and whitish, and they have less weeping and blanching than superficial partial thickness wounds. These may have less pain than expected depending on the extent of damage to nerve endings in the skin. Full-thickness burns extend through the epidermis and entire dermis and destroy nerves and other deep structures. These wounds are insensate, stiff, white or tan in color, and they do not blanch. Wounds of this depth cannot heal spontaneously and will have significant scarring and contracture if not surgically managed.

Areas of burn that have extensive or circumferential deep partial thickness or full-thickness burns are at risk for development of restrictive eschars. Eschars can restrict circulation, leading to compartment syndrome in extremities and can decrease respiration if on the chest or neck. Ideally, burn patients can reach burn centers before these complications arise, but an escharotomy could be required urgently in some cases.

Inhalation injury is a source of significant morbidity in burn patients. The initial injury may not seem particularly severe, but edema can develop rapidly in the airway, which makes delayed airway management perilous. Early intubation may be necessary.

Special Situations

Ocular Injuries

Patients with any signs of burns to the face, complaints of eye pain, or inability to communicate should undergo eye examinations with fluorescein staining. If corneal burns are identified, appropriate antibiotic ointment should be started, and consultation with an eye specialist should be obtained.

Nonaccidental Trauma

Clinicians should have a high index of suspicion for nonaccidental trauma (NAT) in burns occurring in pediatric patients. NAT has been shown to be present in up to 25% of pediatric burn

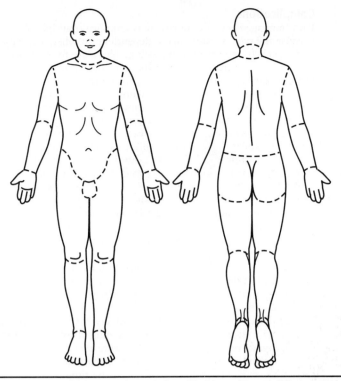

	Birth 1 yr.	1–4 yrs.	5–9 yrs.	10–14 yrs.	15 yrs.	Adult	Burn size estimate
Head	19	17	13	11	9	7	
Neck	2	2	2	2	2	2	
Anterior trunk	13	13	13	13	13	13	
Posterior trunk	13	13	13	13	13	13	
Right buttock	2.5	2.5	2.5	2.5	2.5	2.5	
Left buttock	2.5	2.5	2.5	2.5	2.5	2.5	
Genitalia	1	1	1	1	1	1	
Right upper arm	4	4	4	4	4	4	
Left upper arm	4	4	4	4	4	4	
Right lower arm	3	3	3	3	3	3	
Left lower arm	3	3	3	3	3	3	
Right hand	2.5	2.5	2.5	2.5	2.5	2.5	
Left hand	2.5	2.5	2.5	2.5	2.5	2.5	
Right thigh	5.5	6.5	8	8.5	9	9.5	
Left thigh	5.5	6.5	8	8.5	9	9.5	
Right leg	5	5	5.5	6	6.5	7	
Left leg	5	5	5.5	6	6.5	7	
Right foot	3.5	3.5	3.5	3.5	3.5	3.5	
Left foot	3.5	3.5	3.5	3.5	3.5	3.5	

Total BSAB _____

Figure 2 Lund-Browder classification of burn size.

Because burned tissue increases insensible fluid losses, burn victims have increased fluid requirements. Various formulas are available for calculating approximate fluid requirements, but all require careful monitoring of the results and progress of fluid resuscitation. Patients who receive more than 250 mL/kg in the first 24 hours are at increased risk of developing fluid-related complications. The American Burn Association Consensus Statement formula is used to guide initial fluid management. The starting fluid requirements are 2 to 4 mL/kg of lactated Ringer's solution per TBSA percent value, with half given in the first 8 hours and the rest over the next 16 hours (Box 2). Urine output should be monitored hourly and maintained between 0.5 and 1 mL/kg/h. If a patient's urine output is greater than 1 mL/kg/h, the rate of fluid administration should be decreased by 20% and continued to be monitored hourly. If the urine output is less than 0.5 mL/kg/h, the rate of fluid administration should be increased by 20% and continued to be monitored.

Unfortunately, ensuring adequate urine output does not necessarily guarantee adequate fluid resuscitation. In addition to using urine output as an indicator of resuscitation adequacy, other modes of monitoring can be used to help guide fluid resuscitation (hemodynamic monitoring, echocardiography, gastric tonometry, or other devices). Whether they lead to any increased improvement or survivability is not clear, however.

Burn Center Referral Criteria and Transfer
It is important to identify the regional burn referral center and to establish a line of communication with it before a burn patient is encountered in order to know of the center's suggested criteria

---

BOX 2   Fluid Administration and Calculation

80-kg male patient with a burn of 35% TBSA full-thickness and partial thickness burns:

80 kg × 35 × 3 mL/kg = 8400 mL in first 24 hours

8400 mL/24 hours ÷ 2 = 4200 mL in first 8 hours, 4200 mL in next 16 hours

Initial rate of 525 mL/h over first 8 hours, then switching to a rate of 265 mL/h over next 16 hours

Expected urine output is 0.5–1 mL/kg/h

80 kg × 0.5 mL/kg/h = 40 mL/h

80 kg × 1 mL/kg/h = 80 mL/h

So, for our 80-kg patient, we would expect 40–80 mL of urine every hour. In hours 1 and 2 of resuscitation, the patient has 65 mL of urine per hour. In hour 3 of resuscitation, the patient has 90 mL of urine per hour. We would then decrease the fluid administration rate by 20%, or

525 mL/h–(0.20 × 525) = 420 mL/h

Thus, the rate of administration of lactated Ringer's solution would change from 525 mL/h to 420 mL/h and continue to be monitored and recorded hourly, with continued adjustments based on hourly urine output.

TBSA, Total body surface area.

BOX 3   Burn Center Referral Criteria

Partial thickness burns greater than 10% TBSA

Full-thickness burns

Burns to high-risk areas, such as the face, hands, feet, genitals, perineum, or major joints

Circumferential burns

Electrical burns, including lightning strikes

Chemical burns

Inhalation injury

Preexisting conditions known to impair healing and increase risk of mortality

Burns in combination with traumatic injury (e.g., fracture, traumatic brain injury) whereby the burn is the leading risk for patient mortality

Burn injury in patients who will require special social, emotional, or long-term rehabilitative intervention

Burns in a setting unequipped (personnel, equipment, or unit) to care for critically ill children

---

TBSA, Total body surface area.
Available from https://ameriburn.org/public-resources/burn-center-referral-criteria/. Accessed May 1, 2021.

---

for transfer (Box 3). Burn centers typically manage more than 200 burn patients annually and have specially trained physicians, nurses, and ancillary personnel who are focused on treating burn patients. Severely burned patients who are treated at specialized centers have better outcomes. It is recommended that hospitals and clinics have agreements with burn centers for the management of complicated patients and patients who meet criteria for burn center transfer.

In general, the following criteria are recommended for transfer to a burn center: burns greater than 10% of TBSA; inhalation injury; burns with significant associated mechanical injury; burns of the face, hands, feet, perineum, or genitalia or across major joints; full-thickness burns of any size; and circumferential burns. Burns that warrant a discussion with a burn center for possible transfer or outpatient follow-up include burns in children; patients with comorbid conditions that will impact healing; and patients with special social, emotional, psychological, or rehabilitative needs.

Complications

Pain management for burns may require multiple modalities because the type of pain varies, depending on where the patient is in the cycle of treatment and healing. There are four types of pain that need to be treated during the care of a burn patient: background pain, breakthrough pain, procedural pain, and long-term pain. Background pain is present from the onset of the injury, and the pain is typically intensified during procedures. There will also be episodes of breakthrough pain. Depending on the severity of the injury, initial pain and background pain may be treated with multimodal therapy including acetaminophen, NSAIDs (e.g., ibuprofen, naproxen sodium), or opioids. Low-dose ketamine (Ketalar)[1] is increasingly used in addition to opioids for background and breakthrough pain. Procedural pain may require bolus dosing of opioids or other adjunctive medications such as ketamine (0.1–0.2 mg/kg IV). Long-term pain may respond to medications such as gabapentin (Neurontin),[1] clonidine (Catapres),[1] or others.

Psychosocial recovery from burns is impacted by the preexisting conditions and the resilience of the patient. Preexisting mental health, substance abuse, and other medical and psychosocial issues complicate the patient's recovery from burns. Risk factors for burn injury include poverty, a history of abuse or neglect, substance abuse, serious mental illness, and risk for suicide or assault. Psychiatric recovery is negatively affected by posttraumatic stress disorder, depression, learning disorders, substance abuse, stigma, and disability. Individual resilience, social support, and education or occupation also impact patient outcomes.

The patient's age and stage of life at the time of injury impact recovery as well. Younger victims have a longer remaining lifespan to live with persistent scarring and disfigurement. Pediatric patients often have fewer comorbid medical conditions, which can speed their recovery and limit disability, and they tend to heal more quickly. However, their injuries may have a significant impact on their body image development, self-confidence, and interpersonal relationship building. The family may be of assistance in recovery from the injury, but family members, too, may experience stress and psychological concerns related to the child's injury. Adults and older patients have to deal with the impact of the injury on their identity and their ability to return to their preinjury roles.

Some patients and caregivers may develop posttraumatic stress disorder related to the injury or to postinjury treatment. It is thought that early multidisciplinary interventions may decrease this risk, but the research is unclear. Some patients will require long-term, continued outpatient treatment.

Hypertrophic scarring is the most common complication related to healing of burn wounds, but scar contracture and pruritus are common complications as well. It is thought that hypertrophic scarring may be decreased with early, appropriate surgical repair, but it still can occur. The development of hypertrophic scarring is multifactorial; it is likely a result of a complex interplay of humoral and cellular immunity causing an inappropriate response to healing tissue. Multiple host and injury factors contribute, but protracted healing of a partial thickness injury is a common theme. There are some experimental therapies for manipulating different components of the host response, but none has clearly proven to be beneficial.

Scar contracture results from tissue loss at the time of injury and tissue-healing properties. Burn injuries are more complicated than other traumatic wounds because the destroyed tissue is surrounded by profoundly damaged tissue. As a result of this tissue injury, there is increased collagen deposition resulting from changes in inflammation, proliferation, and remodeling at the cellular and extracellular matrix levels. Hypertrophic scars tend to form within the first month after injury and may improve over the first 6 months but then tend not to show significant changes after that time. Burn treatment and scar prevention consist of tissue replacement, tissue rehabilitation, and tension release. Early and existing scars are often treated with compression garments and silicone sheets. It is thought that these may alter and improve

---

[1]Not FDA approved for this indication.

remodeling of the extracellular matrix and thereby improve scarring. In some cases, surgical release of tension may be necessary.

References

Akelma H, Karahan ZA: Rare chemical burns: review of the literature, *Int Wound J* 16(6):1330–1338, 2019, https://doi.org/10.1111/iwj.13193.

Barrett W, Buxhoeveden M, Dhillon S: Ketamine: a versatile tool for anesthesia and analgesia, *Curr Opin Anaesthesiol* 33(5):633–638, 2020, https://doi.org/10.1097/aco.0000000000000916.

Bitter CC, Erickson TB: Management of burn injuries in the wilderness: lessons from low-resource settings, *Wilderness Environ Med* 27(4):519–525, 2016, https://doi.org/10.1016/j.wem.2016.09.001.

Bizrah M, Yusuf A, Ahmad S: An update on chemical eye burns, *Eye* 33(9):1362–1377, 2019, https://doi.org/10.1038/s41433-019-0456-5.

Burn Incidence and Treatment in United States: 2016, American Burn Association, 2016.

Carboni RM, Santos GL, Carboni Júnior IC, et al: Therapy for patients with burns—an integrating review, *Rev Assoc Med Bras* 65:1405–1412, 2019.

Cartotto R, Greenhalgh DG, Cancio C: Burn state of the science: fluid resuscitation, *J Burn Care Res* 38(3):e596–e604, 2017, https://doi.org/10.1097/bcr.0000000000000541.

Culnan DM, Craft-Coffman B, Bitz GH, et al: Carbon monoxide and cyanide poisoning in the burned pregnant patient: an indication for hyperbaric oxygen therapy, *Ann Plast Surg* 80(3 Suppl 2):S106–S112, 2018, https://doi.org/10.1097/sap.0000000000001351.

Culnan DM, Farner K, Bitz GH, et al: Volume resuscitation in patients with high-voltage electrical injuries, *Ann Plast Surg* 80(3 Suppl 2):S113–s118, 2018, https://doi.org/10.1097/sap.0000000000001374.

Dyamenahalli K, Garg G, Shupp JW, Kuprys PV, Choudhry MA, Kovacs EJ: Inhalation injury: unmet clinical needs and future research, *J Burn Care Res* 40(5):570–584, 2019, https://doi.org/10.1093/jbcr/irz055.

Friedstat J, Brown D, Levi B: Chemical, electrical, and radiation injuries, *Clin Plast Surg* 44(3):657–669, 2017, https://doi.org/10.1016/j.cps.2017.02.021.

Gigengack RK, Cleffken BI, Loer SA: Advances in airway management and mechanical ventilation in inhalation injury, *Curr Opin Anaesthesiol* 33(6):774–780, 2020, https://doi.org/10.1097/aco.0000000000000929.

Griggs C, Goverman J, Bittner EA, Levi B: Sedation and pain management in burn patients, *Clin Plast Surg* 44(3):535–540, 2017, https://doi.org/10.1016/j.cps.2017.02.026.

Hall AH, Mathieu L, Maibach HI: Acute chemical skin injuries in the United States: a review, *Crit Rev Toxicol* 48(7):540–554, 2018, https://doi.org/10.1080/10408444.2018.1493085.

ISBI Practice guidelines for burn care, Part 2, *Burns* 44(7):1617–1706, 2018, https://doi.org/10.1016/j.burns.2018.09.012.

Jeschke MG, Peck MD: Burn care of the elderly, *J Burn Care Res* 38(3):e625–e628, 2017, https://doi.org/10.1097/bcr.0000000000000535.

Jeschke MG, Shahrokhi S, Finnerty CC, Branski LK, Dibildox M: Wound coverage technologies in burn care: established techniques, *J Burn Care Res* 39(3):313–318, 2018, https://doi.org/10.1097/BCR.0b013e3182920d29.

Jeschke MG, van Baar ME, Choudhry MA, Chung KK, Gibran NS, Logsetty S: Burn injury, *Nat Rev Dis Primers* 6(1):11, 2020, https://doi.org/10.1038/s41572-020-0145-5.

Kim DE, Pruskowski KA, Ainsworth CR, Linsenbardt HR, Rizzo JA, Cancio LC: A review of adjunctive therapies for burn injury pain during the opioid crisis, *J Burn Care Res* 40(6):983–995, 2019, https://doi.org/10.1093/jbcr/irz111.

Partain KP, Fabia R, Thakkar RK: Pediatric burn care: new techniques and outcomes, *Curr Opin Pediatr* 32(3):405–410, 2020a, https://doi.org/10.1097/mop.0000000000000902.

Porter C, Tompkins RG, Finnerty CC, Sidossis LS, Suman OE, Herndon DN: The metabolic stress response to burn trauma: current understanding and therapies, *Lancet* 388(10052):1417–1426, 2016, https://doi.org/10.1016/s0140-6736(16)31469-6.

Shah A, Pedraza I, Mitchell C, Kramer GC: Fluid volumes infused during burn resuscitation 1980–2015: a quantitative review, *Burns* 46(1):52–57, 2020, https://doi.org/10.1016/j.burns.2019.11.013.

Shpichka A, Butnaru D, Bezrukov EA, et al: Skin tissue regeneration for burn injury, *Stem Cell Res Ther* 10(1), 2019, https://doi.org/10.1186/s13287-019-1203-3.

Smolle C, Cambiaso-Daniel J, Forbes AA, et al: Recent trends in burn epidemiology worldwide: a systematic review, *Burns* 43(2):249–257, 2017, https://doi.org/10.1016/j.burns.2016.08.013.

Sofia J, Ambardekar A: Pediatric burn resuscitation, management, and recovery for the pediatric anesthesiologist, *Curr Opin Anaesthesiol* 33(3):360–367, 2020, https://doi.org/10.1097/aco.0000000000000859.

Soussi S, Dépret F, Benyamina M, Legrand M: Early hemodynamic management of critically ill burn patients, *Anesthesiology* 129(3):583–589, 2018, https://doi.org/10.1097/aln.0000000000002314.

Stapelberg F: Challenges in anaesthesia and pain management for burn injuries, *Anaesth Intensive Care* 48(2):101–113, 2020, https://doi.org/10.1177/0310057x20914908.

Walls R, Hockberger R, Gausche-Hill M: *Rosen's emergency medicine—concepts and clinical practice E-Book*, Vol 2, 9 ed, Elsevier Health Sciences, 2018.

Yeroshalmi F, Sidoti EJ, Adamo AK, Lieberman BL, Badner VM: Oral electrical burns in children—a model of multidisciplinary care, *J Burn Care Res* 32(2):e25–e30, 2011, https://doi.org/10.1097/bcr.0b013e31820ab393.

Yoshino Y, Ohtsuka M, Kawaguchi M, et al: The wound/burn guidelines—6: guidelines for the management of burns, *J Dermatol* 43(9):989–1010, 2016, https://doi.org/10.1111/1346-8138.13288.

Method of
Jerrold B. Leikin, MD; Scott Leikin, DO; Frederick Korley, MD; and Ernest Wang, MD

CURRENT DIAGNOSIS

- Accidental hypothermia may be classified as mild, moderate, or severe.
- The temperature measured should be core body temperature.
- The method of rewarming depends on the severity of the temperature drop.
- Complications of rewarming include arrhythmias, rewarming-related hypotension, core temperature after drop, and rhabdomyolysis.
- Patients can be declared dead only after they are warm.

CURRENT THERAPY

Mild Hypothermia: 32.2°C to 35°C (90°F to 95°F)
- Begin passive external rewarming; remove wet clothing.
- Ambient temperature should exceed 21°C (70°F).
- Cover the patient with insulating material.

Moderate Hypothermia: 28°C to 32.2°C (82.4°F to 90°F)
- Begin active external rewarming; use radiant heat.
- Use thermal mattresses and electric heating blankets.
- Use forced-air heating blankets.
- Perform active core rewarming; use warmed humidified oxygen.
- Give warmed intravenous saline solution.
- Give bladder, colonic, and gastric irrigation.
- Start pleural cavity lavage.
- Avoid alcohol, caffeine, and nicotine (tobacco).

Severe Hypothermia: Less than 28°C (82.4°F)
- Begin aggressive active core rewarming; use warmed, humidified oxygen.
- Give warmed intravenous saline solution.
- Give bladder, colonic, and gastric irrigation.
- Begin pleural cavity lavage.
- Perform peritoneal lavage or dialysis.
- Perform extracorporeal warming or heated cardiopulmonary bypass.

Frostnip
- Begin gentle rewarming, generally in a water bath of 104°F to 108°F (40°C to 42°C).
- It is usually self-resolving.

Frostbite
- Immerse in warm (not hot) water.
- Débride broken vesicles.
- Do not débride hemorrhagic or intact blisters.
- Apply topical aloe or antibiotic ointment.
- Use nonsteroidal antiinflammatory drugs (NSAIDs) for pain.
- Update tetanus status.
- Do not rub or massage the affected area.
- Do not use a heating pad or heat lamp; affected areas can be easily burned.
- Avoid alcohol and tobacco products.

Chilblain
- Rewarm gently.
- Nifedipine (Procardia)[1] may be useful.

BOX 1   Prevention of High-Altitude Illness

Ascent above 2500 m (8200 ft) should be at a gradual rate of 300 m per 24 hours, with an additional rest day for every 1000 m (3280 ft) gain. With rapid ascent above 2500 m (8200 ft), light activity may be helpful with acclimatization, but strenuous activity should be avoided for at least 48 hours.

Avoid respiratory depressants such as alcohol until acclimatized.

For AMS:

- Acetazolamide (Diamox) 125 mg PO every 12 hours (adult); 2.5 mg/kg (maximum single dose 125 mg) PO every 12 hours (children). Begin 24 hours prior to ascent and stop 2 days after maximum altitude has been achieved or once descent has commenced.
- Alternative: dexamethasone (Decadron)[1] 2 mg PO every 6 hours or 4 mg PO every 12 hours (adult); do not use it for prophylaxis in children.

For persons with a history of HAPE:

- Nifedipine[1] 30 mg ER PO every 12 hours[3] (adult and children ≥50 kg). Begin 24 hours prior to ascent and continue for 5 days after reaching maximum altitude. Acetazolamide 2.5 mg/kg (maximum single dose 125 mg) PO every 12 hours (children ≥50 kg). Begin 24 hours prior to ascent and continue 4 to 5 days at maximum altitude.
- Consider the following alternatives for adults, although data are limited:
  - Tadalafil (Cialis)[1] 10 mg PO every 12 hours.[3] Start day of ascent and continue 3 to 5 days at maximum altitude.
  - Sildenafil (Viagra)[1] 50 mg PO every 8 hours.[3] Start day of ascent and continue 3 to 5 days at maximum altitude.
  - Dexamethasone[1] 8 mg PO every 12 hours. Start day of ascent and continue 2 to 3 days at maximum altitude.
  - Acetazolamide 125 to 250 mg PO every 12 hours. Begin 24 hours prior to ascent and continue 2 to 3 days at maximum altitude.

---

[1] Not FDA approved for this indication.
[3] Exceeds dosage recommended by the manufacturer.
AMS, Acute mountain sickness; *HAPE,* high altitude pulmonary edema.

After 24 to 48 hours, the kidneys excrete excess bicarbonate, normalizing the elevated pH.

The cardiac response to hypoxia includes an initial increase in heart rate and pulmonary perfusion with a goal to optimize oxygenation in the lungs and supply well-oxygenated blood to the brain, heart, and other tissues. Norepinephrine is released and results in increased cardiac output, heart rate, peripheral vascular tone, blood pressure, and pulmonary perfusion. Once acclimatized, heart rate normalizes and plasma volume decreases (diuresis), and cardiac output subsequently decreases. Hypoxia causes generalized pulmonary arterial vasoconstriction and a slight increase in pulmonary arterial pressure independent of the increase in cardiac output. It may initially improve the ventilation-perfusion ratio (V/Q) by redistributing blood flow to less-perfused areas of the lung. Unfortunately, this offers little adaptive advantage over the pathogenesis of HAPE.

Approximately 25% of people who ascend to 3500 m (11,500 ft) and >50% of people who ascend to greater than 6000 m (19,700 ft) develop HAI. The occurrence of HAI relies upon several variables, including the speed of ascent, the overall altitude, sleep quality and quantity, the amount of time spent at high altitude, low temperature, increased ultraviolet radiation, preacclimatization, previous history of HAI, and history of preexisting illnesses. Because of the many factors affecting HAI risk, incidence is highly variable. Globally, the reported incidence for AMS ranges from 10% to 90%; for HAPE and HACE, the range is from <0.01% to 31%. An individual who has a history of HAPE is 10% to 60% more likely to experience a subsequent episode at similar altitude with a similar rate of ascent.

Susceptibility to HAI is highly variable, and there are no reliable measures to predict the risk of developing HAI prior to ascent. Although gender does not appear to be a risk factor, age does play a role. The risk of developing HAI is two times lower in individuals over the age of 50, and HAPE occurs with greater frequency and severity in children and young adults. Fitness level does not appear to be protective against HAI, nor does a high fitness level improve the ability to acclimatize. Conditions that impair ventilation and the ventilatory response can increase the risk of HAI, including sedating medications, alcohol, moderate to severe chronic obstructive pulmonary disease, absence of carotid bodies (radiation, surgical resection), and neuromuscular diseases affecting the diaphragm. Conditions such as interstitial lung disease and cystic fibrosis, congenital cardiac anomalies involving right-to-left shunts, and obstructive sleep apnea are also likely to increase the risk of HAI, although data are limited. Pulmonary hypertension is known to increase the risk of HAPE, and tobacco smoking and asthma do not confer any additional risk. Chronic conditions such as hypertension and diabetes do not appear to be associated with increased risk of HAI.

When evaluating a patient for hypoxemia, it is essential to consider the limitations of current clinical tools. Pulse oximeter devices are widely used to evaluate peripheral blood oxygen saturation; however, there is growing evidence that pulse oximeters are less accurate in patients with dark skin tones at lower saturation (<80%), resulting in overestimation of SpO_2 and higher rates of clinically unrecognized hypoxemia. Awareness of potential limitations of pulse oximeter devices in patients with dark skin tones is essential to avoid treatment delays and mitigate health disparities.

High-Altitude Headache

HAH is recognized as a standalone diagnosis, even though it is a symptom of other AMS. HAH is a result of decreased barometric pressure seen with ascension into higher altitudes. This results in a lower percentage of oxygen molecules per breath. The body's immediate response is to increase respiration. Approximately 80% of people report a headache while ascending to high altitudes, particularly when the ascent is rapid and if altitude is >15,000 ft (4500 m). By definition, HAH can occur within 1 hour after ascent but typically occurs within 6 to 10 hours of ascent to altitudes >8200 ft (2500 m); it resolves within 24 hours of descent to <8200 ft (2500 m). Additionally, the headache should have at least two of the following characteristics: (1) the headache must be bilateral, (2) mild to moderate in intensity, and (3) aggravated by activities such as exertion, movement, straining, or bending. An HAH is often worse in the morning; photophobia and phonophobia are atypical for pure HAH. Treatment of the patient with mild HAH consists of medication, such as acetaminophen or ibuprofen, and implementing descent if the initial strategies are not successful. See the Current Therapy Box and Box 2 for a complete listing.

High-Altitude Syndromes

Acute Mountain Sickness

The most common form of altitude illness is AMS and typically occurs in unacclimatized individuals with rapid ascension to altitudes greater than 2500 m (8200 ft). Similar to HAH, onset can occur within 1 hour but usually begins within 6 to 10 hours after ascent. This condition is a result of exposure to hypobaric hypoxia. Symptoms include headache as well as anorexia, nausea, or vomiting; fatigue or weakness; dizziness or lightheadedness; and decreased urine output.

Early recognition of AMS is essential to promptly initiating treatment that may prevent evolution to the potentially fatal HACE, which exists along the same spectrum. Treatment for mild AMS includes the use of analgesics and antiemetics without further ascent. Acetazolamide is recommended for mild AMS; dexamethasone[1] is recommended for moderate to severe symptoms. For moderate to severe symptoms, low-flow supplemental oxygen and

---

[1] Not FDA approved for this indication.

Acetazolamide

Acetazolamide (Diamox) is a central-acting respiratory stimulant that stimulates bicarbonate diuresis and causes a metabolic acidosis to facilitate acclimatization. It is effective in preventing and treating HAI. Patients should be warned about side effects, including paresthesias, flat taste of carbonated beverages, and polyuria. Persons with a history of asthma, sulfonamide allergy, anaphylaxis, or penicillin allergy should try this medication under the supervision of a medical professional prior to departure. It should not be used in patients with type 1 diabetes due to the risk for acidosis and diuresis resulting in dehydration. It also should not be used in chronic lung disease if FEV_1 is less than 25% predicted or in patients on potassium-wasting diuretics or long-term high doses of aspirin.

Dexamethasone

Dexamethasone (Decadron)[1] is also effective in the prevention of AMS and treatment of AMS and HACE, though its mechanism is not completely understood. Unlike with acetazolamide, it does not facilitate acclimatization. It is not recommended for prophylaxis of AMS unless acetazolamide is contraindicated, though it is the drug of choice for treatment of HACE. Use is cautioned in patients with diabetes due to risk of hyperglycemia. Side effects can include insomnia, irritability, gastrointestinal upset, and euphoria.

Nifedipine

Nifedipine (Procardia)[1] is a calcium channel blocker that inhibits pulmonary vasoconstriction secondary to hypoxia at high altitude and is used in prevention and treatment of HAPE.

Caution should be used with other antihypertensives due to the risk for hypotension. Medications that inhibit the cytochrome P450 3A4 pathway, including macrolides, doxycycline, and azoles, may increase plasma concentrations and also precipitate hypotension. Ginkgo biloba[7] may also increase levels of nifedipine and cause hypotension and should be avoided.

Tadalafil (Cialis)[1] and Sildenafil (Viagra)[1]

Phosphodiesterase inhibitors that cause pulmonary vasodilation can be considered in the prevention or treatment of HAPE, although data are limited. They should not be used in conjunction with nitrates due to risk for significant hypotension or with alpha blockers due to orthostatic hypotension. Medications that inhibit the cytochrome P450 3A4 pathway, including macrolides, doxycycline, and azoles, may increase plasma concentrations and also precipitate hypotension.

---

[1] Not FDA approved for this indication.

[7] Available as a dietary supplement.

AMS, Acute mountain sickness; *FEV₁,* forced expiratory volume; *HACE,* high altitude cerebral edema; *HAPE,* high altitude pulmonary edema.

---

hyperbaric chambers can also be used. Descent is recommended if symptoms do not improve or worsen after 24 hours of rest or treatment. Graded ascent can be resumed once symptoms resolve. However, immediate descent should be undertaken for ataxia, altered mental status, or any signs of pulmonary edema. Refer to the Current Therapy Box and Box 2 for dosing and summary.

High-Altitude Cerebral Edema

HACE is a neurologic disorder characterized by headaches, impaired coordination and muscle weakness as well as impairments of consciousness. It is considered a separate disease from acute mountain sickness and typically progresses over 1 to 3 days. Established risk factors for HACE include rapid ascent, inadequate acclimatization, extreme altitudes, physical exertion, and a prior history of HAI. Clinical signs of HACE typically appear 3 to 5 days after ascension above 2750 m (9022 ft) and include declining neurologic function, such as altered mental status, slurred speech, cranial nerve palsies, papilledema, and ataxia. Truncal ataxia, implying impaired coordination between the trunk and the extremities, is a common sign. If computed tomography or magnetic resonance imaging is available acutely, findings would be consistent with vasogenic edema. If a lumbar puncture is performed, increased opening pressure is typically present. Differential diagnosis is similar to that for AMS but would also include diabetic ketoacidosis, hypoglycemia, electrolyte imbalances, brain tumor, stroke, acute psychosis, and seizure. If symptoms appear when at elevation, early recognition is crucial to prevent evolution to irreversible disease. The most important element of treatment is descent of at least 1000 m (3280 ft). Supplemental oxygen and hyperbaric bags may be used during descent and are imperative if descent is not possible. Dexamethasone[1] should be initiated as soon as possible and continued after descent until symptoms resolve. Currently, there is no evidence to support the use of acetazolamide as monotherapy in treating HACE.[1] Dosages are listed in the Current Therapy Box and details on pharmacology can be found in Box 2.

High-Altitude Pulmonary Edema

HAPE is a potentially lethal pulmonary disorder defined as noncardiogenic (left ventricular function is preserved) pulmonary edema caused by pulmonary blood gas barrier leak in the lung. It is typically diagnosed with at least two of the following: resting dyspnea, cough, weakness or decreased exercise performance, and chest tightness or congestion, in addition to two of the following: wheezing or rales, tachypnea, tachycardia, or central cyanosis. Cough is initially dry but in late stages is productive of pink or bloody sputum. This condition does not typically manifest itself until 2 to 3 days after ascension and rarely presents after 4 days. The physiologic response includes increased pulmonary arterial pressure, hypoxic pulmonary vasoconstriction, and hypoxemia. Physical examination is significant for rales that can begin in the right axilla and progress diffusely along with low-grade temperature elevation. Hypoxia, often very pronounced, is noted on pulse oximetry; oxygen levels will be disproportionately low for a given elevation. Plain films of the thorax show pulmonary thickening but no cardiomegaly; imaging may also include unilateral or bilateral patchy fluffy opacities predominantly in the dependent zone of the lungs. Differential diagnosis includes heart failure, acute myocardial ischemia, pulmonary embolus, asthma, bronchitis, and pneumonia. Although HAPE is associated with the highest rate of mortality of altitude conditions, it is unlikely to cause long-term sequelae if treated appropriately. Treatment includes immediate descent and supplemental oxygen or a hyperbaric chamber. If available, supplemental oxygen and bedrest may be sufficient. If the pulmonary edema is severe, though, descent is the definitive treatment and should be undertaken without delay. Exertion and cold stress should be avoided during descent. Nifedipine (Procardia)[1] may be of benefit in treatment of HAPE but is not as effective as oxygen or descent and should be used as an adjunct.

High-Altitude Retinopathy

Hypoxia is known to cause hyperemia and engorgement of the retinal vessels at any elevation and will be seen above 2500 m (8200 ft) in the setting of hypobaric hypoxia. Macular or vitreous hemorrhage, disc edema, and cotton wool spots can be seen in more severe high-altitude retinopathy (HAR). There may be a delay between ascent and onset of hemorrhage. The retinopathy is generally asymptomatic; however, scotomas and visual field deficits may occur, particularly with macular hemorrhage. Lower oxygen saturation, higher ascent, strenuous exertion, and longer duration at high altitude are associated with HAR. Higher baseline intraocular pressure, hypercoagulable disorders, and aspirin and nonsteroidal antiinflammatory drug (NSAID) use also appear

---

[1] Not FDA approved for this indication.

TABLE 5 Initial Doses of Antidotes for Common Poisonings—cont'd

ANTIDOTE	USE	DOSE	ROUTE	ADVERSE REACTIONS/COMMENTS
	Cyanide Hydrogen sulfide (nitrites are given only) Do not use sodium thiosulfate for hydrogen sulfide Individual portions of the kit can be used in certain circumstances (consult PCC)	Sodium nitrite: *Child:* 0.33 mL/kg of 3% solution if hemoglobin level is not known, otherwise based on tables with product. *Adult:* up to 300 mg (10 mL). Dilute nitrite in 100 mL 0.9% saline, administer slowly at 5 mL/min. Slow infusion if fall in BP.	IV	If methemoglobinemia occurs, do not use methylene blue to correct this because it releases cyanide.
	Do not use sodium thiosulfate for hydrogen sulfide Individual portions of the kit can be used in certain circumstances (consult PCC)	Sodium thiosulfate: *Child:* 1.6 mL/kg of 25% solution, may be repeated q30–60 min to a maximum of 12.5 g or 50 mL in adult. Administer over 20 min.	IV	Nausea, dizziness, headache. Tachycardia, muscle rigidity, and bronchospasm (rapid administration).
Dantrolene Sodium (Dantrium): Stock level to treat 70 kg adult for 24 h: 700 mg, 35 vials (20 mg/vial)	Malignant hyperthermia	2–3 mg/kg IV rapidly. Repeat loading dose every 10 min. If necessary up to a maximum total dose of 10 mg/kg. When temperature and heart rate decrease, slow the infusion 1–2 mg/kg q6h for 24–28 h until all evidence of malignant hyperthermia syndrome has subsided. Follow with oral doses 1–2 mg/kg four times a day for 24 h as necessary.	IV/PO	Hepatotoxicity occurs with cumulative dose of 10 mg/kg. Thrombophlebitis (best given in central line). Available as 20 mg lyophilized dantrolene powder for reconstitution, which contains 3 g mannitol and sodium hydroxide in 70-mL vial. Mix with 60 mL sterile distilled water without a bacteriostatic agent and protect from light. Use within 6 hours after reconstituting.
Deferoxamine (Desferal): Stock level to treat 70 kg adult for 24 h: 17 vials (500 mg/amp)	Iron	IV infusion of 15 mg/kg/h (3 mL/kg/h: 500 mg in 100 mL D₅W) max 6 g/d Rates of >45 μg/kg/h if conc >1000 μg/dL.	Preferred IV: avoid therapy >24 h	Hypotension (minimized by avoiding rapid infusion rates) DFO challenge test 50 mg/kg is unreliable if negative.
Diazepam (Valium): Stock level to treat 70 kg adult for 24 h: 200 mg, 5 mg/mL; 2, 10 mL	Any intoxication that provokes seizures when specific therapy is not available (e.g., amphetamines, PCP, barbiturate and alcohol withdrawal) Chloroquine poisoning	*Adult,* 5–10 mg IV (max 20 mg) at a rate of 5 mg/min until seizure is controlled. May be repeated 2 or 3 times. *Child,* 0.1–0.3 mg/kg up to 10 mg IV slowly over 2 min.	IV	Confusion, somnolence, coma, hypotension. Intramuscular absorption is erratic. Establish airway and administer 100% oxygen and glucose.
Digoxin-Specific Fab Antibodies (Digibind): Stock level to treat 70 kg adult for 24 h: 20 vials	Digoxin, digitoxin, oleander tea with the following: (1) Imminent cardiac arrest or shock (2) Hyperkalemia >5.0 mEq/L (3) Serum digoxin >5 ng/mL (child) at 8–12 h post ingestion in adults (4) Digitalis delirium (5) Ingestion over 10 mg in adults or 4 mg in child (6) Bradycardia or second- or third-degree heart block unresponsive to atropine (7) Life-threatening digitoxin or oleander poisoning	(1) If amount ingested is known total dose × bioavailability (0.8) = body burden. The body burden ÷ 0.6 (0.5 mg of digoxin is bound by 1 vial of 38 mg of Fab) = # vials needed. (2) If amount is unknown but the steady state serum concentration is known in ng/mL: Digoxin: ng/mL: (5.6 L/kg Vd) × (wt kg) = μg body burden. Body burden ÷ 100 = mg body burden/0.5 = # vials needed. Digitoxin body burden = ng/mL × (0.56 L/kg Vd) × (wt kg) Body burden ÷ 1000 = mg body burden/0.5 = # vials needed. (3) If the amount is not known, it is administered in life-threatening situations as 10 vials (400 mg) IV in saline over 30 min in adults. If cardiac arrest is imminent, administer 20 vials (adult) as a bolus.	IV	Allergic reactions (rare), return of condition being treated with digitalis glycoside. Administer by infusion over 30 min through a 0.22-μ filter. If cardiac arrest imminent, may administer by bolus. Consult PCC for more details.

Antidote	Indications	Dose	Route	Comments
Sodium Bicarbonate (NaHCO3): Stock level to treat 70 kg adult for 24 h: 10 ampules or syringes (500 mEq)	Tricyclic antidepressant cardiotoxicity (QRS >0.12 sec; ventricular tachycardia, severe conduction disturbances); metabolic acidosis; phenothiazine toxicity *Salicylate:* to keep blood pH 7.5–7.55 (not >7.55) and urine pH 7.5–8.0. Alkalinization recommended if salicylate conc. >40 mg/dL in acute poisoning and at lower levels if symptomatic in chronic intoxication, 2 mEq/kg will raise blood pH 0.1 unit	*Ethylene glycol:* 100 mg IV daily. 1–2 mEq/kg undiluted as a bolus. If no effect on cardiotoxicity, repeat twice a few minutes apart *Adult* with clear physical signs and laboratory findings of acute moderate or severe salicylism: Bolus 1–2 mEq/kg followed by infusion of 100–150 mEq NaHCO3 added to 1 L of 5% dextrose at rate of 200–300 mL/h *Child:* Bolus same as adult followed by 1–2 mEq/kg in infusion of 20 mL/kg/h 5% dextrose in 0.45% saline Add potassium when patient voids Rate and amount of the initial infusion, if patient is volume depleted: 1 h to achieve urine output of 2 mL/kg/h and urine pH 7–8 In mild cases without acidosis and urine pH >6, administer 5% dextrose in 0.9% saline with 50 mEq/L or 1 mEq/kg NaHCO3 as maintenance to replace ongoing renal losses. If acidemia is present and pH <7.2, add 2 mEq/kg as loading dose followed by 2 mEq/kg q3–4h to keep pH at 7.5–7.55. If acidemia is present, recommend isotonic NaHCO3, 3 ampules to 1 L of D5W at 10–15 mL/kg/h or sufficient to produce normal urine flow and a urine pH of 7.5 or higher	IV	Monitor sodium, potassium, and blood pH because fatal alkalemia and hyponatremia have been reported. Monitor both urine and blood pH. Do not use the urine pH alone to assess the need for alkalinization because of the paradoxical aciduria that may occur. Adjust the urine pH to 7.5–8 by NaHCO3 infusion. After urine output established, add potassium 40 mEq/L.
	Long-acting barbiturates: Phenobarbital and primidone (Mysoline). *Note:* Alkalinization is ineffective for the short- or intermediate-acting barbiturates	NaHCO3: 2 mEq/kg during the first hour or 100 mEq in 1 L of D5W with 40 mEq/L potassium at a rate of 100 mL/h in adults Adequate potassium is necessary to accomplish alkalinization	IV	Additional sodium bicarbonate and potassium chloride may be needed. Adjust the urine pH to 7.5–8 by NaHCO3 infusion.
Thiamine: 100 mg/mL, 2 vials	Thiamine deficiency, ethylene glycol poisoning, alcoholism	100 mg IV followed with 100 mg V/IM for 5–7 days in an alcoholic and followed by 100 mg/d orally	IV/IM	
Vitamin K1 (Aqua Mephyton): 10 mg/1–5 mL; 5-mg tablets	Warfarin anticoagulant or rodenticide toxicity	Oral 0.4 mg/kg/dose child, 10–25 mg adults. If evidence of bleeding, administer vitamin K1 SC, IV 0.6 mg/kg/dose child and up to 25–50 mg adults for 6 hours depending on severity	PO/SC, IV	Give vitamin K daily until PT/INR are normal. Examine stools and urine for evidence of bleeding.

Abbreviations: ALT = alanine aminotransferase; amp = ampule; AST = aspartate aminotransferase; BAL = British anti-Lewisite; BP = blood pressure; conc. = concentration; ECG = electrocardiogram; ET = endotracheal; G6PD = glucose-6-phosphate dehydrogenase; IM = intramuscular; IV = intravenous; PCC = poison control center; PO = oral; PT = prothrombin time; SC = subcutaneous.

TABLE 6	Plasma Concentrations Above Which Removal by Extracorporeal Measures Should Be Considered			
DRUG	PLASMA CONCENTRATION	PROTEIN BINDING (%)	VOLUME DISTRIBUTION (L/KG)	METHOD OF CHOICE
Amanitin	NA	25	1.0	HP
Ethanol	500–700 mg/dL	0	0.3	HD
Ethchlorvynol	150 µg/mL	35–50	3–4	HP
Ethylene glycol	25–50 µg/mL	0	0.6	HD
Glutethimide	100 µg/mL	50	2.7	HP
Isopropyl alcohol	400 mg/dL	0	0.7	HD
Lithium	4 mEq/L	0	0.7	HD
Meprobamate (Equanil)	100 µg/mL	0	NA	HP
Methanol	50 mg/dL	0	0.7	HD
Methaqualone	40 µg/dL	20–60	6.0	HP
Other barbiturates	50 µg/dL	50	0–1	HP
Paraquat	0.1 mg/dL	poor	2.8	HP > HD
Phenobarbital	100 µg/dL	50	0.9	HP > HD
Salicylates	80–100 mg/dL	90	0.2	HD > HP
Theophylline		0	0.5	
Chronic	40–60 µg/mL			HP
Acute	80–100 µg/mL			HP
Trichlorethanol	250 µg/mL	70	0.6	HP

Abbreviations: HD = hemodialysis; HP = hemoperfusion; HP > HD = hemoperfusion preferred over hemodialysis.
Data from Winchester JF: Active methods for detoxification. In Haddad LM, Winchester JF (eds). Clinical Management of Poisoning and Drug Overdose, 2nd ed. Philadelphia, WB Saunders, 1990; Balsam L, Cortitsidis GN, Fienfeld DA: Role of hemodialysis and hemoperfusion in the treatment of intoxications. Contemp Manage Crit Care 1:61, 1991.
Note: Cartridges for charcoal hemoperfusion are not readily available anymore in most locations. So hemodialysis may be substituted in these situations. In mixed or chronic drug overdoses, extracorporeal measures may be considered at lower drug concentrations.

nephrologist should be notified immediately), and cases involving a compound that is ingested in a potentially lethal dose and the rapid removal of which may improve the prognosis. Examples of the latter are ethylene glycol 1.4 mL/kg 100% solution or equivalent and methanol 6 mL/kg 100% solution or equivalent. Common dialyzable substances include alcohol, bromides, lithium, and salicylates.

The patient-related criteria for dialysis are (a) anticipated prolonged coma and the likelihood of complications; (b) renal compromise (toxin excreted or metabolized by kidneys and dialyzable chelating agents in heavy metal poisoning); (c) laboratory confirmation of lethal blood concentration; (d) lethal dose poisoning with an agent with delayed toxicity or known to be metabolized into a more toxic metabolite (e.g., ethylene glycol, methanol); and (e) hepatic impairment when the agent is metabolized by the liver, and clinical deterioration despite optimal supportive medical management. Table 6 gives plasma concentrations above which removal by extracorporeal measures should be considered.

The contraindications to hemodialysis include the following: (a) substances are not dialyzable; (b) effective antidotes are available; (c) patient is hemodynamically unstable (e.g., shock); and (d) presence of coagulopathy because heparinization is required.

Hemodialysis also has a role in correcting disturbances that are not amenable to appropriate medical management. These are easily remembered by the "vowel" mnemonic:
A—refractory acid-base disturbances
E—refractory electrolyte disturbances
I—intoxication with dialyzable substances (e.g., ethanol, ethylene glycol, isopropyl alcohol, methanol, lithium, and salicylates)
O—overhydration
U—uremia

Complications of dialysis include hemorrhage, thrombosis, air embolism, hypotension, infections, electrolyte imbalance, thrombocytopenia, and removal of therapeutic medications.

Hemoperfusion

Hemoperfusion is the parenteral form of oral activated charcoal. Heparinization is necessary. The patient's blood is routed extracorporeally through an outflow arterial catheter with a filter-adsorbing cartridge (charcoal or resin) and returned through a venous catheter. Cartridges must be changed every 4 hours. The blood glucose, electrolytes, calcium, and albumin levels; complete blood cell count; platelets; and serum and urine osmolarity must be carefully monitored. This procedure has extended extracorporeal removal to a large range of substances that were formerly either poorly dialyzable or nondialyzable. It is not limited by molecular weight, water solubility, or protein binding, but it is limited by a volume distribution greater than 400 L, plasma concentration, and rate of flow through the filter. Activated charcoal cartridges are the primary type of hemoperfusion currently available in the United States.

The patient-related criteria for hemoperfusion are (a) anticipated prolonged coma and the likelihood of complications; (b) laboratory confirmation of lethal blood concentrations; (c) hepatic impairment when an agent is metabolized by the liver; and (d) clinical deterioration despite optimally supportive medical management.

The contraindications are similar to those for hemodialysis.

Limited data are available as to which toxins are best treated with hemoperfusion. Hemoperfusion has proved useful in treating glutethimide intoxication, phenobarbital overdose, and carbamazepine, phenytoin, and theophylline intoxication.

Complications include hemorrhage, thrombocytopenia, hypotension, infection, leukopenia, depressed phagocytic activity of granulocytes, decreased immunoglobulin levels, hypoglycemia, hypothermia, hypocalcemia, pulmonary edema, and air and charcoal embolism.

Hemofiltration
Continuous arteriovenous or venovenous hemodiafiltration (CAVHD or CVVHD, respectively) has been suggested as an alternative to conventional hemodialysis when the need for rapid removal of the drug is less urgent. These procedures, like peritoneal dialysis, are minimally invasive, have no significant impact on hemodynamics, and can be carried out continuously for many hours. Their role in the management of acute poisoning remains uncertain, however.

Plasmapheresis
Plasmapheresis consists of removal of a volume of blood. All the extracted components are returned to the blood except the plasma, which is replaced with a colloid protein solution. There are limited clinical data on guidelines and efficacy in toxicology. Centrifugal and membrane separators of cellular elements are used. It can be as effective as hemodialysis or hemoperfusion for removing toxins that have high protein binding, and it may be useful for toxins not filtered by hemodialysis and hemoperfusion.

Plasmapheresis has been anecdotally used in treating intoxications with the following agents: paraquat (removed 10%), propranolol (removed 30%), quinine (removed 10%), L-thyroxine (removed 30%), and salicylate (removed 10%). It has been shown to remove less than 10% of digoxin, phenobarbital, prednisolone, and tobramycin. Complications include infection; allergic reactions including anaphylaxis; hemorrhagic disorders; thrombocytopenia; embolus and thrombus; hypervolemia and hypovolemia; dysrhythmias; syncope; tetany; paresthesia; pneumothorax; acute respiratory distress syndrome; and seizures.

Supportive Care, Observation, and Therapy for Complications
Altered Mental Status
If airway protective reflexes are absent, endotracheal intubation is indicated for a comatose patient or a patient with altered mental status. If respirations are ineffective, ventilation should be instituted, and if hypoxemia persists, supplemental oxygen is indicated. If a cyanotic patient fails to respond to oxygen, the practitioner should consider methemoglobinemia.

Hypoglycemia
Hypoglycemia accompanies many poisonings, including with ethanol (especially in children), clonidine (Catapres), insulin, organophosphates, salicylates, sulfonylureas, and the unripe fruit or seed of a Jamaican plant called ackee. If hypoglycemia is present or suspected, glucose should be administered immediately as an intravenous bolus. Doses are as follows: in a neonate, 10% glucose (5 mL/kg); in a child, 25% glucose 0.25 g/kg (2 mL/kg); and in an adult, 50% glucose 0.5 g/kg (1 mL/kg).

A bedside capillary test for blood glucose is performed to detect hypoglycemia, and the sample is sent to the laboratory for confirmation. If the glucose reagent strip visually reads less than 150 mg/dL, one administers glucose. Venous blood should be used rather than capillary blood for the bedside test if the patient is in shock or is hypotensive. Large amounts of glucose given rapidly to nondiabetic patients may cause a transient reactive hypoglycemia and hyperkalemia and may accentuate damage in ischemic cerebrovascular and cardiac tissue. If focal neurologic signs are present, it may be prudent to withhold glucose, because hypoglycemia causes focal signs in less than 10% of cases.

Thiamine Deficiency Encephalopathy
Thiamine is administered to avoid precipitating thiamine deficiency encephalopathy (Wernicke-Korsakoff syndrome) in alcohol abusers and in malnourished patients. The overall incidence of thiamine deficiency in ethanol abusers is 12%. Thiamine 100 mg intravenously should be administered around the time of the glucose administration but not necessarily before the glucose. The clinician should be prepared to manage the anaphylaxis that sometimes is caused by thiamine, although it is extremely rare.

Opioid Reactions
Naloxone (Narcan) reverses CNS and respiratory depression, miosis, bradycardia, and decreased gastrointestinal peristalsis caused by opioids acting through μ, κ, and δ receptors. It also affects endogenous opioid peptides (endorphins and enkephalins), which accounts for the variable responses reported in patients with intoxications from ethanol, benzodiazepines, clonidine (Catapres), captopril (Capoten), and valproic acid (Depakote) and in patients with spinal cord injuries. There is a high sensitivity for predicting a response if pinpoint pupils and circumstantial evidence of opioid abuse (e.g., track marks) are present.

In cases of suspected overdose, naloxone 0.1 mg/kg is administered intravenously initially in a child younger than 5 years of age. The dose can be repeated in 2 minutes, if necessary up to a total dose of 2 mg. In older children and adults, the dose is 2 mg every 2 minutes for five doses up to a total of 10 mg. Naloxone can also be administered into an endotracheal tube if intravenous access is unavailable. If there is no response after 10 mg, a pure opioid intoxication is unlikely. If opioid abuse is suspected, restraints should be in place before the administration of naloxone, and it is recommended that the initial dose be 0.1 to 0.2 mg to avoid withdrawal and violent behavior. The initial dose is then doubled every minute progressively to a total of 10 mg. Naloxone may unmask concomitant sympatho-mimetic intoxication as well as withdrawal.

Larger doses of naloxone may be required for more poorly antagonized synthetic opioid drugs: buprenorphine (Buprenex), codeine, dextromethorphan, fentanyl and its derivatives, pentazocine (Talwin), propoxyphene (Darvon), diphenoxylate, nalbuphine (Nubain), and long-acting opioids such as methadone (Dolophine).

Indications for a continuous infusion include a second dose for recurrent respiratory depression, exposure to poorly antagonized opioids, a large overdose, and decreased opioid metabolism, as with impaired liver function. A continuous infusion has been advocated because many opioids outlast the short half-life of naloxone (30 to 60 minutes). The hourly rate of naloxone infusion is equal to the effective dose required to produce a response (improvement in ventilation and arousal). An additional dose may be required in 15 to 30 minutes as a bolus. The infusions are titrated to avoid respiratory depression and opioid withdrawal manifestations. Tapering of infusions can be attempted after 12 hours and when the patient's condition has been stabilized.

Although naloxone is safe and effective, there are rare reports of complications (less than 1%) of pulmonary edema, seizures, hypertension, cardiac arrest, and sudden death.

Agents Whose Roles Are Not Clarified
Nalmefene (Revex), a long-acting parenteral opioid antagonist that the FDA has approved, is undergoing investigation, but its role in the treatment of comatose patients and patients with opioid overdose is not clear. It is 16 times more potent than naloxone, and its duration of action is up to 8 hours (half-life 10.8 hours, versus naloxone 1 hour).

Flumazenil (Romazicon) is a pure competitive benzodiazepine antagonist. It has been demonstrated to be safe and effective for reversing benzodiazepine-induced sedation. It is not recommended to improve ventilation. Its role in cases of CNS depression needs to be clarified. It should not be used routinely in comatose patients and is not an essential ingredient of the coma therapeutic regimen. It is contraindicated in cases of co-ingestion of cyclic antidepressant intoxication, stimulant overdose, and long-term benzodiazepine use (may precipitate life-threatening withdrawal) if benzodiazepines are used to control seizures. There is a concern about the potential for seizures and cardiac dysrhythmias that may occur in these settings.

Laboratory and Radiographic Studies

An electrocardiogram (ECG) should be obtained to identify dysrhythmias or conduction delays from cardiotoxic medications. If aspiration pneumonia (history of loss of consciousness, unarousable state, vomiting) or noncardiac pulmonary edema is suspected, a chest radiograph is needed. Electrolyte and glucose concentrations in the blood, the anion gap, acid-base balance, the arterial blood gas (ABG) profile (if patient has respiratory distress or altered mental status), and serum osmolality should be measured if a toxic alcohol ingestion is suspected. Table 7 lists appropriate testing on the basis of clinical toxicologic presentation. All laboratory specimens should be carefully labeled, including time and date. For potential legal cases, a "chain of custody" must be established. Assessment of the laboratory studies may provide a clue to the etiologic agent.

Electrolyte, Acid-Base, and Osmolality Disturbances

Electrolyte and acid-base disturbances should be evaluated and corrected. Metabolic acidosis (usually low or normal pH with a low or normal/high $Paco_2$ and low HCO_3) with an increased anion gap (AG) is seen with many agents in cases of overdose.

The AG is an estimate of those anions other than chloride and HCO_3 necessary to counterbalance the positive charge of sodium. It serves as a clue to causes, compensations, and complications. The AG is calculated from the standard serum electrolytes by subtracting the total CO_2 (which reflects the actual measured bicarbonate) and chloride from the sodium: $(Na - [Cl + HCO_3]) = $ AG. The potassium is usually not used in the calculation because it may be hemolyzed and is an intracellular cation. The lack of anion gap does not exclude a toxic etiology.

The normal gap is usually 7 to 11 mEq/L by flame photometer. However, there has been a "lowering" of the normal AG to 7 ± 4 mEq/L by the newer techniques (e.g., ion selective electrodes or colorimetric titration). Some studies have found AGs to be relatively insensitive for determining the presence of toxins.

It is important to recognize anion gap toxins, such as salicylates, methanol, and ethylene glycol, because they have specific antidotes, and hemodialysis is effective in management of cases of overdose with these agents.

Table 8 lists the reasons for increased AG, decreased anion gap, or no gap. The most common cause of a decreased AG is laboratory error. Lactic acidosis produces the largest AG and can result from any poisoning that results in hypoxia, hypoglycemia, or convulsions.

Table 9 lists other blood chemistry derangements that suggest certain intoxications.

Serum osmolality is a measure of the number of molecules of solute per kilogram of solvent, or mOsm/kg water. The osmolarity is molecules of solute per liter of solution, or mOsm/L water at a specified temperature. Osmolarity is usually the calculated value and osmolality is usually a measured value. They are considered interchangeable where 1 L equals 1 kg. The normal serum osmolality is 280 to 290 mOsm/kg. The freezing point serum osmolarity measurement specimen and the serum electrolyte specimens for calculation should be drawn simultaneously.

The serum osmolal gap is defined as the difference between the measured osmolality determined by the freezing point method and the calculated osmolarity. It is determined by the following formula (BUN is blood urea nitrogen):

$$(Sodium \times 2) + (BUN/3) + (Glucose/20)$$

TABLE 7	Patient Condition/Systemic Toxin and Appropriate Tests
CONDITION	**TESTS**
Comatose	Toxicologic tests (acetaminophen, sedative-hypnotic, ethanol, opioids, benzodiazepine), glucose.
Respiratory toxicity	Spirometry, FEV_1, arterial blood gases, chest radiograph, monitor O_2 saturation
Cardiac toxicity	ECG 12-lead and monitoring, echocardiogram, serial cardiac enzymes (if evidence or suspicion of a myocardial infarction), hemodynamic monitoring
Hepatic toxicity	Enzymes (AST, ALT, GGT), ammonia, albumin, bilirubin, glucose, PT, PTT, amylase
Nephrotoxicity	BUN, creatinine, electrolytes (Na, F, Mg, Ca, PO_4), serum and urine osmolarity, 24-hour urine for heavy metals if suspected, creatine kinase, serum and urine myoglobin, urinalysis and urinary sodium
Bleeding	Platelets, PT, PTT, bleeding time, fibrin split products, fibrinogen, type and match

Abbreviations: ALT = alanine transaminase; AST = aspartate transaminase; BUN = blood urea nitrogen; ECG = electrocardiogram; FEV_1 = forced expiratory volume in 1 second; GGT = γ-glutamyltransferase; PT = prothrombin time; PTT = partial thromboplastin time.

TABLE 8	Etiologies of Metabolic Acidosis

NORMAL ANION GAP HYPERCHLOREMIC	INCREASED ANION GAP NORMOCHLOREMIC	DECREASED ANION GAP
Acidifying agents	Methanol	Laboratory error[†]
Adrenal insufficiency	Uremia*	Intoxication—bromine, lithium
Anhydrase inhibitors	Diabetic ketoacidosis*	Protein abnormal
Fistula	Paraldehyde,* phenformin	Sodium low
Osteotomies	Isoniazid	
Obstructive uropathies	Iron	
Renal tubular acidosis	Lactic acidosis[†]	
Diarrhea, uncomplicated*	Ethanol,* ethylene glycol*	
Dilutional	Salicylates, starvation solvents	
Sulfamylon		

*Indicates hyperosmolar situation. Studies have found that the anion gap may be relatively insensitive for determining the presence of toxins.
[†]Lactic acidosis can be produced by intoxications of the following: carbon monoxide, cyanide, hydrogen sulfide, hypoxia, ibuprofen, iron, isoniazid, phenformin, salicylates, seizures, theophylline.

TABLE 9	Blood Chemistry Derangements in Toxicology
DERANGEMENT	**TOXIN**
Acetonemia without acidosis	Acetone or isopropyl alcohol
Hypomagnesemia	Ethanol, digitalis
Hypocalcemia	Ethylene glycol, oxalate, fluoride
Hyperkalemia	β-Blockers, acute digitalis, renal failure
Hypokalemia	Diuretics, salicylism, sympathomimetics, theophylline, corticosteroids, chronic digitalis
Hyperglycemia	Diazoxide, glucagon, iron, isoniazid, organophosphate insecticides, phenylurea insecticides, phenytoin (Dilantin), salicylates, sympathomimetic agents, thyroid vasopressors
Hypoglycemia	β-Blockers, ethanol, insulin, isoniazid, oral hypoglycemic agents, salicylates
Rhabdomyolysis	Amphetamines, ethanol, cocaine, or phencyclidine, elevated creatine phosphokinase

TABLE 10	Conversion Factors for Alcohols and Glycols		
ALCOHOLS/ GLYCOLS	**1 MG/DL IN BLOOD RAISES OSMOLALITY MOSM/L**	**MOLECULAR WEIGHT**	**CONVERSION FACTOR**
Ethanol	0.228	40	4.6
Methanol	0.327	32	3.2
Ethylene glycol	0.190	62	6.2
Isopropanol	0.176	60	6.0
Acetone	0.182	58	5.8
Propylene glycol	NA	72	7.2

Example: Methanol osmolality. Subtract the calculated osmolality from the measured serum osmolarity (freezing point method) = osmolar gap × 3.2 (one-tenth molecular weight) = estimated serum methanol concentration.

Note: This equation is often not considered very reliable in predicting the actual measured blood concentration of these alcohols or glycols.

This gap estimate is normally within 10 mOsm of the simultaneously measured serum osmolality. Ethanol, if present, may be included in the equation to eliminate its influence on the osmolal gap (the ethanol concentration divided by 4.6; Table 10).

The osmolal gap is not valid in cases of shock and postmortem state. Metabolic disorders such as hyperglycemia, uremia, and dehydration increase the osmolarity but usually do not cause gaps greater than 10 mOsm/kg. A gap greater than 10 mOsm/mL suggests that unidentified osmolal-acting substances are present: acetone, ethanol, ethylene glycol, glycerin, isopropyl alcohol, isoniazid, ethanol, mannitol, methanol, and trichloroethane. Alcohols and glycols should be sought when the degree of obtundation exceeds that expected from the blood ethanol concentration or when other clinical conditions exist: visual loss (methanol), metabolic acidosis (methanol and ethylene glycol), or renal failure (ethylene glycol).

A falsely elevated osmolar gap can be produced by other low molecular weight un-ionized substances (dextran, diuretics, sorbitol, ketones), hyperlipidemia, and unmeasured electrolytes (e.g., magnesium).

Note: A normal osmolal gap may be reported in the presence of toxic alcohol or glycol poisoning, if the parent compound is already metabolized. This situation can occur when the osmolar gap is measured after a significant time has elapsed since the ingestion. In cases of alcohol and glycol intoxication, an early osmolar gap is a result of the relatively nontoxic parent drug and delayed metabolic acidosis, and an anion gap is a result of the more toxic metabolites. The serum concentration is calculated as

$$\text{mg/dL} = \text{mOsm gap} \times \text{MW of substance divided by } 10.$$

Radiographic Studies

Chest and neck radiographs are useful for suspected pathologic conditions such as aspiration pneumonia, pulmonary edema, and foreign bodies and to determine the location of the endotracheal tube. Abdominal radiographs can be used to detect radiopaque substances.

The mnemonic for radiopaque substances seen on abdominal radiographs is CHIPES:
C—chlorides and chloral hydrate
H—heavy metals (arsenic, barium, iron, lead, mercury, zinc)
I—iodides
P—PlayDoh, Pepto-Bismol, phenothiazine (inconsistent)
E—enteric-coated tablets
S—sodium, potassium, and other elements in tablet form (bismuth, calcium, potassium) and solvents containing chlorides (e.g., carbon tetrachloride)

Toxicologic Studies

Routine blood and urine screening is of little practical value in the initial care of the poisoned patient. Specific toxicologic analyses and quantitative levels of certain drugs may be extremely helpful. One should always ask oneself the following questions: (a) How will the result of the test alter the management? and (b) Can the result of the test be returned in time to have a positive effect on therapy?

Owing to long turnaround time, lack of availability, factors contributing to unreliability, and the risk of serious morbidity without supportive clinical management, toxicology screening is estimated to affect management in less than 15% of cases of drug overdoses or poisonings. Toxicology screening may look specifically for only 40 to 50 drugs out of more than 10,000 possible drugs or toxins and more than several million chemicals. To detect many different drugs, toxic screens usually include methods with broad specificity, and sensitivity may be poor for some drugs, resulting in false-negative or false-positive findings. On the other hand, some drugs present in therapeutic amounts may be detected on the screen, even though they are causing no clinical symptoms. Because many agents are not sought or detected during a toxicologic screening, a negative result does not always rule out poisonings. The specificity of toxicologic tests is dependent on the method and the laboratory. The presence of other drugs, drug metabolites, disease states, or incorrect sampling may cause erroneous results.

For the average toxicologic laboratory, false-negative results occur at a rate of 10% to 30% and false-positives at a rate of 0% to 10%. The positive screen predictive value is approximately 90%. A negative toxicology screen does not exclude a poisoning. The negative predictive value of toxicologic screening is approximately 70%. For example, the following benzodiazepines may not be detected by some routine immunoassay benzodiazepine screening tests: alprazolam (Xanax), clonazepam (Klonopin), temazepam (Restoril), and triazolam (Halcion).

The "toxic urine screen" is generally a qualitative urine test for several common drugs, usually substances of abuse (cocaine and metabolites, opioids, amphetamines, benzodiazepines, barbiturates, and phencyclidine). Results of these tests are usually available within 2 to 6 hours. Because these tests may vary with each hospital and community, the physician should determine exactly which substances are included in the toxic urine screen of his or her laboratory. Tests for ethylene glycol, red blood cell cholinesterase, and serum cyanide are not readily available.

For cases of ingestion of certain substances, quantitative blood levels should be obtained at specific times after the ingestion to avoid spurious low values in the distribution phase, which result from incomplete absorption. The detection time for drugs is influenced by many variables, such as type of substance, formulation, amount, time since ingestion, duration of exposure, and half-life. For many drugs, the detection time is measured in days after the exposure.

Common Poisons

Acetaminophen (Paracetamol, *N*-Acetyl-Paraaminophenol)

Toxic Mechanism

At therapeutic doses of acetaminophen, less than 5% is metabolized by P450-2E1 to a toxic reactive oxidizing metabolite, *N*-acetyl-p-benzoquinoneimine (NAPQI). In a case of overdose, there is insufficient glutathione available to reduce the excess NAPQI into nontoxic conjugate, so it forms covalent bonds with hepatic intracellular proteins to produce centrilobular necrosis. Renal damage is caused by a similar mechanism.

Toxic Dose

The therapeutic dose of acetaminophen is 10 to 15 mg/kg, with a maximum of five doses in 24 hours for a maximum total daily dose of 4 g. An acute single toxic dose is greater than 140 mg/kg, possibly greater than 200 mg/kg in a child younger than age 5 years. Factors affecting the P450 enzymes include enzyme inducers such as barbiturates and phenytoin (Dilantin), ingestion of isoniazid, and alcoholism. Factors that decrease glutathione stores (alcoholism, malnutrition, and HIV infection) contribute to the toxicity of acetaminophen. Alcoholics ingesting 3 to 4 g/d of acetaminophen for a few days can have depleted glutathione stores and require *N*-acetylcysteine therapy at 50% below hepatotoxic blood acetaminophen levels on the nomogram.

Kinetics

Peak plasma concentration is usually reached 2 to 4 hours after an overdose. Volume distribution is 0.9 L/kg, and protein binding is less than 50% (albumin).

Route of elimination is by hepatic metabolism to an inactive nontoxic glucuronide conjugate and inactive nontoxic sulfate metabolite by two saturable pathways; less than 5% is metabolized into reactive metabolite NAPQI. In patients younger than 6 years of age, metabolic elimination occurs to a greater degree by conjugation via the sulfate pathway.

The half-life of acetaminophen is 1 to 3 hours.

Manifestations

The four phases of the intoxication's clinical course may overlap, and the absence of a phase does not exclude toxicity.

- Phase I occurs within 0.5 to 24 hours after ingestion and may consist of a few hours of malaise, diaphoresis, nausea, and vomiting or produce no symptoms. CNS depression or coma is not a feature.
- Phase II occurs 24 to 48 hours after ingestion and is a period of diminished symptoms. The liver enzymes, serum aspartate aminotransferase (AST) (earliest), and serum alanine aminotransferase (ALT) may increase as early as 4 hours or as late as 36 hours after ingestion.
- Phase III occurs at 48 to 96 hours, with peak liver function abnormalities at 72 to 96 hours. The degree of elevation of the hepatic enzymes generally correlates with outcome, but not always. Recovery starts at about 4 days unless hepatic failure develops. Less than 1% of patients with a history of overdose develop fulminant hepatotoxicity.
- Phase IV occurs at 4 to 14 days, with hepatic enzyme abnormalities resolving. If extensive liver damage has occurred, sepsis and disseminated intravascular coagulation may ensue.

Transient renal failure may develop at 5 to 7 days with or without evidence of hepatic damage. Rare cases of myocarditis and pancreatitis have been reported. Death can occur at 7 to 14 days.

Laboratory Investigations

The therapeutic reference range is 10 to 20 μg/mL. For toxic levels, see the nomogram presented in Figure 1.

Appropriate and reliable methods for analysis are radioimmunoassay, high-pressure liquid chromatography, and gas chromatography. Spectroscopic assays often give falsely elevated values: bilirubin, salicylate, salicylamide, diflunisal (Dolobid), phenols, and methyldopa (Aldomet) increase the acetaminophen level. Each 1 mg/dL increase in creatinine increases the acetaminophen plasma level 30 μg/mL.

If a toxic acetaminophen level is reached, liver profile (including AST, ALT, bilirubin, and prothrombin time), serum amylase, and blood glucose must be monitored. A complete blood cell count (CBC); platelet count; phosphate, electrolytes, and bicarbonate level measurements; ECG; and urinalysis are indicated.

Management

Gastrointestinal Decontamination. Although ipecac-induced emesis may be useful within 30 minutes of ingestion of the toxic substance, we do not advise it because it could result in vomiting of the activated charcoal. Gastric lavage is not necessary. Studies have indicated that activated charcoal is useful within 1 hour after ingestion. Activated charcoal does adsorb *N*-acetylcysteine (NAC) if given together, but this is not clinically important. However, if activated charcoal needs to be given along with NAC, separate the administration of activated charcoal from the administration of NAC by 1 to 2 hours to avoid vomiting.

N-Acetylcysteine (Mucomyst). NAC (Table 11), a derivative of the amino acid cysteine, acts as a sulfhydryl donor for glutathione synthesis, as surrogate glutathione, and may increase the nontoxic sulfation pathway resulting in conjugation of NAPQI. Oral NAC should be administered within the first 8 hours after a toxic amount of acetaminophen has been ingested. NAC can be started while one awaits the results of the blood test for acetaminophen plasma concentration, but there is no advantage to giving it before 8 hours. If the acetaminophen concentration result after 4 hours following ingestion is above the upper line on the modified Rumack-Matthew nomogram (see Figure 1), one should continue with a maintenance course. Repeat blood specimens should be obtained 4 hours after the initial level is measured if it is greater than 20 mg/mL, which is below the therapy line, because of unexpected delays in the peak by food and co-ingestants. Intravenous NAC (see Table 11) is approved in the United States.

There have been a few cases of anaphylactoid reaction and death by the intravenous route.

Variations in Therapy

In patients with chronic alcoholism, it is recommended that NAC treatment be administered at 50% below the upper toxic line on the nomogram.

If emesis occurs within 1 hour after NAC administration, the dose should be repeated. To avoid emesis, the proper dilution from 20% to 5% NAC must be used, and it should be served in a palatable vehicle, in a covered container through a straw. If this administration is unsuccessful, a slow drip over 30 to 60 minutes through a nasogastric tube or a fluoroscopically placed nasoduodenal tube can be used. Antiemetics can be used if necessary: metoclopramide (Reglan) 10 mg per dose intravenously 30 minutes before administration of NAC (in children, 0.1 mg/kg; maximum, 0.5 mg/kg/d) or ondansetron (Zofran) 32 mg (0.15 mg/kg) by infusion over 15 minutes and repeated for three doses if necessary. The side effects of these antiemetics include anaphylaxis and increases in liver enzymes.

Some investigators recommend variable durations of NAC therapy, stopping the therapy if serial acetaminophen blood

or she must be admitted
se was intentional, psyc
tient can be discharged.

lockers)
treatment of hypertensi
ithalmologic disorders.
s listed in Table 12.
CNS effects, active met
interactions (e.g., propr
dose. Intrinsic partial a
produce tachycardia a
pressive effect (quinidin
at therapeutic doses (e.g.
g effect is weak (e.g.,)

he catecholamines for
n the bronchi, the vas
n.

twice the maximum
i considered toxic (se
inolol in a child may p
een reported in adults
agent is sotalol, and

lol (Corgard), and sot
lation. The duration
o 6 hours, but in cas
The duration of action
with the longest half-li
with the shortest half
urs.

Table 12.
ts produce coma and
the major cardiac sy
intrinsic partial agoni
ertension. ECG chang
y or asystole. Memb
QRS and QT inter
Sotalol produces a
may occur in patier
blocker because the
ations include hypog
mine counter-regulatd

vels are not readily
iitoring should be
olytes, BUN, and
well as ABG if there

Disposition

Symptomatic patients should be observed on a monitored unit until the symptoms resolve and then observed for a short time after resolution for relapse.

Anticholinergic Agents

Drugs with anticholinergic properties include antihistamines (H_1 blockers), neuroleptics (phenothiazines), tricyclic antidepressants, antiparkinsonism drugs (trihexyphenidyl [Artane], benztropine [Cogentin]), ophthalmic products (atropine), and a number of common plants.

The antihistamines are divided into the sedating anticholinergic types and the nonsedating single daily dose types. The sedating types include ethanolamines (e.g., diphenhydramine [Benadryl], dimenhydrinate [Dramamine], and clemastine [Tavist]), ethylenediamines (e.g., tripelennamine [Pyribenzamine]), alkyl amines (e.g., chlorpheniramine [Chlor-Trimeton], brompheniramine [Dimetane]), piperazines (e.g., cyclizine [Marezine], hydroxyzine [Atarax], and meclizine [Antivert]), and phenothiazine (e.g., Phenergan). The nonsedating types include astemizole (Hismanal), terfenadine (Seldane), loratadine (Claritin), fexofenadine (Allegra), and cetirizine (Zyrtec).

The anticholinergic plants include jimsonweed (*Datura stramonium*), deadly nightshade (*Atropa belladonna*), henbane (*Hyoscyamus niger*), and antispasmodic agents for the bowel (atropine derivatives).

Toxic Mechanism

By competitive inhibition, anticholinergics block the action of acetylcholine on postsynaptic cholinergic receptor sites. The toxic mechanism primarily involves the peripheral and CNS muscarinic receptors. H_1 sedating-type agents also depress or stimulate the CNS, and in large overdoses some have cardiac membrane–depressant effects (e.g., diphenhydramine [Benadryl]) and α-adrenergic receptor blockade effects (e.g., promethazine [Phenergan]). Nonsedating agents produce peripheral H_1 blockade but do not possess anticholinergic or sedating actions. The original agents terfenadine (Seldane) and astemizole (Hismanal) were recently removed from the market because of the severe cardiac dysrhythmias associated with their use, especially when used in combination with macrolide antibiotics and certain antifungal agents such as ketoconazole (Nizoral), which inhibit hepatic metabolism or excretion. The newer nonsedating agents, including loratadine (Claritin), fexofenadine (Allegra), and cetirizine (Zyrtec), have not been reported to cause the severe drug interactions associated with terfenadine and astemizole.

Toxic Dose

The estimated toxic oral dose of atropine is 0.05 mg/kg in children and more than 2 mg in adults. The minimal estimated lethal dose of atropine is more than 10 mg in adults and more than 2 mg in children. Other synthetic anticholinergic agents are less toxic, and the fatal dose varies from 10 to 100 mg.

The estimated toxic oral dose of diphenhydramine (Benadryl) in a child is 15 mg/kg, and the potential lethal amount is 25 mg/kg. In an adult, the potential lethal amount is 2.8 g. Ingestion of five times the single dose of an antihistamine is toxic.

For the nonsedating agents, an overdose of 3360 mg of terfenadine was reported in an adult who developed ventricular tachycardia and fibrillation that responded to lidocaine and defibrillation. A 1500-mg overdose produced hypotension. Cases of delayed serious dysrhythmias (torsades de pointes) have been reported with doses of more than 200 mg of astemizole. The toxic doses of fexofenadine (Allegra), cetirizine, and loratadine (Claritin) need to be established.

Kinetics

The onset of absorption of intravenous atropine is in 2 to 4 minutes. Peak effects on salivation after intravenous or intramuscular administration are at 30 to 60 minutes.

Onset of absorption after oral ingestion is 30 to 60 minutes, peak action is 1 to 3 hours, and duration of action is 4 to 6 hours, but symptoms are prolonged in cases of overdose or with sustained-release preparations.

The onset of absorption of diphenhydramine is in 15 minutes to 1 hour, with a peak of action in 1 to 4 hours. Volume distribution is 3.3 to 6.8 L/kg, and protein binding is 75% to 80%. Ninety-eight percent of diphenhydramine is metabolized via the liver by N-demethylation. Interactions with erythromycin, ketoconazole (Nizoral), and derivatives produce excessive blood levels of the antihistamine and ventricular dysrhythmias.

The half-life of diphenhydramine is 3 to 10 hours.

The chemical structure of nonsedating agents prevents their entry into the CNS. Absorption begins in 1 hour, with peak effects in 4 to 6 hours. The duration of action is greater than 24 hours.

These agents are metabolized in the gastrointestinal tract and liver. Protein binding is greater than 90%. The plasma half-life is 3.5 hours. Only 1% is excreted unchanged; 60% of that is excreted in the feces and 40% in the urine.

Manifestations

Anticholinergic signs are hyperpyrexia ("hot as a hare"), mydriasis ("blind as a bat"), flushing of skin ("red as a beet"), dry mucosa and skin ("dry as a bone"), "Lilliputian type" hallucinations and delirium ("mad as a hatter"), coma, dysphagia, tachycardia, moderate hypertension, and rarely convulsions and urinary retention. Other effects include jaundice (cyproheptadine [Periactin]), dystonia (diphenhydramine [Benadryl]), rhabdomyolysis (doxylamine), and, in large doses, cardiotoxic effects (diphenhydramine).

Overdose with nonsedating agents produces headache and confusion, nausea, and dysrhythmias (e.g., torsades de pointes).

Laboratory Investigations

Monitoring of ABG (in cases of respiratory depression), electrolytes, glucose, and the ECG should be undertaken. Anticholinergic drugs and plants are not routinely included on screens for substances of abuse.

Management

For patients in respiratory failure, intubation and assisted ventilation should be instituted. Gastrointestinal decontamination can be instituted. Caution must be taken with emesis in cases of diphenhydramine (Benadryl) overdose because of the drug's rapid onset of action and risk of seizures. If bowel sounds are present for up to 1 hour after ingestion, activated charcoal can be given. Seizures can be controlled with benzodiazepines (diazepam [Valium] or lorazepam [Ativan]).

The administration of physostigmine (Antilirium) is not routine and is reserved for life-threatening anticholinergic effects that are refractory to conventional treatments. It should be administered with adequate monitoring and resuscitative equipment available. The use of physostigmine should be avoided if a tricyclic antidepressant is present because of increased toxicity. Urinary retention should be relieved by catheterization to avoid reabsorption of the drug and additional toxicity.

Supraventricular tachycardia should be treated only if the patient is hemodynamically unstable. Ventricular dysrhythmias can be controlled with lidocaine or cardioversion. Sodium bicarbonate 1 to 2 mEq/kg IV may be useful for myocardial depression and QRS prolongation. Torsades de pointes, especially when associated with terfenadine and astemizole ingestion, has been treated with magnesium sulfate 4 g or 40 mL 10% solution intravenously over 10 to 20 minutes and countershock if the patient fails to respond.

Hyperpyrexia is controlled by external cooling. Hemodialysis and hemoperfusion are not effective.

Disposition

Antihistamine H_1 Antagonists. Symptomatic patients should be observed on a monitored unit until the symptoms resolve, then

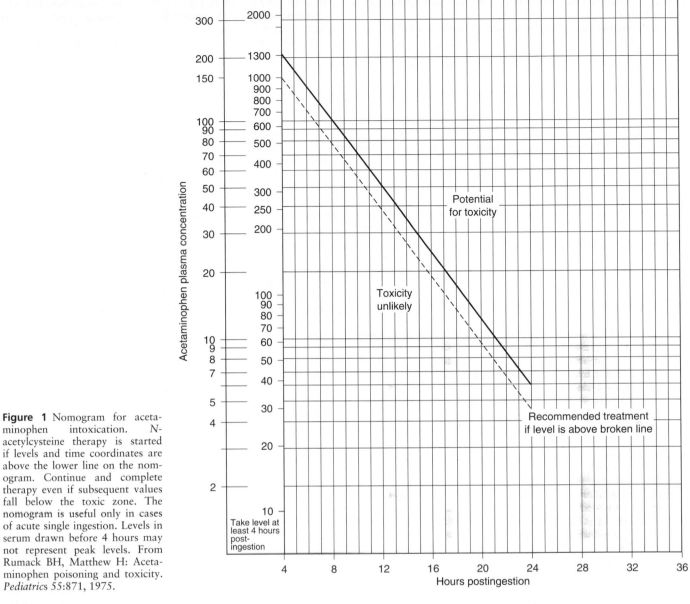

Figure 1 Nomogram for acetaminophen intoxication. N-acetylcysteine therapy is started if levels and time coordinates are above the lower line on the nomogram. Continue and complete therapy even if subsequent values fall below the toxic zone. The nomogram is useful only in cases of acute single ingestion. Levels in serum drawn before 4 hours may not represent peak levels. From Rumack BH, Matthew H: Acetaminophen poisoning and toxicity. *Pediatrics* 55:871, 1975.

		Potential for toxicity
	Toxicity unlikely	
		Recommended treatment if level is above broken line

Take level at least 4 hours postingestion

TABLE 11   Protocol for N-Acetylcysteine Administration

ROUTE	LOADING DOSE	MAINTENANCE DOSE	COURSE	FDA APPROVAL
Oral	140 mg/kg	70 mg/kg every 4 h	72 h	Yes
Intravenous	150 mg/kg over 15 min	50 mg/kg over 4 h followed by 100 mg/kg over 16 h	20 h	Yes

concentrations become nondetectable and the liver enzyme levels (ALT and AST) remain normal after 24 to 36 hours.

There is a loss of efficacy if NAC is initiated 8 or 10 hours postingestion, but the loss is not complete, and NAC may be initiated 36 hours or more after ingestion. Late treatment (after 24 hours) decreases the rates of morbidity and mortality in patients with fulminant liver failure caused by acetaminophen and other agents.

Extended relief formulations (*ER* embossed on caplet) contain 325 mg of acetaminophen for immediate release and 325 mg for delayed release. A single 4-hour postingestion serum acetaminophen concentration can underestimate the level because ER formulations can have secondary delayed peaks. In cases of overdose of the ER formulation, it is recommended that additional acetaminophen levels be obtained at 4-hour intervals after the initial

level is measured. If any level is in the toxic zone, therapy should be initiated.

It is recommended that pregnant patients with toxic plasma concentrations of acetaminophen be treated with NAC to prevent hepatotoxicity in both fetus and mother. The available data suggest no teratogenicity to NAC or acetaminophen.

Indications for NAC therapy in cases of chronic intoxication are a history of ingestion of 3 to 4 g for several days with elevated liver enzyme levels (AST and ALT). The acetaminophen blood concentration is often low in these cases because of the extended time lapse since ingestion and should not be plotted on the Rumack-Matthew nomogram. Patients with a history of chronic alcoholism or those on chronic enzyme inducers may also present with elevated liver enzyme levels and should be considered for NAC therapy if they have a history of taking acetaminophen on a chronic basis, because they are considered to be at a greater risk for hepatotoxicity despite a low acetaminophen blood concentration.

Specific support care may be needed to treat liver failure, pancreatitis, transient renal failure, and myocarditis.

Liver transplantation has a definite but limited role in patients with acute acetaminophen overdose. A retrospective analysis determined that a continuing rise in the prothrombin time (4-day peak, 180 seconds), a pH of less than 7.3 2 days after the overdose, a serum creatinine level of greater than 3.3 mg/dL, severe hepatic encephalopathy, and disturbed coagulation factor VII/V ratio greater than 30 suggest a poor prognosis and may be indicators for hepatology consultation for consideration of liver transplantation.

Extracorporeal measures are not expected to be of benefit.

Disposition

Adults who have ingested more than 140 mg/kg and children younger than 6 years of age who have ingested more than 200 mg/kg should receive therapy within 8 hours postingestion or until the results of the 4-hour postingestion acetaminophen plasma concentration are known.

Amphetamines

The amphetamines include illicit methamphetamine ("Ice"), diet pills, and formulations under various trade names. Analogues include MDMA (3,4 methylenedioxymethamphetamine, known as "ecstasy," "XTC," or "Adam") and MDA (3,4-methylenedioxyamphetamine, known as "Eve"). MDA is a common hallucinogen and euphoriant "club drug" used at "raves," which are all-night dances. Use of methamphetamine and designer analogues is on the rise, especially among young people between the ages of 12 and 25 years. Other similar stimulants are phenylpropanolamine and cocaine.

Toxic Mechanism

Amphetamines have a direct CNS stimulant effect and a sympathetic nervous system effect by releasing catecholamines from α- and β-adrenergic nerve terminals but inhibiting their reuptake.

Hallucinogenic MDMA has an additional hazard of serotonin effect (refer to serotonin syndrome in the SSRI section). MDMA also affects the dopamine system in the brain. Because of its effects on 5-hydroxytryptamine, dopamine, and norepinephrine, MDMA can lead to serotonin syndrome associated with malignant hyperthermia and rhabdomyolysis, which contributes to the potentially life-threatening hyperthermia observed in several patients who have used MDMA.

Phenylpropanolamine stimulates only the β-adrenergic receptors.

Toxic Dose

In children, the toxic dose of dextroamphetamine is 1 mg/kg; in adults, the toxic dose is 5 mg/kg. The potentially fatal dose of dextroamphetamine is 12 mg/kg.

Kinetics

Amphetamine is a weak base with pKa of 8 to 10. Onset of action is 30 to 60 minutes, and peak effects are 2 to 4 hours. The volume distribution is 2 to 3 L/kg.

Through hepatic metabolism, 60% of the substance is metabolized into a hydroxylated metabolite that may be responsible for psychotic effects.

The half-life of amphetamines is pH dependent—8 to 10 hours in acid urine (pH <6.0) and 16 to 31 hours in alkaline urine (pH >7.5). Excretion is by the kidney—30% to 40% at alkaline urine pH and 50% to 70% at acid urine pH.

Manifestations

Effects are seen within 30 to 60 minutes following ingestion.

Neurologic manifestations include restlessness, irritation and agitation, tremors and hyperreflexia, and auditory and visual hallucinations. Hyperpyrexia may precede seizures, convulsions, paranoia, violence, intracranial hemorrhage, psychosis, and self-destructive behavior. Paranoid psychosis and cerebral vasculitis occur with chronic abuse.

MDMA is often adulterated with cocaine, heroin, or ketamine, or a combination of these, to create a variety of mood alterations. This possibility must be taken into consideration when one manages patients with MDMA ingestions, as the symptom complex may reflect both CNS stimulation and CNS depression.

Other manifestations include dilated but reactive pupils, cardiac dysrhythmias (supraventricular and ventricular), tachycardia, hypertension, rhabdomyolysis, and myoglobinuria.

Laboratory Investigations

The clinician should monitor ECG and cardiac readings, ABG and oxygen saturation, electrolytes, blood glucose, BUN, creatinine, creatine kinase, cardiac fraction if there is chest pain, and liver profile. Also, one should evaluate for rhabdomyolysis and check urine for myoglobin, cocaine and metabolites, and other substances of abuse. The peak plasma concentration of amphetamines is 10 to 50 ng/mL 1 to 2 hours after ingestion of 10 to 25 mg. The toxic plasma concentration is 200 ng/mL. When the rapid immunoassays are used, cross-reactions can occur with amphetamine derivatives (e.g., MDA, "ecstasy"), brompheniramine (Dimetane), chlorpromazine (Thorazine), ephedrine, phenylpropanolamine, phentermine (Adipex-P), phenmetrazine, ranitidine (Zantac), and Vicks Inhaler (L-desoxyephedrine). False-positive results may occur.

Management

Management is similar to management for cocaine intoxication. Supportive care includes blood pressure and temperature control, cardiac monitoring, and seizure precautions. Diazepam (Valium) can be administered. Gastrointestinal decontamination can be undertaken with activated charcoal administered up to 1 hour after ingestion.

Anxiety, agitation, and convulsions are treated with diazepam. If diazepam fails to control seizures, neuromuscular blockers can be used and the electroencephalogram (EEG) monitored for nonmotor seizures. One should avoid neuroleptic phenothiazines and butyrophenone, which can lower the seizure threshold.

Hypertension and tachycardia are usually transient and can be managed by titration of diazepam. Nitroprusside can be used for hypertensive crisis at a maximum infusion rate of 10 μg/kg/min for 10 minutes followed with a lower infusion rate of 0.3 to 2 mg/kg/min. Myocardial ischemia is managed by oxygen, vascular access, benzodiazepines, and nitroglycerin. Aspirin and thrombolytics are not routinely recommended because of the danger of intracranial hemorrhage. It is important to distinguish between angina and true ischemia. Delayed hypotension can be treated with fluids and vasopressors if needed. Life-threatening tachydysrhythmias may respond to an α-blocker such as phentolamine (Regitine) 5 mg IV for adults or 0.1 mg/kg IV for children and a short-acting β-blocker such as esmolol (Brevibloc) 500 μg/kg IV over 1 minute for adults, or 300 to 500 μg/kg over 1 minute for children. Ventricular dysrhythmias may respond to lidocaine or, in a severely hemodynamically compromised patient, immediate synchronized electrical cardioversion.

Rhabdomyolysis and myoglobinuria are treated with fluids, alkaline diuresis, and alkaline urine. Hyperthermia is treated with external cooling and cool 100% humidified oxygen. More extensive therapy may be needed in severe cases. If focal neurologic symptoms are present, the possibility of a cerebrovascular accident should be considered and a CT scan of the head should be obtained.

Paranoid ideation and threatening behavior should be treated with rapid tranquilization using a benzodiazepine. One should observe for suicidal depression that may follow intoxication and may require suicide precautions.

Extracorporeal measures are of no benefit.

observed for a short time (3 to 4 hours) after resolution for relapse.

Nonsedating Agents. All asymptomatic children who acutely ingest more than the maximum adult dose and all symptomatic children should be referred to a health care facility for a minimum of 6 hours' observation as well as cardiac monitoring. Asymptomatic adults who acutely ingest more than twice the maximum adult daily dose should be monitored for a minimum of 6 hours. All symptomatic patients should be monitored for as long as there are symptoms present.

Barbiturates

Barbiturates have been used as sedatives, anesthetic agents, and anticonvulsants, but their use is declining as safer, more effective drugs become available.

Toxic Mechanism

Barbiturates are γ-aminobutyric acid (GABA) agonists (increasing the chloride flow and inhibiting depolarization). They enhance the CNS depressant effect of GABA and depress the cardiovascular system.

Toxic Dose

The shorter-acting barbiturates (including the intermediate-acting agents) and their hypnotic doses are as follows: amobarbital (Amytal), 100 to 200 mg; aprobarbital (Alurate), 50 to 100 mg; butabarbital (Butisol), 50 to 100 mg; butalbital, 100 to 200 mg; pentobarbital (Nembutal), 100 to 200 mg; secobarbital (Seconal), 100 to 200 mg. They cause toxicity at lower doses than long-acting barbiturates and have a minimum toxic dose of 6 mg/kg; the fatal adult dose is 3 to 6 g.

The long-acting barbiturates and their doses include mephobarbital (Mebaral), 50 to 100 mg, and phenobarbital, 100 to 200 mg. Their minimum toxic dose is greater than 10 mg/kg, and the fatal adult dose is 6 to 10 g. A general rule is that an amount five times the hypnotic dose is toxic and an amount 10 times the hypnotic dose is potentially fatal. Methohexital and thiopental are ultrashort-acting parenteral preparations and are not discussed.

Kinetics

The barbiturates are enzyme inducers. Short-acting barbiturates are highly lipid-soluble, penetrate the brain readily, and have shorter elimination times. Onset of action is in 10 to 30 minutes, with a peak at 1 to 2 hours. Duration of action is 3 to 8 hours. The volume distribution of short-acting barbiturate is 0.8 to 1.5 L/kg; pKa is about 8. Mean half-life varies from 8 to 48 hours.

Long-acting agents have longer elimination times and can be used as anticonvulsants. Onset of action is in 20 to 60 minutes, with a peak at 1 to 6 hours. In cases of overdose, the peak can be at 10 hours. Usual duration of action is 8 to 12 hours. Volume distribution is 0.8 L/kg, and half-life is 11 to 120 hours. The pKa of phenobarbital is 7.2. Alkalinization of urine promotes its excretion.

Manifestations

Mild intoxication resembles alcohol intoxication and includes ataxia, slurred speech, and depressed cognition. Severe intoxication causes slow respirations, coma, and loss of reflexes (except pupillary light reflex).

Other manifestations include hypotension (vasodilation), hypothermia, hypoglycemia, and death by respiratory arrest.

Laboratory Investigations

Most barbiturates are detected on routine drug screens and can be measured in most hospital laboratories. Investigation should include barbiturate level; ABG; toxicology screen, including acetaminophen; glucose, electrolyte, BUN, creatinine, and creatine kinase levels; and urine pH. The minimum toxic plasma levels are greater than 10 μg/mL for short-acting barbiturates and greater than 40 μg/dL for long-acting agents. Fatal levels are 30 μg/mL for short-acting barbiturates and 80 to 150 μg/mL for long-acting

agents. Both short-acting and long-acting age[...] in urine 24 to 72 hours after ingestion, and lo[...] be detected up to 7 days.

Management

Vital functions must be established and mainta[...] portive care including intubation and assisted[...] dominate the management. All stuporous an[...] should have glucose (for hypoglycemia), thia[...] alcoholic), and naloxone (Narcan) (in case [...] tion) intravenously and should be admitted t[...] unit. Emesis should be avoided especially in c[...] the shorter-acting barbiturates. Activated c[...] MDAC (0.5 g/kg) every 2 to 4 hours has been [...] serum half-life of phenobarbital by 50%, but [...] course is undetermined.

Fluids should be administered to corre[...] hypotension. Vasopressors may be necessar[...] hypotension, and hemodynamic monitoring [...] patient must be observed carefully for fluid [...] zation (ion trapping) is used only for phen[...] but not for short-acting barbiturates. Sodiu[...] 2 mEq/L IV in 500 mL of 5% dextrose in ad[...] kg in children during the first hour, followed [...] bonate to keep the urinary pH at 7.5 to 8.0, en[...] phenobarbital and shortens the half-life by 5[...] advocated because of the danger of cerebral o[...]

Hemodialysis shortens the half-life to 8 to [...] coal hemoperfusion shortens the half-life to 6 [...] acting barbiturates such as phenobarbital. Be[...] be effective in patients with both long-actin[...] barbiturate ingestion. If the patient does n[...] portive measures or if the phenobarbital plas[...] greater than 150 μg/mL, both procedures may [...] the half-life.

Bullae are treated as a local second-degre[...] thermia should be treated.

Disposition

All comatose patients should be admitted to[...] unit. Awake and oriented patients with an [...] acting agents should be observed for at lea[...] hours; overdose of long-acting agents warran[...] least 12 asymptomatic hours because of the p[...] absorption. In the case of an intentional ov[...] clearance is needed before the patient can be [...] use can lead to tolerance, physical dependen[...] and necessitates follow-up.

Benzodiazepines

Benzodiazepines are used as anxiolytics, seda[...]

Toxic Mechanism

The GABA agonists produce CNS depressio[...] ride flow, inhibiting depolarization.

Flunitrazepam (Rohypnol; street name "[...] acting benzodiazepine agonist sold by prescri[...] 60 countries worldwide, but it is not lega[...] United States.

Toxic Dose

The long-acting benzodiazepines (half-life >[...] maximum therapeutic doses are as follow[...] (Librium), 50 mg; clorazepate (Tranxene), [...] (Klonopin), 20 mg; diazepam (Valium), 10 m[...] kg in children; flurazepam (Dalmane), 30 [...] 20 mg.

The short-acting benzodiazepines (half-life [...] their doses include the following: alprazola[...] and lorazepam (Ativan), 4 mg in adults or 0.0[...] which act similar to the long-acting benzodia[...]

TABLE 14 Routes and Kinetics o[...]

TYPE	ROUTE
Cocaine leaf	Oral, chewing
Hydrochloride	Insufflation
	Ingestion
	Intravenous
Freebase/crack	Smoking
Coca paste	Smoking

it blocks the presynaptic reuptake [...] blocks the sodium channels along [...] increases platelet aggregation. Long[...] of dopamine.

Toxic Dose

The maximum mucosal local ane[...] cocaine is 200 mg or 2 mL of a 10[...] effects can occur at relatively low l[...] 95 mg), they are more common wi[...] kg; cardiac effects can occur with [...] The potential fatal dose is 1200 m[...] occurred with 20 mg parenterally.

Kinetics

Cocaine is well absorbed by all rou[...] tion, and oral, dermal, and inhalatio[...] binding is 8.7%, and volume distrib[...]

Cocaine is metabolized by plasma [...] the inactive metabolites ecgonine [...] gonine. Plasma pseudocholinesteras[...] 3% of the population and decrease[...] the elderly, pregnant people, and [...] These enzyme-deficient individuals [...] threatening cocaine toxicity.

Ten percent of cocaine is excrete[...] ethanol undergo liver synthesis to fo[...] lite with a half-life three times longe[...] account for some of cocaine's cardi[...] more lethal than cocaine or ethanol [...]

Manifestations

The CNS manifestations of cocaine i[...] activity, agitation, convulsions, an[...] Mydriasis and septal perforation ca[...] dysrhythmias, hypertension, and hy[...] dose). Chest pain is frequent, but onl[...] myocardial ischemia and infarction. C[...] vasoconstriction, hyperthermia (bec[...] rate), ischemic bowel perforation i[...] rhabdomyolysis, myoglobinuria, and [...] users, premature labor and abruptio[...]

Body cavity packing should be sus[...] toxicity.

Mortality can result from cerebrov[...] artery spasm, myocardial injury, or l[...]

Laboratory Investigations

Monitoring of the ECG and cardiac [...] ration, electrolytes, blood glucose, B[...] kinase levels should be maintained. [...] fraction if the patient has chest pain[...] and the urine for myoglobin. Intrave[...] HIV and hepatitis virus testing.

Urine should be tested for coc[...] other substances of abuse, and [...]

to control seizures will reduce temperature. Dantrolene and anti-pyretics are not recommended. Rhabdomyolysis and myoglobin-uria are treated with fluids, alkaline diuresis, and diuretics.

If the patient is pregnant, the fetus must be monitored and the patient observed for spontaneous abortion.

Paranoid ideation and threatening behavior should be treated with rapid tranquilization. The patient should be observed for suicidal depression that may follow intoxication and may require suicide precautions. If focal neurologic manifestations are present, one should consider the possibility of a cerebrovascular accident and obtain a CT scan.

Extracorporeal clearance techniques are of no benefit.

Disposition

Patients with mild intoxication or a brief seizure that does not require treatment who become asymptomatic may be discharged after 6 hours with appropriate psychosocial follow-up. If cardiac or cerebral ischemic manifestations are present, the patient should be monitored in the intensive care unit. Body packers and stuffers require care in the intensive care unit until passage of the contraband.

Cyanide

Hydrogen cyanide is a byproduct of burning plastic and wools in residential fires. Hydrocyanic acid is the liquefied form of hydrogen cyanide. Cyanide salts can be found in ore extraction. Nitriles, such as acetonitrile (artificial nail removers), are metabolized in the body to produce cyanide. Cyanogenic glycosides are present in some fruit seeds (such as amygdalin in apricots, peaches, and apples). Sodium nitroprusside, the antihypertensive vasodilator, contains five cyanide groups.

Toxic Mechanism

Cyanide blocks the cellular electron transport mechanism and cellular respiration by inhibiting the mitochondrial ferricyto-chrome oxidase system and other enzymes. This results in cellular hypoxia and lactic acidosis. *Note:* Citrus fruit seeds form cyanide in the presence of intestinal β-glucosidase (the seeds are harmful only if the capsule is broken).

Toxic Dose

The ingestion of 1 mg/kg or 50 mg of hydrogen cyanide can produce death within 15 minutes. The lethal dose of potassium cyanide is 200 mg. Five to 10 mL of 84% acetonitrile is lethal. Infusions of sodium nitroprusside in rates above 2 μg/kg per minute may cause cyanide to accumulate to toxic concentrations in critically ill patients.

Kinetics

Cyanide is rapidly absorbed by all routes. In the stomach, it forms hydrocyanic acid. Volume distribution is 1.5 L/kg. Protein binding is 60%. Cyanide is detoxified by metabolism in the liver via the mitochondrial thiosulfate-rhodanase pathway, which catalyzes the transfer of sulfur donor to cyanide, forming the less toxic irreversible thiocyanate that is excreted in the urine. Cyanide is also detoxified by reacting with hydroxocobalamin (vitamin B_{12a}) to form cyanocobalamin (vitamin B_{12}).

The cyanide elimination half-life from the blood is 1.2 hours. The elimination route is through the lungs.

Manifestations

Hydrogen cyanide has the distinctive odor of bitter almonds or silver polish. Manifestations of cyanide intoxication include hypertension, cardiac dysrhythmias, various ECG abnormalities, headache, hyperpnea, seizures, stupor, pulmonary edema, and flushing. Cyanosis is absent or appears late.

Laboratory Investigations

The examiner should obtain and monitor ABGs, oxygen saturation, blood lactate, hemoglobin, blood glucose, and electrolytes. Lactic acidemia, a decrease in the arterial-venous oxygen difference, and bright red venous blood occurs. If smoke inhalation is the possible source of cyanide exposure, CoHB and methemoglobin (MetHb) concentrations should be measured.

Cyanide levels in whole blood, red blood cells, or serum are not useful in the acute management because the determinations are not readily available. Specific cyanide blood levels are as follows: smokers have less than 0.5 μg/mL; a patient with flushing and tachycardia has 0.5 to 1.0 μg/mL, one with obtundation has 1.0 to 2.5 μg/mL, and one in coma or who has died has more than 2.5 μg/mL.

Management

If the cyanide was inhaled, the patient must be removed from the contaminated atmosphere. Attendants should not administer mouth-to-mouth resuscitation. Rescuers and attendants must be protected. Immediate administration of 100% oxygen is called for and oxygen should be continued during and after the administration of the antidote. The clinician must decide whether to use any or all components of the cyanide antidote kit.

The mechanism of action of the antidote kit is twofold: to produce methemoglobinemia and to provide a sulfur substrate for the detoxification of cyanide. The nitrites make methemoglobin, which has a greater affinity for cyanide than does the cytochrome oxidase enzymes. The combination of methemoglobin and cyanide forms cyanomethemoglobin. Sodium thiosulfate provides a sulfur substrate for the rhodanese enzyme, which converts cyanide into the relatively nontoxic sodium thiocyanate, which is excreted by the kidney.

The procedure for using the antidote kit is as follows:

Step 1: Amyl nitrite inhalant perles is only a temporizing measure (forms only 2% to 5% methemoglobin) and it can be omitted if venous access is established. Alternate 100% oxygen and the inhalant for 30 seconds each minute. Use a new perle every 3 minutes.

Step 2: Sodium nitrite ampule is indicated for cyanide exposures, except for cases of residential fires, smoke inhalation, and nitroprusside or acetonitrile poisonings. It is administered intravenously to produce methemoglobin of 20% to 30% at 35 to 70 minutes after administration. A dose of 10 mL of 3% solution of sodium nitrite for adults and 0.33 mL/kg of 3% solution for children is diluted to 100 mL 0.9% saline and administered slowly intravenously at 5 mL/min. If hypotension develops, the infusion should be slowed.

Step 3: Sodium thiosulfate is useful alone in cases of smoke inhalation, nitroprusside toxicity, and acetonitrile toxicity and should not be used at all in cases of hydrogen sulfide poisoning. The administration dose is 12.5 g of sodium thiosulfate or 50 mL of 25% solution for adults and 1.65 mL/kg of 25% solution for children intravenously over 10 to 20 minutes.

If cyanide symptoms recur, further treatment with nitrites or the perles is controversial. Some authorities suggest repeating the antidotes in 30 minutes at half of the initial dose, but others do not advise this for lack of efficacy. The child dosage regimen on the package insert must be carefully followed.

One hour after antidotes are administered, the methemoglobin level should be obtained and should not exceed 20%. Methylene blue should not be used to reverse excessive methemoglobin.

Gastrointestinal decontamination of oral ingestion by activated charcoal is recommended but is not very effective because of the rapidity of absorption. Seizures are treated with intravenous diazepam. Acidosis should be treated with sodium bicarbonate if it does not rapidly resolve with therapy. There is no role for hyperbaric oxygen or hemodialysis or hemoperfusion.

Other antidotes include hydroxocobalamin (vitamin B_{12a}) (Cyanokit), which has proven effective when given immediately after exposure in large doses of 4 g (50 mg/kg) or 50 times the amount of cyanide exposure with 8 g of sodium thiosulfate. Hydroxocobalamin has FDA orphan drug approval.

Disposition

Asymptomatic patients should be observed for a minimum of 3 hours. Patients who ingest nitrile compounds must be observed

Patients with acute poisoning may be asymptomatic, with an early high serum lithium concentration of 9 mEq/L, and deteriorate as the serum lithium concentration falls by 50% and the lithium distributes to the brain and the other tissues. Nausea and vomiting may occur within 1 to 4 hours, but the systemic manifestations are usually delayed several more hours. It may take as long as 3 to 5 days for serious symptoms to develop. Acute toxicity and acute on chronic toxicity are manifested by neurologic findings, including weakness, fasciculations, altered mental state, myoclonus, hyperreflexia, rigidity, coma, and convulsions with limbs in hypertension. Cardiovascular effects are nonspecific and occur at therapeutic doses, flat T or inverted T waves, atrioventricular block, and prolonged QT interval. Lithium is not a primary cardiotoxin. Cardiogenic shock occurs secondary to CNS toxicity. Chronic intoxication is associated with manifestations at lower serum lithium concentrations. There is some correlation with manifestations, especially at higher serum lithium concentrations. Although the levels do not always correlate with the manifestations, they are more predictive in cases of severe intoxication. A serum lithium concentration greater than 3.0 mEq/L with chronic intoxication and altered mental state indicates severe toxicity. Permanent neurologic sequelae can result from lithium intoxication.

Laboratory Investigations
Monitoring should include CBC (lithium causes significant leukocytosis), renal function, thyroid function (chronic intoxication), ECG, and electrolytes. Serum lithium concentrations should be determined every 2 to 4 hours until levels are close to therapeutic range. Cross-reactions with green-top Vacutainer specimen tubes containing heparin will spuriously elevate serum lithium concentration 6 to 8 mEq/L.

Management
Vital function must be established and maintained. Seizure precautions should be instituted and seizures, hypotension, and dysrhythmias treated. Evaluation should include examination for rigidity and hyperreflexia signs, hydration, renal function (BUN, creatinine), and electrolytes, especially sodium. The examiner should inquire about diuretic and other drug use that increase serum lithium concentration, and the patient must discontinue the drugs. If the patient is on chronic therapy, the lithium should be discontinued. Serial serum lithium concentrations should be obtained every 4 hours until serum lithium concentration peaks and there is a downward trend toward almost therapeutic range, especially in sustained-release preparations. Vital signs should be monitored, including temperature, and ECG and serial neurologic examinations should be undertaken, including mental status and urinary output. Nephrology consultation is warranted in case of a chronic and elevated serum lithium concentration (>2.5 mEq/L), a large ingestion, or altered mental state.

An intravenous line should be established and hydration and electrolyte balance restored. Serum sodium level should be determined before 0.9% saline fluid is administered in patients with chronic overdose because hypernatremia may be present from diabetes insipidus. Although current evidence supports an initial 0.9% saline infusion (200 mL/h) to enhance excretion of lithium, once hydration, urine output, and normonatremia are established, one should administer 0.45% saline and slow the infusion (100 mL/h) for all patients.

Gastric lavage is often not recommended in cases of acute ingestion because of the large size of the tablets, and it is not necessary after chronic intoxication. Activated charcoal is ineffective. For sustained-release preparations, whole-bowel irrigation may be useful but is not proven. Sodium polystyrene sulfonate (Kayexalate), an ion exchange resin, is difficult to administer and has been used only in uncontrolled studies. Its use is not recommended.

Hemodialysis is the most efficient method for removing lithium from the vascular compartment. It is the treatment of choice for patients with severe intoxication with an altered mental state, those with seizures, and anuric patients. Long runs are used until the serum lithium concentration is less than 1 mEq/L because of extensive re-equilibration. Serum lithium concentration should be monitored every 4 hours after dialysis for rebound. Repeated and prolonged hemodialysis may be necessary. A lag in neurologic recovery can be expected.

Disposition
An acute asymptomatic lithium overdose cannot be medically cleared on the basis of single lithium level. Patients should be admitted if they have any neurologic manifestations (altered mental status, hyperreflexia, stiffness, or tremor). Patients should be admitted to the intensive care unit if they are dehydrated, have renal impairment, or have a high or rising lithium level.

Methanol (Wood Alcohol, Methyl Alcohol)
The concentration of methanol in Sterno fuel is 4% and it contains ethanol, in windshield washer fluid it is 30% to 60%, and in gas-line antifreeze it is 100%.

Toxic Mechanism
Methanol is metabolized by alcohol dehydrogenase to formaldehyde, which is metabolized to formate. Formate inhibits cytochrome oxidase, producing tissue hypoxia, lactic acidosis, and optic nerve edema. Formate is converted by folate-dependent enzymes to carbon dioxide.

Toxic Dose
The minimal toxic amount is approximately 100 mg/kg. Serious toxicity in a young child can be produced by the ingestion of 2.5 to 5.0 mL of 100% methanol. Ingestion of 5-mL 100% methanol by a 10-kg child produces estimated peak blood methanol of 80 mg/dL. Ingestion of 15 mL 40% methanol was lethal for a 2-year-old child in one report. A fatal adult oral dose is 30 to 240 mL 100% (20 to 150 g). Ingestion of 6 to 10 mL 100% causes blindness in adults. The toxic blood concentration is greater than 20 mg/dL; very serious toxicity and potential fatality occur at levels greater than 50 mg/dL.

Kinetics
Onset of action can start within 1 hour but may be delayed up to 12 to 18 hours by metabolism to toxic metabolites. It may be delayed longer if ethanol is ingested concomitantly or in infants. Peak blood methanol concentration is 1 hour. Volume distribution is 0.6 L/kg (total body water).

For metabolism, see *Toxic Mechanism*.

Elimination is through metabolism. The half-life of methanol is 8 hours; with ethanol blocking it is 30 to 35 hours; and with hemodialysis 2.5 hours.

Manifestations
Metabolism creates a delay in onset for 12 to 18 hours or longer if ethanol is ingested concomitantly. Initial findings are as follows:
- 0 to 6 hours: Confusion, ataxia, inebriation, formaldehyde odor on breath, and abdominal pain can be present, but the patient may be asymptomatic. *Note:* Methanol produces an osmolal gap (early), and its metabolite formate produces the anion gap metabolic acidosis (see later). Absence of osmolar or anion gap does not always exclude methanol intoxication.
- 6 to 12 hours: Malaise, headache, abdominal pain, vomiting, visual symptoms, including hyperemia of optic disc, "snow vision," and blindness can be seen.
- More than 12 hours: Worsening acidosis, hyperglycemia, shock, and multiorgan failure develop, with death from complications of intractable acidosis and cerebral edema.

Laboratory Investigation
Methanol can be detected on some chromatography drug screens if specified. Methanol and ethanol levels, electrolytes, glucose, BUN, creatinine, amylase, and ABG should be monitored every 4 hours. Formate levels correlate more closely than blood

methanol concentration with severity of intoxication and should be obtained if possible.

Management

One should protect the airway by intubation to prevent aspiration and administer assisted ventilation as needed. If needed, 100% oxygen can be administered. A nephrologist should be consulted early regarding the need for hemodialysis.

Gastrointestinal decontamination procedures have no role.

Metabolic acidosis should be treated vigorously with sodium bicarbonate 2 to 3 mEq/kg intravenously. Large amounts may be needed.

Antidote therapy is initiated to inhibit metabolism if the patient has a history of ingesting more than 0.4 mL/kg of 100% with the following conditions:

- Blood methanol level is greater than 20 mg/dL
- The patient has osmolar gap not accounted for by other factors
- The patient is symptomatic or acidotic with increased anion gap and/or hyperemia of the optic disc.

The ethanol or fomepizole therapy outlined below can be used.

Ethanol Therapy. Ethanol should be initiated immediately if fomepizole is unavailable (see *Fomepizole Therapy*). Alcohol dehydrogenase has a greater affinity for ethanol than ethylene glycol. Therefore, ethanol blocks the metabolism of ethylene glycol.

Ethanol should be administered intravenously (oral administration is less reliable) to produce a blood ethanol concentration of 100 to 150 mg/dL. The loading dose is 10 mL/kg of 10% ethanol administered intravenously concomitantly with a maintenance dose of 10% ethanol at 1.0 mL/kg/h. This dose may need to be increased to 2 mL/kg/h in patients who are heavy drinkers. The blood ethanol concentration should be measured hourly and the infusion rate should be adjusted to maintain a concentration of 100 to 150 mg/dL.

Fomepizole Therapy. Fomepizole (Antizol, 4-methylpyrazole) inhibits alcohol dehydrogenase more reliably than ethanol and it does not require constant monitoring of ethanol levels and adjustment of infusion rates. Fomepizole is available in 1 g/mL vials of 1.5 mL. The loading dose is 15 mg/kg (0.015 mL/kg) IV, maintenance dose is 10 mg/kg (0.01 mL/kg) every 12 hours for 4 doses, then 15 mg/kg every 12 hours until the ethylene glycol levels are less than 20 mg/dL. The solution is prepared by being mixed with 100 mL of 0.9% saline or D_5W. Fomepizole can be given to patients requiring hemodialysis but should be dosed as follows:

Dose at the beginning of hemodialysis:
- If less than 6 hours since last Antizol dose, do not administer dose
- If more than 6 hours since last dose, administer next scheduled dose

Dosing during hemodialysis:
- Dose every 4 hours

Dosing at the time hemodialysis is completed:
- If less than 1 hour between last dose and end dialysis, do not administer dose at end of dialysis
- If 1 to 3 hours between last dose and end dialysis, administer one half of next scheduled dose
- If more than 3 hours between last dose and end dialysis, administer next scheduled dose

Maintenance dosing off hemodialysis:
- Give the next scheduled dose 12 hours from the last dose administered

Hemodialysis increases the clearance of both methanol and formate 10-fold over renal clearance. A blood methanol concentration greater than 50 mg/dL has been used as an indication for hemodialysis, but recently some toxicologists from the New York City Poison Center recommended early hemodialysis in patients with blood methanol concentration greater than 25 mg/dL because it may be able to shorten the course of intoxication if started early. One should continue to monitor methanol levels and/or formate levels every 4 hours after the procedure for rebound. Other indications for early hemodialysis are significant metabolic acidosis and electrolyte abnormalities despite conventional therapy and if visual or neurologic signs or symptoms are present.

A serum formate level greater than 20 mg/dL has also been used as a criterion for hemodialysis, although this is often not readily available through many laboratories. If hemodialysis is used, the infusion rate of 10% ethanol should be increased 2.0 to 3.5 mL/kg/h. The blood ethanol concentration and glucose level should be obtained every 2 hours.

Therapy is continued with both ethanol and hemodialysis until the blood methanol level is undetectable, there is no acidosis, and the patient has no neurologic or visual disturbances. This may require several days.

Hypoglycemia is treated with intravenous glucose. Doses of folinic acid (Leucovorin) and folic acid have been used successfully in animal investigations to enhance formate metabolism to carbon dioxide and water. Leucovorin 1 mg/kg up to 50 mg IV is administered every 4 hours for several days.

An initial ophthalmologic consultation and follow-up are warranted.

Disposition

All patients who have ingested significant amounts of methanol should be referred to the emergency department for evaluation and blood methanol concentration measurement. Ophthalmologic follow-up of all patients with methanol intoxications should be arranged.

Monoamine Oxidase Inhibitors

Nonselective monoamine oxidase inhibitors (MAOIs) include the hydrazines phenelzine (Nardil) and isocarboxazid (Marplan), and the nonhydrazine tranylcypromine (Parnate). Furazolidone (Furoxone) and pargyline (Eutonyl) are also considered nonselective MAOIs. Moclobemide,[22] which is available in many countries but not the United States, is a selective MAO-A inhibitor. MAO-B inhibitors include selegiline (Eldepryl), an antiparkinsonism agent, which does not have similar toxicity to MAO-A and is not discussed. Selectivity is lost in an overdose. MAOIs are used to treat severe depression.

Toxic Mechanism

Monoamine oxidase enzymes are responsible for the oxidative deamination of both endogenous and exogenous catecholamines such as norepinephrine. MAO-A in the intestinal wall also metabolizes tyramine in food. MAOIs permanently inhibit MAO enzymes until a new enzyme is synthesized after 14 days or longer. The toxicity results from the accumulation, potentiation, and prolongation of the cate-cholamine action followed by profound hypotension and cardiovascular collapse.

Toxic Dose

Toxicity begins at 2 to 3 mg/kg and fatalities occur at 4 to 6 mg/kg. Death has occurred after a single dose of 170 mg of tranylcypromine in an adult.

Kinetics

Structurally, MAOIs are related to amphetamines and catecholamines. The hydrazine peak levels are at 1 to 2 hours; metabolism is hepatic acetylation; and inactive metabolites are excreted in the urine. For the nonhydrazines, peak levels occur at 1 to 4 hours, and metabolism is via the liver to active amphetamine-like metabolites.

The onset of symptoms in a case of overdose is delayed 6 to 24 hours after ingestion, peak activity is 8 to 12 hours, and duration is 72 hours or longer. The peak of MAO inhibition is in 5 to 10 days and lasts as long as 5 weeks.

Manifestations

Manifestations of an acute ingestion overdose of MAO-A inhibitors are as follows:

Phase I. An adrenergic crisis occurs, with delayed onset for 6 to 24 hours, and may not reach peak until 24 hours. The crisis starts as hyperthermia, tachycardia, tachypnea, dysarthria, transient hypertension, hyperreflexia, and CNS stimulation.

Phase II. Neuromuscular excitation and sympathetic hyperactivity occur with increased temperature greater than 40°C (104°F), agitation, hyperactivity, confusion, fasciculations, twitching, tremor, masseter spasm, muscle rigidity, acidosis, and electrolyte abnormalities. Seizures and dystonic reactions may occur. The pupils are mydriatic, sometimes nonreactive with "ping-pong gaze."

Phase III. CNS depression and cardiovascular collapse occur in cases of severe overdose as the catecholamines are depleted. Symptoms usually resolve within 5 days but may last 2 weeks.

Phase IV. Secondary complications occur, including rhabdomyolysis, cardiac dysrhythmias, multiorgan failure, and coagulopathies.

Biogenic interactions usually occur while the patient is on therapeutic doses of MAOI or shortly after they are discontinued (30 to 60 minutes), before the new MAO enzyme is synthesized. The following substances have been implicated: indirect acting sympathomimetics such as amphetamines, serotonergic drugs, opioids (e.g., meperidine, dextromethorphan), tricyclic antidepressants, specific serotonin reuptake inhibitors (SSRIs; e.g., fluoxetine [Prozac], sertraline [Zoloft], paroxetine [Paxil]), tyramine-containing foods (e.g., wine, beer, avocados, cheese, caviar, chocolate, chicken liver), and L-tryptophan. SSRIs should not be started for at least 5 weeks after MAOIs have been discontinued.

In mild cases, usually caused by foods, headache and hypertension develop and last for several hours. In severe cases, malignant hypertension and severe hyperthermia syndromes consisting of hypertension or hyperthermia, altered mental state, skeletal muscle rigidity, shivering (often beginning in the masseter muscle), and seizures may occur.

The serotonin syndrome, which may be a result of inhibition of serotonin metabolism, has similar clinical findings to those of malignant hyperthermia and may occur with or without hyperthermia or hypertension.

Chronic toxicity clinical findings include tremors, hyperhidrosis, agitation, hallucinations, confusion, and seizures and may be confused with withdrawal syndromes.

Laboratory Investigations

Monitoring of the ECG, cardiac monitoring, CPK, ABG, pulse oximeter, electrolytes, blood glucose, and acid-base balance should be maintained.

Management

In the case of MAOI overdose, ipecac-induced emesis should not be used. Only activated charcoal alone should be used.

If the patient is admitted to the hospital and is well enough to eat, a nontyramine diet should be ordered.

Extreme agitation and seizures can be controlled with benzodiazepines and barbiturates. Phenytoin is ineffective. Nondepolarizing neuromuscular blockers (not depolarizing succinylcholine) may be needed in severe cases of hyperthermia and rigidity. If the patient has severe hypertension (catecholamine mediated), phentolamine (Regitine), a parenteral β-blocking agent, 3 to 5 mg intravenously, or labetalol (Normodyne), a combination of an α-blocking agent and a β-blocker, 20-mg intravenous bolus, should be given. If malignant hypertension with rigidity is present, a short-acting nitroprusside and benzodiazepine can be used. Hypertension is often followed by severe hypotension, which should be managed by fluid and vasopressors. *Caution:* Vasopressor therapy should be administered at lower doses than usual because of exaggerated pharmacologic response. Norepinephrine is preferred to dopamine, which requires release of intracellular amines.

Cardiac dysrhythmias are treated with standard therapy but are often refractory, and cardioversion and pacemakers may be needed.

For malignant hyperthermia, dantrolene (Dantrium), a nonspecific peripheral skeletal relaxing agent, is administered, which inhibits the release of calcium from the sarcoplasm. Dantrolene is reconstituted with 60 mL sterile water without bacteriostatic agents. Glass equipment must not be used, and the drug must be protected from light and used within 6 hours. Loading dose is 2 to 3 mg/kg intravenously as a bolus, and the loading dose is repeated until the signs of malignant hyperthermia (tachycardia, rigidity, increased end-tidal CO_2, and temperature) are controlled. Maximum total dose is 10 mg/kg to avoid hepatotoxicity.

When malignant hyperthermia has subsided, 1 mg/kg IV is given every 6 hours for 24 to 48 hours, then orally 1 mg/kg every 6 hours for 24 hours to prevent recurrence. There is a danger of thrombophlebitis following peripheral dantrolene, and it should be administered through a central line if possible. In addition one should administer external cooling and correct metabolic acidosis and electrolyte disturbances. Benzodiazepine can be used for sedation. Dantrolene does not reverse central dopamine blockade; therefore, bromocriptine mesylate (Parlodel) 2.5 to 10 mg should be given orally or through a nasogastric tube three times a day.

Rhabdomyolysis and myoglobinuria are treated with fluids. Urine alkalinization should also be treated.

Hemodialysis and hemoperfusion are of no proven value.

Biogenic amine interactions are managed symptomatically, similar to cases of overdose. For the serotonin syndrome cyproheptadine (Periactin), a serotonin blocker, 4 mg orally every hour for three doses, or methysergide (Sansert), 2 mg orally every 6 hours for three doses, should be considered. The effectiveness of these drugs has not been proven.

Disposition

All patients who have ingested more than 2 mg/kg of an MAOI should be admitted to the hospital for 24 hours of observation and monitoring in the intensive care unit because the life-threatening manifestations may be delayed. Patients with drug or dietary interactions that are mild may not require admission if symptoms subside within 4 to 6 hours and the patients remain asymptomatic. Patients with symptoms that persist or require active intervention should be admitted to the intensive care unit.

Opioids (Narcotic Opiates)

Opioids are used for analgesia, as antitussives, and as antidiarrheal agents and are illicit agents (heroin, opium) used in substance abuse. Tolerance, physical dependency, and withdrawal may develop.

Toxic Mechanism

At least four main opioid receptors have been identified. The μ receptor is considered the most important for central analgesia and CNS depression. The κ and δ receptors predominate in spinal analgesia. The σ receptors may mediate dysphoria. Death is a consequence of dose-dependent CNS respiratory depression or secondary to pulmonary aspiration or noncardiac pulmonary edema. The mechanism of noncardiac pulmonary edema is unknown.

Dextromethorphan can interact with MAOIs, causing severe hyperthermia, and may cause the serotonin syndrome (see *Selective Serotonin Reuptake Inhibitors*). Dextromethorphan inhibits the metabolism of norepinephrine and serotonin and blocks the reuptake of serotonin. It is found as a component of a large number of non-prescription cough and cold remedies.

Toxic Dose

The toxic dose depends on the specific drug, route of administration, and degree of tolerance. For therapeutic and toxic doses, see Table 24. In children, respiratory depression has been produced by 10 mg of morphine or methadone, 75 mg of meperidine, and 12.5 mg of diphenoxylate. Infants younger than 3 months of age are more susceptible to respiratory depression. The dose should be reduced by 50%.

Kinetics

Oral onset of analgesic effect of morphine is 10 to 15 minutes; the action peaks in 1 hour and lasts 4 to 6 hours. With

TABLE 24 Doses and Onset and Duration of Action of Common Opioids

DRUG	ADULT ORAL DOSE	CHILD ORAL DOSE	ONSET OF ACTION	DURATION OF ACTION	ADULT FATAL DOSE
Camphored tincture of opium	25 mL	0.25–0.50 mL/kg (0.4 mg/mL)	15–30 min	4–5 h	NA
Codeine	30–180 mg	0.5–1 mg/kg	15–30 min	4–6 h	800 mg
	>1 mg/kg is toxic in a child, above 200 mg in adult >5 mg/kg fatal in a child				
Dextromethorphan	15 mg 10 mg/kg is toxic	0.25 mg/kg	15–30 min	3–6 h	NA
Diacetylmorphine; street heroin is less than 10% pure	60 mg	NA	15–30 min	3–4 h	100 mg
Diphenoxylate atropine (Lomotil)	5–10 mg	NA	120–240 min	14 h	300 mg
	7.5 mg is toxic in a child, 300 mg is toxic in adult				
Fentanyl (Duragesic)	0.1–0.2 mg	0.001–0.002 mg/kg	7–8 min	Intramuscular: ½–2 h	1.0 mg
Hydrocodone with APAP (Lortab)	5–30 mg	0.15 mg/kg	30 min	3–4 h	100 mg
Hydromorphone (Dilaudid)	4 mg	0.1 mg/kg	15–30 min	3–4 h	100 mg
Meperidine (Demerol)	100 mg	1–1.5 mg/kg	10–45 min	3–4 h	350 mg
Methadone (Dolophine)	10 mg	0.1 mg/kg	30–60 min	4–12 h	120 mg
Morphine	10–60 mg	0.1–0.2 mg/kg	<20 min	4–6 h	200 mg
	Oral dose is 6 times parenteral dose, MS Contin sustained-release prep				
Oxycodone APAP (Percocet)	5 mg	NA	15–30 min	4–5 h	NA
Pentazocine (Talwin)	50–100 mg	NA	15–30 min	3–4 h	NA
Propoxyphene (Darvon)	65–100 mg	NA	30–60 min	2–4 h	700 mg

sustained-release preparations, the duration is 8 to 12 hours. Opioids are 90% metabolized in the liver by hepatic conjugation and 90% excreted in the urine as inactive compounds. Volume distribution is 1 to 4 L/kg. Protein binding is 35% to 75%. The typical plasma half-life of opiates is 2 to 5 hours, but that of methadone is 24 to 36 hours. Morphine metabolites include morphine-3-glucuronide (inactive) and morphine-6-glucuronide (active) and normorphine (active). Meperidine (Demerol) is rapidly hydrolyzed by tissue esterases into the active metabolite normeperidine, which has twice the convulsant activity of meperidine. Heroin (diacetylmorphine) is deacetylated within minutes to 6-monacetylmorphine and morphine. Propoxyphene (Darvon) has a rapid onset of action, and death has occurred within 15 to 30 minutes after a massive overdose. Propoxyphene is metabolized to norpropoxyphene, an active metabolite with convulsive, cardiac dysrhythmic, and heart block properties. Symptoms of diphenoxylate overdose appear within 1 to 4 hours. It is metabolized into the active metabolite difenoxin, which is five times more active as a regular respiratory depressant agent. Death has been reported in children after ingestion of a single tablet.

Manifestations

Initially, mild intoxication produces miosis, dull face, drowsiness, partial ptosis, and "nodding" (head drops to chest then bobs up). Larger amounts produce the classic triad of miotic pupils (exceptions below), respiratory depression, and depressed level of consciousness (flaccid coma). The blood pressure, pulse, and bowel activity are decreased.

Dilated pupils do not exclude opioid intoxication. Some exceptions to the miosis effect include dextromethorphan (paralyzes iris), fentanyl, meperidine, and diphenoxylate (rarely). Physiologic disturbances including acidosis, hypoglycemia, hypoxia, and postictal state, or a co-ingestant may also produce mydriasis.

Usually, the muscles are flaccid, but increased muscle tone can be produced by meperidine and fentanyl (chest rigidity). Seizures are rare but can occur with ingestion of codeine, meperidine, propoxyphene, and dextromethorphan. Hallucinations and agitation have been reported.

Pruritus and urticaria are caused by histamine release by some opioids or by sulfite additives.

Noncardiac pulmonary edema may occur after an overdose, especially with intravenous heroin abuse. Cardiac effects include vasodilation and hypotension. A heart murmur in an intravenous addict suggests endocarditis. Propoxyphene can produce delayed cardiac dysrhythmias.

Fentanyl is 100 times more potent than morphine and can cause chest wall muscle rigidity. Some of its derivatives are 2000 times more potent than morphine.

Laboratory Investigations

For patients with overdose, one should obtain and monitor ABG, blood glucose, and electrolyte levels; chest radiographs; and ECG. For drug abusers, one should consider testing for hepatitis B, syphilis, and HIV antibody (HIV testing usually requires consent). Blood opioid concentrations are not useful. They confirm diagnosis (morphine therapeutic dose, 65 to 80 ng/mL; toxic, <200 ng/mL), but are not useful for making a therapeutic decision. Cross-reactions can occur with Vick's Formula 44, poppy seeds, and other opioids (codeine and heroin are metabolized to morphine). Naloxone 4 mg IV was not associated with a positive enzyme multiplied immunoassay technique urine screen at 60 minutes, 6 hours, or 48 hours.

Management

Supportive care should be instituted, particularly an endotracheal tube and assisted ventilation. Temporary ventilation can be provided by a bag-valve mask with 100% oxygen. The patient should be placed on a cardiac monitor, have intravenous access established, and have specimens for ABG, glucose, electrolytes, BUN, and creatinine levels, CBC, coagulation profile, liver function, toxicology screen, and urinalysis taken.

For gastrointestinal decontamination, emesis should not be induced, but activated charcoal can be administered if bowel sounds are present.

If it is suspected that the patient is an addict, he or she should be restrained first and then 0.1 mg of naloxone (Narcan) should be administered. The dose should be doubled every 2 minutes until the patient responds or 10 to 20 mg has been given. If the patient is not suspected to be an addict, then 2 mg every 2 to 3 minutes to total of 10 to 20 mg is administered.

It is essential to determine whether there is a complete response to naloxone (mydriasis, improvement in ventilation), because it is a diagnostic therapeutic test. A continuous naloxone infusion may be appropriate, using the "response dose" every hour. Repeat doses of naloxone may be necessary because the effects of many opioids can last much longer than naloxone does (30 to 60 minutes). Methadone ingestions may require a naloxone infusion for 24 to 48 hours. Half of the response dose may need to be repeated in 15 to 20 minutes, after the infusion has been started.

Acute iatrogenic withdrawal precipitated by the administration of naloxone to a dependent patient should not be treated with morphine or other opioids. Naloxone's effects are limited to 30 to 60 minutes (shorter than most opioids) and withdrawal will subside in a short time.

Nalmefene (Revex), an FDA-approved long-acting (4 to 8 hours) pure opioid antagonist, is being investigated, but its role in cases of acute intoxication is unclear and it could produce prolonged withdrawal. It may have a role in place of naloxone infusion.

Noncardiac pulmonary edema does not respond to naloxone, and the patient needs intubation, assisted ventilation, positive end-expiratory pressure, and hemodynamic monitoring. Fluids should be given cautiously in patients with opioid overdose because opioids stimulate the antidiuretic hormone.

If the patient is comatose, 50% glucose (3% to 4% of comatose opioid overdose patients have hypoglycemia) and thiamine should be given prior to naloxone. If the patient has seizures that are unresponsive to naloxone, one administers diazepam and examines for metabolic (hypoglycemia, electrolyte disturbances) causes and structural disturbances.

Hypotension is rare and should direct a search for another etiology. If the patient is agitated, hypoxia and hypoglycemia must be excluded before opioid withdrawal is considered as a cause. Complications to consider include urinary retention, constipation, rhabdomyolysis, myoglobinuria, hypoglycemia, and withdrawal.

Disposition

If a patient responds to intravenous naloxone, careful observation for relapse and the development of pulmonary edema is required, with cardiac and respiratory monitoring for 6 to 12 hours. Patients requiring repeated doses of naloxone or an infusion, or those who develop pulmonary edema, require intensive care unit admission and cannot be discharged from the intensive care unit until they are symptom free for 12 hours. Intravenous overdose complications are expected to be present within 20 minutes after injection, and discharge after 4 symptom-free hours has been recommended. Adults with oral overdose have delayed onset of toxicity and require 6 hours of observation. Children with oral opioid overdose should be admitted to the hospital for observation because of delayed toxicity. Some toxicologists advise restraining a patient who attempts to sign out against

medical advice after treatment with naloxone, at least until the patient receives psychiatric evaluation.

Organophosphates and Carbamates

Cholinergic intoxication sources are insecticides (organophosphates or carbamates), some medications, and some mushrooms, Examples of organophosphate insecticides are malathion (low toxicity, median lethal dose [LD_{50}] 2800 mg/kg), chlorpyrifos, which has been removed from market (moderate toxicity), and parathion (high toxicity, LD_{50} 2 mg/kg). Carbamate insecticides include carbaryl (low toxicity, LD_{50} 500 mg/kg), propoxur (moderate toxicity, LD_{50} 95 mg/kg), and aldicarb (high toxicity, LD_{50} 0.9 mg/kg). Pharmaceuticals with carbamate properties include neostigmine (Prostigmin) and physostigmine (Antilirium). Cholinergic compounds also include the "G" nerve war weapons tabun (GA), sarin (GB), soman (GB), and venom X (VX).

Toxic Mechanism

Organophosphates phosphorylate the active site on red cell acetylcholinesterase and pseudocholinesterase in the serum, neuromuscular and parasympathetic neuroeffector junctions, and in the major synapses of the autonomic ganglia, causing irreversible inhibition. There are two types of organophosphate intoxication: (a) direct action by the parent compound (e.g., tetraethylpyrophosphate), or (b) indirect action by the toxic metabolite (e.g., parathoxon or malathoxon).

Carbamates (esters of carbonic acid) cause reversible carbamylation of the active site of the enzymes. When a critical amount, greater than 50%, of cholinesterase is inhibited, acetylcholine accumulates and causes transient stimulation at cholinergic synapses and sympathetic terminals (muscarinic effect), the somatic nerves, the autonomic ganglia (nicotinic effect), and CNS synapses. Stimulation of conduction is followed by inhibition of conduction.

The major differences between the carbamates and the organophosphates are as follows: (a) carbamate toxicity is less and the duration is shorter; (b) carbamates rarely produce overt CNS effects (poor CNS penetration); (c) carbamate inhibition of the acetylcholinesterase enzyme is reversible and activity returns to normal rapidly; (d) pralidoxime, the enzyme regenerator, may not be necessary in the management of mild carbamate intoxication (e.g., carbaryl).

Toxic Dose

Parathion's minimum lethal dose is 2 mg in children and 10 to 20 mg in adults. The lethal dose of malathion is greater than 1375 mg/kg and that of chlorpyrifos is 25 g; the latter compound is unlikely to cause death.

Kinetics

Absorption is by all routes. The onset of acute ingestion toxicity occurs as early as 3 hours, usually before 12 hours and always before 24 hours. Lipid-soluble agents absorbed by the dermal route (e.g., fenthion) may have a delayed onset of more than 24 hours. Inhalation toxicity occurs immediately after exposure. Massive ingestion can produce intoxication within minutes.

Metabolism is via the liver. With some pesticides (e.g., parathion, malathion), the effects are delayed because they undergo hepatic microsomal oxidative metabolism to their toxic metabolites, the -oxons (e.g., paroxon, malaoxon).

The half-life of malathion is 2.89 hours and that of parathion is 2.1 days. The metabolites are eliminated in the urine and the presence of p-nitrophenol in the urine is a clue up to 48 hours after exposure.

Manifestations

Many organophosphates produce a garlic odor on the breath, in the gastric contents, or in the container. Diaphoresis, excessive salivation, miosis, and muscle twitching are helpful clues to diagnosis.

Early, a cholinergic (muscarinic) crisis develops that consists of parasympathetic nervous system activity. DUMBELS is the mnemonic for defecation, cramps, and increased bowel motility; urinary incontinence; miosis (mydriasis may occur in 20%); bronchospasm and bronchorrhea; excess secretion; lacrimation; and seizures. Bradycardia, pulmonary edema, and hypotension may be present.

Later, sympathetic and nicotinic effects occur, consisting of MATCH: muscle weakness and fasciculation (eyelid twitching is often present), adrenal stimulation and hyperglycemia, tachycardia, cramps in muscles, and hypertension. Finally, paralysis of the skeletal muscles ensues.

The CNS effects are headache, blurred vision, anxiety, ataxia, delirium and toxic psychosis, convulsions, coma, and respiratory depression. Cranial nerve palsies have been noted. Delayed hallucinations may occur.

Delayed respiratory paralysis and neurologic and neurobehavioral disorders have been described following certain organophosphate ingestions or dermal exposure. The "intermediate syndrome" is paralysis of proximal and respiratory muscles developing 24 to 96 hours after the successful treatment of organophosphate poisoning. A delayed distal polyneuropathy has been described with ingestion of certain organophosphates, such as triorthocresyl phosphate, bromoleptophos, and methomidophos.

Complications include aspiration, pulmonary edema, and acute respiratory distress syndrome.

Laboratory Investigations

Monitoring should include chest radiograph, blood glucose (nonketotic hyperglycemia is frequent), ABG, pulse oximetry, ECG, blood coagulation status, liver function, hyperamylasemia (pancreatitis reported), and urinalysis for the metabolite alkyl phosphate paranitrophenol. Blood should be drawn for red blood cell cholinesterase determination before pralidoxime is given. The red blood cell cholinesterase activity roughly correlates with clinical severity. Mild poisoning is 20% to 50% of normal, moderate poisoning is 10% to 20% of normal, and severe poisoning is 10% of normal (>90% depressed). A postexposure rise of 10% to 15% in the cholinesterase level determined at least 10 to 14 days after the exposure confirms the diagnosis.

Management

Protection of health care personnel with clothing (masks, gloves, gowns, goggles) and respiratory equipment or hazardous material suits, as necessary, is called for. General decontamination consists of isolation, bagging, and disposal of contaminated clothing and other articles. Vital functions should be established and maintained. Cardiac and oxygen saturation monitoring are needed. Intubation and assisted ventilation may be needed. Secretions should be suctioned until atropinization drying is achieved.

Dermal decontamination involves prompt removal of clothing and cleansing of all affected areas of skin, hair, and eyes. Ocular decontamination involves irrigation with copious amounts of tepid water or 0.9% saline for at least 15 minutes. Gastrointestinal decontamination, if the ingestion was recent, involves the administration of activated charcoal.

Atropine sulfate can be given as an antidote. It is both a diagnostic and a therapeutic agent. Atropine counteracts the muscarinic effects but is only partially effective for the CNS effects (seizures and coma). Preservative-free atropine (no benzyl alcohol) should be used. If the patient is symptomatic (bradycardia or bronchorrhea), a test dose should be administered, 0.02 mg/kg in children or 1 mg in adults, intravenously. If no signs of atropinization are present (tachycardia, drying of secretions, and mydriasis), atropine should be administered immediately, 0.05 mg/kg in children or 2 mg in adults, every 5 to 10 minutes as needed to dry the secretions and clear the lungs. Beneficial effects are seen within 1 to 4 minutes and maximum effect in 8 minutes. The average dose in the first 24 hours is 40 mg, but 1000 mg or more has been required in severe cases. Glycopyrrolate (Robinul) can

be used if atropine is not available. The maximum dose should be maintained for 12 to 24 hours, then tapered and the patient observed for relapse. Poisoning, especially with lipophilic agents (e.g., fenthion, chlorfenthion), may require weeks of atropine therapy. An alternative is a continuous infusion of atropine 8 mg in 100 mL 0.9% saline at rate of 0.02 to 0.08 mg/kg/h (0.25 to 1.0 mL/kg/h) with additional 1 to 5 mg boluses as needed to dry the secretions.

Pralidoxime chloride (Protopam) has both antinicotinic and antimuscarinic effects and possibly also CNS effects. Successful treatment with pralidoxime chloride may allow a reduction in the dose of atropine. Pralidoxime acts to reactivate the phosphorylated cholinesterases by binding the phosphate moiety on the esteritic site and displacing it. It should be given early before "aging" of phosphate bond produces tighter binding. However, recent reports indicate that pralidoxime chloride is beneficial even several days after the poisoning. Improvement is seen within 10 to 40 minutes. The initial dose of pralidoxime chloride is 1 to 2 g in 250 mL 0.89% saline over 5 to 10 minutes, maximum 200 mg/min, in adults or 25 to 50 mg/kg, maximum 4 mg/kg/min, in children younger than 12 years of age. The dose can be repeated every 6 to 12 hours for several days. An alternative is a continuous infusion of 1 g in 100 mL 0.89% saline at 5 to 20 mg/kg/h (0.5 to 12 mL/g/h) up to 500 mg/h and titrated to desired response. Maximum adult daily dose is 12 g. Cardiac and blood pressure monitoring is advised during and for several hours after the infusion. The end point is absence of fasciculations and return of muscle strength.

Contraindicated drugs include morphine, aminophylline, barbiturates, opioids, phenothiazine, reserpine-like drugs, parasympathomimetics, and succinylcholine.

Noncardiac pulmonary edema may require respiratory support. Seizures may respond to atropine and pralidoxime chloride but often require anticonvulsants. Cardiac dysrhythmias may require electrical cardioversion or antidysrhythmic therapy if the patient is hemodynamically unstable. Extracorporeal procedures are of no proven value.

Disposition

Asymptomatic patients with normal examination findings after 6 to 8 hours of observation may be discharged. In cases of intentional poisoning, the patients require psychiatric clearance for discharge. Symptomatic patients should be admitted to the intensive care unit. Observation of milder cases of carbamate poisoning, even those requiring atropine, for 6 to 8 hours symptom-free may be sufficient to exclude significant toxicity. In cases of workplace exposure, OSHA should be notified.

Phencyclidine (Angel Dust)

Phencyclidine is an arylcyclohexylamine related to ketamine and chemically related to the phenothiazines. Originally a "dissociative" anesthetic banned in United States since 1979, it is now an illicit substance, with at least 38 analogues. It is inexpensively manufactured by "kitchen chemists" and is mislabeled as other hallucinogens. Improper phencyclidine synthesis may release cyanide when heated or smoked and can cause explosions.

Toxic Mechanism

The mechanism of phencyclidine is complex and not completely understood. It inhibits some neurotransmitters and causes a loss of pain sensation without depressing the CNS respiratory status. It stimulates α-adrenergic receptors and may act as a "false neurotransmitter." The effects are sympathomimetic, cholinergic, and cerebellar.

Toxic Dose

The usual dose of phencyclidine mixed with marijuana joints is 100 to 400 mg of phencyclidine. Joints or leaf mixtures contain 0.24% to 7.9% of PCP, 1 mg of PCP/150 leaves. Tablets contain 5 mg (the usual street dose). CNS effects at doses of 1 to 6 mg include hallucinations and euphoria, 6 to 10 mg produces toxic urine tests using human chorionic gonadotropin as an indicator, and give false-positive results for urine porphyrins, indirect Coombs test, urobilinogen, and amylase.

Management

Vital functions must be established and maintained. All overdose patients require venous access, 12-lead ECG (to measure intervals), cardiac and respiratory monitoring, and seizure precautions. One should monitor core temperature to detect poikilothermic effect. If the patient is comatose, intubation and assisted ventilation may be required, as well as 100% oxygen, intravenous glucose, naloxone (Narcan), and thiamine.

Emesis is not recommended. Activated charcoal can be administered if ingestion was within 1 hour. MDAC has not been proven beneficial. A radiograph of the abdomen may be useful, if the phenothiazine is radiopaque. Haloperidol (Haldol) and trifluoperazine (Stelazine) are most likely to be radiopaque. Whole-bowel irrigation may be useful when a large number of pills are visualized on radiograph or if sustained-release preparations were taken, but whole-bowel irrigation has not been evaluated in patients with phenothiazine overdose.

Convulsions are treated with diazepam or lorazepam (Ativan). Loxapine (Loxitane) overdose may result in status epilepticus. If nondepolarizing neuromuscular blockade is required, pancuronium (Pavulon) or vecuronium (Norcuron) should be used (not succinyl-choline [Anectine], which may cause malignant hyperthermia), and EEG should be monitored during paralysis.

Patients with dysrhythmias should be monitored with serial ECGs. Unstable rhythms can be treated with electrical cardioversion. Class 1a antidysrhythmics (procainamide, quinidine, and disopyramide [Norpace]) must be avoided.

Hypokalemia predisposes to dysrhythmias and should be corrected aggressively. Supraventricular tachycardia with hemodynamic instability is treated with electrical cardioversion. The role of adenosine has not been defined. Calcium channel and β-blockers should be avoided.

Prolongation of the QRS interval is treated with sodium bicarbonate 1 to 2 mEq/kg by intravenous bolus over a few minutes. Torsades de pointes is treated with magnesium sulfate IV 20% solution 2 g over 2 to 3 minutes. If there is no response in 10 minutes, the dose is repeated and followed by a continuous infusion of 5 to 10 mg/min or given as an infusion of 50 mg/min for 2 hours followed by 30 mg/min for 90 minutes twice a day for several days, as needed. The dose in children is 25 to 50 mg/kg initially and maintenance dose is 30 to 60 mg/kg per 24 hours (0.25 to 0.50 mEq/kg per 24 hours) up to 1000 mg per 24 hours. Serum magnesium levels should be monitored.

To treat ventricular tachydysrhythmias in a stable patient, lidocaine is used. If the patient is unstable, electrical cardioversion is used. Patients with heart block with hemodynamic instability should be managed with temporary cardiac pacing.

Hypotension is treated with the Trendelenburg position and 0.9% saline. If the condition is refractory to treatment or there is a danger of fluid overload, vasopressors are administered. The vasopressor of choice is α-adrenergic agonist norepinephrine (Levophed), titrated to response. Epinephrine and dopamine should not be used because β-receptor stimulation in the presence of α-receptor blockade may provoke dysrhythmias and phenothiazines are antidopaminergic.

Hypothermia and hyperthermia are treated with external warming and cooling measures, respectively. Antipyretic drugs must not be used.

Management of the neuroleptic malignant syndrome includes the following actions:
- Immediately discontinuing the offending agent
- Hyperventilating the patient, using 100% humidified, cooled oxygen at high gas flows (at least 10 L/min) because of rapid breathing
- Administering a benzodiazepine to control convulsions and facilitate cooling measures
- Initiating appropriate mechanical cooling measures, which may include intravenous cold saline (not lactated Ringer's), ice baths, cold lavage of the stomach, bladder, and rectum, and a hypothermic blanket
- Correcting acid-base and electrolyte disturbances and treating significant hyperkalemia with hyperventilation, calcium, sodium bicarbonate, intravenous glucose, and insulin; hemodialysis may be necessary

In addition, dysrhythmias usually respond to correction of the underlying acid-base disturbances and hyperkalemia. If antidysrhythmic agents are required, calcium channel blockers must be avoided because they may precipitate hyperkalemia and cardiovascular collapse. Dantrolene sodium (Dantrium), which is a phenytoin derivative, inhibits calcium release from the sarcoplasmic reticulum and results in decreased muscle contraction. Dantrolene acts peripherally and does not reverse the rigidity or psychomotor disturbances resulting from the central dopamine blockade; it therefore is often used in combination with bromocriptine. Bromocriptine mesylate (Parlodel) acts centrally as a dopamine agonist, as does amantadine hydrochloride (Symmetrel). Bromocriptine and dantrolene have been reported to be successful in combination with cooling and good supportive measures in malignant hyperthermia.

Dosing for these agents is as follows: dantrolene sodium at 2 to 3 mg/kg IV as a bolus, then 1 mg/kg/min to a maximum of 10 mg/kg or until the tachycardia, rigidity, increased end-tidal CO_2, and temperature elevation are controlled. *Note:* Hepatotoxicity occurs with doses greater than 10 mg/kg. To prevent symptom recurrence, 1 mg/kg should be administered every 6 hours for 24 to 48 hours after the episode. After that time, oral dantrolene can be used at a dose of 1 mg/kg every 6 hours for 24 hours as necessary. The patient should be observed for thrombophlebitis following intravenous dantrolene. It is best administered via a central line. Bromocriptine mesylate at 2.5 to 10 mg orally or via a nasogastric tube, three times a day, should be used in combination with dantrolene.

Idiosyncratic dystonic reaction can be treated with diphenhydramine (Benadryl) 1 to 2 mg/kg/dose intravenously over 5 minutes up to maximum of 50 mg intravenously; a response is noted within 2 to 5 minutes. This can be followed with oral doses for 4 to 6 days to prevent recurrence.

Extracorporeal measures (hemodialysis, hemoperfusion) are not effective in removing these agents.

Disposition

Asymptomatic patients should be observed for at least 6 hours after gastric decontamination. Symptomatic patients with cardiotoxicity, hypotension, and convulsions should be admitted to the intensive care unit and monitored for 48 hours.

Salicylates (Acetylsalicylic Acid, Salicylic Acid)

Toxic Mechanism

The primary toxic mechanisms include (a) direct stimulation of the medullary chemoreceptor trigger zone and respiratory center; (b) uncoupling oxidative phosphorylation; (c) inhibition of the Krebs cycle enzymes; (d) inhibition of vitamin K dependent and independent clotting factors; (e) alteration of platelet function; and (f) inhibition of prostaglandin synthesis.

Toxic Dose

Acute mild intoxication occurs at a dose of 150 to 200 mg/kg, moderate intoxication at 200 to 300 mg/kg, and severe intoxication at 300 to 500 mg/kg. Acute salicylate plasma concentration greater than 30 mg/dL (usually >40 mg/dL) may be associated with clinical toxicity. Chronic intoxication occurs at ingestions greater than 100 mg/kg/d for more than 2 days because of accumulation kinetics. Methyl salicylate (oil of wintergreen) is the most toxic form of salicylate. A dose of 1 mL of 98% contains 1.4 g of salicylate. Fatalities have occurred with ingestion of 1 teaspoonful in children and 1 ounce in adults. It is found in topical ointments and liniments (18% to 30%).

Kinetics

Acetylsalicylic acid and salicylic acid are weak acids with a pKa of 3.5 and 3.0, respectively. Acetylsalicylic acid is absorbed from the stomach, from the small bowel, and dermally. Onset of action is within 30 minutes. Methyl salicylate and effervescent tablets are absorbed more rapidly. Salicylate plasma concentration is detectable within 15 minutes after ingestion and peaks in 30 to 120 minutes. The peak may be delayed 6 to 12 hours in cases of large overdose, overdose with enteric-coated or sustained-release preparations, and development of concretions. The therapeutic duration of action is 3 to 4 hours but is markedly prolonged in cases of overdose.

Volume distribution is 0.13 L/kg for salicylic acid but increases as the salicylate plasma concentration increases. Protein binding is greater than 90% for salicylic acid at pH 7.4 and a salicylate plasma concentration of 20 to 30 mg/dL, 75% at a salicylate plasma concentration greater than 40 mg/dL, 50% at a salicylate plasma concentration of 70 mg/dL, and 30% at a salicylate plasma concentration of 120 mg/dL.

The half-life for salicylic acid is 3 hours after a 300 mg dose, 6 hours after a 1 g overdose, and greater than 10 hours after a 10 g overdose. Elimination includes Michaelis-Menten hepatic metabolism by three saturable pathways: (a) glycine conjugation to salicyluric acid (75%); (b) glucuronyl transferase to salicyl phenol glucuronide (10%); and (c) salicyl aryl glucuronide (4%). Nonsaturable pathways are hydrolysis to gentisic acid (<1%). Ten percent is excreted unchanged.

Acidosis increases the severity of the intoxication by increasing the non-ionized salicylate that can cross membranes and enter the brain cells. In kidneys, the unionized salicylic acid undergoes glomerular filtration, and the ionized portion undergoes tubular secretion in proximal tubules and passive reabsorption in the distal tubules. Renal excretion of salicylate is enhanced by alkaline urine.

Manifestations

The ingestion of concentrated topical salicylic acid preparations (e.g., wart remover) can cause mucosal caustic injury to the gastrointestinal tract. Occult salicylate overdose should be considered in any patient with unexplained acid-base disturbance.

The manifestations of acute overdose of salicylates are as follows:

Minimal Symptoms. Tinnitus, dizziness, and deafness may occur at high therapeutic salicylate plasma concentrations of 20 to 30 mg/dL. Nausea and vomiting may occur immediately because of local gastric irritation.

Phase I. Mild manifestations occur at 1 to 12 hours after ingestion with a 6-hour salicylate plasma concentration of 45 to 70 mg/dL. Nausea and vomiting followed by hyperventilation are usually present within 3 to 8 hours after acute overdose. Hyperventilation, an increase in both rate (tachypnea) and depth (hyperpnea), is present but it may be subtle. It results in a mild respiratory alkalosis with a serum pH greater than 7.4 and urine pH greater than 6.0. Some patients may have lethargy, vertigo, headache, and confusion. Diaphoresis may be noted.

Phase II. Moderate manifestations occur at 12 to 24 hours after ingestion with a 6-hour salicylate plasma concentration of 70 to 90 mg/dL. Serious metabolic disturbances, including a marked respiratory alkalosis with anion gap metabolic acidosis, dehydration, and urine pH less than 6.0, may occur. Other metabolic disturbances include hypoglycemia or hyperglycemia, hypokalemia, decreased ionized calcium, and increased BUN, creatinine, and lactate. Mental disturbances (confusion, disorientation, hallucinations) may occur. Hypotension and convulsions have been reported.

Phase III. Severe intoxication occurs more than 24 hours after ingestion with a 6-hour salicylate plasma concentration of 90 to 130 mg/dL. In addition to the above clinical findings, coma and seizures develop and indicate severe intoxication. Pulmonary edema may occur. Metabolic disturbances include metabolic acidemia (pH <7.4) and aciduria (pH <6.0). In adults, alkalosis may persist until terminal respiratory failure.

In children younger than 4 years of age, a mixed metabolic acidosis and respiratory alkalosis develop earlier (within 4 to 6 hours) than in adults because children have less respiratory reserve and accumulate lactate and other organic acids. Hypoglycemia is more common in children.

Fatalities occur at 6-hour salicylate plasma concentrations greater than 130 to 150 mg/dL and result from CNS depression, cardiovascular collapse, electrolyte imbalance, and cerebral edema.

Chronic salicylism is more serious than acute intoxication and the 6-hour salicylate plasma concentration does not correlate well with the manifestations in both acute and chronic cases of intoxication. Chronic intoxication usually occurs with therapeutic errors in young children or the elderly with underlying illness, and the diagnosis is delayed because it is not recognized. Noncardiac pulmonary edema is a frequent complication in the elderly. The mortality rate is about 25%. Chronic salicylate poisoning in children may mimic Reye syndrome. It is associated with exaggerated CNS findings (hallucinations, delirium, dementia, memory loss, papilledema, bizarre behavior, agitation, encephalopathy, seizures, and coma). Hemorrhagic manifestations, renal failure, and pulmonary and cerebral edema may occur. The metabolic picture is hypoglycemia and mixed acid-base derangements. A chronic salicylate plasma concentration greater than 60 mg/dL with metabolic acidosis and an altered mental state is very serious.

Laboratory Investigations

All patients with intentional salicylate overdoses should have acetaminophen plasma level measured after 4 hours.

One should continuously monitor ECG, urine output, urine pH, and specific gravity. Every 2 to 4 hours in cases of severe intoxication, salicylate plasma concentration, glucose (in a case of salicylism, CNS hypoglycemia may be present despite normal serum glucose), electrolytes, ionized calcium, magnesium and phosphorus, anion gap, ABGs, and pulse oximeter should be monitored. Daily monitoring of BUN, creatinine, liver function tests, and prothrombin time should take place.

The therapeutic salicylate plasma concentration is less than 10 mg/dL for analgesia and 15 to 30 mg/dL for antiinflammatory effect. Cross-reaction with diflunisal (Dolobid) will give a falsely high salicylate plasma concentration. The Done nomogram is not considered accurate in evaluating acute or chronic salicylate intoxications.

Management

Treatment is based on clinical and metabolic findings, not on salicylate levels. Continuous monitoring of the urine pH is essential for successful alkalinization treatment. One should always obtain an acetaminophen plasma level.

Vital functions must be established and maintained. If the patient is in an altered mental state, glucose, naloxone, and thiamine are administered in standard doses. Depending on the severity, the initial studies include an immediate and a 6-hour postingestion salicylate plasma concentration, ECG and cardiac monitoring, pulse oximeter, urine (analysis, pH, and specific gravity), chest radiograph, ABGs, blood glucose, electrolytes and anion gap calculation, calcium (ionized), magnesium, renal and liver profiles, and prothrombin time. Gastric contents and stool should be tested for occult blood. Bismuth and magnesium salicylate preparations may be radiopaque on radiographs. Consultation with a nephrologist is warranted in cases of moderate, severe, or chronic intoxication.

For gastrointestinal decontamination, activated charcoal is useful (each gram of activated charcoal binds 550 mg of salicylic acid) if a toxic dose was ingested up to 4 hours postingestion. MDAC is not recommended for salicylate intoxication.

Concretions may occur with massive (usually >300 mg/kg) ingestions. If blood levels fail to decline, prompt contrast radiography of the stomach may reveal concretions that have to be removed by repeated lavage, whole-bowel irrigation, endoscopy, or gastrostomy.

Pfizer/Wyeth coral snake antivenom is not currently being manufactured at this time. Endemic areas such as Florida, Georgia, Texas, Alabama, and Louisiana have stockpiles; however, the stockpiles are currently being depleted. Pfizer has successfully applied for extensions for expiring lots of NACSA; however, new antivenom vials have not yet entered circulation. An experimental F(ab′)$_2$ antivenom has completed a phase III clinical trial but is not currently available. Foreign-produced antivenoms against related coral snake species may also have efficacy against U.S. snakes but should be used only when a drug that is approved by the U.S. Food and Drug Administration (FDA) is not available and, ideally, with prior FDA approval.

An even more difficult situation results from exotic envenomations for which the appropriate antivenom (if one exists) is certain to be a non–FDA-approved product and must be located at a zoo or other non-healthcare source potentially distant from the location of the envenomation.

Antivenom, local wound care, and symptomatic and supportive care are the mainstays of envenomation management. A regional poison control center should be contacted for information and assistance in managing any venomous snake exposure, including locating an appropriate antivenom. Poison control centers have personnel who are experienced at assessing and managing envenomations and have access to the Antivenom Index, an updatable online database that lists sources of antivenoms for nonnative species. Poison control centers can be contacted from anywhere in the United States by calling 1-800-222-1222.

Snake Identification

The major branch point in native North American snake envenomation is to determine whether the victim has been bitten by a coral snake or a crotalid. Identification of the specific species can help predict some species-specific challenges; however, more important is to determine if the envenomation was caused by a Crotalinae or Elapidae snake. Crotaline snakes are easily differentiated from coral snakes by virtue of the latter's distinctive color pattern of red, yellow, and black bands. It can be difficult to differentiate a coral snake from nonvenomous snakes that have similar markings. The rhyme "red touches yellow, kills a fellow; red touches black, venom lack," which describes the red band being surrounded on either side by yellow or black, is accurate only for coral snakes in the United States and Canada. Mexican and South American coral snakes may have the opposite pattern. Crotalids, or pit vipers, can be distinguished from non-venomous snakes by the presence of vertically elliptical pupils, a triangular-shaped head, and the presence of temperature-sensing pits behind the nostrils.

Physical findings, laboratory evaluation, and geographic location of the envenomation is typically all that is required to determine that the snake is venomous and to guide therapy. Attempting to kill or capture the snake is unlikely to add additional information to treatment decisions and may result in further injury.

Factors Affecting Toxicity and the Severity of Envenomation

Many factors govern whether an envenomation occurs after a bite, the signs and symptoms that develop, and the overall severity of the effects. Up to 25% of crotalid bites and up to 50% of elapid bites do not result in an envenomation. Barriers to fang penetration and other factors may result in no venom being injected. Patients must be watched for a sufficient length of time (i.e., 8 to 12 hours for a crotalid bite and 24 hours for a coral snakebite) to ensure that this is the case.

If an envenomation has occurred, the family and species of snake generally determines the spectrum of symptoms and signs. The amount of venom, specific venom components, and underlying health status of the victim determine severity.

Crotalid Envenomations

Epidemiology

Crotalid snakes are distributed throughout North America, with the exception of Maine, Alaska, and Hawaii. Bites are more common in southern states and during summer months, but they occur year-round and may occur at any time and in any location with captive collections. The various genera and species of crotalids in the United States have relatively stable geographic ranges, with much overlap. Many different species of venomous snakes may inhabit any given area. Nonvenomous or mildly venomous colubrid snakes are also native to the United States.

Pit vipers have large front, mobile fangs through which venom is injected into the victim. Because the fangs are curved, venom is usually injected subcutaneously rather than into deeper muscle compartments. Because of anatomic and other physical factors, bite wounds may appear as scratches or as one or more punctures. Envenomation may occur with any break in the skin.

Crotalid venom is complex, consisting of proteolytic enzymes, small peptides, phospholipases, and other elements responsible for the spectrum of clinical effects seen. There is great variability of venom composition among species, within species, and even within a single specimen over the course of a season and its entire life span.

Clinical Effects

The spectrum of clinical effects is based on the specific genus or species of crotalid and is unpredictable, ranging from non-envenomation (a "dry bite"; up to 25% of bites) to life-threatening reactions. Crotalid snake envenomation typically results in tissue injury and hematologic effects. Local effects are typically pain and progressive swelling, and may include ecchymosis, tissue necrosis, or tissue loss. The complete absence of local effects cannot be used as a reliable marker of non-envenomation in a crotalid bite. We recommend a period of observation of 8 to 12 hours with serial blood draws to monitor for coagulopathy or thrombocytopenia.

Systemic effects including hematologic, neurologic, cardiovascular, and nonspecific findings may occur after crotalid envenomations. Rattlesnake (genera *Crotalus* and *Sistrurus*) envenomations are more likely to result in hematologic effects compared with copperhead or cottonmouth (genus *Agkistrodon*) envenomation. Hematologic abnormalities commonly include thrombocytopenia, hypofibrinogenemia, or prolonged prothrombin time (PT). Rattlesnake envenomations are much more likely to produce neurologic effects, such as muscle fasciculation or weakness, compared with copperhead or cottonmouth envenomations; however, these effects can be seen with any crotalid snake. Acute hypersensitivity can occur from any envenomation, which can result in hypotension, airway compromise, ECG changes, and/or coma. Nausea, vomiting, diaphoresis, anxiety, and other nonspecific effects may be seen.

Duration of Clinical Effects

Local effects may develop rapidly or may not be apparent for many hours. Progression may occur for days, with resolution of tissue injury occurring over 1 to 6 weeks. Complications of tissue necrosis or infection have their own time frame of resolution. Hematologic effects usually begin within 1 to 2 hours of envenomation. If antivenom is given within this time frame, the detection of these effects may be masked and become apparent only after unbound antivenom has been eliminated from the body, usually within 1 week after treatment. Untreated or recurrent/delayed (after antivenom) hematologic effects may persist for up to 3 weeks after an envenomation. Neurologic and other systemic effects tend to occur within a few hours of envenomation and resolve over 24 to 36 hours.

Severity of Envenomation

Untreated, local injury worsens over time, with proximal progression of tissue injury. Hematologic effects can be profound, resulting in spontaneous hemorrhage. Hypotension may be severe and can result in death. Neurologic and other systemic effects are rarely life-threatening events. As a result of changes in basic medical care and healthcare systems, it is not directly applicable to compare case-fatality rates before the introduction of antivenom (1950) with what can be expected today. Currently, there are approximately five deaths from crotalid snakebites per year in the United States.

- Remove jewelry.
- Splint and elevate the extremity in extension.
- Expeditiously transport the patient to a healthcare facility.
- Obtain intravenous access in a non-envenomated extremity.
- Do not use cutting, sucking, tourniquets, heat, cold, or other local "therapies."

- Remove jewelry.
- Obtain intravenous access in a non-envenomated extremity, and use crystalloid as indicated.
- Obtain CBC with platelet count, PT, and fibrinogen level every 6 to 12 hours until normalizing.
- Determine whether an envenomation has occurred.
- Determine severity based on the family or species of snake, age and health status of the victim, and development and rate of progression of signs and symptoms (e.g., local injury, hematologic abnormalities, hypotension, and other systemic effects).
- Determine the patient's tetanus vaccination status, and update if necessary.
- Seek consultation from a poison control center: 1-800-222-1222.
- Determine whether antivenom is indicated, and administer per protocol.
- Provide basic wound care, and determine whether local injury requires specific management.
- Determine whether hematologic or other systemic effects require specific management.

Management

Determining Whether Envenomation Has Occurred and Its Severity

Because of the unpredictability of envenomation and the variability of possible clinical effects, each crotalid bite must be assessed and responded to individually (Box 1). It is important to determine whether an envenomation has occurred. If there are no signs or symptoms of envenomation, there is no indication for antivenom or other specific treatment. The severity of the envenomation helps determine the amount of antivenom required to counter and neutralize venom effects, but this may not be immediately apparent because envenomations tend to progress over time, and what may at first appear to be mild venom effects may progress to a severe envenomation.

Initial Hospital Management

On arrival at the hospital, jewelry should be removed and the bitten extremity loosely splinted in an extended position. The wound should be cleansed (Box 2), and tetanus status should be updated if required. The extremity should be elevated to limit distal edema and pain. Patients often require opioid analgesics for pain relief.

At least one large intravenous line should be placed, avoiding the envenomated extremity, and crystalloid should be infused as required. Initial hospital therapy, including a first dose of antivenom, should be provided in an area capable of close monitoring of vital signs and capable of managing life-threatening reactions; this usually is an emergency department. Whether an intensive care unit or similar patient care area is used for subsequent management depends on the clinical situation.

Indications for Antivenom

Because of the safety of the current FDA-approved antivenoms and their ability to stop proximal progression of local tissue injury, all patients with signs of progressive local envenomation effects as well as those with significant systemic effects are candidates for treatment with antivenom.

Depending on the original indication for treatment (local effects, systemic effects, or both), initial control of envenomation effects is the goal of the loading dose of antivenom. Currently, there are two FDA-approved crotalid antivenoms for North American pit viper envenomation: CroFab and Anavip. The incidence of acute hypersensitivity reactions with CroFab and Anavip are low and generally mild and were found to be similar between products in a comparative trial. Pretreatment sensitivity testing is not required or recommended. There are rare reports of IgE-mediated type I hypersensitivity reactions on repeat exposure in individuals who were previously treated with CroFab, but most people who have been previously treated do not develop an adverse reaction to subsequent administration. The incidence of type III hypersensitivity reaction ("serum sickness") with both antivenoms was approximately 2.5% in the comparative trial.

The half-life of CroFab is approximately 18 to 24 hours, which is considerably shorter than IgG or F(ab′)$_2$ antivenoms, and it is believed to be responsible for increased late hemotoxicity compared with Anavip. Anavip has a longer half-life (approximately 133 hours) and a lower risk of late coagulopathy or thrombocytopenia.

For treatment of envenomations, antivenom is administered as an intravenous solution, with 4 to 6 vials of CroFab, or 10 vials of Anavip diluted into 250 mL of normal saline. The infusion should start at 25 to 50 mL/hour over the first 5 to 10 minutes, and then the rate is increased to finish by 1 hour if there is no reaction. Acute reactions are usually anaphylactoid (rate-related, not IgE-mediated) in nature, but they may reflect true anaphylaxis (IgE-mediated). Anaphylaxis is usually, but not always, more severe, and distinguishing between them is mostly based on a history of prior exposure or reaction.

If an acute hypersensitivity reaction occurs, the infusion should be slowed or stopped, depending on the severity, and appropriate symptomatic treatment should be started with H_1 and H_2 blockers, epinephrine, corticosteroids, and other supportive measures, as required. It should be determined whether antivenom is still required; if so, it should be restarted at a slower rate or higher dilution, or both, and consideration should be given to using an antivenom from a different source animal. CroFab is raised in sheep, and Anavip is raised in horses. Additionally, CroFab uses papain, an enzyme derived from papaya, during production, which may lead to an allergic reaction in those with papaya allergy.

Treatment of Local Tissue Injury

Monitoring the circumference in three locations along the envenomated extremity is usually sufficient to document progressive local injury. If the antivenom is given exclusively for local findings, the envenomation is deemed to be controlled if measurements stabilize or decrease. Pain in the inguinal or axillary lymph nodes is indicative of spreading envenomation, which may be an indication for further doses of antivenom. There is often some redistribution of existing tissue edema, but uncontrolled proximal progression is usually seen as an indication that the envenomation is not under control. If antivenom is being given for hematologic effects, cessation of worsening or reversal should be seen. Often, thrombocytopenia rebounds dramatically. Hypofibrinogenemia may not rebound as quickly or merely stabilize because the liver must manufacture new fibrinogen. Although an elevated D-dimer value indicates fibrinogenolytic activity, it is not an independent indicator for antivenom treatment; therefore we do not recommend routinely obtaining this value.

Other systemic effects may serve as indicators for antivenom use, and they should show improvement by the end of the initial shows signs of neurotoxicity was not associated with poor outcomes. Recent case series of Texas coral snake envenomation reported to the North American Snakebite Registry over a 5-year period demonstrated that a "wait and see" approach for NACSA administration was acceptable as no patients received antivenom, and all patients recovered. NACSA stockpiles still exist; however, it does not appear that any new doses of antivenom have been produced. Pfizer has applied to extend the expiration date on lots of antivenom with the FDA.

When paralysis has progressed to significant airway compromise, complete or partial reversal with antivenom may not be possible. Aggressive respiratory support, including intubation and ventilation, may be needed for days or weeks. If an FDA-approved coral snake antivenom is not readily available, there are reports of coral snake antivenoms from Mexico, Costa Rica, and Brazil, and of tiger snake antivenom from Australia, reversing the neurotoxicity of *M. tener*. The use of foreign non–FDA-approved antivenoms should be reserved for circumstances in which an FDA-approved product is not available in a timely manner and, if possible, with prior approval by the FDA Center for Biologics Evaluation and Research (240-402-8020; after-hours emergency: 866-300-4374; 301-796-8240; email is industry.biologics@fda.hhs.gov). Because these drugs are imported into the United States as Investigational New Drugs, institutional investigational review boards will also have notification requirements.

Exotic Snakebite

Epidemiology and Clinical Effects

In the United States, most exotic snake envenomations occur in private collections. These are not usually known to authorities or healthcare providers until an envenomation occurs, and they may involve the collection owner or family members, including children. They may occur in any locale, and victims may present to any healthcare facility.

Crotalid and elapid snakes, which account for the bulk of venomous bites worldwide, have patterns of venom activity similar to those of their North American counterparts, with some variation and with generally greater toxicity for some non-U.S. species. Some nonnative elapids, such as cobras, mambas, black snakes, or taipans, produce much higher rates of respiratory paralysis and may produce much greater local tissue injury than U.S. coral snakes. Similarly, envenomation from some nonnative crotalids, such as *Bothrops*, *Echis*, or *Bitis* species, or from an African colubrid, such as the boomslang, results in a greater risk of bleeding. Some of these species may directly activate prothrombin (e.g., *Echis* species, *Bothrops* species) and factor X (e.g., *Vipera*

species, *Dispholidus* species), leading to a venom-induced consumptive coagulopathy with intravascular thrombosis, marked organ dysfunction, and, potentially, death.

Management

The specific management of exotic envenomations is beyond the scope of this chapter. Not all venomous exotic snakes have antivenoms. Even for snakes with antivenoms, they may not be available in the United States, although zoos stock antivenoms for snakes in their collections. As discussed earlier, the Antivenom Index lists these antivenoms and is accessible to regional poison control centers. For information on exotic antivenoms and assistance in managing an exotic snake envenomation, the regional poison control center should be contacted.

References

Bush SP, Ruha AM, Seifert SA, et al: Comparison of F(ab')2 versus Fab antivenom for pit viper envenomation: a prospective, blinded, multicenter, randomized clinical trial, *Clin Toxicol (Phila)* 53(1):37–45, 2015, https://doi.org/10.3109/15563650.2014.974263.

Greene S, Ruha AM, Campleman S, Brent J, Wax P, Tox ICSSG: Epidemiology, Clinical Features, and Management of Texas Coral Snake (Micrurus tener) Envenomations Reported to the North American Snakebite Registry, *J Med Toxicol* 17(1):51–56, 2021, https://doi.org/10.1007/s13181-020-00806-3.

Greene SC, Folt J, Wyatt K, Brandehoff NP: Epidemiology of fatal snakebites in the United States 1989-2018, *Am J Emerg Med* 45:309–316, 2021, https://doi.org/10.1016/j.ajem.2020.08.083.

LoVecchio F, Klemens J, Welch S, Rodriguez R: Antibiotics after rattlesnake envenomation, *J Emerg Med* 23(4):327–328, 2002, https://doi.org/10.1016/s0736-4679(02)00563-2.

Ruha AM, Padilla-Jones A, Canning J, Spyres MB, Curry SC: Early Experience with Crotalidae Immune F(ab')2 Antivenom to Treat Arizona Rattlesnake Envenomations, *J Med Toxicol* 18(1):38–42, 2022, https://doi.org/10.1007/s13181-021-00859-y.

Ruha AM, Kleinschmidt KC, Greene S, Spyres MB, Brent J, Wax P, Padilla-Jones A, Campleman S, Tox ICSSG: The Epidemiology, Clinical Course, and Management of Snakebites in the North American Snakebite Registry, *J Med Toxicol* 13(4):309–320, 2017, https://doi.org/10.1007/s13181-017-0633-5.

Spyres MB, Skolnik AB, Moore EC, Gerkin RD, Padilla-Jones A, Ruha AM: Comparison of Antivenom Dosing Strategies for Rattlesnake Envenomation, *Crit Care Med* 46(6):e540–e544, 2018, https://doi.org/10.1097/CCM.0000000000003079.

Spyres MB, Padilla GK, Gerkin RD, Hoyte CO, Wolk BJ, Ruha AM: Late hemotoxicity following North American rattlesnake envenomation treated with Crotalidae immune F(ab')2 (equine) antivenom and Crotalidae immune polyvalent Fab (ovine) antivenom reported to the North American Snakebite Sub-registry, *Clin Toxicol (Phila)* 1-5, 2022https://doi.org/10.1080/15563650.2022.2042550.

Walter FG, Stolz U, Shirazi F, McNally J: Temporal analyses of coral snakebite severity published in the American Association of Poison Control Centers' Annual Reports from 1983 through 2007, *Clin Toxicol (Phila)* 48(1):72–78, 2010, https://doi.org/10.3109/15563650903430944.

Wood A, Schauben J, Thundiyil J, et al: Review of Eastern coral snake (Micrurus fulvius fulvius) exposures managed by the Florida Poison Information Center Network: 1998-2010, *Clin Toxicol (Phila)* 51(8):783–788, 2013, https://doi.org/10.3109/15563650.2013.828841.

Preventive Health

21

IMMUNIZATION PRACTICES

Method of
Beth Damitz, MD

CURRENT DIAGNOSIS

- Single-agent and polyagent variety vaccines are available in the United States.
- Vaccine-preventable diseases are occurring in the United States despite efforts.
- Vaccine registries and office-based strategies can increase vaccination rates.

CURRENT THERAPY

- Vaccination schedules are available through various sources such as the Centers for Disease Control and Prevention, including catch-up dosing.
- Vaccines can prevent diseases that are still occurring in the United States.
- Vaccination registry participation can increase vaccination rates.
- Each office visit should be used as an opportunity to review and offer vaccines.
- Providers need to be aware of special populations such as breastfeeding and pregnant women, immunosuppressed persons, and healthcare workers who could need different vaccines.

Definitions and Background

Vaccination is one of the most successful and cost-effective ways to prevent infectious diseases. Immunization is the process of inducing immunity artificially by either active immunization or passive immunization. It also occurs naturally through transplacental transmission of antibodies to a fetus, which provides protection against many infectious diseases for the first few months of life.

Physiology of Vaccines

Vaccines prevent disease in the people who receive them and protect those who come into contact with unvaccinated individuals, such as children too young to receive vaccines, those who cannot be immunized for medical reasons, and those who cannot make an adequate response to vaccination. Vaccines are preparations of proteins, polysaccharides, or nucleic acids of pathogens that are delivered to the immune system as single entities, as part of complex particles, or by live, attenuated agents to induce specific responses that inactivate, destroy, or suppress the pathogen.

Immunization Recommendations

The Advisory Committee on Immunization Practices (ACIP), sponsored by the Centers for Disease Control and Prevention (CDC) (https://www.cdc.gov/vaccines/schedules/hcp/index.html), the American Academy of Pediatrics, and the American Academy of Family Physicians work together to issue a national schedule for routinely recommended vaccinations.

They recommend routine vaccination to prevent 17 vaccine-preventable diseases that occur in infants, children, adolescents, or adults. These recommendations are reviewed and revised periodically. These immunization schedules give ranges of target ages for vaccines to be given (Figures 1–3). They include single and combination vaccine products. Catch-up dosing and schedules for special populations are also available (for updated immunization schedules see https://www.cdc.gov/vaccines/schedules/downloads/child/0-18yrs-child-combined-schedule.pdf).

Disease Prevention

Since the development of vaccines, we have seen a dramatic decrease in both cases and deaths from vaccine-preventable diseases. For example, in 1950, there were 319,124 cases and 468 deaths from measles. This dramatically decreased to 43 cases and zero deaths in 2007. Obviously, decrease in disease and death is paramount, but it is also important to decrease the cost burden to our healthcare system. For every $1 spent on measles, mumps, and rubella (MMR) vaccine, $21 is saved in direct medical costs of treating a case of measles.

COVID-19 Vaccines

COVID-19 is a respiratory disease caused by SARS-CoV-2, a virus in the coronavirus family, discovered first in China in December of 2019. It spread rapidly across the world, causing a pandemic. Pharmaceutical companies immediately pursued the development of vaccines to COVID-19. Within the next year, several vaccines were authorized for emergency use. Currently, there are three types of COVID-19 vaccine authorized for emergency use in the United States: mRNA (Pfizer-BioNTech and Moderna), protein subunit (Novavax), and viral vector vaccines (Johnson & Johnson/Janssen. As of May 6, 2023, J&J/Janssen COVID-19 vaccine has expired and is no longer available for use in the United States. Currently, four vaccines are available in the United States from these manufacturers: Pfizer-BioNTech, Moderna, Johnson & Johnson/Janssen and Novavax.

The Pfizer-BioNTech and Moderna COVID-19 vaccines are mRNA-derived vaccines. On April 18, 2023, the U.S. Food and Drug Administration (FDA) amended the emergency use authorization (EUA) of mRNA-derived COVID-19 vaccines. Only the Moderna and Pfizer-BioNTech COVID-19 bivalent vaccines (original and omicron BA.4/BA.5 strains) are authorized to be used for all doses administered to individuals 6 months of age and older. Monovalent mRNA COVID-19 vaccines (Moderna and Pfizer-BioNTech) are no longer authorized for emergency use in the United States. The CDC recommends that all persons 6 months of age and older receive at least one age-appropriate bivalent mRNA COVID-19 vaccine.

The bivalent Pfizer-BioNTech COVID-19 vaccine is authorized for use in unvaccinated children 6 months through 4 years as a three-dose primary series (at 0, 3–8, and 11–16 weeks). For individuals 5 years of age or older, the vaccine is given as a two-dose series (at 0 and 3–8 weeks). The bivalent Moderna vaccine is authorized for use in individuals 6 months of age or older as a two-dose primary series (at 0 and 4–8 weeks). For adults 65 years or older, an additional bivalent mRNA vaccine dose may be administered at least 4 months after the first dose of a bivalent mRNA vaccine.

Bivalent Pfizer-BioNTech COVID-19 vaccine:* Monovalent Pfizer-BioNTech vaccine is no longer recommended and should not be used. Vaccine type: mRNA			
Age	**Vaccination history**	**Bivalent vaccine schedule†**	**Administer**
6 months through 4 years‡§	Unvaccinated: 0 doses	3 doses. Administer: • Dose 1 now • Dose 2 at least 3–8 weeks¶ after Dose 1 • Dose 3 at least 8 weeks (2 months) after Dose 2	0.2 mL/3 µg from the vial with a maroon cap
	1 dose of bivalent vaccine	2 doses. Administer: • Dose 2 at least 3–8 weeks¶ after Dose 1 • Dose 3 at least 8 weeks (2 months) after Dose 2	
	2 doses of bivalent vaccine	1 dose. Administer: • Dose 3 at least 8 weeks (2 months) after Dose 2	
	At least 3 doses of bivalent vaccine	No dose	No dose
	Previously vaccinated with monovalent mRNA COVID-19 vaccine		
	1 dose of monovalent vaccine	2 doses. Administer: • Dose 2 at least 3–8 weeks¶ after Dose 1 • Dose 3 at least 8 weeks (2 months) after Dose 2	0.2 mL/3 µg from the vial with a maroon cap
	2 doses of monovalent vaccine	1 dose. Administer: • Dose 3 at least 8 weeks (2 months) after Dose 2	
	3 doses of monovalent vaccine	1 dose. Administer: • Dose 4 at least 8 weeks (2 months) after Dose 3.	
	At least 2 doses of monovalent vaccine and 1 dose of bivalent vaccine	No dose	No dose.
5 years and older‡	Unvaccinated: 0 doses	1 dose now**	**5 through 11 years:** 0.2 mL/10 µg from the vial with an orange cap **12 years and older:** 0.3 mL/30 µg from the vial with a gray cap
	1 dose or more doses of monovalent vaccine§	1 dose. Administer: • Vaccine at least 8 weeks (2 months) after the previous dose**	
	At least 1 dose of bivalent vaccine	No dose**	No dose**

* Refer to CDC's Interim Clinical Considerations for specific guidance on children who turn from 4 to 5 years of age before completing the vaccination series with Pfizer-BioNTech COVID-19 Vaccine and interchangeability of vaccine products for all ages.

† Persons with a recent SARS-CoV-2 infection may consider delaying vaccination by 3 months from symptom onset or positive test (if infection was asymptomatic).

‡ CDC recommends bivalent vaccine doses from the same manufacturer for children 6 months through 5 years of age who are unvaccinated (no previous doses of COVID-19 vaccine) if more than 1 dose is recommended. In the following exceptional situations, a different age-appropriate COVID-19 vaccine may be administered when FDA authorization requires that a vaccine from the same manufacturer be used and a VAERS report is not required: Same vaccine not available; or previous dose unknown; or person would otherwise not complete the vaccination series; or person starts but unable to complete a vaccination series with the same COVID-19 vaccine due to a contraindication

§ Children ages 6 months through 4 years who received bivalent vaccines from different manufacturers for the first 2 doses of an mRNA COVID-19 vaccine series should follow a 3-dose schedule. A third dose of either mRNA vaccine (Moderna or Pfizer-BioNTech) should be administered at least 8 weeks after the second dose.

¶ An 8-week interval between the first and second doses of COVID-19 vaccines might be optimal for some people ages 6 months–64 years, especially for males ages 12–39 years, as it may reduce the small risk of myocarditis and pericarditis associated with these vaccines.

** Adults 65 years of age and older: May receive 1 additional bivalent mRNA vaccine dose at least 4 months after the first dose of a bivalent mRNA vaccine.

Figure 5 Pfizer-BioNTech COVID vaccine interim immunization schedule for persons aged 6 months and older.

date the vaccine was administered, the vaccine manufacturer, the vaccine lot number, and the name, address, and title of the person administering the vaccine. In addition, the provider is required to record the edition date of the VIS distributed and the date those materials were provided. Patients should also keep a record of the immunizations their children receive, when they were received, and at what facility they received them. A permanent vaccination record card should be established for each newborn infant and maintained by the parent or guardian.

Immunization information systems (IIS), formerly referred to as immunization registries, are confidential population-based computerized information systems that collect and consolidate vaccination data from multiple healthcare providers within a geographic area. The CDC oversees a network of 64 IIS programs distributed throughout all 50 states, the District of Columbia, and eight U.S. territories. A fully operational IIS can prevent duplicate vaccinations, provide a complete record of immunizations if the patient has received vaccines from multiple sites, and offer catch-up and needed vaccine information. Although participation of a provider is voluntary, it is highly encouraged.

Special Populations
Children

Although infants are born with some level of immunoglobulin (Ig)G that is contributed from the mother via passive immunity, these levels decrease by 9 months of age, leaving them vulnerable to many infectious diseases. Infants begin developing IgG shortly after birth; these levels continue to increase throughout the first year of life, but children remain susceptible to infection until they achieve adult levels of IgG at 10 years of age. Therefore this age group is especially important to vaccinate.

Breastfeeding

Neither inactivated nor live virus vaccines administered to a lactating woman affect the safety of breastfeeding for women or their infants. Breastfeeding is a contraindication for smallpox vaccination of the mother because of the theoretical risk for contact transmission from mother to infant. Yellow fever vaccine should be avoided. Breastfed infants should be vaccinated according to the recommended schedule.

Pregnancy

No evidence exists of risk to the fetus from vaccinating pregnant women with inactivated virus or bacterial vaccines or toxoids. Live vaccines, such as smallpox, MMR, and varicella (Varivax), pose a theoretical risk to the fetus and therefore are contraindicated during pregnancy. New recommendations from ACIP advise to give all pregnant women a Tdap vaccine during every pregnancy. New data indicate that maternal antipertussis antibodies are short-lived; therefore Tdap vaccination in one pregnancy will not provide high levels of antibodies to protect newborns during subsequent pregnancies. Alternatively, if Tdap is not administered during pregnancy, the woman should receive a dose of Tdap as soon as possible after delivery to ensure pertussis immunity and reduce the risk for transmission to the newborn regardless of when she last received a tetanus booster. Routine influenza vaccination is recommended for all women who are or will be pregnant (in any trimester) during influenza season, which usually occurs early October through late March. The live attenuated influenza vaccine (LAIV4) should be avoided because it is contraindicated in pregnancy.

Altered Immunocompetence

Persons with altered immunocompetence include those with primary and secondary causes of immunodeficiency, as well as those with asplenia, chronic kidney disease, treatments with therapeutic monoclonal antibodies, and prolonged administration of high-dose corticosteroids. In general, this population should receive inactivated influenza virus (Afluria, Fluad, Fluarix, Fluzone) and age-appropriate polysaccharide-based vaccines (PCV [Prevnar], PPSV [Pneumovax 23], meningococcal conjugate [MCV4, Menactra], meningococcal polysaccharide [MPSV4, Menomune], and *Haemophilus* B conjugate [Hib, ActHIB, PedvaxHIB]). Persons with most forms of altered immunocompetence should not receive live vaccines (MMR, varicella, MMRV [ProQuad], LAIV, zoster [Zostavax], yellow fever, oral typhoid, BCG, and rotavirus).

Healthcare Personnel

Healthcare personnel are at substantial risk for acquiring or transmitting hepatitis B, influenza, measles, mumps, rubella, pertussis, and varicella and should be counseled on appropriate vaccinations.

◼ TRAVEL MEDICINE

Method of
Matthew Lambert, MD; and Dawd S. Siraj, MD, MPH, TM

The affordability and ease of cross-border travel combined with the growing world population is increasing the number of individuals traveling internationally. According to the United Nations World Tourism Organization (UNWTO), the number of arriving international tourists in 2018 in all countries exceeded 1.4 billion individuals, and the number of arrivals to countries with emerging markets has surpassed the number of arrivals to developed countries (UNWTO; https://www.e-unwto.org/doi/pdf/10.18111/9789284419876). This increase in international

travel has created a need for the specialty of travel medicine, which focuses on the unique and location-dependent health-related needs of travelers.

An estimated 22% to 64% of travelers report some type of illness while abroad. Most of these illnesses are mild and self-limiting, requiring minimal intervention. Approximately 4% of travelers who seek medical help have an acute, potentially life-threatening disease, and about 1 in 100,000 of these travelers die from complications related to their travel.

The goal of a travel medicine visit is to maximize health and prevent illness while traveling by offering travelers specific structured advice, malaria prophylaxis, and immunization recommendations. Disease risks, current outbreaks, and local health conditions are destination dependent and constantly change; thus the use of current, up-to-date resources is essential for providing travel medicine care (Table 1). Unfortunately, 20% to 80% of international travelers do not undergo a health consultation or receive location-specific pretravel advice before traveling. Travelers visiting friends and relatives in their country of origin, pregnant mothers, children, and travelers who are staying abroad for a long period are at particularly high risk for morbidity and mortality during their trip, requiring special attention to pretravel medical planning. Ideally, pretravel health consultations should take place 4 to 6 weeks before departure to give travelers adequate time to complete the required vaccination series. Pretravel health consultations should be structured and comprehensive. Table 2 lists items that require consideration and discussion during the consultation according to the type of travel and destination. Patients should arrive to their consultation with documentation of their vaccination history. A useful travel history form is available on the Shoreland Travax website (www.travax.com).

Vaccinations

Travel clinics often provide travelers the opportunity to update routine vaccinations that they missed. Additionally, travel medicine provides vaccinations that are recommended or required because of country-specific or ongoing outbreak-specific risks. When deciding which vaccination to recommend, several factors must be considered, including any specific potential risks associated with the travel itinerary, length of stay, and activities. For each vaccine-preventable disease (VPD), one should consider the prevalence and impact of the disease in question.

Routine Vaccines

Routine vaccines are those that are administered at a regular interval for all individuals regardless of travel plans. As the risk of acquisition of these diseases increases during international travel, travel medicine providers should confirm that travelers are up to date on their routine vaccinations before departure. The recent importation of diseases such as measles and mumps, which has resulted in outbreaks of these diseases in the travelers' country of origin, are reminders of the importance of updating routine vaccinations before travel. Travelers are advised to bring documentation of all prior vaccinations to confirm vaccination status and determine the need for booster doses.

Measles-Mumps-Rubella Vaccine

Measles remains a serious cause of morbidity and mortality in the non-Western world. Importation of measles by unvaccinated travelers from regions that report endemic disease, such as Europe, Africa, and parts of Asia, remains a concern for countries where disease transmission has been interrupted (like the Americas). Indeed, several cases have been associated with exposure during air travel itself. All travelers born after 1957 (United States) and 1970 (Canada and the United Kingdom) must have two documented vaccinations or evidence of immunity as confirmed by antibody titer. Infants who are 6 to 11 months of age and are traveling to a measles-endemic area should be given one dose of measles-mumps-rubella (MMR) vaccine before departure. Individuals who have no documented vaccination and a negative antibody titer should receive two doses of MMR vaccine at least

TABLE 1 Information Resources for Risk Assessment of Travel

Centers for Disease Control and Prevention	Comprehensive travel reports and travel vaccination and preparation information including the Yellow Book with information on country-specific risks and travel advice	www.cdc.gov/travel/
Travax (Shoreland)	Commercial software–generated reports combining itinerary-specific recommendations on recommended travel vaccines and risks. Requires a fee.	www.shoreland.com
U.S. Department of State	Travel warnings	https://travel.state.gov/content/passports/en/alertswarnings.html
World Health Organization	General travel health information and access to its international travel guide and alerts	www.who.int/ith/en/

TABLE 2 Checklist of Items to Address in the Pretravel Consultation

CATEGORY	ISSUES THAT SHOULD BE ADDRESSED
Patient risk assessment	Obtain history: itinerary, type of travel, personal medical history, age, underlying diseases, allergies, current medications, pregnancy status, previous vaccination status
Immunizations	Update routine immunizations Provide routine travel immunizations Provide destination-specific immunizations
Malaria prophylaxis	If indicated: Provide malaria education and advice; discuss bite-avoidance measures Prescribe antimalaria prophylaxis
Traveler's diarrhea	Prescribe oral rehydration therapy and loperamide (Imodium) 4 mg initially and 2 mg after each loose stool, not to exceed 16 mg/day Prescribe appropriate antibiotic (see Table 4)
Prevention against mosquito bites	Give advice regarding mosquito-borne disease Discuss personal protection measures
Rabies prevention	Give advice regarding behavior near animals Discuss measures to take if bitten or scratched by an animal—seek urgent medical advice Administer vaccine when indicated
Altitude sickness	Provide education Prescribe acetazolamide (Diamox) 125 mg orally twice a day for 1 day before ascent and continuing for 2 to 3 days on arrival at maximum altitude
Prevention of sexually transmitted diseases	Provide education regarding safe sex
Zika virus	Discuss potential risk of congenital Zika syndrome for pregnant women or women/men planning to conceive after return from an endemic area
Others	Deep venous thrombosis prevention Accident prevention Motion sickness prevention

Some of the recommendations are indicated only for specific destinations or specific at-risk groups.

4 weeks apart. Those who have two documented doses are considered immune for at least 20 years.

Poliovirus Vaccine

As a result of successful efforts to eradicate poliomyelitis, most of the world is now polio free. As of 2019, a few developing countries, particularly Afghanistan and Pakistan, have reported endemic wild-type poliovirus (WPV) outbreaks. In addition, as of February 2022, a small number of developing countries continue to report cases of circulating vaccine-derived poliovirus (cVDPV; www.polioeradication.org).

The injectable, inactivated poliovirus vaccine (IPV, IPOL) is the only polio vaccine available in the United States. All children must have four doses of IPV. Travelers who are traveling to countries with WPV or cVDPV and who have completed the age-appropriate series are recommended to receive a single lifetime adult booster dose before travel. The recommendation also applies to travelers to bordering countries and those who have a high risk of exposure, such as individuals working in healthcare, refugee camps, or humanitarian aid settings (U.S. Centers for Disease Control and Prevention [CDC] health information for international travel, 2019). As the list of countries with WPV or VDPV circulation and recommendations for vaccine is dynamic, providers are encouraged to refer to the CDC's Travelers' Health web page (https://wwwnc.cdc.gov/travel) for up-to-date advice.

A small number of countries require proof of polio vaccination upon entry or before departure, thus administration should be documented on a vaccination certificate.

Tetanus-Diphtheria-Pertussis Vaccine

Unvaccinated or inadequately vaccinated travelers are at risk of contracting diphtheria in developing countries, as well as tetanus and pertussis anywhere in the world. The potential risk of exposure to pertussis is worldwide, with the highest rates of disease in developing countries where vaccine coverage is low. In recent decades, countries with high vaccination rates, including the United States, have seen a resurgence of pertussis despite adequate vaccination programs. Immunity from natural disease or childhood vaccination wanes over time, thus adolescent and adult travelers who have completed their childhood series should receive a booster dose of tetanus-diphtheria-pertussis (Tdap) vaccine (Adacel, Boostrix). Once one documented Tdap booster is given, a subsequent booster can be a tetanus-diphtheria (Td) or Tdap vaccine. If more than 5 years have elapsed since the last booster dose, a tetanus-containing booster should be considered for persons going to remote areas where tetanus boosters may not be readily available after a contaminated trauma.

Varicella Vaccine
Varicella infection remains prevalent worldwide. Infection can occur via inhalation of aerosols or contact of vesicular fluid from a skin lesion. Exposure to active herpes zoster lesions poses a risk of varicella infection to a susceptible traveler. In children, disease is generally mild and self-limiting. However, serious complications can occur in infants, adults, and immunocompromised individuals. Travelers who have not completed age-appropriate vaccination or do not have laboratory evidence of immunity should receive the varicella vaccination (Varivax) before travel. Those older than 13 years of age should receive two doses at least 4 weeks apart.

Influenza Vaccine
Influenza is the most common VPD among travelers. Travelers 6 months of age and older should receive the most up-to-date influenza vaccine available in their countries annually if they are traveling to an area where influenza is circulating at the time of their travel (year-round in tropical and subtropical areas and winter months in temperate areas). Travelers who are 65 years of age and older should receive the high-dose influenza vaccine (Fluzone High-Dose) to elicit higher levels of antibody response.

Pneumococcal Vaccine
The prevalence of pneumococcal disease is highest in developing countries. In 2022, the Advisory Committee on Immunization Practices of the CDC recommended administration of pneumococcal conjugate vaccine (PCV15; Vaxneuvance) to all individuals 65 years of age and older who did not receive a pneumococcal vaccine in the past, followed by a dose of pneumococcal polysaccharide vaccine (PPSV23; Pneumovax) given 1 or more years later for immunocompetent patients and 8 or more weeks later for immunocompromised patients. Another alternative is for travelers to get PCV20 once without the need for a follow-up PPSV23.

Recommended Travel Vaccines
Hepatitis A Vaccine
Hepatitis A viral infection is transmitted through ingestion of contaminated food or water. The virus remains viable in ice and frozen foods. Travelers who visit rural areas, trek in the back country, and often eat in a poor sanitary environment are at high risk of hepatitis A infection. Among men who have sex with men, outbreaks have been reported when traveling to endemic areas. Hepatitis A vaccination is recommended for travel to any developing country and some industrialized countries where sanitary conditions are variable.

Two hepatitis A vaccine preparations are available (Havrix, Vaqta), which are approved for administration in those 12 months of age and older. For infants traveling to high-risk endemic countries, vaccination is recommended for all children older than 6 months of age. A combination of hepatitis A and B vaccines (Twinrix) is also available and is approved for travelers 18 years of age and older. For those who are traveling on short notice, an accelerated schedule is approved. A single dose of hepatitis A vaccine given any time before travel will provide adequate protection in an immunocompetent traveler. A booster dose given 6 to 12 months after the first dose will ensure lifetime protection. Infants who received one dose before travel should receive two more doses of the vaccine for long-term protection. Immunoglobulin for hepatitis A virus prophylaxis (GamaSTAN

S/D), which can be administered to travelers who are not immune and will be traveling in less than 2 weeks, is rarely recommended considering the immunogenicity of the vaccine and long incubation period of hepatitis A. A study comparing hepatitis A vaccine with immunoglobulin to prevent postexposure hepatitis A infection did not show a difference between the two, suggesting the efficacy of the vaccine as an alternate considering its ease and safety compared with immunoglobulin.

Typhoid Vaccine
Although hepatitis A and typhoid fever are both transmitted through ingestion of contaminated food and water, hepatitis A is 100 times more common than typhoid fever in travelers. The Indian subcontinent seems to be a key focus of typhoid fever in travelers, accounting for more than 80% of travel-related typhoid cases in the United States. The efficacy of typhoid vaccines ranges from 50% to 80% in various published studies.

The typhoid vaccine is protective against *Salmonella enterica* serotype typhi, but not against paratyphoid fever, which is caused by strains of *S. enterica* paratyphi A, B, and C. The typhoid vaccine is recommended for long-term travelers to developing countries, short-term travelers to South Asia, and high-risk travelers to other destinations, such as individuals visiting friends and relatives in their country of origin and food adventurers.

Two unconjugated vaccines are available in the United States: the oral live, attenuated typhoid vaccine (Ty21A, Vivotif Berna), which is approved for all travelers older than 6 years of age, and the injectable typhoid Vi polysaccharide vaccine (Typhim Vi) for those older than 2 years of age. The oral vaccine, which consists of four capsules (one taken every other day), is protective for 5 years, whereas the injectable vaccine is only effective for 2 years. Ideally, either vaccine should be given at least 2 weeks before departure.

Hepatitis B Vaccine
The hepatitis B virus (HBV) is endemic worldwide, with a high prevalence in Asia and sub-Saharan Africa. Infection is transmitted through contact with blood, blood products, and body fluids and therefore poses a limited risk to most travelers; however, healthcare professionals traveling to endemic areas are at high risk.

Travelers should be counseled on HBV transmission and minimizing exposure. All patients who are traveling to intermediate- to high-prevalence countries (>2% prevalence of HBV surface antigen) should receive the vaccination. The vaccines (Engerix-B, Recombivax HB, Twinrix [hepatitis A and hepatitis B vaccine]) are approved as a series of three doses given at day 0, 1 month, and 6 months. For those traveling on short notice, Twinrix is approved for an accelerated schedule of day 0, 7, and 21 to 30 days. For long-term immunity, a booster dose of Twinrix is recommended at 12 months. Two doses of this regimen completed in a 1-week interval provides adequate immediate protection for travel. A new conjugate (adjuvanted) vaccine (Heplisav-B) with two doses 1 month apart has been approved for all travelers 18 years of age and older. Protective immunity of Heplisav-B is robust, with over 95% of those who complete the series achieving immunity, and it will likely replace the vaccines that are currently available.

Cholera Vaccine
Most cases of cholera are reported from sub-Saharan Africa, Asia, and the island of Hispaniola (Haiti and the Dominican Republic). The risk of cholera to an average traveler is extremely low. The vaccine is indicated for emergency relief workers, healthcare workers traveling to an endemic area, and travelers going to an area with a declared outbreak. The vaccine is not required for entry to any country. In 2016, a single dose, oral, live-attenuated vaccine (Vaxchora) was approved for adults older than 18 years of age.

Japanese Encephalitis Vaccine
Japanese encephalitis (JE) is a mosquito-borne neurologic disease endemic to China, Korea, the Indian subcontinent, Southeast

Asia, and the Western Pacific. The risk varies according to destination, length of stay, season, and activities being undertaken. In early 2022, an outbreak of JE was reported from rural areas of Australia. The risk is highest for travelers to rural areas, especially with nighttime outdoor activities. The overall incidence of JE cases among persons from nonendemic countries traveling to Asia is estimated to be less than 1 per 1 million, though this could be much higher depending on the type, time, and duration of travel. Though less than 1% of those infected develop neurologic illness, the sequela from such infection is devastating. Among those who develop encephalitis, 20% to 30% die and 30% to 50% of the survivors exhibit long-term neurologic symptoms. Vaccination should be considered for all frequent travelers and those who are planning to stay longer than 1 month in an endemic country.

An inactivated, cell culture–derived vaccine (IXIARO) is licensed in the United States for use in individuals 2 months of age and older. Children 2 months to 2 years of age are given one-half the dose used for adults. The vaccine is given as a two-dose series at 0 and 28 days. An accelerated vaccination schedule of two doses 1 week apart has been approved for travelers who do not have enough time to complete the series before departure.

Rabies Vaccine

Rabies is a fatal viral infection that is transmitted through exposure to saliva of a rabid animal. The virus is neurotropic and results in progressive encephalomyelitis that is often fatal. It has a worldwide distribution with the highest prevalence in Asia, Africa, and South and Central America. Dog bites remain the primary source of infection, though bat exposure is increasingly identified as a common risk factor for disease acquisition. There were 66 cases of rabies documented in travelers from 1990 to 2013 (40% from Asia and 85% after canine exposure). Animal bites are common during travel. Approximately 2700 travelers received care for animal-related exposures and required rabies postexposure prophylaxis at GeoSentinel clinics during a 15-year period (1997 to 2012). Clinical illness follows a variable incubation period ranging from days to months from exposure. Early symptoms include pain and paresthesia at the site of the bite, which is invariably followed by paresis, paralysis, and fatal encephalitis. Hydrophobia, delirium, and convulsions are classic presentations that often are followed by coma and death. Symptomatic and supportive care, including aggressive wound care and postexposure prophylaxis, may improve survival in patients with this uniformly fatal disease.

Veterinarians, animal handlers, field biologists, laboratory workers who handle animals, and children are at high risk and recommended to receive the preexposure vaccination.

In the event of an exposure, vaccinated individuals require two additional doses of vaccine 3 days apart, whereas unvaccinated travelers require four doses of vaccine and additional human rabies immune globulin (HRIG [HyperRab, Imogam Rabies]), which may be expensive, unavailable, or unreliable in the traveler's locale. In light of the devastating consequences of rabies, the fact that animal bites, scratches, or licks over mucous membranes are common among travelers, even during short trips; the difficulties in receiving rabies immune globulin in the developing world; and the fact that a one-time preexposure vaccination course is likely protective "for life" suggest that the threshold for recommending rabies vaccination to travelers to the developing world should be low.

A two-dose preexposure rabies vaccine (Imovax Rabies, RabAvert) has replaced the old three-dose vaccine and is protective for up to 3 years. High-risk individuals should have their rabies titer checked every 6 months to maintain adequate protection.

Tick-Borne Encephalitis Vaccine

Tick-borne encephalitis (TBE) is an arboviral zoonosis transmitted primarily through the bite of *Ixodes* species ticks. It is endemic in many popular tourist destinations in Europe, Eastern Europe, and parts of Asia including China, Japan, Russia, and Siberia. Symptoms include fever, body aches, headache, and arthralgia. Up to 20% to 30% of individuals who are infected will develop encephalitis. Human infections are usually seen in the spring and summer months in temperate zones and in the fall and winter months in the Mediterranean region. A TBE vaccine (TicoVac) is available in Europe, Canada, and now the United States and is considered immunogenic and safe. Vaccination is recommended for travelers with extensive outdoor exposures such as camping in endemic regions during the transmission season. TicoVac is approved by the U.S. Food and Drug Administration (FDA) for 1 year and older travelers. The primary vaccine is a three-dose series that takes a minimum of 5 months to finish the series. In addition, travelers should be advised to use insect repellents and avoid tick bites to protect themselves from tick-borne encephalitis.

Required Vaccines

Yellow Fever Vaccine

Yellow fever (YF) is a mosquito-borne disease endemic to parts of sub-Saharan Africa and tropical South America. Though most patients with YF are asymptomatic, about 15% develop severe disease, with a reported case fatality rate of 20% to 60%. The YF vaccine (YF-VAX) is a live-attenuated vaccine that travelers should receive at least 10 days before arriving to an endemic country. A large YF outbreak was documented in eastern Brazil in 2016 to 2018, which expanded the previously known endemic area within Brazil. The World Health Organization (WHO) and the CDC are now recommending YF vaccination for all travelers to Brazil except for a few sites around Recife. There has been an ongoing outbreak of YF in parts of Nigeria, and the CDC recommends vaccination to everyone traveling to Nigeria. The risk of a traveler acquiring YF varies with season, location, activities, and duration of travel. Since January 2018, 10 travel-related cases of YF, including 4 deaths, have been reported in travelers returning from Brazil. None of the 10 travelers received the YF vaccination before their travel.

Vaccination is recommended for personal protection of travelers to endemic areas. In addition, under WHO rules, any given country may routinely require YF vaccination for entry into its territory. The aim of the regulation is to protect countries that have the mosquito vector from reintroduction of YF by asymptomatic viremic travelers.

The yellow fever vaccine (YF-VAX) is rarely associated with severe and fatal adverse reactions, which generally follow the first dose. The overall rate of serious adverse reaction is about 1 event per 250,000 doses. The likelihood of serious adverse events increases with age, with patients older than 60 years of age having a much higher risk for a severe adverse reaction.

A change in the International Health Regulations in July 2016 now considers a valid YF vaccination to be effective for life, with no need for booster vaccination at 10-year intervals. This also applies retroactively to YF vaccinations given any time before 2016. The new policy extends the validity of the vaccination for personal protection, with no need for booster doses among healthy, immunocompetent individuals. Per this recommendation, countries cannot require proof of vaccination (booster) against YF as a condition of entry to travelers whose YF vaccination was over 10 years prior. A booster vaccine after 10 years is still recommended for specific high-risk individuals: long-term travelers, travelers to West Africa, and travelers to an area where there is a current outbreak. Travel clinics should confirm the requirements of each country when they advise travelers.

Meningococcal Vaccine

Meningitis is caused by the bacteria *Neisseria meningitidis*. It is acquired by exposure to nasopharyngeal droplets during close contact. The disease spectrum ranges from fever and bacteremia to meningitis. There are eight serogroups of meningococci, but most travel-related diseases are caused by the A, C, X, and W135 serogroups. Disease is endemic worldwide, but the highest risk area is the sub-Saharan region, which is loosely named the *meningitis belt.* There is seasonality to disease incidence, with seasonal epidemics occurring during the dry season (December to June).

Meningococcal disease is rare in travelers (1:100,000 to <1:1,000,000 per month of travel). A quadrivalent conjugated vaccine that protects against serogroups A, C, Y, and W135 (Menactra, Menveo, MenQuadfi, and Nimenrix[2]) is recommended for travelers to endemic areas. Travelers to countries in the meningitis belt who anticipate close contact with crowds or the local population, as well as aid workers in refugee camps are considered at high risk and are recommended to receive the vaccine before travel. Vaccination is required for entry to Saudi Arabia during the Hajj or Umrah seasons. Travelers returning to Saudi Arabia or high-risk zones should receive a booster vaccination every 5 years.

Malaria

Reports of malaria cases in the United States have been steadily increasing over the past few decades, largely due to infection in travelers to geographic areas with ongoing malaria transmission. Over half of the cases reported (59.3%) had a travel history to West Africa. In 2018, there were 1823 cases of malaria reported in the United States. Only 24.5% of U.S. residents who developed malaria that year reported taking any malaria prophylaxis, and 95% did not complete an appropriate chemoprophylactic regimen. Of those who reported a reason for travel, most cases were in travelers visiting friends and relatives (77%) (source: https://www.cdc.gov/mmwr/volumes/71/ss/ss7108a1.htm).

Before travel, a risk assessment should be performed to determine if malaria chemoprophylaxis is indicated. Malaria transmission can vary greatly, even within a country, based on the region and season of travel. The traveler's specific itinerary should be reviewed for the cities visited, type of accommodations (bed nets, window screens, air conditioning), reason for travel, and special activities while traveling. Mosquito avoidance measures should be recommended in addition to chemoprophylaxis. Up-to-date travel notices and advisories specific to the destination of travel may be found on the CDC website (https://wwwnc.cdc.gov/travel).

The life cycle of malaria in humans involves an initial asymptomatic liver stage followed by a later symptomatic erythrocytic stage. Malaria chemoprophylaxis is used to prevent the development of clinical malaria if a person is infected. Certain chemoprophylactic agents (chloroquine [Aralen], mefloquine [Lariam], and doxycycline [Vibramycin]) only work on the later erythrocytic stage of malaria parasites and are therefore recommended to be taken for a longer time (4 weeks) after leaving a malaria-endemic area. Atovaquone-proguanil (Malarone) can act on the earlier nondormant liver parasite stage; therefore a shorter posttravel duration is recommended (1 week). Unlike other *Plasmodium* species, *Plasmodium vivax* and *Plasmodium ovale* have dormant liver stages known as *hypnozoites,* which are responsible for disease relapse with these species months or years after an acute infection. Tafenoquine (Arakoda) and primaquine[1] are the only available chemoprophylactic medications effective against all liver stages of the malaria parasite, including the liver hypnozoites of *P. vivax* and *P. ovale.*

Malaria Chemoprophylaxis

All malaria chemoprophylactic options should be started before travel, taken throughout travel, and continued for a period posttravel (Table 3). When choosing a chemoprophylactic agent, factors to consider include the traveler's age and medical history, pregnancy status, length of the trip, cost of the drug, drug allergies, drug interactions, and drug resistance at the destination. Up-to-date information regarding local drug resistance in areas of planned travel can be found on the CDC website (https://wwwnc.cdc.gov/travel).

Chloroquine (Aralen) may only be used for malaria prophylaxis in areas of the world with chloroquine-sensitive *Plasmodium falciparum.* Resistance is found worldwide except in Central America west of the Panama Canal, Haiti, and the Dominican Republic, where *P. vivax* is the dominant species. Chloroquine is used once a week for prophylaxis. It should be started 1 to 2 weeks before travel, taken weekly during travel, and continued for 4 weeks after leaving the malaria zone. The most common side effects are gastrointestinal discomfort, nausea, vomiting, or headache. Serious adverse effects are rare and are more likely to occur with prolonged and high doses of therapy. Retinopathy is associated with high doses and when used for more than 5 years. An overdose of chloroquine could be fatal, and the medication

[2] Not available in the United States.

[1] Not FDA approved for this indication.

TABLE 3	Medication Options for Chemoprophylaxis of Malaria		
DRUG	**USE IN PROPHYLAXIS**	**ADULT DOSE**	**LENGTH OF TREATMENT**
Chloroquine	Areas with chloroquine-sensitive *Plasmodium falciparum*	500 mg (300 mg base) weekly	Start 1 to 2 weeks before exposure. Continue weekly while in the malaria zone and for 4 weeks after leaving
Mefloquine (Lariam)	Areas with mefloquine-sensitive *P. falciparum*	250 mg weekly	Start ≥2 weeks before exposure. Continue weekly while in the malaria zone and for 4 weeks after leaving
Atovaquone-proguanil (Malarone)	All malaria zones	250 mg/100 mg once daily	Start 1 to 2 days before exposure. Continue daily while in the malaria zone and for 7 days after leaving
Doxycycline	All malaria zones	100 mg daily	Start 1 to 2 days before exposure. Continue daily while in the malaria zone and for 4 weeks after leaving
Tafenoquine (Arakoda)	All malaria zones	200 mg	A loading dose is 200 mg taken daily for 3 days before exposure. Then continue 200 mg weekly while in the malaria zone and for 1 week after leaving
Primaquine[1]	Areas with >90% *P. vivax*	30 mg base daily	Start 1 to 2 days before exposure. Continue daily while in the malaria zone and for 7 days after leaving

[1] Not FDA approved for this indication.

should be stored in childproof containers. If a traveler is already taking hydroxychloroquine (Plaquenil) chronically for a rheumatologic condition, they may not have to take additional malaria prophylaxis.

Four potential options are approved by the FDA for malaria chemoprophylaxis in areas with chloroquine-resistant malaria: atovaquone/proguanil (Malarone), doxycycline (Vibramycin), mefloquine (Lariam), and tafenoquine (Arakoda). Primaquine may be used off-label (not FDA approved) for malaria chemoprophylaxis in areas of the world with predominantly *P. vivax* malaria.

Mefloquine should only be used for malaria prophylaxis in areas of the world with mefloquine-sensitive *P. falciparum*. Mefloquine-resistant *P. falciparum* malaria is found in parts of Southeast Asia (along the borders of Thailand with Cambodia and Burma, western Cambodia, eastern Burma, and southern Vietnam), and mefloquine should not be used for malaria prophylaxis in these areas. Mefloquine is used once a week for prophylaxis. It should be started 2 or more weeks before travel, taken weekly during travel, and continued for 4 weeks after leaving the malaria zone. Adverse effects tend to be noted within the first weeks of mefloquine initiation; therefore the medication can be started 2 to 4 weeks before travel to ensure that it will be tolerated during travel. Mefloquine may be associated with sleep disturbances, strange dreams, and insomnia. The FDA also has issued a black-box warning that mefloquine may cause neuropsychiatric adverse effects that can persist after the medication has been discontinued. Mefloquine is contraindicated in those with neurologic and psychiatric disorders and should be avoided in travelers with a significant family history of seizures or major psychiatric disorders. It is also recommended to avoid mefloquine in travelers with cardiac conduction abnormalities. A traveler who is prescribed mefloquine must receive a copy of the FDA medication guide for mefloquine, which can be found online (www.accessdata.fda.gov/drugsatfda_docs/label/2008/019591s023lbl.pdf).

Atovaquone-proguanil can be used for malaria prophylaxis in any malaria zone worldwide. Atovaquone-proguanil is a daily prophylactic drug. It should be started 1 to 2 days before travel, taken daily during travel, and continued for 7 days after leaving a malaria zone. The drug is usually well tolerated, with the most common adverse effect being gastrointestinal upset.

Doxycycline can be used for malaria prophylaxis in any malaria zone worldwide. Doxycycline is a daily prophylactic drug. It should be started 1 to 2 days before travel, taken daily during travel, and continued for 4 weeks after leaving a malaria zone. An added benefit of doxycycline is that it may also provide some protection against rickettsial infections and leptospirosis. However, photosensitivity is a common adverse effect of doxycycline. Patients should also be forewarned about the possibility of pill esophagitis with this medication.

Tafenoquine (Arakoda) can be used for malaria prophylaxis in any malaria zone worldwide. Tafenoquine is used once a week for prophylaxis. It should be started 1 to 2 weeks before travel, taken weekly during travel, and continued for 1 week after leaving the malaria zone. G6PD deficiency must be ruled out by laboratory testing before prescribing this medication because fatal hemolysis could occur in individuals with G6PD deficiency. Tafenoquine should be avoided in those with a history of a psychotic disorder because rare psychiatric events have been observed. The most common adverse events include nonsignificant decreases in hemoglobin, gastrointestinal discomfort, and headache. Tafenoquine is the only FDA-approved medication for malaria prophylaxis that has activity on the hypnozoite stage of the malaria parasite. Note that another tafenoquine-based antimalarial (Krintafel) is approved for radical cure of *P. vivax* infections in those older than 16 years of age.

Primaquine is very effective against *P. vivax* and is an option for travel to areas with greater than 90% *P. vivax* malaria.[1] It is taken daily starting 1 to 2 days before exposure. It is continued daily while in the malaria zone and until 7 days after leaving. It cannot be used in those with G6PD deficiency and may cause gastrointestinal upset.

Posttravel
No prophylaxis is 100% effective. Travelers should be advised to seek medical attention during travel if malaria symptoms occur. They should also be told to notify their physician of their travel history if they develop a febrile illness for up to 1 year posttravel.

COVID-19
Since COVID-19 was identified in late 2019, there have been more than 750 million confirmed cases worldwide with almost 7 million deaths (source: https://covid19.who.int/). Travel requirements during this time have been frequently revised. As of April 30, 2023, the CDC no longer requires air passengers traveling from a foreign country to the United States to show a negative COVID-19 viral test or documentation of recovery from COVID-19 before boarding their flight. All non-immigrant, non–U.S. citizen air travelers to the United States are required to be fully vaccinated and to provide proof of vaccination status before boarding, with limited exceptions. As of April 27, 2023, the CDC updated the list of accepted vaccine series; it can be found at https://www.cdc.gov/coronavirus/2019-ncov/travelers/proof-of-vaccination.html. Any of the accepted vaccine series must be completed at least 2 weeks, or 14 days, before traveling, for a traveler to qualify as fully vaccinated. Proof of vaccination records must include at least two personal identifiers matching the traveler's passport or other documents, the name of the official source issuing the records, and the vaccine manufacturer and date(s) of vaccination. The CDC continues to recommend, but not require, masks during public transportation and at transportation hubs.

Travelers to other countries should also be aware of travel health notices and arrival restrictions at their destination. Persons should not travel if they are sick or experiencing symptoms, have recently been exposed to COVID-19 and are recommended to isolate by current CDC guidance, or have recently tested positive for COVID-19 and are within the isolation period recommended by current CDC guidance. Asymptomatic persons who recently tested positive for COVID-19 and persons recently exposed to COVID-19, who are not recommended to isolate by CDC guidance, should only travel if they are willing and able to wear a high-quality, well-fitted mask during travel. More information on international travel during COVID-19 can be found on the CDC Travel Recommendations by Destination website (https://www.cdc.gov/coronavirus/2019-ncov/travelers/map-and-travel-notices.html).

Personal Protection Measures
Risk for vector-borne disease depends on many factors, including the traveler's destination, season of travel, and length of stay. Viral diseases that may be of concern include JE, Zika virus, dengue, and chikungunya virus. Rickettsial diseases are found worldwide on all continents apart from Antarctica. Malaria is the parasite of greatest concern, but leishmaniasis, trypanosomiasis, and filariasis are other potential parasitic diseases spread by arthropod vectors.

The type of accommodation can affect the traveler's risk of vector-borne diseases. An air-conditioned room for sleeping, effective window screens, and/or bed nets are protective. Wearing long-sleeved shirts, long pants, and socks can also decrease risk. For added protection, a clothing insect repellent, such as permethrin, is recommended. Permethrin activity is maintained on treated clothes despite several wash cycles.

Insect repellents for use on skin have variable efficacy depending on the repellent type and form, concentration, frequency of application, and vector. Typically, a higher concentration of insecticide will provide a longer duration of protection. However, there is a peak at which no further protection is seen, and more toxicity could result. DEET, at a concentration of 20% to 25%, has efficacy against all mosquito species and some tick species, biting flies, chiggers, and fleas. Concentrations above

---

[1] Not FDA approved for this indication.

DEET 50% do not appear to provide added benefit. Products containing picaridin (icaridin outside the United States) are also good options. Potential benefits of picaridin over DEET are that it is odorless and does not damage plastic. Products containing IR3535 are another option and appear to have particularly good activity against *Ixodes scapularis* ticks (commonly known as *deer ticks* or *black-legged ticks*).

Traveler's Diarrhea

During a 2-week trip, traveler's diarrhea has an incidence between 10% and 40%. Higher-risk areas include parts of Asia and Central/West Africa. Certain behaviors may affect the risk of developing diarrhea. Practicing hand hygiene measures before eating has been shown to reduce the incidence of diarrhea. Other potentially beneficial measures include avoiding food that has not been properly cooked, avoiding ice, and drinking only bottled or treated water in resource-poor settings.

Traveler's diarrhea is predominantly caused by bacterial pathogens. However, antibiotic prophylaxis to prevent traveler's diarrhea is rarely indicated, given both the cost and potential for adverse events. Bismuth subsalicylate (BSS [Pepto-Bismol])[1] has shown efficacy in decreasing the risk of traveler's diarrhea and may be considered for prevention. However, BSS requires frequent dosing, causes blackening of the tongue, and has the potential for drug-drug interactions.

Treatment

Treatment recommendations for traveler's diarrhea depend on the severity of illness. Ensuring adequate hydration is always a mainstay of treatment. In the case of severe diarrhea, the WHO recommends oral rehydration therapy, which is available at most pharmacies. An antimotility agent such as loperamide (Imodium) can also provide symptomatic benefit for mild to severe traveler's diarrhea. Loperamide is not recommended to be used alone in travelers with dysentery.

When antibiotics are used for self-treatment of traveler's diarrhea, they may reduce the duration of diarrhea by 1 to 3 days. Several effective antibiotic options are available (Table 4). A combination of an antibiotic with loperamide further shortens the duration of diarrhea. However, the benefits of antimicrobial treatment of traveler's diarrhea must be weighed against the potential risks. Each antibiotic option has the potential for specific side effects, such as tendinopathies in the case of fluoroquinolones. Antibiotic use also increases the risk of developing *Clostridioides difficile* diarrhea. Further, multiple studies have shown that antibiotic use for the self-treatment of traveler's diarrhea increases the risk of developing colonization with antibiotic-resistant bacteria, including extended-spectrum B-lactamase–producing *Enterobacteriaceae* and carbapenemase-producing *Enterobacteriaceae*.

Given the potential risks, antimicrobial therapy is not recommended for acute diarrhea that is tolerable and does not interfere with planned activities. Loperamide or BSS can be used alone for these mild cases. Loperamide, with or without an antibiotic, may be used in the case of moderate diarrhea that is distressing or interferes with planned activities. An antibiotic is recommended to treat severe traveler's diarrhea, which includes all dysentery cases, as well as diarrhea that is incapacitating or prevents planned activities. Single-dose antibiotic treatment regimens are as effective as 3-day regimens for most cases of traveler's diarrhea.

Fluoroquinolones, such as ciprofloxacin (Cipro)[1] and levofloxacin (Levaquin)[1], have long been used to treat traveler's diarrhea. However, there has been increasing resistance to fluoroquinolones among diarrheal pathogens, especially *Campylobacter* isolates in South and Southeast Asia. In this area of the world, azithromycin (Zithromax)[1] is preferred for empiric treatment of traveler's diarrhea. Azithromycin is also the preferred treatment for dysentery[1]. Rifaximin (Xifaxan) is approved to treat traveler's diarrhea caused by noninvasive strains of *Escherichia coli*. Rifamycin SV (Aemcolo) is a nonabsorbable antibiotic with an enteric coating, and it has the same mechanism of action as rifaximin. Because rifamycin SV and rifaximin are not recommended for treatment of invasive diarrhea, their role in the self-treatment of diarrhea is limited.

High-Altitude Illness

High-altitude illnesses (HAIs) caused by hypoxia can occur during travel to high-elevation areas, typically areas with an elevation greater than 8000 feet above sea level. There are three syndromes that may comprise altitude illness: acute mountain sickness (AMS), high-altitude cerebral edema (HACE), and high-altitude pulmonary edema (HAPE).

AMS is the most common form of HAI, and symptoms may include headache, nausea, and fatigue. If left untreated, AMS can progress to HACE, which is a more serious condition. Manifestations of HACE can include ataxia, drowsiness, confusion, and even death. Acute hypoxia may also lead to HAPE. The pathophysiology of HAPE is different from that of AMS/HACE and is presumably caused by pulmonary vasoconstriction that leads to

---

[1] Not FDA approved for this indication.

[1] Not FDA approved for this indication.

TABLE 4	Treatment Options for Empiric Treatment of Traveler's Diarrhea		
ANTIBIOTIC	**ADULT DOSE**	**DURATION**	**COMMENTS**
Rifaximin (Xifaxan)	200 mg tid	3 days	Not recommend in patients with fever or bloody diarrhea
Rifamycin SV (Aemcolo)	388 mg bid	3 days	Not recommend in patients with fever or bloody diarrhea
Azithromycin (Zithromax)[1]	1000 mg	Single dose (or two divided doses on the same day to reduce nausea)	Preferred empiric option in Southeast Asia, and preferred treatment for dysentery
	500 mg daily	3 days	
Ciprofloxacin (Cipro)[1]	750 mg	Single dose	
	500 mg bid	3 days	
Levofloxacin (Levaquin)[1]	500 mg daily	1 to 3 days	

[1] Not FDA approved for this indication.
bid, Twice daily; *tid,* three times daily.

pulmonary edema. Cough, dyspnea on exertion, and pulmonary congestion can progress to death if ascent is continued.

Prevention of High-Altitude Illnesses

Certain individuals are more susceptible to HAI, but it is not possible to reliably predict who may develop symptoms. Rate of ascent, ultimate elevation, underlying medical conditions, and degree of physical exertion are all potential factors in determining risk of developing HAI. The body's ability to acclimate to a high elevation typically takes 3 to 5 days. A slow ascent that allows time for acclimatization is helpful in preventing the development of all forms of HAI; however, this is not always possible. There are several popular high-altitude tourist destinations that may be reached via direct flights from areas of low elevation. Examples include Cuzco, Peru, located at 11,000 feet; La Paz, Bolivia, at 12,000 feet; and Lhasa, Tibet, at 12,000 feet.

Acetazolamide (Diamox) is a nonantibiotic sulfonamide that was developed as a diuretic to treat hypertension. Its efficacy for this purpose was limited. However, multiple studies have since shown that the preemptive use of acetazolamide can decrease the risk of developing AMS. Acetazolamide blocks carbonic anhydrase, primarily in the kidney. This decreases reabsorption of bicarbonate and leads to the development of metabolic acidosis, compensating for the respiratory alkalosis associated with high elevations. Acetazolamide is associated with an increased risk of paresthesia and diuresis. The recommended dose of acetazolamide to prevent AMS while minimizing adverse effects is 125 mg orally twice a day. It is generally recommended to start 1 day before ascent and continue through the first 2 days at peak elevation.

A number of other medications have been studied to prevent AMS, but the benefits of alternative therapies are less clear. Dexamethasone (Decadron)[1] is one of the more commonly used alternatives. The typical dose for prophylaxis is 2 mg every 6 hours or 4 mg every 12 hours. Inhaled budesonide (Pulmicort)[1] was found to be ineffective in preventing AMS in a recent randomized controlled study and is not recommended.

Treatment

Symptomatic travelers should not continue to ascend further until all symptoms resolve, and they should descend to a lower elevation immediately if symptoms progress. Acetazolamide can be considered for treatment of AMS, but it is better at preventing than treating this disorder. Dexamethasone is more reliable for treatment of moderate to severe AMS. However, descent is the most effective therapy and should occur immediately in cases of HACE or HAPE.

Summary

A pretravel consultation should include a health assessment, interventions, and counseling to decrease travel-related risks and improve the likelihood of a safe and enjoyable travel experience.

---

[1] Not FDA approved for this indication.

References

Air Passenger Forecasts. Global Report. https://www.iata.org/publications/Documents/global-report-sample1.pdf. Accessed on 01.09.2017.

Centers for Disease Control and Prevention: *CDC yellow book 2020: health information for international travel*, New York, 2017, Oxford University Press.

Cullen KA, Mace KE, Arguin PM: Malaria surveillance - United States, 2013, *MMWR Surveill Summ* 65:1–22, 2016.

Freedman DO: Protection of travelers. In Bennett JE, Raphael D, Blaser MJ, editors: *Mandell, douglas, and bennett's principles and practice of infectious diseases*, ed 8, Philadelphia, 2015, Saunders Elsevier, pp 3559–3567.

Freedman DO, Chen LH, Kozarsky PE: Medical considerations before international travel, *N Engl J Med* 375:247–260, 2016.

Freedman DO, Weld LH, Kozarsky PE: Spectrum of disease and relation to place of exposure among ill returned travelers, *N Engl J Med* 354:119–130, 2006.

Gautret P, Harvey K, Pandey P: Animal-associated exposure to rabies virus among travelers, 1997-2012, *Emerg Infect Dis* 21:569–577, 2015.

Gautret P, Parola P: Rabies in travelers, *Curr Infect Dis Rep* 16:394, 2014.

Giddings SL, Stevens AM, Leung DT: Traveler's diarrhea, *Med Clin North Am* 100(2):317–330, 2016.

Grobusch MP: Malaria chemoprophylaxis with atovaquone-proguanil: is a shorter regimen fully protective? *J Travel Med* 21(2):79–81, 2014.

Jelinek T, Burchard GD, Dieckmann S, et al: Short-term immunogenicity and safety of an accelerated pre-exposure prophylaxis regimen with Japanese encephalitis vaccine in combination with a rabies vaccine: a phase III, multicenter, observer-blind study, *J Travel Med* 22:225–231, 2015.

Jensenius M, Han PV, Schlagenhauf P, et al: Acute and potentially life-threatening tropical diseases in western travelers–A GeoSentinel multicenter study, 1996-2011, *Am J Trop Med Hyg* 88:397–404, 2013.

Kantele A, Laaveri T, Mero S: Antimicrobials increase travelers' risk of colonization by extended-spectrum betalactamase-producing Enterobacteriaceae, *Clin Infect Dis* 60:837–846, 2015.

Kantele A, Mero S, Kirveskari J: Increased risk for ESBL-producing bacteria from co-administration of loperamide and antimicrobial drugs for travelers' diarrhea, *Emerg Infect Dis* 22(1):117–120, 2016.

Leshem E, Meltzer E, Stienlauf S: Effectiveness of short prophylactic course of atovaquone-proguanil in travelers to sub-Saharan Africa, *J Travel Med* 21(2):82–85, 2014.

Leshem E, Pandey P: Clinical features of patients with severe altitude illness in Nepal, *J Travel Med* 15:315–322, 2008.

Luks AM, Auerbach PS, Freer L: Wilderness medical society clinical practice guidelines for the prevention and treatment of acute altitude illness: 2019 Update, *Wilderness Environ Med* 30(4S):S3–S18, 2019.

Lupi E, Hatz C, Schlagenhauf P: The efficacy of repellents against Aedes, Anopheles, Culex and Ixodes spp.—a literature review, *Travel Med Infect Dis* 11(6):374–411, 2013.

Mace KE, Lucchi NW, Tan KR: Malaria surveillance – United States, 2018, *MMWR Surveill Summ* 71(No. SS-8):1–29, 2022.

Meltzer E, Paran Y, Lustig Y: Travel-related tick-borne encephalitis, Israel, 2006-2014, *Emerg Infect Dis* 23:119–121, 2017.

Menachem M, Grupper M, Paz A: Assessment of rabies exposure risk among Israeli travelers, *Travel Med Infect Dis* 6:12–16, 2008.

Novitt-Moreno A, Ransom J, Dow G, Smith B, Read LT, Toovey S: Tafenoquine for malaria prophylaxis in adults: an integrated safety analysis, *Travel Med Infect Dis* 17:19–27, 2017.

Riddle MS, Connor BA, Beeching NJ, et al: Guidelines for the prevention and treatment of travelers' diarrhea, *J Travel Med* 24:S63–S80, 2017.

Shlim David R: The use of acetazolamide for the prevention of high-altitude illness, *J Travel Med* 1–6, 2020.

Steffen R: Epidemiology of tick-borne encephalitis (TBE) in international travellers to Western/Central Europe and conclusions on vaccination recommendations, J Travel Med 23(4).

Steffen R, Hill DR, DuPont HL: Traveler's diarrhea: a clinical review, *JAMA* 313:71–80, 2015.

Victor JC, Monto AS, Surdina TY, et al: Hepatitis A vaccine versus immune globulin for postexposure prophylaxis, *N Engl J Med* 357(17):1685, 2007.

Yezli S, Alotaibi B: Meningococcal disease during the Hajj and Umrah mass gatherings: A, C, W, Y may be covered but don't forget the B and X factors, *Travel Med Infect Dis* 15:5–7, 2017.

22 Emerging Therapies

GENOMIC TESTING

Method of
Gregory A. Plotnikoff, MD, MTS

In 2021, the National Institutes of Health's National Human Genomic Research Institute (HGRI) proclaimed that by the year 2030, "The regular use of genomic information will have transitioned from boutique to mainstream in all clinical settings, making genomic testing as routine as complete blood counts (CBCs)." In many ways, we are on our way to fulfilling this bold prediction. Affordable testing now exists that strengthens our diagnostic capacities and optimizes our therapeutic strategies. Testing that cost $100 million in 2001 could be performed for less than $1000 in 2021. As costs continue to plummet, clinically meaningful genomic testing will be increasingly available, both in clinical settings as well as in direct-to-consumer product offerings. Our challenge as clinicians is to keep up to date with the implications for prescribed therapies.

Genotyping

The new world of clinical genomics refers to the study of the entire genome of an organism. Genotyping is the clinical application of genomics in which molecular assays are used to detect the presence or absence of a specific variant (or variants) in DNA. *Variants* in coding DNA is the key operative term here. Three types of genomic variations exist: (1) single-nucleotide variants (SNVs; 1 base pair, e.g., A to G); (2) indels (small; <50 base pair insertions, e.g., GC to GAAC) and deletions (e.g., ATGC to AC); and (3) structural variants (SVs). Of the latter, two types occur: copy-number variability (CNV) and others (non-CNV). Two subcategories of genotyping apply to current clinical practice: pharmacogenomic testing and widely advertised direct-to-consumer genetic testing.

Pharmacogenomics

Pharmacogenomics is the study and clinical application of genetic determinants of both drug efficacy (dose response) and drug toxicity including reactions caused by impaired or rapid clearance as well as drug-drug, drug-herb, or drug-nutrient interactions. Pharmacogenomic testing identifies clinically important genetic variations that may affect the safety and efficacy of any prescribed medication. Knowledge of a patient's baseline variation in the metabolism of pharmaceuticals can guide both optimal drug choice and optimal dosing and thus minimize both toxicity and time to effect.

Pharmacogenomic testing results demonstrate that standard doses may not be appropriate for all patients. Clinically meaningful genetic variations can occur in any of the genes involved in absorption, distribution, metabolism, translocation, binding, or clearance (excretion). This leads to a new clinical competency. Prescribers now must understand how genetic variations influence both the pharmacokinetics and pharmacodynamics of drug effects and responses.

Commonly seen examples of pharmacogenomic variability include genetically determined variations in INR response to warfarin dosing, variations in risk for chemotherapy-associated side effects, and variations in antidepressant drug response by ethnicity. Additional pharmacogenomic concerns include the additive epigenetic induction or inhibition of drug clearance by such commonly prescribed medications such as clarithromycin (Biaxin), diltiazem (Cardizem), erythromycin, fluconazole (Diflucan), or verapamil or by uncommonly prescribed medications such as rifampin (Rifadin) or ritonavir (Norvir).

In 2023, physicians can readily order pharmacogenomic testing for their patients. Testing companies include focused pharmacogenomic laboratories such as OneOme, GenoMind, GeneSight, and TruGenX; large genetic testing companies such as Invitae; and large national testing laboratories such as ARUP, LabCorp, and Quest Diagnostics.

Moreover, physicians and healthcare team members including nurses and pharmacists can readily access evidence-based guidelines that synthesize information relevant to genomic/pharmacogenomic tests and selection of drug therapy (see the resources provided at the end of this chapter).

To navigate effectively requires a fluency in both genetic concepts and nomenclature. To begin, *genotype* refers to the combination of the two alleles (one maternal, one paternal) of a gene at a particular location on a chromosome. The non-variant or usual type of allele is referred to as the *wild-type*. Most variations are in a single nucleotide. If this variant is found in >1% of the population, it is termed a *single-nucleotide polymorphism* (SNP, pronounced "snip"). Variants found in less than 1% of the population are termed *mutations*. One variant allele is termed a *heterozygous variant*. When both alleles are variants, the patient is deemed to have a homozygous variant.

Variations and mutations are described by either the "rs" identifying number (for the reference SNP) or by the "star" nomenclature for one or both alleles. To illustrate the importance of nomenclature, for the cytochrome P450 (CYP450) enzyme termed *CYP2C19,* approximately 25 genetic variants in the exonic region of the *CYP2C19* gene have been identified. Of these 25 variations, a change in guanine (G) to adenine (A) at position 681 in exon 5 will result in an aberrant splice cite that alters the metabolism of several medications including the antiplatelet medication clopidogrel (Plavix). For precise communication, this variation can be described by its rs identifying number (rs4244285) or by its star nomenclature (CYP2C19*2). In pharmacogenomic reporting for *CYP450* genes, the star nomenclature is most often used. However, the genomic nomenclature is not always easy because nucleotide position and nucleotide change are often used to report other pharmaceutical metabolizing genes. Examples of the nomenclature complexity include the ATP-binding cassette, subfamily B, member 1 variation termed *ABCB1 3435C>T.* This is also known as *multidrug resistance gene 1 (MDR1)* and encodes for P-glycoprotein (P-gp). Likewise, catechol O-methyltransferase (COMT) rs4680 is also reported as COMT Val158Met. To further the nomenclature challenge, haplotypes refer to a simultaneously linked set of SNPs in an individual. For example, for the thiopurine S-methyltransferase gene, *TPMT*3A* refers to a haplotype composed of two non-synonymous SNPs (rs1800460 and rs1142345).

Within the human genome, several million SNPs have been identified. Of these, most are termed *synonymous* and do not alter the protein products of the gene expression and have no measurable

TABLE 1	Polymorphisms That Adversely Affect Drug Metabolism		
POLYMORPHISM	**STAR NAME**	**ACTIVITY CHANGE**	**EXAMPLE MEDICATIONS AFFECTED**
Premature stop codon	*CYP2C19*2, CYP2C19*3*	Blocked enzyme activity	Clopidogrel (Plavix), omeprazole (Prilosec)
Variable number tandem repeats	*TMPT*2, TMPT*3*	Enhanced active metabolite production	Mercaptopurine (Purinethol)
Gene deletion	*CYP2D6*5*	Gene absence	Antidepressants, beta blockers, antihistamines, numerous prodrugs, others
Copy number variants	*CYP2D6*2XN*	Gene amplification and ultra-rapid function	Antidepressants, beta blockers, antihistamines, numerous prodrugs, others

effects. The consequences of other sequence variants can result in altered structure and function of the encoded proteins or altered level of gene expression. Inheritance of these alleles means that standard doses of a drug therapy can lead to an adverse drug reaction or chemotherapy failure. Several types of polymorphisms can adversely affect drug metabolism. These are illustrated in Table 1. Patients with reduced function of CYP2C19 metabolism who are prescribed clopidogrel have significantly lower levels of its active metabolite and therefore diminished platelet inhibition. Clinically, this translates to a higher rate of major adverse cardiovascular events including stent thrombosis after stent placement for coronary artery disease. Patients with *TMPT* impairment who are prescribed mercaptopurine will have reduced nonactive metabolite production, which in turn results in enhanced active metabolite production and a significantly increased risk of toxicity, including leukopenia. Surprisingly, *CYP2D6* variations can result in a 200-fold effect on drug metabolism (from poor to ultra-rapid metabolism). The amplified activity with copy number variants such as in *CYP2D6*2XN* results in faster clearance. The *N* refers to the number of copies of the gene on a single chromosome. For *CYP2D6*2*, this can range from 2 to 13.

Reported pharmacogenomic CYP450 data are often presented as one of four phenotypic categories: (1) *ultra-rapid*, (2) *extensive* (normal), (3) *intermediate*, and (4) *poor*. A tragic example of ultra-rapid CYP2D6 metabolism of the prodrug codeine into its active metabolite morphine has been seen in children who received codeine following a routine tonsillectomy. The rapid transformation of codeine to morphine results in rapid systemic delivery of a morphine bolus. As a result, children have died from the sudden onset of opioid-induced central respiratory depression, increased sedation, and decreased supraglottic airway tone. Tragic examples of poor CYP2D6 metabolism of the prodrug hydrocodone into its active metabolite hydromorphone has been seen in patients with insufficient analgesia being labeled as drug-seekers. This risk of insufficient analgesia despite "normal" dosing would be worsened with concomitant administration of CYP2D6-inhibiting medications such as bupropion (Wellbutrin), fluoxetine (Prozac), paroxetine (Paxil), quinidine, or terbinafine (Lamisil).

The latter point emphasizes why prescribers must also understand the numerous medications and natural products that can modify existing pharmacogenomic function via either induction or inhibition of CYP450 drug-metabolizing enzymes or drug transporters such as P-glycoprotein, BCRP (breast cancer resistance protein), OAT family proteins (solute carrier organic anion transporters), MATE1 and MATE2 (multidrug and toxin extrusion proteins 1 and 2), and OCT1 and OCT2 (organic cation transporters 1 and 2). Helpful information can be found on the U.S. Food and Drug Administration (FDA) website (https://www.fda.gov/drugs/drug-interactions-labeling/drug-development-and-drug-interactions-table-substrates-inhibitors-and-inducers#table5-2).

Despite existing knowledge, the presence of clinically significant adverse drug-drug interactions may be high in cardiology, oncology, and psychiatry. Likewise, natural product–drug interactions also exist. For example, medicinal cannabis (THC) and cannabidiol (CBD)[7] appear to inhibit multiple CYP450 enzymes including CYP2D6. Saint John's wort *(Hypericum perforatum)*[7] induces CYP3A4 activity, the liver enzyme responsible for metabolizing the vast majority of currently available prescription medications. Berberine, an active ingredient in several herbal medicines such as goldenseal *(Hydrastis canadensis)*[7] and also sold as an isolated, purified, and concentrated ingredient, can inhibit CYP2D6 and CYP3A4 as well as increase P-glycoprotein function.

Future clinical practice will undoubtedly bring pharmacogenomic data to the point of care either via the electronic medical record and/or further incorporation of specially trained pharmacists. The future will likely see calls for each person, perhaps starting at birth, to be tested for clinical variations that are relevant to optimal prescribing and dosing. To support enhanced clinician competency in pharmacogenomics, several excellent resources are noted later in this chapter.

Direct-To-Consumer Genotyping

At this time, the primary genotyping service used in clinics is for pharmacogenomic data to guide therapy. However, since at least 2006, the lay public has seen advertising for home genetic testing for genealogical purposes. Indirectly, direct-to-consumer genomic testing such as 23andme.com and ancestry.com introduced to the public microarray genotyping and single-nucleotide variants. Soon afterward, clinicians and others recognized the potential value of the information found in the common (>1% of the population) SNPs that is found in the unreported raw data in the genomic testing. Consumer-empowering websites that could upload 23andme.com raw data and then sort, organize, and prioritize SNPs for interpretative health reasons quickly appeared (e.g., MTHFRsupport.com, livewello.com, geneticgenie.com). Consumers suddenly had access to their genetic information outside of a physician's office, and patients had the capacity to ask very sophisticated health questions that could overwhelm unprepared physicians.

The greatest value in 23andme.com and related consumer-directed SNP analysis services may be in generating hypotheses relevant to guiding therapeutic recommendations. Clinically relevant categories that can be addressed include the following:
- Vitamin activation (e.g., Beta-Carotene Oxygenase 1 [BCO1] for vitamin A, Vitamin K Epoxide Reductase Complex Subunit 1 [VKORC1] for vitamin K)
- Neurotransmitter production impairment (e.g., L-DOPA decarboxylase [DDC] for dopamine and serotonin; glutamate decarboxylase 1 [GAD1] for gamma aminobutyric acid [GABA])

---

[7] Available as dietary supplement.

- Metabolic pathway analyses (e.g., genes for methylation, trans-sulfonation, and nicotinamide adenine dinucleotide [NAD+] production)
- Detoxification capacity (e.g., paraoxonase 1 [PON1], glucuronidation capacity, glutathione-production genes)
- Apolipoprotein E (APOE) status (genetic risk of Alzheimer disease)

The predictive value and clinical utility of such genotyping services has yet to be validated. However, the future will see tremendous growth in nutrigenomics (the study of the bidirectional interaction of nutrition and genes), intestinal microbiomics, and the combination of the two perspectives. In 2022, the National Institutes of Health announced $170 million in funding for 11 significant new initiatives to provide insight into personalized nutrition. The NIH has acknowledged how poorly understood the intestinal microbiome, metabolism, nutritional status, genetics, and the environment interact to affect health. For healthcare professionals, this initiative promises to catalyze significant scientific advances to generate an evidence base beyond "one-size-fits-all" diets toward precision in dietary guidance for optimal health.

Cell-Free DNA

Cell-free DNA (cfDNA) refers to non-encapsulated DNA fragments released into the blood or other body fluids as a result of secretion, apoptosis, and/or necrosis. Technology now allows separation of circulating fetal DNA, mitochondrial DNA, tumor DNA, and microbial DNA. This breakthrough has resulted in profound changes in diagnostic capacities in both obstetrics with non-invasive prenatal testing (NIPT) and primary care with multi-cancer early detection (MCED). This breakthrough has also led to identification of cell-free mitochondrial DNA (cf-mtDNA) as a marker of trauma, inflammation, acute psychological distress, as well as physiologic distress. Elevated levels are clearly linked to an increase in hospital mortality. Elevated levels also appear to be linked to cognitive and neurodegenerative disorders. Unlike NIPT and MCED, however, meaningful translation to clinical therapies has yet to be defined.

For oncologic therapy guidance, the capacity to separate tumor DNA from germline DNA from a simple blood draw (referred to as a *liquid biopsy*) means that surgery is no longer required to obtain tumor tissue for tumor mutation profiling with any solid advanced-stage malignant neoplasm. Such testing can reliably and rapidly determine clinically pertinent DNA point mutations, indels, amplifications, and fusions. Identification of tumor genomic status (e.g., *EGFR, ALK, BRAF*) can guide optimal selection of targeted chemotherapy for non–small cell lung cancer or colon cancer. At this time, Medicare covers this testing for all solid advanced-stage tumors. In the future, the simultaneous mapping of multiple biomarkers of genomic alterations will drive a deeper understanding of multitargeted therapies and resistance mechanisms. Additionally, I believe these data will lead us to a better understanding of the optimal use of off-label pharmaceuticals and specific dietary interventions as adjunctive therapies for patients with cancer.

In infectious disease, another form of liquid biopsy is available for microbial cell-free DNA sequencing on plasma. This has revolutionized the non-invasive and rapid identification of more than 1000 pathogens including bacteria, fungi, DNA viruses, and protozoans. In this process, cell-free DNA fragments are extracted from the specimen, converted to shotgun DNA sequencing libraries, and then sequenced. The concentration of cell-free DNA molecules from any potential pathogen is then calculated.

An April 2022 report in the Case Records of the Massachusetts General Hospital demonstrated the great value of this testing for targeted and precise treatment of an unknown pathogen. The authors described the clinical challenges of diagnosing a 56-year-old male patient with myalgias, fever, bradycardia, and inflammatory changes in the epicardial fat abutting the non-coronary sinus of the aortic valve. In this case, testing detected *Listeria monocytogenes* at a concentration of 42 cell-free DNA molecules per microliter (reference value <10). This finding confirmed the diagnosis of listeriosis. The authors noted that these results were associated with a 95% sensitivity (at 41 molecules per microliter) and a 98% to 99.99% specificity for the diagnosis of listeriosis.

Such testing means that culture-based methods for microbial identification are likely to be replaced by cfDNA-based methods. The advantages are clear in terms of identifying difficult-to-culture pathogens, the time to results, and the non-invasive sampling. The advantage over rapid multiplex polymerase chain reaction (PCR) tests is that a presumptive diagnosis of a single pathogen is not needed. The bottom-line implication of microbial cfDNA testing is that presumptive or empiric antipathogen therapies will be less necessary for acute illness. Likewise, such testing, similar to interferon-gamma release assays, may clarify the length of treatment required for clearance. And to speculate boldly, microbial cfDNA testing may help define the presence of an unexpected chronic infectious disease driving perplexing chronic illness.

Whole-Exome Sequencing/Genome Sequencing

As a result of the profound reduction in cost and the marked increase in the capacity to manage huge databases, advanced sequencing is now readily available for diagnostic purposes in clinical settings. Whether termed *whole-exome sequencing* (WES) or *whole-genome sequencing* (WGS), next-generation sequencing (NGS) represents numerous advancements over the previously available Sanger sequencing. NGS not only detects the aforementioned DNA changes of interest (e.g., single-nucleotide changes, indels, copy number variants) but also detects RNA alterations such as transcriptional abundance and fusion transcripts. The greatest challenge to widespread implementation after cost include management of the massive amount of data generated and the intensive process of annotation, which involves marking specific features in a DNA, RNA, or protein sequence with descriptive information about structure or function. Specific challenges include lengthy turn-around time as well as the interpretation of both incidental findings unrelated to the initial reason for which the sequencing tests were ordered and variants in a gene of phenotypic significance but of unknown clinical significance (variants of unknown significance [VUS]).

In the clinic, such advanced testing is primarily used for diagnostic purposes. This includes nonfocused or whole-genome sequencing for rare illnesses as well as focused testing for phenotypic patterns such as hypermobility or genetic risk for cancer. Of great interest is the potential presence or absence of incidentally found "actionable" gene mutations relevant to the avoidance of significant morbidity or mortality. In 2013, the American College of Medical Genetics and Genomics (ACMG) released a recommendation suggesting that known pathogenic or expected pathogenic constitutional variants detected in 56 genes, representing 24 conditions with well-known guidelines for prevention or treatment, should be reported to patients sequenced in a clinical setting. In 2017, four genes were added, and in 2021 an additional nine such genes were added. Examples include mutations in the *RYR1* gene, which are causally linked to malignant hyperthermia with administration of halothane gas anesthesia or succinylcholine, and the *BRCA1, BRCA2,* and *PALB2* genes, which are demonstrably connected with breast and ovarian cancers.

Most important for future therapies will likely be the creation of genome-wide polygenic risk scores for an individual's susceptibility to disease. The focus on single-gene causality appears to have blinded us to the networked or polygenic nature of most noncommunicable diseases including cancer and heart disease. Single variants are too often insufficient for assessing disease risk. Even traits thought be the result of single genes, such as eye color, are actually highly polygenic. And for a trait such as height, approximately 80% of an individual's height requires contribution of more than 700 genomic variants. To move beyond single-variable science with a polygenic risk score requires the merger of classic genomic sequencing for monogenic variants with artificial intelligence programming. The goal is to enable early recognition and treatment of high-risk individuals before the onset of disease. An additional benefit may be to uncover new causal disease pathways. The future will bring us a deeper understanding of the clinical utility of such scores.

Conclusion

In the future, genomic testing will be as common as ordering a CBC. Advances in genotyping, cfDNA testing, and whole-genome sequencing will clearly transform multiple dimensions of patient care in every subspecialty. With such changes will also come new insights into the multiple forms of noncoding RNA as well as the role of imprinting and transgenerational epigenetic changes. Whereas current genomic testing may only describe what cards one has been dealt, the secondary "-omics" revolution (e.g., in transcriptomics, metabolomics, and proteomics) will allow us to know not only what cards one has been dealt but also how they are being played. This will undoubtedly completely transform the practice of medicine.

Genomic Resources

General

ClinGen

http://clinicalgenome.org

An NIH-funded resource that defines the clinical relevance of genes and variants for use in medicine and research.

ClinVar

http://www.ncbi.nlm.nih.gov/clinvar/

A public archive of reports about the relationship between specific genetic variants and associated phenotypes (symptoms).

dbSNP

https://www.ncbi.nlm.nih.gov/snp/

A database for human single-nucleotide variations, microsatellites, and small-scale insertions and deletions along with publication, population frequency, molecular consequences, and genomic and RefSeq mapping information for both common variations and clinical mutations.

GeneReviews

http://www.ncbi.nlm.nih.gov/books/NBK1116/

A collection of chapters written by experts in the field for healthcare providers, with each chapter focused on an individual genetic condition or disease.

OMIM

https://www.omim.org/ or https://www.ncbi.nlm.nih.gov/omim

Information on genes and diseases. The entries on genes are particularly useful.

PharmGKB (PharmacoGenomicsKnowledgeBase)

http://www.pharmgkb.org/

A database of pharmacogenomic research findings. This includes free access to the peer-reviewed Clinical Pharmacogenetics Implementation Consortium (CPIC) Guidelines (https://cpicpgx.org/guidelines/) for prescribing decisions from genetic laboratory results with supplemental information and updates.

Pharmacogenomic Testing

Laboratories that offer pharmacogenomic testing include OneOme, GenoMind, GeneSight, TruGenX, and Invitae. Large laboratories that also offer genetic testing include ARUP, LabCorp, and Quest Diagnostics.

Education

Genetics/Genomics Competency Center

https://www.genome.gov/G2C2/resources

Categorized educational resources in genetics/genomics and pharmacogenomics for healthcare educators and clinicians

National Human Genome Research Institute

https://www.genome.gov/For-Health-Professionals/Provider-Genomics-Education-Resources

Information for healthcare professionals and patients on genetics, pharmacogenomics, direct-to-consumer testing, and more including terminology, videos, and illustrations.

PharmGenEd

http://pharmacogenomics.ucsd.edu/

Free educational materials (including recorded lectures and handouts) focused on clinical applications of pharmacogenomics for healthcare students and practitioners.

Medical-Legal

GeneReviews: Resources for Genetics Professionals—Direct-to-Consumer Genetic Testing

https://www.ncbi.nlm.nih.gov/books/NBK542335/#dtc_testing.For_general_predictions_about

Anticipate and Communicate: Ethical Management of Incidental and Secondary Findings in the Clinical, Research, and Direct-to-Consumer Contexts, from the Presidential Commission for the Study of Bioethical Issues

https://pubmed.ncbi.nlm.nih.gov/25150271/

Coalition for Genetic Data Protection: Privacy Best Practices for Consumer Genetic Testing Services

https://geneticdataprotection.com/

Genetic Alliance: Genetic Discrimination

https://geneticalliance.org/policy; then scroll down to Genetic Discrimination

National Human Genome Research Institute: Genetic Discrimination

https://www.genome.gov/about-genomics/policy-issues/Genetic-Discrimination

References

https://www.genome.gov/event-calendar/Bold-Predictions-for-Human-Genomics-by-2030. Accessed March 27, 2022.

https://www.genome.gov/about-genomics/fact-sheets/Sequencing-Human-Genome-cost. Accessed March 27, 2022.

Sanborn D, Sugrue A, Amin M, et al: Outcomes of direct oral anticoagulants co-prescribed with common interacting medications, *Am J Cardiol* 162:80–85, 2022.

Shugg T, Ly RC, Rowe EJ, et al: Clinical opportunities for germline pharmacogenetics and management of drug-drug interactions in patients with advanced solid cancers, *JCO Precis Oncol* 6:e2100312, 2022.

Hefner G, Wolff J, Hahn M, et al: Prevalence and sort of pharmacokinetic drug-drug interactions in hospitalized psychiatric patients, *J Neural Transm (Vienna)* 127(8):1185–1198, 2020.

Doohan PT, Oldfield LD, Arnold JC, Anderson LL: Cannabinoid interactions with cytochrome P450 drug metabolism: a full-spectrum characterization, *AAPS J* 23(4):91, 2021.

Nasrin S, Watson CJW, Perez-Paramo YX, Lazurus P: Cannabinoid metabolites as inhibitors of major hepatic CYP450 enzymes, with implications for cannabis-drug interactions, *Drug Metab Dispos* 49(12):1070–1080, 2021.

Wanwimolruk S, Prachayasittikul V: Cytochrome P450 enzyme mediated herbal drug interactions (Part 1), *EXCLI J* 13:347–391, 2014. eCollection 2014.

Nguyen JT, Tian DD, Wanna RS, et al: Assessing transporter-mediated natural product-drug interactions via in vitro-in vivo extrapolation: clinical evaluation with a probe cocktail, *Clin Pharmacol Ther* 109(5):1342–1352, 2021.

https://www.nih.gov/news-events/news-releases/nih-awards-170-million-precision-nutrition-study. [Accessed 27 March 2022].

Park SS, Jeong H, Andreazza AC, et al: Circulating cell-free mitochondrial DNA in brain health and disease: A systematic review and meta-analysis, *World J Biol Psychiatry* 23(2):87–102, 2022.

Trumpff C, Michelson J, Lagranha CJ, et al: Stress and circulating cell-free mitochondrial DNA: A systematic review of human studies, physiological considerations, and technical recommendations, *Mitochondrion* 59:225–245, 2021.

Para ML, Khurshid S, Folding B, et al: Case 13-2022: A 56-year-old man with myalgias, fever, and bradycardia, *N Engl J Med* 386:1647–1657, 2022.

Green RC, Berg JS, Grody WW, et al: American College of Medical Genetics and Genomics. ACMG recommendations for reporting of incidental findings in clinical exome and genome sequencing, *Genet Med* 15:565–574, 2013.

Miller DT, Lee K, Chung WK, et al: ACMG SF v3.0 list for reporting of secondary findings in clinical exome and genome sequencing: a policy statement of the American College of Medical Genetics and Genomics (ACMG), *Genetic Med* 23:1381–1390, 2021.

MONOCLONAL ANTIBODIES

Method of
Michael Dougan, MD, PhD; and Crystal M. North, MD, MPH

CURRENT DIAGNOSIS

- Monoclonal antibodies are unique, specific, and homogeneous antibodies manufactured by immortalizing and copying an antibody secreting B cell of interest.
- Monoclonal antibodies have a wide variety of applications in diagnostic medicine including identification of pathogens, tissue typing, cancer diagnosis, enzyme-linked immunosorbent assay, radioimmunoassay, and other laboratory testing methods.

CURRENT THERAPY

- Monoclonal antibodies have tremendous applications in the field of therapeutic medicine for treatment of numerous diseases affecting every organ system in the body.
- Monoclonal antibodies can be used alone or to carry drugs, cytotoxic agents, or radioactive substances to targeted cells.
- Monoclonal antibodies are useful as drug-reversal agents (e.g., digoxin and dabigatran).
- Monoclonal antibodies are far superior to polyclonal antibodies because of their highly specific and reproducible affinity for target antigens as well as their controlled manufacturing processes.
- The "humanization" of monoclonal antibodies significantly reduces drug side effects.
- Monoclonal antibodies are delivered via injection or infusion.
- Because of the proliferation of monoclonal therapeutic agents, full prescribing information should be reviewed before administration.

Introduction

Antibodies are key components of the adaptive immune system and are produced by B cells. Antibodies provide protection from infections in two broad ways. They bind tightly to their targets, sometimes inhibiting or neutralizing target activity, and they activate other components of the immune system that can recognize antibody-bound structures.

In the setting of a typical infection, the natural immune response develops dozens of antibodies that recognize the invading microbe. These antibodies typically bind at multiple sites and with varying levels of affinity. As an immune response evolves over the course of weeks or on subsequent exposure to the same infection, these antibodies are further refined, typically targeting a distinct region of the infectious organism with increasingly higher-affinity antibodies. This response, termed a *polyclonal response*, is also what happens in the setting of a vaccine.

Each antibody is genetically encoded at the DNA level and produced by a distinct B cell (termed a *clonotype*). These B cells can proliferate and produce multiple progeny cells that manufacture the antibody that we detect in the blood. B cells can also differentiate into plasma cells, which reside in the bone marrow and are responsible for the production of the most high-affinity antibodies.

By isolating specific B cells and determining the affinity and binding specificity of the antibodies they make, genomic technologies can be used to produce unique antibodies that have medically useful binding properties. These are termed *monoclonal antibodies*. After the DNA encoding them is sequenced and cloned into an expression vector that introduces the specific gene into a target cell that directs the cell's ability to synthesize proteins, large quantities of antibodies can be produced at pharmaceutical grade. These antibodies can be used for the diagnosis and treatment of disease.

Properties of Antibodies as Drugs

Antibodies have several features that make them excellent drugs. The first is that they naturally evolve to bind to their targets with exquisite specificity and high affinity, generally exceeding that of typical receptor-ligand interactions. In theory, antibodies can bind to any structure, including carbohydrates, proteins, DNA, and small-molecule drugs that are covalently bound to proteins. This means that they can be used to selectively bind to any target of interest including human proteins, drugs and other small molecules, or infectious organisms. Their high affinity means that they are unlikely to dissociate from their target after binding. Antibodies have two binding arms, increasing their avidity for targets with recurrent structural motifs or with multiple copies of the binding target.

Monoclonal Antibody Structure

Classic antibodies are composed of four polypeptides, two heavy chains, and two light chains that are bound to the N-terminal region of the heavy chains (Figure 1A). The complex of two heavy chains and two light chains produces two broad structural domains: the target (antigen)-binding regions that are fixed at the ends of the antibody arms and the antibody stalk, which attaches to each binding arm through a flexible linker (see Figure 1A). The antibody arms are referred to as *Fab domains* and are made up of a variable region that binds the target and a constant region that connects to the stalk. The heavy chain and the light chain both contribute to the Fab domains. The amino acid sequence in each arm of a naturally occurring antibody is identical to the sequence in the other arm, but the sequence within the variable region differs from all other antibody clones. The unique sequences in these antibody arms confer the binding properties of the antibody. Antibodies can be bioengineered to have nonidentical arms, generating synthetic bispecific antibodies, an area of increasing therapeutic interest.

The antibody stalk is referred to as the *Fc domain* and is responsible for most antibody effector functions through interactions with Fc receptors. The effector functions conferred by the Fc domain include activation of complement, facilitated phagocytosis (opsonization), activation of NK cells, secretion across mucosal barriers (IgA in particular), and activation of mast cells and eosinophils (IgE in particular). The Fc domain is part of the constant region of the antibody, but it comes in multiple classes that define the distinct "isotypes" of antibodies: IgM, IgG1 to IgG4, IgA, and IgE. For IgG, the Fc domain also dramatically extends the half-life of antibodies through interactions with the serum protein FcRn. This half-life extension can be modified through point mutations, allowing for infrequent dosing of antibody drugs.

The size of monoclonal antibodies prevents efficient absorption across mucosal barriers or the skin. Consequently, all monoclonal antibodies are administered either as injections or as infusions.

Antibodies are produced as part of a normal immune response in all vertebrates, and much of their sequence is highly conserved. Although some important differences exist between human antibody genes and the coding sequence of other animals, modification of antibody sequences to generate "humanized" antibodies is now routinely used to generate drugs from antibodies that were initially identified in other animals. These humanized antibodies have been generated in model organisms such as mice and in culture systems using viruses and bacteria such as *Escherichia coli*. More recent pharmaceutical-grade antibodies have been identified directly in patients. These newer techniques have replaced older techniques for generating antibodies such as the construction of animal-human chimeric antibodies (see Figure 1B), where significant sections of animal sequence remained in the therapeutic antibody, increasing the risk of hypersensitivity reactions during infusion or loss of function caused by antidrug antibodies.

Figure 1 Structure of classic antibodies.

Antibodies are recycled from the serum through protein turnover in a process that is independent of hepatic and renal clearance mechanisms. Consequently, antibodies rarely interact with other drugs.

Interestingly, a subset of antibodies produced by camelids (e.g., alpacas, llamas, and camels) are formed without a light chain. These heavy-chain-only antibodies still retain the same variable antigen-binding domains and constant regions found in conventional antibodies, and they demonstrate approximately the same binding affinities for their targets.

Therapeutic Uses of Monoclonal Antibodies

Monoclonal antibodies have been used for a wide variety of therapeutic purposes. Most antibodies in clinical use neutralize the activity of their target, which is often a protein. This has been especially successful when targeting circulating self-proteins that have been dysregulated as part of a disease process. Most of these neutralizing monoclonal antibodies belong to the IgG4 isotype. This isotype retains the ability to bind to FcRn, but lacks engagement with other Fc receptors, reducing the risk of unintended side effects as discussed in more detail later in this chapter.

Cytokines and their receptors are the targets of many monoclonal antibodies that are used for the treatment of autoimmune and allergic diseases. These targets are particularly amenable to monoclonal antibody targeting because they are secreted and are often present in the interstitial fluid and in circulation, making them accessible to infused antibodies. Multiple other immune receptors have been successfully targeted by monoclonal antibodies, resulting in inhibition of receptor-ligand interactions and blockade of essential functions such as cell trafficking (e.g., to treat autoimmunity) or immune regulation (e.g., to treat cancer).

Monoclonal antibodies are also used to inhibit several serum proteins including components of the complement cascade, receptors involved in platelet activation, and more recently a key regulator of the low-density lipoprotein (LDL) receptor. Similar to cytokines, these factors are ideally suited to monoclonal antibody neutralization because of the accessibility of the target in circulation.

Multiple monoclonal antibodies have been developed that enhance phagocytosis of target-expressing cells and activation of cell-mediated immunity and/or complement. These monoclonal antibodies are often IgG1 antibodies and are often used in cancer treatments, binding directly to the malignant cells. Antitumor antibodies are now incorporated into standard treatment regimens for a wide variety of hematologic and solid tumors, resulting in substantial improvements in outcomes. Similar depletion strategies can be used to treat a variety of autoimmune diseases by depleting the immune cells responsible for the disease.

Although the majority of monoclonal antibody therapies target self proteins, an important class of therapeutics has been developed against infectious targets. These antibodies can be highly specific for their targets with minimal or no effects in uninfected people. Antibodies have been developed against viral and bacterial infections, target cell surface proteins, and secreted toxins. Monoclonal antibodies have had some important successes in viral therapy, as discussed later, but they are generally used less frequently than small-molecule antimicrobial drugs.

Monoclonal Antibody Side Effects

Most side effects associated with monoclonal antibodies relate directly to their mechanism of action. Inhibition of self proteins can lead to deficiencies in function that may overcorrect the disease process; this is most evident with antibodies that inhibit the immune system to treat autoimmunity. The infection-related side effects are common, though often less severe than with broader forms of immune suppression such as systemic glucocorticoids. Antibodies can also improve a disease in one organ system while damaging another. Antibodies that deplete target cells can lead to side effects related to the loss of those cells or to damage to the tissues that express the target. This can occur with some of the antitumor antibodies in which the targets are often expressed on healthy cells in addition to malignant ones.

Because of their specificity and target affinity, off-target side effects of monoclonal antibodies are rare. This is a considerable advantage when comparing monoclonal antibodies to other classes of drugs, such as small-molecule inhibitors. Side effects related to hepatic metabolism or renal clearance are also unlikely with monoclonal antibodies because they are not eliminated through these organs, leading to a relatively good safety profile in patients with multiple comorbid conditions.

Infusion reactions and the formation of antidrug antibodies are significant limitations to all monoclonal antibody treatments. The risk of these reactions is related to the fraction of nonhuman sequence present in the antibody structure. The highest-risk monoclonal antibodies currently in use are the few drugs that are chimeric mouse-human antibodies with human constant regions and mouse variable regions. As a result, few chimeric antibodies are still being developed. Most next-generation antibodies are either humanized, with the animal sequence mutated to resemble the human sequence, or human, the result of antibody identification techniques that start from the human antibody genes either inserted into the mouse genome or produced through in vitro techniques. Monoclonal antibodies have been identified directly in patients, and these antibodies have substantial clinical safety value.

Monoclonal Antibody Nomenclature

The naming of monoclonal antibodies is determined by the World Health Organization International Nonproprietary Names (INN) program, which was established in 1991. Each name consists of a prefix, a target substem (also called an *infix*), a source substem (if named before 2018), and a stem (Figure 2). The prefix does not carry any specific meaning. It is a combination of letters that, when combined with the stem and substems, results in an easily pronounced name. The target substem, also called the infix, indicates the target of the monoclonal antibody. It is composed of a consonant, a vowel, and a final consonant that is sometimes dropped if the name of the monoclonal antibody would otherwise not be easily pronounced. Examples include *-ci-* for agents that target the cardiovascular system and *-vi-* for agents that target viral products. The source substem indicates the animal from which the antibody was derived but was removed from the nomenclature starting in 2017. Examples include *-u-* for human-derived antibodies, *-o-* for mouse-derived antibodies, and *-xi-* for chimeric antibodies composed of both human and nonhuman components. The stem for all monoclonal antibodies named before 2021 is *-mab*. Starting in late 2021, monoclonal antibodies are given one of four stems: *-tug* (unmodified immunoglobulins) *-bart* (antibody **art**ificial), *-mig* (**m**ulti-**i**mmuno**g**lobulin), or *-ment* (frag**ment**).

Examples of Monoclonal Antibodies Used in Clinical Practice

Monoclonal antibodies have been developed for an ever-expanding number of clinical conditions. Included in the following sections are representative examples of monoclonal antibodies used in a variety of disease processes. This list is not meant to be exhaustive; the pace of monoclonal antibody production would make a comprehensive list outdated by the time of publication. We have grouped these examples by body system or shared mechanism, but many monoclonal antibodies are used for several clinical indications. Not all of the clinical uses described are approved by the U.S. Food and Drug Administration (FDA), but they represent common clinical practice. Side effects that are common to most monoclonal antibodies

are highlighted in the previous section, and additional side effects that are of special interest for a given monoclonal antibody are highlighted here. The list of side effects is also meant to be illustrative rather than comprehensive, and full prescribing information should be reviewed before administration of these drugs clinically.

Oncology

Rituximab (Rituxan)
Target: The CD20 antigen on the surface of B cells, leading to depletion of these cells
Similar monoclonal antibodies: Ocrelizumab (Ocrevus), ofatumumab (Arzerra, Kesimpta), obinutuzumab (Gazyva)
Adverse effects of interest: Infusion reactions are quite common, particularly during the first infusion; new and reactivated infections caused by immunosuppression
Initial clinical indication: Relapsed or refractory low-grade or follicular, B-cell non-Hodgkin lymphoma. Rituximab was one of the first monoclonal antibodies developed clinically and the first monoclonal antibody used in oncology.
Other clinical indications: Various lymphomas (non-Hodgkin lymphoma, diffuse large B-cell lymphoma, follicular lymphoma), chronic lymphocytic leukemia, various autoimmune conditions (e.g., rheumatoid arthritis, systemic lupus erythematosus,[1] granulomatosis with polyangiitis)

Bevacizumab (Avastin)
Target: Vascular endothelial growth factor (VEGF), impairing microvascular growth
Similar monoclonal antibodies: Ranibizumab
Adverse effects of interest: Hemorrhage, gastrointestinal perforation (rarely)
Initial clinical indication: First-line treatment, in combination with 5-fluorouracil, of metastatic colon and rectal carcinoma
Other clinical indications: Macular degeneration,[1] diabetic retinopathy[1]

Cetuximab (Erbitux)
Target: Epidermal growth factor receptor (EGFR), impairing cell growth and proliferation, depletion of target-expressing cells
Similar monoclonal antibodies: Panitumumab (Vectibix)
Adverse effects of interest: IgE-mediated allergic reactions, dermatologic reactions
Initial clinical indication: EGFR-expressing metastatic colorectal carcinoma
Other clinical indications: *BRAF* V600E+ metastatic colorectal carcinoma, squamous cell carcinoma of the head and neck

Ipilimumab (Yervoy)
Target: Cytotoxic T lymphocyte antigen (CTLA)-4, an immune checkpoint receptor
Similar monoclonal antibodies: Ipilimumab is considered a "checkpoint inhibitor" along with drugs targeting PD-1 and PD-L1
Adverse effects of interest: Multiple inflammatory toxicities referred to as *immune-related adverse events* (irAEs); these resemble autoimmune diseases and most commonly affect the skin, gastrointestinal tract, and endocrine organs
Initial clinical indication: Metastatic or unresectable melanoma
Other clinical indications: Malignant mesothelioma, hepatocellular carcinoma, metastatic colorectal carcinoma, metastatic non–small cell lung cancer, renal cell carcinoma

Nivolumab (Opdivo)
Target: Programmed cell death-1 (PD-1) receptor, blocking the ligands PD-L1 and PD-L2 from binding with the receptor, enhancing T-cell–mediated antitumor responses
Similar monoclonal antibodies: Pembrolizumab (Keytruda), cemiplimab (Libtayo), atezolizumab (PD-L1, Tecentriq), durvalumab (PD-L1, Imfinzi), avelumab (PD-L1, Bavencio)

Target substem (infix)
-ci(r)-
-li(m)-
-ne(r)-
-t(u)-
-vi(r)-

Stem
-mab
-tug
-bart
-mig
-ment

Rituximab

Prefix

Source substem
-o-
-xi-
-zu-
-xizu-
-u-

Figure 2 An example of the nomenclature used to name a monoclonal antibody.

[1] Not FDA approved for this indication.

effects of umbilical cord MSCs in a randomized study of patients with COVID-19 complicated by ARDS. This use does not have FDA-approval.

References

Beltrami AP, et al: Adult cardiac stem cells are multipotent and support myocardial regeneration, *Cell* 114(6):763–776, 2003.

Burt RK, et al: Effect of nonmyeloablative hematopoietic stem cell transplantation vs continued disease-modifying therapy on disease progression in patients with relapsing-remitting multiple sclerosis: a randomized clinical trial, *J Am Med Assoc* 321(2):165–174, 2019.

Center for International Blood and Marrow Transplant Research: https://www.cibmtr.org/ReferenceCenter/SlidesReports/SummarySlides/pages/index.aspx.

Chen SL, et al: Effect on left ventricular function of intracoronary transplantation of autologous bone marrow mesenchymal stem cell in patients with acute myocardial infarction, *Am J Cardiol* 94(1):92–95, 2004.

Chugh AR, et al: Administration of cardiac stem cells in patients with ischemic cardiomyopathy: the SCIPIO trial: surgical aspects and interim analysis of myocardial function and viability by magnetic resonance, *Circulation* 126(11 suppl 1):S54–S64, 2012.

Cyranoski D: Japan's approval of stem-cell treatment for spinal-cord injury concerns scientists, *Nature* 565(7741):544–545, 2019.

FDA: https://www.fda.gov/vaccines-blood-biologics/cellular-gene-therapy-products/approved-cellular-and-gene-therapy-products, F.a.s.c.t.

Fisher SA, et al: Stem cell therapy for chronic ischaemic heart disease and congestive heart failure, *Cochrane Database Syst Rev* (4):CD007888, 2014.

Gao LR, et al: Intracoronary infusion of Wharton's jelly-derived mesenchymal stem cells in acute myocardial infarction: double-blind, randomized controlled trial, *BMC Med* 13:162, 2015.

Hare JM, et al: Randomized comparison of allogeneic versus autologous mesenchymal stem cells for nonischemic dilated cardiomyopathy: POSEIDON-DCM trial, *J Am Coll Cardiol* 69(5):526–537, 2017.

Henry TD, et al: The Athena trials: autologous adipose-derived regenerative cells for refractory chronic myocardial ischemia with left ventricular dysfunction, *Catheter Cardiovasc Interv* 89(2):169–177, 2017.

Henry TD, Moye L, Traverse JH: Consistently inconsistent-bone marrow mononuclear stem cell therapy following acute myocardial infarction: a decade later, *Circ Res* 119(3):404–406, 2016.

Jayaraj JS, et al: Efficacy and safety of stem cell therapy in advanced heart failure patients: a systematic review with a meta-analysis of recent trials between 2017 and 2019, *Cureus* 11(9):e5585, 2019.

Jo CH, et al: Intra-articular injection of mesenchymal stem cells for the treatment of osteoarthritis of the knee: a proof-of-concept clinical trial, *Stem Cell* 32(5):1254–1266, 2014.

Lanzoni G, et al: Umbilical cord mesenchymal stem cells for COVID-19 acute respiratory distress syndrome: a double-blind, phase 1/2a, randomized controlled trial, *Stem Cells Transl Med* 10(5):660–673, 2021.

Lee JW, et al: A randomized, open-label, multicenter trial for the safety and efficacy of adult mesenchymal stem cells after acute myocardial infarction, *J Korean Med Sci* 29(1):23–31, 2014.

Makkar RR, et al: Intracoronary cardiosphere-derived cells for heart regeneration after myocardial infarction (CADUCEUS): a prospective, randomised phase 1 trial, *Lancet* 379(9819):895–904, 2012.

Orlic D, et al: Bone marrow cells regenerate infarcted myocardium, *Nature* 410(6829):701–705, 2001.

Park YB, et al: Cartilage regeneration in osteoarthritic patients by a composite of allogeneic umbilical cord blood-derived mesenchymal stem cells and Hyaluronate hydrogel: results from a clinical trial for safety and proof-of-concept with 7 Years of extended follow-up, *Stem Cells Transl Med* 6(2):613–621, 2017.

Pelletier JP, Martel-Pelletier J, Abramson SB: Osteoarthritis, an inflammatory disease: potential implication for the selection of new therapeutic targets, *Arthritis Rheum* 44(6):1237–1247, 2001.

Perin EC, et al: Adipose-derived regenerative cells in patients with ischemic cardiomyopathy: the PRECISE Trial, *Am Heart J* 168(1):88–95.e2, 2014.

Richter DL, et al: Knee articular cartilage repair and restoration techniques: a review of the literature, *Sports Health* 8(2):153–160, 2016.

Robinton DA, Daley GQ: The promise of induced pluripotent stem cells in research and therapy, *Nature* 481(7381):295–305, 2012.

Schachinger V, et al: Intracoronary bone marrow-derived progenitor cells in acute myocardial infarction, *N Engl J Med* 355(12):1210–1221, 2006.

Soder RP, et al: A phase I study to evaluate two doses of Wharton's jelly-derived mesenchymal stromal cells for the treatment of De Novo high-risk or Steroid-refractory acute graft versus host disease, *Stem Cell Rev Rep* 16(5):979–991, 2020.

Stamm C, et al: Autologous bone-marrow stem-cell transplantation for myocardial regeneration, *Lancet* 361(9351):45–46, 2003.

ter Huurne M, et al: Antiinflammatory and chondroprotective effects of intraarticular injection of adipose-derived stem cells in experimental osteoarthritis, *Arthritis Rheum* 64(11):3604–3613, 2012.

Thomas ED, et al: Intravenous infusion of bone marrow in patients receiving radiation and chemotherapy, *N Engl J Med* 257(11):491–496, 1957.

Thomson JA, et al: Embryonic stem cell lines derived from human blastocysts, *Science* 282(5391):1145–1147, 1998.

Wollert KC, et al: Intracoronary autologous bone-marrow cell transfer after myocardial infarction: the BOOST randomised controlled clinical trial, *Lancet* 364(9429):141–148, 2004.

Yubo M, et al: Clinical efficacy and safety of mesenchymal stem cell transplantation for osteoarthritis treatment: a meta-analysis, *PloS One* 12(4):e0175449, 2017.

23 Appendix

BIOLOGIC AGENTS REFERENCE CHART

Method of
Laurie A.M. Hommema, MD; and Kevin Hommema, BSME

Biological weapons are devices used intentionally to cause disease or death through dissemination of microorganisms or toxins in food and water, by insect vectors, or by aerosols. Potential targets include human beings, food crops, livestock, and other resources essential for national security, economy, and defense. Unlike nuclear, chemical, and conventional weapons, the onset of a biological attack will probably be insidious. For some infectious agents, secondary and tertiary transmission could continue for weeks or months after the initial attack. In the United States, anthrax has been used in 2001 and ricin in 2003, 2004, and 2013 to target individuals. The Department of Homeland Security leads a national strategy to prevent, detect, respond to, and recover from acts of bioterrorism.

Initial detection of an unannounced biological attack will likely occur when an astute health professional notices an unusual case or disease cluster and reports his or her concerns to local public health authorities. Due to the incubation period of most biologic agents, subjects may have traveled from site of exposure to other geographic locations. Physicians and other health professionals should be alert to the following:
- Unusual temporal or geographic clustering of illnesses in humans, as well as animals
- Increase in specific lab testing or prescription drugs
- Sudden increase of illness in previously healthy persons
- Sudden increase in nonspecific illnesses such as pneumonia; flulike illness; bleeding disorders; unexplained rashes, particularly in adults; neuromuscular illnesses; and gastrointestinal syndromes

To enhance detection and treatment capabilities, physicians and other health professionals in acute care settings should be familiar with the clinical manifestations, diagnostic techniques, isolation precautions, treatment, and prophylaxis for likely causative agents (e.g., smallpox, pneumonic plague, anthrax, viral hemorrhagic fevers). Table 1 provides a quick summary of diagnostic and treatment considerations for various infectious and toxic biological agents. For some of these agents, delay in medical response could result in a potentially devastating number of casualties. To mitigate such consequences, early identification and intervention are imperative. Frontline physicians must have an increased level of suspicion regarding the possible intentional use of biological agents as well as an increased sensitivity to reporting those suspicious to public health authorities, who, in turn, must be willing to evaluate a predictable increase in false-positive reports.

Medical response efforts require coordination and planning with emergency management agencies, law enforcement, health care facilities, and social services agencies. Due to the criminal nature of the act, samples need to be collected and handled as evidence. Healthcare agencies should ensure that physicians know whom to call with reports of suspicious cases and clusters of infectious diseases, and they should work to build a good relationship with the local medical community. Resource integration is absolutely necessary to:
- Establish adequate capacity to initiate rapid investigation of an outbreak
- Establish and ensure decontamination protocols are in place
- Educate and protect healthcare workers and the public
- Coordinate mass distribution of antibiotics and vaccines
- Address psychological consequences

In an epidemic, overwhelming numbers of critically ill patients will require acute and follow-up medical care. Both infected persons and the worried well will seek medical attention, with a corresponding need for medical supplies, diagnostic tests, and hospital beds. The impact—or even the threat—of an attack can elicit widespread panic and civil disorder, overwhelm hospital resources, and disrupt social services.

Any suspicious or confirmed exposure to a biological weapons agent should be reported immediately to the local health department, local Federal Bureau of Investigation office, National Response Center (800-424-8802), and the Centers for Disease Control and Prevention Operation's Center (770-488-7100).

HERB OR NUTRITIONAL SUPPLEMENT	COMMON USES	REASONABLE ADULT ORAL DOSAGE*	PRECAUTIONS AND DRUG INTERACTIONS
Soy	Commonly used for cholesterol reduction in combination with a low-fat diet. Used for menopausal symptoms and for prevention of osteoporosis and cardiovascular disease in postmenopausal women	For lowering cholesterol, 25–50 g/d of soy protein. For hot flashes, 20–60 g/d of soy protein. For osteoporosis, 40 g/d of soy protein containing 90 mg isoflavones	Soy, when consumed as whole foods (e.g., tofu or soy milk), has minimal adverse effects. Consumption of large amounts of soy can cause gastric complaints such as constipation, bloating, and nausea. Long-term use of soy tablets containing isoflavones (150 mg/d for 5 years) has been shown to cause endometrial hyperplasia
St. John's wort	Used for treatment of mild to moderate depression. May have antiinflammatory and antiinfective activities	300 mg tid of hypericum extract standardized to 0.3% hypericin	St. John's wort should not be used in pregnancy. Side effects include dry mouth, GI upset, dizziness, fatigue, and constipation. St. John's wort can induce photosensitivity, especially in fair-skinned individuals. It can cause serotonin syndrome if used with other antidepressants, including SSRIs, or other serotonergic drugs. It has been shown to induce CYP3A4 and decrease blood levels of many drugs such as indinavir, nevirapine, cyclosporine, digoxin, theophylline, simvastatin, oral contraceptive pills, and warfarin. St. John's wort should be discontinued at least 5 d before surgery to avoid any potential drug interactions
Stinging nettle root	Approved in Germany for difficulty in urination in BPH stage 1 and 2	4–6 g/d of cut root; can be taken as tea (1.5 g in 150 mL boiling water for 10–20 min, tid), fluid extract 1:1 (1.5 mL tid), tincture 1:5 (5–7.5 mL tid), or dry extract 5.4–6.6:1 (0.22–0.33 g tid)	Occasionally, mild GI upsets may occur. No known interactions with drugs
Turmeric root	Approved by the German Commission E for dyspeptic conditions. Used extensively in Ayurveda medicine for its antiinflammatory and antiarthritic effects. Other uses include allergic rhinitis, depression, nonalcoholic fatty liver disease, osteoarthritis and cancer	For dyspeptic conditions: 1.5–3 g/d of cut root as tea infusion or equivalent preparations (e.g., powder, extract, tincture). The Commission E monograph requires turmeric to contain not less than 3% curcuminoids, calculated as curcumin and not less than 3% volatile oil	Side effects are uncommon and are generally limited to mild stomach distress. Topical curcumin can cause allergic contact dermatitis. Individuals with bile duct obstruction or gallstones should avoid curcumin due to its stimulating effects on the gallbladder
Valerian root	Used as a mild sedative for insomnia and anxiety	2–3 g of dried root or 1–3 mL of tincture, qd to several times per day. Two clinical trials found 400–450 mg of the root extract effective for insomnia	Valerian has a bad odor and can cause morning drowsiness. Long-term administration can lead to paradoxical stimulation, including restlessness and palpitations. Because of the risk of benzodiazepine-like withdrawal, valerian should be tapered over a period of several weeks before surgery. It can potentiate the sedative effect of CNS depressants (e.g., benzodiazepines, alcohol) and other herbal tranquilizers

*Doses presented in the table are adapted from the German Commission E Monographs and/or data from clinical trials. Products from different manufacturers vary considerably. A reliable product should have a label clearly stating the botanical name of the herb and milligram amount contained in the product. Standardized extracts should be used whenever possible and are often disclosed on the label of quality products.

AMD, Age-related macular degeneration; *BPH*, benign prostatic hyperplasia; *CFU*, colony-forming unit; *CHD*, coronary heart disease; *CNS*, central nervous system; *CYP3A4*, cytochrome P450 3A4; *DHA*, docosahexaenoic acid; *EPA*, eicosapentaenoic acid; *FDA*, Food and Drug Administration; *GI*, gastrointestinal; *HMG-CoA*, 3-hydroxy-3-methylglutaryl coenzyme A; *INR*, international normalized ratio; *LDL*, low-density lipoprotein; *MAOI*, monoamine oxidase inhibitor; *PMS*, premenstrual syndrome; *SLE*, systemic lupus erythematosus; *SSRIs*, selective serotonin reuptake inhibitors; *UTIs*, urinary tract infections.

References

Ang-Lee MK, Moss J, Yuan C: Herbal medicines and perioperative care, *JAMA* 286:208–216, 2001.

Bent S: Herbal medicine in the United States: Review and efficacy, safety, and regulation, *J Gen Intern Med* 23:854–859, 2008.

Blumenthal M, editor: *Herbal Medicines: Expanded Commission E monographs*, Austin, TX, 2000, American Botanical Council.

Blumenthal M, editor: *The ABC Clinical Guide to Herbs*, Austin, TX, 2003, American Botanical Council.

Ernst E: The risk-benefit profile of commonly used herbal therapies: Ginkgo, St John's wort, ginseng, Echinacea, saw palmetto, and kava, *Ann Intern Med* 136:42–53, 2002.

Gregory PJ, Worthington M, Shkayeva M, et al, editors: Natural Medicines (database online), Stockton, CA: 2018 Therapeutic Research Center. Available at https://naturalmedicines.therapeuticresearch.com/. (Assessed July 7, 2019).

Holland S, Silberstein SD, Freitag F, et al: Evidence-based guideline update: NSAIDs and other complementary treatments for episodic migraine prevention in adults: report of the Quality Standards Subcommittee of the American Academy of Neurology and the American Headache Society, *Neurology* 78(17):1346–1353, 2012.

Kligler B, Cohrssen A: Probiotics, *Am Fam Physician* 78:1073–1078, 2008.

Kronenberg F, Fugh-Berman A: Complementary and alternative medicine for menopausal symptoms: A review of randomized controlled trials, *Ann Intern Med* 137:805–813, 2002.

National Center for Complementary and Integrative Health: Herbs at a Glance. Available at https://nccih.nih.gov/health/herbsataglance.htm. Accessed 19 March 2018.

Smet P: Herbal remedies, *N Engl J Med* 347:2046–2056, 2002.

TOXIC CHEMICAL AGENTS REFERENCE CHART

Method of
Laurie A.M. Hommema, MD; and Kevin Hommema, BSME

Toxic chemical agents are poisonous vapors, aerosols, gases, liquids, or solids that have toxic effects on people, animals, or plants. Most of these agents are liquid at room temperature and are disseminated as vapors and aerosols. They may be released as bombs, sprayed from aerosolizing devices, through ventilation systems or introduced to food or water supply. Some of these agents are highly toxic and persistent, features that can render a site uninhabitable and require costly and potentially hazardous decontamination and remediation. Health effects range from irritation and burning of skin and mucous membranes to rapid cardiopulmonary collapse and death.

Efficient deployment of hazardous materials (HazMat) teams is critical to control a chemical agent attack. Although all major cities and emergency medical systems have plans and equipment in place to address this situation, physicians and other health professionals must be aware of principles involved in managing a patient or multiple patients exposed to these agents. Chemical weapon agents have a high potential for secondary contamination from victims to responders. This requires that medical treatment facilities have clearly defined procedures for handling contaminated casualties, many of whom will transport themselves to the facility. Precautions must be used until thorough decontamination has been performed or the specific chemical agent is identified. Healthcare professionals must first protect themselves (e.g., by using protective suits, respiratory protection, and chemical-resistant gloves) because secondary contamination with even small amounts of these substances (particularly nerve agents such as VX) may be lethal.

Primary detection of exposure to chemical agents is based on the signs and symptoms of the potential victim (Table 1). Confirmation of a chemical agent, using detection equipment or laboratory analyses, takes considerable time and will not likely contribute to the early management of mass casualty victims. Several patients presenting with the same symptoms should alert physicians and hospital staff to the possibility of a chemical attack. If a chemical attack occurs, most victims will likely arrive within a short time. This situation differentiates a chemical attack from a biological attack involving infectious microorganisms, which can take days for symptom onset. Additional diagnostic clues include the following:

- Unusual temporal or geographic clustering of illness
- Any sudden increase in illness in previously healthy persons
- Sudden increase in nonspecific syndromes (e.g., sudden unexplained weakness in previously healthy persons; dimmed or blurred vision; hypersecretion, inhalation, or burn-like syndrome)

A coordinated communication network is critical for transmitting reliable information from the incident scene to treatment facilities. Any suspicious or confirmed exposure to a chemical weapons agent should be reported to the local health department, local Federal Bureau of Investigation office, National Response Center (800-424-8802), and the Centers for Disease Control and Prevention (770-488-7100).

TABLE 1 Quick Reference Chart on Chemical Weapon Agents

CHEMICAL AGENT	DIAGNOSTIC CONSIDERATIONS					TREATMENT CONSIDERATIONS*		
	SIGNS AND SYMPTOMS	SYMPTOM ONSET	ODOR	ACTION	TESTING	TREATMENT	ANTIDOTE	COMMENTS
Cyanides—Asphyxiant/Blood								
Cyanogen chloride (CK) Hydrogen cyanide (AC)	"Cherry red" skin Resp: SOB, chest tightness, hyperventilation, resp arrest GI: nausea, vomiting CV: ventricular arrhythmias, hypotension, cardiac arrest, shock CNS: anxiety, headache, drowsiness, weakness, apnea, convulsions, seizure, coma Metabolic acidosis and increased concentration of venous oxygen (possibly also cyanosis)	Rapid, seconds to minutes	Bitter almond, musty, or chlorine-like	Binds cellular cytochrome oxidase, causing chemical asphyxia	Cyanide, thiocyanate, serum lactate levels Venous and arterial partial oxygen pressure	Immediate treatment of symptomatic patients is critical. Hydroxocobalamin (vitamin B_{12a} [Cyanokit]) administered IV with sodium thio sulfate[5],[†] Activated charcoal[1] for oral exposure Mechanical ventilation as needed Circulatory support with crystalloids and vasopressors Metabolic acidosis corrected with IV sodium bicarbonate Seizures controlled with benzodiazepines	Sodium nitrite and sodium thiosulfate (Nithiodote); repeat one-half initial doses of both agents in 30 min if inadequate clinical response; amyl nitrite[1] capsules are available for first aid until intravenous access is achieved. Hydroxocobalamin (vitamin B_{12a}, Cyanokit)	Cyanide antidote kits are commercially available. CNS effects may be confused with carbon monoxide and hydrogen sulfide poisoning. Nonpersistent, not contact hazard.
Incapacitating Agents								
Agent 15 3-quinuclidinyl benzilate (BZ)	May appear as drug intoxication with erratic behaviors; hallucinations. Mydriasis, blurred vision, dry mouth, dry skin, possible atropine-like flush, initial rise in heart rate, hyperthermia, decreased level of consciousness, confusion, disorientation, impaired memory.	Hours—up to 36 h if only on skin 0–4 h: parasympathetic blockade and mild CNS effects 4–20 h: stupor with ataxia and hyperthermia 20–96 h: full-blown delirium Resolution phase: paranoia, deep sleep, reawakening, crawling, climbing automatisms, eventual reorientation	Odorless	Competitive inhibitor of acetylcholine muscarinic receptor		Support, intravenous fluids	Physostigmine salicylate (Antilirium)[1]	Persistent in soil and water and on contact surfaces. Contact hazard.

TABLE 1 Quick Reference Chart on Chemical Weapon Agents—cont'd

| CHEMICAL AGENT | DIAGNOSTIC CONSIDERATIONS | | | | | TREATMENT CONSIDERATIONS* | | | |
	SIGNS AND SYMPTOMS	SYMPTOM ONSET	ODOR	ACTION	TESTING	TREATMENT	ANTIDOTE	COMMENTS
Nerve Agents								
Cyclohexyl sarin (GF) Sarin (GB) Soman (GD) Tabun (GA) VX	Most toxic of known chemical agents May be confused with organophosphate and carbamate pesticide poisoning Eyes: excessive lacrimation, miosis may be present and blurred vision Resp: rhinorrhea, bronchospasm, resp failure GI: hypersalivation, nausea, vomiting, diarrhea Skin: localized sweating Cardiac: sinus bradycardia Skeletal muscles: fasciculations followed by weakness, flaccid paralysis CNs: loss of consciousness, convulsions, apnea, seizures	Vapor: seconds Liquid: minutes or hours Symptom onset may be delayed up to 18 h, particularly for localized exposures.	GB, VX: none GA: fruity GD: camphor-like	Irreversible acetylcholinesterase inhibitors	Erythrocyte or serum cholinesterase activity to confirm exposure	Rapid establishment of patent airway Early administration of 2-PAM (pralidoxime [Protopam]) is critical to minimize permanent agent inactivation of acetylcholinesterase (i.e., "aging"). Benzodiazepines to control nerve agent–induced seizures Airway and ventilatory support as needed	Atropine and 2-PAM Additional doses until bronchial secretions are cleared and ventilation improved	Atropine, 2-PAM, and diazepam[1] are available in autoinjector kits through the US military. VX is a contact hazard.

Continued

1533

Toxic Chemical Agents Reference Chart

HEIGHT IN FEET

HEIGHT IN CENTIMETERS

SURFACE AREA IN SQUARE METERS

WEIGHT IN POUNDS

WEIGHT IN KILOGRAMS

HEIGHT IN FEET

7'
10"
8"
6"
4"
2"
6'
10"
8"
6"
4"
2"
5'
10"
8"
6"
4"
2"
4'
10"
8"
6"
4"
2"
3'
10"
8"
6"

HEIGHT IN CENTIMETERS

220
215
210
205
200
195
190
185
180
175
170
165
160
155
150
145
140
135
130
125
120
115
110
105
100
95
90
85
80
75

SURFACE AREA IN SQUARE METERS

3.00
2.90
2.80
2.70
2.60
2.50
2.40
2.30
2.20
2.10
2.00
1.95
1.90
1.85
1.80
1.75
1.70
1.65
1.60
1.55
1.50
1.45
1.40
1.35
1.30
1.25
1.20
1.15
1.10
1.05
1.00
.95
.90
.85
.80
.75
.70
.65
.60
.55
.50

WEIGHT IN POUNDS

440
420
400
380
360
340
320
300
290
280
270
260
250
240
230
220
210
200
190
180
170
160
150
140
130
120
110
100
90
80
70
60
50
40
15

WEIGHT IN KILOGRAMS

200
190
180
170
160
150
140
130
120
110
100
95
90
85
80
75
70
65
60
55
50
45
40
35
30
25
20